W9-AWT-307

Principles of Practice for the

ACUTE CARE NURSE PRACTITIONER

Principles of Practice for the

ACUTE CARE NURSE PRACTITIONER

Paul Logan, MSN, CRNP, CS, CCRN
Cardiovascular Nurse Practitioner
Norristown Cardiovascular Associates
Cardiovascular Associates of Southeastern Pennsylvania
Norristown, Pennsylvania

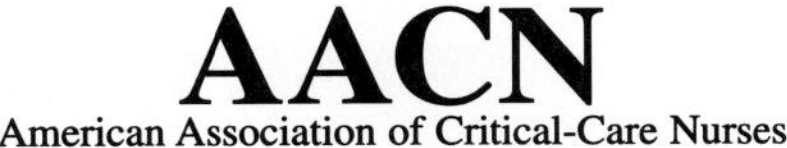

The material contained in this book is endorsed by AACN as a useful component in the ongoing education process of acute care nurse practitioners.

APPLETON & LANGE
Stamford, Connecticut

www.appletonlange.com

99 00 01 02 / 10 9 8 7 6 5 4 3 2 1

Prentice Hall International (UK) Limited, *London*
Prentice Hall of Australia Pty. Limited, *Sydney*
Prentice Hall Canada, Inc., *Toronto*
Prentice Hall Hispanoamericana S.A., *Mexico*
Prentice Hall of India Private Limited, *New Delhi*
Prentice Hall of Japan, Inc., *Tokyo*
Simon & Schuster Asia Pte. Ltd., *Singapore*
Editora Prentice Hall do Brasil Ltda., *Rio de Janeiro*
Prentice Hall, *Upper Saddle River, New Jersey*

Library of Congress Cataloging-in-Publication Data

Logan, Paul.
Principles of practice for the acute care nurse practitioner / by Paul Logan.
p. cm.
ISBN 0-8385-8125-0 (alk. paper)
1. Intensive care nursing. 2. Nurse practitioners. I. Title.
[DNLM: 1. Acute Disease—nursing. 2. Nurse Practitioners. WY 150L831p 1999]
RT120.I5L63 1999
610.73'61—dc21
DNLM/DLC
for Library of Congress 98-26249
CIP

Acquisitions Editor: David P. Carroll
Production Service: Tage Publishing Service, Inc.
Designer: Mary Skudlarek

ISBN 0-8385-8125-0

90000

9 780838 581254

PRINTED IN THE UNITED STATES OF AMERICA

To Jeanne—my friend, my confidante, my foundation, my partner, my wife.

Contents

Contributors

Christine Alberts, MSN, CRNP
Nurse Practitioner
Division of Cardiology
Hahnemann University Hospital
Philadelphia, Pennsylvania
Chapter 32 Coronary Artery Disease

Catherine LaMattina Allen, MS, RN, CS, CRNP
Nurse Practitioner
Department of Anesthesiology
Medical College of Pennsylvania Hospital
Philadelphia, Pennsylvania
Chapter 23 Preoperative Evaluation and Cardiac Risk Assessment

Roberta Anding, MS, RD, LD, CDE
Assistant Clincal Professor
University of Houston
Houston, Texas
Chapter 17 Nutritional Problems

Joanne Angstadt, MSN, CRNP
Faculty, Acute Care Nurse Practitioner Program
School of Nursing
University of Pennsylvania
Philadelphia, Pennsylvania
Chapter 1 The Emergence, Maturation, and Future of the Acute Care Nurse Practioner Role

Barbara Asorian, MSN, CRNP, CS, CCRN
Former Nurse Practitioner and Senior Clinical Coordinator
University of Southern California Cardiothoracic Surgeons
Los Angeles, California
Chapter 34 Cardiac Surgery

Pamela A. Bergmann, MSN, RN
Data Analyst
Quality Improvement
University of Pennsylvania Health System
Philadelphia, Pennsylvania
Chapter 3 Business Considerations for the ACNP

Janet Bienkowski, RN, MSN, ANP
Nurse Practitioner
Plastic and Reconstructive Surgery
Stony Brook Hospital
Stony Brook, New York
Chapter 25 Plastic and Reconstructive Surgery

Nancy P. Blumenthal, MSN, CRNP, CS, CCTC
Lung Transplant Nurse Practitioner
Multiorgan Transplant Unit
Hospital of the University of Pennsylvania
Philadelphia, Pennsylvania
Chapter 37 Pulmonary Problems

Catherine Borkowski-Benoit, RN-C, MSN
Nurse Practitioner
Department of Neurosurgery
Beth Israel Deaconess Medical Center
Brookline, Massachussets
Chapter 40 Neurological Problems

Susan Bradford, RN
Department of Vascular Surgery
Medical College of Pennsylvania Hospital
Philadelphia, Pennsylvania
Chapter 31 Vascular Disease

Suzanne M. Burns, RN, MSN, RRT, CCRN
Clinician 5—MICU and Associate Professor of Nursing
School of Nursing
University of Virginia
Charlottesville, Virginia
Chapter 9 The ACNP as Researcher: Strategies for Practice

David J. Callans, MD
Associate Professor of Medicine
Division of Cardiology, Electrophysiology Section
University of Pennsylvania Medical Center
Philadelphia, Pennsylvania
Chapter 36 Arrhythmias

Linda A. Carrick, PhD, RN
Chief Operating Officer
Mercy Health System
Scranton, Pennsylvania
Chapter 3 Business Considerations for the ACNP

Judy Cavanaugh, RN-C, MS
Nurse Practitioner
Department of Surgery
University of Rochester Medical Center
Rochester, New York
Chapter 41 Gastrointestinal Problems

Milton Coll, MD
Senior Attending Surgeon
Urologic Associates, PC
Philadelphia, Pennsylvania
Chapter 43 Genitourinary Problems

Catherine Congdon, MSN, CRNP
Cardiology Nurse Practitioner
Division of Cardiology
Hahnemann University Hospital
Philadelphia, Pennsylvania
Chapter 30 Hypertension

Daniel G. Deschler, MD
Department of Otolaryngology, Head and Neck Surgery
Hahnemann University Hospital
Philadelphia, Pennsylvania
Chapter 50 Head and Neck Problems

Verdi J. DiSesa, MD
Chairman of Cardiovascular-Thoracic Surgery
Mary and John Bent Prof. of Cardiovascular Surgery
Rush-Presbyterian-St. Lukes Medical Center
Chicago, Illinois
Chapter 27 Organ Donation and Transplantation

Phyllis M. Dubendorf, MSN, CS-ACNP
Faculty, Acute Care Nurse Practitioner Program
School of Nursing
University of Pennsylvania
Philadelphia, Pennsylvania
Chapter 2 Scope and Standards of Clinical Practice

Kim Marie Falk, MSN, RN
Instructor
School of Nursing
Northeastern Hospital
Philadelphia, Pennsylvania
Chapter 26 Cancer Treatment

Neil O. Fishman, MD
Assistant Professor of Medicine
Division of Infectious Disease
University of Pennsylvania Medical Center
Philadelphia, Pennsylvania
Chapter 16 Fever and the Hospitalized Patient
Chapter 44 Infectious Diseases

Leonard Friedland, MD
Director, Pediatric Emergency Department
Temple University Children's Medical Center
Philadelphia, Pennsylvania
Chapter 52 The Hospitalized Child

Sandra L. Gomberg, MSN, RN
Chief Operating Officer
Temple University Children's Medical Center
Philadelphia, Pennsylvania
Chapter 52 The Hospitalized Child

Stephanie Green, MD
Former Assistant Professor of Medicine
Division of Infectious Disease
University of Pennsylvania Medical Center
Philadelphia, Pennsylvania
Chapter 16 Fever and the Hospitalized Patient
Chapter 44 Infectious Diseases

Patricia Baehser Griffith, MSN, CRNP
Faculty, Acute Care Nurse Practitioner Program
School of Nursing
University of Pennsylvania
Philadelphia, Pennsylvania
Chapter 4 Licensure, Certification, and Institutional Credentialing

Robin M. Haskell, MSN, RN, ACNP-CS, CCRN
Trauma Nurse Practitioner
Department of Traumatology
University of Pennsylvania
Coatesville, Pennsylvania
Chapter 24 Trauma

Paula F. Henry, RN, BSN, NP-C, JD
Attorney at Law
R. W. Harlan & Associates
Newport Beach, California
Chapter 6 Legal Considerations for Practice

Janet M. Hines, MD
Assistant Professor of Medicine
Division of Infectious Disease
University of Pennsylvania Medical Center
Philadelphia, Pennsylvania
Chapter 16 Fever and the Hospitalized Patient
Chapter 44 Infectious Diseases

Susan Hoch, MD
Hahnemann University Hospital
Philadelphia, Pennsylvania
Chapter 48 Rheumatic Problems

Kay Huber, DEd, CRNP
Asssociate Professor
Department of Nursing
Messiah College
Grantham, Pennsylvania
Chapter 53 The Hospitalized Older Adult

Melinda Jenkins, PhD, RN
Director, Family Nurse Practitioner Program
School of Nursing
University of Pennsylvania
Philadelphia, Pennsylvania
Chapter 15 Health Promotion and Illness Prevention

Anne Keane, EdD, FAAN, CRNP
Associate Professor
School of Nursing
University of Pennsylvania
Philadelphia, Pennsylvania
Chapter 1 The Emergence, Maturation, and Future of the Acute Care Nurse Practitioner Role

Arlene W. Keeling, PhD, RN
Assistant Professor and Director, ACNP Program
School of Nursing
University of Virginia
Charlottesville, Virginia
Chapter 9 The ACNP as Researcher: Strategies for Practice

Ruth M. Kleinpell, PhD, RN, CCRN
Associate Professor and Faculty, ACNP Program
College of Nursing
Rush University
Chicago, Illinois
Chapter 11 Approach to the Hospitalized Patient

JoAnne Konick-McMahon, MSN, CCRN
Clinical Nurse Specialist, CHF Study
School of Nursing
University of Pennsylvania
Philadelphia, Pennsylvania
Chapter 8 The Acute Care Nurse Practitioner as Educator
Chapter 18 Fluid, Electrolyte, and Acid-Base Abnormalities

Susan L. W. Krupnick, MSN, RN, CARN, CS
Psychiatric Liaison Nurse Specialist
Staff Development
Bay State Medical Center
Springfield, Massachusetts
Chapter 54 The Hospitalized Patient's Psychological Response to Illness

Judi Kuric, MSN, RN, CCRN, CRRN, CNRN
Clinical Nurse Specialist, Adjunct Assistant Professor
School of Nursing
University of Southern Indiana
Evansville, Indiana
Chapter 28 Rehabilitation

William G. Kussmaul III, MD, FACC, FACP, FSCAI
Associate Professor of Medicine
Division of Cardiology
Hahnemann University/MCP
Philadelphia, Pennsylvania
Chapter 13 Medical Reasoning

Mildred Lam, MD
Associate Professor of Medicine
Nephrology Division
University of Virginia
Charlottesville, Virginia
Chapter 42 Renal Problems

Sarah Layman, ACNP, MN, RN
Clinical Nurse Specialist
University of Washington Medical Center
Seattle, Washington
Chapter 21 Wound Management

Margaret Levy, MD, FACS
Department of Surgery
Elkins Park Hospital
Philadelphia, Pennsylvania
Chapter 45 Breast Problems

Hugh Lipshutz, MD
Norristown Cardiovascular Associates
Cardiovascular Associates of Southeastern Pennsylvania
Norristown, Pennsylvania
Chapter 29 Lipid Problems

Paul Logan, MSN, CRNP, CS, CCRN
Cardiovascular Nurse Practitioner
Norristown Cardiovascular Associates
Cardiovascular Associates of Southeastern Pennsylvania
Norristown, Pennsylvania
Chapter 4 Licensure, Certification, and Institutional Credentialing
Chapter 5 Professional Resources for the ACNP
Chapter 12 The History and Physical Examination
Chapter 14 Communication and Documentation
Chapter 33 Valvular and Congenital Heart Disease
Chapter 35 Heart Failure and Cardiomyopathy

Linda M. Lord, NP, MS, CNSN
Nurse Practitioner
Department of Surgery
University of Rochester Medical Center
Rochester, New York
Chapter 41 Gastrointestinal Problems

Mary Malitas, MSN, CRNP, CCRN
Cardiology Nurse Practitioner
Hahnemann University Hospital
Philadelphia, Pennsylvania
Chapter 32 Coronary Artery Disease

Russ Mazda, DO
Associate Faculty Philadelphia College of Osteopathic Medicine
Department of Emergency Medicine
St. Joseph Hospital
Lancaster, Pennsylvania
Chapter 22 Poisoning and Drug Toxicity

Dianne Wasser Monreal, MN, RN
Harrison Memorial Hospital
Bremerton, Washington
Chapter 20 Pain Management

Cheryl Monturo, MSN, CNSN
Lecture
University of Pennsylvania
School of Nursing
Philadelphia, Pennsylvania
Chapter 2 Scope and Standards of Clinical Practice

Carina Knowlton Moravec, ARNP, MA
Nurse Practitioner
Long-Term Follow-Up Program
Fred Hutchison Cancer Research Center
Seattle, Washington
Chapter 46 Hematologic Problems

Koki Niibori, MD
Instructor, Thoracic and Cardiovascular Surgery
Tohoku University School of Medicine
Sendai, Japan
Chapter 19 Shock

Margaret A. O'Connell, MSN, CRNP
Cardiology Nurse Practitioner
Division of Cardiology
Hahnemann University Hospital
Philadelphia, Pennsylvania
Chapter 32 Coronary Artery Disease

Carol A. Offutt, RN, MSN, ANP-C, CS
Nurse Practitioner
Kaiser Permanente
Washington, District of Columbia
Chapter 39 Endocrine Problems

Mary Zemyan Polito, MSN, CRNP
Adult Nurse Practitioner
Ophthalmic Associates
Johnstown, Pennsylvania
Chapter 49 Eye Problems

Joseph R. Polito, MD
Ophthalmic Associates
Johnstown, Pennsylvania
Chapter 49 Eye Problems

Kathleen M. Powers, RN, BSN, CNP
Nurse Practitioner
University of Virginia
Charlottesville, Virginia
Chapter 42 Renal Problems

Sally Boyle Quinn, MSN, RN
Clinical Nurse Specialist
Temple University Hospital
Philadelphia, Pennsylvania
Chapter 52 The Hospitalized Child

Therese S. Richmond, PhD, CRNP, CS, FAAN
Assistant Professor of Trauma and Critical Care Nursing
School of Nursing
University of Pennsylvania
Philadelphia, Pennsylvania
Chapter 2 Scope and Standards of Clinical Practice

Juanita Reigle, RN, MSN, ACNP-CS, CCRN
Practitioner/Teacher
University of Virginia Health Sciences Center
Charlottesville, Virginia
Chapter 7 Ethical Decision Making

Andrew B. Roberts, MD
Professor of Surgery
Department of Vascular Surgery
Medical College of Pennsylvania Hospital
Philadelphia, Pennsylvania
Chapter 31 Vascular Disease

Yvonne A. Ruddy-Stein, MSN, RN, CS, ANP
Nurse Practitioner
The Children's Heart Center
Egleston at Emory University
Atlanta, Georgia
Chapter 12 The History and Physical Examination
Chapter 33 Valvular and Congenital Heart Disease

Joanne Sandberg-Cook, MS, ARNP, CS, CRRN
Gerontological Nurse Practitioner
Lahey-Hitchcock Clinic
Hanover, New Hampshire
Chapter 48 Rheumatic Problems

Ellen Schmidt, RN-C, MS
Nurse Practitioner
University of Rochester Medical Center
Rochester, New York
Chapter 41 Gastrointestinal Problems

C. Beth Staudenmayer, MSN, CRNP, CS, CRNP
Nurse Practitioner
Thomas Jefferson University
Philadelphia, Pennsylvania
Chapter 32 Coronary Artery Disease
Chapter 33 Valvular and Congenital Heart Disease

Eileen M. Sullivan-Marx, PhD, FAAN
Director, Primary Care Nurse Practitioner Program
School of Nursing
University of Pennsylvania
Philadelphia, Pennsylvania
Chapter 3 Business Considerations for the ACNP

Debra Tribett, MS, RN, CS, LNP
Adult and Acute Care Nurse Practitioner
Infectious Disease Physicians, Inc.
Annandale, Virginia
Chapter 47 Immunologic Problems

Carol Twomey, MSN, CRNP
Nurse Practitioner
Hahnemann University Hospital
Philadelphia, Pennsylvania
Chapter 35 Heart Failure and Cardiomyopathy

Marie Uberti-Benz, MD
Presbyterian Medical Center
Philadelphia, Pennsylvania
Chapter 51 Skin Problems

Kathleen A. Walsh, MSN, CRNP
Nurse Practitioner
Hahnemann University Hospital
Philadelphia, Pennsylvania
Chapter 50 Head and Neck Problems

Glenn J. R. Whitman, MD
Department of Cardiothoracic Surgery
University of Maryland
Baltimore, Maryland
Chapter 19 Shock

JoAnne D. Whitney, RN, PhD
Assistant Professor
University of Washington
Seattle, Washington
Chapter 21 Wound Management

Diana J. Wilkie, PhD, RN, AOCN, FAAN
Associate Professor
Department of Biobehavioral Nursing and Health Systems
University of Washington, School of Nursing
Seattle, Washington
Chapter 20 Pain Management

Anne W. Wojner, RN, MSN, CCRN
President
Health Outcomes Institute, Inc.
The Woodlands, Texas
Chapter 10 Outcomes Management and the ACNP

Angela B. Wurster, RN, MSN, CRNP
Nurse Practitioner, Thoracic Surgery
Hospital of the University of Pennsylvania
Philadelphia, Pennsylvania
Chapter 38 Thoracic Surgery

Reviewers

Patricia K. Abbott, AB, MHS, PA-C
Senior Physician Assistant
Thoracic Surgery
University of Pennsylvania Medical Center
Philadelphia, Pennsylvania

Tom Ahrens, DNS, RN, CCRN, CS
Clinical Specialist
Critical Care
Barnes-Jewish Hospital
St. Louis, Missouri

Mary Beth Alder, RN, MSN, DNSc (candidate), LNP
Nurse Practitioner
Infectious Diseases Physicians, Inc.
Annandale, Virginia

Christine L. Archer-Chicko, MSN, RN, CCRN, CCTC
Lung Transplant Coordinator
University of Pennsylvania Medical Center
Philadelphia, Pennsylvania

Saroj Bahl, PhD, RD, LD
Associate Professor of Nutrition
University of Texas
Houston School of Allied Health Sciences
Sugar Land, Texas

John W. Becker, DO
Professor and Chair
Department of Emergency Medicine
Philadelphia College of Osteopathic Medicine
Newtown Square, Pennsylvania

Howard W. Blume, MD, PhD
Beth Israel-Deaconess Medical Center
Brookline, Massachusetts

Karen Calabro, MS, RD, LD, MPH
Coordinator of Health Promotion and Health Education
University of Texas
Houston Health Science Center
Houston, Texas

Marianne Chulay, RN, DNSc, FAAN
Director
Nursing Research and Practice
Moses Cone Health System, Greensboro, NC
Chapel Hill, North Carolina

Mary Cwiertniewicz, RN, MSN, CRNP, CNN
Level III Nephrology Nurse
University of Pennsylvania Medical Center
Brookhaven, Pennsylvania

Joseph deJunco, MD
Lovejoy Heart and Medical Clinic
Lovejoy, Georgia

Patchen Dellinger, MD
Professor and Vice Chairman
Department of Surgery
University of Washington Medical Center
Seattle, Washington

Jeffrey Edelman, MD
Assistant Professor of Medicine
Pulmonary/Critical Care
Hospital of the University of Pennsylvania
Philadelphia, Pennsylvania

Jeffrey M. Feldman, MD
Associate Professor of Anesthesiology
Allegheny University of the Health Sciences
Philadelphia, Pennsylvania

Marianne Ferrin, MSN, ACNP, CS, CCRN
Clinical Nurse Specialist
Pulmonary/Critical Care
Hospital of the University of Pennsylvania
Philadelphia, Pennsylvania

Sally Frese, RN, MSN, CS
Psychiatric Consultation Liaison Nurse
St. Louis University Health Sciences Center
St. Louis, Missouri

Samuel L. Glass, MD
Opthamologist
Johnstown, Pennsylvania

Bruce Hoffman, MD
Medical College of Pennsylvania Hospital
Philadelphia, Pennsylvania

Marilyn Hravnak, RN, MSN, ACNP-CS, CCRN
Coordinator, Acute Care Nurse Practitioner Program
University of Pittsburgh
Pittsburgh, Pennsylvania

Lynette W. Jack, RN, PhD, CARN
Psychiatric Nurse Practitioner
School of Nursing
University of Pittsburg
Pittsburg, Pennsylvania

Venerando G. Jaurigue, MD, FACS
Acting Chief
Department of Surgery
Jeanes Hospital
Philadelphia, Pennsylvania

Pamela S. Johnson, MSN, FNP-C
Family Nurse Practitioner
Lovejoy Heart and Medical Clinic
Hampton, Georgia

Larry R. Kaiser, MD
Director
General Thoracic Surgery
University of Pennsylvania Medical Center
Philadelphia, Pennsylvania

Morris D. Kerstein, MD
Professor of Surgery
Allegheny University of the Health Sciences
Philadelphia, Pennsylvania

Lee L. Konecke, MD
Norristown Cardiovascular Associates
Cardiovascular Associates of Southeastern Pennsylvania
Norristown, Pennsylvania

Robert M. Kotloff, MD
Medical Director
Lung Transplant Program
University of Pennsylvania Medical Center
Philadelphia, Pennsylvania

Theresa Kuczynski, RN, MSN
President
Targeting Transitions
Scranton, Pennsylvania

Amelia Langston, MD
Medical Oncologist
Marrow and Stem Cell Transplantation
Fred Hutchinson Cancer Research Center
Seattle, Washington

Ann Letourman, MD
Plastic and Reconstructive Surgeon
Port Tuffuson, New York

Karen Mahoney, MD
Endocrine and Diabetes Group of Washington
Washington, District of Columbia

Richard Martorelli, MBA, CPA
Director, Clinical Effectiveness
Mercy Health Partners
Scranton, Pennsylvania

Barbara J. Maschak-Carey, RN, MSN, CDE
Diabetes Clinical Nurse Specialist
Hospital of the University of Pennsylvania
Philadelphia, Pennsylvania

Dennis McCullough, PhD, MD, ABFP
Chief Clinical Officer
Community and Family Medicine
Dartmouth Hitchcock Medical Center
Lebanon, New Hampshire

Douglass L. McGee, DO
Associate Director
Emergency Medicine Residency Program
Albert Einstein Medical Center
Philadelphia, Pennsylvania

Susan Mueller, BSN, RN, CRRN, CCM
Case Manager/Marketing Coordinator
Evansville Cancer Center
Evansville, Illinois

Steven Nagelberg, MD
Endocrine and Metabolic Associates
Bala Cynwyd, Pennsylvania

Lynn Noland, RN, PhD, NP
Assistant Professor of Nursing and Nurse Practitioner
Kidney Center
University of Virginia
Charlottesville, Virginia

Harold T. Palevsky, MD
Director
Pulmonary Vascular Disease Program
University of Pennsylvania Medical Center
Philadelphia, Pennsylvania

Melinda Patience, RN, MSN
Research Nurse
Fred Hutchinson Cancer Research Center
Seattle, Washington

Benoit Paul R., Jr., MD
Harvard Combined Orthopedic Surgery Program
Boston, Massachusetts

Lori Ratliff, RN, MSN, ANP, CDE
Nurse Practitioner
University of Virginia Kidney Center
Charlottesville, Virginia

John R. Roberts, MD
Chief, Thoracic Surgery
Vanderbilt University School of Medicine
Nashville, Tennessee

Martin S. Sawson, MD
Clinical Instructor of Medicine
Division of Cardiology
Allegheny University Hospitals: Hahnemann Division
Maple Shade, New Jersey

Cynthia Scalzi, PhD
Associate Professor
School of Nursing
University of Pennsylvania
Philadelphia, Pennsylvania

Steven Shoen, MD
Plastic and Reconstructive Surgeon
University Medical Center
Stony Brook, New York

Barry L. Singer, MD
Hematologist and Oncologist
Norristown, Pennsylvania

Vaughn A. Starnes, MD, FACS
Professor and Chief
Cardiothoracic Surgery
University of Southern California School of Medicine
Los Angeles, California

Eileen M. Sullivan-Marx, PhD, RN
Assistant Professor
University of Pennsylvania School of Nursing
Philadelphia, Pennsylvania

Bory Sumyk, MD
Norridge Medical Center
Norridge, Illinois

Suzanne Tirado, RN, MSN, CRNP, RNFA, CNOR
Surgical Nurse Practitioner
Valley Forge Surgical Associates
Bechtelsville, Pennsylvania

Ann B. Townsend, RN, MSN, CNSC, NPC
Critical Care Clinical Specialist
Cardiovascular Associates
Moorestown, New Jersey

Wendy Valentine, RN, MSN
Surgical Clinical Nurse Specialist
University of Washington Medical Center
Seattle, Washington

Gwyn M. Vernon, MSN, CRNP
Nurse Practitioner and Clinical Faculty
Crozer Keystone Family Practice
University of Pennsylvania SON
Wallingford, Pennsylvania

Holly Watson-Evans, RN, MSN
Director, Neurospine and Orthopedic Service
Central Dupage Hospital
Winfield, Illinois

David Wheeler, MD
Infectious Diseases Physicians, Inc.
Annandale, Virginia

Michael J. Wilkowski, MD
Associate Professor of Medicine
University of Virginia
Charlottesville, Virginia

Rebekah M. Wilmes, APRN, MSN, CS
Transplant Coordinator
Heart Failure and Transplant Cardiology Program
Yale University School of Medicine
New Haven, Connecticut

Robert P. Witherspoon, MD
Associate Professor of Medicine
Fred Hutchinson Cancer Research Center
Seattle, Washington

Preface

ACNPs are an interesting hybrid. We are nurse practitioners, but do not practice primary care. We are expert nurse clinicians, but do not function as clinical nurse specialists. We are responsible for knowing much of what physicians know, but have less foundation in basic science. Textbooks for nurse practitioners, therefore, are not terribly useful to ACNPs. Textbooks for clinical nurse specialists also fail to meet our unique needs, as do medical textbooks. It occurred to me that there is a need for a textbook written specifically for ACNPs; one that combines nursing knowledge with medical knowledge. Hence, here is *Principles of Practice for the Acute Care Nurse Practitioner.*

▶ THE CURRENT ENVIRONMENT

It is unclear how many ACNPs there are, but it is clear that ACNP roles are being created in hospitals, extended care facilities, clinics, rehabilitation facilities, and outpatient settings. Educational programs that prepare ACNPs are rapidly growing in number. There are now over sixty known ACNP programs in the United States, and the number grows annually.

Prior to January 1, 1998, nurse practitioners could not bill Medicare unless they provided services in designated rural areas or qualified under other Federal programs. Since passage of the 1997 Balanced Budget Act that expanded Medicare reimbursement to nurse practitioners in every practice setting, it is likely that nurse practitioners will be viewed by potential employers more positively. That is, they can generate income to support their salary. Additionally, for those employers who value it, nurse practitioners bring to the practice the personalized attention to patients, the patient educational services, and the clinical resourcefulness that characterize nurse practitioners. Employers understand that nurse practitioners are reliable and committed professionals with a good understanding of patients and their physiologic and psychosocial problems.

But we should face facts. Nurse practitioners would not be enjoying their current popularity were it not for the recent changes in the health care delivery system. The government, insurers, hospitals, and physicians no longer have unlimited resources. Everyone is cutting back. Government agencies and insurers are cutting back reimbursement. Hospitals and private practice physicians are cutting back staff. The days of "doing more with less" are here to stay.

Had the current environment not appeared, it is doubtful that nurse practitioners would be making the impact that they are. Nurses realize the benefit that nurse practitioners bring to health care, but frequently physicians and health systems do not value these contributions. What these entities value is the "bottom line."

It is a credit to our profession that nursing leaders foresaw the coming "big business era" of health care and prepared nurse practitioners to fill the voids created by diminishing reimbursement, and that they were able to simultaneously improve the quality of patient care. Patients would have been cared for regardless of nursing's contributions, but nurse practitioners bring their unique perspective to the practice arena and we do so in a way that makes a difference. We make a difference to patients, we make a difference to their families, and we make a difference to the "bottom line."

▶ THE BOOK

This textbook is intended for both graduate students and practicing ACNPs. The goal of the textbook, therefore, is not to provide learning exercises or activities for classroom study. Rather, the book is intended to concisely present the principles integral to competent clinical practice. Gerontological, adult, and family nurse practitioners, clinical nurse specialists, and physician assistants practicing in acute care settings will also find this book useful.

The book is divided into five sections:

Part I: The Role of the Acute Care Nurse Practitioner
Part II: Essentials of Practice
Part III: Clinical Situations in Acute Care
Part IV: Approach to the Patient with an Acute Illness
Part V: Approach to the Patient with Specialized Needs

Part I provides an introduction to the ACNP role. Part II introduces the components of clinical practice that are shared by all ACNPs, including history taking, physical examination, and clinical decision making. Part III presents common acute care problems and multisystem problems such as shock, cancer treatment, wound management, and organ donation and transplantation. Part IV contains a system-by-system approach to patient management. Here, topics such as coronary artery disease, hypertension, and neurological, breast, orthopedic, and eye problems are presented. Lastly, Part V addresses specialized health care needs for the pediatric patient, the older adult patient, and the patient with psychiatric and substance abuse problems.

Throughout the book, emphasis is on clinical management of patients with acute health problems. Each of the clinical chapters is organized similarly. Because it is assumed that readers possess a basic understanding of normal anatomy and physiology, only a brief overview of appropriate anatomy and physiology is given. Then, for each particular disorder, the pathophysiology, history and physical findings, laboratory and diagnostic tests, management, and follow-up are discussed.

Contributors were given these instructions:

- Remember the diversity of ACNP practice settings as you write.
- Assume that the reader has an understanding of normal anatomy and physiology, and give a concise overview of pathophysiology.
- Emphasize diagnosis and treatment of acute problems, but also include appropriate clinical information for management of stable/chronic problems.
- Make the chapter "readable." Write in plain language, be concise, and use no "fluff."

Some of the contributors to this textbook are nationally recognized experts. Others, like me, are clinicians who make no representation of national authority. Rather, they are expert clinicians whose job is caring for patients with acute health problems. They have real-world experience and broad expertise. These traits are indispensable.

It is the hope of each contributor and me that the book will serve you both as a student and as a practicing clinician.

Paul Logan

Acknowledgments

It was December 1995 that I first seriously considered putting together a textbook for a fledgling specialty. Carol Weingarten was kind enough to meet me at the Villanova Diner. We sat, and over breakfast, discussed the garguantuan task of editing a textbook. Carol had a successful maternal-child nursing textbook in its third edition, so I figured she knew what she was talking about. I did not fully appreciate, though, the gravity of her admonitions. She warned me that I should be well prepared to work harder than ever before. But she also told me that completing the project would be the most rewarding accomplishment to date. She was correct on both counts. I thank her for her honesty, encouragement, advise, and cheering.

Without Marianne Chulay's guidance and encouragement, I would never have been in a position to tackle this project. As a new college graduate—and very "green" nurse—I went to work at the National Institutes of Health. Naturally, as a recent nursing graduate I knew everything there was to know and could rarely be persuaded otherwise. Still, Marianne was gracious enough to put up with me. It was Marianne who introduced me to the idea of becoming an Acute Care Nurse Practitioner. She subsequently put me in touch with my two principle mentors. I am deeply indebted to Marianne for her thoughtful guidance at a time when I could very easily have been persuaded down another path.

At the University of Pennsylvania I met two individuals who later became important mentors. Referred by Marianne, Terry Richmond was the person with whom I first spoke about the tertiary nurse practitioner program at Penn. I was immediately hooked. I scheduled an interview with Anne Keane several weeks later and was admitted to the program. I have Terry and Anne to thank for the opportunities they provided, for the lessons they taught, and for the encouragement they continue to give.

Never before have I met, nor do I expect to meet in the future, a clinican as skillful, grounded, and compassionate as Bill Kussmaul. Bill was my physician-preceptor for an eight-month clinical rotation. I am not certain how I was lucky enough to have him for a mentor, but I am eternally grateful for his contributions to my education. In addition to being an outstanding clinician, he is a terrific role model from whom I was privileged to learn.

I am fortunate to now work with three expert cardiologists: Andrea Becker, Lee Konecke, and Hugh Lipshutz. They offered me the perfect ACNP job and allowed me to develop it into a role that is both professionally rewarding to me and beneficial to the practice. They trust my clinical judgement and value my contributions to patient care. In addition to being terrific clinicians, they are also extraordinarily compassionate people with some of the best senses of humor I have witnessed. I learn from them daily and always look forward to going to work.

At the beginning of this venture I knew absolutely nothing about publishing a book. Hopefully, that is not too obvious as you read it. If it is obvious, it is Dave Carroll's fault. It must have been a heinous and unforgivable act that he committed to have been assigned to my book. Nevertheless, Dave has been a terrific help to me and a great friend. I may never be able to repay him for his help, but I do not expect him to ask, either.

Editing 54 chapters is not an easy task, particularly given my toddler-like attention span. So, when Yvonne Ruddy-Stein offered to help with some editing—an offer she no doubt regrets—I was delighted to send her several manuscripts. Her work, and that of Janet Foltin, is appreciated.

Other valuable timesavers were the expert reviewers who kindly reviewed the chapters for content. Although they did not have to, they also made changes in grammar, punctuation, and style. This helped both the contributors and me.

The time that I devoted to this book was meaningless compared to the effort made by the contributors. Without the contributors who wrote the book, there would be no book. They were kind enough to write in return for only my profound gratitude, minimal remuneration, and a copy of the book. I am indebted to them for their hard work and appreciate their dedication to excellence.

Once the novelty of writing a book wore off and the real work began, there were countless moments when I doubted my ability to finish the task that I undertook. As with any big project, there comes a point at which you just want it to be finished. That point came far too early in the process for it to be motivational. With at least seven months remaining until the dreaded deadline, my wife and I found out that we were pregnant with our first child. I am certain that no work was done on the book that month, making it all the more difficult to meet the final deadlines. Through it all, my wife, Jeanne, supported me, encouraged me, and left me alone enough to finish. It is to her that I dedicate this book.

I

The Role of the Acute Care Nurse Practitioner

1

The Emergence, Maturation, and Future of the Acute Care Nurse Practitioner Role

Anne Keane
Joanne Angstadt

Change in health care is ongoing, but these changes have become front-page news that also have obvious social, economic, and political implications. Health care in the late 1990s has been characterized by efforts to contain costs, yet to provide care that is excellent and universally available—goals not yet fully achieved. The development of acute care nurse practitioner (ACNP) roles is a response both to advances in health care and to changing social, economic, and political realities.

The growth of advanced practice nursing roles reflects nursing's efforts to fulfill its social contract with patients and their needs for responsible, comprehensive, yet cost-effective care. Advanced practice nursing roles have evolved steadily over the past century and the development of the ACNP is one part of the ongoing evolution of professional nursing.

ACNP roles have their historical basis in the development of other advanced practice nursing roles, including the emergence of nurse midwives and nurse anesthetists in the beginning of the twentieth century and of clinical nurse specialists (CNSs) and primary care nurse practitioners (NPs) in the latter half of the twentieth century. While these other advanced practice nursing roles and their related responsibilities may seem quite different from those of today's ACNPs, social forces and realities that supported their development are similar and their development resulted in early professional and legislative recognition of advanced practice nursing roles.

Nurse midwife and nurse anesthetist roles were developed in response to the neglected obstetrical needs of poor, immigrant, urban women and to the unmet anesthesia and perioperative care needs of rural patients. More recently the CNS role was developed in the mid-1960s to meet the specialized needs of very ill hospitalized patients, while NP roles were developed in the late 1960s and early 1970s in response to a shortage of physicians that was limiting access to care in primary care settings. In all of these situations unmet needs or unacceptable health care delivery patterns encouraged the development of these advanced practice nursing roles. The creation of these roles also provided advanced practice nurses with more direct access to patients and increased their decision-making scope, authority, and accountability and essentially expanded the boundaries of professional nursing practice (Freund, 1993, p. 310).

▶ DEVELOPMENT OF THE ROLE OF THE ACUTE CARE NURSE PRACTITIONER

The development of the ACNP role in the early 1990s was directly influenced by the responsibilities, successes, and limitations of the existing CNS and NP roles. While these roles were originally differently conceptualized to provide acute, inpatient specialized care versus generalized, outpatient care to well patients, a blurring of responsibilities and sites of practice gradually evolved. As early as 1986 the American Nurses' Association (ANA) Council of Clinical Nurse Specialists and the Council of Primary Health Care Nurse Practitioners identified that the CNS and NP roles were more similar than different (Sparacino & Durand, 1986). The work of Elder and Bullough (1990) supported this position. In 1990 they surveyed the CNS and NP graduates of a university-based graduate nursing program and found that CNS and NP roles differed in only eight of the 25 role-related activities measured. Not surprisingly NPs were more likely than CNSs to conduct histories and physicals and to order diagnostic tests, medications, and treatments and to make referrals (Elder & Bullough, 1990, p. 81). Teaching the clinical staff and conducting support groups were more commonly reported activities of the CNS, but both groups were likely to be involved in teaching patients and their families and in providing counseling and psychosocial assessments. Clinical nurse specialists, however, were more likely to leave clinical practice for administrative or education responsibilities, and even when remaining in clinical settings, they were more than twice as likely as NPs to participate in indirect versus direct patient care activities.

Changing clinical realities, increasing financial pressures, and evolving population demographics have also contributed to the emergence of the ACNP. These increasing pressures on the health care setting have not permitted a "business as usual" approach to the delivery of care in the acute care setting on the part of nurses or other health care providers. Advances in technology and medical science, a growing aging population with concurrent chronic illnesses, and the growth of populations who have survived previously fatal illnesses have produced changes in patient care mixes resulting in highly vulnerable populations requiring specialized care. At the same time, the high cost of health care has produced limitations in the allowable length of hospital stay, a focus on the preparation of primary care versus specialty physicians, and increased pressures to decrease the cost related to the high numbers of specialist physicians. These concerns have produced a more fluid clinical environment in which solutions to these issues can be tested. The emergence of the ACNP has been recognized as one such response to these concerns.

▶ MODELS FOR PRACTICE

A review of the recent literature provides several discussions of the role of the ACNP and includes descriptions of roles as case managers (Soehren & Schumann, 1994), as unit- or service-based practitioners (Richmond & Keane, 1992; Keane, Richmond, & Kaiser, 1994), and as nurse practitioner members of a physician-based plan or group. Richmond and Keane (1992) described two major models in which the ACNP might function: the joint professional practice model and the nursing-based model. In the former model ACNPs practice collaboratively within a specialty physician practice plan, with direct reporting lines to the physician partners in the practice plan and an indirect reporting line to the nursing staff and nursing organization. In the nursing-based model the ACNP may have unit- or service-based responsibilities, perhaps serving as the ACNP in charge of the postcardiothoracic surgery unit or the outpatient heart failure clinic. In this model ACNPs may have dual reporting responsibilities to both the nursing service organization for nursing care issues and to the physician who is responsible for the medical management of unit- or service-based patients. As Richmond and Keane note (1992), the growth of either of these two ACNP organizational patterns depends on the success of the organization in dealing with authority for admission, transfer and discharge, prescription privileges, financial incentives, and reimbursement (p. 235).

Other writers have described evolving aspects of the ACNP role. Taking over house staff responsibilities was described in a recent editorial by Mallison (1993); serving as the "attending nurse" is an idea described by Aiken (1990); expanding care and collaborative roles in critical care settings was described by Dracup and Bryan-Brown (1994); and both hospital and nonhospital-based critical care nurse practitioner roles have been described by Watts and colleagues (1996). Acute care nurse practitioner roles are clearly evolving at a steady pace.

Ackerman, Norsen, Martin, Wiedrich, and Kitzman (1996) described the domains of practice that constitute the parts of the ACNP role. These mutually exclusive domains include: provision of direct, comprehensive care; support of systems that promote innovative patient care and facilitate optimal progression of the patient through the health care system; enhanced patient care through the dissemination of current knowledge; generation of knowledge and integration of research findings into clinical practice; and involvement in professional activities, including publishing that results in a sharing of individual expertise and that promotes nursing and health care (p. 70). Essential to the operation of these five domains are the concepts of: empowerment to establish the ACNP's responsibility for decisions affecting practice; scholarship to promote intelligent, thoughtful, competent, confident care; and collaboration to reflect an awareness that care cannot be effectively provided by a single care provider (pp. 70–73).

These models of ACNP practice are evolving and require ongoing analysis. They can however provide some direction for programs that prepare ACNPs and for organizations or institutions that employ them.

PREPARATION OF THE ACUTE CARE NURSE PRACTITIONER

Educational programs that prepare ACNPs must constantly evolve as they must reflect both current practice expectations and opportunities and the anticipated scope of future practice (Keane & Richmond, 1993, p. 283). Current practice guidelines require that the ACNP be prepared to provide direct care to acutely ill patients in a holistic manner. Hravnak and colleagues (1995) identify three beliefs to guide ACNP programs: content should be driven by patient care needs regardless of the setting; graduates should be able to promote health as well as manage disease; and graduates should be able to view the patient as a whole and not isolate assessment and disease-related interventions (p. 180).

Many forces influence the actual content of ACNP curricula, including the ANA/American Association of Critical Care Nurses' statement on the scope of ACNP practice (1995), the American Association of Colleges of Nursing position on the Essentials of Master's Education for Advanced Practice Nurses (1995), the expectations of potential employing institutions or practice settings and relevant personnel, and the philosophical beliefs and guidelines of the graduate-level nursing program in which the ACNP is prepared.

Content in these programs is generally divided into several areas, including general master's core content, advanced practice core content, and specialty content (AACN Task Force on the Essentials of Master's Education, 1995). Schools differ in their identification of general content, but common areas include preparation as a clinical researcher or research consumer, as a leader capable of critical thinking, able to conceptualize and problem-solve, and as a leader with preparation in health policy, ethics, cultural diversity, finance, systems organization, and role development (O'Flynn, 1995).

General Core Content

The general core provides a base of nursing expertise and an understanding of the range of advanced practice nursing functions (King & Ackerman, 1995). King and Ackerman suggest that general core content include three areas: (1) concepts and theories to provide the ACNP with a grasp of conceptual frameworks and theories from nursing and other disciplines; (2) ethics and public policy to provide a base for clinical, administrative, and public policy decision making; and (3) patient advocacy, consultation, and collaboration; and research content that includes both the use of research and participation in the conduct of research (pp. 2–3).

Advanced Practice Core

Content in this area informs advanced nursing practice, regardless of the area of specialization. It includes advanced physical and clinical assessment of the individual, diagnostic thinking and ability, management of health and common chronic illnesses, pharmacology, physiology, and pathophysiology (Standards for Educational Programs: Preparing Students as Acute Care Nurse Practitioners, 1993; Keane & Richmond, 1993; Clochesy et al., 1994; King & Ackerman, 1995). Content and experiences designed to prepare advanced practice nurses with generic psychomotor versus advanced psychomotor skills probably also belong in the advanced practice core, as consensus grows about common areas for these skills. Such skills might include the ability to suture and safely perform minimally invasive treatments, interpret chest x-rays, and 12-lead electrocardiograms, and deal with common diagnostic and treatment-related technology. There are few practice settings in which these competencies are not required of all health care providers. More advanced preparation in psychomotor skills is found in the specialty core.

Specialty Core Content

Content in the acute care specialty area provides the ACNP with the knowledge needed to care for patients with the full spectrum of high-acuity needs. Both didactic information about acute health problems and guided experience in the management of these problems and concurrent chronic illnesses are essential content. Some programs are organized under the broad acute care label, while others focus more on subspecialty areas such as critical, cardiopulmonary, or acute surgical care. These decisions, and the resultant content, reflect the demands of the practice setting, the beliefs and strengths of the faculty, the ANA/AACN (1995) guidelines on scope of practice, the need to include content found in national certification examinations, and the requirements of the various states that recognize program graduates as ACNPs.

INFLUENCE OF EDUCATIONAL PROGRAMS ON THE MATURATION OF THE ROLE OF THE ACNP

The recent growth in ACNP programs has been noticeable and has contributed to the growth of practicing ACNPs in this country. From 1992 to 1995 the number of nurse practitioner programs in the nation doubled, and the greatest increase was seen in post-master's programs in which master's-prepared nurses can "retool" for changing practice requirements, in family nurse practitioner programs, and in specialty nurse practitioner programs such as ACNP programs. In supporting this growth, faculties and schools of nursing have responded to what Booth (1995) calls the need for curricular reform, as one response to the nation's need for health care reform. By launching credible ACNP programs, developing national certification examinations and national standards for curriculum development, and gaining broad support for the role from nurses, physicians, and others, nursing educators have provided a vision for ACNP practice. This vision is empowered by preparing credible practitioners who can negotiate effective roles in today's unsettled acute care setting.

There are, however, considerable restraints to the ongoing development of these master's-level educational programs. There is little federal financial support for curriculum development training grants to assist nursing faculty members in their efforts to develop or expand ACNP programs, and the money that is available is constantly threatened by congressional budget reduction economies. In addition, while the federal government through Title VIII and through Medicare Graduate Education (GME) funds, provides support for nursing education, these funds are directed disproportionately to diploma-based nursing programs, versus baccalaureate or advanced practice nursing programs (Aiken & Salmon, 1994). For example, only $10.4 million of federal funding available through Title VIII was distributed to baccalaureate nursing programs in 1994, versus a lopsided $220,000 million of GME funds distributed to hospital-based diploma nursing programs (Aiken & Salmon, 1994). Diploma-level nurses are not prepared for the growth and major shifts in health care delivery, or for advanced practice nursing roles. Ill-conceived federal decisions about which type and level of nursing programs to support do not reflect current health care needs or provide for future growth of ACNP and other advanced practice nursing roles. A shortfall or inadequate supply of well-prepared ACNPs and other advanced practice nurses could seriously jeopardize the ongoing expansion of advanced practice nursing roles and compromise this educational reform effort. This concern could become a reality as estimates from the U.S. Department of Health and Human Services (1991) suggest that by the year 2000, there will be half as many baccalaureate and higher degree nurses as are needed.

▶ INFLUENCE OF REGULATION ON THE MATURATION OF THE ROLE OF THE ACNP

Educational Regulation

Professions are regulated on several levels by schools, professional organizations, employing institutions, and the state. These regulations are society's way to ensure that professional care givers are adequately prepared to deliver care, monitor patient progress, and facilitate favorable patient care outcomes. Whelan (1995) calls the regulation provided by educational institutions the most critical aspect of regulation, as the provision of a specialized body of knowledge is essential in controlling entry into the profession and in identifying who is eligible to practice (p. 12).

Advanced practice nursing students, including ACNP students, are prepared in accredited, master's-level graduate nursing programs. Graduates of these programs are then eligible to take national certification examinations that attest to a level of professional competence through successful completion of these examinations.

The effectiveness of educational regulation on ACNP practice largely depends on the resources and quality of the graduate program, the opportunity for guided clinical practice with a range of appropriate patient experiences, and the preparation of the program faculty and clinical preceptors. Considerable regulation by accrediting bodies exists to ensure program quality.

Institutional Regulation

In addition to educational and professional regulation, organizations, practices, or institutions that employ advanced practice nurses also regulate practice by defining the scope of the practice permitted within the employing organization or institution. This regulation is done by reviewing the individuals' credentials and by identifying the scope of practice deemed permissible. A description of permissible practice is then generally described in a practice protocol. As part of the review of credentials, there is a growing tendency for institutions to require evidence of national certification in an appropriate area, within the first 6 to 12 months of employment.

Currently, the scope of practice identified by the credentialing review may have less to do with the preparation and capabilities of the individual than with the policies enforced by the medical board of the organization. As yet, there are few advanced practice nurses appointed to these boards, and as a result there is little direct opportunity to describe the possible range of advanced practice nursing roles and the potential contributions of these nurses to the organization.

State Regulation

Finally, states are the most important influence on the regulation of advanced nursing practice (Whelan, 1995). Through regulations states, with the force of law, define professional practice and related activities within their jurisdictions. Because the authority to regulate professional practice rests at the state level, there is little uniformity in the recognition of the legal status of ACNPs and other advanced practice nurses throughout the United States. States vary in their tendency to recognize or restrict advanced nursing practice. They range from endorsement of independent advanced practice with full prescription privileges to the requirement for direct physician supervision, and finally, even to a lack of acknowledgment of advanced practice nursing status in some state statutes. This range in the recognition of advanced practice nurses and endorsement of their scope of practice is a result of political considerations and barriers to practice rather than a reflection of advanced practice nurses' capabilities.

The first state nurse practice acts were enacted in the early 1900s, and by 1923 every state had enacted nurse licensure laws (Safreit, 1992; Whelan, 1995). These acts did not address the expanded roles and responsibilities of advanced practice nurses, especially those related to diagnosis and treatment, and it became increasingly difficult to describe these activities, already being performed by nurses, as complementary to physician services (Whelan, 1995). As a result, the states began a process, still ongoing today, of amending the nurse practice acts. In 1971 Idaho became the first state to recognize diagnosis and treatment as part of the scope of practice of advanced practice or specialty nurses (Safreit, 1992, p. 445).

Today 25 states and the District of Columbia have nurse practitioner title protection and the board of nursing as the sole authority for scope of practice, and no requirement in the law for physician collaboration or supervision. An additional 16 states have similar title protection and board of nursing authority for the scope of practice, but a requirement for physician collaboration or supervision of the role. An additional six states have nurse practitioner title protection, but both the boards of nursing and medicine have authority for advanced nursing practice. Finally, three states still have no title protection, and the nurse practitioner must function under the broad nurse practice act in that state (Pearson, 1997, p. 18).

Clearly there are more or less severe restrictions on advanced nursing practice resulting from state regulations or the lack of them. Safreit (1992) calls the present situation of advanced nursing practice regulations a "crazy quilt" of regulations with confusing and disabling provisions (p. 454). Still, in the past 26 years, all but three states have recognized the legal status of nurse practitioners, and as a result, have provided some direction for the development of ACNP roles.

According to Safreit (1992), at least several reasons account for the legal mandates for physician supervision of advanced practice nurses: many of the state practice acts were written before the voluminous studies were published demonstrating that advanced practice nurses are competent, autonomous providers of care; and second, legislators may have relied unduly on advice from physicians, who knew no more than the legislators about the capabilities of advanced practice nurses, but who were unsure of the longer-range structural impact of these new providers on their medical practice (pp. 454–456). On the one hand, undue restrictions on advanced practice nurses was a result of a lack of knowledge of their capabilities. On the other hand, these restrictions evolved as physicians attempted to protect their monopolistic control over health care.

The concept of physician supervision identified in the regulations of at least 26 states is very different from the supervision, collaboration, and coordination of care required of all care givers in busy, demanding acute care settings. The mandated requirements in state regulations for supervision of advanced practice nurses are ongoing and do not reflect the growing competencies of ACNPs or other advanced practice nurses, and these regulations are inadequate for the range of clinical decisions required in current practice settings. Whelan (1995) calls physician supervision often unnecessary, inconvenient, and costly (p. 28).

Rather than requiring mandated permanent supervision, ACNPs and other advanced practice nurses require, as do other professionals, a system of supervision and mentoring characterized initially by direct supervision, demonstration, and feedback, and later by opportunities to discuss clinical decisions and review the implications related to new treatments or changing patient situations and to reflect on knowledge, experience, and growing professional competence. Snyder and colleagues (1994) have described the phased periods of supervision for recent ACNP graduates employed in intensive care settings as they progress through the phases of direct, proximate, and general supervision and move toward independent functioning. Supervision and mentoring are necessary for the growth of all health care providers. This is particularly true in acute care settings where appropriate and timely interventions to support critically ill patients are essential.

Regulation of Prescription Authority

The regulation of prescription authority is a special type of regulation that has supported or limited the clinical decision-making ability of advanced practice nurses. Currently, 18 states and the District of Columbia permit nurse practitioners to prescribe medications, including controlled substances independently. An additional 18 states permit this activity with some degree of physician involvement or delegation of prescription writing. Thirteen states permit nurses to prescribe medications, excluding controlled substances, but require some degree of physician involvement or delegation. Currently, only Illinois has no statutory prescribing authority for nurse practitioners (Pearson, 1997, p. 18).

Similar to advanced practice nursing title protection, there is little logic for the wide-ranging pattern of prescribing authority permitted or restricted by the various state regulations. The mandated requirement in state laws for physician supervision of prescription authority artificially restricts advanced practice nurses' scope of practice, resulting in inefficient use of health care resources and limited patient access to care (Safreit, 1992, p. 463).

Pharmacological management in acute care settings requires careful coordination by the multiple care givers, including both nurses and physicians. The use of institutionally based practice protocols in critical care settings is one way in which ACNPs have assumed responsibility for the pharmacological management of their patients. Many acute care settings have developed unit-based protocols that identify the accepted pharmacological management of common patient situations. Critical care pathways also provide guidelines for appropriate pharmacological management. Still, the dynamic nature of critically ill patients requires that existing pharmacological management protocols be further developed.

Only 31% of intensive care units in the United States reported 24-hour coverage by medical residents in 1992, ranging from 95% in large hospitals to only 6% in small hospitals (Groeger, et al., 1992). With the anticipated downsizing of residents' programs, these percentages can be expected to continue to change, and the ACNP's role in pharmacological management of acutely ill patients will expand further.

Mahoney's survey of nurse practitioners (1995) suggests that even when authority to write prescriptions has been legalized, there are administrative barriers to this activity. Barriers to prescribing activities identified in her survey included the perceived need for additional malpractice insurance for the supervising physician, the need to develop new practice policies and procedures, the time-consuming nature of modifying guidelines to include prescribing medications, administrative delays in implementing this new activity, and lack of third-party reimbursement (pp. 59–60).

Second Licensure

A controversy exists about the need for a second license for advanced practice nurses. Because the states vary widely in their recognition of advanced practice nurses and their scope of practice, the National Council of State Boards of Nursing has proposed the need for a second license as a clear, unequivocal authorization for advanced nursing practice (National Council of State Boards of Nursing, 1993). The rationale for this added requirement for practice reflects their belief that advanced practice nursing exceeds the scope of practice permitted in the registered nurse licensing laws of the various states. The American Nurses' Association and other specialty professional organizations oppose this position, arguing that scope of practice and responsibilities of advanced practice nurses is based on registered nurse licensure and that the necessary authority for practice exists, based on that license (Greco, 1995, p. 36). Regulation of advanced nursing practice by requiring a second license would transfer the control of advanced practice from the professional nursing bodies to the political arena. If this is done, decisions made in the various states could be expected to continue to reflect the concerns of political groups and their lobbies, rather than the actual competencies of advanced practice nurses.

Reimbursement

Restriction of public or private third-party payer reimbursement for advanced practice nursing services has sometimes limited the expansion of the role and available services, especially to vulnerable, underserved groups. These barriers are beginning to crumble in the outpatient sector, but they remain strong in inpatient practice settings where reimbursement for nursing services is still largely lumped with the room bill. Currently, nurse midwives and nurse anesthetists are the only advanced practice nurses directly reimbursed for services provided in inpatient settings. Even though ACNPs and other advanced practice nurses who practice in inpatient settings are denied reimbursement, Griffith and Robinson (1991) have demonstrated that critical care nurses are performing procedural terminology-coded services for which physicians are reimbursed. Their survey found that more than 70% of the nurses performed 28 codes, often with little or no supervision.

The federal government's longstanding limitation of advanced practice nursing reimbursement through Medicare is important when considering barriers to practice, as other insurers have looked to the Medicare program to determine their policies for reimbursement. An important change in federal reimbursement policies occurred with the signing by the president of a budget bill passed by Congress. With the passage of this budget bill, which took effect in January, 1998, direct Medicare reimbursement has been extended to NPs and CNSs, regardless of the geographic area in which they practice (Vanderbilt & Keepnews, 1997). Medicare provisions already permitted reimbursement for NP services delivered in nursing homes, for NP and CNS services delivered in designated rural areas, and for reimbursement for services provided "incident to" those of covered services of NPs and CNSs (p. 1).

The new provisions remove the restriction that limited reimbursable services solely to those delivered in rural areas. They also explicitly recognize the clinical nurse specialist as eligible for reimbursement and provide a definition of this title. They maintain the provision for collaboration with a physician, however, and they restrict coverage on some advanced practice nursing services, "but only if no facility or other provider charges or is paid any amounts with respect to the furnishing of such services," a phrase that is confusing and requires further interpretation (Vanderbilt & Keepnews, 1997, p. 3).

The ANA's position on these issues resulting from the recent expansion of Medicare coverage is that NP and CNS services will be covered on a fee-for-service basis by Medicare reimbursement, as long as hospitals or other facilities do not bill Medicare for the cost of the NP or CNS's salaries. The ANA further argues that since part B of Medicare services provided by NPs and CNSs are not reflected in hospital's DRG payments, these services should be reimbursable. Finally, their position is that services delivered by NPs and CNSs in their own practices, in physician practices, or in free-standing clinics, or in nonhospital faculty practices are covered (Vanderbilt & Keepnews,

1997, p. 3). Their rationale for this position is that as long as these services are not billed for by or paid to a facility or other provider, they should be covered (p. 3).

These changes in reimbursement practices represent important progress for advanced practice nurses, but they do not directly address services delivered by most ACNPs who are usually employed by hospitals or other practices that directly bill Medicare and other third-party payers. The opportunity for hospitals or hospital-employed advanced practice nurses to bill for services delivered in inpatient settings is still an unknown, and an area in which further progress is necessary.

FUTURE OF THE ROLE OF THE ACNP

Opportunities, perceived need, and supply will be powerful influences on the future growth of the ACNP role. Opportunities will require that barriers to practice, such as restrictive laws and discriminatory reimbursement practices, be removed. Opportunities will also require that an attitude of acceptance of these new care givers exist or be created. Because ACNP roles are so new, few research studies exist that demonstrate their productivity or capability. Anecdotal evidence exists and many studies of NP effectiveness in the primary care setting and in some specialty settings conclusively demonstrate the capabilities of these advanced practice nurses.

Perceived need requires the development of favorable perceptions on the part of patients, the general public, other health care providers, and hospital administrators. If the role is to flourish, the ACNP must be seen as productive, competent, cost-effective, and providing safe care. There is a pressing need to describe this advanced practice role to patients, their families, and the public, especially to insurers, legislators, and other policymakers. There is also a need to reach out to physicians and administrators to describe the benefits. Finally, there is a need to encourage nursing administrators to develop places for ACNPs within the formal nursing organization of their institutions. Nursing administrators are under tremendous pressure to contain costs and to cut or downsize nursing personnel. As a result, ACNPs can be understood as merely an added budget cost, not an opportunity to develop a new model to provide care. If this occurs, ACNPs will not identify with the organized nursing leadership in the clinical settings.

An adequate supply of ACNPs is essential if the role is to survive. The importance of available, accessible programs to prepare these nurses has been described, as has the need to eliminate reimbursement barriers and unduly restrictive laws that restrict advanced practice nursing roles. In addition to actual numbers of available ACNPs, an adequate supply will demand that these nurses be socialized as professional leaders who are accountable for their practice and who assume responsibility for lifelong learning. Inevitably, the future of ACNP roles will rest with the future of nursing and its ability to respond to the ongoing changes in health care.

REFERENCES

Ackerman, M., Norsen, L., Martin, B., Wiedrich, J., & Kitzman, H. (1996). Development of a model of advanced practice. *American Journal of Critical Care, 5,* 1, 68–73.

Aiken, L. (1990). Charting the future of hospital nursing. *Image: Journal of Nursing Scholarship, 22,* 72–78.

Aiken, L., & Salmon, M. (1994). Health care workforce priorities: What nursing should do now. *Inquiry, 31,* 318–329.

American Association of Colleges of Nursing. (1995). *The Essentials of Master's Education for Advanced Practice Nurses.* Report from the Task Force on the Essentials of Master's Education for Advanced Practice Nursing. Washington, DC: Author.

American Nurses Association & American Association of Critical Care Nurses. (1995). *Standards of clinical practice and scope of practice for the acute care nurse practitioner.* Washington, DC: American Nurses Publishing Company.

Booth, R. (1995). Leadership challenges for nurse practitioner faculty. *Nurse Practitioner, 20,* 4, 52–58.

Clochesy, J., Daly, B., Idemoto, B., Steel, J., & Fitzpatrick, J. (1994). Preparing advanced practice nurses for acute care. *American Journal of Critical Care, 3,* 255–259.

Dracup, K., & Bryan-Brown, C. (1994). The advanced practice nurse in critical care: Yes or no? *American Journal of Critical Care, 3,* 3, 163–164.

Elder, R., & Bullough, B. (1990). Nurse practitioners and clinical nurse specialists: Are the roles merging? *Clinical Nurse Specialist, 4,* 2, 78–84.

Freund, C. (1993). Nurse practitioners in primary care. In M. Mezey & D. McGivern, *Nurse, nurse practitioners. The evolution of primary care.* Boston: Little Brown, 305–333.

Greco, K. (1995). Regulation of advanced nursing practice: Part one-Second licensure. *ONF, 22,* 8, 35–38.

Griffith, H., & Robinson, K. (1991). Survey of the degree to which critical care nurses are performing current procedural terminology-coded services. *American Journal of Critical Care, 1,* 91–98.

Groeger, J., Strosberg, M., Halpern, N., Raphaely, R., Kaye, W., Guntupalli, K., Bertram, D., Greenbaum, D., Clemmer, P., & Gallagher, T. (1992). Descriptive analysis of critical care units in the United States. *Critical Care Medicine, 20,* 846–863.

Hravnak, M., Kobert, S., Risco, K., Baldisseri, M., Hoffman, L., Clochesy, J., Rudy, E., & Snyder, J. (1995). Acute care nurse practitioner curriculum: Content and development process. *American Journal of Critical Care, 4,* 179–188.

Keane, A., & Richmond, T. (1993). Tertiary nurse practitioners. *Image: Journal of Nursing Scholarship, 25,* 4, 281–284.

Keane, A., Richmond, T., & Kaiser, L. (1994). Critical care nurse practitioners: Evolution of the advanced practice nursing role. *American Journal of Critical Care, 3,* 232–237.

King, K., & Ackerman, M. (1995). An educational model for the acute care nurse practitioner. *Advanced Practice Nursing, 7,* 1, 1–7.

Mahoney, D. (1995). Employer resistance to state authorized prescriptive authority for NPs. Results from a pilot study. *Nurse Practitioner, 20,* 1, 58–61.

Mallison, M. (1993). Nurses as house staff. *American Journal of Nursing, 93,* 3, 65–69.

National Council of State Boards of Nursing. (1993). *Position Paper on the Regulation of Advanced Nursing Practice.* Chicago: Author.

O'Flynn, A. (1995). The preparation of advanced practice nurses. Current issues. *Advanced Practice Nursing, 31,* 3, 429–438.

Pearson, L. (1997). Annual update of how each state stands on legislative issues affecting advanced nursing practice. *The Nurse Practitioner, 22,* 1, 18–86.

Richmond, T., & Keane, A. (1992). The nurse practitioner in tertiary care. *Journal of Nursing Administration, 22,* 11–12.

Safreit, B. (1992). Health care dollars and regulatory sense: The role of advanced practice nursing. *Yale Journal on Regulation, 9,* 2, 417–488.

Snyder, J., Sirio, C., Angus, D., Hravnak, M., Kobert, S., Sinz, E., & Rudy, E. (1994). Trial of nurse practitioners in intensive care. *New Horizons, 2,* 296–304.

Soehren, P., & Schumann, L. (1994). Enhanced role opportunities available to the CNS/nurse practitioner. *Clinical Nurse Specialist, 8,* 3, 123–127.

Sparacino, P., & Durand, B. (1986). Editorial on specialization in advanced nursing practice. *Momentum, 4,* 2, 1–4.

Standards for educational programs: Preparing students as acute care nurse practitioners. (1993). *AACN Clinical Issues, 4,* 4, 593–598.

U.S. Department of Health and Human Services (USDHHS), Health Resources and Services Administration, Bureau of Health Professions. (1991). *Health Personnel in the United States: Seventh report to Congress, 1990.* Washington, DC: U.S. Printing Office.

Vanderbilt, M., & Keepnews, D. (August 6, 1997). *Passage of Medicare Reimbursement: What Next?* Washington, DC: American Nurses Association.

Watts, R., Hanson, M., Burke, K., Gallagher, S., & Foster, D. (1996). The critical care nurse practitioner: An advanced practice role for the critical care nurse. *Dimensions of Critical Care Nursing, 15,* 1, 48–56.

Whelan, E. (1995). Regulation of health professions. A concept analysis. Unpublished manuscript. University of Pennsylvania, School of Nursing.

2

Scope and Standards of Clinical Practice

Therese S. Richmond
Phyllis Dubendorf
Cheryl Monturo

The profound changes in health care in the United States have created opportunities for advanced practice nurses to strengthen the foundation of their practice and to implement their scope of practice fully. This is particularly true in acute care where acute care nurse practitioners (ACNPs) provide comprehensive care to medically vulnerable patients throughout the continuum of acute care services. The health care environment has been characterized by a mismatch between provider type and provider characteristics and the actual needs of patients with acute illness or injury. The evolution of ACNPs is the proactive response by the profession to meet the changing needs of society and of the health care system. There is evidence that nurse practitioners who manage patients in acute care settings provide a safe, cost-effective alternative to physician services in the provision of care to acutely ill patients (Goksel, Harrison, Morrison, & Miller, 1993; Mitchell-DiCenso, Guyatt, Marrin, et al., 1996; Riportella-Muller, Libby, & Kindig, 1995; Spisso, O'Callaghan, McKennan, & Holcroft, 1990).

This chapter explores the scope of practice of ACNPs and the standards that serve as a guide for practice. The theoretical discussion of the scope and standards of practice for ACNPs is extended by a description of the actual practices of ACNPs that exemplify this evolving role in a changing health care system. To this end ACNPs and their professional colleagues were interviewed to furnish advice, insight, and direction on how best to implement the role in a variety of acute care specialties and settings.

▶ SCOPE OF PRACTICE

The ACNP role can be viewed as a natural evolution of advanced practice nursing. The challenge for ACNPs is to delineate the scope of practice in a continually evolving health care system. The scope of practice is a broad statement that provides the boundaries and framework for professional practice. The scope of practice as articulated by the profession is important since it serves to inform or direct state nurse practice acts (Keane, Richmond, & Kaiser, 1994). Although the scope of practice may appear static, in reality it is a dynamic statement that provides opportunities for continued evolution. The driving philosophy underlying all professional scope of practice statements is the belief that the needs of patients drive the complexion, boundaries, and nature of nursing practice (Ball, 1997). The boundaries of ACNP practice as defined within the scope are not intended to be confining but rather to provide parameters for practice that are expected to evolve to meet the ever-changing needs of patients and of their families.

The ACNP role falls within the broader context of advanced nursing practice, indicating that ACNPs are prepared at the master's level. Specialization, the acquisition of additional practice skills, and the ability to integrate additional knowledge and research are central to the ACNP role (ANA & AACN, 1995). The scope indicates that ACNPs have a broad repertoire of knowledge and skills in specialty practice that positions them effectively to manage medically complex patients in high-acuity settings.

"The purpose of the ACNP is to provide advanced nursing care across the continuum of acute care services to patients who are acutely and critically ill" (ANA & AACN, 1995, p. 11). It is important to recognize that while many ACNPs have practices that are based in acute care, inpatient settings, practice is not setting dependent, but takes place wherever patients have acute health needs. Restorative care is the foundation of practice and includes initial stabilization, minimization of complications, and comprehensive management of the primary injury or illness and comorbid conditions. Furthermore, the ability to address the physical and psychosocial ramifications of the illness for the patient's and family's lives is central to ACNP practice. Key functions of the ACNP role are listed in Table 2–1.

It is clear that the core of the ACNP role is evidence-based and research-based clinical expertise with commensurate accountability and authority for patient outcomes. To this end, ACNPs are responsibile for integrating care throughout the continuum of acute care services in collaboration with other health care providers. In addition, ACNPs serve as patient advocates. This advocacy extends beyond individual patients to systems of care, through the surveillance of care practices and systems management. ACNPs are responsible to support, maintain, and adapt systems to meet patient and families needs.

STANDARDS OF ACNP PRACTICE

The Standards of Practice for ACNPs include both standards of clinical care and standards for professional performance (Tables 2–2 and 2–3). These standards describe a competent level of performance common to ACNPs and thus serve as a template from which ACNP practice can be judged (ANA & AACN, 1995). These standards are firmly grounded in the philosophic values of the profession and hence, are relatively broad and can be expected to remain constant over time (ANA & AACN, 1995). Although the standards, at first, appear general and non-specific to ACNP practice, these standards are accompanied by criteria that are specific and measurable. Unlike the standards, these specific criteria are expected to change over time to reflect changing knowledge, science, and health care systems.

The standards of practice recognize the importance of respecting the patient's unique cultural, ethnic, and spiritual heritage and beliefs. ACNP practice is typified by critical thinking with the clear incorporation of theoretical knowledge and research. ACNPs must be able to prioritize data collection, synthesize data from a variety of resources to effectively design care, and link practice to specific outcomes. Practice occurs at sufficient breadth and depth to manage patients with complex health care needs within the multidisciplinary health care team. Mutually agreed upon

TABLE 2–1. Key Role Components of the ACNP in Providing Care to High-Acuity Patients

Obtain health history
Conduct comprehensive physical examination
Appraise health risk profile
Perform differential diagnosis based on a logical diagnostic reasoning
Plan and implement advanced therapeutic interventions
Consult with and refer to other health care providers

ANA and AACN (1995).

TABLE 2–2. Standards of Care

Standard I	The ACNP collects patient data
Standard II	The ACNP analyzes the assessment data in determining diagnoses
Standard III	The ACNP identifies expected outcomes individualized to the patient
Standard IV	The ACNP develops a plan of care that prescribes interventions to attain expected outcomes
Standard V	The ACNP implements the interventions identified in the multidisciplinary plan of care
Standard VI	The ACNP evaluates the patient's progress toward attainment of expected outcomes

ANA and AACN (1995).

TABLE 2–3. Standards of Professional Performance

Standard I	The ACNP systematically evaluates the quality and effectiveness of acute care nursing practice
Standard II	The ACNP facilitates the use of organizational resources in caring for the patient
Standard III	The ACNP evaluates his/her clinical practice in relation to professional practice standards and relevant statutes and regulations
Standard IV	The ACNP acquires and maintains current knowledge in advanced nursing practice
Standard V	The ACNP contributes to the professional development of peers, colleagues, and others
Standard VI	The ACNP's decisions and actions on behalf of patients are determined in an ethical manner
Standard VII	The ACNP collaborates with the patient, significant others, and other health care providers in patient care
Standard VIII	The ACNP uses research findings in practice
Standard IX	The ACNP considers factors related to safety, effectiveness, and cost in planning and delivering patient care

ANA and AACN (1995).

outcomes are determined and evaluated in an ongoing and systematic manner (ANA & AACN, 1995).

The standards extend beyond clinical practice to include standards of professional performance that "describe a competent level of behavior in the professional role, including activities related to the quality of care, performance appraisal, education, collegiality, ethics, collaboration, research, and resource utilization" (ANA & AACN, 1995, p. 23). ACNP performance is typified by the self-initiated and self-directed progression toward professional development.

IMPLEMENTING THE SCOPE OF PRACTICE

The scope of practice can be examined by looking at the general competencies central to ACNP practice. These competencies, as identified by our currently practicing ACNPs, are listed in Table 2–4. As the ACNPs told us, these individual competencies are not necessarily unique to ACNP practice. Certain competencies are shared with other professional nurses, advanced practice nurses, and medical colleagues (Watts, Hanson, Burke, Gallagher, & Foster, 1996). Thus, although it is helpful to identify core competencies of ACNP practice, it is important not to define the scope solely through a list of tasks or skills. For this reason, we asked ACNPs and other health care providers to provide us with exemplars of the typical day of ACNPs in practice. This helps to demonstrate how individual competencies and tasks come together with knowledge and advanced clinical decision making to form a cohesive patient-oriented practice.

TABLE 2–4. Competencies Identified as Central to the ACNP Scope of Practice

Have a broad and deep working knowledge base
Possess good communication skills
Perform history and physical examination
Apply general assessment skills
Diagnose medical problems
Order laboratory and diagnostic tests
Interpret laboratory and diagnostic tests
Perform invasive procedures
Remove invasive drains, staples, and provide wound care
Prescribe drugs and medical interventions
Act as liaison between patient/family and physician
Coordinate the interdisciplinary team
Have good organizational skills
Collaborate with other disciplines
Educate staff nurses
Monitor for untoward effects of therapy
Serve as first surgical assist
Manage multisystem problems that extend beyond the primary disease
Be able to take the initiative
Possess intuition beyond common sense
Be enthusiastic
Show respect for patient and family

The scope of practice delineates the boundaries of ACNP practice but should not be considered constrictive of the continuing development of this relatively new role. By the nature of its unique scope, ACNPs' practice is different from that of their primary care NP colleagues as well as that of their acute care clinical nurse specialist colleagues. Moreover, there is no one typical form of ACNP practice. The scope is broad enough to allow and even encourage diversity in practice so that ACNPs can design their roles to meet the driving needs of patients, of their families, and of the health care system. For this reason, we asked several ACNPs to describe a typical day to bring to light actual practices that illustrate the ACNP scope of practice. Furthermore, we asked colleagues (clinical nurse specialists and physician collaborators) of ACNPs to describe the practices that they see to further highlight the scope of practice.

Today's health care system is typified by increasing numbers of patients with complex, specialized health care needs coupled with disease trajectories that have the potential to outstrip the resources of providers to provide acute care in a cost-effective manner (Keane & Richmond, 1993). This fact was a driving force in the evolution of ACNPs. Thus, we typically expect ACNPs to practice in hospital settings and to manage patients with specialized health care needs within the confines of the multidisciplinary team. As the following ACNPs emphasize, their practice is crucial for the smooth running of the system.

> I make rounds with the vascular team . . . take care of any immediate problems. Every day there is something to do after early morning rounds (i.e., educational meetings). The rest of the day, I write all the notes, write the orders to take care of all the day-to-day problems (i.e., IVs, pain medicine, dressings). I cover for them [the residents] when they are in the operating room. But I am always in contact with them. I also do H&Ps on patients who are admitted, we all share this responsibility. . . . At the end of the day we all sit together and we go over everything and if there is anything left to do we go out and do it. I also do consultations.

However, ACNP practice is not setting dependent. As the following exemplar demonstrates, ACNPs manage patients with specialized needs in the outpatient setting as well. In fact, the ACNP provides a bridge for patients during the transition from hospital to home and from illness to health. This typical day demonstrates the very important notion that practice is not setting dependent, but driven by the needs of patients.

> I think the unique thing about being an ACNP is that your day varies from moment to moment and day to day. A typical day would involve seeing patients in the hospital, evaluating them, doing their physical assessment, writing their progress notes. All during this time you are paged several times by different referring physicians, nurses on the floor, social workers. So you have to

> readily be able to change your focus on a moment's notice and organize your time well. Also, the outpatients, patients who have had problems after surgery, or just have some questions and need to come in and talk with you. You really have to change your focus from inpatient to outpatient at a moment's notice.

This capacity to juggle various activities is shared by other ACNPs.

> My typical day includes office hours. When Dr. X is in the OR all day, I always see the patients in the hospital on my own and make sure things are being managed properly on the floors. I answer a lot of phone calls from people who call with questions about surgery and about what they are experiencing. I do a lot of teaching.

In 1990 Aiken suggested that one of nursing's greatest challenges was to achieve a balanced relationship with physicians and hospitals. She proposed that this relationship must provide the opportunity for nurses to grow personally and professionally. The ACNP role is one way by which nurses have broadened professional boundaries to become central players as expert clinicians and decision makers for medically vulnerable patients.

> A typical day starts at 7:00 A.M. with patients rounds from 7:00 to 8:00 A.M. Rounds are in the ICU where we see our post-ops and up on the cardiac floor. We have an average of about 10 patients to see. Then the surgeon goes into the OR and I manage the service while he is in the OR. I go back and reassess the patients because [early] rounds are rushed. I review what's been happening with other services in the chart and then get a plan for the day. That is my inpatient role, managing the patients. The NPs are the primary caregivers for the service; the residents are in the OR and the physician assistants are also in the OR.

Sometimes the scope of practice is seen and articulated most clearly not from the ACNPs themselves, but from other members of the health care team with whom they work. This statement from a clinical nurse specialist (CNS) who works with a group of neurosurgical ACNPs demonstrates the true value of ACNP practice

> NPs bring continuity—this is the first thing. I am very pro-NP. The residents are non-existent. NPs provide visibility for patients and families. They coordinate care and follow-up with results of tests and procedures. They follow up on consultant suggestions, which we had a problem with before. They look at the entire picture, to see where we are and what we need to do. They take all the bits of information floating around and put it all together. The residents don't have the time—they have one particular focus, like temperature or wound management, and they don't look at discharge status. NPs have a broad base and bring in all facets of care.

The continuity of care extends beyond the hospital walls. The following exemplar by a surgical ACNP demonstrates how the continuity benefits the patient, the system, and the collaborating physician.

> All of our patients have some type of chronicity to them, but the patient I actually saw this morning is in his late 30s. He has a long history of diabetes. He needed a fem-distal bypass because he had gangrene in his toes. I worked with him the whole way—pre-op, post-op in the hospital. But now I see him on my own every two weeks for management of his chronic wound, his coumadin, and his overall care right now. I change the management of the wound as I think necessary, I change his coumadin if I think it's necessary. Dr. X comes in every once in a while, every month or so, to see if everything is stable. There are several people I see on my own. Some one like this patient, is the ideal person where I think it's important to follow. There is no way Dr. X can manage him on his own.

By virtue of their education and professional background, ACNPs are distinctly different from their medical colleagues. ACNPs are prepared to provide nursing care as well as what has classically been viewed as medical care. We choose to view this from the perspective that ACNPs are prepared to provide health care that is driven by the illness and injury needs of patients as well as addressing the needs of patients that are driven by the effects of illness or injury on the fabric of their lives. One physician colleague highlights this unique background as a valuable asset to patients.

> With the level of training she [ACNP] has, she is able to handle a lot of different medical situations on top of being able to interact from a social standpoint. This is in terms of rehab or whatever else is necessary. She can handle many different facets [of the care] because of her training. There are multiple examples, but mostly from my standpoint . . . she is able to interact with patients and their families. This is a life saver, in terms of their mental attitude and our ability to keep them with a good attitude for healing. I think that is really one of the pluses that she has brought to our team.

Since ACNPs are distinctly different from their medical colleagues, one issue that surfaces is whether ACNPs are managing groups of patients that are identical to those seen by physicians or whether patients with differing needs are delegated to ACNPs because of their unique knowledge and preparation. In this complex day and age, it is too simplistic to say that medicine focuses on cure and nursing on care (Nolan, 1995). ACNPs incorporate both curing and caring in their practice and that practice occurs on a multidimensional continuum where the cure and care aspects take place simultaneously and certainly enhance the effectiveness of one another. As this exemplar highlights, this differential delegation of patients can benefit all parties.

> In the beginning, as physicians designated patients to our [ACNP] service, I thought it was because they were the easier patients. In fact, they were often the more complex patients, both medically and psychosocially. For example, we are talking about patients with cardiomyopathy or poor ejection fractions who are dealing with major life issues. These are the patients we are getting. Because we can help patients to identify the multifaceted problems they are having. And sometimes the very important problem of meeting end of life issues. Doctors appreciate what we can offer to these very complex patients.

There has been some discussion within the profession that by becoming ACNPs, advanced practice nurses are leaving nursing, selling out the profession. The argument arises that ACNPs are no more than eternal mini-residents, that this role only serves to reinforce the "handmaiden" relationship (Nolan, 1995). Through the description of her practice, a seasoned ACNP elucidates why this is not true. Furthermore, the following exemplar provides a concrete example of the wonderful nature of ACNP practice. This exemplar is not intended to minimize the importance of medical practice, but rather to highlight the different paradigms of practice and the difference between the focus of residencies (teaching) and the focus of ACNP practice (bringing expert practice to the bedside).

> You have to be able to have a good patient relationship and know how to approach your patient. I think that the strongest point for nurse practitioners is not all that medical. It is bringing [together] the medical and the strong nursing philosophy with a strong patient interaction and holistic approach. That is what makes nurse practitioners unique. I don't find that with the residents. They don't approach the patient and they don't look at them the same way that we do. They don't think about the whole picture, from start to home . . . their [resident and intern] focus is what am I getting out of this patient, as opposed to what can I do for this patient.

As we discussed the scope of practice with physician colleagues, they also described the importance of the unique blending of the medical and nursing paradigms. In addition, as this physician colleague identifies, ACNPs provide the continuity that is so necessary for quality patient care.

> They perform several important roles. In our service, they provide a lot of medical care to the patients during the day. Prescribing medications, pulling out ties and tubes. They provide a source of contact and a source of continuity for the patients before surgery, during surgery, and after surgery. And that is especially important, [providing] the inpatient and outpatient interface. A lot more of our patients are same day admission for surgery, a lot of them go home quicker than they used to. First of all, planning just to make that happen, then making it work by providing the patient and his family with someone calm, when the issues come up. . . . Nurses have always done better than doctors or doctors in training in terms of communicating with patients, nurturing patients.

As ACNPs become established in acute care settings, the scope of practice will continue to evolve. All health care professionals should be open to the evolutionary changes that, by necessity, will occur. ACNPs will not "turn into doctors" nor do they strive for this. In reality, both will benefit from the ability of ACNPs and acute care physicians to work together in an interdependent, respectful relationship. As DeAngelis (1994) states, "the NP's clinical decision-making responsibilities are strengthened, and the physician's depth of knowledge about health teaching, family needs, and community resources are augmented" (p. 870).

IMPLEMENTING THE STANDARDS OF CLINICAL PRACTICE

The standards of clinical practice are based on the advanced application of the nursing process to acutely ill and injured patients. The standards indicate that ACNPs are expected to collect and analyze data to derive diagnoses, identify expected outcomes, develop and implement a plan of care that prescribes interventions to achieve expected outcomes, and evaluate attainment of expected outcomes. The exemplars verify that ACNPs have practices in which the components of the standards of clinical practice are in constant interplay. Furthermore, the clinical practice exemplars indicate that the practice extends well beyond the performance of specific tasks or skills: "Physical assessment skills are essential. That's what comes into play all the time, because you are constantly assessing the patient. But a holistic approach is important."

As the ACNPs identified, competent practice is based on assessment skills that extend beyond the physical.

> Not only the physical assessment, but we also have the psychosocial and emotional assessment skills. I think that this is very vital. I don't see that happening with the medical model. I think [we do] a lot more discharge planning and patient advocacy. Just being there and listening, you find out a lot about their home environment, just by small exchanges of conversation.

A physician colleague recognizes the broad preparation of ACNPs and the value to the patient when ACNPs are key members of the multidisciplinary team.

> They [ACNPs] give us the ability to have first rate providers on the scene, while we are in the operating room . . . whatever they are doing, they are right there on the front lines . . . really interacting with patients and their families. That is sometimes not possible for us. A top role I see is that they are giving care, really being there for any immediate problems that could arise.

Both technical and clinical reasoning are critical skills that ACNPs must acquire during the early development of their roles (Shah, Bruttomesso, Sullivan, & Lattanzio, 1997). As the following statement from a novice ACNP highlights, practice derived by ACNP design as well as driven by patient's and system's needs, extends well beyond the technical aspects of the role.

> In clinical I learned a lot of technical things, but unfortunately I don't use them in my practice, I do minimal suturing. I've lost a lot of technical skills, but I'm sure I could pick them up again. It's not where my biggest need is here at the hospital. I use assessment, diagnosis, and management—formulating the management plan are the big issues. My collaborating physician relies on me to do that.

In fact, as a seasoned ACNP states: "You have to have good strong assessment skills. History taking is 90% of your problem solving. You really need to know what questions to ask. This is supplemented by a strong clinical knowledge base."

Assessment is dynamic and continues over time. Patients benefit from this as ACNPs are able to focus on identifying problems early in their evolution: "By interacting with patients more than once or twice daily, NPs frequently pick up on subtle indications of problems."

Although patients are commonly admitted with a known diagnosis by the ACNP's collaborating physician, this does not alleviate the ACNP of the responsibility of diagnosing complications and unexpected health problems: "Determining the diagnosis is essential to be able to run down the differential diagnoses and sort them out."

As another ACNP puts it:

> Because of our presence on the floor, we can pick up when patients are not doing well and when patients are having problems. I actually had a plastic surgery patient who had cardiac problems after his plastic surgery procedure and went down pretty quickly from a cardiac standpoint. I was right there to pick it up, to intervene quickly. He did much better than he probably would have.

ACNPs are prepared to manage acutely ill patients with a variety of acute and chronic health problems. The complexity and progression of the acutely ill patient's status requires an effective multidisciplinary approach to care (Piano, Kleinpell, & Johnson, 1996). From a physician colleague who routinely works with an ACNP service, a different view of assessment and management arises.

> They [ACNPs] are another pair of eyes looking at the patient. They are mobile and they can get there usually faster than I can get there to assess a [critical] situation. Usually I am doing something and I can't break away, but I can send another professional [the ACNP] to gather things, assess, determine medications the patient is on, what is happening . . . what are the drips . . . what is the blood pressure. By the time I get there, they present it to me in a nutshell. The acute situation is controlled because they usually beat me there by 10 minutes or so. I know the nurse practitioner. I know his capabilities. I trust his assessment.

As an integral member of the multidisciplinary team, the ACNP participates in developing the management plan. This often occurs in a give and take manner between disciplines.

> Typically, I see patients first and go over the plan, do a physical assessment and I speak with the physician about the different issues that I feel we should resolve that particular day. And then we sort of just bounce things off of each other . . . come up with a plan for the patient. If there are any other problems that come up and would involve a referring physician or consult service—I would just talk to them directly.

The ACNP holds clear responsibility for implementing the plan of care. This implementation encompasses the performance of procedures, the ongoing assessment of patients, and working with patients and their families to ensure that they are fully integrated in the plan of care.

> A patient who was just discharged yesterday had come in from another hospital on Friday for an electrophysiology study. I was sitting down with him and his family on Friday night, going over everything that had happened to him to that point and reviewing what we wanted to do. He [the patient] said it was the first time anyone had ever explained anything to him clearly . . . I had contact with him throughout the weekend. He continued to reiterate thank-yous for the explanation. He said "I really feel comfortable with everything that is going on. I understand what is happening . . . why my medications are important for me to take."

Nolan (1995) has suggested, that professional reductionism is likely to occur and is evidenced by the tendency to restrict the legitimate professional focus to an area faithful to a given professional paradigm. He further suggests that this is one of the primary reasons multidisciplinary approaches to practice have often remained rhetoric. Yet, ACNP practice incorporates many tasks that demonstrate the expanded boundaries of practice. The boundaries of practice between professional groups comprising the multidisciplinary team have become increasingly blurred (English, 1997). Several activities include those that previously were squarely in the realm of our medical colleagues: "First, I see patients in the ICU, write notes, perform any invasive procedures (i.e., pulling lines, IABPs), and write transfer orders."

Many propose that effective and efficient patient care can be achieved only by a smooth-running multidisciplinary team. A clear understanding of the ACNP scope and boundaries of practice that is formalized by departmental and hospital policies and protocols is important to success, but not the sole criterion (Genet, et al., 1995). While privileging and credentialing protocols often delineate the boundaries of each discipline's practice, the interdisciplinary boundaries of practice are overlapping and are, in fact, constantly changing. Because of this, there is a need for the multidisciplinary team to determine the division of responsibilities and tasks to ensure the smooth running of a multidisciplinary service. Often times, this discussion occurs on a daily basis.

> I guess the real beginning of collaboration is rounds. This is when we talk about what we are going to do and often who is going to be doing it. Who is best suited to carry something out. Probably, I end up getting more involved in discharge planning and not exclusively but working with families and that kind of thing just because the doctors feel it is more of the nurse thing, and that is something that I kind of like.

Evaluating the progress of patients toward expected outcomes is ongoing and occurs in the hospital setting and throughout the specialized follow-up. As with all other components of clinical practice, the evaluation of progress toward or away from expected outcomes often requires ACNPs to act immediately. The following exemplar provided by a CNS colleague of a group of ACNPs demonstrates the importance of combining knowledge, assessment, and decision making with the authority to act.

> Once a patient came in, he was a postop craniotomy who neuro'd down, couldn't wake him up. The NPs ordered an immediate CT scan, were accessible to the patient, and got things ordered. It was faster than calling the MD, because they were right on the floor—they could see, do, and act.

▶ IMPLEMENTING THE STANDARDS OF PROFESSIONAL PERFORMANCE

Implementing the standards of profession practice includes such professional responsibilities as quality of care, systems management, performance appraisal, education, collegiality, ethics, collaboration, research, and research utilization (ANA & AACN, 1995). These standards of professional practice provide the framework for a professional practice model and delineate the broader professional responsibilities of the ACNP to groups of patients. Contributions to patient care within the system partially stem from the availability of the knowledgeable ACNP to health care colleagues: "The NPs have all been well received here. The cardiologists are thrilled to have someone to talk to. They don't have to wait until the surgeon is out of the OR. They feel good about having someone to discuss the case with."

This value of the ACNP is reinforced by a surgeon colleague of a group of ACNPs: "They [ACNPs] provide a form of communication . . . Cardiologists are constantly frustrated about making rounds when the surgeons are in the operating room. There is no way we can tell them about what is going on. Having a nurse practitioner, who is available during the day to discuss the issues of patient management is crucial."

ACNPs have the potential to enhance the continuity of care patients receive in a fragmented health care system (Gates, 1993). The accessibility to and collegiality with fellow health care providers are key roles of ACNPs who help to provide safe passage as well as rapid transit through a system that continues to be challenged with fragmentation of care: "The ACNP has the unique ability to be the center point of a patient's care . . . a conductor, to orchestrate everything. I think we are a lot better at that than our medical colleagues."

The following exemplar indicates that ACNPs take this coordination role seriously.

> My patient today was admitted for a valve replacement. He had a very recent stroke and now has a new diagnosis of Crohn's disease. I needed to get old records of his most recent admission and then consult the most appropriate specialty groups (i.e., GI, neuro, & CT surgery). So, there will be a lot of interaction. I do this initially and then follow through with the fellow and attending.

ACNPs facilitate the appropriate use of resources for the patients in their care. Part of this is by following institutional policies that are specifically developed to enhance the efficiency, safety, and effectiveness of patient care. A CNS colleague recognizes that worth of having a group of health care providers who understand the importance of complying with system policies: "They comply with rules and regulations of the institution. They reorder meds, reorder restraints, reevaluate nutritional status. These things make us look better as a unit and hospital."

ACNPs bring more to the system than just coordinating care. They make the system work for patients and their families. In addition to their preparation as advanced practice clinicians, ACNPs bring an understanding of systems management. As a CNS who works with the ACNPs pointed out,

> NPs serve RNs, patients, families, and the institution. For RNs they answer questions about OOB, braces, feeding tubes, advancing diet, ordering pain meds—all the nitty gritty. For the family, they answer questions about what do tests show, follow up, and the home situation. For the hospital, they complete issues. They are timely. And they practice the way they are supposed to.

Effective orchestration of care cannot occur in the absence of collaboration. Collaboration occurs in many ways throughout the day: "At some point during the day, usually after the first OR case, the surgeon and I round together and develop a collaborative plan of care." "Typically, collaboration means seeing the patient independently, then rounding with the physician to review the case."

For ACNPs who work with a group of ACNP colleagues, collaboration within the group is essential for designing care.

> In the morning, I collaborate with the other nurse practitioners and we divide up the patients that are to be admitted. It is more of a collaborative thing, to a degree we all work with each other to make it best for the patients. . . . Through the day, we follow the patients, do their initial assessment and everything, then follow up with the physician. We round with each physician as far as what their plan of care is and interact and collaborate with them to do what is best for the patient.

This collaboration with other ACNPs and health care providers proceeds beyond the goals of achieving a smooth-running system and extends to professional development and verification of assessments and of decisions made: "I collaborate most often with my peers, the other nurse practitioners. I can bounce ideas off them, get their ideas for differential diagnoses. They have a lot of different experiences and knowledge. [The collaboration] can bring together a lot of their experiences to help each other."

As one ACNP who recently changed positions states, collaboration is not necessarily a given within a system. In this exemplar, collaboration is absent and the ACNP has not been able to fully implement his or her scope of practice.

> In a previous position I was at XXX in the preadmission testing center. There was not a lot of collaboration. I was mostly doing history and preoperative clearances. You didn't have much collaboration with your fellow nurse practitioner peers. Collaboration with the physicians was almost nonexistent. You did what you needed to do and they [the physicians] would follow up, if there was an abnormal lab. They would make the decision. There was no communication or exchange of ideas as far as what you thought would be best for that patient.

It became quite clear that effective collaboration does not occur as soon as ACNPs enter the system. Collaboration takes time to build and time to trust as the following exemplar shows.

> Within the last 6 months, it has gotten better, maybe because of time and exposure to me and our service. For the initial several months it seemed that it was an attending-to-attending dialogue, which was frustrating because I'd be the one primarily responsible for ordering what was needed to enact the plan. Not being made part of that loop directly and getting things third party was frustrating. But, now it seems that I've either learned the system better or they [the attendings] are more familiar with our role. That an attending or consultant dialogue with the nurse practitioner directly now seems more common and it is definitely more beneficial for the patients.

Even when ACNPs identify their physician colleagues as their primary collaborator, it is clear from their examples that collaboration takes place with a variety of providers both within the hospital system and beyond the hospital walls.

> The way we have our service set up, we pretty much work with one individual surgeon, so that would be my collaborating person. The role is unique. All referrals come to us [ACNPs]. Preoperative discussions are with the NPs. This is a nice aspect of my role, the referring cardiologists talks to me. Then I present the information to the surgeon.

Given the complexities of managing medically vulnerable patients in the complex health care system, ACNPs clearly need to collaborate with a variety of health care providers.

> If you look at the person who comes for a cardiac catheterization, I see them and then talk to the physician to facilitate the procedure. I speak with the physician about what we are doing after reviewing the films with him or her and deciding what the next step is. If the next step is surgery, then I need to call the nurse practitioner from CT surgery, the surgeon, anesthesia. If the patient has a diabetic problem or an endocrine problem, then I coordinate with the specialists to make sure that everything is prepared for surgery. Sometimes we need to bring in physical therapy.

While collaboration with one's physician colleague may be excellent, that does not necessarily mean that collaborative relationships occur with ease throughout the multidisciplinary team.

> I collaborate most with Dr. X and to a certain extent with the residents and nurses who take care of the patients. I'm very happy with the collaboration that my attending and I have. We have a mutual respect for each other. We respect each other's clinical decisions. The area that I think needs improvement is with the chief resident. He'll say, "what kind of background do you have to make these decisions?" That gets frustrating. It's like I always have to prove myself. I think a lot of it is just that it's a new role and not widely publicized and not accepted 100% across the board.

In creating a seamless system of care from the present fragmented system, ACNPs will benefit from maintaining an allegiance to their native nursing culture (Daly, 1997). As with all types of health care providers, ACNPs, by the nature of their role interact routinely with a variety of professionals as they work to create a seamless system of care: "Collaboration pretty much occurs across the board with physicians, nurses, and different social service people. For nurses, it is mostly nursing staff, but a lot of the time, if you want to review a disease process you run it by another NP."

Given the rapidity with which patients move through the acute care health system, ACNPs must develop ongoing and effective collaboration with colleagues in the community and home setting.

> I take all of the VNA phone calls. I collaborate with a lot of home health care nurses. They call me to get an order for dressing change or they'll call if they think someone needs to be seen right away, or they'll call about a change in the patient's progress to see if this is OK or normal. We agree on a plan or I'll offer suggestions from my nursing background to changes in a client's care.

Effective collaboration depends on mutual respect and excellent communication skills. A competency identified by several ACNPs is the ability to communicate with a variety of health care providers, in terms of both relaying information and listening and accepting input: "Excellent communication skills and the ability to communicate well with your fellow nurse practitioners along with the physician staff. Being open to suggestion."

This mutual respect and ability to trust communication are highlighted by a physician colleague of a group of ACNPs.

> I know I can trust him [an ACNP]. I know how he talks and how he presents things. When he called me with this patient as I was going out the door, I knew something was wrong. I went up there. He presented everything and cut the time to intervention in half. The problem was assessed. They [ACNPs] reassure the patient, they talk to them. Patients are more calm, they feel like something is being done.

The standards of professional performance require that ACNPs evaluate their practice in relation not just to professional standards, but also to relevant statutes and regulations. As we discussed this particular standard with ACNPs, it became quite clear that relevant statutes and regulations are often viewed as significant barriers to practice. It is important to note that these barriers vary from state to state. Regardless of the type of barrier ACNPs face in their individual states, these barriers to practice interfere with fully achieving the standards of clinical and professional practice: "While the level of collaboration is wonderful, having to be dependent in getting orders co-signed or prescriptions signed is less than ideal."

Not only do some obstacles engender interprofessional dependency, but also overcoming them create logistical challenges to creating a smooth-operating and seamless system.

> I think my greatest barrier to practice is that we cannot write prescriptions. It is extremely difficult because I think a lot of NPs are involved in the discharge practice and part of the discharge practice from the hospital is writing a prescription. . . . So that is one of the biggest barriers now. The other is having to have a lot of our orders cosigned in a relatively short time.

The limitations on practice created by confining state statutes and regulations directly affects the system of care. As Safriet (1992) states, one small step that would directly improve access and provide quality care at a lower cost is to remove the barriers to practice. The effect of barriers on the smooth running of a system is clearly demonstrated in the following exemplar.

> One of the most frustrating barriers that I have is that I cannot write prescriptions. When I do my discharge, I spend a good half hour of everyday tracking down a physician to sign those prescriptions. I think that is my biggest barrier. I can order lab work and the lab will honor that. I can order nuclear studies. I can schedule outpatient studies. But I cannot write a [medication] prescription.

In addition to state statutes and regulations, institutional credentialing and privileging can serve to further hamper or perhaps to enhance ACNP practice. For this reason, ACNPs are well advised to negotiate for protocols that are appropriately broad to provide latitude for professional judgment and decision making but also safety for patients.

> The biggest barrier to practice is the prescriptive privileges. This hospital has been wonderful about that. I was one of the first NPs here so we developed a protocol of appropriate meds I can prescribe and the situations in which I can prescribe them. In-house there are no problems with pharmacy or medical colleagues. Outpatient prescriptions are most frustrating. I manage the patient and then I have to track someone down to sign my outpatient scripts.

According to the Standards, ACNPs are obligated to provide care that is congruent with patient's needs and values and to practice in a manner that is consistent with the *Code for Nurses.* ACNPs participate in determining the direction of care that is consistent with patient's values and beliefs, even if those goals of care are different from what we ourselves would choose.

> We had a patient who had a bypass 15 years ago and developed angina in the past year. He had such a poor quality of life that he was willing to have surgery again—even though he had no graftable veins. We weren't sure we could give him the results he came for. Two months postop, he developed a recurrence of angina, but not as severe as before. He had an angioplasty then. Later he said he really felt we were there for him, thanking us for all the attention—and for walking him and his family through a rough time, even though he's not perfect now. We call our patients' families every day that the patient is in the hospital to give them an update. This is pretty unique to us.

ACNPs have the knowledge, skills, and professional responsibility to assist patients in exploring their values and beliefs and in incorporating these values and beliefs in their plan of care. To advocate for patients, ACNPs must know the patient. Knowing the patient is based on the ACNPs' knowledge of the patient and their willingness to treat the patient as a distinctly unique person (Radwin, 1995). As Tanner, Benner, Chesla, and Gordon (1993) report, this requires knowing the person's typical pattern of responses and knowing the patient as a person. ACNPs come to know the patient through skilled clinical judgment coupled with ongoing involvement with the patient.

> A woman came in with hypertension and over 5 months we worked up every system in her body. She probably had five admissions along the span until her death. It wasn't so much that her scleroderma advanced, but that she ended up on dialysis. I had a significant role in her care and family dynamics, in helping her to ultimately decide to let herself die. My first impression and the role I ended up with in this situation were overwhelming, but I think I had a good role in her ultimate death . . . going through all these complications and multisystem failure . . . keeping the family informed and the communication organized. It was overwhelming at times but very satisfying ultimately.

Ethical practice has many dimensions. Creating an ethical milieu is not just creating one that can effectively deal with such life-changing issues as code status and withholding and withdrawing life-sustaining treatment, but rather creating a practice that views patients as individuals with their own values, beliefs, and needs.

> I've made a lot of difference with a lot of our postops. They come back to the office after their surgery and rave about how attentive I was and how I answered their phone calls. They sort of feel that's how they got through the entire system and feel that they were not just a number. On most of these operative patients I make a difference. I can tell these patients what to expect at home—things that others would not have thought of. They are the sort of questions that they call back with a week later, after they go home.

A clinical nurse specialist colleague places a different twist on ACNP practice. Making the time, repeatedly to "be with" and "discuss with" rather than "to do" and "to inform" serves to create the foundation of ethical practice.

> Value is also from contact. For the families—they are available and accessible to families. If it takes a couple of sessions, they do it. NP follow-up is wonderful. They get back to patients with information. Patients get answers to questions. I love them. They have made such a difference on this unit.

The focus on the rights and responsibilities of patients to make choices concerning their own lives and health has required that the patient's status in medical discourse be elevated (Reiser, 1993). This cannot take place in the absence of a system of care that cultivates information flow and information sharing. As the following exemplar suggests, ACNPs can change the entire paradigm of information flow:

> One of the compliments patients who have had a previous catheterization say is that they have never been told things before. They were not aware and informed of the meaning of the catheterization by the attending prior to this admission. It is rewarding to know that we are making a positive difference in a system. . . . Patients repeatedly say "thank you, I didn't realize what was involved" . . . or "It never was explained to me in that way" . . . This is satisfying.

Many ACNPs speak about patient satisfaction, but looking below the more superficial level of patient satisfaction, one realizes that this satisfaction stems from the partnership that develops between the ACNP and the patient.

> I think the way that myself and other NPs make a difference is with patient satisfaction. I have had many patients call me or send me letters, saying that because I was available at the time that they needed me, they could talk to me at a moment's notice. I kept them [the families] abreast of what was going on with the patient through the whole hospital stay. That made all the difference in the world. It could be a terrible experience or it could be a good experience.

Because ACNPs focus on individuals within the context of their lives, satisfaction is enhanced.

> We had a patient who was ordered NPO. The nurse made a mistake and gave him his breakfast. So we had to postpone his cardioversion. He had a business meeting, a business trip that he had to be on. He had to postpone his air flight 24 hours. He was extremely upset, he was angry at the institution. He wasn't coming back. He didn't care. I was just sitting there, listening. I called the airline and got special arrangements. . . . Later he called us and thanked us . . . he was looking forward to seeing us again. Any form of social service—I think is part of your role.

Satisfaction with ACNP services can translate into the development of services in the complex health care system.

> I have patients who request my services again. We are actually developing a service here. We are an identified commodity to the patients and even to the attendings. . . . They will direct patients back to our service. . . . Patients will come back to an individual nurse practitioner who has made a positive impact on them and their family. They want to come back to you. It is good. It is rewarding.

ACNPs prescribe interventions that take into consideration the appropriate use of resources: "NPs tend to order less labs and are more likely to order less expensive drugs." Eliminating needless tests is not just cost-effective, but also contributes to patient comfort: "Routinely when a patient comes in here, the house staff will just order anything and everything. The lab work . . . we know that unnecessary lab work is very expensive. It is taxing on the patient, because you get blood drawn and you don't really need it."

How exactly might ACNPs more efficiently use resources? The following exemplar describes how resources can be more efficiently used.

> Everyone comes in with the carte blanche order for every blood test and every this, that and the other thing if they are on the regular service [house staff service]. . . . We use a lot more forethought in saying "Do I really need this at this time?" We tend to call the primary care physicians and find out whether the patient had a liver function or cholesterol screening in the recent past. If so, we won't do that study. These are simple things. But they are simple things that by rote the residents seem to order. We tend to have more effective communications with outside physicians and referrals to see what has been done and what needs to be done. We coordinate that care. For example, in the situation with a patient who had a recent hospitalization, who is going to surgery on Monday, I will supplement but not duplicate the whole lot. I am very conscientious about it. Not just ordering for the sake of ordering.

Choice of drugs is another area through which ACNPs can directly influence the cost of care.

> We try to use a lot of medications that are generic. You know, we have been asking for nonformulary and generic medications to be brought into the hospital . . . you know they are cheaper. The pharmacy and the pharmaceutical companies have been very receptive to that.

Another way that ACNPs efficiently use resources is through effective discharge planning. In this changing health care system with highly variable insurance regulations, this can be challenging at best.

> Prescriptions—finding out what insurance the patient has and making sure this is something they can afford. If their pharmacy is not open, providing them with samples to get them through. If they can't afford prescriptions, helping them gain some type of access so that they can get their drug filled. Basically . . . getting the patient through the system as quickly as possible and making sure that every need is met before they are discharged, so they don't come back in.

ACNPs facilitate efficient care in office settings as well. The following exemplar is from a busy cardiologist: "Even in the office setting, if I am late (which everyday I am), patients feel something is being done. The history is gotten. [ACNPs go over] the medications. Patients are not just sitting in a room looking at their toes. Patients love it."

ACNPs incorporate research- and evidence-based decision making to achieve optimal outcomes for the least amount of burden. In the following exemplar, the ACNP has shifted a service's practice away from the use of central lines with their attendant problems to an alternative. One that achieves the same level and quality of vascular access but that has potentially less significant and costly complications: "Frequently, CT surgery patients require and have central venous access. I am often able to prevent that risk exposure by suggesting a PICC line. The next step is to prove that that is beneficial."

As this ACNP identifies, acquiring data to support the change in practice is an important part of the advanced practice paradigm: "That our practice contributes to cost-effective quality care will be a very big issue. We (ACNPs) do contribute because we move patients through the system more efficiently and we provide very good quality care, but I don't think enough of us have documented it. . . . We really need to have some data supporting what we have done."

ACNPs themselves can have a direct effect on the cost of acute health care services.

> NPs are good here at decreasing LOS [length of stay]. We track all of that. We have a four-page data sheet on all operative patients, looking at LOS and complications. Statistics have shown that we have decreased LOS by two hospital days.
>
> They have done some specific analysis of LOS. Since I have come, the LOS has decreased. This is just due to follow-through with discharge, and the continuity I provide even as the house staff services change. I am the common denominator for the patient, and it has made a difference as far as patient satisfaction and family satisfaction.

As ACNP services develop, effective organization of practices has the potential for improving effective resource utilization. The organization of practice should be driven by patient needs rather than system needs only.

> I have two groups of patients. One group from whom I need to get a history, physical, and consent in 30 minutes or less (a cardiac catheterization service). And then I have patients who have needs for and deserve quality long-term time and teaching for a diagnosis of new heart failure or new coronary artery disease. It is very difficult to divide your time in that system. We [the cardiology NP group] are effectively making changes . . . hopefully to divide our services into two groups—a medical management team and a cath team. We will rotate between those two services, so that we hopefully will have much more satisfied patients with higher quality of care.

To provide optimal patient care, ACNPs are accountable to maintain current knowledge and skills relevant to their practice. Given the relatively new nature of this role, ACNPs strive for continual knowledge acquisition through a variety of mechanisms.

> I keep myself up to date through informal discussions with other NPs, professional meetings, asking questions of the physicians with whom I work, attending clinical conferences at work, reading medical and advanced practice nursing journals, and attending national conventions.
>
> I try to go to as many CE classes as I can, through journals, tons of conferences here that I am getting better at attending, cardiology and CT lectures, bigger conferences outside the hospital.

The experienced ACNPs recognize that they are constantly learning, that it is a lifelong process: "At this point, knowing how secure I am with my knowledge of cardiology, it amazes me how I learn something new every single day."

Developing and building on one's knowledge occur daily. As advanced practitioners, ACNPs must constantly augment their knowledge: "I read every night. Something I have never heard of before, I go home and read."

In settings where there is a group of ACNPs, this can focus on patient cases: "We also have little case presentations. One of the nurse practitioners will present a patient and then we discuss this. That helps a lot."

Certainly in academic medical centers, ACNPs have access to a variety of multidisciplinary specialty conferences. However, since ACNPs hold direct clinical responsibility for acutely ill patients, finding the time to attend conferences while running a clinical service can be challenging at best: "We have a number of conferences that are offered here. To be honest, these are not very convenient to the nurse practitioner service. In the reorganization of the ACNP service, we have made every effort to identify this as an issue and to make positive scheduling changes."

The scope of practice and standards of care are the foundations on which acute care nurse practitioners practice. The broad strokes of the scope of practice provide sufficient structure to describe practice but are coupled with a latitude that will allow for the necessary and inevitable evolution of the ACNP role. The standards for clinical practice and professional performance provide a template against which ACNP practice can be evaluated. This chapter has provided exemplars to bring to life the diversity and dynamic nature of ACNP practice.

REFERENCES

Aiken, L. H. (1990). Charting the future of hospital nursing. *Image: The Journal of Nursing Scholarship, 22,* 72–78.

American Nurses Association & American Association of Critical Care Nurses. (1995). *Standards of clinical practice and scope of practice for the acute care nurse practitioner.* Washington, DC: American Nurses Publishing Company.

Ball, C. (1997). Planning for the future: Advanced nursing practice in critical care. *Intensive & Critical Care Nursing, 13,* 17–25.

Daly, B. J. (1997). Acute care nurse practitioners: "Strangers in a strange land." *AACN Clinical Issues, 8,* 93–100.

DeAngelis, C. (1994). Nurse practitioner redux. JAMA, *271,* 868–871.

English, T. (1997). Personal paper: Medicine in the 1990s needs a team approach. *British Medical Journal, 314,* 661–663.

Gates, S. J. (1993). Continuity of care: The orthopaedic nurse practitioner in tertiary care. *Orthopaedic Nursing, 12,* 48–50.

Genet, C. A., Brennan, P. F., Ibbotson-Wolff, S., Phelps, C., Rosenthal, G., Landefeld, C. S., & Daly, B. (1995). Nurse practitioners in a teaching hospital. *Nurse Practitioner, 20,* 47–52.

Goksel, D., Harrison, C. J., Morrison, R. E., & Miller, S. T. (1993). Description of a nurse practitioner inpatient service in a public teaching hospital. *Journal of General Internal Medicine, 8,* 29–30.

Keane, A., & Richmond T. S. (1993). Tertiary nurse practitioners. *Image: The Journal of Nursing Scholarship, 25,* 281–284.

Keane, A., Richmond, T. S., & Kaiser, L. (1994). Critical care nurse practitioners: Evolution of the advanced practice nursing role. *American Journal of Critical Care, 3,* 232–237.

Mitchell-DiCenso, A., Guyatt, G., Marrin, M., Goeree, R., Willan, A., Southwell, D., Hewson, S., Paes, B., Rosenbaum, P., Hunsberger, M., & Baumann, A. (1996). A controlled trial of nurse practitioners in neonatal intensive care. *Pediatrics, 98,* 1143–1148.

Nolan, M. (1995). Has nursing lost its way? Towards an ethos of interdisciplinary practice. *The British Medical Journal, 311,* 305–307.

Piano, M. R., Kleinpell, R., & Johnson, J. A. (1996). The acute care nurse practitioner and management of common health problems: A proposal. *American Journal of Critical Care, 5,* 289–292.

Radwin, L. E. (1995). Knowing the patient: A process model for individualized interventions. *Nursing Research, 44,* 364–370.

Reiser, S. J. (1993) The era of the patient: Using the experience of illness in shaping the missions of health care. *JAMA, 269,* 1012–1017.

Ripportella-Muller, R., Libby, D., & Kindig, D. (1995). The substitution of physician assistants and nurse practitioners for physician residents in teaching hospitals. *Health Affairs, 14,* 181–191.

Safriet, B. J. (1992). Health care dollars and regulatory sense: The role of advanced practice nursing. *Yale Journal on Regulation, 9,* 417–488.

Shah, H. S., Bruttomesso, K. A., Sullivan, D. T., & Lattanzio, J. (1997). An evaluation of the role and practice of the acute care nurse practitioner. *AACN Clinical Issues, 8,* 147–155.

Spisso, J., O'Callaghan, C., McKennan, M., & Holcroft, J. W. (1990). Improved quality of care and reduction of housestaff workload using trauma nurse practitioners. *Journal of Trauma, 30,* 663–665.

Tanner, C. A., Benner, P., Chesla, C., & Gordon, D. R. (1993). The phenomenology of knowing the patient. *Image: The Journal of Nursing Scholarship, 25,* 273–280.

Watts, R. J., Hanson, M. J. S., Burke, K. G., Gallagher, S. M., & Foster, D. E. (1996). The critical care nurse practitioner: An advanced practice role for the critical care nurse. *Dimensions of Critical Care Nursing, 15,* 48–56.

3

Business Considerations for the ACNP

Linda A. Carrick
Pamela A. Bergmann
Eileen M. Sullivan-Marx

Dramatic economic changes in health care have reshaped how care is provided. The primary focus in today's health care environment is to preserve or to enhance quality while delivering services in a more efficient and cost-effective manner. Fagin (1992) stated that these will be "more powerful efforts to examine alternatives for quality health care at a reduced cost in the 1990's." This chapter examines the reimbursement mechanisms affecting nurse practitioners and also explores the essential components of business planning that are becoming a necessary tool for nurse practitioners.

▶ REIMBURSEMENT ISSUES

Innovative health care delivery models using nurse practitioners improve access and quality of services for patients and are cost effective. To maintain models of care using acute care nurse practitioners (ACNP), services provided by ACNPs need to be included in payment systems and financial databases. The traditional role of nurses as employees in hospital systems has contributed to their "invisibility" in health systems. This lack of visibility has made nurses vulnerable to job elimination during health care system restructuring. Acute care nurse practitioners (ACNPs) are usually employees of hospital systems or physician groups rather than solo practitioners. As employees, ACNPs must use business strategies to ensure that their salaries are commensurate with the revenues that they generate in the practice. In addition, ACNPs may contract directly with hospital systems as sole proprietors or independent contractors. In either case, ACNPs must be cognizant of all payment and reimbursement mechanisms currently in place for funding their services. Reimbursement is a complex process for all health care providers in today's changing health care environment. Health care professionals need to understand a myriad of concepts and terms, including managed care, integrated delivery systems, fee-for-service reimbursement, and contract negotiation, to provide services and to be paid for those services.

Because of nursing's traditional employment relationship, nurses and nurse practitioners (NPs) have not kept pace with reimbursement and payment systems for their services. A 1993 American Nurses Association (ANA) survey of nurses providing services by the Current Procedural Terminology (CPT) coding system found that most were unaware of how their services were charged and reimbursed in their practice (ANA, 1994). The following sections outline various payment mechanisms for ACNP practice.

Managed Care

Managed care, initially developed in the 1970s as a cost containment model for employees of industry, uses a prospective payment structure in which providers or plans are paid for "covered lives" of their patients on a prorated basis, called capitated payment. These monthly fees remain the same regardless of the number of visits provided to the patient (ANA, 1995). Hence, a plan or provider with a panel of patients who are relatively healthy may incur a profit. However, the same fee is paid for those patients who may require frequent, lengthy visits or hospitalization. A major criticism of managed care is that incentives exist to underserve patients, as opposed to fee-for-service payment systems in which providers determine the number of patient services needed and are paid a fee for each service. The high costs of fee-for-service visits, however, have led to a rapid increase in the utilization of private and public funded managed care plans. Many states are in the process of converting state Medicaid plans to managed care systems. Medicare, largely a fee-for-service system, now has approximately 11% of their beneficiaries in managed care plans with enrollments growing rapidly each month (PPRC, 1997).

Managed care includes a wide variety of health delivery structures that blend payment and service models. Health maintenance organizations (HMOs) are entities that provide an organized system for health delivery in a geographic area with an agreement to cover specified preventive and treatment services to individuals who voluntarily enroll in the group plan. Models vary by level of financial risk incurred. The most typical HMO is a group model in which a health plan contracts with a large health professional generalist or specialty group to provide care to plan members and assumes the greatest financial risk and responsibility for outcomes. An independent practice association (IPA) assumes less risk by contracting with a managed care plan for a negotiated fee while continuing to provide services to patients other than those in the HMO. The preferred provider organization (PPO) contracts with independent health care providers for negotiated fees for services provided to members of the managed care plan. A growing version of all these models in the point of service option (POS) in which members can opt to use the managed care plan or providers out of the plan by paying a higher monthly premium or a fee at the time they choose to go outside the plan (ANA, 1995).

Nurse practitioners, clinical specialists, certified nurse midwives, and certified registered nurse anesthetists have been used in managed care models to provide preventive services, primary care, and coordination of care and to manage the care of high-risk and high-need members in a health plan. Their contributions have led to reductions in complications, in readmissions following discharge, in use of emergency services, and in length of hospital stay (Lang, Sullivan-Marx, & Jenkins, 1996). Such outcomes are attractive to managed care plans interested in using ACNPs who can both provide direct tertiary services and emphasize preventive care.

Employment relationships for ACNPs with managed care plans may range from employees in PPOs to direct negotiation for fees as a provider for a panel of members. Since ACNPs most commonly provide care in tertiary settings or for limited periods following acute illness, it is likely that most ACNPs will be employed in health systems or by multispecialty groups.

For hospital services, managed care plans negotiate payment rates with hospitals or health systems. Salaries for ACNPs employed in health systems may be covered as part of the payment made to the hospital by the managed care plan. For ACNPs employed by physician groups, revenue for salaries may be generated from the capitated payment for "covered lives" of patients or from a prenegotiated payment made for a procedure or hospital service. As employees, ACNPs must be certain that their contributions are being recognized in the managed care data system. It is common for services provided by nurse practitioners to be accounted for under the physician's name or provider I.D. Productivity in managed care is often measured by outcomes achieved, visits provided, or patient satisfaction surveys. If ACNPs are not clearly identified in these managed care databases, their contributions will either be ignored or attributed to physician practice by default. ACNPs need to document their contributions themselves if the managed care plan is not doing so.

Medicare

Over 38 million Americans receive health insurance through the federal Medicare program, which guarantees insurance to those over 65 years of age, to individuals with kidney disease, and to disabled persons. Part A of Medicare covers hospitalization, skilled nursing facilities, hospice, and home health care and is paid for by federal payroll tax. Part B of Medicare covers physician and other provider services and is paid for by voluntary supplement insurance through Medicare beneficiary premiums. Services provided by nurses in hospitals are covered as part of Medicare Part A. Physicians bill Medicare Part B for services provided in all settings, including hospital visits.

Since the inception of nurse practitioners in the 1960s, efforts to obtain direct Medicare reimbursement for nurse practitioners led to incremental changes in Medicare law at the federal level. Most recently landmark legislation in the Balanced Budget Act of 1997 now provides direct reimbursement for nurse practitioners and clinical nurse specialists regardless of geographic setting at 85% of the prevailing physician rate. Effective January 1998 ACNPs may be able to bill Medicare directly for services provided under Part B of Medicare ***provided that their services are not***

already covered by Medicare Part A payment to hospitals. Billing under Part B of Medicare requires that ACNPs (1) obtain a provider number from Medicare, (2) work in collaboration with a physician ***but the physician does not need to be on the premises in which the service was provided or directly supervise the service provided,*** and (3) practice according to the regulations of the state in which the service is provided.

Prior to this long-sought legislation, nurse practitioners could only bill for Medicare Part B services in rural areas, skilled nursing facilities, or when services were provided "incident to" physician services. "Incident to" reimbursement was paid at 100% of the prevailing physician rate, but created barriers to practice and impinged on the autonomy of nursing practice because it required that the physician be present in the suite in which service was provided and implied the need for direct supervision of the nurse practitioner's service although state practice regulations may not have required such a provision.

The new legislation pays 15% less per service but has the advantage of increasing access to community-based care for Medicare beneficiaries and enhances the ability for ACNPs to bill for outpatient services when the collaborating physician is off-site. More important, this legislation brings payment for nurse practitioner services into mainstream payment systems, making the NP visible in federal and public databases. Ultimately, services provided by nurse practitioners can be linked to financial and clinical outcomes. Such data ultimately provide support for all nursing practice.

It is incumbent upon salaried ACNPs who are considering billing for Medicare Part B services to ensure that they are not already receiving Medicare Part A services for hospital care. Medicare Part A covers nursing services in hospitals and some outpatient settings. If an ACNP's salary comes from Part A payment, then that ACNP is precluded from also billing Medicare under Part B. Understanding the intricacies of the sources of an ACNP's salary is crucial to avoid legal and financial penalties under federal law.

Medicaid

In 1989 the U.S. Congress established direct Medicaid payment for pediatric and family nurse practitioners to increase access to health care services for children. As a federally mandated program, states have discretion in how Medicaid funds are disseminated. Consequently, some states interpret language regarding nurse practitioner payment broadly and provide direct Medicaid payment to all nurse practitioners in their state, with varying rates of 70–100% of the prevailing physician rate (Pearson, 1997).

States have increasingly adopted managed care methods for their Medicaid programs through the federal government waiver plan, part of Sections 1115 and 1915(b) of the Social Security Act (White, 1995). Nurse practitioners are not necessarily included in state "waiver" plans as primary providers. Political action has been needed in many states to ensure inclusion of nurse practitioners in state Medicaid managed care plans.

As salaried employees in acute care facilities, ACNPs may receive salaries from Medicaid payment to hospitals for inpatient services, or they may bill Medicaid as providers in outpatient settings. There is tremendous regional flux currently in Medicaid payment, and ACNPs need both to be cognizant of local variation in Medicaid structures, and understand the hybrid of managed care plans that may be contributing to their practice.

Traditional Indemnity Plans

Although less prevalent in recent years, private fee-for-service indemnity plans (e.g., Blue Shield plans) continue as a viable alternative to managed care plans. Payment for nurse practitioners through private indemnity plans is regulated at the state level. Currently, 37 states have legislation covering nurse practitioner reimbursement (Pearson, 1997).

In states where ACNPs receive private fee-for-service reimbursement, they are able to obtain a billing provider number from the indemnity plan and to submit a fee-for-service bill to the provider. Often such plans pay a percentage of the prevailing physician rate. Business managers may be concerned about the reduced rate obtained for nurse practitioner services and prefer that billing to be done under the physician's provider number. Billing under a physician provider number when the nurse practitioner actually is doing the work (or the majority of the clinical work) for that visit undermines services provided by nurse practitioners and may constitute fraudulent billing practice.

CONTRACT AND SALARY NEGOTIATION

When addressing salary and employment issues, ACNPs need to step into the arena of the business world. Financial negotiations and business plans will likely be unfamiliar to nurses. A good first step is to learn business terms and basic contract issues. General "how to" books on small business planning and entrepreneurial viewpoints are quite informative. Whether ACNPs are approaching a position as employees or independent contractors, they should be ready to discuss basic mechanisms of payment and reimbursement in addition to the usual issues of benefits, malpractice, and salary. Knowledge of business planning enables them to evaluate the core delivery model using a business or financial perspective in addition to a quality or outcomes perspective and to implement appropriate changes.

Buppert (1997) notes that salaries for ACNPs should be based on the income that the ACNP brings to the practice or health system, removing 10% for unpaid bills, another 20–50% for practice expenses, and another 10–20% for physician consultation. In addition, an employer profit percentage may also be deducted. Revenue generated by the ACNP comes from various sources: (1) prospective payments for patient admissions made to a hospital or health system, (2) fee-for-service reimbursements made directly to the ACNP or employer, and (3) capitated payment made to a multispecialty group practice.

Acute care nurse practitioners have many resources for further information. In addition to networking with colleagues at regional and national meetings, ACNPs can hire business consultants such as accountants, health care managers, or attorneys; attend seminars conducted by Medicare carriers and insurance companies; develop a working knowledge of reimbursement manuals used by practice managers; and seek information from business managers in the settings where they practice. Although the current complexity in health care financing is daunting, a step-by-step approach to understanding payment systems and the relevance of business planning will lead to greater dissemination of ACNP practice throughout the health care system.

BUSINESS PLANNING

The starting point for cultivating financial skills is to familiarize yourself with business terminology. You need to understand and speak the same language as potential clients, investors, and administrators. It is also important to network with business or financially minded people both in and outside the profession. These individuals can serve as valuable resources instrumental to your learning. Last, it is important to be able to create and express your plans for any new venture or redesign of an existing service in an organized and professional manner. This is accomplished through a business plan. Business plans should not be viewed as only being applicable for top-level administrators and managers, but as an effective business tool or framework for nurse administrators.

Evaluating the profitability of a practice, opening a new wing, proposing a new program, or even starting a new business are now becoming career opportunities for ACNPs. Advanced practice nurses are remarkably adaptable as witnessed by their practice in many different work environments outside the traditional hospital setting. The remainder of this chapter is a discussion of the purpose and elements of sound business planning.

The Business Plan

Used to communicate ideas about the development of a practice or the expansion of a service, a business plan serves as an internal blueprint for a practice or business. Business plans are also used externally as a financing proposal for prospective investors. Questions answered by the business plan include who you are, what you do, where you are headed, how and when you expect to get there, and why you will be successful.

A business plan can be tailored to reflect the uniqueness of a specific business or program. However, several essential components must be included. These include a title page, table of contents, executive summary, statement of purpose, business description, market analysis and plan, location, organization and management, SWOT (strengths, weaknesses, opportunities and threats) analysis, financial data, and supporting documents.

Executive Summary

The executive summary provides the overview of the plan. Although it appears in the beginning of a plan, it is typically written last by the author. It is a brief summary, usually no more than two pages, introducing the practice or service, anticipated costs, goals and objectives, and strategies used to accomplish the desired results. The executive summary should be concise, insightful and captivating. The use of medical jargon is discouraged, and the anticipated readers should be able to understand the major components.

Statement of Purpose

The statement of purpose clearly and concisely describes the goal(s) of the proposal. It sets the stage for the ensuing planning process.

Business Description

In the description of the business the nature of the practice or service and of the projected consumer interest is defined. This section identifies the targeted consumers and anticipates the needs that will be satisfied. Potential obstacles and strategies to overcome these obstacles are specified. Long-term opportunities and business goals are also defined.

Market Analysis. The market analysis is a key component of your business plan. Pivotal to the success of a new or expanded service is research that scrutinizes your target market. You may assume that there is a need for your service or product; market analysis may prove otherwise. According to Ginny L. Kuebler (1996), there are five questions you need to ask:

1. Who are your potential customers?
2. Where are they located?
3. How large is your target market?
4. What are the needs and wants of your potential customers?
5. What criteria do they use in making buying decisions?

Kuebler goes on to provide the following examples of customer needs: convenience, education, recreation, safety, and concern about personal appearance. She cautions the creator of a business plan to discern between a consumer's needs and wants. In doing so, you'll be better able to predict the value of your product. The desired outcome of your research is finding a market niche.

Competition. Do not enter into a market with naïveté. Know your competitors. Determine who they are, where they are, what they do, and what they charge. Examine their strengths and weaknesses. Ascertain their potential impact on the success of your venture. After sizing up your competitors, embrace an attribute that gives you a competitive advantage, such as quality, variety, uniqueness, convenience, performance, or price.

Marketing Plan

In this section of your business plan, you need to outline the effective strategies and tactics you will use to sell your product or service successfully. A marketing plan would not be complete without addressing all four P's: product, promotion, price, and place.

Product

As you launch your marketing campaign, you first need to answer three questions. (1) What is your business? (2) What is being sold? (3) How will you best meet the customer's needs? While these questions seem simple, your answers need to be provocative. Illustrate how you plan to capture a segment of the market. What differentiates your service? Many entities employ a tactic called *branding,* in other words, identifying a selling point. For instance, imagine a medical center that recruits world-renowned cardiac surgeons, invests in cutting-edge cardiac monitors and equipment, performs innovative cardiac procedures, and caters to the sickest of cardiac patients. Clearly, this medical center is identifying itself as a premier cardiac care center.

Promotion

Timidity and complacency in marketing your idea or expanded service are not the name of the game; confidence and ambition are. Distributing flyers, posting signs, handing out business cards, and networking are some simple, yet successful, marketing strategies employed by many entrepreneurs. Advertising schemes need to be creative (e.g., Nike: "Just do it!" Bell Atlantic: "Let your fingers do the walking."). Selling strategies need to be competitive. Your public relations efforts need to be aggressive. Examples of tactics specific to health care are follow-up a physician referral to your service with a personal letter; promote your service by having a health fair; offer free parking; have a postop nurse call the day or week after surgery to assess the patient's recovery. Keep in mind that although these gimmicks/slogans/tactics may seem small and insignificant, their impact may be great.

Price

Without question, you must know what you are charging, to whom, who's paying, and who is not. Establishing a price for your service can often be complex. On the one hand, a higher price can generate revenue with a fewer number of visits, but limit your pool of customers. On the other hand, a lower price attracts customers, thereby increasing your market share. However, with a lower price, will you be able to meet expenses and still make a profit? When you are the owner of a business, a negative profit margin correlates with the inability to pay your bills and yourself. Overall, the best indicator for pricing is the value perceived by potential customers. Unfortunately, the merit of an idea does not always guarantee a profit. For example, a service that offers in-home nursing care after surgery would probably be more attractive to a customer than an in-home preop teaching nursing service. Realistic predictions can often prevent the disappointment and financial loss associated with the discovery that customers tend to pay less or not at all when the expense is out of pocket.

Place

The last component of your marketing plan is the distribution of your service. You must determine if you will sell directly or indirectly to the customer. That is, are you providing the service directly to the client or contracting your services to a physician's provider group. You must also decide how much inventory you need and where to store it. Having too large an inventory in an attempt to meet all demands can waste valuable space and money. In contrast, you will also bear the cost of having too little and of running out.

Location

As most business owners would agree, the location of your business can either make or break you. For example, if a geriatric nurse practitioner chooses a site for his or her venture in a community comprised of mostly young families, the customer base will be sparse. Find out where your target market is located and if you are easily accessible to them. Prioritize the location characteristics most important to your business, such as safety, cost, visibility, convenience, and proximity to competitors.

Organization and Management

According to Dun and Bradstreet, approximately 98% of all business failures are attributed to managerial weakness. Management may not be your forte, so you would be wise to invest in the professional help of an accountant and/or lawyer as you plan this piece of your venture. You can begin by formatting an organizational chart, illustrating the various personnel, their responsibilities, and lines of communication and authority. Standards have to be identified. Policies and procedures need to be written. You also need to evaluate your tax structure, necessary insurance policies, and your financial condition.

SWOT Analysis

Your business plan is not complete without the identification of your venture's Strengths, Weaknesses, Opportunities, and Threats (SWOT). The advantages of doing so are twofold. First, it reveals to your reader your insight into potential obstacles and your methods of minimizing them. Second, it allows you to internally benchmark your business. It is paramount to the ongoing success of your business that you periodically evaluate whether or not you are meeting your goals and objectives. "Failure to reassess and reset goals and revise plans as dictated by the realities that unfold is another reason planning fails" (Kuebler, 1996).

Financial Data and Analysis

As a clinician you may lack the experience necessary to calculate and analyze the financial aspects of your business plan. Your budget may not allow for an accountant on staff; however, utilizing their services temporarily in the start-up phase could be well worth the additional cost. Thereafter, the acquisition of these skills will be necessary to meet the ongoing demands of your venture and to make sound business decisions. Essentially, the financial plan demonstrates whether or not your business will be a viable one both short-term and long-term. The components of a thorough financial plan are: summary of sources and uses of funds, capital equipment, beginning inventory, start-up costs, working capital, projected income statement, projected cash flow statement, and projected balance sheets.

Be alert to avoid the following financial traps: (1) not having enough money on the front end to cover bad debt in the beginning, (2) assuming that your buyers will be prompt in making payments, (3) underestimating the number and cost of resources (e.g., staff, capital equipment, inventory), (4) overestimating your market share, and (5) setting up a practice based on a grant without the foresight that you will need a secondary source of revenue once the grant runs out. A point also worth mentioning is that nurses provide exemplary care for the underprivileged. This certainly is an admirable feature, but if you focus exclusively on this segmented population, will your profit margin be one to keep you afloat?

As a clinician you have many sanctions that can work in your favor. Investors typically like to finance small businesses. Bankers also like to finance clinicians. It is assumed that in the event the business should fail, the health care professional can easily find something else to do to pay back the loan. In the same respect, many clinicians opt to retain their current position as they build a new practice. This ensures a steady revenue stream even if the business does not initially make a profit. Never be afraid to take advantage of the relationships you have formed with colleagues, the networks you have established, and the people you know.

Supporting Documents

The last piece to your business plan is any relevant information that supports and completes your proposal. This may include organizational charts, résumés of key personnel, recruiting and training programs, marketing tools and findings, letters of reference, operational details, financial details, and any explanatory charts, tables, graphs, and documents.

During times of great change and chaos, natural leaders are born. We are part of the health care revolution. Nurse practitioners must assume a leadership role in charting the future of health care delivery. By combining outstanding clinical competence with business planning skills, nurse practitioners can demonstrate efficient and effective care delivery methods. As reimbursement for nurse practitioners becomes stronger, new roles and independent clinical business opportunities will continue to emerge.

REFERENCES

American Nurses Association. (1994). American Nurses Association/National Organization Liaison Forum Current Procedural Terminology (CPT) Survey. Washington, DC: Author.

American Nurses Association. (1995). *Managed care: Challenges and opportunities for nursing.* Washington, DC: Author.

Buppert, C. K. (1997, July/August). Negotiating salary. *NP World News.*

Fagin, C. M. (1992). *Cost-effectiveness of nursing care revisited: 1981–1990, Charting nursing's future.* Philadelphia: Lippincott.

Hollreiser, E. (1996). Physicians, not hospitals, are key for Penn Health. *Philadelphia Business Journal.*

Kuebler, G. L. (1996). *Let's write your business plan* (5th ed.). New York: GLK Management Consulting.

Lang, N. M., Sullivan-Marx, E. M., & Jenkins, M. (1996). Advanced practice nurses and success of organized delivery systems. *American Journal of Managed Care, 2,* 129–135.

Levit, K. R., Lazenby, H. C., & Sivarajan, L. (1996). Health care spending in 1994: Slowest in decades. *Health Affairs, 15*(2), 130–153.

Pearson, L. J. (1997). Annual update of how each state stands on legislative issues affecting advanced nursing practice. *Nurse Practitioner, 22,* 18–86.

Physician Payment Review Commission. (1997). *Annual report.* Washington, DC: Author.

Sharp, N. (1993). Mothers, infants and children: What's happening now? *Nursing Management, 24,* 17–20.

Turini, N. N. (1995). Business Plans: An effective tool for making decisions. *Nursing Leadership Forum, 1*(4), 116–120.

White, K. M. (1995). The fate of Medicaid waivers. *Nursing Policy Forum, 1*(3), 37–39.

Whitmire, R. (1995). Infant death rates drops, but racial differences widen, report says. *Gannett News Service.*

4

Licensure, Certification, and Institutional Credentialing

Patricia Baehser Griffith
Paul Logan

To practice, nurse practitioners must first obtain a license and, frequently, certification from a professional organization. The process of state licensure is generally well understood. Institutional credentialing, however, is a process with which nurse practitioners have not dealt extensively. Because of their practice environment, acute care nurse practitioners (ACNPs) must understand the complexities of institutional credentialing. Included are reviews of the licensing and certification processes and a detailed discussion of the institutional credentialing process.

▶ LICENSURE

Licensure is permission granted by a competent authority to an individual to engage in an activity that is otherwise illegal. The purpose of licensure is to protect the health, safety, and well-being of the public, not to benefit the individual being licensed. Generally, licensure is granted on the basis of education and examination. Licensure can be revoked by the granting agency for incompetence, criminal acts, and other reasons provided in the rules regulating the specific license (Anderson, Anderson, & Glanze, 1994). All Registered Nurses (RNs) are required to have state licenses to practice in the United States. Licensure of RNs is the responsibility of the state boards of nursing (SBON).

Each of the 50 states, U.S. territories, and the District of Columbia has a SBON responsible for the licensure of all registered nurses, implementation of the state's nurse practice act, and regulation of educational programs for nursing students. Each SBON is unique and its specific responsibilities vary. The exact makeup of the SBON varies from state to state. Most state boards of nursing are composed of governor-appointed RNs, licensed practical nurses (LPNs), and consumers. Some states require a nurse practitioner (NP) to be on the SBON.

The SBON is a regulatory agency, not a law-making body. The SBON, therefore, cannot make changes to the nurse practice act. Rather, changes to the nurse practice act must be made through the legislative process. Proposed changes to the nurse practice act are frequently brought to the legislature by interested parties such as the state nurses association, but changes can be proposed by the SBON as well (Dalton, Speakman, Duffey, & Carlson, 1994; Rosen, 1995).

The National Council of State Boards of Nursing (NCSBN) is an organization of all the state boards of nursing. The NCSBN's mission is to protect the public by regulating the safe and effective practice of nursing. The NCSBN is composed of two members of each SBON (House of Delegates). The NCSBN holds an annual convention to vote on policies and positions of common interest and concern affecting public health, safety, and welfare. After a proposal is adopted by the delegates, the members attempt to implement these proposals within their nurse practice act by promulgating the rules and regulations or through legislature. The NCSBN can only make proposals to the state boards of nursing, it cannot implement the proposal into law (Havens & Hannan, 1996).

Regulation of Advanced Practice Nurses

Nurse Practitioners require licensure as RNs. Currently, no state requires second licensure to practice as a nurse practitioner. Many states, however, do require NPs to provide proof of additional training or education to practice. This is specified in a certification or registration statute. This statute both defines "nurse practitioner" and provides title protection for the NP. It does not limit practice, as does licensure statute (Hall, 1993).

Nurse practitioners are legally bound to practice within the range that is defined and regulated by the state, called the scope of practice. The scope of practice defined by each state's nurse practice act includes a definition of the role of the nurse practitioner, the criteria for legal recognition, the use of the title of NP (title protection), and the criteria for termination of function as an NP. Some states include in their scope of practice reimbursement regulations and prescriptive authority (Hravnak, Rosenzweig, & Baldisseri, 1996). There is much diversity in state recognition of NP scope of practice, ranging from very restrictive to unrestrictive (Table 4–1).

▸ CERTIFICATION

Certification is a credentialing process granted by a nongovernmental organization to an individual who demonstrates competence based on specific criteria. The purpose of certification is to demonstrate that a professional has mastered the minimum skills necessary to practice a particular specialty and has acquired the body of knowledge common to that specialty (Geolot, 1986). Certification also provides the opportunity for acknowledgment by one's profession, by other health care professionals, and by patients (Nicholas, 1995).

TABLE 4–1. Legal Authority for Advanced Nursing Practice

Nurse practitioner title protection and SBON as sole authority in scope of practice	AK, AR, CO, CT, DE, DC, HI IA, IN, KS, ME, MI, MT, ND, NH, NJ, NM, OK, OR, RI, TX, UT, VT, WA, WV, WY
Nurse practitioner title protection and SBON as sole authority in scope of practice, but scope of practice has a requirement for physician collaboration/supervision	AL, AZ, CA, FL, GA, KY, LA, MA, MD, MO, NE, NY, NV, OH, SC, WI
Nurse practitioner title protection and scope of practice is authorized by the Board of Nursing and the Board of Medicine	ID, MS, NC, PA, SD, VA
No nurse practitioner title protection: APNs function under a broad Nurse Practice Act	IL, MN, TN

Used with permission from the January, 1997, issue of Nurse Practitioner, *p. 18, Springhouse Corporation.*

Currently, the only certifying agency for acute care nurse practitioners is the American Nurses Credentialing Center (ANCC) in conjunction with the American Association of Critical Care Nurses (AACN) certification corporation. To obtain ACNP certification, the candidate must have graduated from a master's level ACNP program or a formal postgraduate ACNP program in a school granting graduate-level academic credits. The candidate must also pass the certification examination. A "grandfather" accommodation permits graduates of master's-level adult or family NP programs to sit for the ACNP certification examination, but only if they fulfill specific clinical and academic criteria. This option for graduates of non-ACNP programs is available only until the end of 1999 (ANCC, 1995).

Advanced practice certification is also offered in many other clinical specialty areas by organizations such as the ANCC; American Academy of Nurse Practitioners; National Certification Board of Pediatric Nurse Practitioners; National Certification Corporation for the Obstetric, Gynecologic, and Neonatal Nursing Specialties; and Oncology Nursing Certification Corporation (Spencer-Cisek & Svengingson, 1995). Each organization and specialty has different eligibility requirements. The eligibility requirements and recertification criteria are based on education, experience, and practice.

State Recognition

Certification is intended to be a voluntary process, but becomes compulsory in states where certification is necessary to achieve recognition as a nurse practitioner. Individual states grant recognition in the form of registration or certification based on criteria set forth in their nurse practice acts. Passing a national certification examination in an individual's area of specialty practice is a requirement in many states' nurse practice acts for recognition of nurse practitioners (Bullough, 1982; Edmunds, 1992; Geolot, 1986; Nicholas, 1995; Spencer-Cisek & Sveningson, 1995). The incorporation of voluntary national certification into the requirements for state recognition (in some states) has essentially made certification equal to licensure.

Second Licensure versus Certification

Since the late 1980s the NCSBN has actively attempted to standardize advanced practice nurses under one title and to develop a second license for advanced practice nurses. NCSBN's rationale is that the NP's scope of practice exceeds the legal boundaries of a RN. The NCSBN maintains that NPs would benefit from a second license by (1) providing clear legal authority to practice and preventing others who are not licensed from practicing as NPs, (2) improving reimbursement eligibility by clearly defining NPs to legislators and insurers as direct health care providers, and (3) enhancing NP mobility across state lines (assuming states had similar licensing requirements, this could be a form of reciprocity) (Greco, 1995; Sheets, 1993).

The NCSBN addressed the issue of second licensure due to concerns voiced by the state boards of nursing. The state boards feel there is great difficulty determining whether a nurse practitioner is competent to be granted licensure because of confusion created with so many types of voluntary certification. Certification examinations differ with regard to their requirements among organizations and within specialties. The NCSBN has also questioned whether various certification examinations are legally defensible and psychometrically sound for regulatory purposes. The NCSBN delegates believe that the exam subject matter may not be harmonious with the scope of practice being regulated and that it is not designed to measure competence for the purpose of regulation. They maintain that only subject matter directly related to public safety be included in a core examination as public safety is the purpose of professional regulation (NCSBN, 1993).

The American Nurses Association (ANA) has contested the proposal of second licensure for NPs. ANA has stated that (1) the scope of practice and responsibilities of the NP are based on RN licensure and that regulatory authority exists with this license, (2) states provide protection of public safety through the regulation of RNs, (3) second licensure sends a message to legislators that NPs need more regulation than any other health care profession, (4) disciplinary action is difficult if there is multiple licensing of individuals, and (5) second licensure increases costs (Greco, 1995; Malone, 1993). The ANA states that any examination developed to assess the core competence of all NPs would be unable to assess competence in any single area of specialization, thus offering no assurance as to the competency of an individual within his or her area of specialization. They also point to the precedent of only single licensure for other health care professions. For example, physicians use voluntary certification to designate specialists, as is the current system for NPs. Therefore, second licensure for NPs would vary from this single licensure model (Havens & Hannan, 1996; Spatz, 1996).

The controversy between certification versus second licensure has been present for many years and probably will continue for many more. As these ideas are debated, individuals and organizations will need to voice their concerns and opinions to their state boards of nursing and state legislators to ensure that their ideas are considered.

► INSTITUTIONAL CREDENTIALING

Whether the ACNP is employed by the institution or a private practice, the nurse practitioner must be "credentialed" by the institution. Institutional credentialing grants permission to perform certain acts within the institution. Institutional credentialing is the process by which an institution verifies the competence of an NP to perform these acts (Hravnak & Baldisseri, 1997).

The institutional credentialing process typically begins by writing to the chief of the department to which the ACNP wishes to apply for privileges. In the letter, the ACNP requests an application for staff privileges. Providing the medical staff bylaws allow credentialing of nurse practitioners, the department head then writes a letter on behalf of the applicant to the chair of the credentials committee requesting that an application be released to the applicant. Once this is accomplished, the process of institutional credentialing begins.

In addition to the application itself, many other documents are typically required (Table 4–2). Once submitted, this information is reviewed by the credentialing committee, which evaluates each applicant and reviews matters concerning the clinical and ethical conduct of health care providers (Hravnak, Rosenzweig, & Baldisseri, 1996; Smith, 1993). The credentialing committee is generally comprised of physicians who are members of the medical staff. If other advanced practice nurses are on staff at the institution, it is possible that one or more of them may be committee members, although they may have limited or no voting privileges. The director of medical affairs and legal counsel may also be present at the meetings of the committee.

Particularly if there are no other ACNPs on staff at the institution, the credentialing committee may require a lot of other information. ACNPs should be prepared to clearly articulate the ACNP scope of practice and what privileges are necessary to fulfill the duties of the ACNP role.

Delineation of Privileges

The "delineation of privileges" is a document that lists the privileges for which the practitioner is applying. If the institution has credentialed other ACNPs before, there may be a standardized form that the applicant can complete. If not, it

TABLE 4–2. Documents Frequently Required for Institutional Privileges

Current license as a RN and as a NP for the state in which the hospital is located
Certification in your specialty
Sponsorship of a physician on staff at the hospital
Recommendations from colleagues
Proof of liability insurance and description of any malpractice claims made against you
Curriculum vitae or résumé
Current certification in basic CPR and/or advanced life support
Proof of immune or vaccination status
Description of requested privileges
Completed application

is wise for the applicant to submit a delineation of privileges for the committee to consider (Table 4–3). Doing so meets at least three important needs. First, it ensures that the ACNP has requested all of the privileges that are necessary to practice effectively. Second, submitting a comprehensive delineation of privileges form speeds up the approval process. Last, people like self-starters. The committee may look more favorably on an applicant who knows the role of the ACNP and helps the committee to understand it.

The applicant usually completes the delineation of clinical privileges, selecting those privileges that are necessary for the completion of their duties, and sends the form to the department chairperson for review and comment. Occasionally, applicants will be asked to provide some documentation that they have shown competency in the listed procedures. If the ACNP has kept a list of procedures performed, either during their education or in a previous job, it is easy to document proficiency. Otherwise, the ACNP may be required to perform certain procedures under the direct supervision or the collaborating physician or another member of the medical staff credentialed to perform the procedure.

Included in the credentialing document must be a statement of the ACNP's intended scope of practice within the institution. The scope of practice describes function and general job responsibilities of the ACNP in the hospital. The ACNP's reporting mechanisms must also be delineated. The ACNP should then provide a list of all the clinical privileges being sought within the hospital.

If the ACNP is denied hospital privileges after submitting all of the necessary documents, the reason should be sought and a solution should be pursued. Initially, the credentialing committee may not wish to grant an ACNP all privileges that were requested, but some compromises might be made to develop privileges and protocols that are amenable to both the committee and the ACNP. Some hospitals do not currently employ or recognize nurse practitioners and may, therefore, deny an ACNP privileges. It may be beneficial to have the sponsoring physician speak to the credentialing committee on the ACNP's behalf. The physician may be able to encourage the committee to grant an ACNP privileges on a trial basis.

Despite an ACNP's best efforts, however, some hospitals may still deny privileges. In this instance it is wise for the ACNP to collect information and implement a strategy to obtain privileges. If, for instance, it is learned that privileges were denied because pharmacy services objected, then a meeting with the pharmacy director, vice president for nursing, the ACNP, and a staff member of the credentialing office should be called. Other individuals can be present too, depending on the specific needs. Last, the services of a health care attorney familiar with nursing laws and reimbursement issues would be a valuable asset.

Once granted, privileges are reviewed periodically, according to the institution's medical staff bylaws. At the time of review, the ACNP is required to forward updated documents such as licenses, certifications, malpractice insurance, and CPR recertification to the credentialing committee. This is also an ideal time to request additional privileges, if necessary. Again, the ACNP should provide some evidence of expertise, certification and/or letters of recommendation that can assist in the approval process.

Clinical Practice Guidelines

Clinical practice guidelines, commonly referred to as protocols, are required for ACNP practice in many states. Institutions typically require that clinical practice guidelines be reviewed by the credentialing committee. If the institution has previously credentialed other ACNPs in identical positions, there may be standardized clinical practice guidelines. At institutions where ACNPs are a new concept, the ACNP has the challenge of creating clinical practice guidelines. To a motivated and innovative ACNP, this challenge is also a golden opportunity to create a unique practice environment that is both legal and effective.

Each institution has different expectations regarding the specificity of clinical practice guidelines. Some may want very detailed documentation of how the ACNP functions in a given situation. Other institutions may be less stringent. Because each patient and each clinical situation is unique, it is recommended that (if possible) the clinical practice guidelines be written broadly. Rarely, for instance, should absolutes be included in the guidelines. That the ACNP will obtain a stat vascular surgery consult for a pulseless extremity following cardiac catheterization, however, is probably appropriate to include, providing the ACNP and collaborating physician agree that this should be the standard for handling such a situation.

One common complaint from ACNPs is that they don't want to regurgitate a textbook to represent their clinical practice guidelines. Some ACNPs have obtained approval from the credentialing committee to use as their clinical practice guidelines a one-page letter that briefly describes the rules and regulations for nurse practitioners in their state, then lists several standard references that can be consulted in clinical practice. Such digest-format clinical practice guidelines may read: "The acute care nurse practitioner (ACNP) will practice according to the rules and regulations for nurse practitioners of the state of X and the medical staff bylaws of the Y Hospital. Practice will, at all times, be within the scope of practice for the ACNP, as defined by the American Nurses Association and the American Association of Critical-Care Nurses and will be in line with the community standard for ACNPs. The following clinical references (e.g., textbooks) will be used. . . ." The advantages of this digest format are that there is relatively little to update and it does not limit the ACNPs practice. Unfortunately, the brevity is often not satisfactory to credentialing committees.

An alternative to the use of digest format clinical prac-

TABLE 4–3. Example of Delineation of Clinical Privileges for a Cardiovascular Nurse Practitioner

Task/Procedure	Level of Supervision Required[a]	Requested by Applicant	Recommended by Service Chief	Not Recommended by Service Chief
Obtain patient history and perform physical examination	3			
Record pertinent patient data in the medical record	3			
Write orders in the medical record	3			
Document patient discharge summaries in accordance with the policies and procedures of the institution	3			
Order common laboratory and diagnostic studies	3			
Perform independent patient rounds with assessment of patient's physical status, overall progress, and current laboratory evaluation	3			
Initiate consultations and implement recommendations of consultants	3			
Institute emergency treatment for life-threatening patient situations	3			
Supervise exercise and pharmacological stress tests	3			
Perform electrical cardioversion	1			
Initiate, maintain, and discontinue transcutaneous pacing	3			
Adjust temporary pacemaker settings	3			
Remove temporary intravenous pacing wires	2			
Remove central venous catheters and introducer sheaths (all sites)	3			
Insert, maintain, and remove central venous catheters and introducer sheaths (femoral site)	3			
Insert, maintain, and remove pulmonary artery catheters	1			
Insert, maintain, and remove arterial lines	2			
Draw arterial blood samples by arterial puncture	3			
Draw femoral arterial and venous blood samples	3			

[a] Level of supervision key: 3 = Collaborating physician is immediately accessible, either in person or by electronic means (e.g., telephone, pager, fax). 2 = Collaborating physician is in the facility. 1 = Collaborating physician is in the room.

Adapted from Hravnak & Baldisseri. (1997).

TABLE 4–4. Example of Expanded Clinical Practice Guidelines for Acute Myocardial Infarction

Diagnosis

1. Perform history and physical
2. Consider chest x-ray
3. Perform EKG
   - ST elevation of ≥1 mm in at least 2 limb leads
   - ST elevation of ≥2 mm in at least 2 precordial leads
   - Diminuation of R waves throughout precordial leads
   - Evolving Q waves
   - Simultaneous presence of reciprocal ST depression
4. If acute inferior myocardial infarction (MI), consider right-sided EKG
5. Consider echocardiogram for the following indications:
   - Cardiogenic shock
   - To distinguish acute severe MR from papillary muscle rupture
   - Atypical EKG pattern and clinical features of MI
   - Suspected RV infarction vs. cardiac tamponade
   - To identify high-risk patients with multivessel disease
   - In patients with persistent congestive heart failure (CHF) after at least two doses of diuretic
6. Consult with physician regarding placement of pulmonary artery catheter for the following indications:
   - Cardiogenic shock or signs of systemic hypoperfusion
   - Severe CHF
   - Suspected mechanical complications (VSD, papillary muscle rupture/dysfunction, tamponade)
   - Diagnosis of right ventricle infarct in the presence of left ventricle failure
   - Progressive or unexplained hypotension failing to respond to fluid administration in patients without pulmonary congestion
7. Consider diagnostic cardiac catheterization

Treatment

1. Administer aspirin 324 mg
2. Consult attending regarding thrombolytics vs. primary angioplasty
3. Consider morphine IV
4. Transfer to ICU or CCU
5. Consider pharmacological interventions
   - Beta-blockers
   - Nitroglycerine
   - Heparin—according to anticoagulation protocol to maintain PTT 60–80 seconds
6. For MI complicated by CHF, consider:
   - Morphine sulfate
   - Nitroglycerine
   - Diuretics
   - Digoxin
   - ACE inhibitors
   - Intubation and mechanical ventilation
7. For MI complicated by cardiogenic shock, consider:
   - Dobutamine
   - Dopamine
   - Amrinone
   - Milrinone
   - Nitroprusside
   - Intraaortic balloon pump
8. For right ventricle infarct, consider:
   - Administration of IV fluids to maintain adequate hemodynamic function
   - Dobutamine
   - Intraaortic balloon pump

Discharge

1. Consult with the attending physician regarding discharge medications:
   - Beta-blockers
   - Aspirin
   - ACE inhibitors
   - Antilipid agents
2. Ensure that patient understands discharge and follow-up instructions

tice guidelines is to construct expanded clinical practice guidelines that are both broad in scope and nonspecific in nature. Because medical diagnostic modalities and therapeutic interventions change frequently, and, because each patient situation is unique, it is impractical to write guidelines that provide "recipes" for patient care in given clinical situations. Rather, expanded clinical practice guidelines facilitate the clinician's decision making. Table 4–4 provides an example of expanded clinical practice guidelines. Although, at first glance, the example seems overly detailed, it is, instead, very broad and generous.

Recommendations

The following are recommendations that may aid the ACNP in gaining state recognition, certification, and institutional credentialing:

- Obtain applications for RN licensure and NP recognition or certification from the states in which you intend to work. Collect the necessary documents to complete these applications. If the cost is not prohibitive, apply for RN licensure. This alone takes several weeks. If you intend to work in a state where you are already licensed as an RN, then you will only need to wait for NP recognition or certification to be processed. Not already having RN licensure may mean the difference between beginning a job in 2 months as opposed to 1 or not getting a position that needs to be filled immediately.
- Take the national certification examination for ACNPs. Many states and job positions will require this for state recognition or employment. Even in states where passing a national certification examination is not required, doing so documents mastery and improves marketability.
- Keep current of any changes regarding second licensure. Most changes do not take effect immediately, and you may be able to be "grandfathered" under the current law.
- Upon acceptance of a position, call the human resources department or the medical staff director of the hospital in which you will be credentialed and granted practice privileges. An application for credentialing should be requested along with a list of any necessary documents. Begin working on this immediately to avoid any delays in practicing. The credentialing committee should be informed of the date on which you plan to start work. It may be possible to have the application processed within that time frame so that you will have privileges when you start.

If you must develop your own practice privileges, but are unsure what will be necessary, find out from other ACNPs on staff or affiliated with the hospital what information is necessary. Also, work closely with your collaborating physician to determine together how you both envision the ACNP's role and the types of clinical privileges needed to perform successfully. It may be advantageous to have the privileges reviewed in 6 months, rather than 1 year, so that other privileges may be added as the role develops.

The terminology and understanding of certification and licensure can be quite confusing to physicians, patients, employers, insurance companies, and NPs themselves. In this chapter the terminology of licensure, certification, credentialing, and privileging was outlined. Knowledge of these terms and the materials necessary to provide for them will assist NPs in gaining state recognition, legal defensibility, employment, and institutional credentialing.

REFERENCES

American Nurses Association & American Association of Critical Care Nurses. (1995). *Acute care nurse practitioner examination.* Washington, DC: American Nurses Credentialing Center.

Anderson, K., Anderson, L., & Glanze, W. (Eds.). (1994). *Mosby's medical, nursing, and allied health dictionary* (4th ed.). St Louis, MO: Mosby.

Bullough, B. (1982). State certification of the nursing specialties: A new trend in nursing practice law. *Pediatric Nursing, 8*(2), 121–124.

Dalton, J., Speakman, M., Duffey, M., & Carlson, J. (1994). The evolution of a profession: Where do boards of nursing fit in? *Journal of Professional Nursing, 10*(5), 319–325.

Edmunds, M. (1992). Council's pursuit of national standardization for advanced practice nursing meets with resistance. *Nurse Practitioner, 17*(10), 81–83.

Geolot, D. (1986). The relationship between certification and practice. *Nurse Practitioner, 11*(3), 55–58.

Greco, K. (1995). Regulation of advanced nursing practice: Part one—Second licensure. *Oncology Nursing Forum, 22*(8 suppl.), 35–38.

Hall, J. K. (1993). How to analyze nurse practitioner licensure laws. *Nurse Practitioner, 18*(8), 31–34.

Havens, D. H., & Hannan, C. (1996). The National Council of State Boards of Nursing's movement toward second licensure: Questioning the competency of nurse practitioners again? *Journal of Pediatric Health Care, 10*(5), 234–238.

Hravnak, M., & Baldisseri, M. (1997). Credentialing and privileging: insight into the process for acute care nurse practitioners. *AACN Clinical Issues, 8*(1), 108–115.

Hravnak, M., Rosenzweig, M., & Baldisseri, M. (1996). Current questions with regard to acute care nurse practitioner preparation and role implementation. *AACN Clinical Issues, 7*(2), 289–299.

Malone, B. (1993, September). Second licensure: ANA and

NCSBN debate the issue: American Nurses Association. *The American Nurse,* 8.

National Council of State Boards of Nursing. (1993). *Position paper on the regulation of advanced nursing practice.* Chicago, IL: Author.

Nicholas, P. (1995). Issues in certification versus advanced practice licensure. *Nurse Practitioner, 20*(3), 12.

Pearson, L. (1997). Annual update of how each state stands on legislative issues affecting advanced nursing practice. *Nurse Practitioner, 22*(1), 18–86.

Rosen, L. (1995). A brief discussion of nurse practice acts. *Today's O.R. Nurse, 17*(4), 42.

Sheets, V. R. (1993, September). Second licensure: ANA and NCSBN debate the issue: National Council of State Boards of Nursing. *The American Nurse,* 8–9.

Spatz, D. (1996). Women's health: The role of advanced practice nurses in the 21st century. *Nursing Clinics of North America, 31*(2), 269–277.

Spencer-Cisek, P., & Sveningson, L. (1995) Regulation of advanced nursing practice: Part two—Certification. *Oncology Nursing Forum, 22*(8 suppl.), 39–42.

Smith, S. A. (1993). Obtaining hospital privileges for the advanced practice nurse. *Journal of Pediatric Health Care, 7*(6), 292–293.

5

Professional Resources for the ACNP

Paul Logan

The role of the nurse practitioner in primary care has existed for more than 25 years. During that time many supports for nurse practitioners have evolved. Organizations, journals, national conferences, and technological resources now support primary care nurse practitioners. The role of the acute care nurse practitioner (ACNP), however, is relatively new and the supports for ACNPs are few. What follows is an overview of some of the organizational, educational, and online computer resources available to ACNPs. Admittedly, the contents are influenced by my experiences and biases.

▶ ORGANIZATIONAL RESOURCES

The role of the ACNP is an interesting hybrid. ACNPs are both acute care nurses and nurse practitioners. Because the patients for whom ACNPs care are typically in acute care facilities, ACNPs are well served by the organization that represents the interests of acute and critical care nurses. ACNPs, however, also function as members of the nurse practitioner dimension. This requires that ACNPs be active participants in nurse practitioner organizations.

The following organizations have been important players in the early development of the ACNP role. Their contributions to date and their current programs are discussed.

Disclosure: The author is one of the founding members of the Association of Acute Care Nurse Practitioners and is a member of the editorial board of *Nurse Practitioner.*

American Association of Critical-Care Nurses

The American Association of Critical-Care Nurses (AACN) was founded in 1969, in part, as a result of the rapid technological changes in health care. Nurses were challenged with more responsibility at the bedside and greater expectations from physicians. AACN was founded as an educational resource for nurses practicing in the newly founded specialty of critical care. The services offered by the organization grew rapidly. By 1972 AACN produced the first critical care journal for nurses, *Heart & Lung.* The first National Teaching Institute™ was held in 1974 and critical care registered nurse certification was offered the following year. Today AACN is the professional association for acute and critical care nurses. Table 5–1 describes the mission, vision, and values adopted by AACN.

Despite the small percentage of total AACN members that acute care nurse practitioners represent, AACN continues to take an active role in the advancement of the ACNP role. AACN has committed to providing support to ACNPs through publications such as *AACN Clinical Issues* and educational offerings such as the Advanced Practice

TABLE 5–1. Mission, Vision, and Values of the American Association of Critical-Care Nurses (AACN)

Mission

Building on decades of clinical excellence, the American Association of Critical-Care Nurses provides and inspires leadership to establish work and care environments that are respectful, healing, and humane. The key to AACN's success is through its members. Therefore, AACN is committed to providing the highest quality resources to maximize nurses' contribution to caring for critically ill patients and their families.

Vision

AACN is dedicated to creating a healthcare system driven by the needs of patients and families where critical care professionals make their optimal contribution.

Values

As AACN works to promote its mission and vision, it is guided by values which are rooted in, and arise from, the Association's history, traditions and culture. Therefore, AACN, its members, volunteers, and staff will:

- Be accountable to uphold and consistently act in concert with ethical values and principles.
- Advocate for organizational decisions that are driven by the needs of patients and families.
- Act with integrity by communicating openly and honestly, keeping promises, honoring commitments, and promoting loyalty in all relationships.
- Collaborate with all essential stakeholders by creating synergistic relationships to promote common interests and shared values.
- Provide leadership to transform thinking, structures, and processes to address opportunities and challenges.
- Demonstrate stewardship through fair and responsible management of resources.
- Embrace lifelong learning, inquiry, and critical thinking to enable each to make optimal contributions.
- Commit to quality and excellence at all levels of the organization, meeting and exceeding all standards and expectations.
- Promote innovation through creativity and calculated risk taking.
- Generate commitment and passion to the organization's causes and work.

Reprinted with permission from the American Association of Critical-Care Nurses. AACN Member Benefits Directory.

Institute™. Discussions are ongoing to provide more services for the growing ACNP contingent of AACN. For more information about membership and programs, contact AACN: American Association of Critical-Care Nurses, 101 Columbia, Aliso Viejo, CA 92656; tel: (800) 899-2226; Internet: www.aacn.org.

American Nurses Association

The American Nurses Association (ANA) is the professional organization for nurses and is comprised of state constituents. ANA does not allow individual members to join the organization. Rather, members join the state nurses association and, then, receive the benefits of membership in the ANA. ANA is also the parent organization to the American Nurses Credentialing Center, the American Nurses Foundation, the American Academy of Nursing, and the Ethnic/Racial Minority Fellowship Program. Table 5–2 lists some of the ANA member benefits. Information about ANA and related organizations is available at: American Nurses Association, 600 Maryland Avenue, SW, Suite 100 West, Washington, DC 20024-2571; tel: (202) 651-7000, (800) 274-4ANA; fax (202) 651-7001; Internet: www.nursingworld.org.

American Nurses Credentialing Center

The role of the ACNP was first considered by professional nursing organizations in 1993 by the American Nurses Association Council of Nurses in Advanced Practice. The council appointed the Task Force on Acute Care Nurse Practitioners. What followed was a collaborative effort by the American Nurses Association (ANA) and the American Association of Critical-Care Nurses (AACN) that culminated in the publication of the *Standards of Clinical Practice and Scope of Practice for the Acute Care Nurse Practitioner* in 1995.

In December 1995 AACN and the American Nurses Credentialing Center (ANCC; a branch of the ANA) offered the acute care nurse practitioner certification examination.

TABLE 5–2. Benefits of Membership in the American Nurses Association

Information
- *American Nurse* newsletter
- *American Journal of Nursing*
- Internet site

Representation to the American Public
- News releases
- Public education efforts
- Involvement with media

Patient's rights and quality of care
- Center for Ethics and Human Rights
- Influencing national health policy
- Code for Nurses with Interpretive Statements
- Nursing's Safety and Quality Initiative

Political voice for nursing
- Lobbying
- Nurses Strategic Action Team
- ANA Political Action Committee
- Testimony on behalf of Nursing
- International representation for United States (e.g., World Health Organization)

Workplace rights
- Labor relations

The examination is still offered jointly by AACN and ANCC. Information about ANCC and the certification examination is available at American Nurses Credentialing Center, 600 Maryland Avenue, SW, Suite 100 West, Washington, DC 20024-2571; tel: (202) 651-7251, (800) 284-CERT; Internet: www.nursingworld.org.

American College of Nurse Practitioners

The American College of Nurse Practitioners is a consortium of organizations and individuals with an interest in legislative issues that impact nurse practitioners. The College played a vital role in the passage of the 1997 Balanced Budget Amendment that expanded Medicare reimbursement to nurse practitioners in all practice areas. Table 5–3 contains facts about the College. For information, contact American College of Nurse Practitioners, 1090 Vermont Avenue, NW, Suite 800, Washington, DC 20005; tel: (202) 408-7050; fax: (202) 408-0902; E-mail: ACNP@aol.com; Internet: http://www.nurse.org/acnp.

▶ EDUCATIONAL RESOURCES

Journals

AACN Clinical Issues

Although not exclusively devoted to ACNPs, *AACN Clinical Issues: Advanced Practice in Acute and Critical Care* is

TABLE 5–3. Facts About the American College of Nurse Practitioners

Founded in 1993, the American College of Nurse Practitioners, previously titled the National Nurse Practitioner Coalition (NNPC), is a national non-profit membership organization. The College is focused exclusively on advocacy, lobbying and keeping you current on the legislative, regulatory and practice issues that affect you in this era of health care reform.

Mission

The mission of the College is to unite, galvanize, and represent politically nurse practitioners across this nation. These efforts are to ensure an appropriate, prevention-based health care system with nurse practitioners as essential health care providers.

Objectives

- Unite nurse practitioner organizations and individuals who represent, support, or practice as nurse practitioners
- Advocate for the professional and political interests of nurse practitioners
- Increase the visibility and viability of nurse practitioners as primary care providers with the goal of increasing access to primary health care
- Formulate and influence health care policy to improve the health of the nation
- Provide leadership for timely action by nurse practitioners in a rapidly changing health care system
- Provide rapid information dissemination and effective communication networks to and on behalf of nurse practitioners
- Provide individuals, government, and organizations with a centralized office to access all nurse practitioner resources

Government Relations Activities

ACNP contracts with the American Nurse Association as its government affairs liaison. Services include direct lobbying activities on behalf of ACNP; monitoring federal and regulatory issues related to NPS; provision of initial analyses on legislative/regulatory proposals; provision of documents (bills, regulations, reports) related to current issues; assistance with written and oral testimony for Congressional hearing, making Congressional visits and developing grassroots strategies and implementation plans.

Membership

- Individual nurse practitioners
- State nurse practitioner organizations
- National organizations with nurse practitioner members
- Student nurse practitioners
- Friends of the College
- Corporate members

Membership Benefits

- Political representation in Washington, DC
- Legislative alerts and timely communication with late-breaking news affecting NPs and other advanced practice nurses
- Fact sheets on NP Issues (i.e., reimbursement, prescriptive authority, admitting privileges)
- *ACNP On the Hill*—quarterly report
- Representation on national Board of Directors
- Special member rate for annual NP Summit
- Assistance with professional and job-related issues
- Information on availability of liability insurance
- Discounts on publications and educational conferences
- Referral network for assistance with state and national issues
- Access to the College's Library of Resources

Reprinted with permission from the fact sheet of the American College of Nurse Practitioners.

perhaps the preeminent scholarly publication for ACNPs. It is published quarterly by Lippincott for the American Association of Critical-Care Nurses and is intended for advanced practice nurses such as ACNPs and clinical nurse specialists. Each issue contains several related articles that deal with advanced practice issues and specialty care. In addition, continuing education modules are offered in each issue for a small fee.

Past topics for the journal have included "Diagnostic Approach to Common Medical Problems in the Hospitalized Adult"; "Outcomes Management"; "Oncologic Critical Care"; and "Cardiac Surgery." The articles are evidence based (i.e., research based) and have clinical relevance.

Periodically, the topic is "Advanced Practice." In these issues the role of the ACNP has been celebrated and challenged. Thoughtful debate has been instigated by articles in the journal. Subscription information is available at: Lippincott-Raven Publishers, 12107 Insurance Way, Hagerstown, MD 21740; tel: (800) 638-3030.

Nurse Practitioner: The American Journal of Primary Health Care

As the name implies, *Nurse Practitioner: The American Journal of Primary Health Care* has traditionally been for nurse practitioners who practice in primary health care settings. In 1997, however, the journal took an important step in recognizing acute care nurse practitioners by appointing two ACNPs to the editorial review board. There are now more articles of interest to ACNPs.

Among the features that ACNPs find useful is the "Annual Update of How Each State Stands on Legislative Issues Affecting Advanced Nursing Practice." This annual report, published in the January issue, describes the status of legal authority to practice, reimbursement issues, and prescriptive authority for each state and the District of Columbia. Another valuable tool is "NP Abstracts," which concisely reviews selected articles from the nursing and medical research literature. Discounted subscription rates are available for members of the American College of Nurse Practitioners and other organizations. Subscription information is available from The Nurse Practitioner, PO Box 5053, Brentwood, TN 37024–9739; tel: (800) 490-6580.

Conferences

National Nurse Practitioner Summit

The National Nurse Practitioner Summit is an annual meeting that is traditionally held in Washington, DC. The Saturday and Sunday meeting typically includes topics on legislation, politics, health policy, computer and telehealth technology, and practice issues. The Monday following the meeting, participants have the opportunity to meet legislators and lobby on Capitol Hill. Continuing education units are included in the registration fee. For more information contact the American College of Nurse Practitioners.

AACN Advanced Practice Institute

Offered for the first time at AACN's 1998 National Teaching Institute, the Advanced Practice Institute (API) addresses the learning needs of AACN's such advanced practice nurses as clinical nurse specialists and acute care nurse practitioners. At the first API 36 sessions were included in the program, many of which targeted the ACNP. AACN plans to hold the API in conjunction with the National Teaching Institute each year. Continuing education credits offered to participants are included in the registration fee. More information can be obtained from American Association of Critical-Care Nurses, 101 Columbia, Aliso Viejo, CA 92656; tel: (800) 899-2226; Internet: www.nti.org.

Annual Acute Care Nurse Practitioner Consensus Conference

The Annual Acute Care Nurse Practitioner Consensus Conference is sponsored by a different educational institution each year. The purpose of this national meeting is to "bring together clinicians and educators from around the country to focus upon issues relevant to the educational preparation, clinical practice, professional development, and role definition of ACNPs" (conference brochure, 1998). Since no individual or organization hosts the meeting, there is no standard mailing list. In the past information has been posted online on the ANPACC listserv (see "Online Computer Resources").

▶ ONLINE COMPUTER RESOURCES

A plethora of clinically useful information exists on the Internet if users are savvy enough to find and retrieve it. Some information is free and some is available with a subscription or a one-time fee.

ANPACC Listserv

Listservs are automated E-mail programs that regularly send messages to subscribers. Responses to listserv messages are posted for other subscribers to view and respond to. Listservs are generally run by corporations or other organizations and are almost always free.

One electronic listserv that appeals to many ACNPs around the world is the "Advanced Nursing Practice in Acute and Critical Care (ANPACC) Listserv." This listserv is sponsored by the Nursing Section of the Society of Critical Care Medicine and the University of Pennsylvania School of Nursing. The objective of the listserv is to enhance communication and networking among advanced practice nurses and other health care professionals in the fields of acute and critical care. Frequent discussion items include clinical, administrative, and role issues. Worldwide educational and career opportunities are also included in the postings.

Since 1997 the ANPACC listserv has become an invaluable tool for communicating with other ACNPs around the world. To subscribe to the ANPACC listserv do the following:

1. Send an E-mail message to: LISTSERV@lists.upenn.edu
2. Type the following exactly in the body of the message: SUBscribe ANPACC
3. Send the E-mail message.

The listserv computer typically responds immediately, but certainly within 24 hours, with a message welcoming you to the listserv. In this message is important information for unsubscribing and posting messages to the listserv. It is a good idea to save this information for future reference.

Once subscribed to the listserv, you begin to receive messages addressed to ANPACC. To contribute a message to the listserv, address an E-mail message to ANPACC@lists.upenn.edu. Or, if you want to respond to one of the messages that you receive, use the "reply" function of your E-mail software. Either of these methods delivers your message to the listserv, which in turn delivers it to each subscriber's mailbox. If, however, you want to send a personal reply, you must address the E-mail message to the individual, not to the listserv. Even experienced users have made the embarrassing mistake of posting personal messages for all the listserv subscribers to read.

Note that the address for sending commands (such as subscribe or signoff) to the listserv is different from the address for posting messages for all listserv subscribers to view. This is a point that separates the listserv neophytes from the experienced users. Knowing this will help you to avoid embarrassing faux pas and great frustration. Further details and Netiquette rules of the listserv can be found on the ANPACC web page: http://pobox.upenn.edu/~jtv/button8.html.

World Wide Web Sites

The Internet is a confusingly dynamic tool. By now many educational institutions that prepare ACNPs require students to have computers and access to the Internet for E-mail and research. Many ACNPs, therefore, already know the pros and cons of the Internet and have used it to find valuable information.

Apart from its often slow responsiveness, one of the major disadvantages of the Internet is the necessity of "surfing" to find what you're looking for. Surfing requires the user to log onto the Internet, contact sites, sift through the potentially absurd amount of information, and retrieve what is valuable. The problems with this system are many. First, the user must know where to find the desired information. If the Internet site is unknown, a search must be performed (e.g., www.yahoo.com or www.excite.com). Often, the internet connection, particularly when connecting from home, can be very slow. Together, these facts sometimes make the Internet cumbersome and frustrating.

Also frustrating is the variety in quality of information on the Internet. Some sites are both useful and informative. They are updated regularly—perhaps even daily—and contain essential information that is well organized, exhaustive, and easily retrievable. Other sites are less user friendly. Because of the complex nature of the Internet and the expenses of hiring staff and maintaining equipment, many organizations do not update the content of their web site frequently enough. Such is the nature of the Internet.

The computer innovators have promised improvements in the Internet and in the ways that it is used. One of the more impressive ideas is "push technology." Push technology alleviates the need to surf the web. Based on your preferences—and perhaps from personal information that you did not even know existed—large "servers" deliver information to your computer at specified times. The *New England Journal of Medicine* web site (www.nejm.com), for instance, allows users to have the journal's table of contents delivered by E-mail every Thursday. Further refinements are required before clinical or educational information is reliably delivered. Overviews of web sites that may appeal to ACNPs follow.

American Nurses Association

The American Nurses Association (ANA) web site holds valuable information about the nursing profession. News is updated regularly and links to the full text are provided. There are also links to The American Academy of Nursing, The American Nurses Credentialing Center, The American Nurses Foundation, and the *Online Journal of Issues in Nursing,* a journal for nursing leaders that is both informative and exceptionally written. The American Nurses Association web site can be found at www.nursingworld.org.

American Association of Critical-Care Nurses

The American Association of Critical-Care Nurses (AACN) web site contains information about the organization. Information about upcoming educational programs such as the National Teaching Institute™ and the Advanced Practice Institute™ is provided. Descriptions of the AACN journals and publications are also included, along with instructions for ordering. The AACN web site is at www.aacn.org.

Agency for Health Care Policy and Research

The Agency for Health Care Policy and Research (AHCPR) web site contains information about the agency and instructions for applying for funding. Full-text AHCPR guidelines can be downloaded directly from the site. The web address for AHCPR is www.ahcpr.gov.

National Institutes of Health

The National Institutes of Health (NIH) web site contains news and events, health information, and information about grants and contracts, scientific resources, institutes, and offices. There are links to other Department of Health and Human Services sites such as the Centers for Disease Control and Prevention. Visitors can subscribe to the mailing list of the *Morbidity and Mortality Weekly Report.* The NIH web site address is www.nih.gov.

National Library of Medicine

Among the most valuable resources on the Internet is the National Library of Medicine site. The site allows free searches of databases, such as MEDLINE. There are also links to consumer health information resources. The National Library of Medicine web address is www.nlm.nih.gov.

Specialty Medical Organizations

It is not practical to include descriptions of web sites for each medical specialty in this chapter. Nevertheless, many specialty organizations such as the American Heart Association and physician groups such as the American College of Cardiology have developed web sites that contain informative and pertinent information for ACNPs.

REFERENCE

American Association of Critical Care Nurses & American Nurses Association. (1995). *Standards of clinical practice and scope of practice for the acute care nurse practitioner.* Washington, DC: American Nurses Publishing Company.

6

Legal Considerations for Practice

Paula F. Henry

The fastest growing specialty area of practice for the nurse practitioner (NP) is in acute care. The acute care nurse practitioner (ACNP) possesses the knowledge and skills to provide medical care to the acutely ill patient. These responsibilities range from immediate life-and-death decisions to establishing the continuity of care after the acute crisis has resolved. While assuming these increased responsibilities, the ACNP is exposed to an increased risk of liability. An important aspect of the ACNP's practice is a thorough understanding of the legal aspects of that role. This chapter provides an overview of the legal relationships and legal issues pertaining to the ACNP. With knowledge of these principles the ACNP is capable of providing competent and quality health-care services to the acutely ill patient, while minimizing the risks of liability.

▶ LEGAL ACCOUNTABILITY

Liability for One's Own Actions

The key legal principle that the ACNP must remember is: The NP is legally accountable at all times for the NP's own actions (*Sermchief v. Gonzales*, 1983). Regardless of the practice setting or the type of collaborative relationship, the ACNP as a licensed health-care provider is now recognized by the courts as a professional who is held accountable to the patient and to society. The ACNP is held liable for professional negligence when the ACNP fails to conform to the conduct required of a reasonable ACNP acting in the same or similar circumstances (McCella, 1994). The ACNP will not be held liable for a mistake in judgment as long as the ACNP's clinical judgment was reasonable under the circumstances and supported by sound scientific principles. The law does not expect the ACNP to be perfect, nor to function at the highest standard of practice. The ACNP must function, however, within his or her scope of practice.

The ACNP has assumed many of the responsibilities and tasks that traditionally had been performed by physicians and previously defined as the practice of medicine. The evolution of health care, however, has resulted in the legal recognition of the overlap of these functions between physicians and advanced practice nurses. With any increase in responsibility there is a parallel increase in legal accountability. The ACNP must take seriously this increased exposure to liability to avoid a malpractice claim.

One of the hallmarks of being recognized as a professional is the acknowledgment that the NP is legally accountable for the NP's own actions. In the past, the legal community failed to understand the role of the nurse practitioner and thus a legal claim was not usually pursued directly against the NP, but focused instead on the physician and facility as the responsible parties. That strategy, however, is no longer used as NPs have become the direct target of the allegations in a malpractice claim. In the past there were relatively few reported legal cases in which the NP was named as the party being sued. Over the past seven years, however, there has been a definite increase in the number of reported cases (Pearson & Birkholz, 1995). It has been, and continues to be, difficult to determine the exact number of cases in which an NP has been held legally liable because there is a lack of uniform tracking or data collecting regarding NP-involved cases. Since the role of the ACNP is fairly new, reported legal cases involving ACNPs are relatively scarce. Legal recognition of the ACNP will generally lag several years behind the medical community's recognition of the role of the ACNP.

There are several reasons for this lack of reporting of cases involving NPs. Failing to name the NP as a party may be the result of legal counsel's decision to focus on the deeper financial pocket (generally, the NP's employer) or may be the result of the lack of understanding by lawyers of the role that NPs occupy in health care, and especially the role of the NP in the acute care setting. Also, if a claim is settled and thus no action has been filed in court, then the settlement may go unreported and the NP's involvement may never be made public. Based upon a current review of the reported legal cases, only a few cases were found that involved allegations against an NP functioning in an acute care setting. None of the reported cases, to date, specifically identified the NP as an ACNP.

The ACNP must remember that if the ACNP's care is at issue in the lawsuit but the ACNP is not a named party, the ACNP can still be found negligent. The named party (the physician, hospital, or medical plan), however, will be liable for paying the judgment. In a separate action, the named party who has paid the judgment may seek indemnification from the ACNP for the judgment amount. Indemnification actions against NPs are rare, but not unheard of.

Several recent surveys have indicated that nurse practitioners are at a low risk for having a malpractice claim brought against them (Birkholz, 1995). With the expansion of the NP role into the high-risk acute care area, and the legal recognition of that role, it is inherent that there will be medical malpractice claims being brought against ACNPs.

Therefore, it is imperative that the ACNP has a thorough understanding of the legal principles pertaining to the standard of care and scope of practice of the ACNP, and the common legal issues that may arise within that role.

Vicarious Liability

Due to the nature of the ACNP's practice setting, in most situations the ACNP will be providing health-care services in conjunction with other coproviders. To fully understand the legal aspects of the ACNP's practice, the ACNP should be knowledgeable about the legal accountability of coproviders involved with the ACNP's practice.

The legal principle of vicarious liability arises when liability for the actions of another is imposed due to the existence of a special relationship. This legal principle should only be applied in fact-specific circumstances. Unfortunately, it is often applied improperly due to a lack of understanding of the dynamics of this principle (Jenkins, 1994). As stated previously, the ACNP is directly responsible for the ACNP's own actions. Whether additional liability is imposed on a coprovider as a result of the ACNP's negligence depends on the legal relationship between the ACNP and the coprovider.

The most common example of the application of vicarious liability is in the situation involving the employer–employee. Vicarious liability is applied based upon the doctrine of *respondeat superior,* the Latin term meaning: "let the Master speak" (Brent, 1997, pp. 39–64). Liability is imputed upon the employer when, in the course and scope of the employee's duties, the employee causes harm to an individual. Thus the employer of an ACNP, which may be a hospital, medical group, or individual physician, can be held liable for any negligent acts committed by the ACNP that causes harm to a patient. Public policy has established that the employer (also known to have the deeper financial pocket) is in the better position to bear the financial responsibility to the injured patient (Andrews, Goldberg, & Kaplan, 1996, pp. 198–235). Under the doctrine of *respondeat superior,* the employer is held vicariously liable for the employee's negligent acts, even though the employer had no direct contact with the patient and despite the fact that the employer had properly evaluated the employee's credentials.

The employer can, however, avoid liability if the ACNP's actions were beyond the ACNP's scope of practice, beyond the scope of employment, or were in violation of the employer's policies and procedures. An example is when the ACNP is employed part-time in the Emergency Room of a local hospital and also moonlights as an independent contractor at the Urgent Care Center down the street. The hospital would not be held liable for any claim against the ACNP that arose out of the care rendered at the Urgent Care Center, as the ACNP's actions would be beyond the scope of employment with the hospital. It is important to note that the best way the ACNP's employer can reduce the risk of exposure to liability is if the ACNP functions within the standard of care and scope of practice (Henry, 1996, pp. 5–6).

The ACNP should be aware that in certain circumstances vicarious liability is applied in the absence of a true employer–employee relationship. Under the doctrine of apparent agency (also known as ostensible agency), if a patient reasonably believes, as a result of the ACNP's actions or representations, that the ACNP is an agent or employee of another, then the injured party may be able to hold the principle (employer) vicariously liable for the ACNP's negligent acts (Jenkins, 1994, p. 100). Two of the essential elements in apparent/ostensible agency are: (1) the principle also must have knowingly participated in the representation (directly or indirectly); and (2) the patient relied on that representation. An illustration of apparent agency is the situation in which an Emergency Room Nurse Practitioner, who was employed by a separate and independent practice group that staffed the local hospital's Emergency Room, was identified to the patient as the "Memorial Hospital E.R. Nurse Practitioner"; the hospital failed to give notice to the patient that the NP was not an employee or agent for the hospital; and in the course and scope of the ACNP's duties, the ACNP failed to properly diagnose the patient's condition that resulted in harm to the patient. Under the doctrine of apparent agency, the court may allow the patient to recover against the hospital, even though the ACNP was not an employee. Liability is based on the fact that the representation to the patient inferred that the ACNP was acting as an employee or agent of the hospital and the patient could have reasonably relied on that representation, believing that the NP was an employee or agent of the hospital. Thus it is important that all patients be given notice of the true legal relationship of the ACNP with a coprovider or facility in order to avoid claims based on apparent/ostensible agency.

Vicarious liability, however, should not be applied in a supervisory relationship, unless the supervisor has direct and absolute control of another's actions (Jenkins, 1994, p. 100). One of the most frequent fears of physicians who supervise an ACNP is that the physician will be held liable for the ACNP's actions. In most circumstances, the ACNP's "supervisory" physician is actually functioning as a consultant to the ACNP or functioning in a collaborative role and that physician does not directly control the ACNP's actions (Jenkins, 1994, pp. 100, 101). Any vicarious liability claim against the supervising physician who does not have direct control of the ACNP's action would then be inappropriate. The supervising physician, however, can be held personally liable for failing to provide the proper supervision or for providing improper advice that resulted in the harm to the patient (Jenkins, 1994, pp. 100, 101).

It is therefore imperative that the ACNP understands when and under what circumstances vicarious liability may be applied properly. It is also important for the ACNP to understand that vicarious liability of a coprovider can be created as a result of contractual agreements and policies within a facility. If a practice agreement, policy, or protocol implies that a physician or entity has the right of control over the ACNP's actions, then an injured party may assert that the physician or entity should be vicariously liable for the negligent acts of the ACNP. It is imperative that the role of the supervising physician be clearly defined, and that vicarious liability is not improperly created as a result of a contractual agreement or by a written policy. Any claim that involves the ACNP's care and treatment and is based upon the theory of vicarious liability should be scrutinized for direct evidence that a special relationship exists between the ACNP and a coprovider and should only apply to the appropriate fact-specific case.

The ACNP should also be aware that if the ACNP is a partner in a group practice or in partnership with another individual, each partner is considered, under the laws governing partnerships, to be the agent of the other partner and each will be held vicariously liable for each other's negligent conduct (Jenkins, 1994, p. 101). In a collaborative practice arrangement, in which the ACNP joins other health-care providers in providing care in a collaborative and collegial manner, each member is liable for its own actions and will not be held vicariously liable for another member's action unless the collaborative practice agreement creates a partnership or an agent–principle relationship (Henry, 1996, p. 5).

The ACNP should, therefore, be diligent in clarifying the bylaws, policies, protocols, and contractual agreements that govern the ACNP's practice and could create vicarious liability unnecessarily. These documents may create a supervisory relationship that could be interpreted as giving authority and direct control of the ACNP's actions, when true supervision may not be occurring in the acute care setting. The use of the correct terminology and a clear definition of the ACNP's relationships with other health-care providers can minimize the risk and decrease the anxiety of a possible vicarious liability claim.

Joint and Several Liability

In the ordinary course of providing acute care, it is not unusual for the ACNP to provide care in conjunction with other health-care providers during the various stages of a patient's illness. In fact, acute care is generally provided within a team concept. The general rule is that two independent health-care providers treating the same patient are not vicariously liable for the other provider's negligence (Jenkins, 1994, p. 102). When a claim of joint liability is brought, generally the patient is alleging that two or more providers have caused the patient's injuries and that both providers should be held jointly liable. The ACNP can, however, be held jointly liable for an injury to a patient, even though the ACNP did not directly harm the patient (McMahon, 1993). In those specific circumstances, if the ACNP observes or is aware of another provider's negligence and fails to intervene, then the ACNP can be found jointly liable with a negligent coprovider and severally (independently) liable for the harm to the patient (Jenkins, 1994, p. 102). Joint and several liability is applied when the harm to the patient cannot be apportioned among two or more negligent providers. If, however, the jury is able to determine the harm that occurred was separate and apart from the other provider's actions, then each provider will be liable for his or her proportionate share of the damages (Hoffman, 1995).

Corporate Liability

Another theory of legal accountability the ACNP should be aware of is corporate liability. When the allegations assert that the ACNP's negligence caused harm to the patient, corporate liability may be asserted directly against the entity responsible for determining if the ACNP is competent to render acute care medical services. Under the theory of corporate liability, the entity that allows or authorizes the ACNP to provide care to acutely ill patients has an affirmative duty to exercise reasonable care in the selection of competent health-care providers and must have in place a mechanism for the ongoing evaluation of the ACNP's skills and competency level (Hollowell & Block, 1995). If the entity (hospital, HMO, health plan, managed care organization) is negligent by failing to properly investigate the ACNP's credentials or level of competency and, as a result of the ACNP's incompetence, the patient is injured, that entity could be held directly liable for the patient's injuries. It should be noted, however, that in order to succeed in a claim under the theory of corporate liability, actual or constructive knowledge by the entity of the ACNP's incompetence must be proven. Additionally, the entity's negligence in allowing an incompetent ACNP to care for the patient must have substantially contributed to or caused the harm to the patient (MacDonald, 1992).

The entity's credentialing policies and procedure manuals will be reviewed to determine the level of skill necessary to provide the acute care services. Thus the ACNP should anticipate that the entity (it may be more than one) that authorizes, selects, or grants privileges to an ACNP will be required to scrutinize, on an ongoing basis, the ACNP's skills and level of competency in providing acute care. It is extremely important, therefore, that the ACNP document any expansion in that role, the achievement of new skills, or the acquisition of additional knowledge. Since the ACNP's level of skills and education in acute care will increase with time and experience, it is recommended that written documentation regarding credentialing, mentoring, and proctoring be completed and maintained throughout the ACNP's career to clearly define the ACNP's capabilities to function within the acute care role (McClosky, 1997). This documentation is also beneficial as evidence to support the defense of the ACNP charged with negligence and in the defense of an entity charged with negligence under a corporate liability theory.

▶ LEGAL PROCESS

Participants in a Lawsuit

Parties

Understanding who the parties are in a civil lawsuit helps the ACNP to have a better working knowledge of the overall legal process. The patient who allegedly has been injured—or, when the patient has died, then the family of the patient—has the right to file a lawsuit to recover monetary damages. The injured patient or the patient's legal representative is known as the plaintiff. When the injured patient is a child, the court appoints a guardian *ad litem* to represent the child's interest. In most circumstances, the guardian is one of the parents. The provider and/or entity that is being sued, who allegedly caused the harm to the patient, is known as the defendant.

Each party to the lawsuit is generally represented by an attorney. A party has the right to represent himself or herself and is considered to be "in pro per" or acting as his or her own attorney. It is, however, strongly recommended, due to the complexity of the legal process, that a party has legal representation by an attorney.

Trier of Fact

The trier of fact, which is generally a jury, determines whether the defendant was negligent and whether that negligence caused or substantially contributed to the harm alleged by the plaintiff. The judge, pursuant to the applicable law and rules of evidence, instructs the jury regarding what facts, documents, and testimony are admissible as evidence and how to apply the law to the evidence in order to reach a decision regarding liability.

Under certain circumstances, either party may waive its right to a jury trial and then the judge acts as the trier of fact. This is known as a bench trial. Certain medical malpractice claims are submitted to arbitration, a different forum, and then the trier of fact is the arbitrator or panel of arbitrators, since there is no jury in an arbitration proceeding.

Witnesses

All parties involved in a lawsuit are entitled to call witnesses during trial or arbitration. A precipitent witness is an individual who has personal knowledge of the events or circumstances surrounding the alleged incident. Treating health-care providers are often called as precipitent witnesses to testify to the patient's medical condition or state of mind during a specific time period. Each health-care provider involved in the treatment of the patient, including the ACNP, may be called as a precipitent witness to establish the level and degree of care that was given, establish the patient's condition, and describe the effect or response to the care that was provided at a specific point in time. This time frame can encompass the minute-to-minute details, which is particularly applicable in the acute care setting, or involve months or even years of medical services. Often the actual event has taken place several years before the case goes to trial, and a witness's recollection of the events can be dimmed with the passage of time. Thus the medical record is an important legal document that is used to refresh the witness's recollection.

Expert witnesses are required in medical malpractice cases since the majority of the subject matter that relates to medical care is beyond the common knowledge and experience of a lay person sitting on a jury. At the time of a medical malpractice trial, the expert witness's role is to educate the trier of fact (generally the jury) regarding the relevant standards of care that the provider's action should be measured against (Brent, 1997, pp. 65–85). Expert witnesses also provide testimony regarding the nature and extent of the injury to the patient and regarding the need for future medical care and the cost of that treatment.

It is very important that an NP expert be retained to provide consultation and expert testimony on behalf of any NP whose care is the focus of a medical malpractice claim. Unfortunately, the courts have allowed physicians to offer expert opinions regarding the standard of care of an NP. In a 1980 case in which an NP was held liable for negligence, the court allowed a physician to testify that the NP breached the standard of care when she failed to properly instruct the patient on the known risk of infection associated with IUD (intrauterine device) and for the NP's failure to institute timely and proper treatment for the patient's pelvic infection (*Guigino v. Harvard Community Health Plan*, 1980).

Other courts, however, have recognized that physicians are not qualified to testify as an expert regarding the NP's standard of care because the physician has never been licensed as an NP nor functioned in the role of an NP (*Dolan v. Galluzo*, 1979). The majority of attorneys do not have any understanding of the role of the NP or the scope of the NP's practice. Often the attorney assumes that a physician's expert testimony, either in support of or against the NP, should be deemed credible as the attorney believes the physician has the superior knowledge, and thus believes the physician's testimony would be sufficient to establish the NP's standard of care. The NP is entitled to and should have a qualified NP expert, who thoroughly understands the role and the applicable standard of care, to provide expert testimony on behalf of the NP anytime the NP's care is at issue. This issue is particularly important for the ACNP, whose role and scope of practice includes assuming responsibility for acutely ill patients, a domain that traditionally has been steadfastly held by physician specialists. The court will need assistance in understanding the ACNP role in acute care and the scope of practice. It is therefore strongly advocated that a qualified ACNP expert be retained as a consultant and testifying expert on any case involving an ACNP's care and treatment.

Forum

State Court/Federal Court

A civil action alleging medical malpractice is filed with the court that has jurisdiction (authority) to hear the action. This type of action is generally filed with the State's trial court, which then schedules the trial (jury or bench) to determine if any liability exists for the plaintiff's alleged injuries. Each State has established rules of civil procedure and evidence that governs the legal process required to resolve the dispute. In which State trial court the action will be filed depends on where the injury occurred, and where each party resides. The plaintiff selects the venue (the geographic location) based upon which court has jurisdiction to hear the case, although the defendant can request a hearing, seeking a change in venue (Brent, 1997, pp. 15–37).

In certain instances, a case may be filed in Federal Court if the NP is employed by the Federal government; is a member of the Armed Forces; if one of the parties resides in another State or country; or if the allegation also involves a violation of the civil rights of the patient (Brent, 1997, p. 22). An illustration of a medical malpractice case that was filed in Federal Court is the case of *Beckom v. United States of America,* which involved a negligence allegation against a surgeon and an Air Force NP for failing to properly diagnose and treat Mrs. Beckom's breast cancer (*Beckom v. United States*, 1984).

In *Beckom,* the plaintiff, the husband of Linda Beckom who died as a result of metastatic breast cancer, alleged that in July of 1977 the nurse practitioner failed to properly examine his wife, and failed to timely diagnose that his wife had infiltrating ductile carcinoma that was diagnosed three months after the NP had seen his wife. At the time of the NP exam, it was alleged that Mrs. Beckom was complaining of a breast lump and nipple retraction for several months and had been previously examined by the co-defendant, a surgeon, who had informed her that she had fibrocystic breast disease. The Federal Court eventually dismissed the allegations against the NP because the plaintiff failed to submit any expert testimony that the NP had breached the standard of care (Beckom, 1984, pp. 1477, 1478). In *Beckom,* the allegations against the NP were based upon the fact that the NP had relied on the history given by the patient that her surgeon had previously diagnosed her problem as fibrocystic breast disease and the NP did not perform any diagnostic tests to confirm or, more important, to determine if Mrs. Beckom had breast cancer. Although this cause of action occurred in the State of New York, both defendants were members of the Armed Forces and had provided care to Mrs. Beckom due to her military status, thus this case was filed in Federal District Court instead of State Court.

Alternative Forums

Due to the increased cost and volume of medical malpractice claims, legislation was enacted in several States to establish different forums, known as Alternative Dispute Resolution (ADR), to handle these claims. Various States have recognized the alternative forums of binding arbitration, nonbinding arbitration, and mediation as the mechanism in which the claim may be heard and resolved rather than the claim being tried in the State trial court.

Under some States' statutes, and pursuant to certain contractual agreements, the patient's legal claim may be submitted to arbitration. In arbitration, there is no jury and the arbitrator (or panel of arbitrators) acts as the judge and jury. Arbitration is generally an informal process, though the applicable law and rules of evidence still apply. Since 1969, a large health maintenance organization (HMO) has required that all claims against the health plan or against a health plan provider be submitted to binding arbitration on the basis that this forum results in a fair resolution of the disputes, while reducing the time and costs of litigation (Ladimer, 1995, pp. 78–86). When a claim is submitted to binding arbitration based upon a contractual agreement, the decision of the arbitrator(s) is final. If the claim is submitted to nonbinding arbitration, then after the Arbitrator'(s) award is made, either party may request a trial *de novo* (new trial) and have the matter heard before a jury.

Mediation is a different process that encourages the parties in a dispute to resolve it themselves with the assistance of an expert facilitator (mediator) (Ladimer, 1995, p. 80). In the medical malpractice area, some States have established pretrial screening or mediation panels. The panel initiates a fact-finding process that includes a review by medical experts and makes recommendations for resolution. The panel's recommendations, however, are not binding upon the parties, and the parties still maintain the right to seek recovery in a court of law.

The ACNP should be aware of the various alternative forums that exist for resolution of a medical malpractice claim. Whether a claim against an ACNP is heard in Federal, State, or one of the ADR forums depends on the State statutes and contractual agreements that impact upon the provider–patient relationship.

Administrative Hearing

Another part of the legal process in which the ACNP may become involved is an administrative hearing involving a disciplinary action. Each State has established the administrative agency that has the authority to investigate and determine whether the ACNP's license to practice should be restricted, suspended, or revoked as a result of an allegation of professional negligence. The right to practice as an ACNP is not an absolute right but is conditioned upon meeting the specific licensing regulations that govern the ACNP's practice within that State (Henry, 1991, pp. 144–145). A disciplinary hearing is separate and apart from any civil or criminal action and may occur even if the NP is not held legally liable for malpractice. At the time of a disciplinary hearing, the NP has the fundamental right to due process—that the NP be given notice and an opportunity to be heard prior to any permanent action being taken against the NP's right to practice. Grounds for a disciplinary hearing include, but are not limited to, allegations of incompetence, professional negligence, exceeding the scope of practice, and unauthorized practice (Henry, 1991, pp. 144, 145). The ACNP must be cognizant of the regulations governing the ACNP's practice and the parameters of the scope of practice in acute care in order to be aware of the potential issues that could result in a disciplinary hearing.

▶ LEGAL THEORIES

A clear understanding of the various legal theories that could be brought against an ACNP is essential for reducing or avoiding the risk of exposure to liability. Civil actions are based upon torts, which in simplistic terms, means any action or omission by an individual that causes injury or harm to another person (Anderson, et al., 1996, p. 202). Tort claims are divided into two categories: negligence (unintentional) and intentional torts. The following is an overview of the common tort claims that are frequently brought against health-care providers and are applicable to the ACNP's practice.

Professional (Medical) Negligence

The most well known of the tort claims is medical negligence, also known as medical malpractice (Flamm, 1995, pp. 118–128). Health-care providers have a legal duty to act with reasonable care and in good faith in providing health-care services to each patient. The law requires that each ACNP must possess and use the skills, knowledge, and degree of care that a reasonable ACNP would ordinarily possess and use under similar or the same circumstances. This is known as the standard of care and is the legal yardstick that is used to measure whether an individual provider's actions conforms to the conduct of similar-situated providers in the community (Feutz, 1989, pp. 13–28).

The ACNP is held legally responsible to act within the standard of care that exists at the time the care is being rendered (Feutz, 1989, p. 17). The 1986 California case of *Fein v. Permanente* established that a nurse practitioner should be held to the standard of care of a nurse practitioner, and not to a physician's standard of care (*Fein v. Permanente*, 1985). Therefore, the ACNP must continually update the ACNP's skills, knowledge, and training to meet the appropriate standards of care that is constantly evolving as health care progresses.

The standard of care is established from several different sources. Expert testimony is an essential part of a medical malpractice claim. The expert testifies regarding the applicable standard of care—the minimum level of skills and knowledge required to provide competent and safe treatment necessary for the patient's specific medical problem—and whether the provider who is being sued met the standard of care. It is extremely important that an NP expert be retained and testify regarding the NP's standard of care. This ensures that the correct standard is being applied in the determination of whether the ACNP is negligent. Permitting a physician to testify to the standard of care of an ACNP is inappropriate since the ACNP's liability is determined by whether the ACNP met the applicable standard care within the NP community. The ACNP's actions should not be compared with, or measured against, a physician standard. An ACNP is a better-qualified expert than a physician expert because the physician's training and knowledge is different from an ACNP's and does not encompass the ACNP's education and experience (Eccard & Guinn, 1994). It is well accepted that the ACNP approaches the acutely ill patient in a more wholistic manner and, although there are overlapping functions, the ACNP's standard of care is different and separate from the physician's standard (Knaus, Felter, Burton, et al., 1997, pp. 20–27).

The standard of care can be derived from several different sources including the standards of practice established jointly by the American Nurses Association (ANA) (1994) and the American Association of Critical Care Nurses (AACN). These standards have set forth the minimum level of skills and knowledge required to be certified as an acute care nurse practitioner and involve continuing education requirements, peer review, and ethics (Aiken & Catalano, 1994, pp. 57–75). The standards of practice drafted by ANA also advocate the development of practice guidelines (also known as protocols or standardized procedures). These guidelines recommend a course of action and are not meant to require mandatory compliance. Despite ANA's intentions, however, the practice guidelines are being used by the legal system as evidence of the standard of care and any deviation is considered to be a breach of the standard of care (Aiken, 1994, p. 61).

Another source used to establish the standard of care is the hospital's bylaws that may govern the ACNP's clinical privileges and authorize the ACNP to render care—within the ACNP's level of competency and scope of practice—to acutely ill patients in the hospital (Knaus, 1997, p. 23). A health-care facility's policies and procedures can also be introduced as evidence to establish the standard of care. If the facility's policies and procedures establish the standard of care at a higher level than the standard that exists within the community, and the ACNP deviates from the facility's own policies, then the ACNP can be held to the higher standard (Aiken, 1994, p. 63). It should be noted that complying with a facility's policies and procedures may still expose the ACNP to liability if those policies and procedures require conduct that are below the standard of practice within the community. It is therefore imperative that the ACNP be aware of the content of policies, procedures, bylaws, and regulations that establish a standard of care that the ACNP may be held to when there is a claim of negligence.

The terms "reasonable care" and "competency" are used in the legal arena to define the level of practice, whereas the terms "incompetence," "negligence," and "malpractice" are used to claim a breach of the standard of care (Aiken, 1994, p. 64). Although written standards may be introduced as evidence of the standard of care, it does not mean that these documents are conclusive evidence that the ACNP is negligent (Aiken, 1994, p. 68). Malpractice is more than a mere mistake or an error in judgment. Additionally, a poor patient outcome by itself is insufficient to support a claim of medical negligence. To prevail in a medical malpractice action, the plaintiff must prove all four of the essential elements of medical negligence: (1) duty; (2) breach of the duty; (3) that the breach of that duty proximately (legally) caused, or was a substantial factor in causing, the patient's injury; and (4) that the patient suffered economic, emotional, or physical injury (Brent, 1997, p. 43).

Essential Elements

Duty. The first element, "duty," arises when a provider–patient relationship is created. Once a provider–patient relationship is established, the ACNP has the affirmative duty to act in a reasonable manner and within the standard of care. In most situations, there is no question whether a provider–patient relationship exists, as the ACNP initiates direct care to the patient in an acute care setting. The ACNP, however, should be aware that a provider–patient relationship can be established when there is indirect interaction with patients, family members, and even colleagues.

An example of indirect interaction is the situation in which the ACNP provides telephone advice to a family member for the benefit of a patient with whom the ACNP has not been directly involved prior to the telephone call (Henry, 1994, pp. 124–125). The legal issue that arises is whether or not a provider–patient relationship has been created such that the ACNP would be held liable to the patient. In the few legal cases that have addressed this issue, the courts have considered certain facts in determining if a duty exists. The courts have generally held that if the advice being given would be the type that the patient may reasonably rely on, and thus make decisions about medical treatment, then the court has found that a provider–patient relationship does exist and the provider has a duty to the patient to provide complete and appropriate advice (Henry, 1994, p. 124). Documentation of the advice given, and to whom, is very important and can be used as evidence in support of a defense to a negligence claim.

Another situation that may give rise to a provider–patient relationship is when the ACNP is informally consulted by a colleague, staff member, or other health-care professional regarding a patient for whom the ACNP is not directly caring or is not the primary provider for the patient. Since the ACNP is often viewed as a resource person, the ACNP must be cognizant of the legal duty that may arise when the ACNP assumes the role of consultant, especially during the informal "curbside consults" that occur in the course of the ACNP's practice (Knaus, 1997, p. 25). In a case-by-case basis, the court examines the interaction between the consultant and consultee to determine if the consultant's actions reach the level of establishing a duty to the patient. Facts—such as the type of advice being sought, how patient-specific was the advice that was given, the information given, and whether the consultee relied on the advice to make a clinical decision or to initiate treatment for a specific problem—are carefully considered by the trier of fact.

The ACNP who is involved in a patient-specific consultation must be sure to obtain all the facts of the case and provide appropriate advice within the ACNP's scope of practice. The ACNP should document in the patient's medical record the advice that was given. The ACNP should also be aware that the consultee has the option to accept or reject the advice given by the ACNP consultant. In general, if there is no risk of harm to the patient, then the consultant does not have any direct responsibility to insure that the consultee follows the consultant's recommendations or advice (Monicken, 1995, pp. 183–195). If the ACNP accepts the role of consultant, then exposure to liability is higher when the consultee is seeking advice for a patient-specific situation. When the consultee is only seeking general information for educational purposes or for administrative problem-solving matters, then the exposure to liability is less, but the ACNP is not totally immune to a negligence claim.

The ACNP must be aware that indirect interaction with patients, patients' family members, and other staff members may give rise to a provider–patient relationship requiring an affirmative duty of due care.

Breach of the Duty. The second element of a medical negligence claim that must be proven is whether there has been a breach of the duty owed to the patient. Any deviation from the standard of practice can result in a negligence claim being filed against that provider (Mezez & McGiven, 1993, pp. 281–310). A breach of the duty may occur when there is a failure to act (omission) in accordance with the standard of practice within the community, or when the provider acts in such a manner that would be considered to be below the standard of care. In a malpractice claim the plaintiff must establish by the evidence that a duty to the patient by the defendant–provider existed, and establish the standard of care at the time of the alleged injury. Expert testimony is presented by both parties that either supports or defeats the plaintiff's allegations that there is a breach of the duty by the provider.

Causation. Even though there may have been a breach of the duty owed to the patient, the plaintiff must establish a causal connection between the breach and the injuries that occurred. Legal causation differs from medical causation (Flamm, 1995, p. 119). In medicine, there may be several causes for the patient's medical condition or death since multiple medical problems can contribute to illness or death. In determining legal causation, the legal principle that is generally applied is: "'but for' the provider's action or inaction, the patient's injuries would not have occurred." Some States, however, felt there was some confusion in the application of this principle (also known as proximate cause) because of the tendency to relate proximate cause with a temporal or a closeness in time between the neglect act and the injury (McDonald, 1992, p. 292). However, since the patient's injury may be discovered later than when the negligence actually occurred, or the negligent act may set in motion a chain of events that ultimately results in the patient's injuries, legal causation may be established if the plaintiff proves the defendant's actions substantially contributed to or caused the plaintiff's injuries *(Morgenroth v. Pacific Care Medical Center*, 1976). A mere possibility that a causal nexus exists is not sufficient evidence to hold the defendant liable to the plaintiff. In order to obtain a verdict of negligence against the defendant, there must be sufficient expert testimony and factual evidence to establish a causal connection between the defendant's actions and the alleged injury to the plaintiff.

The causation element is the most difficult element for the plaintiff to prove and often is the one essential element out of the four that defeats plaintiff's claim. The ACNP should understand that although a breach of the duty to the patient has occurred, that breach must have a causal connection to the patient's injuries, either directly causing the injury or by substantially contributing to (greater than 51%) the cause of the patient's injuries.

Harm/Damages. The fourth essential element that the plaintiff must prove is that the defendant's actions caused the plaintiff to suffer some type of harm. If there is no harm, then the plaintiff cannot recover any monetary award, also known as damages (Flamm, 1995, p. 120). The harm to the patient (his or her injuries) can encompass a variety of types of injuries including physical injury, emotional injury, and past and future financial loss. Damages are divided into two categories: (1) general damages (noneconomic) that cover the pain and suffering the patient experiences as a result of the defendant's actions, and (2) special damages (economic) that include actual monetary losses sustained by the injured patient, such as a loss of income, medical expenses, and funeral expenses. Economic damages also include any future losses or expenses and includes the loss of future earning capacity due to the inability to work, future medical and rehabilitative costs, and the costs for vocational training, if applicable.

A third category of damages is punitive damages that may be awarded to punish or make an example of the defendant for very egregious conduct, generally when there has been an intentional disregard for human life or fraudulent behavior. Punitive damages are usually triple the amount of the damage award in the negligent action and are in addition to that award. Recovery of punitive damages rarely occurs in medical malpractice claims. When there is a battery claim (an unconsented touching), a claim for lost or altered records (spoliation), or an allegation of gross negligence, however, punitive damages are often requested by the plaintiff.

Related Legal Concepts

Two other concepts that are important in understanding the legal process, and which are associated with a negligence claim, are the concepts of: "negligence per se" and *res ipsa loquitor.* Negligence per se is a legal theory that creates a presumption that the defendant was negligent. This presumption arises when the defendant's actions are in violation of a statute, regulation, or the defendant's own policies and procedures that have established a standard of conduct (Henry, 1997, pp. 491–515). This is particularly relevant to the ACNP whose actions are assessed against the ACNP's standardized procedures (Henry, 1997, p. 500). Any deviation from the standardized procedures or protocols may give rise to an assertion of negligence per se. A failure to have the proper protocols or standardized procedures in place can also result in a negligence per se claim.

In a negligence per se allegation, if there is a violation of a statute, regulation, or policy by the defendant, then it is presumed that there has been a breach of the duty to the patient. The burden of proof then shifts to the defendant to prove that no breach occurred, and, if successful, then the presumption is rebutted. The ACNP should be aware, however, that in a negligence per se allegation, the plaintiff must still prove the remaining two elements of causation and damages.

Res ipsa loquitor is a Latin phrase meaning "the thing speaks for itself" (Henry, 1997, p. 501). This is a legal principle involving the rules of evidence that allow the plaintiff to prove his or her case based upon circumstantial evidence in the situation where the defendant was solely and exclusively in control at the time of the plaintiff's injury (Andrews, 1996, p. 207). The burden of proof shifts to the defendant when this principle is applied and requires that the defendant prove that the plaintiff's injuries were caused by someone or something other than the defendant's actions.

For the plaintiff to be allowed to introduce circumstantial evidence under the doctrine of *res ipsa loquitor,* the following three elements must be present: (1) the plaintiff's injury would not have occurred under normal circumstances if someone had not been negligent; (2) the plaintiff was under the exclusive control of the defendant when the injury occurred; and (3) the plaintiff's actions did not contribute to his or her injury (Henry, 1997, p. 501). An example of a case in which *res ipsa loquitor* would be applied is where a patient had developed an abscess as a result of a retained portion of a packing in a wound that obviously should have been removed entirely at the time of the removal. The plaintiff would assert that, based upon the doctrine of *res ipsa loquitor,* the defendant was negligent for failing to remove the entire packing. Thus the plaintiff would not have developed an abscess had it been completely removed. The application of a *res ipsa loquitor* doctrine would be successful as all three elements would be met. In general, expert testimony is not required to establish a breach of the standard of care that is presumed when the three elements of *res ipsa loquitor* are established by circumstantial evidence.

Lack of Informed Consent/Refusal

In medical malpractice actions, the plaintiff frequently alleges that there is a lack of informed consent. This allegation can be brought as part of the negligence cause of action or as a separate and additional cause of action. Since the ACNP is involved in providing acute care, which may include the use of invasive procedures (such as chest tube insertions, etc.) or diagnostic tests (such as bone marrow aspirations, etc.) that require an informed consent or make recommendations for treatment in which an informed decision is required (El-Sherif, 1995); the ACNP should be knowledgeable regarding the legal issues of informed consent and informed refusal in order to limit the ACNP's risk of liability.

The informed consent process is more than just having the patient sign a consent form. Under the doctrine of informed consent, the health-care provider who is performing the procedure or test, or who is recommending a course of treatment, has an affirmative duty to disclose and discuss all material facts necessary for the patient to make an informed decision regarding the proposed treatment or test. This is a duty that cannot be delegated to anyone else (Bianco & Hirsch, 1995, pp. 274–296).

The courts have long recognized the patient's right to self determination, which is the right of the patient to determine whether or not to undergo any recommended treatment based upon the information the patient was given at the time of the decision (*Schloendorff v. Society of New York Hospitals*, 1914). The consent process consists of two parts: the informed aspect relates to the information that should be provided to the patient in order for the patient to make an informed decision, and the patient, who has the capacity to consent voluntarily and with sufficient knowledge, agrees to undergo the recommended treatment (Andrews, 1996, pp. 60–100).

Most cases involving the allegation of a lack of informed consent are determined on a case-by-case basis. There are, however, certain essential elements that need to be established to determine if an informed consent did occur (Brent, 1997, pp. 237–268). The first element is that the health-care provider has fully explained the nature and extent of the proposed treatment or procedure and the reason that such treatment or procedure is necessary, and for what medical condition or problem. The second element is that the health-care provider has disclosed the benefits of the proposed treatment/procedure and the likelihood of success. The third element is a full disclosure by the provider of all the material risks and complications that would be pertinent to the patient in making an informed decision. The fourth element is that all reasonable alternative treatments, if any exist, have been discussed with the patient.

The last essential element of the informed consent process is a full discussion regarding the consequences that may occur if the recommended treatment or procedure is refused (Bianco, 1995, p. 283).

Two legal standards have developed under the doctrine of informed consent regarding the scope of disclosure that is required of a health-care provider. The first standard is known as the "professional standard" which focuses on the content of the disclosure that a reasonable provider in the community according to the applicable standard of care would be required to disclose for a specific procedure or treatment (Brent, 1997, p. 243). Expert testimony is necessary to establish this standard.

The second standard is the "reasonable patient standard." The requirements of a full disclosure sufficient to obtain an informed consent is measured by the amount of information needed by a reasonable patient in order to make an informed decision (Brent, 1997, p. 243). If the information that is important and necessary for a reasonable patient to make an informed decision is within the knowledge of a lay person, then expert testimony is not required (Bianco, 1995, p. 285).

It should be remembered that investigational or experimental treatments or procedures require a more specific consent process and the scope of disclosure may be established by statute, regulations, or protocols (*Medical Liability Reporter,* 1997, pp. 61–62). Expert testimony is required to establish the material facts that should be disclosed during the informed consent process for any investigational or experimental procedure, since a lay person lacks sufficient knowledge of facts that should be disclosed for an informed consent.

In the landmark case of *Canterbury v. Spence,* which involved the issue of whether the surgeon should have disclosed a 1% risk of paralysis in undergoing a laminectomy procedure, the court applied the reasonable patient standard to determine if there was a lack of informed consent. The court held the physician liable in this case and in making its determination. The court focused on the serious nature of the risk, not the 1% chance of occurrence. The court determined that this serious of a risk would be the type that a reasonable patient would have wanted to be informed about to make an informed decision (*Canterbury v. Spence*, 1972). It should also be noted, however, that in *Cobb v. Grant* the California Supreme Court held that a provider did not have to disclose all possible complications or provide the patient with a mini course in medicine (*Cobb v. Grant*, 1972). The key fact in the scope of disclosure is what information is material to the patient, not what information the provider believes is important to disclose.

In a recent 1997 case, *Daum v. Spinecare Medical Group,* the California Appellate Court held that when a statute or regulation establishes the scope of disclosure, expert testimony is not required to establish that the standard of care was breached (*Daum v. Spinecare*, 1997). The plaintiff in the *Daum* case filed a medical malpractice claim when he developed complications related to the fixation device utilized during his spine surgery. The issue of the scope of disclosure arose when the plaintiff alleged that he was not informed that the fixation device being used during his spinal fusion was part of an investigational study. Although there was a signed consent form, the plaintiff rebutted that evidence by establishing that he had signed the consent form right before his surgery and after a preanesthetic drug—which had blocked his memory of signing the form—had been given. It should be noted that the defendant physician had failed to document during the preoperative visit that he had disclosed that the fixation device was part of an investigational study. In this case, the plaintiff also overcame the causation defense argument by testifying that had he been informed of the investigational nature of the fixation device, he would have chosen to undergo the traditional spinal fusion surgery and would not have agreed to participate in a clinical trial (*Daum v. Spinecare*, 1997).

Evidence was presented in the *Daum* case that established there were specific statutes that had been incorporated into the manufacturer's clinical protocol for the use of the fixation device which required the patient be informed of the investigational status of the device as part of the required consent process. Thus, the court held that these statutes established the standard of care to be met for the consent process for the investigational study (*Medical,* 1997, pp. 61–62).

Legal issues that may arise for the ACNP regarding the consent process is when there is an issue of whether the patient has the capacity to consent to the recommended treatment or procedure and, if not, who has the legal status to consent for the patient. There is a legal presumption that adults are competent to make decisions pertaining to themselves and, therefore, an adult has the right to consent to any treatment being proposed for himself or herself (Bianco, 1995, p. 282). Minors, who are below the age of majority (generally, age 18), lack the capacity to consent to medical treatment. Exceptions to the age limitations to consent to treatment have been established for minors in certain specific circumstances, such as pregnancy and related care; sexually transmitted disease treatment; psychiatric, drug, and alcohol treatment; or, in situations when the minor is considered to be emancipated (Bianco, 1995, p. 245).

An adult patient who is incapacitated due to a physical or mental illness to the extent that the patient cannot fully understand the nature of the proposed treatment or procedure, even though that state may only be temporary, is deemed incompetent and thus cannot give a valid informed consent (Bianco, 1995, p. 282). The ACNP is certain to encounter patients in the acute care setting whose decision-making capacity is compromised due to the patient's acute medical condition. The ACNP should, therefore, be aware of the legal procedure to obtain the court's determination regarding the capacity of the patient to give a valid consent.

If the patient lacks the capacity to consent, then the ACNP should be aware of the procedure for seeking the appointment of a guardian or agent to make health-care decisions. Consent to treatment by a patient's spouse or family member is not legally valid unless that person was designated by the patient as his or her agent to make health-care decisions or has been appointed the legal guardian (Bianco, 1995, pp. 276, 277).

In addition, the ACNP should be aware of the emergency situation in which the patient is unable to give consent and that may require immediate intervention to protect the health and life of the patient, especially where any delay increases the risk of harm to the patient (Bianco, 1995, pp. 283, 284). Emergency exception to the consent process and the doctrine of an implied consent may be applicable in the acute care setting. The ACNP is encouraged to be familiar with each individual State's regulations and community practice regarding emergency consent. All emergency exceptions to the consent process must be clearly documented regarding the facts that support any exception to the consent process. It is important to understand, however, that if the proposed treatment is only medically advisable and not medically necessary to protect the patient's health or life, or if the necessity will occur sometime in the future, then the exception does not apply (Bianco, 1995, pp. 283, 284).

To have a valid consent, the patient must also have given that consent voluntarily without any undue influence or coercion by the provider or family members. The patient should be informed of his or her right to refuse the proposed treatment and be informed that his or her medical care will not, and cannot, be withdrawn due to that refusal (Andrews, 1996, p. 71).

The courts have recognized the legal right of a person to refuse treatment, and the legal analysis of the doctrine of informed refusal is similar to that of informed consent. It is important that the ACNP understands and accepts that the patient has the right to determine his or her own life's course, and even though the patient's refusal may compromise the patient's health or result in the patient's death, the patient has the legal right to refuse treatment (Brent, 1997, p. 246). The elements to establish a valid informed refusal are the same as those required for an informed consent. The patient must have the capacity to refuse, be informed of all material facts necessary to make an informed decision, be informed of the risks of refusal, and be informed that medical care and treatment will continue to be provided within the parameters of the patient's refusal (Brent, 1997, p. 247).

The patient's right to refuse treatment may be challenged, either by establishing that the patient is incompetent to make an informed decision or by establishing a compelling reason to override the patient's decision, such as when refusing treatment would endanger the life of another or when the public interest outweighs the individual's interest (e.g., vaccinations). Absent a court's order overriding the refusal, the patient's wishes must be honored by the ACNP, despite the ACNP's personal or professional feelings regarding the matter. Additionally, neither the patient's spouse nor the patient's family members can override a competent patient's decision. The ACNP will often be involved with the patient's decision-making process and must be prepared to work within the parameters of those decisions.

The ACNP should at all times clearly and completely document any refusal by the patient to undergo a treatment or proposed procedure. There also must be clear documentation of the ACNP's disclosure of the material facts required to establish a valid informed refusal. The patient should not be asked to sign a waiver of the right to sue or to sign a "hold harmless clause." These attempts to avoid liability are generally not upheld by the courts because it gives the appearance that the patient had no choice but to sign the waiver in order to continue to receive care (Brent, 1997, p. 248).

Since the patient's right to consent or to refuse care and treatment is not absolute, the ACNP should therefore be cognizant of the legal issues pertaining to informed consent/refusal doctrines and keep abreast of any changes or special circumstances that may apply to the ACNP's practice.

Battery

Another cause of action related to the issue of consent that can be filed against a health-care provider is the intentional tort of battery. Battery is the unconsented touching of another (Flamm, 1995, p. 120). A battery claim may arise when the patient alleges that a procedure or treatment has occurred in the absence of the proper consent or exceeds the scope of the consent given. It can also arise in situations where the patient's refusal of treatment is not honored. The ACNP should be aware that a battery claim may be alleged even in situations where there has been no direct contact with the patient (Bianco, 1995, p. 275). This is known as constructive touching and, when it occurs without consent, a battery allegation can be filed. An example of constructive touching is where the provider orders the wrong treatment, but did not administer the treatment directly to the patient. Although the injurious agent may have been a medication or radiation, the provider who ordered the treatment is liable even though there was no direct patient–provider contact.

An important issue that may arise in the acute care setting is when the police requests that the ACNP collect blood, hair, tissue, or fluid samples from a patient for a criminal investigation. In these situations, especially if the patient is a suspect in a crime, that patient will not want to give consent for obtaining the samples. The ACNP should be knowledgeable of the individual State's statutes dealing with this issue. Most statutes permit the collection of samples and testing to be performed in the absence of an expressed consent from the patient as long as it is done in a medically accepted manner and unreasonable force is not used to obtain the samples (Bianco, 1995, p. 289).

Although a technical battery has occurred in these types of situations, most States have granted immunity from liability to health-care providers who are responding to a valid and reasonable request from police officials. In situations that may require more invasive procedures, such as pumping a patient's stomach or surgical removal of an object, the courts have held that the method of extraction and the associated conduct (i.e., pumping of the stomach to obtain the drugs ingested at the time of arrest) cannot be done in such a manner as to shock the conscience of the average person (Bianco, 1995, p. 29). In the case of *Rochin v. California* the court held that the forcible extraction of the plaintiff's stomach contents to obtain evidence of illegal possession of a drug went beyond the bounds of reasonable conduct (*Rachin v. Calif.*, 1952). Although the court did not specifically address the provider's liability in pumping the patient's stomach, the court's ruling placed limits on what would be accepted as reasonable medical conduct. Later, cases involving the drawing of a blood alcohol on a patient involved in a vehicle accident who was suspected of driving under the influence, even though the patient may object to the withdrawal of his blood, were upheld by the courts as this conduct was considered a minor intrusion of the patient's privacy and was warranted under the circumstances (*Breithaupht v. Abram*, 1996). In general, each State's court considers the issue of obtaining evidence without express consent on a case-by-case basis.

The ACNP must be aware of the exposure to liability in the acute care setting of a battery claim and never make the assumption that there is an exception to consent. The only defense to a battery claim is to establish that a valid informed consent was obtained or a valid exception applied to the situation. Limited immunity pursuant to a statute may be applied but all the criteria for the immunity must be met.

Withholding/Withdrawal of Treatment

In conjunction with the principles pertaining to informed consent and informed refusal, the ACNP in the acute care setting may become involved with the legal issues regarding the withholding or withdrawal of life-sustaining treatment. A competent adult has the legally recognized right to refuse treatment and the legal right to discontinue treatment (Paola & Anderson, 1995, pp. 404–423). The legal recognition of these rights is based upon the fundamental right of self determination, the right of the patient to control and make decisions regarding medical treatment. There is also the recognition that a health-care provider has no duty to provide care that has been declined by a competent patient (Paola, 1995, p. 410). The legal and medical literature contains multiple publications addressing these issues (Gostin, 1993, pp. 94–101), and several well-known legal cases—such as *Cruzan v. Director, Bouvia v. Riverside General Hospital, In the Matter of Quinlan,* and *Barber and Nejdl v. Superior Court*—addressed the issues of abatement of treatment and the patient's or the patient's agent's right to make that decision (*Cruzan v. Director*, 1990, 1986, 1983, 1976).

The *Cruzan* case dealt with the fact that clear and convincing evidence of the patient's wishes prior to becoming incapacitated was necessary in order to stop life-sustaining treatment (Paola, 1995, p. 412). The *Bouvia* case established the right of a severely handicapped patient, who was not terminally ill, to refuse medical treatment—specifically, the removal of a nasogastric tube that would prevent her from receiving nutrition and fluids for hydration (Paola, 1995, p. 412). The *Quinlan* case involved the doctrine of substituted judgment, which permits an incapacitated patient's guardian or family to make the decision to withdraw life-support in substitution for the decision of the patient (Paola, 1995, p. 412).

The *Barber and Nejdl v. Superior Court* case, however, had slightly different issues. This was a criminal case in which the physicians (Drs. Barber and Nejdl) were convicted for withdrawing life support in accordance with the family's wishes (*Barber v. Superior Court*, 1983). The Appellate Court overturned the conviction on the basis that there was no legal duty to continue life support in the presence of the express wishes of the family and that the patient's death was caused by his underlying disease and not the action of the physician (Gostin, 1993, p. 95). It should be noted that the *Barber and Nejdl* case was initiated by the complaint of a staff nurse—not the family—who believed that the doctors had acted wrongly.

The ACNP should also be aware that the courts do not always uphold the wishes of a patient's family or parent. In 1988 the New York Court of Appeals, in the *Matter of Westchester County Medical Center,* held that the refusal by the family of a 78-year-old woman, incapacitated by dementia, to consent to the insertion of a nasogastric tube to provide nutrition to the patient would not be honored as there was no clear evidence that the patient would have declined treatment (*Matters of Westerchester,* 1988). Another case decided by the same Court of Appeals held that a mother of a 52-year-old mentally retarded man who had the mental age of a 5-year-old could not withhold consent for a blood transfusion needed to treat her son's anemia, which was secondary to his bladder cancer (Paola, 1995, p. 413). Only twenty States have enacted laws recognizing the right of the next of kin to make health-care decisions, in the absence of any legal document designating an agent, when a patient is unable to personally decide (Paola, 1995, p. 412). Awareness by the ACNP of the State's regulations governing who can legally consent to withdrawal or withholding treatment for an incapacitated patient is very important in order that the ACNP may avoid the risk of liability.

A slightly different fact scenario occurred in the case of *In re Wanglie.* In this case the patient's health-care provider requested that the court appoint a conservator for Mrs. Wanglie, an 86-year-old ventilator-dependent woman who was in a persistent vegetative state, and whose family refused to allow the physicians to terminate her life support. The physician treating Mrs. Wanglie made the request because the physician believed that the life support was no longer beneficial (In *Re Helga,* 1991). Whether the physician had a legal right or duty to discontinue treatment—and whether the life-support treatment provided any benefit to the patient—was never addressed as Mrs. Wanglie died three days after her husband was appointed conservator (Paola, 1995, pp. 414, 415).

Multiple legal and ethical issues will be encountered by the ACNP due to the nature of the acute care setting and the acuity of the patient's medical condition. Medical futility issues and the issuance of "do not resuscitate" orders may lead to close legal scrutiny of the ACNP's actions. Any decision regarding withholding or withdrawal of treatment should never be done unilaterally by the ACNP or any provider. It is, therefore, imperative that the ACNP concisely and completely document the patient's and family's wishes and the basis for any decision made by the ACNP in determining to withdraw or withhold any treatment. The ACNP should be knowledgeable of the legal ramifications and legal debates associated with voluntary passive euthanasia (VPE), provider-assisted suicide (PAS), and the evolving legal issues of patient refusal of hydration and nutrition (PRHN) (Paola, 1995, pp. 415, 416). Compliance with a patient's advance directives is also necessary to avoid liability. The ACNP has the affirmative duty to educate the patient in an acute care setting regarding his or her right to make decisions regarding medical care, including the right to accept or refuse treatment.

In several cases, the courts have recognized that an incompetent or incapacitated patient has the right to forego treatment and that right may be asserted by way of a living will, as in the case of *John F. Kennedy Memorial Hospital v. Bludworth* (*John F. Kennedy Hospital v. Bludworth,* 1984) or in instances where there is a designated agent and an advanced directive indicating the patient's wishes. An immunity, although not absolute, to criminal or civil liability does exist for any individual, including a conservator, guardian, or agent, who in good faith participates in the decision to withhold or withdraw treatment (Brent, 1997, pp. 143–170). That immunity, however, is not available to the ACNP who decides on his or her own to withdraw or withhold treatment particularly when the patient, the patient's family or legally designated agent for the patient, or other treating health-care providers did not participate in the decision made by the ACNP. The ACNP should keep in mind that these issues continually evolve and the ACNP needs to keep abreast of the changes.

Another practice area that gives rise to liability regarding withholding or withdrawal of treatment is in emergency care. Failing to provide emergency care has recently resulted in increased legal scrutiny and resulted in the enactment of Federal antidumping legislation, known as the Consolidated Omnibus Budget Reconciliation Act, (COBRA) (Brent, 1997, pp. 403–422). Criminal and civil charges, in addition to a medical negligence claim, can be alleged against the ACNP for failing to render emergency care to a patient who presents in an emergency state or if the ACNP transfers an unstable patient.

The ACNP who practices in any emergency or urgent care setting has the duty to evaluate a patient to determine if a true emergency exists and determine if nontreatment would result in a threat of harm to the patient's well-being or life. If there is no "true" emergency and a delay in treatment will not cause any harm, then there is no obligation to provide immediate care. Absent any unnecessary delay, the patient can be referred to another facility or provider. In order to avoid violating Federal law, the ACNP who provides emergency medical services in a hospital must be aware of The Emergency Medical Treatment and Active Labor Act (EMTALA) which provides the definitions of an emergency medical condition and active labor (Hollowell, 1995, p. 643). Violations of EMTALA result in civil penalties being assessed against the facility, the loss of the contract to provide services to Medicare and Medicaid patients, and can result in a personal injury civil action.

False Imprisonment

The ACNP may also be faced with an allegation of false imprisonment by a patient whose ability to move freely was allegedly unjustly or unreasonably restricted (Feutz, 1989, pp. 111–193). A false imprisonment allegation is one of the intentional tort actions that can be brought in conjunction with a medical malpractice claim or as a single action by itself. A false imprisonment allegation generally arises when the patient wants to leave the facility but is not allowed to, when the patient is admitted voluntarily and is not allowed to leave pending an evaluation, or in situations in which restraints (physical and chemical) are used. An action for false imprisonment may be filed when there is an actual threat of force to restrict a patient's movement or when there is a show of authority (i.e., the appearance of a security guard) (Blouin & Brent, 1995, pp. 11–12, 55). Threats of restriction in the future and the use of moral pressure or influence to restrict or confine a patient's movement are not actionable under a claim of false imprisonment (Brent, 1997, pp. 105–125).

False imprisonment is an intentional tort. Thus, if the plaintiff is to succeed in this claim, the plaintiff must prove two essential elements: that the defendant had the intent to restrict or confine the patient's movement and that there was an awareness by the patient of the involuntary restriction or confinement (Blouin, 1995, p. 11). If the plaintiff is successful in proving a false imprisonment claim, then he or she is entitled to recover monetary damages for any emotional distress as a result of being confined and recover for any loss of time, physical injury (although actual harm is not required for recovery), or damage to reputation as a result of the confinement (Brent, 1997, p. 110). In fact, nominal damages may be awarded when no actual damages have occurred (Hoffman, 1995, p. 132). Also, since a claim for false imprisonment is an intentional tort, the plaintiff may seek to recover punitive damages (Blouin, 1995, p. 11).

In the ACNP's expanded role, determining the medical necessity of restraints may be one of the ACNP's responsibilities. Restraints are lawful when there is a clearly documented medical necessity to protect the patient from personal injury or from injuring another person and that medical necessity outweighs the patient's right to independence. The least restrictive restraint and for the minimum amount of time should be used to meet the goal of patient safety (Feutz, 1989, pp. 150, 151). Comprehensive policies and procedures should exist in all practice settings in which restraints are used. The policies should identify which provider can order restraints, under what situations, (i.e., combativeness, confusion, or when sedated) and what to do if a competent or incompetent patient refuses to be restrained. The patient's right to refuse treatment applies in restraint situations unless there has been a legal determination that the medical necessity outweighs the patient's right. The courts make such a determination on a case-by-case basis.

In 1988, the Colorado Court of Appeals in *Blackman for Blackman v. Rifkin* held that an emergency room staff was not liable for false imprisonment as there was a medical necessity to physically restrain an intoxicated and combative patient while being treated for a scalp laceration and head trauma (*Blackman for Blackman v. Rifkin*, 1988). The Court of Appeals in *Blackman* ruled that the staff's specific actions of holding the patient's head while suturing her laceration, and placing her in restraints when she became combative, did not constitute unreasonable acts of restraint. The false imprisonment allegation was brought in conjunction with a medical negligence claim as the patient had suffered permanent brain damage when she went into cardiac and respiratory arrest subsequent to the aspiration of vomitus (Blackman, 1988).

ACNPs who practice in emergency settings may be involved in assessing patients for the medical necessity of a 72-hour involuntary admission to a psychiatric treatment facility. Frequently in the emergency department, the ACNP is involved in caring for patients who have indicated that they are suicidal, or who are contemplating harming themselves or another person. The ACNP has the affirmative and statutory duty to detain that patient for a psychiatric evaluation. Complete documentation of the evaluation and the basis for the confinement must be done to avoid liability for false imprisonment.

The acute care setting is a common practice area that could give rise to a false imprisonment claim. Any inappropriate or improper restraint or confinement exposes the ACNP to liability. Again, the ACNP must recognize the patient's legal right to refuse medical care, even if it is against the ACNP's advice. The only exception is if the patient presents a harm to self or others and there is the legal authority to detain the patient.

Breach of Confidentiality

Another intentional tort that can be brought against the ACNP occurs when there has been a breach of confidentiality. Breach of confidentiality occurs when confidential information has been disclosed without the consent of the patient or a disclosure beyond the scope of accepted disclosure to other treating providers in the course of caring for the patient. The ACNP has the affirmative duty to keep confidential all information pertaining to the patient that was obtained within the provider–patient relationship. Confidentiality is one of the primary patient rights recognized by Federal and State laws and most medical organizations (i.e., JCAHO) (Feutz, 1989, pp. 93–109).

The ACNP has the legal authority to release medical information regarding a specific patient to other providers involved in the care and treatment of the patient; and in life-threatening emergencies certain information necessary to treat the patient can be released even if the patient is unaware or unable to consent to the disclosure (Flemm, 1995, p. 122). Any other disclosure of information must be with the consent of the patient, preferably in writing. Although consent for disclosure may have been given by the patient, the ACNP must be aware of any limits or restrictions that may exist. There may be specific limits on the information that may be disclosed, which were placed by the patient or there may be legal limits regarding the type of information to be disclosed. If the ACNP exceeds the scope of consent or the legal limits pertaining to certain types of confidential information, then the ACNP is liable for a breach of confidentiality. If the ACNP violates any disclosure statutes, the ACNP can be subjected to civil penalties and fines in addition to being held liable for a breach of confidentiality.

Concerns regarding a breach of the confidentiality have been raised when the provider is using computer documentation, also known as the electronic medical record or electronic medical charting. Specific guidelines must be in place to safeguard any unauthorized access or disclosure of confidential patient information. If the ACNP is using computer documentation in the acute care setting, the ACNP needs to ensure the accuracy of the information imputed and obtain the patient's written consent for the use or the release of the stored information.

In the mental health arena, the ACNP must be familiar with the Federal and State laws governing patient confidentiality and disclosure of confidential information. Most States have enacted specific statutes requiring the written consent of an individual prior to any disclosure of information regarding drug, alcohol, or psychiatric treatment (Firestone, 1995, pp. 585–614). An example is the State of Illinois, which has seventeen sections in the Mental Health and Developmental Disabilities Act pertaining to the duty of confidentiality and which sets forth the legal procedures for authorized disclosure of confidential information and the penalties for unauthorized disclosure (Firestone, 1995, p. 601). Additionally, there are Federal statutes regarding disclosure of information of drug abuse and alcohol treatment that the ACNP must be aware of in order to avoid liability (Feutz, 1989, pp. 398–99).

Strict confidentiality and disclosure statutes exist regarding HIV status and treatment (Royal, 1995, pp. 516–530). Due to the high risk for discrimination, confidentiality issues are of primary concern and statutory safeguards mandating confidentiality regarding HIV test results and treatment have been instituted by several States. Examples are Pennsylvania's Confidentiality of HIV-Related Information ACT and California's Health and Safety Code, Section 199.21, Unauthorized Disclosure statute (Royal, 1995, fnt.).

The HIV positive status of a health-care provider has also become a complex and controversial issue in both the legal and medical fields. Legal issues pertaining to confidentiality, privacy rights, and scope of disclosure have been raised and have necessitated a balancing of the public's concerns for safety and the provider's right to privacy and consent to disclosure. The acute care setting is a practice area that is more closely scrutinized due to the seriousness and potentially life-threatening status of that particular patient population.

Due to the increased public concern and anxiety, employers of health-care providers have attempted to institute policies regarding HIV screening and disclosure of HIV status and a diagnosis of AIDS (Brent, 1997, pp. 359–401). Legal challenges to these policies have occurred as well as patients' suing health-care providers for failing to disclose the provider's HIV status (Brent, 1997, pp. 394–395). Unfortunately, the court decisions that have addressed the issue of provider disclosure and employee mandatory testing have not been uniform. It is, therefore, important for the ACNP to become knowledgeable regarding each State's regulations and court decisions regarding provider disclosure and employee mandatory testing, which govern the individual ACNP's practice.

The American Nurses Association (ANA) recommends that confidential or anonymous testing be done and recommends that providers who are HIV positive voluntarily disclose their status when necessary. ANA also recommends voluntary avoidance of participating in or the performance of any invasive procedures that may place the patient at risk (Brent, 1997, p. 394).

The ACNP should also be aware of the exceptions to the confidentiality statutes that require disclosure to third parties, even in the absence of a patient's consent. These exceptions were established to protect the public's health and safety and thus outweigh the individual's rights. In the emergency room setting, as well as other practice areas, some of the more common conditions that are required to be reported to a State agency include: child abuse and neglect, elder abuse and neglect, communicable diseases (TB, sexually transmitted disease), gunshot or stab wounds, sexual assault, food poisoning, work-related injuries, and toxic exposures (Brent, 1997, pp. 403–422). In other settings, patients who have been diagnosed with a seizure disorder are reported to the State agency that regulates driving and patients diagnosed with cancer are reported to Tumor Registries (Feutz, 1989, p. 96). All States require the reporting of individuals by name who have been diagnosed with AIDS, whereas only thirty-five States that require the reporting of the diagnosis of an HIV infection can be done either by name or anonymously (Royal, 1995, p. 530).

A qualified immunity for a breach of confidentiality is available to any health-care provider who in good faith, and pursuant to statutory requirements, complies with a reporting requirement (Feutz, 1989, p. 95). The ACNP should understand that failing to report as required by law may subject the ACNP to civil and criminal liability (Feutz, 1989, p. 95).

Another exception to the duty of confidentiality is where the health-care provider has knowledge that a third party is at risk of harm. In the 1976 California Supreme Court decision in *Tarasoff v. Regents of University of California* a duty to warn a third person of impending danger was established as an exception to the duty of confidentiality (Firestone, 1995, pp. 601, 602). In *Tarasoff,* the defendant health-care providers were held liable for failing to notify a woman who was subsequently killed, despite the fact that the treating psychologist had notified the local police that his client had expressed an intent to harm the victim (*Tarasoff v. Regents*, 1976). Several States subsequent to the *Tarasoff* case enacted statutes, with varying applications, that addressed the affirmative duty to warn and in general require warning to a potential, identifiable victim of any threat or potential harm (Firestone, 1995, p. 601).

Several other exceptions to the doctrine of confidentiality have been recognized by the medical and legal fields. In the event of a medical emergency, patient information may be released without a patient's consent to the appropriate authorities or health agencies. Medical information can also be disclosed without the patient's authorization for scientific research, management audits, financial audits, and program evaluation as long as that information does not contain any patient identification (Feutz, 1989, p. 99).

As stated previously, in the absence of an exception to the doctrine of confidentiality, disclosure of confidential medical information to a third party must be done with the written consent of the patient or legal representative. There are, however, certain legal situations in which confidential medical information is released to a third party without the patient's written consent. Such releases are done by a court order, known as a *subpoena duces tecum,* for the release of records or a subpoena issued to compel testimony in person, either for a deposition or at a trial or arbitration (Feutz, 1989, pp. 102, 103). Although under a subpoena a patient's written authorization is not necessary, most States require notification of the individual whose records or information is being sought so that the individual has an opportunity to object before the information is released. Compliance with a proper subpoena is required and failure to do so results in a contempt charge by the court (Feutz, 1989, p. 102).

In order for a subpoena to be valid, the information being sought must be relevant to the subject matter of the lawsuit and not be privileged. Additionally, it must meet any procedural requirements established for subpoenas in that jurisdiction. The ACNP should seek legal counsel regarding the appropriateness of the subpoena as disclosure in the face of an improper or invalid subpoena is actionable for a breach of confidentiality.

Confidentiality is the cornerstone of the provider–patient relationship as it establishes a trust relationship and gives rise to an affirmative duty of nondisclosure. The ACNP must be knowledgeable regarding the legal issues that can arise regarding confidentiality, authorized disclosure, and the associated risks of liability for unauthorized disclosures.

Discrimination

Although the ACNP does not have a legal duty to treat all persons, once a provider–patient relationship has been established, the ACNP cannot discriminate against any person on the basis of race, color, religion, national origin, or disability. Refusal to care for a patient because of a particular disability (such as AIDS or TB) violates the 1990 Title III of the Americans with Disabilities ACT (ADA) (Brent, 1997, p. 396). Some case examples that are illustrative of patient discrimination are discussed in the following paragraphs.

In 1997, the Federal Appellate Court in *Abbott v. Bragdon* held a dentist liable under the Americans with Disabilities Act for refusing to treat an asymptomatic HIV positive patient in his office, even though the dentist had offered to treat the patient in the hospital, causing the patient to incur additional expenses (*Medical,* 1997, pp. 50–53). The court ruled that the dentist's actions were in violation of ADA because the dentist had discriminated against this patient on the basis of the patient's disability. In the 1994 case of *Armstrong v. Flowers Hospital,* the 11th Circuit Court of Appeals upheld the employer's (the Hospital's) right to terminate an employee—a pregnant nurse working in home health care—for refusing to care for AIDS patients, on the grounds that the employer's policy applied equally to nonpregnant and pregnant employees (*Armstrong v. Flowers Hospital*, 1994). In another case the court ruled that the employer's firing of a lab technician for refusing to test lab specimens labeled with a biohazard warning label was proper on the basis that the technician's refusal was discriminatory (*Stepp v. Review Board*, 1988). The lab technician's refusal was based upon the religious belief that AIDS was a plague from God, and therefore the lab technician felt it was wrong to perform tests on the lab specimens of AIDS patients. The court held that the employer had the proper procedural guidelines and policies in place in compliance with the Centers for Disease Control and Prevention and that there was no risk of exposure for the lab technician.

The courts, however, hold an employer liable for negligence when a provider's health is placed at risk when there are insufficient safeguards to protect the provider from harm. An example is the 1993 case in which the court awarded $5 million to a State correctional facility nurse who tested positive for HIV one year after receiving a needle stick that occurred during a struggle with an HIV positive inmate/patient (*Doe v. N.Y. State*, 1992).

Prior to refusing to care for any patient, the ACNP must be aware of the legal and professional consequences resulting from the refusal. Refusal on the basis of a patient's race, color, religion, ethnic origin, or disability is discriminatory and the ACNP is liable for violating the patient's rights, possibly facing disciplinary action.

Abandonment

Another cause of action, in addition to a medical malpractice claim, that can be brought against the ACNP is the tort claim of abandonment. Abandonment is defined as the unilateral nonconsensual termination of the provider–patient relationship, without notice, when continued medical care is still necessary (Howard & Vogt, 1995, pp. 265–273). An allegation of abandonment may arise when: there is a failure to respond; there has been inattentiveness; there has been insufficient treatment, an improper transfer, or a premature discharge (Feutz, 1998, pp. 11–193). A claim for abandonment can also occur when the provider terminates the relationship without sufficient time for the patient to make other arrangements for care.

The ACNP's affirmative duty of due care continues until the provider–patient relationship is properly terminated. Proper termination can occur when: care has been completed and no further care is necessary; the ACNP discharges the patient from the ACNP's care; by mutual consent of the provider and patient, the patient's care is transferred to another provider; the ACNP formally withdraws from the case (Howard, 1995, p. 270). It is noted, however, that patients frequently, unilaterally, and without notice, terminate the relationship when they fail to return for continued care.

The provider–patient relationship can be formally terminated by the ACNP for any reason (except based upon discrimination) as long as there is sufficient written notice to the patient, and that notice includes an explanation of the patient's condition, any need for future care, and the likely consequences if the patient fails in obtaining continued care (Howard, 1995, p. 270). The ACNP needs to continue to treat the patient for a reasonable length of time to allow the patient sufficient time to establish a different provider–patient relationship.

Allegations of abandonment can occur if there is a lack of proper follow-up for a medical condition requiring continued care. An example is if the ACNP failed to follow-up on an abnormal laboratory test, either by failing to repeat the test or initiate a further diagnostic evaluation. Another example is where the patient should have been seen more frequently due to the medical condition, but the ACNP failed to evaluate the patient on a timely basis. Timelines of care is a frequent issue in the acute care setting and can lead to a claim for constructive abandonment, where there is an inference that due to the infrequent care that was provided to a patient, the provider abandoned the patient (Howard, 1995, p. 270). The ACNP must be diligent in following up on abnormal lab tests, and in responding to any changes in the patient's medical condition.

In the on-call situation, abandonment issues may rise if the ACNP is slow to respond, or fails to respond, to a change in the patient's condition or a request by the staff nurse. In the presence of the right fact scenario, a claim for abandonment can lead to a punitive damages (triple damages) claim, as well as disciplinary actions against the ACNP's license.

APPLICATIONS TO PRACTICE

The most common allegations asserted in malpractice claims are discussed in the context of the ACNP's practice. Several of the legal theories have been previously discussed, but the ACNP should understand how those theories are applied in the acute care setting and the role of the ACNP.

Failure to Adequately Assess/Obtain Adequate History

A significant number of malpractice actions are brought for the alleged failure to adequately assess a patient's medical condition. The ACNP's educational preparation includes specific courses in physical assessment and diagnostic reasoning (Alexander, et al., 1996). Assessment of a patient's medical condition is one of the primary skills used by the ACNP in evaluating an acutely ill patient (Richard & Keane, 1996, pp. 316–326). The ACNP's ability to adequately assess a patient decreases the ACNP's exposure to liability.

Assessment encompasses multiple skills and a thorough analysis of a variety of information from different sources by the ACNP in a practice setting that requires immediate decision-making. Thus, this type of practice leads to a higher risk of liability for failing to properly assess the patient's continually changing condition. It is, therefore, extremely important that the ACNP has the ability to obtain a detailed patient and family history and perform a careful, comprehensive examination in a relatively short period of time. To avoid liability for the failure to adequately assess, the ACNP should have a systematic method of evaluation that has been developed over the course of the ACNP's practice and that should have evolved into the usual and customary practice for that individual ACNP. Part of the ACNP's educational experience is learning the right questions to ask—gathering data, both historical and present, from multiple sources, (patient, family, coproviders)—and from performing a physical exam and diagnostic tests, then analyzing that information to develop a differential diagnosis, then a definitive diagnosis. This assessment process then should result in the ACNP's ability to initiate the appropriate treatment for the patient's condition.

One of the key strategies in a claim for the failure to adequately assess is for the injured plaintiff to present evidence that the provider failed to carry out one of the essential steps in the assessment process. An example is when the plaintiff presents evidence that there was a failure to obtain an adequate history, perform a complete exam, or obtain significant prior medical records. Documentation becomes a key piece of evidence that can be used to support the provider's actions. Or, it can be used to point out the provider's lack of due care or raise the inference that the provider failed to properly assess the patient. Several small omissions by the ACNP can have the cumulative effect of influencing a jury to ultimately decide that the ACNP was negligent.

The ACNP is cautioned against placing too much reliance on another provider's history, assessment, or conclusions. As discussed previously in the *Beckom* case, one of the allegations against the NP was that the NP relied on the history (as provided by the patient) that the patient's previous provider (the surgeon) had diagnosed her breast problem as fibrocystic breast disease, when in fact the patient had infiltrating ductal carcinoma. That reliance resulted in the NP failing to initiate any further workup (Beckom, 1984). The ACNP should personally perform the necessary examination of the patient and insure that all pertinent information is obtained, including requesting prior medical records, before the ACNP makes a clinical decision for the treatment of the patient. Failing to follow these steps in the assessment process can lead to the patient being harmed and result in liability for the ACNP.

Failure to adequately document the ACNP's assessment can also lead to an allegation of the failure to adequately assess. Plaintiffs' lawyers frequently use the old adage "if it was not documented, then it was not done" to support the plaintiff's claim against the provider (Aiken,

1994, pp. 234–250). A 1990 study regarding the role that documentation factors into determining the outcome of malpractice suits indicated that the medical record played a significant role in one case out of four, and an indirect role in all cases (Brent, 1997, pp. 65–84). Thus, it is imperative that the ACNP comprehensively document any and all assessments of the patient's condition and include all pertinent positive and negative findings.

Failure to Diagnose/Misdiagnosis

Within the health-care community, the art of diagnosing a patient's medical condition has long been recognized. The process encompasses the collection of data from multiple sources, the analysis of that data, the consideration of the more likely and remote causes of the patient's complaints and signs and symptoms, and culminates in determination of the most likely cause (i.e., the diagnosis).

In the legal cases that allege a failure to diagnose, the plaintiff may assert that the defendant–provider failed to correctly diagnose the patient's medical condition, delayed making the correct diagnosis, misdiagnosed the patient (a loss of a chance of treatment). A failure to properly diagnose and a delay in correctly diagnosing the patient's problem are the two leading allegations asserted in medical malpractice claims, with the failure to diagnose cancer twice as common as the failure to diagnose other health problems (Schiffman, 1995, pp. 494–508). Traditionally, the medical profession has claimed that the art of diagnosing a patient's medical condition is a medical function and it has been in the exclusive domain of physicians. Currently, however, both the legal and medical communities have recognized that nurse practitioners, as a part of their scope of practice, have the responsibility of diagnosing and implementing the proper treatment for their patients (Smith & Kelly, 1987; Richard, 1996, pp. 316–326). With this recognition also comes the legal accountability if the NP fails to properly diagnose the patient's medical condition.

A survey of a specific group of NPs conducted in 1994 reported that 50% of the reported malpractice claims brought against NPs contained an allegation for the failure to properly diagnose a patient's condition (Pearson & Berkholz, 1995, pp. 18, 21, 24–26, 29–30). Although the survey contained a relatively small sample of NPs who reported having negligence claims filed against them, it indicates that failure to diagnose is the most common allegation asserted against the responding NPs. It has been acknowledged in the past that there has been an underreporting of claims against NPs and a lack of adequate data and uniformity in NP claim reporting. Recently, there has been an effort on the part of various NP organizations to change this trend.

Failure by the ACNP to properly diagnose a problem in the acute care setting can have a devastating effect on the course of the patient's condition and the outcome of treatment. The ACNP is legally accountable to possess and maintain the minimum level of skills and knowledge necessary to make a reasonable clinical decision that is based upon sound scientific principles and valid data, thus enabling the ACNP to make the proper diagnosis in a timely manner and implement the appropriate treatment. In the acute care setting, even a short delay in making the proper diagnosis may result in liability of the ACNP if the patient is harmed by that delay. In *Fein v. Permanente* the NP was charged with the failure to timely diagnose the cause of the plaintiff's chest pain (a myocardial infarction) which resulted in a delay in treatment (*Fein v. Permanente*, 1985). For the plaintiff to have succeeded in its action for a delay in diagnosis, the plaintiff had to prove that the delay materially affected the ultimate treatment and outcome for the patient (Schiffman, 1995, p. 494).

The legal issue that needs to be determined in a misdiagnosis claim is whether, based upon a reasonable medical certainty, there has been a loss of the chance for effective treatment and survival that was caused by the misdiagnosis, or whether that lost chance would have occurred as part of the natural progression of the patient's medical condition (Schiffman, 1995, p. 494).

Frequently in cases involving a failure to diagnose or a misdiagnosis, the issues of what did the provider consider in the differential diagnosis and what was the basis for each differential are frequently raised by the plaintiff. These issues are raised to determine if the provider even considered the alleged correct diagnosis at all, and to determine if the provider possessed the proper knowledge and diagnostic reasoning to reach the proper diagnosis. As the ACNP is aware, a differential diagnosis reflects the most probable causes of the patient's problem and are generally ranked in descending order of probability. It is common knowledge in the medical community, and accepted practice, that providers do not customarily document all of the potential differential diagnoses. Unfortunately, at the time of a lawsuit, the provider will be expected to recall all of the thought processes at the time of treatment. Again, documentation is a key factor in medical malpractice suits and pertinent differential diagnoses should be documented.

Similar factors discussed in the section regarding how to avoid an allegation for failure to adequately assess can be applied to minimize the risk of liability for failing to properly diagnose or a misdiagnosis allegation. The ACNP needs to obtain a complete history, not only of the presenting complaint but also regarding prior medical problems, any prior or current treatment, and any relevant family and social history. If the ACNP, due to the time constraints of the acute care setting, takes short cuts in obtaining a complete history or in performing a thorough exam, then the ACNP may miss relevant information that would lead the ACNP to consider other conditions in the differential diagnosis. A subsequent history obtained by another provider that contains relevant information may be used to support an allegation of a misdiagnosis or a delay in diagnosis. It is difficult to overcome such evidence. Over-reliance on certain historical facts, and failing to verify historical facts, can mislead the ACNP and result in a misdiagnosis or a failure to properly diagnose the patient's condition.

Clearly, a complete and thorough physical examination is essential to reaching the appropriate diagnosis. Equally important is the performance of a follow-up exam to determine any change, improvement, or new findings. Ordering a diagnostic test in place of performing a physical exam (i.e., ordering a mammogram without performing a breast exam) is considered a breach of the standard of care, and that provider could be held liable, even though the mammogram had been improperly interpreted as negative (Schiffman, 1995, p. 502). Additional ways to avoid a failure to diagnose allegation include: (1) ordering, in a timely manner, the proper diagnostic tests, and, (2) obtaining the proper referral to insure that a complete evaluation is accomplished to ascertain the cause of the patient's problem and the correct diagnosis is reached.

Failure to Properly Treat or Intervene

The second major allegation asserted in medical malpractice claims is negligent treatment—the failure to properly treat (omission), or initiation of the wrong treatment (commission), or a delaying treatment (Brent, 1997, p. 42). In the acute care setting, the failure of the ACNP to respond to a change in the patient's physical condition (such as developing hypovolemic shock, or congestive heart failure), a change in the patient's level of consciousness, or failing to note an abnormal lab test results can result in an allegation for the failure to properly treat or intervene if the ACNP's inaction causes harm to the patient. Responding quickly and competently to certain situations is a primary duty of the ACNP. The ACNP must develop the ability to perform a careful assessment and analysis of the patient in a relatively short period of time while avoiding a hurried conclusion and initiating improper treatment.

The fact that the ACNP did not intend to harm the patient is of little consequence in a malpractice suit. Proof of the intent to harm is not an essential element of a malpractice claim (Brent, 1997, p. 42).

An allegation for the failure to properly treat is based upon the principle that the ACNP knew or should have known the proper treatment and the ACNP breached the ACNP's duty in failing to initiate the proper treatment, which resulted in harm to the patient. Several cases illustrative of this allegation are discussed.

In the 1980 case of *Gugino v. Harvard Community Health Plan,* one of the reasons for holding the NP liable for negligence was that the NP failed to properly and timely treat the patient's pelvic infection. In fact, the NP had prescribed the incorrect treatment when she advised the patient to douche with yogurt (*Gugino v. Harvard*, 1980). In *Fein v. Permanente,* in addition to a failure to diagnose allegation, the plaintiff also alleged that the NP, as well as the physician, failed to properly treat the patient's chest pain, which was subsequently diagnosed as a myocardial infarction (Fein, 1985).

Another case that is illustrative of improper treatment is the 1992 case of *Callahan v. Cardinal Glennon Hospital* in which the Missouri Court of Appeal upheld a $16 million judgment for the minor plaintiff (*Callahan v. Cardinal*, 1992). In this case, it was alleged that a pediatric nurse practitioner (PNP) on an acute care unit failed to properly treat the patient's perirectal abscess. The PNP had properly diagnosed the patient's problem but failed to incise and drain the abscess or obtain any bacterial cultures, and prescribed the incorrect antibiotic (Oxacillin) which is effective for gram positive bacilli, but not gram negative (Callahan, 1992). The minor continued over the next three days with an elevated fever and was seen by another health-care provider who continued the treatment prescribed by the PNP. The minor developed neurological deficits, and ultimately developed paralysis of his left arm and both legs. Expert testimony was presented that the improperly treated infection had significantly suppressed the patient's immune system, resulting in the patient developing paralysis as a complication of receiving a polio vaccine two weeks prior to the abscess diagnosis. The minor's abscess was finally incised and drained and the cultures showed four different types of gram negative bacteria, but no gram positive bacteria. Expert testimony was presented to establish that the abscess should have been incised and drained and cultures obtained at the time of the initial visit with the PNP and that the antibiotic prescribed by the PNP was the incorrect treatment for this patient's condition (Callahan, 1992).

Another case also illustrative of the failure to properly treat and intervene is a 1994 case in California that was settled for $1 million (*Confidential Report for Attorneys,* 1994). This case involved an obstetric nurse practitioner who evaluated a pregnant woman complaining of leaking clear fluid from her vagina. At the time of the evaluation, the NP did not perform any diagnostic tests to determine if the patient had premature rupture of membranes. Nor did the NP consult with a physician, thus failing to initiate the office protocol for possible premature rupture of the membranes. The patient was, instead, sent home with reassurances that there was no premature rupture of membranes. Four days later the patient was admitted with signs of infection and choriamnionitis. The baby was born with sepsis and developed cerebral palsy, quadriparesis, and severe development delays. At the time of the NP's deposition, the NP testified that since she did not observe any fluid leaking from the cervical os, she did not want to do a nitrazine or ferning test as she knew of many false positives. The NP acknowledged, however, that she didn't think to do the test to look for a negative result that could potentially rule out the issue of premature rupture (*Confidential,* 1994). The medical malpractice allegation in this case was that the NP failed to initiate the proper diagnostic workup and consultation with a physician for possible premature rupture of the membranes and thus resulted in a delay of the proper treatment for the patient's condition, and would have prevented harm to her baby (*Confidential,* 1994).

To avoid liability for the failure to properly treat or intervene, the ACNP must use accepted community standards of treatment and be sure to fully investigate and evaluate the nature of the patient's condition before initiating treatment. Although it is human nature to want to quickly relieve a patient's discomfort and give the patient reassurance, administering treatment before determining the correct diagnosis, or delaying treatment because of an incorrect diagnosis, will result in harm to the patient and the ACNP is held liable for that harm.

Failure to Obtain a Timely Consult or Referral

One of the hallmarks of a competent ACNP is knowing the limits of the ACNP's scope of practice, recognizing the necessity for a consultation or referral, and obtaining it in a timely manner. Since the role of the ACNP is fairly new, challenges to the ACNP regarding the scope of practice may occur frequently until the role becomes more known and accepted within the medical and legal communities. A part of that challenge may be the legal allegation that the ACNP failed to obtain a physician consultation in a timely manner. Another allegation may be that, due to the acuteness of the patient's condition, the patient should have been treated by a physician or the ACNP should have consulted with a physician, if not referred the patient. If the ACNP functions under a set of protocols, standardized procedures, or clinical guidelines, these documents are frequently used by the court to establish the ACNP's standard of care. A presumption of negligence is raised if the ACNP fails to comply with the protocols, standardized procedures, or clinical guidelines.

In the case of *Sermchief v. Gonzales,* the Court of Appeals reversed the lower court's decision and held that the two nurse practitioners were functioning within their scope of practice in providing gynecological and family planning services (Sermchief, 1983). The allegation against the NPs in this case was that the NPs should have referred their patients to physicians since the NPs were performing services that were within the domain of the practice of medicine. In a case that resulted in a $750,000 settlement for the wrongful death of a mother and child, a certified nurse midwife was charged with a breach of the statutory duty to consult a physician when there was a significant change in either the mother's or child's condition (Sermchief, 1983). The nurse midwife allegedly failed to recognize that the mother's condition was consistent with preeclampsia.

The duty to refer to another provider who possesses a higher level of skill and knowledge than the ACNP arises when the ACNP recognizes or should recognize that the ACNP lacks the sufficient knowledge or skills to provide competent care for the patient's problem or when the patient is not responding to treatment. Failure to obtain a timely consult or make a timely referral may compromise the patient's health and, especially in the acute care setting, can threaten the patient's survival. The fact that the ACNP obtains a consultation or makes a referral is not in any way an indication of incompetence, but rather the act of a professional who understands his or her limitations.

AVOIDING EXPOSURE TO LIABILITY

One of the primary goals of this chapter is to provide the ACNP some insight into the potential issues that can give rise to the exposure to liability. Understanding the legal principles and the various allegations that may be filed against the ACNP assists the ACNP in establishing good practice habits and improves the quality of the ACNP's care to patients and interactions with other providers.

Key factors in avoiding liability were discussed throughout this chapter. Maintaining competency is, and should continue to be, one of the ACNP's primary goals. The ACNP must keep abreast of the legal changes that will effect health care in general, and more specifically, the ACNP's practice. Thus, continuing education is imperative.

Proper documentation is another primary factor in avoiding liability. Without the proper documentation, a legal case against the ACNP may be lost or result in a settlement. Proper documentation validates the care by the ACNP and represents the quality of care that is provided. Documentation can establish that the ACNP has met the affirmative duty of due care and reflects the basis for the ACNP's clinical decisions. The ACNP's documentation of today can be the best defense against any litigation brought in the future against the ACNP or in a matter involving the ACNP's care.

Another important factor in avoiding liability is the ACNP's understanding the limits of the ACNP's knowledge and skills, and thus enabling the ACNP to function within the ACNP's scope of practice. With time and experience, the ACNP's knowledge and skills increase and there is less need for supervision and perhaps a decrease in the number of consultations and referrals. The ACNP is cautioned, however, to document any expansion of the ACNP's knowledge and skills, and any mentoring or proctoring, to demonstrate the ACNP's ability to perform a new procedure or manage a more complex patient problem.

Finally, the ACNP should participate in a peer review that evaluate the ACNP's practice to determine if the ACNP is practicing within the standards of the community. If the

ACNP is functioning under standardized procedures or protocols, these documents must reflect the ACNP's actual practice and be revised on a periodic basis to keep them current. The ACNP is encouraged to participate and be an active member in the professional organizations, not only for the benefits of networking and for the ACNP's personal growth, but also for the ACNP's valuable input regarding the development of the ACNP role and its legal recognition.

The role of the ACNP is evolving. Associated with that is the legal accountability of the ACNP. The ACNP must understand the legal principles that are applicable to the ACNP's standard of care, scope of practice, and the potential legal theories and allegations that may arise in the acute care setting. The ACNP will then be well prepared to continue to provide competent care to patients and withstand any legal challenge to the ACNP's practice.

REFERENCES

Aiken, T. & Catalano, J. (1994). Documentation. *Legal, Ethical and Political Issues in Nursing* (pp. 234–250). Philadelphia: F.A. Davis Company.

Aiken, T. & Catalano, J. (1994). Standard of care. *Legal, Ethical, and Political Issues in Nursing.* (pp. 57–75). Philadelphia: F.A. Davis Co.

Alexander, M., Bourgeois, A., Goodman, L. & Higgs, M. (1996). An acute/critical care nurse practitioner program. *Nursing Management* (28B-28C).

American Nurses Association (1994). Scope of acute care advanced nursing practice and the standard of acute care advanced nursing practice. Washington DC: American Nurses Association.

Andrews, M., Goldberg, K. & Kaplan, H. (Eds.). (1996). Malpractice liability. *Nurses Legal Handbook, 5* (3rd edition). (pp. 198–235). Springfield, PA: Springfield Corporation.

Andrews, M., Goldberg, K. & Kaplan, H. (Eds.) (1996). Patient's rights. *Nurses Legal Handbook.* (3rd edition). (pp. 60–100). Springhouse, PA: Springhouse Co.

Armstrong v. Flowers Hospital, Inc., 812 F. Supp. 1183 (M.D. Ala. 1993), Call No. 93–6502 (October 3, 1994).

Barber v. Superior Crt. (1983).

Beckom v. United States, 584 F.Supp. 1471, 1477, 1478 (1984).

Bianco, E. & Hirsch, H. (1995). Consent to and refusal of medical treatment. *Legal Medicine* (3rd edition). (pp. 274–296). St. Louis: Mosby.

Birkholz, G. (1995). Malpractice data from the national data bank. *Nurse Practitioner, 20* (3), 22–35.

Blackman for *Blackman v. Rifkin,* 759 P.2d 54 (Colo. Ct. App. 1988).

Blouin, H. & Brent, N. (1995) Selected causes of action beyond professional negligence. *Journal of Nursing Administration,* 25 (3), 11–12, 55.

Breithaupht v. Abram, 352 U.S. 432 (1957) and *Schmerber v. Calif.,* 384 U.S. 757 (1966) as discussed by Bianco, E., & Hirsch, H. (1995). 290–291.

Brent, N. (Ed.) (1997) (2) The nurse and the judicial system. *Nurses and the Law* (pp. 15–37). Philadelphia: W.B. Saunders.

Brent, N. (1997). Concepts of negligence, professional negligence and liability. In Brent, N. (Ed), *Nurses and the Law* (pp 39–64). Philadelphia: W.B. Saunders.

Brent, N. (1997). (Ed.) (3) Professional negligence: Prevention and defense. *Nurses and the Law* (pp. 65–85). Philadelphia: W. B. Saunders.

Brent, N. (Ed.) (1997). Other torts and civil rights. *Nurses and the Law.* (pp 105–125). Philadelphia: W.B. Saunders & Co.

Brent, N. (Ed.) (1997) Criminal law. *Nurses and the Law* (pp. 143–170). Philadelphia: W. B. Saunders.

Brent, N. (Ed.) (1997). Informed consent and refusal of treatment. *Nurses and the Law.* (pp. 237–268). Philadelphia: W. B. Saunders.

Brent, N. (Ed.) (1997). Nurse as an Employee. *Nurses and the Law* (pp. 359–401). Philadelphia: W. B. Saunders.

Brent, N. (Ed.) (1997). The nurse in acute care setting. *Nurses and the Law* (pp. 403–422). Philadelphia: W. B. Saunders.

Callahan v. Cardinal Glennon Hosptial, 1561 Lexus 80 (Ct. of App., Mo. E. Dist., Div. 3) (1992).

Canterbury v. Spence, 464 F. 2d 772 (D.C. 1972).

Cobb v. Grant, 502 P.2d 1 (Calif. 1972).

Cruzan v. Director, 100 S. Ct. 2851 (1990); *Bouvia v. Riverside General Hosp.,* 225 Cal. Rptr. 287 (1986); *Barber v. Superior Crt.,* 147 Cal. App. 3d 1006, 196 Cal. Rptr. 484 (1983); and *In Re the Matter of Karen Quinlan* 429 U.S. 922, crt.denied, 335 A.2d 679, 70 N.J. 10 (1976).

Daum v. Spinecare Medical Group, 52 C.A. 4th 1285 (1997).

Dentist's refusal to treat HIV positive patient in his office violated Americans with Disabilities Act, citing *Abbott v. Bragdon,* No. 96–1643 (1st Cir., March 5, 1997), *Medical Liability Reporter, 19,* (3), 50–53.

Doe v. N. Y. State, 588 N.Y.S. 2d 698 (Ct. Cl. 1992), 595 N.Y. S 2d 592 (N.Y. Appellate Div., 1993) rev. in part 588 N.Y.S.2d 698 (Ct. Cl. 1992).

Dolan v. Galluzo, 396 N. E. 2d 13 (Ill. 1979).

Eccard, W. & Guinn, E. (1994). Legal ramifications for expanded practice. *Legal, Ethical and Political Issues in Nursing* (pp. 281–308). Philadelphia: F. A. Davis Co.

El-Sherif, C. (1995). Nurse practitioners, where do they belong in the organizational structure of the acute care setting. *Nurse Practitioner, 20,* (1). 62, 64–65.

Federal regulations require disclosure of medical device's investigational status; expert testimony not required to establish informed consent claim where duty of disclosure was imposed by statute or regulation. (1997). *Medical Liability Reporter, 19,* (3), 61–62.

Fein v. Permanente, 695 P. 2d 665, 38 Cal.3d 137. 211 Cal. Rptr. 368 (1985).

Feutz, S. (Ed.) (1989). Common sources of liability. *Nursing and the Law.* (3rd edition). (pp. 111–193). Eau Claire: Professional Education Systems, Inc.

Feutz, S. (Ed.) (1989). Confidentiality and privacy issues. *Nursing and the Law,* (3rd edition). (pp. 93–109). Eau Claire: Professional Education Systems, Inc.

Feutz, S. (Ed.) (1989). Professional negligence and intentional torts. *Nursing and the Law* (3rd edition). (pp. 13–28). Eau Claire: Professional Education System Inc.

Firestone, M. (1995). Psychiatric patients and forsenic psychiatry. *Legal Medicine.* (3rd edition). (pp. 585–614). St. Louis: Mosby.

Flamm, M. (1995). Health care provider as a defendant. *Legal Medicine* (3rd edition). (pp. 118–128). St. Louis: Mosby.

Gostin, L. (1993). Drawing a line between killing and letting die. The law, and law reform on medically assisted dying. *The Journal of Law, Medicine, & Ethics, 21* (1), 94–101.

Guigino v. Harvard Community Health Plan, 403 N.E. 2d 1166, 380 Mass. 464 (1980).

Henry, P. (1997). Legal issues in advanced practice. *Nurses and the Law.* (pp. 491–515). Philadelphia: W.B. Saunders.

Henry, P. (1996). Analysis of the nurse practitioner's legal relationships. *Nurse Practitioner Forum, 7* (1), 5–6.

Henry, P. (1994). Legal principles in providing telephone advice. *Nurse Practitioner Forum, 5* (3) 124–125.

Henry, P. (1991) Disciplinary action by the nursing board. *Nurse Practitioner Forum, 2,* 144–145.

Hoffman, A. (1995). Medical malpractice. *Legal Medicine* (3rd edition). (pp. 129–140). St. Louis: Mosby.

Hollowel, E. & Block, B. (1995). Coproviders and institutional practice. *Legal Medicine* (3rd edition). (pp. 635–661). St. Louis: Mosby.

Howard, M. & Vogt, L. (1995). Physician–patient relationship. *Legal Medicine* (3rd edition) (pp. 265–273). St. Louis: Mosby.

In *Re Helga Wanglie Fourth Judicial District* (Dist, Crt. Probate Crt. Div.) PX-91-283, Hennepin Cty, Minn. (1991).

Jenkins, S. (1994). The myth of vicarious liability. *Journal of Nurse–Midwifery, 39* (2), 98–106.

John F. Kennedy Hospital v. Bludworth, 452 S. 2d 921 (Florida 1984).

Knaus, V., Felter, S., Burton, S., Forbes, P. & Davis, K. (1997). The use of nurse practitioner in acute care setting. *Journal of Nursing Administration, 27* (2), 20–27.

Ladimer, I. (1995). Alternative dispute resolution in health care. *Legal Medicine* (3rd Edition). (pp. 78–86). St. Louis: Mosby.

MacDonald, George (Ed.) (1992). Initial case presentation. *California Medical Malpractice.* (pp. 177–301). St. Paul: West Publishing Co.; citing *Robinson v. Duszynski,* 243 S.E.2d 148,151–152, 36 N.C. App. 103 (1978), and *Fridena v. Evans,* 622 P.2d 463, 466, 127 Ariz. 516 (1980).

Matter of Westchester County Medical Center, 531 N.E.2d 607, 534 N.Y.S. 2d 886, 72 N.Y.2d 517 (1988).

McCella, F. (1994) The common law of medical malpractice. *Medical Malpractice* (pp. 24–44). Philadelphia: Temple University Press.

McClosky, J. (1997, May 15) The role of the ACNP. Symposium conducted at Long Beach Memorial Medical Center, Long Beach, California for California State University, Los Angeles students enrolled in the ACNP program.

McMahon, M., (1993), Joint and several liability of physicians whose independent negligence in treatment of patient causes indivisible injury. *American Law Reports, 9,* 746–825. (5th edition). Rochester: Lawyers Cooperative Publishing.

Mezez, M. & McGiven, D. (Eds.) (1993). Nurses, nurse practitioner, evolution to advanced practice. *Advanced Practice Nursing, A Guide to Professional Development.* (pp. 281–310). Springhouse, PA: Springhouse Publishing Co.

Monicken, D. (1995). Consultation in advanced practice nursing. *Advanced Practice Nursing, A Guide to Professional Development* (pp. 183–195). New York: Springhouse Publishing.

Morgenroth v. Pacific Care Medical Center, 54 Cal. App. 3d 521, 533, 126 Cal. Rptr. 681 (1976).

Nurse Practitioner blamed for bad baby; cerebral palsy, spastic quadriparesis. (1994). *Confidential Report for Attorneys, 19,* 21–22.

Paola, F. & Anderson, J. (1995) The process of dying. *Legal Medicine.* (3rd edition). (pp. 404–423). St. Louis: Mosby.

Paola, F. & Anderson, J. (1995). 413, citing *Matter of Storar,* 454 U.S. 858, cert. denied, 420 N.E.2d 64, 438 N.Y.S. 2d 266 (1976).

Pearson, L. & Birkholz, G. (1995). Report on the 1994 readership survey on NP experience with malpractice issues. *Nurse Practitioner, 20* (3), 18, 21–30.

Richard, T. & Keane, A. (1996). Acute care nurse practitioners. *Advanced Practice Nursing* (pp. 316–326). Philadelphia: Lippincott.

Rochin v. Calif., 342 U.S. 165 (1952).

Royal, M. (1995) Patients with human immunodeficiency virus (HIV) infection and acquired immunodeficiency syndrome (AIDS). *Legal Medicine* (3rd edition). (pp. 516–530); footnote #366 citing PA Confidentiality Information Act, 35 P.S. section 7601 et seq. Act No. 1990–148; California Health and Safety Code section 199.21 (West 1991); Appendix 36–4, Reporting requirements for HIV infections. *Legal Medicine* (3rd edition) (p. 530). St. Louis: Mosby.

Schiffman, M. (1995) Oncology patients. *Legal Medicine* (3rd edition) (pp. 494–508). St. Louis: Mosby.

Schloendorff v. Society of New York Hospitals, 105 N.E. 92 (1914).

Sermchief v. Gonzales, 660 S.W. 2d 683 (Mo. banc. 1983).

Smith, J. & Kelly, M. (1987). Nurses employed as practitioners, anesthetists, midwives, clinical specialists. *Legal Issues in Nursing.* (pp. 363–378). Philadelphia: Mosby.

Stepp v. Review Board of the Indiana Employment Security Division, 521 N.E. 2d 350 (Ind. App. Crt. 1988).

Tarsoff v. Regents of the University of California, 551 P2d 334, 131 Cal. Rptr. 14, 529 P2d 334, 17 Cal. 3d 425 (1976).

7

Ethical Decision Making

Juanita Reigle

The health-care environment is one in which acute care nurse practitioners (ACNPs) practice changes constantly. Increased economic pressures, expanded medical technologies, and the changing roles of health-care professionals present new clinical challenges and diverse moral issues. Although ethics have always been central to nursing, now more than ever, a general knowledge of biomedical ethics and decision-making theory is essential to navigate moral issues.

As an advanced practice nurse, the ACNP must develop ethical sensitivity and an ability to engage in moral reasoning. Ethical sensitivity is an awareness of the moral aspects of a position or situation. An individual's ethical sensitivity is distinct and is influenced by values, culture, religion, and education. Moral reasoning, on the other hand, is a cognitive and deliberate process. It involves analyzing a moral dilemma, determining what ought to be done and formulating an ethically sensible plan of action. To develop these processes, both knowledge and experience are essential (Fry, 1994).

The purpose of this chapter is to provide the ACNP with some fundamental information that contributes to the development of ethical sensitivity and moral reasoning. The chapter explores the various roles of values, ethical theories and principles, and approaches to conflict resolution. The concepts of shared decision making and informed consent are discussed as frameworks to enhance moral reasoning. The chapter concludes with a discussion of ethical resources for the ACNP. A comprehensive discussion of particular clinical issues is beyond the scope of this chapter; however, the information provided will assist the ACNP in framing moral issues and developing a plan of action for most dilemmas encountered in practice.

▶ THE ROLE OF VALUES

Values are beliefs or attitudes that have motivational power and guide an individual's behavior. Values provide a frame of reference from which an individual can evaluate and synthesize new ideas and concepts (Uustal,1987). An individual's personal value system is influenced by his or her culture, religion, education, and life experiences.

Professional values are those beliefs respected and honored by a professional group. The American Nurses Association's *Code for Nurses* delineates both the professional values and ethical principles prized by the profession. Other professional groups, such as the American Association of Critical-Care Nurses, provide insight into professional values through position papers and standards of practice.

Value Clarification

Value clarification enables one to uncover beliefs and values that influence behavior, but of which we may not be consciously aware. By raising the value to our awareness, we can choose to retain it or prioritize it in a different manner.

Personal and professional values can be in opposition and create an internal conflict for the ACNP. In addition, the ACNP will encounter situations in which his or her personal or professional values are in conflict with the patient's or another health-care professional's values. Because values influence decisions and actions on both personal and professional levels, it is important for the ACNP to be aware of the underlying values that uphold a specific position. Although professional codes provide some guidance in these situations, value clarification exercises assist individuals in the identification of central values that guide life choices (Uustal, 1987).

ETHICAL THEORIES

A general understanding of ethical theories provides insight into the various frameworks for approaching ethical dilemmas. Because individuals involved in the decision-making process often consider their positions from different theoretical frameworks, it is important for the ACNP to have a basic knowledge of the more dominant bioethical theories.

Utilitarian Theory

Utilitarianism, or consequentialism, is a theory maintaining that the moral rightness of actions are determined by the balance of their good or bad consequences. A general guideline for a utilitarian is to produce the "greatest good for the greatest number." Act utilitarians morally assess their decisions and actions on the principle of utility. In other words, if an action produces maximal value it is justified to the act utilitarian. Rule utilitarians, on the other hand, conform to rules that promote utility. Rather than disregard particular rules, the rule utilitarian respects rules even if it does not always maximize the general good (Beauchamp & Childress, 1994).

Deontological Theory

A deontological approach, also referred to as Kantianism or Formalism, argues that the moral rightness of an action is determined by particular features of the act in addition to the consequences. Embracing particular rules, such as maintaining confidentiality, or upholding a particular duty or obligation, such as parent–child relationships, are basic features in a deontological approach to moral reasoning. For example, a deontologist is more apt to believe that lying is inherently wrong. The consequences are incidental; it is the act of lying, in itself, that is wrong. On the other hand, a pure utilitarian also may agree that lying is wrong, but only because of the consequences, not because of the action (Beauchamp & Childress, 1994).

Virtue Ethics

Virtue ethics, or character ethics, emphasize the individual and the moral choices expressed in the individual's actions. Moral character is evident in the manner in which the individual displays good judgment, such as demonstrating courage, generosity, or temperance. When ethical dilemmas arise, virtue ethics rely on the individual character to make the best judgments, rather than relying on rules or calculating consequences (Beauchamp & Childress, 1994).

Ethic of Care

The ethical theory of caring has emerged as a critique of traditional, western approaches to biomedical ethics. This approach, first introduced in feminist literature, argues that the traditional approach to ethical problems reflects a male bias. The ethic of care maintains that viewing moral problems from a perspective of impartiality and distance does not acknowledge the intricacy of human relationships and the resulting moral responsibilities (Gilligan, 1982). Indeed, other ethical theories do not emphasize the role of intimate personal relationships and other values such as love, compassion, or fidelity when approaching ethical issues. A "caring" perspective argues that individuals are not islands, and the resolution of issues must consider the contextual aspects of the situation, such as current relationships and responsibilities (Beauchamp & Childress, 1994; Cooper, 1989; Gilligan, 1982).

Casuistic Theory

In a casuistic theory, individual cases and the reasoning behind these cases set the stage for moral decision making and reflection. A casuistic approach involves using "paradigm cases" and identifying elements of the current case that conform to aspects of analogous cases. Paradigm cases are grounded in experience, tradition, and a thoughtful and rationale approach to resolution (Ahronheim, Moreno, & Zuckerman, 1994). For example, classic cases, such as the cases of Karen Ann Quinlan or Nancy Cruzan, serve to advance the decision-making process surrounding end-of-life care.

Principle-Based Theory

A principle-based theory relies on ethical principles and rules to guide moral action. The principles and rules are derived from common morality and are used to shape moral arguments. Four general principles are used to identify, define, discuss, and analyze the moral elements of a dilemma. A principle-based theory emphasizes principles of obligation and, thus, suggests that particular actions ought (or ought not) to be supported (Beauchamp & Childress, 1994).

The four main principles embraced in clinical decision making are respect for autonomy, beneficence, nonmaleficence, and justice. These principles have two common features. First, the principles are prima facie binding. This means that principles are neither expendable nor absolute. However a principle should not be violated unless there is a compelling reason to do so. Second, principles are universally important and can be applied across all cultures. There is no defined hierarchy of principles and no one particular principle that trumps all others. An appeal to principles does not result in the answer to a moral dilemma; instead, principles and rules serve to guide an individual in moral reasoning (Beauchamp & Childress, 1994).

Respect for Autonomy

The principle of autonomy maintains that individuals ought to be free to make choices without undue controlling forces and to act according to these choices. To respect a person's autonomy is to acknowledge his or her right to have opinions, make choices, and act in accordance with personal values and beliefs (Beauchamp & Childress, 1994). One does not have to agree with another's choices to respect autonomy. In fact, respecting another's autonomy means that we respect their good choices as well as the decisions with which we disagree.

The key to respecting autonomy is to assure that the individual is functionally capable of making a decision. The fundamental elements of decision-making capacity are: the ability to understand the problem and the consequences; the ability to reason and deliberate about the problem; the ability to communicate the decision; and the ability to make a free and independent choice (Applebaum & Grisso, 1988).

In the clinical setting, there are certain constraints on autonomy that, whenever possible, should be minimized to enhance an individual's free choice. The hospital environment, the amount and manner in which information is provided, or lack of financial resources can suppress an individual's autonomy. Patients may lack capacity to make independent decisions during the course of an illness, such as patients requiring neuromuscular blockade, or due to an illness, such as patients with advanced Alzheimer's disease. Respect is still owed such patients, and other ethically justified approaches, such as reliance on surrogate decision makers, may be used to uphold the patient's previously defined values.

Beneficence

The principle of beneficence is a central theme in the professional values and practice of nursing. Beneficence requires us to act in ways that benefit or contribute to the welfare of others. Several rules of beneficence have been identified. These rules are to: (1) protect and defend the rights of others, (2) prevent evil or harm, (3) remove evil or harm, (4) help others with disabilities, and (5) rescue others in danger (Beauchamp & Childress, 1994). Clearly these rules reflect a range of moral requirements and they should not be interpreted as morally obligatory on all occasions. Some actions, such as donating one's kidney to a stranger in need, are supererogatory acts of extreme generosity and are morally praiseworthy, but not obligatory. The obligation to act becomes more compelling when the relationship changes. For example, most would agree that the duty of a father to donate a kidney to his daughter suggests a more positive requirement for action than the act of donating to a stranger.

There are, of course, limits to beneficence. We could become so consumed with an unqualified obligation to do good for others that we neglect our primary responsibilities. We have an obligation to act in a beneficent manner when the action does not significantly interfere with our life plans or pose serious personal risk. Therefore, limits to beneficence generally are distinguished by the sacrifices incurred by the moral agent (Beauchamp & Childress, 1994).

The special relationship between the ACNP and the patient depicts a powerful commitment and understanding that upholds the moral obligations of beneficence. Clinical decisions and interventions are directed toward doing good and preventing harm. Unfortunately, confusion and uncertainty surface when there is a misunderstanding or misinterpretation of what is good. The patient's values and the preferences of the ACNP may be incongruent, and the question becomes not "What is good?" but "Who should decide what is good?" (Beauchamp & Childress, 1994). This clash between autonomy and beneficence is not uncommon and is the undercurrent in many well-known court cases, such as the Bouvia case. Balancing the duty of beneficence with respect for personal autonomy is a major objective of the strategies used in conflict resolution.

Nonmaleficence

Nonmaleficence is the obligation not to inflict evil or harm intentionally (Beauchamp & Childress, 1994). Some of the earliest medical and nursing documents defend this principle openly. The Nightingale Pledge states that the nurse ". . . will abstain from whatever is deleterious and mischievous, and will not take or knowingly administer any harmful drug" (Gretter, 1893). Other rules of nonmaleficence include: do not kill, do not inflict pain, and do not disable (Beauchamp & Childress, 1994).

The difference between preventing harm or evil (beneficence) and not inflicting harm or evil (nonmaleficence) lies in the need for action. Duties of nonmaleficence, such as prohibiting killing or disablement, require refraining from a particular action. Obligations of beneficence—the duties to prevent and remove harm or promote good—require one to take action (Beauchamp & Childress, 1994).

The principle of nonmaleficence is not absolute and examples of inflicting harm for the patient's benefit are numerous. A patient with a gangrenous leg requiring amputation is entitled to the necessary surgery, even though the surgeon is obligated by the principle of nonmaleficence not to intentionally disable. The key is to focus on a risk–benefit analysis. Certainly, if the patient agrees, the loss of a limb outweighs the risk of foregoing the surgery and the probable sepsis and death that would follow.

In addition to appealing to a risk–benefit analysis, the rule of double effect is invoked to justify claims that an act with foreseeable harmful effects is not always morally prohibited (Beauchamp & Childress, 1994). Some of the most common examples of the use of this rule are situations in which a terminally ill patient in extreme pain requires high doses of morphine sulfate that may cause respiratory depression. If the ACNP does not prescribe or administer the medication, the patient will suffer. Yet if the medication is administered, respiratory depression may ensue and the patient may die.

Four conditions must be met to morally justify an act with a double effect. These conditions are: (1) the act must be good or at least morally neutral, (2) the agent intends only the good effect, even though the harmful effect is foreseen and permitted, (3) the harmful effect cannot be a means to the good effect, and (4) the good effect outweighs the bad effect (Beauchamp & Childress, 1994). In the previous example, the ACNP did not intend to cause the patient's death, but rather meant to alleviate suffering. However, the foreseeable consequence of respiratory depression should be discussed with the patient or appropriate surrogate so all parties recognize the potential consequence and tolerate or permit its presence. If the goals of treatment are directed toward promoting comfort and minimizing suffering, the aggressive use of morphine to realize this goal is appropriate. On the other hand, if the patient expresses a desire to live in any state and willingly tolerates extreme pain to prolong life, the good effect would be interpreted as extending life, and any medication that foreseeably could hasten death would be unacceptable.

Justice

The principle of justice suggests an appreciation of fairness, equity, and entitlement. There are many theories of justice, each with its own philosophical perspective of moral life. However, the most common application of this principle in health care is in the area of distributive justice. Distributive justice focuses on the fair, equitable, and appropriate allocation of goods and services. Usually, issues of distributive justice arise when there is competition for scarce resources. For example, issues surrounding the distribution of scarce organs for transplantation reflect problems in distributive justice (Beauchamp & Childress, 1994).

There are five commonly held material principles of distributive justice. The material principles of distributive justice are: (1) to each person an equal share, (2) to each person according to need, (3) to each person according to effort, (4) to each person according to contribution, (5) to each person according to merit, and (6) to each person according to free market exchanges. It is easy to see how each principle could be applied to the issue of organ transplantation, and result in several different methods to allocate the scarce resource. Although each material principle has merit, they cannot be exercised independent of the contextual features of a particular situation (Beauchamp & Childress, 1994). For example, choosing to allocate scarce organs for transplantation on the basis of contribution or merit raises questions about whether this approach has relevance in this situation. Does a physician in need of a heart transplant present a more compelling case than a janitor with the same level of need? Society has determined that individual contributions are not valid considerations in a fair system of allocating scarce organs. However, distribution based on merit and societal contribution is appropriate when considered for distributing limited research funds.

Many issues of justice that occur in the clinical setting are not answered by societal decisions. Triage decisions often reflect the material principles of justice. The last ICU bed may be allocated, based on need, to a severely ill patient being transferred from another hospital. Or, perhaps the decision is influenced by factors other than need, such as merit or contribution. In that case the preferred decision may be to admit a philanthropist, with a lesser need, but who has contributed to the development of a new cancer center for the hospital. In some cases there are clear clinical guidelines that define how and when particular resources are to be provided. But in many situations, it is the clinician who makes the case-by-case decision. The ACNP must remember not to abandon the central commitment to the patient when confronting issues with broad societal implications. However, in some institutions the decision in this particular example may be beyond the control of the ACNP. Even if the ACNP is not in a position to make the admission decision, he or she must be prepared to address any decision that appears nonethical or unethical and that effects the safety or well-being of others.

There remains considerable debate about what constitutes a decent minimum of health care and what makes a just system for the allocation of limited resources. Even the issue of access to health care has not been resolved for millions of Americans. These issues of justice will haunt the health-care system for many years. Maintaining an active voice in the political arena is one way in which the values of nursing will remain in the forefront.

▶ RESOLVING ETHICAL CONFLICTS

An understanding of personal and professional values, ethical theories, and principles and rules helps develop the framework for ethical analysis and decision making. This framework should help clarify the dilemma and illuminate specific features of the issue or situation. However, to move effectively toward resolution, it is important to realize the variety of mechanisms for resolving disagreement. A deliberate decision to employ one approach for problem resolution will enable the process to proceed in a more efficient manner, whereas, a random approach to resolution is inefficient, frustrating, and may intensify the conflict rather than resolve it.

The following methods of conflict resolution reflect a range of approaches to the decision-making process. Each technique has advantages and disadvantages associated with the process. The ACNP should understand each approach and consciously choose the manner to proceed toward resolution. By deliberately choosing one technique, the ACNP is clear about the process and expectations, and can effectively facilitate decision making.

Variables in Conflict Resolution

In all of the following approaches to conflict resolution, four variables have crucial roles in determining how to address the conflict. These elements are commitment to the relationship, moral certainty, time available, and cost–benefit ratio (Spielman,1993).

Commitment to the Relationship

Whether the clinician or patient has a high or low degree of commitment to the relationship will effect the technique used in conflict resolution. A high degree of commitment, as seen in patients who have longstanding relationships with their caregivers, tends to increase the individual's commitment to move toward decisions that reflect mutual acceptance of the decision (Spielman, 1993). For example, an ACNP who practices in a specialty area in which patients have a chronic illness is more likely to establish relationships with a high degree of commitment than an ACNP in an emergency setting in which most patients are seen for episodic and infrequent interventions.

Moral Certainty

Moral certainty, or the opinion that one is correct in his or her moral view, increases one's commitment to resolving the dilemma. When one is uncertain about the moral accuracy of a position, techniques such as accommodation or avoidance may be employed. Moral uncertainty may arise from incomplete information, inaccurate information, or a genuine indistinct moral position (Spielman, 1993).

Time Available

Avoidance, coercion, and accommodation are techniques in conflict resolution that require little time. There are some "ethical emergencies" in the clinical setting that may require immediate action regardless of the caregiver's commitment to the relationship. A child of Jehovah's Witnesses who requires an emergent blood transfusion presents a situation in which little time is available to reach a decision. When more time is available, other techniques such as compromise or collaboration are desirable to resolve the problem in a mutually satisfactory way (Spielman, 1993).

Cost–Benefit Ratio

Several factors influence the calculation of the cost–benefit analysis in the strategies for moral decision making. The benefit to the patient or health-care professional, the risk of disrupting professional relationships, and the negotiability of each party's position will influence the strategy used in conflict resolution (Spielman, 1993). If one party holds a position that is nonnegotiable, such as the Jehovah's Witnesses parents, techniques such as collaboration are unattainable. An intentional examination of the cost–benefit variables will enable the ACNP to identify the most effective strategies to conflict resolution.

Strategies to Resolve Conflicts

Avoidance

To deny, ignore, withdraw, or flee from confronting a moral dilemma is to engage in avoidance. This technique is most common when there is little commitment to the relationship, time is limited, the cost–benefit ratio is unfavorable, the issue is trivial, or the individual is uncertain about the moral rightness of his or her position (Spielman, 1993). An example of avoidance occurred when the ACNP working on a cardiology unit noticed that a cardiac surgeon consistently visited the CCU late at night to obtain patients' written consent for cardiac surgery the following day. Often the patients were asleep and in some cases they had received some sleep medication. The ACNP was concerned that consent was obtained without family members present and that the patients' ability to comprehend the complexity of the surgery was compromised from the sleep medication. Because the ACNP was uncertain of her moral position and was not committed to preserving her relationship with the physician, she avoided confronting the issue.

Although avoidance can be an appropriate approach to conflict, it is not a technique to practice regularly. Occasionally, issues that at first appear trivial become more significant as the frequency of the problem increases. When an individual cares about an issue or when the individual ignores the conflict but has lingering negative feelings, the use of avoidance is inappropriate. Moreover, an individual who habitually retreats from conflict should be advised and guided through other effective conflict-resolution approaches (Spielman, 1993).

Coercion

The use of coercion to resolve a dilemma is evident when one party insists on one's own way at the expense of others. This approach often results in open competition and ends with a win–lose situation. Coercion is used when time is short, there is little commitment to the relationship, and one feels a strong sense of moral rightness in the position (Spielman, 1993). Coercion may be appropriate in some emergency situations, such as administering a blood transfusion to a child of Jehovah's Witnesses. However, this approach often diminishes others' self-respect and is destructive to long-term relationships.

At times there seems to be a fine line between coercion and presenting a strong and persuasive argument. Many patients feel vulnerable and sense a loss of control in the health-care environment. Patients may perceive recommendations from the health-care team as absolute, controlling, and authoritative. In this relationship, patients feel powerless to negotiate or collaborate effectively and they respond with avoidance or anger. It is imperative that whenever possible, health-care recommendations be presented as proposed directions for care to be discussed and negotiated, rather than absolutes.

Accommodation

Accommodation occurs when one party agrees to the other party's position. This technique tends to take place when time is short, when the issue is not important to one party, or if the moral rightness of one's position is uncertain. One is more likely to appease or accept the other party's position if the relationship is valued and there is considerable concern for the other party (Spielman, 1993).

For example, a cardiologist discussed with the wife of a 30-year-old man suffering from an end-stage viral cardiomyopathy the futility of continuing aggressive treatment. The patient was receiving maximal interventions but the mean arterial pressure could not be raised above 45 mm Hg, and secondary complications including renal and hepatic failure had resulted. Despite this information, the wife insisted that her husband receive CPR. The cardiologist was uncertain of his moral position because the patient had recently become ill and the patient's wishes were unknown. The cardiologist agreed to the wife's request because she had little time to adjust to her husband's critical illness and this additional effort could provide some comfort to her during her bereavement.

Compromise

Engaging in compromise to resolve conflicts is effective when both parties do not wish to relinquish completely their positions, yet they are willing to bargain and reduce expectations. Thus, each party gives up some piece of their viewpoint in order to reach a solution. This "win some, lose some" outcome is useful when cooperation is important but time is somewhat limited. The willingness to compromise suggests that each party holds a strong loyalty to the relationship as well as a sincere moral commitment to their positions (Spielman, 1993).

An example of resolving a conflict using compromise occurred when J.T., a 42-year-old woman with type II diabetes mellitus continued to present to the emergency room with hyperglycemia. The ACNP who followed J.T. in clinic was frustrated with the patient's refusal to follow dietary and medication instructions provided to her on previous clinic visits. When it was clear that J.T. would not limit her intake of certain foods, the ACNP opted to bargain with J.T. to find a solution that could satisfy elements of each of their positions. J.T. agreed to increase the frequency of testing her blood sugar and adjusting her medication accordingly if the ACNP would agree not to dwell on J.T.'s dietary indiscretion.

Collaboration

In many situations collaboration is the ideal method to resolve conflict because both parties succeed in achieving a mutually satisfactory solution. Effective problem solving using a collaborative approach can only occur if the issue and relationship are important to both parties. Collaboration magnifies the creative potential of each party and leads to strengthened and improved relationships. Collaboration is not appropriate when time is short because this process requires time to gather information, identify alternative solutions, discuss the options, and formulate a decision (Spielman, 1993).

One of the keys to successful collaboration is that each party must focus on understanding the other's point of view and the beliefs and values that underlie the other's perceptions. This step in collaboration underscores the mutual respect between the parties because the varying viewpoints are discussed and carefully examined. This approach also emphasizes individual accountability, as each party must articulate his or her position as well as listen to the other's perspective (Krouse & Roberts, 1989). Because there is much dialogue involved with a collaborative approach, both parties must be willing to invest the time and energy necessary for successful resolution.

The following case illustrates a dilemma successfully resolved through a collaborative approach.

> M.J. was an 80-year-old widow with a history of emphysema and coronary artery disease who was admitted to the Medical Intensive Care Unit (MICU) with severe pneumonia. She required mechanical ventilation and was receiving IV antibiotic therapy. On the third day of her hospitalization she developed acute ECG changes consistent with a large anterior myocardial infarction. Despite attempts to limit the extent of the infarction, an echocardiogram at day six revealed severe global hypokinesis of the left ventricle.
>
> As the MICU nurses cared for M.J., they were uncertain that she wanted aggressive care to continue. M.J. had to be restrained to prevent her from pulling out the endotracheal and nasogastric tubes. She avoided making eye contact with the nurses and was often tearful when they talked with her. When provided pencil and paper to enable her to communicate with the staff, M.J. would write "Let me die" or "Take these tubes out." The nurses struggled with imposing care on a competent patient who was resisting the treatment plan.
>
> The physician's assessment of the situation was that M.J. could recover from the pneumonia. The heart failure could be managed medically and M.J. could return to a functional life. The physician wrote an order for additional pain medication because she believed that M.J.'s agitation was evidence of discomfort from the invasive tubes.
>
> The ACNP decided to facilitate a resolution to the problem by having all parties discuss their positions and agree on the issue in conflict. First the nurses and physician discussed their differing perspectives and concerns. Both parties agreed that the issue was the treatment plan and goals for M.J. Because M.J. had capacity to make decisions, the nurses and physician agreed to discuss their perspectives with her. The ACNP explained to M.J. that the physician and nurses were trying to create a

plan of care that best met M.J.'s needs. However, it was important to understand M.J.'s values and know how she wanted her care to proceed. M.J. was able to communicate her values of a functional and active life. She did not want to remain on life support for an indefinite amount of time and she was concerned that she would die before having an opportunity to complete a photograph album for her grandchildren.

During this collaborative approach to resolving the dilemma, some important information surfaced. First, the staff uncovered some meaningful aspects of M.J.'s life. M.J. had been very involved in community events and maintained an active presence with her friends and family. Her commitment and responsibilities to her family and friends were an important value to her. Furthermore, the staff was able to clarify some of M.J.'s misconceptions about being placed on life-sustaining technologies. M.J. was informed, to the best of the health-care team's abilities, about the likelihood of her recovery and what life would be like when she returned home. A discussion about future deterioration of her health and the impact the disease would have on her life were presented in an honest and caring manner.

Once M.J. understood the implications of her illness and was a recognized and involved member of the treatment discussions, the decision-making process moved forward. The physician and nurses, being clearer of M.J.'s interests, constructed a treatment plan with M.J. that was agreeable to all parties. Because the collaborative approach fostered open communication and established trust between M.J. and the health-care team, future issues were addressed as they occurred.

As described, successful outcomes to resolving moral dilemmas require a keen sense of the importance of the relationship to both parties, the amount of time available for resolution, and each party's moral conviction on the issue at hand (Spielman, 1993). In the case of M.J., seeking the patient's participation and discovering the underlying values were the initial steps that resulted in an effective collaborative process. The health-care team and M.J. shared responsibility for creating a mutually acceptable solution for a perceived dilemma. An environment in which shared decision making is valued and practiced cultivates trust and open communication.

▶ SHARED DECISION MAKING

Shared decision making is a model for open communication that is grounded in the principles of respect for personal autonomy and beneficence. The concept refers to an ongoing dialogue between the caregiver and patient in which the patient's information needs become known and are addressed by the primary providers of care (Karlawish, 1996). The decisions that emerge from this environment are informed choices that advance the values and beliefs of the particular patient (President's Commission, 1982). Shared decision making does not suggest that the family is distant from the decision. Instead, this comprehensive model acknowledges the many contextual features that influence decisions and it invites the perspectives of other involved parties into the process. Moreover, a collaborative and shared approach to decision making can neutralize the internal and external pressures that constrain moral action (Cooper, 1991).

There are several strategies to involve the patient and others in the decision-making process. Because patients and families often feel overwhelmed and exceedingly vulnerable in a health-care setting, these barriers must be identified and transcended before a collaborative environment is developed. The ACNP has a primary role in creating this relationship with individual patients as well as generating a practice environment in which shared decision making is supported.

As discussed earlier in this chapter, values play an important role in how individuals make decisions. The ACNP can help patients clarify values by asking directed questions such as "What are your thoughts about chronic illness?" or "What aspects of your life make it worth living at all costs?" Patients should be encouraged to complete values histories to distinguish preferences and reaffirm individual beliefs (Doukas & McCullough, 1991; Kielstein & Sass, 1993).

Although values guide an individual's decisions, patients are unable to make informed decisions without adequate information. However, caregivers often assume that patients want particular pieces of information and the caregiver may unintentionally omit information important to the individual patient. The ACNP should ask questions such as "What additional information do you need or want to make a decision?" or "What are your thoughts about what is going on with your illness?" These questions can reveal misconceptions or gaps of information that the patient may need to make an informed choice.

Generally, it is presumed that the patient wants full involvement in the decision-making process. The interpretation of this involvement varies with the individual caregiver. For example, some caregivers assume that the patient wants to know all the possible diagnoses in the differential. Other caregivers presume that patients prefer a more definitive diagnosis and will withhold information until some certainty is established. Unless patients are asked directly, the degree of individual patient involvement will be uncertain and ambiguous. The ACNP can ask the patient "How do you want to be involved in the decision-making process?" and "Do you want to know what we are thinking about when we order particular tests, or do you only want to know when we find something significant?"

In addition to clarifying how the patient wants to be involved, it is important for the ACNP to increase patient involvement by tempering the patient's feelings of vulnerability. The ACNP can empower patients to be active participants in the decision-making process by providing information and helping patients understand the health-care environment (Rushton, 1988). Clear explanations of each health-care professional's role will enable the patient to discuss pertinent issues with the appropriate professional. In addition, patients feel less vulnerable if they have control over the most basic aspects of their care such as toileting or food selection.

These strategies demonstrate how a model of shared decision making can satisfy the emotional and informational needs of patients and their families. Caregivers also benefit from this environment of mutual trust and support. As providers gain an understanding of the patient's perspectives, new insights, energy, and creativity surface that advance patient and family care (Pike, 1991). Shared decision making between the patient and primary providers contributes to a humane and caring environment in which healing and recovery are possible (Karlawish, 1996).

Informed Consent

The practice of informed consent, in which the patient and primary caregiver contribute to the process, exemplifies the model of shared decision making. The theory of informed consent is central to the practice of ACNPs. Whether obtaining consent for the insertion of a central line or enrolling a patient in a research study, the basic principles of providing the necessary information for an informed decision apply. Unfortunately, obtaining informed consent is often thought of as an event in which the caregiver provides the information to the patient and obtains consent at the same time. An alternative model, the process model, illustrates a collaborative approach and portrays a model more consistent with the concept of shared decision making. In the process model, the caregiver and patient establish the overall goals of treatment and select the appropriate treatment accordingly (President's Commission, 1982).

There are both legal and moral purposes of informed consent. If an ACNP fails to obtain a patient's consent, he or she may be subject to a charge of battery or neglect (White, 1991). Therefore, the legal intent of the informed consent process is to protect the patient from nonconsensual touching or harm.

From the moral perspective, informed consent upholds the values of respect for autonomy and personal well-being (President's Commission 1982). The informed consent process allows the individual to voluntarily choose a course of action that best reflects his or her beliefs and values (Faden & Beauchamp, 1986).

The Elements of Informed Consent

The four aspects of an ethically valid consent are disclosure, comprehension, competence, and voluntariness. Each of these concepts is an essential element of good decision making and together they advance the patient's interests in self-determination and personal well-being (President's Commission, 1982).

The concept of disclosure conveys that an individual has a right to information that is pertinent to the decision. Generally, the disclosure should include the nature, purpose, risks, benefits, and alternatives of the proposed therapy. It is unnecessary and inappropriate to attempt to disclose every possible rare or theoretical risk. Instead, most clinicians are guided by a reasonable person standard. This standard asserts that the caregiver must disclose information that would be relevant to a reasonable person's decision (Faden & Beauchamp, 1986).

As the information is disclosed, the patient must be able to comprehend and understand the relevant facts. First, the information must be disclosed in a manner that reinforces understanding. Medical jargon or extensive technical facts may obscure the information relevant to the patient's understanding (Faden & Beauchamp, 1986). Asking patients to describe the proposed therapy in their own words will help the ACNP discern the patient's perceptions and comprehension. The patient should demonstrate a clear understanding of the benefits and risks of the proposed treatment, and the risks and benefits of alternative treatments (Reigle, 1990).

In order for a patient to consent to a treatment, he or she must demonstrate competence, or the capacity to participate in the decision-making process. Several standards of capacity have evolved; however, the most widely accepted is the functional standard. In this standard, the capacity of an individual is based on the functional ability of the decision maker, rather than the status of the individual or the outcome of the decision. Capacity is determined by the ability of the patient to understand relevant information, communicate the choices, and to reason about relevant alternatives (President's Commission, 1982).

The fourth element, voluntariness, is sometimes difficult to achieve in a clinical setting. An individual is able to make a choice voluntarily only when free from coercion and controlling forces (Faden & Beauchamp, 1986). The subtle coercion sometimes present from the patient's family or caregiver can threaten this element of the informed consent process. Of course, various factors, such as family responsibilities or financial obligations, will influence decisions. However, the ACNP must be aware of situations in which the patient is experiencing pressure from family members, religious groups, or others that threatens the voluntariness of the consent (Beauchamp & Childress, 1994).

The goal of the informed consent process is to assure that the individual makes an informed decision. Although the term "consent" is used, the concept is about making a choice based on information about the risks and benefits of proposed treatments and alternatives. The patient, after understanding and considering the information, may choose to refuse the proposed therapy. This informed choice is a valid refusal, and should be respected as such. Although the ACNP should explore the reasoning underlying the refusal of beneficial treatment, a competent patient has a right to refuse even worthwhile treatments (President's Commission, 1982).

RESOURCES IN ETHICS

Professional Codes and Guidelines

Professional codes of ethics function to delineate the values and ethical position of a professional group. The American Nurses Association (ANA) code identifies the ethical conduct expected from nurses in the professional, patient, or societal domains (American Nurses Association, 1985; Fry, 1994). Many other nurses associations have developed guidelines or codes that also define the parameters of ethical responsibility. Often these codes provide a general overview of ethical practice, but are difficult to apply to specific dilemmas in clinical practice. It is important for the ACNP to understand the core values of the profession and the moral positions affirmed by the organization.

Some professional groups, such as the ANA or the American Association for Critical-Care Nurses (AACN), develop position statements on ethical issues. These statements often provide clear direction for moral action on specific issues. For example, the ANA position statement on foregoing artificial nutrition and hydration outlines the nurse's position (American Nurses Association, 1992). These statements can be valuable resources to an ACNP confronted with such complex issues.

Legal and Regulatory Guidelines

Although law and ethics are distinct disciplines, the interface of law and biomedical ethics is a reality in clinical practice. There are some cases in clinical ethics that have reached federal courts; however, the majority of these cases have been litigated on local or state levels. This fact is made evident in how laws may differ from State to State (White, 1991). The ACNP must understand the effect and influence of statutes and laws that influence clinical decision making and individual practice. For example, the Federal guidelines on withholding or withdrawing treatment outlined in the Child Abuse Amendment Act of 1984 should be understood by an ACNP practicing in a pediatric setting. Information on State statutes and regulations can be obtained from State boards of nursing.

Organizational Policies

Health-care institutions develop policies that guide ethical practice within the organization. These policies define the organization's values, the professional's responsibilities, and the rights of patients. The obligations of the ACNP and other professionals to the organization are reflected in the policies. Although policies often are revised to reflect contemporary practice, it is important for the ACNP to consider the implications of organizational policies on his or her practice before choosing a place to work. Once employed by an institution, the ACNP should actively be involved in developing and revising policies to uphold the moral elements of practice.

Ethics Committees

Many organizations have institutional ethics committees, but the manner in which the committees function varies significantly. The purpose of some ethics committees is to develop organizational policies and guidelines. Ethics committees in other institutions may fulfill the policy responsibilities and provide education within and external to the institution. In still other situations, an ethics committee will develop policies, provide education, and offer consultation services.

Despite the manner in which the ethics committee functions, committee members often are valuable resources for the ACNP. Discussing a perplexing case with a committee member can provide additional insight into the issue and lead to resolution (Rushton, 1988). The committee member also may suggest other resources to help frame the dilemma. If the ethics committee provides consultation or reviews cases, the ACNP should present difficult ethical dilemmas in this format. This process may not only lead to resolution of the particular case, but institutional policies could be developed to prevent recurrence of the dilemma.

It is inevitable that the ACNP will encounter ethical dilemmas in clinical practice. The manner in which the issue is confronted should be a conscious and purposeful choice for the ACNP. This chapter provides the ACNP a vocabulary and some strategies to initiate the resolution of ethical problems in the clinical setting. Upholding the values of shared decision making and acknowledging the essential contributions of all involved individuals will help the ACNP advance a humanistic and caring environment.

REFERENCES

Ahronheim, J. C., Moreno, J., & Zuckerman, C. (1994). *Ethics in clinical practice.* Boston: Little, Brown.

American Nurses Association (1985). *Code for nurses with interpretive statements.* Kansas City, MO: ANA.

American Nurses Association (1992). Position statement on foregoing artificial nutrition and hydration. Washington DC: ANA.

Applebaum, P. S., & Grisso, T. (1988). Assessing patient's capacities to consent to treatment. *New England Journal of Medicine, 319*(25), 1635–1638.

Beauchamp, T. L., & Childress, J. F. (1994). *Princples of biomedical ethics* (4th ed.). New York: Oxford University Press.

Cooper, M. C. (1989). Gilligan's different voice: A perspective for nursing. *Journal of Professional Nursing, 5*(1), 10.

Cooper, M. C. (1991). A response to Pike A. W. Moral outrage and moral discourse in nurse–physician collaboration. *Journal of Professional Nursing, 7*(6), 351–363.

Doukas, D. J., & McCullough, L. B. (1991). The values history. *The Journal of Family Practice, 32*(2), 145–150.

Faden, R. R., & Beauchamp, T. L. (1986). *A history and theory of informed consent.* New York: Oxford University Press.

Fry, S. (1994). *Ethics in nursing practice.* Geneva, Switzerland: International Council of Nurses.

Gilligan, C. (1982). *In a different voice.* Cambridge, MA: Harvard University Press.

Gretter L. The Florence Nightingale Pledge, 1893.

Karlawish, J. H. T. (1996). Shared decision making in critical care: A clinical reality and an ethical necessity. *American Journal of Critical Care, 5*(6), 391–396.

Kielstein, R., & Sass, H. M. (1993). Using stories to assess values and establish medical directives. *Kennedy Institute of Ethics Journal, 3*(3), 303–352

Krouse, H. J., & Roberts, S. J. (1989). Nurse–patient interactive styles: Power, control, and satisfaction. *Western Journal of Nursing Research, 11*(6), 717–725.

Pike, A. W. (1991). Moral outrage and moral discourse in nurse–physician collaboration. *Journal of Professional Nursing, 7*(6), 351–363.

President's Commission for the Study of Ethical Problems in Medicine and Biomedical and Behavioral Research (1982). *Making healthcare choices.* Washington, DC: U.S. Government Printing Office.

Reigle, J. (1990). A study of variance between written and oral consent in four invasive procedures. *Virginia Nurse, 58*(3), 37–40.

Rushton, C. H. (1988). Ethical decision making in critical care, Part 1: The role of the pediatric nurse. *Pediatric Nursing, 14*(5), 411–412.

Spielman, B. J. (1993). Conflict in medical ethics cases: Seeking patterns of resolution. *The Journal of Clinical Ethics, 4*(3), 212–218.

Uustal, D. (1987). Values: The cornerstone of nursing's moral art. In Fowler M.D.M., & Levine-Ariff J. (Eds.), *Ethics at the bedside* (pp. 136–153). Philadelphia: J.B. Lippincott.

White, M. L. (1991). Informed consent. In Fletcher J.C., (Ed.), *Introduction to clinical ethics and health care law.* Charlottesville, VA: The Center for Biomedical Ethics.

8

The Acute Care Nurse Practitioner as Educator

JoAnne Konick-McMahon

The role of educator carries the ACNP to many arenas. ACNPs educate patients and their families about self-care related to an acute or chronic illness. This may occur in a "teachable moment" during rounds or clinic or in a group process for a lay organization. Education of patients and families may come through a pamphlet, audiotape, or videotape the ACNP develops. The ACNP may be asked to be a consultant for patient education in formulating a care path or teaching plan for a group of patients for whom he or she provides expert advanced practice care.

The role of educator of colleagues may be carried out in a formal way such as a presentation to an organizational or professional group. The ACNP may informally educate other professionals to appropriate care, including house staff and/or nursing staff. The ACNP may serve as a preceptor for a single student or a group of students. All of these situations require knowledge of the educational and teaching process to increase the potential for a positive outcome. This chapter illustrates the theoretical frameworks for education of patients and families, colleagues, and students.

▶ ADULTS AS LEARNERS

Patients and colleagues of the ACNP have common ground in being adult learners. According to Knowles (1984), the ACNP must be consistently aware of, and use in planning a teaching/learning process, the characteristics of adult learners. Use of principles of teaching based on these characteristics enhances learning and, ultimately, produces behavior change in adults.

Knowles's study of teaching adults, or andragogy, examines conditions necessary for adult learning, assumptions of adult teaching, and general techniques of the adult teaching–learning process based on conditions and assumptions (Table 8–1).

TABLE 8–1. Teaching–Learning Process According to Andragogy

Conditions necessary for teaching adults

1. Climate of collaboration—trust, respect, support
2. Learner is involved in needs assessment, planning, and evaluating learning

Assumptions of adult teaching

1. As we grow, we move to self direction
2. Personal experiences establish self-identity
3. Readiness to learn is related to social roles
4. Adults want immediate application, problem-centered, of knowledge

General techniques for teaching/learning with adults

1. Use past experiences of learners to build new knowledge
2. Use problem-oriented activities such as case studies
3. Share responsibility for teaching/evaluations
4. Use a variety of teaching strategies, not just one

Knowles, M. (1970). The modern practice of adult education.

Conditions necessary for adult learning, according to andragogy, include a climate of collaboration. This climate, set forth by the teacher as facilitator, includes trust, respect, and support of the learner. The learner is involved in all areas of the teaching–learning process, including needs assessment, planning, and evaluating the process. These mutual activities of the teacher and learner help to assure a positive outcome of the educational effort for both parties involved.

Knowles, in his study of adult learners, proposes four assumptions that provide a basis for adult teaching–learning. The first assumption states that as adults grow, they move to self-direction. Therefore, adult learners, unlike children, have ideas about what they need to know. They may have had a relevant situation in their life (i.e., the surgical patient whose brother had the same surgery). Adult learners are also aware of the methods by which they learn best and should have the opportunity to make the teacher aware of those preferences.

A second assumption underlying andragogy states that the learner's identity has been established by personal experiences. Those experiences include other adult teachers as well as other health-care providers. A negative experience in the past with teaching–learning in the health-care setting may greatly influence the ACNP's interaction with the adult patient/colleague learner today. Those patients with low literacy skills may be especially apprehensive about any learning situation (Doak, Doak & Root 1996). Both assumptions call for assessment of the learner's prior knowledge and experiences, and his or her perceived learning needs.

Readiness to learn is related to social roles, and is a third assumption of the teaching–learning process for adults. Motivation to change behavior through an educational process must be part of the way that an individual perceives him- or herself in his or her own world view. If an individual's social role does not include the activity or behavior being taught, the behavior will be less likely to be integrated by that adult.

The fourth and final assumption of adult teaching–learning delineates the need of adults for immediate application of knowledge. A problem-solving approach to teaching and learning, such as case studies, encourages the immediate use of learned information. That immediate application increases the potential for behavior change for the learner.

Knowles (1984) calls for general techniques or tips to be incorporated in the teaching–learning process for adults based on his assumptions. He recommends the use of past experiences of learners attained through an oral or written needs assessment. The teaching–learning process is more effective when it is a shared responsibility with a variety of strategies developed to meet the learner's style. The strategies might include printed materials, group discussion, audiotapes, videotapes, computer-guided instruction, or others. The adult learner, in Knowles's view, should share the responsibility for teaching and evaluation of the process.

Another general technique for teaching adults is the use of problem-oriented activities. The use of this method assists in application of the material to the learner's world. Active learning increases the likelihood of retention of the information taught. Always aim for the learner to use the "need to know" information in an active way.

▶ THEORIES OF LEARNING

A basis for the teaching–learning process can be established through examination of the learning theories (Redman, 1997). Two categories of current learning theories exist: behaviorist theories and cognitive theories. A third theory, social learning theory, combines elements of the behaviorist and cognitive theories of learning (Table 8–2).

Behaviorist learning theories are based on the concept that learning is conditioning or behavior reinforcement. The act of observing the desired behavior is the criterion to evaluate for a successful teaching–learning process. Behavioristic theorists consider learners to be motivated to change their behavior because of a lack of something in their environment. Positive reinforcement (such as praise or another reward) after a behavior increases the chance of repeated behavior.

Cognitive theory is based on the concept that learning may occur with or without behavior change. Instead, the learner may develop understanding about an issue or topic. That understanding or learning may guide behavior, but not necessarily so. Motivation, according to cognitive theorists, is a result of learner disequilibrium associated with life goals or purpose. Using cognitive learning theory, the teacher determines the learner's existing knowledge and experience with a topic and provides the appropriate level of information and teaching strategies.

Social cognitive theory, also known as social learning theory or self-efficacy theory, combines elements of cognitive and behaviorist theories (Doak, Doak & Root 1996). Bandura, who developed this theory, considered observation of others to be a major method or strategy that learners use to get information, learn about values, and make judg-

TABLE 8–2. Overview of Learning Theories

Behaviorist Theory Learning is conditioning or behavior reinforcement. Positive reinforcements, such as teacher praise and success, are powerful reinforcers.
Cognitive Theory Learning may occur with or without behavior change. Motivation results from a need associated with life goals.
Social Cognitive Theory Role modeling is a major source of behavior modification. Belief in one's ability to perform is critical to success.

ments. After observing others, humans model that behavior. Humans, however, have the ability to hold onto learned behavior for a time without using it, as long as they see a need for that behavior in the future.

Social cognitive theory of learning sees extrinsic rewards as necessary initially during a behavior development, until the behavior becomes self-rewarding. Additionally, this learning theory includes the concept that learners must have a belief in their ability to perform a behavior, called self efficacy. Complicated, multi-step processes may be broken down and approached step-by-step to provide successful achievement by the learner. In this way, the complicated process becomes achievable.

The teacher, using this social cognitive theory of learning, facilitates the learner's success to provide the reward, thereby encouraging new behavior. Learners judge their own performance. A belief in one's ability to perform a behavior is lowered with each failure. Therefore, the teacher, using social cognitive theory as a base, uses teaching strategies to ensure learner success to increase the likelihood of ongoing belief in ability to perform.

The theories of learning as briefly described create a basis for an educational process for adult learners. Major principles that emerge from Knowles's work, and that are relevant to the ACNP's practice, include the following:

- Effective education starts with a learner who sees a need for education about a health-care problem and a teacher who views him- or herself as a facilitator of learning and behavior change. Assisting adults to see a need for specific education is a function of the educator.
- A change in behavior requires an adult's belief in his or her ability to do that behavior. This requires step-by-step progression through complex behaviors, repetition, active learning guided by the teacher, and praise.

▶ THE ACNP AS PATIENT EDUCATOR

"The goal of educating the patient and family is to improve patient health outcomes by promoting recovery, speeding return to function, promoting health behavior and appropriately involving the patient in his or her own health care decisions" (Joint Commission on the Accreditation of Healthcare Organizations, 1994).

"The patient has the right to, and is encouraged to obtain from his physician and other direct caregivers, relevant, current, and understandable information concerning diagnosis, treatment, and prognosis" (American Hospital Association, *A Patient's Bill of Rights,* 1992).

Patient education is the "deliberative process of creating behavioral and cognitive change in patients" (Redman, 1993, p. 10). Patient education includes teaching, counseling, and behavior modification.

Teaching can be defined as those "activities that allow the teacher to help students learn" (Redman, 1993, p. 8). "Active learner" is the key phrase in any teaching process for adults. The educational process for adult patients in health care includes needs assessment, planning teaching–learning activities, implementing those activities, and follow-up evaluation of learning and behavior change by the learner and teacher. Each of these areas is addressed separately.

Needs Assessment

Assessment of the patient and family, prior to initiating the teaching–learning process, is essential to set the tone for a successful outcome. Important questions to ask are outlined in Table 8–3. The key question for the ACNP is: What is the "need to know" information for this patient?

This is the most important question and is the target for teaching. If it isn't "need to know" behaviors and information, it is fluff. Nonessential behaviors and information should not be included in the educational process in an acute care environment.

During acute hospitalization, focus on three or four critical objectives. Observe or evaluate through oral questioning—and document—the patient's ability to meet those objectives (Rankin & Stalling, 1996, p. 280). Follow-up phone calls at home by the ACNP provide the opportunity for learning after discharge. Frequently, the ACNP can refer patients to outpatient learning opportunities such as home-care agencies or other community health education sources.

Motivation to change or take on new health behaviors, such as weighing oneself daily or taking medicines on a regular basis, is a factor to consider throughout the educational process. Teaching in the setting of acute illness or chronic illness with an acute flare is most effective after the initial impact has passed. Behavior change is most likely to result as the patient begins to acknowledge and think about lifestyle changes necessary to prevent recurrence or to deal with the results of an illness or trauma (Belcher, 1993).

The *Health Belief Model* (Rosenstock et al., 1994) states that patients respond best to information about health promotion when they see themselves at risk. Changing patient behavior, such as adherence to a medication schedule or limiting sodium in the diet, is more likely to occur if the

TABLE 8–3. Questions to Answer for Patient Needs Assessment

1. What do this patient and support person already know?
2. What experiences have they had with this kind of health-care problem?
3. How will the patient's cultural belief affect their willingness to take on new behaviors?
4. How does the patient like to learn?
5. Can this patient read?
6. What teaching materials and equipment are available?
7. What is the teacher's style and preference for learning?
8. How will learning/behavior change be evaluated?
9. What motivates this patient to change current health behaviors and/or take on new behaviors?
10. Is the patient ready to learn? What are barriers to behavior change?

patient sees that the risk of not changing behavior is serious. In the patient's mind, the benefits of such activity must outweigh the barriers to the behavior change (Doak, Doak & Root, 1996). Applying the Health Belief Model to patient education, the ACNP focuses the key teaching activities on the behaviors that put the patient at risk and the ways to change those behaviors. The outcomes of nonadherence to prescribed behavior, such as medications and diet, must be presented to assure patient understanding of risk.

The ACNP can provide an educational process that motivates patients and other adults in an educational setting. Guidelines to promote learner motivation are summarized in Table 8–4 and include:

1. **Use the environment to focus and motivate the learner.** Make it accepting but with a clear purpose. Visual aids that grab a learner's interest and curiosity are part of a motivating environment.
2. **Rewards, including praise, motivate learners.** The motivation that produces the longest lasting results is internal, not external. Acutely ill patients may need guidance and external rewards from the ACNP initially, but should progress to internal or self motivation as time passes. Some adults have little internal motivation and require ongoing reinforcement of needed behaviors. These learners need extra help from the ACNP, family, and community resources to maintain behaviors over time.
3. **Learning is most likely to occur when the learner wants to know something.** Thus, responding to patient questions promptly and as close as possible to the time of asking is important. It is the "teachable moment."
4. **Organization of material to be learned should progress from known to unknown, from easy to complex.** Start material presentation at a point that the learner knows to provide a basis. Add new ideas or techniques when a behavior has been achieved.
5. **Goals should be achievable to ensure success.** Success motivates the learner to try new behaviors.

Along with assessment of motivation to take on new or revised health behaviors, the ACNP should assess the patient's literacy level to plan appropriate teaching strategies. The National Adult Literacy Survey, published in 1993, found that 22%, or 40 to 44 million adult Americans, function at the lowest skill levels in ability to use reading, writing, and computation skills in daily life. These abilities are essential to using medications, making appointments, reading over-the-counter drug labels correctly, and following directions for home care.

TABLE 8–4. Guidelines for Motivating Patients as Learners

1. Use the environment to focus the learner
2. Rewards, including praise, motivate learners
3. Learning, or behavior change, is most likely to occur when the learner is ready
4. Organize the material from known to unknown, simple to complex
5. Set up the learner for success by being realistic

Adapted from Redman, B. K. (1993). The process of patient education. *Philadelphia: Mosby*

Two reading skill tests can be used to determine the appropriate reading level for educational materials. The Wide-Range Achievement Test, or WRAT 3, has been used in school systems for years (Doak, Doak & Root 1996). The patient reads a list of words until 10 errors are made in pronunciation. The number of words correctly pronounced is converted to a reading grade level.

The Rapid Estimate of Adult Literacy in Medicine (REALM) test uses a list of health/medical-related words to estimate a grade range (Doak, Doak & Root 1996). It may be more acceptable in the health-care setting to patients than the WRAT. The REALM can be used with acknowledgment of the copyright without charge. Figure 8–1 shows the REALM test and scoring guide.

Understanding health-care instructions is an ability that is more important to validate than reading alone. An instrument that measures functional health literacy, the TOFLA (Test for Functional Health Literacy in Adults), has been developed to measure the ability of patients in the areas of reading comprehension and numerical ability in the area of health care (Parker et al., 1995). A study of the instrument in two urban settings found that significant percentages of patients were not able to understand prescription directions. Using real text from patient education materials, as well as prescriptions and directions for follow-up, the TOFLA currently requires up to 22 minutes to administer. The need for a more concise screening tool for functional health literacy is evident to assure appropriate teaching–learning strategies while being time-efficient.

Doak, Doak & Root (1996) suggest an indirect method of assessing a patient's ability to comprehend health-care instructions. The teacher uses a graded health instruction, has the patient read several paragraphs or a short section, and then asks several questions about the content. If the patient answers the questions, then materials written at that grade level are appropriate. If the patient is unable to answer questions, a lower grade level of material should be used or alternative methods such as audiotapes should be used. Specific teaching–learning strategies for patients with low literacy skills are included later in this chapter.

Following the assessment, the ACNP is ready to begin to plan for appropriate learning strategies and evaluation. That plan begins with the formulation of objectives to guide the educational process.

Objective Writing

Objectives are merely goals for the teaching–learning process. The objectives are closely linked to the needs assessment data. They reflect the teaching strategies and the method of evaluation to be used.

Objectives state what the learner is to be like after a learning experience based on the learner's goals. They denote an observable change in behavior. Although objectives are not necessarily written as in a formal teaching plan (see Table 8–5), the learner should hear the objective as the teacher sees it to assure agreement for the outcome of learning. The purpose of objectives is to provide a measure of how the teaching–learning process will change the learner.

Objectives should be written with the learner's goals as their basis. What behavior does the learner desire as an outcome of teaching? For example, if the patient with heart failure wants to avoid hospitalization for fluid overload, the ACNP would build objectives based on the patient behaviors necessary to achieve that goal. An example of such objectives is:

> After listening to the heart failure audiotape and discussion with the ACNP, the learner will be able to:
>
> 1. Weigh himself at the same time daily;
> 2. Recall that a two-pound weight gain overnight or a five-pound weight gain in a week means that the patient should call the ACNP the same day before noon.

In this example, the objectives or desired behaviors are weigh and recall. The conditions are listening to an audiotape and discussing the information. These conditions are also the teaching strategies in this case. The evaluation process will be: A record of daily weights either returned to the ACNP on a follow-up visit or phoned in; and questioning by the teacher to obtain the correct answers for weight gain and how soon to call. This example illustrates the flow of a plan from objectives through evaluation.

Three domains of behavioral objectives were developed by Bloom and his colleagues to provide consistency in the educational process (Redman, 1997). The three domains are cognitive, affective, and psychomotor. The cognitive domain outlines behaviors in the knowledge area of learning. The affective domain includes feelings, attitudes, and values, while the psychomotor domain deals with motor skills. Each of the three domains are ordered from simple to complex behaviors in the taxonomy (Table 8–6). The learner with basic knowledge needs objectives at a higher level on the taxonomy to avoid repetition and learner frustration with the teaching-learning process.

The Rapid Estimate of Adult Literacy in Medicine (REALM) is a screening instrument to assess an adult patient's ability to read common medical words and lay terms for body parts and illnesses. It is designed to assist medical professionals in estimating a patient's literacy level so that the appropriate level of patient education materials or oral instructions may be used. The test takes 2 to 3 minutes to administer and score. The REALM has been correlated with other standardized tests.

Correlation of REALM with SORT, PIAT-R, and WRAT-R

	PIAT-R Recognition	SORT	WRAT-R
Correlation Coefficient	.97	.96	.88
P Value	p<.0001	p<.0001	p<.0001

Reliability Studies

Test-Retest	Inter-Rater
(n=100)	(n=20)
.99	.99

DIRECTIONS

1. Give the patient a laminated copy of the REALM and score answers on an unlaminated copy that is attached to a clipboard. Hold the clipboard at an angle so that the patient is not distracted by your scoring procedure. Say:
   "I want to hear you read as many words as you can from this list. Begin with the first word on List 1 and read aloud. When you come to a word you cannot read, do the best you can or say 'blank' and go on to the next word."
2. If the patient takes more than five seconds on a word, say "blank"and point to the next word, if necessary, to move the patient along. If the patient begins to miss every word, have him/her pronounce only known words.
3. Count as an error any word not attempted or mispronounced. Score by marking a plus (+) after each correct word, a check ($\surd$) after each mispronounced word, and a minus (–) after words not attempted. Count as correct any self-corrected word.
4. Count the number of correct words for each list and record the numbers in the "SCORE" box. Total the numbers and match the total score with its grade equivalent in the table below.

Figure 8–1. Rapid estimate of adult literacy in medicine (REALM). *(Continued)*

Rapid Estimate of Adult Literacy in Medicine (REALM) ©

Terry Davis, PhD • Michael Crouch, MD • Sandy Long, PhD

Reading Level ____________

Patient Name/ Subject# ______________ Date of Birth __________ Grade Completed ____________

Date______________ Clinic ______________ Examiner________________

List 1		List 2		List 3	
fat	____	fatigue	____	allergic	____
flu	____	pelvic	____	menstrual	____
pill	____	jaundice	____	testicle	____
dose	____	infection	____	colitis	____
eye	____	exercise	____	emergency	____
stress	____	behavior	____	medication	____
smear	____	prescription	____	occupation	____
nerves	____	notify	____	sexually	____
germs	____	gallbladder	____	alcoholism	____
meals	____	calories	____	irritation	____
disease	____	depression	____	constipation	____
cancer	____	miscarriage	____	gonorrhea	____
caffeine	____	pregnancy	____	inflammatory	____
attack	____	arthritis	____	diabetes	____
kidney	____	nutrition	____	hepatitis	____
hormones	____	menopause	____	antibiotics	____
herpes	____	appendix	____	diagnosis	____
seizure	____	abnormal	____	potassium	____
bowel	____	syphilis	____	anemia	____
asthma	____	hemorrhoids	____	obesity	____
rectal	____	nausea	____	osteoporosis	____
incest	____	directed	____	impetigo	____

SCORE	
List 1	____________
List 2	____________
List 3	____________
Raw Score	____________

GRADE EQUIVALENT

Raw Score	*Grade Range*
0–18	**3rd Grade and Below** Will not be able to read most low literacy materials; will need repeated oral instructions, materials composed primarily of illustrations, or audio or video tapes.
19–44	**4th to 6th Grade** Will need low literacy materials; may not be able to read prescription labels.
45–60	**7th to 8th Grade** Will struggle with most patient education materials; will not be offended by low literacy materials.
61–66	**High School** Will be able to read most patient education materials.

Figure 8–1. *(Continued)*

Contracts use objectives as the basis for behavior change. This tool clearly identifies the behaviors needed to achieve a goal. Learning contracts between patient and ACNP provide a written outline for discussion and may provide insight about reasons for nonadherent behavior in the past.

Criticisms exist for the use of objectives to guide the teaching–learning process in patient education. Objectives, as outlined or written by the teacher, may not use the individual patient's needs. Rigid objectives may defeat their own purpose of helping learning if the teacher is not willing

TABLE 8–5. Teaching Plan

Objectives	Topical Outline	Strategies	Resources	Evaluation
Behavioral terms to the student's level	Content specific to objectives, introduction. Body in a logical sequence with frequent summaries	Choose active strategies; devise questions to ask and where. Include activity	Refer to written or audio materials as resource	Be sure each objective is measured

or unable to adapt them to the patient's goals and level of ability. Certainly, objectives in patient education should be changed to meet the true needs of the individual. Objectives should be added if they are important to the outcome and are achievable during the educational process.

The needs assessment has provided information to guide the formulation of objectives for the teaching–learning process. In some situations those objectives may be written in a clinical progress note or a patient education record. In other situations the objectives may be in the ACNP's mind as the teaching strategies or methods take place.

Teaching Strategies

The ACNP who teaches patients should remember the following statement (Patterson, 1962) as activities for learning are planned.

> *Adults remember 10% of what they read,*
> *20% of what they hear,*
> *30% of what they see,*
> *50% of what they see and hear,*
> *80% of what they say,*
> *90% of what they say and do.*

Multiple teaching strategies exist in health care. The most common method is the use of written material such as a pamphlet or instructional leaflet. Unless this is followed up with demonstration and actual patient practice, the chance for retention is small. Active learning by the patient is the "gold standard" in adult education.

Using Multimedia for Patient Education

Doak, Doak & Root (1996) formulated guidelines for health education methods and materials (Table 8–7). All instruction should be simple and easy to understand. A key criterion for a written information sheet, audiotape, or videotape is the correct reading level. To reach a wide range of patients, the reading level of instructional material should be fifth to sixth grade. A reading formula is used to calculate the reading level.

A wide variety of reading formulas exist to calculate the reading level of a health instruction. The SMOG formula (McLaughlin, 1969) is simple to use and predicts grade level within 1.5 grades 68% of the time. See Figure 8–2 for the instructions and conversion table for the SMOG grade-level readability. Many computer word-processing programs calculate the reading level of text.

Choosing or producing materials to accompany discussion or demonstration of needed health-care information includes additional factors. Print size should be large enough to be read by older patients. A color contrast should exist between the ink and paper to make reading easier. Graphics and/or pictures help to increase the appeal of an instructional medium. Address a single objective or concept per paragraph. Education materials should be culturally appropriate and in the appropriate language. These factors should be considered when analyzing patient education materials for use.

Methods of Teaching

Direct methods of teaching are those with face-to-face teacher–learner interaction. This category includes discussion, demonstration, role-playing, games, and simulation. Lecture is appropriate when used for groups of patient learners, such as a lay organization. A time for discussion should follow lectures. Lecture is not the most effective strategy or method of teaching in a one-on-one situation where actively engaging the learner is more appropriate.

TABLE 8–6. Behavioral Objectives from Bloom's Taxonomy

Domain	Level	Verbs
COGNITIVE	Knowledge	Define, label, match, name, select
	Comprehension	Defend, distinguish, explain, summarize, give example
	Application	Demonstrate, prepare, relate, use, change
	Analysis	Diagram, illustrate, discriminate, break down
	Synthesis	Compose, create, devise, design, organize, explain
	Evaluation	Compare, conclude, criticize, interpret, justify
AFFECTIVE	Receiving	Ask, follow, reply, use
	Responding	Assist, comply, help, practice, cooperate
	Valuing	Complete, invite, share, select, desire, accept
	Organization	Adhere, alter, modify, generalize, organize, choose
	Characterization	Display, use, solve, revise, act, model
PSYCHOMOTOR	Perception	Be aware of, relate, identify, recognize
	Set	Perform, demonstrate, discriminate, adjust, prepare
	Guided Response	Initiate, try, test, solve, discover
	Mechanism	Administer, control, guide, perform regularly
	Complex Overt Response	Perform with ease, perform accurately
	Adaptation	Alter, adapt, generalize, design, modify

Adapted from Redman, B. K. (1997). The practice of patient education, *8th ed. Philadelphia: Mosby.*

TABLE 8–7. Guidelines for Health Education Methods and Materials

1. Set realistic objectives
   - Limit the objective to what the majority of the target population needs now
   - Use a planning sheet to write down the objective and key points
2. To change health behaviors, focus on behaviors and skills
   - Emphasize behaviors and skills rather than facts
   - Consider placing key points first and last

     OR
   - Consider establishing risk for the patient first, ways to reduce risk and belief in ability to practice those behaviors
3. Present context or purpose for new information before presenting it
   - Relate new information to the context of patient's life
4. Break down complex instructions
   - Provide opportunities for small successes by achieving parts of the big picture
5. Make it interactive
   - Consider including an interaction with the material after each key topic. The patient must write, tell, show, demonstrate, select, or solve a problem

From Doak, C. C., Doak, L. G., & Root, J. H. (1996). Teaching patients with low literacy skills. *Philadelphia: Lippincott.*

Indirect methods of teaching are those that substitute experiences through means other than direct interaction of the teacher and learner. These include readings, audiotapes, storyboards, modular self-learning, videotapes, and computer methods.

Table 8–8 correlates teaching strategies for patients and families with the type of learning by objective domain and active learner involvement. Each strategy is described with considerations for the teacher and learner outlined.

Discussion is a direct, active learner strategy using the patient's questions and input for direction. The discussion may come before or after an indirect strategy such as reading pertinent handouts or listening to an audiotape. These strategies provide reinforcement for one another to enhance learner retention of information.

Group teaching using a discussion format with the educator as facilitator is a cost-effective strategy that may have the advantage of providing group support and peer influence. For patients who like groups for learning, this strategy may enhance behavior change. This method, ideally occurring in the acute care setting for a captive patient audience, may not be feasible in today's health-care market where patients are discharged to recuperate at home. Devel-

SMOG Testing

The SMOG formula was originally developed by G. Harry McLaughlin in 1969. It will predict the grade-level difficulty of a passage within 1.5 grades in 68% of the passages tested. That may be close enough for your purposes. It is simple to use and faster than most other measures. The procedure is presented below.

Instructions

1. You will need 30 sentences. Count out 10 consecutive sentences near the beginning, 10 consecutive from the middle, and 10 from the end. For this purpose, a sentence is any string of words puncuated by a period (.), an exclamation point (!), or a question mark (?).
2. From the entire 30 sentences, count the words containing **three or more syllables,** including repetitions.
3. Obtain the grade level from the table below, or you may calculate the grade level as follows: Determine the nearest perfect square root of the total number of words of three or more syllables and then add a constant of 3 to the square root to obtain the grade level.

Example

Total number of multisyllabic (3 or more syllables) words	67
Nearest perfect square	64
Square root	8
Add constant of 3	11 This is the grade level

TABLE A. SMOG CONVERSION TABLE

Word count	Grade level
0–2	4
3–6	5
7–12	6
13–20	7
21–30	8
31–42	9
43–56	10
57–72	11
73–90	12
91–110	13
111–132	14
133–156	15
157–182	16
183–210	17

Developed by Harold C. McGraw, Office of Educational Research, Baltimore County Public Schools, Towson, Maryland.

Figure 8–2. SMOG testing for reading grade level. *(From Doak, C.C., Doak L.G., & Root, J.H. [1996]; McLaughlin, G.H. [1969].)*

TABLE 8–8. Teaching Strategies Correlated with Type of Objective

Teaching strategy	Domain[a]	Active learning
1. Discussion		
a. one on one	c, a	Usually
b. group	c, a	Usually
2. Demonstration	c, a, p	Usually
3. Case study/critical incident	c, a	Yes
4. Instructional game	c	Yes
5. Role play	c, a, p	Yes
6. Lecture	c, a	No
7. Independent study	c, p with practice	Usually
8. Media	c, p with practice	Usually
a. Reading/Instruction sheet		
b. Audiotape	also a	
c. Videotape	also a	
d. Computer		
e. Modular self-learning		

[a] c = cognitive
a = affective
p = psychomotor

oping a group educational process as part of a community outreach may be an alternative to the in-hospital format. Referral to an existing group known to the ACNP to be a valid teaching–learning process may be another alternative for the patient who learns best in a group format.

Demonstration is a direct teaching strategy for psychomotor skills such as injecting medication or changing a dressing. The teacher is the model of the skill and provides immediate feedback during the return demonstration by the patient. Provide written instructions to follow during demonstration to provide additional stimulation for learning as well as a reference for home. The written instructions also serve as an evaluation tool for the educational process. Use equipment similar to the equipment the patient will use at home for the demonstration and return demonstration.

If demonstration is a group process, the teacher needs to ensure that all learners can see the demonstration. A videotape is useful in this setting. Videotapes have the advantage of consistent instructions. Purchasing or producing a videotape for those ongoing target populations seen by the ACNP may be an alternative to repeated teacher instruction. The educator reviews the tape ahead of time and begins the demonstration by asking the learner to focus on key points in the video related to objectives. Allow time for questions and clarification following the demonstration.

Sufficient space, equipment, and teachers for patient–learners must be present for the return demonstration in a group setting. As mentioned above, the written instructions provided can also serve as the evaluation tool during return demonstration.

Case studies or critical incidents can be used with patients in a discussion or demonstration format. This direct teaching strategy focuses the patient on key points derived from the objectives. The case study presents a real-life situation, such as hypoglycemic symptoms or angina symptoms, and asks the patient to apply the information they have previously learned to manage the symptoms at home. The key to success with this strategy is to focus on "need to know" information to avoid learner overload. The case study method, written or verbal, is used to stimulate discussion or as an evaluation tool to find out what the patient has learned.

Instructional games and role playing are direct strategies that may be used for individuals groups (Backer et al., 1995). Games provide an active, innovative strategy for teaching cognitive or knowledge objectives. Examples include crossword puzzles or a game-show format to reinforce group learning. The ACNP as educator needs to assure the participant(s) that the game format is not intended to decrease the seriousness of a health problem. Rather it is one more strategy to learn the information necessary to deal with the health problem.

Role-playing is a strategy especially effective for affective, or feeling, objectives. One example for use of role-play would be discussing symptoms with the patient's health-care provider. The teacher sets the stage by giving each learner information about a situation and characters. After the scene is played out, the patients, as a group, critique the behaviors and interactions in a debriefing session.

The ACNP must be able to deal with groups to facilitate learning through role-playing. Group facilitator skills are outlined in Table 8–9. Observation of an expert group facilitator along with practice with feedback are methods for fine tuning group skills.

Lecture, a direct teaching strategy, is not pertinent to patient education except as an invited guest speaker for a large lay organization. In the setting of a large group, lecture is a way of disseminating large amounts of information in a cost-effective, time-efficient way. The drawbacks of

TABLE 8–9. Group Facilitator Skills

The group discussion leader provides structure to a group activity by:

1. arranged seats so all participants may see and converse with one another
2. providing the purpose and rationale for the session
3. identifying the topic to be addressed by the group
4. providing instructions for the way discussion should occur and the amount of time available
5. facilitating the exchange of information by asking questions of the group, providing answers when appropriate, resolving problems, and redirecting members to the focus
6. encouraging, in a kind and gentle way, quiet group members to join the discussion
7. controlling talkative group members to allow all a chance to speak
8. providing a summary and closure of the discussion session findings

Adapted from Alspach, G. (1995). The educational process in nursing staff development. *Philadelphia: Mosby, p.75.*

this method include the learner's inactivity and the inability to meet other learning styles or preferred methods. Handouts and a question–answer time help to deal with these problems. Guidelines for preparing a lecture are found in Table 8–10 and in the section for professional education.

Modular self-study or independent study meets the needs of adults who like to learn on their own. The teacher serves as facilitator by suggesting and/or giving printed or audiovisual material. The learner proceeds at his or her own pace with the teacher serving as a guide and evaluator of learning (O'Brien, 1995).

Multiple media are used in patient education. The use of videotapes as a part of a patient learning channel on hospital television continues to grow in popularity. With this format, the teacher should be available to answer questions, reinforce key points through discussion and other media, and evaluate patient learning.

The use of audiotapes increases knowledge and produces greater numbers of self-care behaviors when used for a population undergoing radiation therapy (Hagopian, 1996). Audiotapes can be used at a time convenient to patients and at a pace that meets their needs. Audiotapes can be used for those who have low reading abilities, provided the reading level is in the fifth- to seventh-grade range. Discussion of key concepts should follow to reinforce that material. Oral questioning after discussion can be used as an evaluation tool for patient learning.

Cohen (1993) suggests bibliotherapy, the use of literature, for those who enjoy reading to provide a method for coping with and learning about an illness. In some situations, the book or selection may be used as a discussion point for teaching–learning. At other times, bibliotherapy may serve as a self-learning tool for coping for both the patient and family.

Keep note cards of those selections that are helpful in particular situations and/or file folders with short selections or poetry. Librarians at the local public library could be invaluable resources for suggesting materials. Read suggested selections to know the content before recommending literature to patients. Ask patients to identify particular selections that were helpful in learning about or coping with their illness.

Computer-based learning for patients is a technology in its beginning stages. Advantages of this medium include active learning and self-paced instruction. Immediate feedback and reinforcement from the media to the learner are additional positive characteristics of computer-based learning. Learning outcomes or evaluation can be built into the program. These features, along with individualization of instruction, increase the potential for prolonged retention.

Computer programs for patient education are available, but infrequently used. A study of diabetes educators found a majority of respondents felt lack of computer availability for patients was a barrier to the use of computer-based patient education. Financial constraints (the cost of hardware and software) and time for patients to learn computer skills were additional barriers to this mode of education (Lewis, 1996).

The ACNP as patient educator should be aware of the computer software available in her or his area of practice and begin to use it for those patients who are computer literate.

If software does not exist, consider developing a program in collaboration with computer programmers in the workplace or a publishing house. Learners with a computer background as part of their education may see software as their preferred method of learning. Using and developing software for health and illness patient education provides an additional active learning strategy.

An innovative method of meeting family needs for information in acute care is the storyboard. Described by Westphal (1995), the storyboard uses pictures with few words to describe an environment such as an ICU. Visual images provide key points of information to teach and relieve anxiety for anxious families. Because distractions can be overwhelming during an ICU admission, a family's ability to focus on needed information is limited. Vivid pictures with key word phrases of what to expect provide small chunks of information in a stimulating and memorable manner. This method has potential for use in same-day surgical areas, pre-admission areas, clinic waiting areas, and others.

Multiple teaching–learning strategies for patient education are available to the ACNP to meet various learning styles and needs of individuals. Use objective-focused strategies that correlate with the patient's desired outcome for his or

TABLE 8–10. Guidelines for Lecture Presentation

1. Assess the audience and program goals by asking the group organizer.
2. Write objectives for the content; usually one to two in a one-hour presentation is adequate. Make sure objectives are at the appropriate level for the audience to avoid boredom.
3. Prepare an introduction that establishes why they need to know information.
4. Prepare a body of information that proceeds simple to complex.
5. Stop every 15 minutes to address questions and summarize. Allow time for questions and answers at end to increase learner activity.
6. Prepare a conclusion that points to key information as outlined in objectives.
7. Practice the presentation outloud twice to hear how the words sound.
8. Write times on the outline or cards. FINISH ON TIME. Be prepared to pass over information if time runs out. Direct the learners to another source.
9. Prepare handouts as a visual strategy for learners to use.
10. Audiovisual aids such as slides or transparencies will add a visual dimension as well. Be prepared to do without the aids if the machinery should fail.
11. Be enthusiastic, motivated to teach, and approachable to the learner.
12. Questions will be asked that are unfamiliar information. Be honest and admit that. Follow up after a break or by mail with the answer.

her health-care education. Focus on "need to know" information. The next step in the process is evaluation of patient learning and evaluation of teacher and methods.

Evaluation

While measuring the performance or achievement of an objective is a key step in the teaching–learning process, it is not the final step. It may be viewed as a step in the circle of patient education. Evaluation may lead to revised objectives, revised teaching strategies, or a next level of learning for the patient. That next level may be home in the case of a hospitalized patient if objectives of patient education are achieved.

The purposes of evaluation are threefold:

- to reinforce correct behavior or knowledge
- to help the learner realize how to change incorrect behavior
- to determine adequacy of teaching

Two types of evaluation occur in education. Formative evaluation is ongoing measurement of knowledge or behavior before proceeding to the next step in the process. Summative evaluation is the final measurement of learner achievement. An example of formative evaluation is questioning the patient's ability to recall signs of wound infection before proceeding to the next step in instruction. Summative evaluation, in this case, includes recall of the signs along with "who to call, when to come back, and what medications to take."

Two methods of evaluation can be used in adult education. The first is direct evaluation or observation of the learned behavior. An example is self-administration of medications in the hospital setting prior to discharge. The evaluation should occur after initial instruction with written reinforcement and a learning time is provided. In the case of a psychomotor objective such as medication administration, the acceptable level of performance needs to be decided. Does the patient need to be 100% accurate? For how many observational periods?

Two problems or potential errors can occur with direct evaluation (Redman, 1997, p. 70). One is observer bias or the fact that behavior may be open to the evaluator's interpretation or human error. A second potential error is sampling error. This may be exemplified in the self-administration of medications in acute care. The number of observational evaluations may be too few to actually document acceptable behavior.

Symptom management of angina or an asthma flare may not occur when direct evaluation is possible. Indirect evaluation becomes the appropriate method. Indirect evaluation involves the learner responding to substitute situations such as oral or written questions. A source of measurement error in this case lies in the fact that what people say they would do and what they may actually do may be two different behaviors entirely. This form of evaluation is the method to use to assure adequate knowledge of emergency care.

Direct and indirect evaluations must be objectively based. Measurable objectives based on accurate patient assessment data supply the evaluation criteria. An objective for the transplant patient who is self-administering medications in the acute care setting might be: *Using a written medication schedule, the patient will take all doses of medications at the correct time (within one hour) in the correct amounts for 24 hours.* Direct evaluation via an observation must occur as the patient takes each medication at the appropriate time. Documentation can be a copy of the patient's medication schedule with "yes" or "no" boxes for correct behaviors. This objective, as written, requires 100% compliance.

Indirect evaluation should also be objective based. An example of an objective is: *After reading the instructional sheet on hypoglycemia, watching the video "Hypoglycemia and Insulin," and discussing with the ACNP, the patient will relate the symptoms to appropriate actions to take.* This cognitive objective suggests an evaluation question such as a case scenario with symptoms of hypoglycemia, with the focus on recognizing the symptoms, what to do, and why. The case scenario increases the real-life applicability of the "need to know" action. Incorporating aspects of the patient's life into the question improves the chance of retaining knowledge and, hopefully, appropriate behavior.

If evaluation reveals inadequate behavior or knowledge to meet the objectives, the educational process should be examined for flaws and reworked. Does the patient see the need for knowledge regarding what to do in the case of hypoglycemia? Does he or she understand the life-threatening nature of this problem and the ability to correct it on his or her own? Were the teaching materials at the right level? Was the process hurried? Was the patient physically ready to learn? Was the teacher able to provide a comfortable atmosphere for learning? Answers to these questions, which evaluate the process of teaching–learning, are crucial to a successful outcome.

Special Populations

Patients with Low Literacy Skills

The number of adults with low literacy skills is one out of three or four. JCAHO requires that patient records reflect an assessment of learning level and that appropriate materials be provided (JCAHO, 1995). Grade level achieved does not correlate with literacy level. Those most likely to have low literacy skills are those who live in poverty, have fewer years of education, are older, or were born outside of the United States (Office of Educational Research and Improvement, 1993). Multiple suggestions for meeting the needs of these patients have been made in this chapter. In-depth strategies can be found in Doak, Doak & Root's *Teaching the Patient with Low Literacy Skills.*

Objectives should be limited to "need to know" information; that is, survival techniques. The patient must agree that the objectives are important to his or her life and meet his or her goals. In other words, the patient must "buy into" the learning process. This is the job of the ACNP as educator at the beginning of patient education. Present the reasons why the patient needs to change his or her behavior. Discuss the risks if he or she doesn't take on the new behaviors or drop old behaviors that are not healthy.

Effective written materials include many visuals, symbols, and pictures (Mayeaux et al., 1996). Materials used should be tested for reading level using a reading-level formula. All media should be written for a fifth-grade reading level. Audiotapes and easy-to-use highly visual computer programs provide mediums to meet the learning needs of patients with low literacy skills. Adherence to health-care prescriptions may be improved by including a family member or significant other in the teaching–learning process.

The use of discussion in a one-on-one format or with a group in combination with visual media reinforces and provides a method for answering patient questions particular to his or her situation. The use of return demonstration as a teaching method is a valid method of assuring patient understanding (Alspach, 1996). Repetition is an important teaching technique to reinforce key behaviors. Patient demonstration is the only way to verify learned behavior. These strategies are applicable to all learners, but especially those with low literacy skills.

Patients Who Are Older Adults

Application of learning theories, Knowles's study of teaching adults, and health belief theory is critical when the ACNP is working with older adults. As the largest consumers of health care, older adults present the challenge of multiple-disease states frequently requiring multiple-health prescriptions. Economic and social support issues play a huge role in the way older adults adapt to a teaching–learning situation.

Ahroni (1996) sees recognition of the life experiences of older persons as a way of acknowledging their self identity or uniqueness. Such recognition provides a way of opening lines of communication and assessing methods of dealing with illness situations in the past. Assessment of important social support systems and how much the older adult can count on them is important. Visual or hearing deficits need to be determined to devise appropriate teaching strategies.

The ACNP works with older adult patients to fit new habits and rituals into the patient's life. Directions and information must be specific and concrete with initial instructions focusing on survival skills. Include a spouse or child in the process if at all possible to provide reinforcement and clarification. Addition of more complex behaviors can occur after survival skills are in place. Reinforcement of psychomotor skills is important, as skills decline over time. Regular review of key points at office visits is important teaching–learning practice for older adults and other learners.

Medication adherence is an area of concern for health-care practitioners working with older adults. Written medication schedules increase adherence according to a study done by Esposito (1995). Forty-two patients were randomized to four groups: standard education; standard education with verbal instruction; standard education with medication schedule; and standard education with medication schedule and verbal instruction. Both groups with a medication schedule had less errors at two-week visits, one- and two-month visits. An observation by several patients was made concerning confusion on the day of discharge. This pilot study recommended medication education with a written medication schedule beginning prior to hospital discharge day.

Older adults require the basic steps (needs assessment, objectives writing, teaching strategies, evaluation) of the educational process to assure knowledge and behavior change. The ACNP must pay attention to individual sensory changes, such as hearing or vision loss, that may require alternative teaching strategies. Complex medication regimens must be carefully reviewed and a written schedule created with each patient to fit into his or her unique lifestyle. Adapt the times to decrease the number of times pills are taken to increase adherence.

Patients of Another Culture

The effect of culture on health-care patient education will be increasingly important as the population of the United States continues to diversify. The influence of learned beliefs about health and individual responsibility for healthy behaviors is culturally based. Each individual member of that culture, however, cannot be categorized to a particular way of behaving based on his or her cultural background alone. The ACNP uses assessment skills to gain knowledge about the patient's health beliefs, recommend behavior changes in a sensitive manner, and negotiate with the patient for the behaviors that fit into his or her cultural pattern (Magnus, 1996; Keenan, 1996).

Cultural differences in language make pamphlets and handouts in the appropriate language a necessity. Doak, Doak & Root (1996) recommend using professionals from the culture to develop written instructions. In the absence of this resource, a simplified version in English with illustrations as the main guide may meet the needs of patients of that culture. Members of the culture working along with the ACNP can assure cultural correctness. Since children in some cultures are not accepted as authority figures, use an adult translator whenever possible.

Patients with Disabilities

The Americans with Disabilities Act of 1990 ensures equal opportunity for all citizens with disabilities. The ACNP must be prepared to provide necessary adjustments in teaching strategies to meet this law for those patients with visual impairment, hearing impairment, spinal cord injury, cerebral palsy, and mental retardation.

King & Cheatham (1995) provide general and specific guidelines for each patient population. The general guidelines for interactions with patients with disabilities are:

- Maintain eye contact.
- Address the person, not a partner or caregiver.
- Encourage expression of opinion through writing or computer if needed.
- Speak in a normal tone of voice.
- Ask if assistance is needed before giving it.

Assuring equal access to the teaching–learning process using a variety of teaching strategies is the goal for the ACNP working with a patient with a disability.

Meeting the educational needs of many different patients requires a team approach to the process. Use the experts in the practice system to help with challenging situations. Consult with colleagues about tools and means of meeting patients' learning needs.

One interesting proposal to meet the challenge of multiple educational needs is a Patient Learning Center (PLC). This is a separate service in cooperation with hospital and clinic providers. Patients are referred to the PLC for specific education provided by professional educators who are nurses with expertise in teaching for behavior change. Goldstein et al. (1996) compared outcomes for lung and heart–lung transplant patients taught to use a home spirometer for daily monitoring in the clinic setting versus the PLC. The patients taught in the PLC setting demonstrated a 30% better adherence to spirometer use and recording. This service, designed specifically to provide the most effective patient education, is a method of improving outcomes. Support and input for this design is within the realm of the ACNP.

COLLEAGUE AND STUDENT EDUCATION

The educational process for colleagues and professional students involves the assessment, planning, implementation, and evaluation components as discussed in patient education (Alspach, 1995). The ACNP who is asked to present a lecture for a professional or student group should obtain particular information: Who is the target audience? What level of learner should the lecture be prepared to address? Are objectives developed by the organizer? What audiovisual equipment is available? What is the learning evaluation process? Answers to these questions assist in preparing a presentation that motivates and meets the needs of the audience. Key points for a speaker–educator are to practice aloud, look confident, and finish on time.

Clinical teaching is an area of the ACNP educator role that provides stimulation and challenge. Benner's framework in the book *From Novice to Expert* (1984) provides strategies for teaching clinical students and colleagues based on their stage of professional development. DeTornyay & Thompson (1993) see a clinical teacher as a role model, consultant, and support person for students and staff.

In a formal preceptor relationship, responsibilities and objectives are provided by the institution in writing. Provide structure for daily learning based on the learner's and course objectives. Daily objectives written by the learner and reviewed by the preceptor give purpose to clinical time. They also provide an evaluation tool for the end of the day and for the course. Perhaps the biggest challenge for a clinical teacher is scheduling time for discussion of learning that is occurring. This one-on-one discussion is critical to providing ongoing feedback (formative evaluation) to maintain appropriate behaviors or to correct inappropriate ones. Document in writing this ongoing communication about progress to provide a basis for the final, summative evaluation.

The ACNP as educator brings advanced practice skills to a role requiring many talents. Learning theories and adult teaching theory provide principles to use when working with adult patients, colleagues, or students. The teaching–learning process gives a structure of assessment, planning, implementation, and evaluation to achieve the outcome of education desired by the adult learner and the teacher. The science found in educational theories and processes plus the art of nursing builds a system meeting the needs of its consumers.

REFERENCES

Ahroni, J. H. (1996). Strategies for teaching elders from a human development perspective. *Diabetes Educator, 22*(1), 47–52.

Alspach, G. (1996). Reading and bleeding: An insidious link. *Critical Care Nurse, 16*(4), 12–14.

Alspach, J. G. (1995). *The educational process in nursing staff development.* Philadelphia: Mosby.

American Hospital Association (1992). *A Patient's Bill of Rights.* Chicago: AHA.

Backer, L., Deck, M., & McCallum, D. (1995). *The presenter's survival kit.* Philadelphia: Mosby.

Bandura, A. (1986). Foundations of thought and action: A social cognitive theory. Englewood Cliffs, NJ: Prentice-Hall.

Belcher, A. E. (1993). Teaching and learning. In Kinney, M.R., Pacha, D.R., & Dunbar, S. B.(Eds.). *Clinical reference for critical care nursing.* Philadelphia: Mosby.

Benner, P. (1984). *From novice to expert.* Menlo Park, CA: Addison-Wesley.

Cohen, L. J. (1993). Discover the healing power of books. *American Journal of Nursing,* October, 70–80.

de Tornyay, R., & Thompson, M. A. (1987). *Strategies for teaching nursing.* New York: John Wiley & Sons.

Doak, C. C., Doak, L. G., & Root, J. H. (1996). *Teaching patients with low literacy skills.* Philadelphia: Lippincott.

Esposito, L. (1995). The effects of medication education on adherence to medication regimens in an elderly population. *Journal of Advanced Nursing, 21,* 935–943.

Goldstein, N. L., Snyder, M., Edin, C., Lindgren, B., & Finkelstein, S. M. (1996). Comparison of two teaching strategies: Adherence to a home monitoring system. *Clinical Nursing Research, 5*(2), 150–166.

Hagopian, G. H. (1996). The effects of informational audiotapes on knowledge and self-care behaviors of patients undergoing radiation therapy. *Oncology Nursing Forum, 23*(4), 697–700.

Joint Commission on the Accreditation of Healthcare Organizations (1995). Education of the patient: Standards and scoring guidelines. In *Comprehensive Accreditation Manual for Hospitals.* Chicago: JCAHO.

Keenan, D. P. (1996). In the face of diversity: Modifying nutrition education delivery to meet the needs of an increasingly multicultural consumer base. *Journal of Nutrition Education, 28*(2), 86–91.

King, E. H., & Cheatham, D. (1995). Health teaching for people with disabilities. *Home Healthcare Nurse, 13*(6), 52–58.

Knowles, M. (1970) *The modern practice of adult education.* New York: Association Press.

Knowles, M. (1973). *The adult learner: A neglected species.* Houston, TX: Gulf Press.

Knowles, M. (1984). *Andragogy in action.* San Francisco: Jossey-Bass.

Lewis, D. (1996). Computer-based patient education: Use by diabetes educators. *Diabetes Educator, 22*(2), 140–145.

Magnus, M. H. (1996). What's your I.Q. on cross-cultural nutrition counseling? *Diabetes Educator, 22*(1), 59-62.

Mayeaux, E. J., Murphy, P. W., Arnold, E., Davis, T. C., Jackson, P. H., & Sentell, T. (1996). Improving patient education for patients with low literacy skills. *American Family Physician, 53*(1), 205–211.

McLaughlin, G. H. (1969). SMOG grading: A new readability formula. *Journal of Reading, 12*(8), 639–646.

O'Brien, J. M. (1995) Developing and implementing a self-learning packet on epidural analgesia. *Med-Surg Nursing, 4*(6), 438–444.

Office of Educational Research and Improvement (1993). Adult literacy in America: A first look at the results of the National Adult Literacy Survey. Washington, DC: U.S. Department of Education.

Parker, R. M., Baker, D. W., Williams, M. V., & Nurss, J. R. (1995). The test of functional health literacy in adults: A new instrument for measuring patients' literacy skills. *Journal of General Internal Medicine, 10,* 537–541.

Patterson, O. (1962). *Special tools for communication.* Chicago: Industrial Audiovisual Association.

Rankin, S. H., & Stallings, K.D. (1996). *Patient education: Issues, principles, and practices.* Philadelphia: Lippincott.

Redman, B. K. (1993). Patient education at twenty five years: Where we have been and where we are going. *Journal of Advanced Nursing, 18,* 725–730.

Redman, B. K. (1993). *The process of patient education.* Philadelphia: Mosby.

Redman, B. K. (1997). *The practice of patient education.* Philadelphia: Mosby.

Rosenstock, I. M., Strecher, V. J., & Becker, M. H. (1994). The health belief model and HIV risk behavior change. In DiClemente, R. J., & Peterson, J. L., (Eds.), *Preventing AIDS: Theories and methods of behavioral interventions.* New York: Plenum Press.

Westphal, C. G. (1995). Storyboards: A teaching strategy for families in critical care. *Dimensions of Critical Care Nursing, 14*(4), 214–221.

9

The ACNP as Researcher: Strategies for Practice

Suzanne M. Burns
Arlene W. Keeling

It is widely accepted that patient care should be based on the latest scientific research (Briones, 1990). It is also often assumed that leadership in the area of linking research and practice should come from advanced practice nurses who work in clinical settings. Based on these assumptions, it can be logically concluded that the ACNP, an advanced practice clinician, would be an excellent candidate for the job of enhancing both the utilization and conduct of nursing research in the practice setting. Unfortunately, the researcher role of the acute care nurse practitioner has yet to be actualized to its fullest potential. In reality, ACNPs struggle with the problem of how to incorporate the researcher component into their job. This chapter addresses the issues related to the ACNP as a researcher and describes strategies for the development of a research-based practice.

▶ REALITIES OF EDUCATIONAL PREPARATION AND CLINICAL PRACTICE

Too often the role of the acute care nurse practitioner (ACNP) as a researcher is the least emphasized aspect of educational preparation and, later, of clinical practice. During the educational experience, particularly in post-Master's programs, little emphasis may be placed on the researcher role due to time constraints in the curriculum. Instead of research, what is emphasized is the acquisition of new knowledge about diagnostic reasoning and patient-care management. Of necessity, the ACNP curriculum focuses on providing the advanced practice nurse with skills necessary for successful transition to the new role. These include critical thinking, skills in taking patient histories and performing physical examinations, and expertise in diagnostic decision-making. This focus is essential since the advanced practitioner is once again joining the ranks of novice (Benner, 1984) in a role that challenges the nurse to practice in a manner that has been traditionally considered to be within the realm of medicine. In addition, emphasis is placed on the acquisition of technical skills such as intubation, suturing, and the insertion of central venous lines. In contrast, less time is devoted to learning research methodology and developing the expertise needed to critique research for use in the clinical setting.

In the practice setting, the constraints inherent in the clinical nature of the ACNP role may conflict with the ACNP's desire and/or ability to participate in research activities. ACNP roles have evolved as one means of meeting the needs of a [illegible]lly changing health-care system (Kleinpell, 1997). With[illegible]ocus on efficiency and cost containment in the provisi[illegible]re, the emerging ACNP role may be quite narrow in scope, yet exceptionally time and effort intensive. Examples include the utilization of ACNPs to "replace housestaff" (Hravnak, 1996; Mallison, 1993; Mitchell-

DiCenso et al., 1996; Snyder et al., 1994; Spisso et al., 1990), to serve as "case managers" for high-risk patient populations, and to manage large numbers of patients (such as those with congestive heart failure) in clinic settings (Anderson, 1997; Lorenz, 1994; Moore, 1993). With the current emphasis on accountability for direct patient care, the broader, traditional "advanced practice" domains of teaching, research, and consultation may be underemphasized except as they relate to specific patient-management questions.

While numerous clinical and bench research studies have been published that provide scientific justification for practice decisions (Hanson & Ashley, 1994; Ohman, 1996; Paladichuk, 1997; Polit & Hungler, 1991), too often, in the fast-paced practice arena, nurses turn to tradition-based practice or experiential knowledge as rationale for practice changes. Several trends seem to be emerging in this regard. Some nurses rely on institution-based protocols for information about practice decisions. The ease with which information about protocols can be exchanged on the Internet may be a factor here, as numerous practitioners sign onto server lists and ask someone from another country/region/state what the "usual protocol" for a given procedure is at their health-care facility. This practice, while easy and quick, may result in "consensus-based" practice, rather than "research-based" practice.

Yet another common and alarming trend in institutional initiatives that appears to be contributing to the devaluing of scientific methodology is the assertion that data, collected in the process of case or outcomes management, is "scientific" evidence of cause and effect. In this process, liberties are taken with the research design (i.e., controlled experimental designs are lacking), and it is common for retrospective data to be compared with prospective data. Unfortunately, the associations that may be discovered retrospectively are rarely causal, and the bias inherent in these "studies" results in clinical applications that may be ineffective or even detrimental to patients' welfare. In fact, relationships may have had little to do with the variable of interest. Unfortunately, there is often little interest in designing studies to test the relationships.

The realities of both the educational process and the development of these trends in the clinical setting explain, in part, why a "theory/practice gap" (Brock, 1990; Janken, Dufault & Yean, 1988) exists. However, the acknowledgment that a gap exists, or explanations of the realities of education and practice, do little to help us establish "research-based practice."

▶ THE THEORY–PRACTICE GAP

For decades, scholars have lamented the "theory–practice" gap (Brock, 1990; Janken et al., 1988). More recently, Rafferty (1996, p. 685) has argued that "the persistence of the [theory–practice] gap would suggest that it is either inevitable or much more complex than we have hitherto thought." Rafferty goes on to say that "We need to understand the power relations that regulate the resources devoted to nursing education and practice, and to address the political and organizational factors that promote or constrain the development of nursing practice at any given time. Only by doing so can we set ourselves realistic goals and move beyond self-blame and self-recrimination in crafting solutions to the theory–practice divide" (1996, p. 685). In fact, according to Rafferty, it may well be that "it is only when the theory–practice gap is held in dynamic tension that change can occur" (1996, p. 689). In other words, the gap is a healthy, necessary part of what triggers knowledge development and change. Others, like Chulay (Paladichuk, 1997) focus on demystifying the research process and providing a practical approach to the attainment of research-based practice. It is Chulay's conclusion that the concept of clinical research is made needlessly complex and confusing by academicians' use of scientific jargon and insistence on methodologic strategies that are at odds with the reality of the clinical practice arena. These two positions need not be in opposition. Indeed, we support Rafferty's position that the "theory–practice" gap is inevitable and important. However, we also agree with Chulay that the gap need not be quite so wide, and that much may be done by advanced clinicians to narrow it.

In fact, it may be that central to the existence of the "gap" is the inherent belief that science and practice are somehow separate. In reality, science is not separate from what we do: science defines nursing. Advanced practice nursing must embrace and emulate this philosophy in practice. Indeed, role modeling may be the key to the true emergence of the ACNP's research-based practice and serve as a method to bridge the theory–practice gap. As noted by Hanneman (1997), the presence of a unit-based clinical expert is necessary for the "catalytic-conversion" of others. "Expert nurses methodically build non-expert nurse expertise through flexible, context-dependent strategies" (1997, p. 334). Specific to the implementation of research-based practice, experts in the clinical setting can foster the dissemination of research findings, identify clinical problems, design and initiate clinical studies, and make system changes based on scientific research. To that end, some practical approaches for developing and promoting a research-based practice follow.

▶ APPROACHES TO DEVELOPING AND PROMOTING A RESEARCH-BASED PRACTICE

Critical-Decision Making and "Clinical Challenging"

The ACNP's clinical presence provides opportunities for regular inquiry about the research basis for practice routines. Opportunities for "clinical challenging" are present on a daily basis while the ACNP makes clinical rounds with other members of the health-care team, or when he or she is present at the bedside.

"Clinical challenging," the process of questioning clinicians about the scientific basis for their decision-making, may be thought of as a method to increase clinical decision-making by developing the critical-thinking skills of clinicians rather than having them depend on intuitive nursing practice (Paul & Heaslip, 1995). By using the technique of "clinical challenging" while making patient care rounds, the ACNP can focus on the latest scientific research to answer a specific patient problem, rather than allowing a solution to be reached by "consensus" or "tradition." Moreover, by questioning the research base related to a specific practice, further exploration of the topic in the form of literature reviews and/or clinical research projects may result as clinicians attempt to find appropriate answers to clinical questions. The ACNP's role is to stimulate scientific inquiry, to identify and delineate the research questions, and to help clinicians decide how to pursue the answers.

It is important—in fact, integral to the process of clinical challenging—that critical thinking be valued. It is also important that nurses be able to accept the role of the ACNP as one who *should* be challenging their clinician decision-making. Unfortunately, assuring this acceptance may be difficult since few clinical practice environments nurture this type of critique. Too often, such clinical challenging is viewed as threatening and hostile. However, ACNPs can change this cultural nursing norm. Since ACNPs are relative newcomers in the acute care setting, yet are trained in scientific reasoning and clinical decision-making, they can use their newly acquired skills to teach other nurses the elements of critical thinking as well. Consistent regular role-modeling of the "clinical challenging" technique with students and staff is essential if desensitization of nurses related to scientific-based reasoning and decision making is to occur.

Using Available Resources

Often, practicing clinicians have little "protected time" to accomplish literature reviews and/or find information related to potential practice changes. Thus, it is important to consider the numerous resources that are available to provide information. For example, professional organizations like the Centers for Disease Control and Prevention (CDC), the National Institutes of Health (NIH), the American Association of Critical Care Nurses (AACN), and others provide information free of charge (or at a nominal cost) in the form of guidelines and/or practice recommendations. Some organizations (e.g., AACN) will do a focused literature review upon request and/or provide "research-based practice protocols" for a small fee. In addition, vendors of supplies, equipment, and drugs all have research reviews on selected topics, and are generous when requests for the information are made.

Experts on selected topics are also an excellent source of information. These physicians, nurses, and other health-care colleagues can often identify immediately whether or not information exists on the topic of inquiry and can make recommendations about locating it. In addition, their "national" perspective can provide important information on the most recent (and sometimes unpublished) research findings.

Partnerships with Educators

While the development of partnerships between academicians and clinicians has long been touted as a means of accomplishing a research-based practice and narrowing the theory practice gap, the paucity of successful partnerships makes such a strategy less than believable to practicing clinicians. There are many reasons for the underutilization of this strategy, including the perception of clinicians that academicians "don't understand the practice setting," and a similar perception held by academicians that clinicians "don't understand research." However, there are some partnerships that do work. These may be useful models for the development of similar relationships. An example follows.

ACNP students at the University of Virginia, many of whom already worked in advanced practice roles at the Medical Center, were assigned by the course professor to identify a clinical nursing question from their own advanced practice, review the scientific literature available on the topic, and write a paper making recommendations for practice changes. One ACNP student who followed surgical patients in her advanced practice reviewed the literature on topical cleansing antiseptics for surgical drain exit sites (Sims, 1997, unpublished). Another ACNP student who worked in Coronary Care reviewed the literature on pulmonary artery catheter manipulation by nurses versus physicians (Zavachy, 1997, unpublished). Under the direction of the course professor, these clinicians and other members of the ACNP cohort are currently moving forward with institutional practice changes and/or studies to further explore the topics. While this innovative partnership was initiated by the educator, similar research applications might be initiated by the ACNP in his or her own institution.

Though quite simple in approach, the application is practical and efficient. Central, however, to such a partnership is the careful selection of the partner. The belief by both the ACNP and educator that such a partnership is valuable (i.e., access to clinical practice in the case of the educator, and a "research resource" for the clinician), is essential.

It is important that we begin to think of partnerships with educators in a more practical manner than we have in the past. Traditionally, we have spoken about these partnerships solely related to the development of studies. This narrow focus has limited our understanding of one another. In fact, academicians need to understand the realities of practice so that they can adequately prepare students for their new roles. One way of promoting this understanding is by having the course professor make clinical rounds with both ACNP students and practicing ACNPs. Involving both students and faculty in a partnership where issues of clinical importance are discussed can decrease the gap between the "Ivory Tower" of academia and the realities of the practice setting. Clinical rounds also attract the attention of other nurses and physicians and promote collaborative practice.

Partnerships with Administrators

Projects that result in positive quality and cost outcomes are important from clinical and institutional perspectives and are more likely to be supported administratively than research that does not focus on such outcome measures. This is not to say that studies that do not link financial outcomes to clinical practice changes are not important or valued by administrators, but "buy-in" will happen more quickly if science-based practice is viewed as a common goal. By linking cost outcomes to science-based practice changes, administrative acknowledgment of the ACNP's "system perspective" is assured. ACNPs should actively work with administrative partners to determine quality practice initiatives and take lead roles in establishing the research base (or lack thereof) associated with the potential change.

Institutions across the country are scrambling to find "cost effective," "quality" solutions to care delivery. Numerous changes in clinical practice have occurred in an effort to accomplish such outcomes. Though many of these changes have been quite costly and disruptive, it is evident that few of the initiatives have been based in science or tested for efficacy. The premise appears to be that there is "no time" to test the initiatives; that immediate action is essential for survival. ACNPs must be cautious in adopting such changes for use in practice.

Many of the current managed-care initiatives, such as the design and use of critical pathways and different forms of care management (e.g., case or outcomes), require the input of experts like ACNPs who have knowledge of specific diseases and patient populations, and understand not only the systems in which care is managed but also how to interpret the scientific findings. For critical pathways to be effective, a scientific base must be used to establish "best practice" indicators, and an understanding of how the indicators may best be monitored (and by whom), is essential. ACNPs must critically evaluate these findings based on their clinical knowledge and understanding of research methodology. In so doing, they may discover that data derived from the "care management" models are compared with retrospective data in an attempt to determine "effect." Rarely, if ever, may these findings be considered *causal.* ACNPs, especially those who fill care-management roles, are in key positions to help clinicians and administrators interpret the data and to appropriately focus future initiatives.

Designing Clinical Studies

The development of clinical studies to answer specific clinical questions is a likely and natural progression of scientifically based clinical inquiry. Practice traditions that have little or no scientific basis will be identified and challenged. Many of these questions may be answered with a literature review; however, some practice questions may have no answers. In that situation, the initiation of a clinical research project may be needed.

The decision to initiate a research project to answer a practice question is first and foremost one of feasibility within the practice setting and "buy-in" [by the clinicians who will be involved]. To this end the researcher should determine the feasibility of answering the specific question in a given period of time, thoroughly understand the complexity of the methods (e.g., data collection, requirement for informed consent) and attain administrative support for instituting the project. These steps are essential if the project is to be a success. Of these, administrative and clinician acceptance and participation in the project is the most important element. The science must be able (in most cases) to take place during work hours and staff involvement should be encouraged. While numerous research textbooks exist on the topic of conducting research, few are designed for practicing clinicians. Instead, as noted by Chulay (Paladichuk, 1997), they are designed for students of research and written by educators and academicians. Some of the proposed tenants in these books are overwhelming and clearly at odds with the realities of clinical practice. For example, the concept of using a data collector (separate from staff) who is hired and trained to collect data in a specific practice environment immediately separates the practicing clinician from the research process. In addition, such a solution is costly and unlikely to be successful; it promotes the concept that research is a separate endeavor and not an essential part of a science-based practice. When the ACNP is guiding and conducting a study in a clinical setting, data collection should rarely be considered a task that an "outsider" accomplishes.

The UVA Experience

In our own institution, a science-based practice is alive and well; numerous studies and resultant publications exist to attest to the success of the projects (Burns et al., 1994; Burns et al., 1995; Burns et al., 1997; Keeling et al., 1994; Keeling et al., 1996). While the studies are quite focused in nature, they have answered, in part, the clinical questions from which they emerged. In addition, the projects have helped to develop a milieu of scientific inquiry. Advanced practice nurses, including those with Master's and Doctoral degrees, collaborate with other clinicians in the process of joining research and practice. Staff nurses have been involved with the formation of the research questions and study design, participated in data collection, and have participated in data entry and analysis. The research process is considered to be a part of practice; it is not separate. The following clinical projects varied in effort and intensity but all demonstrate a focus on research-based practice while considering both quality and cost outcomes.

Ventilator Tubing (Circuit) and Intravenous Line Changes

Some practice changes can be initiated by implementing research findings that have been evaluated and adopted as standards of care at the national level. For example, frequent ventilator circuit and intravenous line changes are linked to increased infection risk. Though the Centers for Disease Control and Prevention have published guidelines related to these practices in an effort to prevent nosocomial pneumonias and line infections, many institutions have not implemented the guidelines. The ACNP can use such "expert" scientific resources to help identify "best practice" goals for his or her own institution. Related practice changes, while requiring coordination and excellent communication to implement, are relatively easy to accomplish and cost-effective. In this example, thousands of dollars may be saved by instituting such "quality" practice changes. In addition, the practice changes demonstrate that "research" is practical and feasible.

Naso/Orogastric Tube Study

Another level of research-based practice includes projects that emanate from unit or service line data. Quality-improvement monitoring frequently yields data that may be difficult to interpret since causality is unable to be determined. However, these data may be used to identify clinical issues of importance that require further investigation through well-designed studies. For example, in our Medical Intensive Care Unit (MICU), clinicians noted that 33% of all naso/orogastric tubes (NG) were "accidentally" being removed. This trend was of concern since tube replacement is associated with complications, can be uncomfortable for the patient, and results in increased hospital costs. Unfortunately, it was unclear if the problem of displaced NG tubes was secondary to decreased monitoring (i.e., staffing levels), tube size or type, patients' mental status, or the methods used to secure the tubes in place. However, since we had been using a standard method for securing the tubes, a study that compared the standard method with experimental methods was seen as a valuable first step in exploring the problem.

Clinicians interested in the project worked with the ACNP to design a study comparing tube securing methods and tube types (Burns, Martin, Robbins, Friday et al., 1995). The study was accomplished in approximately three months and the results suggested that our standard securing method was inferior (highest incidence of failure) to an alternate method tested in the study. A practice change was implemented immediately. To date, the method continues to be our preferred method and considerable cost savings have been associated with the quality-improvement practice change.

Weaning Study

An example of yet a more sophisticated unit-based study is one that focused on patients who require prolonged mechanical ventilation. In this example, a large MICU multidisciplinary team, headed by the ACNP, worked together to identify "best practice" for patients requiring prolonged ventilation. The purpose of the project was to design a clinical pathway (or critical pathway) for the patients who would be managed by the ACNP ("outcomes manager"). Since previous work in the MICU had focused on weaning patients from prolonged ventilation (Burns, Truwit, Burns, 1994; Burns, Carpenter, Harris, 1995; Burns, Egloff, Ryan, Carpenter, Burns, 1994; Burns, Barton, Fahey, Slack, 1991), interest in designing a project that would further improve the care of these patients was very high. To that end, we designed a prospective study to test the efficacy of a comprehensive, standardized, systematic model of care delivery (Burns, Marshall, Burns et al., 1998). The project required a high degree of administrative support since we were asking for a dedicated advanced clinician to be assigned to "manage" the patients three days per week on alternate months for one year. We hypothesized that better outcomes (cost, successful wean, etc.) would be present for those patients managed by the outcomes manager than for those who were not. While the advantage of such an approach seemed obvious from a clinical perspective, few studies supported such an approach to care delivery (especially in such a complex patient population), despite widespread national interest in "critical pathways" and "care management models." In our own institution, multidisciplinary groups were in the process of developing clinical pathways to manage care for numerous patient categories. A scientific approach to the design and testing of such a model was seen as potentially helpful to the institution and might guide the development of future care systems as well.

Though the results of our study did not demonstrate a statistically significant difference in outcomes between outcomes-managed and non-outcomes-managed groups, a trend (which continues today) of cost savings ($3000/case) and shorter ventilator duration (1.2 days) between the groups existed. The true value of the project was related to the systematic, comprehensive multidisciplinary approach guided by an experienced expert (the ACNP).

Cardiac Catheterization Time-In-Bed Studies (TIBS I and II)

In a final example of research-based practice, a service line perspective is used. In an effort to decrease length of stay while maintaining quality of care and promoting comfort in patients following cardiac catheterization, a series of studies have been conducted involving collaboration among cardiologists, staff nurses, advanced practice clinicians, and the primary investigator (a nurse researcher). These studies were randomized, clinical trials reducing requisite time-in-bed for patients who had undergone cardiac catheterization using a femoral artery approach. While the nurse researcher initiated and directed the studies, clinical nurses on all levels of the career ladder (Clinicians I to V) participated in identifying patients for inclusion into the studies, obtaining written consent, randomizing patients to control or experimental group, completing the study protocol, and recording the data. As a result of these studies (Keeling, Knight, Dura et al., 1994; Keeling, Taylor, Nordt, Powers et al., 1996), practice changes reducing requisite time-in-bed for patients postcardiac catheterization from 12 to 6 hours and subsequently from 6 to 4 hours, were made. Moreover, the studies generated new questions for further research (Keeling, Nordt, Haugh et al., 1997) and heightened the awareness of cardiac nurses about the value of clinical research to their practice.

In many institutions the role of ACNP is fairly narrow and limited to patient care management. Applications of the ACNP role to fill the gaps left by the downsizing of staff and to serve as case managers are reasonable and valuable ways to meet care needs of patients and families; they are likely to be common in the future. Though these applications are well suited to the qualifications of the ACNP, this narrow focus, especially related to the use of research, may not serve us well long term.

If we are to be viewed historically as "advanced clinicians," our practice must reflect the application of science and the development of a knowledge base for nursing rather than simply reflecting the limited applications of research findings to solve specific patient-care problems. If ACNPs are to distinguish themselves from others whose focus is to "extend the practice" of physicians, then a research-based practice is essential.

Given the fact that ACNPs are in positions designed to improve processes of care, and outcomes for patients, families, and institutions, it is essential that they use a scientific approach to the development and evaluation of such initiatives. It is the role of the ACNP and other advanced practice nurses to continually challenge the assumptions of practice, identify research issues, and encourage this dynamic tension within the practice arena if a research-based practice is to be established.

REFERENCES

Anderson, R. (1997). Managed care: Increased opportunities for acute-care nurse practitioners. *AACN Clinical Issues, 8*(1), 101–107.

Barton, D., Burns, S. M., & Fahey, S. (1992). Computer application of program to assist patients in weaning from mechanical ventilation. *Computers in Nursing, 10*, 65–71.

Benner, P. (1984). *From Novice to Expert: Excellence and Power in Clinical Practice.* Philadelphia: W. B. Saunders.

Bower, F. L. (1994). Research utilization: Attitude and value. Sigma Theta Tau *Reflections,* (Summer issue), 4–5.

Briones, T., & Bruya, M. (1990). The professional imperative: Research utilization in the search for scientifically based nursing practice. *Focus on Critical Care, 17*(1), 78–81.

Brock, L. R. (1990). From research to utilization: Bridging the gap. *Nursing Management, 21*(3), 50–51.

Burns, S. M., Barton, D., Fahey, S., & Slack, D. (1991). Weaning from mechanical ventilation: A method for assessment and planning. *AACN Clinical Issues in Critical Care Nursing, 2,* 372–387.

Burns, S. M., Burns, J. E., & Truwit, J. D. (1994). Comparison of five clinical weaning indices. *American Journal of Critical Care, 3,* 342–352.

Burns, S. M., Carpenter, R., Harris, R., & Bascle, M. (1995). Developing a team approach to weaning. *Nursing, 95,* May, 32TT-32WW.

Burns, S. M., Egloff, M. B., Ryan, B., Carpenter, R., & Burns, J. E. (1994). Effect of body position on spontaneous respiratory rate and tidal volume in patients with obesity, abdominal distention, and ascites. *American Journal of Critical Care, 3,* 102–106.

Burns, S. M., Marshall, M., Burns, J. E., Ryan, B., Wilmoth, D., Carpenter, R., Aloi, A., Wood, M., & Truwit, J. D. (1998). Design, testing and results of an outcomes managed approach to patients requiring prolonged mechanical ventilation. *American Journal of Critical Care, 7,* 45–57.

Burns, S. M., Martin, M., Robbins, V., Friday, T., Scarborough, M., Burns, S., & Burns, J.E. (1995). Comparison of nasogastric securing methods and tube types in medical intensive care patients. *American Journal of Critical Care, 4,* 198–203.

Cesar, N. S. (Sept. 1988). Nursing rounds: A method to facilitate patient care conferences. *Critical Care Nursing Quarterly, 11*(2), 85–88.

Funk, S. G., Tornquist, E. M., & Champagne, M. T. (1989). A model for improving the dissemination of nursing research. *Western Journal of Nursing Research, 11*(3), 361–367.

Ganong, L. H. (1987). Integrative reviews of nursing research. *Research in Nursing & Health, 10*(1), 1–11.

Hanneman, S. K. (1996). Advancing nursing practice with a unit-based clinical expert. *Image: Journal of Nursing Scholarship, 28*(4), 331–338.

Hanson, J., & Ashley, B. (1994). Advanced practice nurses' application of the Stetler Model for research utilization: Improving bereavement care. *Oncology Nursing Forum, 21*(4), 720–723.

Hravnak, M., Rosenzweig, M. Q., & Baldisseri, M. (1996). Current questions with regard to acute care nurse practitioner preparation and role implementation. *AACN Clinical Issues, 7*(2), 289–299.

Huber, G. L. (1994). Clinical nurse specialist and staff nurse colleagues in integrating nursing research with clinical practice. *Clinical Nurse Specialists, 8*(3), 118–121.

Janken, J. K., Dufault, M., & Yean, E. (1988). Increasing student/staff nurse awareness of the relevancy of research to practice. *Journal of Professional Nursing, 4*(3), 186–191.

Keeling, A., Knight, D., Dura, A., Taylor, V., & Nordt, L. A. (1994). Post cardiac catheterization time in bed study: Enhancing patient comfort through nursing research. TIBS I. *Applied Nursing Research, 7*(4), 14–17.

Keeling, A., Taylor, V., Nordt, L. A., Powers, E., & Fisher, C. (July 1996). Reducing time in bed after cardiac catheterization. *American Journal of Critical Care, 5*(4), 277–281.

Keeling, A., Nordt, L. A., Haugh, K., Taylor, V., Fisher, C., & Powers, E. (1997). *Abstract:* Post-angioplasty time-in-bed study (TIBS 3). *American Journal of Critical Care, 6*(3), 246.

Kleinpell, R. M. (1997). Acute-care nurse practitioner: Roles and practice profiles. *AACN Clinical Issues, 8*(1), 156–162.

Linquist, R., Brauer, D. J., Lekander, B. J., & Foster, K. (1990). Research utilization: Practical considerations for applying research to nursing practice. *Focus on Critical Care, 17*(4), 342–347.

Lorenz, B. T. (1994). Advanced practice nursing in the acute care setting. *Journal of Vascular Nursing, 22*(4), 117–120.

Mallison, M. B. (1993). *Editoral:* Nurses as house staff. *AJN, 3*(7).

Mitchell-DiCenso, A., Guyatt, G., Marrin, M., Goeree, R., Willan, A., Southwell, D., Hewson, S., Paes, B., Rosenbaum, P., Hunsberger, M., & Bauman, A. (1996). A controlled trial of nurse practitioners in neonatal intensive care. *Pediatrics, 98*(6), 1143–1148.

Moch, S., Robie, D., Bauer, K., Pederson, A., Bowe, S., & Shaddick, K. (1997). Linking research and practice through discussion. *Image: Journal of Nursing Scholarship, 29*(2), 189–191.

Moore, S. M. (1993). Promoting advanced practice nursing. *AACN Clinical Issues, 4*(4), 603–608.

Ohman, K. (1996). Expanding collaborative ANS efforts for research utilization. *Clinical Nurse Specialist, 10*(2), 58–61.

Olson, K. (1993). Creating the impetus for research-based practice. *The Canadian Nurse, 89*(1), 36–39.

Paladichuk, K. A. (1997). Marianne Chulay, DNSc: Bridging the research practice gap. *Critical Care Nurse, 17,* 81–85.

Paul, R., & Heaslip, P. (1995). Critical thinking and intuitive nursing practice. *Journal of Advanced Nursing, 22,* 40–47.

Pettengill, M., Gilles, D., & Clark, C. (1994). Factors encouraging and discouraging the use of nursing research findings. *Image: Journal of Nursing Scholarship, 26*(2), 143–147.

Polit, D., & Hungler, B. (1991). *Nursing research.* (4th ed.). Philadelphia: J. B. Lippincott

Rafferty, A. M., Allcock, N., & Lathlean, J. (1996). The theory/practice "gap": Taking issue with the issue. *Journal of Advanced Nursing, 23,* 685–691.

Rudisill, P. T. (1995). Unit-based advanced practice nurse in critical care. *Critical Care Nursing Clinics of North America, 7*(1), 53–59.

Sims, T. (1997). Topical antiseptics as cleansing agents for surgical drain exit sites: A review of the literature (unpublished).

Snyder, J. V., Sirio, C. A., Angus, D. C., Hravnak, M. T., Robert, S. N., Sinz, E. H., & Rudy, E. B. (1994). Trail of nurse practitioners in intensive care. *New Horizons, 2*(3), 296–304.

Spisso, J., O'Callaghan, C., McKennan, M., & Holcroft, J.W. (1990). Improved quality of care and reduction of housestaff workload using trauma nurse practitioners. *The Journal of Trauma, 3*(6), 660–665.

Stetler, C. B. (1985). Research utilization: Defining the concept. *Image: The Journal of Nursing Scholarship, 17*(2), 40–44.

Tibbles, L., & Sanford, R. (1994). The research journal club: A mechanism for research utilization. *Clinical Nurse Specialist, 8*(1), 23–26.

Titler, M., Kleiber, C., Steelman, V., Goode, C., Rakel, B., Barry-Walker, J., Small, S., & Buckwalter, K. (1994). Infusing research into practice to promote quality care. *Nursing Research, 43*(1), 307–313.

White, J., Nativio, D., Kobert, S., & Engberg, S. (1992). Content and process in clinical decision-making by nurse practitioners. *Image: Journal of Nursing Scholarship, 24*(2), 153–158.

Zavacky, B. (1997). Pulmonary artery catheter manipulation by critical care nurses (unpublished).

10

Outcomes Management and the ACNP

Anne W. Wojner

The startling costs of United States health care generated during the former era of provider-driven services are largely responsible for the emergence of today's payer-empowered system. Payers began rewriting the rules for health-care reimbursement in 1982 with the advent of diagnostic related groups (DRGs). Yet, provider change was slow, not becoming a reality until the appearance of managed health care in the late 1980s. Payers have now empowered themselves as the gatekeepers for treatment decision-making, selection of medical providers, health-care institutions, and health-service utilization through control of the almighty U.S. dollar (Wojner, 1999).

As practice professions, the health-care disciplines maintain a contract with the public, and must respond to societal demands for high quality, cost-efficient care with innovative, holistic health processes. Health-care institutions and interdisciplinary providers must prove their value to consumers, preparing for increased accessibility to performance "track" records or report cards. The products of care delivery, namely "outcomes," will be scrutinized by consumers as decision trees are formed to determine *best* provider practices for specific health conditions. Without question, the success of future care delivery models will be judged not by the health disciplines, but by the payers and consumers of health services (Wojner, 1999).

While utilization of nurse practitioners has been viewed positively by both payers and consumers, NPs, like other providers, must position themselves for continued success by constantly reevaluating their care processes through assessment of patient and familial outcomes. This chapter will examine the role of the acute care nurse practitioner (ACNP) as a health outcomes manager, identifying methods that document continuous quality improvement (CQI) of clinical care, enhance research utilization, and foster an ongoing pursuit of *best practice*.

▶ OUTCOMES MANAGEMENT

Outcomes management (OM) is the "enhancement of physiologic and psychosocial patient outcomes through development and implementation of exemplary health practices and services, as driven by outcomes assessment" (Wojner, 1997a, p. 5). Outcomes management was first theorized by Paul Ellwood who suggested that quality measures should be anchored to outcome analyses. Ellwood (1988, p. 1549) defined OM as a "technology of patient experience designed to help patients, payers and providers make rational medical care-related choices based on better insight into the effect of these choices on the patient's life." Four key components were cited by Ellwood for inclusion in an OM initiative:

1. Emphasis on standards that physicians can use to select appropriate interventions
2. Measurement of patient functioning and well-being along with disease-specific clinical outcomes
3. Pooling of clinical and outcome data on a massive scale
4. Analysis and dissemination of the database to appropriate decision makers (Ellwood, 1988)

Figure 10–1 illustrates the four phases of OM. The need for continuous restructuring and refinement of health-care delivery systems becomes evident through OM. As outcomes are measured, interdisciplinary care processes are reevaluated for their appropriateness and benefit to a specific patient aggregate. Providers are lured toward moving care delivery closer to achievement of best practice through a living CQI process that fosters interdisciplinary collaboration and collegiality (Wojner, 1997a & 1997b).

▶ OUTCOMES RESEARCH AND OUTCOMES MANAGEMENT

OM programs must be supported by a strong research arm to enable quantification of outcomes within specified patient populations. Ongoing outcomes research facilitates the study of interdisciplinary interventions (care processes) aimed at achievement of specified goals (physiologic and psychosocial outcomes). Masters-prepared ACNPs are prepared with a basic research foundation to begin the process of outcomes measurement, but are well advised to seek the support of doctorally prepared health science researchers and statisticians to lend ongoing guidance and mentorship (Wojner, 1997b).

Outcomes Defined

Outcomes are the result of specific processes. A favorable outcome is defined as one that results in achievement of a defined goal (Davies, Doyle, Lansky, Rutt, Stevic, & Doyle, 1994). What defines an "acceptable" or "desirable" outcome varies by patient, payer, and provider. At the start of an outcomes initiative, providers must agree upon the health outcomes to be measured and how each outcome marker will be defined (Wojner, 1999).

Selecting an Outcomes Research Strategy

Health care is delivered to diverse patient populations by a variety of provider disciplines. The heterogeneity of both providers and patients challenges the measurement and validity of health outcomes research. Heterogeneity can be overcome through use of tightly controlled, experimental research studies capable of yielding cause-and-effect relationships about hypothetical best practices, but the generalizability of findings becomes questionable when considering the diversity of real-life patients and providers. While experimental research remains the gold standard for outcomes analysis, it may not provide a realistic framework to answer questions about an aggregate's health-care experience within a particular institution and community (Wojner, 1999; Wojner, 1996). Acute care nurse practitioners should

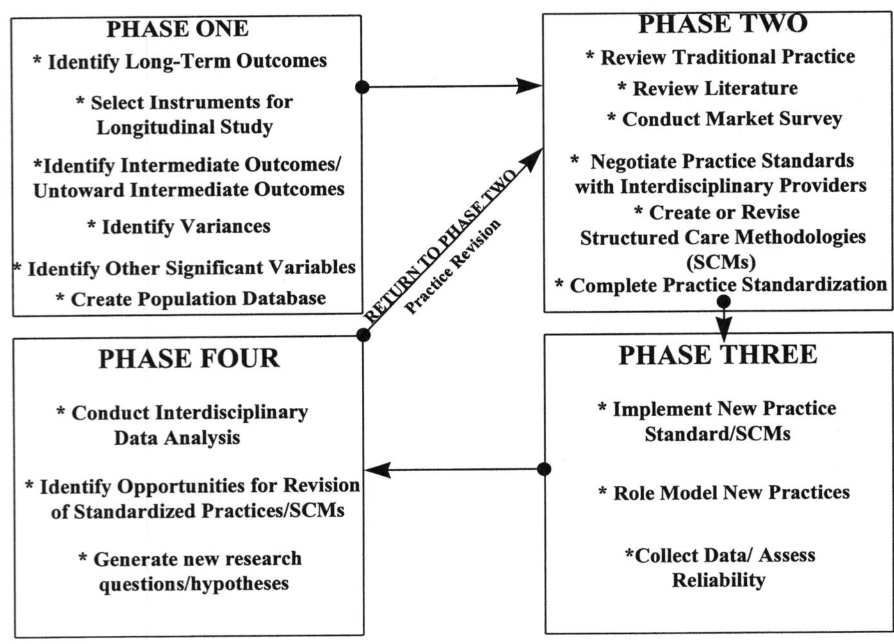

Figure 10–1. Outcomes management quality model.

therefore consider a number of analytical research strategies when developing an OM program.

Analytical research is a rigorous type of study involving the use of a study group and a carefully selected comparison group to test hypotheses. In epidemiological research, two analytic research design categories exist: observational and interventional. Experimental designs are interventional analytic studies that are limited by their artificiality as previously discussed. Observational studies, however, provide a sound model for testing hypotheses and may be integrated into routine practice with much less rigor (Wojner, 1999; Wojner, 1996).

Case-control and cohort studies constitute the two types of observational research that allow hypothesis testing. In case-control studies, a series of patients *with a specific health outcome* (dependent variable), and a comparison group, *without a specific health outcome* are compared. Differences between the groups and varying degrees of risk (odds) for the occurrence of the dependent variable are calculated. Case-control studies are conducted retrospectively, which may limit the power of their findings and the ability to persuade providers toward a change in practice (Wojner, 1999; Wojner, 1996).

Cohort studies classify subjects into two groups: those who *received a specific intervention* (independent variable) and those in which *the intervention was withheld.* The dependent variable is the *health outcome* of interest. Cohort studies may be conducted prospectively or retrospectively depending upon the time of study initiation (Wojner, 1999; Wojner, 1996).

In a retrospective cohort study, the *intervention of interest has occurred* within a group of patients prior to initiation of the research. Subjects are classified into the study group if they received the intervention, or the control group if the intervention was withheld. Differences in the occurrence of the *health outcome* of interest (dependent variable) between the two groups would then be measured. Similar to the case-control design, retrospective cohort studies are conducted by working backwards, thereby limiting their power (Wojner, 1999; Wojner, 1996).

In a prospective cohort design, subjects are placed into two groups: study group *(those who will receive an intervention)* and control group *(those who will have the intervention withheld).* Both groups are followed over a specified period of time and occurrence of a specific *health outcome* (dependent variable) within the two groups is measured. The time over which a prospective cohort study is conducted varies according to the questions or hypotheses generated, but may range from a month to several years. Prospective cohort studies lend themselves well to OM for testing of protocol or algorithmic structured care methodologies (SCMs) (Wojner, 1999; Wojner, 1996).

Outside the typology of epidemiological research, quasiexperimental research designs may also serve the outcomes research effort. Quasiexperiments are similar to true experiments in that they involve manipulation of an independent variable, but they lack at least one of the two other properties that categorize a true experiment, namely, randomization or use of a control group. Similar to a prospective cohort design, quasiexperiments may be readily integrated into the OM process. The disadvantage of using a quasiexperimental design is its relative weakness compared with experimental research in drawing causal inferences (Wojner, 1999; Wojner, 1996).

A Model for Outcomes Management

Figure 10–1 illustrates an OM model that provides a framework for describing the steps taken by an interdisciplinary team in the process of OM. Acute care nurse practitioners should select populations from within their practice settings to study. After organizing a collaborative practice team (CPT) consisting of all interdisciplinary providers that care for the aggregate, the ACNP and team members begin to work through the phases represented in the model (Wojner, 1999).

In phase one, the interdisciplinary team defines population goals and begins construction of a database to support ongoing study of the aggregate. The process then progresses to phases two through four, recycling through the last three phases when the need for revision in clinical practice standards is made evident through outcomes measurement (Wojner, 1999).

Phase One. In phase one, population goals, namely intermediate and long-term outcomes, are defined for measurement. Long-term outcomes are measured longitudinally at specified points following a health-care intervention—for instance, 3, 6, 12, and 24 months following hospital discharge. Long-term outcomes are typically assessed through use of instruments that measure quality of life, resource utilization, functional status, and/or consumer satisfaction (Wojner, 1999).

Intermediate outcomes are measured proximally—for instance, at the time of discharge from the hospital. Intermediate outcomes can be captured through documentation of outcomes attainment, or through documentation by exception. In documentation by exception, the occurrence of untoward intermediate outcomes (UIOs) is captured, providing data rich in unsatisfactory occurrences that prevented outcome attainment within the cohort. Each UIO must be supported by a rigorous definition to ensure the validity and reliability of the data retrieved (Wojner, 1999).

Identification of the UIOs that will be assessed occurs through a sharing of interdisciplinary provider knowledge and review of the literature. Two categories of UIOs may be organized: physiologic UIOs and psychosocial UIOs. An example of a physiologic UIO might be development of deep vein thrombosis following total hip replacement. Valid, measurable operational definitions must be written by team members for each UIO selected for study (Wojner, 1999).

Team members must also identify and define variances that will be tracked for the selected patient cohort. Variances are provider or system "process-problems" that may contribute to unsatisfactory patient outcomes. System variances usually relate to inefficiencies in the system that prohibit or slow patient progression through the facility. An example of a system variance would be inability to transfer the patient out of the intensive care unit due to a lack of intermediate care unit bed space. Provider variances usually pertain to inability to follow through with a needed medical order, care efficiency, practice errors, or inappropriate level of care designation. An example of a provider variance might be failure to order nutrition for a patient within a prescribed time interval. Variances may be best captured by case managers well versed in insurance and institutional regulations and procedures (Wojner, 1999).

Once outcome targets have been defined, interdisciplinary team members identify other variables of interest for the selected patient population that will allow them to distinguish significant differences in outcome within the cohort, relationships among variables of interest, and predictive risk for untoward occurrences. All of these variables are organized into a database to support ongoing descriptive study and outcomes measurement (Wojner, 1999).

To more accurately define patients at risk, team members must identify disease or surgery specific variables that are believed to contribute to differences in patient outcomes. For example, within a stroke patient population, the following variables would be appropriate for collection: age, gender, location and number of brain infarcts, hemorrhagic versus ischemic infarction, stroke severity as measured by a standardized instrument, the presence of dysphagia, and the existence of common co-morbid conditions, to name but a few. Collection of these data enable the team to identify high-risk subgroups of patients such as tube feeding-dependent dysphagia cases at risk for aspiration pneumonia within the stroke cohort that could benefit from additional interventions that may not be necessary for all stroke patients (Wojner, 1999).

Once the database is organized, the CPT begins descriptive study of the cohort. Descriptive research is generally viewed as the least powerful form of outcomes research. This type of research "describes" the general characteristics of an aggregate in relation to an intervention. Variables of interest are usually readily available fostering timeliness and ease in study completion (Wojner, 1999; Wojner, 1996).

While this form of research lacks the rigor of analytical research, use of a descriptive design should not be overlooked. Descriptive studies often pave the road for development of hypotheses or more sophisticated research questions about the aggregate. Through descriptive study, team members are able to define what the cohort "looks like," including the incidence of specific UIOs that may signal the need for practice improvement. Descriptive research often fosters analytical research by identifying opportunities to develop and implement new interventions that may enhance health outcomes within the aggregate (Wojner, 1999; Wojner, 1996).

During descriptive analysis, team members may ask questions of the data such as:

- "What is the incidence of Y event among the population?"
- "Is there a relationship between the occurrence of Y and characteristic X in the population?"
- "Is there a difference in the occurrence of Y between subgroups of patients within the population?"
- "What are the risk factors for Y within the population? (Wojner, 1999).

Findings from the descriptive analysis are used in phase two to identify areas for practice enhancement through standardization of care (Wojner, 1999; Wojner, 1996).

Phase Two. The development of interdisciplinary practice standards designed to achieve a specified health outcome occurs in phase two. Using the findings from the descriptive study, team members develop structured care methodologies (SCM) such as critical pathways, protocols, algorithms, and preprinted order sets that will be used to standardize practice for the cohort, and/or a subgroup of patients within the cohort. Each type of SCM varies in both specificity and degree of provider practice flexibility (Table 10–1). Structured care methodologies should be derived from a combination of research, successful existing practices, published guidelines, and expert opinion. In keeping with the OM model (refer to Figure 10–1), SCMs should be viewed as dynamic, not static, in that they are never a final product, but are continuously enhanced as indicated by the outcomes measured (Wojner, 1999).

Critical pathways usually serve as the foundation for layered SCM application. Pathways should represent a minimum, interdisciplinary practice standard that is broad enough to apply to patients of the same diagnosis, with varying ranges of disease severity (Wojner, 1999). Figure 10–2 illustrates a stroke pathway. Note that regardless of stroke severity, on the day of admission patients in coma, as well as those that are alert and oriented, may be managed using the practices listed on the pathway.

Because of their broad characteristics and minimalistic approach to practice standardization, pathways cannot be credited for a change in outcomes. In other words, team members are unable to measure a cause-and-effect relationship between use of a pathway and achievement of a specified health outcome within the cohort. When outcomes improve following implementation of a pathway, it is not the result of the pathway, but instead the result of enhanced team collaboration among a group of providers that formerly practiced in isolation (Wojner, 1999).

TABLE 10–1. Characteristics of Structured Care Methodologies (SCMs)

Structured Care Methodology	Characteristics
Critical Pathway	Represents a sequential, interdisciplinary, minimal practice standard for a specific patient population. Provider flexibility to alter care to meet individualized patient needs. Abbreviated format, broad perspective. Phase- or episode-driven. Lack of control prohibits ability to measure cause-and-effect relationship, between pathway and patient outcomes; changes in patient outcome are directly attributable to the efforts of the Collaborative Practice Team.
Algorithm	Binary decision trees that guide stepwise assessment and intervention. Intense specificity; no provider flexibility. Useful in the management of high-risk subgroups within the cohort. May be "layered" on top of a pathway to highly control care practices used to manage a specific problem. May utilize analytical research methods to measure cause and effect.
Protocol	Prescribes specific therapeutic interventions for a clinical problem unique to a subgroup of patients within the cohort. Multifaceted; may be used to drive practice for more than one discipline. Broader specificity than an algorithm; allows for minimal provider flexibility by way of treatment options. May be "layered" on top of a pathway to control care practices used to manage a specific problem. May utilize analytical research methods to measure cause and effect.
Order Set	Preprinted provider orders used to expedite the order process once a practice standard has been validated through analytical research. Complements and increases compliance with existing practice standards. Can be used to represent the algorithm or protocol in order format.
Guideline	Broad, research-based practice recommendations. May or may not have been tested in clinical practice. Practice resources helpful in the construction of SCMs. No mechanism for assuring practice implementation.

Reprinted with permission from the Health Outcomes Institute, Inc., The Woodlands, Texas.

Throughout the pathway in Figure 10–2, providers are prompted to consider additional layers of SCMs that may be useful in the management of high-risk subgroups of patients. When used to standardize provider practice, SCMs should be complementary and interrelated, so that practitioners may add layers of care appropriate to manage high-risk subgroups of patients (Wojner, 1999).

It is also important to note that some diagnoses (e.g., multiple traumatic injury) possess such a high degree of patient heterogeneity that the ability to write meaningful and functional pathways is prohibited. When this is the case, team members should move to the next level of SCMs—namely, protocols, algorithms, and order sets—to standardize specific aspects of patient management (Wojner, 1999; Wojner, 1997a). SCMs of this nature might focus, for example, on ventilator weaning, provision of enteral nutrition, or the management of sepsis (Wojner, 1999).

Use of protocols and algorithms enable team members to apply an individualized intervention toward enhancing a specific health outcome within the cohort or a high-risk subgroup, marking the ability for analytical study. Figure 10–3 provides an example of a protocol for use of pentobarbital coma in patients with increased intracranial pressure. Protocols and algorithms are highly specific and limit provider flexibility, enabling team members to measure cause and effect. Often protocols and algorithms lend themselves to conversion to an order set, as illustrated in the rtPA administration order set presented in Figure 10–4. Order sets enhance provider compliance and reduce workload, but because of their cost, should not be utilized until team members have refined the process to one that they believe to be best practice (Wojner, 1999).

It is all too common for providers to mistakenly write SCMs, such as critical pathways, without first defining what they wish to accomplish for a patient cohort. Structured care methodologies written outside an outcomes framework lack the vision and direction necessary to effectively support improved patient health experiences. Additionally, SCMs are of no value when commitment to their implementation is lacking among members of the interdisciplinary team. The people behind the SCM are the most important part of any OM quality initiative. Generally, team support for the development and implementation of an SCM is increased when outcomes measurement identifies the need to restructure care delivery. In other words, outcomes data are powerful at producing commitment to change (Wojner, 1999).

Phase Three. Phase three of the OM process centers around SCM implementation by CPT members. New practices are role modeled and data collection begins. Staff education and credentialing on the new practice standard occurs, followed by collection of outcomes data over a defined period of time. Should the new practice standard in-

HEALTH OUTCOMES INSTITUTE, INC. *Interdisciplinary Critical Pathway* *DRG 014: Ischemic or Non-Operative Hemorrhagic Stroke*				Addressograph	
DATE	**DAY 1:** ____	**DAY 2:** ____	**DAY 3:** ____	**DAY 4:** ____	**DISCHARGE TARGET DAY 5:** ____
CONSULTS	Neurology; Social Service; Dietitian; Physical & Occupational Therapists; Consider Speech and Language Pathologist	Physical Medicine & Rehabilitation (PM&R)			Consider Consult for Percutaneous Gastrostomy Tube (PEG)
DIAGNOSTICS	Chest x-ray C. Brain CT Scan C. 12 Lead ECG C. Chemistry 7 & 12 C. CBC and platelets C. PT/PTT C. Consider prealbumin	Consider Carotid Doppler C. Anticoagulated: PT/PTT C. Consider trans-esophageal echocardiogram	Consider modified barium swallow study Anticoagulated: PT/PTT	Anticoagulated: PT/PTT C. Consider prealbumin	* Anticoagulated: PT/PTT
ASSESSMENTS	Calculate National Institutes of Health Stroke Scale score Calculate Dysphagia Risk Score Neuro assessment q2-4 hr C. Intake & Output q8hr	Complete PM&R therapy plan Neuro assessment q2-4 hr C. Intake & Output q8 hr	C. Neuro assessment q4 hr C. Intake & Output prn	Neuro assessments q4-8 hr C. Intake & Output prn	C. Neuro assessment q8 hr and at discharge
TREATMENTS	Consider Weight-Based Heparin Protocol Consider rt-PA Protocol C. Consider Dysphagia Protocol	Consider Continency Protocol	Consider Warfarin therapy		Discontinue Heparin
ACTIVITY	Begin Stroke Activity Protocol; advance as directed by physical therapist	Stroke Activity Protocol C. Begin ADL Retraining Protocol; advance as directed by occupational therapist	Stroke Activity Protocol C. ADL Retraining Protocol	C. Stroke Activity Protocol C. ADL Retraining Protocol	C. Stroke Activity Protocol C. ADL Retraining Protocol
NUTRITION	Nutrition Risk Screening Consider Nutritional Assessment Order diet to suit swallow competency and nutritional needs	C. Diet as ordered by registered dietitian	Diet as ordered by registered dietitian	C. Diet as ordered by registered dietitian	C. Diet as ordered by registered dietitian
PT/FAMILY EDUCATION	Introduction to stroke disease process	Individual care routine: ADLs	Nutritional management	Prevention of complications	Collaborate with patient/family to generate discharge care plan
DISCHARGE PLANNING	Complete Patient Assessment Profile Assess for advance directive and durable power of attorney Notify payer	Patient and family counseling regarding discharge options Referral made to discharge site		Transfer/discharge plans finalized	Provide contact numbers for nursing, registered dietitian, speech & language pathologist, physical therapist, occupational therapist, physician, social worker Discharge

Figure 10–2 Clinical pathway for stroke.

1. Anesthesia consult: Intubation, oximetric pulmonary artery catheter insertion, jugular bulb catheter insertion and initiation of pentobarbital protocol.
2. Clinical pharmacist consult for ongoing medication/interaction monitoring.
3. Registered dietitian consult for comprehensive enteral nutritional support.
4. Ventilator and intubation setup to bedside.
5. Place warming blanket on bed; continuous temperature monitoring and automatic blanket temperature adjustments to maintain patient temperature between 97 to 100°.
6. a. Administer loading dose of pentobarbital 10 mg/kg over 30 minutes IV.
   b. Follow with pentobarbital 5 mg/kg/hr x 3 hours to achieve a serum pentobarbital concentration greater than 2 mg/dL.
   c. Follow with a maintenance dose of 2.5 mg/kg/hr.
   d. If ICP increases above 20 mm Hg, and the serum pentobarbital concentration is < 3 mg/dL, administer an additional pentobarbital 5 mg/kg IV over 30 minutes to reduce ICP.
7. Administer morphine sulfate ____ mg IV q2 hours for duration of pentobarbital therapy.
8. Administer _________(paralytic agent) ___ mg IV _____(frequency) for duration of pentobarbital therapy; assess depth of neuromuscular blockade q15 until 1-2 twitch response is achieved; follow with q8 hour assessments of depth of neuromuscular blockade.
9. Obtain baseline ABGs, H&H, serum osmo and cardiac output with calculated hemodynamic profile within 1 hour of loading dose administration.
10. Draw serum pentobarbital levels at 4, 8, 12 and 24 hours after initial loading dose administered; (therapeutic range = 2-4 mg/dL).
11. Continuous SvO_2, SpO_2, JvO_2 and temperature monitoring.
12. Repeat cardiac output q8 hrs for first 24 hours, then qday and prn for duration of pentobarbital therapy.
13. Serum pentobarbital levels qday for duration of therapy; maintain level between 2-4 mg/dL.
14. Set ventricular drain at an overflow level of ____ mmHg/cmH_2O; document ICP, CPP and ventricular drainage hourly.

Figure 10–3. Pentobarbital coma protocol. *(Reprinted with permission from the Health Outcomes Institute, Inc., The Woodlands, Texas.)*

volve use of expensive technology, CPT members should be prepared to conduct a cost:benefit analysis to document cost savings related to reduced complications, prevented readmissions, decreased intensive care use, and length of stay (Wojner, 1999).

Phase Four. In phase four, CPT members review the outcomes measured within the cohort. Opportunities for further enhancement of clinical practice are identified, returning the process to phase two where practice standards are renegotiated, and new SCMs are generated for implementation (Wojner, 1999).

THE ACNP AS "OUTCOMES MANAGER"

Acute care nurse practitioners should actively facilitate the OM process for interdisciplinary providers. Acting as "outcomes managers," ACNPs are well prepared to function as

1. Complete inclusion/exclusion criteria checklist.

2. Call Stroke Response Team STAT.

3. Start 2 IV lines as follows:
   a. Dedicated rtPA infusion line
   b. KVO line for other fluid and medication administration

5. Insert foley catheter if unable to void prior to start of rtPA infusion.

6. Calculate dosage of rt-PA 0.9 mg/kg:

   Step A. Patient weight ______ kg X 0.9 mg = ______ **mg total rtPA dose.**
   (Stop: Check dose; if greater than 90 mg by calculation, give total of 90 mg only).

   Step B. Administer 10% of total rtPA dose as an initial bolus:

   ______ mg total rtPA dose X .10 = ______ **mg bolus dose.**

   Step C. Administer the balance of the rtPA over the next 60 minutes

   ______ mg total rtPA - ______ mg bolus dose = ______ **mg infusion dose.**

7. Neuro vital signs q15 minutes x 1 hour; then begin q1 hour x 5 hours, and then q2 hours for 18 hours. Increase frequency of neuro vital signs as indicated by patient's clinical status. Notify MD STAT of signs and symptoms of deterioration.

8. Cardiac monitoring x 24 hours.

9. *Following rtPA infusion*, no nasoenteric/nasogastric tube insertions, foley catheter insertions, or invasive lines/procedures x 24 hours unless clinically indicated.

10. STAT brain CT for signs and symptoms of clinical deterioration.

11. Stop anticoagulant or antiplatelet medications until further notice.

Figure 10–4. rtPA order set. *(Reprinted with permission from the Health Outcomes Institute, Inc.,The Woodlands, Texas.)*

leaders supporting achievement of excellence in clinical practice through clinical inquiry (Wojner, 1999; Wojner & Kite-Powell, 1997).

Several prerequisite professional and personal characteristics are necessary to support success of the ACNP as an outcomes manager: recognized hands-on clinical expertise, the ability to act as a leader and change agent, sound teaching and consultation skills, experience in research conduct, a collaborative practice philosophy, tenacity, political astuteness, and a willingness to take risks. A commitment to continuous self-reflection, evaluation, and role improvement are necessary to foster effective team relationships and improved clinical outcomes management (Wojner, 1999; Wojner & Kite-Powell, 1997).

Figure 10–5 illustrates a model that represents the two main roles of the ACNP as an outcomes manager: clinical practice and clinical inquiry. Extending from the clinical roles are subroles that are driven by the clinical role components. For example, interdisciplinary education provided by the ACNP should be the result of clinical inquiry into patient outcomes produced by the team. As untoward outcomes are measured, the ACNP develops and participates in the provision of interdisciplinary staff education aimed at use of a newly proposed practice standard targeted to improve patient outcomes within the cohort (Wojner, 1999; Wojner & Kite-Powell, 1997).

Table 10–2 identifies performance criteria to support role development and evaluation of position effectiveness for the ACNP–outcomes manager. Again, the clinical practice and clinical inquiry roles are used to support the

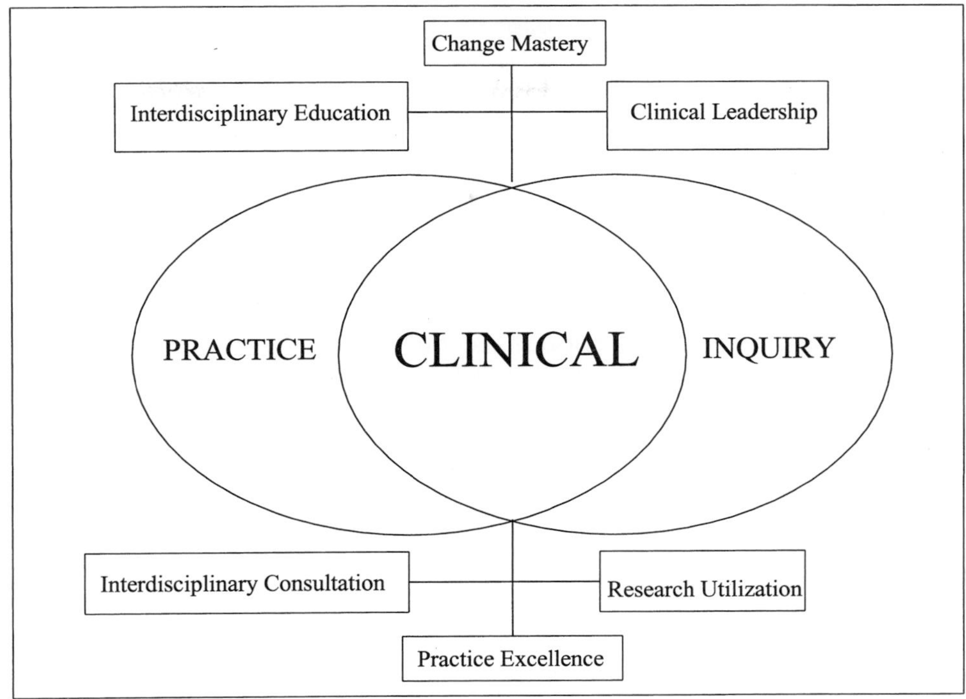

Figure 10–5. Clinical practice and clinical inquiry components of the role of the outcomes manager.

process of OM and position development/implementation (Wojner, 1999; Wojner & Kite-Powell, 1997).

Outcomes management enhances patient care. Patients and their families benefit from ongoing evaluation and commitment to the provision of best practice. Providers benefit from the use of interdisciplinary outcomes measures that enable them to continuously improve care, use research, and contribute to the body of knowledge that supports health care. Payers benefit from an ability to benchmark provider and institutional performance, and the establishment of predictive models that may be used to foster realistic, severity-based payment systems (Wojner, 1999; Wojner, 1997a).

Outcomes management is here to stay, placing the

TABLE 10–2. Performance Criteria for Outcomes Managers

The Clinical Domain

Expert Clinical Practice*—Analyses practice and designs interdisciplinary interventions for implementation and testing toward achievement of best practice for an assigned patient population.*

Effective (10)	Exceeds Effective (15)	Highly Effective (20)
1. Demonstrates and communicates clinical expertise in an assigned patient population, role modeling application of clinical practice standards. 2. Responds to interdisciplinary requests for evaluation and management of complex patients as they move across the continuum. 3. Analyzes contributors to variable cost, making recommendations for change in clinical practice to facilitate cost effective, quality care. 4. Provides informal education to interdisciplinary providers and consumers as indicated by patient outcomes.	1. Supports development of business and marketing plans for assigned patient population. 2. Provides formal educational programs to interdisciplinary providers and/or consumers. 3. Practices beyond the boundaries of his/her assigned patient population as requested, to enhance quality and financial outcomes. 4. Mentors graduate nursing students in the provision of expert, research-based, clinical care. 5. Supports the ongoing proffessional growth of his/her peer group within the outcomes management department.	1. Demonstrates increased efficiency and quality in clinical practice. 2. Impacts community wellness through development and implementation of continuum-based services. 3. Achieves a balance between clinical quality and financial outcomes that positively impacts the institution's bottom line. 4. Develops service and/or divisional policy and procedures as driven by outcomes measured.

(Continued)

TABLE 10–2. Performance Criteria for Outcomes Managers *(Continued)*

The Clinical Inquiry/Research Domain

Researcher*—Facilitates enrichment of the body of science and research-based care, leading to the identification of best practice for the assigned patient population.*

Effective (10)	Exceeds Effective (15)	Highly Effective (20)
1. Facilities development, implementation and ongoing revision of structured care methodologies based on scientific evidence. 2. Establishes outcomes measures and methods for data collection. 3. Builds an outcomes management database to describe quality and efficiency of care. 4. Participates in the development of descriptive research. 5. Engages members of the interdisciplinary team in the generation of research questions or hypotheses for study within the population of interest. 6. Shares findings from outcomes management database with interdisciplinary grassroots providers.	1. Participates as a co-investigator in the development of research proposals suitable for submission to the IRB. 2. Implements well-conducted observational studies related to assigned population. 3. Implements a research-based change in practice that results in improved quality and/or financial outcomes. 4. Provides formal education regarding the research process to interdisciplinary providers.	1. Serves as a principal investigator in the development of research proposals. 2. Implements well-conducted randomized controlled trials or cohort studies. 3. Serves as an administrator for funded research project. 4. Submits grant proposal(s) for funding of proposed research study. 5. Publishes original research in peer-reviewed journal. 6. Mentors interdisciplinary providers in the process of research proposal development. 7. Coordinates a service-based journal club charged with research utilization for assigned patient population.

Reprinted with permission from the Health Outcomes Institute, Inc., The Woodlands, Texas.

ACNP in an unique position to facilitate program development and implementation. Movement away from tradition-based practice toward practice that embraces outcomes-driven care has become a reality. Acute care nurse practitioners are challenged to bring the richness of OM to life through a commitment to research-based continuous quality improvement.

REFERENCES

Davies, A. R., Doyle, M. A., Lansky, D., Rutt, W., Stevic, M. O., & Doyle, J. B. (1994). Outcomes assessment in clinical settings: A consensus statement on principles and best practices in project management. *Journal on Quality Improvement, 20*(1), 6–16.

Ellwood, P. M. (1988). Outcomes management. A technology of patient experience. *New England Journal of Medicine, 318*(23), p 1549–1556.

Wojner, A. W. (1996). Outcomes management: Driving enhancement of interdisciplinary practice with outcomes research. *Seminars in Perioperative Nursing, 5*(1), 3–11.

Wojner, A. W. (1997a). Outcomes management: From theory to practice. *Critical Care Nursing Quarterly, 19*(4), 1–15.

Wojner, A. W. (1997b). Widening the scope: From case management to outcomes management. *The Case Manager, 8*(2), 77–82.

Wojner, A. W. & Kite-Powell, D. (1997). Outcomes manager: A role for the advanced practice nurse. *Critical Care Nursing Quarterly, 19*(4), 16–24.

Wojner, A. W. (1999). *Outcomes Management: Applications for Clinical Practice.* St. Louis: Mosby.

II

Essentials of Practice

11

Approach to the Hospitalized Patient

Ruth M. Kleinpell

Unpredicted illness and hospitalization are stressful life events. The approach to the hospitalized patient, therefore, must be with the knowledge that the patient and his or her family members may be experiencing extreme stress and anxiety.

Hospitalization disrupts family roles and often creates crisis. Families of critically ill patients may experience high levels of emotional distress not only because the patient is critically ill, but also because the illness or injury is unexpected, and may have a critical phase that may be prolonged for days (King & Gregor, 1985).

Health crises are critical events in families' lives, and the hospitalization of a family member in a critical care setting has immense potential for creating a family crisis (Leavitt, 1984). The degree of stress experienced by patients and family members, as well as the responses to the stress, are highly variable. King & Gregor (1985) maintain that emotional distress—stress that is emotionally or psychologically uncomfortable or unpleasant—increases when the person:

- is exposed to a source of stress, or "stressor," with little or no time for anticipatory preparation,
- experiences a stressor for a prolonged period of time,
- experiences multiple stressors concurrently,
- is exposed to an ambiguous or uncertain event, or
- is exposed to an event that involves an important aspect of life, such as health or survival.

Hospitalization in an acute or critical care unit is certainly a stressful experience, that often initially has an uncertain outcome. Family members of the hospitalized patient are also exposed to this stressful event and, depending on how they interpret it, can also experience a stress response.

▶ PHYSIOLOGICAL AND BEHAVIORAL RESPONSES TO STRESS

Stress is the nonspecific response of the body to any demand (Selye, 1978). While hospitalization itself is a stressor, additional stressors such as prolonged state of illness prior to hospitalization, sudden trauma, intense pain, and fear can compound the state of stress for the hospitalized patient.

The physiological response to stress includes a local adaptation syndrome (LAS) in tissues directly affected by a stressor, which constitutes the inflammatory response, and a general adaptation syndrome (GAS) of neuroendocrine responses (Selye, 1978). The stress response is initiated by the activation of the hypothalamus, pituitary, and adrenal glands, with subsequent release of catecholamines (epinephrine, norepinephrine, and dopamine) and a variety of hormones, including antidiuretic hormone, prolactin, growth hormone, adrenocorticotropin hormone, and cortisol (Fig. 11–1). The circulating catecholamines result in

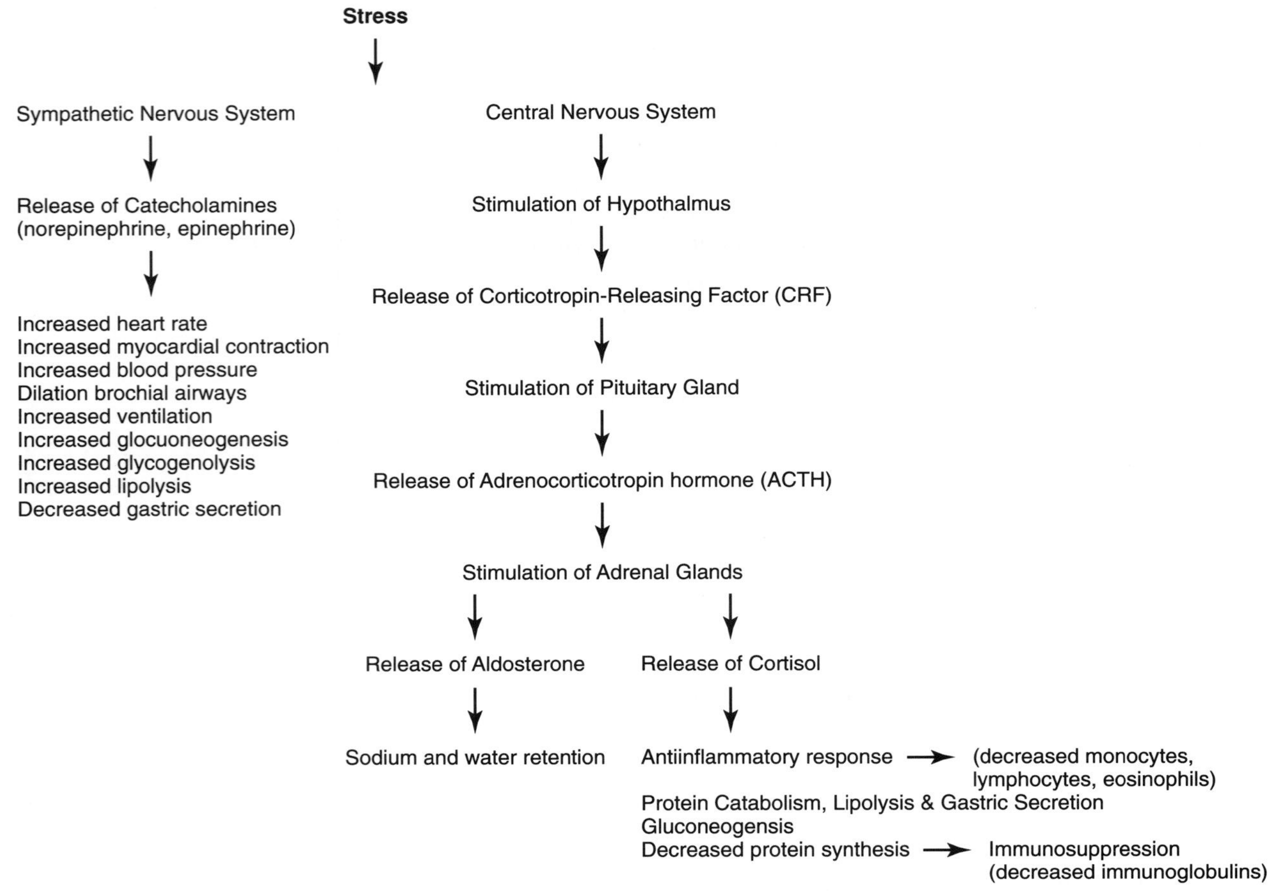

Figure 11–1. Mechanisms of the stress response.

increased heart rate, increased myocardial contractility, increased venous return, peripheral vasoconstriction, brochodilation, increased ventilation, dilation of skeletal muscle vasculature, hyperglycemia, lipolysis, gluconeogenesis, glycogneolysis, and decreased protein synthesis (McCance & Shelby, 1994). Increased gastric secretion, immunosuppression, and antiinflammatory effects result from the secretion of cortisol. Cortisol-induced effects are initially adaptive as a stress response, but can be destructive to target cells with prolonged exposure. Stress-induced alterations of the nervous, endocrine, and immune systems are protective in nature, but prolonged stress responses can result in maladaptive cellular and organ system changes and may potentiate the risk for disease (McCance & Shelby, 1994). Many diseases and immune-related conditions are associated with stress including infection, hypertension, stroke, irritable bowel syndrome, ulcerative colitis, allergy, autoimmune diseases, depression, and insomnia (Table 11–1). However, the specific mechanisms causing stress-induced illnesses are not clearly known. Additionally, the effect of psychological factors in minimizing physiologic stress responses is acknowledged, but continues to be researched.

STRESS, COPING, AND ILLNESS

Stressful life events may cause illness, affect the course of illness, or may affect response to treatment. Whether a stressful life event produces distress or illness depends on a person's appraisal of the event and the coping strategies

TABLE 11–1. Examples of Stress-Related Conditions/Diseases
Hypertension
Myocardial Infarction
Cerebrovascular Accident
Peptic Ulcers
Migraine Headaches
Asthma
Autoimmune Diseases
Irritable Bowel Syndrome
Ulcerative Colitis
Eczema
Alcholism
Obesity
Depression
Insomnia

used. Coping, or the process of managing stressful demands, involves using strategies to deal with stress arising from perceived threats to psychological integrity (Aquilera & Messick, 1993).

Lazarus (1964) highlighted the importance of the mediating cognitive process, appraisal, to assess coping methods used by individuals. Appraisal is an ongoing perceptual process that helps one to distinguish potentially harmful from beneficial events in one's life. When a threatening situation occurs, an initial primary appraisal is made to judge the perceived outcome of the event (Aguilera & Messick, 1993). A secondary appraisal follows, which allows one to consider potential coping strategies to counter the threat. As coping mechanisms are used, ongoing reappraisals help one to adjust coping behaviors.

The use of effective positive coping strategies can prove beneficial in successfully combating stress. Alternatively, ineffective negative coping behaviors may compound the effects of distress on health. Mediating factors that may influence stress susceptibility include age, gender, past experience, current health, social economic status, social support, personality, self-esteem, and genetics (McCance & Shelby, 1994).

Recognizing that critical illness is a stressful event for the hospitalized patient, the acute care nurse practitioner (ACNP) can directly impact the experience to minimize the effects of stress and promote coping strategies. In providing information, offering explanations, teaching, being empathetic, and providing reassurance, the ACNP can help to allay the patient's anxiety and promote acceptance of the hospitalization. Recognizing and addressing increasing anxiety in the patient prevents escalating stress responses. Ensuring that comfort measures and, if needed, anxiolytic medication are provided helps to combat the stress of critical illness.

FAMILY/SIGNIFICANT OTHER RESPONSE TO STRESS AND ILLNESS

Family and significant other responses to the stress of hospitalization and illness also can affect the patient. The emotional distress of a critical illness taxes the usual coping mechanisms of the family and, when threatening, can lead to a family crisis. In developing a conceptual framework for viewing families in crisis, the crisis model offered an equation to reflect the interaction of important variables: **A** (the event) → interacting with **B** (the family's crisis–meeting resources) → interacting with **C** (the definition the family makes of the event) → produces **X** (the crisis) (McCubbin & McCubbin, 1992). The crisis framework has since been cited in numerous subsequent work dealing with family members experiencing a sudden and critical illness. In understanding how the family may interpret a critical illness, interventions can be made to prevent a crisis situation. In other situations, should a family crisis occur, strategies for dealing with the event—or crisis intervention—may be warranted.

Crisis-intervention activities are aimed at influencing the course or development of a crisis through providing support and guidance. The goal of crisis intervention for families is to strengthen the adaptive and problem-solving capabilities of the family (Braulin, Rook, & Sills, 1982; Hoff 1995). A crisis is a state of homeostatic imbalance, and interventions by the ACNP can assist the family in crisis to move toward homeostatic balance. Interventions may involve clarifying aspects of the hospitalization, problem solving, or referral to other health-care professionals. Through providing information, assessing social support systems and counseling or therapy needs, and encouraging life style changes (such as diet, rest, exercise, relaxation), the ACNP can assist the family to manage the crisis of hospitalization. The acknowledgment of the role of the family, and of the importance in addressing and meeting family members' needs, can assist the family in crisis toward adaptive coping. Consequently, the family is better able to provide support to the hospitalized patient.

Family Assessment

The "Standards of Clinical Practice and Scope of Practice for the Acute Care Nurse Practitioner" (American Nurses Association, 1995) identifies family assessment as a key element of the ACNP role. Family assessment models are of value in analyzing family dynamics and providing direction for interventions. Three commonly used family assessment models include Structural–Functional, Family Systems, and Family Stress (Friedman, 1992). Each provides a framework for assessing and dealing with aspects of family functioning.

Structural–Functional Model

The Structural–Functional model proposes that relationships between and within the family are dependent on the structure or organization of the family. Assumptions of the model include that the family is a social system that serves to meet family functions including meeting the affective, socialization, coping, economic, physical, and health needs of the family (Artinian, 1994). The focus of the model is the family structure, and how well the family functions are met. Critical illness results in alterations in the family structure that can impact family functioning. The Structural–Functional model highlights important assessment criteria in families during critical illness, including family coping, affective functioning, and physical and health needs of the family. Interventions that can be used when a change in family structure alters functioning include assisting the family to modify role responsibilities, identify effective coping skills, and recognize their own health needs to strengthen family functioning (Artinian, 1994).

Family Systems Model

The Family Systems model focuses on the interaction of family members as a system, wherein a change in one member affects the entire family as a system. A family system is interrelated and interdependent, so that critical illness has the potential to impact the entire system. Interventions are aimed at assisting the whole family system in adapting and include facilitating family communication, interaction, and decision making (Artinian, 1994).

Family Stress Model

The Family Stress model views the family as a system that can be disrupted by a stressful event. Resources available to the family and perceptions of the stressful event impact the degree of disruption that can occur due to critical illness. Understanding the family's perception of hospitalization, clarifying misconceptions, and identifying resources available to the family can help to promote family coping.

The ACNP can use family assessment models to determine the impact of hospitalization on the family. Interventions can then be structured to assist the family in coping with the patient's critical illness and hospitalization, and to meet specific family needs.

Family Needs

Identifying family needs during critical illness has been explored in a variety of studies since the late 1970s. Numerous studies have examined important needs and concerns of families. One of the first studies that identified the needs relatives of critically ill patients was done by Molter (1979). In this descriptive study, 45 statements of possible needs were rated by level of importance by 40 relatives of critically ill patients. The most important needs identified were: (1) to feel there was hope, (2) to feel that hospital personnel cared about the patient, (3) to have a waiting room near the patient, (4) to be called at home about changes in the condition of the patient, and (5) to know the patient's progress.

Molter's research was used as a prototype for additional nursing research studies on family needs. In 1983, the Critical Care Family Needs Inventory (CCFNI) (Molter & Leske, 1983) was developed based on the original research of Molter. The CCFNI is a structured questionnaire of 45 need statements that has since been used and adapted in numerous studies examining important family needs (Bouman, 1984; Daley, 1984; Hickey, 1990; Leske, 1986; Molter, 1979; Norheim, 1989; Norris & Grove, 1986; Rodgers, 1983; Simpson, 1989; Spatt et al., 1986; Stillwell, 1984).

From these studies, it became evident that family members of critically ill patients identified similar important needs, regardless of ICU setting (Table 11–2). The need for information has consistently been a top priority need. Other needs—to know the prognosis, to feel there is hope, to have questions answered honestly, to have explanations given in terms that are understandable, and to know what is being done for the patient—have also been identified as priority needs to family members. In empirically analyzing 27 studies of family needs, Leske (1991) found that five categories of family needs emerged. These included the need for information, assurance, proximity, comfort, and support.

TABLE 11–2 Important Family Needs
To know how the patient is being treated medically
To know specific facts about the patient's progress
To know why things are done for the patient
To have explanations given in terms that are understandable
To recieve information about the patient once a day
To know the prognosis
To see the patient frequently
To have questions answered honestly
To feel there is hope
To be assured that the best care possible is being given to the patient
To feel that hospital personnel care about the patient
To be called at home about changes in the patient's condition
To have directions as to what to do at the bedside
To know the occupational identity of staff members

Although much research has addressed identifying family needs during critical illness, only a few studies have examined interventions aimed at meeting family needs. Interventions that have been explored include changing visiting hours to flexible or open hours, providing visitor pamphlets that outline ICU care and general hospital-related information, providing an ICU orientation for family members, conducting family support groups, and calling family members with patient updates (Chavez & Faber, 1987; Cray, 1989; Daly et al., 1994; Dracup & Breu, 1978; Freismuth, 1986; Gillis et al., 1990; Halm, 1990; Halm & Titler, 1990; Henneman et al., 1992; Kirchoff, 1982; Makielski et al., 1986; Simpson et al., 1996; Schwartz & Brenner, 1979) (Table 11–3). The need for continued study on interventions to best meet family needs during critical illness remains.

▶ ROLE OF THE ACNP

In a recent survey examining roles and practice components of ACNPs, the most frequently performed element of care was discussing care with family members (Kleinpell, 1997).

TABLE 11–3 Interventions to Meet Family Needs
Flexible/open visiting hours
Visitor pamphlets
Education/orientation sessions
Family group meetings
Family contact person with whom daily contact is made
Calling family at home to report patient changes

The role of the ACNP in assisting patients and families in adapting to critical illness involves several components. These include providing information, helping to meet family needs, providing support, promoting coping strategies, and providing referrals.

The need for information has been identified as a top priority need for patients and family members during critical illness. In providing information regarding diagnosis, planned treatment, response to treatment, prognosis, and likely outcomes, ACNPs can meet families' informational needs and promote acceptance of and coping with a critical illness event. The ACNP can intervene and provide for family needs in a timely manner to prevent adverse family occurrences such as increased stress or altered coping.

Strategies that can be used by the ACNP in assisting the patient include helping the patient to recognize the presence of stress and identifying coping behaviors. Working to minimize environmental related stress such as decreasing noise levels, preventing sleep and rest interruptions, and scheduling tests and treatments at convenient times whenever possible can also help ease the effects of stress on the patient.

Physiologically, the ACNP can institute measures to prevent harmful effects of stress, such as stress ulcer prophylaxis, monitoring oxygenation and perfusion status, minimizing exposure to infection, ensuring adequate nutritional intake, and initiating sedation and anxiolytic medications as indicated.

The ACNP's role in helping patients' and family members' transitions during critical illness involves interrupting or minimizing stress, assisting to cope with hospitalization, and promoting adaptation to the stressors of critical illness.

REFERENCES

Aguilera, D. & Messick, J. (1993). *Crisis Intervention: Theory and Methodology.* St. Louis: Mosby.

American Nurses Association (1995). *Standards of Clinical Practice and Scope of Practice for the Acute Care Nurse Practitioner.* Washington DC: American Nurses Publishing.

Artinian, N. (1994). Selecting a model to guide family assessment. *Dimensions of Critical Care Nursing, 14*(1), 4–12.

Bouman, C. (1984). Identifying priority concerns of families of intensive care unit patients. *Dimensions of Critical Care Nursing, 3*(5), 313–319.

Braulin, J., Rook, J., & Sills G. (1982) Families in crisis: The impact of trauma. *Critical Care Quarterly, 5*(3), 38–46.

Chavez, C. & Faber, L. (1987). Effect of an education–orientation program on family members who visit their significant other in the ICU. *Heart & Lung, 16*(1), 92–99.

Cray, L. (1989). A collaborative project: Initiating a family intervention program in a medical intensive care unit. *Focus on Critical Care Nursing, 16*(3), 212–218.

Daley, L. (1984). The perceived immediate needs of families with relatives in the intensive care setting. *Heart & Lung, 13*(3), 231–237.

Daly, K., Kleinpell, R., Lawinger, S., & Casey, G. (1994). The effect of two nursing interventions on families of ICU patients. *Clinical Nursing Research, 3*(4), 414–422.

Dracup, K. & Breu, C. (1978). Using nursing research findings to meet the needs of grieving spouses. *Nursing Research, 27*(4), 212–216.

Freismuth, C. (1986). Meeting the needs of families of critically ill patients: A comparison of visiting policies in the intensive care setting. *Heart & Lung, 15*(3), 309–310.

Friedman, M. (1992). *Family Nursing: Theory and Practice.* Norwalk, CT: Appleton & Lange.

Gillis, C., Neuhaus, J., & Hauck, W. (1990). Improving family functioning after cardiac surgery: A randomized trial. *Heart & Lung, 19*(6), 648–654.

Halm, M. (1990). Effects of support groups on anxiety of family members during critical illness. *Heart & Lung, 19*(1), 62–71.

Halm, M. & Titler, M. (1990). Appropriateness of critical care visitation: Perceptions of patients, families, nurses, and physicians. *Journal of Nursing Quality Assurance, 51*(1), 25–37.

Hampe, S. (1975). Needs of the grieving spouse in a hospital setting. *Nursing Research, 24*(2), 113–120.

Henneman, E., McKenzie, J., & Dewa, C. (1992). An evaluation of interventions for meeting the information needs of families of critically ill patients. *American Journal of Critical Care, 1*(3), 85–93.

Hickey, M. (1990). What are needs of families of critically ill patients? A review of the literature since 1976. *Heart & Lung, 19(4)*, 401-415.

Hoff, L. (1995). *People in Crisis: Understanding and Helping.* San Francisco: Jossey-Bass.

King S. & Gregor F. (1985) Stress and coping in families of the critically ill. *Critical Care Nurse, 5*(4), 48–51.

Kirchoff, K. (1982). Visiting policies for patients with myocardial infarction: A national survey. *Heart & Lung, 11*(6), 571–576.

Kleinpell, R. (1991). Needs of families of critically ill patients: A literature review. *Critical Care Nurse, 11*(8), 34–40.

Kleinpell, R. (1997). Acute-care nurse practitioners: Roles and practice profiles. *AACN Clinical Issues in Acute and Critical Care, 8*(1), 156–162.

Lazarus, R. (1964). *Psychological Stress and the Coping Process.* New York: McGraw-Hill.

Leavitt, M. (1984). Nursing and family-focused care. *Nursing Clinics of North America, 19*(1), 83–86.

Leske, J. (1986) Needs of relatives of critically ill patients: A follow-up. *Heart & Lung, 15*(2), 189–193.

Leske, J. (1991). Overview of family needs after critical illness: From assessment to intervention. *AACN Clinical Issues in Acute and Critical Care, 2*(2), 220–226.

Makielski, M., Winet, E., Kaufman, M., Gerbasich, K., Meert, S., & Galbraith, G. (1986). The effects of open visitation on the stress perceptions of cardiac care patients. *Heart & Lung, 15*(3), 312–313.

McCance, K. & Shelby, J. (1994). Stress and disease. In McCance, K. and Huether, S. (Eds.). (pp 219–317). *Pathophysiol-*

ogy: The Biologic Basis for Disease in Adults and Children. St. Louis: Mosby.

McCubbin, M. & McCubbin, H. (1992). Families coping with illness: The resiliency model of family stress, adjustment, and adaptation. In Danielson, C., Hammel-Bissell, B., and Winstead-Fry, P. (Eds.) (pp 21–63). *Families, Health & Illness: Perspectives on Coping and Intervention.* St. Louis; Mosby.

Molter, N. (1979). Needs of relatives of critically ill patients: A descriptive study. *Heart & Lung, 8*(2), 332–339.

Molter, N. & Leske, J. *Critical Care Family Needs Inventory.* Copyright 1983.

Norheim, C. (1989). Family needs of patients having coronary artery bypass graft surgery during the intraoperative period. *Nursing Research, 18*(6), 622–626.

Norris, L. & Grove, S. (1986). Investigation of selected psychosocial needs of family members of critically ill adult patients. *Heart & Lung, 15*(2), 194–199.

Rodgers, C. (1983). Needs of relatives of cardiac surgery patients during the critical care phase. *Focus on Critical Care Nursing, 10*(5), 50–55.

Selye, H. (1978). *The Stress of Life.* New York: McGraw-Hill.

Schwartz, L. & Brenner. Z. (1979). Critical care unit transfer: Reducing patient stress through nursing interventions. *Heart & Lung, 8*(3), 540–546.

Simpson, R. (1989). Needs and concerns of families of critically ill adults. *Focus on Critical Care Nursing, 16*(5), 388–397.

Simpson, T., Wilson, D., Mucken, N., Martin, S., West, E., & Guinn, N. (1996). Implementation and evaluation of a liberalized visiting policy. *Americal Journal of Critical Care, 5*(6), 420–426.

Spatt, L., Ganas, E., Hying, S., Kirsch, E., & Koch, M. (1986). Informational needs of families of intensive care patients. *Qualitative Review Bulletin, 12*(1), 16–21.

Stillwell, S. (1984). Importance of visiting needs as perceived by family members of patients in the intensive care unit. *Heart & Lung, 13*(3), 238–242.

12

The History and Physical Examination

Yvonne A. Ruddy-Stein
Paul Logan

THE PATIENT HISTORY

The Initial Encounter

Obtaining the history is the first contact you have with the patient, and your conduct greatly affects the quality of information you obtain during the interview. There are several ways to make a positive initial impression on the patient.

The history is best obtained in a quiet room without distractions. In an acute care situation, the environment is often noisy and chaotic. In this case, make the patient comfortable by displaying a calm demeanor.

A simple introduction with a handshake identifies who you are and what you will be doing with the patient: "Hello, Mr. Jones, I am Ellen Smith, a cardiology nurse practitioner. I would like to talk with you for a few minutes about the symptoms you have been having." Maintain good eye contact to convey your interest in the patient's problems.

It is crucial that you appear comfortable and attentive. If you are not comfortable, it is likely the patient will not be either, and the fact-gathering process may be affected. It may be tempting to cut the interview short because of time constraints, but both you and the patient benefit if there is no rush during the history-taking process. As a result, the patient will be satisfied knowing that you have listened fully and you will know where to focus your physical examination.

The goal of the interview is to obtain the account of symptoms in the patient's own words. You will use this account to formulate a diagnosis and treat the patient's illness. There are several communication techniques that facilitate this process.

Communication Techniques

The way you ask questions of a patient can encourage the patient to elaborate on the presenting symptoms. Your first questions should be general and get more specific as the patient gives you additional information.

Open-ended questions do not bias the patient's account of the story: "What were the pains like?" not "Were you having sharp pains?" If the patient cannot or will not answer an open-ended question, give the patient choices: "Were the pains sharp? dull? burning? or pressure-like?"

Closed-ended questions may be appropriate when the patient has given you the account of the symptoms and you need specific information: "Did you have palpitations?" or "Did you break into a sweat?"

Do not group questions together so that the patient does not know which one to answer: "Were you nauseated, sweaty, or short of breath?"

Many times a patient does not understand a question as asked, due to differences in education or regional dialect. Rephrase the question, keeping in mind these differences:

"Were you nauseated?"
Silence.
"Did it feel like you were going to throw up?"

Do not use medical terms unless you are certain the patient knows the terms: "Were you sweaty?" instead of "Were you diaphoretic?"

Even when you are not asking a question, you can gather additional information by simply encouraging the patient to say more: "Go on . . ." or "Then what happened?"

It is often helpful to repeat the last thing the patient said. This will confirm the patient's story and also encourage elaboration:

"The pain first started after I ate."
"After you ate?"
"Yes, I had just eaten a slice of pepperoni pizza. I took some Maalox but that didn't help."
"That didn't help?"
"No. My father has an ulcer and that's what he does when he has pain after he eats spicy foods."

Clarification is essential during the history. The words the patient uses to describe the symptoms are especially meaningful. Chest pain described as "tearing" suggests a different etiology than "burning" chest pain.

When a patient uses a medical term such as "ulcer" or "heart attack," ask, "Did a health-care provider call it an 'ulcer'?" or "Did your cardiologist tell you that you had a heart attack?" The patient may have self-diagnosed him- or herself with an ulcer or heart attack without actually having had either.

If the patient uses ambiguous terms, such as "I feel bad," it is your obligation to find out what the patient means by "bad." One patient may mean "fatigued," another may mean "achy." These symptoms require different approaches for diagnosis. "When you say you felt 'bad,' what did you feel like?"

Remember that there may be regional and educational differences when patients describe their symptoms or history. What one patient calls "heartburn," another calls "reflux." A patient from the Southern United States may describe an episode of "falling out," whereas those from other regions of the United States may use the term "fainting." If you are uncertain about a term the patient uses, ask for clarification of the term.

Be careful when using the word "pain." Many patients do not admit having "pain." They use the terms "discomfort" or "funny feeling." It is best to ask if a patient is having "pain or discomfort," or "aches or pains." When asking about angina I often ask, "Do you get chest pain, pressure, tightness, heaviness, or burning?"

When the patient has stopped talking and you think you understand the reasons for the visit, you can summarize the patient's account:

"This is what I heard you say. Tell me if there is something I forgot. You were carrying in groceries from the car, when suddenly you got a dull, aching pain in the middle of your chest. You sat down, took a nitroglycerine, and the pain went away in about 2 minutes."

The patient sometimes adds additional information.

Components of the History

Elements of a comprehensive history are shown in Table 12–1.

Age, Sex, Race

The likelihood of having a disease varies with age, sex, and race. For instance, men typically develop coronary artery disease in their 50s, whereas women typically develop it after menopause. Knowing the age, sex, and race of the patient allows you to determine the probability of a certain medical problem. For example, generalized muscle aches and pains in a 35-year-old woman might lead you to suspect an autoimmune disorder as opposed to a 75-year-old woman with the same symptoms in whom you may suspect arthritis. Assessment of periodic painful episodes of joints in an African-American patient would have to include the possibility of sickle cell anemia, whereas this disorder is almost nonexistent in Caucasian patients. Pain involving the toe or lower extremity joints is more likely to be gout in a man than a woman. Because disease prevalence varies so much between populations, it is valuable to know which diseases are most prevalent in each group.

Source of Referral

If another provider referred the patient, the patient might have undergone one or more work-ups that did not reveal a diagnosis for the presenting symptoms. Any negative work-ups should be reviewed and noted in the medical record.

Sometimes significant information is revealed in a subtle way through the source of referral. If you find out during the history that a concerned friend or relative made the patient seek treatment, you have identified part (or all) of the patient's support systems. You have also learned about the response to their own illness; perhaps the patient was too frightened by the symptoms to initiate the visit for him- or herself.

TABLE 12–1. Components of the History

Demographic characteristics
Source of referral (if applicable)
Source of history (if applicable)
Chief complaint
History of present illness
Past medical problems
Past surgeries/diagnostic tests
Allergies
Social practices
Family medical problems and surgeries
Medications (both prescription and over-the-counter)
Review of systems

Source of the History

If the patient is unable to give the history for any reason, the history giver should be recorded. If someone is translating because the patient and nurse practitioner do not share a common language, care should be taken to ask the translator not to paraphrase the questions or answers.

If the patient comes in with his or her spouse and the spouse has observations to contribute, this should be added to the history, too.

If the patient is accompanied by a history from a referring provider, it is prudent to verify it with the patient: "Mr. Jones, you told Dr. Lewis that the pain started yesterday, and continued on and off until this morning. It felt like cramping in your stomach. Is this correct? Is there anything else you'd like to add?" Then obtain the additional details you need to complete the history.

Chief Complaint

The patient's reason for the visit, in the patient's own words, is the chief complaint. The reason for the visit can be ascertained simply by asking, "What brings you to the hospital today?" or "Why are you being seen today?" The patient can then explain what brought him or her to see you.

History of Present Illness

The history of the present illness provides additional details about the chief complaint, including a description of the symptom and its chronology. Every illness has a "typical" set of features. For this reason it is important to inquire about each of the features listed in Table 12–2.

Onset, Duration, and Timing. Onset and duration help differentiate acute problems from exacerbations of chronic problems. These features can also help determine whether the problem is progressive, and how rapidly it is progressing. Timing may help identify a pattern to the symptom.

Location. Location helps you determine which body systems are affected and directs you to where to pay particular attention during the physical examination. For instance, upper epigastric pain is suggestive for either gastrointestinal or cardiovascular disorders. The physical examination concentrates on these systems. The exception to this is referred pain. Certain types of pain occur in an area removed from the body part that is actually affected. For example, the pain of a kidney stone often occurs in the back or flank, and may radiate to the testicles in a male. Remember common patterns of pain radiation when a patient tells you where the pain is located. Ask the patient to point with one finger to the area of most concern.

TABLE 12–2. Features of a Symptom

Onset: When did the symptom first occur? What were you doing?
Location: Where is the symptom located? Point to it. Does it radiate?
Duration: How long does it last? How often does it occur? Is it continuous or intermittent? How long has it been occurring?
Characteristics: Describe the symptom. What does it feel like? How bothersome is it? Has this ever happened before? Is it the worst you ever had?
Associated Symptoms: Are there any other symptoms that accompany this symptom?
Aggravating factors: Does anything make it worse?
Relieving factors: Does anything make it better?
Treatment: Did you do anything to treat the problem? What have you done to try to relieve it?

Characteristics. Characteristics communicate the patient's subjective sensations to the provider. The words the patient uses to describe the sensations can provide important clues that may aid in diagnosis. For example, chest pain that feels like someone is sitting on the patient's chest suggests myocardial ischemia. Ask the patient to rate the severity of the pain on a numeric or visual scale. This allows you to monitor the progression or relief of the pain over time.

Patients who have acute symptoms with a history of similar symptoms should be asked if their current symptoms are like their usual symptoms. For example, after determining that the patient has had a medically diagnosed gastric ulcer and is complaining of abdominal pain, ask, "Is this the same pain you had with your ulcer, or is it different?"

Patients who have chronic medical problems should be asked what prompted them to come for evaluation. People who are used to pain often present if their pain is worse or different than usual. Others present if their pain is reminiscent of past pain that indicated a medical problem. Others still present if their symptoms are getting in the way of their daily activities. Ask the patient, "Are you able to do the things you usually do?" For example, to assess complaints of dyspnea, muscle weakness, and heartburn, ask respectively, "Are you able to walk to the mailbox? Pick up your grandchild? Eat spicy food?" Mention specific activities and assess whether the patient has stopped doing them over time.

Associated Symptoms. Associated symptoms are those that typically accompany another symptom. For example, chest pain is often accompanied by dizziness, nausea, vomiting, shortness of breath, or arm/neck/jaw pain or numbness.

Aggravating and Relieving Factors. Aggravating and relieving factors either exacerbate the problem or alleviate it. For instance, abdominal pain relieved with eating suggests a gastric ulcer whereas abdominal pain exacerbated by eating suggests duodenal ulcer.

Treatment. Treatments can ease, aggravate, or have no effect on the patient's symptoms. The discovery of the patient's self-treatment may provide an opportunity for teaching. For example, after the patient with established coronary artery disease reveals that Tylenol was taken for chest pain, a note should be made to educate the patient about nitroglycerine that would have treated the chest pain more appropriately. Self-treatment also tells you about the patient's response to illness. If the pain has been present for three days and the patient has not tried to treat it, either the patient has a high tolerance for pain or he or she was not worried enough about the pain to make it go away. This information may also reveal how compliant the patient is likely to be with the treatment you prescribe.

Past Medical History/Past Surgical History/Diagnostic Tests

The presence of preexisting medical problems may help identify the patient's current problems. It is possible that the patient may describe already-diagnosed problems that exacerbate the current problems or vice versa. For example, newly diagnosed bronchitis exacerbates chronic obstructive pulmonary disease (COPD), and longstanding COPD, in turn, compromises the body's ability to cope with bronchitis.

There are many approaches to obtaining the patient's past history. You may go through a list of medical problems, specifically asking the patient if he or she has one or more of them. This is thorough, but unnecessarily time consuming. Alternatively, you may ask if the patient has any problems with each body system. This is less time consuming, but also less thorough. Often, asking a combination of system-based questions plus specific questions to assess for significant medical problems gives you a timely yet thorough past medical history. See Table 12–3 for system-based questions with a list of significant diseases to assess for. First ask the patient general questions, then more specific questions. If a system-based problem is identified, ask the patient about pertinent disease entities in that system. You are identifying diagnosed medical conditions. If the patient tells you about symptoms that have not been worked up or diagnosed, these can be included in the review of systems.

A good opening question is, "Do you have any medical problems?" or "Are you being treated for any medical conditions?" This may bring out some of the patient's diagnosed problems, but usually patients need to be prompted further for their full past medical history.

You may ask if the patient has ever been hospitalized or treated in the emergency room. This often identifies a chronic medical problem that has not been mentioned before.

Ask if the patient has had any operations. For example, finding out whether the patient has had a cholecystectomy while evaluating right lower quadrant abdominal pain is extremely helpful. Ask specifically about tonsillectomy/adenoidectomy. Patients often exclude this in their surgical history.

Knowing whether diagnostic tests have been performed can help confirm or refute whether the patient has a certain medical problem. If the patient tells you of a past ulcer but never had any gastrointestinal testing done, you may need to clarify what the patient means by an "ulcer."

Childhood Illnesses. Ask if the patient has had any childhood illnesses when it is relevant to the chief complaint. For example, if the patient relates a history of a heart murmur, ask if he or she had rheumatic fever as a child. See Table 12–4 for a list of common childhood illnesses.

Immunizations. Inquire whether the patient has received the appropriate immunizations when it is relevant. For instance, if the patient is being seen for evaluation of a penetrating wound, ask if he or she has received a tetanus immunization in the last five years. See Table 12–5 for a list of immunizations.

Screening Tests. Ask the patient about any screening tests that have been performed when it is appropriate to the chief complaint. For example, when a woman presents with bleeding after intercourse, you should find out the date and

TABLE 12–3. Past Medical History

Questions	Look especially for
Do you have any skin problems?	Skin cancer
Do you have any head/eye/ear/nose/throat problems?	Glaucoma, headaches, vertigo
Do you have any problems with your breasts?	Breast cancer
Do you have any heart problems?	Hypertension, murmurs, existing coronary artery disease, congestive heart failure, arrhythmias
Do you have any lung problems?	Emphysema, asthma, tuberculosis
Do you have any stomach problems?	Ulcers, gastroesophageal reflux disease
Do you have any liver or gallbladder problems?	Hepatitis, gallstones
Do you have any kidney or bladder problems?	Renal failure, kidney stones
Do you have any sexual problems?	Bleeding, impotence
Do you have any problems with your blood vessels?	Deep vein thrombosis, clotting problems, anemia
Do you have any muscle or joint problems?	Arthritis, gout
Do you have any neurological problems?	Seizures, syncope, stroke
Do you have any thyroid problems?	Hypo/hyperthyroidism
Do you have any psychological problems?	Depression, suicide attempts

TABLE 12–4. Chilhood Illnesses
Measles
Mumps
Rubella
Whooping cough
Varicella
Rheumatic fever
Scarlet fever
Polio

result of her last Papincolau smear. See Table 12–6 for a partial list of common screening tests.

Allergies

It is essential to document all allergies. Knowing what prescription and over-the-counter medication allergies the patient has prevents treatment with those or related medications.

Identification of allergens like dust, plants, and animal dander aids in the identification and treatment of allergic rhinitis, asthma, rashes, and other allergy-mediated disorders.

Allergies to shellfish can indicate an allergy to iodine dye that may be used for contrast in angiograms and computerized tomography scans. The allergic reaction can be prevented by premedication if the allergy is identified before the administration of contrast. Additionally, because of the ubiquitous use of latex and the severity of some reactions, it is important to note a history of allergies to this substance.

Often, allergic reactions to insect bites like bee stings can be fatal. These reactions can be quickly treated if they are identified. See Table 12–7 for common allergies that should be assessed in every patient.

Social Practices

Inquire whether the patient is single, married, divorced, or widowed. Knowing this information can indicate what type of support the patient has or needs. Another way to ascertain the patient's support at home is to ask, "Is there anyone at home to help you do the things you need to do?"

Tobacco abuse predisposes the patient to gastroesophageal reflux disease, frequent upper respiratory infections, emphysema, and lung cancer. Knowing how much the patient smokes can help you design a smoking cessation plan. If there is a history of cigarette smoking, quantify the amount in packs per day, then multiply that by the years the patient has been smoking for pack-years. Forced expiratory volume in one second has been inversely correlated with pack-years of smoking. Ask the patient specifically about cigars, snuff, and chew tobacco.

TABLE 12–5. Immunizations
Diphtheria/tetanus/pertussis
Measles/mumps/rubella
Influenza
Hepatitis B
Pneumococcal vaccine

TABLE 12–6. Screening Tests
Cholesterol
Hemoglobin
Blood sugar
HIV testing
Dental examination
Eye examination
Blood pressure
Electrocardiogram
Chest roentogram
Mammogram
Papincolau smear
Urinalysis
Sigmoidoscopy
Stool guaiac testing
Tuberculosis skin test

The excessive use of alcohol can interact with medications, deplete the body's vitamin supplies, and affect the functioning of the liver. Accurate assessment of alcohol use is vital when a patient is admitted to the hospital and therefore at risk for acute alcohol withdrawal. By asking about alcohol intake in a nonthreatening way as if you expect that the patient does drink, you are more likely to get a true assessment of his or her alcohol usage. "How much beer, wine, or liquor do you drink in an average week?" If this is a large number, ask how much the patient drinks in an average day. Some patients state that they drink "only socially." Try to quantify this in number of drinks per week, month, or holiday.

To verify whether the patient uses drugs, do not ask in a judgmental way. Instead of asking "Do you do drugs?" that has a negative connotation, ask specifically, "Do you use marijuana? Cocaine? Heroin?" Find out how much and how often the patient uses each.

It is often helpful to know what the patient does for a living. Certain occupations put the patient at a higher risk for certain health problems. For example, health-care workers have a higher risk of contracting hepatitis. Examples of environmental hazards that may affect a patient's current or future health status include asbestos, smoke, pesticides, radiation, and chemicals.

TABLE 12–7. Allergies
Prescription medicine
Over-the-counter medicine
Food
Dust
Animal dander
Plants
Insects

When relevant to the chief complaint, the type of diet the patient follows can be assessed by asking "What is a typical breakfast for you? Lunch? Dinner? Any snacks?" If this recall does not identify the information you need, ask specifically about the food intake in which you are interested. For example, when assessing for sodium in the diet, ask "How many times a week do you eat soup? Canned vegetables? Frozen dinners? Potato chips? How much salt do you use in cooking? At the table?" Certain foods can exacerbate certain medical conditions. For example, a diet high in caffeine can exacerbate palpitations or symptoms of gastroesophageal reflux disease. If a diet high in cholesterol is identified and the patient has other risk factors for the development of coronary artery disease, teaching can be done at a later time.

When appropriate, determine the amount of traveling the patient does and to where. This is essential when the patient presents with symptoms of a febrile illness, pulmonary embolism, heart failure, or deep venous thrombosis.

It is often helpful to learn the patient's health-care practices, such as exercise patterns and frequency of physical exams. See Table 12–8 for the social practices that should be ascertained in each patient.

Family Medical/Surgical History and Diagnostic Tests

The familial medical and surgical history contributes important information to the patient history. Certain diseases, such as cardiovascular disease, can be inherited. Include the patient's parents' and siblings' past medical problems and surgeries. It is usually sufficient to ask, "Does your mother have any medical problems? Your father? What about your sisters and brothers?" If the family history of a certain disease is strong, include maternal and paternal grandparents and siblings. If a narrative format is used, list each relative, with age, medical problems or surgeries, and age at death if applicable. See Table 12–9 for an example of the narrative family history format. The pedigree format provides a visual summary of the family's medical problems and relationships. See Figure 12–1 for the pedigree format for the family history.

Medications

The medications the patient is taking can help identify the medical problems the patient has. Include each medication's name, dose, frequency, and indications. It is essential to determine whether the patient is taking any over-the-counter medicines such as laxatives, Tylenol, or antiinflammatories, that can precipitate, respectively, bowel obstruction, liver damage, or gastrointestinal bleeding. Many patients take vitamins such as magnesium or vitamin E, that can precipitate, respectively, diarrhea or clotting disorders. See Table 12–10 for types of medicines that should be recorded.

TABLE 12–8. Social Practices

Marital status
Cigarette use
Alcohol use
Drug use
Profession
Diet
Traveling
Health practices

Review of Systems

After you have determined the primary reason for the patient's visit along with the past medical and surgical problems, you need to determine if the patient has any additional problems. It is usually sufficient to go through each body system and if there are any problems identified, to probe further into that system for symptoms. See Table 12–11 for a list of common symptoms and questions that help you identify them.

Each symptom identified needs to be followed up with questions on features: onset, location, duration, timing, characteristics, associated symptoms, aggravating/relieving factors, and treatment. Tables 12–12 through 12–16 list common symptoms and thorough questioning about the features of each.

Patients with Specialized Needs

The Hospitalized Child

The acutely ill child is likely to be frightened at being in the hospital. Although much of the history is obtained from the child's accompanying parent or guardian, it is important to address the child directly, to establish trust and allay fear.

Approach the child in the same way you would approach an adult. An introduction with a handshake for the child who is old enough to shake hands tells the child that he or she is the focus of the interview. "Hi, Jane, my name is Paul. I'm a nurse practitioner and I want to ask you some questions."

An open-ended question is best when obtaining the child's chief complaint, and should be asked of the patient directly. "Why did you come see me today?" or "How come you came to the hospital today?" Usually the child gives a very simple reason: "My tummy hurts" or "It hurts to swallow."

Some of the symptom features can be obtained from the younger patient. For example, "When did it start to hurt?" determines the onset. "Show me where it hurts" describes the location. The other features can be obtained from the parent or guardian who accompanies the younger child: "Does he have a fever? Has she been pulling her ears? Have you noticed a pattern to the pain? What did you do to treat the problem? Did it work?"

Obtain the allergies, past medical and surgical history, medications, diet and travel history, health practices, family history, and review of systems from the parent or guardian of the younger child patient.

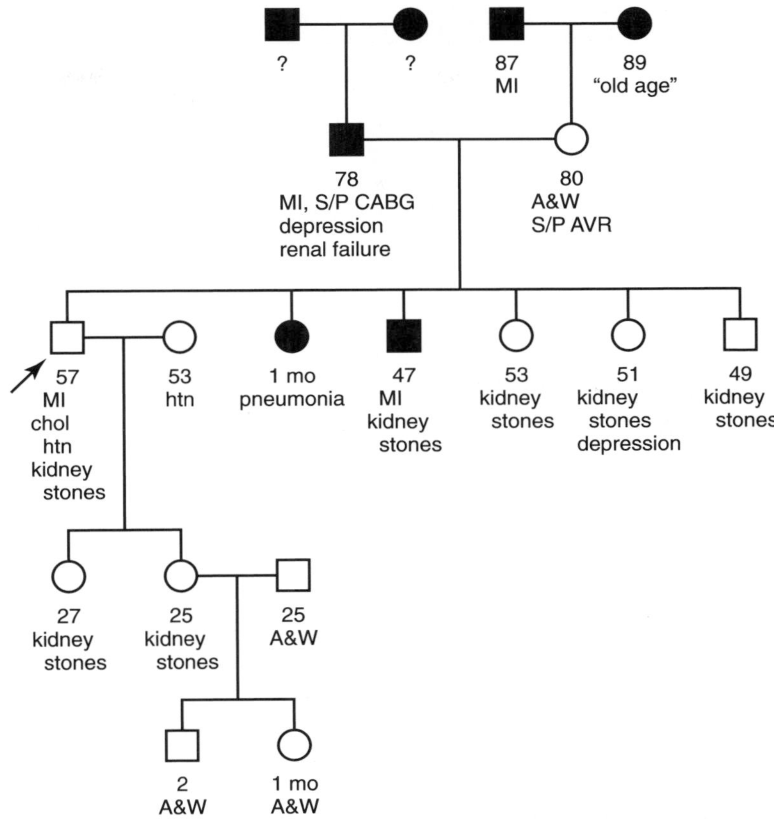

Figure 12–1. Genogram format for family history.

The following additional information should be ascertained, particularly in the younger child patient, when appropriate: problems with conception or delivery of the child; problems with the pregnancy or labor of the mother; age when developmental milestones were met; age at development of appropriate language, motor, and social skills.

The hospitalized older child should be approached in the same way as the adult patient. Older children and adolescents usually respond appropriately and favorably when you ask them directly about their complaints.

The older child can describe the chief complaint, all features of the complaint, social practices, and the review of systems. Older children should be asked directly about cigarette, alcohol, and drug use. The parent or guardian usually provides the past medical and surgical history, allergies, medications, and family history.

By addressing both the younger and older child patient personally, you include them in their own diagnostic and healing processes.

TABLE 12–9. Narrative Format for Family History

Mother, 54, alive and well.
Father, 56, myocardial infarction at age 51, bypass at age 51.
Sister, 30, alive and well.
Brother, 32, recently had "failed stress test," no workup done yet.
Paternal brother, 52, alive and well.
Maternal sister, 51, alive and well.
Paternal grandfather, died at 87, cardiac catheterization at age 67 which revealed "one blocked artery."
Paternal grandmother, 82, gastroesophageal reflux disease.
Maternal grandfather, died at 79.
Maternal grandmother, died at 81.

The Hospitalized Older Patient

Obtaining the history from the older patient is modified slightly from obtaining the younger adult patient's history. Many older patients have decreased hearing. Therefore it is easiest for the patient to hear when there is minimal background noise. Additionally, the older patient frequently has decreased visual acuity and decreased peripheral vision, so be sure to sit directly in front of the patient during the interview so that the patient can see you when you speak. Also, enunciate clearly and allow more time for the older adult to

TABLE 12–10. Medication Use

Prescription medicine
Over-the-counter medicine
Vitamins

TABLE 12–11. Review of Systems

General symptoms	Weight gain/weight loss	Have there been any changes in appetite or weight? Have there been any changes in your diet?
	Fatigue/loss of energy	Have you felt tired? Do you feel that it's due to lack of sleep?
	Weakness	Do you feel weak?
	Fever	Have you had fevers?
	Chills/sweats	Have you had any sweats or chills?
Skin	Changes in skin/hair/nails	Have you noticed any changes in your skin? Your hair? Your nails?
	Rashes	Do you have any rashes?
	Sores	Do you have any sores?
	Lumps	Do you have any lumps?
	Itching	Have you been itching?
Head	Headache	Do you get headaches?
	Trauma	Have you had any injuries to your head?
Eyes	Visual changes or disturbances	Do you have blurred vision? Double vision? Flashing? Spots? Specks? Episodes of blindness?
	Pain/irritation	Do you have any pain or irritation in your eyes?
	Redness	Do you have any redness of your eyes?
	Tearing	Do your eyes tear excessively?
Ears	Hearing changes or loss	Do you have any trouble with your hearing?
	Tinnitus	Do you have any ringing in your ears?
	Vertigo	Do you ever feel like the room is spinning around you?
	Earache/ear pain	Do you have an earache or pain in your ears?
	Discharge	Do you have drainage from your ears?
Nose/sinuses	Rhinorrhea/nasal stuffiness	Do you have a runny nose? Do you have a stuffy nose?
	Sneezing/itching	Do you sneeze a lot? Does your nose itch?
	Sinus pain/tenderness	Do you have any tenderness or pain over your sinuses?
	Epistaxis	Do you get nosebleeds?
Mouth/throat/neck	Dental problems	Do you have any problems with your teeth?
	Bleeding gums	Do your gums bleed?
	Mouth sores	Do you have any sores in your mouth?
	Sore tongue	Is your tongue sore?
	Sore throat	Do you have a sore throat?
	Hoarseness	Does your voice get hoarse?
	Swollen glands	Do you have any swollen glands?
	Neck pain/stiffness	Do you have any neck pain or stiffness?
	Goiter	Do you have a goiter?
Breasts	Pain/tenderness	Do you have any pain or tenderness in your breasts?
	Lumps	Do you have any lumps in your breasts? Do you examine your breasts monthly?
	Discharge	Have you noticed any discharge from your nipples?
Cardiac	Chest pain/discomfort	Do you have any discomfort in your chest?
	Palpitations	Have you had palpitations?
Respiratory	Wheezing	Do you wheeze when you breathe?
	Cough	Do you have a cough? Does anything come up when you do?
	Hemoptysis	Do you ever cough up blood?
	Dyspnea	Do you get short of breath? How far can you walk on level ground before you get short of breath? How many stairs can you climb before you get short of breath?
	Orthopnea	How many pillows do you sleep on? Are you able to breathe if you lay flat on your back?
	Paroxysmal nocturnal dyspnea	Do you ever wake up in the middle of the night gasping for breath?
	Edema	Do you have swelling in your feet, ankles, or legs?
	Pleurisy	Does it hurt in your chest when you inhale?
Gastrointestinal	Dysphagia	Do you have any trouble swallowing? Do you ever feel like food sticks in your throat? Do liquids stick in your throat?
	Odontophagia	Does it hurt to swallow?
	Indigestion/heartburn	Do you have an upset stomach? Do you have heartburn?
	Abdominal pain	Do you have stomach pain?
	Nausea	Are you nauseous?

(Continued)

TABLE 12–11. Review of Systems *(Continued)*

	Vomiting	Do you vomit? What does it look like?
	Regurgitation	After you eat, do you feel the food coming back up?
	Changes in bowel habits	Has there been anything different about your bowels?
	Diarrhea	Do you have diarrhea? Are your stools frequent? Are they watery? Are they soft?
	Constipation	Are you constipated? Are your stools hard? How often do you have a bowel movement?
	Hematochezia	Do you have blood in your stool? Is the blood in the toilet, or is it on the tissue? Do you have black stools?
	Jaundice	Has your skin been yellow?
Urinary tract	Pain/burning	Does it hurt or burn when you urinate?
	Frequency	Do you urinate very often?
	Urgency	Do you feel you won't make it to the bathroom in time?
	Hesitancy	Do you feel like you have to urinate, but when you try, nothing comes out?
	Reduced force	Is your stream less strong than usual?
	Dribbling	Do you dribble when you urinate?
	Nocturia	Do you ever get up in the middle of the night to urinate?
	Polyuria	Do you urinate in abnormally large amounts?
	Hematuria	Do you have blood in your urine?
	Incontinence	Do you lose urine? Is it when you cough or sneeze? Is it when you can't make it to the bathroom?
Female genitalia	Metrorraghia	Do you bleed between your periods?
	Post coital bleeding	Do you bleed after intercourse?
	Dysmenorrhea	Do you have discomfort before or during your period?
	Amenorrhea	Have you skipped a period?
	Post-menopausal bleeding	Have you bled since you went through menopause?
	Hot flashes	Do you have hot flashes?
	Discharge	Do you have any discharge?
	Itching	Do you have any itching?
	Discomfort during intercourse	Do you have any pain during intercourse?
Male genitalia	Discharge	Do you have any discharge?
	Sores	Do you have any sores?
	Growths	Do you have any growths?
	Scrotal swelling	Do you have any swelling in your scrotum?
	Scrotal pain	Do you have any pain in your scrotum?
	Hernia	Do you have any hernias?
Peripheral vascular	Leg pain	Do you have any pain in your legs?
	Edema	Do you have any swelling in your legs?
	Temperature changes	Do your arms or legs get cold? Warm?
	Intermittent claudication	Do you get pain in the back of your legs when you walk? Does it get better when you stop walking?
	Variocosities	Do you have any varicose veins?
Musculoskeletal	Muscle/joint pain/tenderness	Do you have pain or tenderness in any muscles or joints?
	Cramps	Do you get muscle cramps?
	Swelling	Do you have swelling in any of your joints?
	Stiffness	Do you have any stiff muscles?
	Decreased range of motion	Do your joints move like they should?
Nervous system	Loss of consciousness	Have you ever fainted?
	Dizziness	Are you dizzy?
	Seizures	Do you have seizures?
	Paralysis	Is any part of your body paralyzed?
	Tremors/involuntary movement	Do you ever shake or tremble without meaning to?
	Parasthesias	Do you have numbness or tingling?
Hematologic	Bruising	Do you bruise easily?
	Bleeding	Do you bleed excessively?
Endocrine	Diabetes	Do you urinate in excessive amounts? Do you eat excessively? Do you drink excessively? Do you have sores that don't heal?
	Thyroid disorders	Do you get excessively hot? Cold? Have you had a weight loss or gain without a change in diet? Do you have a goiter?

TABLE 12–12. Headache

Where is the pain? Point to it.
Have you ever had a headache before? If so, is this the worst one you've ever had? Rate the pain on a scale of 1 to 10.
What does the pain feel like? (Throbbing? Dull? Aching? Sharp?)
Do you have any numbness or tingling anywhere?
Have you had any loss of vision? Does it hurt to look at light?
Have you had any slurring of your speech?
Does anything make the pain better?
Does anything make the pain worse? (Specifically, coughing? sneezing? bending over?)
What have you tried to treat the headache?
If the headache is gone:
How long did it last?
What made it go away, or did it go away by itself?

TABLE 12–13. Chest Pain

Where is the pain? Point to it.
Does the pain radiate anywhere?
When did it start? What were you doing when it started?
Is it continuous or intermittent?
Have you ever had pain like this before? If so, is this the worst it has ever been? Rate the pain on a scale of 1 to 10.
What does the pain feel like? (Sharp? Dull? Pressure? Stabbing?)
Do you have any arm numbness or tingling? Do you have any palpitations? Dizziness? Nausea? Vomiting? Diaphoresis?
Does anything make the pain better? (Specifically, rest? nitroglycerine?)
Does anything make the pain worse? (Specifically, exertion? emotional upset?)
What have you tried to treat the chest pain?
If the chest pain is gone:
How long did it last? What made it go away, or did it go away by itself?

respond to your questions. Degenerative joint changes in the older patient may preclude the patient from sitting for long periods of time.

Most of the time the history of the older patient takes longer than the younger patient's history because there have been more hospitalizations, illnesses, and medical problems in the older patient. Since there are so many medical problems, it is common that multiple symptoms are mentioned as the chief complaint. Keep the patient focused by asking which of the symptoms is most troubling, address that symptom first, then address the rest of the symptoms one at a time.

The older patient appreciates the modifications to your interview, so that he or she can more fully participate in the data-collection process.

TABLE 12–14. Dyspnea

When did you get short of breath? What were you doing when it started?
Is it that you feel like you can't get a deep breath or that you're smothering?
How long have you been short of breath?
Have you ever been short of breath before? Is this the worst your breathing has ever been?
How many stairs can you climb before you get short of breath?
How far can you walk on level ground before you get short of breath?
If you lie flat, are you able to breathe? If not, how many pillows do you need to sleep on?
Do you ever wake up in the middle of the night not able to breathe?
Does anything make the shortness of breath better? (Specifically, inhalers? diuretics? oxygen?)
Does anything make the shortness of breath worse?
Have you tried anything to make your breathing easier?
If the shortness of breath is relieved:
How long did it last?
What made it go away, or did it go away by itself?

The Hospitalized Patient with a Psychiatric Disorder

When a patient with a psychiatric disorder enters the hospital for an acute medical problem, additional information must be gathered to address the patient's psychological as well as medical needs.

To assess for a past history of a psychiatric problem, the question, "Have you ever seen a psychiatrist, psychologist, or counselor for any reason?" is a good starting point. If the patient has had treatment of this nature, ask, "Why?" or "What was going on in your life at that time?" It may be helpful to ask the patient if he or she was diagnosed with any psychiatric illnesses at that time. Obtain the features of the disorder, just as with a medical disorder. In addition, when the patient discusses treatment, ask if the patient con-

TABLE 12–15. Abdominal Pain

Where is the pain? Point to it.
Does the pain radiate anywhere?
When did it start? What were you doing when it started?
Is it continuous or intermittent?
Have you ever had pain like this before? If so, is this the worst it has ever been? Rate the pain on a scale of 1 to 10.
What does the pain feel like? (Sharp? Dull? Crampy?)
Are you nauseous? Have you vomited?
Do you have diarrhea? Are you constipated?
Are you jaundiced?
Does anything make the pain better? (Specifically, eating? bowel movement? antacids?)
Does anything make the pain worse? (Specifically, eating?)
What have you tried to treat the pain?
If the abdominal pain is gone:
How long did it last?
What made it go away, or did it go away by itself?

TABLE 12–16. Syncope

When did you faint? What were you doing when you fainted? Did you lose consciousness completely, or were you partially awake?
How long were you out?
Have you fainted before? When? Did you ever see someone about it? What did they find out?
Did you know you were going to faint?
Did you have palpitations before you fainted? Chest pain? Did you smell or taste anything funny?
Did anyone see you faint? Did they say you had any seizure-like movements? Did you lose control of your bladder or bowels?
When you woke up, did you know where you were and what had happened?

sidered it successful. "Did you notice a change for the better after your sessions? Do you feel this was a good treatment for you?" This helps identify the patient's feelings towards treatment and may suggest future treatments.

During the family history, ask specifically whether there are relatives with psychiatric illnesses because some psychiatric illnesses can be inherited. Also ask if any relatives have committed suicide. Patients with relatives who have committed suicide may be at a higher risk for suicide themselves because suicide may be seen as a possible way to cope with problems.

During the review of systems, be aware of symptoms that may mask a medical disorder or indicate an exacerbation of the psychiatric disorder. Feelings of unhappiness, sadness, irritability, apathy, helplessness, or hopelessness may occur in persons with depression. The patient with depression may also have difficulty concentrating or remembering, inability to enjoy activities, change in sleeping habits, change in appetite, or a lack of energy.

Patients with anxiety may describe a sense of dread or impending harm, vulnerability, or lack of control over unpleasant events. For this reason, they may avoid situations they consider unpleasant.

Patients who describe hallucinations may have a psychotic disorder. Ask, "Do you ever see/hear/smell/taste things that other people may not be able to see/hear/smell/taste?"

Patients with delirium and dementia may be disoriented and have impaired memory. Delirium is usually an acute process, whereas dementia can be a long, insidious process. The memory and orientation problems make it very difficult to assess patients with these disorders.

Recognizing the presence and extent of a psychiatric disorder allows you to incorporate counseling, psychological, or psychiatric treatment into your plan of medical treatment.

The Hospitalized Patient with a Disability

The history of a patient with a disability is identical to the history of a patient without one. The disabled patient should have additional items assessed in the history. "How did your disability happen? When did it happen?" Disability resulting from an accident at 40 years old has different implications than disability at birth from a congenital defect. If the disability is recent, ask, "How are you coping?" or "How are you dealing with your disability?" If the disability is not recent, ask, "How did you cope?" or "How did you deal with your disability?"

Assess how the patient has been affected by the disability: "Do you have any limitations?" Ask specifically about the ability to change from a sitting to a standing position, walk (indoors and outdoors), climb stairs, use the toilet (bladder and bowel), get in and out of bed, get in and out of the car, dress his or her upper body, dress his or her lower body, eat, and bathe.

Ask if there are any problems with hearing, sight, or communication. Patients with hearing problems should be asked whether they have a hearing aid. Make every attempt to obtain it and make sure it is working. If the hearing impaired patient reads lips, speak slowly and clearly while obtaining the history. You can also obtain the history by writing down your questions and the patient's answers.

Blind patients need an explanation of who you are and what you are doing while you do it. "Tell me what brought you here today, Mr. Jones. I'm going to write as we talk." Try to make the area you are in as quiet as possible, to avoid any difficulties the patient may have in hearing you.

Patients with speech disorders also need a modified interview. Aphasic patients can be frustrating to interview, but they can be just as frustrated by the interview. In a patient with expressive aphasia, ask as many yes-or-no questions as possible, and ask the patient to nod "yes" or shake the head "no" to your questions. If family members are present, they may be able to supplement the history or translate the patient's words to you. In a patient with receptive aphasia, rely on the patient's family for history.

Knowing the patient's limitations allows you to adapt the environment in such a way that the patient has maximum autonomy.

The Hospitalized Pregnant Patient

An acute medical problem in a pregnant patient has implications for the patient and her fetus. Thus it is important to assess for certain conditions in her history.

Ask, "How do you feel about being pregnant?" This can indicate whether the pregnancy was desired and the attitude towards the child. Also ask, "How is your life going to change by having a baby?" A negative response to either of these questions can warn you of a harmful attitude towards the baby.

The patient's past obstetrical history is particularly important, whether there have been any problems with conception, during pregnancy, labor or delivery of previous children, or any medical problems of previous children. Problems with previous pregnancies may repeat themselves with subsequent pregnancies.

During the past medical and surgical history, ask particularly about diabetes and hypertension, as these conditions are well-known causes of fetal morbidity and mortality. Previous uterine or pelvic surgery may require that the current birth method be by cesarean section. Previous spinal surgery may contraindicate epidural anesthesia.

While obtaining the social practices of the patient, be aware of any behaviors that may adversely affect the fetus (particularly tobacco and alcohol usage) and educate the patient about their possible harmful effects.

While obtaining the review of systems, be aware that symptoms of nausea, fatigue, breast tenderness, constipation, heartburn, backache, weight gain, and urinary frequency are very common during pregnancy. These symptoms may be due to an underlying medical problem or the pregnancy itself.

Knowing that an acutely ill patient is pregnant changes her options for treatment. A thorough history helps identify potential problems and possible treatments.

Acute Care

In acute care it is especially important to obtain a timely yet complete medical history. If the history is thorough you avoid an unfocused physical exam, unnecessary diagnostic testing, and wasting valuable time.

As a nurse practitioner, you are in a distinctive position. You have the skills to obtain a thorough medical history, perform a comprehensive physical examination, all the while building a relationship with the patient. Utilizing the information obtained from the history, physical examination, and knowledge of the patient allows you to diagnose and treat the patient's acute medical problem. Without the ability to obtain a comprehensive medical history, the nurse practitioner does not have a foundation to use the rest of the diagnostic process. See Table 12–17 for an example of a completed health history.

▶ THE PHYSICAL EXAMINATION

Approach to the Physical Examination

The physical examination is an intimate experience between the provider and the patient. It is often surprising how open and uninhibited patients are with health-care pro-

TABLE 12–17. Completed Health History

H.R. is a 57-year-old caucasian male.

Chief complaint: Chest pain

History of present illness: Patient has had chest pains that are pressure-like, located midsternally, occurring only when patient exerts himself (playing tennis). It lasts 2 to 3 seconds and is relieved immediately with rest. No radiation to arm/neck/jaw, shortness of breath, palpitations, nausea, vomiting, or diaphoresis. No PND or edema.

Past medical history: Myocardial infarction at age 40, angina from 35 years old to present, hypertension, hypercholesterolemia, gout, kidney stones, myopia, and presbyopia

Past surgical history: Removal of kidney stone at age 22

Past diagnostic tests: Yearly stress tests, all negative

Allergies: No known diagnosed allergies

Social practices: Married, two daughters, mechanical engineer. Denies smoking (ever); alcohol: four glasses of wine per week; diet: low fat, low cholesterol since MI, wife shops and cooks (uses 1% milkfat milk, part skim cheese, low-cholesterol/low-fat brands whenever possible, no fried foods, eats red meat 1 or 2 days per week). Eats lunch out on business 3 days/week, usually orders fish and a salad. Caffeine: two cups hot herbal tea/day, coffee 1 or 2 times/week, no soda or iced tea. Travel: takes about three business trips each year: last year—Wisconsin, Boston, Chicago; none in last 3 months. Exercise: none. Health practices: bi-annual cardiology visit.

Family history: Mother, 80, alive and well, status post aortic valve replacement at age 76; father died at age 78, myocardial infarction at age 51 and 60, coronary artery bypass grafting at age 74, renal failure, depression. Brother, died at age 47 of myocardial infarction, kidney stones. Sister, died at 1 month of pneumonia. Sister, 53, alive and well, kidney stones. Sister, 51, alive and well, kidney stones, depression. Brother, 49, alive and well, kidney stones. Maternal grandfather, died at age 87 of myocardial infarction. Maternal grandmother died at 89 of "old age." Paternal grandfather, unknown. Paternal grandmother, unknown. Daughter, 27, kidney stones. Daughter, 25, kidney stones. See Figure 12–2 for the genogram format for the family history.

Medications: Procardia XL 60 mg p.o. QD (blood pressure), Tenormin 50 mg p.o. QD (blood pressure), Mevacor 20 mg p.o. QD (cholesterol), Nitroglycerine 0.4 mg patch QD (angina), aspirin 81 mg p.o. QD (heart), vitamin E, vitamin C, garlic tablet, magnesium, selenium, occasional ibuprofen for headache.

Review of systems: General: denies weight changes, fatigue, weakness, fever, chills, sweats. Skin: denies skin/hair/nail changes, rashes, sores, lumps, itching. Head: + occasional headache, relieved within 1 hour with ibupofen, no workup done. Denies trauma. Eyes: + redness, + tearing, denies visual changes, eye pain. Ears: denies hearing changes, tinnitus, vertigo, ear pain, discharge. Nose/sinuses: + nasal stuffiness/sneezing, denies sinus pain, tenderness, epistaxis. Mouth/throat: denies dental problems, gum problems, tongue/mouth soreness, sore throat, swollen glands, neck pain, goiter. Cardiac: see HPI. Respiratory: denies wheezing, cough, hemoptysis, pleurisy. Gastrointestinal: + constipation, drinks apple juice each morning which regulates him, denies dysphagia, odontophagia, heartburn, abdominal pain, nausea, vomiting, regurgitation, diarrhea, rectal bleeding, jaundice. Urinary: + hesitancy and reduced force of stream, + nocturia once/night, denies dribbling, urinary pain, frequency, urgency, polyuria, hematuria, incontinence. Genital: denies discharge, sores, growths, scrotal pain/swelling, hernia. Peripheral Vascular: denies leg pain, claudication, temperature changes, varicosities, edema. Musculoskeletal: denies muscle/joint tenderness, cramps, swelling, stiffness, decreased range of motion. Neurological: denies loss of consciousness, dizziness, seizures, paralysis, involuntary movements, numbness, tingling. Hematological: denies easy bruising/bleeding. Endocrine: denies symptoms of diabetes/thyroid problems.

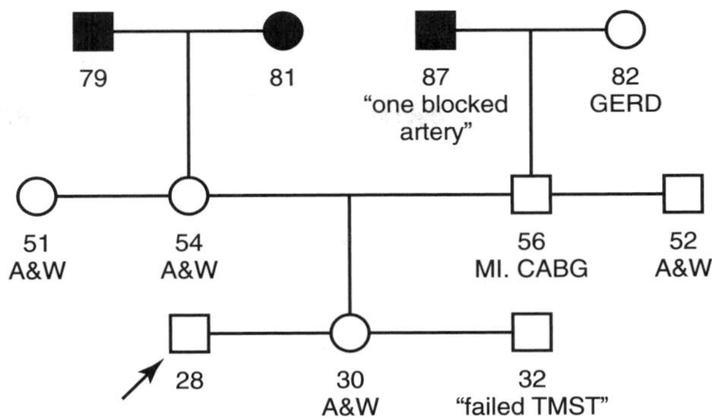

Males are represented by squares.
Females are represented by circles.
A darkened symbol indicates that the person is dead.
The number below the symbol indicates the person's current age or age at death.
An arrow designates the patient.

Figure 12–2. Genogram format for H. R.'s family history.

fessionals. Apart from an encounter with a health-care provider, there is no other instance in which people voluntarily allow strangers to explore their most intense fears and examine their entire physical being. This requires exceptional trust on the patient's part, and the highest human and professional standards on the provider's part.

There may also be patients who are anxious or fearful about undergoing a physical examination conducted by a virtual stranger. Reasons may include fear of pain induced by the examination, fear of discovering an abnormality, or fear of being physically exposed to a stranger. Be aware that the patient may not be open to or accepting of you for these or other reasons. Try to allay their fears.

If done correctly the physical examination can provide the clinician with valuable information and allow the patient to maintain his or her dignity, a commodity that need not wontedly be forfeited upon admission to the hospital. If done improperly, however, the physical examination can be awkward for the patient and examiner, make the patient resistant to later examinations, and yield few diagnostic clues.

Patient Comfort

As with the patient history, every effort should be made to make the patient comfortable for the examination. It's often the "little things" that make the deepest impact. Especially when mechanically ventilated, or pharmacologically paralyzed and sedated, patients are at their most vulnerable and are unable to communicate effectively. In such circumstances it is particularly important to explain to the patient that you are going to examine him or her. Never assume that a sedated patient is entirely unaware of what is happening around him or her. Every patient should receive an explanation of what you are doing.

Be careful not to shout needlessly when speaking to a patient. No patient wants his or her confidential conversation with the provider to be heard by the staff, patients, and visitors of the unit, particularly when the patient hears without difficulty. Do not assume that because a patient is older, he or she cannot hear. Speak only as loudly as is necessary to be clearly understood.

Similarly, provide as much privacy as possible for the examination. In outpatient settings or in private hospital rooms it is easy to close the door to the examination room. Curtains in emergency departments and critical care units do not provide the best level of privacy. Making the effort to ensure the patient's privacy, however, is important. Regardless of the actual degree of privacy, the patient perceives your attempt at providing privacy.

Make certain that the patient is warm enough and that he or she is comfortably positioned. Also, allow the patient to remain clothed for as much of the examination as possible. Sitting scantly clothed before a stranger, regardless of the stranger's professional role, must be extraordinarily dehumanizing. It is also completely unnecessary. Expose only the area that you are examining. There are few, if any, situations in which patients must be exposed more than briefly for an elective examination.

Order of Physical Examination

Typically, the history taking precedes the physical examination. In addition to guiding the physical examination, the history provides the opportunity to interact with the patient in a nonthreatening way and allows a segue into the more vulnerable part of the experience.

When examining children it is recommended that clinicians perform the least threatening components of the examination first, and the most threatening last. This is a good routine to use for adults, too. In patients with abdominal discomfort, for instance, it is generally best to reserve deep abdominal palpation and the digital rectal examination for the end of the interaction. Develop a system for yourself to follow when examining patients, and don't stray from it. It is less likely, then, that important parts of the examination will be omitted.

Positioning for the Physical Examination

The position of the patient is largely dependent upon the setting in which he or she is examined. Outpatients generally meet the clinician while seated on the examination table. This may also be appropriate for many hospitalized patients. Critically ill or injured patients, those with severe pain, and others may not be able to be so accommodating. It is in these situations where patient-centered care is defined. Try to remain at the patient's eye-level, whether he or she is seated, lying, or standing. Anticipatory guidance, insightful planning, and ingenuity are helpful assets.

Generally, the physical examination is started from the sitting position. Here the ACNP can examine the head, neck, and chest. Much of the neurologic examination is done with the patient seated, but parts that require the patient to stand or walk are conveniently done at this point. The patient can then be positioned supine with the head of the bed at about 30 degrees and the legs flat. The heart and extremities are easily examined in this position. The abdomen can be examined with the head of the bed flat. The patient is then easily rolled onto his or her side for the rectal examination.

Levels of Physical Examination

It is neither appropriate nor necessary for the ACNP to perform a complete history and physical at each encounter. The comprehensive exam, the interim exam, and the focused exam are three types of physical examinations that are clinically useful and frequently used in inpatient settings.

The Comprehensive Examination

Every new patient—whether admitted to the hospital or seen in an outpatient setting—must have a comprehensive health history and physical examination documented in the medical record. The purposes of this comprehensive examination are to: evaluate the chief complaint in detail; elicit evidence of comorbid conditions; and discover other health conditions that could place the patient, fellow patients, or health-care workers at risk (e.g., substance abuse, communicable diseases, etc.).

There are ten essential components of the comprehensive examination: skin, head/eyes/ears/nose/throat, neck, chest, cardiac, abdomen, genitourinary, rectal, extremities, and neurological. Each component should be performed and documented. No portion of the initial examination should be deferred or omitted unless there is a medically valid reason.

Tables 12–18 through 12–27 list the normal and abnormal findings of each component of the comprehensive physical examination. More detailed information can be found in appropriate chapters.

The Interim Examination

The interim examination is performed daily or more frequently to assess the effectiveness of treatment and discover complications. Although it is most commonly performed in the hospital, it can also be useful in the outpatient setting for serial evaluations of acute illnesses.

The interim examination is ideal for a hospitalized patient who is seen once or twice daily. Naturally, it is not necessary to perform a comprehensive exam at each encounter. Consider, for example, a woman with congestive heart failure hospitalized for intravenous diuresis. The initial comprehensive examination is performed at the time of admission. Subsequent examinations of the patient should evaluate her response to treatment and monitor for development of complications. So, review of the intake and output, weight and vital signs, examination of the jugular veins, carotid pulses, and degree of peripheral edema and auscultation of the heart and lungs are warranted. Additionally, because the patient has an IV it is essential that the site be examined for evidence of infection or infiltration at least

TABLE 12–18. Examination of the Skin

	Normal Findings	Abnormal Findings	Explanation
Appearance			
Color	Pink, brown	Vitiligo	Absence of melanin
		Jaundice	Yellow appearance of skin due to serum bilirubin levels above 2–2.5 mg/dL (Kaplan and Isselbacher, 1994)
		Cyanosis	Low oxygen saturation
Lesions	Absent	Macules, patches	Flat lesions (in ascending order of size)
		Papules, plaques, nodules, tumors	Raised lesions (in ascending order of size)
		Vesicles, bullae	Fluid-filled lesions (in ascending order of size)
		Erosion, ulcer	Absence of skin surface (in ascending order of size)
Palpation			
Moistness	Dry	Diaphoretic	Generalized cool, clammy feeling
Turgor	Normal	Delayed	Poor skin turgor can indicate dehydration (not reliable in older adults)

TABLE 12–19. The HEENT Examination

	Normal Findings	Abnormal Findings	Explanation
Head			
Inspection of head and face	Hair normally distributed	Abnormal hair growth	Hirsutism may suggest underlying endocrinopathy or be due to adverse drug effects
Palpation of skull	Smooth skull	Swelling, fracture	
Palpation of lymph nodes	Nontender, nonpalpable	Tender, enlarged	Lymphadenopathy suggests infection or cancer
Eyes			
Lids	Pupil visible when lid open	Ptosis	Indicates neurologic impairment (e.g., Horner's syndrome, cranial nerve lesions)
	Dry	Drainage	Purulent drainage suggests infection; serous drainage indicates irritation
Conjunctiva	Translucent	Edematous	Common following cardiopulmonary bypass
		Red, inflamed	Suggests infection or irritation
Sclera	Firm, white, spherical	Soft, nonspherical	Trauma
Retina	Red reflex, no retinal lesions	Exudates, hemorrhages, papilledema, cotton-wool patches	Hypertensive retinopathy
		Microaneurysms, neovascularization, yellow macular exudates	Diabetic retinopathy
Pupils	Equal, round, reactive to light	Unequal	Neurological problem
		Irregular	Surgical iridectomy
		Nonreactive to light	Blindness, neurological disorders
		Pinpoint	Narcotics, miotics
		Fixed and dilated	Anticholinergics, neurologic catastrophe
Ears			
Tympanic membrane	Clear, light reflex	Bulging, fluid visible	Serous otitis media
		Red, inflamed, bulging	Otitis media
Hearing	Equal acuity (Weber)	Unilateral acuity	Conduction deafness
	Air conduction > bone conduction (Rinne)	Bone conduction > air conduction	Nerve deafness
Nose			
Nares	Patent	Unilateral blockage	Deviated septum, tumor, mucous accumulation
Turbinates	Moist, deep red		
Mouth and Throat			
Gums	Pink	Red, inflamed	Infection
Teeth	Smooth, white	Dental carries	
Tongue	Smooth, pink		
Palate	Pink, smooth	High and arched	Classic finding in Marfan's syndrome
Pharynx	Pink	Red	Postnasal drip
		Red, injected, inflamed tonsils, tonsilar exudate	Pharyngitis/tonsilitis
		Deviated uvula and swollen tonsilar pillar	Peritonsilar abcess

daily. If on bedrest, the patient should be examined for evidence of skin breakdown.

Because of the potential complications of hospitalization, it is important that the ACNP thoroughly examine each patient at least daily. The clinician should especially keep in mind common hospital-acquired infections such as pneumonia, cellulitis (at IV sites), and urinary tract infection. Other potential complications of hospitalization include gout flare, skin breakdown, and falls. Table 12–28 lists the components of the interim physical examination that should be part of every hospitalized patient's daily examination.

TABLE 12–20. Examination of the Neck

	Normal Findings	Abnormal Findings	Explanation
Neck Veins			
a and v waves	a wave > v wave	Absent a waves	Atrial fibrillation
Jugular venous pressure	Less than 10 cm water	Greater than 10 cm water	Right heart failure
Carotid Arteries			
Intensity and duration of carotid impulse	Single, rapid rising impulse	Hyperdynamic impulse Pulsus tardus Pulsus alternans Pulsus paradoxus	High output states, AR Aortic stenosis Left ventricular failure Cardiac tamponade, restrictive pericarditis
Thyroid			
Palpation	Barely palpable, nonpalpable Free of nodules	Enlarged Palpable nodules	Goiter Tumors

The Focused Examination and Differential Diagnosis

The focused examination—perhaps the most critical to the patient's care—is performed when there is a change in the patient's baseline health status. Outpatients who present with a concise complaint and who are known to the provider often do not require a comprehensive examination. Much of the information necessary to treat the patient is available from the medical record.

Focused exams are also well suited to emergency department settings. It matters little, for example, what are a patient's cardiac risk factors when they present with a simple laceration. Similarly, in life-threatening situations the only examination required is one that facilitates saving the patient's life.

The focused examination is generally guided by symptoms. The patient presents with a complaint. It is the job of the clinician, then, to evaluate the chief complaint. As

TABLE 12–21. Examination of the Chest

	Normal Findings	Abnormal Findings	Explanation
Appearance			
Work of breathing	Comfortable	Respiratory distress	Respiratory or cardiovascular disease
General health	Healthy	Cachectic	Chronic disease, cancer
Shape of chest		Increased AP diameter	COPD
Trachea	Midline	Deviated	Tumor, pneumothorax, atelectasis
Chest movement	Symmetric	Asymmetric	Pneumothorax, flail chest
Percussion			
	Resonance	Flatness/dullness	Pleural effusion, pneumonia
		Hyperresonance/tympany	Emphysema, pneumothorax
Palpation			
Subcutaneous emphysema	Absent	Palpable over thorax	Ruptured bullae, pneumothorax, barotrauma secondary to positive pressure ventilation
Tactile fremitus	Present	Absent	Pneumothorax
		Decreased	Pleural effusion, atelectasis
		Increased	Consolidation
Auscultation			
Breath sounds	Vesicular	Bronchial	Suggests consolidation
Transmitted voice sounds	Garbled/muffled	Distinct	Egophony, bronchophony, and whispered pectoriloquy suggest consolidation
Adventitious sounds	None	Early inspiratory crackles	Chronic obstructive pulmonary disease
		Late inspiratory crackles	Congestive heart failure, interstitial lung disease
		Rhonchi	Pulmonary edema, poor pulmonary toilet
		Pleural friction rub	Pulmonary infarction, pleuritis, hemothorax

TABLE 12–22. Examination of the Heart

	Normal Findings	Abnormal Findings	Explanation
Palpation			
PMI	Single impulse, 4th–5th ICS, MCL	Diffuse and sustained impulse	Left ventricular hypertrophy
		Lateral displacement	Left ventricular dilation
		Presystolic impulse	Left ventricular noncompliance
RV impulse	Absent	Lower left sternal border	Right ventricular dilation, pulmonary hypertension
Auscultation			
S_1 (M_1, T_1)	Single sound		Split S_1 has no pathological significance
S_2 (A_2, P_2)	Single sound or physiological splitting	Paradoxical splitting	LBBB
		Wide splitting	RBBB
		Wide fixed splitting	Atrial septal defect, pulmonary embolism
		Increased A_2	Hypertension
		Decreased P_2	Aortic stenosis
S_3	Absent (may be normal in children and young adults)	Heard at PMI	Left ventricular failure, fluid volume overload
		Heard at lower left sternal border	Right-sided failure
S_4	Absent	Heard at lower left sternal border	Hypertension, aortic stenosis, left ventricular hypertrophy
Mid-systolic clicks	Absent	Heard at apex	Mitral valve prolapse
Ejection sound	Absent	Precedes systolic ejection murmur	Aortic stenosis
Opening snap	Absent	Heard at apex	Mitral stenosis
Systolic murmur	Absent, "functional" murmur	Late-peaking systolic ejection murmur	Aortic stenosis, pulmonic stenosis
		Holosystolic murmur	Mitral regurgitation, ventricular septal defect
Diastolic murmur	Absent	Early diastolic, decrescendo	Aortic regurgitation
		Presystolic, crescendo	Mitral stenosis
Pericardial friction rub	Absent	3-component rub heard throughout precordium	Pericarditis, mediastinal tumor

Key: PMI = point of maximum intensity, ICS = intercostal space, MCL = midclavicular line, LBBB = left bundle branch block, RBBB = right bundle branch block

stated earlier, the history produces clues that guide the physical examination. But, the clinician must also consider the differential diagnoses. That is, what are the *potential causes* of the patient's chief complaint?

Consider, for instance, the complaint of chest pain. From the history, the clinician learns that the patient suddenly developed retrosternal chest pain, described as "heaviness," that occurred while shoveling snow. The pain radiated to the neck and jaw, and has persisted for the last 45 minutes. He has come to the emergency department because he is concerned that he is having a heart attack.

Before examining the patient and ordering laboratory and diagnostic tests, the clinician must first consider the possible causes of chest pain (Table 12–29). The history that the patient reports is suspicious of acute myocardial infarction. Naturally, this complaint deserves urgent consideration since myocardial infarction is potentially life threatening. Since there are no physical findings that absolutely confirm acute myocardial infarction, physical examination in this circumstance should not delay emergency treatment.

But, what if the symptoms are more vague? Consider this example. A normally healthy 28-year-old man known to the clinician complains of constant chest pain for the past week and increasing orthopnea over the last two days. Careful history taking reveals that he also had a viral upper respiratory infection about ten days before. At first, the history may not clearly define the etiology of the symptoms. But, reviewing the differential diagnoses of chest pain, the clinician is prompted to consider pericarditis. In this instance focused physical examination is extremely helpful. Careful auscultation of the heart reveals a three-component pericardial friction rub. Pulsus paradoxus also is diagnostic.

In neither of these examples is it imperative that the patient have a comprehensive physical examination. Comprehensive physical examination does not yield additional useful data for the diagnosis or management of acute pericarditis.

Chest Pain. The focused physical examination for the patient with acute chest pain is necessarily aimed at determining whether the pain represents life-threatening pathology. As mentioned previously, there are no physical findings that are, by themselves, diagnostic of acute myocardial ischemia. The patient history and electrocardiogram are the

TABLE 12–23. The Abdominal Examination

	Normal Findings	Abnormal Findings	Explanation
Inspection			
	Flat, no visible masses	Masses	Splenomegaly, hepatomegaly, tumor, aneurysm
		Midline mass with abdominus contraction	Ventral hernia
Auscultation			
Bowel sounds	5–35 sounds per min	Absent, hypoactive	Ileus, peritonitis
		Hyperactive	Bowel obstruction
Vascular sounds	Absent	Bruits	Occlusive arterial disease (stenosis of aorta or renal, iliac, or hepatic arteries)
		Venous hums	Cirrhosis
Percussion			
Right upper quadrant	Liver span 6–12 cm	Liver span > 12 cm	Hepatomegaly
Left upper quadrant	Tympany, hyperresonance (gastric air bubble)	Flatness	Splenomegaly
Lateral abd. wall	Tympany	Dullness, fluid wave	Ascites
Palpation			
Epigastrum	Nontender	Tender	Pancreatitis, peptic ulcer
Periumbilicus	Nonpulsatile	Pulsatile mass	Aortic aneurysm
Right upper quadrant	Soft, nontender, liver edge nonpalpable	Tender, positive Murphy's sign	Cholelithiasis, cholecystitis
		Palpable liver edge	Hepatomegaly
Left upper quadrant	Soft, nontender	Palpable/percussable mass	Splenomegaly
Left lower quadrant	Soft, nontender	Tender	Diverticulitis
Right lower quadrant	Soft, nontender	Tender; abdominal guarding; rebound tenderness; referred rebound tenderness; positive psoas or obturator signs	Appendicitis (Bates, 1991)

TABLE 12–24. The Genitourinary Examination

	Normal Findings	Abnormal Findings	Explanation
Male			
Testes	Firm, nontender, smooth	Tender, swollen epididymis	Epididymitis
		Nontender, palpable mass	Tumors
Penis	No lesions	Lesions, drainage	Sexually transmitted diseases, cancer
Inguinal canal	Pelvic/abdominal contents nonpalpable	Palpable abdominal contents with cough/strain	Inguinal hernia
Female			
External genitalia	Pink, no lesions, no drainage	Visible lesions, drainage	Sexually transmitted diseases, cancer
Vaginal wall	Pink, no lesions, no drainage	Visible lesions, drainage	Sexually transmitted diseases, cancer
Cervix	Smooth, no visible lesions	Lesions	Cancer
Uterus	Smooth, firm	Palpable mass	Uterine tumor
		Nonpalpable	Hysterectomy
Ovaries	Smooth, firm, nontender	Palpable mass	Ovarian cyst, tumor
		Tender	Pelvic inflammatory disease

TABLE 12–25. The Rectal Examination

	Normal Findings	Abnormal Findings	Explanation
External Perineum			
	Smooth, pink	Hemorrhoids	
		Warts	Genital warts
Rectum			
	Smooth, no palpable masses, stool heme-negative	Heme-positive	Cancer, GI bleeding
		Masses	Internal hemorrhoids, cancer, polyps
Prostate			
	Smooth, nontender, walnut-sized	Nodules/masses	Cancer
		Enlarged, tender	Prostatitis
		Enlarged	Prostatic hypertrophy

most useful tools for diagnosing ischemia. Nevertheless, other important causes of chest pain may be overlooked unless a careful focused physical examination is performed (Table 12–30).

Dyspnea. The potential causes of acute dyspnea are many. Common pulmonary causes of dyspnea such as reactive airway diseases and pneumonia are most common. Other pulmonary causes include pneumothorax, pulmonary embolism, solid tumor, and pleural effusion, which are less common. Extra-pulmonary causes of dyspnea such as congestive heart failure, arrhythmia, cardiomyopathy, and pericarditis must also be considered. To adequately identify the cause and definitely exclude other potential causes of dyspnea, careful physical examination is required (Table 12–31).

Syncope. There are numerous causes of syncope; vasodepressor syncope and orthostatic hypotension are the most common causes. Pure cardiac causes of syncope include arrhythmia, vaso–vagal syndrome, aortic stenosis, hypertrophic cardiomyopathy, and neurocardiogenic syncope. Cough and voiding (micturition) are also causes of syncope. The components of the focused physical examination for syncope are listed in Table 12–32.

Abdominal Pain. Because of the innervation of the visceral organs, diagnosing abdominal pain is challenging.

TABLE 12–26. Examination of the Extremities

	Normal Findings	Abnormal Findings	Explanation
Skin			
	Warm, pink	Erythematous, swollen	Cellulitis
		Cool, ruboric (red), hairless, thin and shiny; ulcers at pressure points	Arterial insufficiency
		Warm, edematous, darkly pigmented, ulcers near medial maleolous	Venous insufficiency
Edema			
	None–trace	Symmetrical pitting edema	Congestive heart failure, fluid volume overload
		Unilateral edema	Venous insufficiency, lymphedema
Bruits			
	Absent	Present	Atherosclerosis or aneurysm; following invasive procedure could be due to clot, pseudoaneurysm, arteriovenous fistula
Pulses			
	2+ throughout	Absent or diminished	Arterial insufficiency
		Accentuated	Atherosclerosis, aneurysm, aortic regurgitation
Musculoskeletal			
	Extremities symmetrical	Asymmetry	Fracture, hematoma
	Joints move smoothly	Crepitus	Degenerative joint disease

TABLE 12–27. The Neurological Examination

	Normal Findings	Abnormal Findings	Explanation
Mental Status			
Level of consciousness	Alert; oriented to person, place and time; follows commands	Obtunded, stuporous, comatose	Trauma, CVA, hypoglycemia, increased ICP, infection/sepsis, hepatic failure, poisoning/intoxication, hypoxemia, fluid/electrolyte/acid–base abnormalities, seizure disorder
Speech	Clear, well-articulated	Inarticulate	Aphasia, sedation, drug/alcohol effects
Mood/affect	Appropriate to situation	Depressed, elated	Depression, bipolar disorder, drug/alcohol effects
Thought	Coherent thought processes	Delusions, hallucinations, psychosis	Drug/alcohol effects, ICU psychosis, hepatic failure
Memory and attention	Serial 7's, remember three objects	Unable to perform	Dementia, psychosis
Cognition	Able to calculate simple mathematical problems and interpret proverbs	Unable to perform higher cognitive functions	Dementia, psychosis
Cranial Nerves			
Olfactory (I)	Intact sense of smell		Inability to perform tasks suggests lesion (e.g., tumor, ischemia/stroke) involving corresponding cranial nerve
Optic (II)	Visual acuity intact		
Oculomotor, Trochlear, Abducens (III, IV, and VI)	Extraocular movements intact (EOMI)		
Trigeminal (V)	*Motor:* Able to clench jaw *Sensory:* Light touch and temperature sensation intact		
Facial (VII)	*Motor:* Facial movements intact *Sensory:* Taste and touch sensations of tongue intact		
Acoustic (VIII)	Hears whispered voice		
Glossopharyngeal and Vagus (IX and X)	Soft palate rises, voice free of hoarseness, gag intact		
Spinal Acc. (XI)	Shrugs shoulders		
Hypoglossal (XII)	Speech articulate		
Motor Function			
	Appropriate muscle bulk, tone and strength	Muscle atrophy	LMN lesions
		Diminished muscle tone and strength	Guillian Barre syndrome, LMN lesions
	No involuntary movements	Tremors	Parkinson's disease, multiple sclerosis, hyperthyroidism, anxiety
	Gait steady	Unsteady gait	Stroke or other UMN lesions, LMN lesions, Parkinson's disease
		Ataxia	Cerebellar or posterior column lesions
Sensory Function			
	Light touch, pain, and vibratory sensation intact and symmetrical	Asymmetric sensation of light touch and pain	UMN lesion
		Absence of vibratory sense	Posterior column lesion
Reflexes			
	Deep tendon reflexes 2+ throughout	Absent or diminished reflexes on affected side	LMN lesion
		Babinski reflex, clonus and accentuated reflexes on affected side	UMN lesion

Key: CVA = cerebrovascular accident, ICP = intracranial pressure, LMN = lower motor neuron, UMN = upper motor neuron

TABLE 12–28. Components of the Interim Examination of Hospitalized Patients

System	Physical Examination Component	Check for
General appearance		Ill appearance
Vital signs	Temperature	Fever
	Blood pressure	Hypertension, hypotension
	Heart rate	Rate, regularity
	Respirations	Labored breathing, tachypnea
Chest	Auscultation and percussion of lungs	Nosocomial pneumonia
Heart	Auscultation of heart	New murmurs, particularly in patients at risk for endocarditis
Extremities	Inspection and palpation of joints	Gout
Skin	Inspection of incisions and wounds	Healing, infection
	Inspection of dependent areas	Skin breakdown
	Inspection of IV/drain sites	Cellulitis
Neurologic	Mental status	Oriented to person, time, place (especially important in elderly)

TABLE 12–29. Differential Diagnosis of Chest Pain

Acute myocardial infarction
Unstable angina
Aortic stenosis
Mitral valve prolapse
Pericarditis
Dissecting aortic aneurysm
Hypertrophic cardiomyopathy
Pneumonia
Pulmonary embolism
Pneumothorax
Musculoskeletal injury
Esophageal spasm
Esophageal reflux, peptic ulcer disease

TABLE 12–30. The Focused Physical Examination in Acute Chest Pain

System	Physical Examination Component	Check for
General appearance		Ill appearance
Vital signs	Blood pressure	Hypertensive, hypotensive
	Heart rate	Tachycardia, bradycardia, irregular rhythm
Neck	Palpation of carotid arteries	Pulsus tardus, pulsus alternans
	Inspection of jugular veins	Jugular venous distention
Chest	Auscultation and percussion of the lung fields	Pneumonia, pneumothorax
Heart	Auscultation	Murmurs, gallops
	Palpation	Displaced or diffuse and sustained PMI
Extremities	Palpation of pulses	Pulse deficit (e.g., dissecting thoracic aneurysm)
	Palpation of legs	Edema

TABLE 12–31. The Focused Physical Examination in Acute Dyspnea

System	Physical Examination Component	Check for
General appearance		Ill appearance
Vital signs	Respiratory rate	Tachypnea, hyperpnea
	Heart rate	Tachycardia, bradycardia, irregular rhythm
Neck	Palpation of carotid arteries	Pulsus paradoxus
	Inspection of jugular veins	Jugular venous distention
Chest	Auscultation and percussion of the lung fields	Pneumonia, pneumothorax
Heart	Auscultation	Murmurs, gallops
	Palpation	Displaced or diffuse and sustained PMI
Extremities	Palpation of legs	Edema

TABLE 12–32. The Focused Physical Examination in Syncope

System	Physical Examination Component	Check for
General appearance		Ill appearance
Vital signs	Blood pressure	Orthostatic hypotension
	Heart rate	Tachycardia, bradycardia
Neck	Palpation of carotid arteries	Pulsus tardus
Heart	Auscultation	Murmurs, gallops
	Palpation	Displaced or diffuse and sustained PMI
Neurologic	Mental status	Comatose, confused, post ictal state, etc.

TABLE 12–33. The Focused Physical Examination for Abdominal Pain

System	Physical Examination Component	Check for
General appearance		Mild, moderate, or severe distress
Vital signs	Temperature	Fever
	Blood pressure	Hypotension, hypertension
	Heart rate	Tachycardia
Abdomen	Observation	Distended
	Bowel sounds	Absent, increased, decreased
	Palpation	Tender, guarded
	Maneuvers	Psoas sign, rebound tenderness, referred pain, etc.
Rectal	Palpation	Constipation, occult blood

Abdominal pain may emanate from multiple juxtaposed organs. Among the differential diagnoses of abdominal pain are enteritis, ileus, pancreatitis, hepatitis, cholangeitis, appendicitis, peritonitis, retroperitoneal bleed, intraabdominal hemorrhage, diverticulitis, dissecting aneurysm, and mesenteric ischemia. Table 12–33 lists the components of the focused examination for abdominal pain.

The history and physical examination are among the most important tasks performed by the ACNP. A carefully conducted history and examination allows the clinician to develop an appropriate treatment plan, anticipate patient needs, prevent complications of hospitalization, and return the patient to his or her previous functional level.

Acknowledgment: I am grateful for the assistance that Nelson Wolf, MD provided in conceptualizing the physical examination content of this chapter and for all that he taught me, a neophyte clinician, about the art of physical examination. *(PL)*

REFERENCES

Bates, B. (1991). *A Guide to Physical Examination and History Taking* (5th edition). Philadelphia: J.B. Lippincott.

Batzer, E. S. (1991). Psychiatric evaluation. In G. W. Stuart & S. J. Sundeen (Eds.), *Principles and Practice of Psychiatric Nursing,* pp. 182–188. St. Louis: Mosby-Yearbook.

Billings, J. A. & Stoeckle, J. D. (1989). *The Clinical Encounter.* Chicago: Year Book Medical Publishers, Inc.

Burchfiel, C. M., Marcus, E. B., Sharp, D. S., Enright, P. L., Rodriguez, B. L., Masaki, K. H., Hwang, L. & Curb, J. D. (1996). Characteristics associated with rapid decline in forced expiratory volume. *Annals of Epidemiology, 6* (3), 217–227.

Kaplan, L. M. & Isselbacher, K. J. (1994). Jaundice. In Isselbacher, K. J., Braunwald, E., Wilson, J. D., Martin, J. B., Fauci, A. S. & Kasper, D. L. (Eds.), *Harrison's Principles of Internal Medicine* (13th edition), p. 226. New York: McGraw-Hill.

Kemp, B. J. (1993). Psychologic care of the older rehabilitation patient. *Clinics in Geriatric Medicine, 9* (4), 841–857.

13

Medical Reasoning

William G. Kussmaul III

Medical reasoning is the process of collecting data and arriving at diagnostic and therapeutic conclusions. Medical diagnostic reasoning answers the question, "What's wrong with this patient?" Therapeutic reasoning deals with the questions, "How should this patient be treated?" and "Is the treatment working?" The answer to the last question, if negative or uncertain, leads to a new round of diagnostic reasoning. The medical thought process is essentially iterative: it cycles back again and again, always seeking to reduce uncertainty and reach the correct conclusion.

Uncertainty is characteristic of the medical reasoning process. Patients and their families do not like uncertainty. They want to know what is wrong, what caused it, what to do about it, and what will happen. Health practitioners also want to be (or at least want to appear to be) certain about their recommendations and decisions. Even the way we use language shows how uncomfortable health practitioners are with uncertainty and imprecision (Carleton, 1997). However, reality is seldom clear-cut. Practioners must be prepared to deal with uncertainty as logically as possible, reaching the most "reasonable" conclusions available, and should then be able to explain their reasoning to the patient. Uncertainty can be viewed as a positive, in that it leads to alternatives that can be evaluated in collaboration with the patient and his or her environment. Much of this chapter is devoted to organizing the medical thought process in the face of uncertainty.

An example of medical diagnostic uncertainty frequently encountered in critical care practice is the evaluation of chest pain. Suppose a 63-year-old man develops retro sternal burning pain two days after an aortic aneurysm repair. Other than diffuse abdominal tenderness, there are no important physical findings. The ECG shows "nonspecific" ST segment abnormalities. The patient is a long-term smoker. Is this pain caused by angina, heartburn, postoperative pain, or previously undiagnosed gallstones?

The evaluation of this diagnostic problem would take into account the patient's risk factors for the various possibilities (high risk for postoperative pain: he just had an operation; fairly high risk for angina: he is a 63-year-old male smoker). You would also consider the relative importance of the diagnostic possibilities: heartburn is not life-threatening; angina could be. The choice of possible diagnostic maneuvers (for example, stress testing) and therapeutic maneuvers (for example, a trial of sublingual nitroglycerin) would be guided by the priority you set on this list of differential diagnostic possibilities.

Therapeutic uncertainty can also be illustrated from this patient's course. Suppose he underwent a pharmacological stress/nuclear study that was abnormal, suggesting multivessel coronary disease. He then underwent cardiac catheterization, revealing three-vessel disease in which none of the major trunks (anterior descending, circumflex, or right coronary) were severely narrowed, but several sizable diagonal and marginal branches had stenoses varying in severity from 50% to 100% occlusion. Some of these were amenable to angioplasty, others were not. A discussion would then need to be held regarding the relative risks and benefits, both short term and long term, associated with the three options of medical therapy, angioplasty, and bypass surgery. We will return to this discussion later in the chapter.

DATA GATHERING

Clinical data are summarized in the written History and Physical with which all are familiar. The sources from which this information is gathered are worth pondering: direct patient interview; family members; previous office or hospital charts; notes and records supplied by other physicians or hospitals; physical examination; laboratory tests; the results of procedures. In the age of information, it is easier than ever to obtain the records of tests, procedures, or hospital admissions elsewhere, though patient confidentiality must be respected in this process. Patients are now able to carry with them their own electronic copies of medical records.

Recording the available data in an organized format makes it easier to apply the subsequent steps of data evaluation and differential diagnosis.

DATA EVALUATION

Before deciding on a list of possible diagnoses, it is necessary to evaluate the clinical data. How reliable is the source? Are the data current? Are the data complete?

A "reliable history" sometimes seems difficult to elicit, but the fault may lie more often with the history-taker than the history-giver. Whether the historical data comes spontaneously or in answer to questions, rarely do patients provide a linear timeline of all relevant events, and rarely are their recollections of events complete on the first try. It is the history-taker's challenge to assemble the pieces of the story in order, decide what gaps need to be filled, and gather additional data if needed. Only then can a coherent history of the illness be recorded.

Previous records are essential. The patient may report having a "heart attack" 5 years ago. This may be the best recollection of what he or she was told at the time. But was it, in fact, an admission for undiagnosed chest pain? Or for an uncomplicated small infarction? Or was the patient in cardiogenic shock?

The patient may report, and hospital records may also seem to confirm, the diagnosis of "heart failure," but this phrase may merely have been copied from history to history over the years. Evaluating this important piece of data might involve searching for an ejection fraction measurement, a catheterization or echocardiogram report, or a chest radiograph report. Furthermore, even if heart failure is confirmed, the question remains: due to what? Thus the iterative process of medical reasoning unfolds, as data lead to new hypotheses, the evaluation of which requires more data.

Certain historical details can only be gleaned from detailed records. For example, a patient who has had previous bypass surgery may require cardiac catheterization for evaluation of chest pain or for an acute cardiac event. In this case, it is important to know exactly how many grafts were constructed at the time of surgery, of what type, and to what coronary arteries the grafts were connected. These data can come only from a surgeon's report; "CABG × 3 in 1988" is not sufficient. Similarly, the type of heart valve implanted in a patient with rheumatic heart disease could have a major impact on the management of an episode of gastrointestinal bleeding.

Diagnostic Tests

All diagnostic tests are subject to uncertainty. Consider a test with a "Yes/No" type of result, such as a pregnancy test. If completely reliable, such a test represents the ideal kind of information on which to base a related diagnostic decision, such as the answer to the question, "What is causing nausea and vomiting in this 23-year-old sexually active female?"

Unfortunately, most tests are not ideal in this sense. First, a test result can be inaccurate. An inaccurate test gives a wrong answer through error (e.g., running the wrong patient's blood sample; drawing a blood sample above an IV site) or incorrect adjustment of testing parameters (e.g., a nonfasting lipid panel). Second, a test result may seem imprecise. Many diagnostic tests do not return binary results like a pregnancy test, but rather a numeric value that has to be interpreted further. A 45-year-old male has a hemoglobin of 12.5 g/dL. Is this anemia? The answer to this question requires knowledge of the normal range of hemoglobin for males of this age. The fact that there is a normal range indicates not a lack of precision in the measurement of hemoglobin, but a normal degree of variability compatible with a healthy state.

In addition, abnormal states such as gastritis with associated bleeding may not cause a hemoglobin below the normal range in their early stages. Put differently, the range of hemoglobin values associated with normality overlaps with the range of hemoglobin values seen in patients with peptic ulcer disease. Therefore, some patients with "normal" values might have ulcers, while others with "low" values might be normal, or might have another cause for their anemia.

False-Positive and False-Negative Tests

These examples illustrate the critically important concept of false–positive and false–negative test results. It is vital to realize that no test is perfect, i.e., devoid of false–positive and false–negative results. This fact may be disturbing to patients, who are told after a normal cardiac catheterization test that the previous abnormal noninvasive test was wrong. How can this happen? Possibilities include under-interpretation of the coronary angiogram, over-interpretation of the noninvasive test, or an alternative explanation for the abnormal stress test other than fixed obstruction of radiologically visible, epicardial vessels. For the purposes of this discussion, we will examine the ways in which the noninvasive test may have been inaccurate, assuming that the catheterization results were correct.

Sensitivity and Specificity

The terms *sensitivity* and *specificity* describe the behavior of a diagnostic test in situations where false-positive and false-negative tests are possible. Stress testing for myocardial ischemia is a paradigm of such a test. Suppose 100 people have coronary disease. If all 100 undergo stress testing, only 90 will have abnormal or "positive" results. The other ten have false–negative results. The sensitivity of stress testing for ischemia is about 90%. We will miss the diagnosis of coronary artery disease in 10 of every 100 patients tested.

Consider another 100 individuals, none of whom have coronary disease. If they undergo stress testing, about 80 will have normal results ("true–negative"), while the other 20 will have false–positive test results for any of several reasons: concomitant medications, unrelated ECG abnormalities, electrolyte disturbances. The specificity of stress testing for the exclusion of coronary disease is in fact about 80%.

To illustrate these numbers, it is useful to construct what is known as a "two-by-two figure." (See Fig. 13–1.)

Put differently: Sensitivity answers the question, "Among patients who have the disease, what percent will have an abnormal test and be diagnosed?" Specificity answers the question, "Among patients who do not have the disease, what percent will have a negative test and be correctly classified as normal?"

Positive Predictive Value and Negative Predictive Value

Unfortunately, these are not clinically useful questions. Patients do not present to the office already specified as to whether or not a given disease is present. Rather, the practitioner is presented with the results of a diagnostic test in a particular patient, and must then answer the question, "Given the results of the test, does this patient have disease?" More accurately, what is the *probability* of disease? (Thinking in terms of probabilities is central to medical reasoning. Probabilities quantify uncertainty. The reasoning process seeks to arrive at the most probable answer, by minimizing the uncertainty inherent in the situation.) Returning to the use of stress testing in diagnosing coronary disease, the clinically appropriate questions are:

1. "Given a positive stress test, what is the probability that this patient has coronary disease?" And,
2. "Given a negative stress test, what is the probability that this patient does not have coronary disease?"

The answers to these questions are, respectively, termed the Positive Predictive Value (PV+) and the Negative Predictive Value (PV–).

The same two-by-two figure may be used to calculate these values. (See Fig. 13–2.)

It can be seen that of all patients with a positive stress test (110), 90 actually have coronary disease. The Positive Predictive Value is 90/110 = 82%.

Of all those with a negative test (90), 80 actually do not have coronary disease. The Negative Predictive Value is 80/90 = 89%.

While these figures are far from the 100% that would represent the ideal, consider that the original population from which the example was drawn—100 patients with and 100 patients without coronary disease—had an overall 50% incidence of disease. In this group, an abnormal stress test raised the probability of coronary disease from 50% to 82%. A normal stress test lowered the probability of coronary disease from 50% to 11%. Not bad.

Standard abbreviations exist for all of the above terms. Patients with disease who have abnormal tests are True–Positives (TP); those with normal test results are False–Negatives (FN). Among patients who do not have disease, those with negative tests are True–Negative (TN), while those with positive tests are False–Positives (FP).

$$\text{Sensitivity} = \frac{\text{TP}}{(\text{TP} + \text{FN})}$$

	Coronary Disease Present	Coronary Disease Absent
Stress Test Normal	10	80
Stress Test Abnormal	90	20
Totals:	100	100

Sensitivity = $^{90}/_{100}$ = 90%
Specifity = $^{80}/_{100}$ = 80%

Figure 13–1.

			Totals
Stress Test Normal	10	80	90
Stress Test Abnormal	90	20	110
Totals:	100	100	

PV+ = $^{90}/_{110}$ = 82%
PV– = $^{80}/_{90}$ = 89%

Figure 13–2.

$$\text{Specificity} = \frac{\text{TN}}{(\text{TN} + \text{FP})}$$

$$\text{Positive Predictive Value} = \frac{\text{TP}}{(\text{TP} + \text{FP})}$$

$$\text{Negative Predictive Value} = \frac{\text{TN}}{(\text{TN} + \text{FN})}$$

Overall predictive accuracy is the number of patients in whom the correct (positive or negative) diagnosis is made. The following equation, where n is the total number of patients, defines predictive accuracy.

$$\text{Predictive Accuracy} = \frac{(\text{TP} + \text{TN})}{\text{n}}$$

More on Predictive Values

A further property of predictive values is that they vary depending on the population to which they are applied. This is not true of sensitivity and specificity, which are characteristics of the test itself (there are exceptions to this generalization). Because this concept is not always intuitive, some additional examples may help.

In the above example of the use of stress testing, we applied the test to a population with a 50% pretest probability of disease. Let's try it in two other populations frequently encountered in practice.

Chest pain may occur in young females, particularly under conditions of stress. Very few of these individuals have coronary atherosclerosis, although a few may have coronary ischemia due to familial hyperlipidemias, coronary spasm, or congenital coronary artery abnormalities. Overall, let us assume that 10% of 200 patients have coronary disease. What will stress testing tell us? (See Table 13–1.)

The population of 200 patients has now been constructed of 20 patients with and 180 patients without coronary disease. The same sensitivity and specificity values (90% and 80%) have been applied as before. However, look at what has happened to the predictive values: PV+ = 18/54 = 33%; PV− = 144/146 = 99%. In other words, our positive test raised the probability of disease from 10% to only 33%—not very certain. A negative test lowered the probability of disease from 10% to 1%—not very helpful. In this low-risk population, the chance of a positive test being false is higher than the chance of it being positive.

Consider another population consisting of 200 70-year-old hypertensive men with typical angina. By history alone, at least 80% of these men have coronary disease as the cause of their pain. What will stress testing tell us here? (See Table 13–2.)

The population of 200 patients has now been constructed of 160 patients with and 40 patients without coronary disease. The same sensitivity and specificity values (90% and 80%) have been applied as before. However, now look at what has happened to the predictive values: PV+ = 144/152 = 95%; PV− = 32/48 = 67%. In other words, our positive test raised the probability of disease from 80% to 95%—not very helpful. We already knew these men were likely to have disease. A negative test lowered the probability of disease from 80% to 67%—again, not very helpful in ruling out disease in this at-risk population. In these men, a negative test is more likely to be false than true.

These calculations illustrate two universal principles of the use of diagnostic tests.

1. The positive and negative predictive values of a test vary depending on the population to which the test is applied. This is usually not true of sensitivity and specificity, which are properties of the test itself.
2. When a test is imperfect (and all are), it has its greatest utility in patients with *intermediate pretest probabilities of disease.* In patients already known to have very high or very low probabilities of disease, the results of a further test may not influence our diagnostic estimate very much.

A third central principle of diagnostic testing is this: If the characteristics of a test are adjusted to increase sensitivity, specificity must decrease; if specificity is improved, sensitivity must decrease.

We can illustrate this trade-off by returning to the example of anemia given at the beginning of this chapter. Suppose we draw a line at 12.0 g/dL, defining "anemia" as any adult male with a hemoglobin level lower than this. Most healthy adult males have hemoglobin values higher than this; so almost all with hemoglobins lower than 12 will have some disease process causing it. The specificity of the test as defined is very high. However, a great many men with earlier stages of disease will not yet have fallen to the level of 12 g/dL; our criterion will miss the diagnosis of disease in all of them. The sensitivity of the test is low.

On the other hand, taking 14 g/dL as the lower limit of normal, suppose we set a hemoglobin of 13.9 as the limit for diagnosing disease. Now, we will catch most of the men

TABLE 13–1. Stress Testing in Low-Probability Populations

	Have Coronary Disease	No Coronary Disease	Total
Stress Test Normal	2	144	146
Stress Test Abnormal	18	36	54
Total	20	180	

TABLE 13–2. Stress Testing in High-Probability Populations

	Have Coronary Disease	No Coronary Disease	Total
Stress Test Normal	16	32	48
Stress Test Abnormal	144	8	152
Total	160	40	

who have disease (high sensitivity). However, by random variability many men without disease will also have "anemia" by this definition—low specificity. These characteristics of high sensitivity but low specificity are typical of tests used for screening, where it is important not to miss any cases, and when further testing can be done to separate the true from the false positives.

For further reading, a classic article by Diamond and Forrester (1979) may be consulted in which these principles are further developed, as applied to the diagnosis of coronary artery disease.

▶ DATA SYNTHESIS AND DIFFERENTIAL DIAGNOSIS

Having gathered data from all relevant sources and evaluated its precision and accuracy as the circumstances permit, it is time to put the data together and make a list of diagnostic possibilities, as we did earlier in the postoperative patient experiencing chest pain. Barbara Bates, in her textbook on physical examination and history taking (1991), includes an excellent chapter on clinical thinking. Her description of the differential diagnostic process includes the following suggested steps.

1. Identify the abnormal findings in the data base. (In our earlier example, the postoperative patient had chest pain and a recent abdominal surgical incision.)
2. Localize these findings anatomically. (Chest—heart, esophagus; abdomen—stomach, gallbladder, surgical repair area)

Interpret the findings in terms of possible disease states that could cause them, resulting in a list of diagnostic hypotheses. (Angina; esophageal reflux; ulcer disease; gallstones; postoperative pain; a leak from the aortic repair site)

Bates then goes on to suggest evaluating, refining, and sorting the list of hypotheses using other considerations, including:

1. Select the most specific and central findings that seem to fit together.
2. Match your findings against all the conditions that can produce them.
3. Eliminate the possibilities that fail to explain all the findings.
4. Select the most likely diagnosis, using information such as the patient's age, sex, habits, locality, and the timing of the illness.
5. Give special attention to diagnoses that are potentially life-threatening and treatable, even if they do not seem especially likely.

Be aware that the process can be made more difficult by the existence of multiple conditions; psychosocial considerations; and concerns about the quality of the data, as we have discussed at length above.

Differential diagnosis is another iterative process, because the practitioner is constantly forming hypotheses from the moment the patient is first encountered. As data are gathered, hypotheses are revisited, reevaluated, and resorted. Some are discarded, while new ones are added. The steps listed above continue to be useful, but it may be necessary to repeat them mentally many times. Even when a probable diagnosis is selected and treatment begun, one should keep an open mind about differential diagnosis. Perhaps the patient will not respond as was expected. This raises a new list of possibilities: wrong diagnosis; another confounding diagnosis; more advanced stage of disease than was expected; not enough (or too much) treatment; unexpected adverse reaction to treatment. The process always continues. This is one of the things that makes medical practice so interesting, although at times frustrating too.

▶ RISK/BENEFIT RATIOS

The phrase "evidence-based medicine" is gaining popularity. The phrase encapsulates the notion that medical actions should be based on studies that show effectiveness of treatments. Some have criticized the phrase because it implies that one should not act at all unless there is evidence to support the action. Of course, action is required in a situation where there is, as yet, no definitive evidence for or against a treatment option; an example is found in the proliferation of new technology for the treatment of coronary artery stenoses. Yet it seems self-evident that thoughtful consideration of everything that *is* known about a course of action should be a part of a medical therapeutic decision.

The meaning of this phrase can be broadened to further imply that the practitioner understands and can explain the potential positive effects (benefits) and the possible negative consequences (risks) that may result from a treatment plan. One way to crystallize this process is through consideration of the risk/benefit ratio. Every option carries potential benefit, which can be described in terms of the probability of cure. Each option also carries potential risks, the probabilities of which may be known from published literature. The recommendation we make to a patient represents our best estimate of which among many courses of action provides the greatest potential for benefit with the least potential for harm. When one of the options provides great probability of benefit at minimal risk, the choice is easy. When a series of options presents varying kinds of benefits at varying levels of risk, the choice can become more difficult. There is room for discussion. The patient's preferences can and should be part of the decision.

The calculation of risk/benefit ratios can be done mathematically based on published data and is used in a form of logical reasoning known as decision analysis. (See Goldman, 1994.) Such considerations are beyond the scope of this text. Nevertheless, the concept remains that varying risks and benefits need to be balanced when making therapeutic decisions.

MORE ON UNCERTAINTY

Kassirer (1989a) has analyzed the causes of excessive use of diagnostic tests. He attributes this phenomenon, which has contributed to the uncontrolled upward spiral of health-care costs in the recent past, to a familiar foe: uncertainty, and our discomfort with it. He goes on to list other contributing factors: pressure from peers and supervisors, the convenience with which tests may be ordered, the desires and demands of patients and families, "defensive" anticipation of potential lawsuits, and personal habits and whims.

Once an acceptable degree of certainty exists, the use of further testing provides little incremental value and merely adds to costs and risks. Worse, further tests may provide inconsistent results, leading to even more testing to resolve the disagreement.

Kassirer (1989b) has also analyzed and catalogued the ways that reasoning proceeds in the quest to reduce uncertainty. He lists three types of diagnostic reasoning: probabilistic, causal, and deterministic. Most of this chapter has described the workings of probabilistic reasoning. Causal reasoning draws on knowledge of pathophysiology: what causes chest pain? What is the differential diagnosis of hypokalemia? Deterministic reasoning makes use of "unambiguous rules" derived from previous knowledge. Clinical algorithms or "critical pathways" are examples of such reasoning processes, which also have produced computerized expert systems that attempt to replicate the process of diagnostic and therapeutic reasoning.

USING PROBABILITY IN PRACTICE

Once we realize that diagnostic possibilities are really probabilities, it is possible to place this information back into context in order to decide whether a further iteration, or refinement, is necessary. An 11% chance of a patient having a nonthreatening disease about which nothing needs to be done immediately (such as mild asthma) may be adequate reassurance. An 11% chance of an airline pilot having significant coronary disease is not adequate certainty, and catheterization would certainly be recommended.

Therapeutic options require greater diagnostic certainty to the extent that they are either marginally effective, dangerous, or have significant consequences. Prescribing an oral antibiotic for a child with a sore throat carries relatively little risk (although the risk is certainly not nil), and is based on a probability estimate that the sore throat may be due to streptococcal infection. There is no need for a high degree of diagnostic certainty. On the other hand, prescribing radical mastectomy for breast cancer demands great diagnostic certainty, as does recommending coronary bypass surgery for a patient with symptoms suggesting unstable angina. There are risks involved in such procedures, and even if no unexpected events occur, there will be long-term consequences for the patient.

Intuitively, providers and patients alike desire high degrees of certainty. The legal atmosphere in which medicine is practiced in the United States today seems to assume a degree of certainty in diagnostic and therapeutic decision making that is usually unrealistic. At the same time, the attempt to achieve certainty, if pushed beyond reasonable limits, leads to excessive costs and risks to patients. Kassirer (1989a) has discussed the search for certainty and its pitfalls in detail. When a reasonable degree of certainty has been achieved, this may become clearer when the next test is considered in the context of what has already been learned. If the abdominal ultrasound test shows gallstones, do we need a CT scan to further confirm the diagnosis (additional test safe, but unnecessary)? If a student with an aortic stenosis murmur has an echocardiogram showing a congenitally bicuspid valve, do we need a catheterization to confirm the diagnosis (additional test unnecessary, and carries additional risk)? Probably not; but a 65-year-old man with critical aortic stenosis might need catherization to rule out coexistent coronary disease that should be addressed at the time of surgery. In this case, the additional risk provides the potential for an additional benefit to the patient.

To return to our earlier example of a patient with angiographically documented coronary disease involving only branch vessels: the patient had three options. The least risky, in the short term, was medical therapy; of medium short-term risk was angioplasty; and the course associated with the highest short-term risk was coronary bypass surgery. Each of these options actually carries a complex series of possible risks and benefits, as summarized in Table 13–3.

TABLE 13–3. Risks and Benefits Associated with Treatment Options

Option	Benefits	Risks
Medical therapy: aspirin, beta blocker, lipid-reducing diet and drugs	Lowered risk of myocardial infarction	Continued risk of myocardial infarction; drug side effects; will continue to have some angina
Angioplasty: balloon, stents, etc.	At least partial relief of angina; requirement for less medication	Risk of MI from procedure (3–5%); risk of restenosis (20–40%); if all vessels cannot be treated, risk of continued angina; continued risk of MI
Coronary bypass surgery	Relief of angina, chance of complete revascularization	Risk of MI or stroke from procedure (4–8%); longer hospital stay and recovery time

This list is not complete, but gives a flavor of the range of risks and benefits that both the practitioner and the patient must consider. In this case, because the major coronary trunks were not involved and left ventricular function was normal, there was no evidence to suggest a survival benefit from bypass surgery. If these characteristics had been present, they would have tipped the balance towards surgery. The patient also did not have proximal single vessel disease, which would likely have led to a recommendation for angioplasty/stenting. The patient should therefore be advised to proceed with medical therapy, with the other two options as future possibilities in case symptoms were not controlled. This is the lowest risk short-term course, while future options are maximized. Of course, the patient may prefer to accept the risk of a procedure in the hope of better relief of symptoms, and the choice would ultimately be his.

REFERENCES

Bates, B. (1991). Clinical thinking: From data to plan. In B. Bates, *A Guide to Physical Examination and History Taking* (5th ed.), pp. 637–650. Philadelphia: J. B. Lippincott Co.

Carleton, R. A. (1997). Dichotomous disservice? *Annals of Internal Medicine, 126,* 589–591.

Diamond, G. & Forrester, J. S. (1979). Analysis of probability as an aid in the clinical diagnosis of coronary artery disease. *New England Journal of Medicine, 300,* 1350–1358.

Goldman, L. (1994). Quantitative aspects of clinical reasoning. In K. J. Isselbacher, E. Braunwald, J. D. Wilson, J. B. Martin, A. S. Fauci, & D. L. Kasper (eds.), *Harrison's Principles of Internal Medicine* (13th ed.), pp. 43–48. New York: McGraw-Hill.

Kassirer, J. P. (1989a). Diagnostic reasoning. *Annals of Internal Medicine, 110,* 893–900.

Kassirer, J. P. (1989b). Our stubborn quest for diagnostic certainty: A cause of excessive testing. *New England Journal of Medicine, 320,* 1489–1491.

14

Communication and Documentation

Paul Logan

ORGANIZATION AND CLARITY OF WRITING

Organization and clarity are essential when writing in the medical record. The medical record is the source of all patient information and is used by other clinicians, institutional reviewers, payers, and courts to determine what assessments were made, what treatments were instituted, and what results were achieved.

Every ACNP has once read a note in the medical record and been unable to understand what the author was trying to communicate. Ambiguous or poorly written notes can endanger the health of the patient. Additionally, the importance of legible handwriting goes without saying.

The organization of a note in the medical record is, perhaps, as important as the contents of the note. Nurses, physicians, consultants, social workers, case managers, and other clinicians rely on the medical record to facilitate the patient's care. We are all asked to "do more with less" in the current health-care delivery environment. It only makes sense to be organized and concise when documenting in the medical record.

Many clinicians abbreviate their notes extensively, using frequent abbreviations and phrases rather than complete sentences. Although neither is necessarily incorrect, I prefer to write notes in narrative form, foregoing the temptation to write terse, abbreviated notes. A note can be both concise and well-written.

One feature of concise, well-written notes is omission of the word "patient." There are very few instances in which the reader is uncertain to whom you are referring. Consider, for example, this note.

> Patient states, "I'm sick of being in the hospital." Patient informed of need for continued treatment. Patient understands and consents to continued treatment. Patient also displeased about the quality of the food.

There is no need to use the word "patient" at all. Equally as detailed and informative is:

> "I'm sick of being in the hospital." Discussed, at length, the need for continued treatment. He is willing to stay, but requests that his wife bring food from home.

Not only is it less redundant and clearer, it is also more concise. The patient's own words are indicated by the quotation marks, eliminating the need to use the word "patient." Also, the contents of the interaction are condensed, while not adversely affecting the objectivity.

THE MEDICAL RECORD

The History and Physical

The comprehensive history and physical examination (H&P) is generally written on a standard H&P form, though in some institutions it is dictated and later placed in the chart. Regardless of the documentation method, the components of the H&P are the same. The typical outline of the H&P is shown in Table 14–1.

The history of present illness (HPI) is a critical component of the H&P. Time and again, one of my mentors stressed that "no patient is ever admitted to the CCU because of their EKG. It's their story (e.g., HPI) that gets them a bed in the unit." Among other things, this means that the very sickest patients in the hospital—those at greatest risk of dying from an MI—are not identified by elaborate laboratory or diagnostic tests. Rather, a detailed history of present illness—their "story"—is the best screening tool in a clinician's arsenal.

Since the HPI is a story, it should be written like a story. It should have an introduction, a climax, and a resolution. It should also cover the essential components described in Chapter 12 and listed in Table 14–1. Figure 14–1 is a sample HPI.

TABLE 14–1. Outline of the History and Physical

Chief complaint (generally quoted in patient's own words)
History of present illness
- Onset
- Duration
- Timing
- Location
- Characteristics
- Associated symptoms
- Aggravating/relieving factors
- Treatment

Past medical history
- Illnesses (childhood/adult)
- Surgery
- Hospitalizations
- Immunizations
- Medications
- Allergies

Social History
- Occupation
- Family relationships
- Tobacco/alcohol/drug use
- Diet
- Exercise
- Sleep pattern
- Recreational activities

Family history
Review of systems
- General symptoms
- Skin
- Head
- Eyes
- Ears
- Nose/sinuses
- Mouth/Throat/Neck
- Breasts
- Cardiac

Progress Notes

The findings of the interim or focused examination can be documented in the progress notes. Typically, the progress note is written in the "SOAP" format: **S**ubjective data, **O**bjective data, **A**ssessment, and **P**lan. If well-written, there is no need to label the subjective data with an "S," for example—it will be clear to the reader whether the data is objective or subjective.

The subjective data are those that the patient describes. Often, direct quotes are used to indicate the patient's mood and current health status. Narrative form is used to describe symptoms and other subjective data. Figure 14–2 is an example of a progress note in SOAP format.

The objective data are those that are observed by the examiner and include the physical examination and laboratory and diagnostic tests. It is unnecessary (and awkward) to write the objective data in narrative form, though when dictated narrative format may save space and improve the flow.

The assessment (e.g., impressions) and plan should ideally be separated, particularly when first learning to write concise and accurate notes. With practice, however, the two components can be combined. Doing so makes the note less repetitious and can improve the clarity (refer to Figure 14–2).

It is important to remember that for each impression, there should be a plan. If combining the impressions and plan, be certain to clearly indicate each. The plan may be as simple as consulting a specialist or as elaborate as listing the entire plan for hospitalization.

Consults

It is usually sufficient to use the SOAP format to document consults. Included in the document, then, are the subjective

> Mr. Glenny is a 52-year-old white man with DM and HTN. He was in his usual state of health until 1 week ago when he began having left-sided chest discomfort while gardening. The discomfort recurred with exertion several times over the past week. This morning he awoke with similar retrosternal "pressure" that was accompanied by diaphoresis and nausea, and radiated to the left arm. He took an antacid without relief and now presents to the ED with continuing "6/10" discomfort.

Figure 14–1. History of present illness in narrative format.

"I feel much better today. I can finally breathe." Slept soundly for 6 hours with head of bed flat. No PND, orthopnea, dyspnea, or chest pain.
Exam: BP 96/68 T-P-R 98.8-60-16
Skin. IV site free of erythema and swelling.
Neck. No JVD. Carotids 2+ without bruits.
Chest. Lungs clear to auscultation and percussion.
Cardiac. PMI laterally displaced. No murmurs or rub. Soft S3.
Abdomen. Bowel sounds positive. Soft and nontender, nondistended.
Extremities. Warm, 1+ pitting pretibial edema.
Labs/Diagnostics:
Chem-7 pending.
Echo (preliminary)—Severely reduced LV systolic function, moderate MR, RVSP 35 mm Hg. No AS or AI.
Impression/Plan:
1. CHF. Symptoms improving. Continue IV diuresis. Monitor weight. Await chem-7. Replace K+ as needed.
2. Discharge plan. Begin PO diuretic tomorrow. If stable on PO medications, D/C the following day. Coordinate D/C with family and social worker. Will need home care follow-up for heart failure teaching.

Figure 14–2. "SOAP" Note documenting an interim examination of a patient hospitalized for congestive heart failure.

and objective findings. Generally, consultants do not direct care. Rather, they make recommendations to the team primarily caring for the patient. It is generally best for consultants to use the term "recommendation," rather than "plan." Figure 14–3 is an example of a consult for preoperative evaluation.

Discharge Summaries

The discharge summary summarizes the events of the patient's hospitalization. Typically, if the patient is discharged in 48 hours, the discharge instruction sheet suffices for the discharge summary. If the patient is hospitalized longer than 48 hours, or if his or her hospitalization has been complicated, a dictated summary of the hospitalization is generally required. Every institution has specific guidelines for discharge summaries.

The discharge summary, too, should be written in narrative form. A typical outline is shown in Table 14–2.

▶ ORDERS

The privilege of writing orders at an institution is protected by the medical staff bylaws or other policies of the institution. In the past, this privilege was granted only to physicians. Because of recent changes in the health-care delivery system, other health professionals such as podiatrists, psy-

Mr. D'Arcangelo is a 78-year-old white man with a history of previous MI. He was well until this morning when he tripped and fell. There was no syncope—"I was just a klutz." He complained of left hip pain and was brought to the hospital. Shortening of the left leg and external rotation were noted on physical examination. X-ray revealed a left intertrochanteric femoral fracture and he is now for ORIF.
PMH: inferior MI 1989, dyslipidemia, GERD, appendectomy age 14.
Meds: Aspirin 325 mg daily, metoprolol 50 mg BID, simvistatin 40 mg daily HS.
Allergies: NKDA
Social History: Married, lives with wife in 2-story home. Has three grown children and 7 grandchildren, all of whom live locally. Quit smoking 25 years ago, 50 pack-year history previously. Has 1 glass red wine with dinner each evening. Plays golf 3 days/wk.
R.O.S.: No chest pain, dyspnea, PND, orthopnea, palpitations, dizziness, light-headedness, or syncope.
Physical Exam: BP 120/80 T-98.4 HR-60 RR-18
HEENT. PERRL. EOMI.
Neck. No JVD. Carotids 2+ without bruits.
Chest. Lungs clear to auscultation and percussion.
Cardiac. RRR. PMI 5th ICS/MCL, diffuse and sustained. S4. II/VI mid-peaking-SEM, preserved S2. No S3.
Abdomen. + BS, no bruits. Soft and nontender, nondistended. No palpable masses.
Extremities. Warm, no edema. DPs and PTs 2+.
Neuro. AAO. Speech clear, thought coherent. Strength 5/5 throughout, tactile sensation intact throughout. DTRs 2+ throughout.
Laboratory and Diagnostic Tests: EKG—SR at 60/min, LVH with repolarization abnormalities, inferior MI of undetermined age. Sodium 142, potassium 4.1, chloride 103, CO2 27, BUN 48, creatinine 1.6, glucose 110. WBC 6.7, Hb 14.7, Hct 44.1, plts 230,000. PT 12.3, PTT 33. Stress echo (last month)—exercised 7:30 on the Bruce protocol, achieved 85% predicted max HR, had no chest pain or dyspnea, and stopped for fatigue. Echo showed fixed inferior akinesis, no EKG or echocardiographic evidence of ischemia.
Impressions/Recommendations: CAD, previous MI. Asymptomatic, recent negative stress-echo. No cardiac contraindications to proposed surgery. Should remain on metoprolol—may use IV if necessary, otherwise resume PO when eating/drinking. Also, resume ASA when OK with surgery. Will follow with you.

Figure 14–3. Preoperative evaluation consult.

TABLE 14–2. Components of the Discharge Summary

Patient name and medical record number
Attending physician
Admission and discharge dates
Admission diagnosis
Discharge diagnoses
Procedures/operations
Consultants
Hospital course
  Chief complaint
  History of present illness
  Past medical history
  Admission medications
  Physical examination
  Laboratory and diagnostic tests
  Clinical course (summary of hospitalization events)
Discharge medications
Discharge instructions
Follow-up
Disposition

chologists, and physician assistants have been credentialed to write orders. The newest category of provider to be granted order-writing privileges is the ACNP. As with anything new, there can be varying degrees of resistance from patients, physicians, staff nurses, administrators, and other health-care providers. ACNPs who are credentialed to write orders must, therefore, be particularly cognizant of the rules of the institution.

The delineation of privileges and clinical practice guidelines are the framework that guide the ACNP when writing orders (see Chapter 4, Licensure, Certification, and Institutional Credentialing). These documents can be referenced by staff nurses and other health professionals to verify the privileges of the ACNP writing orders. Ideally, there should be a central location that health professionals can access these documents, whether on each nursing unit or in the medical staff office. In reality, once a trusting relationship has been established with the staff the documents may be a mere formality.

Admission Orders

After the history and physical have been performed, the plan is instituted by writing orders in the patient chart. Table 14–3 lists the essential components of the admission orders.

Daily Orders

Following the patient assessment each day, the previous orders should be reviewed and adjustments made as warranted. Many institutions have rules that require orders for certain medications or treatments to be renewed regularly. Restraint orders, for instance, may need to be renewed every 24 hours, or antibiotics may need to be renewed every three days. It is important that the ACNP know the rules of the institution to avoid inadvertent discontinuation of necessary treatments and medications.

TABLE 14–3. Admission Orders

1. Admitting provider (e.g., physician, ACNP)
2. Floor/unit
3. Diagnosis
4. Condition (e.g., guarded, critical, stable)
5. Vital sign frequency
6. Diet
7. Activity level
8. Allergies
9. Nursing (e.g., daily weights, I&O, cardiac monitor, dressings, etc.)
10. IVs
11. Medications
12. Laboratory and diagnostic tests
13. Consults

Prescriptions

The laws and rules and regulations in each state regulate the way in which nurse practitioners must write prescriptions. So, it is important that ACNPs know the law of the state in which they practice.

All prescriptions require the date, patient's name, and the provider's phone number, license number, and signature. Ideally, the patient's address should also be included.

The prescription is traditionally written in Latin (Table 14–4). The medication, strength, quantity, administration instructions, and number of refills must all be written. In many states, unless the words "brand medically necessary" are written, the pharmacist may substitute the generic equivalent of the drug. Figure 14–4 shows a completed prescription.

When writing for controlled substances, many clinicians prefer to use few abbreviations. Abbreviations and numerals can easily be altered by unscrupulous patients. If numerals are written—especially the quantity to be dispensed and the number of refills—the numeral should be written out. A prescription for lorazapam, 30 tablets should be written as "lorazapam 1 mg, # 30 (thirty)."

Alleviating Errors

The importance of legible handwriting is paramount. There is, perhaps, no other instance in which legible handwriting is as important as when writing orders or prescriptions. Particularly in hospitals where copies of original order sheets or faxed order sheets are used by the pharmacy to dispense medications, legible handwriting is critically important. Even the best handwriting, however, may not prevent some medication errors. Table 14–5 shows additional precautions recommended by The Institute for Safe Medication Practices (www.ismp.org) to prevent medication errors.

TABLE 14–4. Terminology and Abbreviations Commonly Used in Prescriptions

Latin/Abbreviation	Translation
Sig	Take
PO	By mouth
PR	By rectum
$\bar{c}$	With
$\bar{s}$	Without
$\bar{a}$	Before
$\bar{p}$	After
q	Every
°	Hour/s
′	Minute/s
prn	As needed
OD or QD	Daily
BID	Twice daily
TID	Three times daily
QID	Four times daily
AC	Before meals
HS	At bedtime
PC	After meals

▶ MEDICARE DOCUMENTATION GUIDELINES

The Health Care Financing Administration (HCFA) recently released documentation guidelines that were to be effective July 1, 1998. These guidelines require that specific documentation guidelines be followed. The guidelines were to apply to all providers who bill Medicare for evaluation and management (E/M) services. Failure to follow the guidelines would result in fines up to three times the reimbursement amount, plus up to a $10,000 fine for each occurrence, plus exclusion from Medicare and other federal health-care programs (Sarraille, W. A., 1998). As of January 1999 implementation of the rules has been postponed indefinitely.

Table 14–6 lists the HCFA general principles of medical record documentation. The components of the list are common-sense to most ACNPs. Nevertheless, failure to abide by them may lead to serious consequences if the rules are implemented.

The proposed rules also require that the encounter level meet certain minimum documentation requirements. An outpatient visit for hypertensive medication adjustment, for instance, is billed at level two. The HCFA regulations require that an "expanded problem-focused" examination (Table 14–7) be documented. The required components of the examination, then, are found in the table that corresponds to the appropriate body system (Tables 14–8 to 14–17, each of which is available at *www.hcfa.gov/medicare/mcarpti.htm* under "Documentation Guidelines for Evaluation and Management Services").

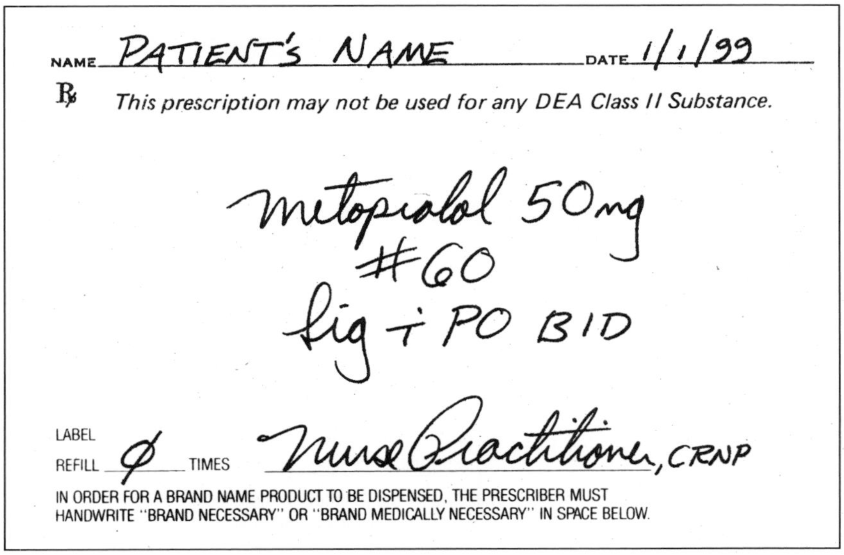

NAME PATIENT'S NAME DATE 1/1/99

℞ *This prescription may not be used for any DEA Class II Substance.*

metoprolol 50 mg
#60
Sig $\bar{i}$ PO BID

LABEL
REFILL ∅ TIMES Nurse Practitioner, CRNP

IN ORDER FOR A BRAND NAME PRODUCT TO BE DISPENSED, THE PRESCRIBER MUST HANDWRITE "BRAND NECESSARY" OR "BRAND MEDICALLY NECESSARY" IN SPACE BELOW.

Figure 14–4. Example of completed prescription.

TABLE 14–5. Methods for Reducing Medication Errors

Example	Improvement	Explanation
Sig one PO Q.D.	Sig one PO daily	Handwritten "Q.D." can be mistaken for "QID"
Ativan 1.0 mg	Ativan 1 mg	The decimal point is unnecessary. The dosage can be misread as a ten-fold overdose.
Midazolam .5 mg	Midazolam 0.5 mg	If the dose is less than 1, a zero should precede the decimal point. A ten-fold overdose could result if the decimal point is not seen.
Epinephrine 0.3 mL	Epinephrine 0.3 mg	The concentration of epinephrine is not indicated in the example. A ten-fold overdose could result if the patient is given 0.3 mL of epinephrine 1:1,000 versus 0.3 mL of 1:10,000 solution.
Regular insulin 10U	Regular insulin 10 units	Regular insulin "10U" could be misread as "100." Always write out the word "units."

Adapted from the Institution for Safe Medication Practices (www.ismp.org).

TABLE 14–6. General Principles of Medical Record Documentation

1. The medical record should be complete and legible.
2. The documentation of each patient encounter should include:
   reason for the encounter and relevant history, physical examination findings, and prior diagnostic test results
   assessment, clinical impression, or diagnosis
   plan for care
   date and legible identity of the observer.
3. If not documented, the rationale for ordering diagnostic and other ancillary services should be easily inferred.
4. Past and present diagnoses should be accessible to the treating and/or consulting physician.
5. Appropriate health-risk factors should be identified.
6. The patient's progress, response to and changes in treatment, and revision of diagnosis should be documented.
7. The CPT and ICD-9-CM codes reported on the health insurance claim form or billing statement should be supported by the documentation in the medical record.

TABLE 14–7. Levels of Examination

Encounter Level	Examination Level	Explanation
1	Problem focused	A limited examination of the affected body area or organ system.
2	Expanded problem focused	A limited examination of the affected body area or organ system and any other symptomatic or related body area(s) or organ system(s).
3	Detailed	An extended examination of the affected body area(s) or organ system(s) and any other symptomatic or related body area(s) or organ system(s).
4	Comprehensive	A general multisystem examination, or complete examination of a single organ system and other symptomatic or related body area(s) or organ system(s).

TABLE 14–8. General Multisystem Examination

System/Body Area	Elements of Examination
Constitutional	• Measurement of **any three of the following seven** vital signs: (1) sitting or standing blood pressure; (2) supine blood pressure; (3) pulse rate and regularity; (4) respiration; (5) temperature; (6) height; (7) weight (May be measured and recorded by ancillary staff) • General appearance of patient (e.g., development, nutrition, body habitus, deformities, attention to grooming)
Eyes	• Inspection of conjunctivae and lids • Examination of pupils and irises (e.g., reaction to light and accommodation, size, and symmetry) • Ophthalmoscopic examination of optic discs (e.g., size, C/D ratio, appearance) and posterior segments (e.g., vessel changes, exudates, hemorrhages)
Ears, nose, mouth, and throat	• External inspection of ears and nose (e.g., overall appearance, scars, lesions, masses) • Otoscopic examination of external auditory canals and tympanic membranes • Assessment of hearing (e.g., whispered voice, finger rub, tuning fork) • Inspection of nasal mucosa, septum, and turbinates • Inspection of lips, teeth, and gums • Examination of oropharynx: oral mucosa, salivary glands, hard and soft palates, tongue, tonsils, and posterior pharynx
Neck	• Examination of neck (e.g., masses, overall appearance, symmetry, tracheal position, crepitus) • Examination of thyroid (e.g., enlargement, tenderness, mass)
Respiratory	• Assessment of respiratory effort (e.g., intercostal retractions, use of accessory muscles, diaphragmatic movement) • Percussion of chest (e.g., dullness, flatness, hyperresonance) • Palpation of chest (e.g., tactile fremitus) • Auscultation of lungs (e.g., breath sounds, adventitious sounds, rubs)
Cardiovascular	• Palpation of heart (e.g., location, size, thrills) • Auscultation of heart with notation of abnormal sounds and murmurs Examination of: • carotid arteries (e.g., pulse amplitude, bruits) • abdominal aorta (e.g., size, bruits) • femoral arteries (e.g., pulse amplitude, bruits) • pedal pulses (e.g., pulse amplitude) • extremities for edema and/or varicosities
Chest (breasts)	• Inspection of breasts (e.g., symmetry, nipple discharge) • Palpation of breasts and axillae (e.g., masses or lumps, tenderness)
Gastrointestinal (abdomen)	• Examination of abdomen with notation of presence of masses or tenderness • Examination of liver and spleen • Examination for presence or absence of hernia • Examination (when indicated) of anus, perineum, and rectum, including sphincter tone, presence of hemorrhoids, rectal masses • Obtain stool sample for occult blood test when indicated
Genitourinary	
Male	• Examination of the scrotal contents (e.g., hydrocele, spermatocele, tenderness of cord, testicular mass) • Examination of the penis • Digital rectal examination of prostate gland (e.g., size, symmetry, nodularity, tenderness)
Female	Pelvic examination (with or without specimen collection for smears and cultures), including • Examination of external genitalia (e.g., general appearance, hair distribution, lesions) and vagina (e.g., general appearance, estrogen effect, discharge, lesions, pelvic support, cystocele, rectocele) • Examination of urethra (e.g., masses, tenderness, scarring) • Examination of bladder (e.g., fullness, masses, tenderness) • Cervix (e.g., general appearance, lesions, discharge) • Uterus (e.g., size, contour, position, mobility, tenderness, consistency, descent, or support) • Adnexa/parametria (e.g., masses, tenderness, organomegaly, nodularity)
Lymphatic	Palpation of lymph nodes in **two or more** areas • Neck • Axillae • Groin • Other

(Continued)

TABLE 14–8. General Multisystem Examination *(Continued)*

System/Body Area	Elements of Examination
Musculoskeletal	• Examination of gait and station • Inspection and/or palpation of digits and nails (e.g., clubbing, cyanosis, inflammatory conditions, petechiae, ischemia, infections, nodes) Examination of joints, bones and muscles of **one or more of the following six** areas: (1) head and neck; (2) spine, ribs, and pelvis; (3) right upper extremity; (4) left upper extremity; (5) right lower extremity; and (6) left lower extremity. The examination of a given area includes • Inspection and/or palpation with notation of presence of any misalignment, asymmetry, crepitation, defects, tenderness, masses, effusions • Assessment of range of motion with notation of any pain, crepitation, or contracture • Assessment of stability with notation of any dislocation (luxation), subluxation, or laxity • Assessment of muscle strength and tone (e.g., flaccid, cog wheel, spastic) with notation of any atrophy or abnormal movements
Skin	• Inspection of skin and subcutaneous tissue (e.g., rashes, lesions, ulcers) • Palpation of skin and subcutaneous tissue (e.g., induration, subcutaneous nodules, tightening)
Neurologic	• Test cranial nerves with notation of any deficits • Examination of deep tendon reflexes with notation of pathological reflexes (e.g., Babinski) • Examination of sensation (e.g., by touch, pin, vibration, proprioception)
Psychiatric	• Description of patient's judgment and insight Brief assessment of mental status including • orientation to time, place, and person • recent and remote memory • mood and affect (e.g., depression, anxiety, agitation)

Content and Documentation Requirements

General Multisystem Examination

Content and Documentation Requirements for General Multisystem Examination

Level of Exam	Perform and Document
Problem Focused	**One to five** elements identified by a bullet.
Expanded Problem Focused	**At least six** elements identified by a bullet.
Detailed	**At least two** elements identified by a bullet **from each of six areas/systems** OR **at least twelve** elements identified by a bullet **in two or more areas/systems.**
Comprehensive	Perform **all elements** identified by a bullet in **at least nine** organ systems or body areas and document **at least two** elements identified by a bullet **from each of nine areas/systems.**

TABLE 14–9. Cardiovascular Examination

System/Body Area	Elements of Examination
Constitutional	• Measurement of **any three of the following seven** vital signs: (1) sitting or standing blood pressure; (2) supine blood pressure; (3) pulse rate and regularity; (4) respiration; (5) temperature; (6) height; (7) weight (May be measured and recorded by ancillary staff) • General appearance of patient (e.g., development, nutrition, body habitus, deformities, attention to grooming)
Head and Face	
Eyes	• Inspection of conjunctivae and lids (e.g., xanthelasma)
Ears, Nose, Mouth, and Throat	• Inspection of teeth, gums, and palate • Inspection of oral mucosa with notation of presence of pallor or cyanosis
Neck	• Examination of jugular veins (e.g., distension; a, v, or cannon a waves) • Examination of thyroid (e.g., enlargement, tenderness, mass)
Respiratory	• Assessment of respiratory effort (e.g., intercostal retractions, use of accessory muscles, diaphragmatic movement) • Auscultation of lungs (e.g., breath sounds, adventitious sounds, rubs)
Cardiovascular	• Palpation of heart (e.g., location, size, and forcefulness of the point of maximal impact; thrills; lifts; palpable S3 or S4) • Auscultation of heart including sounds, abnormal sounds, and murmurs • Measurement of blood pressure in two or more extremities when indicated (e.g., aortic dissection, coarctation) Examination of: • Carotid arteries (e.g., waveform, pulse amplitude, bruits, apical–carotid delay) • Abdominal aorta (e.g., size, bruits) • Femoral arteries (e.g., pulse amplitude, bruits) • Pedal pulses (e.g., pulse amplitude) • Extremities for peripheral edema and/or varicosities
Chest (Breasts)	
Gastrointestinal (Abdomen)	• Examination of abdomen with notation of presence of masses or tenderness • Examination of liver and spleen • Obtain stool sample for occult blood from patients who are being considered for thrombolytic or anticoagulant therapy
Genitourinary (Abdomen)	
Lymphatic	
Musculoskeletal	• Examination of the back with notation of kyphosis or scoliosis • Examination of gait with notation of ability to undergo exercise testing and/or participation in exercise programs • Assessment of muscle strength and tone (e.g., flaccid, cog wheel, spastic) with notation of any atrophy and abnormal movements
Extremities	• Inspection and palpation of digits and nails (e.g., clubbing, cyanosis, inflammation, petechiae, ischemia, infections, Osler's nodes)
Skin	• Inspection and/or palpation of skin and subcutaneous tissue (e.g., stasis dermatitis, ulcers, scars, xanthomas)
Neurological/ Psychiatric	Brief assessment of mental status including • Orientation to time, place, and person • Mood and affect (e.g., depression, anxiety, agitation)

Cardiovascular Examination

Content and Documentation Requirements for Cardiovascular Examination

Level of Exam	Perform and Document
Problem Focused	**One to five** elements identified by a bullet.
Expanded Problem Focused	**At least six** elements identified by a bullet.
Detailed	**At least twelve** elements identified by a bullet.
Comprehensive	Perform **all** elements identified by a bullet; document every element in each screened area and at least one element in each unscreened area.

TABLE 14–10. Ear, Nose, and Throat Examination

System/Body Area	Elements of Examination
Constitutional	• Measurement of **any three of the following seven** vital signs: (1) sitting or standing blood pressure; (2) supine blood pressure; (3) pulse rate and regularity; (4) respiration; (5) temperature; (6) height; (7) weight (May be measured and recorded by ancillary staff) • General appearance of patient (e.g., development, nutrition, body habitus, deformities, attention to grooming) • Assessment of ability to communicate (e.g., use of sign language or other communication aids) and quality of voice
Head and Face	• Inspection of head and face (e.g., overall appearance, scars, lesions, and masses) • Palpation and/or percussion of face with notation of presence or absence of sinus tenderness • Examination of salivary glands • Assessment of facial strength
Eyes	• Test ocular motility including primary gaze alignment
Ears, Nose, Mouth, and Throat	• Otoscopic examination of external auditory canals and tympanic membranes including pneumo-otoscopy with notation of mobility of membranes • Assessment of hearing with tuning forks and clinical speech reception thresholds (e.g., whispered voice, finger rub) • External inspection of ears and nose (e.g., overall appearance, scars, lesions, and masses) • Inspection of nasal mucosa, septum, and turbinates • Inspection of lips, teeth, and gums • Examination of oropharynx: oral mucosa, hard and soft palates, tongue, tonsils, and posterior pharynx (e.g., asymmetry, lesions, hydration of mucosal surfaces) • Inspection of pharyngeal walls and pyriform sinuses (e.g., pooling of saliva, asymmetry, lesions) • Examination by mirror of larynx including the condition of the epiglottis, false vocal cords, true vocal cords, and mobility of larynx (Use of mirror not required in children) • Examination by mirror of nasopharynx including appearance of the mucosa, adenoids, posterior choanae, and eustachian tubes (Use of mirror not required in children)
Neck	• Examination of neck (e.g., masses, overall appearance, symmetry, tracheal position, crepitus) • Examination of thyroid (e.g., enlargement, tenderness, mass)
Respiratory	• Inspection of chest including symmetry, expansion, and/or assessment of respiratory effort (e.g., intercostal retractions, use of accessory muscles, diaphragmatic movement) • Auscultation of lungs (e.g., breath sounds, adventitious sounds, rubs)
Cardiovascular	• Auscultation of heart with notation of abnormal sounds and murmurs • Examination of peripheral vascular system by observation (e.g., swelling, varicosities) and palpation (e.g., pulses, temperature, edema, tenderness)
Chest (Breasts)	
Gastrointestinal (Abdomen)	
Genitourinary	
Lymphatic	• Palpation of lymph nodes in neck, axillae, groin and/or other location
Musculoskeletal	
Extremities	
Skin	
Neurological/ Psychiatric	• Test cranial nerves with notation of any deficits Brief assessment of mental status including • Orientation to time, place, and person • Mood and affect (e.g., depression, anxiety, agitation)

Ear, Nose, and Throat Examination

Content and Documentation Requirements for Ear, Nose, and Throat Examination

Level of Exam	Perform and Document
Problem Focused	**One to five** elements identified by a bullet.
Expanded Problem Focused	**At least six** elements identified by a bullet.
Detailed	**At least twelve** elements identified by a bullet.
Comprehensive	Perform **all** elements identified by a bullet; document every element in each screened area and at least one element in each unscreened area.

TABLE 14–11. Eye Examination

System/Body Area	Elements of Examination
Constitutional	
Head and Face	
Eyes	• Test visual acuity (Does not include determination of refractive error) • Gross visual field testing by confrontation • Test ocular motility including primary gaze alignment • Inspection of bulbar and palpebral conjunctivae • Examination of ocular adnexae including lids (e.g., ptosis or lagophthalmos), lacrimal glands, lacrimal drainage, orbits, and preauricular lymph nodes • Examination of pupils and irises including shape, direct, and consensual reaction (afferent pupil), size (e.g., anisocoria), and morphology • Slit lamp examination of the corneas including epithelium, stroma, endothelium, and tear film • Slit lamp examination of the anterior chambers including depth, cells, and flare • Slit lamp examination of the lenses including clarity, anterior and posterior capsule, cortex, and nucleus • Measurement of intraocular pressures (except in children and patients with trauma or infectious disease) Ophthalmoscopic examination through dilated pupils (unless contraindicated) of • Optic discs including size, C/D ratio, appearance (e.g., atrophy, cupping, tumor elevation), and nerve fiber layer • Posterior segments including retina and vessels (e.g., exudates and hemorrhages)
Ears, Nose, Mouth and Throat	
Neck	
Respiratory	
Cardiovascular	
Chest (Breasts)	
Gastrointestinal (Abdomen)	
Genitourinary	
Lymphatic	
Musculoskeletal	
Extremities	
Skin	
Neurological/ Psychiatric	Brief assessment of mental status including • Orientation to time, place, and person • Mood and affect (e.g., depression, anxiety, agitation)

Eye Examination

Content and Documentation Requirements for Eye Examination

Level of Exam	Perform and Document
Problem Focused	**One to five** elements identified by a bullet.
Expanded Problem Focused	**At least six** elements identified by a bullet.
Detailed	**At least nine** elements identified by a bullet.
Comprehensive	Perform **all** elements identified by a bullet; document every element in each screened area and at least one element in each unscreened area.

TABLE 14–12. Genitourinary Examination

System/Body Area	Elements of Examination
Constitutional	• Measurement of **any three of the following seven** vital signs: (1) sitting or standing blood pressure; (2) supine blood pressure; (3) pulse rate and regularity; (4) respiration; (5) temperature; (6) height; (7) weight (May be measured and recorded by ancillary staff) • General appearance of patient (e.g., development, nutrition, body habitus, deformities, attention to grooming)
Head and Face	
Eyes	
Ears, Nose, Mouth, and Throat	
Neck	• Examination of neck (e.g., masses, overall appearance, symmetry, tracheal position, crepitus) • Examination of thyroid (e.g., enlargement, tenderness, mass)
Respiratory	• Assessment of respiratory effort (e.g., intercostal retractions, use of accessory muscles, diaphragmatic movement) • Auscultation of lungs (e.g., breath sounds, adventitious sounds, rubs)
Cardiovascular	• Auscultation of heart with notation of abnormal sounds and murmurs • Examination of peripheral vascular system by observation (e.g., swelling, varicosities) and palpation (e.g., pulses, temperature, edema, tenderness)
Chest (Breasts)	[See Genitourinary (Female)]
Gastrointestinal (Abdomen)	• Examination of abdomen with notation of presence of masses or tenderness • Examination for presence or absence of hernia • Examination of liver and spleen • Obtain stool sample for occult blood test when indicated
Genitourinary **Male**	• Inspection of anus and perineum Examination (with or without specimen collection for smears and cultures) of genitalia including: • Scrotum (e.g., lesions, cysts, rashes) • Epididymides (e.g., size, symmetry, masses) • Testes (e.g., size, symmetry, masses) • Urethral meatus (e.g., size, location, lesions, discharge) • Penis (e.g., lesions, presence or absence of foreskin, foreskin retractability, plaque, masses, scarring, deformities) Digital rectal examination including: • Prostate gland (e.g., size, symmetry, nodularity, tenderness) • Seminal vesicles (e.g., symmetry, tenderness, masses, enlargement) • Sphincter tone, presence of hemorrhoids, rectal masses
Genitourinary **Female**	Includes **at least seven of the following eleven** elements identified by bullets: • Inspection and palpation of breasts (e.g., masses or lumps, tenderness, symmetry, nipple discharge) • Digital rectal examination including sphincter tone, presence of hemorrhoids, rectal masses Pelvic examination (with or without specimen collection for smears and cultures) including: • External genitalia (e.g., general appearance, hair distribution, lesions) • Urethral meatus (e.g., size, location, lesions, prolapse) • Urethra (e.g., masses, tenderness, scarring) • Bladder (e.g., fullness, masses, tenderness) • Vagina (e.g., general appearance, estrogen effect, discharge, lesions, pelvic support, cystocele, rectocele) • Cervix (e.g., general appearance, lesions, discharge) • Uterus (e.g., size, contour, position, mobility, tenderness, consistency, descent, or support) • Adnexa/parametria (e.g., masses, tenderness, organomegaly, nodularity) • Anus and perineum
Lymphatic	• Palpation of lymph nodes in neck, axillae, groin, and/or other location
Musculoskeletal	
Extremities	
Skin	• Inspection and/or palpation of skin and subcutaneous tissue (e.g., rashes, lesions, ulcers)
Neurological/ Psychiatric	Brief assessment of mental status including • Orientation (e.g., time, place, and person) • Mood and affect (e.g., depression, anxiety, agitation)

Genitourinary Examination

Content and Documentation Requirements for Genitourinary Examination

Level of Exam	Perform and Document
Problem Focused	**One to five** elements identified by a bullet.
Expanded Problem Focused	**At least six** elements identified by a bullet.
Detailed	**At least twelve** elements identified by a bullet.
Comprehensive	Perform **all** elements identified by a bullet; document every element in each screened area and at least one element in each unscreened area.

TABLE 14–13. Hematologic/Lymphatic/Immunologic Examination

System/Body Area	Elements of Examination
Constitutional	• Measurement of **any three of the following seven** vital signs: (1) sitting or standing blood pressure; (2) supine blood pressure; (3) pulse rate and regularity; (4) respiration; (5) temperature; (6) height; (7) weight (May be measured and recorded by ancillary staff) • General appearance of patient (e.g., development, nutrition, body habitus, deformities, attention to grooming)
Head and Face	• Palpation and/or percussion of face with notation of presence or absence of sinus tenderness
Eyes	• Inspection of conjunctivae and lids
Ears, Nose, Mouth, and Throat	• Otoscopic examination of external auditory canals and tympanic membranes • Inspection of nasal mucosa, septum, and turbinates • Inspection of teeth and gums • Examination of oropharynx (e.g., oral mucosa, hard and soft palates, tongue, tonsils, posterior pharynx)
Neck	• Examination of neck (e.g., masses, overall appearance, symmetry, tracheal position, crepitus) • Examination of thyroid (e.g., enlargement, tenderness, mass)
Respiratory	• Assessment of respiratory effort (e.g., intercostal retractions, use of accessory muscles, diaphragmatic movement) • Auscultation of lungs (e.g., breath sounds, adventitious sounds, rubs)
Cardiovascular	• Auscultation of heart with notation of abnormal sounds and murmurs • Examination of peripheral vascular system by observation (e.g., swelling, varicosities) and palpation (e.g., pulses, temperature, edema, tenderness)
Chest (Breasts)	
Gastrointestinal (Abdomen)	• Examination of abdomen with notation of presence of masses or tenderness • Examination of liver and spleen
Genitourinary	
Lymphatic	• Palpation of lymph nodes in neck, axillae, groin, and/or other location
Musculoskeletal	
Extremities	• Inspection and palpation of digits and nails (e.g., clubbing, cyanosis, inflammation, petechiae, ischemia, infections, nodes)
Skin	• Inspection and/or palpation of skin and subcutaneous tissue (e.g., rashes, lesions, ulcers, ecchymoses, bruises)
Neurological/ Psychiatric	Brief assessment of mental status including • Orientation to time, place, and person • Mood and affect (e.g., depression, anxiety, agitation)

Hematologic/Lymphatic/Immunologic Examination

Content and Documentation Requirements for Hematologic/Lymphatic/Immunologic Examination

Level of Exam	Perform and Document
Problem Focused	**One to five** elements identified by a bullet.
Expanded Problem Focused	**At least six** elements identified by a bullet.
Detailed	**At least twelve** elements identified by a bullet.
Comprehensive	Perform **all** elements identified by a bullet; document every element in each screened area and at least one element in each unscreened area.

TABLE 14–14. Musculoskeletal Examination

System/Body Area	Elements of Examination
Constitutional	• Measurement of **any three of the following seven** vital signs: (1) sitting or standing blood pressure; (2) supine blood pressure; (3) pulse rate and regularity; (4) respiration; (5) temperature; (6) height; (7) weight (May be measured and recorded by ancillary staff) • General appearance of patient (e.g., development, nutrition, body habitus, deformities, attention to grooming)
Head and Face	
Eyes	
Ears, Nose, Mouth, and Throat	
Neck	
Respiratory	
Cardiovascular	• Examination of peripheral vascular system by observation (e.g., swelling, varicosities) and palpation (e.g., pulses, temperature, edema, tenderness)
Chest (Breasts)	
Gastrointestinal (Abdomen)	
Genitourinary	
Lymphatic	• Palpation of lymph nodes in neck, axillae, groin, and/or other location
Musculoskeletal	• Examination of gait and station Examination of joint(s), bone(s), and muscle(s)/tendon(s) of **four of the following six** areas: (1) head and neck; (2) spine, ribs, and pelvis; (3) right upper extremity; (4) left upper extremity; (5) right lower extremity; and (6) left lower extremity. The examination of a given area includes: • Inspection, percussion and/or palpation with notation of any misalignment, asymmetry, crepitation, defects, tenderness, masses, or effusions • Assessment of range of motion with notation of any pain (e.g., straight leg raising), crepitation, or contracture • Assessment of stability with notation of any dislocation (luxation), subluxation, or laxity • Assessment of muscle strength and tone (e.g., flaccid, cog wheel, spastic) with notation of any atrophy or abnormal movements NOTE: For the comprehensive level of examination, all four of the elements identified by a bullet must be performed and documented for each of four anatomic areas. For the three lower levels of examination, each element is counted separately for each body area. For example, assessing range of motion in two extremities constitutes two elements.
Extremities	(See Musculoskeletal and Skin)
Skin	• Inspection and/or palpation of skin and subcutaneous tissue (e.g., scars, rashes, lesions, cafe-au-lait spots, ulcers) in **four of the following six** areas: (1) head and neck; (2) trunk; (3) right upper extremity; (4) left upper extremity; (5) right lower extremity; and (6) left lower extremity. NOTE: For the comprehensive level, the examination of all four anatomic areas must be performed and documented. For the three lower levels of examination, each body area is counted separately. For example, inspection and/or palpation of the skin and subcutaneous tissue of two extremitites constitutes two elements.
Neurological/ Psychiatric	• Test coordination (e.g., finger/nose, heel/knee/shin, rapid alternating movements in the upper and lower extremities, evaluation of fine motor coordination in young children) • Examination of deep tendon reflexes and/or nerve stretch test with notation of pathological reflexes (e.g., Babinski) • Examination of sensation (e.g., by touch, pin, vibration, proprioception) Brief assessment of mental status including • Orientation to time, place, and person • Mood and affect (e.g., depression, anxiety, agitation)

Musculoskeletal Examination

Content and Documentation Requirements for Musculoskeletal Examination

Level of Exam	Perform and Document
Problem Focused	**One to five** elements identified by a bullet.
Expanded Problem Focused	**At least six** elements identified by a bullet.
Detailed	**At least twelve** elements identified by a bullet.
Comprehensive	Perform **all** elements identified by a bullet; document every element in each screened area and at least one element in each unscreened area.

TABLE 14–15. Neurological Examination

System/Body Area	Elements of Examination
Constitutional	• Measurement of **any three of the following seven** vital signs: (1) sitting or standing blood pressure; (2) supine blood pressure; (3) pulse rate and regularity; (4) respiration; (5) temperature; (6) height; (7) weight (May be measured and recorded by ancillary staff) • General appearance of patient (e.g., development, nutrition, body habitus, deformities, attention to grooming)
Head and Face	
Eyes	• Ophthalmoscopic examination of optic discs (e.g., size, C/D ratio, appearance) and posterior segments (e.g., vessel changes, exudates, hemorrhages)
Ears, Nose, Mouth, and Throat	
Neck	
Respiratory	
Cardiovascular	• Examination of carotid arteries (e.g., pulse amplitude, bruits) • Auscultation of heart with notation of abnormal sounds and murmurs • Examination of peripheral vascular system by observation (e.g., swelling, varicosities) and palpation (e.g., pulses, temperature, edema, tenderness)
Chest (Breasts)	
Gastrointestinal (Abdomen)	
Genitourinary	
Lymphatic	
Musculoskeletal	• Examination of gait and station Assessment of motor function including: • Muscle strength in upper and lower extremities • Muscle tone in upper and lower extremities (e.g., flaccid, cog wheel, spastic) with notation of any atrophy or abnormal movements (e.g., fasciculation, tardive dyskinesia)
Extremities	(See Musculoskeletal)
Skin	
Neurological	Evaluation of higher integrative functions including: • Orientation to time, place, and person • Recent and remote memory • Attention span and concentration • Language (e.g., naming objects, repeating phrases, spontaneous speech) • Fund of knowledge (e.g., awareness of current events, past history, vocabulary) Test the following cranial nerves: • 2nd cranial nerve (e.g., visual acuity, visual fields, fundi) • 3rd, 4th, and 6th cranial nerves (e.g., pupils, eye movements) • 5th cranial nerve (e.g., facial sensation, corneal reflexes) • 7th cranial nerve (e.g., facial symmetry, strength) • 8th cranial nerve (e.g., hearing with tuning fork, whispered voice, and/or finger rub) • 9th cranial nerve (e.g., spontaneous or reflex palate movement) • 11th cranial nerve (e.g., shoulder shrug strength) • 12th cranial nerve (e.g., tongue protrusion) • Examination of sensation (e.g., by touch, pin, vibration, proprioception) • Examination of deep tendon reflexes in upper and lower extremities with notation of pathological reflexes (e.g., Babinski) • Test coordination (e.g., finger/nose, heel/knee/shin, rapid alternating movements in the upper and lower extremities, evaluation of fine motor coordination in young children)
Psychiatric	

Neurological Examination

Content and Documentation Requirements for Neurological Examination

Level of Exam	Perform and Document
Problem Focused	**One to five** elements identified by a bullet.
Expanded Problem Focused	**At least six** elements identified by a bullet.
Detailed	**At least twelve** elements identified by a bullet.
Comprehensive	Perform **all** elements identified by a bullet; document every element in each screened area and at least one element in each unscreened area.

TABLE 14–16. Respiratory Examination

System/Body Area	Elements of Examination
Constitutional	• Measurement of **any three of the following seven** vital signs: (1) sitting or standing blood pressure; (2) supine blood pressure; (3) pulse rate and regularity; (4) respiration; (5) temperature; (6) height; (7) weight (May be measured and recorded by ancillary staff) • General appearance of patient (e.g., development, nutrition, body habitus, deformities, attention to grooming)
Head and Face	
Eyes	
Ears, Nose, Mouth, and Throat	• Inspection of nasal mucosa, septum, and turbinates • Inspection of teeth and gums • Examination of oropharynx (e.g., oral mucosa, hard and soft palates, tongue, tonsils, and posterior pharynx)
Neck	• Examination of neck (e.g., masses, overall appearance, symmetry, tracheal position, crepitus) • Examination of thyroid (e.g., enlargement, tenderness, mass) • Examination of jugular veins (e.g., distension; a, v, or cannon a waves)
Respiratory	• Inspection of chest with notation of symmetry and expansion • Assessment of respiratory effort (e.g., intercostal retractions, use of accessory muscles, diaphragmatic movement) • Percussion of chest (e.g., dullness, flatness, hyperresonance) • Palpation of chest (e.g., tactile fremitus) • Auscultation of lungs (e.g., breath sounds, adventitious sounds, rubs)
Cardiovascular	• Auscultation of heart including sounds, abnormal sounds, and murmurs • Examination of peripheral vascular system by observation (e.g., swelling, varicosities) and palpation (e.g., pulses, temperature, edema, tenderness)
Chest (Breasts)	
Gastrointestinal (Abdomen)	• Examination of abdomen with notation of presence of masses or tenderness • Examination of liver and spleen
Genitourinary	
Lymphatic	• Palpation of lymph nodes in neck, axillae, groin, and/or other location
Musculoskeletal	• Assessment of muscle strength and tone (e.g., flaccid, cog wheel, spastic) with notation of any atrophy and abnormal movements • Examination of gait and station
Extremities	• Inspection and palpation of digits and nails (e.g., clubbing, cyanosis, inflammation, petechiae, ischemia, infections, nodes)
Skin	• Inspection and/or palpation of skin and subcutaneous tissue (e.g., rashes, lesions, ulcers)
Neurological/ Psychiatric	Brief assessment of mental status including • Orientation to time, place, and person • Mood and affect (e.g., depression, anxiety, agitation)

Respiratory Examination

Content and Documentation Requirements for Respiratory Examination

Level of Exam	Perform and Document
Problem Focused	**One to five** elements identified by a bullet.
Expanded Problem Focused	**At least six** elements identified by a bullet.
Detailed	**At least twelve** elements identified by a bullet.
Comprehensive	Perform **all** elements identified by a bullet; document every element in each screened area and at least one element in each unscreened area.

TABLE 14–17. Skin Examination

System/Body Area	Elements of Examination
Constitutional	• Measurement of **any three of the following seven** vital signs: (1) sitting or standing blood pressure; (2) supine blood pressure; (3) pulse rate and regularity; (4) respiration; (5) temperature; (6) height; (7) weight (May be measured and recorded by ancillary staff) • General appearance of patient (e.g., development, nutrition, body habitus, deformities, attention to grooming)
Head and Face	
Eyes	• Inspection of conjunctivae and lids
Ears, Nose, Mouth, and Throat	• Inspection of lips, teeth, and gums • Examination of oropharynx (e.g., oral mucosa, hard and soft palates, tongue, tonsils, posterior pharynx)
Neck	• Examination of thyroid (e.g., enlargement, tenderness, mass)
Respiratory	
Cardiovascular	• Examination of peripheral vascular system by observation (e.g., swelling, varicosities) and palpation (e.g., pulses, temperature, edema, tenderness)
Chest (Breasts)	
Gastrointestinal (Abdomen)	• Examination of liver and spleen • Examination of anus for condyloma and other lesions
Genitourinary	
Lymphatic	• Palpation of lymph nodes in neck, axillae, groin, and/or other location
Musculoskeletal	
Extremities	• Inspection and palpation of digits and nails (e.g., clubbing, cyanosis, inflammation, petechiae, ischemia, infections, nodes)
Skin	• Palpation of scalp and inspection of hair of scalp, eyebrows, face, chest, pubic area (when indicated), and extremities • Inspection and/or palpation of skin and subcutaneous tissue (e.g., rashes, lesions, ulcers, susceptibility to and presence of photo damage) in **eight of the following ten** areas: • Head, including the face and • Neck • Chest, including breasts and axillae • Abdomen • Genitalia, groin, buttocks • Back • Right upper extremity • Left upper extremity • Right lower extremity • Left lower extremity NOTE: For the comprehensive level, the examination of at least eight anatomic areas must be performed and documented. For the three lower levels of examination, each body area is counted separately. For example, inspection and/or palpation of the skin and subcutaneous tissue of the right upper extremity and the left upper extremity constitutes two elements. • Inspection of eccrine and apocrine glands of skin and subcutaneous tissue with identification and location of any hyperhidrosis, chromhidroses, or bromhidrosis
Neurological/ Psychiatric	Brief assessment of mental status including • Orientation to time, place, and person • Mood and affect (e.g., depression, anxiety, agitation)

Skin Examination

Content and Documentation Requirements for Skin Examination

Level of Exam	Perform and Document
Problem Focused	**One to five** elements identified by a bullet.
Expanded Problem Focused	**At least six** elements identified by a bullet.
Detailed	**At least twelve** elements identified by a bullet.
Comprehensive	Perform **all** elements identified by a bullet; document every element in each screened area and at least one element in each unscreened area.

Documentation of an Encounter Dominated by Counseling or Coordination of Care

In the case where counseling and/or coordination of care dominates (more than 50%) of the physician/patient and/or family encounter (face-to-face time in the office or other or outpatient setting, floor/unit time in the hospital or nursing facility), time is considered the key or controlling factor to qualify for a particular level of E/M services. The total length of time of the encounter (face-to-face or floor time, as appropriate) should be documented and the record should describe the counseling and/or activities to coordinate care.

REFERENCES

Sarraille, W. A. (1998). *Selected Billing and Coding Issues for Nurse Practitioners.* Presented at the meeting of the American College of Nurse Practitioners, Washington, DC.

15

Health Promotion and Illness Prevention

Melinda Jenkins

Nurses support the wellness and optimum functioning of individuals, families, and groups (Neuman, 1989). Advanced practice nurses—acute care nurse practitioners (ACNPs) in particular—frequently have wonderful opportunities to support wellness by integrating ongoing public health concerns with episodic personal health care. In so doing, ACNPs promote individual patient/provider and system behavior toward coordinated, continuous, and comprehensive health care.

The challenge to promote health and prevent illness is pervasive. "It is a national tragedy that preventable illness makes up approximately 70% of the burden of illness and associated cost. This has major implications in our debate on health-care reform and the use of our health-care resources. The plain fact is that we Americans do a better job of preventive maintenance on our cars than on ourselves" (Friede, O'Carroll, Nicola, Oberle, & Teutsch, 1997, p. v). Our patients, whether they receive primary, acute, or chronic care, deserve education, intervention, and follow-up on preventive health maintenance.

A nursing perspective on health promotion, the Neuman (1989) framework depicts nursing clients as open systems in dynamic interaction with their internal and external environments. When actual or potential stressors arise, nurses assess and intervene with client systems to assist them in balancing the physiologic, psychologic, sociocultural, developmental, and spiritual aspects of their lives. Individuals, families, groups, or communities may be client systems.

Thorough risk assessment contributes to the identification of actual and potential stressors that guide nursing intervention in primary, secondary, and tertiary prevention strategies (Neuman, 1989). Primary prevention strengthens client defenses against stressors or reduces the risk of an encounter with stressors. Primary prevention may defend against illnesses in general and/or in particular. After symptoms occur, secondary prevention increases resistance to a particular illness through early case-finding and treatment. After treatment begins to take effect, tertiary prevention promotes general readaptation and stability to prevent further reaction to stressors. The most effective interventions depend on our current knowledge base regarding general health and the natural history of a particular disease. The provision of "person-centered care" (Barbour, 1995) in the context of family and community is a unique strength of nursing.

Primary and secondary prevention are the particular focus of community health nurses and primary care NPs (Jenkins & Sullivan-Marx, 1994). According to the Institute of Medicine (IOM), "primary care is the provision of integrated, accessible health care services by clinicians who are accountable for addressing a large majority of personal health care needs, developing a sustained partnership with patients, and practicing in the context of family and community" (IOM, 1996, p. 32). In many managed care environments, primary care clinicians are diagnostic experts who initiate referrals to "involve other health care practitioners for further evaluation or treatment when appropriate" (IOM, 1996, p. 33).

While primary care is quite broad in scope, acute care is focused in depth on a specific physiologic system or a severe episode of illness. ACNPs' specialty expertise and depth of knowledge allows them to invest particularly in secondary and tertiary prevention (Keane & Richmond, 1993). However, ACNPs are well advised to think "primary prevention" while delivering acute care. As our health-care system evolves, it is conceivable that specialty care for some population groups will be delivered by "full service" NPs, fully prepared to provide integrated primary-specialty care for a group of patients with similar needs, while working in partnership with physicians and other disciplines. In the meantime, PCNPs and ACNPs must communicate and work together to increase the coordination of care across practice sites (Vernon & Jenkins, 1995).

POPULATION AND AGE-RELATED RISK ASSESSMENT

In selecting preventive services, "the two most important factors to consider are the potential effectiveness of clinical interventions in improving clinical outcomes and the leading causes of mortality and morbidity" (U.S. Guide to Preventive Services, 1996, p. lvii). Assessment of risk for the leading causes of mortality and morbidity correlates with Neuman's identification of actual or potential stressors and is broadly based on the patient's age and population characteristics. The U.S. Public Health Service's *Healthy People 2000* gives a detailed background on major population and age-related risks (USDHHS, 1990). Objectives for risk reduction, improved health status, and health/protection services are proposed to meet three overall goals for the year 2000:

Increase the span of healthy life for all Americans,
Reduce health disparities among Americans, (and)
Achieve access to preventive services for all Americans (USDHHS, 1990, p. 43).

Population-related risks depend upon the family, group, or community identification of the patient and/or the prevalence of a particular illness in the environment. *Healthy People 2000* focuses on low-income, minority, and disabled populations that are at high risk for many types of morbidity and mortality.

Age-related risks depend on human growth and development, expected behaviors, and common social and family relationships. Preventive recommendations are given by the U.S. Preventive Services Task Force (1996) for pregnant women, children to age 10, ages 11 to 24, 25 to 64, and over age 65; modifications are given for high-risk groups. Recommended interventions are based on published research and guidelines from primary care specialty organizations such as the American Academy of Pediatrics, the American College of Obstetricians and Gynecologists, the American College of Physicians, the American Academy of Family Physicians, and the Canadian Task Force on the Periodic Health Examination.

DATA COLLECTION FOR RISK ASSESSMENT

Subjective and objective data collection for risk assessment includes a comprehensive health history, focused physical assessment, and relevant screening tests. The Neuman framework may be used to guide the health history by addressing individual and family physiologic, psychologic, sociocultural, developmental, and spiritual variables along with attention to healthy behaviors.

A physical assessment appropriately focused for health promotion is informed by patient symptoms and population- and age-related risks. At the present time, the value of a full physical assessment in the absence of risks or symptoms is not known.

Physical assessment and laboratory screening are components of secondary prevention—early case-finding and treatment—which rest on accurate diagnostic thinking. The prevalence of a given illness in the population is a key ingredient in diagnostic thinking. The predictive value of patient symptoms and physical exam findings, in combination with diagnostic test results, depends heavily on the prevalence of the illness within the population and, in lesser part, on the sensitivity and specificity of the data (Bates, 1995).

One important difference between primary care and specialty care is that the probability of a given diagnosis in a general primary care patient group is much less than the probability of that diagnosis in a selected group of specialty patients (Rosenblatt, Hart, Gamliel, et al., 1995; Sox, 1996). Thus, a large part of the work of the primary care NP is focused on data collection and diagnostic thinking. The ACNP often receives a patient referred for a problem in one organ system; possible differential diagnoses for a referred patient are limited (Sox, 1996). Therefore, the work of the ACNP is often focused on treatment. For example, a patient who comes to a primary care NP with a headache may have meningitis, a sinus infection, a cerebral vascular accident, a brain tumor, muscle tension, glaucoma, or any number of diagnoses. The Primary Care NP narrows the list of possible diagnoses, and seeks to rule out life-threatening diagnoses, with a thorough history, exam, diagnostic testing, and knowledge of the predictive value of the observation. After the work-up, if a severe neurological problem is suspected, the patient may be referred to a specialty provider for further identification and complex treatment of the problem.

Although the predictive value of an observation is very useful in theory, in reality it is not always known. We lack data on the prevalence of many illnesses in a given population and on the sensitivity and specificity of many observations. However, *Healthy People 2000* includes data on the prevalence of major causes of morbidity and mortality in general and select populations and age groups. *A Guide to Clinical Preventive Services* (1996) includes data on the burden of suffering for important illnesses, the accuracy of available screening tests, and the effectiveness of primary prevention and early detection.

▶ NURSING INTERVENTIONS FOR HEALTH PROMOTION

Nursing interventions to promote health may be with individuals, families, groups, communities, and large institutional or sociopolitical systems. The range of interventions to promote the health of an individual may expand or contract depending upon the context of family, group, and system. For example, institutionalized individuals and institutional caregivers may benefit from more frequent TB screening than the general population. Patients seeking acute care may not have had appropriate periodic preventive services. Also, they may be at increased risk for certain preventable problems (such as infectious diseases) because of their acute illness, its treatment, or the treatment setting itself.

Individual Interventions for Health Promotion

Health promotion interventions with individual patients include: screening, counseling, immunizations, chemoprophylaxis, documentation, referral, and follow-up. "For many interventions, evidence of an optimal periodicity is lacking. In addition, periodicity for certain interventions varies with patient characteristics (age, gender, risk factors)" (U.S. Preventive Services Task Force, 1996, p. lx). The following recommendations are summarized from the *Guide to Clinical Preventive Services* (U.S. Preventive Services Task Force, 1996). See Tables 15–1 through 15–6.

Screening

Recommended screening for the general population includes: height, weight, blood pressure, vision and hearing,

TABLE 15–1. Birth to 10 Years

Interventions Considered and Recommended for the Periodic Health Examination	Leading Causes of Death
	Conditions originating in perinatal period
	Congenital anomalies
	Sudden infant death syndrome (SIDS)
	Uninentional injuries (non-motor vehicle)
	Motor vehicle injuries

Interventions for the General Population

SCREENING
- Height and weight
- Blood pressure
- Vision screen (age 3–4 yr)
- Hemoglobinopathy screen (birth)[1]
- Phenylalanine level (birth)[2]
- T_4 and/or TSH (birth)[3]

COUNSELING
- Injury Prevention
  - Child safety car seats (age <5 yr)
  - Lap-shoulder belts (age ≥5 yr)
  - Bicycle helmet; avoid bicycling near traffic
  - Smoke detector, flame retardant sleepwear
  - Hot water heater temperature <120–130°F
  - Window/stair guards, pool fence
  - Safe storage of drugs, toxic substances, firearms, and matches
  - Syrup of ipecac, poison control phone number
  - CPR training for parents/caretakers
- Diet and Exercise
  - Breast-feeding, iron-enriched formula and foods (infants & toddlers)
  - Limit fat and cholesterol; maintain caloric balance; emphasize grains, fruits, vegetables (age ≥2 yr)
  - Regular physical activity*
- Substance Use
  - Effects of passive smoking*
  - Anti-tobacco message*
- Dental Health
  - Regular visits to dental care provider*

(Continued)

TABLE 15–1. Birth to 10 Years *(Continued)*

Floss, brush with fluoride toothpaste daily*
Advice about baby bottle tooth decay*

IMMUNIZATIONS

Diptheria-tetanus-pertussis (DTP)[4]
Oral poliovirus (OPV)[5]
Measles-mumps-rubella (MMR)[6]
H influenzae type b (Hib) conjugate[7]
Hepatitis B[8]
Varicella[9]

CHEMOPROPHYLAXIS

Ocular prophylaxis (birth)

Interventions for High-Risk Populations

POPULATION	POTENTIAL INTERVENTIONS (see detailed high-risk definitions)
Preterm or low-birth weight	Hemoglobin/hematocrit (HR1)
Infants of mothers at risk for HIV	HIV testing (HR2)
Low income; immigrants	Hemoglobin/hematocrit (HR1); PPD (HR3)
TB contacts	PPD (HR3)
Native American/Alaska Native	Hemoglobin/hematocrit (HR1); PPD (HR3); hepatitis A vaccine (HR4); pneumococcal vaccine (HR5)
Travelers to developing countries	Hepatitis A vaccine (HR4)
Residents of long-term care facilities	PPD (HR3); hepatitis A vaccine (HR4); influenza vaccine (HR6)
Certain chronic medical conditions	PPD (HR3); pneumococcal vaccine (HR5); influenza vaccine (HR6)
Increased individual or community lead exposure	Blood lead level (HR7)
Inadequate water fluoridation	Daily fluoride supplement (HR8)
Family h/o skin cancer, nevi; fair skin, eyes, hair	Avoid excess/midday sun, use protective clothing* (HR9)

[1] Whether screening should be universal or targeted to high-risk groups will depend on the proportion of high-risk individuals in the screening area, and other considerations. [2] If done during first 24 hr of life, repeat by age 2 wk. [3] Optimally between day 2 and 6, but in all cases before newborn nursery discharge. [4] 2, 4, 6, and 12–18 mo; once between ages 4–6 yr (DTaP may be used at 15 mo and older). [5] 2, 4, 6–8 mo; once between ages 4–6 yr. [6] 12–15 mo and 4–6 yr. [7] 2, 4, and 12–15 mo; no dose needed at 6 mo if PRP-OMP vaccine is used for first 2 doses. [8] Birth, 1 mo, 6 mo; or, 0–2 mo, 1–2 mo later, and 6–18 mo. If not done in infancy: current visit, and 1 and 6 mo later.[9] 12–18 mo; or any child without hx of chickenpox or previous immunization. Include information on risk in adulthood, duration of immunity, and potential need for booster doses.

* The ability of clinician counseling to influence this behavior is unproven.

HR1 = Infants age 6–12 mo who are: living in poverty, black, Native American or Alaska Native, immigrants from developing countries, preterm and low-birth weight infants, infants whose principal dietary intake is unfortified cow's milk.

HR2 = Infants born to high-risk mothers whose HIV status is unknown. Women at high risk include: past or present injection drug use; persons who exchange sex for money or drugs, and their sex partners; injection drug-using, bisexual, or HIV-positive sex partners currently or in past; persons seeking treatment for STDs; blood transfusion during 1978–1985.

HR3 = Persons infected with HIV, close contacts of persons with known or suspected TB, persons with medical risk factors associated with TB, immigrants from countries with high TB prevalence, medically underserved low-income populations (including homeless), residents of long-term care facilities.

HR4 = Persons ≥2 yr living in or traveling to areas where the disease is endemic and where periodic outbreaks occur (e.g., countries with high or intermediate endemicity; certain Alaska Native, Pacific Island, Native American, and religious communities). Consider for institutionalized children aged ≥2 yr. Clinicins should also consider local epidemiology.

HR5 = Immunocompetent persons ≥2 yr with certain medical conditions, including chronic cardiac or pulmonary disease, diabetes mellitus, and anatomic asplenia. Immunocompetent persons ≥2 yr living in high-risk environments or social settings (e.g., certain Native American and Alaska Native populations).

HR6 = Annual vaccination of children ≥6 mo who are residents of chronic care facilities or who have chronic cardiopulmonary disorders, metabolic diseases (including diabetes mellitus), hemoglobinopathies, immunosuppression, or renal dysfunction.

HR7 = Children about age 12 mo who: (1) live in communities in which the prevalence of lead levels requiring individual intervention, including residential lead hazard control or chelation, is high or undefined; (2) live in or frequently visit a home built before 1950 with dilapidated paint or with recent or ongoing renovation or remodeling; (3) have close contact with a person who has an elevated lead level; (4) live near lead industry or heavy traffic; (5) live with someone whose job or hobby involves lead exposure; (6) use lead-based pottery; or (7) take traditional ethnic remedies that contain lead.

HR8 = Children living in areas with inadequate water fluoridation (<0.6 ppm).

HR9 = Persons with a family history of skin cancer, a large number of moles, atypical moles, poor tanning ability, or light skin, hair, and eye color.

U.S. Preventive Services Task Force. (1996).

assessment for substance use, and fecal occult blood and/or sigmoidoscopy (over age 50). Recommended screening for females includes: papanicolaou smear, chlamydia testing (under age 20), rubella serology or vaccination history, and mammogram with or without clinical breast exam (over age 50). Total blood cholesterol is recommended for men aged 35 to 64 and women aged 45 to 64. At the present time, with existing screening tests, evidence is lacking that large-scale laboratory screening for prostate cancer contributes to healthy years of life for the older male population in general. Community standards on prostate screening vary widely.

Additional screening is recommended for pregnant women: hemoglobin, hepatitis B surface antigen, syphilis serology, blood typing/antibody screen, and an offer of hemoglobinopathy screening, HIV screening, and chorionic villi sampling or amniocentesis over age 35. Screening for newborns includes hemoglobinopathy, phenylalanine, and T4 or TSH.

(Text continued on p. 175)

TABLE 15–2. Ages 11–24 Years

Interventions Considered and Recommended for the Periodic Health Examination	Leading Causes of Death
	Motor vehicle/other unintentional injuries Homicide Suicide Malignant neoplasms Heart diseases

Interventions for the General Population

SCREENING

- Height and weight
- Blood pressure[1]
- Papanicolaou (Pap) test[2] (females)
- Chlamydia screen[3] (females <20 yr)
- Rubella serology or vaccination hx[4] (females > 12 yr)
- Assess for problem drinking

COUNSELING

- Injury Prevention
  - Lap/shoulder belts
  - Bicycle/motorcycle/ATV helmets*
  - Smoke detector*
  - Safe storage/removal of firearms*
- Substance Use
  - Avoid tobacco use
  - Avoid underage drinking and illicit drug use*
  - Avoid alcohol/drug use while driving, swimming, boating, etc.*
- Sexual Behavior
  - STD prevention: abstinence*; avoid high-risk behavior*; comdoms/female barrier with spermicide*
  - Unintended pregnancy: contraception
- Diet and Exercise
  - Limit fat and cholesterol; maintain caloric balance; emphasize grains, fruits, vegetables
  - Adequate calcium intake (females)
  - Regular physical activity*
- Dental Health
  - Regular visits to dental care provider*
  - Floss, brush with fluoride toothpaste daily*

IMMUNIZATIONS

- Tetanus-diphtheria (Td) boosters (11–16 yr)
- Hepatitis B[5]
- MMR (11–12 yr)[6]
- Varicella (11–12 yr)[7]
- Rubella[4] (females > 12 yr)

CHEMOPROPHYLAXIS

- Multivitamin with folic acid (females)

Interventions for High-Risk Populations

POPULATION	POTENTIAL INTERVENTIONS (See detailed high-risk definitions)
High-risk sexual behavior	RPN/VDRL (HR1); screen for gonorrhea (female) (HR2), HIV (HR3), chlamydia (female) (HR4); hepatitis A vaccine (HR5)
Injection or street drug use	RPR/VDRL (HR1); HIV screen (HR3); hepatitis A vaccine (HR5); PPD (HR6); advice to reduce infection risk (HR7)
TB contacts; immigrants; low income	PPD (HR6)
Native Americans/Alaska Natives	Hepatitis A vaccine (HR5); PPD (HR6); pneumococcal vaccine (HR8)
Travelers to developing countries	Hepatitis A vaccine (HR5)
Certain chronic medical conditions	PPD (HR6); pneumococcal vaccine (HR8); influenza vaccine (HR9)
Settings where adolescents and young adults congregate	Second MMR (HR10)
Susceptible to varicella, measles, mumps	Varicella vaccine (HR11); MMR (HR12)
Blood transfusion between 1975–1985	HIV screen (HR3)
Institutionalized persons; health care/lab workers	Hepatitis A vaccine (HR5); PPD (HR6); influenza vaccine (HR9)

(Continued)

TABLE 15–2. Ages 11–24 Years *(Continued)*

Family h/o skin cancer; nevi; fair skin, eyes, hair	Avoid excess/midday sun, use protective clothing* (HR13)
Prior pregnancy with neural tube defect	Folic acid 4.0 mg (HR14)
Inadequate water fluoridation	Daily fluoride supplement (HR15)

[1] Periodic BP for persons aged ≥21 yr. [2] If sexually active at present or in the past: q ≤ 3 yr. If sexual history is unreliable, begin Pap tests at age 18 yr. [3] If sexually active. [4] Serologic testing, documented vaccination history, and routine vaccination against rubella (preferably with MMR) are equally acceptable alternatives. [5] If not previously immunized: current visit, 1 and 6 mo later. [6] If no previous second dose of MMR. [7] If susceptible to chickenpox.

* The ability of clinician couseling to influence this behavior is unproven.

HR1 = Persons who exchange sex for money or drugs, and their sex partners; persons with other STDs (including HIV); and sexual contacts of persons with active syphilis. Clinicians should also consider local epidemiology.

HR2 = Females who have: two or more sex partners in the last year; a sex partner with multiple sexual contacts; exchanged sex for money or drugs; or a history of repeated episodes of gonorrhea. Clinicians should also consider local epidemiology.

HR3 = Males who had sex with males after 1975; past or present injection drug use; persons who exchage sex for money or drugs, and their sex partners; injection drug-using, bisexual, or HIV-positive sex partner currently or in the past; blood transfusion during 1978–1985; persons seeking treatment for STDs. Clinicians should also consider local epidemiology.

HR4 = Sexually active females with multiple risk factors including: history of prior STD; new or multiple sex partners; age under 25; nonuse or inconsistent use of barrier contraceptives; cervical ectopy. Clinicians should consider local epidemiology of the disease in identifying other high-risk groups.

HR5 = Persons living in, traveling to, or working in areas where the disease is endemic and where periodic outbreaks occur (e.g., countries with high or intermediate endemicity; certain Alaska Native, Pacific Island, Native American, and religious communities); men who have sex with men; injection or street drug users. Vaccine may be considered for institutionalized persons and workers in these institutions, military personnel, and day-care, hospital, and laboratory workers. Clinicians should also consider local epidemiology.

HR6 = HIV positive, close contacts of persons with known or suspected TB, health care workers, persons with medical risk factors associated with TB, immigrants from countries with high TB prevalence, medically underserved low-income populations (including homeless), alcoholics, injection drug users, and residents of long-term facilities.

HR7 = Persons who continue to inject drugs.

HR8 = Immunocompetent persons with certain medical conditions, including chronic cardiac or pulmonary disease, diabetes mellitus, and anatomic asplenia. Immunocompetent persons who live in high-risk environments or social settings (e.g., certain Native American and Alaska Native populations).

HR9 =Annual vaccination of: residents of chronic care facilities; persons with chronic cardiopulmonary disorders, metabolic diseases (including diabetes mellitus, hemoglobinopathies, immunosuppression, or renal dysfunction; and health care providers for high-risk patients.

HR10 = Adolescents and young adults in settings where such individuals congregate (e.g., high schools and colleges), if they have not previously received a second dose.

HR11 = Healthy persons aged ≥13 yr without a history of chickenpox or previous immunization. Consider serologic testing for presumed susceptible persons aged ≥13 yr.

HR12 =Persons born after 1956 who lack evidence if immunity to measles or mumps (e.g., documented receipt of live vaccine on or after the first birthday, laboratory evidence of immunity, or a history of physician-diagnosed measles or mumps).

HR13 = Persons with a family or personal history of skin cancer, a large number of moles, atypical moles, poor tanning ability, or light skin, hair, and eye color.

HR14 = Women with prior pregnancy affected by neural tube defect who are planning pregnancy.

HR15 = Persons aged < 17 yr living in areas with inadequate water fluoridation (<0.6 ppm).

U.S. Preventive Services Task Force. (1996).

TABLE 15–3. Ages 25–64 Years

Interventions Considered and Recommended for the Periodic Health Examination	Leading Causes of Death
	Malignant neoplasms
	Heart diseases
	Motor vehicle and other unintentional injuries
	Human immunodeficiency virus (HIV) infection
	Suicide and homicide

Interventions for the General Population

SCREENING

- Blood pressure
- Height and weight
- Total blood cholesterol (men age 35–64, women age 45–64)
- Papanicolaou (Pap) test (women)[1]
- Fecal occult blood test[2] and/or sigmiodoscopy (≥50 yr)
- Mammogram ± clinical breast exam[3] (women 50–69 yr)
- Assess for problem drinking
- Rubella serology or vaccination hx[4] (women of childbearing age)

COUNSELING

- Substance Use
  - Tobacco cessation
  - Avoid alcohol/drug use while driving, swimming, boating, etc.*
- Diet and Exercise
  - Limit fat and cholesterol; maintain caloric balance; emphasize grains, fruits, vegetables
  - Adequate calcium intake (women)
  - Regular physical activity*

(Continued)

TABLE 15–3. Ages 25–64 Years *(Continued)*

Injury Prevention
- Lap/shoulder belts
- Motorcycle/bicycle/ATV helmets*
- Smoke detector*
- Safe storage/removal of firearms*

Sexual Behavior
- STD prevention: avoid high-risk behavior*; condoms/female barrier with spermicide*
- Unintended pregnancy: contraception

Dental Health
- Regular visits to dental care provider*
- Floss, brush with fluoride toothpaste daily*

IMMUNIZATIONS

Tetanus-diptheria (Td) boosters
Rubella[4] (women of childbearing age)

CHEMOPROPHYLAXIS

Multivitamin with folic acid (women planning or capable of pregnancy)
Discuss hormone prophylaxis (peri- and postmenopausl women)

Interventions for High-Risk Populations

POPULATION	POTENTIAL INTERVENTIONS (See detailed high-risk definitions)
High-risk sexual behavior	RPR/VDRL (HR1); screen for gonorrhea (female) (HR2), HIV (HR3), chlamydia (female) (HR4); hepatitis B vaccine (HR5); hepatitis A vaccine (HR6)
Injection or street drug use	RPR/VDRL (HR1); HIV screen (HR3); hepatitis B vaccine (HR5); hepatitis A vaccine (HR6); PPD (HR7); advice to reduce infection risk (HR8)
Low income; TB contacts; immigrants; alcoholics	PPD (HR7)
Native Americans/Alaska Natives	Hepatitis A vaccine (HR6); PPD (HR7); pneumococcal vaccine (HR9)
Travelers to developing countries	Hepatitis B vaccine (HR5); hepatitis A vaccine (HR6)
Certain chronic medical conditions	PPD (HR7); pneumococcal vaccine (HR9); influenza vaccine (HR10)
Blood product recipients	HIV screen (HR3); hepatitis B vaccine (HR5)
Susceptible to measles, mumps, or varicella	MMR (HR11); varicella vaccine (HR12)
Institutionalized persons	Hepatitis A vaccine (HR6); PPD (HR7); pneumococcal vaccine (HR9); influenza vaccine (HR10)
Health care/lab workers	Hepatitis B vaccine (HR5); hepatitis A vaccine (HR6); PPD (HR7); influenza vaccine (HR10)
Family h/o skin cancer; fair skin, eyes, hair	Avoid excess/midday sun, use protective clothing* (HR13)
Previous pregnancy with neural tube defect	Folic acid 4.0 mg (HR14)

[1] Women who are or have been sexually active and who have a cervix: q ≤ 3 yr. [2] Annually. [3] Mammogram q1–2 yr, or mammogram q1–2 yr with annual clinical breast examination.
[4] Serologic testing, documented vaccination history, and routine vaccination (preferably with MMR) are equally acceptable.
* The ability of clinician counseling to influence this behavior is unproven.
HR1 = Persons who exchange sex for money or drugs, and their sex partners; persons with other STDs (including HIV); and sexual contacts of persons with active syphilis. Clinicians should also consider local epidemiology.
HR2 = Women who exchange sex for money or drugs, or who have had repeated episodes of gonorrhea. Clinicians should also consider local epidemiology.
HR3 = Men who had sex with men after 1975; past or present injection drug use; persons who exchange sex for money or drugs, and their sex partners; injection drug-using, bisexual, or HIV-positive sex partner currently or in the past; blood transfusion during 1978–1985; persons seeking treatment for STDs. Clinicians should also consider local epidemiology.
HR4 = Sexually active women with multiple risk factors including: history of STD; new or multiple sex partners; nonuse or inconsistent use of barrier contraceptives; cervical ectopy. Clinicians should also consider local epidemiology.
HR5 = Blood product recipients (including hemodialysis patients), persons with frequent occupational exposure to blood or blood products, men who have sex with men, injection drug users and their sex partners, persons with multiple recent sex partners, persons with other STDs (including HIV), travelers to countries with endemic hepatitis B.
HR6 = Persons living in, traveling to, or working in areas where the disease is endemic and where periodic outbreaks occur (e.g., countries with high or intermediate endemicity; certain Alaska Native, Pacific Island, Native American, and religious communities); men who have sex with men; injection or street drug users. Consider for institutionalized persons and workers in these institutions, military personnel, and day-care, hospital, and laboratory workers. Clinicians should also consider local epidemiology.
HR7 = HIV positive, close contacts of persons with known or suspected TB, health care workers, persons with medical risk factors associated with TB, immigrants from countries with high TB prevalence, medically underserved low-income populations (including homeless), alcoholics, injection drug users, and residents of long-term care facilities.
HR8 = Persons who continue to inject drugs.
HR9 = Immunocompetent institutionalized persons aged ≥50 yr and immunocompetent persons with certain medical conditions, including chronic cardiac or pulmonary disease, diabetes mellitus, and anatomic asplenia. Immunocompetent persons who live in high-risk environments or social settings (e.g., certain Native American and Alaska Native populations).
HR10 = Annual vaccination of residents of chronic care facilities; persons with chronic cardiopulmonary disorders, metabolic diseases (including diabetes mellitus), hemoglobinopathies, immunosuppression or renal dysfunction; and health care providers for high-risk patients.
HR11 = Persons born after 1956 who lack evidence of immunity to measles or mumps (e.g., documented receipt of live vaccine on or after the first birthday, laboratory evidence of immunity, or a history of physician-diagnosed measles or mumps).
HR12 = Healthy adults without a history of chickenpox or previous immunization. Consider serologic testing for presumed susceptible adults.
HR13 = Persons with a family or personal history of skin cancer; a large number of moles, atypical moles, poor tanning ability, or light skin, hair, and eye color.
HR14 = Women with previous pregnancy affected by neural tube defect who are planning pregnancy.
U.S. Preventive Services Task Force. (1996).

TABLE 15–4. Age 65 and Older

Interventions Considered and Recommended for the Periodic Health Examination	Leading Causes of Death
	Heart diseases Malignant neoplasms (lung, colorectal, breast) Cerebrovascular disease Chronic obstructive pulmonary disease Pneumonia and influenza

Interventions for the General Population

SCREENING
- Blood pressure
- Height and weight
- Fecal occult blood test[1] and/or sigmoidoscopy
- Mammogram ± clinical breast exam[2] (women ≤69 yr)
- Papanicolaou (Pap) test (women)[3]
- Vision screening
- Assess for hearing impairment
- Assess for problem drinking

COUNSELING
- Substance Use
  - Tobacco cessation
  - Avoid alcohol/drug use while driving, swimming, boating, etc.*
- Diet and Exercise
  - Limit fat and cholesterol; maintain caloric balance; emphasize grains, fruits, vegetables
  - Adequate calcium intake (women)
  - Regular physical activity*
- Injury Prevention
  - Lap/shoulder belts
  - Motorcycle and bicycle helmets*
  - Fall prevention*
  - Safe storage/removal of firearms*
  - Smoke detector*
  - Set hot water heater to <120–130°F*
  - CPR training for household members
- Dental Health
  - Regular visits to dental care provider*
  - Floss, brush with fluoride toothpaste daily*
- Sexual Behavior
  - STD prevention: avoid high-risk sexual behavior*; use condoms*

IMMUNIZATIONS
- Pneumococcal vaccine
- Influenza[1]
- Tetanus-diphtheria (Td) boosters

CHEMOPROPHYLAXIS
- Discuss hormone prophylaxis (peri- and postmenopausal women)

Interventions for High-Risk Populations

POPULATION	**POTENTIAL INTERVENTIONS** (See detailed high-risk definitions)
Institutionalized persons	PPD (HR1); hepatitis A vaccine (HR2); amantadine/rimantadine (HR4)
Chronic medical conditions; TB contacts; low income; immigrants; alcoholics	PPD (HR1)
Persons ≥75 yr; or ≥70 yr with risk factors for falls	Fall prevention intervention (HR5)
Cardiovascular disease risk factors	Consider cholesterol screening (HR6)
Family h/o skin cancer; nevi; fair skin, eyes, hair	Avoid excess/midday sun, use protective clothing* (HR7)
Native Americans/Alaska Natives	PPD (HR1); hepatitis A vaccine (HR2)
Travelers to developing countries	Hepatitis A vaccine (HR2); hepatitis B vaccine (HR8)
Blood product recipients	HIV screen (HR3); hepatitis B vaccine (HR8)
High-risk sexual behavior	Hepatitis A vaccine (HR2); HIV screen (HR3); hepatitis B vaccine (HR8); RPR/VDRL (HR9)

(Continued)

TABLE 15–4. Age 65 and Older *(Continued)*

Injection or street drug use	PPD (HR1); hepatitis A vaccine (HR2); HIV screen (HR3); hepatitis B vaccine (HR8); RPR/VDRL (HR9); advice to reduce infection risk (HR10)
Health care/lab workers	PPD (HR1); hepatitis A vaccine (HR2); amantadine/rimantadine (HR4); hepatitis B vaccine (HR8)
Persons susceptible to varicella	Varicella vaccine (HR11)

[1] Annually. [2] Mammogram q1–2 yr, or mamogram q1–2 yr with annual clinical breast exam. [3] All women who are or have been sexually active and who have a cervix. Consider discontinuation of testing after age 65 yr if previous regular screening with consistently normal results.

* The ability of clinican counseling to influence this behavior is unproven.

HR1 = HIV positive, close contacts of persons with known or suspected TB, health care workers, persons with medical risk factors associated with TB, immigrants from countries with high TB prevalence, medically underserved low-income populations (including homeless), alcoholics, injection drug users, and residents of long-term care facilities.

HR2 = Persons living in, traveling to, or working in areas where the disease is endemic and where periodic outbreaks occur (e.g., countries with high or intermediate endemicity; certain Alaska Native, Pacific Island, Native American, and religious communities); men who have sex with men; injection or street drug users. Consider for institutionalized persons and workers in these institutions, and day-care, hospital, and laboratory workers. Clinicians should also consider local epidemiology.

HR3 = Men who had sex with men after 1975; past or present injection drug use; persons who exchange sex for money or drugs, and their sex partners; injection drug-using; bisexual, or HIV-positive sex partner currently or in the past; blood transfusion during 1978–1985; persons seeking treatment for STDs. Clinicians should also consider local epidemiology.

HR4 = Consider for persons who have not received influenza vaccine or are vaccinated late; when the vaccine may be ineffective due to major antigenic changes in the virus; for unvaccinated persons who provide home care for high-risk persons; to supplement protection provided by vaccine in persons who are expected to have a poor antibody response; and for high-risk persons in whom the vaccine is contraindicated.

HR5 = Persons aged 75 years and older; or aged 70–74 with one or more additional risk factors including: use of certain psychoactive and cardiac medications (e.g., benzodiazepines, antihypertensives); use of ≥4 prescription medications; impaired cognition, strength, balance, or gait. Intensive individualized home-based multifactorial fall prevention intervention is recommended in settings where adequate resources are avalable to deliver such services.

HR6 = Although evidence is insufficient to recommend routine screening in elderly persons, clinicians should consider cholesterol screening on a case-by-case basis for persons ages 65–75 with additional risk factors (e.g., smoking, diabetes, or hypertension).

HR7 = Persons with a family or personal history of skin cancer, a large number of moles, atypical moles, poor tanning ability, or light skin, hair, and eye color.

HR8 = Blood product recipients (including hemodialysis patients), persons with frequent occupational exposure to blood or blood products, men who have sex with men, injection drug users and their sex partners, persons with multiple recent sex partners, persons with other STDs (including HIV), travelers to countries with endemic hepatitis B.

HR9 = Persons who exchange sex for money or drugs and their sex partners; persons with other STDs (including HIV); and sexual contacts of persons with active syphilis. Clinicians should also consider local epidemiology.

HR10 = Persons who continue to inject drugs.

HR11 = Healthy adults without a history of chickenpox or previous immunization. Consider serologic testing for presumed susceptible adults.

U.S. Preventive Services Task Force. (1996).

Added screening for institutionalized persons and health-care workers includes a tuberculosis test (U.S. Preventive Task Force, 1996).

Counseling

Recommended counseling is based on research that demonstrates its effectiveness in preventing morbidity and mortality from prevalent risky behaviors. Behavior change is the desired outcome of counseling and is most likely if readiness to change and self-efficacy are evident. A personalized, detailed plan, in line with the patient's physiologic, psychologic, sociocultural, developmental, and spiritual situation, and followed-up periodically, is most likely to succeed (Wagner, Austin, & Von Korff, 1996). In addition, patients should be held accountable for healthy behaviors and follow-up. The Preventive Services Task Force has delineated counseling for injury prevention, diet and exercise, substance use, dental health, and sexual behavior.

Counseling on injury prevention is age-specific. Motor vehicle injuries may be prevented by encouraging all patients to use safety belts (safety seats for children), to refrain from driving after using alcohol or drugs, and to wear a helmet while riding a motorcycle. Common household and recreational injuries may be prevented by encouraging patients to protect against falls, hot water burns, fires, firearms, poisoning, drowning, suffocation/choking, and bicycling accidents. Elderly persons at increased risk for falls include those aged 75 or above and those aged 70 to 74 using benzodiazepines or antihypertensives, using four or more medications daily, and/or having neurological impairments.

Physical activity may help prevent obesity, heart disease, hypertension, and diabetes. Regular, moderate-level exercise that can be incorporated into a daily routine is to be encouraged for everyone. A gradual increase of activity over a period of months should lead to an ideal routine of about 30 minutes of brisk walking each day.

Diet counseling is recommended for everyone over age 2 to limit fat and cholesterol intake, balance caloric intake and expenditure, and emphasize fiber intake in fruits, vegetables, and whole grains. Women should consume at least 1 gram of calcium per day and up to 11/2 grams if adolescent, pregnant/nursing, or postmenopausal. To prevent congenital neural tube defects, women of childbearing age should take daily multivitamins including folic acid. Breastfeeding of infants is to be encouraged. Referral to a registered dietician or other qualified provider is recommended if providers' time or skills are lacking for a comprehensive dietary assessment and intervention.

Substance use counseling is recommended for everyone. Substance use contributes to violence, accidents, birth defects, and a host of diseases. All pregnant women should

TABLE 15–5. Pregnant Women**

Interventions Considered and Recommended for the Periodic Health Examination

Interventions for the General Population

SCREENING

First visit
- Blood pressure
- Hemoglobin/hematocrit
- Hepatitis B surface antigen (HBsAg)
- RPR/VDRL
- Chlamydia screen (<25 yr)
- Rubella serology or vaccination history
- D(Rh) typing, antibody screen
- Offer CVS (<13 wk)[1] or amniocentesis (15–18 wk)[1] (age ≥35 yr)
- Offer hemoglobinopathy screening
- Assess for problem or risk drinking
- Offer HIV screening[2]

Follow-up visits
- Blood pressure
- Urine culture (12–16 wk)
- Offer amniocentesis (15–18 wk)[1] (age ≥35 yr)
- Offer multiple marker testing[1] (15–18 wk)
- Offer serum α-fetoprotein[1] (16–18 wk)

COUNSELING

- Tobacco cessation; effects of passive smoking
- Alcohol/other drug use
- Nutrition, including adequate calcium intake
- Encourage breastfeeding
- Lap/shoulder belts
- Infant safety car seats
- STD prevention: avoid high-risk sexual behavior*; use condoms*

CHEMOPROPHYLAXIS

- Multivitamin with folic acid[3]

Interventions for High-Risk Populations

POPULATION	**POTENTIAL INTERVENTIONS** (See detailed high-risk definitions)
High-risk sexual behavior	Screen for chlamydia (1st visit) (HR1), gonorrhea (1st visit) (HR2), HIV (1st visit) (HR3); HBsAg (3rd trimester) (HR4); RPR/VDRL (3rd trimester) (HR5)
Blood transfusion 1978–1985	HIV screen (1st visit) (HR3)
Injection drug use	HIV screen (HR3); HBsAg (3rd trimester) (HR4); advice to reduce infection risk (HR6)
Unsensitized D-negative women	D(Rh) antibody testing (24–28 wk) (HR7)
Risk factors for Down syndrome	Offer CVS[1] (1st trimester), amniocentesis[1] (15–18 wk) (HR8)
Prior pregnancy with neural tube defect	Offer amniocentesis[1] (15–18 wk), folic acid 4.0 mg[3] (HR9)

[1] Women with access to couseling and follow-up services, reliable standardized laboratories, skilled high-resolution ultrasound, and, for those receiving serum marker testing amniocentesis capabilities. [2] Universal screening is recommended for areas (states, counties, or cities) with an increased prevalence of HIV infection among pregnant women. In low-prevalence areas, the choice between universal and targeted screening may depend on other considerations. [3] Beginning at least 1 mo before conception and continuing through the first trimester.

* The ability of clinician counseling to influence this behavior is unproven.

** See Tables 15–2 and 15–3 for other preventive services recommended for women of this age group.

HR1 = Women with history of STD or new or multiple sex partners. Clinicians should also consider local epidemiology. Chlamydia screen should be repeated in 3rd trimester if at continued risk.

HR2 = Women under age 25 with two or more sex partners in the last year, or whose sex partner has multiple sexual contacts; women who exchange sex for money or drugs; and women with a history of repeated episodes of gonorrhea. Clinicians should also consider local epidemiology. Gonorrhea screen should be repeated in the 3rd trimester if at continued risk.

HR3 = In areas where universal screening is not performed due to low prevalence of HIV infection, pregnant women with the following individual risk factors should be screened: past or present injection drug use; women who exchange sex for money or drugs; injection drug-using, bisexual, or HIV-positive sex partner currently or in the past; blood transfusion during 1978–1985; persons seeking treatment for STDs.

HR4 = Women who are initially HBsAg negative who are at high risk due to injection drug use, suspected exposure to hepatitis B during pregnancy, multiple sex partners.

HR5 = Women who exchange sex for money or drugs, women with other STDs (including HIV), and sexual contacts of persons with active syphilis. Clinicians should also consider local epidemiology.

HR6 = Women who continue to inject drugs.

HR7 = Unsensitized D-negavitve women.

HR8 = Prior pregnancy affected by Down syndrome, advanced maternal age (≥35 yr), known carriage of chromosome rearrangement.

HR9 = Women with previous pregnancy affected by neural tube defect.

U.S. Preventive Services Task Force. (1996).

TABLE 15–6. Conditions for Which Clinicians Should Remain Alert

Condition	Population
Symptoms of peripheral arterial disease	Older persons, smokers, diabetic persons
Skin lesions with malignant features	General population, particularly those with established risk factors
Symptoms and signs of oral cancer and premalignancy	Persons who use tobacco, older persons who drink alcohol regularly
Subtle or nonspecific symptoms and signs of thyroid dysfuntion	Older persons, postpartum women, persons with Down syndrome
Signs of ocular misalignment	Infants and children
Symptoms and signs of hearing impairment	Infants and young children (<3 yr)
Large spinal curvatures	Adolescents
Changes in functional performance	Older persons
Depressive symptoms	Adolescents, young adults, persons at increased risk for depression
Evidence of suidical ideation	Persons with established risk factors for suicide
Various presentations of family violence	General population
Symptoms and signs of drug abuse	General population
Obvious signs of untreated tooth decay or mottling, inflamed or cyanotic gingiva, loose teeth, and severe halitosis	General population
Evidence of early childhood caries, mismatching of upper and lower dental arches, dental crowding or malalignment, premature loss of primary posterior teeth (baby molars) and obvious mouth breathing	Children

U.S. Preventive Services Task Force. (1996).

be counseled to avoid alcohol, drugs, and tobacco. All children, adolescents, and young adults should be counseled to avoid tobacco, alcohol, and drug use. Research supports the effectiveness of health-care provider counseling to prevent and decrease tobacco use. Parents and providers are to be encouraged to support community- and school-based programs to prevent tobacco use. Effective counseling strategies for smoking cessation include: give direct advice about the benefits of quitting; set a date to stop; follow-up with repeated support within the first 2 weeks; highlight smokers' charts for repeated encouragement; provide medications, referrals to community programs, and written materials as needed.

Counseling is recommended to prevent dental and periodontal disease. All patients over age 3 should be encouraged to floss and brush with fluoride toothpaste daily, and visit a dentist regularly. Parents should be discouraged from giving infants a bottle in bed. Fluoride supplements are recommended for children where water is not fluoridated.

The prevention of HIV infection and other sexually transmitted diseases (STDs) is important counseling. All adolescent, adult, and pregnant patients should be assessed for risks and informed of risk-reduction measures for STDs. Those at risk for STDs should be encouraged to abstain from sex, maintain a monogamous relationship, use condoms, and/or avoid anal intercourse, and should be appropriately tested. Proper use of condoms should be discussed.

Counseling is recommended to prevent unintended pregnancy. Adolescent and adult patient assessment should include a history of sexual preferences, activity, use of contraception, and risk of pregnancy. Counseling for sexually active patients and those considering sexual activity should include information about various effective contraceptive measures. Follow-up should include assessment of patient satisfaction with the chosen contraceptive method.

Immunizations

Children and adults without contraindications should be offered immunizations in the recommended schedule. Childhood immunizations include diphteria–tetanus–pertussis (DTP), oral poliovirus (OPV), inactivated poliovirus (IPV), measles–mumps–rubella (MMR), *H influenza* type b (Hib), hepatitis B, and varicella. See Table 15–1 for the recommended schedule.

In addition, high-risk children (over age 2) and adolescents should be offered hepatitis A vaccine. Individuals traveling to, living, or working in areas with endemic hepatitis A, and those in chronic care institutions are considered at high risk. Children over 6 months and adolescents who live in institutions or who have chronic diseases should receive influenza vaccine annually. Children/adolescents over age 2 should received pneumococcal vaccine if they have chronic disease or live with high-risk groups. Evidence does not clearly support pneumococcal vaccine for immunocompromised children.

Adult immunizations include influenza vaccine, pneumococcal vaccine, tetanus–diphtheria (Td), MMR, hepatitis B, hepatitis A, and varicella (see Tables 15–3 and 15–4). Influenza vaccine is recommended annually for everyone aged 65 and over, living in chronic care facilities, having chronic disease, or providing health care to high-risk groups. In case of institutional outbreaks of influenza A, amantadine or rimantadine, 200 mg/day by mouth, may be given with immunization and continued for 2 weeks.

A one-time vaccination for pneumococcus is recommended for adults aged 65 and over, and younger adults living in chronic care facilities, having chronic disease, or living with high-risk groups. It may be useful to revaccinate those over 75, with severe chronic disease, or immunocompromised conditions after 5 years. Clear evidence is lacking on the value of pneumococcal vaccination in immunocompromised adults.

Td immunization is usually recommended every 10 years but in the United States, those fully immunized in childhood may be protected with every 15- to 30-year boosters. International travelers should receive boosters every 10 years.

MMR is recommended for everyone born after 1956 who have negative laboratory evidence of immunity, have no record of childhood immunization, or have never been diagnosed with measles. A second dose should be given to adolescents who have not had a second dose in childhood and who are in school or college.

Three doses of hepatitis B vaccine should be given to young adults (not previously immunized) and to susceptible adults in high-risk groups. High-risk groups include homosexual men, intravenous drug users/partners, travelers to areas with endemic hepatitis B, those with a history of multiple sex partners or recent STD, those receiving blood products (including patients on hemodialysis), and health-care workers with exposure to blood/blood products. Three doses are recommended at 0, 1 month, and 6 months.

Hepatitis A vaccine should be offered to high-risk adults. Individuals traveling to/living in/working in areas with endemic hepatitis A, homosexual men, street drug users, military/hospital/laboratory/day care workers, and those in chronic care institutions are considered at high risk. Hepatitis A vaccine is given in two doses 6 to 12 months apart.

Varicella vaccine is recommended for all adults with no evidence of the disease and no previous vaccination. Two doses are given 4 to 8 weeks apart. Those particularly in need of the vaccine are health care/day care/institutional workers and families of immunocompromised individuals.

Chemoprophylaxis

In certain circumstances, chemoprophylaxis—pharmaceutical treatment to prevent disease or infection—may be provided. Postmenopausal women should be counseled about the risks and benefits of hormonal replacement. At the present time, each woman must weigh potential benefits due to personal and family medical history, and potential risks of iatrogenic problems to decide whether, and when, to take hormonal replacement. If women choose replacement therapy, the minimum effective dose of conjugated estrogen is 0.625 mg per day. Progestin should be added for women with intact uteri; the dose is medroxyporgesterone acetate 2.5 mg daily **OR** 5 to 10 mg for each of 10 to 14 days per month.

Chemoprophylaxis is recommended after exposure to H influenza type B, hepatitis A and B, meningococcal infection, rabies, and tetanus. Chemoprophylaxis after institutional outbreaks of influenza A is recommended. *H influenza* type B prophylaxis with rifampin is indicated for patients with the disease, and for all household contacts if even one of the contacts is a child younger than 4 who has not been immunized fully against Hib. Day care contacts should also receive rifampin and exposed children should be brought up to date with Hib vaccine.

Hepatitis A immune globulin, .02 mL/kg intramuscularly, is indicated within 2 weeks of sexual, household, day care, or contaminated food contacts. Hepatitis B immune globulin is recommended for infants born to mothers positive for hepatitis B surface antigen, for those with skin or mucosal contact to infected blood, for those with sexual contact to a hepatitis B surface antigen positive person, and for infants with primary caretakers who are hepatitis B surface antigen positive.

Rifampin prophylaxis is recommended for close contacts of patients with meningococcal infection. Meningococcal vaccine is recommended in addition to antibiotics (Ceftriazone) for outbreaks of serogroup A strain. Serogroups C, Y, and W-135 strains should be treated with vaccination.

Unprovoked bites by a carnivorous wild animal should be treated with rabies prophylaxis. Human rabies immune globulin is given (20 IU/kg), half at the wound, and half intramuscularly elsewhere. If the patient has never been immunized, HDCV or RVA 1.0 mL is given intramuscularly on days 0, 3, 7, 14, and 28. Previously immunized individuals should receive only two doses, days 0 and 3. Preexposure prophylaxis may be done with three doses on days 0, 7, and 21. Those with frequent exposure should check antibody levels every 6 months and boost them if necessary.

Tetanus vaccination should be given with human tetanus immune globulin (250 units IM) to those with major wounds or wounds contaminated with dirt or feces if their immunization was incomplete. If the immunization was complete but more than 5 years earlier, Td alone is sufficient.

In case of institutional outbreaks of influenza A, amantadine or rimantadine, 200 mg/day by mouth, may be given with immunization and continued for 2 weeks.

Documentation, Referral, and Follow-Up

In a perfect world, comprehensive patient records would be available to inform the acute care provider of which preventive services each patient has received. Then, additional services provided in the acute care setting would be added to the record that would go with the patient to the next provider.

Often, data that are collected as a normal part of acute care have value for health promotion if the data are used in a thoughtful way. For example, blood pressure and weight are commonly monitored after surgical procedures. If either is elevated over time, counseling and treatment or referral for health promotion are warranted. "Data not recorded are data lost" (Bates, 1995, p. 650). Similarly, referral visits not kept are referrals lost. Documentation, data transfer, and follow-up are required to provide effective referrals and to ascertain whether referrals were kept. Timely communication between acute and primary care providers is essential for efficient, effective care. Monitoring key measures documented for the delivery of preventive services and/or referral enhances quality of care.

Remember that the internal environment of mind and body work together; patients with emotional distress are at risk for injuries, substance use, risky sexual behavior, and unhealthy diet/activity patterns. Patient priorities for behavior change and follow-up are likely to follow a hierarchy of needs: from basic, safety, belongingness, ego status, growth, to self-actualization (Maslow, 1954). A large challenge for nurses is to link individuals and support networks. ACNPs should consider follow-up or mental health referral for emotional stressors that may adversely affect health or self-care.

Family, Group, Community, and System Interventions

Just as patient population characteristics relate to individual risk factors, population characteristics may support or detract from nursing interventions on behalf of individual patients. Nursing interventions for individuals are sometimes most effective when directed at the psychosocial, sociocultural, or environmental context. Many of the interventions suggested above will only be effective with individual behavioral change that is supported by family, community, and system.

Pender (1996) has developed the Health Promotion Model for nurses from a social learning theory base. In her model, prior behavior and personal factors contribute to interpersonal, situational, and behavioral influences that lead to a commitment to a plan for health promoting behavior. Immediate demands and preferences of the patient and family may compete with the actual implementation of the planned behavior.

For example, it is common for nurses to educate both patient and significant other about dietary recommendations. An educated couple may commit to changing their diet but may have few food choices due to financial or geographical limitations. A community intervention would be the next step; perhaps a church group or a local store could arrange for the proper foods to be available.

ACNPs may develop patient support/education groups to address needs common to a group of patients. Starting computer newsgroups is a new way of enhancing patient support. ACNPs may present information to established groups that focus on a single disease, such as diabetes or Parkinson's disease (Vernon & Jenkins, 1995). Broadening the discussion to health promotion and prevention of other serious problems may be well received.

ACNPs in institutional settings have the opportunity to influence those systems to promote patient health. For example, a specialty clinic that gives appointments in a block, rather than individual appointments, may discourage patient follow-up visits. Attending to transportation services for patients or linking patients to providers near to home are other helpful nursing interventions that recognize the individual in context.

ACNPs may support community-level health promotion such as school-based education on substance abuse and sexual behavior. ACNPs who vote may monitor services that are provided via tax dollars for Medicare and Medicaid. For example, some states do not include preventive dental care in Medicaid. Of those states that do, many regions may lack sufficient participating providers to meet the need. It is short-sighted for a nurse to refer a patient for dental care (or any other care) that does not exist or that cannot be afforded.

NURSES' CONTRIBUTIONS TO CONTINUOUS, COMPREHENSIVE CARE

Continuous, comprehensive care is the goal of integrated delivery systems. Identification of risks, early detection and treatment of disease, and case management are key ingredients of seamless care. Nurse-to-nurse referrals are an important method of effective case management (Jenkins & Sullivan-Marx, 1994). Before offering comprehensive preventive services, ACNPs are wise to consider their specific accountability and their cost and time pressures, especially in expensive, acute care institutional settings. Appropriate and comprehensive discharge planning is likely to include primary care as well as tertiary care follow-up. Financial incentives for primary care–acute care provider teams are needed to facilitate comprehensive care.

ACNPs are encouraged to integrate ongoing public health concerns with episodic personal health care. A thorough risk assessment identifying actual and potential stressors guides nursing intervention in primary, secondary, and tertiary prevention strategies (Neuman, 1989). Interventions to promote health and prevent illness in individuals, families, groups, and communities will assist them in balancing the physiologic, psychologic, sociocultural, developmental, and spiritual aspects of health.

REFERENCES

Barbour, A. (1995). *Caring for patients: A critique of the medical model.* Stanford, CA: Stanford University Press.

Bates, B. (1995). *A guide to physical examination and history taking* (6th ed.). Philadelphia: Lippincott.

Friede, A., O'Carroll, P. W., Nicola, R. M., Oberle, M. W., & Teutsch, S. M. (1997). *CDC Prevention guidelines: A guide for action.* Baltimore: Williams & Wilkins.

Institute of Medicine (1996). *Primary care.* Washington, DC: National Academy Press.

Jenkins, M. L. & Sullivan-Marx, E. M. (1994). Nurse practitioners and community health nurses: Partnerships and future visions. *Nursing Clinics of North America, 29,* 459–470.

Keane, A. & Richmond, T. (1993). Tertiary nurse practitioners. *Image, 25(4),* 281–284.

Maslow, A. (1954). *Motivation and personality.* New York: Harper & Row.

Neuman, B. (1989). *The Neuman systems model: Application to nursing education and practice* (2nd ed.). East Norwalk, CT: Appleton & Lange.

Pender, N. J. (1996). *Health promotion in nursing practice* (3rd ed.). Stamford, CT: Appleton & Lange.

Rosenblatt, R. S., Hart, J., Gamliel, S., et al. (1995). Identifying primary care disciplines by analyzing the diagnositic content of ambulatory care. *Journal of the American Board of Family Practice, 8,* 34–45.

Sox, H. C., Jr. (1996). Decision-making: A comparison of referral practice and primary care. *Journal of Family Practice, 42,* 155–160.

U.S. Department of Health and Human Services. (1990). *Healthy People 2000: National health promotion and disease prevention objectives.* Washington, DC: U.S. Government Printing Office.

U.S. Preventive Services Task Force. (1996). *Guide to clinical preventive services* (2nd ed.). Baltimore: Williams & Wilkins.

Wagner, E. H., Austin, B. T., & Von Korff, M. (1996). Improving outcomes in chronic illness. *Managed Care Quarterly, 4*(2), 12–24.

Vernon, G. & Jenkins, M. L. (1995). Health maintenance behaviors in advanced Parkinson's disease. *Journal of Neuroscience Nursing, 27*(4), 229–235.

III

Clinical Situations in Acute Care

16

Fever and the Hospitalized Patient

Janet M. Hines
Neil O. Fishman
Stephanie Green

APPROACH TO THE HOSPITALIZED PATIENT WITH FEVER

Because infection can sometimes progress rapidly, when fever occurs in the hospitalized patient it is important to do a complete workup until the source is found. The evaluation should focus on two necessary outcomes: namely, identifying

1. the degree of acuity of illness
2. the source of infection.

In other words, although your evaluation may not yield information about the source of infection, you must still decide how aggressively to treat the presentation. Since the administration of antibiotics should always be considered as a treatment with its own very significant risks, the safest course is not necessarily empiric antibiotic coverage.

The workup of fever in the hospitalized patient needs to be thorough, but if the guidelines are followed, then the workup can be done efficiently. The history, physical examination, and laboratory studies should be performed as recommended. The data should then be synthesized according to the outcomes listed above (identifying the degree of acuity of the illness and the source of infection). The outcomes will be discussed in the next section.

History

The traditional elements of the history (illnesses, surgeries, medications, family and social history, and review of systems) should be included. In the hospitalized patient, often the most significant part of the history is that of the present illness, most of which occurs *in* the hospital. Often patients may have been hospitalized for weeks or months. If the clinician has not been caring for the patient during this time, chart review can be a daunting task. Chart review must be treated as an art, or else it will act as a sedative. The essence is to look for only what is important, and to throw away (figuratively) everything else. It is often helpful to remember that the chart review is only being performed to ascertain the reason for the present situation, namely, factors that may have contributed to infection. Other important facts that are gleaned from the review that do not pertain to the work-up of fever should be set aside or marked to be dealt with at another time. Systematically, the review should progress, more or less in a chronological order, as shown in Table 16–1.

It is also important to consider that the hospitalized patient may have had exposures to infectious agents prior to admission; if the patient cannot provide this history, a family member should be sought to complete the history. The

TABLE 16–1. Data Collection for the Work-up of Fever

From the progress notes:	Date and reason for admission Major events, such as surgeries and other invasive procedures Clinical impressions from the progress notes (often the only thing worth reading); the problem list is also helpful, to keep an eye on preexisting diagnoses that might help clarify the source or presence of infection (for example, altered mental status)
From the graphic sheets:	Dates and duration of fever Dates of placement of indwelling devices (often this part of the chart will have descriptions of the device's function, which is key) Usual blood pressure range (if patient currently hemodynamically unstable)
From the medication administration records	Dates and duration of adminstration of antibiotics Times of administration of amphotericin, when given (it elevates temperature after its administration) Administration of antipyretics (tylenol, aspirin, nonsteroidal anti-inflammatory agents, and steroids) Administration of other drugs that commonly cause fever (see below)
From the lab sheets	WBC trend Creatinine trend
From the culture sheets	Dates, sites, and results of all cultures, including susceptibility testing
From the imaging section	Most recent chest x-ray report, and baseline chest x-ray on admission Results of any CT or MRI imaging

exposure history is an important element of the infection history, and though more traditionally associated with outpatients, it may come into play in the inpatient setting. The list of exposures that may lead to unusual infections is extensive. Even so, it is helpful to determine if there is a history of certain exposures in the hospitalized patient.

Physical Exam

The physical exam should be performed keeping in mind that some aspects of the exam will yield specific information regarding the presence of an infection (i.e., cellulitis around an IV site); others will yield information about the degree of acuity of illness (i.e., use of accessory muscles to indicate respiratory distress). In the patient with fever, the physical exam should pay special attention to the following areas. If all of these areas are assessed, there is little that will be missed.

Vital Signs

Vital signs are often overlooked, though they still reveal the most important information about the ability of the patient to stay ahead of the infection. Though abnormal signs are not specific for any given abnormality, they still are a good indicator of the intensity of the underlying process.

General Appearance

The degree of distress and the presence of increased work of breathing should be noted, as should evidence of perfusion to the extremities. These also point to the intensity of the underlying process.

Devices and Lines

Note should be made of the presence of all indwelling devices (such as endotracheal tubes, nasogastric tubes, rectal tubes, foley catheters, and all intravenous lines). All such devices violate barriers to infection. The date of placement of central lines (which is less important for other indwelling devices), can be conveniently recorded here, though it is generally determined during the chart review.

Head, Eyes, Ears, Nose, and Throat

Tubes entering the nasopharynx may block the eustachian tube or the sinus ostia, leading to otitis media, sinusitis, or mastoiditis. The presence of sinus or mastoid tenderness to percussion should be noted, and the tympanic membranes should be examined for fluid, dullness, and loss of the normal architecture. Often imaging is necessary to confirm these areas are normal.

Conjunctival injection, particularly in the presence of petechiae elsewhere, may signify a drug reaction, such as Stevens-Johnson syndrome. This syndrome generally occurs in conjunction with redness of other mucous membranes and the classic target lesion on the skin.

Facial asymmetry may be a sign of deep pharyngeal space infection, which may originate in a tooth infection. Such an infection may track easily down anatomic planes into the deeper structures of the base of the skull, ultimately compressing the pharyngeal opening or extending down to the mediastinum, where serious mediastinitis may result.

Thrush may be noted in exam of the oral mucosa. While it may occur in the absence of HIV infection (in patients on antibiotics, or patients on steroid inhalers who do not flush the mouth out properly), the presence of HIV should at least be considered in patients with thrush.

Tooth abscesses can be responsible for fever, or, as mentioned, can be the only sign of a deep pharyngeal space infection. They do not always cause abnormalities visible to external exam, but in some cases, the tooth can be broken and black (with caries), and the surrounding gum is inflamed. Percussion on the affected tooth with a tongue blade should cause pain.

Pharyngitis is simply redness of the posterior aspect of the pharynx, which may be associated with Group A streptococcal infection (strep throat). More commonly it is related to excessive secretion related to allergies or dryness related to debility.

Neck

The neck should be passively flexed to determine whether it is supple. A neck that cannot be passively flexed is defined as having "meningismus." The presence of meningismus is difficult to determine in some patients with cervical degenerative joint disease, who may have decreased flexibility at baseline. When present, meningismus should raise concern for meningitis.

If lymph nodes are present (in the neck, as well as in the axillae and groins), their location and characteristics should be described. Benign lymph nodes are mobile, firm, and smooth.

Chest

Accurate examination of the chest in a hospitalized patient is quite difficult, particularly in a patient that is unable to cooperate or one that is on mechanical ventilation. The degree of voluntary respiratory excursion often is not enough to ventilate affected areas, leading to false signs of consolidation (atelectasis) or the false absence of signs of consolidation. The sounds of the ventilator tubing can also interfere with the exam. Under ideal circumstances, signs of consolidation and pleural effusion should be sought, as discussed in Chapter 37, Pulmonary Problems.

Cardiac

When searching for a cause of fever, the presence of murmurs is the most important element of the heart exam, as they are helpful in the ascertainment of the presence of *endocarditis.* The presence of regurgitant murmurs (mitral and tricuspid regurgitation, and aortic insufficiency) are the only ones that are supportive of a diagnosis of endocarditis. However, stenotic murmurs are indicative of the presence of underlying valvular disease, such as rheumatic valve disease. It is important to realize that such valve abnormalities are a risk factor for endocarditis, rather than proof of the presence of endocarditis. It is also important to realize that in the absence of murmurs, endocarditis cannot be ruled out.

Signs of *pericarditis* may include a pericardial friction rub or a pericardial knock; additionally, the heart sounds may sound muffled due to the volume of the fluid.

Abdomen

The absence of bowel sounds may signify an obstruction or an ileus, either of which may point to or be the cause of fever. Abdominal rigidity or rebound may result from a ruptured bowel or ruptured abscess, and is a surgical emergency.

Abdominal tenderness that is mild in intensity is quite unhelpful, and while it is not a specific sign for any abdominal pathology, in a patient in whom there are no other suggestive findings, it may be reason enough to image the abdomen.

Hepatosplenomegaly may be seen in certain infections or malignancies, as well as in cirrhosis and right heart failure. It is thus not of itself a specific finding, though it is significant and its cause should be determined.

When ascites is present in the patient with fever, it may also be a source of infection (even when the abdomen is nontender). In the absence of clear evidence for infection elsewhere, the patient with ascites and fever should undergo paracentesis.

Back

Tenderness along the spine may be indicative of a spinal abscess or epidural abscess (or a tumor). In the presence of *any* neurologic deficits in the lower extremities, the presence of such tenderness is a surgical emergency.

Costovertebral angle (CVA) tenderness may be a sign of pyelonephritis; however, occasionally its presence is quite dependent on the degree to which the examiner exerts pressure (or in some cases, blunt force). It should be kept in mind that CVA tenderness is not necessary for the diagnosis of pyelonephritis.

The back and buttock area should also be searched for decubitus ulcers. Such ulcers, when kept clean, are not likely to be the source of fever. However, the amount of infection that can be present under an eschar can be impressive, so the evaluation of all decubiti include adequate debridement. Occasionally such decubiti will be surrounded by a broad rim of redness and swelling consistent with cellulitis; this is not required to consider deep debridement. Clean ulcers without cellulitis do not require antibiotic therapy.

Genitals

Genital herpes may be associated with fever. The presence of typical lesions (cloudy vesicles on a red base, scattered in a serpiginous fashion on in the genital or rectal area, particularly when associated with the inguinal adenopathy) suggests herpes simplex virus (HSV).

Diabetics may be predisposed, particularly when a foley catheter is present, to a form of necrotizing fasciitis known as *Fournier's gangrene.* It may start as an area of erythema anywhere in the groin area, but it progresses rapidly to skin and soft tissue necrosis. Such a finding should be considered an emergency, with surgical evaluation promptly arranged.

The rectal area should not only be examined for the presence of HSV lesions, it should be examined for the presence of perirectal fluctuance, tenderness, or induration. Such findings are indicative of a perirectal abscess. An abscess may be palpated more readily by introducing a gloved finger into the rectum. There is a traditional concern that neutropenic patients, who are particularly predisposed to perirectal abscesses, should not undergo such a digital rectal exam in the course of evaluation for fever, for fear of inducing bacteremia. However, the risk of bacteremia is not superceded by the benefit from diagnosing such a condition, so gentle digital rectal exam may be undertaken in neutropenics.

The prostate should be examined for fluctuance, swelling, and tenderness. Indwelling bladder catheterization is a risk factor for prostatitis. Prostatitis requires a longer period of treatment than simple urinary tract infection (UTI).

Pelvic inflammatory disease (PID) can cause fever in women who are sexually active. Findings of cervical motion tenderness or adnexal tenderness by pelvic exam are very suggestive of PID.

Extremities

The joints should be examined for effusions or erythema. Such findings could be indicative of septic arthritis or gout. Gout is an important noninfectious cause of fever. Intravenous sites should be examined for tenderness, induration, erythema, and lymphangitis (i.e., streaks of erythema extending proximally from the IV site). Calf swelling or tenderness may be a sign of deep vein thrombosis.

Neurologic

Abnormalities in the neurologic exam do not generally help differentiate infectious causes from each other or from noninfectious causes. However, a full neurologic exam should always be performed on the patient who has no other identified source for fever.

Skin

A maculopapular rash located only in pressure areas may simply be a folliculitis due to heat and moisture, but it conversely may be the beginning of a more generalized eruption characteristic of a drug rash.

Findings of generalized xerosis or seborrheic dermatitis may be indicative of previously undiagnosed or undisclosed HIV infection. In general, a sick patient with a rash with a hemorrhagic or bullous component should undergo dermatologic evaluation.

Signs of endocarditis include Osler's nodes, Janeway lesions, petechiae, and splinter hemorrhages. These findings are discussed in more detail in the endocarditis section of Chapter 44.

Laboratories

Lab tests can be prioritized into those that should always be ordered, and those that should only be performed in specific situations. The following should always be ordered:

- White blood cell count: while leukocytosis is suggestive of the presence of infection, it is neither sensitive nor specific. Leukocytosis may occur in response to noninfectious stresses. The "left shift," refers to the appearance in the blood of premature forms of neutrophils (known as "bands"). There is no formally accepted range for a normal number of bands. Traditionally, a left shift is taken to mean that the leukocytosis is due to infection; however, the positive and negative predictive values of this finding are not sufficient to be able to exclude or define diagnoses. The trend of the WBC count helps to establish a baseline for recovery.
- BUN/creatinine: to determine the presence of renal insufficiency, which would potentially alter either the type of antibiotic given or the dosage.
- Urinalysis: the presence of pyuria, particularly in the presence of bacteriuria, is suggestive of UTI. Other abnormalities may help in the diagnosis of endocarditis.
- Chest radiograph: for the presence of an infiltrate (which suggests pneumonia), as well as atelectasis, an important noninfectious cause of fever. There are multiple other possible findings on a chest radiograph which can be helpful in the determination of the source of infection, the discussion of which is beyond the scope of this review.

The following tests should be ordered in certain situations:

- Arterial blood gas: while not specific for infection, it may help to stratify the patient according to intensity of illness, as evidenced by acidosis or respiratory failure.
- Prothrombin Time (PT) and Partial Thromboplastin Time (PTT). The PT and PTT may be elevated in disseminated intravascular coagulation (DIC); fibrin split products will also help in this evaluation.
- Liver function tests: should be ordered in the presence of any right upper quadrant tenderness, or in situations in which hepatitis may be present. If such is the case, hepatitis serologies should be ordered as indicated.
- Computerized Tomography (CT) and Magnetic Resonance Imaging (MRI): CT scans and MRI scans have changed the landscape of medicine, however, it is important to be familiar with their indications and limitations. Imaging for an infectious source of fever usually entails imaging the chest, abdomen, and pelvis. CT seems to remain superior to MRI here. If intracranial abscess is suspected, MRI is preferred. Both oral and intravenous contrast should be used, if possible. There are protocols to decrease the likelihood of allergic reaction if the patient gives a history of dye allergy.

Cultures

In general, blood and urine cultures should always be drawn on a febrile patient; sputum should be obtained in any patient with a cough or abnormal chest x-ray. Any other abnormal finding or collection (joint, pleural, pericardial) should also be sampled for culture. Such drainage may also be necessary to treat the infection.

For patients remaining continuously febrile, there is a point beyond which the likelihood of culture contamination exceeds the likelihood of a meaningful positive result. If daily blood cultures are obtained for 2 weeks, the likelihood of obtaining a result consistent with contamination by skin flora increases. In other words, consider a patient who has fever for 2 weeks due to a noninfectious cause, such as a drug reaction, that is unbeknownst to the clinician. If this patient, with an indwelling central venous catheter, has coagulase negative staph grow from more than one culture, the clinician is likely to treat the patient with vancomycin for suspicion of line-associated bacteremia, though it may not, in fact, exist. Contaminant blood cultures may contribute to excess cost for the hospitalized patient by increasing the number of tests performed to determine whether the culture isolate is meaningful, and by increasing the amount of unnecessary antimicrobial use. They also contribute to excess morbidity and mortality. A more in-depth discussion of the use of blood cultures is given in the section on bloodstream infections.

DEVELOPMENT OF A DIFFERENTIAL DIAGNOSIS: SYNTHESIS OF THE DATA

Determination of the Site of Infection

For some patients, determination of the site of infection is easy, based on their complaints or physical exam (e.g., complaint: diarrhea; conclusion: gastroenteritis). For others, particularly those who are sick enough to be hospitalized, the complexity of the coexistent illness may obscure the etiology of the fever. In those cases, determining the source of a fever must be based on characterizing the patient as a host with a normal or abnormal immune system, as well as characterizing the exposures the patient may have had.

Immune Status

Immune status of the host determines the ability of the patient to fight off infection. Different immune deficiencies will predispose to different infections. Certain medical conditions, which are less clearly associated with immune deficiency, may also predispose to certain infections.

Immune Deficiencies. *Neutropenia* is defined as an absolute neutrophil count (ANC) of less than 1000 (though different studies quote different numbers). Neutropenia should be suspected in any patient who has undergone intensive chemotherapy, though not all chemotherapeutic agents will cause it. It may also be seen in the less common situation of aplastic anemia. ANC counts below 100 pose significantly more danger than do those above 100. However, the more rapidly the neutropenia develops, and the longer it lasts, the more likely the patient is to get a serious infection.

TABLE 16–2. Pathogens to Which the Neutropenic Host Is Susceptible

Gram-Positive Cocci	Gram-Negative Rods	Fungi
Staphylococcus aureus Coagulase negative *staphylococci* Viridans streptococci, pneumococci (alpha-hemolytic strep)	*E coli* *Pseudomonas aeruginosa* *Klebsiella pneumoniae*	*Candida albicans* Other *Candida* spp. *Aspergillus* spp. Mucor

When the neutropenic patient develops a fever, it is felt to be an infectious disease emergency. Because such patients do not have a sufficient number of neutrophils, the usual signs of inflammation are often absent. Fever is still able to develop, but localizing the site is very difficult. Therefore, such patients will also be subject to more rapid development of complications, such as septic shock. Table 16–2 lists the pathogens to which the neutropenic host is susceptible.

Cell-Mediated Immune Dysfunction. Macrophages and monocytes, which are responsible for defense against intracellular pathogens (Table 16–3), are the arm of the immune system affected in patients with AIDS (mentioned elsewhere), Hodgkin's disease, organ transplantation, and long-term moderate to high-dose steroid treatment (the equivalent of 20 mg prednisone daily).

Among patients with defects in their cell-mediated immunity, infections actually tend to be rare. Empiric antibiotic therapy recommendations do not exist for such hosts when they develop fever, as it is much more difficult to predict the organism (given the range of organisms), and since such patients tend to manifest more signs of infection. Patients with connective tissue diseases (systemic lupus erythematosis and rheumatoid arthritis) may also be at risk for infections caused by cell-mediated defects, though possibly not entirely due to the immunosuppressive therapy.

Humoral Immune Dysfunction. Patients with multiple myeloma, B-cell lymphoma, AIDS, or who have under-

TABLE 16–3. Macrophages and Monocytes for Defense Against Intracellular Pathogens

Bacteria	Fungi	Viruses	Protozoa	Worms
Listeria monocytogenes *Legionella* spp. *Salmonella* spp. *Mycobacterium tuberculosis* *Mycobacterium avium-intracellular* (MAC) *Nocardia* spp.	*Cryptococcus neoformans* *Histoplasma capsulatum* *Coccidioides immitis*	Herpes simplex virus Varicella-zoster virus Cytomegalovirus Epstein-Barr virus	*Pneumocystis carinii* *Toxoplasma gondii* *Cryptosporidium* spp.	*Strongyloides stercoralis*

gone splenectomy, may have defects in their humoral immune system (meaning the antibodies themselves). While other arms of the immune system can generally make up for the loss of antibodies, organisms with capsules (*Streptococcus pneumoniae* and *Haemophilus influenzae*) may pose a particular threat. Antibodies are required to effectively defend against these organisms because the remainder of the immune system cannot sufficiently compensate. It is important to recognize that, although not all patients with multiple myeloma will have this defect (it depends on the degree of advancement of the disease), those patients who do have such a defect can become ill quite rapidly. Fever in a patient with multiple myeloma should always be taken seriously, until it is clear that a source is found.

Medical Conditions Predisposing to Certain Types of Infection

Diabetes Mellitus. Diabetics are at increased risk for infection for a number of reasons. Peripheral sensory neuropathy predisposes to trauma, and the vascular disease prevents adequate repair of such trauma. Other poorly defined factors are responsible for the predisposition to rhinocerebral mucormycosis and "malignant" otitis externa (an aggressive infection caused by *Pseudomonas*). Diabetics also seem to be at risk for colonization by *Candida,* probably due to glycosuria.

Chronic Renal Failure. The predisposition to bacterial infection seen in patients with renal failure is not entirely due to the frequent access required by hemo- and peritoneal dialysis. However, the role such access plays in intravascular infection and prosthetic device (e.g., peritoneal catheter) infection is clear. Additionally, patients with renal failure have diminished antibody responses as well as cell-mediated immunity. The hemodialysis membrane may activate complement, causing a transient neutropenia during dialysis (Arnaout, Hakim, Todd, et al., 1985). It is not clear to what extent this is responsible for the predisposition to bacterial infection in renal failure.

The Elderly. The elderly are at increased risk of infection due to changes in their humoral and cell-mediated immunity, as well as certain physiologic changes, such as immobility and vascular disease. Diagnosis is occasionally difficult because signs in the elderly are more subtle. Urinary tract infection, pneumonia, infection of decubitus ulcers, and bacteremia (usually secondary to infection at another site) are important infections in the elderly. When the elderly have fever but no clear source identified after several days, only about one third of the time is it due to infection; the remainder of the time it is due to either neoplasm or connective tissue disease (a third each) (Esposito & Glickman, 1978). It is also important to note that even though many of the elderly have lower body temperatures than normal, 95% of the time that they are infected, they will be able to manifest a fever (McAlpine, Martin, Lennox, et al., 1986).

Sickle Cell Anemia. Because of repeated infarcts of the spleen (functional splenectomy), patients with sickle cell disease have poor humoral immunity, and are thus at increased risk for serious infection with both *Streptococcus pneumoniae* and *Salmonella.* Pneumococcal vaccine still has some efficacy in these patients.

Alcoholism. The depressed consciousness that corresponds to intoxication places a person at risk for aspiration pneumonia. The lifestyle (poverty, crowded conditions) that some alcoholics experience places them at risk for tuberculosis. There is a generally increased risk of bacterial infections in severe alcoholism; malnutrition may contribute to this deficiency.

Liver Disease. Patients with cirrhosis are at increased risk for septicemia and spontaneous bacterial peritonitis, at least partly due to poor hepatic blood flow with resultant impaired clearance of antigens.

Spinal Cord Injury. Patients with spinal cord injury are predisposed to infection for mechanical reasons. Such infection includes pneumonia (intercostal muscle paresis in high-cord lesions), urinary tract infection (neurogenic bladder), and infection of the skin, soft tissue, and bone (pressure and immobility, combined with loss of sensation). Evaluation of the spinal cord injured patient for infection can be difficult by the lack or alteration of sensation of pain, dysuria, or dyspnea.

Exposure History

The exposure history is essential to the clinician addressing infectious diseases, and one that generally is unique to the discipline. It is, however, necessary for any clinician facing an unknown.

Certain conditions or situations predispose to certain infections. An essential part of the infectious disease history is identification and characterization of such situations. For clarity, these can be divided into hospital (nosocomial), geographical, and animal exposures, substance use/abuse, sexual habits, and occupational exposures.

Nosocomial Infections. All patients who have been in the hospital for more than 48 hours are at risk for such infections; in fact, these are some of the most commonly encountered infections in acute care. The timing (48 hours) is arbitrary, and mainly serves to help categorize infections from an epidemiologic standpoint. Thus, it does not mean that patients hospitalized for less than 48 hours never get these infections (for example, a line-associated infection in a patient receiving home IV antibiotics). It is estimated that approximately 4.5% of all patients admitted to the hospital will develop a nosocomial infection (Haley et al., 1985). The most common nosocomial infections are:

- Urinary tract infection
- Surgical wound infection
- Respiratory tract infection

- Bacteremia
- Infectious gastroenteritis (*Clostridium difficile*)

In other words, a patient is at risk for these infections just by residing in a hospital. Clinical information can help guide whether these should be considered: in other words, most patients who are at risk for UTIs have indwelling urinary catheters; most who develop bacteremia have venous catheters in place. Patients who have not had surgery during the course of their hospitalization obviously would not have surgical wound infections. Respiratory tract infections are more likely to occur in association with mechanical ventilation, or in patients unable to protect their own airway. The patients most likely to get *C difficile* infection are those who have been on antibiotics, particularly cephalosporins or ampicillin.

In any given hospital, certain nosocomial infections may be more likely to be found in a patient; for example, rates of sternal wound infections may exist at widely varying rates from hospital-to-hospital. Determining whether a nosocomial infection is occurring at rates that are higher than acceptable is a complicated task. While the infection control section takes responsibility for such determinations, it is sometimes impossible to have the first-hand knowledge that clinicians have. Therefore, perception that a certain infection is occurring at an unacceptable rate should prompt discussion with infection control.

Because nosocomial infections are caused by a different range of organisms than community acquired infections, management of each of these disorders should be considered separately. It is important, though, to mention a few complicating factors in the management of nosocomial infection.

Indwelling Devices. Any device that is placed into the patient, crossing the natural barriers, places the patient at risk for infection at that site (Table 16–4).

Note that generally, tubes that are in place to drain fluid out of the body (e.g., thoracostomy tubes, Jackson-Pratt drains, etc.) should not result in infection in that site, *as long as the tube is functioning correctly.* Studies to determine if a catheter or drainage tube is functioning may be necessary in the appropriate evaluation for the source of fever.

TABLE 16–4. Indwelling Devices

Endotracheal tube	Ventilator-associated pneumonia Sinusitis (occlusion of the sinus ostia)
Nasogastric tube	Sinusitis (occlusion of the sinus ostia)
Central venous catheter	Bacteremia Septic thrombophlebitis Tunnel infection Exit site infection
Urinary catheter	Urethritis Cystitis Pyelonephritis Prostatitis Epididymo-orchitis

Contact Transmission. Because the process of caring for patients in the hospital often requires significant hands-on contact, caregivers may be the reason for a given infection. For example, Mr. Jones may have soiled his bed with feces. Medical student Orville did not feel it was his job to clean it up, so he performed his daily, albeit brief, exam without addressing the presence of feces. He then proceeded to do his exam on Mrs. Lovely, after washing his hands but not his stethoscope. Mrs. Lovely had had recent abdominal surgery, and had not yet gotten her bowel function back. Medical Student Orville listened for a very long time to her abdomen to see if bowel sounds had returned. In fact, by the time her bowel function did return, she could not go home because she had developed a wound infection with *Klebsiella,* and then Mrs. Lovely really wasn't lovely anymore. Proper and sufficient handwashing and decontamination of devices used between different patients cannot be overemphasized. This is particularly important in the era of multiple drug resistance, when factors that are responsible for resistance can be transmitted from one patient to the next by contact. Thus, in this sense, every hospitalized patient is at risk for being colonized with organisms found almost exclusively in the hospital, even if they have not resided there very long. Because hospital stays are shorter than in the past, many of these patients take such organisms home with them. These organisms do not pose a threat to healthy active people in the home situation.

Habits, Exposures, and Occupation. An essential part of the infectious disease history is determination of exposures of the patient to various infectious hazards. For clarity, these can be divided into geographical, animal exposures, and habitats.

Geographical Exposure. An extensive branch of the discipline of infectious diseases pertains to diseases that can be obtained from other countries. Discussion of fever in a returning traveler is beyond the scope of this chapter. In general, though, travel histories which are recent (i.e., within the past 2-3 months) are the most important, particularly those to underdeveloped countries. Malaria, tuberculosis, hepatitis A, dengue fever, typhoid fever, and typhus are the most notable infectious diseases acquired by travel. However, they are not necessarily the most likely to present in a patient having recently returned from an endemic area. Infectious disease consultation is entirely appropriate in a febrile patient who has recently traveled.

Travel within the United States can also predispose to certain infections. It is less important to define the geography than the type of travel: wooded, mosquito infested, desert, or aquatic. Table 16–5 lists briefly the risk of infection by type of travel.

Animal Exposure. Zoonoses, or infections acquired from animals, are not terribly common in the United States. Very seldom do they present in a patient already hospitalized for other reasons. However, some rare but serious in-

TABLE 16–5. Infection Risk by Type of Travel

Type of Travel	Infection Risk
Wooded areas	Lyme disease Ehrlichia Rocky Mountain Spotted Fever Babesiosis
Mosquito-infested areas	Viral encephalitis
Desert southwest	*Coccidioides immitus* (fungal pathogen that may cause pneumonia or other systemic symptoms)
Rivers and streams	*Giardia lamblia*
Ocean areas	Hepatitis A Infectious gastroenteritis (seafood ingestion)

fections would only be suspected based on the history of animal exposure, so this history is sometimes helpful.

The patient should be characterized in terms of exposure to (1) farms and livestock; (2) outdoor recreational activities; (3) veterinary or research animal lab workers; (4) fishing or exposure to fresh or salt water; and (5) household pets (Table 16–6).

Intravenous Drug Use. The injection drug user is at risk for infection of the skin, soft tissues, and bloodstream. *Staphylococcus aureus,* streptococci, enteric gram negative rods and *Pseudomonas aeruginosa* are the most common pathogens. However, injection drug users sometimes self-administer antibiotics in an attempt to prevent infection. Thus they are at risk for resistant organisms. Because HIV is transmitted by sharing of injection paraphernalia, the index of suspicion must be high that this disease exists in injection drug users, and may be advanced enough to be contributing to the fever. It is not uncommon for persons at risk for HIV to have well-developed systems of denial, so the history of being HIV uninfected may not be a reliable one. Hepatitis B and C are transmitted by sharing needles as well, and may cause fever during acute infection. Finally, the injection drug user is at risk for tuberculosis, as it is seen in lower socioeconomic groups and crowded situations. TB is transmitted by aerosolization (coughing, for example), not by sharing body fluids.

Sexual Habits. In the past, a history of homosexuality prompted concern for HIV infection; today, HIV is just as important in the heterosexual population. A history of multiple partners should prompt concern for HIV. A patient who is monogamous may not volunteer that his or her partner either is an injection drug user or is sexually promiscuous. The sexual history may suggest diagnoses in addition to HIV that pertain to the hospitalized febrile patient. For example, disseminated gonococcal infection is characterized by fever, inflamed tendons or joints, and a pustular rash with a hemorrhagic component. It thus may resemble infective endocarditis, but will not necessarily be suspected without the sexual history. Because Hepatitis B is transmitted sexually, it should also be considered as a reason for fever.

Determination of the Acuity of Infection

Principles used to guide determination of the acuity of infection are the same as determining the acuity of illness in general. In other words, a high fever, though it is neither sensitive nor specific for infection, connotes a sense of urgency. Abnormalities of other vital signs can "triage" a patient to a higher level of acuity: particularly the respiratory rate. This is especially true when it is accompanied by evidence that breathing is requiring a higher than normal expenditure of energy. For example, use of the accessory muscles in the setting of tachypnea is a much more worrisome sign than is tachypnea that seems effortless. In general, signs of mental distress and confusion distinguish the patient in whom illness is acute as well. Such distress may in fact even be subtle; this is evidenced when one considers the appearance of a patient who is at ease versus one who is in pain. It is also helpful when one discovers that fever, in one who has no source identified and who also has no immune defects, has been present for several days. Such a fever is unlikely to be a manifestation of sepsis, and the evaluation may preceed at a more humane pace.

TABLE 16–6. Notable Zoonoses

Organism	Presentation	Animal
Brucellosis (*Brucella spp.*)	Fever without a source	Livestock
Capnocytophaga canimorsus	Sepsis after a bite, particularly in liver disease	Dogs (especially), cats
Cat-scratch disease (*Bartonella spp.*)	Fever, lymphadenopathy	Cats
Leptospirosis (*Leptospira spp.*)	Fever with jaundice, organ failure	Dog or rat urine
Pasteurella multocida	Rapid infection of a bite	Cats (especially), dogs
Plague (*Yersinia pestis*)	Fever, lymphadenopathy, occurring with eschar at site of flea bite	Ground rodents in desert southwest
Psittacosis (*Chlamydia psittaci*)	Pneumonia (atypical pattern)	Birds
Toxoplasmosis (*Toxoplasma gondii*)	Fever, lymphadenopathy (brain abscesses if AIDS)	Cat feces; undercooked meat
Tularemia (*Francisella tularensis*)	Various: fever, pneumonia, pharyngitis, abdominal pain, lymphadenopathy, cutaneous ulcer	Rabbits or other small wild animals

Fever is a common problem in the hospitalized patient. Because it can represent a serious infection that may rapidly worsen, it challenges the practitioner to perform a rapid and thorough evaluation. Most fevers are not serious, so it is not advantageous to treat all fevers with antibiotics. In fact, such a practice has directly contributed to the escalating problem of multidrug resistance among both hospital- and community-acquired organisms. Distinguishing between those patients who need antibiotics and those who do not requires an understanding of certain key concepts, an attention to detail in obtaining the history and physical, and an awareness of what constitutes an infectious disease emergency.

This chapter address critical concepts in the management of infectious diseases, including distinction between colonization and infectious disease, importance of using narrow spectrum antibiotics, and the importance of draining pus. A microbiology primer introduces the reader to key organisms encountered in inpatient practice, the use of the microbiology laboratory, and the pharmacology of antibiotics. Infection control issues also are covered. Chapter 44 discusses the care of patients with fever and infection.

INFECTION CONTROL ISSUES

Infection control practitioners perform a number of vital functions in the hospital. In essence, their role is to decrease

TABLE 16–7. Clinical Syndromes or Conditions Warranting Additional Empiric Precautions to Prevent Transmission of Epidemiologically Important Pathogens Pending Confirmation of Diagnosis[a]

	Clinical Syndrome or Condition[b]	Potential Pathogens[c]	Empiric Precautions
Diarrhea	Acute diarrhea with a likely infectious cause in an incontinent or diapered patient	Enteric pathogens[d]	Contact
	Diarrhea in an adult with a history of recent antibiotic use	Clostridium difficile	
Meningitis		Neisseria meningitidis	Droplet
Rash or exanthems, generalized, etiology unknown	Petechial/ecc hymotic with fever	Neisseria meningitidis	Droplet
	Vesicular	Varicella	Airborne and Contact
	Maculopapular with coryza and fever	Rubeola (measles)	Airborne
Respiratory infections	Cough/fever/upper lobe pulmonary infiltrate in an HIV-negative patient or a patient at low risk for HIV infection	Mycobacterium tuberculosis	Airborne
	Cough/fever/pulmonary infiltrate in any lung location in a HIV-infected patient or a patient at high risk for HIV infection (23)	Mycobacterium tuberculosis	Airborne
	Paroxysmal or severe persistent cough during periods of pertussis activity	Bordetella pertussis	Droplet
	Respiratory infections, particularly bronchiolitis and croup, in infants and young children	Respiratory syncytial or parainfluenza virus	Contact
Risk of multidrug-resistant microorganisms	History of infection or colonization with mulitdrug-resistant organisms[e]	Resistant bacteria[e]	Contact
	Skin, wound, or urinary tract infection in a patient with a recent hospital or nursing home stay in a facility where multidrug-resistant organisms are prevalent	Resistant bacteria[e]	Contact
Skin or wound infection	Abscess or draining wound that cannot be covered	Staphylococcus aureus, group A streptococcus	Contact

[a] Infection control professionals are encouraged to modify or adapt this table according to local conditions. To ensure that appropriate empiric precautions are implemented always, hospitals must have systems in place to evaluate patients routinely according to these criteria as part of their preadmission and admission care.

[b] Patients with the syndromes or conditions listed below may present with atypical signs or symptoms (e.g., pertussis in neonates and adults may not have paroxysmal or severe cough). The clinician's index of suspicion should be guided by the prevalence of specific conditions in the community, as well as clinical judgment.

[c] The organisms listed under the column "Potential Pathogens" are not intended to represent the complete, or even most likely, diagnoses, but rather possible etiologic agents that require additional precautions beyond Standary Precautions until they can be ruled out.

[d] These pathogens include enterohemorrhagic *Escherichia coli* 0157:H7, Shigella, hepatitis A, and rotavirus.

[e] Resistant bacteria judged by the infection control program, based on current state, regional, or national recommendations, to be of special clinical or epidemiological significance.

Source: Taken verbatim from http://www.cdc.gov/ncidod/hip/isolat/isotab_2.htm.

the likelihood that a hospitalized patient will acquire an infection by virtue of being in the hospital. This requires intense information-gathering, or surveillance, often in the form of chart review, but certainly also observations from clinicians. The definition of an epidemic is the development of a number of infections above the level of what is normally expected. It is thus implied that surveillance must be performed initially to see what is normally expected. The clinician plays a key role in determining whether an epidemic is at hand, by contacting infection control practitioners when unusual observations are noted.

The understanding and use of isolation guidelines (Table 16–7) can minimize the occurrence of nosocomial infections. These are based on the Centers for Disease Control (CDC) criteria. More information is available at the CDC website for the Hospital Infections Program (http://www.cdc.gov/ncidod/hip).

REFERENCES

Arnaour, M. A., Hakim, R. M., Todd III, R. F., et al. (1985). Increased expression of an adhesion promoting surface glycoprotein in the granulocytopenia of hemodialysis. *New England Journal of Medicine, 312,* 457.

Esposito, A. L. & Glickman, R. A. (1978). Fever of unknown origin in the elderly. *Journal of the American Geriatric Society, 26,* 498].

Haley, R. W. et al. (1985). The nation-wide nosocomial infection rate: A new need for vital statistics. *American Journal of Epidemiology 121,* 182.

McAlpine, C. H., Martin, B. J., Lennox, I. M., et al. (1986). Pyrexia in infection in the elderly. *Age and Ageing, 15,* 230.

17

Nutritional Problems

Roberta Anding

▶ INTRODUCTION

Medical nutrition therapy is an integral component of the management of many chronic and acute diseases. Nutritional intervention has been shown to promote favorable outcomes and to be cost effective in a variety of clinical conditions (Gallagher-Allred, Voss, Finn, & McCamish, 1996). Nurse practitioners should have a solid foundation in the principles of nutrition in order to provide patients with optimum care. Central to the delivery of care is the understanding of nutritional alterations during starvation versus stress, the nutritional assessment process, and the incorporation of this data into an effective nutritional care plan for patients with common metabolic disorders.

Nutritional Alterations in Starvation

During starvation, physiologic sources of calories include glycogen, somatic (skeletal) and visceral (organ) protein, and fat. In the early hours of a fast, glycogen serves as the primary source of energy. Metabolism favors glucose stability to support tissues that are dependent on glucose as the sole energy source, such as the brain, nerves, red blood cells, and renal medulla. During the initial stages of starvation, a fall in arterial blood glucose causes a decrease in insulin, a major anabolic hormone. As insulin levels fall, the levels of the counter-regulatory or catabolic hormones increase. The major catabolic or opposing hormone to insulin is glucagon. The decrease in the insulin:glucagon ratio stimulates glycogenolysis and the release of hepatic and somatic stores of glucose. Depending on caloric requirements, glycogenolysis is the major source of glucose for the first 16 to 24 hours. Gluconeogenesis from protein serves as the major source of glucose after the initial stage of starvation. As there are no "reserves" of protein, loss of protein can result in loss of physiological function. Urinary losses of nitrogen from protein catabolism can be measured and losses of 12 grams of nitrogen per day become common. As the fast continues, the decreased level of insulin allows lipolysis and the release of free fatty acids (FFA), oxidation of fatty acids, and the synthesis of ketones. The brain cannot use FFA as they do not cross the blood–brain barrier. Free fatty acids condense into ketones and ketoacids can cross the blood–brain barrier and serve as an alternative energy source for the brain, a major consumer of glucose. Ketoadaptation allows protein breakdown to slow and urinary nitrogen losses become approximately 3 to 5 grams per day. Serum proteins such as albumin are relatively well preserved at the expense of somatic protein until the individual is close to death and fat reserves are exhausted. At this point, gluconeogenesis increases, nitrogen excretion increases, and death is imminent.

Concomitantly, a decrease in metabolic rate reduces the caloric needs of the body and slows the rate of deterioration. A decrease in voluntary work and a loss of lean mass from the metabolically active pancreas and gut may also contribute to this hypometabolic state. Additionally, cardiac workload decreases and bradycardia lowers the basal metabolic rate. The classic example of simple starvation, or marasmus, exists in the patient with anorexia nervosa. However, there are also modified implications for the patient on a weight-reduction diet. The caloric value for the pound of lean body mass is approximately 2000 kcal whereas the caloric value of a pound of adipose tissue is 3500 kcal. Therefore, a patient losing weight initially experiences rapid weight loss signaling a loss of lean body mass and fluid. As ketoadaptation ensues, weight loss levels off and patients get discouraged as the calories needed to "lose a pound" increases.

Nutritional Alterations in Stress

Stressed starvation, or hypoalbuminemic malnutrition, has a profound and different effect on body composition, protein utilization, and organ function when compared with simple starvation. During physiologic stress, there is rapid mobilization of body fuels. Glycogen stores are readily exhausted and provide limited caloric support. Protein, through gluconeogenesis, becomes the obligatory source of glucose. Nitrogen losses can be as high as 35 grams per day, significantly greater than simple starvation. Neuroendocrine controls are altered and mediate the changes in nutritional status. Through the actions of catecholamines, glucagon, and cortisol, an abundance of glucose is produced. Glucose serves as the preferred energy source of the brain, fibroblasts, macrophages, and leukocytes. Hyperglycemia results, and insulin release is stimulated, albeit blunted by epinephrine. Elevations in cortisol contribute to the insulin resistance and allow the hyperglycemia to persist. This condition is often referred to as "stress diabetes." The proteinaceous process of gluconeogenesis continues and the loss of protein is more severe and accelerated when compared with unstressed or simple starvation. In this hypermetabolic state, lipolysis mobilizes free fatty acids but there is no significant condensation of FFAs into ketones to serve as an alternate fuel. Significant ketosis does not develop, probably due to the abundance of the anabolic effects of insulin. Consequently, gluconeogenesis continues at a rapid rate at the expense of both somatic and visceral proteins; but no significant ketoadaptation occurs. Endogenous protein continues to be a major source of calories causing a loss of vital lean body mass, which results in the loss of essential immunologic, enzymatic, organ, and structural protein. This failure to ketoadapt has numerous clinical applications. Obese clients are often viewed as having ample caloric reserves. While this is true, the major fuel in stressed starvation is protein, not fat, and therefore these patients are often overlooked or not perceived as being at nutritional risk. Indeed, fat stores are relatively well preserved although the patient loses weight at the expense of lean body mass.

Another clinical application centers around the use of intravenous dextrose as the sole caloric source for physiologically stressed patients. Intravenous dextrose, usually in the form of D_5W, is inadequate caloric support, and indeed, provides only 510 calories and no protein in three liters. Dextrose may also contribute to the insulin surge seen in stress and potentially decrease the body's ability to ketoadapt. A clear understanding of this process also directs the clinician to appropriate decision making regarding the nutritional assessment data needed and in formulating nutritional goals and interventions.

▶ NUTRITIONAL ASSESSMENT

The process of nutritional assessment consists of a dietary history or nutritional intake evaluation, anthropometric measurements, physical examination, and nutritional lab studies. This process should be integrated into any history and physical and the information collected depends on the patient's medical condition and acuity.

Dietary History

In the management of chronic disease, a dietary history is a relatively straightforward, although subjective, process. Clinical dieticians, trained in interviewing, may choose to use a more time-consuming tool, such as food records or food frequency questionnaires. The expertise of a trained dietician improves the accuracy and increases the assurance that the information obtained reflects true intake.

Nurse practitioners and physicians often incorporate into the history and physical an informal 24-hour recall that is designed to provide crude data on dietary intake. The patient is asked to recall all food eaten and beverages consumed over the last 24 hours. Careful open-ended questioning, with attention to portion size, can give a reasonable assessment of intake. Most patients are unable to quantify portions and often underestimate the amount eaten. A rough estimation of a 3-oz. piece of meat is the size of a deck of cards and a 1/2-cup measure is equal to the size of the palm of the hand. Visual aids and food models can assist in this area.

The 24-hour recall is subject to criticism as many individuals may not be able to remember foods eaten and report a "good" or "healthy" diet to please the practitioner, and omit foods perceived as unacceptable such as alcohol and desserts (Dwyer, Krall, & Coleman, 1987). Strategies to enhance the accuracy and reliability of this being a true intake pattern include using open-ended questions, obtaining several random recalls, and providing ample time to obtain the recall. The evaluation of the dietary history obtained can be done by comparing the intake against the Food Pyramid, the Basic Four, or by using a computer software program. Table 17–1 compares the differences in the Basic Four and Food Pyramid.

The Food Pyramid is a wellness or health promotion tool. Because the intent of the Pyramid is wellness, the tool provides the best population guide for the prevention of chronic illness through diet while ensuring nutritional adequacy. The Basic Four can be used as a minimalist approach. This tool represents the minimum amount of food

TABLE 17–1. Recommended Servings

	Basic Four	Food Pyramid
Milk	2	2-3
Bread	4	6-11
Fruits	2	2-4
Vegetables	2	3-5
Meat	2	2-3
Fats/Sugars	Use sparingly	Use sparingly

needed from each group to prevent protein, vitamin/mineral deficiencies, and—with careful food selection—the RDA for vitamins and minerals can be met. This assessment tool may be appropriate to use in geriatrics as many of the elderly cannot consume the amount of food outlined in the Food Pyramid. The RDAs are listed in Table 17–2.

Vitamin and mineral status can be determined by a variety of factors. Fat-soluble vitamins A, D, E, and K are absorbed together with dietary fat and are readily stored in fatty tissues; deficiency states are uncommon, but do occur in fat malabsorption states. Table 17–3 lists the fat-soluble vitamins, function sources, and clinical factors influencing deficiency and toxicity. Due to the storage of these vitamins in fat deposits, toxicity can occur. Toxicity symptoms of vitamin A can occur as little as ten times the RDA.

Water-soluble vitamins are most influenced by dietary intake as they are not stored in appreciable amounts by the body. Disease states significantly alter the physiological demand for water-soluble vitamins. Table 17–4 summarizes the water-soluble vitamins, their functions, sources, and clinical factors influencing deficiency and toxicity.

The assessment of diet takes on a different connotation in the critically ill patient. Frequently it is not feasible to obtain a dietary history from the patient. In these situations, past medical history and pre-existing disease can provide clues as to intake and the likelihood of malnutrition. Patients with a history of alcoholism, pressure sores, inflammatory bowel disease, advanced liver disease, and certain cancers carry an inherent risk of poor dietary intake, and hence malnutrition.

Nutritional intake in the critically ill population is often delivered via either enteral or parenteral nutrition support. In enteral support, product type, strength, volume rate, and tolerance are major contributors to nutritional adequacy. Critically ill patients require increased calories and protein. The calorie/protein content of commonly used enteral products and the volume of the product needed to meet the RDA is given in Table 17–5. There is no RDA for vitamins/minerals in critically ill patients.

Anthropometric Measurements

Anthropometry is the measurement of a part or whole of the body. The most common of these measures is height and weight. These values are extremely important as most estimates of ideal body weight and calorie and protein requirements are based upon height and weight. Determination of desired or ideal body weight can be done numerous ways. Body mass index (BMI) (wt/ht^2) is the current accepted standard. A normal body weight is a BMI of 21-25 and the greatest risk of obesity-related diseases is in patients with a BMI greater than 27. Table 17–6 outlines BMI.

Other estimates of ideal body weight do exist and the Hamwi equation shown in Table 17–7 is one such formula. The advantage of this equation is its simplicity and its clinical utility. Clinicians can use the Hamwi equation as a "ballpark" figure for ideal body weight. However, BMI and estimates of ideal body weight are inadequate alone to determine desired body weight in its relationship to the development of chronic disease. The waist-to-hip ratio is an invaluable clinical anthropometric measure and triage tool to determine the risk or existence of cardiovascular disease, noninsulin dependent diabetes, and hypertension.

In this approach to classifying body fat distribution, the android or upper body fat distribution is characterized by excess fat being stored in the neck region, upper back, and abdomen. It is often referred to as the "apple" body type. Conversely, lower body fat is characterized by body fat accumulation below the waist, generally in the hips and thighs. This type of fat distribution is known as the "pear" body type. A waist-to-hip ratio (WHR) of greater than .8 for women and 1.0 for men is associated with an increased risk of the above-mentioned diseases (Seidel, 1992). The actual numerical calculation is simplistic (W/H) but obtaining the measurement requires diligence. Waist circumference should be obtained at the natural waist or at the level of the umbilicus and the hip measurement at the widest portion of the buttocks (Van Itallie, 1988). Identifying patients at high risk can help the practitioner prioritize those individuals who may require additional diagnostic testing and education. Table 17–8 provides guidelines for evaluating health risks of obesity using both BMI and WHR.

Fat accumulation in the abdominal region occurs in part due to hyperinsulinemia and insulin resistance. Research over the last decade has focused on the link between android obesity and hyperinsulinemia. The role of insulin and insulin resistance in the development of chronic illness is well established. Hyperinsulinemia does not imply diabetes. Hyperinsulinemia may be present in the absence of diabetes or impaired glucose tolerance as a result of overcompensation by the endocrine pancreas. However, there are distinct physiological consequences of hyperinsulinemia. There is a direct relationship between increasing plasma insulin concentration and elevations of blood pressure. Additionally, patients with hyperinsulinemia often have elevations in triglycerides and a decrease in high density lipoprotein, both risk factors in the development of coronary artery disease (Reaven, 1988). This anthropometric guideline provides insight as to the appropriate screening needed.

TABLE 17–2. Food and Nutrition Board, National Academy of Sciences—National Research Council Recommended Dietary Allowances (RDAs)

Age (Years) and Sex Group	Weight		Height		Fat-Soluble Vitamins					Water-Soluble Vitamins		
	kg	*lb*	*cm*	*in.*	*protein*	*vitamin A*	*vitamin B*	*vitamin E*	*vitamin K*	*vitamin C*	*thiamin*	*riboflavin*
					gm	μg Re	μg	mg α-TE	μg	mg	mg	mg
Infants												
0.0-0.5	6	13	60	24	13	375	7.5	3	5	30	0.3	0.4
0.5-1.0	9	20	71	28	14	375	10	4	10	35	0.4	0.5
Children												
1-3	13	29	90	35	16	400	10	6	15	40	0.7	0.8
4-6	20	44	112	44	24	500	10	7	20	45	0.9	1.1
7-10	28	62	132	52	28	700	10	7	30	45	1.0	1.2
Males												
11-14	45	99	157	62	45	1000	10	10	45	50	1.3	1.5
15-18	66	145	176	69	59	1000	10	10	65	60	1.5	1.8
19-24	72	160	177	70	58	1000	10	10	70	60	1.5	1.7
25-50	79	174	176	70	63	1000	5	10	80	60	1.5	1.7
51+	77	170	173	68	63	1000	5	10	80	60	1.2	1.4
Females												
11-14	46	101	157	62	46	800	10	8	45	50	1.1	1.3
15-18	55	120	163	64	44	800	10	8	55	60	1.1	1.3
19-24	58	128	164	65	46	800	10	8	60	60	1.1	1.3
25-50	63	138	163	64	50	800	5	8	65	60	1.1	1.3
51+	65	143	160	63	50	800	5	8	65	60	1.0	1.2
pregnant					60	800	10	10	65	70	1.5	1.6
lactating												
1st 6 months					65	1300	10	12	65	95	1.6	1.8
2nd 6 months					62	1200	10	11	65	90	1.6	1.7

Skinfold thicknesses are another anthropometric measure used in clinical nutrition. Skinfold thicknesses provide an indirect measure of body fat and somatic protein pool. These measures commonly include tricep skinfold thickness, midarm muscle circumference, and the calculated midarm muscle mass. These anthropometric measures may be used in comparison with others of the same sex, and age group. Clinically, the best use of the skinfold measures is to evaluate change in body composition over time. A clinical scenario interpreting skinfold data is given in Table 17–9. Arm circumference and triceps skinfold thickness are measured values. A nomogram for estimating midarm muscle circumference is given in Figure 17–1.

Nutritional Labs

Biochemical markers of nutritional status are a vital component of the nutrition assessment process. Visceral (organ) protein status can be assessed using albumin, transferrin, pre-albumin, and retinol binding protein. These are considered proteins of wellness or homeostasis. Therefore, these proteins are, to a certain degree, affected by physiological stress. During stress, acute phase proteins are synthesized in response to a physiologic insult. These acute phase reactants include interlukin-1, tumor necrosis factor (cachetin), haptoglobin, complement C_3, ceruloplasmin, and clotting factors. The production of acute phase reactants alters the synthesis of the proteins of homeostasis. The redirection in protein synthesis from the proteins of homeostasis to acute phase reactants, coupled with a shift of protein to the interstitial space and often inadequate nutritional support, contributes to the hypoalbuminemia often seen in acutely ill or stressed patients. Albumin levels can decline by 1.0 to 1.5 g/dL within 3 to 5 days of a catabolic illness (Patyek & Blackburn, 1984).

Care must be used when interpreting serum proteins in the differential diagnosis of malnutrition as many non-nutritional factors can influence these proteins. Albumin is the most commonly measured serum protein and the most often affected. Factors influencing albumin levels include hydration status, liver disease, infection, sepsis, cancer, and nephrotic syndrome (Doweiko & Nomgleggi, 1991). Whether albumin is a marker of poor protein intake, injury, or both, it has prognostic value. Mortality risk increases 12-fold with albumin levels of 2.0 g/dL or less (Boosalis & Levine, 1989). Albumin level is also a predictor of immunosuppression. As serum albumin levels decline, there is an increased risk of infection. There is a threefold greater likelihood of pneumonia in older patients with albumin levels of less than 3 g/dL (Garibaldi, Brittmore & Coleman,

TABLE 17–2. *(Continued)*

				Minerals						
niacin	***vitamin*** B_6	***folate***	***vitamin*** B_{12}	***calcium***	***phosphorus***	***magnesium***	***iron***	***zinc***	***iodine***	***selenium***
mg NE	mg	μg	μg	mg	mg	mg	mg	mg	μg	μg
5	0.3	25	0.3	400	300	40	6	5	40	10
6	0.6	35	0.5	600	500	60	10	5	50	15
9	1.0	50	0.7	800	800	80	10	10	70	20
12	1.1	75	1.0	800	800	120	10	10	90	20
13	1.4	100	1.4	800	800	170	10	10	120	30
17	1.7	150	2.0	1200	1200	270	12	15	150	40
20	2.0	200	2.0	1200	1200	400	12	15	150	50
19	2.0	200	2.0	1200	1200	350	10	15	150	70
19	2.0	200	2.0	800	800	350	10	15	150	70
15	2.0	200	2.0	800	800	350	10	15	150	70
15	1.4	150	2.0	1200	1200	280	15	12	150	45
15	1.5	180	2.0	1200	1200	300	15	12	150	50
15	1.6	180	2.0	1200	1200	280	15	12	150	55
15	1.6	180	2.0	800	800	280	15	12	150	55
13	1.6	180	2.0	800	800	280	10	12	150	55
17	2.2	400	2.2	1200	1200	320	30	15	175	65
20	2.1	280	2.6	1200	1200	355	15	19	200	75
20	2.1	260	2.6	1200	1200	340	15	16	200	75

Reprinted with permission from National Academy of Sciences. (1989). Recommended dietary allowances *(10th ed.). Washington, DC: National Academy Press.*

1981). Pinchocofsky-Devin & Kaminsky (1986) demonstrated a relationship between decreasing albumin levels and the development of decubitus ulcers. Research by Brinson and Kolts (1987) suggests that an albumin level of less than 2.6 g/dL may increase the likelihood of tube-feeding intolerance.

In an era of cost containment and an emphasis on decreased length of stay, hypoalbuminemia is a predictor of health-care costs. Reilly and others (1988) demonstrated that patients with a likelihood of malnutrition had an increased cost per patient of $1738; when complications occurred, malnutrition increased costs by $2996 per patient. Of the indicators used in this study, hypoalbuminemia was significantly correlated with increased cost per day, higher total costs, greater number of days in intensive care, and prolonged hospitalization. Drug toxicity can also occur from protein-bound drugs as albumin levels decline. Delirium can be an adverse outcome of hypoalbuminemia, particularly in the elderly. An increase in unbound drug results in greater concentration of drug crossing the blood–brain barrier, contributing to acute neurological changes (Dickson, 1991).

As predictive as low albumin levels can be of morbidity and mortality, they are a relatively poor marker of nutritional repletion. Albumin has a long half-life (20 days) and has a low sensitivity for acute changes in protein status. More sensitive markers of nutritional repletion are available. Transferrin, with a half-life of 8 to 10 days, is a more sensitive marker of protein repletion. Transferrin levels are, however, inversely related to iron stores; concentrations are high with iron deficiency anemia and low when excess iron is being stored. Pregnancy, hypoxia, and chronic blood loss can elevate transferrin levels. Prealbumin and retinol-binding protein are short turnover proteins with half-lives of 1 to 2 days and 10 to 12 hours respectively. These proteins quickly detect changes in protein status and respond promptly to refeeding. Practitioners may be able to avoid unnecessary increase in protein and calorie intake via nutrition support by using these clinical tools (Erstad, Campbell, Rollins & Rappaport, 1994).

Levels of prealbumin are also predictors of morbidity and mortality. Low levels of prealbumin are a predictor of mortality and morbidity in patients undergoing hemodialysis or continuous peritoneal dialysis (Avram, Goldwasser Erroa, & Fein, 1994; Goldwasser et al., 1993). Levels of prealbumin of less than 125 mg/dL carried the highest risk. Retinol binding protein, the transport protein for the retinol form of vitamin A, is in a complex with prealbumin. In healthy individuals the concentrations are very stable, with mean values slightly higher in men (Vahlquist, Peterson, &

(Text continued on p. 200)

TABLE 17–3. Functions and Alterations in Fat-Soluble Vitamins

Vitamin	Function	Food Sources	Deficiency	Factors Influencing Requirements	Signs and Symptoms	Toxicity
Vitamin A (retinoids) beta carotene (precursor)	Visual adaptation adrenal hormone biosynthesis, mucopolysaccharide and glycoprotein synthesis, maintenance of epithelial structure, wound healing, immunocompetence	Whole milk, butter, carrots	Xerophthalmia	Preterm infants, gastrointestinal dysfunction, respiratory ailments, burns, trauma	Night blindness, keratinization of epithelial cells, diarrhea	Nausea, vomiting, alopecia, hypercalcemia, long bone tenderness, pregnant women and persons with chronic renal disease may be more susceptible
Vitamin D cholecalciferol, synthesized via ultraviolet light	Absorption of calcium and phosphorus, calcium reabsorption from kidney, removal of calcium and phosphorus from bone, immunoregulatory	Milk, dairy products	Rickets, osteomalacia	Tropical sprue, regional enteritis, pancreatic insufficiency, gastric resection, jejunoileal bypass, chronic renal failure, hypoparathyroidism, medications (anticonvulsants, cimetidine, isoniazid), total parenteral nutrition	Bone pain, increased serum alkaline phosphatase, decreased serum calcium levels, bone demineralization	Nausea, vomiting, anorexia, headache, diarrhea, confusion, calcification of soft tissue
Vitamin E (tocopherols)	Antioxidant, cell membrane integrity, immunoregulatory	Vegetable oil	Hemolytic anemia	Increased intake of polyunsaturated fats, steatorrhea, protein calorie malnutrition, infancy, cystic fibrosis, short bowel syndrome, respiratory distress syndrome, retrolental fibroplasia, bronchopulmonary dysplasia, smoking	Increased platelet aggregation, neurological abnormalities, decreased serum creatinine, excessive creatinuria	Nausea, headache, antagonist to vitamin K
Vitamin K (phylloquinone) diet (menaquinone) gut flora	Clotting factors	Greens, broccoli, cauliflower	Hemorrhagic disease	Stage of life cycle (newborn, elderly), renal failure, ulcerative colitis, chronic pancreatitis, biliary dysfunction, medications (antibiotics, coumadin, cholestyramine)	Prolonged bleeding times	With prescription menadione, jaundice, anemia

Reprinted with permission from Bullock, B. L. (1996). Pathophysiology: Adaptations and alterations in function *(4th ed.). Philadelphia: Lippincott.*

TABLE 17–4. Functions and Alterations in Water-Soluble Vitamins

Vitamin	Function	Food Sources	Deficiency	Factors Influencing Requirements	Signs and Symptoms	Toxicity
Thiamine	Metabolism through oxidative reaction	Pork, whole grains, organ meats	Beri beri, chronic alcoholism	Alcoholism, fever, infection, hyperthyroidism, burns, trauma, chronic antacid use	Anorexia, fatigue, peripheral neuropathy, foot-drop, cardiomegaly, depression	Nausea and vomiting
Riboflavin	Coenzyme flavin, mononucleotide, citric acid, beta-oxidation	Milk, diary products	Cheilosis, ariboflavinosis	Thyroid dysfunction, burns, trauma, diabetes, alcoholism, oral contraceptives, tricyclic antidepressants	Seborrheic dermatitis, scrotal dermatitis, growth failure, photophobia	None known
Niacin	Coenzyme NAD, NADP, formation of ATP, oxidation/reduction, reactions, immune competence	Mushrooms, enriched grain products, tuna, chicken, can be synthesized from dietary tryptophan	Pellegra	Alcohol, thyroid disorders, neoplasia, isoniazid for TB, burns	Diarrhea, dermatitis, dementia, weakness, fatigue	In large amounts, nicotinic acid functions as a vasodilator; nausea, vomiting, hypo-cholesterolemic effect
Pyridoxine (B_6)	Coenzyme form, pyridoxical phosphate, transamination of amino acids, synthesis of hemoglobin, neurotransmitter synthesis	Meat, fish, poultry, bananas, cantaloupe, broccoli	Irritability, depression	Uremia, burns, advancing age, neoplastic disease, liver disease, medication, uremia, isoniazid, hydralazine, high protein diets, asthma, degenerative diseases	Stomatitis, glosstitis, cheilosis, anemia (after prolonged deficiency)	Irreversible nerve damage, ataxia
Folic acid	One carbon transfer reaction, synthesis of RBC, nucleotides, RNA, DNA, proteins	Orange juice, liver, green leafy vegetables	Megalobastic anemia/ macrocytic anemia	Fevers, burns, alcoholism, ileal disease, inflammatory bowel disease, gluten-induced enteropathy, gastrectomies, periods of increased growth, medications, methotrexates, common deficiency in elderly and adolescent females	Smooth, sore tongue; dementia; diarrhea; weight loss	May mask B_{12} deficiency
B_{12}	Coenzyme transfer of methyl (CH_3) groups, synthesis of nucleic acids and choline, RBC formation	Animal protein	Megaloblastic anemia, pernicious anemia	Vegetarian, gastrectomy patients, ileal resection, gastric bypass surgery, intestinal parasites, medications such as neomycin, potassium chloride	Loss of appetite, weight loss, glossitis, leukopenia, thrombocytopenia, tingling in extremities, dementia	None known
Ascorbic acid (vitamin C)	Collagen formation, cartilage formation, synthesis of bile, acts as a reducing agent, wound healing	Green peppers, citrus fruit, strawberries, broccoli, cabbage	Scurvy	Cigarette smoking, alcoholic, oral contraceptive users, cancer, surgical patients, burns	Capillary fragility, hemorrhagic disorders, fatigue, anorexia, muscle, pain gingivitis	Diarrhea, nausea, excess converted to oxalate and form kidney stones, interfere with urine glucose tests, rebound scurvy

Reprinted with permission from Bullock, B. L. (1996). Pathophysiology: Adaptations and alterations in function *(4th ed.). Philadelphia: Lippincott.*

TABLE 17–5. Enteral Products: Polymeric, High Calorie, High Protein

Product Name	Product Parameters			Vol Needed to Meet RDA
	cal/mL	*Protein g/L*	*mOsm/kg*	
Ensure Plus HN	1.5	62.6	650	947
Pulmocare	1.5	62.6	490	946
Trauma Cal	1.5	82.4	490	1964
Two Cal HN	2.0	83.7	690	946
Polymeric, High Calorie				
Nutren 1.5	1.5	60	530	1400
Nutren 2.0	2.0	80	800	1000
Resource Plus	1.5	55	600	1600
Sustacal HC	1.5	61	650	1183
Ensure Plus	1.5	54.2	690	1425
Isocal HCN	2.0	74.8	690	986
Magnacal	2.0	70	590	1000
Polymeric, High Nitrogen				
Ensure HN	1.06	44	470	1329
entrition HN	1.00	44	300	1300
Isocal HN	1.06	44	300	1183
Isosource HN	1.20	53	330	1500
Osmolite HN	1.06	44.4	300	1330
Polyumeric with Fiber				
Enrich	1.10	39.7	480	1392
Jevity	1.06	44.4	310	1324
Pro Fiber	1.00	40	300	1500
Sustacal with Fiber	1.06	46	450	1391
Fibersource	1.20	43	390	1500
Defined/Elemental Diets				
Criticare HN	1.06	38	650	1893
Peptumen	1.00	40	240	2000
Pepti-2000	1.00	40	490	1600
Precision Isotonic	1.00	29	300	1560
Precision HN	1.05	44	525	2850
Reabilan	1.00	31.5	350	2250
Reabilan HN	1.33	58	490	2494
Tolerex	1.00	20.6	550	1800
Traum-AID HBC	1.00	56	760	3000
Travasorb HN	1.00	45	560	2000
Vital HN	1.00	42	500	1500
Vivonex T.E.N.	1.00	38	630	2000
Periative	1.30	67	385	1155
Alitraq	1.00	52.5	575	1500

Reprinted with permission from Ruppert, S. D., Kernicki, J. G., & Dolan, J. T. (1996). Dolan's critical care nursing clinical management through the nursing process *(2nd ed.). Philadelphia: F. A. Davis.*

Wilbell, 1973). Concentrations of retinol binding protein are decreased in liver disease, hyperthyroidism, and cystic fibrosis (Rask et al., 1980). Table 17–10 gives a guide to the classification of protein depletion.

Cholesterol values have two distinct and opposing functions as an assessment of nutritional status. In young adults, cholesterol values of greater than 200 mg/dL are associated with an increased risk of cardiovascular disease (CAD) and should alert the practitioner to focus on family history of cardiovascular disease and perhaps obtain a lipoprotein analysis. Figure 17–2 provides a risk classification scheme for evaluating lipoprotein analysis data (Expert Panel, 1993). Hypocholesterolemia, however, should also warrant investigation. Low cholesterol values are often found in patients with inflammatory bowel disease, reflecting the severity of bile malabsorption. Bile, which is 70% cholesterol, is normally recycled via enterohepatic circulation. Malabsorption of bile, therefore, represents a loss of recycled cholesterol. As with albumin, cholesterol levels decline with malnutrition and are under the influence of cytokines. Low cholesterol values in the geriatric population are indicative of poor health status and requires further investigation and assessment of nutrition status (Goichot, Schlienger, Grunenberger, Pradignac, & Aby, 1995).

Physical Examination

Physical exam encompasses both the gross assessment of nutritional deficiencies outlined in Tables 17–3 and 17–4, but also the assessment of muscular function. This assessment includes hand grip strength, respiratory muscle strength, and response of the adductor pollices to electrical stimulation. Changes in muscular strength occur rapidly and can be used to evaluate the effectiveness of nutritional support (Russell, Lester, & Whitwell, 1983). These assessment tools have been shown to have a greater predictive value of postoperative complications than weight loss (Windsor & Hill, 1988).

Nutrition Assessment Tools

Screening tools encompassing most of the individual components listed above can be used to assess a patient's nutritional status. Those most commonly used in hospitalized patients include the Subjective Global Assessment (SGA) and Prognostic Nutritional Index (PNI). The SGA combines historical data with symptoms, such as nausea, vomiting, diarrhea, and physical parameters (Baker, Detsky, Wesson, & Wolman, 1982). The SGA has been shown to give reproducible results with more than an 80% agreement among double-blinded observers (Baker et al., 1982). The SGA is a good predictor of malnutrition in surgical patients and those undergoing dialysis (Enia, Sicuso, Alti, & Zocalli, 1993). The Prognostic Nutritional Index incorporates objective measurements of serum proteins, tricep skinfold, and immunologic function. It predicts risk of postoperative complications in patients undergoing surgery (Mullen, Buzby, & Matthews, 1980). Table 17–11 compares these tools.

▶ COMMON METABOLIC DISTURBANCES

Obesity

Obesity is a cause or contributor to many chronic illnesses facing Americans. Many of the medical conditions managed by nurse practitioners have obesity as an underlying factor. A recent survey indicates that the incidence of obesity in the United States is rising from 25% in 1980 to 33.4% in 1992. Obesity is a multifactorial disorder influenced by genetics, inactivity, and inappropriate dietary habits. Minority populations and the poor may be particularly affected (Kuzmarski, Flegal, Campbell, & Johnson, 1994). Inactivity may be the major contributor to the increase in obesity. Calorie intake has decreased by 10% in the last century but the incidence of obesity has doubled during that time span (Pi-Sunyer, 1988). Even more troubling is the fact that since 1975, obesity in children ages 6 to 11 has increased by 54% and by 39% in the 12- to 17-year-old group. Approximately 40% of children who are obese at age 7 will be obese adults (Morgan, 1988). Clearly, obesity is a major public health problem and despite the fact Americans spend more than $33 billion on weight control products, we are clearly getting heavier (Foreyt & Goodrich, 1995).

Obesity is generally defined as being 20% above ideal body weight (IBW), and severely obese as 40% above IBW. Ideal body weight estimates are found in Table 17–7. A body mass index of greater than 27 may also be used and is the preferred method. Although these definitions are relatively well accepted, the treatment approach used for the management of obesity must assess readiness to diet and integrate lifestyle, culture, age, activity, and body fat distribution. The treatment of obesity has a high recidivism rate and, therefore, initial goals should not be overly ambitious. Prevention of weight gain, particularly in women, should be of paramount importance. Weight gain of as little as ten pounds for women carries an increased risk of mortality from all causes (Manson et al., 1995). Many chronic conditions associated with obesity, such as non-insulin dependent diabetes, may benefit from as little as a 10 to 20 pound weight loss.

Caloric prescription for weight loss can be determined using a variety of approaches. Weight-reduction diets can be prescribed by reducing daily intake by approximately 500 kcal/day, which provides a 1-pound-per-week loss. This approach requires the practitioner to have a thorough knowledge of calories in foods. An alternate approach allows 25 kcal/kg of ideal body weight. A third approach uses the ideal body weight multiplied by 10. For example, a woman 5′4″ who weighs 180 lb (IBW = 120) is allowed 1200 kcal per day. This approach is simple and easy to use. Adjustments may be necessary to enhance compliance, but this prevents picking a "one size fit all" method to prescribing calories.

The Harris–Benedict Equation (Table 17–12), often used for the critically ill, can also provide resting energy expenditure (REE) that can be used to provide a caloric level for weight reduction. This equation may be technically the most accurate but also the most time consuming. The distribution of the calories prescribed may be equally important.

Most popular weight-reduction programs, such as the American Heart Association diet plans, provide a high-carbohydrate, low-fat approach that are appropriate for most individuals. However, obesity is often accompanied by an increase in beta cell production of insulin and a peripheral resistance to insulin, resulting in hyperinsulinemia. This condition is manifested in those individuals with an elevated waist-to-hip ratio. High carbohydrate diets may ag-

TABLE 17–6. Body Weight (in pounds) According to Height (in inches) and Body Mass Index

	19	20	21	22	23	24	25	26	27	28	29	30	31	32	33	34
Height								***Body Weight***								
58	91	95	100	105	110	114	119	124	129	133	138	143	148	152	157	162
59	94	99	104	109	114	119	124	129	134	144	144	149	154	159	164	169
60	97	102	107	112	117	122	127	132	138	148	148	153	158	163	168	173
61	101	106	111	117	122	127	132	138	143	154	154	159	164	169	175	180
62	103	109	114	120	125	130	136	141	147	158	158	163	168	174	179	185
63	107	113	119	124	130	135	141	147	152	164	164	169	175	181	186	192
64	111	117	123	129	135	141	146	152	158	170	170	176	182	187	193	199
65	114	120	126	132	138	144	150	156	162	174	174	180	186	192	198	204
66	118	124	131	137	143	149	156	162	168	180	180	187	193	199	205	212
67	121	127	134	140	147	153	159	166	172	185	185	191	198	204	210	217
68	125	132	139	145	152	158	165	172	178	191	191	198	205	211	218	224
69	128	135	142	149	155	162	169	176	182	196	196	203	209	216	223	230
70	133	140	147	154	161	168	175	182	189	203	203	210	217	224	231	237
71	136	143	150	157	164	171	179	186	193	207	207	214	221	229	236	243
72	140	148	155	162	170	177	185	192	199	214	214	221	229	236	244	251
73	143	151	158	166	174	181	189	196	204	219	219	226	234	241	249	257
74	148	156	164	171	179	187	195	203	210	226	226	234	242	249	257	265
75	151	159	167	175	183	191	199	207	215	231	231	239	247	255	263	271
76	156	164	172	181	189	197	205	214	222	238	238	246	255	263	271	279

gravate the hyperinsulinemia. A moderate-carbohydrate, higher unsaturated fat diet may be desirable (Kaplan, 1989). Table 17–13 provides a comparison between these dietary distributions.

Health-care professionals often label patients noncompliant when, in fact, the calorie prescription and distribution are inaccurate. The above strategies enable the patient to lose 1 to 2 pounds per week enhanced with an exercise program. Calorie levels less than 1200 require a multivitamin–mineral supplement. Patients who are severely obese, BMI > 30, may ideally require a more aggressive approach. Very low calorie diets are indicated for those individuals who are severely overweight (American Dietetic Association, 1990). Very low calorie diets (VLCDs) are defined as diets consisting of 400 to 800 kcal per day. Protein intake is usually set at 1.5 gm/kg/IBW and is enriched with vitamins, minerals, and electrolytes. These diets are usually administered in a liquid form and commercially prepared formulas are available. Typically, the VLCD is used for a period of 12 to 16 weeks with a gradual refeeding program that lasts 4 to 8 weeks. A behavioral and nutritional counseling program is recommended as part of the program. Short-term results can be dramatic with an average weight loss of 20 kg in 12 weeks (*Journal of the American Medical Association* [*JAMA*], 1993). In comparison, patients on traditional low-calorie diets lose 8 to 10 kg in a 20- to 24-week program (Wadden, Foster, Letizia, & Stunkard, 1992). Few longitudinal studies exist regarding the long-term results of the VLCD. Research by Wadden et al., compared the results of a VLCD with a traditional weight-loss program for 7-8 weeks with long-term follow-up. Although the initial losses were greater on the VLCD, there were no significant differences in the groups at the end of the study (Wadden, Foster, & Letizia, 1994). Therefore, although initial losses are substantial, VLCDs may not provide significant long-term advantages and may indeed be more costly.

Contraindications to the VLCD include renal disease, liver disease, cerebrovascular disease, and insulin dependent diabetes (American Diabetic Association, 1997; *JAMA*, 1993). Blood chemistries and electrocardiograms must be obtained at regular intervals to monitor electrolytes and cardiac function. VLCDs have not been found to produce cardiac abnormalities when used for up to 12 weeks, nor do they cause a permanent decrease in metabolic rate or lean body mass as is often reported (*JAMA*, 1993). Currently, no weight-loss program has shown consistently favorable results over the long-term, indicating that diet alone may not control obesity. Certainly, physical activity is an essential component of a weight-management program and the key element in the prevention of obesity. Research suggests that exercise may produce moderate weight loss in comparison to diet alone, but positively impact central body fat accumulation, thereby reducing cardiovascular risk factors (Pritchard, Nowson, & Wark, 1997).

Diabetes

Diabetes is one of the most common metabolic disturbances facing Americans. Approximately 6% of Americans have diabetes with an estimated 8 million yet to be diagnosed. Of the individuals with diabetes, 95% have type 2 diabetes (American Diabetes Association, 1997). Approximately 80 to 90% of these patients are obese. The remainder of these

TABLE 17–6. *(Continued)*

Height	35	36	37	38	39	40	41	42	43	44	45	46	47	48	49	50
								Body Weight								
58	167	172	176	181	186	191	195	200	205	210	214	219	224	229	233	238
59	174	179	184	188	193	198	203	208	213	218	223	228	233	238	243	248
60	178	183	188	194	199	204	209	214	219	224	229	234	239	244	250	255
61	85	191	196	201	207	212	217	222	228	233	238	244	249	254	260	265
62	90	196	201	206	212	217	223	228	234	239	245	250	255	261	266	272
63	198	203	209	214	220	226	231	237	243	248	254	260	265	271	277	282
64	205	211	217	223	228	234	240	246	252	258	264	269	275	281	287	293
65	210	216	222	228	234	240	246	252	258	264	270	276	282	288	294	300
66	218	224	230	236	243	249	255	261	268	274	280	286	292	299	305	311
67	223	229	236	242	248	255	261	268	274	280	287	293	299	306	312	319
68	231	238	244	251	257	264	271	277	284	290	297	304	310	317	323	330
69	236	243	250	257	263	270	277	284	290	297	304	311	317	324	331	338
70	244	251	258	265	272	279	286	293	300	307	314	321	328	335	342	349
71	250	257	264	271	279	286	293	300	307	314	321	329	336	343	350	357
72	258	266	273	281	288	295	303	313	317	325	332	340	347	354	362	369
73	264	272	279	287	294	302	309	317	324	332	340	347	355	362	370	377
74	273	281	288	296	304	312	319	327	335	343	351	358	366	374	382	390
75	279	287	294	302	310	318	326	334	342	350	358	366	374	382	390	398
76	287	296	304	312	320	328	337	345	353	361	370	378	386	394	402	411

individuals have type 1 (insulin dependent) diabetes. Diabetes has a major social and economic impact. Fifteen percent of health-care costs or $105 billion annually is spent on diabetes, primarily in acute care settings. In 1992, the cost of treating each person with diabetes per year was more than $11,000 (Rubin & Altman, 1994). It is the leading cause of blindness, renal failure, and nontraumatic amputations in adults (Harris, 1995). The incidence of diabetes is increasing with 625,000 new cases being diagnosed yearly (Rubin & Altman, 1994). Although hyperglycemia is a central feature to both types of diabetes, the nutritional goals and the medical nutritional therapy are quite different.

Type 1 Diabetes

The goals of medical nutritional therapy have changed dramatically over the last 5 years. Currently, there is no "one" diet for the control of type 1 diabetes. In fact, the American Diabetes Association (Schafer et al., 1997) has recommended the abandonment of the term "ADA" diet. The term "ADA" diet generally implied that a practitioner prescribed a calorie level that was translated into an exchange-diet format. Instead, the nutritional care for patients with type 1 diabetes has been revolutionized by the multicenter results from the Diabetes Control and Complications Trial. This study provided the evidence that the control of blood glucose levels to near normal values can prevent retinopathy, neuropathy, and nephropathy associated with diabetes. With the results of the DCCT as a guide, many patients are striving for tighter control or are being urged by practitioners towards that goal. A variety of dietary approaches can be used to obtain optimal glycemic control. Most practitioners agree that diet constitutes the biggest barrier to comprehensive diabetes control. Patients are often labeled noncompliant or not motivated when, in fact, they have not received appropriate nutrition education (Arnold, Stephen, Jess, & Hiss, 1993). Therefore, individual assessment is critical in guiding patients toward improved control.

The most commonly recognized dietary approach for the management of type 1 diabetes is still the Exchange System for Meal Planning. The exchange lists were developed in the 1950s as a method of classifying commonly used foods by their carbohydrate, protein, and fat contents.

TABLE 17–7. Quick Estimation of Ideal Body Weight

Men

For 5 feet, consider 106 pounds a reasonable weight
For each inch over 5 feet, add 6 pounds
Subtract 6 pounds for each inch under 5 feet
Add 10 percent for a large-framed individual; subtract 10 percent for a small-framed individual
Example: A man 5 feet 8 inches tall (medium frame) would start at 106 pounds, add 48, and arrive at a reasonable weight of 154 pounds

Women

For 5 feet, consider 100 pounds a reasonable weight
For each inch over 5 feet, add 5 pounds
Subtract 5 pounds for each inch under 5 feet
Add 10 percent for a large-framed individual; subtract 10 percent for a small-framed individual
Example: A woman 5 feet 6 inches tall (medium frame) would start at 100 pounds, add 30, and arrive at a reasonable weight of 130 pounds

U. S. Department of Agriculture and U. S. Department of Health and Human Services. (1990). Nutrition and your health. Dietary guidelines for Americans *(3rd ed.).*

TABLE 17–8. Health Risks of Obesity

	Body Mass Index (BMI)									
	25	26	27	28	29	30	31	32	33	...
No Comorbidities WHR not Elevated	◄ Slight	►	◄	Moderate		►	◄	High		...
Comorbidities and/or WHR Elevated	◄ Moderate	►	◄	High		►	◄	Very High		...

Reprinted with permission from Thomas, P. R. (Ed.). (1995). Criteria for evaluating weight management programs. *Washington, DC: National Academy Press.*

In the 1950s, mixed dishes, convenience foods, and frequent dining out were rare as opposed to eating patterns of today. Recently revised, the 1995 exchange groups have been divided into three major groups: carbohydrates, meat and meat substitutes, and fat. Table 17–14 gives an overview of the exchange groups.

The traditional use of the exchange system for patients with type 1 diabetes relies on an accurate assessment of caloric needs and weighing/measuring food. As most patients with type 1 diabetes are lean, caloric prescription provides a significant challenge for practitioners. The Harris–Benedict Equation is one approach using adults and the formula is listed in Table 17–12. It is not essential, however, that initially a precise calorie level be determined by the practitioner. Carbohydrate control is of primary importance as protein and fat have a negligible effect on blood glucose. Prescribing total carbohydrate and matching it to the insulin given have replaced rigid systems of the past. During the follow-up period, one can estimate the calories needed, and adjustments can be made, realizing that protein and fat consumption may be loosely controlled. The focus is on matching total amount of carbohydrate or exchanges to insulin, and not prescribing a set number of meat or fat exchanges. An estimate of caloric needs for lean individuals can be determined by the formula in Table 17–15.

After the determination of calories, the distribution of calories into carbohydrate, protein, and fat is the next step. In general, for patients with type 1 diabetes carbohydrate percentage should be approximately 50 to 60%, protein 20%, and fat between 20 to 30%. There is no evidence that simple sugars aggravate hyperglycemia more than complex carbohydrates; therefore, it is the total carbohydrate content that is important rather than the source (Loghmani et al., 1991). Caution should be used to incorporate individual nutrition assessment and preferences into applying the above percentages. After the calculation of calories and distribution of nutrients, the food is systematically matched to the peak and duration of insulin. In general terms, clients with type 1 diabetes require three meals per day and two to three snacks.

Carbohydrate counting is a tool that is specifically focused on the techniques to optimize blood glucose levels and is less rigorous than an exchange approach. In type 1 diabetes, carbohydrate counting matches pre-meal insulin doses to the carbohydrate content of the food to be consumed. A quick estimate of the insulin demand created by a meal or snack can be calculated by counting the grams of carbohydrate a food contains. This can be done precisely through a food label and accurate determination of portion size or estimated through the use of the exchange system. In clinical practice, it is preferable to teach patients the carbohydrate content of foods via the exchange system so that a method of estimating carbohydrate becomes ingrained. This allows for greater flexibility and accuracy when dining out or when food labels are unavailable.

For an individual patient, there is an identifiable ratio between the grams of carbohydrate consumed and the amount of insulin required to metabolize them. In general, this ratio is one unit regular insulin per 15 grams of carbohydrate. Factors that influence this ratio include the patient's body size and activity level. Athletic patients require less insulin, thereby increasing the ratio. Overweight patients require more insulin, thereby decreasing the ratio. Intermediate insulin is given to cover the endogenous production of glucose and the moderate amount of glucose derived from dietary protein and fat. Boluses of regular insulin do not need to be given with CHO intake of less than 15 grams, but rather should be used to cover specific meals and snacks. Care must be exercised to not give too many boluses, as regular insulin does have a discernable peak and duration, and peaks may inadvertently overlap producing hypoglycemia. Carbohydrate counting requires patients with type 1 diabetes to perform self-glucose monitoring, but allows more flexibility than an exchange approach. Registered dieticians, with advanced certification as diabetes educators, are an essential component of a carbohydrate

TABLE 17–9. Case Study–Interpretation of Skinfold Data

J.T. is an 85-year-old woman who is 5′4″ and weighs 210 lb. She was recently in a motor vehicle accident and sustained multiple broken bones and soft tissue trauma. Upon admission to the ICU, her triceps' skinfold (TSF) was 38 mm (95th%), her arm circumference (AC) was 39 cm, and her midarm muscle circumference (MAMC) was 25 cm (76th%). Three weeks later J.T. is serially reassessed and the following data was obtained: TSF, 36 mm (90th%); AC, 33 cm; and MAMC, 20.5 (62nd%). Clearly, the data show that there has been a loss of lean body mass or somatic protein stores while the fat stores have been relatively well preserved. J.T. was obese upon admission, but the physiological stress has caused an obligatory loss of lean body mass as indicated by a change in the skinfold measure.

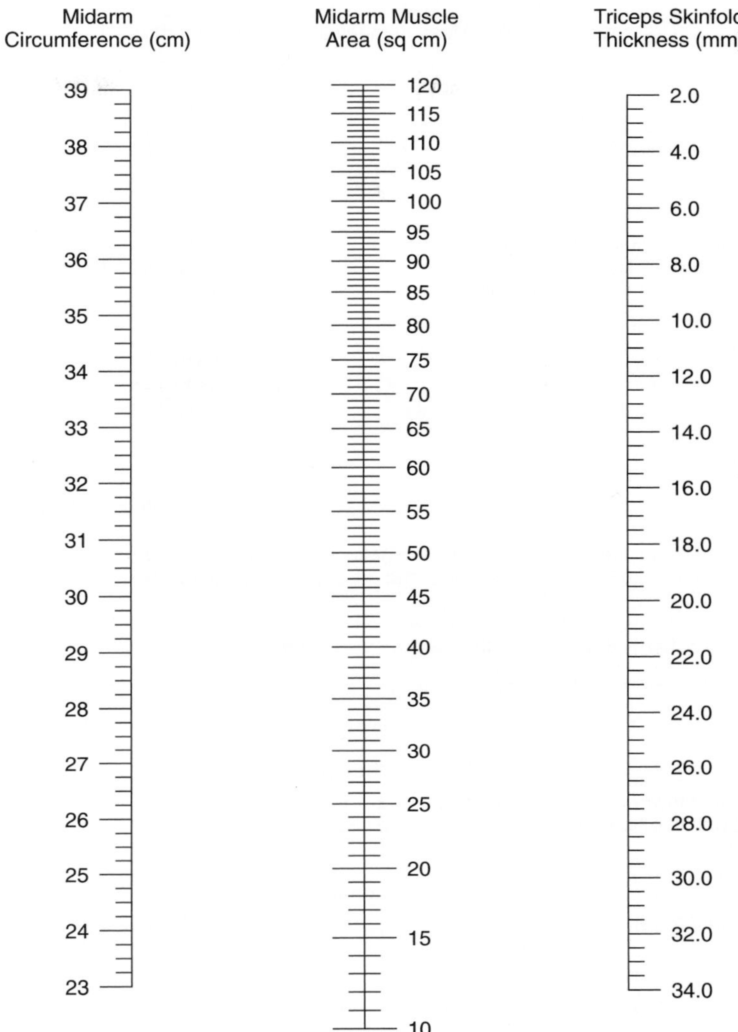

Figure 17–1. Nomogram for the determination of mid-upper-arm muscle area for adults.

counting regimen and are an integral part of any diabetes team.

Caring for patients with type 1 diabetes in the acute care setting provides a challenge for practitioners. Changes in routine, diet, exercise, infection, and surgical procedures make optimal blood glucose control difficult. Infection, catabolic illnesses, and physiological stress can cause significant hyperglycemia independent of food intake. Diligent monitoring of blood glucose levels is critical and insulin requirements should be adjusted accordingly. Decreasing the caloric intake to control hyperglycemia is inappropriate; insulin adjustments must be made. Postsurgical diets should be initiated quickly and progression from clear liquids to full liquids should occur as rapidly as tolerated. Clear liquid

TABLE 17–10. Relationship Between Nutritional Depletion and Serum Proteins

		Degree of Depletion		
Indicator	**Normal**	***Mild***	***Moderate***	***Severe***
Albumin (g/dL)	3.5–5.5	2.8–3.4	2.1–2.7	<2.1
Transferrin (mg/dL)	180–260	150–200	100–149	<100
Prealbumin (mcg/dL)	200–300	100–150	50–90	<50
Retinol-binding protein (mcg/dL)	40–50	—	—	—

Reprinted with permission from Whitney, E. N., Cataldo, C. B., & Rolfes, S. R. (1994). Understanding normal and clinical nutrition *(4th ed.). Minneapolis, MN: West.*

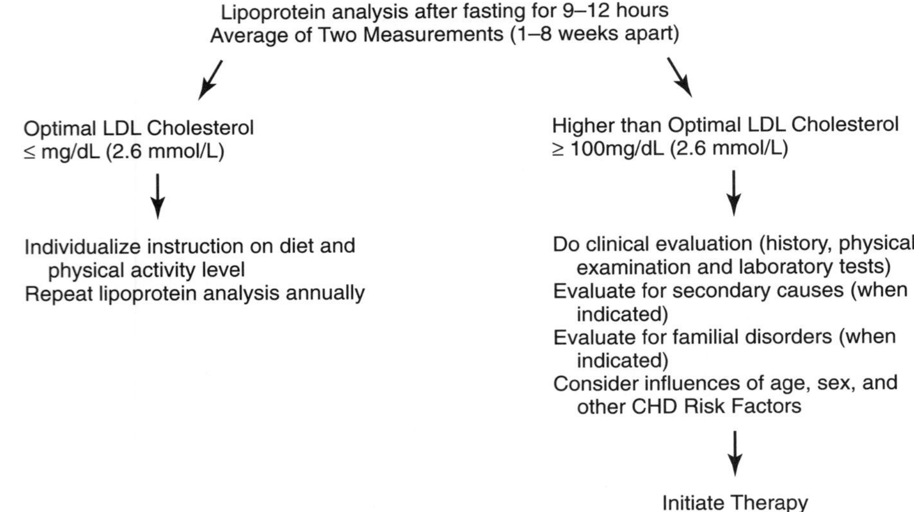

- Lipoprotein analysis should be performed when the patient is not in the recovery phase from an acute coronary or other medical event that would lower the usual LDL-cholesterol level.
- If the first two LDL-cholesterol test results differ by more than 30 mg/dL (0.7 mmol/L), a third test result would be obtained within 1–8 weeks and the average value of the three tests used.

Patient Category	Initiation Level	LDL Goal
Dietary Therapy		
Without CHD and with fewer than two risk factors	≥ 160 mg/L (4.1 mmol/L)	< 160 mg/L (4.1 mmol/L)
Without CHD and with two or more risk factors	≥ 130 mg/L (3.4 mmol/L)	< 130 mg/L (3.4 mmol/L)
With CHD	> 100 mg/L (2.6 mmol/L)	≤ 100 mg/L (2.6 mmol/L)
Drug Treatment		
Without CHD and with fewer than two risk factors	≥ 190 mg/L (4.9 mmol/L)	< 160 mg/L (4.1 mmol/L)
Without CHD and with two or more risk factors	≥ 160 mg/L (4.1 mmol/L)	< 130 mg/L (3.4 mmol/L)
With CHD	≥ 130 mg/L (3.4 mmol/L)	≤ 100 mg/L (2.6 mmol/L)

Figure 17–2. Classification and treatment decisions based on LDL cholesterol level. *(Reprinted with permission from Expert Panel on Detection, Evaluation and Treatment of High Blood Cholesterol in Adults. [1993].)*

or full liquid diets should consist of approximately 200 grams of carbohydrate per day, equally divided into three meals and three snacks. Sugar-free liquids are inappropriate other than for hydration (American Diabetes Association, 1997).

The majority of patients have type 2 or non-insulin dependent diabetes. Weight reduction is the cornerstone of therapy for obese patients with type 2 diabetes. Although the DCCT was conducted to evaluate the risk and benefits of tight control on type 1 diabetes, it is generally accepted that the results are applicable to type 2 diabetes. Indeed, research has suggested that intensive insulin therapy in type 2 diabetes may be more effective in lowering glycosolated hemoglobin than diet or oral agents (Colwell, 1996).

TABLE 17–11. Screening Tools for Hospitalized Patients

Screening Tools	Parameters Assessed
Subjective Global Assessment (SGA)	Weight change, dietary intake, gastrointestinal symptoms (nausea, vomiting diarrhea) edema, muscle wasting
Prognostic Nutritional Index	Albumin, transferrin, tricep skinfold thickness, delayed cutaneous hypersensitivity

The principles of weight loss outlined for the obese patient certainly apply to obese patients with type 2 diabetes. A recent metaanalysis suggests that dietary interventions are the most effective strategy in the reduction of fasting blood glucose, glycosolated hemoglobin, and cardiovascular risk factors. Interestingly, although the exchange system historically has been the most commonly prescribed dietary strategy, little clinical research has been conducted to evaluate its effectiveness as a weight-loss tool (Brown, Upchurch, Anding, Winter, & Ramirez, 1996).

TABLE 17–12. Harris Benedict Equation with Long Adjustment Factors

Resting energy expenditures is equal to:

Women:
$655 + (9.6 \times w) + (1.7 \times h) - (4.7 \times a)$

Men:
$66 + (13.7 \times w) + (5 \times h) - (6.8 \times a)$
w = actual weight in kilograms
h = height in centimeters
a = age in years

Activity factor:
BEE × 1.2 = sedentary
BEE × 1.3 = active

Stress factor:
Skeletal trauma × 1.35
Sepsis × 1.60
Severe thermal injury × 2.10

Reprinted with permission from Long, C. L., Schaffel, N., & Gerger, J. W. (1979). Metabolic response to injury and illness: Estimation of energy and protein needs from indirect calorimetry and nitrogen balance. Journal of Parenteral and Enteral Nutrition, 3, *452–456.*

This meta-analysis validates the findings of others indicating that a weight loss of as little as 10 to 20 pounds improves blood glucose control, even if ideal body weight has not been achieved (American Diabetic Association, 1997). Weight loss has a positive effect on B-cell function and insulin sensitivity that characterizes the insulin resistance often associated with the obesity of diabetes. Breaking the cycle of chronic hyperglycemia through caloric restriction is critical as unchecked hyperglycemia has toxic effects on the pancreas impairing further insulin secretion and sensitivity (Yki-Järvinen, 1992). However, in order for caloric restriction and possible weight loss to be effective, the patient's input, readiness to change, and the development of a meal plan and exercise program is crucial.

Many patients with type 2 diabetes remain undiagnosed for a number of years and therefore, at presentation, may already have developed complications. Cardiovascular disease remains the leading cause of death in patients with type 2 diabetes and it is two to six times more common in people with diabetes than in the general population (Wingard & Barrett-Connor, 1995). Arteriosclerosis in diabetes is multifactorial. Diabetic dyslipidemia is somewhat unique and the modification of the guidelines of the National Cholesterol Education Program have been suggested (Garg & Grundy, 1990). The lipid abnormalities seen in type 2 diabetes include elevation of very low density lipoprotein (VLDL) triglycerides/low density lipoproteins (LDL) and a decrease in high density lipoprotein (HDL). In a given patient, total cholesterol may only be mildly elevated, but coupled with high triglycerides and low HDL, a significant cardiovascular risk is present. A total cholesterol alone, therefore, is inadequate for assessment of cardiovascular risk.

TABLE 17–13. Caloric Distribution Based on Body Composition

	Gynoid Obesity	Android Obesity
Carbohydrate	50–60%	35–40%
Protein	20%	20%
Fat	20–30%	40–45%
Less than 10% saturated fat		

Adequate control of hyperglycemia, as measured by hemoglobin A_1C, may also reduce cardiovascular risk. Elevations in HgA_1C are a significant risk factor for CHD particularly in women (Singer, Nathan, Anderson, Wilson, & Evans, 1992). Hyperglycemia leads to a glycosolation of serum proteins including LDL and HDL, which has harmful effects (Bierman, 1992).

Dyslipidemia in diabetes is also associated with a procoagulant state linked with hypertriglyceridemia. There is an increase in clotting activities of thrombogenic factors such as factor VII and factor X that may lead to thrombosis.

Microalbuminuria and renal disease are also a risk factor or predictive of CHD in type 2 diabetes. Dietary strategies to manage type 2 diabetes with CHD focus on weight control as a means to control hyperglycemia and manage dyslipidemia. A comprehensive overview of dietary man-

TABLE 17–14. Exchange List Overview

Exchange List	Carbohydrate (g)	Protein (g)	Fat (g)
Carbohydrate Containing:			
Starch	15	3	1 gram or less
Fruit	15	—	—
Vegetables	5	2	—
Milk			
Skim	12	8	0–3
Low-fat	12	8	5
Whole	12	8	8
Other (chips, biscuits)	15	Varies	Varies

TABLE 17–15. Estimate of Caloric Requirements in Lean Individuals

IBW × 10 = BEE		
Plus	30%	for sedentary
	50%	for moderately active
	100%	for vigorously active

TABLE 17–16. General Guidelines for Exercise in Diabetes

Summary of Guidelines
- Avoid exercise in extremes of temperature
- Inspect feet daily
- Avoid exercise if metabolic control is poor

Type 1	Type 2
Benefits • Improvement in cardiovascular function • Improvement in well-being	*Benefits* • Reduction of cardiovascular risk factor • Potential weight loss
Risk • Hypoglycemia • Hyperglycemia/ketosis • Cardiovascular ischemia • Traumatic/repetitive use injury	Risk • Pre-exercise evaluation needed to assess for undiagnosed complications • Cardiovascular ischemia • Traumatic/repetitive use injury

agement of cardiovascular disease is covered in the following section. The importance of physical activity in preventing and managing type 2 diabetes and its associated coexisting disease states cannot be minimized. Clinical practice recommendations for exercise prescriptions are summarized in Table 17–16 (American Diabetes Association, 1997).

Diabetic Nephropathy

Diabetic nephropathy, a microvascular complication, is most often associated with type 1 diabetes. However, given the incidence of type 2 diabetes being ten times that of type 1 diabetes, the economic, physiological, and psychological burden of end stage renal disease is equally distributed between type 1 diabetes and type 2 diabetes (Alzaid, 1996). Recent developments in the detection of early nephropathy through the measurement of microalbuminuria has allowed for earlier dietary and pharmacological intervention. Angiotensin converting enzyme (ACE) inhibitors have been shown to be effective in controlling microalbuminuria (Clark & Guiterrez, 1992) and delaying the onset and progression of diabetic nephropathy. Earlier detection of renal impairment has led to renewed interest in dietary manipulations designed to preserve renal function. In principle, the reduction of dietary protein, phosphorus, and sodium are the mainstays of medical nutrition therapy. Protein allowances are restricted to the RDA of .8 gm/kg IBW, phosphorus to 8 to 12 mg/kg IBW, and sodium to 1000 to 3000 mg. In practice, this represents a significant deviation from most dietary intakes (American Diabetes Association, 1994). Diligent control of hyperglycemia is an integral part of the dietary management of early diabetic nephropathy. Results from the DCCT indicate that intensive diabetes treatment delays both the onset and the progression of nephropathy indicated by the assessment of microalbuminuria and hemoglobin A_1C. Table 17–17 provides prescriptive information on diets for the management of renal dysfunction in diabetes.

Cardiovascular Disease

Coronary artery disease (CAD) is the major cause of death in the United States. Contributing factors include genetics, smoking, inactivity, obesity, and dietary habits. Although *Healthy People 2000* has set population guidelines and nutritional goals to reduce heart disease, more than 80% of American children exceed the recommended amount of total fat and cholesterol. Medically underserved children are at an increased risk of obesity and lipid abnormalities, indicating future generations are at an enhanced risk of CAD (Bronner, 1996). The National Cholesterol Education has developed screening protocols for the assessment of cardiovascular risk based on total cholesterol levels, as well as the assessment of very low density lipoprotein (primarily in the form of triglycerides), low density lipoprotein (LDL), and high density lipoprotein (HDL). Both primary and secondary prevention protocols have been developed. These

TABLE 17–17. General Diet Recommendations for Renal Patients

Treatment	Pre-ESRD	Hemodialysis	Peritoneal Dialysis
Protein (g/kg IBW	0.6–0.8	1.1–1.4	1.2–1.5
Nephrotic syndrome	0.8–1.0		
Energy (kcal/kg IBW)	35–40	30–35	25–35
Phosphorus (mg/kg IBW)	8–12	<17	<17
Sodium (mg/d)	1000–3000 if necessary	2000–3000	2000–4000
Potassium (mg/kg IBW)	Typically unrestricted	Approximately 40	Typically unrestricted
Fluid (mL/d)	Typically unrestricted	500–700 + daily urine output or 1000 mL if anuric	2000+
Calcium (mg/d)	1200–1600	Depends on serum level	Depends on serum level

Reprinted with permission from National Renal Diet. Copyright 1993. The American Dietetic Association.

protocols are summarized in Figure 17–2. Recently, other risk factors have emerged and may warrant investigation. Elevations of lipoprotein (a) has been implicated as a marker of genetic risk of coronary artery disease. Lipoprotein (a) is generally not modifiable by diet, but can be affected by nicotinic acid or estrogen therapy (Berglund, 1995). Elevated homocysteine is an identified marker for thrombolytic disorders and coronary artery disease. Homocysteine accumulates as a result of dietary deficiencies of folic acid and/or vitamin B_{12}. Patients with abnormalities of clotting function or deep vein thrombosis should have homocysteine levels assessed. Microalbuminuria is also predictive of CAD, particularly in patients with type 2 diabetes.

After an initial assessment, dietary strategies focus on weight reduction and assessment of waist-to-hip ratio. Weight loss not only improves the lipid profile, particularly triglycerides and LDL, but reduces plasma viscosity and platelet activity. Very low calorie diets appear most effective in reducing plasma viscosity (Poggi et al., 1994; Toplak & Wascher, 1994). Lowering of LDL cholesterol is accomplished most effectively by reducing dietary saturated fat. The level of plasma LDL, which transports 60 to 70% of total plasma cholesterol, is directly related to the development of coronary artery disease. Despite the abundance of information available, many patients are confused about the dietary sources of saturated fat. Saturated fat can come from plants or animals. Simplistically, it is any fat solid at room temperature. Table 17–18 gives the saturated fat content of commonly eaten foods. The major source of saturated fat for adults is animal products, specifically meats. For children, saturated fats come primarily from whole milk dairy products.

The American Heart Association and the NCEP have developed a stepped approach to the dietary management of coronary artery disease, focusing on the control of LDL cholesterol. The Step 1 diet is currently used in population-based diet for the prevention of heart disease and is the diet promoted by *Healthy People 2000.* For those patients with pre-existing coronary artery disease, the Step 2 diet is indicated. Table 17–19 summarizes the differences in the two-step approach. A registered dietician is needed for the successful implementation of a Step 2 diet.

The major difference between the Step 1 and 2 diets is the level of dietary saturated fat and cholesterol. The cholesterol-lowering effect of a Step 1 diet is approximately 30 to 40 mg/dL and an additional reduction of 15 mg/dL can be achieved if the diet is advanced to a Step 2 diet. Most of the cholesterol lowering is in the LDL fraction. Elderly patients in good health should not be excluded from dietary therapy, though caution must be exercised to prevent malnutrition. Medically complicated elderly patients, including those with congestive heart failure, dementia, advanced cerebrovascular disease, and malignancy, should be excluded from aggressive cholesterol lowering therapy (Expert Panel on Detection, Evaluation, and Treatment of High Blood Cholesterol in Adults, 1993).

TABLE 17–18. Saturated Fats in Foods

Food Item	Portion Size	Grams of Saturated Fat
Milk, whole	1C	5.1
Ice cream	1C	9.0
Butter	1T	7.1
Margarine	1T	2.2
Canola oil	1T	1.0
Olive oil	1T	1.9
Mayonnaise	1T	1.6
Hamburger	4 oz	7.9
Flounder	4 oz	0.4
Chicken breast	4 oz	0.9
Sausage	3 oz	12.2
Cheese	1 oz	6.0

Intensive diet therapy is recommended for a minimum of six months before the initiation of drug therapy, with the exception of patients with an LDL cholesterol of 220 mg/dL or greater. LDL levels of this magnitude may require pharmacological intervention as part of the initial first step. The substitution of saturated fat by monounsaturated fat has a cholesterol-lowering effect. Monounsaturated fat (MUFA) is found in olive, peanut, and canola oils. Patients can substitute these oils for butter or lard in cooking rather than eliminating all dietary fat. Many patients eliminate all added fat, which may have provided a balance of fat sources. The fat consumed, therefore, is often of animal origin and primarily saturated fat.

The issue of polyunsaturated fat deserves attention. Polyunsaturated fat (PUFA) includes two major classes: W6 and W3 fatty acids. These two families of fatty acids have distinct physiological functions. Omega 6 fatty acids, when substituted for saturated fats, can lower LDL but can adversely affect HDL levels. Omega 6 fatty acids can be found in vegetable oils, specifically corn oil and safflower oil (Kuske & Feldman, 1987). Omega 3 fatty acids found in cold water fish, soy bean, and canola oil work as antithrombetic agents by altering production of specific prostaglandins. These fatty acids can also reduce inflammation and have a clinical use in the management of inflammatory disorders,

TABLE 17–19. Step 1 vs Step 2 Diet

Calories: to achieve ideal body weight
Protein: to meet requirements/up to 20%
Total Fat: 30%

	STEP 1	STEP 2
Saturated Fat	<10%	<7%
Polyunsaturated Fat	up to 10%	up to 10%
Monounsaturated Fat	10–15%	10–15%
Cholesterol	<300 mg	<200 mg

such as arthritis. Omega 3 fatty acids increase the clearance of chylomicrons and probably very low density (VLDL) lipoproteins from the plasma, thereby reducing the levels of triglycerides. However, these fatty acids do not significantly affect LDL cholesterol (Schaefer, Lichenstein, & Lamon-Fava, 1996). The cardioprotective effects of fish oils is derived through the modification of non-lipid risk factors. The modification of prostaglandin synthesis by fish oils is similar to that of aspirin therapy. Because clotting times may be prolonged, it is advisable for patients to discontinue fish oil supplements prior to surgery.

Antioxidant Therapy

Over the past few years, there have been numerous studies, both experimental and epidemiological, that provide strong evidence that antioxidant vitamins, particularly vitamins C and E, can reduce the risk of coronary heart disease, in both men and women across age groups (Losconczy, Harris, & Havlik, 1996; Stephens et al., 1996). The mode of action appears to be via the reduction of the highly atherogenic oxidized low density lipoprotein (LDL). Native or "unoxidized" LDL does not have the same atherogenic potential as does the oxidized particle. There is debate in the literature as to whether the vitamin E should come from food or in the form of supplements (Kushi et al., 1996). Dietary sources include nuts, vegetable oils (excluding coconut oil), and seeds. The consumption of many of these foods is reduced by individuals on a low-fat diet. The benefits of supplementation with vitamin E appears to outweigh the benefit of increasing dietary fat as very low-fat diets have been shown as well to increase the resistance of LDL to the effects of oxidation (Beard, Barnard & Robbins, 1996). The amount of vitamin E should be 400 IU and vitamin C 1000 mg. Inclusion of antioxidants should be considered in the prevention/management of CHD.

Hypertension

Hypertension is a major public health issue in the United States. Recent data indicate that only 47% of adult Americans have normal blood pressure (BP) (120/80) and the percentage of those with normal BP decreases with age (Burt, Whelton, & Roccella, 1995). The cornerstone of medical nutritional therapy has been the sodium-restricted diet. While effective for sodium-sensitive individuals, not all patients respond to sodium restriction in a similar manner. Predicting those who are sodium sensitive versus those who are sodium resistant is clinically challenging and difficult (Zoccali, Mallamaci, Cuzzola, & Leonardis, 1996). The variability of the response to a sodium load may not be related to sodium intake per se, but the hypertensive effects of insulin on sodium sensitivity and the overall mineral adequacy of a diet. A decrease in dietary sodium may increase vascular insulin resistance and perpetuate the adverse effects on glucose and lipid abnormalities on blood pressure (Feldman, Logan, & Schmidt, 1996).

Considerable data exist in both human and animal studies suggesting the protective effects of calcium, magnesium, and potassium in the prevention/management of sodium chloride induced hypertension (McCarron, 1997). Sodium restriction, when employed, may be of most benefit in the hypertensive geriatric patient, but may be of limited use in the prevention of hypertension in a normotensive population (Midgley, Matthew, Greenwood, & Logan, 1993). However, the safety of low-sodium diets in treated hypertensives is questionable and indeed may be a risk factor for myocardial infarction (Fleet, 1995). Sodium restriction poses a difficult clinical problem in that 80% of sodium intake is obtained from processed or easy to prepare foods. Table 17–20 gives the average sodium content of foods by group. The two most common levels of restriction are the 2-gram NA (low sodium) or 4 to 6 gram NA (no added salt).

Initially, prior to the selection of a sodium level, it is recommended to assess current intake levels. A patient consuming eight grams of NA per day may benefit from no added salt versus the highly restrictive 2-gram sodium. A teaspoon of salt contains 2000 mg of sodium. Therefore, a patient who salts food heavily may need no further restriction.

Obesity, particularly central obesity, is a risk factor for the development of hypertension and weight loss is a valued nonpharmacologic intervention in the management of HTN. Obesity contributes to hypertension via increase in SNS activity, insulin resistance, hyperinsulinemia, and enhanced vascular reactivity (Hsueh & Buchanan, 1994). Insulin resistance and hyperinsulinemia seen in obesity may contribute to the development of hypertension. Insulin has a sodium retaining effect on the kidney and can enhance the vascular sensitivity to vasoconstrictors. Hyperinsulinemia indeed may be a causative factor in salt-sensitive hypertension (Zavaroni, et al., 1995; Hsueh & Buchanan, 1994). Weight reduction can reduce hyperinsulinemia and improve blood pressure (Mediratta, Fozailoff, & Friskman, 1995). Weight loss as modest as 2.8 kg can decrease systolic blood pressure by 7.5 mm Hg and diastolic pressure by 6.5 mm Hg. Weight loss in treated hypertensives can reduce the needs for medication by 50% (Darne et al., 1993).

Recently, a clinical trial entitled Dietary Approaches to

TABLE 17–20. Average Sodium Content of Foods by Group

Food Exchanges	Approximate Sodium Content[a]
Milk (8 oz)	120 mg
Fresh Meat (1 oz) [no process or cured meat]	25 mg
Fresh Vegetables [no canned or frozen in sauce]	10 mg
Bread	150 mg
Fruit	2 mg
Fat	50 mg

[a] Convenience foods are generally higher in sodium

Stop Hypertension (DASH) was conducted to investigate the effect of a diet high in fruits and vegetables and rich in low-fat dairy products on blood pressure. Sodium intake and body mass index were maintained. A diet rich in fruits and vegetables (nine servings) and calcium (two servings) was associated with a decrease in systolic/diastolic blood pressure by 11.4 mm Hg and 5 mm Hg respectively in hypertensive individuals. The composition of the diet is listed in Table 17–21 (Appel et al., 1997). The DASH diet represents a significant deviation from the traditional American diet. Patients require education and support in implementing this approach, but this approach may be more acceptable than the traditional low-sodium diet.

Other dietary components can influence blood pressure. Omega 3 fatty acids, such as those found in cold water fish, can decrease both systolic and diastolic pressures. The dose most effective in lowering blood pressure is 3 g/day, a relatively high dose. Care must be exercised with this dose as fish oils decrease platelet aggregation and potential drug/drug interaction exists with aspirin and anticoagulant therapies (Appel, Miller, Seidler, & Whelton, 1993).

Alcohol has a dual role in hypertension. Reduction of alcohol intake can lower blood pressure in patients with hypertension. Alcohol consumption greater than two drinks per day increases the risk of hypertension. Although alcohol consumption can increase the risk of hypertension, the acute effects of alcohol include a vasodilatory effect and light drinking (< 2 drinks per day) appears to protect against coronary disease and ischemic stroke (Beilin, Puddey, & Burke, 1996).

NUTRITION SUPPORT

The determination of caloric requirements for the critically ill patient depends on a variety of clinical parameters including severity of stress, comorbid disease, age, and nutritional/physical status. Formulas can be used to estimate caloric requirements with the most common being the Harris–Benedict equation. The Harris–Benedict equation and the Long Correction Factors include the physiological parameters of height, weight, age, activity, and extent of injury. The formula with activity and stress factors is listed in Table 17–12. This equation or any other formula should be used as a guideline for initiating nutritional support but should be constantly reevaluated for adequacy. The Harris–Benedict equation may underestimate the caloric need of mechanically ventilated, surgical patients (Weisman, Kempner, & Askanzi, 1986), patients with chronic obstructive pulmonary disease (Branson, Hurst, & Warner, 1987), and overestimate caloric requirements in sedated patients. The problematic area in the use of this formula is the subjectively applied stress factor that estimates the increase in energy required for various degrees of physiological stress. Overfeeding should be avoided and is associated with fluid overload, respiratory compromise, hepatic steatosis, immunosuppression, and increased cost (Tapers, 1992).

TABLE 17–21. DASH Diet Composition Using the Food Pyramid

	Servings
Milk	2.7
Fruit	5.2
Vegetables	4.4
Grains	7.5
Meats (Beef, Chicken, Pork, Nuts, Seeds, Legumes)	2.3
Fats, Oils	2.5
Sweets, Snacks	0.7

Another method for estimating caloric requirements is to provide 30 to 35 kcal/kg as a general rule of thumb and monitor response to therapy via serial nutritional assessment. However, medically complex or obese patients in whom caloric requirements are often difficult to predict may benefit from the measurement of caloric need via indirect calorimetry. Indirect calorimetry measures oxygen consumption and carbon dioxide production utilizing an automated metabolic cart. Although indirect calorimetry can predict caloric need, it provides a "snapshot" view and requires that the patient be rested. Stressful or painful procedures, such as suctioning, can have a short-term influence on caloric need. Caloric requirements are not static in the critically ill and, as with other measures, should be serially reassessed. It is often recommended to have repeat measures of indirect calorimetry throughout the day and obtain the average.

The determination of protein need is dependent on current medical condition and, often times, protein tolerance supersedes protein requirements. A patient in multisystem organ failure (MOS) may have protein requirements of 2 gm/kg/IBW, but only tolerate 1 gm/kg/IBW. A starting point of 1.5 to 2.0 gm/kg/IBW is recommended. This increase in requirements above the 0.8 gm/kg/IBW for healthy individuals is due to the alteration or imbalance in protein catabolism and protein synthesis exhibited during stress. Protein catabolism rates exceed synthesis resulting in a net nitrogen loss (O'Keefe, Sender, & James, 1974). The goal, therefore, of protein provision via nutrition support is to improve nitrogen balance, rather than reducing protein catabolism. Provision of nutrition support, altering fuel sources, or types of products do not alter the protein physiology of stress (DeChalain, Mitchell, & O'Keefe, 1992).

Enteral Nutrition

Enteral nutrition is the preferred mode of delivery of nutritional support. The use of the gastrointestinal tract can be problematic as physiologic stress can cause sphlanic vasoconstriction, gut mucosal damage, a decrease in gastric barrier function, and partial gut immotility (Charney & Martindale, 1994). Paradoxically, the provision of early enteral nutrition may improve blood flow to the gut, thereby stabilizing the villus structure and maintaining barrier function.

Early enteral nutrition has demonstrated in clinical trials to blunt hypermetabolism after burns and promote enhanced wound healing (Chiarelli, Enzi, & Casadei, 1990; Schroeder, Gillanders, Mahrs, & Hill, 1991). Enteral support improves immune function and markers of nutritional repletion after major abdominal surgeries (Braga et al., 1996). A metaanalysis by Moore, Feliciano, and Andrassy (1992) indicates that the rate of septic complications was twice as high in those trauma patients receiving TPN versus enteral support. Additionally, TPN is between 4 to 12.5 times more expensive than enteral nutritional (Trice, Melnik, & Page, 1997). Criteria exist for the provision of early enteral support. Criteria includes adequate resuscitation, adequate blood flow, and oxygen administration. The patient must be hemodynamically stable with the primary concern being the avoidance of the hypovolemic state (Andrassy, Deitch, Booth, & Moore, 1991). Enteral feeding is contraindicated in patients with complete bowel obstruction, paralytic ileus, severe vomiting or diarrhea, peritonitis, and short bowel syndrome (ASPEN Board of Directors, 1993). Zaloga (1990) defines early enteral nutrition as support introduced with the first 36 hours, whereas other clinical studies have demonstrated safe and effective enteral support within 12 to 18 hours postoperatively. Decision trees exist for the selection and progression of nutrition support as in Figure 17–3.

The benefits of enteral support and attempting early introduction of this form of nutrition support are numerous. Preservation of gut mucosa is of primary concern. The intestinal tract, in addition to absorbing nutrients, provides an immunological barrier. Approximately 70 to 80% of the immunological cells are found in the intestine. Collectively known as gut associated lymphoid tissue (GALT), this tissue includes lymphocytes, macrophages, and mast cells, and defends against foreign antigenic material in the intestine (Langkemp-Henken, Glezer, & Kudsk, 1992; Phillips & Olson, 1993). The primary immunoglobin in the intestinal mucosal cells is secretory IGA. The secretion of this immunoglobin is dependent, to a large degree, on an oral diet or the provision of enteral nutrition (Keithley & Eisenberg, 1993). Total parenteral nutrition, bowel rest, and steroid and immunosuppressive therapy negatively affect the production of secretory IGA. A decrease in secretory IGA allows the presentation of antigens to GALT, thereby stimulating a systemic inflammatory response (Minard & Kudsk, 1994). Early enteral nutrition, therefore, provides a stimulus to the gut's own immune system.

Gut barrier function and immune defenses can be impaired through a variety of clinical conditions and treatments. These include intestinal ischemia and obstruction, hemorrhagic and septic/endo toxic shock, anesthesia, and surgery (Keithley & Eisenberg, 1993; Langkamp-Henken et al., 1992). The breakdown of the gut barrier function has been implicated in the translocation of bacteria or endotoxins from the lumen of the intestine to systemic circulation. This invasion triggers the production of cytokines and prostaglandins, which may result in hypermetabolism and progressive organ dysfunction (McMahon, Farnell, & Murray, 1993). The bacteria most frequently associated with translocation are *Escherichia coli*, *Klebsiella pneumoniae*, *Pseudomonas aeruginosa*, *Staphylococcus epidermidis*, and *Candida albicans* (Alexander, 1990). These aerobic bacteria are those often implicated in the development of sepsis in the ICU patient. Bacterial translocation (BT) is estimated to occur in approximately 10% of patients (Sedman et al., 1994). Recently, prostacyclin has been demonstrated to have a protective effect against bacterial translocation. Further work is needed to validate this effect and possibly modify the production of endogenous prostacyclin (Brinkmann et al., 1996).

Research is inconclusive as to whether the form of nutrition support, enteral versus parenteral, is causative or protective against bacterial translocation. In most studies, the provision of polymeric enteral nutrition, particularly products enriched with water-soluble fiber, arginine, glutamine, and omega 3 fatty acids appear to be the most beneficial in the prevention of bacterial translocation (Adawi, Kasravi, Molin, & Jeppsson, 1996; Buchman, 1996; Frankel et al., 1995; Gennari, Alexander & Eaves-Pyles, 1995). Elemental or predigested enteral feedings have been implicated as a potential contributor to bacterial translocation (Deitch et al., 1995). Enteral nutrition may also have a positive effect on immune function because of unique nutrients inherent or added to the formula. Research has indicated that glutamine, a nonessential amino acid in the absence of disease, may be an essential nutrient in the critically ill (Buchman, 1996; Smith, 1990). Arginine and omega 3 fatty acids, in addition to being essential nutrients, function as immunomodulators. Arginine has been shown to enhance nutritional repletion and enhance the immune system by increasing the number of T-helper cells (Kirk & Barkul, 1990). Arginine may also have a positive impact on wound healing via secretagogue activity of growth hormone, which has been shown to stimulate wound healing and by stimulating collagen synthesis (Kirk & Barkul, 1990; Charney, 1994). Arginine and the probiotic bacteria, Lactobacillus, may protect against the BT associated with acute liver failure (Adawi, Kasravi, Molin, & Jeppsson, 1997). The optimal amount of arginine required is not known, but clinical studies using 15 to 30 g/day appear safe and effective (Kirk & Barkul, 1990; Charney, 1994). Arginine is a component of most commercial enteral products, but at relatively low levels. Products formulated to be immune-enhancing contain arginine levels of 15.4 g/liter.

Omega 3 fatty acids (fish oils), long chain polyunsaturated fats, are also considered an immunomodulator. Traditional enteral products have a predominance of omega 6 fatty acids. Omega 6 fatty acids are precursors to prostaglandins (PGE_2) and leukotrienes (LTB_4) that can be immunosup-

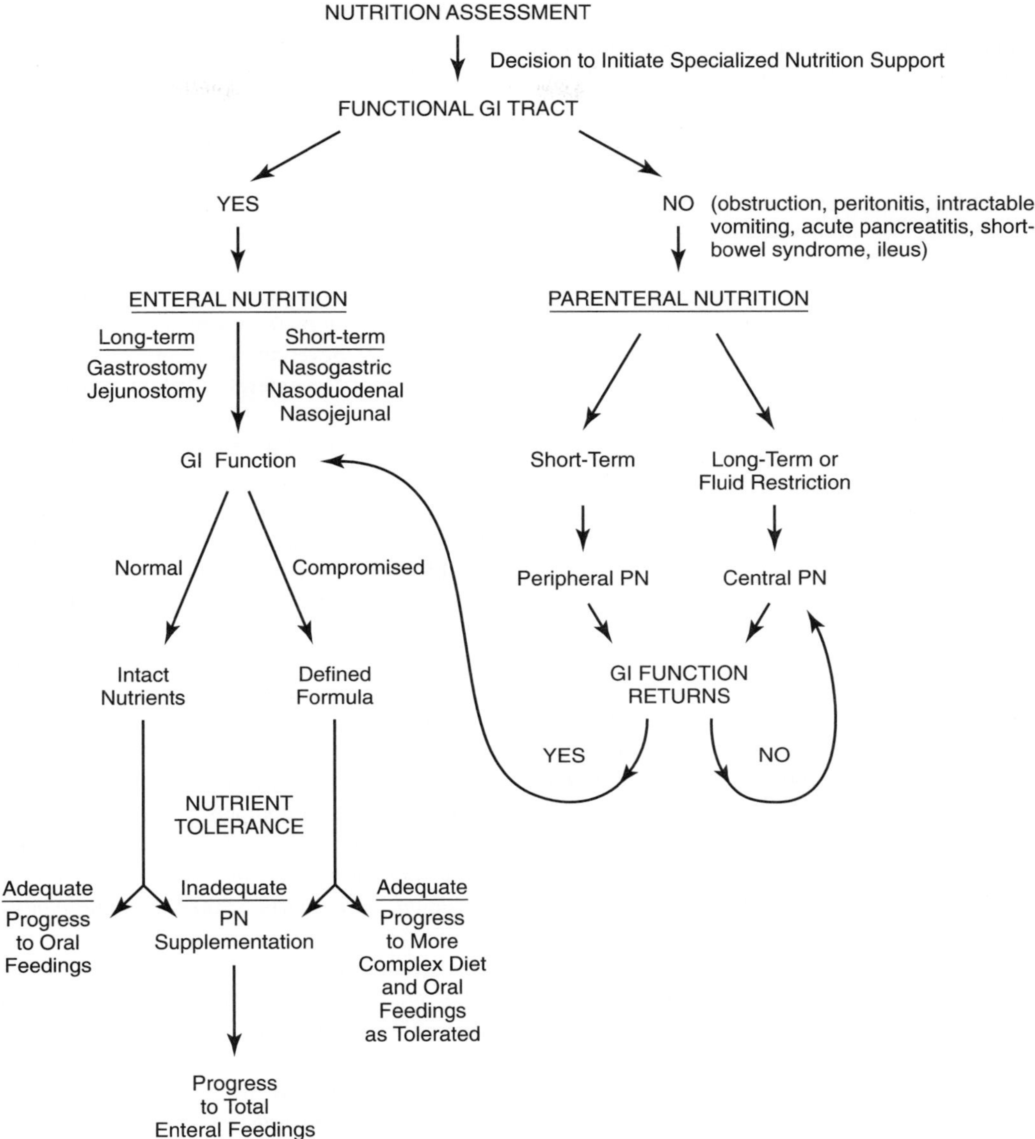

Figure 17–3. Nutrition assessment selection and progression of nutritional support. *(Reprinted with permission from ASPEN Board of Directors. [1993].)*

pressive, inhibiting lymphocytes and macrophage activity (Phillips & Olson, 1993). Omega 3 fatty acids serve to selectively inhibit the production these immunosuppressive mediators. Omega 3 fatty acids also have the ability to support immune function and have anti-inflammatory properties (Seidner, 1994).

Short-chain fatty acids are a metabolic product from the metabolism of dietary fiber. Short-chain fatty acids, in addition to providing energy, have a trophic effect on the intestinal tract and may aid in the prevention of bacterial translocation (Mao et al., 1996). In clinical practice, fiber-enriched formulas may provide benefits for patients with intestinal dysfunction such as inflammatory bowel disease. The role of fiber-enriched products in the ICU patient remains unclear. Although in theory the fermentation byproducts of fiber may have beneficial effects, there have been few studies demonstrating the efficacy of fiber. Banana flakes, a source of pectin, have been demonstrated to reduce the severity of diarrhea and can be used during the work-up for *Clostridium difficile.* One to two tablespoons mixed with 60 to 120 cc of water per 8 hours can be administered in a bolus fashion through the feeding tube as an adjunct to medical therapy (Emery et al., 1997). The use of fiber-enriched formulas does not pose a risk to patients, but exogenous fiber should be added with care to enteral feeding as it is likely to clump and clog feeding tubes.

Branch-Chain Amino Acids

The branch-chain amino acids (BCAA)—leucine, isoleucine, and valine—have unique metabolic properties that may be of clinical utility to the critically ill patient. These amino acids are metabolized primarily in skeletal tissue rather than the liver. Branch-chain amino acids also compete with aromatic amino acids (AAA) for transfer across the blood—brain barrier and may be able to influence the rate of some monoamine neurotransmitters. The potential benefit of BCAA is for the patient with hepatic failure. In hepatic failure, the amino acid profile shifts with an increase in the AAA:BCAA ratio. BCAA are selectively taken up by the muscle and AAA are unable to be effectively metabolized by the liver. Alterations in this amino acid profile may be a contributing factor to the development of encephalophy. The clinical use of BCAA indicates the potential effect of these amino acids in patients who are protein intolerant secondary to chronic or latent hepatic encephalopathy (Marsano & McClain, 1991). However, BCAA have failed to consistently prove to be efficacious in septic patients (Garcia-DeLorenzo, Planas, & Ortiz-Lebya, 1994; von Meyenfeldt, Soeters, & Vente, 1990).

Obstacles to Successful Enteral Support

Clinicians must recognize and be able to prevent or manage problems associated with enteral support. Recognizing that enteral support is the preferential nutrition delivery system for the ICU patient, there are, however, contraindications for its use. Contraindications include gastrointestinal hemorrhage, complete bowel obstruction, paralytic ileus, severe vomiting, or diarrhea (ASPEN Board of Directors, 1993). Assessment of gut function is a prerequisite to successful enteral feeding. Research suggests that the gut is the first organ system to be affected by hypoxia. Low cardiac output is the major nonocculsive cause of intestinal ischemia with malabsorption of protein and carbohydrate appearing approximately within one hour. Gastric intramucosal pH decreases with hypoperfusion and can be assessed using gastrointestinal tonometry. This assessment may be used as an early marker in predicting tolerance to enteral feedings (Clark & Guitierrez, 1992).

Although enteral nutrition is considered the preferred method of nutritional support, barriers to this form of support, real and perceived, must be evaluated and overcome. Paralytic ileus is often cited as a reason to delay or withhold enteral support. Traditionally, the presence of bowel sounds signaled the initiation of enteral support. Ileus commonly occurs in critically ill patients as the result of the underlying pathology or secondary to treatment regimens. However, the small intestine, the major absorptive site of nutrients, regains motility within the first 24 hours after the insult. In the majority of patients, if it is possible to deliver nutrition directly to the intestinal mucosa, absorption can occur without significant bloating or discomfort (Gottschlich, Alexander, & Bower, 1990). Aspiration is a risk in the enterally fed patient and can be life-threatening. Numerous risk factors for aspiration exist including advanced age, level of consciousness, neurological disorders, enteral tube positioning and feeding schedule, and body positioning (Elpern, 1997). The risk of aspiration can minimized by proper assessment and feeding tube positioning. Advancing age is the major risk factor associated with aspiration (Mullan, Roubenoff, & Roubenoff, 1992). The aging of America is changing the population in ICUs. In the 1980s, half of all patients admitted to the intensive care units were over the age of 65, although patients in this age group represent only 12% of the population (Fedullo & Sevenburne, 1983). Patients over the age of 65 receive half the enteral nutrition delivered in the acute care setting. Therefore, aspiration is emerging as a major clinical concern (United States Congress, Office of Technology Assessment, 1987). Tube positioning can reduce, but not eliminate, the risk of aspiration. Postpyloric positioning of feeding tubes is the standard of care when the risk of aspiration is high or when previous aspiration has been documented (Strong, Condon, & Solinger, 1992). The semirecumbent position with head elevated at 45° is also recommended (Elpern, 1997). Large-bore feeding tubes should be avoided as the tube renders the gastroesophageal sphincter incompetent and increases the risk of reflux and aspiration (Forlaw & Guenter, 1990).

Diarrhea remains the major physiological barrier to the delivery of enteral support. The causes of diarrhea are multifactorial in the critically ill. Hypertonic tube feeding is often implicated as a cause of diarrhea. The osmolality of the product, particularly >500 Mosm/kg, can cause an osmotic shift. However, hypertonic solutions are more likely to cause osmotic diarrhea if the feeding tube is placed distal to the pyloric sphincter. When the tube is placed gastrically, the pyloric sphincter controls the rate of emptying and prevents a dumping syndrome reaction. Indeed, common beverages such as soft drinks and juices have osmolalities exceeding 800 Mosm/kg and are well tolerated by those with competent sphincter function. Positioning of the feeding tube may be the most significant determinant of osmotic diarrhea in critically ill patients. In the assessment of osmotic diarrhea, stool volume decreases in patients when the tube feeding is stopped. It is obligatory to use a continuous feeding via pump when feeding into the small intestine to avoid these fluid shifts. To prevent problems, hyperosmolar feedings should be started at a smaller volume, then advanced at a fairly rapid rate. Dilution is not recommended. Although hypertonic tube feedings are often thought of as a major cause of osmotic diarrhea, medications can also contribute to osmotic load and indeed contribute substantially to osmotic load. Many elixirs are formed from a sorbitol base and sorbitol itself can cause osmotic diarrhea. The osmolalities of selected drugs are listed in Table 17–22.

Hypoalbuminemia may contribute to the development of diarrhea in the critically ill patient. Colloid osmotic pressure decreases with hypoalbuminemia and results in mu-

TABLE 17–22. Osmolalities of Commonly Prescribed Medications

Drug	Osmolality
Acetaminophen elixir, 65 mg/mL	5400
Cimitidine	5500
Potassium chloride 10%	3500
Digoxin 50 ug/mL	1350
Furosemide solution 10mg/mL	2050

cosal edema and impaired absorption resulting in a secretory or malabsorptive disorder. Research documenting hypoalbuminemia as a potential cause of diarrhea is conflicting. Albumin levels of less than 2.5 g/dL have been reported to increase the likelihood of diarrhea (Brinson & Kolts, 1987). However, other authors have found hypoalbuminemia not to be a risk factor for the development of diarrhea in the critically ill population (Gottschlich, Warden, & Michel, 1988). The management of hypoalbuminemia is also controversial. Peptide-based or partially hydrolyzed protein formulas may be useful in avoiding diarrhea in the hypoalbuminemia patient (Brinson & Kolts, 1988). However, conflicting research has indicated no significant improvement in diarrhea or nutritional status using a peptide-based formula versus standard, polymeric formula (Mowatt-Larssen, Brown, & Wjotysiak, 1992). Certainly, there is no harm in ordering a peptide-based formula as an attempt to modulate diarrhea. Resurrecting serum albumin via intravenous albumin is a costly measure that only provides temporary elevation in albumin levels and should not be routinely used.

Clostridium difficile is also a potential cause of diarrhea. Broad spectrum antibiotics ordered for infections attack susceptible species of bacteria and may allow the overgrowth of pathogenic bacteria species such as *C difficile* or its endotoxin. *C difficile* can cause pseudomembranous colitis. The incidence of pseudomembranous colitis may be as high as 1:100 patients (Andrejack, Schmitt, & Tondriaux, 1991). The most common antibiotics associated with pseudomembranous colitis include clindamycin, ampicillin, and the cephalosporin. Other risk factors for pseudomembranous colitis diarrhea include burns, duration of hospitalization, and advanced age (Grube, Heimbach, & Marvin, 1987). Candida albicans is also a pathogenic cause of diarrhea in the critically ill with elderly, malnourished patients at greatest risk. Symptoms include frequent, watery stools without blood or abdominal pain (Gupta & Ehrinpreis, 1990). Retrograde contamination of tube feeding can also be a potential cause of diarrhea. Prescription of histamine antagonists and antacids to reduce stress ulceration and bleeding is a common practice. Buffering the acidic nature of the gut reduces the bacteriostatic capacity of the stomach. Bacteria, normally killed in an acidic pH, are able to grow and proliferate when the stomach pH is 3.5 to 4. The remaining bacteria in the stomach are able to migrate up the feeding tube and contaminate the enteral product and where further bacterial multiplication can occur (Payne-James, 1992). The enteral product, even in a closed system, is as likely to become contaminated and contribute to the development or continuation of diarrhea (Donius, 1993). Additionally, the buffered pH of the stomach can contribute to bacterial ventilator-associated pneumonia seen in critically ill patients. Another factor in the development of diarrhea is lactose intolerance. Secondary lactose intolerance may develop via medical treatments or prolonged bowel rest. While the vast majority of products are lactose free, a quick product check can help avoid lactose-containing products (Torres et al., 1996).

Even with the best clinical management, oftentimes patients are unable to tolerate the full complement of calories and protein via enteral support. Although controversy exists, a portion of the calories should be delivered enterally with the bulk of nutrition provided by parenteral support. As little as 25% of total calories as enteral nutrition can prevent gut atrophy and possibly BT (McCauley, Heel, Christiansen, & Hall, 1996; Sax, Illig, Ryan, & Hardy, 1996).

Initiation of Enteral Support

Early protocols for tube feeding promoted the use of isotonic/hypotonic formulas or dilution of the product to prevent a dumping syndrome reaction. However, research has demonstrated that "starter regimens" and dilution of formula is not indicated. Dilution of formula is associated with an increased risk of bacterial contamination from the water used, mixing utensils, and from the provider (Kohn & Keithley, 1989). The gastrointestinal tract can tolerate full-strength hypertonic solutions administered intragastrically or intraduodenally at rates up to 150 ml/hr without gastrointestinal complications (Zarling, Parmer, & Mobarhan, 1986). However, in critical illness or prolonged periods of NPO, slower initial rates of 30 to 50 ml can be initiated without dilution. Gradual advancement is needed with reduction in rate if intolerance develops.

Product selection is driven primarily via formulary restrictions. Calculation of caloric and protein needs should be the primary consideration. Products containing 1.5 kcal/ml and high in nitrogen (HN) are often the best match for the critically ill patient. Table 17–5 gives a concise list of products meeting these requirements. The registered dietician should be consulted for product selection and availability.

Parenteral Support

In the era of nutritional support, parenteral nutrition is a relatively new modality. Popularized in the 1970s, it quickly became the mainstay of nutritional therapy for critically ill patients or in patients with a nonfunctional gastrointestinal tract. However, with the abundance of research demonstrating the safety, efficacy, and cost savings of enteral support, the pendulum has swung back favoring enteral support. Nevertheless, there are patients who are not able to tolerate enteral therapy or those in whom operative procedures, diagnostic tests, or mechanical or metabolic complications limit the effectiveness of enteral therapy.

As with enteral therapy, assessment of prior nutritional and medical status calorie and protein requirements are required before the initiation of parenteral support. After the initial assessment of need is made, the division of macronutrients is determined. Carbohydrate is given primarily as dextrose which, because it is a hydrous form, yields 3.4 kcal per gram. Preparations of dextrose solutions range from 2.5 to 70%. Maximal oxidative capacity of stressed patients is approximately 5 mg of glucose/kg/minute. Higher concentrations of dextrose are beneficial in the fluid-restricted patient.

Conventional protein solutions are supplied as crystalline amino acids in concentrations ranging from 7 to 15% and special formulations exist that are high in BCAA for liver disease or high in essential amino acids for acute renal failure. Amino acids solutions provide 4.0 kcal/gram. The calories from amino acids are often not calculated as a caloric source in TPN solutions. Amino acids should be available for protein synthesis and not oxidized as a caloric course.

The function of fat in the TPN solution is to serve as a source of kcal and essential fatty acids. The concentrations of fat emulsions is 10 to 20%. Calories supplied by fat emulsions should be between 10 to 40%. The provision of at least 10% fat is needed to supply essential fatty acids (EFA) needs of 2 to 4% of total calories. Lipid emulsions are made from either soybean or safflower oil. Although both types of emulsions can meet EFA requirements, soybean oil emulsions are preferred as they contain a higher percentage of W3 fatty acids. Recent interest has developed in the clinical use of a fish oil emulsion that would be rich in omega 3 fatty acids. Omega 3 fatty acids, beneficial to the immune system, would have clinical application in the stressed population. Contraindications to the use of fat emulsions include lipoid nephrosis, acute pancreatitis with hyperlipidemia, and severe egg allergy. Egg lecithin is used as an emulsifying agent in lipid emulsions. Caloric density of lipid emulsions is 1.1 kcal per 10% emulsion and 2.0 kcal/ml per 20% emulsion. Lipid emulsions should not exceed 2.5 g/kg per day in adults.

Vitamins and Minerals

Vitamin requirements may vary based on substrate composition, prior nutritional status, and medical diagnosis. Parenteral vitamin formulations are based on the RDA with adjustments made for the mildly malnourished patient. Parenteral solutions with a high level of dextrose may require additional thiamin, a cofactor in carbohydrate metabolism. Patients receiving a high percentage of calories from a lipid emulsion may require supplemental vitamin E, the antioxidant that protects polyunsaturated fats. Certain medical diagnoses necessitate careful attention to vitamin/mineral status. Malabsorption states including HIV, alcohol abuse, burns, and dialysis may initially require adjusted levels.

It is critical for the practitioner to realize that standard vitamin formulations may not meet an individual patient's needs. The unique delivery of parenteral vitamins also allows for unique losses. Adsorption of vitamins to the tubing or losses upon exposure to ultraviolet light may predispose the patient on TPN to vitamin deficiencies. Trace elements considered to be essential are iron, zinc, copper, manganese, selenium, chromium, iodine, molybdenum, fluoride, and cobalt. Of the trace elements routinely added, iron has been linked with toxicity reactions. Zinc requirements are the most labile. Requirements for zinc are increased with gastrointestinal losses, particularly with diarrheal or ileostomy losses. Increases of 2.0 mg of zinc per day above baseline are needed for physiological stress (American Medical Association [AMA], 1979).

Electrolytes

The greatest variability in the parenteral solution exists in electrolyte concentrations. Electrolyte homeostasis is affected by many clinical conditions. Needs decrease in renal failure and congestive heart failure. Increased need can occur in diarrheal or malabsorptive disorders, ostomies, vomiting, nasogastric suctioning, diabetic ketoacidosis, and anabolism. Monitoring electrolytes is critical to avoid abnormalities.

Mode of Access

Peripheral parenteral nutrition (PPN) is indicated when the need for parenteral nutrition is estimated to be 2 weeks or less. Few suitable peripheral veins and limited tolerance to osmolarity made long-term support impractical. Clinically, parenteral solutions with an osmolarity of 250 to 600 Mosm/L can be used in peripheral veins. Relative contraindications include severely malnourished patients and those with increased needs for nutrients and electrolytes and the fluid-restricted patients (ASPEN, 1993).

Total parenteral nutrition (TPN) is designed to provide large volumes of hypertonic nutrients in restricted volumes. Due to the unique nature of TPN, complications can be related to the catheter itself (mechanical and infectious) or metabolic derangements. Table 17–23 provides an overview of common complications and treatment approaches.

Nurse practitioners, functioning as part of interdisciplinary teams, should possess a basic knowledge of the principles of nutrition in acute and chronic conditions. This knowledge, partnered with referrals to registered dieticians, can enhance patient care and have a positive impact on outcomes.

TABLE 17–23. Complications of Parenteral Nutrition

Complication	Prevention	Treatment
	Catheter Related	
Pneumothorax	• Place patient in Trendelenburg position prior to central line insertion.	• A small pneumothorax may be self-limiting. • Insertion of chest tube with underwater seal drainage.
Air Embolus	• Place patient in Trendelenburg position prior to central line insertion.	• Should a disconnection occur, immediately place a finger over the exposed end of the catheter until the tubing can be reconnected.
	• Check the intravenous connections periodically during shift to be certain they are secure. Tape connections for added protection against disconnection. • Change intravenous tubing during expiratory phase of respiratory cycle. • Apply an occlusive dressing over the site after the catheter has been removed.	• Place patient in Trendelenburg in a left-side lying position.
Subclavian Vein Thrombosis	• Use a catheter that has proven to be the least thrombogenic (Silicone). • Administer heparin as ordered by a physician.	• Remove catheter. • Administer heparin.
Catheter Position Displacement	• Securely tape intravenous dressing and tubing in place.	• Notify NP/physician immediately if catheter is displaced.
	• Check dressing at least every 4 hr for signs of inadvertent displacement. • Assist with obtaining periodic chest x-rays for visualization of catheter placement.	
Catheter Occlusion	• Check intravenous fluid for proper infusion rate at least every 2 hr.	• Have patient cough and/or change body position. • Attempt to aspirate clot with a syringe.
	• Check intravenous tubing for any kinks or bends in the tubing every 2 hr. • Do not give blood transfusions through a catheter that is also being used for TPN infusion. • Do not withdraw blood through catheter for blood specimens.	• Notify NP/physician if the above measures do not alleviate the problem.
Infection	• Do not add any additives to the TPN solution on the nursing unit. • Avoid the intravenous injection or "piggyback" of any medications to the TPN set-up.	• Obtain blood cultures. • Administer antibiotics
	• Avoid the use of stopcocks. • Tape all connections securely. • Use a biocclusive dressing. • Change dressing and tubing every 48 hr.	• Remove catheter if so necessitated. • Send catheter for culture upon its removal.
	Metabolic	
Hyperglycemia	• Monitor serum glucose levels frequently. • Do not increase the rate of infusion even if it is behind schedule.	• Order sliding scale insulin. • Adjust flow rate of infusion.
Hypoglycemia	• Monitor serum glucose levels frequently. • Do not discontinue the infusion suddenly.	• Administer dextrose.
Allergic Reaction	• Administer a test dose of lipid emulsions prior to initiating the infusion at the rate ordered.	• Administer benadryl and/or steroids.
	• Monitor patient closely during the first 30 minutes of infusion of TPN (allergic reactions have been lipids, iron dextran, heparin, and insulin).	• Avoid the use of TPN products to which the patient demonstrates reported with hypersensitivity.
Burns	• Administer fluids based on patient's clinical status.	• Thermal injury results in destruction of the skin barrier leading to evaporative water loss.

(Continued)

TABLE 17–23. Complications of Parenteral Nutrition *(Continued)*

Complication	Prevention	Treatment
	Metabolic *(continued)*	
	• Administer electrolytes based on patient's clinical status, especially sodium, potassium, chloride, calcium, magnesium, and phosphorus.	• Electrolytes are depleted along with water via evaporative and renal losses. • Some substances used in burn wound care deplete electrolytes (e.g., silver nitrate, mafenide acetate). • Increased carbohydrate intake necessitates higher quantities of phosphorus.
Sepsis	• Administer formulas high in branched-chain amino acids (BCAA).	• Sepsis increases energy needs. BCAA supply energy to the heart, liver, and skeletal muscle.
	• Administer lipids as 30–50% of the total nonprotein calories.	• Lipid administration is vital during sepsis as there is an increased breakdown of this substrate.
	• Administer insulin based on patient's clinical status.	• Hyperglycemia occurs in response to stress. • Insulin may inhibit protein breakdown and stimulate its synthesis.
	• Restrict the administration of iron.	• Iron is essential for the growth of numerous bacteria. • Iron administration during the acute phase of sepsis may increase its severity.

Reprinted with permission from Ruppert, S. D., Kernicki, J. G. & Dolan, J. T. (1996). Dolan's critical care nursing clinical management through the nursing process *(2nd ed.). Philadelphia: F. A. Davis.*

REFERENCES

Adawi, D., Kasravi, F. B., Molin, G., & Jeppsson, B. (1996). Oral arginine supplementation in acute liver injury. *Nutrition, 12,* 529–533.

Adawi, D., Kasravi, F. B., Molin, G., & Jeppsson, B. (1997). Effect of lactobacillus supplementation with and without arginine on liver damage and bacterial translocation in an acute liver injury model in the rat. *Hepatology, 25* (3), 642–647.

Alexander, J. W. (1990). Nutrition and translocation. *Journal of Parenteral and Enteral Nutrition, 14,* 455–505.

Alzaid, A. A. (1996). Microalbuminuria in NIDDM: An overview. *Diabetes Care, 19,* 79–89.

American Diabetes Association. (1994). Nutrition recommendations and principles for people with diabetes mellitus. *Diabetes Care, 17,* 519–522.

American Diabetes Association. (1997). Clinical practice recommendation: Translation of the diabetes nutrition recommendations of health care institutions. *Diabetes Care, 20* (Suppl. 1), S37–S40.

American Diabetes Association. (1997). Position statement on: Nutrition recommendations and principles for people with diabetes mellitus. *Diabetes Care, 20* (Suppl. 1), S14–S17.

American Dietetic Association. (1990). Position statement on: Very low calorie weight loss diets. *Journal of the American Dietetic Association, 90,* 722–726.

American Dietetic Association. (1997). Position statement on: Screening for diabetes. *Diabetes Care, 20* (Suppl. 1), S22–S23.

American Medical Association. (1979). Guidelines for essential trace element preparations for parenteral use. *Journal of Parenteral and Enteral Nutrition, 2,* 263–267.

Andrassy, R. J., Deitch, E. A., Booth, F. V., & Moore, F. A. (1991). Current concepts in postoperative feeding. *Contemporary Surgery, 39,* 37–46.

Andrejak, M., Schmitt, J., & Tondriaux, A. (1991). The clinical significance of antibiotic associated pseudomenbranous colitis in the 1990s. *Drug Safety, 6,* 339–349.

Appel, L. J., Miller, E. R., Seidler, A. J., & Whelton, P. K. (1993). Does supplementation of diet with "fish oil" reduce blood pressure? A meta-analysis of controlled clinical trials. *Archives of Internal Medicine, 153* (12), 1429–1438.

Appel, L. J., Moore, J. J., Obarzaner, E., Vollmer, W. M., Svetkey, L. P., Sacks, F. M., Bray, G. A., Vogt, T. M., Cutler, J. A., Windhauser, M. M., Lin, P. H., & Karanja, N. (1997). A clinical trial of the effects of dietary patterns on blood pressure. *New England Journal of Medicine, 336,* 1117–1123.

Arnold, M. S., Stephen, C. J., Jess, G. E., & Hiss, R. G. (1993). Guidelines versus practice in the delivery of diabetes nutrition care. *Journal of the American Medical Association, 93,* 34–39.

ASPEN Board of Directors. (1993). Guidelines for the use of parenteral and enteral nutrition in adult and pediatric patients. *Journal of Parenteral and Enteral Nutrition, 17* (Suppl. 4), 1SA–23SA.

Avram, M. M., Goldwasser, P., Erroa, M., & Fein, P. A. (1994). Predictors of survival in continuous ambulatory peritoneal dialysis patients: The importance of pre-albumin and other nutritional and metabolic markers. *American Journal of Kidney Diseases, 23,* 91–98.

Baker, J. P., Detsky, A. S., Wesson, D. E., & Wolman, S. L. (1982). A comparison of clinical judgment and objective measurements. *New England Journal of Medicine, 306,* 969–972.

Beard, C. M., Barnard, R. J., & Robbins, D. C. (1996). Effects of diet and exercise on qualitative and quantitative measures of LDL and its susceptibility to oxidation. *Arteriosclerosis, Thrombosis & Vascular Biology, 16,* 201–207.

Beilin, L. J., Puddey, I. B., & Burke, V. (1996). Alcohol and hypertension—kill or cure? *Journal of Human Hypertension, 10S* (2), S1–S5.

Bennett, W. (1995). Beyond overeating. *New England Journal of Medicine, 332,* 672–674.

Berglund, L. (1995). Diet and drug therapy for lipoprotein (a). *Lipidology, 6*(1), 48–56.

Bierman, E. L. (1992). Atherogenesis in diabetes. *Arteriosclerosis and Thrombosis, 12,* 647–656.

Boosalis, M. G. & Levine, A. S. (1989). Relationship of visceral protein to nutritional status in chronic and acute stress. *Critical Care Medicine, 17,* 741–747.

Braga, M., Vignali, A., Giariotti, L., Cestar, A., Profel, M., & Carlo, V. D. (1996). Immune and nutritional effects of early enteral nutrition after major abdominal operations. *European Journal of Surgery, 162,* 105–112.

Branson, R. D., Hurst, J. M., & Warner, B. W. (1987). Measured versus predicted energy expenditure in mechanically ventilated patients with chronic obstructive pulmonary disease. *Respiratory Care, 32,* 748–756.

Brinkmann, A., Wolf, C. F., Berger, D., Kneitinger, E., Neumeister, B., Buchler, M., Radermacher, P., Seeling, W., & Georgieff, M. (1996). Perioperative endotoxemia and bacterial translocation during major abdominal surgery: Evidence for the protective effect of endogenous prostacyclin? *Critical Care Medicine, 24* (8), 1293–1301.

Brinson, R. R., & Kolts, B. (1987). Hypoalbuminemia as an indicator of diarrheal incidence of critically ill patients. *Critical Care Medicine, 15* (5), 506–509.

Brinson, R. R., & Kolts, B. (1988). Diarrhea associated with severe hypoalbuminemia: A comparison of a peptide-based chemically defined diet and standard alimentation. *Critical Care Medicine, 16,* 130–136.

Bronner, Y. L. (1996). Nutritional status outcomes for children: Ethnic, cultural and environmental contexts. *Journal of the American Dietetic Association, 96* (9), 891–903.

Brown, S., Upchurch, S., Anding, R., Winter, M. & Ramirez, E. (1996). Promoting weight loss in type 2 diabetes. *Diabetes Care, 19* (6), 613–624.

Buchman, A. L. (1996). Glutamine: Is it a conditionally required nutrient for the human gastrointestinal tract. *Journal of the American College of Nutrition, 15,* 195–196.

Burt, V. L., Whelton, P., & Roccella, E. J. (1995). Prevelance of hypertension in the U.S. adult population. *Third National Health and Nutrition Examination Survey 1988–1991, 25,* 305–313.

Charney, P. (1994). Arginine support line. *Dietitians in Nutrition Support Practice Group of the A.D.A., 16,* 15–17.

Charney, P. & Martindale, R. (1994). Early enteral nutrition support in metabolic stress. *Nutrition, 14,* 1–9.

Chiarelli, A., Enzi, G., & Casadei, A. (1990). Very early nutrition supplementation in burned patients. *American Journal of Clinical Nutrition, 51,* 1035–1039.

Clark, C. & Guitierrez, G. (1992). Gastric intramucosal ph: A noninvasive method for the indirect measurement of tissue oxygenation. *American Journal of Critical Care, 1,* 53–60.

Colwell, J. A. (1996). Intensive insulin therapy in type 2 diabetes; Rationale and collaborative clinical trail results. *Diabetes Care, 19,* 896–898.

Darne, B., Nivarong, M., Tugaye, A., Safar, M., Plouin, P. F., Guillanneuf, M. T., Cubeau, J., Pannier, B., Pequignot, F., & Cambien, F. (1993). Hypocaloric diet and antihypertensive drug treatment. A randomized controlled clinical trial. *Blood Pressure, 2* (2), 130–135.

DeChalain, T. M. B., Mitchell, W. L., & O'Keefe, S. J. (1992). The effect of fuel source on amino acid metabolism in critically ill patients. *Journal of Surgical Research, 52,* 167–180.

Deitch, E. A., Xu, D., Naruhn, M. B., Deitch, D. C., Lu, Q., & Marino, A. A. (1995). Elemental diet and IV TPN induced bacterial translocation is associated with loss of intestinal mucosal barrier function against bacteria. *Annals of Surgery, 221* (3), 229–307.

Dickson, L. R. (1991). Hypoalbuminemia in delirium. *Psychosomatics, 32,* 317–323.

Donius, M. A. (1993). Contamination of a prefilled ready to use enteral feeding system compared with a refillable bag. *Journal of Parenteral and Enteral Nutrition, 17* (5), 461–464.

Doweiko, J. P. & Nomgleggi, M. D. (1991). The role of albumin in human physiology and pathophysiology, III. Albumin and disease states. *Journal of Parenteral and Enteral Nutrition, 15,* 476–483.

Dwyer, J., Krall, E. A., & Coleman, K. A. (1987). The problem of memory in nutritional epidemology research. *Journal of the American Dietetic Association, 87,* 1509–1512.

Elpern, E. H. (1997). Pulmonary aspiration in hospitalized patients. *Nutrition in Clinical Practice, 12,* 5–13.

Emery, E. A., Ahmed, S., Koethe, J. D., Skipper, A., Perlmutter, S., & Paskin, D. L. (1997). Banana flakes control diarrhea in enterally fed patients. *Nutrition in Clinical Practice, 12,* 72–77.

Enia, G., Sicuso, C., Alti, G., & Zocalli, C. (1993). Subjective global assessment of nutrition in dialysis patients. *Nephrology, Dialysis, Transplantation, 8,* 1094–1098.

Erstad, B. L., Campbell, D. J., Rollins, C. J., & Rappaport, W. D. (1994). Albumin and pre-albumin concentrations in patients receiving post-operative parental nutrition. *Pharmacotherapy, 14* (4), 458–462.

Expert Panel on Detection, Evaluation, and Treatment of High Blood Cholesterol in Adults. (1993). Summary of the second report of the National Cholesterol Education Program (NCEP) on detection, evaluation and treatment of high blood cholesterol in adults. *Journal of the American Medical Association, 269* (23), 3015–3023.

Fedullo, A. J. & Sevenburne, A. J. (1983). Relationship of patient age to cost and survival in a medical ICU. *Critical Care Medicine, 11* (3), 155–159.

Feldman, R. D., Logan, A. G., & Schmidt, N. D. (1996). Dietary salt restriction increases vascular insulin resistance. *Clinical Pharmacology & Therapeutics, 60,* 444–451.

Fleet, J. C. (1995). Are low sodium diets appropriate for treated hypertensive men? *Nutrition Reviews, 53* (10), 296–298.

Foreyt, J. P. & Goodrich, G. K. (1995). The ultimate triumph of obesity. *Lancet, 346,* 135.

Forlaw, L. & Guenter, P. (1990). Enteral delivery systems. In J. Rombeau & M. S. Caldwell, (Eds.), *Clinical nutrition: Enteral and tube feeding* (2nd ed.). Philadelphia: W. B. Saunders.

Frankel, W., Zhang, W., Singh, A., Bain, A., Satchithanandam, S., Klurfield, D., & Rombeau, J. (1995). Fiber: Effect on bacterial translocation and intestinal mucin content. *World Journal of Surgery, 19,* 144–148.

Gallagher-Allred, C. R., Voss, A. C., Finn, S. C., & McCamish, M. A. (1996). Malnutrition and clinical outcomes. *Journal of the American Dietetic Association.* 361–366.

Garcia-DeLorenzo, A., Planas, M., & Ortiz-Lebya, C. (1994). Effects of different amounts of branch chain amino acids in septic patients: A multicenter trial. *Journal of Parenteral and Enteral Nutrition, 18,* 21–24S.

Garg, A. & Grundy, S. M. (1990). Management of dyslipidemia in NIDDM. *Diabetes Care, 13,* 153–169.

Garibaldi, A., Brittmore, M. R., & Coleman, M. L. (1981). Risk factors for post-operative pneumonia. *American Journal of Medicine, 70,* 677–680.

Gennari, R., Alexander, J. W., & Eaves-Pyles, T. (1995). Effect of different combinaitons of dietary additives on bacterial translocation and survival in gut related sepsis. *Journal of Parenteral and Enteral Nutrition, 19,* 319–325.

Goichot, B., Schlienger, J. L., Grunenberger, F., Pradignac, A., & Aby, M. A. (1995). Low cholesterol concentrations in free living elderly subjects: Relations with dietary intake and nutritional status. *American Journal of Clinical Nutrition, 62* (3), 547–553.

Goldwasser, P., Michael, M. A., Collier, J., Mittman, N., Fein, P. A., Gusik, S. A., & Avram, M. M. (1993). Pre-albumin and lipoprotein (a) in hemodialysis: Relationships with patient and vascular access survival. *American Journal of Kidney Diseases, 22* (1), 215–225.

Gottschlich, M. M., Alexander, J. W., & Bower, R. H. (1990). Enteral nutrition in patient with burns and trauma. In J. Rombeau & M. D. Caldwell (Eds.), *Clinical nutrition: Enteral and tube feeding* (2nd ed.). Philadelphia: W. B. Saunders.

Gottschlich, M., Warden, G., & Michel, M. (1988). Diarrhea in tube-fed burn patients: Incidence, etiology, nutritional impact and prevention. *Journal of Parenteral and Enteral Nutrition, 12,* 338–345.

Grube, B., Heimbach, D., & Marvin, T. (1987). Clostridium difficile in critically ill burned patients. *Archives of Surgery, 122,* 655–661.

Gupta, T. & Ehrinpreis, M. (1990). Candida associated diarrhea in hospitalized patients. *Gastroenterology, 98,* 780–785.

Harris, M. (1995). *Diabetes in America* (2nd edition) (NIH Publication No. 95–1468, Chapter 1). Washington, DC: U.S. Department of Health and Human Services.

Hsueh, W. A. & Buchanan, T. A. (1994). Obesity and hypertension. *Endocrinology & Metabolism Clinics of North America, 23* (2), 405–727.

Kaplan, N. M. (1989). The deadly quartet: upper body obesity, glucose intolerance, hypertriglyceridemia and hypertension. *Archives of Internal Medicine, 149* (7), 1514–1520.

Keithley, J. K. & Eisenberg, P. (1993). The significance of enteral nutrition in the intensive care unit patients. *Critical Care Nursing Clinics of North America, 5,* 23–29.

Kirk, S. J. & Barbul, A. (1990). Role of arginine in trauma, sepsis and immunity. *Journal of Parenteral and Enteral Nutrition, 14,* 2265–2295.

Kohn, C. L. & Keithley, J. K. (1989). Enteral nutrition. Potential complications and patient monitoring. *Nursing Clinics of North America, 24,* 339–353.

Kuske, H. & Feldman, E. B. (1987). Hyperlipoproteinemia, atherosclerosis risk and dietary management. *Archives of Internal Medicine, 147,* 357–362.

Kushi, L. H., Folsom, A. R., Prineas, R. J., Mink, P. J., Wu, Y., & Bostick, R. M. (1996). Dietary antioxidant vitamins and death from coronary disease in post-menopausal women. *New England Journal of Medicine, 334,* 1156–1162.

Kuzmarski, R. J., Flegal, K. M., Campbell, S. M., & Johnson, C. L. (1994). Increasing prevalence of overweight among U.S. adults: The National Health & Nutrition Examination Surveys, 1960-1991. *Journal of the American Medical Association, 272,* 205–211.

Langkamp-Henken, B., Glezer, J. A., & Kudsk, K. A. (1992). The immunologic structure and function of the gastrointestinal tract. *Nutritional Clinical Practice, 7,* 100–108.

Loghmani, E., Richard, K., Washburne, L., Vandagriff, H., Fineberg, N., & Golden, M. (1991). Glycemic response to sucrose-containing mixed meals in diets of children with insulin dependent diabetes mellitus. *Journal of Pediatrics, 119,* 531–537.

Losconczy, K. G., Harris, T. B., & Havlik, R. J. (1996). Vitamin E and vitamin C supplement use and risk of all cause mortality in older persons: The established populations for epidemiological studies of the elderly. *American Journal of Clinical Nutrition, 64* (2), 190–196.

Manson, J. E., Nathan, D. M., Krowlewski, A. S., Stampfer, M. J., Willett, W. C., & Hennekens, C. H. (1992). A prospective study of exercise and incidence of diabetes among U.S. male physicians. *Journal of the American Medical Association, 268,* 63–67.

Manson, J. E., Rimm, E. B., & Stampfer, M. J. (1991). Physical activity and incidence of non-insulin dependent diabetes mellitus in women. *Lancet, 338,* 774–778.

Manson, J. E., Willett, W. C., Stempfer, M. J., Colditz, G. A., Hunter D. J., Hankinson, S. E., Hennekens, C. H., & Sperzer, F. E. (1995). Body weight and mortality among women. *New England Journal of Medicine, 333* (11), 677–724.

Mao, Y., Kasravi, B., Nobaek, S., Wang, L. Q., Adawi, D., Roos, G., Stenram, U., Molin, G., Bengmark, S., & Jeppsson, B. (1996). Pectin supplemented enteral diet reduces the severity of methotrexate induced enterocolitis in rats. *Scandinavian Journal of Gastroenterology, 31* (6), 558–567.

Marsano, L. & McClain, C. T. (1991). Nutrition and alcoholic liver disease. *Journal of Parenteral and Enteral Nutrition, 15,* 337–344.

McCarron, D. A. (1997). Role of adequate dietary calcium intake in the prevention and management of salt sensitive hypertension. *American Journal of Clinical Nutrition, 65* (25), 712S–716S.

McCauley, R. D., Heel, K. A., Christiansen, K. J., & Hall, J. C. (1996). The effect of minimum luminal nutrition on bacterial translocation and atrophy of the jejunum during parenteral nutrition. *Journal of Gastroenterology and Hepatology, 11* (1), 65–70.

McMahon, M. M., Farnell, M. B., & Murray, M. J. (1993). Nutrition support of critically ill patients. *Mayo Clinic Proceedings, 68,* 911–920.

Mediratta, S., Fozailoff, A., & Friskman, W. H. (1995). Insulin resistance in systemic hypertension: Pharmacotherapeutic implications. *Journal of Clinical Pharmacology, 35* (10), 943–956.

Midgley, J. P., Matthew, A. G., Greenwood, C. M., & Logan A. G. (1993). Effect of reduced dietary sodium on blood pressure: A meta-analysis of randomized controlled trials. *Journal of the American Medical Association, 275* (20), 1590–1597.

Minard, G. & Kudsk, K. A. (1994). Is early enteral nutrition beneficial? How early is early? *New Horizons, 2* (2), 156–163.

Moore, F. A., Feliciano, D. V., & Andrassy, R. J. (1992). Early enteral feeding compared with parenteral reduces postoperative septic complications. *Annals of Surgery, 216,* 172–173.

Morgan, B. L. G. (1988). Obesity. *Nutrition and Health, 8,* 1–7.

Mowatt-Larssen, C., Brown, R., & Wojtysiak, S. (1992). Comparison of tolerance and nutritional outcome between a peptide and a standard enteral formula in critically ill, hypoalbuminemic patients. *Journal of Parenteral and Enteral Nutrition, 16,* 20–24.

Mullan, H., Roubenoff, R. A., & Roubenoff, R. (1992). Risk of pulmonary aspiraiton among patients receiving enteral nutrition. *Journal of Parenteral and Enteral Nutrition, 16,* 160–164.

Mullen, J. L., Buzby, G. P., & Matthews, D. C.(1980). Reduction of operative morbidity and mortality by combined preoperative and postoperative nutritional support. *Annals of Surgery, 192,* 604–613.

National HLBI. (1989). *Detection, evaluation, and treatment of high blood cholesterol in adults.* In National Cholesterol Education Program, Expert Panel (NIH Publication No. 89-2925, pp. 1–23). Washington, DC: U.S. Department of Health and Human Services.

National Task Force on the Prevention and Treatment of Obesity. (1993). Very low calorie diets. *Journal of the American Medical Association, 270,* 967–974.

O'Keefe, S. J., Sender, P. M., & James, W. P. T. (1974). Catabolic loss of body nitrogen in response. *Lancet, 2,* 1035–1042.

Patyek, J. A. & Blackburn, G. L. (1984). Goals of nutritional support in acute infections. *American Journal of Medicine, 76,* 81–87.

Payne-James, J. J. (1992). Retrograde (ascending) bacterial contamination of enteral diet administration systems. *Journal of Parenteral and Enteral Nutrition, 16,* 369–373.

Phillips, M. C. & Olson, L. R. (1993). The immunologic role of the gastrointestinal tract. *Critical Care Nursing Clinics of North America, 5,* 107–120.

Pinchocofsky-Devin, G. D. & Kaminsky, M. V. (1986). Correlation of pressure sores and nutritional status. *Journal of American Geriatric Society, 34,* 435–440.

Pi-Sunyer, F. X. (1988). Exercise in the treatment of obesity. In F. T. Frankle & M. U. Yang (Eds.), *Obesity and Weight Control.* Rockville, MD: Aspen.

Poggi, M., Palareti, G., Biagi, R., Legnani, C., Parenti, M., Babini, A. C., Baraldi, L., & Coccheri, S. (1994). Prolonged very low calorie diet in highly obese subjects reduces plasma viscosity and red cell aggregation but not fibrinogen. *International Journal of Obesity & Related Metabolic Disorders, 18* (7), 490–496.

Pritchard, J. E., Nowson, C. A., & Wark, J. D. (1997). A worksite program for overweight middle-aged men achieves lesser weight loss with exercise than with dietary change. *Journal of the American Dietetic Association, 97,* 37–42.

Rask, L., Arundi, H., Bohme, J., Eriksson, U., Fredriksson, A., & Nilsson, S. F. (1980). The retinol binding protein. *Scandinavian Journal of Clinical and Laboratory Investigation, 154,* 45–61.

Reaven, G. M. (1988). Role of insulin resistance in human disease. *Diabetes, 37,* 1595–1607.

Reilly, J. J., Hull, S. F., Albert, N., Waller, A., & Bringardener, T. (1988). Economic impact of malnutrition: A model system for hospitalized patients. *Journal of Parenteral and Enteral Nutrition, 12,* 871–875.

Rubin, R. J. & Altman, W. M. (1994). 1992 Estimates of health care expenditures from people with diabetes. *Journal of Clinical Endocrinology Metabolism, 78,* 809A–809F.

Russell, D., Lester, L. A., & Whitwell, J. (1983). Skeletal muscle function during hypocaloric diets and fasting: A comparison with standard nutritional assessment parameters. *American Journal of Clinical Nutrition, 37,* 133–139.

Sax, H. C., Illig, K. A., Ryan, C. K., & Hardy, D. J. (1996). Low dose enteral feeding is beneficial during total parenteral nutrition. *American Journal of Surgery, 171* (6), 587–590.

Schafer, R., Bohammon, B., Franz, M. J., Freeman, J., Holmes, A., McLaughlin, S., Haas, L., Kruger, D., Lorenz, R., & McMahon, M. (1997). Translation of the diabetes nutrition recommendations for health care institutions. *Diabetes Care, 20,* 96–105.

Schaefer, E. J., Lichenstein, A. H., & Lamon-Fava, S. (1996). Effects of the National Cholesterol Education Program Step 2 diets relatively high or relatively low in fish derived fatty acids on plasma lipoproteins in middle aged or elderly subjects. *American Journal of Clinical Nutrition,* .

Schroeder, D., Gillanders, L., Mahrs, K., & Hill, G. L. (1991). Effects of immediate postoperative enteral nutrition on body composition, muscle function and wound healing. *Journal of Parenteral and Enteral Nutrition, 15,* 376–383.

Sedman, P. C., Macfie, J., Sagar, P., Mitchell, C. J., May, J., Mancey-Jones, B., & Johnstone, C. (1994). The prevelance of gut translocation in humans. *Gastroenterology, 107,* 643–649.

Seidel, J. C. (1992). Regional obesity & health. *Internal Journal of Obesity, 16,* 531–534.

Seidner, D. L. (1994). Clinical uses for omega 3 polyunsaturated fatty acids and structured lipids. *Support Line, 16,* 7–11.

Singer, D. E., Nathan, D. M., Anderson, K. M., Wilson, P. N., & Evans, J. C. (1992). Association of HgA_1C with prevalent cardiovascular disease in the original cohort of the Framingham Heart Study. *Diabetes, 41,* 202–208.

Smith, R. J., (1990). Glutamine metabolism and its physiologic importance. *Journal of Parenteral and Enteral Nutrition, 14,* 945–995.

Stephens, N. G., Parsons, A., Schofield, P. M., Kelly, F., Cheeseman, K., & Mitchenson, M. J. (1996). Randomized controlled trial of vitamin E in patients with coronary disease: Cambridge Heart Antioxidant Study (CHAOS). *Lancet, 347,* 781–786.

Strong, A. M., Condon, S. C., & Solinger, M. R. (1992). Equal aspiration rates from postpylorus and intragastric placed nasoenteric feeding tubes: A randomized, prospective study. *Journal of Parenteral and Enteral Nutrition, 16,* 59–63.

Tapers, S. S. (1992). Nutritionally associated increased carbon dioxide production: Excess total calories vs high proportion of carbohydrate calories. *Chest, 102,* 551–555.

Toplak, H. & Wascher, T. G. (1994). Influence of weight reduction on platelet volume: Different effects of a hypocaloric diet and a very low calorie diet. *European Journal of Clinical Investigation, 24* (11), 778–780.

Torres, A., El-Ebiary, M., Soler, N., Monton, C., Fabregas, N., & Hernandez, C. (1996). Stomach as a source of colonization of the respiratory tract during mechanical ventilation: Association with ventilator associated pneumonia. *European Respiratory Journal, 9* (8), 1729–1735.

Trice, S., Melnik, G., & Page, C. P. (1997). Complications and costs of early postoperative parenteral versus enteral nutrition in trauma patients. *Nutrition in Clinical Practice, 12,* 114–119.

United States Congress, Office of Technology Assessment. (1987). *Life sustaining technologies and the elderly.* Washington, DC: U.S. Government Printing Office.

Vahlquist, A., Peterson, P. A., & Wilbell, L. (1973). Metabolism of the vitamin A transporting protein complex I: Turnover studies in normal persons and in patients with chronic renal failure. *European Journal of Clinical Investigation, 3,* 352–362.

Van Itallie, T. B. (1988). Topography of body fat: Relationship to risk of cardiovascular disease and other diseases. In T. G. Lohman, A. F. Roche & R. Martovell (Eds.), *Anthropometric Standardization Manual* (pp. 143–149). Champaign, IL: Human Kinetic.

von Meyenfeldt, M. F., Soeters, P. B., & Vente, J. P. (1990). Effect of branch chain amino acid enrichment of total parenteral nutrition on nitrogen sparing and clinical outcome of sepsis and trauma: A prospective randomized double blind trial. *British Journal of Surgery, 77,* 924–929.

Wadden, T. A., Foster, D. G., & Letizia, K. A. (1994). One year behavioral treatment of obesity: Comparison of moderate and severe caloric restriction and the effects of weight maintenance therapy. *Journal of Consulting and Clinical Psychology, 62,* 165–171.

Wadden, T. A., Foster, D. G., Letizia, K. A., & Stunkard, A. J. (1992). A multicenter evaluation of a proprietary weight reduction program for the treatment of marked obesity. *Archives of Internal Medicine, 152,* 961–966.

Weisman, C., Kempner, M. C., & Askanzi, J. (1986). Resting metabolic rate of critically ill patients: Measured vs predicted. *Anesthesiology, 64,* 673–678.

Windsor, J. A. & Hill, G. L. (1988). Weight loss with physiologic impairment. A basic indicator of surgical risk. *Annals of Surgery, 207,* 290–296.

Wingard, D. L. & Barrett-Connor, E. (1995). Heart disease and diabetes. *Diabetes in America* (NIH Publication No. 95-1468, 2nd ed.). Washington, DC: National Institute of Health.

Yki-Järvinen, H. (1992). Glucose toxicity. *Endocrinology Reviews, 13,* 415–431.

Zaloga, G. P. (1992). Enteral nutrition in hospitalized patients: A summary. In a report of the Twelfth Ross Roundtable on Medical Issues, *Enteral nutrition support for the 1990s: Innovations in nutrition, technology & techniques* (pp. 177–183). Columbus, OH: Ross Laboratories.

Zarling, E. J. Parmer, J. R. & Mobarhan, S. (1986). Effect of enteral formula infusion rate, osmolatity and chemical composition upon clinical tolerance and carbohydrate absorption in normal subjects. *Journal of Parenteral and Enteral Nutrition, 10,* 588–590.

Zavaroni, I., Coruzzi, P., Bonini, L., Mossini, G. L., Musiari, L., Gasparini, P., Fantuzzi, M. & Reaven, G. M. (1995). Associations between salt sensitivity and insulin concentrations in patients with hypertension. *American Journal of Hypertension, 8* (8), 855–858.

Zoccali, C., Mallamaci, F., Cuzzola, F. & Leonardis, D. (1996). Reproducibility of the response to short term low salt intake in essential hypertension. *Journal of Hypertension, 14* (2), 1455–1459.

18

Fluid, Electrolyte, and Acid–Base Abnormalities

JoAnne Konick-McMahon

This chapter deals with the complex topic of fluid, electrolyte, and acid–base imbalances. The ACNP frequently encounters abnormalities—usually in combination with one another—in the hospital and follow-up settings. Surgical and medical patients have multiple reasons for these clinical problems which, if not recognized and corrected promptly, may cause unwanted patient outcomes.

▶ FLUID BALANCE

Two major compartments exist for fluids in the body: the extracellular and intracellular. Two-thirds of body fluid is intracellular fluid (ICF) in adults while the remainder is extracellular fluid (ECF). An important note for the ACNP is that the decrease in the relative size of the ECF in older adults provides little reserve for fluid deficit situations (O'Donnell, 1995).

The ECF consists of three compartments (Table 18–1): the interstitial fluid (ICF), intravascular fluid (IVF), and transcellular fluid (TCF). Fluids and solutes move across compartments through osmosis, filtration, diffusion, and active transport (Table 18–2).

The ICF provides a stable environment for the cells with little change in composition of the fluid. The ECF, however, requires continuous change of fluids and solutes in response to changes in intake of nutrients. Regulation of the vascular volume and composition of the ECF occurs via several mechanisms (Table 18–3). These mechanisms serve to maintain a balance of fluid as well as electrolytes.

TABLE 18–1. Fluid Compartments and Volumes for a 70-kg Man

Intracellular fluid (ICF) = 27 liters
Extracellular fluid (ECF) = 15 liters
  Interstitial fluid = 11–121
  Intravascular fluid = 3 liters of plasma + 2–3 liters of red blood cells, white blood cells, platelets
  Transcellular fluid = 1 liter

TABLE 18–2. Transport Processes for Water and Solutes Between Compartments

1. Osmosis	Water movement across semipermeable membrane from area of lower solute (particle) concentration to higher concentration.
2. Filtration	Water/solute movement from area of high hydrostatic pressure (created by weight of fluid) to area of low hydrostatic pressure.
3. Diffusion	Movement of particles through solution or gases from area of high concentration to area of low concentration (e.g., diffusion of oxygen from lung to blood).
4. Active transport	Movement of solutes (electrolytes, glucose, hydrogen) requiring energy to move from area of lesser or equal concentration to area of equal or higher concentration.

TABLE 18–3. Mechanisms Regulating ECF Volume

Volume Stretch Receptors	Carotid sinuses, aortic arch, cardiac atria, renal vessels, change in cardiac output, vascular resistance, thirst, and renal wasting or retaining of sodium and water
Sympathetic Nervous System	Release of epinephrine
Renin Angiotensin System	Renal perfusion decreased leads to vasoconstriction and aldosterone release
Aldosterone	Saves sodium and water
Atrial Natriuretic Factor (ANF)	Increased atrial pressure leads to reduced blood pressure and vascular volume
Antidiuretic Hormone	Responds to decreased ECF volume or increased plasma osmolality by kidney water conservation
Thirst	Hypothalamus causes sensation as a result of decreased volume or increased osmolality

These seven mechanisms provide protection for the cells. Changes in the ECF osmolality (concentration of particles to fluid) cause changes in the ICF. The brain cells, in particular, respond to sudden changes by changing the number of intracellular particles to prevent swelling or shrinking of the brain cells. This points to the need for cautious correction of ECF volume and osmolality abnormalities to avoid sudden changes in brain cell volume.

Fluid Abnormalities

Hypovolemia

Hypovolemia is a deficit of extracellular fluid volume (ECF). Three pathophysiologic processes can lead to hypovolemia (Baer, 1993). The first is excessive loss of fluids and electrolytes through vomiting, diarrhea, draining wounds, burns, or excess diuretics. Bleeding as a result of trauma or injury may also lead to hypovolemia through this process.

The second process leading to hypovolemia is decreased intake of fluids and electrolytes. Examples include patients who are unable to swallow and those in whom fluids and electrolytes are not adequately replaced. The third pathophysiologic process causing hypovolemia is movement of fluid and electrolytes into areas that are not available for body use. Commonly called "third spacing," clinical examples include ascites, peritonitis, and pancreatitis.

Clinical history to support a diagnosis of hypovolemia includes fluid loss through the gastrointestinal system, skin (diaphoresis because of fever or exercise), renal system (osmotic diuresis or polyuric diseases), third spacing processes, or hemmorhage, and lack of fluid intake.

Subjective findings for the patient with hypovolemia can include dizziness, fainting, weakness, fatigue, thirst, constipation, and oliguria. Physical findings of hypovolemia include orthostatic blood pressure and pulse changes, tachycardia, decreased skin turgor, dry furrowed tongue, flat neck veins, increased temperature, and weight loss (more than 5% of total body weight). Hemodynamic measurements in hypovolemia include decreased central venous pressure (CVP) and pulmonary artery wedge pressure (PAWP), decreased cardiac output (CO) and mean arterial pressure, and increased systemic vascular resistance (SVR).

Severe hypovolemia, or shock, is characterized by supine hypotension; rapid, weak pulse; cool, clammy skin; and confusion, stupor, or coma. This stage of hypovolemia has been associated with an acute weight loss of more than 10%.

Diagnostic tests include serum, arterial, and urine studies. Serum blood urea nitrogen (BUN) may be increased while serum electrolytes reflect the fluid lost. GI or renal losses lead to hypokalemia while adrenal insufficiency causes hyperkalemia. Hyponatremia is a common finding early in hypovolemia because of sodium dilution due to the normal mechanisms of thirst and increased antidiuretic hormone. Hypernatremia may be present if hypovolemia is related to diabetes insipidus (pure water loss) or diaphoresis. Hematocrit is elevated with dehydration and decreased with bleeding. Serum osmolality varies related to the type of body fluid loss as well as the person's ability to compensate through thirst and ADH.

Arterial blood gas values reflect the fluid loss as well as the perfusion state. Metabolic acidosis (7.35, $HCO_3<22$ mEq/L) is seen with diarrhea, diabetic ketoacidosis, and shock. Metabolic alkalosis ($pH>7.45$, $HCO_3>26$ mEq/L) is seen with vomiting and diuretics.

Urine specific gravity is concentrated (i.e., >1.020), reflecting the kidney's conservation of water. Urine sodium also reflects kidney conservation in hypovolemia and should be less than 10 to 20 mEq/L in the absence of diuretics, renal disease, or osmotic diuresis.

Management of hypovolemia includes treatment of the underlying cause of fluid imbalance as well as replacement of lost fluids and electrolytes. Fluid and electrolyte replacement for hypovolemia may begin, if renal function is in question, with a hydrating solution such as normal saline to challenge the renal system and look for urine response.

With renal response verified, all-purpose solutions or crystalloids such as normal saline are used to replace fluid deficit to improvement of physical signs. Specifically created solutions may be the next step to correct particular fluid and electrolyte imbalances. Colloids including banked or autotransfused blood may be fluid of choice in the anemic or hemmorhaging patient. Table 18–4 illustrates common intravenous solutions and their components.

Follow-up for the patient with hypovolemia includes return of baseline blood pressure and heart rate less than 100 bpm. Urine output increases to 30 or more mL/hr in adults. The ACNP should continue to monitor serum electrolytes, hematocrit and hemoglobin, osmolality, and arte-

TABLE 18–4. Components of Common IV Solutions

Solution	Glucose (gm/L)	Na+ (mEq/L)	Cl−(mEq/L)	Tonicity/mOsm/L
Saline				
0.9%		154	154	Isotonic/308
0.45%		77	77	Hypotonic/154
3.0%		513	513	Hypertonic/1026
Dextrose in Water				
5%	50			Isotonic/278
Dextrose in saline				
5% in 0.225%	50	38.5	38.5	Isotonic/355
5% in 0.45%	50	77	77	Hypertonic/432
5% in 0.9%	50	154	154	Hypertonic/586
Ringer's		147	156	Isotonic/309

Adapted from Horne, et al. (1997). Fluid, electrolyte and acid-base balance.

rial blood gas. Management of the cause of hypovolemia, such as inadequate intake or diabetic ketoacidosis, is useful to prevent recurrence. Provide patients and significant others with verbal and written instructions about signs and symptoms of hypovolemia as well as how to contact the appropriate health-care provider when symptoms occur.

Hypervolemia

Excess extracellular fluid volume, hypervolemia, has three potential pathophysiologic causes. The first is retention or excessive intake of increased amounts of sodium and, thus, water. A second etiology is decreased renal excretion of sodium and water. For example, acute or chronic renal failure. Finally, decreased mobilization of fluid within the intravascular space, as in heart failure, can lead to hypervolemia.

Pertinent clinical history includes heart failure, cirrhosis, excess steroids, excess intravenous fluids (including hypertonics or albumin), and treated burns. Subjective complaints are shortness of breath and orthopnea. Physical exam reveals weight gain, increased BP, edema, ascites, crackles, rhonchi, wheezes, distended neck veins, and tachycardia with S_3. Hemodynamic monitoring reveals CVP 10 mm Hg or greater, PAP greater than 30/15 mm Hg, and pulmonary capillary wedge pressure greater than 15 mm Hg.

If the hypervolemia is isotonic, there may not be any changes in serum electrolytes or blood count. There may be decreased hematocrit, hemaglobin, and red blood cell count related to hypotonia or water dilution. Urine may have increased sodium and decreased specific gravity if kidney function is normal. Arterial blood gas monitoring may indicate hypoxemia if pulmonary congestion is present along with a respiratory alkalosis (pH>7.45 and $PaCO_2$ less than 35 mEq/L). Chest x-ray reveals pulmonary vascular congestion.

Management includes fluid and sodium restrictions, use of diuretics, and dialysis or continuous arteriovenous or venovenous hemofiltration in renal failure or life-threatening fluid overload. Until diuretics remove excess volume, supplemental oxygen via nasal cannula or mask may be needed if hypoxia is present.

Evaluation of treatment outcomes include clear lungs, absence of extra heart sounds (S3 and/or S4), adequate urinary output of 30 mL/hr, normal urine specific gravity (1.010–1.020), baseline weight, and no edema. Normalization of blood pressure, heart rate, CVP, and PAWP indicate correction of hypervolemia. Oxygenation and serum electrolytes (especially potassium) should be monitored.

▶ ELECTROLYTES

The electrolytes are regulated via multiple mechanisms (Table 18–5). Sodium, the primary extracellular cation, is directly related to serum osmolality. Abnormalities of serum sodium indicate changes in water balance more often than changes in the electrolyte.

Potassium, the primary intracellular cation, exists in the serum in small amounts. Movement of potassium between the intracellular and extracellular fluid is regulated by the sodium–potassium pump in the cell membrane.

Calcium, an extracellular and intracellular cation, plays a major role in muscle contraction and cardiac electrophysiology. Changes in acid–base balance and albumin levels affect availability of ionized calcium.

Magnesium is primarily an intracellular cation and leads to enzyme activity involved in carbohydrate and protein metabolism. Magnesium also stimulates the sodium–potassium pump in the intracellular space. Only 1% of total body magnesium is in the ECF. Thirty percent of ECF magnesium is protein bound, a small amount is bound to other substances, and the rest is the active or ionized magnesium. Thus, magnesium levels, like calcium levels, must be evaluated in relation to serum albumin levels.

TABLE 18–5. Electrolyte Regulation and Normal Values

Electrolyte	Mechanism of Regulation
Sodium (135–145 mEq/L)	Kidney excretes or conserves sodium Aldosterone/angiotensin II conserves sodium via kidney ANF cause renal excretion of sodium Thirst serves to dilute excess sodium and decrease serum osmolality ADH saves water via kidney to dilute excess sodium and decrease osmolality
Potassium (3.5–5 mEq/L)	Kidney excretes or conserves Movement in and out of cell influenced by insulin and serum pH
Calcium (8.5–10 mg/dL) Ionized Calcium (4.5 to 5.5 mg/dL)	99% of body calcium is bound with phosphorus in bone/teeth <1% in ECF Parathyroid hormone causes increased bone resorption to correct hypocalcemia Vitamin D causes increased calcium absorption from gut Calcitonin inhibits bone resorption to correct elevated calcium
Magnesium (1.5–2.5 mEq/L)	Excreted by kidney Vitamin D causes increased magnesium absorption from gut

Sodium Abnormalities

Hyponatremia

Hyponatremia (sodium less than 135 mEq/L) is a disorder of water balance in most situations and is the most common electrolyte disorder (Gross & Hensen, 1995). According to Black (1996), hyponatremia occurs either because of abnormal water excretion or increased water ingestion with normal water excretion. Serum hypoosmolality (less particles than normal in solution) is a frequent finding in hyponatremia. Hyponatremia may occur without hypoosmolality in the setting of elevated triglycerides, genitourinary irrigations, or azotemia.

Hyponatremia with impaired water excretion may be due to hypovolemic (decreased ECF) states such as gastrointestinal, skin, or renal losses. This type of hyponatremia may also occur in heart or liver failure in which arterial perfusion pressure falls, causing the hypovolemic hormones (norepinephrine, angiotensin II, and ADH) to turn on and conserve water and sodium.

Diuretics, especially the thiazides, and advanced renal failure may cause *hyponatremia related to impaired water excretion.* Hypothyroidism and hypoadrenalism have also been associated with hyponatremia since both hormone deficiencies may cause decreased cardiac output and, therefore, increased ADH release.

Syndrome of inappropriate antidiuretic hormone (SIADH) is hyponatremia with hypoosmolality related to a variety of causes (Table 18–6). To diagnose SIADH, the ACNP must exclude renal, adrenal, and thyroid disease.

Hyponatremia with normal water excretion and therefore normal ECF volume is seen in primary polydipsia. This may be related to a psychiatric problem such as schizophrenia or a hypothalmic problem (site of the thirst center).

Clinical history in hyponatremia with ECF losses include GI losses through vomiting, nasogastic suction, renal fluid loss (e.g., diuretics), or burns. Hyponatremia with normal or increased ECF volume include a clinical history of those causes of SIADH, heart failure, liver disease, nephrotic syndrome, and primary psychogenic polydipsia associated with schizophrenia and/or phenothiazine use.

Physical findings are based on the level of hyponatremia as well as fluid volume state. A sodium level of 120 mEq/L or less is considered a critical situation because of dangerous neurologic symptoms related to shifting of water to the brain cells. This is especially true in hyponatremia that develops acutely (Freeland & Kruse, 1996). Hyponatremia may lead to signs of increased intracranial pressure such as seizures, papilledema, and coma. Symptoms usually resolve with treatment, although hyponatremia of this degree may be fatal or result in permanent neurologic injury.

A patient with a sodium level of 120-130 mEq/L may present with clinical signs of headache, lethargy, weakness, and confusion related to increased cerebral edema. GI symptoms of nausea and abdominal cramping may also occur with hyponatremia.

Additional findings on physical exam are related to fluid state. The patient with decreased ECF volume and hyponatremia often presents with the neurologic symptoms mentioned above plus postural hypotension, dry mucous membranes, tachycardia, decreased urine output, and decreased CVP and PAP. The patient with normal or increased ECF and hyponatremia, as in SIADH, presents with neurologic manifestations plus weight gain, edema, increased blood pressure, CVP, and PAP if fluid volume is increased.

Laboratory testing includes serum sodium and serum

TABLE 18–6. Causes of SIADH

Central nervous system	Head trauma, intracranial hemorrhage, encephalitis, brain tumor, stroke, Guillain–Barre syndrome
Pulmonary system	Pneumonia, bacterial, viral or fungal, tuberculosis, lung abscess, cystic fibrosis
Neoplastic diseases	Oat cell carcinoma of lung, duodenal carcinoma, pancreatic cancer, thymoma, lymphoma
Drugs	Cyclophosphamide, carbamazepine, chloropropamide, nonsteroidal antiinflammatory drugs
Symptomatic HIV infection	

osmolality. Urine specific gravity is decreased (1.005 or less) if the kidney is excreting excess water. In dehydrated patients or those with SIADH, the urine is concentrated. Urine sodium is decreased (less than 20 mEq/L) except with adrenal insufficiency and SIADH.

The goal for treatment of hyponatremia is to raise sodium to 120-130 mEq/L to prevent life-threatening complications. The sodium should be increased by no more than 1-2 mmol/L/hr and 12-20 mmol/L per day to avoid complications associated with rapid correction (Freeland & Kruse, 1996). Hypertonic saline (3%) may be used if seizures due to hyponatremia are present. The calculation for volume and infusion rate are:

$$\text{Volume of 3\% saline} = \frac{0.6 \times \text{weight (kg)} \times (\text{desired Na} - \text{current Na})}{3 \text{ mmol/L}}$$

$$\text{Infusion rate} = \frac{\text{volume of 3\% saline rate of correction}}{(\text{desired Na} - \text{current Na})}$$

The patient with hypovolemic hyponatremia is treated with isotonic saline. Hold diuretics and replace adrenal hormones if needed. Hypertonic saline should be considered if severe neurologic symptoms are present.

The ACNP dealing with hypervolemic hyponatremia in heart failure, cirrhosis, or renal disease rarely sees severe symptoms. Treatment includes water restriction, diuretics, inotropes in heart failure, and albumin in liver or renal failure.

The patient with hyponatremia because of SIADH is treated with water restriction, low-dose loop diuretic, and high-sodium diet. The drug demeclocycline (300-600 mg orally twice daily) is used to block ADH action on the kidney. Hypertonic saline may be used if life-threatening hyponatremia is present.

Follow-up consists of neurologic assessment to determine return to baseline function as well as continued surveillance of sodium and other electrolyes. Patient and caregiver education for chronic hyponatremia should focus on signs, symptoms, and needed treatment.

Hypernatremia

Sodium levels greater than 145 mEq/L may be related to increased fluid loss (more water than sodium) through GI, skin, or lung; diuretics; or osmotic diuresis (hyperglycemia or urea diuresis). Hypernatremia may also be related to iatrogenic causes such as use of hypertonic saline or sodium bicarbonate. These causes, as well as excess mineralocorticoid (aldosterone) levels, may lead to hypervolemia and hypernatremia. The third situation in which hypernatremia may be found is a normal ECF volume state such as diabetes insipidus in which there is pure water loss.

Hypernatremia is produced only in those individuals who do not have an intact thirst mechanism and/or do not have access to water. Therefore, older adults and those with comorbidities are most likely to develop symptomatic hypernatremia.

Symptoms in hypernatremia are related to the pulling of water from brain cells because of the hypertonic serum. The most dramatic symptoms occur with acute rise in serum sodium. The symptoms may include intense thirst, fatigue, restlessness, agitation, and coma. Fever, nausea, vomiting, muscle weakness, fasiculations, and spasticity may also be seen with hypernatremia. With sodium gain and a hypervolemic state, pulmonary and peripheral edema may be present. With water loss, postural hypotension and the other signs of fluid deficit are present. Diabetes insipidus produces huge volumes of urine.

Serum osmolality is increased because of elevated sodium. Urine specific gravity and osmolality are increased as the kidneys retain water to correct the hyperosmolar state. The urine is dilute (decreased specific gravity and osmolality) if diabetes insipidus is present.

Treatment of hypernatremia is a gradual replacement of free water. The goal is to prevent cerebral edema, which may occur if serum water moves into cerebral cells because of large concentration differences (hypotonic serum versus hypertonic cerebral cells). Free water replacement orally or intravenously is necessary in all forms of hypernatremia. Correction should occur over two days (Horne et al., 1997). Diuretics may be needed to treat sodium gain with fluid lost through diuresis being replaced with free water (Dextrose 5% in water). Desmopressin acetate (DDAVP) is used as ADH replacement in diabetes insipidus along with free water if needed.

Follow-up includes neurologic assessment and laboratory examinations of serum sodium and osmolality. If neurologic symptoms improve and then become worse, suspect cerebral edema and hold free water replacement until status improves. Anticipated outcomes are return to baseline neurologic function and stabilization of cardiovascular status and fluid levels.

Potassium Abnormalities

Hypokalemia

Hypokalemia is frequently related to use of medications that causes potassium loss such as diuretics and certain antibiotics and inadequate replacement during parenteral nutrition and hydration. Additional causes of reduction in total body potassium include gastric losses through vomiting or nasogastric suction, excessive diaphoresis, and malnutrition associated with anorexia or alcoholism.

A second pathophysiologic basis for hypokalemia is intracellular shifts of potassium. This occurs with insulin use and treatment of diabetic ketoacidosis, during alkalosis and after treatment of acidosis, and during tissue repair like burns or trauma.

Clinical history indicative of hypokalemia includes diuretic use, vomiting, diarrhea, intravenous hydration or nutrition, and diabetic ketoacidosis. Symptoms include leg cramps, muscle weakness, nausea, vomiting, and ileus. Physical findings may include weak, irregular pulse; decreased reflexes and muscle tone; and decreased bowel sounds. Neurologic signs of confusion and disorientation may occur with hypokalemia, for unknown reasons (Braxmeyer & Keyes, 1996).

A serum potassium less than 3.5mEq/L constitutes hypokalemia. Arterial blood gas may show alkalosis while EKG findings show ST segment depression, flattened T wave, a U wave, and ventricular dysrhythmias (Fig. 18–1). EKG may also reveal rhythms seen in digoxin toxicity during hypokalemia despite a normal dig level.

Treatment is aimed at correction of underlying cause, such as diabetic ketoacidosis, while repleting potassium. If renal function is questionable, cautious replacement is needed until urine flow and function via creatinine level have been established.

Potassium repletion may occur orally or intravenously usually totalling 40-80 mEq/day. Rate of IV potassium replacement should not be faster than 10-20 mEq/hr or in concentrations greater than 40 mEq/L, unless potassium is very low (less than 2.5 mEq/L). Continuous monitoring of the EKG is needed for the patient receiving 20 mEq/hr to assess peaking of T waves, widening of the QRS, and slowing of the rate, signs of hyperkalemia. Peripheral infusion of potassium supplementation may cause venous irritation and discomfort requiring a decreased rate of infusion. If large doses of potassium are necessary, a central line is required.

Potassium is usually given with chloride to patients with ECF deficit, and therefore chloride loss. Potassium may be given with phosphate in situations such as diabetic ketoacidosis when an intracellular anion is needed.

Evaluation and follow-up include frequent monitoring of potassium levels to avoid over- or under-treatment. Continued hypokalemia in the face of adequate potassium replacement may be related to hypomagnesemia. Low magnesium leads to potassium movement to the intravascular space and then increased wasting in the urine. Outcomes include correction of the underlying cause, normal potassium level, and return to baseline EKG.

Hyperkalemia

Hyperkalemia can be a life-threatening electrolyte finding. It may lead to severe dysrhythmias if not detected and treated quickly. Potassium levels greater than 5.0 mEq/L occur because of three etiologies. The first is decreased excretion by the kidney as in acute or chronic renal failure. A second cause is movement of potassium from the intracellular area as in hyperglycemia or hypernatremia. In these two situations, osmolarity increases in the extracellular space, which causes fluid shifts as well as potassium shifts from the intracellular space. A third pathophysiologic cause of hyperkalemia is acidosis, which leads to entrance of hydrogen ions into the cell and potassium exchange to the extracellular area.

Clinical history for hyperkalemia might include intravenous or oral supplementation of potassium, potassium sparing diuretics, or angiotensin-converting enzyme (ACE) inhibitors, acidosis, and insulin deficiency. Symptoms include abdominal cramping, diarrhea, weakness, irritability, and anxiety. Physical signs of hyperkalemia depend on the level of potassium and how quickly the potassium level rose. With rapid onset of hyperkalemia, there might be a weak, irregular pulse with hypotension.

EKG changes are hallmark findings in hyperkalemia and should be checked as soon as a level above normal is obtained (Fig. 18–1). A level of 6 mEq/L usually produces tall peaked T waves, short QT, and slow rate. The PR lengthens and AV blocks appear as K^+ reaches 7 mEq/L. As the levels rises, the QRS lengthens and bradycardia begins. Cardiac standstill occurs near 8.5 mEq/L, although this depends on how quickly the level rose.

Acute management of the patient with hyperkalemia includes an EKG to check for cardiac signs of hyperkalemia. If no signs are present on EKG and no relevant clinical history exists, a repeat potassium is in order. Hemolyzed specimens as well as prolonged tourniquet use during venipuncture can lead to falsely elevated potassium levels.

If potassium is less than 7 mEq/L with EKG changes (e.g., peaked T waves, widened QRS, prolonged PR interval, or slowing of the rate), a sodium exchange resin, Kaexylate, is used to remove extra potassium via the bowel. This may be given orally or via enema. Kaexylate needs to be in contact with the bowel for 2 minutes to cause exchange, so a large bore catheter may be used as a rectal tube to insert and keep the medicine in the rectum. One gram of Kaexylate removes 1 mEq of K^+.

Life-threatening K^+ levels, greater than 7 mEq/L with EKG changes, necessitates emergency action to prevent cardiac asystole. While Kaexylate is being given, IV calcium is used to counteract the effect of potassium on the heart. IV bicarbonate is used to create an alkalosis to pull potassium into cells. Insulin and glucose are also used to pull potassium into cells. These actions have effect for 15-30 minutes while Kaexylate can work and/or diuretics or dialysis can be administered to remove excess potassium.

Evaluation and follow-up include checking potassium levels to avoid hypokalemia. Desired outcomes are return to normal potassium levels with normal EKG and blood pressure. Follow-up includes patient education to avoid high K^+ foods if this may be a chronic problem, along with the signs, symptoms, and who to call with hyperkalemia.

Calcium Abnormalities

Hypocalcemia

The most common cause of total calcium level less than 8.5 mg/dL, which may occur in as many as 80% of critically ill patients, is hypoalbuminemia (Yucha & Toto, 1994). This

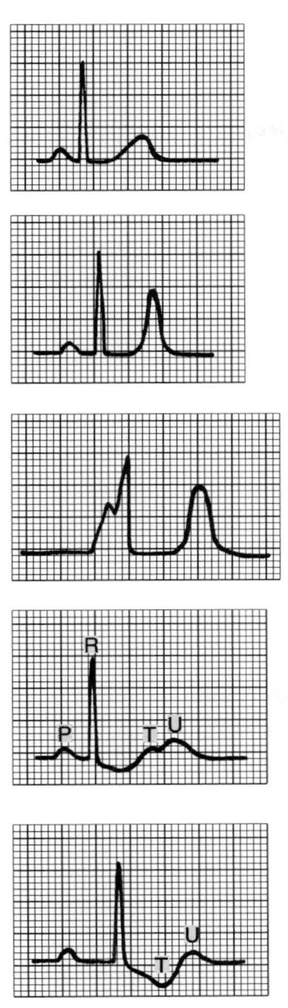

Normal tracing (plasma K^+ 4–5.5 meq/L). PR interval = 0.16 s; QRS interval = 0.06 s; QT interval = 0.4 s (normal for an assumed heart rate of 60).

Hyperkalemia (plasma K^+ ±7.0 meq/L). The PR and QRS intervals are within normal limits. Very tall, slender peaked T waves are now present.

Hyperkalemia (plasma K^+ ±8.5 meq/L). There is no evidence of atrial activity; the QRS complex is broad and slurred and the QRS interval has widened to 0.2 s. The T waves remain tall and slender. Further elevation of the plasma K^+ level may result in ventricular tachycardia and ventricular fibrilation.

Hypokalemia (plasma K^+ ±3.5 meq/L). PR interval = 0.2 s; QRS interval = 0.06 s; ST segment depression. A prominent U wave is now present immediately following the T. The actual QT interval remains 0.4 s. If the U wave is erroneously considered a part of the T, a falsely prolonged QT interval of 0.6 s will be measured.

Hypokalemia (plasma K^+ ±2.5 meq/L). The PR interval is lengthened to 0.32 s; the ST segment is depressed; the T wave is inverted; a prominent U wave is seen. The true QT interval remains normal.

Figure 18–1. Correlation of plasma K^+ level and the ECG, assuming that the plasma calcium level is normal. The diagrammed complexes are left ventricular epicardial leads. *(Reproduced with permission from Goldman, M. J. (1986).* Principles of Clinical Electrocardiography, *(12th ed.) Norwalk, CT: Appleton & Lange.)*

type of hypocalcemia, pseudohypocalcemia, does not require treatment as long as ionized calcium level remains normal (4.0 mg/dL).

Causes of true hypocalcemia with decreased ionized calcium include hypoparathyroidism (especially after neck surgery), elevated phosphate (as in acute renal failure), hypomagnesemia, and lack of calcitrol (as in pancreatitis). Sepsis can lead to hypocalcemia because of mediator supression of the parathyroid gland and impaired calcitrol production. Diuretics cause calcium loss and, in acute illness, may lead to hypocalcemia.

Low ionized calcium may also be caused by calcium chelation or precipitation. This may be caused by the preservative and anticoagulant, citrate, in banked blood or plasmapheresis replacement. Metabolic or respiratory alkalosis increases calcium–albumin binding, thus decreasing ionized calcium and presenting symptoms of hypocalcemia.

Clinical history of hypocalcemia may include multiple blood transfusions or plasmapheresis, sepsis, diuretic use, neck surgery, pancreatitis, acute renal failure, or low magnesium. Complaints, usually seen with ionized levels less than 3.2 mg/dL, include numbness and tingling of fingers and circumorally, hyperactive reflexes, muscles cramping, tetany, and seizures. Physical signs include positive Trousseau's sign and Chvostek's sign. Trousseau's sign is produced by BP cuff inflation on the upper arm to above systolic for 2 minutes to produce carpal spasm. Chvostek's sign is produced with facial nerve percussion in front of the ear leading to unilateral contraction of facial and eyelid muscles because of spasticity related to hypocalcemia.

EKG findings included prolonged QT interval or Torsades de pointes ventricular tachycardia. Decreased cardiac contractility may occur with hypocalcemia, leading to heart failure or pulmonary edema.

Laboratory findings include serum calcium as well as albumin levels. If albumin is low, ionized calcium should be followed. Measurement of parathyroid hormone (normal is 150-350 pg/mL) may show decreased levels in hypoparathyroidism. Serum magnesium and phosphate levels may indicate possible causes of hypocalcemia.

Treatment of true ionized calcium deficit is treated with calcium replacement, either oral or IV. Hypocalcemia = para 7— Tetany is treated with 10-20 mL of 10% calcium gluconate IV or as an *IV drip* over 4 to 6 hours with 100 mL of

10% calcium gluconate in 1000 mL of D5W. IV calcium is best given in a central line to avoid tissue damage with infiltration.

Along with primary electrolyte replacement, treatment consists of magnesium replacement and vitamin D therapy. Reducing hyperphosphatemia in acute or chronic renal failure with aluminum hydroxide antacids or calcium acetate occurs before treating hypocalcemia. Decreasing phosphate first will decrease the production of calcium phosphate crystals in the kidney and heart.

Evaluation and follow-up include normal ionized calcium levels, monitored every 1-4 hours, and return to baseline neuromuscular exam. Patients with chronic hypocalcemia require dietary education for foods high in calcium as well as medication education for calcium supplements and vitamin D supplements. Signs and symptoms of hypocalcemia should be taught to the patient.

Hypercalcemia

Levels of calcium above 10.5 mg/dL total, and 5.5 mg/dL ionized, may produce no symptoms. Calcium levels greater than 13.5mg/dL require emergency treatment. Hypercalcemia may be a life-threatening electrolyte imbalance due to cardiac asystole at levels of 18 mg/dL.

The most common pathophysiology in acutely ill patients is malignancy with bone metastases leading to release of calcium into the serum. Primary hyperparathyroidism with elevated parathormone levels also lead to hypercalcemia. Sarcoidosis and other granulomatous diseases may release excess calcitrol from the granuloma causing hypercalcemia. Other less common causes may be immobilization and renal failure.

Clinical history to raise suspicion of hypercalcemia includes malignancy, hyperparathyroidism, sarcoid, and chronic renal failure. Patient complaints might include polyuria, thirst, lethargy, weakness, nausea and vomiting, bone pain, and flank pain due to kidney stones. Physical signs depend on level and rate of rise in calcium. Hypercalcemia prevents normal depolarization of nerve and muscle cells leading to flaccidity, decreased muscle tone, and depressed reflexes. Confusion, lethargy, and coma may be seen at higher levels.

Cardiac signs include decreased contractility, short QT interval, and rhythm disturbances like bradycardia, heart blocks, and bundle branch blocks. Cardiac asystole may occur with calcium levels greater than 18 mg/dL.

Diagnostic tests include serum calcium, albumin, and ionized calcium. Parathyroid hormone may be increased in primary or secondary hyperparathyroidism. X-ray may indicate fractures, bony metastases, or kidney stones. Examine the EKG for the findings of hypercalcemia mentioned above.

Management of life-threatening hypercalcemia includes intravenous saline to dilute calcium and promote urinary excretion, and furosemide to increase calcium excretion. ECF deficit related to polyuria of hypercalcemia may require large volume replacement usually with saline. Pamidronate, an intravenous infusion, inhibits bone resorption. Dose is 60-90 mg over 24 hours in a continuous infusion (*Nursing IV Drug Handbook,* 1995, p. 461). Calcitonin, to suppress bone resorption, may also be given IV to treat hypercalcemia. Intravenous steroids may be used to decrease intestinal absorption of calcium. The patient must be EKG-monitored to detect cardiac dysrhythmia. Underlying causes such as malignancy require management, if possible, to decrease recurrance of hypercalcemia.

The goals of hypercalcemia treatment are return to normal levels of calcium and baseline neurologic and cardiac functions. Discharge planning includes education about diet, fluid intake, signs and symptoms, pain control, and resuscitation status.

Magnesium Abnormalities

Hypomagnesemia

Serum levels of magnesium remain a very poor indicator of total body magnesium, since 99% of magnesium is intracellular. Serum magnesium level of less than 1.5mEq/L is termed hypomagnesemia, while magnesium deficiency refers to reduced body stores of the electrolyte (Toto & Yucha, 1994). Despite normal serum levels of magnesium, total body stores may be low. Signs and symptoms of low magnesium become important in this situation.

The pathophysiology of magnesium deficiency may be loss of magnesium via the kidneys, as in alcoholism, or kidney loss as a result of a drug such as furosemide (Lasix) or aminoglycosides (Ferrin, 1996). Osmotic diuresis with large urine losses, such as happens in diabetic ketoacidosis or hypercalcemia, may lead to magnesium deficiency. Magnesium deficiency may also be related to decreased dietary intake, such as in the alcoholic; decreased absorption, such as diarrhea, nasogastric suction or vomiting; or pancreatitis. A final cause of magnesium deficiency may be shifts of calcium from the extracellular space to the intracellular space as a result of insulin or catechoamines. Multiple causes of magnesium deficiency are possible in acutely ill patients whom the ACNP may encounter.

Magnesium deficiency has been found in patients with acute myocardial infarction (MI) and sudden death. Magnesium deficiency does occur post-MI, perhaps related to intracellular shifts due to catecholamines. Speculation as to the role of low magnesium pre-cardiac event continues.

Clinical history of alcohol abuse, diuretic or aminoglycoside use, vomiting, or diarrhea raise suspicion of magnesium deficiency. Physical findings of low magnesium are similar to those of low calcium including neuromuscular, cardiac, metabolic, and mental status changes. Chvostek's and Trousseau's signs as well as nystagmus, hyperreflexia, and seizures may be present in magnesium deficiency. Mental status changes seen with magnesium deficiency include confusion, agitation, and hallucinations. Cardiac symptoms include tachycardia, hypertension, digoxin sensitivity, coronary artery spasm, and dysrhythmias such as supraventricular tachycardia (SVT) or ventricular tachycardia (VT). Insulin resistance may be found with magnesium deficiency as well as hypokalemia and hypocalcemia that resist correction until magnesium is corrected. This need to correct magnesium first is related to the kidney's ability to conserve potassium and calcium.

The EKG changes of magnesium deficiency include prolonged PR and QT intervals, U waves, wide QRS, and flattening of the T wave.

Laboratory and diagnostic studies in patients with low serum magnesium (hypomagnesemia) should include calcium and phosphate, since these are frequently altered with magnesium deficiency. Serum ionized magnesium level is a new test available to detect magnesium deficiency, since this level more accurately reflects intracellular magnesium level. Check serum albumin as low levels of albumin may cause a decreased magnesium level. This occurs due to less protein-bound magnesium.

Treatment includes increased intake of magnesium-rich foods like milk, seafood, fruits, and vegetables, if possible, and/or oral supplementation of 200-400 mg/day of magnesium oxide. Use of oral replacement may cause diarrhea. If oral replacement is not sufficient, intravenous magnesium in 100 cc of normal saline may be used. Slow influsion over 4 hours increases the retention of magnesium in the serum.

Rapid infusion of magnesium is used in the case of dysrhythmia, like torsades. Infusion of 1-2 grams over 30 minutes may then be used with close BP checks to detect hypotension.

Evaluation and follow-up include laboratory monitoring of magnesium as well as physical signs and the EKG. Desired outcomes for the patient with magnesium deficiency include return to normal serum levels and correction of neuromuscular, mental status, and cardiac symptoms.

Hypermagnesemia

The kidney is very efficient in excreting extra magnesium even in the face of excess supplementation. Hypermagnesemia is most commonly related to renal failure. The use of excessive amounts of magnesium-containing antacids and/or milk of magnesia and/or magnesium citrate in the elderly combined with declining renal function may lead to hypermagnesemia. The use of magnesium supplementation in parenteral nutrition or as treatment for hypomagnesemia without consideration or knowledge of declining renal function may lead to hypermagnesemia.

Serum levels of magnesium in hypermagnesemia are an accurate reflection of symptoms unlike hypomagnesemia. Signs and symptoms of hypermagnesemia include early symptoms of hyporeflexia with serum levels of 4 mEq/L or greater. Magnesium in this case blocks impulse transmission across the neuromuscular junction. At levels of 9-10 mEq/L, deep tendon reflexes are absent and respiratory depression and arrest may occur at levels greater than 13 mEq/L. Mental-status changes in hypermagnesemia include lethargy and confusion, with coma at high levels. The cardiovascular effects of hypermagnesemia include bradycardia, atrioventricular block and asystole, and hypotension.

Treatment of hypermagnesemia includes stopping the source, and use of saline and loop diuretics to increase renal excretion, if possible. For more severe cases, intravenous calcium chloride can be used to reverse neuromuscular blockade and stabilize the cardiovascular system. Mechanical ventilation may be necessary until magnesium levels decrease. In cases of renal failure, hemodialysis or peritoneal dialysis with magnesium-free dialysate may be required to prevent further deterioration.

▶ ACID–BASE BALANCE

The body's mechanisms for maintaining a balance of hydrogen ion (H^+) to bicarbonate ion (HCO3$^-$) include the buffer systems in the body fluids, the respiratory system, and the renal system (Table 18–7). These systems maintain the pH within a life-sustaining range despite major insults.

Arterial blood gases (ABGs) are the measure used to detect and treat acid base imbalances. Table 18–8 provides the normal range of values for the components of ABGs. The pH measures H^+ concentration while $PaCO_2$ is the measure of partial pressure of carbon dioxide in the blood and reflects the respiratory component of acid base analysis. HCO_3^- is the renal component of acid base analysis. Base excess or deficit measures the amount of blood buffer present, that is, hemaglobin and bicarbonate. PaO_2 and oxygen saturation are measures of oxygenation of the bloodstream and do not play a role in analysis, except to define causes.

Analysis of blood gases to determine acid–base status

TABLE 18–7. Mechanisms to Maintain Acid–Base Balance

1. Buffers—Act within seconds of abnormal pH; combine with excess acid or base in the blood to form substances that do not affect pH.
   a. Bicarbonate—generated by kidneys and helps excrete H^+
   b. Phosphate—excretes H^+ in the renal tubules
   c. Ammonium—Ammonia (NH_3) combines with excess H^+ to form ammonium (NH_4) in the renal tubule to allow excretion of excess H^+
   d. Protein—Buffers in cells, blood, and plasma to maintain acid base balance
2. Respiratory system—Response within minutes; acidemia causes increased respiratory effort to blow off CO_2 while alkalemia causes decreased alveolar ventilation to retain CO_2.
3. Renal system—Response of hours to days; increases or decreases HCO_3^- in body fluids.

TABLE 18–8. Normal Arterial Blood Gas Findings

Component	Normal Range
pH	7.35–7.45
PCO_2	35–45 mm Hg
PO_2	60–100 mm Hg
HCO_3^-	22–28 mEg/L

is a systematic process. Questions to guide analysis include the following:

1. Is the pH normal? Higher than 7.45 is alkalosis, lower than 7.35 is acidosis.
2. Is the PCO_2 normal? Higher than 45 mm Hg is indicative of acidosis as the respiratory system retains CO_2, while lower than 35 mm Hg indicates an alkalosis as the lung blows off CO_2.
3. Is the HCO_3 normal? HCO_3 above 28 mEq/L indicates kidney saving of bicarbonate while below 22 mEq/L shows kidney wasting of bicarbonate or use of bicarbonate to buffer acid.
4. Which value, PCO_2 or HCO_3^-, corresponds to the pH? If the pH is acidotic (below 7.35), is the $PaCO_2$ increased (respiratory) or is there a decreased bicarbonate (metabolic)? This is the primary disturbance.

Consider, for example, the following arterial blood gas results. pH = 7.33, PCO_2 50; HCO_3 25. The pH is acidotic (less than 7.35); the pCO_2 is acidotic (more than 45); the HCO_3 is normal (22-28). The blood gas is an example of respiratory acidosis since the increased pCO_2 is the primary cause of the acidotic pH.

If the bicarbonate in the above example was greater than normal, that would indicate an attempt by the kidney to compensate for the increased pCO_2 by saving HCO_3. If the pH were within normal range because of the increased HCO_3, the blood gas would indicate a respiratory acidosis with compensation. An example is: pH = 7.37, pCO_2 50, HCO_3 30. This blood gas indicates a more chronic process allowing the kidneys time to be activated.

Mixed metabolic (renal) and respiratory disturbances or compensatory mechanisms may be present if both PCO_2 and HCO_3^- are abnormal.

Respiratory Acidosis

The pathophysiology of respiratory acidosis is hypoventilation with excess carbon dioxide in the system. This results in excess carbonic acid in the extracellular fluid. The etiologies of respiratory acidosis revolve around six primary problem areas: pulmonary/thoracic disorders; increased resistance to air flow; mechanical ventilation; central nervous system depression; neuromuscular disorders; and systemic causes. Table 18–9 provides specific clinical examples of each category.

TABLE 18–9. Etiologies of Respiratory Acidosis

Disorder	Examples
Pulmonary/Thoracic Disorders	Severe pneumonia, acute respiratory distress syndrome (ARDS), flail chest, pneumothorax, hemothorax, smoke inhalation, pulmonary embolus, pulmonary edema, chronic obstructive pulmonary disease
Increased Resistance to Air Flow	Upper airway obstruction, aspiration, laryngospasm, bronchspasm, asthma attack
Mechanical Ventilation (Iatrogenic)	Fixed minute ventilation with increased CO_2 production, increased dead space, equipment failure
Central Nervous System (CNS) Depression	Sedative overdose, narcotic or alcohol overdose, anesthesia, cerebral trauma, cerebral infarct, increased intracranial pressure, meningitis
Neuromuscular Disorders	Guillain–Barre syndrome, myasthenia gravis crisis, high cervical cordotomy, drugs, toxins
Systemic Causes	Cardiopulmonary arrest, hypo- or hyperkalemia, hypophosphatemia

Clinical history might include prior disease such as asthma or COPD or may be related to an acute event such as drug and/or alcohol exposure, trauma including chest and cerebral, or cardiac arrest. Clinical findings include dyspnea and restlessness, with exam findings of tachycardia, tachypnea, and diaphoresis. Change in mental status weakness, asterixis, and decreased reflexes may be seen. Cyanosis is a late sign of respiratory acidosis. Signs of increased intracranial pressure with papilledema may be seen with severe acidosis because of cerebral vasodilation.

Laboratory and diagnostic tests include ABG findings of pH less than 7.35 and PCO_2 greater than 45 mm Hg. Bicarbonate may be normal or increased, if the kidney has had the opportunity to respond to the acidosis by retaining bicarb. PO_2 may be normal or decreased. Serum potassium may be increased in acidosis. Chest x-ray and drug screen are used to determine etiology of the respiratory acidosis.

Treatment for respiratory acidosis is support of respiratory function. Supplemental oxygen is indicated for treatment of hypoxemia. Use of mechanical ventilation is indicated if $PaCO_2$ is greater than 50-60 mm Hg with clinical signs of lethargy. This may be accomplished via continuous positive airway pressure (CPAP) masks or intubation. Sodium bicarbonate is usually avoided because of the risks of the sodium load and over-correction. In the case of iatrogenic respiratory acidosis related to mechanical ventilation, increase in rate or volume of breaths delivered or decrease in dead space is needed. Treatment of the underlying disorder, such as pneumonia or asthma, is essential.

Follow-up includes frequent blood gas analysis to assess adequacy of ventilation and treatment. Desired outcome is return to baseline blood gas, which may be normal $PaCO_2$ for most patients. Patients with COPD who live with elevated CO_2s would have that level as their goal. Respiratory rate would return to baseline for that individual as would PaO_2. Additional desired outcomes are clear lung fields and return to baseline mental functioning with acidosis correction.

Respiratory Alkalosis

Any clinical situation that leads to increased depth or rate of breathing and a deficit of carbon dioxide and carbonic acid may lead to respiratory alkalosis. The most common etiology is hyperventilation syndrome due to anxiety. This is related to direct stimulation of the respiratory center. Fever, pain, gram negative sepsis, and stroke may lead to respiratory alkalosis through this path. Clinical events that cause hypoxemia, such as hypotension or heart failure, may lead to respiratory alkalosis. Pulmonary causes, like pulmonary emboli or asthma, stimulate ventilation in mild situations. Iatrogenic overventilation through mechanical ventilators may also lead to respiratory alkalosis.

Physical findings include lightheadedness, anxiety, paresthesias, and circumoral numbness. Extreme alkalosis may produce confusion, tetany, syncope, hypotension, dysrhythmias, and seizures. Tetany in this case may be related to decreased ionized calcium because of increased binding. This may occur despite normal total calcium levels (bound, complexed, ionized).

Arterial blood gas findings show a pH greater than 7.45 with a $PaCO_2$ less than 35 mm Hg. Hypoxemia, PaO_2, less than 60 may indicate potential etiologies. Bicarbonate would be normal or low. Sodium phosphate may fall to less than 0.5 mg/dL (normal is 3-4.5mg/dL) because of increased uptake of phosphate by the cells. EKG may show cardiac dysrhythmias related to alkalosis.

Treatment of the underlying etiology, such as hypoxemia, sepsis, or pain, is the first line management issue for the ACNP. With anxiety, reassurance and a rebreathing bag may be needed with frequent blood gas monitoring during correction to prevent metabolic acidosis because of lowered bicarbonate. Sedatives and tranquilizers may also be needed for anxiety. Mechanical ventilator adjustments to decrease rate or volume or add dead space correct respiratory alkalosis related to overventilation.

Follow-up includes return of pH, $PaCO_2$, and EKG to baseline. Follow-up for anxiety includes psychological counseling and pharmacotherapy as needed.

Metabolic Acidosis

Metabolic acidosis, a deficit of bicarbonate in the ECF, has two causes. The first cause is a loss of bicarbonate from the body while the second is production of excess amounts of nonvolatile acids. Loss of bicarbonate occurs in severe diarrhea, malabsorption syndromes, drainage of biliary and pancreatic secretions, and ileostomy. Increased acid production occurs in diabetic and alcoholic ketoacidosis, renal tubular acidosis, acute and chronic renal failure, and lactic acidosis. Ingestion of salicylates, methanol, ethylene glycol, or toluene provides an external source of excess acids to the system.

Clinical history for metabolic acidosis are renal disease, drug ingestion, cardiac arrest, shock, draining wounds, diarrhea, and out-of-control diabetes. Physical assessment findings depend on the level of acidosis and other disease processes. Changes in level of consciousness may occur, as well as hypotension; tachypnea; Kussmaul's respirations (slow deep breaths to blow off CO_2 to correct acidosis); cold, clammy skin; dysrhythmia; and shock. GI symptoms of nausea, vomiting, and anorexia occur with metabolic acidosis. Severe metabolic acidosis (less than 7.2) can cause cardiovascular collapse and death and demands immediate treatment.

The ABG in metabolic acidosis reveals a pH less than 7.35 with a HCO_3^- less than 22 mEq/L. CO_2 is usually less than 35 mm Hg as the lungs compensate for the acidosis. Serum potassium may be increased during acidosis as the body sends H^+ ion intracellularly to attempt to return to a physiologic acid base balance. This hyperkalemia may be reflected on EKG with peaked T waves and widened QRS.

Anion gap is an analysis of serum electrolytes to define a cause for metabolic acidosis. The equation is:

$$\text{anion gap} = Na - (C1^- + HCO_3^-)$$

Normal anion gap is 10-14 mEq/L and, if found with a metabolic acidosis, indicates a direct loss of bicarbonate, such as occurs in diarrhea. An increased anion gap, greater than 14 mEq/L, indicates increased nonvolatile acids, which occurs in lactic acidosis, renal failure, and diabetic ketoacidosis.

Treatment for pH less than 7.2 in metabolic acidosis may be mechanical ventilation if the patient's own ventilatory effort is failing and lessening effectiveness of the compensatory mechanism of decreasing CO_2. Sodium bicarbonate ($NaHCO_3^-$) may be used cautiously in this setting with 2-3 ampules (44.5 mEq/L) in 1000 mL of dextrose in water in a continuous infusion titrated to ABG response (Horne, et al., 1997). The danger of HCO_3^- is over-correction leading to metabolic alkalosis as well as pulmonary edema due to the sodium load. Potassium replacement is usually needed as acidosis correction forces potassium back into cells and leads to hypokalemia. If hypokalemia exists initially, correction is needed before bicarbonate is given.

In many cases of metabolic acidosis, treatment of the underlying disorder leads to correction. Diabetic ketoacidosis, acute renal failure, drug ingestion, lactic acidosis, and diarrhea all require specific intervention that will reverse the process producing excess acids or causing loss of HCO_3^-.

TABLE 18–10. Summary of Changes in Arterial Blood Gas Results with Primary Acid-Base Abnormalities

	pH	$PaCO_2$	HCO_3^-
Respiratory Acidosis	<7.35	>45 mm Hg	normal, increased
Respiratory Alkalosis	>7.45	<35 mm Hg	normal or decreased
Metabolic Acidosis	<7.35	normal or decreased	< 22 mEq/L
Metabolic Alkalosis	>7.45	normal or increased	>28 mEq/L

Evaluation and follow-up include normal arterial blood gas results and electrolyte panel along with return to baseline mental and cardiovascular functions. The underlying etiology for metabolic acidosis is stabilized.

Metabolic Alkalosis

Elevated serum bicarbonate to levels greater than 28 mEq/L results in metabolic alkalosis. The causative factors may be loss of gastric acid from vomiting or nasogastric suction, diuretic use, excess bicarbonate use, and over-correction of hypercapnea.

Clinical history involves volume/chloride depletion via vomiting or nasogastric suction, bicarbonate use during resuscitation, and prescribed or hidden diuretic use. Physical findings of severe alkalosis might be neuromuscular irritability, seizures, confusion, and coma. Hypovolemia, if present, may exhibit the signs of postural hypotension with tachycardia, decreased jugular venous pressure. Hypokalemia occurs as hydrogen exits the cell to correct the alkalosis, while potassium enters the cells, leading to low serum potassium. Atrial and ventricular dysrhythmias as well as muscular weakness and hyporeflexia are the result of the hypokalemia associated with metabolic alkalosis. GI symptoms of ileus, nausea, and vomiting may occur.

Laboratory and diagnostic findings include arterial blood gas results with a pH greater than 7.45 and HCO_3^- greater than 28 mEq/L. Rising $PaCO_2$ compensates for the increased base. Serum potassium (less than 3.5 mEq/L) and chloride (less than 95 mEq/L) may be low. EKG gives evidence of severe alkalosis or hypokalemia with dysrhythmias.

Treatment of metabolic alkalosis consists of volume repletion with normal saline to correct the deficit if present. This solution repletes chloride to facilitate excretion of HCO_3^- by the kidney. Potassium chloride is used to correct hypokalemia. Carbonic anhydrase inhibitors, such as Diamox, cause increased renal secretion of bicarbonate in patients who cannot tolerate increased volume of saline. Potassium must be corrected first as Diamox causes potassium loss.

Evaluation and follow-up focus on return of pH to less than 7.45 and return of baseline cardiac and neuromuscular function. EKG indicates a normal tracing while potassium, chloride, and volume status return to normal. If related to chronic diuretic use, signs and symptoms of volume depletion and whom to call are important discharge teaching to avoid recurrence of the metabolic alkalosis.

Table 18–10 provides a comparison of the four types of acid–base disturbances. The ACNP is reminded that these disorders may occur in combination with one another, especially metabolic and respiratory acidosis, in the acute care setting.

REFERENCES

Baer, C. L. (1993). Fluid and electrolyte balance. Acid-base balance. In Kinney, M. R., Packa, D. R., & Dunbar, S. B. (Eds). *Clinical reference for critical care nursing* (pp. 173–216). Philadelphia: Mosby.

Black, R. (1996). Disorders of plasma sodium and plasma potassium. In Rippe, J. M., Irwin, R. S., Fink, M. P., & Cerra, F. B. (Eds.). *Intensive Care Medicine.* New York: Little, Brown & Company.

Braxmeyer, D. L. & Keyes, J. L. (1996). The pathophysiology of potassium balance. *Critical Care Nurse; 16*(5); 59–71.

Ferrin, M. S. (1996). Magnesium. *RN;* May; 31–34.

Freeland, M. J. & Kruse, J. A. (1996). Hyponatremia and hypernatremia. In Kruse, J. A., Parker, M. M., Carlson, R. W., & Gehab, M. A. (Eds). *Prinicples and practice of medical intensive care.* Philadelphia: Saunders.

Gross, P. & Hensen, J. (1995). Evaluation of hyponatremia: Is there a rational approach? *Nephrology, Dialysis, Transplantation;* 1789–1791.

Horne, M. M., Heitz, U. E., & Swearingen, P. L. (1997). *Fluid, electrolyte and acid-base balance.* Philadelphia: Mosby Year Book.

Nursing I.V. Drug Handbook (1995). Springhouse, Pennsylvania: Springhouse Corporation.

O'Donnell, M. E. (1995). Assessing Fluid and electrolyte balance in elders. *American Journal of Nursing; 95*(11); 4145.

Toto, K. H. & Yucha, C. B. (1994). Magnesium: Homeostasis, Imbalances, and therapeutic uses. *Critical Care Nursing Clinics of North America;* 6(4); 767–783.

Yucha, C. B. & Toto, K. H. (1994). Calcium and phosphorus derangements. *Critical Care Nursing Clinics of North America;* 6 (4); 747–766.

19

Shock

Koki Niibori
Glenn J. R. Whitman

Shock is a clinical state resulting from inadequate tissue perfusion in which O_2 delivery does not meet O_2 demands. Obviously, this definition encompasses a variety of syndromes. An exact definition of shock has proved elusive. Regardless, the underlying principle of inadequate O_2 supply to meet O_2 demands is the sine qua non of this entity. This theme can be seen in the definitions of shock that span the last three decades.

- " . . . the cardiac output is insufficient to fill the arterial tree with blood under sufficient pressure to provide organs and tissues with adequate blood flow" (Simeone, 1964)
- "Disordered response of organisms to an inappropriate balance of substrate supply and demand at a cellular level" (Cerra, 1983)
- " . . . state in which profound and widespread reduction of *effective* tissue perfusion leads first to reversible, and then, if prolonged, to irreversible cellular injury" (Kumar & Parrillo, 1995)

▶ CLASSIFICATION

Various classifications of shock have been proposed. Blalock (1937) suggested four categories of shock: hematogenic or oligemic (hypovolemic), cardiogenic, neurogenic, and vasogenic (primarily septic shock). Along the same lines, a more recent classification based on cardiovascular and vasomotor characteristics has been accepted by most clinicians. The categories include (1) hypovolemic shock, due to a decreased circulating volume in relation to the total vascular capacity; (2) cardiogenic shock, related to cardiac pump failure (common causes include cardiac arrhythmias or acute myocardial infarction); (3) compressive cardiogenic shock, due to mechanical obstruction of cardiac function (as seen with cardiac tamponade, tension pneumothorax); and (4) distributive shock, due to loss of vasomotor tone resulting in arteriolar and venular dilatation. Neurogenic shock is a form of distributive shock in which spinal anesthesia or spinal injury leads to arteriolar vasodilation. Septic shock is also a form of distributive shock in which loss of arteriolar resistance with an increase in venous capacitance produces a discrepancy between intravascular size and volume. Each of these disorders may lead to inadequate tissue perfusion, a concept underlying all clinical states referred to as *shock* (Table 19–1).

TABLE 19–1. Classification of Shock

Hypovolemic
Traumatic
Cardiogenic
Compressive cardiogenic
Distributive
Neurogenic
Septic
Hypoadrenal
Anaphylatic

▶ BACKGROUND

Neuroendocrine Response to Shock

The neuroendocrine response to shock attempts to restore the circulating blood volume with mobilization of metabolic substrates, and maintenance of central perfusion pressure, in an effort to protect the brain and heart. The mechanisms include (1) autonomic control of cardiac contractility and peripheral vascular tone, (2) hormonal response to stress and volume depletion, and (3) local microcirculatory mechanisms that are organ-specific and regulate regional blood flow (Peitzman et al., 1995). Not only hypovolemia but other stimuli including hypotension, pain, hypoxemia, hypercarbia, acidosis, infection, and emotional state can elicit this neuroendocrine response.

In hemorrhagic shock, the magnitude of the neuroendocrine response is based on the magnitude of the decrease in effective circulating blood volume as well as the rate at which volume of blood is lost. This response to shock may be modified further by associated injuries or conditions such as alcohol, drugs, and prescribed medications, or simply the age of the patient.

The nervous system responds immediately to pain or to loss of circulating blood volume with sympathetically mediated vasoconstriction. This vasoconstriction promptly reduces the capacitance of the circulatory system. The high-pressure baroreceptors in the aortic arch and carotid sinus respond instantly to changes in blood pressure by adjusting the sympathetic tone. The arterial baroreceptors sense decreased stretch of the arterial wall. The low-pressure atrial stretch receptors are sensitive to both stretch and pressure (Peitzman, et al., 1995).

The intense triggering of sympathetic signals is activated when the arterial blood pressure falls below 50 mm Hg and is maximally stimulated when the systolic blood pressure is less than 15 mm Hg (Guyton, 1991). However, metabolic vasoregulation of the heart and brain counteract systemic vasoconstriction in an effort to maintain their regional perfusion in spite of the ongoing systemic catecholamine response. On the other hand, renal blood flow may be reduced to 5% to 10% of normal with acute hypovolemia, and flow to the splanchnic circulation, skin, and skeletal muscle may also decrease significantly. These constrictor responses are mediated by epinephrine and norepinephrine, which are released from the adrenal medulla and through direct effects of local sympathetic activity on blood vessel walls (Peitzman et al., 1995).

Stimulation of peripheral chemoreceptors located in the aortic arch and carotid bodies results in bradycardia, vasodilatation of coronary arteries, and constriction of the arteries in skeletal muscle and the splanchnic circulation (O'Ryan & Majcherczyk, 1982). This stimulation further ensures preservation of blood flow to the heart and the brain at the expense of other organ systems.

In addition to initiating autonomic nervous activity, shock initiates multiple endocrine responses. The hypothalamus secretes releasing hormones, which induce stress hormones to be released by the pituitary. As part of this response, adrenocorticotropic hormone (ACTH) secretion by the anterior pituitary is increased, stimulating cortisol secretion by the adrenal cortex. Cortisol affects cellular metabolism by alterations in substrate usage and protein synthesis. It leads to decreased peripheral uptake of glucose and amino acids, enhanced lipolysis, and increased gluconeogenesis. Glucose intolerance or overt hyperglycemia may result. In conjunction with elevated plasma levels of cortisol, increased pancreatic secretion of glucagon, which accelerates hepatic gluconeogenesis, further enhances glucose intolerance. The hyperglycemia and increased blood osmolarity tend to shift fluid from the intracellular space to the intravascular space and thus help maintain circulating blood volume.

The secretion of renin is increased in response to adrenergic discharge and decreased perfusion of the juxtaglomerular apparatus in the kidney. Renin induces formation of angiotensin from angiotensinogen produced by the liver. This angiotensin I is then converted to angiotensin II in the lung. Angiotensin II is not only a vasoconstrictor but also stimulates aldosterone release by the adrenal cortex as well as vasopressin (ADH) release by the posterior pituitary. Aldosterone serves to maintain intravascular volume by inducing tubular reabsorption of sodium in the distal tubule of the kidney. Aldosterone secretion is increased in response to ACTH stimulation of the adrenal cortex as well as circulating angiotensin II. Similarly, release of vasopressin also occurs, resulting in increased water absorption in the collecting duct of the kidney. Vasopressin also induces splanchnic vasoconstriction.

Cardiovascular Response to Shock

The physiologic response of the patient in shock is to maintain the immediate needs of the two most vital organs—the brain and the heart—since the metabolic rates of the heart and brain are higher and their stores of energy substrates lower than other organs. When circulation is compromised, the continuous supply of nutrients may quickly fall below demand levels in these tissues, a condition not tolerated for more than brief periods (Cerra & Snyder, 1993). Along with mechanisms that maintain central blood pressure, autoregulation attempts to maintain coronary and cerebral perfusion throughout significant degrees of shock. Although protection of the brain and heart during shock is of prime importance, it does occur at the expense of other tissue beds as has been pointed out. As a result, physiologic compensations or therapeutic interventions must optimize effective circulating blood volume to restore peripheral tissue perfusion and halt the progressive and diffuse microcirculatory derangements associated with prolonged shock.

CLINICAL SHOCK SYNDROMES

Hypovolemic Shock

The symptoms and signs of hypovolemic shock depend upon the degree of blood volume depletion, the duration of shock, and the body's compensatory reactions to the shock itself (Holcroft & Blaisdell, 1991).

In mild shock (loss of less than 20% of blood volume), the most sensitive clinical findings are caused by adrenergic constriction of blood vessels to the skin. The extremities, particularly the feet, become pale and cool. The subcutaneous veins collapse. Capillary filling decrease, and the feet may become damp with sweat. Blood pressure with the patient in the supine position usually remains normal, as does the urinary output (although the urine may be concentrated).

Patients in moderate shock (loss of 20 to 40% of blood volume) develop low urinary output (defined as less than 0.5 mL/kg/hr in the adult or less than 2.0 mL/kg/hr in the infant) reflective of circulating aldosterone and vasopressin. The supine blood pressure may remain normal, but the patient will unquestionably be orthostatic.

The patient in severe shock (loss of more than 40% of blood volume) shows signs of adrenergic discharge with the skin being cool and clammy and with urinary output marginal. Supine blood pressure is low. The patient may be agitated, restless, or obtunded (Table 19–2) (Holcroft & Blaisdell, 1991).

It is important to recognize that after acute hemorrhage, hemoglobin and hematocrit values as well as electrolyte concentrations do not change until intrinsic compensatory fluid shifts or exogenous fluid administration has taken place.

Moderately severe and severe shock are easily recognized, but early or mild hypovolemic shock poses a difficult diagnosis as the body may compensate quite well. To help detect mild or progressive hypovolemic shock, urinary output should be monitored and serial hematocrit levels measured. In addition, postural changes in blood pressure should be evaluated. When changing from a supine to a sitting position, a fall in the systolic pressure of 10 mm Hg with a compensatory tachycardia indicates hypovolemia; a lack of orthostatic changes may be misleading, however, as a slow and unresponsive heart rate may reflect myocardial dysfunction, frequently seen in the elderly.

Hypoglycemic shock may present with the same signs and symptoms as hypovolemic shock. A hypoglycemic patient typically is cool, vasoconstricted, pale, and sweaty; with severe hypoglycemia, the patient may be hypotensive, oliguric, irritable, obtunded, or unconscious. Any patient in shock with a history of insulin-dependent diabetes should have the blood glucose measured and should be given an infusion of 25 grams of glucose acutely to treat possible hypoglycemia (Holcroft & Blaisdell, 1991).

The principles of treatment of hemorrhagic and nonhemorrhagic hypovolemic shock are similar. Resuscitation should begin with immediate assurance of adequate ventilation and oxygenation and then point to volume resuscitation. Of course, successful treatment of hemorrhagic shock mandates identification and control of the bleeding source. Intravenous fluid should be administered immediately. Access to the venous system depends on the clinician's assessment of the degree of hypovolemia. If the patient's only sign of hypovolemia is cutaneous vasoconstriction, percutaneously placed venous cannulas in the upper extremities are adequate. If hypovolemia is more severe, two or three large-bore (12-gauge or larger) intravenous catheters may be necessary for adequate volume resuscitation.

The approach to volume resuscitation involves understanding where fluid goes once it is administered intravenously. For example, D5W distributes itself throughout the body; consequently, only one-twelfth remains intravascular. Normal saline or lactated Ringers, on the other hand, remain extracellular, distributing evenly throughout that space. Consequently, 1/4 remains intravascular. Colloid, such as 5% albumin or 6% hetastarch, are physiologically designed to generate approximately the same oncotic pressure as our own serum. Consequently, and with the caveat that the endothelial cells lining the vascular tree maintain

TABLE 19–2. Characteristics of Shock

	Hypovolemic			Septic			
	Mild	*Moderate*	*Severe*	*Hyper-*	*Hypodynamic*	Neurogenic	Cardiogenic
Skin perfusion	Pale	Pale	Pale	Pink	Pale	Pink	Pale
Urinary output	Normal	Low	Low	Low	Low	Low	Low
Blood pressure	Normal	Normal	Low	Low	Low	Low	Low
Mental status	Thirsty	Restless	Obtunded	Abnormal	Abnormal	Normal	Normal
Neck vein	Flat	Flat	Flat	Flat	Flat	Flat	Distended
Cardiac output	Low	Low	Low	High	Low	Low	Low
SVR[a]	High	High	High	Low	High	Low	High

[a] SVR = systemic vascular resistance

their barrier to the extravasation of large oncotically active molecules, administration of a 5 or 6% colloid solution expands the intravascular space by the full amount infused. An ampule of salt-poor albumin which is 50 cc of a 25% albumin solution (12.5 gms albumin) has a greater oncotic pressure than serum and expands the intravascular space by approximately 200-250 cc. In that case, the oncotic pressure generated by the 12.5 gms of albumin infused pulls into the vascular space that amount of fluid required to have it reach equilibrium with serum, i.e., a protein concentration between 5 and 7 gms % (Table 19–3).

Traumatic Shock

The major cause of shock in the setting of trauma, including shock caused by burns, is hypovolemia. Although initially caused by both internal and external volume losses, tissue injury in and of itself may cause broader pathophysiologic changes and potentially a more devastating degree of shock than that produced by hypovolemia alone. The degree of direct organ injury, such as cellular injury, tissue devitalization, ischemia, and bacteremia, contribute to the development of an inflammatory response whose mediators are similar to those seen in sepsis. These mediators lead to a generalized increase in systemic vascular permeability with loss of plasma into the interstitial tissues and worsening of preexisting hypovolemia.

Therapy of traumatic shock involves control of hemorrhage as the major concern with the highest priority over all other injuries. Secondary efforts are aimed at minimizing postshock sequelae, the most devastating being multiple organ failure syndrome, by restoration of blood flow to ischemic areas and debridement of devitalized or contaminated tissues.

Cardiogenic Shock

Cardiogenic shock results from the failure of the heart as a pump. It is the most common cause of in-hospital mortality in patients with myocardial infarction. Cardiogenic shock can be produced by intrinsic cardiac disease, penetrating cardiac trauma, or, rarely, blunt trauma. Intrinsic cardiac disease can include congenital defects, valvular abnormalities, coronary artery disease, cardiomyopathies, and arrhythmias. The major cause of cardiogenic shock is extensive myocardial infarction. Cardiogenic shock occurs when at least 40% of the left ventricular myocardium has been damaged by myocardial infarction (Weber, Ratshin, Janicki, & Russell, 1973). Diminished or ineffective contractility of the right or left side of the heart allows blood to accumulate in the respective venous circulations. Right-sided failure leads to accumulation of blood in the systemic veins and capacitance vessels. If this is severe or chronic, hepatomegaly with hepatojugular reflux develops. In left-sided failure, the pulmonary vasculature initially accommodates blood accumulation by dilatation of the capacious pulmonary veins. If pulmonary capillary permeability is normal, pulmonary interstitial edema develops only after a capillary pressure of 20 mm Hg has been reached. Overt pulmonary alveolar edema develops at greater than 22 to 24 mm Hg. Pulmonary edema impacts on pulmonary function by limiting diffusion of oxygen from alveoli to capillaries and decreasing lung compliance, thereby increasing the fraction of blood shunted past unventilated alveoli with resultant hypoxemia (Cerra & Snyder, 1993).

Patients in cardiogenic shock on the basis of either right or left ventricular dysfunction present with clinical findings associated with discharge of the adrenergic nervous system and generation of angiotensin, aldosterone, and vasopressin. In making the diagnosis of cardiogenic shock, any history of cardiac disease is very important. Associated physical findings include those of hemodynamic instability, peripheral vasoconstriction, and congestive fluid accumulation, as well as findings specific to the underlying cardiac abnormality. Tachycardia, tachypnea, hypotension, and cool, pale, mottled, or cyanotic extremities are commonplace. In shock caused by right ventricular dysfunction, the neck veins are distended. In shock caused by left ventricular dysfunction, the patient has crackles and a third heart sound. An electrocardiogram may provide evidence of preexisting disease as well as acute changes. Chest radiographs may demonstrate abnormalities consistent with the specific underlying heart disease, as well as the presence of pulmonary vascular congestion, pulmonary edema, pleural effusions, and cardiomegaly. Echocardiograms may demonstrate the presence of structural abnormalities or functional cardiac impairment. Hemodynamic findings consistent with cardiogenic shock include a low cardiac output (index less than 2.2 L/min/m^2), a very high systemic vascular resistance (SVR), and elevated cardiac filling pressures. The PCWP is usually 18 mm Hg or greater.

The management of cardiogenic shock rests upon

TABLE 19–3. Impact of IV Fluids on Intravascular Volume Expansion[a]

	D5/W	NSS	5% albumin	6% hetastarch	25% albumin
Amount	***1L***	***1L***	***250 cc***	***250 cc***	***50 cc***
Intravascular volume expansion (cc)	80	250	200–250	200–250	200–250

[a] An understanding of the intravascular impact of intravenous fluid therapy is crucial for a rational approach to the treatment of hypovolemic shock. This table outlines the impact of a variety of typically used IV fluids on intravascular volume expansion.

many of the same principles used to treat other kinds of shock. The initial treatment of cardiogenic shock begins with administration of supplemental oxygen, mechanical ventilation (if needed), and appropriate treatment of dysrhythmias. When acute myocardial infarction is the cause of shock, invasive angiography and aggressive therapy with thrombolytic agents, balloon dilatation, or surgery should be given early consideration (Cerra & Snyder, 1993).

Treatment of cardiogenic shock should be approached sequentially by (1) correcting arrhythmias and optimizing the heart rate, (2) optimizing ventricular end-diastolic volume, (3) assuring adequate peripheral vasodilation, (4) maximizing myocardial contractility, (5) preserving marginal myocardial contractility, (6) assuring adequate perfusion of the coronary vasculature with the use of vasoconstrictors, (7) providing mechanical assistance to the heart, and (8) surgical correction of cardiac lesions (Holcroft & Blaisdell, 1991).

Mechanical circulatory support devices, including the intraaortic balloon pump (IABP) and left ventricular assist devices (VADs), can support patients with severe cardiogenic shock who exhibit an inadequate response to volume expansion and drug therapy for significant periods of time. Circulatory-assist devices are used as a means of temporary support for the patient in cardiogenic shock, either with the hope of recovery of myocardial function or while preparations are made for other intervention. In acute myocardial infarction, Mueller (1994) described that the IABP might decrease the rate of reocclusion and infarct extension after percutaneous transluminal coronary angioplasty (PTCA) and, thus, interrupt the vicious cycle of further myocardial damage with the development of left-ventricular failure and cardiogenic shock. The IABP consists of a sausage-shaped balloon placed in the descending aorta just distal to the subclavian artery. The balloon is inflated and deflated in synchrony with cardiac contraction. A pneumatic device cyclically fills the balloon with helium during diastole and actively deflates it during systole. Inflation of the balloon during diastole augments diastolic pressure and improves coronary perfusion. Deflation during systole provides a degree of afterload reduction. Approximately 15% of patients with IABP suffer a complication—most often vascular, such as thrombus or embolus formation and compromised distal extremity circulation.

Compressive Cardiogenic Shock

Shock from external cardiac compression arises when external pressure on the heart impairs ventricular filling. Diagnosis of compressive cardiac shock can sometimes be difficult, especially in the acutely injured patient. When shock is associated with distended neck veins, one should search for tension pneumothorax, cardiac tamponade, mediastinal hematoma, or diaphragmatic rupture.

Patients with a tension pneumothorax have distended neck veins, tracheal deviation away from the affected thorax, as well as hyperresonant percussion and decreased breath sounds on the involved side. As with all cardiogenic shock, the skin is pale, cool, and clammy. Radiographic findings reveal a pneumothorax with tracheal and mediastinal deviation to the contralateral side, splaying of the ipsilateral ribs, and depression of the diaphragm. All such patients require urgent relief of the ipsilateral increase in intrathoracic pressure. Emergent placement of a 14-gauge needle in the second intercostal space, midclavicular line can be lifesaving. A standard 36F chest tube should be inserted in the fourth intercostal space in the midaxillary line for definitive treatment.

Patients with pericardial tamponade may also present in cargiogenic shock with pale, cool, clammy skin. The classic findings of pericardial tamponade include Beck's triad of hypotension, neck vein distention, and muffled heart sounds. A chest x-ray may show enlargement of the cardiac silhouette or a widened mediastinum. Voltage on the electrocardiogram may be diminished. In many cases the findings on physical examination may be subtle, but the diagnosis can almost always be established by a transthoracic or transesophageal echocardiogram. In patients with pericardial tamponade, a pulsus paradoxus (i.e., a decrease of systolic blood pressure by 10 mm Hg with inspiration) may also be present. Acute pericardial tamponade in an unstable patient should be treated by an immediate left anterolateral thoracotomy or subxyphoid approach with pericardiotomy and decompression of the tamponade. In a stable patient, pericardiocentesis can be accomplished by needle aspiration of the fluid-filled pericardial space.

The specific clinical findings associated with diaphragmatic herniation may be demonstrated on the admission chest film showing a blunted left (most commonly) costophrenic angle and abnormal viscera or a radiopaque nasogastric tube within the left chest. Acute rupture or laceration of the diaphragm requires immediate surgical correction, usually through the abdomen.

Finally, positive pressure ventilation with large tidal volumes can produce low cardiac output and shock. Definitive diagnosis requires documentation of a low cardiac output with modestly elevated right atrial and pulmonary artery wedge pressures. Treatment requires volume expansion combined with adjustment of the ventilator settings, usually with lower tidal volumes, in an effort to produce the highest cardiac output with the lowest cardiac filling pressures.

Distributive Shock

Neurogenic Shock

Neurogenic shock results from interruption of sympathetic vasomotor input and may develop after spinal cord injury, spinal anesthesia, or severe head injury. Ablation of baseline sympathetic activity results in decreased systemic vascular resistance and a dramatic increase in venous capacitance. The increase in venous capacitance decreases venous return and ventricular preload causing cardiac output and blood pressure to fall.

In most cases, the patient has obvious signs of neurologic pathology. Hypotension and tachycardia may be present, but the extremities are warm, not cool and clammy. Central venous pressure, pulmonary wedge pressure, systemic vascular resistance, and cardiac output are all typically decreased. Blood pressure is usually responsive to intravascular volume replacement. Pharmacological intervention with α-agonists is occasionally necessary. In the setting of trauma, hemodynamic instability may not be the sole result of neurogenic injury and occult blood loss or cardiogenic causes of shock must be ruled out.

Body temperature should be monitored and excessive heat loss prevented. If the patient is hypothermic, heating blankets should be used to restore the patient to normothermia.

Septic Shock

The longevity of patients with complex, chronic diseases has increased the number of patients who are at risk for developing severe infection and subsequent complications such as septic shock. Sepsis and septic shock remain huge clinical problems. In-hospital mortality due to septic shock has remained high and has changed little in the last few years despite improvements in intensive management (Lynn & Cohen, 1995). Septic shock is associated with gram-negative bacteremia in the overwhelming majority of cases, although shock can also be seen as a consequence of fulminant gram-positive bacterial, viral, fungal, rickettsial, and parasitic diseases (Jones, Fahey, & Tom Shires, 1993). The clinical presentation of septic shock is variable and depends to a large extent on the status of the patient's health prior to the onset of invasive infection, including preexisting fluid and electrolyte status and cardiovascular reserve. In normovolemic patients, septic shock exhibits a hyperdynamic circulatory pattern characterized by hypotension, increased cardiac output, decreased peripheral vascular resistance, normal central venous pressure with a normal blood volume, and warm, dry extremities (MacLean, Mulligan, MacLean, & Duff, 1967).

In contrast, when septic shock develops in patients who are hypovolemic, it is likely that a hypodynamic circulatory pattern will result characterized by hypotension, decreased cardiac output, increased peripheral vascular resistance, low central venous pressure, and cold, cyanotic extremities. Typically, hyperdynamic septic shock is seen in previously healthy persons who develop a severe infection that leads to sudden bacteremia, such as urosepsis or cholangitis. Hypodynamic septic shock is classically seen in patients who have ongoing fluid losses, such as a patient with infarcted gut and continued third-space losses. Hyperdynamic shock can progress to hypodynamic shock if it is not recognized and treated aggressively at an early stage. Early signs of septic shock include an altered mental status (particularly in the elderly), hyperventilation with a respiratory alkalosis, tachycardia, fever, and rigors. In the critically ill intensive care unit patient, sepsis often presents as a constellation of clinical and laboratory findings with oliguria or increasing fluid requirements, development of insulin resistance, thrombocytopenia, granulocytosis or granulocytopenia with a left shift, acidosis, hypoxemia, and altered mentation (Jones, Fahey, & Tom Shires, 1993).

Whether septic shock presents as hyperdynamic or hypodynamic, the principles of management are similar. These therapeutic principles are restoration of tissue perfusion and oxygenation to meet metabolic demands and a prompt search for the source of infection with therapy aimed at its control (Cerra & Snyder, 1993). If the infectious process requires drainage, operation should be performed as soon as possible after the patient has been stabilized, as some conditions, such as septic shock secondary to ascending cholangitis, respond only briefly to supportive measures (Jones, Fahey, & Tom Shires, 1993). The restoration of tissue perfusion and tissue oxygen delivery is best accomplished through hemodynamic manipulations based on pulmonary artery catheter measurements and oxygen transport calculations. Fluid resuscitation requirements in excess of 10 L of Ringer's lactate solution are commonplace and may sometimes exceed 20 L or more. Resuscitation to a PCWP of 15 mm Hg is a reasonable initial goal. Antibiotic treatment should be based on the results of cultures and sensitivities when possible. If unavailable, broad-spectrum antibiotics should be started immediately and adjusted when culture and sensitivity reports reveal a specific pathogen. Central monitoring intravascular catheters in all intensive care patients should be viewed as possible sources of sepsis and should be removed and replaced unless another source has been identified. When there is doubt as to the source, these lines, including Swan–Ganz catheters, should be changed and the tips cultured.

Adequate fluid resuscitation usually improves renal function. If sepsis continues for more than 24 hours, acute tubular necrosis (ATN) may develop. Renal failure after adequate fluid resuscitation sometimes requires hemofiltration or dialysis.

In the past, steroids were used in the treatment of septic shock. However, clinical trials have failed to show benefit (Bernard et al., 1987; Bone et al., 1987). The only current indication for steroid treatment in septic shock is for stress coverage in patients previously taking steroids for immunosuppression or hypoadrenalism.

Hypoadrenal Shock (Adrenal Crisis)

Shock of a dramatic nature, poorly responsive to resuscitation, may develop as a consequence of adrenal insufficiency. Clinically, this occurs most often when unknown or overlooked adrenal insufficiency complicates the course of another illness. Clinical deterioration in the face of what would otherwise seem to be appropriate treatment is an important sign suggesting the diagnosis. In this country, adrenal insufficiency most commonly arises as the consequence of prior chronic therapeutic administration of exogenous corticosteroids causing adrenal suppression without adequate steroid administration in the acute setting. Other causes include idiopathic adrenal atrophy (Addison disease), tuberculosis, metastatic disease, bilateral adrenal hemorrhage, amyloidosis, and pituitary apoplexy (Cerra & Snyder, 1993).

Findings associated with adrenal insufficiency may be nonspecific but almost always include hypovolemia with spontaneous diuresis and hyperkalemia.

Surgical patients with adrenal insufficiency may develop refractory shock with hyperthermia. Hypotension may be dramatic despite massive volume resuscitation and pressor support. There may be no other findings suggestive of adrenal insufficiency other than a failure to respond to what would appear appropriate therapy. Thus, if vasopressor–refractory shock occurs in patients potentially predisposed to adrenal insufficiency, a cortisol level should be drawn and a trial of steroid therapy begun.

Successful therapy of an Addisonian crisis often requires significant cardiovascular support as well as stress doses of corticosteroids. Hydrocortisone may be given at a dose of 100 mg every 6 to 8 hours. Volume resuscitation and pressor support may be required for hours to days after therapy is initiated. Monitoring with a pulmonary artery catheter should be maintained until hemodynamic stability is achieved (Cerra & Snyder, 1993).

Anaphylactic Shock

Anaphylaxis is an acute and potentially life-threatening allergic reaction that, if severe, may lead to shock. Foreign substances that can act as antigens include drugs (especially penicillin), insect bites/stings, contrast media, blood, anesthetic agents, foods, and vaccines.

▶ THE SYSTEMIC RESPONSE TO SHOCK

Pulmonary Response to Shock

Most of the late deaths after successful resuscitation from shock are caused by pulmonary damage and respiratory failure (Demling & Goodwin, 1989). Pulmonary function may be compromised by not only pathologies intrinsic to the lung itself, including pulmonary contusion, aspiration, airway obstruction, pneumonia, hemothorax, and atelectasis, but also pathology of extrathoracic origin. Recumbency itself may cause a loss of up to 20% of functional residual capacity (FRC) (Alexander & Hechtman, 1988). The pain of either thoracic or abdominal origin contributes to further loss of FRC and the development of atelectasis.

The adult respiratory distress syndrome (ARDS) is a syndrome of acute lung injury that arises after shock, but it may happen as a consequence of various kinds of diseases as well. Characteristic findings of ARDS are the presence of pulmonary edema, hypoxia, and significantly decreased lung compliance. The pulmonary edema is noncardiac in origin and occurs despite normal left atrial pressures. The hypoxemia results from intrapulmonary shunting and diminished lung compliance from the interstitial accumulation of fluid. If ARDS develops, therapy is aimed at eradicating any septic focus while supportive care is maintained (Cerra & Snyder, 1993). Increasing positive end expiratory pressure may improve oxygenation dramatically. Despite improvement in ventilatory management and supportive care, ARDS mortality remains in the 50% range (Krafft et al., 1996).

Renal Response to Shock

In the past, patients in shock almost immediately manifested a fall in urinary output. Recently, renal failure has become less frequent because of aggressive resuscitation. Although renal injury may occur early during shock, clinical manifestations may not be apparent for 1 to 3 days.

When the kidney is subjected to shock, the physiologic response is to conserve salt and water. As a consequence of selective regional vasoconstriction as previously discussed, blood flow to the kidneys and other viscera is limited to preserve central arterial pressure. Sympathetic mediated vasoconstriction increases resistance at the level of the afferent arterioles, as do angiotensin II and circulating catecholamines (Cerra & Snyder, 1993). Increased preglomerular resistance accounts for a diminished glomerular filtration rate (GFR) as well as decreased renal blood flow (Oken, 1984). Decreased filtration in conjunction with the effects of increased circulating levels of ADH (vasopressin) and aldosterone produce oliguria and azotemia.

Acute renal failure (ARF) is a major complication of shock and is a common component of multiple organ failure syndrome (MOFS), the major cause of late ICU mortality. ARF is associated with mortality rates between 35% and 80% (Kumar & Parrillo, 1995).

Gastrointestinal Response to Shock

The gastrointestinal tract is relatively sensitive to shock due to the responsiveness of the splanchnic vasculature to vasoconstrictive stimulation by extrinsic factors. Typical gastrointestinal manifestations associated with shock include ileus, erosive gastritis, pancreatitis, acalculous cholecystitis, and colonic submucosal hemorrhage (Robert & Kaufman, 1989). In addition, recent studies suggest that enteric ischemia produced by shock and free radical injury with resuscitation may breach gut barrier integrity (Deitch, 1990). These studies also suggest that enteric bacteria and associated endotoxin may translocate from the gastrointestinal lumen to the systemic circulation during shock, resulting in an exacerbation of the shock state. Currently enteral feedings are recommended in an effort to enhance perfusion of the GI tract and decrease bacteria and endotoxin translocation.

Mediators of Septic Shock and Immunologic Therapy

The effect of inflammatory mediators known as cytokines on cellular metabolism is very important in the pathogenesis of septic shock and may play a substantial role in other types of shock as well. Many of these inflammatory mediators have just recently been discovered (Table 19–4). Macrophage production of cytokines such as tumor necrosis factor-alpha (TNF) and interleukin-1 (IL-1) appear to be central (Bone, 1991).

TNF is a small polypeptide that is produced by macrophages in response to a variety of inflammatory stimuli, including bacteria and other cytokines. TNF has many effects such as: causing white cell release of IL-1, IL-6, IL-8, platelet activating factor (PAF), leukotrienes, thromboxanes, and prostaglandins; stimulation of production and activity of polymorphonuclear leukocytes; promotion of immune cell adhesion to endothelium; activation of coagulation and complement systems; direct endothelial cell cytoxity; depression of myocardial contractility; and fever production by the hypothalamus (Bone, 1991). Administration of TNF to animals results in a cardiovascular state that is similar to untreated septic shock (Eichenholz et al., 1992). Interestingly, TNF receptor-deficient mice are resistant to the toxic effect of systemically applied endotoxin or gram-negative bacteria, pointing out the important role of TNF in septic shock (Volk et al., 1996). IL-1 can potentiate the *in vivo* effects of TNF. Interferon (INF)-gamma promotes the release of other cytokines, enhances adhesion of immune cells, and promotes macrophage activation (Kumar & Parrillo, 1995). As with TNF deficiencies, INF-gamma receptor-deficient mice are more resistant to gram-negative bacteremia or endotoxin, and also to the toxic effects of systemic TNF-alpha and IL-1 (Volk et al., 1996). Inhibiting the production of other cytokines such as IL-1 or blocking their effect can also modulate the manifestations of septic shock, consistent with the complexity and interrelationship among all of the cytokines.

On the basis of these observations, a strategy of inhibiting the synthesis or activity of mediators was developed to treat sepsis. A number of pharmaceutical companies have developed cytokine antagonists such as anti-TNF monoclonal antibodies and IL-1 receptor antagonists. Unfortunately, this approach has not met with success (Fisher, Opal et al., 1993; Fisher, Dhainut et al., 1994). It may be that neutralizing cytokines at the wrong moment may suppress important intrinsic defense mechanisms with fatal consequences. That may be a reason why antiinflammatory therapy has not succeeded to date. Regardless, knowledge of the cytokine cascade may prove the key to our ultimate treatment of shock and its late sequelae.

TABLE 19–4. Mediators of Sepsis and Multiple-Organ Failure Syndrome

Mediator	Major effects
Cytokines	
Tumor necrosis factor α (TNF)	Release stimulation of the other mediators; activation of PMN[a] cells; toxic effect to vascular endothelial cells (increases microvascular permeability); depression of cardiac monocyte contractility
Interleukin-1	The same as TNF effects
Interleukin-6	Induction of the synthesis of acute-phase protein by hepatocyte
	Inhibition of TNF production
Interleukin-8	Induction of tissue infiltration of both neutrophils and lymphocytes
Interferon-gamma	Promotion of the release of other cytokines; encouragement of PMN cell activation and accumulation; promotion of macrophage activation
Platelet-activating factor	Aggregation of platelets; activation of neutrophils; enhancement of microvascular permeability; coronary artery vasoconstriction
Leukotrienes	Promotion of neutrophil chemotaxis and adhesion of neutrophils to endothelium; enhancement of microvascular permeability; vasoconstriction; bronchoconstriction
Prostaglandins	
Prostaglandin E_2	Vasodilatation; improvement of tissue perfusion
Prostagrandin I_2	Inhibition of platelet aggregation and adhesion; smooth muscle relaxation
Complement C3a, C5a	Neutrophil aggregation; release of toxic oxygen radicals; histamine release; vasodilatation; enhancement of microvascular permeability

[a] PMN = polymorphonuclear

Systemic Inflammatory Response Syndrome

Abnormal host response characterized by generalized inflammation in organs remote from the patient's initial insult can be caused by infectious or noninfectious insults. Systemic inflammatory response syndrome (SIRS) is defined by the presence of two or more of the following signs: (1) body temperature >38°C or <36°C; (2) heart rate >90 bpm; (3) respiratory rate >20 rpm or $PaCO_2$ <32 mm Hg; and (4) WBC >12,000/mm^3 or <4000/mm^3 or "bands" >10%. This definition was generated by the American College of Chest Physicians/Society of Critical Care Medicine Consensus Conference in Chicago in 1991 to improve the clinicians' ability to diagnose this entity and thus provide earlier therapeutic interventions (Bone et al., 1992). Although there is the criticism that the above definition of SIRS appears to be too sensitive as a predictor of multiple-organ failure syndrome (MOFS), its use does provide a standard that provokes the clinician to more thoroughly evaluate patients at risk. From a research point of view, it also provides a framework that can lead to a better evaluation of cellular and immunologic mechanisms that cause sepsis and related organ dysfunction.

Multiple-Organ Failure Syndrome

Defined as progressive failure of two or more organ systems, this now commonplace syndrome has resulted from recent advances in knowledge and technology that have made optimal acute resuscitation routine, thus leading to prolonged survival with resultant long-term sequelae.

Despite appropriate resuscitation and correction of the process precipitating shock, frequently precipitated by earlier recognition of SIRS, gross metabolic and physiologic dysfunction may persist and progress. Transition from a hypermetabolic state to the clinically defined MOFS does not occur suddenly. As discussed above, a variety of insults, including hemorrhage, sepsis, traumatic injury, ischemia, pancreatitis, burns, and major surgery, may precipitate shock and a generalized inflammatory process. The normal physiologic response initiates a systemic inflammatory response that may eventually lead to multiple-organ system failure, despite an adequate initial therapy of the shock state.

Once initiated, the systemic response to shock despite adequate resuscitation follows a typical time course. After the initial insult and resuscitation, there is a 48- to 72-hour period of relative stability, during which time the hypermetabolic response begins. Thereafter, the course of the recovery depends on the extent of the insult and host response. This response typically peaks in 3-4 days and resolves within 2 weeks. However, occasionally and unpredictably, the resolution of the initial response may lead to a progressive host response wherein complications develop, and patients become persistently hypermetabolic with the development of multiple-organ failure.

Shock is a clinical state resulting from inadequate tissue perfusion in which O_2 delivery does not meet O_2 demands. Persistence of this state leads to cellular and metabolic dysfunction while timely restoration of perfusion and oxygen delivery often stops what can be progression of a deadly process. Despite appropriate resuscitation and correction of the process precipitating shock, gross metabolic and physiologic dysfunction is always initiated and may persist and progress to multiple-organ failure syndrome (MOFS), which has increased dramatically in most intensive care units and is now the leading cause of death after sepsis, trauma, and burns. Although some progress has been made in the understanding of the physiologic mechanisms and therapy of shock and the pathway to MOFS, many questions remain. The most advanced experimental therapies involve direct manipulation of gene expression, but it is doubtful whether a single agent or mode of therapy will be successful in treating all patients with shock. For now, the keys to preventing shock from advancing to MOFS seem to be (1) aggressive early resuscitation so that prolonged periods of hypoperfusion are avoided, (2) prevention of sepsis by careful attention to aseptic technique and aggressive debridement of devitalized tissue, and (3) timely and aggressive medical and surgical treatment of sepsis when it is present.

REFERENCES

Alexander, F. & Hechtman, H. B. (1988). Pulmonary and cardiovascular responses. In G. H. A. Clowes, Jr. (Ed.), *Trauma, Sepsis, and Shock: The Physiological Basis of Therapy.* New York: Marcel Dekker.

Bernard, G. R., Luce, J. M., Sprung, C. L., Rinaldo, J. E., Tate, R. M., Sibbald, W. J., Kariman, K., Higgins, S., Bradly, R., Metz, C. A., Harris, T. R., & Brigham, K. L. (1987). High-dose corticosteroids in patients with the adult respiratory distress syndrome. *New England Journal of Medicine, 317* (25), 1565–1570.

Blalock, A. (1937). Shock: Further studies with particular reference to the effects of hemorrhage. *Archives of Surgery, 29,* 837

Bone, R. C. (1991). The pathogenesis of sepsis. *Annals of Internal Medicine, 115* (6), 457–469.

Bone, R. C., Fisher, C. J., Jr., Clemmer, T. P., Slotman, G. J., Metz, C. A., Balk, R. A., & the Methypredonisolone Severe Sepsis Study Group. (1987). A controlled clinical trial of high-dose methylpredonisolone in the treatment of severe sepsis and septic shock. *New England Journal of Medicine, 317* (11), 653–658.

Bone, R. C., Balk, R. A., Cerra, F. B., Dellinger, R. P., Fein, A. M., Knaus, W. A., Schein, R. M., & Sibbail, W. J. (1992). Definitions for sepsis and organ failure and guidelines for the use of innovative therapies in sepsis. *Chest, 101,* 1644–1655.

Cerra, F. B. (1983). Shock. In J. F. Burke (Ed.), *Surgical Physiology* (pp. 497–508). Philadelphia: W. B. Saunders.

Cerra, F. B. & Snyder L. M. (1993). Shock. In L. J. Greenfield (Ed.), *Surgery: Scientific Principles and Practice* (pp. 170–195). Philadelphia: J. B. Lippincott.

Deitch, E. A. (1990). Bacterial translocation of the gut flora. *The Journal of Trauma, 30* (Suppl), 184–189.

Demling, R. H. & Goodwin, C. W. (1989). Pulmonary dysfunction. In D. W. Wilmore, M. F. Brennan, A. H. Harken, J. W. Holcroft, & J. L. Meakins (Eds.), *Care of the Surgical Patient. Vol. 1, Critical Care, A Publication of the Committee on Pre- and Post-operative Care, American College of Surgeons.* New York: Scientific America.

Eichenholtz, P. W., Eichacker, P. Q., Hoffman, W. D., et al. (1992).

Tumor necrosis factor challenges in canines: Patterns of cardiovascular dysfunction. *American Journal of Physiology, 263,* H668–675.

Fisher C. J., Dhainut, J. F., Opal, S. M., Pribble, J. P., Balk, R. A., & Slotman, G. J. (1994). Recombinant human interleukin-1 receptor antagonist in the treatment of patients with sepsis syndrome: Results from a randomized, double-blind, placebo-controlled trial. *JAMA, 217,* 1836–1843.

Fisher C. L., Opal S. M., Dhainut, J. F., Stephens, S., Zimmermann, J. L., & Nightingale, P. (1993). Influence of an anti-tumor necrosis factor monoclonal antibody on cytekine levels in patients with sepsis. *Critical Care Medicine, 21,* 318–327.

Guyton, A. C. (1991). *Textbook of Medical Physiology* (8th ed.). Philadelphia: Saunders.

Holcroft, J. W. & Blaisdell, F. W. (1991). Shock. In D. C. Sabiston (Ed.), *Textbook of Surgery: The Biological Basis of Modern Surgical Practice* (pp. 34–56). Philadelphia: Saunders.

Jones II, W. G., Fahey III, T. J., & Tom Shires, G. (1993). Shock, resuscitation, and fluid management. In P. S. Barie & G. Tom Shires (Eds.), *Surgical Intensive Care* (pp. 309–344). Boston: Little, Brown

Krafft, P., Fridrich, P., Fitzgerald, R. D., Koc, D. & Steltzer, H. (1996). Effectiveness of nitric oxide inhalation in septic ARDS. *Chest, 109,* 489–493.

Kumar, A. & Parrillo, J. E. (1995). Shock. In J. E. Parrillo & R. C. Bone (Eds.), *Critical care medicine* (pp. 291–339). St. Louis: Mosby.

Lynn, W. A. & Cohen, J. (1995). Management of septic shock. *Journal of Infection, 30* (3), 207–212.

MacLean, L. D., Mulligan, W. G., MacLean, A. P. H., & Duff, J. H. (1967). Patterns of septic shock in man—a detailed study of 56 patients. *Annals of Surgery, 166* (4), 543–562.

Mueller, H. S. (1994). Role of intra-aortic counterpulsation in cardiogenic shock and acute myocardial infarction. *Cardiology, 84* (3), 168–174.

Oken, D. E. (1984). Hemodynamic basis for human acute renal failure (vasomoter nephropathy). *American Journal of Medicine, 176* (4), 702–710.

O'Ryan R. G. & Majcherczyk, S. (1982). Role of peripheral chemoreceptors and central chemosensitivity in the regulation of respiration and circulation. *Journal of Experimental Biology, 100,* 23–29.

Peitzman, A. B., Billiar, T. R., Harbrecht, B. G., Kelly, E., Vdekwn, A. O., & Simmons, R. L. (1995). Hemorrhagic shock. *Current Problems in Surgery, 32* (11), 925–1002.

Robert, A. & Kaufman, G. (1989). Stress ulcers, erosions, and gastric mucosal injury. In M. H. Sleisenger & J. S. Fordtran (Eds.), *Gastrointestinal Disease* (pp. 772–792). Philadelphia: W. B. Saunders.

Simeone, F. A. (1964). Shock. In L. Davis (Ed.), *Christopher's Textbook of Surgery.* Philadelphia: W. B. Saunders.

Volk, H. D., Reinke, P., Krausch, D., Zuckermann, H., Asadullah, K., Muller, J. M., Docke, W. D., & Kox, W. J. (1996). Monocyte deactivation—Rationale for a new therapeutic strategy in sepsis. *Intensive Care Medicine, 22* (Suppl), 474–481.

Weber, K. T., Ratshin, R. A., Janicki, J. S., & Russell, R. O. (1973). Left ventricular dysfunction following acute myocardial infarction. A clinicopathologic and hemodynamic profile of shock and failure. *American Journal of Medicine, 54* (6), 697–705.

20

Pain Management

Diana J. Wilkie
Dianne Wasser Monreal

December 10, 1862. Fredericksburg, Virginia. Civil War. Medical Officer's Diary—Several men were injured when a cannon misfired and exploded. The surgeons used saws to amputate the mangled limbs. The men screamed throughout the procedure despite the liberal use of whiskey. Praise be that we had some whiskey and few injuries today. I fear what Lacy House (our make-shift infirmary) will be like if there is a major battle.

Star Date: 2499.27.3. U.S.S. Proceeder, Medical Officer's Log—Fire in Docking Bay 12, three personnel had radiation and chemical burns. I used my new tricorder to diagnose the injuries and the complexities of the pain-related nociception. Two of the men had cellular and chromosomal destabilization secondary to radiation exposure. The third person, Ensign Loz, suffered transdermal searing with ruptured protoplasmic membranes. I was able to abolish the pain totally with direct neural stimuli and to treat the burns with a dermal regenerator. Despite the extent of the injuries and the pain, their recovery was quick. Loz and I will play Domjok tonight, after all.

While amputations are not performed without anesthesia in today's medical arena, neither do acute care nurse practitioners (ACNPs) today have the futuristic technology of a Star Tech Infirmary. Yet, the ACNP's mission is to properly diagnose and treat pain with current levels of knowledge and expertise. ACNPs are in a unique position to use a holistic approach that views pain as a process with physiological, sensory, affective, behavioral, and cognitive dimensions and to provide maximal pain relief with minimal side effects. In this chapter, scientific findings and case studies are used to illustrate how the pain process can be altered using pharmacological and nonpharmacological methods. The focus is on evidence-based practice to achieve patient-centered outcomes. Translation of the current knowledge into current clinical practice allows the ACNP to relieve most of the pain encountered in a twenty-first century practice.

DEFINITIONS

Today the scientific community has begun to understand the anatomy and physiology of pain at the molecular level. This knowledge makes two points clearly evident: (1) the extent of injury does not explain all pain, and (2) unrelieved pain has dire physiologic and psychologic consequences. Unfortunately, the pain-free public, patients, and most health or legal professionals do not share this understanding. Instead, many people call a variety of sensations and emotions painful, which can be an important source of misconception in the management of pain.

A lay person is likely to describe pain in the ways that it effects the body or its function. For example, the person says "my back is out" to describe lumbosacral pain or says "my head hurts so bad I can't see straight" to describe a headache. Often the person does not use the word *pain,* but instead calls it an ache, such as a toothache or headache. Pain also is used by some people to describe emotions of disappointment or loss, closely linking it with suffering. The ACNP must decode the patient's own words or phrases in order to assess the pain.

Health professionals recognize that pain, no matter what the cause, is subjective. The person experiencing the pain is the expert about its existence and severity. One commonly cited definition views pain as "whatever the person experiencing the pain says it is, existing whenever and wherever the person says it does" (McCaffery & Beebe, 1989). A more specific and current view defines pain as "an unpleasant sensory and emotional experience associated with actual or potential tissue damage, or described in terms of such damage" (Merskey & Bogduk, 1994). Based on the recent definition, pain typically is viewed as a multidimensional phenomenon. Anatomical, physiological, affective, behavioral, and cognitive aspects all influence the sensory pain experience.

Despite interchangeable use of the terms *pain* and *suffering* by the legal system and the general public, pain and suffering are distinct but related concepts. Suffering is a state of severe distress associated with events that threaten the intactness of the person (Cassell, 1982). As a threat to personhood, suffering is an emotion. In contrast, pain is associated with threatened tissue integrity and is considered a sensation that sometimes is affected by emotions. Suffering may or may not be associated with pain. Pain, not suffering, is discussed in this chapter, including its mechanisms, assessment, and treatment. The responsibilities of the ACNP in the independent and collaborative management of pain are also addressed and illustrated through case studies.

▶ NEURAL MECHANISMS OF PAIN

The ACNP uses knowledge of the pain mechanisms to interpret assessment data and to prescribe therapies that promote maximum pain relief with minimum side effects. The neural mechanisms by which pain is perceived involve a process that involves four major steps: (1) transduction; (2) transmission; (3) perception; and (4) modulation. The transduction and transmission steps relate to the neurochemical signals of actual or impending tissue damage (nociceptive stimuli). Not all nociceptive stimuli are perceived as pain. If there is sufficient modulation of signals and perception of nociceptive events is prevented, there is no pain. Perception is critical to sensing pain. Modulation, either enhancing or inhibiting nociception, is crucial to pain perception. Most pain-management techniques probably mimic endogenous pain-inhibition processes. Conversely, pain that is difficult to relieve probably results from enhanced nociceptive signals. Additional details about these four steps provide a foundation for ACNP practice.

Transduction

The first step of the pain process is transduction. Transduction is conversion of a mechanical, thermal, or chemical stimulus into a neuronal action potential (Fig. 20–1). Understanding the clinical significance of this important and complex step in the pain process requires knowledge of the anatomy, physiology, and pathophysiology of the peripheral nervous system and its response to tissue injury.

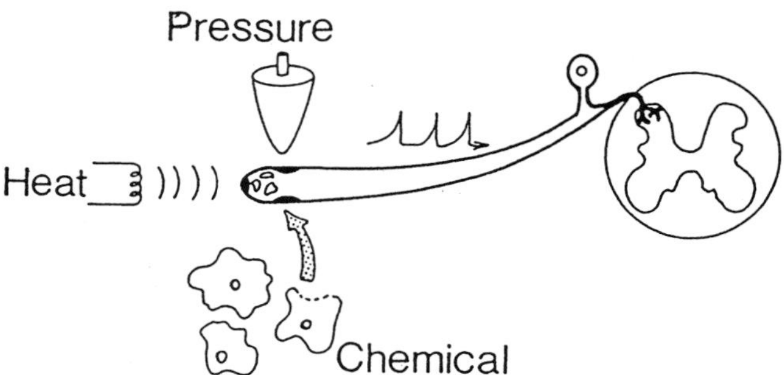

Figure 20–1. Peripheral terminals are sensitive to direct heat, mechanical pressure, and chemicals released in response to tissue damage. *(Reprinted with permission from Fields, H.L. [1987], [p 27].)*

Anatomy and Physiology of Transduction

Peripheral nerve cells are stimulated by tissue damaging (noxious), pressure, heat, or chemical forces. A sufficient stimulus generates an action potential at nociceptors (receptors) on A-delta fibers and C fibers. These cells are known as primary afferent nociceptors (PANs), the first-order neurons in the processing of nociceptive stimuli. PAN fibers traverse through the dorsal root ganglia along with the A-alpha (sensory muscle), A-beta (sensory skin), and sympathetic afferent fibers, into the dorsal horn of the spinal cord where various connections are made (Fig. 20–2).

The A-alpha and A-beta fibers carry the sensation of light pressure to deep muscles, soft touch to skin, and vibration. The A-alpha and A-beta fibers primarily ascend to rostral centers in the dorsal column pathway, but they also make synapses in the spinal dorsal horn close to synapses of the A-delta and C fibers (refer to Fig. 20–2). This dorsal horn connection means that input from touch fibers can enter the spinal cord and synapse or communicate with cells carrying nociceptive input.

The three types of fibers differ in size and speed at which action potentials are conducted (Sidedall & Cousins, 1997). A-alpha or A-beta fibers are large (6-22 microns) with myelin sheaths around them. Because of the myelin sheath and axon size, A-alpha and A-beta fibers conduct at a rapid rate (35-120 meters per sec). In contrast, A-delta fibers are smaller fibers also with myelin sheaths. Because of their size (1-5 microns), A-delta fibers conduct at a slower rate (5-30 meters per sec) than the larger A-alpha and A-beta fibers. C fibers, in comparison, are small (0.2-1.5 microns) and unmyelinated. C fibers occur singly or in clusters, and they conduct at a rate of 0.5 to 2 meters per second. The conduction rates are important because information carried to the spinal cord by the A-alpha and A-beta fibers communicates with dorsal horn cells sooner than in-

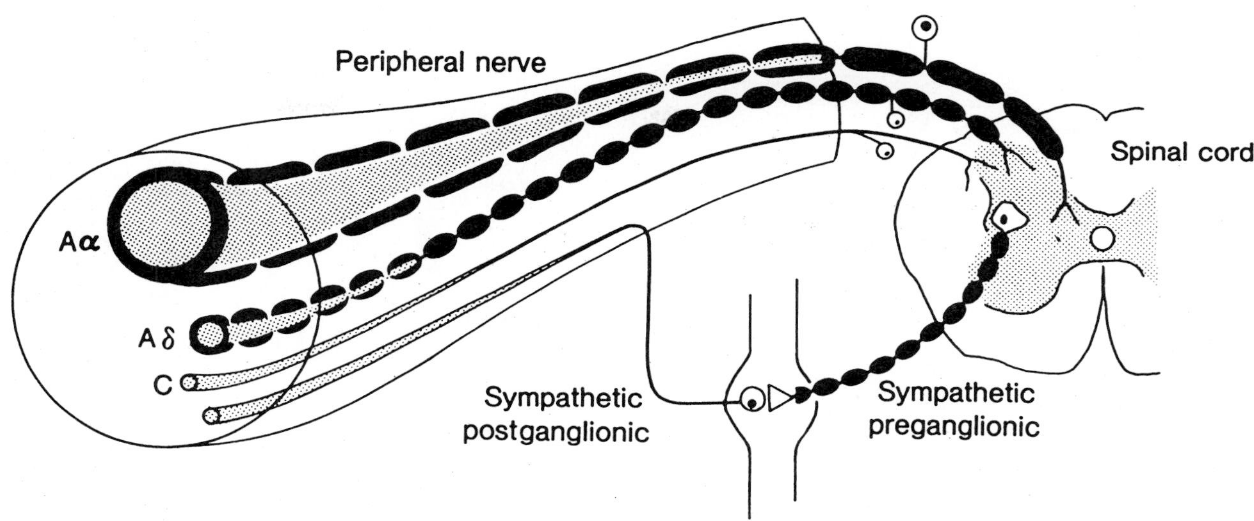

Figure 20–2. Components of a cutaneous nerve: primary afferents fibers with cell bodies in the dorsal root ganglion and sympathetic postganglionic fibers with cell bodies in the sympathetic ganglion. Primary afferents include neurons with large-diameter myleninated (A alpha), small-diameter mylinated (A-delta), and unmylinated (c) axons. All sympathetic postganglionic fibers are unmyelinated. *(Reprinted with permission from Fields, H.L. [1987], [p 14].)*

formation carried by A-delta or C fibers. These conduction rates have important implications for modulation of noxious information from A-delta and C fibers. Because of anatomical proximity, the peripheral environment (physiologic milieu) of the axons and dendrites of one neuron can influence other nearby neurons.

Pathophysiology of Transduction

When a soft tissue mass exerts sufficient pressure on the PAN to cause nerve transduction, the nerve is activated and signals the tissue damage to the CNS. This type of mechanical injury to somatic (skin, muscle, or bone) or to visceral tissues is known as *nociceptive pain.* In contrast, pressure from a mass that encircles and constricts neural tissue (e.g., nerve plexus, nerve root, spinal cord) and that is sufficient to injure the tissue, produces pain known as *neuropathic pain.* Nerve tissue also may be damaged by surgery (postthoracotomy injury to intercostal nerves, postmastectomy interruption of intercosto–brachial nerves, radical neck dissection injury to cervical nerves, or phantom limb syndrome after amputation), chemotherapy (peripheral neuropathy after vinca alkaloid therapy), traumatic events (brachial plexus avulsion), or viral infection (postherpetic neuralgia). These types of injury to neural tissue are examples of neuropathic pain.

Burns are obvious examples of tissue damage from thermal stimuli. Superficial burns injure somatic tissue and result in nociceptive pain. Massive burns, however, are likely to injure peripheral nerve fibers as well as somatic tissues. Therefore, extensive burns may result in neuropathic and nociceptive types of pain.

Tissue damage produces chemicals that cause an action potential (Dickenson, 1995). Although it is intuitively clear how pressure from masses or injury from burns initiate the neuronal action potential, it may be less obvious how chemicals generate an action potential. Therefore, chemical transduction is described in detail because of its importance to pain experienced by acutely ill patients.

When tissue is traumatized and cells are damaged, a number of chemicals are released near the PAN (Fig. 20–3). Some chemicals (bradykinin, serotonin, histamine, potassium ions, norepinephrine) *stimulate,* while others (leukotrienes, prostaglandins, substance P) *sensitize* the PAN to be excitable and to fire an action potential toward the spinal cord. Several details are helpful in fully understanding this process and how analgesics affect it.

All human cells have a two-layer lipid membrane. When a cell is damaged, phosolipids and other substances are liberated from the cell into the intracellular space. The release of phosolipids initiates the arachidonic acid cascade through which 5-lipo-oxygenase and cyclo-oxygenase synthesize leukotrienes and prostaglandins, respectively (Weissman, 1991). These events are displayed in Figure 20–3. Leukotrienes and prostaglandins sensitize the PAN to be activated by a smaller stimulus than when these chemicals are not near the PAN. For example, light pressure is not perceived as painful in normal conditions, but sometimes is sensed as pain (allodynia) if leukotrienes or prostaglandins surround the PAN.

Inhibition of leukotriene and prostaglandin synthesis can improve pain control when tissue damage is known or suspected (Fig. 20–4). A specific inhibitor of leukotrienes is not yet approved for pain control, but ketoprophen, a nonsteroidal antiinflammatory drug (NSAID), appears to have

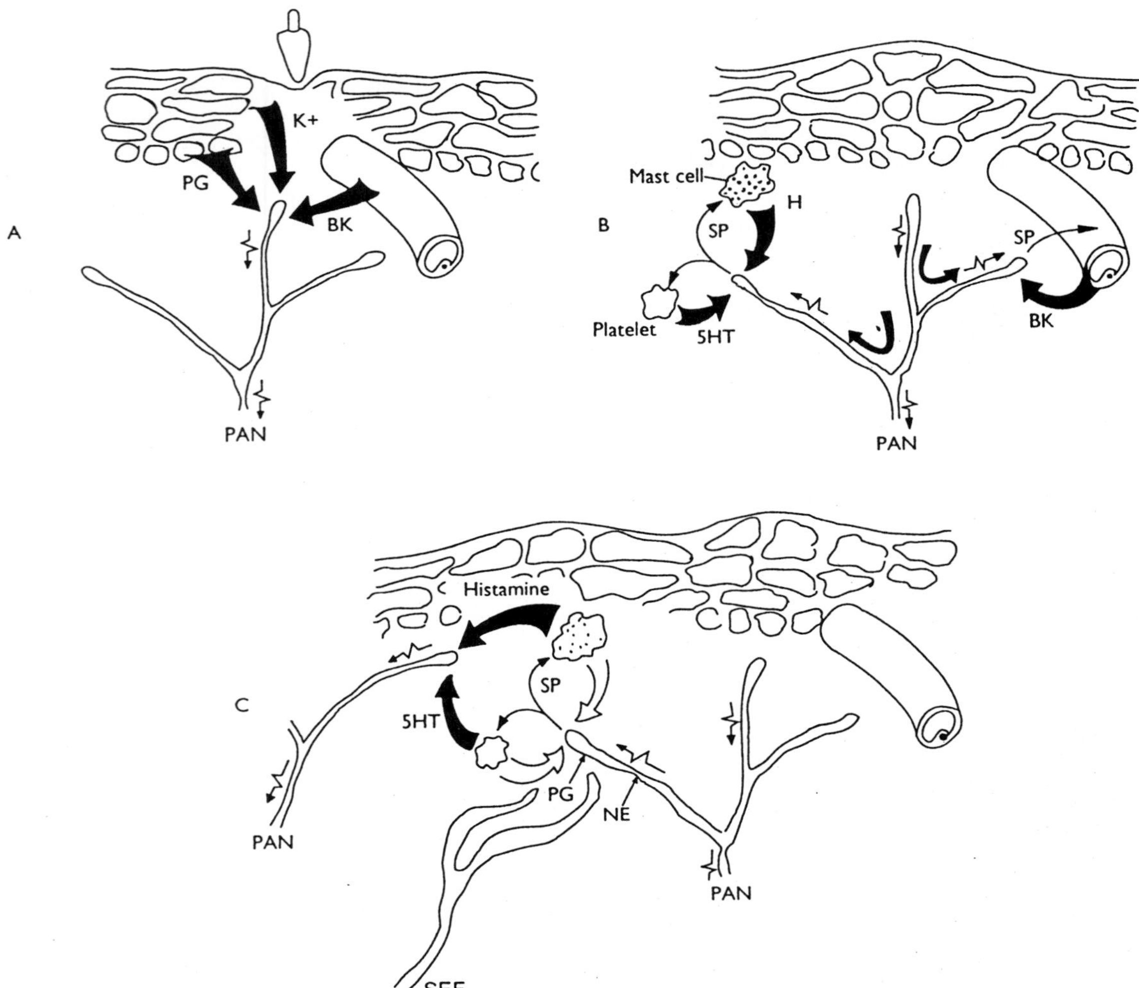

Figure 20–3. Diagram summarizing ingredients of peripheral soup in response to tissue injury. **A.** Direct activation of primary afferent nociceptor (PAN) by intense pressure and consequent cell damage which leads to potassium (K+) leaking from the cell and to prostaglandin (PG) and bradykinin (BK) synthesis. **B.** Secondary activation occurs when impulses generated in the stimulated terminal produce a retrograde release of peptides, such as substance P (SP). SP causes vasodilation, increased accumulation of bradykinin, and release of histamine (H) from mast cells and serotonin (5HT) from platelets. **C.** Histamine and serotonin levels rise in the extracellular space, sensitizing nearby nociceptors. Sympathetic efferent fibers (SEF) release norepinephrine (NE) and additional prostaglandins, which activates the nociceptor if the nerve has been injured. *(Adapted with permission from Fields, H.L. [1987], [p 36].)*

some activity in blocking leukotriene synthesis (Stambaugh & Drew, 1988). Aspirin and other nonsteroidal antiinflammatory drugs block prostaglandin synthesis, and most interfere with platelet aggregation. Choline magnesium trislicylate (Trilisate), however, is an example of a NSAID that does not inhibit synthesis of thromboxane A_2, a necessary factor for platelet aggregation (Cashman, 1996). Steroids act earlier in the cascade and prevent production of arachidonic acid, thus inhibiting synthesis of both leukotrienes and prostaglandins. Any of these drugs (ASA, NSAIDs, steroids) block chemicals that sensitize the PAN and thereby raise the threshold at which the PAN is transduced. These drugs are powerful analgesics, particularly when there is tissue injury such as occurs with excessive peripheral edema, burns, arthritis, and bone metastasis.

In addition to the arachidonic cascade, many chemicals activate the PAN when they leak out of the cell or are released into the intracellular space as part of the inflammatory response (Willis & Westlund, 1997). For example, potassium and histamine exude from damaged cells, and bradykinin is degraded from plasma kininogen, a component of inflammatory exudate. Other chemicals are released from platelets (serotonin) or mast cells (histamine). Sufficient concentrations of any one of these chemicals around the PAN causes the PAN to be activated (transduced), firing an action potential. These chemicals also act in combina-

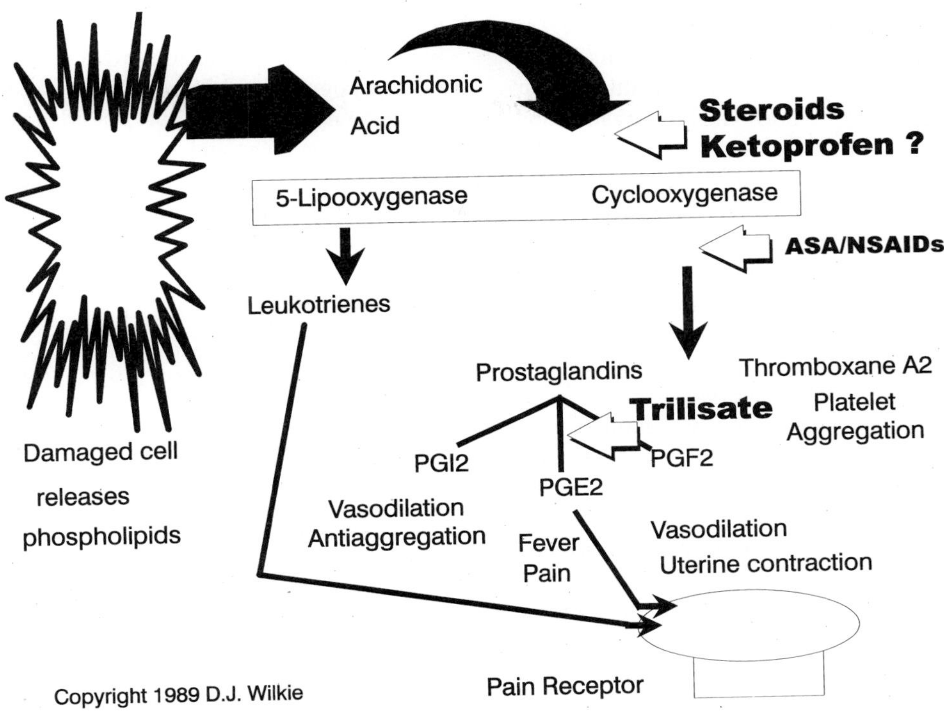

Figure 20–4. Inhibition of the arachidonic acid pathway by several drugs. Steroids inhibit production of arachidonic acid, thereby blocking synthesis of leukotrienes and prostaglandins. Ketoprophen is believed to block production of 5-lipo-oxygenase and cyclo-oxygenase. Aspirin and nonsteroidal anti-inflammatory drugs block conversion of cyclo-oxygenase to prostaglandins and thromboxane A_2. Trilisate blocks production of prostagandins E_2 and F_2, but not I_2 or thromboxane A_2. *(Reprinted with permission. Copyright © 1989. Wilkie, D. J.)*

tion to sensitize the PAN, enabling it to fire with a stimulus smaller than usual. Few drugs inhibit the excitatory actions of these chemicals. Antihistamine drugs are an exception. By blocking the excitatory action of histamine, these drugs have shown analgesic effects in people with cancer (Stambaugh & Lane, 1983).

If the PAN is activated and fires an action potential, the PAN itself releases chemicals, one of which is substance P (Willis & Westlund, 1997). Substance P is stored in the distal terminals of the PAN and is released through a retrograde process. In this way, substance P sensitizes the PAN, dilates nearby blood vessels which leads to local edema, and causes release of histamine from mast cells. Capsaicin (Zostrix), when applied to the skin in the painful area, is believed to deplete the PAN terminal of substance P and, by this action, to block retrograde release of substance P (Willis & Westlund, 1997). In this way capsaicin, a topical analgesic available over the counter (OTC), helps to prevent further sensitization of the PAN.

Finally, activation of the autonomic nervous system contributes to PAN transduction through release of norepinephrine and prostaglandins (Gonzales, Goldyne, Taiwo, & Levine, 1989). Norepinephrine activates a PAN when it comes into contact with the PAN, only if the PAN has been injured (Sato & Perl, 1991). Tumors often invade nerve tissue and surgical incisions cut small peripheral nerves, both of which can produce injured PANs (examples of neuropathic pain). In the context of nerve injury, therefore, it is clear that emotions, which can increase autonomic nervous system release of norepinephrine, can increase pain through physiologic mechanisms. Nonpharmacologic (behavioral) and pharmacologic methods of reducing autonomic nervous system activation can be important analgesic methods. For example, reducing fear, anger, and anxiety through behavioral methods (such as patient education, relaxation, and distraction), theoretically, can reduce activation of the PAN. Anxiolytic agents also can reduce activation of the PAN by reducing autonomic nervous system discharge.

In summary, tissue injury results in production and release of a number of chemicals around the PAN. These chemicals can sensitize or activate the PAN directly (example of nociceptive pain) and through secondary processes (usually an example of nociceptive pain unless neural tissue has been injured, then an example of neuropathic pain). These chemicals are commonly described as ingredients in the peripheral soup surrounding the PAN. If any or all of these ingredients can be eliminated from the peripheral soup, then the PAN may not send an action potential to the CNS. A number of nonopioid analgesics inhibit these chemicals and thereby remove peripheral soup ingredients that contribute to PAN activation. Drugs that block production or release of these chemicals can be powerful analgesics and are the first-line drugs recommended in several published guidelines for acute pain and cancer pain (American Pain Society, 1998; U.S. Department of Health and Human Services, 1992, 1994; World Health Organization, 1996).

In addition to the powerful effect of the drugs inhibiting peripheral soup ingredients, people with pain often engage in behaviors that limit PAN activation. For example, if a certain movement routinely produces pain, a person avoids that movement. Guarding and immobilizing the injured body area are common methods of preventing the onset of pain (Wilkie, Keefe, Dodd, & Copp, 1992; Wilkie, Lovejoy, Dodd, & Tesler, 1988). One way patients guard against pain is to wear loose, unrestrictive clothing when light touch produces pain (allodynia). Use of a foot cradle is another way to remove the pressure of a sheet or blanket when the weight causes pain. Use of a cane, walker, or back brace are examples of ways to prevent PAN activation in a person with vertebral metastasis. These types of devices prevent movement-induced vertebral flexion, a common source of pain in people with vertebral masses (bone metastasis) or vertebral lesions (osteoporosis). Such behavioral methods of pain control can supplement drugs that also prevent transduction.

Some pain control behaviors, however, may have untoward sequella. For example, the person with a chest or abdominal incision who guards the respiratory muscles by taking shallow breaths dramatically increases his or her risk of atelectasis and pneumonia (Cousins, 1994). Long-term immobilization can increase the person's risk of developing a decubitus ulcer. Persons with pain are quite expert at finding behavioral methods to prevent or minimize PAN activation. Recognition of these behavioral pain-control attempts helps the ACNP to avoid the common misconception that a patient lying quiet and still cannot be experiencing pain. When a patient minimizes activity, the ACNP should prescribe regularly scheduled—not p.r.n.—analgesics in order to prevent the undesired sequella of the immobilization.

Transmission

Once the PAN has been transduced, the action potential must be transmitted to the CNS and through the CNS before pain is perceived. Three steps are involved in nociceptive signal transmission: (1) projection to the CNS; (2) processing within the dorsal horn of the spinal cord; and (3) transmission to the brain. Each step in the transmission process is important to pain perception.

Projection to the CNS

Transduction at the PAN terminal causes the PAN membrane to depolarize. In a depolarized cell, sodium ions enter the cell through sodium channels and potassium ions exit the cell through potassium channels to generate a neuronal action potential. The action potential rapidly spreads along the neuron, more rapidly for myelinated than unmyelinated axons because ion exchange occurs only at nodes of Ranvier and jumps between nodes (Garoutte, 1981) (Fig. 20–5). In contrast, ion exchange travels the entire length of the unmyelinated, C fiber axon. The transmission of the action potential to the central terminal of the neuron is neces-

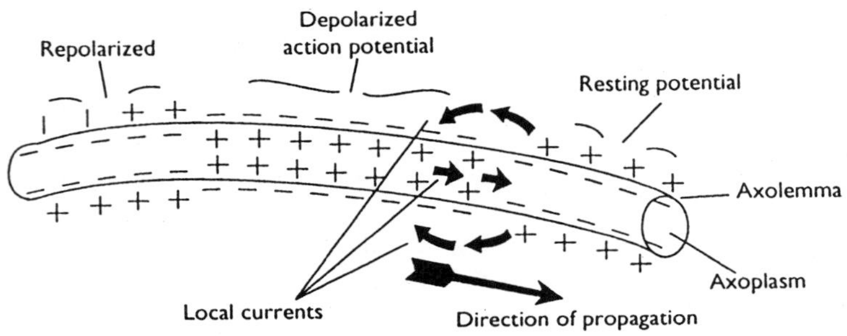

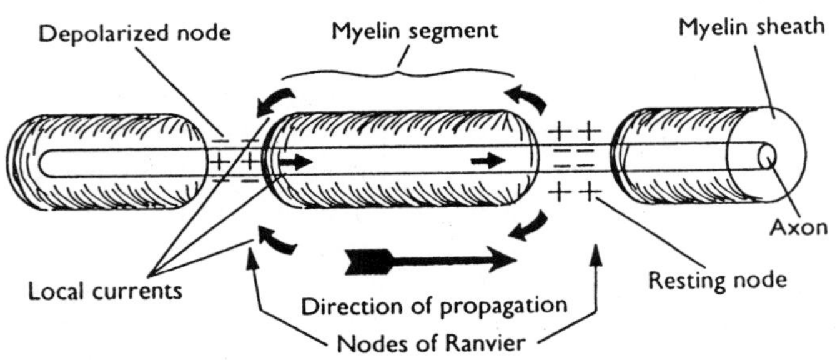

Figure 20–5. Propagation of a neuronal action potential in a C fiber *(top)* and a myelinated fiber (A-alpha, A-beta, or A-delta) *(bottom).* Because of myelinization, ion exchange occurs only at the nodes of Ranvier. *(Reprinted with permission from Garoutte, B. [1981], [p 43].)*

sary for the cell to deliver the nociceptive signal to cells in the spinal cord. This transmission requires more time for C fibers and explains some of the differences in fiber conduction rates described previously.

The action potential can be inhibited, however, if the ion channels are inactivated. Drugs known as membrane stabilizers inactivate the sodium channels and disrupt the transmission of the action potential along the PAN axon (Woolf & Wiesenfield-Hallin, 1985). Some adjuvant drugs, such as local anesthetics (e.g., lidocaine, bupivicane, mexilitine, Emla) and anticonvulsant drugs (e.g., phenytoin, carbamazepine, clonazepam), prevent transmission via this type of mechanism. In dilute concentrations, local anesthetics effectively block small fiber transmission. Larger concentrations of local anesthetics block larger fibers, including the motor fibers (Wilkie, Vivenzio, & Puntillo, 1991).

An important concept to recognize is that one nerve cell extends the entire distance from the periphery to the dorsal horn of the spinal cord. The cell usually makes synapses only at the terminals at the peripheral and central nervous system sites. For example, an afferent fiber from the great toe travels from the toe through the fifth lumbar nerve root into the spinal cord; it is one cell. It does not synapse at the knee or hip. Once an action potential is generated, it travels all the way to the spinal cord. The message is transmitted to the dorsal horn of the spinal cord, unless it is blocked (e.g., by a sodium channel inhibitor) or disrupted (e.g., by a lesion at the central terminal of the fiber such as a dorsal root entry zone lesion [DREZ]). Altering the peripheral soup ingredients at the distal end of the PAN is an important way to prevent pain. Once the first nerve cell in the pain process has fired an action potential, however, the uninhibited message is transmitted to the spinal cord.

The A-alpha, A-beta, A-delta, and C fibers extend from the peripheral tissues through the dorsal root ganglia to the dorsal horn of the spinal cord (refer to Fig. 20–2). The area of skin innervated by a single nerve root is known as a dermatome (Fig. 20–6). Each nerve root innervates typical segments of the body, sometimes far removed from the area where the nerve enters the spinal cord. Although fibers enter the spinal segment associated with the nerve root in which they travel to the spinal cord, the A-delta and C fibers send dendrites rostrally (toward the brain) and caudally (toward the feet) for two to four spinal segments (Willis & Westlund, 1997) (Fig. 20–7). Therefore, one fiber can communicate with as many as nine spinal segments. The innervation expanse is important when transcutaneous nerve stimulators (TENS) are used to block transmission of nociceptive stimuli. If, in positioning TENS electrodes, the ACNP does not take into consideration the full range of spinal segments innervated by a single nerve cell, pain may not be blocked.

Dorsal Horn Processing

Once the nociceptive signal arrives in the CNS, it is processed within the dorsal horn of the spinal cord. This processing includes: (1) release of neurotransmitters from the PAN into the synaptic cleft and (2) binding of neurotransmitters to receptors on nearby cell bodies and dendrites of cells that may be located elsewhere in the dorsal horn. The transmitters include (1) excitatory amino acids, such as glutamate and aspartate; (2) fluoride-resistant acid phosphatase (FRAP); and (3) many peptides, such as substance P, vasoactive intestinal polypeptide (VIP), somatostatin, cholecystokinin (CCK), gastrin-releasing peptide (GRP), angiotensin II, calcitonin gene-related peptide (CGRP), as well as leu-enkephalin and dynorphine, both of which are commonly known as endorphins (Willis & Westlund, 1997). Amino acids are fast transmitters, and peptides are slow transmitters. Some of these PAN neurotransmitters produce activation, perhaps through cooperation of other neurotransmitters, when bound to receptors whereas others inhibit activation of nearby cells. Cells excited by PAN input release other neurotransmitters, such as gamma-amiobutyric acid (GABA) and glycine, which increases the complexity of the neurochemical communication occurring within the dorsal horn. The net effects of the complex neurotransmitter release can either facilitate or inhibit transmission of nociceptive stimuli.

Neurotransmitter release and binding involves several different types of cells located in the dorsal horn (Fig. 20–8). Areas within the gray matter of the spinal cord are represented by laminae numbered between I and X; the dorsal horn is represented by laminae I to V. Cells that receive nociceptive input are located in lamina I (projection cells), lamina II (some projection cells and interneurons), and lamina V (wide dynamic range neurons most of which are projection cells) (Willis & Westlund, 1997). All of the cells in these laminae are important to propagation of the nociceptive signal from the spinal cord to the brain.

Most projection cells (second-order neurons) send axons to the brain in the contralateral anterolateral quadrant. They receive excitatory and inhibitory messages, the net sum of which determines whether the PAN action potential is transmitted to the brain on the opposite side of the stimulus.

Interneurons can be either excitatory or inhibitory. They communicate with other lamina II cells, located within one or two spinal segments, and with dendrites from cells located in laminae I, III, IV, and V (Dickenson, 1995). The concept of excitatory and inhibitory interneurons is important because it helps to explain why some behavioral therapies are effective. Although the exact mechanisms have not been determined, it is known that stimulation of large sensory fibers (A-beta) can have an inhibitory effect on cells that project nociceptive signals to the brain. TENS and massage are examples of nonpharmacologic methods by which rapidly conducting large fibers can be activated. Application of heat or cold are examples of methods by which smaller, less rapidly conducting fibers can be activated by nonnoxious stimuli. All of these methods are known to inhibit transmission of nociceptive stimuli.

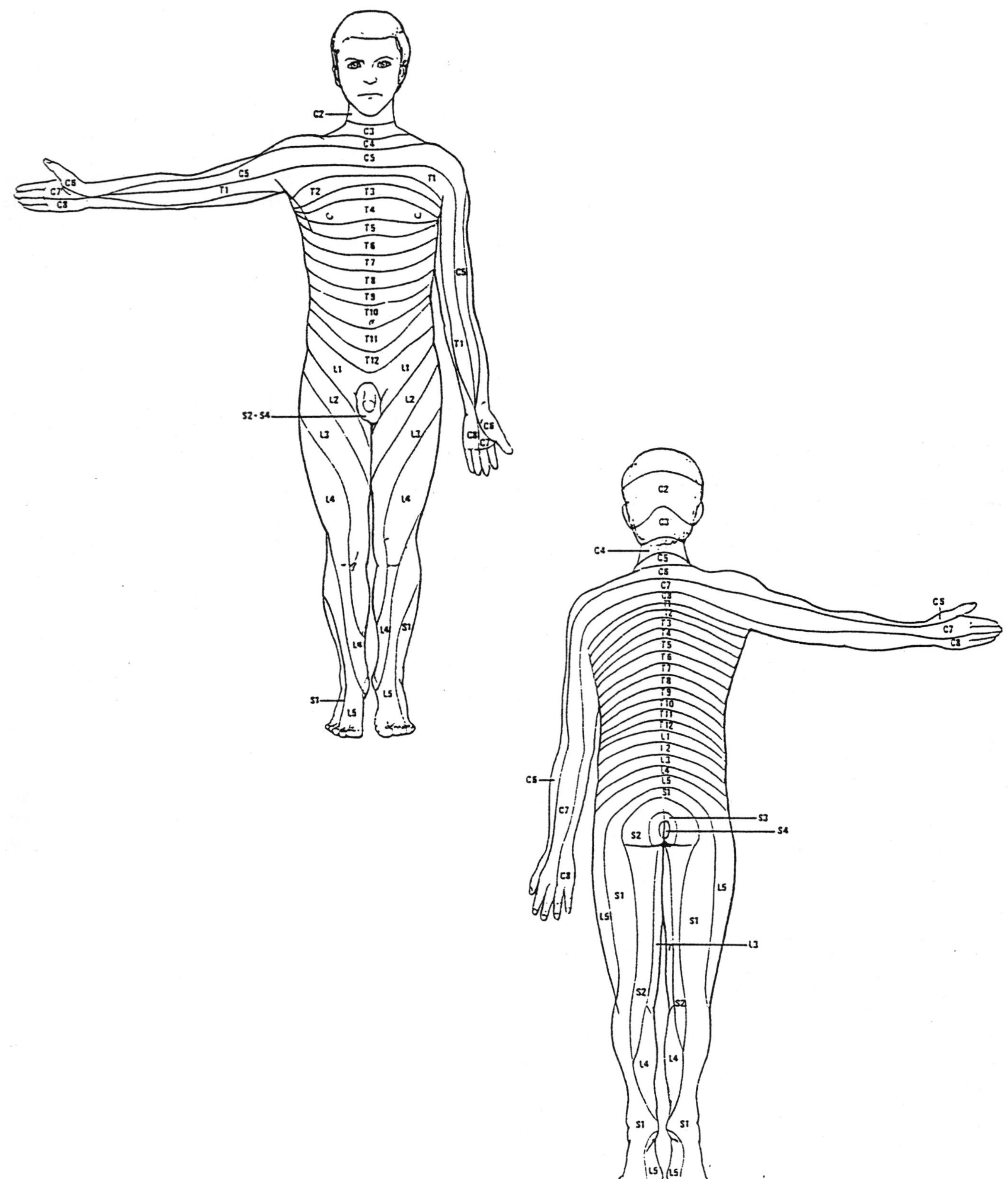

Figure 20–6. Spinal dermatomes represent organized sensory input carried via specific spinal nerve roots. S=sacral, L=lumbar, T=thoracic, C=cervical. (*Reprinted with permission from Martin, J.H. [1985]. Anatomical substrates for somatic sensation. In Kandel, E.R., Schwartz, J.H., (eds.).* Priciples of Neural Science *[2nd ed.], [p 303]. New York: Elsevier.*)

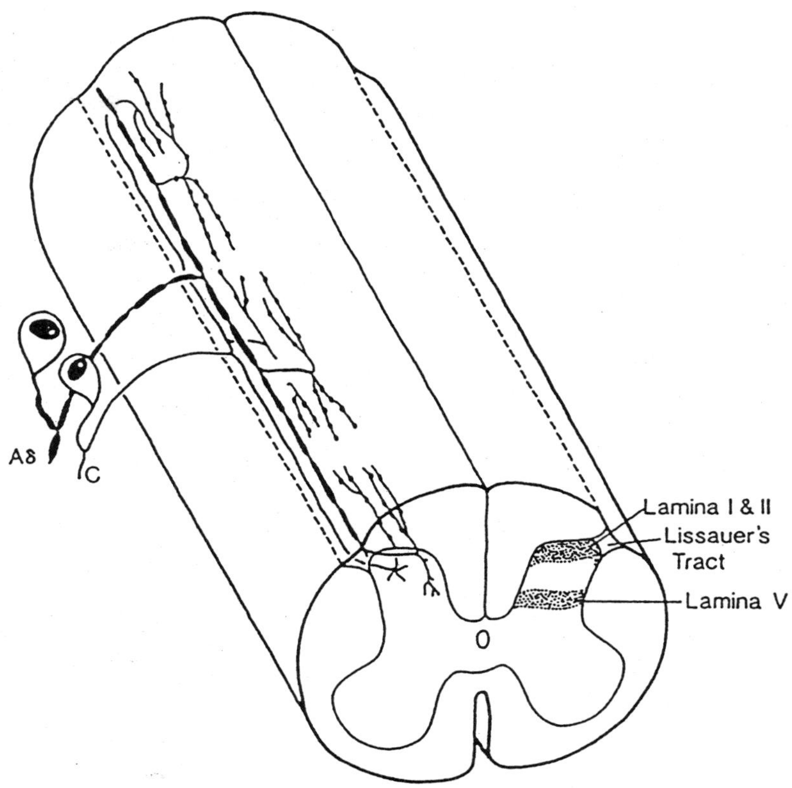

Figure 20–7. A single small-diameter primary afferent nociceptor has an extensive terminal field. After bifurcating at the point of entry into Lissauer's tract, the small-diameter fibers penetrate the spinal gray matter. C fibers terminate predominately in lamina II. A-delta nociceptors terminate in laminae I and V. The terminal axons of both types of small-diameter primary afferents are varicose and have a longitudinal orientation, extending for several millimeters in laminae I and II, contacting hundreds of spinal neurons. *(Reprinted with permission from Fields, H.L. [1987], [p 45].)*

Wide dynamic range (WDR) neurons receive input from noxious stimuli primarily carried by A-delta and C fiber afferents (especially from viscera), nonnoxious stimuli from A-beta fibers, and indirect input from dendritic projections into laminae I, II, III, and IV (Willis & Westlund, 1997). Most lamina V neurons project to the brainstem and to the thalamus (Dickenson, 1995; Sidedall & Cousins, 1997).

Discovery that WDR neurons have large receptive fields and receive inputs from nonnoxious and noxious stimuli provides a neural explanation for referred pain (Fields, 1987; Willis & Westlund, 1997). Inputs from nociceptive fibers innervating visceral organs and nonnoxious somatic fibers innervating the body part to which pain is referred all converge on the same WDR neuron. When the message received by the WDR neuron is transmitted to the brain, the originating location is poorly localized. Pain, therefore, is perceived in the body part presumably innervated by the somatic fiber rather than from the visceral A-delta or C fibers. Since primary and metastatic malignant tumors often involve thoracic, abdominal, and pelvic viscera, the concept of referred pain must be considered when interpreting the location of pain. As indicated in Figure 20–9, the location of the pathology may be quite distant from the pain location reported by the patient. For example, Figure 20–9 shows that pain from liver disease is located in the right upper abdominal quadrant, but also it frequently is referred to the anterior and posterior neck regions and to a posterior flank area. If referred pain is not considered when evaluating a pain location report, therapy could be misdirected.

An important concept related to neural mechanisms of persistent pain is neural plasticity (Coderre, Katz, Vaccarino, & Melzack, 1993). Repetitive transmission of PAN nociceptive signals to the dorsal horn results in several changes in dorsal horn processing, including: (1) enlargement of the receptive field of a peripheral neuron; (2) activation of receptors normally inactive; (3) "wind-up" of C fibers (a phenomenon of progressively increased neural response to repeated noxious stimuli); and (4) allodynia (pain evoked by light tactile stimulation) (Coderre et al., 1993; Dickenson, 1995; Yaksh, 1991). N-methyl-D-aspartate (NMDA) and non-NMDA receptors are excitatory and have been implicated in these changes in dorsal horn processing

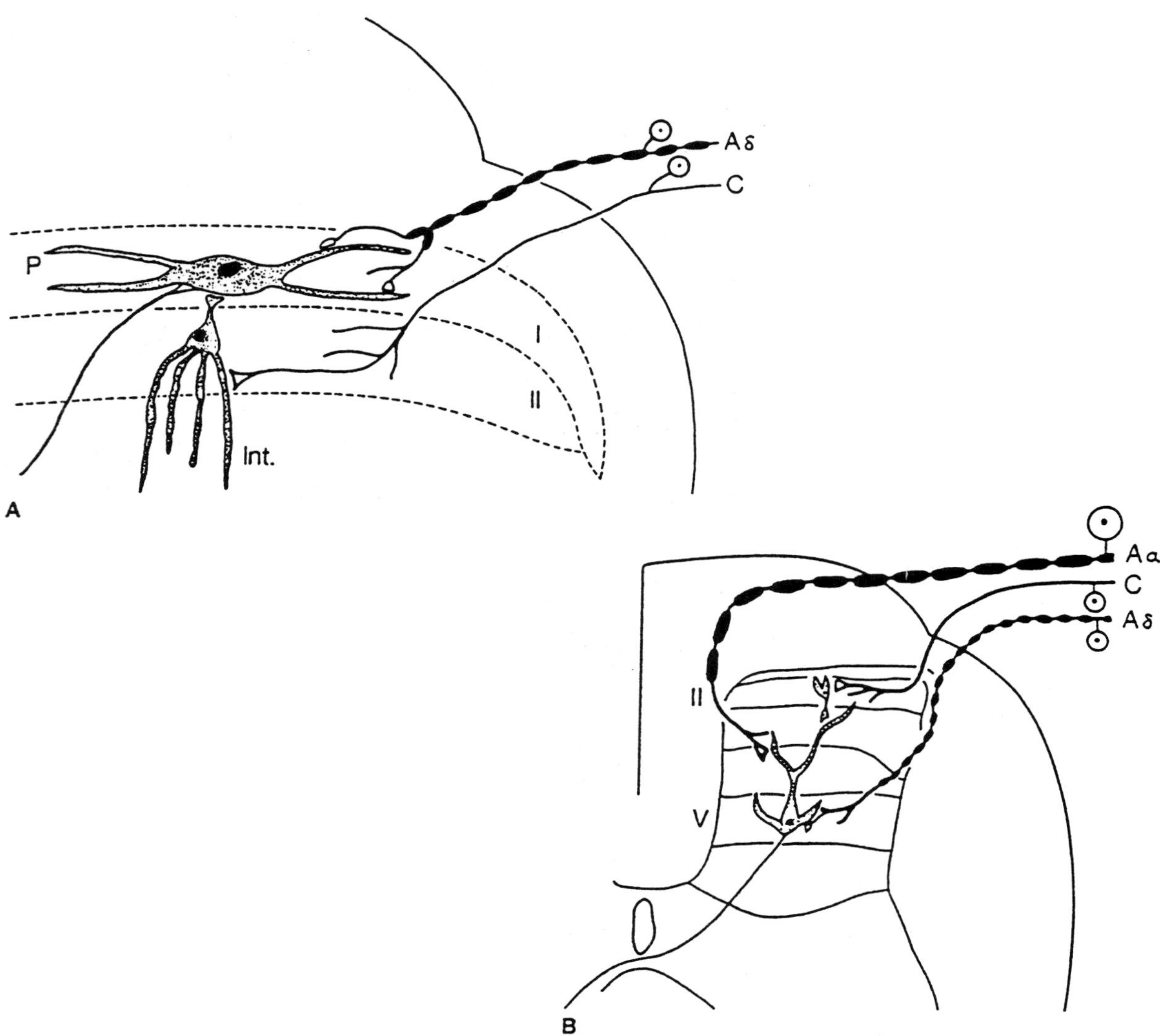

Figure 20–8. Input to dorsal horn projection cells (P). **A.** Lamina I neurons are predominately excited by nociceptive input directly from A-delta fibers and indirectly from C-fibers. **B.** Lamina V neurons are predominately wide dynamic range (WDR) and receive input from low-threshold A-beta fibers as well as direct and indirect input from nociceptive afferents. In addition, the dendrites of WDR neurons contact cells located in laminae II (nociceptive) and III (non-noxious). *(Reprinted with permission from Fields, H.L. [1987], [p. 55].)*

(Coderre et al., 1993). The NMDA receptors are enabled once the neuron has been depolarized and—along with subsequent changes in calcium channel conduction—produce profound alterations in neural processing of afferent stimuli (an example of neuropathic pain) that can persist for long periods of time (Fig. 20–10). For this reason, Sidedall & Cousins (1997) state that current pain-treatment goals are to be preemptive and prevent nociceptive pain and, therefore, the neural changes (causing neuropathic pain) that occur with a persistent barrage of nociceptive stimuli. Although researchers are conducting studies to develop NMDA antagonist drugs for clinical use, two currently available drugs, dextromethorphan (cough suppressant) and ketamine (general anesthetic), block the NMDA receptor-mediated changes.

Propagation Through the CNS

With adequate summation (net excitatory effects) on projection cells, nociceptive stimuli are propagated to the third-order neuron, primarily in thalamus and several other areas of the brain. The axons of the dorsal horn projection cells (second-order neurons) enter the brain through several pathways, including the: (1) spinothalamic tract (STT); (2) spinoreticular tract (SRT); (3) spinomesencephalic tract (SMT); (4) spinocervial tract; (5) second-order dorsal column tract (SDCT); and (6) spinohypothalamic tract (Willis

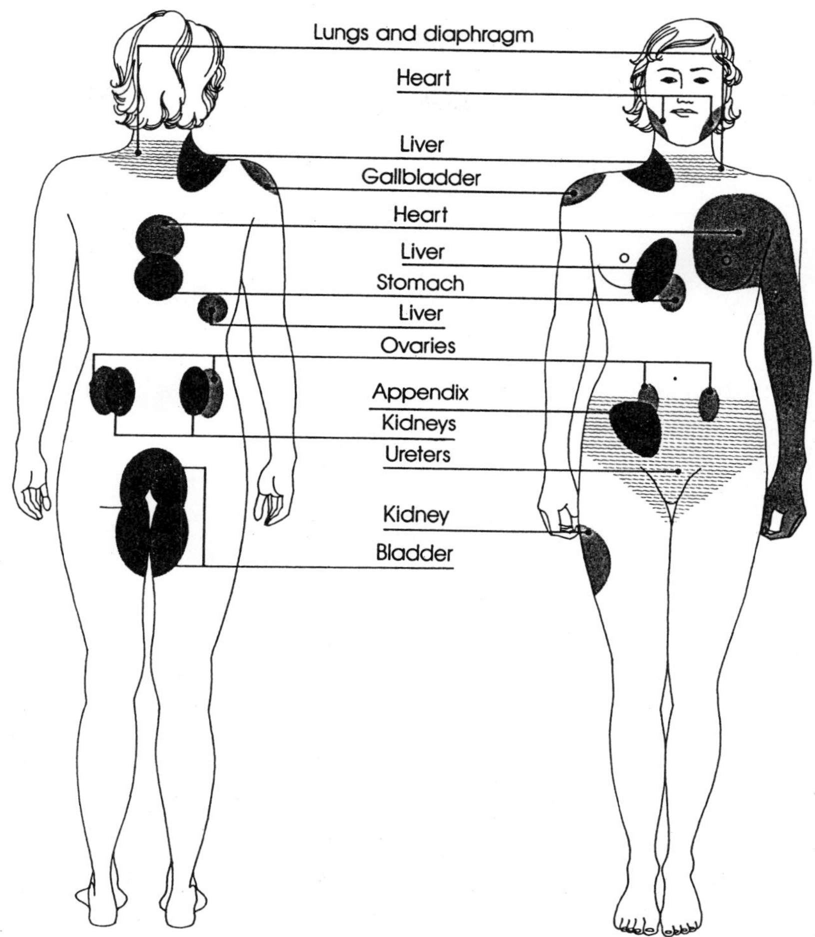

Figure 20–9. Posterior and anterior views showing commonly reported sites where pain is referred from visceral organs. (*Reprinted with permission from Brockrath, M. [1985], [p. 18].* Fundamentals. In Nursing Now. *PA: Springhouse, Springhouse Corp.*)

& Westlund, 1997). The anterolateral quadrant of the spinal white matter contains all but the SDCT, which traverses in the dorsal column pathway (Dickenson, 1995; Willis & Westlund, 1997).

Generally, the STT and SRT are the best understood pathways. The STT segregates into medial and lateral branches near the thalamus with the medial branch terminating in medial thalamus and the lateral branch terminating in lateral thalamus. The lateral branch is known also as the neospinothalamic pathway. The medial branch is known also as the paleospinothalamic pathway or the paramedian pathway. The paleospinothalamic pathway also sends a collateral to the reticular formation and appears functionally similar to the SRT (Willis & Westlund, 1997).

Each of four distinct thalamic nuclei, which receive nociceptive input from the spinal cord, has projections to the cerebral cortex, anterior cingulate cortex, or to the insula. The primary somatosensory cortex has neurons responding selectively to nociceptive input. Recent studies with PET (positron emission tomography) imaging show that the somatosensory cortex is important for interpretation of pain location, pattern, and possibly intensity (Casey, Minoshima, Morrow, & Koeppe, 1996). The frontal cortex receives projections from the central lateral and submedial thalamic nuclei (Sidedall & Cousins, 1997). PET studies show the frontal cortex and especially the anterior cingulate cortex to be involved in affective components of pain. Additionally, the insula has been shown to be involved in the suffering components of pain (Jones, 1997). Recent evidence refutes the common belief that a single brain structure is responsible for pain perception.

Transmission of the action potential in the second-order neuron by way of the anterolateral spinal cord quadrant can be interrupted by anterolateral cordotomy. This procedure can be performed by open surgical or percutaneous techniques, both of which create a spinal cord lesion that transects axons ascending to the brain in the anterolateral quadrant (Sweet, Poletti, & Gybels, 1994). Theoretically the procedure is appealing, but clinical results have been disappointing for many people. Careful preprocedure selec-

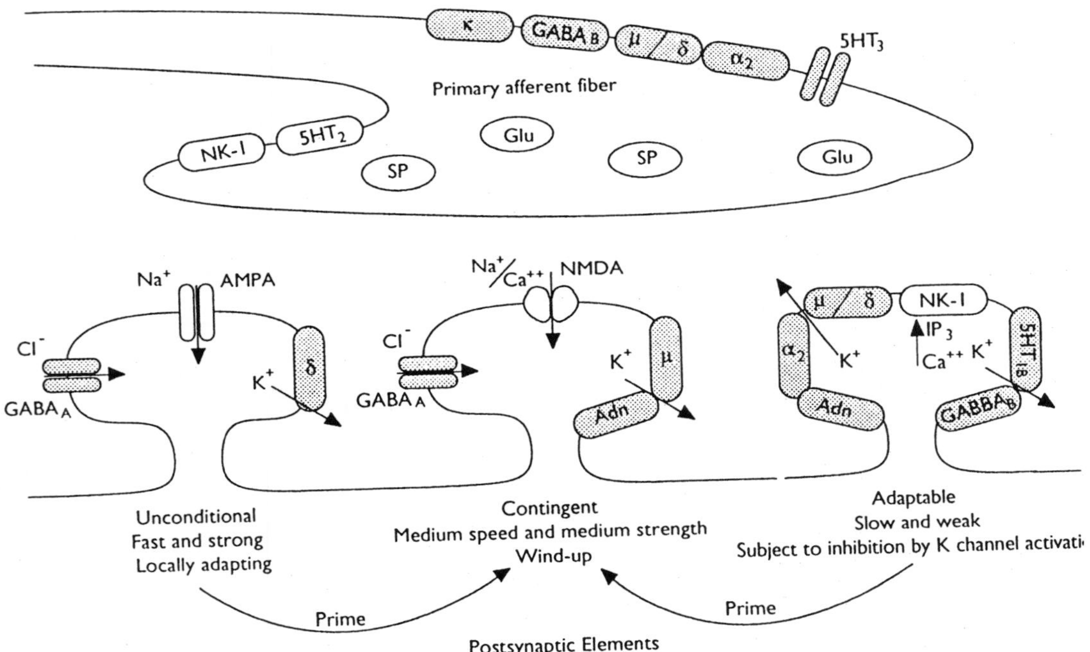

Figure 20–10. A hypothetical spatial arrangement of excitatory *(clear)* and inhibitory *(shaded)* receptors and transmitters in and on pre- and postsynaptic structures in the spinal dorsal horn. Receptors grouped in a substructure have been observed to interact with one another in behavioral, electrophysical or behavioral and electrophysical experiments. *(Reprinted with permission from Wilcox, G.L. [1991]. Excitatory neurotransmitters and pain. In Bond, M.R., Charlton, J.E., Wolf, C.J. (eds.).* Proceedings of the VIth World Congress on Pain *[p 99]. New York: Elsevier.)*

tion improves results. Good pain relief is likely in people with cancer pain characterized by unilateral location below the mandible and with lancinating or toothache qualities rather than burning, pricking, pressure, or crawling qualities (Rosomoff, Papo, & Loeser, 1990). Lack of complete pain relief with cordotomy may be related to sparing of axons in the anterolateral quadrant that overlap into the descending corticospinal tract or creation of a new neuropathic pain. The corticospinal neurons are involved with descending motor input and are crucial to functions such as bowel and bladder control, arm movement, and ambulation. If preservation of these motor functions is important, complete transection of the anterolateral quadrant fibers, which transmit nociceptive information rostrally, generally is not possible.

Pain Perception

In the brain, nociceptive input is perceived as pain. New data suggest that there is no single, precise location where pain perception occurs. Instead pain perception involves several brain structures (Casey et al., 1996; Jones, 1997). It is known that the brain is necessary for pain perception; hence no brain, no pain. Until it is understood clearly where pain is perceived, prudent, advanced nursing practice involves treatment of *any* noxious stimulus as potentially painful, even in the comatose person who does not respond to noxious stimuli. Lack of a behavioral response to a noxious stimulus does *not* indicate that the person lacks pain perception. This notion is extremely important when providing care to the comatose person with massive injuries or the person with cancer who is actively dying. Unless there is some reason for assuming that there has been removal of the nociceptive stimuli, which caused pain when the person was awake, it is crucial that pain therapies be continued, even though the person cannot report pain perception or show behaviors usually considered to be indicative of pain.

Because of the complex neural mechanisms of nociceptive processing, pain is perceived as a multidimensional sensory and emotional experience to which there are cognitive and behavioral responses. Hence the acronym, the ABCs of pain, serves as a means by which the distinctive components easily can be remembered by persons with pain and by health professionals. In particular, the sensory component of pain is paramount in appropriate assessment of pain perception. At minimum, sensory pain elements include **p**attern, **a**rea, **i**ntensity, and **n**ature, which spell the word pain. Persons with pain, when provided with tools, easily report these four sensory pain elements. Sensory pain reports can be indispensable to appropriate diagnosis and treatment when the data are interpreted by an ACNP who is knowledgeable about the pain process. Persons with pain, however, are the most appropriate experts about the effectiveness of therapies prescribed to modulate the pain process and block pain perception.

Modulation

Critical to transmission of nociceptive stimuli and pain perception are the modulatory mechanisms, the final step in the pain process. Evidence has been available for 25 years that nociceptive cells in the spinal dorsal horn are selectively inhibited by brainstem stimulation (Guilbaud, Besson, Oliveras, & Liebeskind, 1973). The dorsolateral funiculus (DLF) also has been shown to be critical to the inhibition of nociceptive responses in animals (Basbaum, Clanton, & Fields, 1976). Today, however, we know that modulation may include both *inhibition* as well as *enhancement* of nociceptive stimuli. Fields & Heinricher (1985) demonstrated that the firing pattern of specific cells in the rostral ventral medulla may be associated with the inhibition of nociception but that other cells may permit transmission of the nociceptive information. The clinical significance of these findings is not clear. It is possible that people with intractable pain experience enhanced modulation of nociceptive stimuli that leads to more intense pain through mechanisms not understood fully.

Fields & Basbaum (1994) proposed a diagram of the structural components of the descending opioid-related pain inhibitory system (Fig. 20–11). Generally, findings indicate that several centers are involved in generating analgesia, three of which have received extensive investigation: the periventricular and periaqueductal grey, the rostral ventral medulla, and the spinal cord. Afferent input to the descending pain modulating system is less well known, but certainly hypothalamic and amygdala inputs are involved and possibly the frontal granular and insular cortex (Sidedall & Cousins, 1997).

Descending inhibition of pain occurs through a complex circuit involving a number of receptor systems, such as mu, delta, and kappa opioid; alpha$_2$ adrenergic; serotonin (5HT); adenosine; GABA; neuropeptide Y; calcitonin; somatostatin; and neurotensin receptors (Sidedall & Cousins, 1997; Yaksh, 1991). Although 5HT, alpha$_2$ agonists, and opioids are known to inhibit nociceptive cells in the spinal dorsal horn, the role of the neurochemicals has not been fully delineated in each of the areas of the CNS that are believed to be involved in pain modulation.

Figure 20–12 provides a graphical summary of the descending inhibitory mechanisms at the level of the spinal cord dorsal horn. Once nociceptive information is perceived as pain, inhibition can occur at any of the synapses in the ascending pathways. A well-studied and important inhibitory synapse is in the spinal dorsal horn. For example, serotonin, norepinephrine, and enkephalin are released by descending fibers and inhibit release of neurotransmitters, such as substance P and CGRP, and thereby diminish excitation of projection cells. The inhibitory neurotransmitters successfully prevent the PAN from communicating its information about the nociceptive stimuli to the second-order neuron and pain is blocked even though the PAN has been activated and has transmitted an action potential to the spinal cord. If the PAN action potential does not result in release of sufficient neurotransmitters to communicate the signal to the projection cell, pain is blocked.

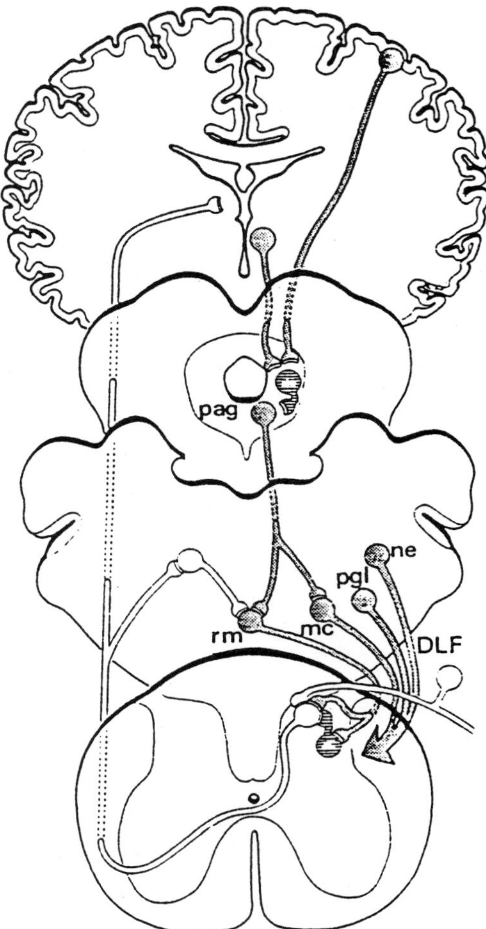

Figure 20–11. Pain-modulation network as proposed by Fields and Basbaum. The network extends from the frontal cortex and hypothalamus through the periaqueductal grey (PGA) to the rostral ventral medulla and then to the spinal dorsal horn. rm = nucleus rahe magnus; mc = reticularis magnocellularis; pgl = paragigantocellularis; ne = noradrenergic pontomedullary cell groups; DLF = dorsolateral funiculus. *(Reprinted with permission from Fields, H.L. & Basbaum, A.I. [1989]. Endogenous pain control mechanisms. In Wall, P.D., Melzack, R. (eds.).* Textbook of Pain (2nd ed.). *New York: Churchill Livingstone, [p 208].)*

Many drug and behavioral therapies provide pain relief through actions involving the descending pain inhibition mechanisms. Opioids, tricyclic antidepressants, alpha$_2$ agonists, placebos, counterirritation, hypnosis, imagery, and distraction act via mechanisms to mimic or enhance descending inhibitory systems (Table 20–1). When these therapies are combined with methods that influence the process of PAN transduction and transmission, impressive analgesia can be obtained (Fig. 20–13).

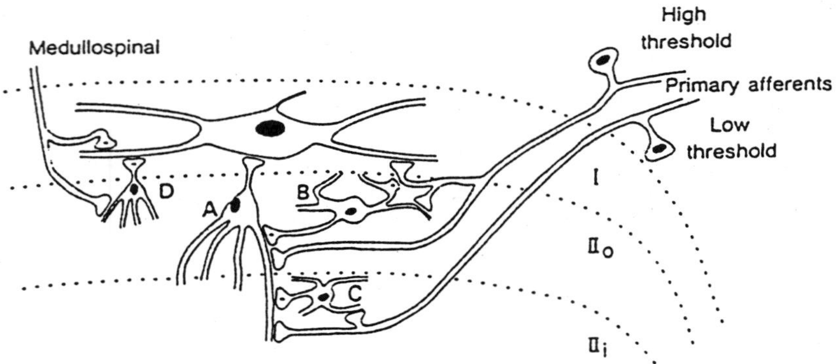

Figure 20–12. Dorsal horn schematic illustration of local circuitry. High-threshold afferents (A-delta and C fibers) excite the nociceptive projection neurons in lamina I. The same afferents excite dendrites of excitatory interneurons (A) and inhibitory interneurons (B) in lamina II_0. The excitatory interneuron provides further excitatory drive to lamina I projection cell whereas the inhibitory interneuron (B) provides a circuit that generates an inhibitory, feed-forward control of the lamina I projection cell by nociceptive inputs. Low-threshold primary afferent fibers provide a non-nociceptive input to lamina I projection cells via their excitatory connections with dendrites of excitatory cells (A) in lamina II_i. In contrast, the non-nociceptive input to inhibitory interneurons in lamina II_i (C) may contribute to the inhibitory control of nociceptive lamina I projection cells. The schema also illustrates some possible descending control mechanisms. These may be exerted directly on dorsal horn lamina I-projection neurons. Alternatively, descending axons (some of which contain serotonin) may excite inhibitory interneurons (e.g., enkephalin-containing (D) cells, which in turn postsynaptically control the nociceptive lamina I-projection neurons. Another possibility not illustrated is that the descending systems inhibit the excitatory cell (A). *(Reprinted with permission from Fields, H.L. & Basbaum, A.I. [1994]. [p.248].)*

Opioids mimic the descending inhibitory system by binding to endogenous endorphin receptors (mu, delta, kappa) in the brain, spinal cord, and peripheral tissues. Opioids act by hyperpolarizing the cell membrane and thereby inhibiting generation of an action potential (Sidedall & Cousins, 1997; Yaksh, 1991). Opioids effectively inhibit A-delta and C fibers, but are less effective in the wind-up state described previously. Administered in small volumes by the intrathecal route, opioids exert powerful analgesic action at spinal cord synapses with limited rostral spread. In contrast, opioids delivered by the epidural route exert action not only at spinal cord sites, but also brain and peripheral sites because a substantial portion of the dose is absorbed by epidural blood vessels and provides access to systemic circulation. Opioids administered systemically (oral, transmucosal, transdermal, rectal, vaginal, subcutaneous, intramuscular, or intravenous) cross the blood–brain barrier, enter the cerebrospinal fluid, and bind to opioid receptors throughout the brain and spinal cord. Discovery of opioid receptors on the PAN suggests that systemically administered opioids may exert analagesic action at peripheral sites in inflamed tissue as well as at central nervous system sites (Herz, 1996). Interdermal injection of opioids at the tissue injury site has shown impressive analgesia (Sidedall & Cousins, 1997). Analgesic effects, side effects, and doses required to produce analgesia all differ based on route of administration, in part because access to opioid-receptors varies by administration route.

In comparison to opioids, tricyclic antidepressant drugs enhance the descending pain inhibitory system by preventing cellular re-uptake of serotonin and norepinephrine (Fig. 20–14). These transmitters typically are released from the cell and rapidly transported back into the cell. Rapid re-uptake limits the time serotonin and norepinephrine are available for receptor binding and thereby to inhibit transmission of nociceptive signals. Tricyclic antidepressants, which have moderate serotonin effects and weak to potent norepinephrine effects (Max et al., 1992; McQuay, Carroll, Jadad, Wiffen, & Moore, 1995), are effective adjuvant analgesics in some neuropathic pain conditions.

$Alpha_2$ agonists (e.g., clonidine), calcitonin, somatostatin, and baclofen are other agents known to provide analgesia. Exact location of action for these agents is known for some but not others. Clonidine, for example, acts pre- and postsynaptically at $alpha_2$ receptors in the dorsal horn to hyperpolarize cell membranes and thereby to inhibit generation of the action potential (Yaksh, 1991). Baclofen also acts pre- and postsynaptically, but does so at GABA-B receptors. It is less clear where calcitonin and somatostatin act. Gabapentin interacts with an $alpha_2$ delta subunit of a voltage-dependent Ca_2+ channel (Gee et al., 1996). These agents also are known as adjuvant analgesics and are especially effective in neuropathic pain states.

The exact mechanisms by which the behavioral therapies exert analgesia are not known. It clearly has been demonstrated, however, that placebo response is mediated by endogenous opioid systems. Placebo response can be reversed by naloxone (Narcan), indicating that its mechanism involves enkephalin systems (Levine, Gordon, & Fields, 1978). It is possible that other behavioral therapies, such as

TABLE 20–1. Neural Mechanisms of Pain: Facilitating and Inhibiting Factors

Anatomical Structure	Neurotransmittors, Neurochemicals or Receptors	Modulatory Effect on Transduction or Transmission (Facilitates [F] Inhibits [I])	Therapy *Enhancing* Effect (Relieves Pain Sensation)	Therapy *Inhibiting* Effect (Relieves Pain Sensation)
Peripheral Nervous System		**Transduction**		
PAN Terminal				Corticosteroids,
	Leukotriene	F, sensitizes		ketoprophen
	Prostaglandins	F, sensitizes		ASA, NSAIDs
	Potassium	F, activates		n/a
	Histamine	F, activates		Antihistamines
	Bradykinin	F, activates		n/a
	Serotonin	F, activates		n/a
	Substance P	F, sensitizes		Capsaisin
	Endorphin	I	opioids	
Fiber	Na+, K+ exchange across the cellular membrane	F, **Transmission** of action potential to CNS		Mexiletine, tocainide, EMLA
Autonomic Nervous System	Norepinephrine	**Transduction** F, sensitizes nociceptive state F, activates neuropathic state		Anxiolytics, relaxation
Spinal Cord	Substance P, glutamate, and others	F, **Transmission** to projection cell (2nd order neuron)		Opioids
	NMDA	F, **Transmission** with wind-up		Ketamine Dextromethorphan
	serotonin ($5HT_{1B}$	I	TCAs	
	and $5HT_3$	I	TCAs	
	norepinephrine	I	TCAs, clonidine	
	mu	I	opioid agonists (e.g., morphine)	
	delta	I	opioid agonists	
	kappa	I	opioid antagonist-agonists	
	$GABA_A$	I	baclophen	
	$GABA_B$	I	benzodiazapines	
Brain	Substance P, glutamate, and others	F, **Transmission** to 3rd or 4th order neuron		Opioids

PAN =primary afferent nociceptor; ASA = aspirin; NSAIDs = nonsteroidal antiinflammatory drugs; n/a = not available or not applicable; Na+ = sodium; K+ = potassium; CNS = central nervous system; TCAs = tricyclic antidepressant drugs or other re-uptake inhibitor drugs.

counter-irritation or descending noxious inhibitory control (DNIC) (LeBar, Dickenson, & Besson, 1979), hypnosis, imagery, and distraction also act via endogenous opioid or possibly nonopioid inhibitory systems throughout the neural axis (e.g., brain and spinal cord).

Many of the inhibitory mechanisms that block pain transmission were initially proposed in general by Melzack & Wall (1965) in their gate control theory of pain. Today some of the details by which inhibition occurs are known and progress is being made to understand those not known. The message important for ACNP practice is that multiple methods can be used simultaneously to prevent transduction or transmission of nociceptive stimuli and therefore to block the perception of pain (refer to Table 20–1). Differentiating nociceptive from neuropathic pain processes is important to therapy decisions. Used together, several pharmacologic and behavioral therapies—each of which block pain perception via different mechanisms—can dramatically improve pain relief.

▶ CLINICAL IDENTIFICATION OF PAIN

Before the recent evidence supporting the notion of neural plasticity, pain was often viewed as a secondary symptom of disease or injury. Acute, chronic, and malignant types of pain were distinguished based on differences in clinical presentations and therapy options available to cure the cause of the pain. Pain related to an acute injury was expected to subside when the tissue damage healed. Relief of

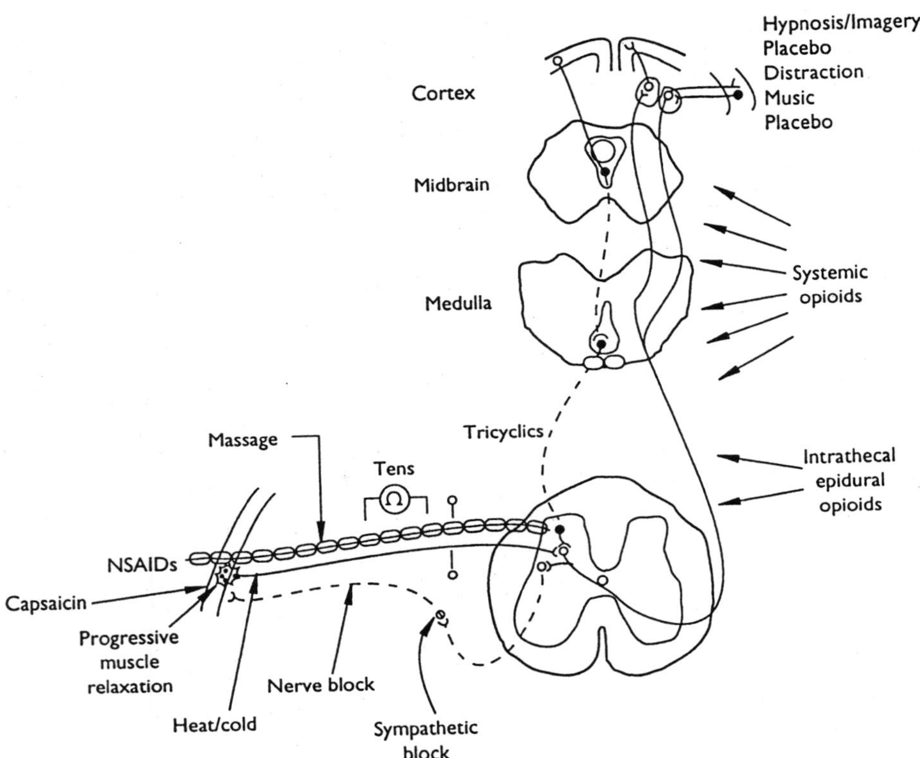

Figure 20–13. Putting the pain process together. A schematic showing sites of action of commonly used pharmacologic and behavioral analgesic therapies. *(Reprinted with permission from Fields, H.L. & Levine, J.D. [1994]. [p. 350].)*

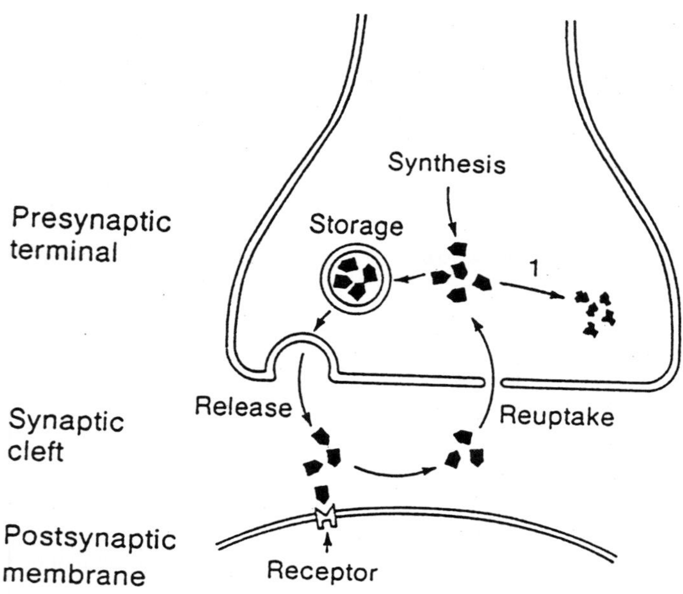

Figure 20–14. Example of mechanism by which tricyclic antidepressant drugs promote analgesia by inhibiting re-uptake of serotonin and norepinephrine. *(Reprinted with permission from Fields, H.L. [1987], [p. 295].)*

acute pain was expected through the curative treatment of the underlying injury or disease. Pain related to chronic disease, which could not be cured, was often considered to be unfortunate but benign and related to psychological rather than physiological processes. Relief of chronic pain was not expected but some comfort was expected to be achieved through use of nonopioid drugs and cognitive behavioral therapies. Opioid and other drugs were expected to provide some relief for people dying of cancer.

Recent findings about the pathophysiological consequences of unrelieved pain (Table 20–2) (Cousins, 1994; Page & Ben Eliyahu, 1997) and increased knowledge of the pain process indicate that health professionals should aggressively treat all pain to prevent a facilitated, neuropathic pain state. Aggressive treatment of pain is provided by either preemptive or palliative analgesia, both of which offer new ideas for advanced nursing practice. The Pain Relief Algorithm is a new model for the ACNP to conceptualize pain (Fig. 20–15). The Pain Relief Algorithm equips the ACNP with an approach for making clinical decisions about pain management.

Pain Relief Algorithm

When a patient presents with a chief complaint that includes pain, the ACNP makes a series of decisions based on subjective and objective data obtained through procedures including interview (history), physical examination, and laboratory and diagnostic tests. As shown by the Pain Relief Algorithm in Figure 20–15, the ACNP's first decision is to diagnose the etiology of the pain; that is, determine the cause of the pain. The second decision is to classify the pain etiology as involving nociceptive or neuropathic pain mechanisms. The third decision is to determine if the cause of the pain can or cannot be eliminated (cured or treated). These decisions are necessary to determine if the treatment is to be directed toward a curative care goal or a palliative care goal. The Pain Relief Algorithm also guides subsequent decisions about the general treatment plan aimed at either goal.

The plan usually should include palliative treatment of the pain sensation and concurrent treatments that either cure the cause of the pain or palliate the disease and other symptoms. The Pain Relief Algorithm helps the ACNP to recognize that different therapies are implemented for palliation of nociceptive and neuropathic types of pain and that these pain-relief therapies also are different from those used to treat the injury or disease from which the pain originated. Research findings from many disciplines guide the data collection and decision-making within the framework of this algorithm. The remaining sections of this chapter summarize current knowledge about assessment and palliative management of nociceptive and neuropathic types of pain. It is beyond the scope of this chapter to describe diagnosis and treatment of the conditions from which all pain originates, but this information is available in several textbooks focused entirely on pain (Bonica, 1990; Fields, 1987; Kanner, 1997; Merskey & Bogduk, 1994; Omoigui, 1995; Patt, 1993; Puntillo, 1991; Raj, 1992; Ramamurthy & Rodgers, 1993; Sevarino & Preble, 1992; Turk & Melzack, 1992; Wall & Melzack, 1994; Warfield, 1991, 1993). Bonica's (1990) two-volume book provides details learned from 50 years of experience and research and is particularly useful to the advanced practice clinician. Wall & Melzack's (1994) book is an excellent resource for the pain researcher and clinician.

TABLE 20–2. Pathophysiologic Consequences of Unrelieved Acute Pain: Pain Can Kill

Body System	Pathophysiologic Responses to Unrelieved Acute Pain	Complications
Respiratory[a]	Reflex muscle spasms and muscle splinting leads to decreased: tidal volume, vital capacity, functional residual capacity, and alveolar ventilation	Atelectasis and impaired oxygen and carbon dioxide exchange lead to hypoxemia and pneumonia
Cardiovascular[a]	Sympathetic overactivity leads to increased: heart rate, peripheral resistence, blood pressure, and cardiac output; decreased diastolic filling time; and coronary vasoconstriction	Increased cardiac work and myocardial oxygen use, and decreased oxygen delivery to myocardium lead to increased risk of hypoxemia, myocardial ischemia, angina, and myocardial infarcation
Gastrointestinal[a]	Increase sympathetic activity leads to increased intestinal secretions and smooth muscle sphincter tone and to decreased intestinal motility	Gastric stasis, paralytic illeus
Immune[b]	Decreased natural killer cell numbers and function	Host resistence decreased especially to cancer metastasis (early deaths have been noted in animal studies)
Neurological[c]	Primary and secondary hyperalgesia with changes in primary afferent nociceptor responses at peripheral terminal and changes in the communication patterns of central nervous system cells	Neuropathic pain can occur and may persist for long periods of time after healing has occured
Musculoskeletal[a]	Muscle spasms increase pain leading to increased sympathetic activity which increases sensitivity of nociceptors	Impaired muscle metabolism and muscle atrophy

Sources: [a] *Cousins, M. (1994);* [b] *Page, G.G. & Eliyahu, B. (1997);* [c] *Willis, W.D. & Westlund, K.N. (1997).*
Reprinted with permission. Copyright © 1998 Wilkie, D.J.

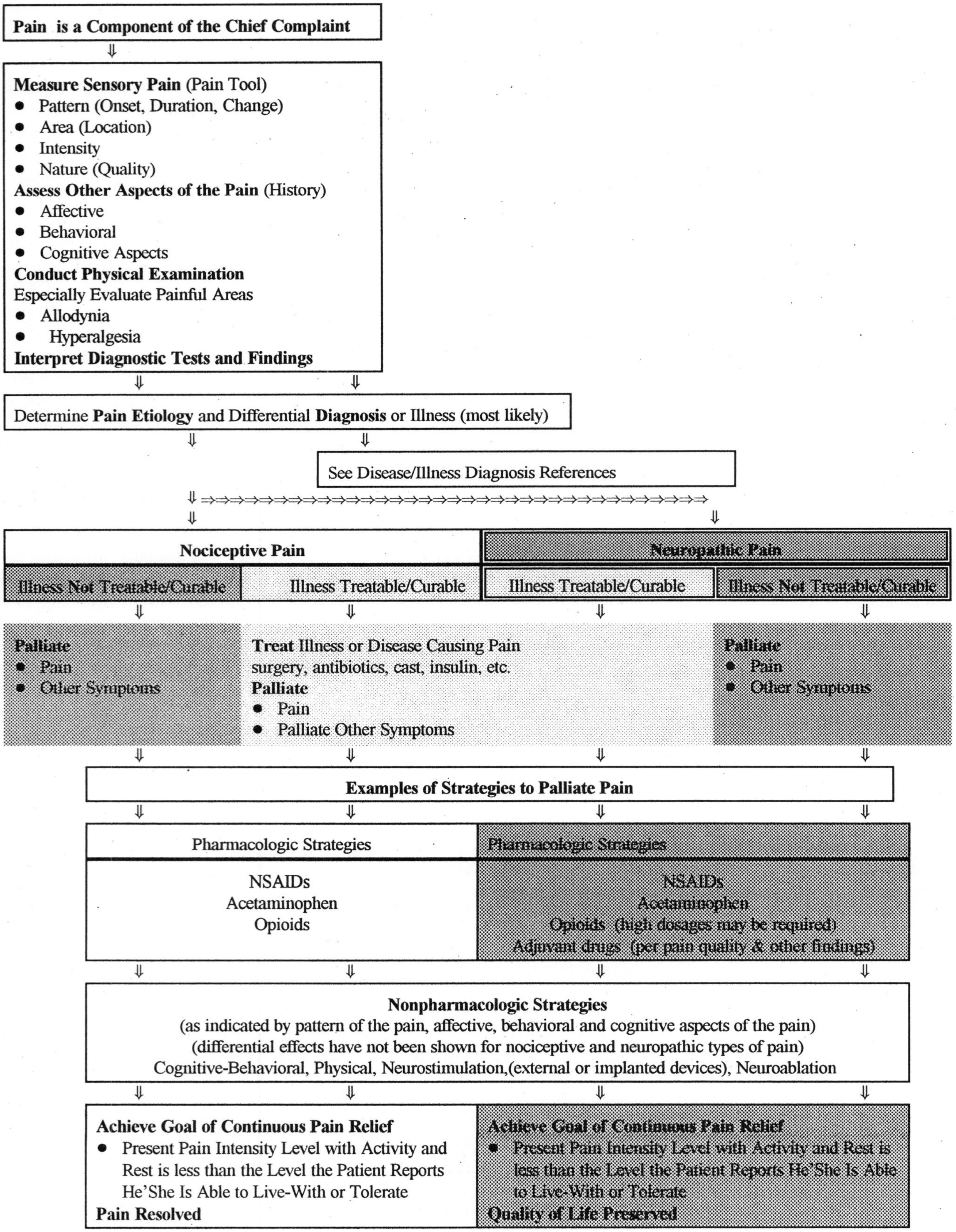

Pain is a Component of the Chief Complaint

⇓

Measure Sensory Pain (Pain Tool)
- Pattern (Onset, Duration, Change)
- Area (Location)
- Intensity
- Nature (Quality)

Assess Other Aspects of the Pain (History)
- Affective
- Behavioral
- Cognitive Aspects

Conduct Physical Examination
Especially Evaluate Painful Areas
- Allodynia
- Hyperalgesia

Interpret Diagnostic Tests and Findings

⇓ ⇓

Determine **Pain Etiology** and Differential **Diagnosis** or Illness (most likely)

⇓ ⇓

See Disease/Illness Diagnosis References

⇓ ⇒⇒⇒⇒⇒⇒⇒⇒⇒⇒⇒⇒⇒⇒⇒⇒⇒⇒⇒⇒⇒⇒⇒⇒⇒⇒⇒⇒⇒⇒⇒⇒⇒

⇓ ⇓

Nociceptive Pain		**Neuropathic Pain**	
Illness Not Treatable/Curable	Illness Treatable/Curable	Illness Treatable/Curable	Illness Not Treatable/Curable
Palliate • Pain • Other Symptoms	**Treat** Illness or Disease Causing Pain surgery, antibiotics, cast, insulin, etc. **Palliate** • Pain • Palliate Other Symptoms		**Palliate** • Pain • Other Symptoms

⇓ ⇓ ⇓ ⇓

Examples of Strategies to Palliate Pain

⇓ ⇓ ⇓ ⇓

Pharmacologic Strategies	Pharmacologic Strategies
NSAIDs Acetaminophen Opioids	NSAIDs Acetaminophen Opioids (high dosages may be required) Adjuvant drugs (per pain quality & other findings)

⇓ ⇓ ⇓ ⇓

Nonpharmacologic Strategies
(as indicated by pattern of the pain, affective, behavioral and cognitive aspects of the pain)
(differential effects have not been shown for nociceptive and neuropathic types of pain)
Cognitive-Behavioral, Physical, Neurostimulation,(external or implanted devices), Neuroablation

⇓ ⇓ ⇓ ⇓

Nociceptive	Neuropathic
Achieve Goal of Continuous Pain Relief • Present Pain Intensity Level with Activity and Rest is less than the Level the Patient Reports He'She Is Able to Live-With or Tolerate **Pain Resolved**	**Achieve Goal of Continuous Pain Relief** • Present Pain Intensity Level with Activity and Rest is less than the Level the Patient Reports He'She Is Able to Live-With or Tolerate **Quality of Life Preserved**

Figure 20–15. Pain relief algorithm. A guide for pain management by the acute care nurse practitioner. *(Reprinted with permission. Copyright © 1998, Wilkie, D.J.)*

Pain Assessment

The ACNP conducts a thorough symptom analysis of the patient's pain by measuring its location, intensity, nature, and temporal pattern, including its onset, duration, and aggravating and alleviating factors, well known as the sacred seven aspects of a symptom. Also the ACNP examines the patient to clarify and provide additional data about the pain problem. The purposes of these assessment procedures are to identify the etiology of the pain in order to make a diagnosis and to understand the patient's sensory, affective, behavioral, and cognitive pain experience in order to implement and evaluate a pain-management plan. Table 20–3 lists examples of data from the symptom analysis that are important in leading the ACNP to diagnose pain as nociceptive, neuropathic, or both.

If tricorder technology were available today, pain assessment would be as simple as reading a number on a screen. The screams of the Civil War soldier during an amputation were an indication that he was in pain, but pain is not always that obvious. Today, the only way an ACNP can accurately assess pain is to ask the person about it. Findings from tests and examination of the painful area may be diagnostic, but not always. Pain is subjective, owned and communicated by the patient. Asking about pain in a systematic, standardized format is the single most important step to diagnosis and treatment (APS Quality of Care Committee, 1995).

A common belief, however, is that pain can be assessed but it cannot be measured. Assessment is the act of determining the importance, size, or value of something. In contrast, measurement is the act or process of applying a

TABLE 20–3. Sensory Characteristics of Selected Nociceptive or Neuropathic Types of Pain

Etiology or Diagnosis	Location	Intensity	Quality	Pattern: (Onset, Duration, and Changes with Time, Activity, Emotions)	Typical Type of Pain
HEAD					
Trigeminal neuralgia (tic douloureux)	Anterior face, unilateral, **distributed along one or more branches of trigeminal nerve:** maxillary, mandibular, or ophthalmic	Extremely intense	**Electrical shocklike, shooting, stabbing**	Intermittent episodes of sudden onset but brief duration pain, pain-free between episodes; increased by nonnoxious stimulation of facial trigger areas, eating, chewing; decreased by minimizing facial stimulation	Neuropathic
Migraine (common) without aura	Unilateral, whole hemicranium (75%) **localized,** starting in frontal areas	Mild to severe	**Pressing, pulsating, throbbing**	1–4 times/month, builds to plateau lasting 4–10 hours, up to 24–48 hours; increased by minimal physical activity, stress, anxiety, depression, conflict, light and noise; reduced by rest, quiet environment, reduced anxiety and stress	Nociceptive (probable)
CHEST					
Acute Myicardial Infarctionl (AMI)	Anterior chest mostly retrosternally, referred to parasternal region, left arm or right arm or both, epigastrium and sometimes lower jaw, neck, and interscapular region	Severe to excruciating	**Dull, heavy, crushing, pressure,** sense of impending death	Sudden onset, lasts 1 to 8 hours; increased by life style factors: smoking, large meal; decreased by oxygen, morphine	Nociceptive
Angina	Anterior chest, referred to medial aspects of left arm, neck, jaw, back, epigastrium	Mild to severe	**Dull, crushing** or **constricting, heavy**	Intermittent, lasts few minutes to hours; increased by stress (physical activity, emotional), large meal; decreased by rest nitroglycerin, rest	Nociceptive
Pulmonary embolism	General thoracic area; **localized in one area**	Severe	Crushing, like AMI pain	Sudden onset, lasts few minutes to hours; increased by deep breathing, coughing	Nociceptive
Herpes Zoster	**Distribution of intercostal nerves, spinal nerve roots**	Severe	**Aching, itching, burning,** bouts of **lancinating** pain	Onset 1–2 days before herpetic vesicles appear, continuous, increased by trunk motion or palpation of vesicles; decreased when rask heals in 1–4 weeks unless it becomes postherpetic neuralgia	Neuropathic

(Continued)

TABLE 20–3. Sensory Characteristics of Selected Nociceptive or Neuropathic Types of Pain *(Continued)*

Etiology or Diagnosis	Location	Intensity	Quality	Pattern: (Onset, Duration, and Changes with Time, Activity, Emotions)	Typical Type of Pain
Postherpetic neuralgia	**Distributin of intercostal nerves, spinal nerve roots**	Moderate to severe	Unrelenting **burning, itching, tearing, stabbing, lancinating**	Continuous and intermittent, persists months to years after rash heals; increased by trunk motion, mechanical contact to affected skin	Neuropathic
ABDOMEN					
Duodenal ulcer	Epigastric area, referred to back, upper right quadrant	Mild to moderate	**Gnawing,** burning, **aching**	Gradual onset, intermittent during day, none in morning, becomes more frequent and lasts longer until **continuous** without pain-free periods; increased 1 to 2 hours after meals; decreased by eating or antacids	Nociceptive
Dysmenorrhea, primary	**Localized** in mid, lower abdomen, referred to lower back, and rarely upper thighs	Moderate to severe	**Cramping**	Cyclic, onset before menses, lasts several days; increased as flow begins	Nociceptive
Dysmenorrhea, secondary	Midline, **localized** deep in pelvis, frequently referred to low back and rectum, and rarely upper thighs	Mild to moderate, can be severe	**Tender**	Constant, lasts longer than menses; increased by intercourse, urination, defecation	Nociceptive
LOW BACK					
Lumbosacral strain or sprain	**Localized** lumbarsacral joint area	Moderate to severe	**Tender, dull, aching**	Sudden onset after injury; increased by motion; decreased by local injection of lumbosacral joint	Nociceptive
Sciatica neuralgia	**Projected** to posterior thigh, calf, and outer and planter side of foot	Moderate to severe	**Burning** or sharp **lancinating**	Continuous; increased by flexion of the thigh with knee extended	Neuropathic

Characteristics listed in bold typically are considered diagnostic for nociceptive or neuropathic types of pain.
Sources: Bonica, J.J. (1990); Merskey H. & Bogduk, N. (1994).
Reprinted with permission. Copyright © 1998 Wilkie, D.J.

metric to gauge something. Health professionals, however, consider other subjective phenomena to be measurable. For example, vision is a subjective phenomenon, yet a metric can be applied to determine visual acuity (e.g., Snellen Eye Chart) and ability to see color. Pain can be measured in a similar way by including valid and reliable metrics (tools or scales) of the pain experience as part of the symptom analysis process.

Many tools are available to measure the sensory components of pain (pattern, area, intensity, and nature). Fewer tools are available to measure the affective, behavioral, and cognitive pain components in clinical practice. Therefore, the ACNP can *measure* pain pattern, area, intensity, and nature with the following tools and *assess* affective, behavioral, and cognitive pain components as the patient's history is obtained, at least until valid and reliable measures also become available for these components.

Pattern

Pain pattern is measured by the use of words such as those listed in Table 20–4 to describe how the pain *changes with time, activity,* or *other factors.* The patient is also asked the date or time that the pain started and how long the pain lasts to measure the onset and duration of a painful episode. Pain-pattern data are crucial for diagnosis of some diseases or illnesses and for appropriate scheduling of analgesic therapies.

Area

The ACNP can determine pain location by asking the patient to mark all painful areas on a drawing of the body,

TABLE 20–4. Pain Pattern Descriptors from the McGill Pain Questionnaire

How does your pain change with time? Circle the words you would use to describe the pattern of your pain.

1	2	3
Continuous	Rhythmic	Brief
Steady	Periodic	Momentary
Constant	Intermittent	Transient

Melzack, R. (1975).

called a body outline (Fig. 20–16). Another method is to ask the patient to point to the places where pain is felt, and the ACNP can document those places on either a body outline or descriptively in the medical record. Of these two methods, the body outline provides data that is more specific and, therefore, more diagnostic than the pointing method. Often patients are not able to reach the specific area where they hurt. Their verbal reports are more general when they point than when they use the body outline to show where their pain is located. The body outline drawings allow the ACNP to identify each pain site as either localized, referred, or projected areas of pain, an inference that is crucial to diagnosing the pain as nociceptive or neuropathic. Monitoring the pain sites on a body outline also is useful to identify new pain sites that may signal complications.

The distribution of nociceptive pain typically is localized to the area in which the pathologic process occurs, for example, near the incision, arthritic joint, or site of cancer. Also, pain referred from the site of pathology to a distant area (refer to Fig. 20–9) usually is a type of nociceptive pain. Marks on the body outline and physical findings often help the ACNP to determine that the pain is localized or referred and hence most likely to be nociceptive pain.

The distribution of neuropathic pain, however, is projected along a single nerve, within a spinal dermatome (refer to Fig. 20–6), or spread diffusely over the whole body or one side of it. When patients have neuropathic types of pain, especially related to nerve damage, the marks on the body outline and other sensory findings usually reflect the anatomy of the peripheral or central nervous system (Fig. 20–17).

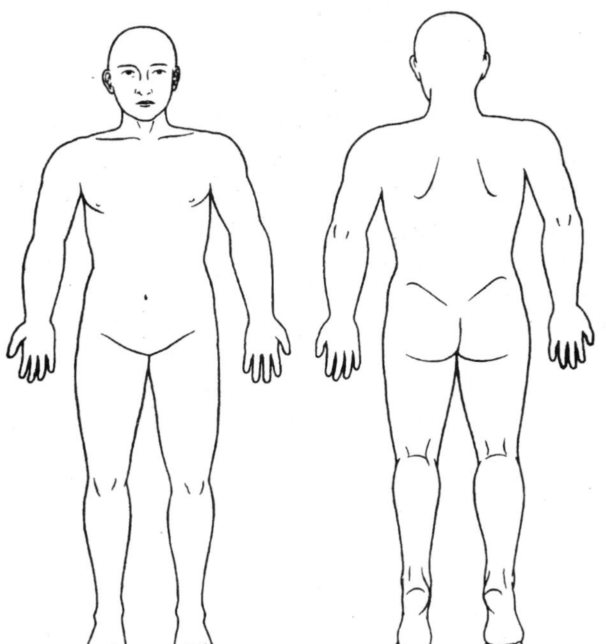

Figure 20–16. Body outline drawing for patients to locate painful areas. *(Reprinted with permission. Copyright © 1989, Wilkie, D.J. & Puntillo, K.A.)*

Intensity

Pain intensity can be measured using the numbers 0 through 10 as a scale to report the pain magnitude. A patient may not intuitively know how to use numbers to measure pain. The script shown in Table 20–5 has been useful in helping children as young as 8 years (Tesler, Savedra, et al., 1991) and elderly patients (Wilkie, Keefe, et al., 1992) to use the 0–10 scale.

Although pain intensity levels do not distinguish between nociceptive and neuropathic types of pain, published practice guidelines (APS, 1998; U.S. Department of Health and Human Services, 1992, 1994; WHO, 1996) recommend that different analgesic drugs be used for pain that is mild (1–3), moderate (4–6), or severe (7–10) in intensity based on previous research findings (Cleeland et al., 1996). Therefore, the pain intensity number can be used to plan and evaluate pain interventions. The 0–10 scale also can be used to help a patient identify goals for pain therapy, for example, the amount of pain desired (usually no pain) and the amount that is acceptable (often a higher number than what is desired) (Berry, Wilke, Huang, & Thomas, submitted 1998). The intensity level reported by the patient for his or her present pain intensity can be compared with the desired and acceptable levels and used to guide additional pain therapies. The present pain intensity level is important data to help the ACNP titrate pain medications to the desired analgesic effect and to monitor the effects of various pain treatments.

Some patients are unable to use the 0–10 scale, but they can use verbal descriptors of pain intensity, such as the Present Pain Intensity (PPI) scale from the McGill Pain Questionnaire (Melzack, 1975). Although these words are commonly used by patients to describe the magnitude of their pain, research indicates that these words mean different levels of pain to individual patients. The most common levels are displayed in Table 20–6 (Mykelbust, Wilkie,

TABLE 20–5. Standardized Instructions for Using the Pain Intensity Number Scale

"I need to know how much pain you have. Because I can't feel your pain, I want you to use a scale to let me know how much pain you have right now. The numbers between 0 and 10 represent *all* the pain a person could have. Zero means no pain and 10 means pain as bad at it could be. You can use any number between 0 and 10 to let me know how much pain you have right now. Call your pain a number between 0 and 10 so I will know the intensity of the pain you feel now."

Note: Use the phrase "call your pain" rather than "rate your pain" because patients have difficulty knowing what is expected of them when asked to rate their pain. They easily "call" their pain a number.

Reprinted with permission. Copyright © 1990, Wilkie, D.J.

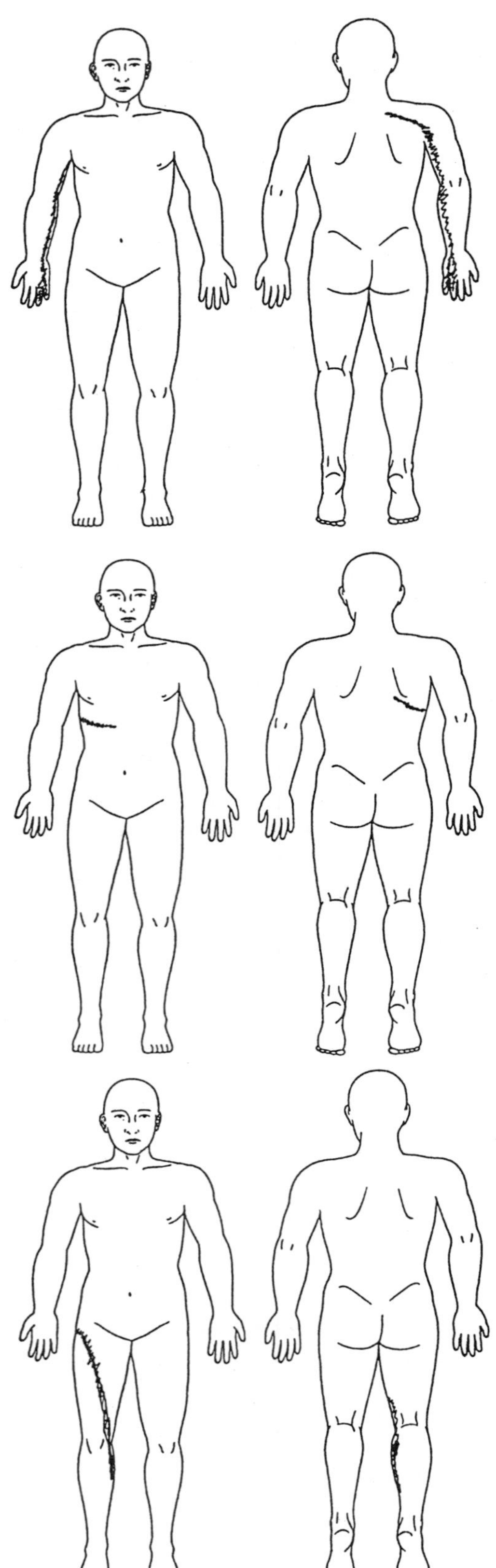

Figure 20–17. Examples of projected pain as drawn by patients with lung cancer pain. *(Reprinted with permission. Copyright © 1998, Wilkie, D.J.)*

Cain, Huang, & Fortner, submitted 1998). The ACNP may use these research-derived values to clarify the ambiguous language of pain intensity and to better understand the pain level the patient is feeling when a particular word is used to describe the pain intensity, and to prescribe the drug appropriate for that level of pain.

Nature

Pain quality is measured using a verbal descriptor list, such as the words listed in Table 20–7. These words are derived from the McGill Pain Questionnaire (Melzack, 1975). The ACNP reads the list, one word per second, and asks the patient to indicate when he hears a word that describes the nature of his pain. This procedure usually takes less than 3 minutes. If the patient is able, he can be asked to read the list and circle the words himself. If the patient has pain in more than one site, often several words per group are selected, and the patient indicates that some words describe one pain site and the other words describe another pain site. The U.S. Department of Health and Human Services (1994) reported that people with neuropathic pain typically select the following words to describe their pain: aching, flashing, burning, electric shock, shooting, stabbing, radiating, tingling, pricking, itching, cold, tight, constricting, and numb; people with nociceptive pain typically select other words to describe their pain: throbbing, pulling, gnawing, heavy, and tender. Since recommended treatments differ for nociceptive and neuropathic types of pain, it is crucial for the ACNP to collect pain-quality data in a systematic format.

The ACNP interprets the selected words to understand the patient's pain in terms of its sensory quality (groups 1–10), affective quality (groups 11–15), evaluative quality (group 16), and miscellaneous quality (groups 17–20). The words that discriminate between nociceptive and neuropathic types of pain are sensory and miscellaneous words, not affective and evaluative words. Affective words help the ACNP to document the level of the patient's distress. Evaluative words help the ACNP to document the patient's coping reserves. The 78 pain quality words provide a system-

TABLE 20–6. McGill Pain Questionnaire Present Pain Intensity Descriptors and Their Research-Based Values

Intensity Verbal Descriptor	Median Value Assigned to Word by 246 Hospitalized Subjects (0–10 Scale)	Range of Values for 80% of 246 Subjects
No Pain	0	0–0.2
Mild	1.4	0.3–3.3
Discomforting	2.8	0.5–6.2
Distressing	5.5	2.2–8.8
Horrible	9.3	6.8–10.0
Excruciating	9.8	8.3–10.0

Present Pain Intensity Words from Melzack, R. (1975).
Values from Myklebust, E.K. et al. (1998).

TABLE 20–7. McGill Pain Questionnaire Pain Quality Descriptors

What Does Your Pain Feel Like?

Some of the words below describe your *present* pain. Circle *ONLY* those words that best describe it. Leave out any category that is not suitable. Use only a single word on each appropriate category—the one that applies best.

1	2	3	4
Flickering Quivering Pulsing Throbbing Beating Pounding	Jumping Flashing Shooting	Pricking Boring Drilling Stabbing Lancinating	Sharp Cutting Lacerating
5	**6**	**7**	**8**
Pinching Pressing Gnawing Cramping Crushing	Tugging Pulling Wrenching	Hot Burning Scalding Searing	Tingling Itchy Smarting Stinging
9	**10**	**11**	**12**
Dull Sore Hurting Aching Heavy	Tender Taut Rasping Splitting	Tiring Exhausting	Sickening Suffocating
13	**14**	**15**	**16**
Fearful Frightening Terrifying	Punishing Grueling Cruel Vicious Killing	Wretched Blinding	Annoying Troublesome Miserable Intense Unbearable
17	**18**	**19**	**20**
Spreading Radiating Penetrating Piercing	Tight Numb Drawing Squeezing Tearing	Cool Cold Freezing	Nagging Nauseating Agonizing Dreadful Torturing

Reprinted with permission from Melzack, R. (1975).

atic method to document the sensory, affective, and cognitive (evaluative) components of the pain experience (Wilkie, Savedra, Holzemer, Tesler, & Paul, 1990).

Several instruments are available to assist the ACNP in measuring all the sensory data needed for analysis of the pain symptom (refer to Table 20–3). The advantages and disadvantages of each tool have been reviewed by several authors (McGuire, 1997; Puntillo & Wilkie, 1991; Wilke, Savedra, et al., 1990). There is no one best tool to measure sensory pain components, although some are easier to use than others. The ACNP should recognize that a tool must be used consistently and that the staff, patient, and family all need to understand it to ensure valid measurements. If different pain tools are used by staff working throughout an organization (e.g., in home care or on an inpatient unit), the patient and family may have difficulty reporting pain to different professionals. Also colleagues may misinterpret pain information unless there is documentation about which tool has been used (Dalton & McNaull, 1997). Researchers are developing computerized tools for pain measurement with hopes of simplifying the process for the patient and health professionals and providing systematic data for decision making about pain therapies.

ANALGESIC THERAPIES

Treatment goals are useful in making decisions about analgesic therapies. As indicated previously, the patient's goal usually is to be free of pain (Berry et al., submitted 1998). Health-care professionals, however, rarely have a similar treatment goal. Instead health-care professionals tend to expect patients to experience mild to moderate levels of pain, levels not expected to interfere with the patient's functional status. As new research findings emphasize the dangers of even mild to moderate levels of pain (refer to Table 20–2) (Page & Ben Eliyahu, 1997), perhaps the ACNP and other health-care professionals will adopt treatment goals consistent with the patient's goal to be as pain-free as possible both *at rest* and *with activity.*

Achieving a pain-free state may not be possible at all times, but current research shows that optimal use of a variety of pain therapies can significantly control most types of pain without excessive side effects (Gottschalk et al., 1998; Pederson, 1997). The ACNP can implement optimal pain therapy plans by using knowledge of pharmaceuticals and other complementary therapies. Choosing the correct analgesic for pain is just as important as choosing the correct antibiotic for an infection.

Several important concepts assist the ACNP in choosing the appropriate analgesic drug for the type of pain experienced by the patient. The ACNP uses the:

- symptom analysis process to determine if the pain is nociceptive or neuropathic;
- analgesic ladder (WHO, 1986, 1996) and drug classifications to select analgesic drugs most likely to relieve the patient's type of pain;
- pharmacokinetic profile (onset, peak effect, duration, half life, metabolism, and excretion) to titrate the drug to the desired effect; equianalgesic doses to change routes or drugs (Omoigui, 1995); and
- a symptom reanalysis process to evaluate the effects of analgesic.

The following sections summarize the analgesic ladder and the classes of analgesics most effective for nociceptive and neuropathic types of pain. Mechanism of action, pharmacokinetics, titration, and equianalgesic dosages are included to assist the ACNP in the critical thinking required to use analgesics in the context of a particular patient's condition and pain problem.

Analgesic Drug Selection

As indicated in the neural mechanism section of this chapter, the many analgesic drugs provide analgesia via different mechanisms. Recent evidence indicates that many of the drugs act in both the PNS and the CNS. For the sake of simplicity, the analgesic drugs have been organized by broad three groups (nonopioids, adjuvants, and opioids) that relate somewhat to the mechanisms by which they produce analgesia. Since 1986 pain experts have recommended a systematic, three-step ladder approach to use of these various drugs (U.S. Department of Health and Human Services, 1992, 1994; WHO, 1986, 1996).

Analgesic Ladder

The WHO analgesic ladder (Fig. 20–18) provides the ACNP with a systematic approach to treating nociceptive and neuropathic pain caused by acute, chronic, or malignant conditions. The systematic plan calls for the concurrent treatment of the cause of pain when possible *and* the use of the three-step ladder approach for palliative management of the pain. As simple as this idea may seem, treating the disease or injury is of paramount importance in pain relief. One would not think to treat an acute appendix with only opioids when surgical removal is mandated. Conversely, one should not deny analgesics for palliation of the abdominal pain while preparations are made for the surgery. The key to successful pain management is curative care (when possible) provided concurrently with palliative pain control. The notion of palliative pain control applies equally to people who will survive their acute illness and to those who are near the end of their lives.

In acute conditions and severe pain intensity (7 to 10 on 0–10 scale), the drug choices start at the third step of the analgesic ladder and go down the steps as the tissue injury heals and the pain subsides. For example, severe postsurgical pain is treated first with intravenous opioids and NSAIDs (U.S. Department of Health and Human Services, 1992). When the patient's GI tract is functioning, the medications are changed to oral preparations. As the incision heals and the pain intensity level decreases, a step 2 drug is prescribed and the nonopioid is continued. As further healing occurs, pain relief can be obtained with only a nonopioid drug until the pain totally resolves.

In conditions of chronic pain or cancer pain and mild pain intensity (1 to 3 on 0–10 scale), the drug choices start at the first rung of the analgesic ladder. Drugs from step 2 are prescribed if the pain increases to a moderate intensity (4 to 6 on 0–10 scale) or the mild pain is not relieved. Step 3 drugs are selected for severe pain (7 to 10 on 0–10 scale).

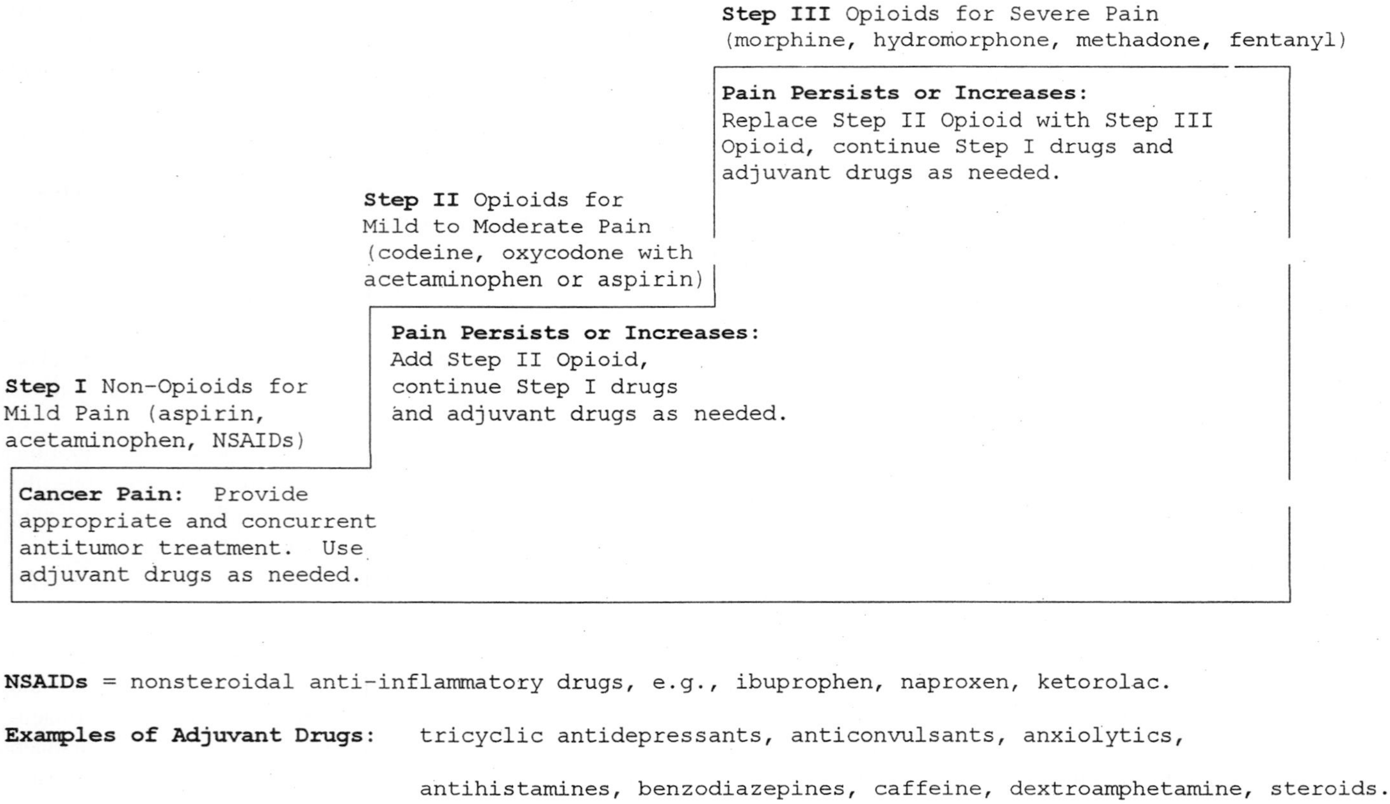

Step III Opioids for Severe Pain (morphine, hydromorphone, methadone, fentanyl)

Pain Persists or Increases: Replace Step II Opioid with Step III Opioid, continue Step I drugs and adjuvant drugs as needed.

Step II Opioids for Mild to Moderate Pain (codeine, oxycodone with acetaminophen or aspirin)

Pain Persists or Increases: Add Step II Opioid, continue Step I drugs and adjuvant drugs as needed.

Step I Non-Opioids for Mild Pain (aspirin, acetaminophen, NSAIDs)

Cancer Pain: Provide appropriate and concurrent antitumor treatment. Use adjuvant drugs as needed.

NSAIDs = nonsteroidal anti-inflammatory drugs, e.g., ibuprophen, naproxen, ketorolac.

Examples of Adjuvant Drugs: tricyclic antidepressants, anticonvulsants, anxiolytics, antihistamines, benzodiazepines, caffeine, dextroamphetamine, steroids.

Figure 20–18. The analgesic ladder proposed by the World Health Organization (1986). *(Reprinted with permission. Copyright © 1993, Wilkie, D.J.)*

Nonopioid and adjuvant drugs are used at any step of the analgesic ladder based on the sensory characteristics of the pain.

Step 1 Drugs

The typical step 1 *nonopioid drugs* include aspirin and other salicylates, other nonsteroidal antiinflammatory drugs (NSAIDs), and acetaminophen. Acetaminophen appears to relieve nociceptive and perhaps neuropathic pain via central mechanisms, possibly involving nitric oxide and NMDA receptors (Bjorkman et al., 1994). Daily doses in excess of 4000 mg have been associated with hepatic toxicity (Eriksson, Broom´e, Kalin, & Lindholm, 1992). Aspirin, other salicylates, and NSAIDs provide analgesia by inhibiting prostaglandin synthesis. These drugs are particularly effective for nociceptive pain but recent evidence also shows that they can relieve neuropathic pain by inhibiting prostaglandins in the CNS (Yaksh & Malmberg, 1993). GI and renal toxicity have limited the use of these drugs, especially in people with a history of GI bleeding or renal failure. New NSAIDs are available to selectively inhibit synthesis of the prostaglandins that are associated with pain (Cox-2) but not those needed for normal GI and renal function (Cox-1). These Cox-2 NSAIDs are expected to increase the therapeutic index of the step 1 drugs (Cashman, 1996).

These nonopioid drugs can be used alone for mild pain or along with adjuvant drugs or opioid drugs to control moderate or severe pain. These drugs can be powerful analgesics. About 27% of cancer patients reported effective control of mild or moderate pain when they used only step 1 drugs before death (Wilkie, 1993). Postoperative pain and musculoskelatal pain are other nociceptive types of pain that can be controlled with step 1 drugs. However, there is a ceiling dose for each of the nonopioid drugs, meaning that dose escalation above the ceiling does not improve analgesia, but contributes significantly to side effects and toxicity. Many of the step 1 nonopioid drugs are available over the counter (OTC) without prescription. Unfortunately, OTC drugs can have serious side effects, toxicities, and drug interactions (Garnett, 1996). The ACNP plays an important role in teaching patients about appropriate use of OTC drugs for pain control. Table 20–8 lists the pharmacokinetic and cost data for some of the nonopioid drugs commonly used in the United States (Omoigui, 1995).

Adjuvant drugs have primary indications other than pain relief but have analgesic properties. Adjuvant drugs (e.g., tricyclic antidepressants, anticonvulsants, and anxiolytics) can be used at all three steps of the analgesic ladder. Baclofen, tricyclic antidepressants, anticonvulsants, steroids, and local anesthetics are examples of adjuvant drugs that often are effective in treating neuropathic pain (Yaksh, 1991). Some types of pain respond to treatment with certain drugs (i.e., burning pain often responds to tricyclic antidepressants; shooting pain often responds to phenytoin or carbamazepine) (Max, et al., 1992; McQuay, Carroll, Jadad, Wiffen, & Moore, 1995). Table 20–9 lists the pharmacokinetic and cost data for some of the adjuvant drugs.

Step 2 Drugs

Step 2 opioid drugs include codeine, hydrocodone, oxycodone, propoxyphene, oral meperidine, and pentazocine. These opioids can be prescribed as preparations of the single agent or in combination with aspirin or acetaminophen. Step 1 drugs can be continued with step 2 drugs as long as the amount of aspirin or acetaminophen does not exceed the recommended daily dose (Wagner & Silberstein, 1996). Step 2 drugs bind to the opioid receptors in the PNS and CNS and block transmission of nociceptive signals.

There are several subtypes of opioid receptors. Mu, delta, and kappa receptors are associated with analgesia. Agonist opioid drugs fit into the receptor sites and activate the intracellular events that inhibit pain. Step 2 agonists (e.g., codeine, hydrocodone, oxycodone, propoxyphene, and meperidine) bind to the mu, delta, and kappa receptor sites and produce effects at each receptor site. The agonist–antagonist drugs (e.g., pentazocine) bind to the mu and kappa receptors, produce an effect at the kappa site (agonist), and block the drug's effect at the mu receptors (antagonist). Table 20–10 lists the pharmacokinetic and cost data for the most common step 2 drugs (Omoigui, 1995).

Step 3 Drugs

Step 3 drugs include agonist drugs (e.g., morphine, oxycodone [single agent], hydromorphone, levorphanol, oxymorphone, methadone, meperidine, and fentynal), agonist–antagonist drugs (e.g., butorphanol, nalbuphine, and dezocine) and partial agonist drugs (e.g., buprenorphine). Like the step 2 opioids, the step 3 drugs produce their effect by binding to the opioid receptor sites in the PNS and CNS. Table 20–11 lists the pharmacokinetic and cost data for the most common step 3 drugs (Omoigui, 1995).

Meperidine is considered a step 2 drug by the oral route and a step 3 drug by the IV or IM routes. The ACNP must consider several limitations in use of meperidine. Reputable guidelines recommend that meperidine be limited to doses less than 600 mg per 24 hours and for less than 48 hours duration (APS, 1998). The major reason for this recommendation is that its active metabolite, normeperidine, has a high incidence of neurotoxicity. Normeperidine is twice as potent as a convulsant and half as potent as an analgesic compared with its parent compound, meperidine. The half life of normeperidine is three to four times that of meperidine, thus accumulation of the metabolite with repeated dosing can result in central nervous system excitability, tremors, multifocal myoclonus, and seizures. Naloxone does not reverse the seizures produced by meperidine. With all its potential side effects, meperidine is not a drug of choice for pain that is expected to persist for more than two days or when the pain is of suf-

TABLE 20–8. World Health Organization Analgesic Ladder Step 1 Analgesics: Pharmacokinetics and Costs

Generic Drug (Trade Drug)	**Typical Dose and (Maximum Dose)**	**Approximately Equivalent to**	**Onset Effect (min)**	**Peak Effect (min)**	**Duration Effect (hr)**	**Plasma Half Life (hr)**	**Cost in Dollars for Typical Dose (daily)**
Acetaminophen (Tylenol, Tempra, others)	600 mg PO 600 mg PR (4000–6000 mg/day)	Aspirin 600 mg	30	60	3–4	1–4	0.02 0.55 (0.14–0.21)
Acetylsalicylic acid (aspirin)	600 mg PO 600 mg PR (5200 mg/day)	Morphine 2 mg IM	30	60	3–4	.25	0.07 (0.64)
Ibuprophen (Motrin, Advil, others)	200 mg PO (3200 mg/day)	Aspirin 650 mg	30	60–120	4	3–4	0.08 (1.34)
Choline magnesium trisalicylate (Trilisate)	2000–3000 mg PO (3000 mg/day)		5–30	60–180	3–6	7–18	1.80–2.71 (2.71)
Diflunisal (Dolobid)	500 mg PO (1500 mg/day)	Aspirin 650 mg	60	120–180	8–12	8–12	1.17 (3.51)
Ketoprofen (Orudis)	25 mg PO (300 mg/day)	Aspirin 650 mg	30	30–120	6	2–3	0.81 (9.68)
Naproxen (Naprosyn)	250 mg PO (1250 mg/day)	Aspirin 650 mg	60	120–240	6–8	13	0.75 (3.73)
Ketorolac Tromethamine (Toradol)	30–60 mg IM initially (120 mg IM/day × 5 day, max 30 mg IM × 20 doses)	Morphine 6–12 mg IM	10	60	3–6	3–9	0.72–0.77 (1.55–1.94)
Nabumetone (Relafen)	1000 mg PO (2000 mg/day)	Aspirin 3600 mg/ day	1–2 days	days–2 wk	Unknown	24	2.04 (4.08)
Etodolac (Lodine)	200–400 mg PO (1200 mg/day)	Aspirin 650 mg	30	60–120	4–12	7	1.09–2.18 (6.54)
Piroxicam (Feldene)	20 mg PO (20 mg/day)		60	180–300	>12	50	(2.47)
Sulindac (Clinoril)	200 mg PO (400 mg/day)	(Aspirin 4800 mg/ day	1–2 days	60–120	Unknown	18	(2.29)
Indomethacin (Indocin)	25 mg PO (100 mg/day)	Aspirin 650 mg	60	60–120	4	4–5	0.03 (0.12)

Key: PO = oral; PR = rectal; IM = intramuscular; IV = intravenous. PO cost is based on least expensive, 100 tablet quantity, generic preparation if available; and IV or IM is based on least expensive.

ficient intensity to require large doses in order for the patient to obtain adequate pain relief (APS, 1998).

Concerns regarding tolerance, dependence, addiction, conscious sedation, assisted suicide, and euthanasia often serve as barriers to effective use of step 2 or 3 drugs. Extensive research shows that these concerns are shared by the patient, family members, and health-care providers (U.S. Department of Health and Human Services, 1992, 1994; WHO, 1986, 1996). The ACNP can play an important role in helping others to understand the differences among these various concepts.

Tolerance occurs with chronic exposure to many drugs. In the case of opioids, tolerance is characterized by the need for an increased opioid dose to maintain the same degree of analgesia. Every patient does not experience tolerance, but patients with a past or current substance abuse history are likely to do so. The need for an increase in the analgesic dose may reflect other factors, such as disease progression (e.g., cancer progression), or a new pathologic condition (e.g., pulmonary embolus), rather than tolerance. The patient's reports of increased pain should not be ignored; the increased pain should be treated while the cause is pursued. One of the ways tolerance is managed is by drug titration to balance desired effects and side effects while maintaining patient comfort. Other approaches include changing to another drug in the same class or adding a nonopioid drug such as ibuprofen. It is important to note that there is no ceiling effect (increased dosing provides additional pain relief) for opioid–agonist drugs. As tolerance increases, doses can be increased. In fact, one of the largest

TABLE 20–9. World Health Organziation Analgesic Ladder Step 1 to 3 Adjuvant Analgesics: Pharmacokinetics and Costs

Generic Drug (Trade Drug)	**Approximate Daily Dose**	**Onset Effect**	**Peak Effect (hr)**	**Duration Effect (hr)**	**Plasma Half Life (hr)**	**Cost in Dollars for Typical Dose**
Carbamazepine (Tegretol, Epitol)	200–1600 mg PO	8–72 hr	2–12	Unknown	14–30	0.35–2.78 0.24–1.92
Phenytoin (Dilantin)	300–500 mg PO	2–24 hr	1.5–3	6–12	22	0.54–0.90
Amitriptyline (Elavil and others)	10–150 mg PO	3–4 days	1–2 weeks	Days–weeks	10–50	0.18–1.57
Doxepin (Sinequan, Adapin)	25–150 mg PO	3–4 days	1–2 weeks	Days–weeks	8–25	0.42–1.78
Imipramine (Tofranil and others)	20–100 mg PO	60 min	2–6 weeks	Weeks	8–16	0.29–1.44
Trazodone (Desyrel and others)	75–225 mg PO	2 weeks	2–4 weeks	Weeks	5–9	0.89–2.67
Hydroxyzine (Vistaril, Atarax, and others)	300–450 mg IM	15–30 min	2–4 hr	4–6 hr	3	2.16–3.24
Lidocaine	5 mg/kg IV	2 min	2 min	10–20 min	90–120 min	0.01 (5 mg)
Mexiletine	450–600 mg PO	30–120 min	2–3 hr	8–12 hr	10–12 hr	1.84–2.45
Tocainide	20 mg/kg PO	30–60 min	0.5–2 hr	8–12 hr	11–23 hr	0.04
Dexamethasone (Decadron and others)	16–96 mg PO/IV	2–4 days	1–2 hr	2.75 days	1.5–3.5	0.84–5.05(PO) 1.20–7.20(IV)
Sumatriptan (Imitrex)	6–12 mg SC	30 min	Up to 2 hr	Up to 24 hr	2hr	33.59–67.19
Gabapentin (Neurontin)	900–1800 mg PO				5–7 hr	2.85–5.70
Paroxetine (Paxil)	20–50 mg PO	1–4 wk			21 hr	1.90–4.75
Nefazodone (Serzone)	200–600 mg PO		1 hr		2–4 hr	0.83–2.49
Dextroamphetamine (Dexedrine and others)	10–15 mg PO	1–2 hr	Unknown	2–10 hr	10–12	0.36–0.54
Methylphenidate	10–15 mg PO	Unknown	1–3 hr	4–6 hr	1–3	0.36–0.54

Key: PO = oral; PR = rectal; IM = intramuscular; IV = intravenous. PO cost is based on least expensive, 100 tablet quantity, generic preparation if available; and IV or IM is based on least expensive.

doses noted in the literature has been **1,568 mg intravenous (IV) morphine per hour, which is 37,632 mg per day** (Miser et al., 1986). Patients often worry about tolerance, especially if they expect their pain to increase or persist. The ACNP can ease this worry by explaining that numerous pain medicines are available and that many have no maximum dose. The ACNP can compare the dose reported by Miser et al. (1986) with the patient's dose in order to ease his or her concern about tolerance.

Dependence is an expected physiologic response to ongoing exposure to pharmacologic agents that produce a withdrawal syndrome when exposure is abruptly stopped. Withdrawal from opioids is characterized by symptoms such as chills alternating with hot flashes, salivation, sweating, runny nose, anxiety, irritability, insomnia, abdominal cramps, vomiting, and diarrhea when the drug dosage is markedly decreased or abruptly discontinued. Dependence appears to be highly individualized. Some patients gradually decrease their use of pain medication as the pain decreases. Other patients require a tapering schedule. For example, to withdraw a patient from morphine, the total 24-hour dose used by the patient is calculated and decreased by 50% (APS, 1998). Of this decreased amount, 25% is given every 6 hours. After 2 days, the daily dose is reduced by an additional 25% every 2 days until the 24-hour oral dose is 30 mg per day. The morphine then is discontinued.

Addiction is a psychologic condition characterized by a drive to obtain and take substances for other than the prescribed therapeutic purpose. Research findings suggest that

TABLE 20–10. World Health Organziation Analgesic Ladder Step 2 Opioid Analgesics for Mild to Moderate Pain: Pharmacokinetics and Costs

Generic Drug (Trade Drug)	**Typical Dose**	**Approximately Equivalent to**	**Onset Effect (min)**	**Peak Effect (min)**	**Duration Effect (hr)**	**Plasma Half Life (hr)**	**Cost in Dollars for Typical Dose**
Step 2 Opioid Agonist Drugs							
Codeine	30–60 mg PO 200 mg PO 120 IM	Aspirin 650 mg Morphine 10 mg IM Morphine 10 mg IM	30–45 10–30	20–120 30–60	4 4	2.5–4	0.27–0.55 1.51 0.90
Oxycodone *Immediate release* (Roxicodone, w/ aspirin—Percodan w/acetaminophen—Percocet)	5 mg PO 30 mg PO	Codeine 60 mg PO Morphine 10 mg IM Morphine 30 mg PO	0–15	60	3–4	2–3	0.25 1.47
Hydrocodone (in Vicodin, Lortab, Lorcet, and others)	30 mg PO	Morphine 10 mg IM	10–30	30–60	4–6	3.8	2.20
Meperidine (Demerol, Pethadol); Causes central nervous system excitation ranging from irritability to seizures	50 mg PO 300 mg PO 75 mg IM 50 mg IV	Aspirin 650 mg Morphine 10 mg IM Demerol 75 mg IM Morphine 10 mg IM Morphine 10 mg IM	15 10–15 1	60–90 30–60 5–7	2–4 2–4 2–3	2.4–4	0.69 3.94 0.39 0.26
Tramadol (Ultram)	50–100 mg	Codeine 60 mg PO		2 hr	4–6 hr	6–11 hr	0.60–1.20
Propoxyphene HCL (Darvon, Dolene) Propoxyphene napsylate (w/aspirin—Darvon N w/acetaminophen—Darvocet N)	65 mg PO 100 mg PO	Aspirin 600 mg Aspirin 600 mg	15–60	120	4–6	6–12	0.31 0.45
Step 2 Agonist–Antagonist Drugs							
Pentazocine HCL (Talwin); may cause abstinence reactions in patients physically dependent on opioids	60 mg IM 30 mg PO 180 mg PO	Morphine 10 mg IM Aspirin 600 mg Morphine 10 mg IM or Talwin 60 mg IM	15–20 15–30	30–60 60–90	2–3 3	2–3	2.53 0.48 2.88

Key: PO = oral; PR = rectal; IM = intramuscular; IV = intravenous. PO cost is based on least expensive, 100 tablet quantity, generic preparation if available; and IV or IM is based on least expensive.

4 out of 12,000 patients (less than 0.1%) who received analgesics as a part of their medical treatment regimen became addicted (Porter & Jick, 1980). Two examples of behavior suggestive of addiction are patients receiving pain medications from multiple physicians, and reporting that pain prescriptions have been lost or stolen. Other types of behavior may be incorrectly interpreted as signs of addiction, such as clock-watching by the person undertreated for the pain. Addiction cannot be verified in the person with pain until the etiology of the pain has been eliminated, physical dependence has been eliminated through detoxification, and the patient seeks and takes the substance again. The patient who is physically dependent on the drug seeks and takes the drug, but may not be addicted. Often the term *addiction* is inappropriately applied to a patient, and the label can be a barrier to pain relief for that person. It is important for the staff, patient, and family to recognize that opioid tolerance and physical dependence are expected with long-term opioid treatment and should not be confused with addiction, which is expected to occur *almost never.*

Conscious sedation implies that the patient can respond to verbal and physical stimuli when sedatives are used. The American Nurses Association (1996) has established practice guidelines for the role of the registered nurse in the management of patients receiving IV conscious sedation for short-term therapeutic, diagnostic, or surgical

TABLE 20–11. World Health Organziation Analgesic Ladder Step 3 Opioid Analgesics for Moderate to Severe Pain: Pharmacokinetics and Costs

Generic Drug (Trade Drug)	Typical Dose	Approximately Equivalent to	Onset Effect (min)	Peak Effect (min)	Duration Effect (hr)	Plasma Half Life (hr)	Cost in Dollars for Dose (Typical)
Step 3 Agonist Drugs							
Morphine sulfate	30[a] mg PO	Morphine 10 mg IM	20–60	120	4–5	2–3	0.27 (tab)
Immediate release	30[a] mg PR	Morphine 10 mg IM					0.60 (liq)
tablets, liquids, and suppositories							1.36 (PR)
Sustained release (MS Contin, Oramorph SR, Kadian)	30 mg PO	Morphine 10 mg IM		210	8–12		1.39
Injectable (Astramorph, Duramorph, Infumorph)	10 mg IM	Morphine 10 mg IM	10–30	60	4–5		0.64
	5 mg IV	Morphine 10 mg IM	5	20	2–4		0.32
Oxycodone	5 mg PO	Codeine 60 mg PO	0–15	60	3–4	2–3	0.25
Immediate release (Roxicodone)	30 mg PO	Morphine 10 mg IM Morphine 30 mg PO					1.47
Controlled release (OxyContin)	30 mg PO	Morphine 30–60 mg PO[b]	30–60	60–420	12	4.5	?
Methadone (Dolophine)	20 mg PO	Morphine 10 mg IM Methadone 10 mg IM	30–60	90–120	4–6	15–25	0.28
	10 mg IM	Morphine 10 mg IM	10–20	60–120	4–5		0.56
	5 mg IV	Morphine 10 mg IM		15–30	3–4		0.28
Hydromorphone (Dilaudid)	7.5 mg PO	Morphine 10 mg IM	30	90–120	4	2.5–4	1.05
	3 mg PR	Hydromorphone 1.5 mg IM	15–30	30–90	4–5		2.91
	1.5 mg IM	Morphine 10 mg IM	15	30–60	4–5		0.50
	1 mg IV	Morphine 10 mg IM	10–15	15–30	2–3		0.33
Oxymorphone (Numorphan)	1 mg IM	Morphine 10 mg IM	10–15	30–90	3–6	2.6–4	2.93
	.5 mg IV	Morphine 10 mg IM	5–10	15–30	3–4		1.47
	10 mg PR	Oxymorphone 1 mg IM	15–30	60	3–6		9.47
Levorphanol (LevoDromoran)	4 mg PO	Morphine 10 mg IM Levorphanol 2 mg IM	10–60	90–120	4–5	15	1.12
	2 mg IM	Morphine 10 mg IM		60	4–5		2.04
	1 mg IV	Morphine 10 mg IM		15	3–4		1.32
Fentanyl (Sublimaze)	0.1 mg IM	Morphine 10 mg IM	7–15	20–30	1–2	3.6	1.73
(Duragesic)	25–50 mcg/hr transdermal	Morphine 30 mg sustained-release q 8 hr	6 hr	12–24 hr	72	17	9.12–13.67
Step 3 Agonist–Antagonist Drugs							
Butorphanol (Stadol)	2 mg IM	Morphine 10 mg IM	10–30	30–60	3–4	2.5–4	6.04
see pentazocine	2 mg IV	Morphine 10 mg IM	2–3	30	2–4		
Nalbuphine (Nubain);	10 mg IM	Morphine 10 mg IM	15	60	3–6	5	1.62
see pentazocine	10 mg IV	Pentazocine 60 mg IM	2–3	30	3–4		
Dezocine (Dalgan)	10 mg IM	Morphine 10 mg IM	30	60–120	3–6	2.4	6.26
Step 3 Partial Agonist Drugs							
Buprenorphine (Buprenex)	.4 mg IM	Morphine 10 mg IM	15	60	6	3	2.92

Key: PO = oral; PR = rectal; IM = intramuscular; IV = intravenous. PO cost is based on least expensive, 100 tablet quantity, generic preparation if available; and IV or IM is based on least expensive. Controversial equivalency: [a] use 60 mg in single-dose situation and 30 mg in repeated-dose situations; [b] use 60 mg as initial conversion and titrate to analgesic effect.

procedure. Although analgesics may produce sedation as a side effect, sedatives generally do not produce analgesia.

Assisted suicide and euthanasia are controversial topics. When large doses of opioids are required to control pain, often health-care providers (both physicians and nurses) hesitate to prescribe and administer the dose, because they are concerned that the actions will be considered performing euthanasia or assisting the patient to commit suicide. Relieving pain, even if it hastens the death of a terminally ill person, is considered the ethical and moral obligation of the professional nurse; it is not euthanasia or assisted-suicide (ANA, 1990, 1992, 1996). When consistent with the patient's wishes, the position of the ANA is: "Nurses should not hesitate to use full and effective doses of pain medication for the proper management of pain in the dying patient. The increasing titration of medication to achieve adequate symptom control, even at the expense of life, thus hastening death, is ethically justified" (ANA, 1996). Relief of pain, not death, is the objective of the intervention.

Unfortunately, inadequate pain relief and intolerable suffering have been cited by many patients as reasons for seeking assisted suicide. The ACNP is responsible for assisting the patient to obtain pain relief satisfactory to him or her. Aggressive management of pain is essential and may limit the number of people who seek assisted suicide. The ANA and other nursing organizations have taken the position that nurses should not participate in assisted suicide or euthanasia (ANA, 1996). Assisting a patient to commit suicide is in violation of the Code for Nurses. The ACNP and other professional nurses, however, have a responsibility to provide analgesia to patients with pain. Meeting this responsibility is facilitated by systematic dose escalation to adequately control the patient's pain.

Analgesic Dose Titration

Doses of all step 3 agonist drugs, except meperidine, can be safely escalated without a ceiling effect by means of titration. *Analgesic titration* is dose adjustment based on the adequacy of analgesic effect and on the side effects produced. The ACNP often assists in titrating analgesics. There is no set amount of an opioid that produces pain relief for every patient. The right dose is the dose that works and helps the patient achieve the pain-intensity goal. The initial dose, however, can be estimated for each patient using a mg/kg formula for each opioid (Fig. 20–19). For example, morphine 0.05 to 0.1 mg/kg IV every 2 hours is used to determine the size of the morphine dose when beginning titration (U.S. Department of Health and Human Services, 1992). Skillful titration results in the optimal dose of an analgesic being given and helps the ACNP to recognize when additional or alternative drugs might be helpful. In some states, the ACNP consults with a physician in order to provide the patient with appropriate prescriptions to effectively continue dose titration.

The dose required to relieve a person's pain can vary tremendously. Differences in pain levels, drug metabolism, drug interactions, and other responses to specific drugs can affect the dose needed to relieve pain. Patients with renal dysfunction are more sensitive to some opioids, such as meperidine and morphine (Christrup, 1997; Portenoy et al., 1991). Larger doses may be required if the pain is out of control or is a neuropathic type of pain. The person with a smoking history may require larger doses of morphine, meperidine, pentazocine, and propoxyphene to obtain pain control (Miller, 1990). Genetic factors can also affect analgesic responses. For example, the analgesic effect of codeine depends on metabolism of codeine to morphine via O-demethylation, which requires sparteine/debrisoquine oxygenation (CYP2D6). Research shows that about 10% of caucasians with Northern European ancestry are not able to metabolize spartine and, therefore, may not obtain *any* pain relief from codeine (Sindrup et al., 1993). Research also shows plasma concentrations of opioids vary tremendously between patients who receive the same dose and have similar diseases. Robison, Wilkie, & Campbell (1995) noted that plasma concentrations of morphine varied from 2.5 ng/mL to nearly 60 ng/mL after a 10-mg dose of oral morphine. Since minimum effective concentration of morphine is about 15 ng/mL, these findings help to explain the different responses observed clinically after opioid administration. The ACNP plays an important role in recognizing the variable responses to pain medications by titrating the analgesic drug to the dose that relieves the patient's pain and prevents excessive side effects.

Equianalgesic Dose

Equianalgesic dose refers to a dose of one analgesic that is equivalent in pain-relieving effects to another analgesic. This equivalence permits substitution of medications to relieve the pain and avoid possible adverse effects of one of the drugs. Refer to Tables 20–10 and 20–11 for equianalgesic data for different opioids administered by oral, IV, and IM routes.

Analgesic Dose Schedule

Scheduling doses of the analgesic drugs should be done to *prevent pain.* The ACNP should verify that the patient is medicated before painful procedures and activities that can be expected to produce pain. The ACNP can help the family and other nurses to plan these procedures or activities so that they occur when the patient's analgesic has reached its peak effectiveness. Then the pain is decreased to its minimal level with that dose and the patient's ability to cooperate with the procedures or activity will be maximized with that dose. Moreover, if the patient is medicated before the pain begins to increase rather than once it has become severe, far less medication is required. This type of scheduling plan can minimize the drug's side effects and eliminate

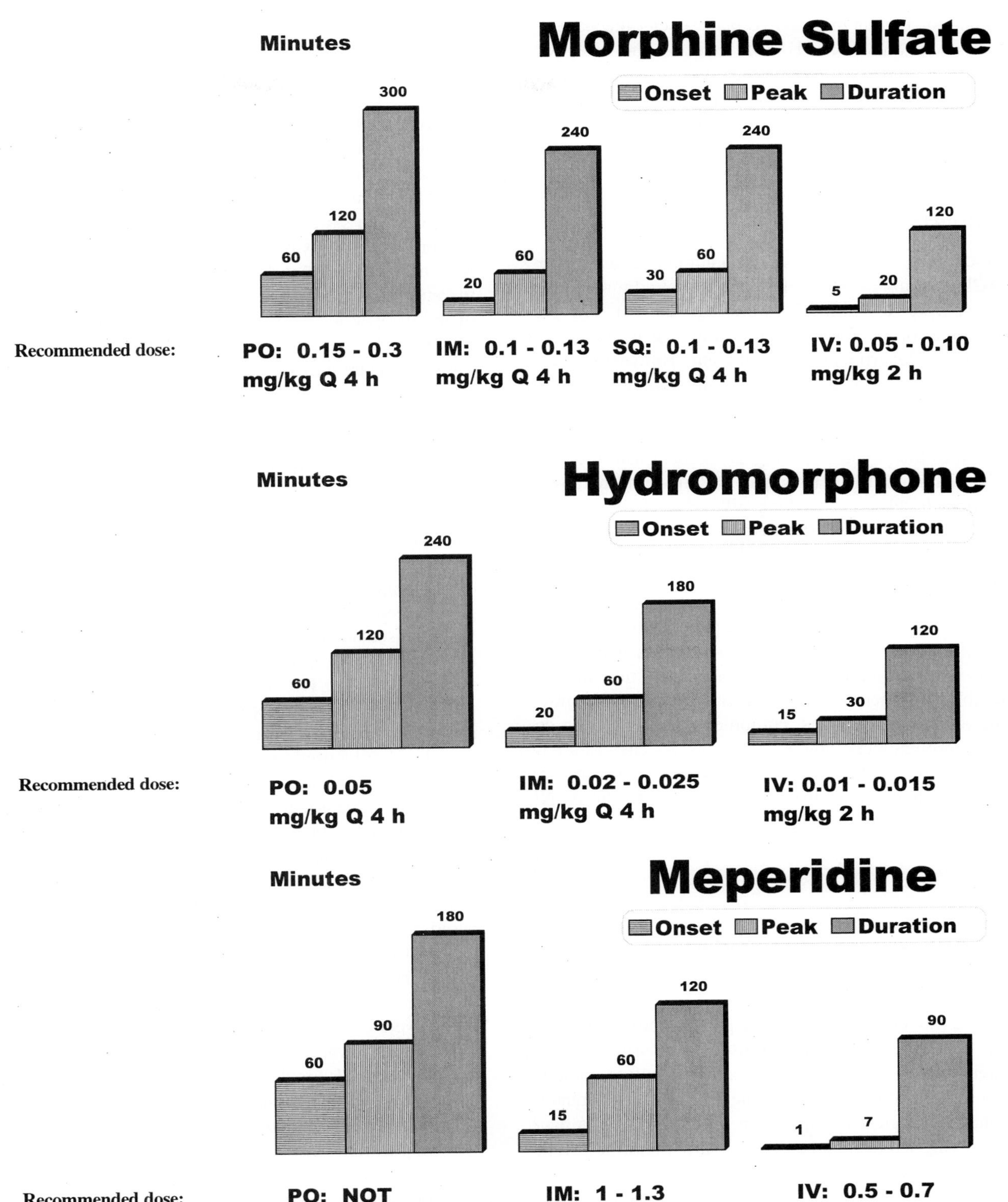

Figure 20–19. Graphical representation of the pharmacokinetics with weight-based dosages for selected opioids. Administered by PO, IM or SQ, and IV routes. *(Reprinted with permission. Copyright © 1998, Wilkie, D.J.)*

an important barrier to effective pain relief—the patient's concerns about uncontrolled side effects. The analgesics may also be scheduled on a time-controlled basis, with the medication given on a set schedule regardless of the presence or absence of pain. Analgesics scheduled around the clock are particularly helpful if the patient has constant pain.

Administration Routes

When choosing a route by which to administer analgesics, the ACNP should consider efficacy, ease of administration, and cost (refer to Tables 20–9 through 20–11). The preferred route for the administration of analgesics is the oral route (U.S. Department of Health and Human Services, 1994). As long as the patient has a functioning GI system and there is no risk of aspiration, oral analgesics provide optimum relief. The ACNP should also consider other factors such as the patient's willingness to deal with the route of administration if it is to be part of long-term therapy. If the patient is adverse to taking pills several times a day, then a long-acting drug that requires dosing fewer times per day is more acceptable to the patient and increases compliance with the medication regime. Long-acting preparations such as MS Contin, Oramorph, Kadia, and Oxycontin must not be crushed. If a patient has highly sensitive skin, then transdermal fentanyl patches may be uncomfortable and another route of administration may be preferable. It is very easy to fall into the trap of wanting the newest drugs and latest equipment that have been developed through technological advances. As easy as a new device may be for the health-care providers to operate, the patient may have great difficulty operating it. The ACNP should keep the pain-management plan simple, cost effective, and manageable for the patient and family when they are at home.

▶ NONPHARMACOLOGICAL AND COMPLEMENTARY THERAPIES

There are numerous ways to treat pain effectively without drugs. The holistic practitioner uses nonpharmacological therapies when appropriate to the situation, often combining them with pharmacological therapies when warranted. Nonpharmacological therapies can be as simple as a back rub, applying ice to inflamed tissue, slow rhythmic breathing, and relaxing and thinking about pleasant things and places. The ACNP can teach the patient and family how to use these techniques.

Ascending nociceptive input can be altered with proper positioning and support of limbs. Patients immobilize or guard painful body parts as an automatic response to pain. Excessive immobilization or guarding can result in pressure ulcers or stiff joints. Therapeutic beds and body pillows can be used to relieve pressure and splint affected limbs. Mechanical supports for injured or atrophied limbs can reduce the level of pain. Active or passive range-of-motion can relieve stiffness and muscle contractures. It is important that all planned activity and range-of-motion exercises coincide with the peak of analgesic effect of prescribed drugs.

Cutaneous or dermal stimulation is noninjurious stimulation of the skin for the purpose of pain relief. Massage and pressure (forms of stimulation) harness the autonomic responses to hold, clutch, and rub the injured area. A recent literature review with pilot study findings describe the many therapeutic effects of massage, including pain control in seriously ill hospice patients (Wilkie et al., submitted 1998). Pressure may be applied using the hand or a smooth hard object such as a sandbag. Acupressure is a technique that involves applying pressure and/or massage to points at which the pain is triggered. Trigger points are hypersensitive areas with taut bands in the muscle or connective tissue and are similar to the traditional acupuncture points. These areas can be injected with normal saline or local anesthetic solutions of lidocaine or bupivacaine to provide temporary relief of myofascial pain. Sometimes extended pain relief can be obtained by breaking the cycle of pain with trigger-point injections.

Transcutaneous electric nerve stimulation (TENS) is another way of stimulating peripheral nerves and blocking nociceptive input. TENS is the delivery of an electrical current through electrodes applied to the skin surface over a peripheral nerve or trigger points in the painful region. This modality can be used in acute postoperative as well as persistent pain syndromes. The TENS has been used in low back pain, arthritis, sciatica, postherpetic neuralgia, peripheral nerve injury, brachial plexus injuries, and during childbirth. The ACNP applies the TENS unit and works with the patient to adjust the electrode placement and frequency to achieve optimal pain relief. Multiple sites of stimulation based on the spinal dermatomes may be tried to determine the most effective site of pain modulation. The TENS can be applied several times a day for 20 to 60 minutes. TENS units are not recommended for use in patients with cardiac pacemakers or a history of ischemia or arrhythmias. TENS is not applied over a fetus, broken skin, or anesthetic areas. Areas to avoid also include the eyes, carotid sinuses, and laryngeal and pharyngeal muscles. A hypoallergenic contact gel may reduce the risk of skin irritation.

Application of therapeutic heat or cold can reduce pain. Either moist or dry heat or cold is applied to the skin for short periods of time. Heat should be used (5 minutes for acute pain, 20-30 minutes for chronic pain) after the initial swelling and inflammation of injury has subsided, usually 24 hours. Acute pain and chronic pain can be relieved by application of cold or massage with ice, with slow up and down strokes for 10 to 30 minutes. Vasocoolant spray also can be used as a type of cold therapy. After spraying with a vasocoolant, painful trigger point areas are gently stretched.

One of the most often overlooked aspects of pain control is allowing the patient to get adequate rest and sleep. A patient deprived of rapid eye movement (REM) and deep sleep becomes irritable and fatigued and has increased sensitivity to pain. The ACNP can recommend that tests and procedures are scheduled to allow the patient to have at least 2-hour blocks of undisturbed sleep and periods of down time during the day. To promote sleep, the use of analgesics, hypnotics, and relaxation techniques are appropriate.

There are several ways to treat pain with behavioral and cognitive strategies. In the helping–teaching role, the ACNP takes time to listen and counsel on lifestyle changes (e.g., smoking cessation for the patient with angina, dietary modification for the interstitial cystitis patient) that would be beneficial to pain management. Eliciting behaviors and thoughts incompatible with pain can help relieve pain. A patient who is applying relaxation techniques cannot tense muscles. Telling all the details about a beautiful place or a favorite activity prevents the patient from focusing on the pain, at least for a while. Relaxed rhythmic breathing is calming and beneficial for control of pain. The ACNP can teach the patient to use these pain-control techniques. Actively listening to music can help the patient relax and be distracted from the pain. Use of headphones can allow the patient to listen to music and simultaneously block out other noises and sounds. The ACNP can use humor to distract the patient from the pain. These cognitive and behavioral strategies work best with patients who are cognitively intact and are mentally alert enough to actively participate. There is also improved benefit if these techniques are taught before the pain begins. For example, breathing exercises are best taught before labor begins, not during advanced stages of labor.

ACUTE CARE NURSE PRACTITIONER RESPONSIBILITY

The ACNP has several roles concerning pain management. The ACNP is responsible for assessment and diagnosis of the pain problem and for prescribing, administering, and monitoring the therapeutic interventions, often in collaboration with physician colleagues. The ACNP is also responsible for consultation, collaboration, and outcome evaluations.

Four case studies are presented in Table 20–12 to show examples of the ACNP's potential role in management of

TABLE 20–12. Case Examples

Case	Diagnosis	Treatment	Analysis
1	Mrs. K, a 42-year-old female, presents to the ER reporting recent onset of waves of lower abdominal pain that radiate to the upper abdomen and back. She tells the ACNP that the pain began 14 hours ago, has been increasing in intensity and duration and is a sharp, cramping sensation not associated with nausea, vomiting, or diarrhea. Lying still helps to reduce the back pain and walking increases the back pain but neither affects the abdominal pain. The waves of pain originally occurred every 15 to 20 minutes, but now occur every 3 to 5 minutes. She has taken Tylenol with little relief. She is afraid that she "has appendicitis or one of those E. coli infections that killed so many people last year." Her past medical history is significant for hypertension and obesity. She has not seen a health-care provider in many years. The ACNP must narrow the list of differential diagnoses regarding the disorder causing Mrs. K's pain. Mrs. K's description reflects a localized, recent onset pain that is increasing in magnitude and the pain quality descriptors are indicative of an acute, nociceptive pain. Unfortunately, the nociceptive process	The pain caused by uterine contractions during the birthing process can be cured by delivery of the fetus and palliated during labor and delivery. The mutually agreed-upon treatment goals were labor pain relief and the safe delivery of the baby. Mrs. K required a C-section; received intraoperative analgesia, and she and the baby experienced no complications.	The curative treatment of the labor pain produced a new pain, acute surgical pain from the abdominal incision. The ACNP recognized the potential for affective, behavioral, and cognitive aspects of the pain to be important considerations in the plan for palliation of incisional pain. Anxiety over the unexpected child may increase her need for analgesia because norepinephrine released from the efferent autonomic nervous system terminals could activate the primary afferent nociceptors that were injured by the surgical incision. Additionally, her pain could be increased if she received insufficient analgesia in the early postoperative period and the NMDA receptors were enabled, producing a neuropathic pain syndrome. Mrs. K may be reluctant to increase her mobility ofter surgery because of her obesity and sedentary lifestyle, especially if postoperative analgesia is suboptimal. This case study demonstrates two different causes of nociceptive pain, one that was treated by delivery of her baby and the other postsurgical was self-limiting. Both types of pain should have been palliated in order to

(Continued)

TABLE 20–12. Case Examples *(Continued)*

Case	Diagnosis	Treatment	Analysis
	causing the pain could be located in several abdominal or pelvic structures. Subjective report is insufficient to determine the etiology. The ACNP needs additional data in order to make a diagnosis. The physical exam is a cost-efficient method for the ACNP to clarify and extend the sensory pain report data provided by Mrs. K. Exam findings reveal that the pain originates from the uterus. The ACNP discovered that Mrs. K is pregnant and experiencing labor pains. Mrs. K is shocked at the news because she and her husband were told they could not have children. She says that her menstrual cycles always have been erratic and that she was not worried when she had not menstruated in a "long time." Abdominal ultrasound findings indicate a 37-week pregnancy.		improve health outcomes for both mother and baby.
2	Paula G, a 48-year-old female, presents to the ER with a complaint of abdominal pain. Paula states the pain has been increasing over several days. The pain is dull and achy and increases when she lies flat. She also has had some shortness of breath and weight loss. The ACNP completes a comprehensive history and physical exam and orders a chest x-ray. The x-ray films show a right pleural effusion, masses in the upper lobes bilaterally, and a mediastinal mass. The ACNP administers local anesthesia and assists the MD with the thoracentesis, which removed 1.5 liters of fluid. Immediately after the procedure, Paula's abdominal pain decreased and her breathing improved. The ACNP refers Paula to an oncologist for work-up of probable lung cancer. The work-up includes a CT scan of the chest and head, fiber optic bronchoscopy for biopsy, bone scan, and blood work that includes CBC, liver profile, BUN, and creatinin. The work-up is positive for metastatic non–small-cell lung cancer.	Paula decides she does not want aggressive treatment and wants to be followed by a hospice team which includes an ACNP, a specialist in palliative treatment of pain and other symptoms. Since Paula's pain after the thoracentesis was 2/10 (mild), the ACNP prescribed a step 1 analgesic, etodolac (Cox-2 specific NSAID), 400 mg q 6 hr for her abdominal pain, a nociceptive type of pain caused by the liver metastasis.	Palliative care goals will address end-of-life issues and the need for pain control, as well as other symptoms such as dyspnea and the side effects of opioids including constipation, dry mouth, and nausea. The ACNP recognizes that the upper lobe lung masses can compress the brachial plexus, causing pancoast syndrome, a neuropathic pain that often responds to tricyclic antidepressants. Paula is also at risk for bone metastasis especially to the spine. Bone metastasis causes a nociceptive type of pain that often responds to corticosteroids, NSAIDs, opioids, and palliative radiation therapy.
3	The nursing staff at a subacute nursing facility calls the ACNP about a 86-year-old man who reports rib pain. The patient is a poor historian and has mild dementia. The staff thinks he may have fallen. He is able to describe the pain as shooting and lancinating. He uses one finger to show that the pain starts in the mid-back and travels along his 7th rib. There are no signs of abrasion or burising. The staff asks the ACNP if this man needs a rib x-ray to rule out a rib fracture. The ACNP thinks the pain he is describing is a neuropathic type of pain and declines the x-ray.	The ACNP prescribes a low-dose tricyclic antidepressant at bedtime and an opioid for mild to moderate pain. Two days later, the staff nurse calls the ACNP and reports the patient has a series of fluid-filled blisters along the painful rib. The ACNP confirms her diagnosis of herpes zoster and prescribes Acyclovir and continues the analgesics.	This man has an acute neuropathic pain related to a treatable etiology, herpes zoster. Unfortunately, this elderly man is at risk for postherpetic neuralgia. Postherpetic neuralgia is not curable, so treatment is for the relief of the pain and hypersensitivity in the area. Treatment may include capsaicin cream, nerve blocks, TENS unit, or acupuncture. Capsaicin cream renders skin insensitive to pain by depleting substance P in the peripheral sensory neurons (Omoigui, 1995).

(Continued)

TABLE 20–12. Case Examples *(Continued)*

Case	Diagnosis	Treatment	Analysis
4	B. A., a 67-year-old with metastatic ovarian CA, was admitted to the hospital with a small bowel obstruction secondary to adhesions and tumor invasion. Prescriptions included NPO status, hydration fluids, anti-emetic medications, and morphine sulfate 2–4 mg IV every 1 hour prn for pain. About two hours after admission, B. A. complained of severe pain in the upper, left quadrant of the abdomen. She described the pain as sharp, piercing, and unlike the pain she had a few hours ago. She called the pain as "200 out of 10."	The ACNP consulted with the physician and the bolus opioid dose range was increased to allow titration to comfort. During the night B. A. became diaphoretic, hypotensive, and tachycardic. Later she became disoriented and confused. The next morning, abdominal x-rays showed a perforated bowel. Because of her underlying medical condition, her family refused surgery. She died 24 hours later.	B. A. reported pain that did not fit the diagnosis of small bowel obstruction. The pain from a small bowel obstruction is dull and steady. B. A.'s ovarian cancer pain was usually well controlled with oral medications. The pain she experienced was very different from her previous pain. The new pain had a sudden onset, was much more intense, and was in a different location. Other physical signs, increased heart rate and diaphoresis, pointed to an acute pain episode. If the ACNP and the physician had considered the potential causes of a new pain, B. A. could have had more aggressive titration to a sufficient comfort level with a morphine infusion, not the prn bolus doses she received during the night. The infusion also would have been much more effective from the perspective of the nursing staff. Furthermore, early recognition of the emergent condition could have allowed B. A. to participate in the end-of-life decisions that her family subsequently made for her, all of which were consistent with B. A.'s wishes that she expressed earlier in the course of her cancer experience.

pain in people with different types of acute conditions or illness. The cases illustrate how the ACNP can use the Pain Relief Algorithm in appropriate management of nociceptive or neuropathic pain. Optimal pain relief with minimal side effects are the outcomes the ACNP is likely to observe when following this algorithm and applying pharmacokinetic principles and the WHO analgesic ladder.

Another important role is that of professional leadership. The ACNP can be a dynamic leader in the role of pain management by being an advocate for the patient and family. The ACNP can lead the effort to see that the acute care setting makes treating pain a high-level priority. As midlevel practitioners, the ACNP can bridge gaps between physicians and staff nurses. The ACNP can encourage all health-care providers to implement a systematic pain-management approach, such as that in the Pain Relief Algorithm and other pain-management guidelines (U. S. Department of Health and Human Services, 1992, 1994, WHO, 1986, 1996).

Educating the patient and family on pain-management strategies is important, yet teaching other health-care providers is equally as important. The nurse practitioner can advocate for a holistic approach to treating pain. Knowing that pain has affective, behavioral, and cognitive aspects as well as physical components, the ACNP can enhance pain management by using complementary approaches to treatment and palliative pain control.

ACNPs do not have futuristic Star Tech equipment for pain management, but tools for practice are better than in the days of the Civil War. Today and into the twenty-first century, the ACNP will be able to use research findings from many disciplines to provide optimal care to seriously ill people who experience pain. This care will focus on appropriate treatment of the illness, disease, or injury causing the pain and on palliative management of the pain to improve patient outcomes.

REFERENCES

American Nurses Association. (1990). Position statement on the role of the registered nurse (RN) in the management of analgesia by catheter techniques (epidural, intrathecal, intrapleural, or peripheral nerve catheters). Washington, DC: ANA.

American Nurses Association. (1992). Compendium of position statements on the nurse's role in end-of-life decisions. Washington, DC: ANA.

American Nurses Association. (1996). ANA's position on assisted suicide. *American Nurse, 28* (4), 9.

American Pain Society. (1998). *Principles of analgesic use in the treatment of acute pain and chronic cancer pain: A concise guide to medical practice* (4th ed.). Skokie, IL: American Pain Society.

American Pain Society Quality of Care Committee. (1995). Quality improvement guidelines for the treatment of acute pain and cancer pain. *JAMA, 274* (23), 1874–1880.

Basbaum, A. I., Clanton, C. H., & Fields, H. L. (1976). Opiate and stimulus-produced analgesia: Functional anatomy of a medullospinal pathway. *Proceedings of the National Academy of Sciences of the United States of America, 73* (12), 4685–4588.

Berry, D. L., Wilkie, D. J., Huang, H. Y., & Thomas, C. R. (submitted, 1998). Patient's goals for cancer pain control and their use of analgesics.

Bjorkman, R., Hallman, K. M., Hedner, J., Hedner, T., & Henning, M. (1994). Acetaminophen blocks spinal hyperalgesia induced by NMDA and substance P. *Pain, 57,* 259–264.

Bonica, J. J. (Ed.). (1990). *The management of pain* (2nd ed.). Philadelphia: Lea & Febiger.

Casey, L., Minoshima, S., Morrow, T. J., & Koeppe, R. A. (1996). Comparison of human cerebral activation pattern during cutaneous warmth, heat pain, and deep cold pain. *Journal of Neurophysiology, 76,* 571–581.

Cashman, J. N. (1996). The mechanisms of action of NSAIDs in analgesia. *Drugs, 52* (suppl. 5), 13–23.

Cassell, E. J. (1982). The nature of suffering and the goals of medicine. *New England Journal of Medicine, 306,* 639–645.

Cleeland, C. S., Nakamura, Y., Mendoza, T. R., Edwards, K. R., Douglas, J., & Serlin, R. C. (1996). Dimensions of the impact of cancer pain in a four country sample: New information from multidimensional scaling. *Pain, 67* (2–3), 267–273.

Coderre, T. J., Katz, J., Vaccarino, A. L., & Melzack, R. (1993). Contribution of central neuroplasticity to pathological pain: Review of clinical and experimental evidence. *Pain, 52* (3), 259–285

Cousins, M. (1994). Acute and postoperative pain. In P. D. Wall, & R. Melzack (Eds.), *Textbook of pain* (3rd ed.). (pp. 357–385). New York: Churchill Livingstone.

Christrup, L. L. (1997). Morphine metabolites. *Acta Anaesthesiologica Scandinavica, 41* (1, pt. 2), 116–122.

Dalton, J. A. & McNaull, F. (1997). A call for standardizing the clinical rating of pain intensity using a 0 to 10 rating scale. *Cancer Nursing, 21* (1), 46–49.

Dickenson, A. H. (1995). Central acute pain mechanisms. *Annals of Medicine, 27,* 223–227.

Eriksson, L. S., Broom´e, U., Kalin, M., & Lindholm, M. (1992). Hepatotoxicity due to repeated intake of low doses of paracetamol. *Journal of Internal Medicine, 231* (5), 567–570.

Fields, H. L. (1987). *Pain.* New York: McGraw-Hill.

Fields, H. L. & Basbaum, A. L. (1994). Central nervous system mechanisms of pain modulation. In P. D. Wall & R. Melzack (Eds.), *Textbook of pain* (3rd ed.). (pp. 243–257). New York: Churchill Livingstone.

Fields, H. L. & Heinricher, M. M. (1985). Anatomy and physiology of a nociceptive modulatory system. *Philosophical Transactions of the Royal Society of London Series B: Biological Sciences, 308* (1136), 361–374.

Garnett W. R. (1996). GI effects of OTC analgesics: Implications for product selection. *Journal of the American Pharmaceutical Association, 36,* 565–572.

Garoutte, B. (1981). *Survey of functional neuroanatomy.* Greenbrae, CA: Jones Medical Publications.

Gee, N. S., Brown, J. P., Dissanayake, V. U., Offord, J., Thurlow, R., & Woodruff, G. N. (1996). The novel anticonvulsant drug, gabapentin (neurontin), binds to the alpha$_2$ delta subunit of a calcium channel. *Journal of Biological Chemistry, 271* (10), 5768–5776.

Gonzales, R., Goldyne, M. E., Taiwo, Y. O., & Levine, J. D. (1989). Production of hyperalgesic prostaglandins by sympathetic postganglionic neurons. *Journal of Neurochemistry, 53* (5), 1595–1608.

Gottschalk, A., Smith, D. S., Jobes, D. R., Kennedy, S. K., Lally, S. E., Noble, V. E., Grugan, K. F., Seifert, H. A., Cheung, A., Malkowicz, S. B., Gutsche, B. B., & Wein, A. J. (1998). Preemptive epidural analgesia and recovery from radical prostatectomy: A randomized controlled trial. *JAMA, 279* (14), 1076–1082.

Guilbaud, G., Besson, J. M., Oliveras, J. L., & Liebeskind, J. C. (1973). Suppression by LSD of the inhibitory effect exerted by dorsal raphe stimulation in certain spinal cord interneurons in the cat. *Brain Research, 61,* 417–422.

Herz, A. (1996). Peripheral opioid analgesia—Facts and mechanisms. *Progress in Brain Research, 110,* 95–104.

Jones, A. K. P. (1997). Pain, its perception, and pain imaging. *IASP Newsletter, 3,* 3–5.

Kanner, R. (1997). *Pain management secrets.* Philadelphia: Hanley & Belfus.

LeBar, D., Dickenson, A. H., & Besson, J. M. (1979). Diffuse noxious inhibitory controls DNIC. Effects on dorsal horn convergent neurons in the rat. *Pain, 6,* 283–304.

Levine, J. D., Gordon, N. C., & Fields, H. L. (1978). The mechanism of placebo analgesia. *Lancet, 2,* 654–657.

Max, M. B., Zeigler, D., Shoaf, S. E., Craig, B. E., Benjamin, J., Li, S. -H., Buzzanell, C., Perez, M., & Ghosh, B. C. (1992). Effects of a single dose of desipramine on postoperative morphine analgesia. *Journal of Pain and Symptom Management, 7,* 454–462.

McCaffery, M. & Beebe, A. (1989). *Pain: A clinical manual for nursing practice.* St. Louis: Mosby.

McGuire, D. B. (1997). Measuring pain. In M. Frank-Stromborg & S. J. Olsen (Eds.), *Instruments for clinical health care research (2nd ed.).* (pp. 528–564). Boston: Jones and Bartlett.

McQuay, H., Carroll, D., Jadad, A. R., Wiffen, P., & Moore, A. (1995). Anticonvulsant drugs for management of pain: A systemic review. *British Medical Journal, 311,* 1047–1052.

Melzack, R. (1975). The McGill Pain Questionnaire: Major properties and scoring methods. *Pain, 1,* 277–299.

Melzack, R. & Wall, P. (1965). Pain mechanisms: A new theory. *Science, 150,* 971–979.

Merskey, H. & Bogduk, N. (1994). *Classification of chronic pain: Descriptions of chronic pain syndromes and definitions of pain terms.* Seattle: IASP Press.

Miller, L. G. (1990). Cigarettes and drug therapy: Pharmacokinetic and pharmacodynamic considerations. *Clincal Pharmacy, 9,* 125–135.

Miser, A. W., Moore, L., Greene, R., Gracely, R. H. & Miser, J. S. (1986). Prospective study of continuous morphine infusions for therapy related or cancer related pain in children and young adults with cancer. *Clinical Journal of Pain, 2,* 101–106.

Myklebust, E. K., Wilkie, D. J., Cain, K., Huang, H. Y. & Fortner, P. (submitted, 1998). Measurement of pain: Quantifying pain intensity word descriptors.

Omoigui, S. (1995). *The Pain Drugs Handbook.* St. Louis: Mosby.

Page, G. G. & Ben Eliyahu, S. (1997). The immune-suppressive nature of pain. *Seminars in Oncology Nursing,13* (1), 10–15.

Patt, R. B. (1993). *Cancer pain.* Philadelphia: J. B. Lippincott.

Pederson, D. C. (1997). Preemptive analgesia. *CRNA, 8,* 110–113.

Portenoy, R. K., Foley, K. M., Stulman, J., Khan, E., Adelhardt, J. & Layman, M. (1991). Plasma morphine and morphine-6-glucuronide during chronic morphine therapy for cancer pain: Plasma profiles, steady-state concentrations, and the consequences of renal failure. *Pain, 47* (1), 13–19.

Porter, J. & Jick H. (1980). Addiction rare in patients treated with narcotics. *New England Journal of Medicine, 302,* 123.

Puntillo, K. A. (1991). *Pain in the critically ill: Assessment and Management.* Gaithersburg, MD: Aspen.

Puntillo, K. A. & Wilkie, D. J. (1991). The assessment of pain in the critically ill. In K. A. Puntillo (Ed.), *Pain in the critically ill: Assessment and management* (pp. 45–64). Gaithersburg, MD: Aspen.

Raj, P. P. (1992). *Practical management of pain.* St. Louis: Mosby.

Ramamurthy, S. & Rogers, J. N. (1993). *Decision making in pain management.* St. Louis: Mosby.

Robison, J. M., Wilkie, D. J., & Campbell, B. (1995). Sublingual and oral morphine administration: Review and new findings. *Nursing Clinics of North America, 30* (4), 725–743.

Rosomoff, H. L., Papo, I., & Loeser, J. (1990). Neurosurgical operations on the spinal cord. In J. J. Bonica (Ed.), *The management of pain: Vol. II* (pp. 2067–2081). Philadelphia: Lea & Febiger.

Sato, J. & Perl, E. R. (1991). Adrenergic excitation of cutaneous pain receptors induced by peripheral nerve injury. *Science, 251,* 1608–1610.

Sevarino, F. B. & Preble, L. (1992). *A manual for acute postoperative pain management.* New York: Raven Press.

Sidedall, P. J. & Cousins, M. J. (1997). Spine update: spinal pain mechanisms. *Spine, 22,* 98–104.

Sindrup S. H., Poulsen, L., Broesen, K., Arendt-Nielsen, L., & Gram, L. F. (1993). Are poor metabolisers of sparteine/debrisoquine less pain tolerant than extensive metabolisers? *Pain, 53* (3), 335–349.

Stambaugh, J. & Drew, J. (1988). A double-blind parallel evaluation of the efficacy of a single dose of ketoprofen in cancer pain. *Journal of Clinical Pharmacology, 28,* S39.

Stambaugh, J. E. & Lane, C. (1983). Analgesic efficacy and pharmacokinetic evaluation of meperidine and hydroxyzine, alone and in combination. *Cancer Investigations, 1,* 111–117.

Sweet, W. H., Poletti, C. E. & Gybels, J. M. (1994). Operations in the brainstem and spinal canal, with an appendix on the relationship of open to percutaneous cordotomy. In P. D. Wall, & R. Melzack (Eds.), *Textbook of pain,* (3rd ed.) (pp. 1113–1135). New York: Churchill Livingstone.

Tesler, M. D., Savedra, M. C., Holzemer, W. L., Wilkie, D. J., Ward, J. A., & Paul, S. M. (1991). The word–graphic rating scale as a measure of children's and adolescents' pain intensity. *Research in Nursing and Health, 14,* 361–371.

Tesler, M. D., Wilkie, D. J., Holzemer, W. L., & Savedra, M. C. (1994). Postoperative analgesics for children and adolescents: Prescription and administration. *Journal of Pain and Symptom Management, 9,* 85–95.

Turk, D. C. & Melzack, R. (Eds.). (1992). *Handbook of pain assessment.* New York: Guilford Press.

U.S. Department of Health and Human Services. (1992). Clinical practice guideline. Acute pain management: Operative or medical procedures and trauma. Rockville, MD: Agency for Health Care Policy and Research.

U.S. Department of Health and Human Services. (1994). Clinical practice guideline. Management of cancer pain. Rockville, MD: Agency for Health Care Policy and Research.

Wagner, M. L. & Silberstein, S. D. (1996). Headache. In E. T. Herfindal & D. R. Gourley (Eds.), *Textbook of therapeutics* (6th ed.). Baltimore: Williams & Wilkins.

Wall, P. D. & Melzack, R. (1994). *Textbook of pain* (3rd ed.). New York: Churchill Livingstone.

Warfield, C. A. (1991). *Manual of pain management.* Philadelphia: J. B. Lippincott.

Warfield, C. A. (1993). *Principles and practice of cancer pain management.* New York: McGraw-Hill.

Weissman, G. (1991). The actions of NSAIDs. *Hospital Practice, 26,* 60–76.

Wilkie, D. J. (1993). Pharmacological management of cancer pain: Summary of the science. *Journal of the National Cancer Institute, 85,* 1117–1120.

Wilkie, D. J., Kampbell, J., Cutshall, S., Halabisky, H., Harmon, H., Johnson, L. P., Weinacht, L., & Rake-Marona, M. (submitted, 1998). Effects of Massage on Pain Intensity, Analgesics and Quality of Life in Patients with Cancer Pain: A Pilot Study of a Randomized Clinical Trial Conducted within Hospice Care Delivery. *Hospice Journal.*

Wilkie, D. J., Keefe, F. J., Dodd, M. J., Copp, L. A. (1992). Behavior of patients with lung cancer: Description and associations with oncologic and pain variables. *Pain, 51,* 231–240.

Wilkie, D., Lovejoy, N., Dodd, M., & Tesler, M. (1988). Cancer pain control behaviors: Description and correlation with pain intensity. *Oncology Nursing Forum, 15,* 723–731.

Wilkie, D. J., Savedra, M. C., Holzemer, W. L., Tesler, M. D., & Paul, S. M. (1990). Use of the McGill Pain Questionnaire to measure pain: A meta-analysis. *Nursing Research, 39,* 36–41.

Wilkie, D. J., Vivenzo, K., & Puntillo, K. (1991). Point: Registered nurses should administer and monitor spinal analgesia within the state-defined scope of practice—The California perspective. *Nurse Anesthesia, 2,* 6–9.

Willis, W. D. & Westlund, K. N. (1997). Neuroanatomy of the pain system and of the pathways that modulate pain. *Journal of Clinical Neurophysiology, 14,* 2–31.

Woolf, C. J. & Wiesenfield-Hallin, Z. (1985). The systemic administration of local anaesthetics produce a selective depression of C-afferent fiber evoked activity in the spinal cord. *Pain, 23,* 361–374.

World Health Organization. (1986). *Cancer pain relief.* Geneva: WHO.

World Health Organization. (1996). *Cancer pain relief* (2nd Edition). Geneva: WHO.

Yaksh, T. L. (1991). The spinal pharmacology of anomalous pain processing. In K. L. Casey (Ed.), *Pain and central nervous system disease: The central pain syndromes* (pp. 243–256). New York: Raven Press.

Yaksh, T. L. & Malmberg, A. B. (1993). Spinal actions of NSAIDs in blocking spinally mediated hyperalgesia: The role of cyclooxygenase products. *Agents Actions, (Suppl), 41,* 89–100.

21

Wound Management

JoAnne D. Whitney
Sarah Layman

Wounds occur when there is a break in the integument or the continuity of soft tissues and underlying structures associated with trauma, surgery, or invasive procedures. Wounds are classified in various ways, including anatomic location of the wound, source of injury, depth of tissue involvement, degree of contamination, and whether the wound is acute or chronic. It is recognized that not all wounds, for a variety of reasons, follow the usual course of healing. It was with this in mind that Lazarus et al. (1994) suggested definitions of wounds and guidelines for assessing and evaluating wound healing. Definitions of healing (Fig. 21–1) and important components of the wound history and physical exam are listed in Table 21–1.

Wounds have common characteristics, including asymmetry, the presence of a center or dead space, and an edge (Hunt, 1988). Regardless of the initiating event, there is a common physiological pathway for healing consisting of specific cellular and tissue responses. Cells that do not normally exist together travel to the area of injury and participate in the steps of the healing process. There is increasing understanding of how tissue repair occurs, made possible by techniques that allow the study of cellular signaling, angiogenesis, matrix formation, epithelialization, contraction, and other healing responses at the molecular level. This developing knowledge guides the application of therapies that are physiologic and promote a local environment that optimizes healing and limits wound complications.

▶ PHYSIOLOGY OF WOUND HEALING

Tissue repair occurs through multiple vascular, cellular, and biochemical responses. A number of cells—polymorphonuclear leukocytes (PMNs), macrophages, fibroblasts, endothelial, and epithelial—function together to restore tissue integrity. Inflammation, cellular proliferation and migration, synthesis of connective tissue, and remodeling are common features of healing. Wounds sustained by critically ill patients heal by these processes, though the healing response and time for healing may differ due to factors such as the extent of the wound, presence of infection, or nutritional status.

Wounds heal by primary intention, secondary intention, or delayed primary closure. Wounds healing by primary intention are closed surgically. In secondary intention healing, the wound is left open, and, in third intention, the wound is left open for several days and closure performed when bacterial contamination is controlled. Typically, wounds that heal by primary intention involve minimal synthesis of connective tissue, while wounds healing by secondary intention require greater synthesis of connective tissue, new vessels, and epithelium to reestablish tissue continuity. Events early in the course of healing (e.g., cell migration) are important to those later in the healing sequence (e.g., synthesis of collagen). Healing is often described in terms of major phases: inflammation, prolifera-

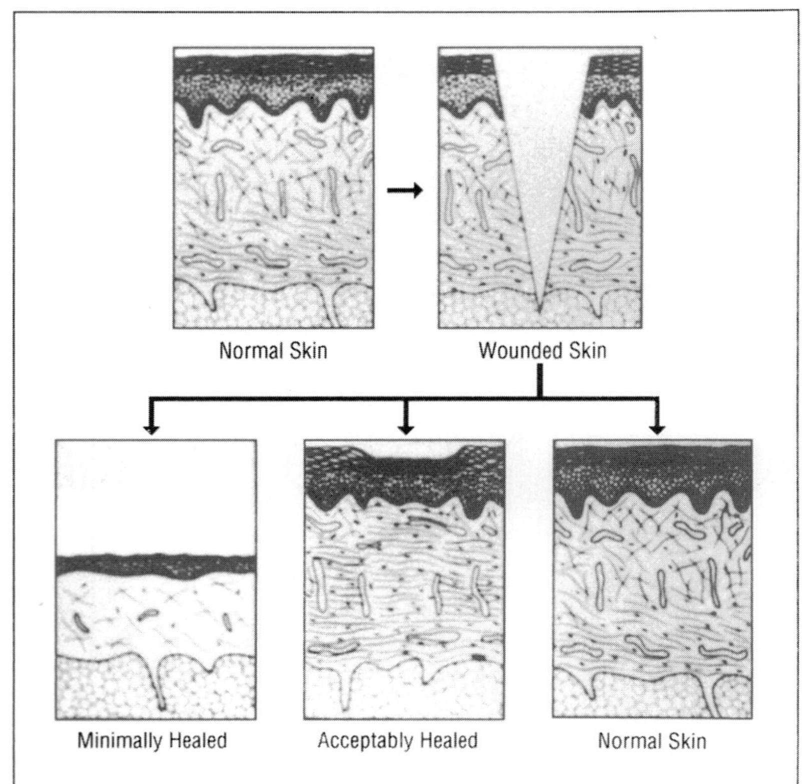

Figure 21–1. Prototypic forms of wound healing. An ideally healed wound results in a return to normal anatomic function, structure, and appearance. A minimally healed wound results in the restoration of anatomic continuity but without a sustained functional result. An acceptably healed wound is characterized by restoration of sustained functional and anatomic continuity. *(From Lazarus, G. S. et al., (1994).* Archives of Dermatology, 130, *p. 490. Copyright American Medical Association. Used with permission.)*

tion (synthesis of collagen, new vessels, and epithelium), and remodeling of the scar. The major phases of healing, cellular, and matrix components are shown in Figure 21–2.

Inflammation and Cellular Migration

Inflammatory responses to injury include vasoconstriction and activation of the coagulation, complement, and kinin cascades that initiate the healing process. Soon after injury, growth factors released by platelets and other inflammatory cells attract macrophages and fibroblasts to the area of injury. The platelet factors serotonin and thromboxane A_2 induce vasoconstriction, while platelet derived growth factor is mitogenic and chemotactic for fibroblasts (Knighton, Fiegel, Doucette, & Fylling, 1989; Seppa, Grotendorst, Seppa, Schiffmann, & Martin, 1982). Others—platelet derived angiogenic factor, platelet derived epidermal growth factor, transforming growth factors alpha and beta, and platelet factor IV—are chemotactic for endothelial cells, epidermal cells, monocytes, and neutrophils, and stimulate the production of collagen by fibroblasts respectively (Deuel, Senior, Chang, Griffin, Heinrikson, & Kaiser, 1981; Knighton, Hunt, Thakral, & Goodson, 1982; Oka & Orth, 1983; Sporn, Roberts, Wakefield, & de Cormbrugghe, 1987). Biologically active molecules from complement activation opsonize and lyse bacteria cause mast cell histamine release and attract PMNs and monocytes to the area of injury (Leibovich, 1984). Monocytes in injured tissue develop into macrophages that influence collagen synthesis through production of cytokines that stimulate fibroblasts (Leibovich & Ross, 1976; Olsen, 1984).

Proliferation

Inflammation is followed by the proliferative phase of healing where the synthesis of collagen by fibroblasts occurs. Fibroblasts also synthesize proteoglycans and elastin. It is collagen that provides strength and support to new tissues as it is deposited and crosslinked. Collagen formation is linked to the enzymes lysl and prolyl hydroxylase and the presence of molecular oxygen, ascorbate, iron, and alpha–ketoglutarate. Because of these requirements, tissue perfusion, pulmonary function, and nutrition are important clinical factors. Procollagen molecules secreted into the extracellular wound space become tropocollagen through enzymatic peptidase cleavage. Tropocollagen fibrils band together, cross link, and overlap to form collagen fibers. Collagen is both synthesized and degraded in a continual

TABLE 21–1. History and Physical Exam Findings Important in Defining Wounds

History	
Wound	***Periwound***
Location	Spontaneous pain
Duration	Induced pain
Spontaneous pain	
Induced pain	
Positional pain	
Prior wound manipulation	
Exudate	
Odor	
Physical Examination	
Location	Erythema
Color: elevated/dependent	Induration
	Edema
Odor	Lymphangitis
Fibrin	Callus
Necrosis	Joint abnormalities
Undermining	Capillary refill
Tunnel/sinus formation	Hair distribution
Exposed tissues	Exposed tissue
Instrument probe	Function and status of surrounding organs

Used with permission from Lazarus G. S. et al., (1994) (p. 491). Copyright American Medical Association.

process of turnover that increases the strength of the final scar (Enquist & Adamson, 1965). Collagen strength increases as fibrils are compressed and as water and mucopolysaccharides are lost from the wound. These processes remodel the newly formed connective tissue into an organized and stronger matrix. By the third week after injury, the wound has its greatest mass and net collagen loss begins.

New capillary growth and connective tissue proliferation are related processes. The new vessels provide a continued supply of cofactors and nutrients for wound healing and formation of the granulation bed that consists of fibroblasts, collagen, new vessels, and macrophages. New capillaries, supported by the collagen matrix, arise from endothelial buds of existing venules in the injured tissues. Tissue hypoxia in the central space of a wound where oxygen levels are low (0-3 mm Hg) act as one stimulus for both collagen synthesis and angiogenesis (Folkman, 1974). Hypoxic wound gradients stimulate macrophages to produce plasminogen activator, mitogenesis factor(s), and angiogenesis factor(s) that, in turn, stimulate angiogenesis (Knighton, Oredsson, Banda, Werb & Hunt, 1982). While the full range of angiogenic cytokines is not known, there are a number of likely factors including lactate and fibroblast growth factors (Folkman & Klagsbrun, 1987). The

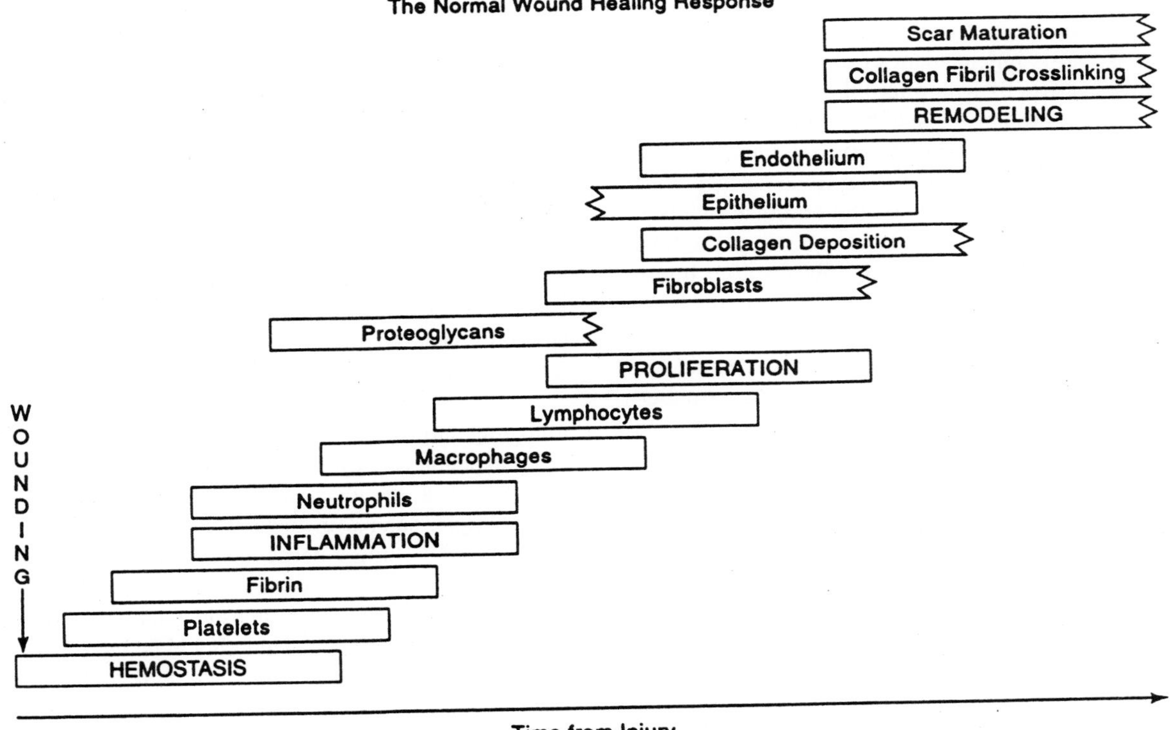

Figure 21–2. Temporal relationship between the multiple processes occurring in dermal wound healing. *(Used with permission from Mast, B. A. [1992]. The skin. In I. K. Cohen, R. F. Diegelmann, & W. J. Lindblad (Eds.).* Wound healing: Biochemical and clinical aspects. *Philadelphia: W. B. Saunders, p. 347.)*

reestablishment of higher oxygen levels in the wound space as healing continues is thought to decrease secretion of macrophage angiogenesis factor (Knighton et al., 1982).

The migration of epithelial cells across wounds protects against entry of bacteria into the wound and wound fluid loss. Possible signals for epithelial cell proliferation and migration, which begins within 24-48 hours after injury, include a "free edge" of tissue created from the injury as well as release of local cytokines (Clark, 1996). When the layer is complete, the cells again divide to form another layer of epithelium. If wounds become dry, eschar forms on the wound surface and limits movement of epithelial cells from the wound edge. In wounds allowed to heal in a moist, protected environment, epithelial cells migrate more easily across the wound. The classic work of Winter (1962) and others demonstrated that the rate of epithelialization in surgical epidermal wounds that were kept moist was twice as fast as wounds exposed to air with scab formation, showing that moisture facilitates tissue repair.

Remodeling

As healing progresses, connective tissue is remodeled and the size of open wounds decreases through contraction of granulation tissue and scar as well, the inward movement of the surrounding skin. Wound location and shape affect contraction. Wounds in areas where tissue is loose contract more and wounds with square edges contract faster than wounds that are circular (Lawrence, 1996). The mechanisms of contraction are not well understood but it appears to be a process that is independent of changes in collagen. Both myofibroblasts (cells with microfibril and microtubule components) and fibroblasts have been proposed as the cells responsible for contraction (Majno, Gabbiani, Hirshal, Ryan, & Statkov, 1971; Ehrlich, 1984). As local metabolic needs of the tissue decrease, edema, the numbers of fibroblasts, and blood vessels also recede. Remodeling, the final tissue repair process, begins about three weeks after injury and continues over many months. The scar tissue loses mass and gradually gains strength as collagen becomes more organized. As scar tissue matures, the red, edematous, firm scar softens, lightens to pink, and becomes smaller. Scar tissue is strengthened through remodeling. Skin and fascia, however, achieve only about 80% of their original strength by 3 to 6 months post injury in wounds closed by primary intention; less than that in wounds that close by secondary intention.

SURGICAL WOUNDS

The majority of surgical wounds heal by primary intention, where wound edges are approximated at the completion of the operative procedure. The method of delayed primary closure (also known as third intention) is used when the wound is highly contaminated and risk of infection believed to be high. In this case the wound is left open for a short time (5-10 days) while wound contamination is reduced and then is closed either with tape or sutures. Wounds that heal by secondary intention are left open and heal by the formation of granulation tissue, epithelial migration, and wound contraction.

Surgical Wound Treatment

In any wound, the purpose of the dressing is to protect the wound from external contamination, to provide material to absorb wound exudate if it is present, and to provide some level of thermal insulation. The choice of surgical wound dressings is based largely on tradition and preference of the provider. Gauze remains the most common surgical wound dressing. Gauze provides absorbency and thermal protection but is not occlusive to the entry of bacteria from external sources. If gauze dressings become wet, they are unable to prevent the entry of bacteria and in fact allow bacteria to be "wicked" toward the wound (Alexander, Gammage, Nichols, & Gaskins, 1992). Dressings that are occlusive, such as the hydrocolloid dressings or semipermeable transparent dressings, are gaining acceptance as postoperative wound coverings. These dressings maintain a moist environment that promotes epithelialization, and provide a more effective barrier to entry of external bacteria than gauze dressings. Concerns about increased infection rates with the use of semiocclusive or occlusive wound coverings have not been substantiated in clinical studies and infection rates have been below levels that occur with gauze dressings (Hulten, 1994; Hutchinson & Lawrence, 1990; Rubio, 1991).

Wounds that heal by primary intention are reepithelialized within 24 to 48 hours. The initial surgical dressing is generally left on for 48 hours while the epithelial seal is established. However, dressings do need to be changed when they become saturated with blood or other body fluids. If bleeding is excessive, the source needs to be located and hemostasis reestablished. In some cases this may require the removal of a hematoma that is preventing wound closure. The wound should be reopened, the clot evacuated, and—if bacterial contamination is not suspected—the wound edges reapproximated (Coit & Sclafani, 1991).

Removal of sutures is usually performed 5 to 15 days following surgery. The length of time that sutures are left in place depends on location of the wound, the amount of tension placed on the incision, and the desired cosmetic result. For example, sutures in facial incisions may be removed a few days after surgery because there is adequate local blood supply, little tension on the forming scar, and minimal scar formation is desired. Suture lines located on the trunk, lower extremities, or in obese patients should be left in longer (7-14 days) to permit greater wound strength to be established, though the wound still has limited tensile strength at this time.

Surgical Wound Infection

Surgical wounds are still the most common site of nosocomial infection (Horan et al., 1993). Wound classification systems for surgical wounds are designed to predict risk of complications; specifically, infection. Correct classification helps the practitioner to identify patients who are most at risk for developing infections and to institute preventive therapies. The traditional classification system proposed by the American College of Surgeons has four categories and is based on level of wound contamination (Table 21–2).

The SCENIC risk index, developed by the Centers for Disease Control and Prevention (CDC) has four factors: the site of the operation, the duration of the surgical procedure, the estimated degree of contamination, and the number of diagnoses when the patient is discharged (Haley, Culver, Morgan, White, Emori & Hooton 1985). Haley et al. (1985) found that abdominal procedures, surgery longer than 2 hours, a classification of contaminated or infected by the traditional system, and having three or more underlying diagnoses were the factors associated with the greatest risk of wound infection. Each of these factors is given a score of one, so that highest risk is equal to 4 and lowest to 0.

Another index, the National Nosocomial Infection Surveillance (NNIS)—a variation of the SCENIC index—is also used to follow wound infection rates and identify patients at risk (Culver et al., 1991). The NNIS rating assigns a risk index score of 0 to 3 depending on assessment of three factors (Table 21–3). Use of any of these assessment methods helps to identify patients at risk of developing wound infections; the SCENIC and the NNIS methods, however, are better predictors than the traditional classification system (Haley et al., 1985; Culver, et al., 1991).

Wound infection occurs when microorganisms overwhelm host defenses, invading tissues and eliciting a response of fever, pain, erythema, induration, and increased tissue temperature. All wounds are contaminated to some degree and have resident bacteria. It is the number of organisms, the virulence of the organism, and the condition of the patient that influences the development of true wound infection. It is recognized that the presence of greater than 10^5 organisms per gram of tissue is associated with impaired healing and/or wound infection. It should also be noted that, although infection is likely with this level of bacterial contamination, some wounds heal (Robson, Duke, & Krizek, 1973). Wounds may be cultured either by biopsy or swab, though currently biopsy is viewed as the more informative method. However, in many settings swab cultures remain the more common method. The technique with which a swab culture is performed is critical to obtaining meaningful results. It is particularly important that the wound be cleansed prior to doing a swab culture. If this is done, swab cultures have been shown to correlate well with tissue biopsy (Thomson & Smith, 1994). With either culture method, the emphasis in quantifying bacteria should be placed on organisms that are invading the tissue and not those that colonize the wound surface.

Common pathogens associated with wound infections vary by anatomical site. The anatomic sites or types of injury and common organisms that are likely to become pathogenic during healing are listed in Table 21–4. Treatment of surgical wound infection once identified or highly suspected may require reexploration of the wound, drainage of any pockets, and dressing of the open wound area with moist saline gauze. Topical antiseptics are usually not necessary and are associated with adverse cellular effects to fi-

TABLE 21–2. Traditional Wound Classification

Wound Class	Wound Description
I	Clean (Elective, noninfected, without drains)
II	Clean-Contaminated (Respiratory, Gastrointestinal, or Genitourinary tracts are entered but contamination is minimal)
III	Contaminated (Traumatic wounds, break in sterile technique)
IV	Infected (Infected tissue entered during surgery)

From Coit, D. G. & Sclafani, L. Care of the surgical wound. Section VI. Chapter 7. In, D. W. Wilmore, L. Y. Cheung, A. H. Harken, et al. (eds.). Scientific American Surgery. *Copyright 1991, Scientific American, Inc. All Rights Reserved.*

TABLE 21–3. National Nosocomial Infection Surveillance (NNIS) Risk Factors

Risk Factor	Description
American Society of Anesthesia Score	Preoperative assessment score of 3, 4, or 5
Level of contamination	Surgery classified as contaminated or infected
Length of surgery	Number of hours above predetermined level, specific to type of surgery

TABLE 21–4. Common Organisms and Their Anatomic Site

Anatomic Site	Organism(s) or Likely Pathogens
Skin	*Staphylococcus aureus;* Streptococcus
Oropharynx	Oral anaerobes: Peptostreptococcus, Fusobacterium, *Bacteroides melaninogenicus,* Peptococcus
Stomach	Oral anaerobes; Enterics *(E coli, Klebsiella, Enterobacter)*
Colon	*Bacteroides fragilis;* Enterics; Enterococcus
Biliary tract	Enterics; Enterococcus; *Bacteroides fragilis,* Clostridium
Vagina	Enterics; Enterococcus, *Bacteroides fragilis;* Streptococcus
Burns	*Staphylococcus aureus;* Pseudomonas
Traumatic wounds	*Staphylococcus aureus;* Group A Streptococcus; Clostridium
Devitalized tissue	*Staphylococcus aureus;* Clostridium
Chronic wounds	Pseudomonas species; Proteus species, *Staphylococcus aureus;* Streptococcus

broblasts (Brown & Zitelli, 1995). Changing the moistened gauze dressings every 6 to 8 hours and irrigating the open wound with sterile normal saline using a 19-gauge needle or angiocatheter and 30-cc syringe decreases wound bacterial counts. Patients who have cellulitis, deep wound infections, or signs of sepsis require treatment with systemic antibiotics. Prior to antibiotic therapy a gram stain is obtained to direct initial therapy with culture and sensitivity results to follow. Antibiotic selection is based on the known/suspected organism, known/suspected sensitivity, patient allergy, associated toxicities, and the cost of the drug.

Factors Influencing Postsurgical Wound Healing

Diabetes

Individuals with either insulin dependent diabetes (IDDM) or non-insulin dependent diabetes (NIDDM) are at risk of healing problems. These problems are attributed to elevated serum glucose levels and changes in the functional ability of neutrophils and lymphocytes, reductions in inflammatory response after injury, and defects in collagen synthesis (Mowat & Baum, 1971). Tissue ischemia related to changes in large and small vessels also contributes to impaired healing (Moran & Colen, 1990). Healing problems can occur in both acute and chronic wounds. Metabolic control in the postoperative period is important for tissue repair. Elevated glucose levels associated with surgery, trauma, or infection require surveillance and treatment. If hyperglycemia is corrected in the first postoperative week, normal healing can be achieved (Goodson & Hunt, 1977). Hemoglobin A1C levels of 9% (mean values) are associated with normal connective tissue formation, suggesting normal production of collagen when serum glucose levels are normalized (Goodson & Hunt, 1984). A maximum preprandial serum glucose level of 11.1 mmol/L (200 mg/dL) and a minimum goal of 6.7 mmol/L (120 mg/dL) are guidelines based on limiting the risks of hyperglycemia or hypoglycemia while supporting wound healing and leukocyte function (Hirsch, Paauw, & Brunzell, 1995).

Control of serum glucose levels in patients with NIDDM may benefit healing but this has not been shown experimentally. Poor healing in genetically obese NIDDM rodents was not improved with either insulin therapy or dietary measures (Goodson & Hunt, 1986). However, case reports of wound infection and delayed healing following plastic surgery have been reported in patients with previously undetected impaired glucose tolerance (Guyuron & Rasqewski, 1990). The presence of diabetes should be investigated when healing complications occur in the absence of other factors such as nutritional deficiencies or known perfusion problems.

Chemotherapy, Corticosteriods, Radiation

Chemotherapeutic agents disrupt the normal cycle of tumor and healthy cells and induce thrombocytopenia and leukopenia. These effects place the patient at risk and unable to mount the normal inflammatory response that is needed for wound healing. While many experimental studies have shown adverse healing effects associated with chemotherapeutic agents, the effects in humans have not been well established. At present, general knowledge suggests that if chemotherapy is needed following surgery that it be delayed several days (Coit & Sclafani, 1991).

Glucocorticoids adversely affect wound healing. Moderate doses within 2 to 3 days of injury delay skin incision healing in animals (Ehrlich & Hunt, 1968). Similarly, the strength of intestinal anastomoses is decreased in steroid-treated animals (Furst, Stromberg, Baltchford, Christensen & Thorson, 1994; Matsusue & Walser, 1992). The inhibitory wound-healing effects of glucocorticoids occur with doses that increase levels above those in the physiologically normal range. The mechanisms underlying the wound-healing effects are not well understood but are believed to be related to the antiinflammatory effects of steroids, and to their effects on fibroblasts and collagen synthesis (Durant & Duval 1986). Delays in wound healing can be counteracted by administration of vitamin A 25,000 IU systemically per day (Lawrence, 1992). Vitamin A in an ointment preparation can also be used topically for 7 to 10 days (Hunt, 1986).

Radiation damages cells and decreases tissue vascularity, leaving tissue vulnerable to poor healing. Fibroblasts, which are critical in healing, are abnormal after radiation exposure (Lawrence, 1992). Because cells are damaged, the levels of growth factors within the wound area are also affected (Tibbs, 1997). Because of these changes patients who have had radiation and subsequent surgery or trauma should be followed closely for impairments in healing.

Nutrition

Wound healing requires protein, carbohydrates, fats, vitamins, and trace elements. Nutrients are particularly important in the inflammatory and proliferative phases of healing when the local wound metabolism is increased. Protein supplies amino acids for enzymes, angiogenesis, and collagen, and maintains oncotic pressure. Carbohydrates provide energy for cells and, if supplies are insufficient, amino acids are supplied by depletion of protein stores. Fats are also an energy source and linoleic acid, which is needed for the synthesis of linolenic and arachidonic acids (cell membrane components), cannot be synthesized so must be supplied dietarily. Vitamin C is required for collagen synthesis, maintenance of capillary integrity, and function of leukocytes (Levenson, Crowley, & Geever, 1964). Plasma levels of vitamin C are rapidly depleted following severe injury and humans are unable to synthesize this vitamin to maintain physiologic levels. While scurvy is rare, patients who are elderly, smokers, and/or have cancer, liver disease, or acute injury are at risk of vitamin C depletion and are likely to need supplementation. Vitamin A is known for its ability to reverse the negative effects of corticosteroids on healing

(Hunt & Ehrlich, 1968). It is also necessary for epithelialization, collagen synthesis and crosslinking, immune function, and avoidance of infections. Vitamin A deficiencies are associated with depletion of liver stores when there has been a prolonged decrease in intake such as gastrointestinal digestive or absorption disturbances. Vitamin D is needed for calcium metabolism and bone healing, and vitamin K is needed for the synthesis of prothrombin and factors VII, IX, and X to avoid negative wound healing effects associated with excessive bleeding. Thiamine, riboflavin, niacin, pyridoxine, folate, and cyanocobalmin are enzyme cofactors, and deficiencies are associated with metabolic disturbances in protein, carbohydrate, and fat. However, their specific roles in wound healing are not well documented.

The trace elements—magnesium, copper, and selenium—serve as enzyme cofactors. Copper is required for crosslinking of collagen. Zinc is also a cofactor for collagen production and is involved in enzymatic reactions and epithelial repair. Deficiency of zinc is likely to disrupt formation of granulation tissue and reduce wound strength (Albina, 1994). However, it should be noted that zinc supplementation to nondeficient patients does not improve healing and can have detrimental effects on phagocytosis and collagen synthesis. Patients who are most likely to be zinc deficient are those with reduced food intake or increased gastrointestinal losses from diarrhea or fistuli drainage. Iron participates in wound healing through its role in binding and transporting oxygen and also is a cofactor for collagen synthesis. A hematocrit of 17% or above is believed to be sufficient for oxygen delivery (LaVan & Hunt, 1990).

Recently, the amino acids arginine and glutamine have been reported to be beneficial to healing (Barbul, Lazarou, Efron, Wasserkrug, & Efron, 1990; Kirk et al., 1993; Nirgiotis, Hennessey, & Andrassy, 1987) though direct evidence in human healing linked to clinical outcomes has not been established. Arginine is a precursor for proline, which is a component of collagen. Glutamine is the primary fuel of the gut mucosa, and is also utilized by fibroblasts, lymphocytes, and epithelial cell migration. The use of glutamine and arginine supplementation in practice remains controversial and further study is needed to demonstrate their efficacy to influence wound healing clinically.

Growth hormone acts to decrease protein catabolism, promote protein synthesis, promote fat mobilization, and stimulate release of insulin-like growth factor (ILGF). ILGF in turn acts to reduce protein degradation, increase amino acid uptake by cells, and cellular proliferation. Growth hormone has increased wound strength in animals (Atkinson, Kosi, Srikanth, Takan, & Costlin, 1992) and been associated with faster healing of skin graft donor sites in burned children with adequate nutritional intake (Gilpin et al., 1994). Adequate protein–calorie repletion is needed in conjunction with growth hormone to achieve maximum anabolic effects.

Malnutrition is well-documented among general surgical, orthopedic, elderly, and critically ill populations (Bistrian, 1974; Haydock & Hill, 1986; Gherini, 1993). Preoperative metabolic state including acute illness prior to surgery or injury are factors that predispose patients to decreased healing (Windsor, Knight, & Hill, 1988; Goodson, Jensen, Granja-Mena, Lopez-Sarmiento, West, & Chavez-Estrella, 1987). Patients with wounds, drains, and secretions have multiple routes of protein loss. Loss of 14 to 20 grams of urea nitrogen per day is not uncommon (Streat, Beddoe, & Hill, 1987).

Despite recognition of the importance of nutrition to healing, therapy for the purposes of wound healing is not well defined. It is useful to screen based on the patient demonstrating evidence of impaired physical function, and in clinical situations where major surgery is planned, or the patient is metabolically stressed (Windsor & Hill, 1991). Specific guidelines for nutrient supplementation related to wound healing are dispersed throughout the literature. Recommendations are summarized in Table 21–5. Correcting deficiencies is desirable, but giving vitamin C or A to achieve above-normal levels does not necessarily accelerate healing (Albina, 1994). Timing of nutritional support is more important than the route by which it is provided. Perioperative starvation and delays in feeding should be avoided, especially for patients in a catabolic state. Wound healing has been promoted by parenteral and enteral feeding, including the nasojejunal route (Daly et al., 1992; Law & Ellis, 1990; Schroeder, Gillanders, Mahr, & Hill, 1991). Providing enteral nutrition requires the presence of normal gut enzymes and motility. Use of the gut helps to maintain the mucosa and its competence. Until guidelines for nutritional support of wound healing are better defined, the statement that "wound nutrition is in fact whole body nutrition" (Hunt & Goodson, 1988, p. 635) serves patients well.

Oxygenation and Perfusion

The delivery of molecular oxygen to the wound is dependent on adequate perfusion. Oxygen is needed for the hydroxylation of proline and lysine on the forming collagen chains, and the quality of collagen is adversely affected if there is insufficient oxygen for this process. Other aspects of healing that require oxygen include angiogenesis and epithelial repair. Control of bacteria in wounds is also largely dependent on levels of oxygen in tissue. Leukocytes use large amounts of oxygen during the respiratory burst and production of oxygen radicals that destroy bacteria. Data available from general surgery patients indicate there is an optimum level of perfusion and oxygen tension in healing tissues that helps to reduce the incidence of wound infections (Hopf, et al., 1997). Based on clinical studies, the patients most likely to suffer from inadequate tissue oxygen levels are those experiencing trauma, and cardiac or vascular surgery (Chang, Goodson, Gottrup, & Hunt, 1983).

Measures to insure an adequate blood flow and supply

TABLE 21–5. Nutrients Recommended for Wound Healing

Nutrient	Role in Healing	Suggested Daily Intake
Protein	Supplies amino acids for enzymes, collagen synthesis, new vessel growth	1.25–3.0 Gm/kg (Bergstrom, et al., 1994; Streat & Hill, 1987)
Carbohydrates	Provide energy for cells	50% of daily calories
Fats	Cell wall components, energy source	5–30% of daily calories (Berger & Adams, 1989)
Vitamin C	Cofactor in collagen synthesis, maintenance of capillary structure, leukocyte function	600 mg up to 2 Gm (severe injury or deficiency) (Bergstrom, et al., 1994; Levenson & Demetriou, 1992)
Vitamin B Complex	Enzyme cofactors	5–10 times the recommended daily allowance (Levenson & Demetriou, 1992)
Vitamin A	Counteracts effects of corticosteroids; collagen synthesis, epithelial repair, immune function	25,000 IU for malnourished, GI dysfunction, or severe injury (Levenson & Demetriou, 1992)
Zinc	Cofactor for collagen synthesis and enzymes	4.5–6.0 mg for acute catabolic state; additional 12.2 mg/L of small bowel fluid loss (Levenson & Demetriou, 1992)

of oxygen to healing tissues are aimed at supporting the vascular and pulmonary systems. Supplemental oxygen can be administered to patients at risk, including those who have had emergent procedures, lengthy and extensive surgeries, or procedures where contamination is likely (Chang et al., 1983; LaVan & Hunt, 1990). Since measuring actual tissue oxygen levels is not possible in most clinical situations, SpO_2 monitoring can be used. An SpO_2 of 94% is likely to be inadequate for healing and can serve as a clinical indicator signaling the need for oxygen administration (Hopf & Sessler, 1994). Adequate vascular volume is needed for supplemental oxygen to reach the wound. Therefore, effective treatment may require supplemental fluids, depending on the patient's hydration status. There is little research on hydration levels that support tissue oxygen; however, existing evidence indicates small volumes (e.g., 250-500 cc bolus) may be helpful in restoring perfusion to peripheral tissues (Chang et al., 1983; Jonsson, Jensen, Goodson, West, & Hunt 1987). An increase in standard fluid replacement levels of 1.1 liter on the day of surgery has been shown to support peripheral tissue oxygen and wound healing in general surgery patients (Hartmann, Jonsson, & Zederfeldt, 1992). Either crystalloid or colloids are effective in supporting perfusion and tissue oxygen (Hartmann, Jonsson, & Zederfeldt, 1993).

Temperature

In recent years there has been better understanding of how control of body temperature and the application of local heat can assist wound healing. As body temperature is lowered in the perioperative period, thermoregulatory responses cause vasoconstriction that impairs perfusion to the skin and subcutaneous tissues. Maintaining normothermia intraoperatively and early postoperatively can reduce the risk of infection. Experimentally, animals with core temperatures of 36°C during anesthesia have shown decreased resistance to *E coli* (Sheffield, Sessler, & Hunt, 1994). In a randomized double-blind study, patients whose core temperatures were kept near 36.5°C during surgery had fewer postsurgical wound infections and were discharged home sooner than those who were hypothermic (core temperature of 34.5°C) (Kurz, Sessler, & Lenhardt, 1996). Application of heat locally to wounds is an effective way to increase local blood flow and oxygen (Rabkin & Hunt, 1986); however, further study is needed of specific therapies using heat to determine the efficacy for wound healing. Existing evidence indicates it is important to maintain normal temperature to protect against infection and preserve blood supply to healing tissues.

PRESSURE ULCERS

First described in the 1800s, pressure ulcers have only recently been identified as a major health-care issue. The cost of treatment has been estimated to be between $14,000 and $40,000 per patient, potentially lengthening a patient's hospital stay by a minimum of 3 to 5 days (Maklebust & Sieggreen, 1996). As money allocated for health care declines, patients with pressure ulcers are moved into primary care settings under the care of practitioners unfamiliar with the variety of dressings and treatment options available today. It is important then that the practitioner has a basic understanding of the causes of pressure ulcers, the goal of treatment, and the tools available to reach that goal.

Pathophysiology

Although not recognized as such, the skin is the largest organ, weighing from 6 to 8 pounds and covering more than 20 square feet (Maklebust & Sieggreen, 1996). It protects other organs from bacterial invasion, facilitates excretion while protecting the body from excessive moisture loss, maintains normal body temperature, and conducts sensations to the brain for immediate evaluation and action. Pressure ulcers interrupt the function of the organ and can be life threatening if enough surface area is damaged and open.

A pressure ulcer is any injury caused by unrelieved or repeated pressure that results in varying levels of damage to underlying tissue (U.S. Department of Health and Human Services, 1992). Although it occurs primarily below the waist, any area compressed against a bony prominence can be injured in a variety of ways: prolonged exposure to external pressure or repeated exposure to pressure without sufficient time for ischemic tissue to reperfuse. Tissues must have adequate circulation for the "transcapillary exchange of oxygen, carbon dioxide, nutrients, wastes and regulatory substrates" (Lee & Thoden, 1985). When the tissues are compressed against bone by an external force for varying lengths of time, capillaries are compressed and become thrombosed. This process leads to tissue ischemia and edema with further circulation compromise and possible hemorrhage. Exchange of oxygen and nutrients abates and metabolic wastes accumulate leading to cell death (Maklebust & Sieggreen, 1996).

The pressure injury is transmitted from the body surface to the bone in a cone-shaped fashion, so the appearance of the size of the wound is deceptive. Seventy percent of the destruction is below the surface where tissue meets bone. Muscle and fat are more susceptible to pressure injury, so what is seen on the surface is the smallest part of the wound. In fact, muscle may be necrotic even before the wound appears on the skin (Maklebust & Sieggreen, 1996).

Risk Factors

Certain populations and conditions have been identified that place the patient at increased risk of pressure ulcers. The elderly and critically ill patients develop ulcers more often than the general population. And, although they vary somewhat from author to author, commonly identified high-risk factors include shearing, friction, moisture, level of consciousness, and nutritional status (U.S. Department of Health and Human Services, 1992; Bryant, Shannon, Pieper, Braden, & Morris, 1992).

Increased age is identified because of the natural changes that take place with aging. There is loss of sweat glands, decreased padding below the surface, thinning of tissue, reduced cohesion between dermis and epidermis, and decreased levels of collagen. Critical care populations are at increased risk because of their multiple medical conditions, poor nutritional status, and decreased level of consciousness.

Shearing injuries occur when the deep tissues attached to bone shift in the opposite direction from stationary surface tissue. This happens, for instance, when a patient is sitting in bed at an angle greater than 30 degrees. The skin sticks to the bed linens, while the deep fascia attached to the bones slides down because of its weight and the forces of gravity. Vessels are then distorted and stretched causing thrombosis and possible hemorrhage. Deprived of oxygen and nutrition, tissue becomes ischemic, edematous, and necrotic, and an ulcer develops. In addition, the tissue then becomes less tolerant of additional injury from even smaller amounts of pressure and injury occurs more rapidly.

Friction injuries also place the patient at risk for injury. As a patient is pulled across bed sheets, or spontaneously rubs bony prominences across coarse surfaces, the stratum corneum is removed. This accelerates the development of pressure ulcers as water is lost and moisture is allowed to accumulate against the skin (Lee & Thoden, 1985).

Moisture through incontinence or perspiration may be one of the greatest identified risk factors, second only to pressure itself (Lee & Thoden, 1985; Maklebust & Sieggreen, 1996; U. S. Department of Health and Human Services, 1992). Urine and feces increase the pH and, together, create ammonia. The activity of fecal proteases and lipases increases and the skin becomes more susceptible to irritants, often burning when exposed to these caustic substances. When macerated by constant exposure to dampness, connective tissues are softened and skin is more easily sloughed (Maklebust & Sieggreen, 1996), altering the skin's ability to protect against bacterial and fungal contamination.

In addition to shearing, friction, and moisture, decreased level of consciousness is a well-documented risk for the development of ulcers. When sedated or restrained, the patient either doesn't feel pain or may be unable to react to discomfort by changing positions. The longer in one position without movement, the more chance for injury. Prolonged pressure is an important factor in the development of pressure ulcers (Bryant et al., 1992; U.S. Department of Health and Human Services, 1992).

Finally, poor nutritional status places the patient at risk for ulcer formation. Low serum albumin levels are associated with protein malnutrition and high levels of mortality. Low protein levels change the oncotic pressures and can lead to edema. There is poor exchange of nutrients and oxygen through edematous tissue (Bryant et al., 1992). This then leads to ischemia and eventually tissue death. Vitamin deficiency slows the production of collagen and reepithelialization, which results in slower healing and increased capillary fragility (Doughty, 1992).

Measurement of Wound Extent

Measurements can be taken in a variety of ways, although most practical methods are deficient in some way. Tracings, photographs using graphing film, and measurements are easily done but do not assess the depth of the wound. Nor can all of these methods be used when there is tunneling. Linear measurements are objective and describe the length and width of the open area. It is sometimes difficult for the practitioner to determine the edges of the wound to maintain accuracy from measurement to measurement. Also, strict measurement says nothing about the wound appearance and must be accompanied by a detailed description. This method is inexpensive, however, and easily done by all health-care providers.

Photographs can provide measurement when developed on graphing film and also provide a visual account of the appearance. This allows for easy comparison over time. It is important, however, that the picture be taken from the same distance so the graphing measurement is accurate. Unfortunately, instant cameras may not have high-quality resolution, so color from picture to picture may be somewhat distorted.

Tracings are done using templates (often provided by dressing manufacturers) or with transparent paper. They can be difficult when wounds are located in awkward areas, but can provide a rough estimate of changes occurring over time when compared with previous tracings (Bryant et al., 1992).

Wound Evaluation

Classification or staging of wounds helps the practitioner determine treatment needed. The extent of the wound should be established when the patient is first seen by the practitioner. A four-stage classification system, based on extent of tissue damage, has been promoted by numerous groups and recently incorporated into the Agency for Health Care Policy and Research (U.S. Department of Health and Human Services, 1992) guidelines. Stage I refers to nonblanchable erythema of the skin. This is the first indicator of skin damage. Stage II is partial thickness injury involving epidermis and/or dermis and appears as an abrasion, blister, or crater. Stage III denotes full thickness injury with damage or necrosis to the subcutaneous tissue and may extend to the fascia. Stage IV refers to extensive destruction and necrosis of deep tissue including muscle, bone, or joints. This presents as a deep crater and may include undermining and sinus tract formation.

It is important to realize that wounds containing eschar and necrotic tissue cannot be staged until the wound base can be seen and evaluated. It is also difficult to stage darkly pigmented patients. Staging does not describe exudate, condition of the wound itself, or the surrounding layers; rather, it relies on the experience of the practitioner at identifying tissue types (Cooper, 1990; Cooper, 1992). As wounds heal they do not progress through earlier stages; for example, an initial stage IV ulcer does not become a stage III ulcer. This has been termed "downstaging" and is not recommended as a way to monitor progress (Rodeheaver & Stotts, 1995). An accurate description must accompany the initial ulcer staging and continue as the wound heals for proper assessment.

A method of classification that incorporates assessment is the Red–Yellow–Black system introduced by Marion Laboratories (Stotts & Washington, 1990). This method of classification, although simplistic, allows the practitioner to look closely at the wound and evaluate it based on the color of the surface. This also allows the practitioner to learn that wounds change in appearance over time and treatments should change accordingly. Black refers to wounds with predominance of eschar at the base that must be removed for proper healing to take place. Yellow refers to slough tissue that again must be removed to enhance healing. Finally, Red refers to healthy, granulating tissue that needs to be kept moist and protected to continue to heal well (Cuzzel, 1990).

A more detailed evaluation of healing can be made using the 15-item Pressure Sore Status Tool (PSST) (Bates-Jensen, 1995). Though more lengthy than the Red–Yellow–Black assessment approach, the PSST allows the practitioner to follow the status of several important wound healing indices (location, shape, size, depth, edges, undermining, necrotic tissue type/amount, exudate type/amount, surrounding skin color, peripheral tissue edema and induration, granulation, and epithelial tissue). Each of the factors are given a score between 1 and 5 based on specific findings on physical examination, providing a total score for the wound that falls between 1 (healthy tissue) and 65 (wound degeneration). This type of evaluation is useful for monitoring wound progress on a weekly basis so that wound status and changes in specific indices can be determined. Reported interrater and intrarater reliability with this instrument have been high, particularly when used by advanced practice nurses (Bates-Jensen, Vredevoe, & Brecht, 1992; Bates-Jensen, 1995).

Once classified, promotion of rapid wound healing with the best functional and cosmetic results becomes the objective (Wiseman, Rovee, & Alvarez, 1992). Therapy is guided by the basic principles dictating (1) removal of necrotic tissue and debris; (2) cleansing the wound, and (3) providing a local wound environment that is physiologic. In the acute stage, it is important to remove any debris and to prevent further damage while controlling infection. Phagocytic action during the initial inflammatory stage assists with cleaning. Scrubbing with betadine and chlorhexidine, and cleansing with hydrogen peroxide should be avoided since these have proven to be cytotoxic to new tissue (Doughty, 1992). The rule of thumb is: place within the wound only what you could place within your eye (Branemark, 1966). Normal saline is sufficient for cleaning. Pressures of between 4 and 15 PSI are considered safe and effective for the removal of bacteria and debris (Bergstrom, Bennett, Carlson, et al., 1994). For example, saline delivered with a 30-cc syringe through a 19-gauge needle or angiocatheter provides sufficient force to remove debris, including bacteria (Edlich, Rodeheaver, & Thacker, 1992), while allowing new epithelial cells to remain in place. Cleaning with higher pressures (water pik) should only be used in heavily contaminated wounds.

Management

The best treatment is prevention. Toward that end, many tools have been developed to aid in assessment and identification of patients at risk. The most widely used tools are the Braden Scale (Table 21–6), Norton Scale (Table 21–7), and

Gosnell Scale, which have been studied extensively. Each identifies mental status or level of consciousness, activity, and continence (moisture) as assessment criteria. The Braden Scale also identifies nutritional status, friction and shear, and spontaneous movements, rating each parameter from 1 to 4. A lower score yields a higher risk for developing pressure ulcers. In addition to level of consciousness, activity, and continence, the Norton Scale recognizes physical conditioning and mobility. It also rates each risk factor on a scale of 1 to 4. Again, the lower the score, the greater the risk for getting an ulcer. Finally, the Gosnell Scale changed the Norton Scale slightly, deleting conditioning and adding nutrition. With this tool, the higher the score, the greater the risk. Each scale can be effective in identifying patients at risk as it ensures systematic evaluation of individuals at risk. Each identifies the need for intervention. However, no tool is of value if it is not used routinely.

There are many common interventions that effectively reduce the risk of ulcers. Most important, to reduce injury by reducing the duration of insult, the patient must be repositioned every two hours even when sitting up (U.S. Department of Health and Human Services, 1992). For some patients, however, even two hours between turns can be too long and tissue damage may occur. Turning schedules should be designed for the individual based on evaluation of skin tolerance in areas that are exposed to pressure. Nonblanchable erythema, or reactive hyperemia (increased, persistent erythema) that lasts longer than three quarters of the amount of time that pressure was applied, are indications that turning frequency needs to be increased.

The need for added cushioning with pillows or other devices that relieve pressure over bony prominences and distribute the pressure more evenly must be considered. Heels should be elevated or cushioned using a heel protector. When turning side to side, the patient should not be placed directly onto the trocanter because of the intense pressure created over that bony area. A lateral position at a 30- to 45-degree tilt works best.

Outdated devices such as donuts and sheepskin should be avoided (Alterescu & Alterescu, 1988). Recent research has shown donuts and ring devices actually increase pressure and cause venous congestion to the surrounding tissue and reduce capillary flow to the injured area (Bryant et al., 1992; Crewe, 1987; U.S. Department of Health and Human Services, 1992). If the patient has many additional risk factors, a support surface, either static or dynamic, such as an air- or fluid-filled overlay may be needed. There are also several mattress replacements now on the market that reduce interface pressures more than conventional mattresses. Finally, high and low air loss beds and beds that provide constant repositioning through passive motion are available, although expensive. These beds provide pressure relief instead of pressure reduction and should be considered in patients with many risk factors and who already have breakdown on more than one surface.

When placing a patient into an upright position, the head of the bed should be less than 30 degrees. Sheets should be loose so they slide with the patient rather than hold the patient in place, which can lead to a shearing injury. Patients should be lifted, not dragged across linens, to prevent friction burns. If seated, the patient should be upright to maintain proper alignment and to keep from sliding downward, which leads to shearing injury. It is also important the pressure be distributed across the posterior thigh, not on the ischial tuberosities.

Other common interventions include keeping the skin clean and dry, preferably using warm water since alkaline soaps reduce the number of stratum corneum cells (Bryant et al., 1992). Excessive rubbing with a harsh towel can cause friction injury and should be avoided. Incontinence should be controlled and, if excessive, a moisture barrier cream should be used to protect the surrounding skin from additional injury.

Nutritional supplements in the form of snacks or formula feedings should be used to correct any nutritional deficits. Caloric needs should be based on ideal weight, not actual weight. All nutritional parameters, i.e., serum albumin, total lymphocyte count, serum cholesterol, electrolytes, hemoglobin, and weight, should be checked routinely every 2 to 4 weeks (Doughty, 1992; Pinchcofsky-Devin, & Kaminiski, 1986; Sanders, 1992).

Even though risk factors are identified and interventions are applied consistently, some patients still develop ulcers. The practitioner must determine the cause and intervene to prevent further damage. Then the wound must be measured and classified so the practitioner can decide whether it can be treated successfully with dressings, or if surgical intervention is needed.

Wound Dressings

Once cleaned, the wound should be covered with a dressing (Norris, Provo, & Stotts, 1990; Doughty, 1992; Maklebust & Sieggreen, 1996; Walker, 1996). In the past, many wounds were kept open to air and allowed to dry out. Exposed wounds, however, become more inflamed and necrotic and develop more scarring (Wiseman et al., 1992). Epithelial cells, proliferating during the inflammatory stage, are forced to move below dry scab to find enough moisture to support migration. Hence, healing is slowed. Now, semiocclusive and occlusive dressings are the treatment choice for wounds as they provide a moist environment that allows for easy cell migration. Pain is also reduced, perhaps because nerve endings are covered (Wiseman et al., 1992). Table 21–8 summarizes information on wound characteristics and appropriate dressing choices.

Transparent Dressings. There are many types of semiocclusive and occlusive dressings that provide for adequate hydration and oxygenation. Whatever the practitioner decides to use, it should be easy to apply and allow freedom of movement. When dressing a stage I or stage II ulcer or

TABLE 21–6. Braden Scale for Predicting Pressure Sore Risk

Patient's Name________________ Evaluator's Name________________ Date of Assessment

SENSORY PERCEPTION ability to respond meaningfully to pressure related discomfort	1. *Completely Limited:* Unresponsive (does not moan, flinch, or grasp) to painful stimuli, due to diminished level of consciousness of sedation. OR Limited ability to feel pain over most of body surface.	2. *Very Limited:* Responds only to painful stimuli. Cannot communicate discomfort except by moaning or restlessness. OR Has a sensory impairment which limits the ability to feel pain or discomfort over 1/2 of body.	3. *Slightly Limited:* Responds to verbal commands, but cannot always communicate discomfort or need to be turned. OR Has some sensory impairment which limits ability to feel pain or discomfort in 1 or 2 extremities.	4. *No Impairment:* Responds to verbal commands. Has no sensory deficit which would limit ability to feel or voice pain or discomfort.
MOISTURE degree to which skin is exposed to moisture	1. *Constantly Moist:* Skin is kept moist almost constantly by perspiration, urine, etc. Dampness is detected every time patient is moved or turned.	2. *Very Moist:* Skin is often, but not always moist. Linen must be changed at least once a shift.	3. *Occasionally Moist:* Skin is occasionally moist, requiring an extra linen change approximately once a day.	4. *Rarely Moist:* Skin is usually dry, linen only requires changing at routine intervals.
ACTIVITY degree of physical activity	1. *Bedfast:* Confined to bed.	2. *Chairfast:* Ability to walk severely limited or non-existent. Cannot bear own weight and/or must be assisted into chair or wheelchair.	3. *Walks Occasionally:* Walks occasionally during the day, but for very short distances, with or without assistance. Spends majority of each shift in bed or chair.	4. *Walks Frequently:* Walks outside the room at least twice a day and inside room at least once every two hours during waking hours.
MOBILITY ability to change and control body position	1. *Completely Immobile:* Does not make even slight changes in body or extremity position without assistance.	2. *Very Limited:* Makes occasional slight changes in body or extremity position but unable to make frequent or significant changes independently.	3. *Slightly Limited:* Makes frequent though slight changes in body or extremity position independently.	4. *No Limitations:* Makes major and frequent changes in position without assistance.

NUTRITION usual food intake pattern	1. *Very Poor:* Never eats a complete meal. Rarely eats more than 1/3 of any food offered. Eats 2 servings or less of protein (meat, dairy products) per day. Takes fluids poorly. Does not take a liquid dietary supplement. OR Is NPO and/or maintained on clear liquids or IVs for more than 5 days.	2. *Probably Inadequate:* Rarely eats a complete meal and generally eats only about 1/2 of any food offered. Protein intake includes only 3 servings of meat or dairy products per day. Occasionally will take a dietary supplement. OR Receives less than optimum amount of liquid diet/tube feeding.	3. *Adequate:* Eats over half of most meals. Eats a total of 4 servings of protein (meat, diary products) each day. Occasionally will refuse a meal, but will usually take a supplement if offered. OR Is on a tube feeding or TPN regimen which probably meets most of nutritional needs.	4. *Excellent:* Eats most of every meal. Never refuses a meal. Usually eats a total of 4 or more servings of meat and dairy products. Occasionally eats between meals. Does not require supplementation.
FRICTION AND SHEAR	1. *Problem:* Requires moderate to maximum assistance in moving. Complete lifting without sliding against sheets is impossible. Frequently slides down in bed or chair, requiring frequent repositioning with maximum assistance. Spasticity, contractures or agitation leads to almost constant friction.	2. *Potential Problem:* Moves feebly or requires minimum assistance. During a move skin probably slides to some extent against sheets, chair, restraints, or other devices. Maintains relatively good position in chair or bed most of the time but occasionally slides down.	3. *No Apparent Problem:* Moves in bed and in chair independently and has sufficient muscle strength to lift up completely during move. Maintains good position in bed or chair at all times.	
				Total Score

Used with permission from Braden, B. & Bergstrom, N. 1989. Decubitus, *p. 45.*

TABLE 21–7. Norton Risk Assessment Scale

		Physical Condition	Mental Condition	Activity	Mobility	Incontinent	Total Score
		Good 4 Fair 3 Poor 2 V. Bad 1	Alert 4 Apathetic 3 Confused 2 Stupor 1	Ambulant 4 Walk/Help 3 Chairbound 2 Bed 1	Full 4 Sl. Limited 3 V. Limited 2 Immobile 1	Not 4 Occasional 3 Usually/urine 2 Doubly 1	
Name	Date						

healthy granulating wound, transparent films (Op-Site, Tegaderm, Bioclusive, etc.) are commonly used. They protect the wound from bacteria and injury. Oxygen can enter, water vapor can escape, but normal wound fluid is contained for a moist healing environment. These dressings should not be used if infection is present or if drainage is heavy. After cleaning the wound and surrounding tissue, transparent dressings should be carefully sealed around the edges to prevent bacterial contamination under wrinkles. Cloudy fluid can accumulate under the dressing and should not be confused with pus if no other signs of infection are present. Drainage can be aspirated from the dressing edges with a small gauge needle, but the edges should again be carefully sealed. Finally, transparent dressings can be left in place for 5 to 7 days and should not be changed more frequently than every third day since their adhesive quality can damage intact skin.

Hydrocolloid Dressings. Hydrocolloids (Duoderm, J&J Ulcer, Comfeel, Tegasorb, etc.) work well with clean stage II and III ulcers and also with healthy granulating wounds and exudative wounds. These dressings are absorptive (although not indicated for heavy drainage) and protect the wound from contamination. They maintain a moist environment and provide slow autolytic debridement as wound fluids interact with the hydrocolloid. The wound must be cleaned with saline before the dressing is applied. Exudative wounds should be flushed with saline through a 19-gauge needle on a 30-cc syringe. The hydrocolloid dressing should extend approximately two inches beyond the edges of the wound for proper adherence. Some hydrocolloids are nonadherent and need additional tape to secure in place. However, even if adherent, edges may need to be secured with transparent tape if the wound is located in an area where the dressing may get rubbed off (heels, sacrum). The dressing should be left in place for 3 to 7 days and ideally allowed to soften and fall off. Expect to see a gelatinous material covering the wound when the dressing is removed; this may be rinsed off with saline.

Hydrogel Dressings. Hydrogels (Carrasyn, Nugel, Vigilon, Elastogel, etc.) are indicated for use with stage II, stage III, and clean stage IV, as well as moderately deep healthy granulating wounds and exudative and necrotic wounds. They come in sheets or as amorphous gels. The sheets are absorbent and nonadherent, maintain a moist environment, and conform easily to the wound while reducing pain. They provide some autolytic debridement since they soften eschar and slough over time. Hydrogel should be placed only on the wound as the high water content can cause maceration of surrounding tissue. Amorphous gels can be used as fillers and to cover deep wound beds. Most hydrogel dressings must be held in place with a secondary dressing, although some have an adhering frame surrounding the gel sheet. If allowed to dry out before removal, dampen with saline to prevent debridement of epithelial cells.

Impregnated Dressings. Impregnated dressings (Adaptic, Xeroform, Vaseline, etc.) are used to protect superficial wounds (stage I) with evidence of infection and to prevent dressing adherence in healthy granulating wounds or new surgical wounds. They are nonadherent, some are antibacterial, and all are easy to use. A secondary dressing should be used to hold the impregnated dressing in place and provide further protection.

Gauze, Foam, and Absorption Dressings. Additional dressings that should be considered in the treatment of pressure ulcers are gauze, polyurethane foams (Allevyn, Lyofoam, Epilock, etc.), and absorption dressings (Bard Absorption, Sorbsan, DuoDerm Paste, Debrisan, etc.). Gauze is absorptive and can autolytically debride exudative and necrotic wounds and clean stage III and IV ulcers using the traditional wet-to-moist method of packing. It is very good for packing sinus tracts. It is important to remember when packing a wound that as little dressing as

TABLE 21–8. Properties of Commonly Used Dressing Materials

Dressing Category	Examples	Indications	Advantages	Disadvantages	Considerations
Polyurethane films	Op-site, Tegaderm, Bioclusive, Blisterfilm, Ensureit, Accuderm, Uniflex, Opraflex, etc.	Protection of partial thickness red wounds. Cover dressing for hydrophillic powder and paste preparations and hydrogels	Transparent; good adhesion, waterproof; reduces pain; minimizes friction forces to wound; time saving; easy to store	Adhesive injury to intact and new skin; nonabsorbent, some products difficult to apply; variable barrier function; can promote wound infection	Protect wound margins; avoid in wounds with infection, copious drainage, or tracts; change only if dressing leaks
Hydrocolloids	Duoderm, J&J Ulcer Dr., Comfeel, Restore, Intact Intrasite, Tegasorb, etc.	Protection of superficial and small, deep red wounds. Autolytic debridement of smali, noninfected yellow wounds[a]	Absorbent; nonadhesive to healing tissue; good barrier; waterproof; reduce pain; easy to apply; time saving; easy to store	Nontransparent; may soften and lose shape with heat or friction; odor and brown drainage on removal (melted dressing material)	Frequency of changes will depend on amount of exudate (change as needed for leakage); avoid in wounds with infection or tracts
Hyrdogel sheets	Nugel, Vigilon, Geliperm, Elastogel, Cutinova, etc.	Protection of superficial and moderately deep red wounds. Autolytic debridement of small, noninfected yellow or black wounds[a]	Absorbent; nonadhesive; reduces pain; compatible with topicals; good conformity; easy to store	Poor barrier; semi-transparent; requires cover dressing to secure; can promote growth of *Pseudomonas* and yeast; expensive	Avoid in infected wound; change every 8 hr or as needed for leakage
Hydrophillic beads, powders, and pastes	Bard Absorbtion dressing, Hydrogran, Hoolister Exudate, Absorber, Duoderm granules, Comfeel Powder, Envisan, Debrisan	Cleansing of draining yellow wounds, protection of deep draining and nondraining red wounds (except Envisan and Debrisan). Autolytic debridement of noninfected black wounds[a] (except Envisan and Debrisan)	Good "filler" for deep wounds; absorbs large amounts of exudate; rapid cleansing of yellow wounds; cost effective; helps control odor	Occasional pain on application; requires cover dressing; dressing material leaks out with position change if outer dressing not sealed; difficult to remove from tracts and deep pockets	Partially fill wound cavities to allow for expansion; avoid in wounds with fistulas or deep tracts. Monitor electrolytes if copious drainage
Gel pastes	Carrington Gel, Geliperm, intrasite, Biolex, etc.	Protection of red wounds. Autolytic debridement of noninfected yellow or black wounds	Good "filler" for small deep red wound; easy to apply	Requires cover dressing; expensive; variable absorbency	Same as hydrogels
Foams	Lyofoam, Epi-Lock, Allivin, Cutinova Plus, etc.	Protection of red wounds. Dressing tracheostomy and drain sites	Insulates wound; provides some padding; nonadherent; easy to use; easy to store	Poor absorbency; poor barrier; nontransparent; requires sealing of edges with tape; poor conformability to deep wounds	Change every 24 hours or as needed for leakage; avoid in draining wounds with viscuous exudate
Impregnated dressings	Adaptic, Xeroforj, Aquaphor, Scarlet Red, Vaseline Gauze, etc.	Protection or superficial infected and noninfected red wounds; "contact layer" for primarily closed wounds	Nonadherent (if gauze cover dressing used); antibacterial if medicated; easy to use; easy to store	Some products will adhere to wound if allowed to dry out; poor barrier if nonmedicated	Change at least every 24 hr (if nonadherent); if adherent, allow to separate spontaneously
Cotton and gauze dressings	Wet to dry→ Wet to damp→ Continuous dry→ Continuous moist→	Mechanical debridement of yellow wounds Mechanical debridement of red/ yellow wounds Heavily exudating red wounds Protection of red wounds. Autolytic debridement of yellow or black wounds[a]; delivery of topical meds	Readily available; good mechanical debridement if properly used; cost effective "filler" for large wounds: effective delivery of topicals if kept moist	Delayed healing if used improperly; pain on removal (wet to dry); labor intensive	Use rolled gauze for packing large wounds (ensures complete removal); pack loosely (tight packing delays healing); use wide mesh gauze for debriding; use fine mesh for protection; do not use cotton-filled on wound surface

[a] Use with caution in critically ill patients who are leukopenic or have poor wound perfusion. Avoid in patients with clinically infected wounds.

Used with permission from Cuzzell, J. (1990), (pp. 574–575).

possible should be used to minimize pain associated with the dressing and to encourage drainage. In addition, minimizing packing may promote good cosmetic results by minimizing scar formation. Gauze should be used with gels to maintain a moist environment in some situations. Foams absorb moderate to large amounts of drainage while protecting the wound from additional trauma. They are nonadherent and must be held in place by some other means. Foams are changed as needed, preferably not more than three times a week. Finally, the absorption dressings are used with draining wounds and to fill dead space while providing some autolytic debridement.

Absorptive dressings can absorb up to twenty times their weight, making them ideal for wounds with heavy drainage. Both foams and absorptive dressings are indicated for use with stage III, IV, and exudative wounds. They should not be used with necrotic wounds or wounds with dry eschar.

Biologic Dressings. Biologic dressings, primarily allografts, have long been used as a temporary substitute for skin over extensive burn injuries, to protect and prevent bacterial invasion. More recently, however, investigators have looked into the use of collagen as a wound dressing. As a principle component of the skin matrix, its use within the wound bed to enhance healing makes sense. Collagen has been incorporated into beads, gels, and sheets (Fibracol, Biocare, etc.,) and has been combined with alginate to further aid with absorption and to provide the moist healing environment necessary for optimum healing. Collagen dressings can be used in the treatment of stage I, II, and healthy granulating wounds. When used in combination with alginate, it is very effective with heavy exudate wounds. When exposed to moist environment, the collagen turns to gel if in bead or sheet form.

Growth Factors

The role that growth factors play in the healing process is an area of intensive study. Growth factors are peptides that are released by many types of cells. Their biologic activity includes the induction of cell growth, replication, and migration (Herndon, Hayward, Rutan, & Barrow, 1992). There are numerous growth factors and basic research has increased our understanding of their regulatory functions. There have been clinical studies of their effects in chronic wounds, though our understanding of their role in wound treatment is far from complete. Growth factors that have been studied in clinical trials are platelet derived growth factor (PDGF), transforming growth factor beta (TGF-β_2 and TGF-β_3), fibroblast growth factor (FGF), interleukin 1β, colony stimulating factor (GM-CSF), and epidermal growth factor (EGF). Table 21–9 lists the wound-healing effects and results of these growth factors shown in clinical studies.

While clinical studies indicate that growth factors have beneficial effects on healing in chronic wounds, not all studies have demonstrated significant clinical effects such as faster wound closure. Aspects of study design such as sample size, healing outcome variables, heterogeneous sample, and dosage of the growth factor may account for some of these results.

PDGF—released by platelets after injury—effects monocytes, neutrophils, and fibroblasts. Several studies have examined different isoforms and preparations of PDGF with variable wound-healing results, though in general results look promising (Knighton, Ciresi, Fiegel, et al., 1990; Mustoe, Gutter, Allman, et al., 1994). A recent paper reviews the results of several clinical trials of growth factors (Choucair & Phillips, 1997). As further information on growth factors becomes available, it will guide their use for the treatment of selected nonhealing wounds.

Despite appropriate conservative treatment, some ulcers do not heal. The wound should be evaluated carefully for evidence of infection, including x-rays and biopsy for osteomyelitis, since this can impede the healing process. Also, the practitioner should be mindful of the impact that

TABLE 21–9. Growth Factors and Cytokines in Clinical Development

Growth Factor/Cytokine	Preclinical Effect	Clinical Trial Results
PDGF-BB	↑Neovessels ↑Reepithelialization ↑Granulation tissue	↑Healing in pressure and diabetic ulcers; Phase III trials in progress
TGF-β_2	↑Collagen-containing granulation tissue	↑Healing in venous stasis ulcers; repair of macular holes not successful
TGF-β_3	↑Healing ↓Scarring	Chronic ulcers, in progress
Basic FGF	↑Neovessels in a provisional matrix, ↑Reepithelialization	Pressure ulcers—biological effect; diabetic and venous stasis ulcers no effect
IL-1β	↑Healing in infected open wounds	Pressure ulcers, Phase I study in progress
GM-CSF	↑Healing in incisions	Chronic ulcers, in progress
Acidic FGF	↑Neovessels, ↑Matrix	Diabetic and venous stasis ulcers, in progress
EGF	↑Reepithelialization	Donor graft sites, chronic ulcers, minimal effects

Used with permission from Pierce, G. F. & Mustoe, T. A. (1995) Annual Review of Medicine, 46.

diabetes, venous insufficiency, alcoholism, cigarette smoking, malnutrition, and medications, as discussed earlier, have on the healing process.

A final consideration for pressure ulcer treatment is surgical intervention. If the ulcer is deep, slow to heal, at risk for infection, or if conservative treatment significantly impacts the patient's quality of life, surgery may be the treatment of choice. It can speed the process of healing and restore function and form (Black, 1996). Not every patient is a candidate for surgical intervention and the plastic surgery team must decide on the appropriateness of surgical intervention and the best surgical approach. The practitioner's role is to optimize the patient's physical condition preoperatively so the best possible surgical results can be realized.

In summary, patients at risk for developing pressure ulcers should be identified and assessed accordingly to prevent ulcer development. If an ulcer develops, it must be evaluated weekly so treatments can be adapted to changes within the wound bed as it heals. When patients are seen daily, changes in wound odor, color, and amount of exudate may be indicative of early infection and should be noted. In general, adjustments in wound dressings are made in accordance with the wound status but not more frequently than every 7 to 10 days. Frequent changes in therapy may actually delay healing and make evaluation of the effect of individual treatments difficult.

BURNS

It is estimated that more than two million burns occur each year, with approximately 80% of those being treated by the provider in an outpatient setting (Greenfield & Jordan, 1996). Burns are caused by exposure to some type of heat source, whether it be liquid, flame, chemical, or electricity. Obviously, the longer the exposure and the hotter the source, the greater the injury. Wounds are classified according to depth and percentage of body area affected. They are often described as partial or full thickness.

Minor thermal injuries or partial thickness injuries involve less than 20% of the total body surface. The changes in capillary permeability and fluid loss are limited to the injured area. There is circulatory disturbance with erythema and edema in first-degree burns. Induration and excoriation occur with second-degree burns, revealing the partial-thickness injury, but no full thickness destruction can be seen. These burns are moist and often painful because of loss of epidermal covering and exposure of nerve endings. In appearance, the wound is bright pink to red. If there is partial dermal loss, the wound may be pink with red islets. These islets aid in the healing process since the epidermal cells are capable of regeneration.

Burns respond to insult in much the same way other skin wounds do. Injury to the epidermis, regardless of the cause, sets into motion a cascade of events that eventually lead to healing. There is an immediate inflammatory response followed by growth of epithelial cells, cell migration across the wound bed, and reestablishment of normal skin function. The wound enters the maturation stage approximately three weeks after injury. This phase can last for weeks to years, depending on the extent of injury. During the initial phases, as with all wound healing, it is important to provide adequate oxygenation and moisture to the wound bed, as well as optimizing the nutritional status of the patient, and reducing risk factors that can impede healing (Greenfield & Jordan, 1996).

Many home remedies have been used to treat burns, similar to the practice mentioned previously of leaving wounds open to air. Oils and butter, commonly used in the past, can be detrimental since both can introduce bacteria to the wound and lead to infection. Application of ice compromises circulation and can increase the area of injury. It is important to remember that the principles of moist and occlusive wound healing should be applied to burn injuries.

Management

As stated earlier, epithelial cells need a moist environment for easy migration across the wound bed. Although large surface area burns drain during the acute stage (24-48 hours), if allowed to dry, scab formation inhibits migration and delays healing. Initially, then, the primary dressing should be nonadherent but absorbent and able to prevent maceration of the surrounding tissues. If the drainage is copious, the surrounding tissue may need a moisture barrier cream for protection.

Dressings

When drainage stops, transparent dressings or polyurethane films (Tegaderm, Op-Site, Bioclusive, etc.) can minimize friction, reduce pain, and allow water vapor and oxygen exchange. Films should be restricted to first-degree burns because improper removal can cause adhesive injury to new tissue. Hydrocolloid dressings absorb minimal amounts of drainage and are nonadherent to the new skin. They may be used with both first- and second-degree burns with few contraindications. Finally, hydrogel sheets also absorb minimal amounts of drainage and reduce pain, but most must be held in place with a secondary dressing. The amorphous gels can be applied frequently and do not need secondary dressings to hold in place.

Topical antibiotics are often recommended in minor burn treatment but it is unclear the benefit of use without evidence of infection. It is thought the antimicrobial vehicle (lotion or ointment) enhances healing rather than the antimicrobial itself (Wiseman, et al., 1992). The ointment or lotion provides a moist healing environment and prevents formation of scab. Epithelialization can then occur more easily and wound healing takes place quickly.

Evaluation and Follow-Up

First-degree burns should require no follow-up after initial treatment and the patient can expect healing to occur within five days. Dressings should stay in place during that time to maintain a moist healing environment. Second-degree burns should be followed more closely so adjustments in treatment can be made as necessary. With more tissue damage, expect to see healing occur over a 21-day course, with minimal scarring (Allwood, 1995). In summary, therapy of superficial burn wounds over limited surface area need not be intimidating if the practitioner remembers to maintain a moist healing environment, provide for adequate oxygenation, and protect the wound and surrounding tissue from additional injury.

INFECTIONS IN TRAUMATIC AND CHRONIC WOUNDS

Although wounds often occur under traumatic, nonsterile conditions, many simple and uncomplicated wounds remain uninfected. The development of infection depends on many things, including the type of injury, its location and size, and the overall condition of the injured patient (Trott, 1991). However, several factors increase the risk for infection.

Time is an important factor in the development of wound infections. The longer the time between injury and cleansing, the greater the risk of infection. According to Trott (1991), studies have shown that wounds repaired after 5 hours have higher levels of bacterial growth. Clean wounds and those located in highly vascular areas, however, have reduced risk of infection despite longer lapses in time before cleaning.

In addition to time, the cause and extent of injury as well as the condition of the patient may impact infection rates significantly. Crush injuries often produce large areas of damaged tissue and expose the area to dirt and debris. This places the patient at greater risk for infection. In addition, wounds occurring below the knee or on an arm or hand are more likely to develop an infection than those wounds occurring elsewhere. Finally, the elderly, diabetic, or malnourished patients, and those patients on steroids have greater potential to develop a wound infection.

Although many wounds, particularly traumatic and chronic wounds, become colonized with bacteria, infection does not usually develop unless there are high levels of bacteria, there is foreign matter within the wound, the patient is immunocompromised, or there are comorbid conditions such diabetes, advanced age, and steroid use. As noted earlier, wound infection is defined as bacterial invasion of tissue that overwhelms host defenses and elicits a response. Quantitatively, wound infection is defined as 10^5 or greater bacteria per gram of tissue.

Although trying to discern between colonization and infection can be difficult, a wound usually is not considered infected unless the classic signs of infection (erythema, fever, odor, purulence, and pain) are present. Remember that the diabetic and steroid-dependent patient may not mount that typical systemic response. In some instances, pain or erythema may be the only evidence of infection.

If infection is suspected or the patient has a fever of unknown origin, an open wound should be examined carefully and a white blood cell count should be obtained. Infections disrupt the normal healing process (Doughty, 1992) and potentially place the patient at risk for bacteremia and even sepsis. Early identification is essential. Noninvasive and easy to do, start with a culture of the wound itself. However, with large levels of colonizing bacteria within the wound, culture alone may not be adequate to determine the presence of infection (Kravitz, Lyder, Luehrs, & Fornek, 1994). It is suggested that cultures be obtained through deep-tissue biopsy or fine-needle aspiration, although even aspiration may not be reliable (Rudensky, Lipschits, Issacsohn, & Sonnenblick, 1994; Sapico, Witte, & Canawati, 1984). If confirmed, systemic antibiotics appropriate for the offending agent should be used. Topical antibiotics, although frequently mentioned in the management of infected burn wounds (Martin, 1990), do not provide the coverage or penetration necessary to prevent secondary bacteremia and sepsis in deep wounds or pressure ulcers. If specimens cannot be obtained, a broad spectrum antibiotic is appropriate for coverage.

In summary, although it is difficult to differentiate between wound colonization and infection, it is important to diagnose and treat wound infections as early as possible to prevent complications.

REFERENCES

Albina, J. E. (1994). Nutrition and wound healing. *Journal of Parenteral and Enteral Nutrition, 18,* 367–376.

Alexander, D., Gammage, D., Nichols, A., & Gaskins, D. (1992). Analysis of strike-through contamination in saturated sterile dressings. *Clinical Nursing Research, 1* (1), 28–34.

Allwood, J. (1995). The primary care management of burns. *Nurse Practitioner, 20* (8), 74, 77–79, 83.

Alterescu, V. & Alterescu, K. (1988). Etiology and treatment of pressure ulcers. *Decubitus, 1* (1), 28–35.

Atkinson, J. G., Kosi, M., Srikanth, M. S., Takano, K., & Costin, G. (1992). Growth hormone reverses impaired wound healing in protein-malnourished rats treated with corticosteroids. *Journal of Pediatric Surgery, 27,* 1026–1028.

Barbul, A., Lazarou, S. A., Efron, D. T., Wasserkrug, H. L., &

Efron, G. (1990). Arginine enhances wound healing and lymphocyte immune responses in humans. *Surgery, 108,* 331–337.

Bistrian, B. R., Blackburn, G. L., Hallowell, E., & Heddle, R. (1974). Protein status of general surgical patients. *JAMA, 230,* 858–860.

Black, J. (1996). Surgical options in wound healing. *Critical Care Clinics of North America, 8* (2), 169–182.

Branemark, P. I. (1966). Local tissue effects of wound disinfectants. *Acta Chirurgica Scandinavica, 357,* 166–176.

Brown, C. D. & Zitelli, J. A. (1995). Choice of wound dressings and ointments. *Otolaryngologic Clinics of North America, 28,* 1081–1091.

Bryant, R., Shannon, M., Pieper, B., Braden, B., & Norris, D. (1992) Pressure ulcers. In R. Bryant (ed.), *Acute and chronic wounds: Nursing management* (pp. 105–163). St. Louis: Mosby.

Chang, N., Goodson, W. H., Gottrup, F., & Hunt, T. K. (1983). Direct measurement of wound and tissue oxygen tension in postoperative patients. *Annals of Surgery, 197,* 470–478.

Choucair, M. M. & Phillips, T. J. (1997). What is new in clinical research in wound healing. *Advances in Clinical Research, 15* (1), 45–58.

Clark, R. A. F. (1996). *The molecular and cellular biology of wound repair* (2nd ed.). New York: Plenum Press.

Coit, D. G. & Sclafani, L. (1991). Care of the surgical wound. In D. W. Wilmore, L. Y. Cheung, A. H. Harken, J. W. Holcroft, & J. L. Meakins (eds.), *Surgery, American College of Surgeons* (sec. VI, pp. 7-1–7-10), New York: Scientific American.

Cooper, D. (1990). Human wound assessment: Status report and implications for clinicians. *AACN Clinical Issues in Critical Care Nursing, 1* (3), 553–565.

Cooper, D. (1992). Wound assessment and evaluation. In R. Bryant (ed.), *Acute and chronic wounds: Nursing management* (pp. 69–90). St. Louis: Mosby.

Crewe, R. (1987). Problems of rubber ring nursing cushions and a clinical survey of alternative cushions for ill patients. *Care and Scientific Practice, 5* (2), 9–11.

Culver, D. H., Horan, T. C., Gaynes, R. P., Martone, W. J., Jarvis, W. R., & Emori, T. G. (1991). Surgical wound infection rates by wound class, operative procedure, and patient risk index. *American Journal of Medicine, 91* (Suppl 3B), 152S–157S.

Cuzzel, J. (1990). Choosing a wound dressing: A systematic approach. *AACN Clinical Issues in Critical Care Nursing, 1* (3), 566–577.

Daly, J. M., Lieberman, M. D., Goldfine, J., Shou, J., Weintraub, F., & Rosato, E. F. (1992). Enteral nutrition supplemental arginine, RNA, and omega-3 fatty acids in patients after operations: Immunologic, metabolic, and clinical outcome. *Surgery, 112,* 56–67.

Deuel, T. F., Senior, K. M., Chang, D., Griffin, G. L., Heinrikson, R. L., & Kaiser, E. T. (1981). Platelet factor 4 is chemotactic for neutrophils and monocytes. *Proc Natl Acad Sci USA, 78,* 4584–4587.

Doughty, D. (1992). Principles of wound healing and wound management. In R. Bryant (ed.), *Acute and chronic wounds: Nursing management* (pp. 31–68). St. Louis: Mosby.

Durant, S., & Duval, D. (1986). Factors involved in the control of fibroblast proliferation by glucocorticoids: A review. *Endocrine Reviews, 7,* 254–269.

Edlich, M., Rodeheaver, G., & Thacker, J. (1992). Surgical devices in wound healing management. In I. K. Cohen, R. Diegelmann, & W. Lindblad (eds.), *Wound healing: Biochemical and clinical aspects* (pp. 581–600). Philadelphia: W. B. Saunders.

Ehrlich, H. P. (1984). The role of connective tissue matrix in hypertrophic scar contracture. In T. K. Hunt, R. B. Heppenstall, E. Pines, & D. Rovee (Eds.), *Soft and hard tissue repair* (pp. 533–553). New York: Praeger.

Ehrlich, P., & Hunt, T. K. (1968). Effect of cortisone and vitamin A on wound healing. *Annals of Surgery, 167,* 324–328.

Enquist, I. F. & Adamson, R. J. (1965). Collagen synthesis and lysis in healing wounds. *Minnesota Medicine, 48,* 1695–1698.

Folkman, J. (1974). Tumor angiogenesis. *Advances in Cancer Research, 19,* 331–358.

Folkman, J. & Klagsbrun M. (1987). Angiogenic factors. *Science, 235,* 442–448.

Furst, M. B., Stromberg, B. V., Blatchford, G. J., Christensen, M. A., & Thorson, A. G. (1994). Colonic anastomoses: Bursting strength after corticosteroid treatment. *Disease of the Colon and Rectum, 37,* 12–15.

Gherini, S., Vaughn, B. K., Lombardi Jr, A. V., & Mallory, T. H. (1993). Delayed wound healing and nutritional deficiencies after total hip arthroplasty. *Clinical Orthopaedics and Related Research, 293,* 188–195.

Gilpin, D. A., Bch, M. B., Barrow, R. E., Rutan, R. L., Broemeling, L., & Herndon, D. N. (1994). Recombinant human growth hormone accelerates wound healing in children with large cutaneous burns. *Annals of Surgery, 220,* 19–24.

Goodson, W. H. & Hunt, T. K. (1977). Studies of wound healing in experimental diabetes mellitus. *J Surg Res, 22,* 221–227.

Goodson, W. H. & Hunt, T. K. (1984). Wound healing in well-controlled diabetic men. *Surgical Forum, 35,* 614–616.

Goodson, W. H. & Hunt, T. K. (1986). Wound collagen accumulation in obese hyperglycemic mice. *Diabetes, 35,* 491–495.

Goodson, W. H., Jensen, J. A., Granja-Mena, L., Lopez-Sarmiento, A., West, J., & Chavez-Estrella, J. (1987). The influence of a brief preoperative illness on postoperative healing. *Annals of Surgery, 205,* 250–255.

Greenfield, E. & Jordan, B. (1996). Advances in burn care. *Critical Care Nursing Clinics of North America, 8* (2), 203–213.

Guyuron, B. & Rasqewski, R. (1990). Undetected diabetes and the plastic surgeon. *Plastic Reconstructive Surgery, 86,* 471–474.

Haley, R. W., Culver, D. H., Morgan, W. M., White, J. W., Emori, T. G., & Hooton, T. M. (1985). Identifying patients at high risk of surgical wound infection. *American Journal of Epidemiology, 121* (2), 206–215.

Hartmann, M., Jonsson, K., & Zederfeldt, B. (1992). Effect of tissue perfusion and oxygenation on accumulation of collagen in healing wounds. *European Journal of Surgery, 158,* 521–526.

Hartmann, M., Jonsson, K., & Zederfeldt, B. (1993). Effects of dextran and crystalloids on subcutaneous oxygen tension and collagen accumulation. *European Surgical Research, 25,* 270–277.

Haydock, D. A. & Hill, G. L. (1986). Impaired wound healing in surgical patients with varying degrees of malnutrition. *JPEN, 10,* 550–554.

Herndon, D. N., Hayward, P. G., Rutan, R. L., & Barrow, R. E. (1992). Growth hormones and factors in surgical patients. *Advances in Surgery, 25,* 65–97.

Hirsch, I. B., Brunzell, J., & Paauw, D. S. (1995). Inpatient management of adults with diabetes. *Diabetes Care, 18,* 870–878.

Hopf, H. W., Hunt, T. K., Blomquist, P., Goodson, W. H., Jensen, J.A., Jonsson, K., Paty, P.G., Rabkin, J.A., von-Smitten, K., West, J., & Whitney, J.D. (1997). Wound tissue oxygen tension predicts the risk of wound infection in surgical patients. *Archives of Surgery, 132,* 997-1004.

Hopf, H. W. & Sessler, D. I. (1994). Routine postoperative oxygen supplementation [letter]. *Anesthesia and Analgesia, 79,* 615–616.

Horan, T. C., Culver, D. H., Gaynes, R. P., Jarvis, W. R., Edwards, J. R., & Reid, C. R. (1993). Nosocomial infections in surgical patients in the United States, January 1986-June 1992. *Infect Control and Hospital Epidemiology, 14,* 73–80.

Hulten, L. (1994). Dressings for surgical wounds. *American Journal of Surgery, 167* (Suppl. 1A), 42S–45S.

Hunt, T. K. (1986). Vitamin A and wound healing. *American Academy of Dermatology, 15,* 817–821.

Hunt, T. K. (1988). Prospective: A retrospective perspective on the nature of wounds. *Progress in Clinical and Biological Research, 266,* xiii–xx.

Hutchinson, J. J. & Lawrence, J. C. (1991). Wound infection under occlusive dressings. *Journal of Hospital Infection, 17,* 883–894.

Jonsson, K., Jensen, J. A., Goodson, W. H., West, J., & Hunt, T. K. (1987). Assessment of perfusion in postoperative patients using tissue oxygen measurements. *British Journal of Surgery, 74,* 263–267.

Kirk, S. J., Hurson, M., Regan, M. C., Holt, D. R., Wasserkrug, H. L., & Barbul, A. (1993). Arginine stimulates wound healing and immune function in elderly human beings. *Surgery, 114,* 155–160.

Knighton, D. R., Fiegel, V. D., Doucette, M. M., Fylling, C. P., & Cerra, F. B. (1989). The use of topically applied platelet growth factors in chronic nonhealing wounds: A review. *Wounds, 1,* 71–78.

Knighton, D. R., Hunt, T. K., Thakral, K. K., & Goodson, W. H. (1982). Role of platelets and fibrin in the healing sequence: An in vivo study of angiogenesis and collagen synthesis. *Annals of Surgery, 196,* 379–384.

Knighton, D. R., Oredsson, S., Banda, M., Werb, Z., & Hunt, T. K. (1982). Hypoxia stimulates production of angiogenesis factor, plasminogen activator and growth factor by rabbit bone marrow macrophages. *Fed Proc, 41,* 270.

Kravitz, R., Lyder, C., Luehrs, S., & Fronek, M. (1994). Dermal cultures: Frequency and associated symptoms. *Journal of Wound, Ostomy, and Continence Nursing, 21* (1), 22–25.

Kurz, A., Sessler, D. I., & Lenhardt, R. (1996). Perioperative normothermia to reduce the incidence of surgical-wound infection and shorten hospitalization. *New England Journal of Medicine, 334,* 1209–1215.

Lavan, F. B. & Hunt, T. K. (1990). Oxygen and wound healing. *Clinics in Plastic Surgery, 17,* 463–472.

Law, N. W. & Ellis, H. (1990). The effect of parenteral nutrition on the healing of abdominal wall wounds and colonic anastomoses in protein-malnourished rats. *Surgery, 107,* 449–454.

Lawrence, W. T. (1992). Clinical management of nonhealing wounds. In I. K. Cohen, R. Diegelmann, & W. Lindblad (eds.), *Wound healing: Biochemical and clinical aspects* (pp. 540–561). Philadelphia: W. B. Saunders.

Lawrence, W. T. (1996). Wound healing biology and its application to wound. In J. P. O'Leary & L. R. Capote (eds.), *The physiologic basis of surgery,* (2nd ed., pp. 118–140). Baltimore: Williams & Wilkins.

Lazarus, G. S., Cooper, D. M., Knighton, D. R., Margolis, D. J., Pecoraro, R. E., & Rodeheaver, G. (1994). Definitions and guidelines for assessment of wounds and evaluation of healing. *Archives of Dermatology, 130,* 489–493.

Lee, B. & Thoden, W. (1985). Surgical management of pressure sores. In B. Lee (ed.), *Chronic ulcers of the skin* (pp. 147–170). New York: McGraw-Hill.

Leibovich, S. J. (1984). Mesenchymal cell proliferation in wound repair: The role of macrophages. In T. K. Hunt, R. B. Heppenstall, E. Pines, & D. Rovee (eds.), *Soft and hard tissue repair* (pp. 329–351). New York: Praeger.

Leibovich, S. J. & Ross, R. (1976). A macrophage dependent factor that stimulates proliferation of fibroblasts in vitro. *American Journal Pathology, 84,* 501–514.

Levenson, S. M., Crowley, L. V., & Geever, E. R. (1964). Some studies on wound healing: Experimental methods, effect of ascorbic acid, and effect of deuterium oxide. *Journal of Trauma, 4,* 543–566.

Majno, G., Gabbiani, G., Hirshcel, B. J., Ryan, G. B., & Statkov, P. R. (1971). Contraction of granulation tissue in vitro: Similarity to smooth muscle. *Science, 173,* 548–550.

Maklebust, J. & Sieggreen, M. (1996). *Pressure ulcers: Guidelines for prevention and nursing management.* Springhouse, PA: Springhouse Corporation.

Martyn, J. (1990). *Acute management of the burned patient.* Philadelphia: W. B. Saunders.

Matsusuc, S. & Walser, M. (1992). Healing of intestinal anastomoses in adrenalectomized rats given corticosterone. *American Journal of Physiology, 263,* R164–R168.

Morain, W. D. & Colen, L. B. (1990). Wound healing in diabetes mellitus. *Clinics in Plastic Surgery, 17,* 493–501.

Mowat, A. & Baum, J. (1971). Chemotaxis of polymorphonuclear leukocytes from patients with diabetes mellitus. *New England Journal of Medicine, 284,* 621–627.

Nirgiotis, J. G., Hennessey, P. J., & Andrassy, R. J. (1991). The effects of an arginine-free enteral diet on wound healing and immune function in the postsurgical rat. *Journal of Pediatric Surgery, 26,* 936–941.

Norris, S., Provo, B., & Stotts, N. (1990). Physiology of wound healing and risk factors that impede the healing process. *AACN Clinical Issues in Critical Care Nursing, 1* (30), 545–552.

Oka, Y. & Orth, D. N. (1983). Human plasma epidermal growth factor/beta-urogastrone is associated with blood platelets. *Journal of Clinical Investigation, 72,* 249–259.

Olsen, C. E. (1984). Macrophage factors effecting wound healing. In T. K. Hunt, R. B. Heppenstall, E. Pines, & D. Rovee (eds.), *Soft and hard tissue repair* (pp. 352–360). New York: Praeger.

Panel for the Prediction and Prevention of Pressure Ulcers in Adults. (1992). *Pressure ulcers in adults: Prediction and prevention. Clinical Practice Guideline, Number 3* (AHCPR Publication No. 92-0047). Rockville, MD: U.S. Department of Health and Human Services.

Pinchcofsky-Devin, G., Kaminski, M., & Williams, S. (1986). Correlation of pressure ulcers and nutritional status. *Journal of the American Geriatric Society, 34* (6), 435–440.

Rabkin, J. & Hunt, T. K. (1987). Local heat increases blood flow and oxygen tension in wounds. *Archives of Surgery, 74,* 263–267.

Robson, M. C., Duke, W. F., & Krizek, T. J. (1973). Rapid bacterial screening in the treatment of civilian wounds. *Journal of Surgical Research, 14,* 420–430.

Rubio, P. A. (1991). Use of semiocclusive, transparent film dressings for surgical wound protection: Experience in 3637 cases. *International Surgery, 76,* 253–4.

Rudensky, B., Lipschits, M., Isaacsohn, M., & Sonnenblick, M. (1992). Infected pressure sores: Comparison of methods for bacterial identification. *Southern Medical Journal, 85* (9), 901–903.

Sanders, S. L. (1992). Pressure ulcers, part two: Management strategies. *Journal of American Academy of Nurse Practitioners, 4,* 101–106.

Sapico, F., Witte, J., & Canawati, H. (1984). The infected foot of the diabetic patient: Quantitative microbiology and analysis of clinical features. *Review of Infectious Disease, 6,* 171–176.

Schroeder, D., Gillanders, L., Mahr, K., & Hill, G. L. (1991). Effects of immediate postoperative enteral nutrition on body composition, muscle function, and wound healing. *JPEN, 15,* 376–383.

Seppa, H., Grotendorst, G. R., Seppa, S., Schiffmann, E., & Martin, G. R. (1982). Platelet-derived growth factor is chemotactic for fibroblasts. *Journal of Cell Biology, 92,* 584–588.

Sheffield, C. W., Sessler, D. I., & Hunt, T. K. (1994). Mild hypothermia during isoflorane anesthesia decreases resistance to E coli dermal infection in guinea pigs. *Acta Anaesthesiolggica Scandinavica, 38,* 201–205.

Sporn, M. B., Roberts, A. B., Wakefield, L. M., & de Cormbrugghe, B. (1987). Some recent advances in the chemistry and biology of transforming growth factor-beta. *Journal of Cell Biology, 105,* 1039–1045.

Stotts, N. & Washington, D. (1990). Nutrition: A critical component of wound healing. *AACN Clinical Issues in Critical Care Nursing, 1* (3), 585–591.

Streat, S. J., Beddoe, A. H., & Hill, G. L. (1987). Aggressive nutritional support does not prevent protein loss despite fat gain in septic intensive care patients. *Journal of Trauma, 27,* 262–266.

Thomson, P. D. & Smith, D. J. (1994). What is infection? *American Journal of Surgery, 167,* 7S–10S.

Tibbs, M. K. (1997). Wound healing following radiation therapy: A review. *Radiotherapy and Oncology, 42,* 99–106.

Trott, A. (1991). *Wounds and lacerations: Emergency care and closure.* St. Louis: Mosby.

Walker, D. (1996). Choosing the correct wound dressing. *American Journal of Nursing, 96* (9), 35–39.

Windsor, J. A., Knight, G. S., & Hill, G. L. (1988). Wound healing response in surgical patients: Recent food intake is more important than nutritional status. *British Journal of Surgery, 75,* 135–137.

Windsor, J. A. & Hill, G. L. (1991). Nutritional assessment: A pending renaissance. *Nutrition, 7* (5), 377–379.

Winter, G. D. (1962). Formation of the scab and the rate of epithelization of superficial wounds in the skin of the young domestic pig. *Nature, 193,* 293–294.

Wiseman, D., Rovee, D., & Alvarez, O. (1992). Wound dressings: Design and use. In I. K. Cohen, R Diegelmann, & W. Lindblad (eds.), *Wound healing: Biochemical and clinical aspects* (pp. 562–580). Philadelphia: W. B. Saunders.

22

Poisoning and Drug Toxicity

Russ Mazda

For the acute care nurse practitioner managing patients in an emergency department setting, knowledge of the principles of treatment of the poisoned patient is mandatory. Poison exposure may involve acute or delayed presentation, toxic versus nontoxic ingestion, and accidental versus deliberate act.

Many potentially harmful exposures to a toxin occur by accident in the home as a result of pediatric curiosity, though the majority are mild. One must always consider possible child abuse, especially in a child over age five. Accidents in the workplace or at home also account for many visits to the emergency department and are usually chemical dermal exposures requiring simple measures to decontaminate. Experimentation and substance abuse for recreation represent the majority of overdose presentations and suicide attempt remains an important consideration in the overall care of the patient presenting with a toxic exposure.

This chapter discusses the basic care of the poisoned patient for exposures due to ingestions, methods of GI decontamination, management of coma, common antidotes available to treat common overdoses, and important drug interactions of which the clinician should be aware. A description of current thoughts regarding the available modalities for treatment of the poisoned patient are provided so that a well-informed, logical, insightful approach may be employed.

▶ PRESENTATION

Assessment of Airway, Breathing, Circulation (the well-known ABC's) must be rapidly accomplished to determine the aggressiveness of the initial management of the poison/overdose victim. A patient who is awake and able to communicate allows more time for obtaining a history, performing a physical exam (including determination of the presence of any toxidromes), ordering laboratory and diagnostic tests, and making treatment decisions. Many ingestions or intravenous exposures are not dangerous and require only supportive care, observation, and perhaps psychiatric referral or detox evaluation (i.e., heroin or cocaine abuse).

In the awake patient, the airway and breathing may be normal, allowing a complete history and physical to direct treatment. Determining the identity of the toxin, quantity, time elapsed since exposure, and the reason for use (recreational/accidental overdose versus suicide attempt/gesture) will assist the clinician in deciding if a threat to the patient's health exists. Ascertaining that the toxin is benign demands a less aggressive response than a truly toxic exposure. Knowledge of the time since exposure and quantity ingested is valuable. A person who is awake and alert several hours after the toxin exposure requires different intervention than someone who presents within minutes. Of course, one must keep in mind the potential unreliability of a history from the patient alone, who may desire to hide illegal drug use or suicide attempt. If family or friends can provide additional history, they should be sought, particularly if the patient is unwilling or unable to provide an adequate history. Some drugs can distort the person's mental states such that a reliable history is not forthcoming from the patient. Importantly, the search for identity of the toxins must be done with care if searching the patient's clothing.

Putting one's hand indiscriminately into the patient's pocket may reward the unsuspecting health care worker with a needle stick from an uncapped, used needle, potentially exposing him or her to hepatitis or HIV. Prehospital personnel may provide valuable history and may have medicine bottles or other paraphernalia collected from the scene.

The physical examination may be brief and focused or more complete, depending on the situation. An alert, coherent, and appropriate patient requires a less detailed neurologic examination than a delirious or comatose patient. Much useful information is obtained while speaking with the patient (i.e., higher cortical functions intact, pupils equal and normal size, airway patent, breathing not compromised, and color normal). Vital signs must be obtained and, if abnormal, accounted for with consideration given to any necessary treatment (i.e., rapid respiratory rate may represent respiratory alkalosis caused by salicylate or ethylene glycol ingestion). The clinician should remain aware of any telltale scents indicative of specific toxins (Table 22–1). Particular attention to the presence of a toxidrome may assist in the diagnosis. The goal is to obviate any life-threatening effects on the cardiovascular or central nervous systems. Medical etiology for altered mental status must be considered if a history of poisoning is not available.

The patient with an altered mental status or coma requires a rapid assessment. Can the person protect his or her airway or is the person at risk for aspiration due to toxin-induced vomiting or loss of the gag reflex? The airway may be opened by any one of the basic life support maneuvers as well as through the use of oral or nasal devices, though these do not protect the airway. The decision regarding airway control is easy in either an alert or comatose patient, whereas the somnolent person who may or may not deteriorate requires careful consideration. If the patient remains obtunded, or becomes so after an initial trial of antidotes, airway control is necessary. Definitive airway management is also indicated in the patient at risk for aspiration, including those in whom lavage is contemplated and those who are not alert. If the patient's trachea is to be intubated, then be aggressive and use paralysis/sedation by rapid sequence technique. Of the many techniques for airway control, rapid sequence orotrachel intubation (RSI) is the safest method to prevent aspiration during the procedure. Simply sedating the patient with a benzodiazepine is insufficient, and vomiting and resistance may still occur, resulting in prolonged at-

TABLE 22–1. Diagnostic Odors

Characteristic Odor	Responsible Drug or Toxin
Acetone (sweet, fruity; pearlike)	Lacquer, ethanol, isopropyl alcohol, chloroform, diabetic ketoacidosis, alcoholic ketoacidosis, trichloroethane, paraldehyde, chloral hydrate, methylbromide, *Pseudomonas* infections
Alcohols	Ethanol, (congeners) isopropyl alcohol
Ammonialike	Uremia
Automobile exhaust	Carbon monoxide (odorless, but associated with exhaust)
Beer (stale)	Scrofula
Bitter almond	Cyanide
Carrots	Cicutoxin (of water hemlock)
Coal gas (stove gas)	Carbon monoxide (odorless, but associated with coal gas)
Disinfectants	Phenol, creosote
Eggs (rotten)	Hydrogen sulfide, carbon disulfide, mercaptans, disulfiram, *N*-acetylcysteine
Feculent	Intestinal obstruction
Fish or raw liver (musty)	Hepatic failure, zinc phosphide, hypermethioninemia, trimethylaminuria
Fruitlike	Nitrites (amyl, butyl, etc.), ethanol, (congeners) isopropyl alcohol
Garlic	Phosphorus, tellurium, arsenic, parathion, malathion, selenium, dimethyl sulfoxide (DMSO), thallium
Halitosis	Acute illness, poor oral hygiene
Hay	Phosgene
Mothballs	Naphthalene, *p*-dichlorobenzene, camphor
Peanuts	*N*-3-pyridyl-methyl-*N*-*p*-nitrophenyl urea (Vacor)
Pepperlike	*O*-chlorobenzylidene malonitrile
Putrid	Anaerobic infections, esophageal diverticulum, lung abscess, scurvy
Rope (burned)	Marijuana, opium
Shoe polish	Nitrobenzene
Sweating feet	Isovaleric acid acidemia
Tobacco	Nicotine
Vinegar	Acetic acid
Vinyl-like	Ethchlorvynol (Placidyl)
Violets	Turpentine (metabolites excreted in urine)
Wintergreen	Methyl salicylate

From Goldfrank, L. R. et al. (1994).

tempts at intubation, risking hypoxia or increased intracranial pressure. Addition of the paralytic agent provides a compliant patient in whom rapid control of the airway may be accomplished. I prefer oral over nasal intubation because of the ability to directly visualize the airway and the avoidance of inducing a nosebleed, which could complicate management. In addition, the endotracheal tube will likely be required only briefly. Once definitive airway control has been established, the rush to use agents in the coma cocktail is alleviated, thereby allowing a thoughtful, rational approach to managing the altered mental status.

Many deaths, as well as morbidity, result from improper management of the airway, allowing aspiration to occur, with subsequent atelectasis, pneumonia, or ARDS. One must be aggressive. Whether or not definitive airway management is required, all patients should receive oxygen in the initial treatment phase.

Obtaining venous access in the patient with altered mental status must be accomplished concurrent with the airway management. Venous access allows infusion of crystalloid to correct hypovolemia (relative or absolute) and also facilitates administration of agents needed for RSI and to treat the coma. Normal saline is the fluid of choice. IV access provides the site for administration of antiarrhythmics, antiseizure medicine, or vasopressors/vasodilators if needed. Central venous access may be considered depending on the clinical picture.

Use of the laboratory depends on the situation, as determined by the history and physical examination and the stability of the patient. A less comprehensive workup may be done if the patient is stable and the exposure is nonthreatening. A more detailed discussion of laboratory studies is presented later.

▶ COMA TREATMENT

When confronted with a patient who has altered mental status, including coma, poisoning is one of many considerations. After attention to the ABC's and accomplishing a physical exam with neurologic evaluation, a standard protocol has traditionally been used to empirically treat the most common causes of altered mental status. This "coma cocktail" has included D50, naloxone, thiamin, and, in the past few years, flumazenil. Conventional thought has been that there is no danger to giving any of these agents and there is the potential for a rapid reversal of an unknown medical problem, thereby obviating the need for extensive and costly tests and invasive procedures. Is this "shotgun" treatment approach—lacking in any knowledgeable thought process regarding the cause of coma—actually safe, as has been believed? Or, is there a potential downside? Research has challenged the universal use of these substances (Browning, 1990; Gueyy, 1996; Hoffman, 1991). The following is a discussion of each agent with current recommendations for use.

Glucose

For years, the administration of D50 had been considered safe, since normoglycemic or hyperglycemic persons suffered no apparent ill consequences. Because delay in treating undiagnosed hypoglycemia may cause brain damage, giving D50 to anyone with altered mental status seemed reasonable. Is D50 harmful in any circumstance? Are we overtreating? Can one tell who may be hypoglycemic? Concern about sudden changes in blood glucose and the resulting increased osmolality with electrolyte shifts has been a focus of investigation. As it turns out, the osmolality only increases about three milliosmols, even with large transient increases in serum glucose levels (Hoffman, 1996).

Another area of controversy has been an apparent adverse effect of high glucose levels on ischemic brain tissue. The current belief regarding the mechanism of harmful effect glucose has on ischemic brain tissue relates to the formation of lactate (Kalimo, 1981). In the absence of adequate oxygen to support aerobic metabolism of glucose, lactate results from the anaerobic pathway and the accumulation of lactate is believed to be detrimental to the injured brain. Many early animal studies demonstrated worse morbidity and mortality outcomes when glucose was administered prior to an ischemic event and mixed results were obtained if glucose was given after the ischemic event (D'Alecy, 1986, Myers, 1976; Welsh, 1980). In humans, most studies have noted a worse outcome from an ischemic stroke if the serum glucose was high (Candelise, 1985; Longstreth, 1984; Pulsinelli, 1983).

Interestingly, Goldfrank and Hoffman point out that the blood glucose rises from the stress of a significant stroke and a bad outcome will likely result anyway. If the person is already hyperglycemic, no further damage will likely result from additional dextrose. In one large study, long-term survival has been unaffected. Goldfrank (1996) believes this concern is not an issue. Certainly, some selective criteria are available. If a person is comatose and has focal neurologic deficit, then there is a greater possibility of stroke than if no focal deficit exists. Hypoglycemia generally produces altered mental status (confusion, agitation, combativeness) but not focal findings, whereas a stroke has focality without altered mental status. The experienced clinician will realize that some patients develop focal findings as a result of hypoglycemia. A stroke is a manifestation of decreased blood flow to an area of the brain. Since an anaerobic state requires a low flow state with resulting hypoxia, hypotension may suggest caution in administering dextrose prior to knowledge of the serum glucose.

With the wide availability of rapid glucose testing devices, this issue seems academic. Dextrose sticks and similar reagent strips are simple to use. Unfortunately, their accuracy is questionable in some hypoglycemic states, where a false normal will result. They are quite accurate if the blood glucose is elevated. Recently, the development of the One Touch machine has raised the accuracy of rapid glucose determination significantly. These test devices must be used under certain conditions (i.e., room temperature, antecubital blood sample [or femoral], and no alcohol at sampling site). Causes of errors may include machine malfunction, outdated reagent/test strip, low or high hematocrit, finger stick in a person with poor circulation to the digit, or extremes of temperature or humidity (Atkin, 1991; Weiner, 1991). Any of these may give a falsely elevated result. Studies have demonstrated an 8% false high with fingerstick method. With awareness of these situations, rapid determination is useful and should be performed. Correlation with the clinical situation remains important.

If there is potential for harm in the administration of dextrose, can the clinician determine who might be hypoglycemic? Generally accepted physical findings associated with low blood glucose are altered mental status, diaphoresis, tachycardia, and a history of diabetes. J. Hoffman (1992) studied these criteria and found that 25% of hypoglycemic patients had no physical manifestations typical of low blood glucose. Also, only 8.5% of ambulance calls were for hypoglycemic patients. Many additional symptoms may occur, including hemiplegia, agitation, mild confusion, and bizarre behavior simulating psychiatric or chemical-induced etiology. In some people with diabetes who live with blood glucose levels of 300 or more, symptoms of hypoglycemia may result at higher than the conventionally-accepted cutoff of 80 mg/dL. So, the treating clinician may have to adjust the threshold for giving dextrose and consider a higher value of 100 or 120.

Since dextrose is inexpensive and no clear evidence regarding negative consequences exists, should we continue as we have done in the past? The clinician will best serve the patient by maintaining a standard for excellent care and developing a selective set of criteria for treating a person with dextrose. Clearly, some form of bedside testing should be available in the treatment setting whether it is an office, emergency department, or prehospital area. Integrate the result into the overall clinical picture and consider a higher threshold for hypoglycemia in the diabetic patient. If a focal neurologic deficit exists, certainly check blood glucose first and correct hypotension, but do not withhold dextrose if it is required. Administer D50 if blood sugar is not hyperglycemic (i.e., greater than 120). In the absence of hypotension and neurologic deficit, dextrose can be safely given. If glucose testing is unavailable, dextrose has not been shown to be clearly harmful, and may be given if the clinician desires.

Naloxone and Newer Agents

Naloxone (Narcan), like dextrose, has been considered safe with no downside to its use in the patient with altered mental status (Rosen, 1992). It is a pure opiod antagonist that reverses respiratory and CNS depression, bradycardia, and any analgesic effect. Notably, naloxone reverses hypotension caused by most narcotics, especially if due to bradycardia (Weisman, 1994). Since its availability in 1976, it has been widely used and given without reserve to anyone with altered mental status. Initially, dosages of 0.2 to 0.4 mg were used, and repeated if needed. In the last 10 years, common practice has been to give an initial 2 mg as the standard dose and then repeat if deemed necessary, especially when given by paramedics. Again, analysis of this practice reveals a need for change. Current thinking supports a more selective use with varying dosages based on the clinical presentation.

It is possible to make an informed decision regarding the use of naloxone based on the history and physical examination. One must ask if there is a benefit in administering this drug to a sleepy patient who is able to protect his or her airway. Benefits may include making the diagnosis based on actual effect or history obtained from a more alert patient, avoiding endotracheal intubation, reducing or eliminating the risk of aspiration, and limiting the need for tests and procedures. On the other hand, risks to be weighed include inducing a withdrawal reaction in an opiate-dependent person, arousing the person enough to cause vomiting if an oral airway is in place or other drugs are present, seizure, arousal to a combative state placing others at risk as well as the patient, and death due to adverse reaction. Additionally, if the history from bystanders leads the clinician to believe that GI decontamination is necessary, an aroused patient may be uncooperative to any further care.

Reports of morbidity and mortality are primarily in the anesthesia and surgical literature where many medications were involved, making the likelihood of naloxone being the causative agent of adverse outcome questionable (Weisman, 1994). Naloxone has been used for years in emergency departments without significant problems, even at 10 mg doses. The most common problem is withdrawal symptoms that are typical of an opiate-dependent person who has not had access to the usual amount of substance. The clinician will note tremors, anxiety, stomach cramps, nausea, and diaphoresis, as well as the possibility of vomiting and diarrhea, if severe withdrawal occurs. If withdrawal occurs, the clinician must not be tempted to give a narcotic as treatment, since this will only compound the problem when the naloxone wears off. Simple reassurance that the effect is short-lived is all that can be done.

Naloxone has been given to acutely agitated individuals with delirium, probably hoping to improve the delirium. This is ill-advised, since the likely result in this mixed picture is a more agitated, combative person, especially if withdrawal occurs. The administration of naloxone in this particular situation will not improve morbidity or mortality, since the primary symptoms of concern (low respiratory rate and poor airway control) normally reversed by naloxone are not present. Therefore, in a polysubstance situation where no clear opiate toxidrome exists and the patient is not comatose, naloxone may be withheld.

Treatment may still include naloxone if opiate dependence is suspected by using low doses such as 0.1 to 0.2 mg. Opiate intoxication presents with a typical toxidrome consisting of CNS depression, miosis, respiratory depression, hypotension, bradycardia, and possibly hypothermia. Results of a study by J. Hoffman (1991) support the concept that clinically-significant opiate intoxication is unlikely in the absence of at least one of the following: miosis, respiratory rate less than 12, history of opiate use based on bystander description, actual presence of the substance or needle, or track marks. In the absence of respiratory depression, waking the patient fully risks elopement. Incremental lower doses such as 0.4 to 0.8 mg may therefore be considered as a diagnostic aid. There is no need to fully arouse the patient before the substance of abuse loses effect, as long as respiratory compromise is not a problem. One dies from airway compromise or poor ventilation. Respiratory adequacy must be evaluated by determining oxygenation rather than simply observing the rate of breathing. The patient may be quite hypoxic despite a respiratory rate of 16 if the effort is shallow. Pulse oximetry aids in determining oxygen saturation and allows a better assessment of breathing. Be aware of cold extremities or hypotension causing a poor reading on the oximeter. If there is doubt, administer the naloxone. In the apneic patient, the conventional 2-mg dose is still recommended.

Naloxone can be given by any route, i.e., IV, IM, SQ, endotrachealy, and sublingually. Be careful if the sublingual method is chosen, since a bite wound from a potentially HIV-positive patient may result while lifting the tongue to inject the naloxone. With the variety of routes available, this method seems the least desirable.

Naloxone has a duration of 60 to 90 minutes and then loses effect quickly. If the patient leaves after having been woken by the naloxone, recurrence of coma is possible when the naloxone's effect abates, especially if additional narcotic is administered by the patient. The patient must be convinced to stay in the emergency department for at least 90 minutes. Use physical restraint prior to arousing the comatose patient, thereby preventing violence or elopement.

Newer alternatives have become available with longer half lives and pure antagonist activity. Nalmefene (Revex) has a duration of action of 4 to 8 hours after IV route and Naltrexone (ReVia) lasts up to 12 hours. Nalmefene may have greater effect against naloxone-resistant narcotics (e.g., Darvon) due to more potent activity at U and K receptors. One study showed the safety and effectiveness of nalmefene (Kaplan, 1993). Advantages of a longer-acting antagonist cited include a decreased chance of recurrent coma in a patient who leaves the emergency department after being aroused, reduced risk of airway difficulties or aspiration from recurrence of opiate effect, and eliminating the need for continuous infusion as sometimes must be used for ongoing effect with naloxone. Since most opiates have longer half lives than naloxone, the longer action of the newer agents is attractive. In the event that an unwanted effect (such as withdrawal) occurs, however, one must wait much longer for this to subside if a newer agent has been used. It makes more sense to use naloxone, at least initially, for treatment or as a diagnostic aid and then, if desired, go to a longer-acting medicine if the opiate has been determined to be long acting.

The clinician will best manage a suspected narcotic overdose with the short-acting naloxone used in low dose if the respiratory rate is less than 12, and a dose of 2 mg if apneic. In the absence of coma or respiratory compromise and no toxidrome, naloxone is unlikely to be of any benefit. For the suspected opiate-dependent patient, use small, incremental doses to avoid inducing a withdrawal reaction. If a long-acting narcotic (e.g., Darvon) is suspected, doses up to 10 mg may be required. Subsequent to the initial trial, a longer-acting agent may be used to eliminate the need for a constant infusion. Use of a constant infusion allows for titration and can be discontinued in the event of any withdrawal symptoms. An infusion is calculated by taking two thirds of the bolus required to reverse respiratory depression and administering it at an hourly rate. An additional bolus of one half the initial dose may be required 15 minutes later to obtain a steady state (Goldfrank, 1986). Dosages of naloxone in the pediatric population are the same. In the neonate, 0.1 to 0.2 mg dose is used. Not every narcotic-overdose patient requires admission; after an adequate period of observation, most can be safely discharged (Smith, 1992).

Thiamin

Misconceptions regarding the role of thiamin persist. Thiamin is a B vitamin (B_1) that acts as a coenzyme in the Krebs cycle and pentose–phosphate pathway. It is necessary for normal functioning of muscle, nerve, vasculature, and brain. Thiamin is a water-soluble vitamin that is easily destroyed in cooking (Garrison, 1995). It is also soluble in alcohol, which prevents absorption from the GI tract. Thiamin is ingested from beef, organ meats, whole wheat products, peas, green leafy vegetables, and eggs. The human body does not store it, so regular consumption of appropriate food sources is mandatory (Garrison, 1995). A thiamin deficiency may result from the absence of foods for the body to absorb, due, for example, to vomiting, poor intake, alcoholism, or dieting, or from disease states affecting the gut's ability to assimilate nutrients (i.e., gastrectomy, AIDS, cancer, or malabsorption syndromes) (Doyon, 1994). Thiamin is poorly absorbed in the presence of alcohol, explaining the common deficiency in the alcoholic population. (This is also a reason for not giving thiamin orally to replete in the treatment setting.)

A deficiency of thiamin may manifest as fatigue, nausea, weakness, tender muscles, and tingling. Beriberi develops from ongoing deficiency, and can be either "wet" or "dry" (R. S. Hoffman, 1996). Wet beriberi presents with edema and peripheral vasodilatation causing high output CHF. Dry beriberi manifests with CNS symptoms including ataxia, peripheral neuropathy, ophthalmoplegia, and confusion known as Wernicke's encephalopathy. Longstanding deficiency can progress to Korsakoff psychosis. Korsakoff's syndrome is characterized by amnesia and confusion or confabulation and has a poor prognosis for recovery. Wet beriberi, as well as the ataxia, ophthalmoplegia, and vomiting of Wernicke's, respond quickly to thiamin, usually within 24 hours. It seems that great concern involving the dosing of thiamin and timing relative to dextrose administration arises from fear of precipitating Wernicke's encephalopathy or causing Wernicke's to progress to Korsakoff's syndrome. Since thiamin is necessary for glucose metabolism, Wernicke's encephalopathy can result from a bolus of dextrose, though this is unlikely to be an immediate occurrence. There is no reason to withhold dextrose while waiting for thiamin to be obtained and slowly given.

Since the most rapid delivery and, therefore, bioavailability is by the IV route, the recommended dosage is 100 mg IV. Reports of such adverse effects as pruritis can be minimized by dilution and slow administration. Anaphylaxis, though rare, can be treated if it occurs and does not preclude IV administration (Goldfrank, 1996). Studies that have been done looking at thousands of IV administrations failed to demonstrate a problem with anaphylaxis or adverse reaction.

Generally, the benefit of thiamin outweighs any risk and should be included in the overall initial care of the patient with altered mental status. Thiamin is cheap, safe, and can be given several minutes following the dextrose (Goldfrank, 1996). For the apparently well-nourished, awake, alert, drug-overdose victim, thiamin may not be necessary unless a history of poor nutrition is elicited. The IM route may be considered in that instance. Pediatric patients may receive IV thiamin at one tenth to one quarter of the adult dose.

Flumazenil

Benzodiazepine-type medications are easily available to many people with liberal prescribing by health-care providers and street marketing. Overdose with benzodiazepines causes sedation, but toxicologists agree that, alone, benzodiazepines cannot produce a fatal overdose. The problem becomes the mixed overdose where the combination could cause enough respiratory depression to be dangerous. Flumazenil (Romazicon) acts as a nearly pure antagonist of CNS benzodiazepine receptor sites with a duration of action that is shorter than any benzodiazepine. This is important because, as with naloxone, the toxin will likely outlast the reversal agent, making recurrence of sedation likely, usually within an hour. Reversal of the respiratory and CNS depression carries the same benefits as reversal of an opiate-induced coma (i.e., diagnosis, decreased testing, decreased invasive procedures, reduced risk of airway problem or aspiration, and ability to more easily rule out other problems or injuries) (Ashton, 1985; Prischl, 1988; Votey, 1991). Despite these significant advantages, there are potential risks of which the clinician must be aware (Doyon & Roberts, 1994). Withdrawal symptoms, including abdominal cramping, tremors, nausea, and other manifestations similar to opiate withdrawal, may occur if the patient is dependent on benzodiazepines. Flumazenil has not been found to shorten length of stay in the hospital. Therefore, selection of appropriate patients for use of this agent is an important part of the decision-making process.

Recent studies have found very limited applicability of flumazenil in an overdose situation. If a mixed overdose is involved, such as with cocaine or TCA, seizures may result that, though typically short lived, can lead to morbidity. An epileptic whose seizures are controlled with a benzodiazepine, or an alcoholic in whom withdrawal seizures are suppressed by a benzodiazepine, may develop seizure activity when the flumazenil blocks the effect of the drug.

In a study by Gueye, Hoffman, et al. (1996), it was found that very few people present with pure benzodiazepine overdose, which is not associated with any mortality anyway. Unquestionably, it is very useful for reversal of conscious sedation where a known amount of a short-acting benzodiazepine has been used and other compounding factors do not exist. In those who did not fit the criteria for uncomplicated benzodiazepine overdose, 16% had seizures after administration of flumazenil, with several of these patients having multiple seizures. The authors concluded that flumazenil should not be given to all comatose patients, but only to those in whom other complicating factors can be eliminated, such as coingestion of a tricyclic antidepressant (TCA), cocaine toxicity, or epileptogenic drug (theophylline, INH, lithium, and others). Though it is sometimes possible to suggest TCA presence using anticholinergic signs or EKG criteria, this is not universal. Among the drugs that most commonly cause seizures in an overdose situation, tricyclic antidepressants and cocaine/stimulants were found to be predominant at 29% each (Olson, 1993). Since TCAs are commonly prescribed for depression, and anxiety frequently complicates this illness, it is not uncommon for a person to be taking both a TCA and a benzodiazepine. Therefore, this type of mixed overdose is common. The newer antidepressants are not so likely to cause seizures, but are not so well studied.

Derlet & Albertson (1994) found that blocking the effect of a benzodiazepine ingestion can unmask seizures when there is concomitant cocaine toxicity and increases the incidence of death in a rat model by nearly 100%. Spivey found that some people will not respond to the usual dosage of flumazenil and require doses of 5 mg or more. Though most responded to 3 mg or less, some did not; so, a benzodiazepine could be involved, but the diagnostic capability of flumazenil may be limited (Spivey, 1993). Also, when a TCA or propoxyphene was present, three patients had seizures. Their recommendation is to use caution in a polydrug situation.

Several other researchers have noted problems (e.g., seizures, ventricular tachycardia) with administering flumazenil in an overdose situation (Lukas, 1982; Marcangt, 1989; Mordel, 1992; Spivey, 1992). R. S. Hoffman (1996) found that mixing flumazenil with chloral hydrate or tegretol could be fatal. Goldfrank (1996) and Hoffman believe that the use of flumazenil is not worth the risk in a patient who is just sleeping.

Clearly, flumazenil has much more limited applicability than the other agents discussed, since one can truly cause harm if it is given to the wrong patient (i.e., certain coingestions, alcoholics, epileptics, etc.). Additionally, it would not make sense to reverse the sedative effects if they are required for a procedure or maintenance on ventilator (Table 22–2). For the patient with no contraindication in whom the clinician would like to confirm the diagnosis, flumazenil is very useful. Once comfortable with the patient's clinical condition, allowing the patient to sleep it off is the most reasonable approach.

Certainly, the ABCs take precedence, and airway must be maintained. The dose recommended is 0.2 mg every 45 to 60 seconds up to 1 mg. Recent literature recommends up to 3 mg, with some patients requiring 5 mg. But, these patients have coingestions, and higher doses risk developing adverse reactions (Doyon, 1994; Spivey, 1993). Though not approved by the FDA for pediatrics, its use has been safe, and is very useful in the typical single substance pediatric overdose.

TABLE 22–2. Considerations for the Use of Flumazenil

Useful	1. Reverse benzodiazepine sedation after conscious sedation protocol.
	2. Diagnostic aid in pure benzodiazepine overdose with no contraindication.
Relative contraindications	1. Benzodiazepine sedation may be needed (i.e., for intubation or management on ventilator).
	2. No coma or apnea (i.e., lethargic but adequate airway protection and satisfactory O_2).
	3. Long-term dependence (i.e., prescribed for anxiety, muscle spasms, known abuser).
Absolute contraindications	1. Benzodiazepine needed or given for seizure control prehospital or in emergency department.
	2. Benzodiazepine prescribed for maintenance of seizure control.
	3. Concomitant tricyclic antidepressant toxicity (EKG changes, anticholinergic finding, dysrhythmias, hypotension, seizures). This may be difficult to diagnose clinically.
	4. Head trauma where seizures are possible.

GI DECONTAMINATION

Once the basic supportive measures have been accomplished and the need for administration of any of the antidotes determined, the clinician must address the need for decontamination. Performing one or more of the decontamination procedures decreases the amount of toxin absorbed, thereby potentially preventing the patient from becoming toxic and requiring more prolonged treatment. It seems reasonable that reducing the available toxin to be absorbed by the gut should reduce morbidity and mortality, thereby improving outcome. This discussion will focus on ingestions, but there are other routes of exposure that could require treatment. Interestingly, there are no good studies demonstrating that gastric and GI decontamination affect outcome. There have been a large number of studies that have looked at the relative effectiveness of the different techniques, but none really direct the clinician as to what might be the best treatment.

Gastric decontamination requires the toxin to be present in the stomach in order for the procedure to have any potential impact on the eventual outcome. In order for gastric emptying of toxin into the intestine to be minimized, it is believed that maintaining the patient in the left lateral decubitus position is best. One study demonstrated decreased absorption of acetaminophen for 2 hours by preventing movement into the duodenum (Vance, 1992). Vance et al., (1992) showed that the left lateral decubitus position with some trendelenburg decreases absorption of toxin from the gut by keeping it in the stomach longer. This may also improve recovery of toxin (Burke, 1972).

Ipecac

Induction of vomiting has been the accepted method of evacuating toxin for centuries. Ipecac is the most effective and reliable emetic agent. Ipecac acts directly on the gastric mucosa as an irritant and also as a stimulant of the emetic chemoreceptors in the brain. Generally, vomiting occurs in 20 to 30 minutes in 88% of people (R. S. Hoffman, 1996; Robertson, 1962). If no emesis occurs in 30 minutes, a repeat dose may be given and 97% of people will then experience emesis. The duration of vomiting can be 2½ hours and occasionally longer, though prolonged emesis is generally believed to be due to the ingested toxin. Nonetheless, if vomiting continues for 2 hours, this can delay other treatment.

Since each ingestion is unique, many items must be considered with each poisoning victim. What is the toxin? Is it a slow release formulation? Is the ingestion toxic at all? Is the amount ingested dangerous? A patient with a nontoxic ingestion requires no intervention (Table 22–3). The length of time since ingestion is very important, as is the age of the person. Some toxins may cause sedation or coma, which would be an undesirable state should emesis

TABLE 22–3. Nontoxic Ingestions

Medications	Antacids Antibiotics (with some exceptions) Birth control pills Calamine lotion Corticosteroids Hydrogen peroxide 3% Laxatives Mineral oil Petrolatum Vitamins without iron Zinc oxide Zirconium oxide
Household products	Adhesives Artificial sweeteners Ball-point pen ink Charcoal Chalk Crayons (Marked AP or CP) Clay Deodorizers Fertilizer Felt-tip pens and magic markers Fish bowl additives Iodophil disinfectants Household bleach (2-5% hyochlorite) Pencils Polaroid picture-coating film Rubber cement Silica Thermometer (mercury) Watercolors White glue
Soaps and baby products	Baby product cosmetics Bar soap Bath foam Bath oils
Soaps and baby products *(cont'd)*	Body conditioner Bubble bath Cologne (low alcohol content) Cosmetics Deodorants Eye make-up Fabric softener Hair products Hair spray Hand lotion Laundry detergent Lipstick Liquid soap (hand and dish) Perfume Rouge Shampoo Shaving cream Suntan lotion Toilet water Toothpaste (with or without fluoride)
Miscellaneous	Abrasives Bathtub floating toys Cigarettes (small amount, no butts) Etch-a-Sketch Grease and motor oil Matches Paint Paste Prussian blue (ferricyanide) Putty and spackle Silly Putty/Play-Doh Incense Lubricating oil Newspaper Toy pistol caps (potassium chlorate)

develop. Wrenn et al., (1993) found that ipecac was administered inappropriately in 20% of cases. Either too much time had elapsed, the patient had altered mental status, or the ingestion was nontoxic. Administering ipecac to induce emesis in a nontoxic ingestion as a matter of habit, or to punish the patient in hopes of preventing a future similar act, shows a lack of thought, understanding, and compassion. If the ingestion was accidental and not dangerous, a physical examination and reassurance may be all that is needed. If it was purposeful, then the clinician should ascertain the underlying problems, determine risk for recurrence, and obtain psychiatric evaluation or refer for outpatient psychotherapy.

Generally, ipecac must be given soon after ingestion of the toxin, since removal from the stomach cannot be accomplished if the toxin has moved into the intestine (Krenzelok, 1994). Time is the single biggest limiting factor in the utility of ipecac, since most people will not present for treatment within one hour of toxin ingestion. The greatest value has become the home setting where ipecac can be administered in a timely fashion (Bond, 1995). Usually, this involves a pediatric ingestion that comes to the immediate attention of a caretaker, and the emetic can be given quickly, if appropriate, after being recommended by a poison control center. Since time is important, even out-of-date ipecac may be used (Krenzelok, 1994). It has been shown effective even four years past its expiration date. A study by Young et al., (1993) showed the superiority of ipecac to lavage if given quickly. They administered ipecac 10 minutes after ingestion of a marker capsule and recovered an average of 54% of marker, compared with 35% with lavage. This demonstrates the importance of early gastric emptying. Bond et al., (1993) found the greatest effect if emesis occurs within 30 minutes and no demonstrable impact when emesis occurs beyond 90 minutes postingestion. Other studies have found maximum benefit from ipecac when given within 60 minutes (Amitai, 1987; Neuvonen, 1983).

An interesting exception to this may be ingestion of a substance that slows gastric emptying, is not well absorbed by charcoal, and will have delayed onset of action such that lethargy should not occur prior to the effect of ipecac (i.e., sustained release lithium). Substances such as narcotics, TCAs, and anticholinergics, such as antihistamines, slow gastric emptying, but also cause decreasing alertness with coma possible, thereby making the use of ipecac contraindicated. Medicines that form concretions and remain in the stomach may by evacuated by emesis despite a time delay over 1 hour.

Though ipecac has excellent efficacy in producing emesis, studies fail to show consistent efficacy in retrieving toxin or in affecting eventual outcome. Some authors believe toxin can be reduced by half if emesis occurs within 90 minutes. But, studies show a range of gastric emptying of 20 to 70%, with an average of 38%. This leaves the majority of toxin available for absorption with vomiting delaying other treatment such as charcoal or specific antidotes, i.e., N-Acetylcysteine (N-AC) for Tylenol overdose.

There are specific contraindications to emesis (Table 22–4) and involve risk of reinjury of the mucosa, sedation prior to emesis, previous emesis, or long delay in presentation. Ingestion of caustics such as acids (HCL) or alkali (lye) cause reexposure of esophageal and oral mucosa to injury, as well as risk pulmonary damage if aspiration occurs. Generally, dilution is all the clinician can do to minimize further damage. Administration of a neutralizing substance risks further damage from the heat of the chemical reaction (Goldfrank, 1994). Hydrocarbons (kerosene, gasoline) are generally not dangerous in quantities below 1 cc/kg; the predominant problem involves aspiration and chemical pneumonitis. Again, emesis risks aspiration and should be avoided. If the patient is obtunded or at risk of becoming less responsive, emesis risks aspiration and creates more problem than benefit. In someone who already vomited, ipecac offers no further benefit except to risk protracted emesis from the combined effect of the toxin and the ipecac.

Even in a situation that seems appropriate for the use of ipecac, some complications of emesis should be kept in mind. Protracted vomiting may hinder more important treatment, Mallory Weiss tears may occur, pneumomediastinum or contaminants in the mediastinum can lead to morbidity or mortality, or diaphragmatic and gastric rupture (rare with only three deaths reported) may occur (Knight, 1987; Robertson, 1979; Tandberg, 1981; Wolowodiuk, 1984). Cardiomyopathy results only from chronic abuse, so the clinician need not worry about cardiotoxicity from 1 or 2 doses of ipecac, even if emesis does not occur.

The dose of ipecac is 30 cc for people over age 12, 15 cc between 1 and 12 years, and 10 cc between 6 months and 1 year. Unless a parent is neglectful, a nonambulatory child should not present with a toxic ingestion. The quantity of fluid to drink is controversial (Grande, 1987; Krenzelok, 1994). Four ounces are adequate, with larger amounts risking transport of dissolved toxin out of the stomach (Borowitz, 1971). Any fluid will do, though milk may obscure pill fragments in the vomitus. Temperature of the fluid has no bearing on development of emesis, nor does rocking the patient (Krenzelok, 1994).

In conclusion, ipecac has limited utility in an emergency setting unless the patient presents within 15 minutes of the ingestion, remains alert and able to protect the airway, and has no contraindication to its use. Ipecac is simple to use, cheap, and generally safe when used appropriately. Most toxicologists believe ipecac has the greatest efficacy at home where a child has a witnessed ingestion. The clinician should remember that much of the toxin may not be evacuated and reconsider its use if more effective treatment can be instituted.

TABLE 22–4. Considerations for the Use of Ipecac

Useful	1. Presentation within 10 minutes of ingestion—usually pediatric patient at home.
	2. Home use—no delay in administration after potentially toxic ingestion.
	3. Tablets too large to come through a lavage tube when presentation is early.
	4. Toxin not adsorbed to charcoal and presentation is early.
	5. May be somewhat effective up to 90 minutes (occurrence of emesis) in some ingestions—slow GI motility, form concretions, sustained release.
Not helpful	1. Over 90 minutes since ingestion.
	2. Liquid ingestion more than 20 minutes time elapsed.
	3. Nontoxic ingestions.
Contraindicated	1. Altered mental status, seizures (occurring or potential).
	2. Emesis already occurred.
	3. Caustic ingestion—acids, alkalis.
	4. Petroleum products—risks aspiration.
	5. Sharp object ingested.
	6. Age less than 6 months.
	7. Emesis will delay use of a specific antidote.
	8. No gag reflex or unable to protect airway.
	9. Risk of hemorrhage, bleeding diathesis.

Gastric Lavage

As with emesis, gastric lavage depends on the presence of toxin in the stomach for evacuation. Therefore, time is of the essence and accomplishing lavage within an hour of the ingestion yields the best results. Most studies demonstrate equal success between ipecac-induced emesis and lavage with an average of 30 to 40% of the toxin being recovered. Young & Bivins (1993) found ipecac more effective, but gave ipecac 10 minutes after ingestions—an unrealistic scenario in most overdose situations, unless ipecac can be given at home. Lavage eliminates the delay to emptying the stomach, though there is delay associated with arrival at the hospital, compared with giving ipecac at home in the alert patient. Lavage is most useful in situations where emesis would not be indicated, such as the patient who is comatose or expected to possibly become less alert and unable to protect the airway. Many toxicologists believe that an overdose victim who requires endotracheal intubation is sick enough to warrant lavage. For any life-threatening or serious ingestion where the possibility of decreased level of consciousness exists, lavage is the method of choice for recovering toxin, if the time factor is appropriate. In addition to eliminating the uncertainty of when gastric emptying may occur, the presence of the tube in place in the stomach provides an easy route for the administration of charcoal or an initial dose of an antidote if indicated, especially since many patients need coercion to drink the unpalatable substances. (Charcoal is gritty and N-AC tastes like rotten eggs.)

To perform gastric lavage, a large tube is passed through the mouth (less often, passage through the nose is possible) and into the stomach. Confirmation of correct placement is performed by aspiration of stomach contents as well as auscultating the gurgling of air in the upper abdomen when air is pushed through the tube. One should choose the largest tube likely to pass through the esophagus so larger fragments may be recovered. In adults, a 36 to 40 F tube is used, and in children a tube as large as 24 F may be passed. It is generally accepted that lavage should be performed until the fluid returning is clear. At least 5 liters of irrigant should be used. In their study, Young and Bivins recovered almost 13% more marker with continued lavage after clear. Generally, 200 to 300 cc volumes may be instilled in adults and 1 cc/kg in children. The fluid should be warmed for use in children and isotonic saline is the irrigant of choice. For adults, tap water is acceptable, as is NSS or LR, and the fluid need not be warmed unless the patient is hypothermic, in which case warmed irrigation will assist in rewarming the patient.

Once lavage is complete, charcoal should be instilled unless the clinician is certain that only a single ingested toxin that is not bound by charcoal is involved. In my practice, I have the nurse instill charcoal prior to lavage and after aspiration of as much gastric contents as possible. After several minutes, the charcoal is recovered and then lavage performed. Once lavage is completed, charcoal is repeated. In this manner, toxin is first bound by the charcoal so any unrecovered toxin does not subsequently get absorbed, especially if lavage causes passage of some toxin into the small bowel. Of course, this method may be messier, but with the newer closed irrigation setups, such as Code Blue EasiLav (Ballard), the possibility of charcoal splattering has been greatly reduced.

Though lavage seems to be efficient, there are contraindications, risks, and problems. If the patient has already vomited, then no benefit has been demonstrated in performing subsequent lavage, though this doesn't mean that no benefit exists. Ingestion of a nontoxic substance or a nontoxic quantity of any substance requires evaluation, but not gastric emptying, since outcome will not be affected (Blake, 1978). Punitive reasons are more unacceptable than with ipecac. If the ingestion involved a caustic (acid/alkali) or a sharp foreign body, the possibility of reinjury to the esophagus exists, both from passage of the tube and from any reflux or emesis that might occur secondary to passage of the tube. If the patient is not completely alert but will not require endotracheal intubation, then this procedure risks aspiration and should not be performed. If gastric emptying is deemed important in the lethargic individual, then control of the airway is mandatory prior to passage of the orogastric tube. As discussed previously, RSI is the procedure of choice to minimize complications. Overdose on beta blockers or calcium channel blockers carries the risk of profound brachycardia if vagal effects from passage of the tube compound bradycardic effects of the drug ingested. Bradycardia can be treated with atropine in the usual dose. Studies have noted a decrease in the PO_2 of 12%, so supplemental oxygen may help. Reflux around the tube may occur, risking aspiration and passage of the tube can traumatize the pharynx, epiglottis, esophagus, or stomach (Mariani, 1993). If the nasal route is chosen, a nosebleed can be a problem. R. S. Hoffman (1996) reports that the tube can kink and get stuck in the stomach. Forceful removal of an impacted tube can tear the esophagus (Wald, 1986). Tracheal intubation may create significant morbidity and mortality if not recognized before lavage or charcoal administration are performed.

Despite the best technique, some factors may limit the effectiveness of lavage. Many pills are larger that the holes in the tube, especially sustained-release preparations, and lavage may simply propel them into the duodenum. Similarly, medications that form concretions can be difficult to recover through the tube. If there is food in the stomach, the tube can become blocked, making lavage difficult and preventing a successful procedure. In the alert patient, intolerance to attempts at passing such a large tube may prevent lavage. Also, vomiting may occur, which is effective in toxin evacuation, but risks aspiration if the patient does not protect the airway.

Clearly, both ipecac and gastric lavage have limitations. In the properly selected patient, however, these procedures have their place. Is gastric emtying worth the risks, given that no effect on outcome has been demonstrated? A frequently cited study by Kulig (1985) looked at the benefit of ipecac versus lavage and charcoal or charcoal alone. Unless lavage was performed within an hour, no benefit was seen. There were limitations to the study, but early gastric emptying is supported. Pond (1995) promotes treatment without gastric emptying since this Australian study found no benefit, even when performed within an hour of the ingestion. Treatment with charcoal alone is promoted by Pond. Again, it is unclear if a benefit exists in situations involving substances where delayed gastric emptying might occur, but intuitively removing toxin in large overdose situations should help.

The asymptomatic patient who is unlikely to develop any significant problems should not be tormented by gastric emptying. Charcoal may be sufficient and may also be unnecessary. In the symptomatic patient, or one who may develop morbidity, gastric emptying should be performed in keeping with the aforementioned indications and contraindications (Table 22–5). Certainly, every poisoning does not automatically require either of these procedures. A thoughtful, logical approach will minimize problems and maximize benefits.

Charcoal

Whether or not gastric emptying is performed, almost every patient with a worrisome ingestion should receive activated charcoal to bind any toxin in the stomach or bowel. Similar to gastric emptying, the sooner charcoal can be given, the better.

Charcoal simply binds the toxin, trapping it in the GI tract and preventing systemic adsorption. Since time is important, induced emesis with ipecac must be considered carefully since vomiting delays administration of charcoal.

TABLE 22–5. Considerations for the Use of Gastric Lavage

Useful	1. Recent ingestion (< 1 hour and emesis not indicated). 2. Expedite administration of activated charcoal. 3. Altered mental status patient in whom the airway is protected. 4. Toxin not well adsorbed to activated charcoal. 5. NG tube can ease administration of repeat doses of antidote (remove large-bore tube and replace with smaller caliber tube).
Not helpful	1. Over 90 minutes since ingestion (unless substance slows GI motility). 2. Liquid ingestion over 20 minutes. 3. Nontoxic ingestion.
Contraindications	1. Emesis already occurred. 2. Caustic ingestion. 3. Petroleum product. 4. Sharp object. 5. Bleeding diathesis. 6. Body packer or body stuffer. 7. Unable to protect airway. (Airway must be secured with a cuffed endotracheal tube; if child, use cuff only during lavage procedure from insertion to removal of tube. 8. Hemodynamic instability (treat hypotension and bradycardia if lavage is to be done). 9. Pills known to be too large to pass through holes in tube.

Emesis may be delayed 20 to 30 minutes after ipecac, and if given 30 to 40 minutes post ingestion, there will be a significant reduction in the recovery of toxin. Add to that the potential for a 2-hour delay prior to the end of emesis and one can see that simply administering charcoal from the start may be more effective. Many studies have compared the two modalities and found that gastric emptying is not better than charcoal alone unless gastric emptying can be accomplished within 30 minutes (Amitai, 1987; Bond, 1993; Neuvonen, 1983; Robertson, 1962). Several researchers have shown the efficacy of charcoal alone (Kulig, 1985; McNamara, 1989; Merigian, 1990). One study comparing charcoal to ipecac and lavage found that charcoal reduced toxin by 50%, while the other modalities averaged 38% (Tenenbein, 1987).

A benefit of charcoal administration is its ability to bind toxin that has passed into the small intestine where ipecac and gastric lavage will have no effect. Charcoal binds toxin still present in the bowel, but an additional benefit also exists. The ability to interrupt readsorption of toxin that has been secreted into the bowel makes charcoal significantly more effective (Chyka, 1995; Goldfrank, 1994; Pond, 1986). Drug secretion into the bowel occurs by entero–entero and entero–hepatic circulation, and the amount secreted depends on the pharmacokinetics of the substance. Many variables include such drug characteristics as intrinsic clearance, distributive phase, protein binding, and volume of distribution. Also, drug kinetics may change in an overdose situation, making more drug available by secretion when blood levels are high, compared with minimal secretion with therapeutic blood levels (Chyka, 1995). Some substances that have lower protein binding and low intrinsic clearance (causing high entero secretion) are acetaminophen, digoxin, theophylline, phenobarbital, tegretol, quinine, dapsone, and salicylate. Tricyclic antidepressants have a large volume of distribution but are well absorbed to charcoal and are secreted into the bowel. Berg (1982) noted accelerated clearance of phenobarbital with the use of charcoal. An interesting study by Beringer (1983) proved that enterosecretion occurs: aminophylline infused intravenously was found to have a half-life 50% less when charcoal was administered orally. This enteric effect of charcoal has been called gastrointestinal dialysis and has been found effective with many drugs (Levy, 1982). Table 22–6 shows drugs that are adsorbed to charcoal. One can see that charcoal serves an important role since the drugs mentioned are among the most commonly involved substances in overdose situations.

Depending on the specific exposure, a single dose of charcoal may be insufficient to bind a significant portion of the toxin. The concept of multi-dose or pulse-dose activated charcoal (MD-AC) has developed. Charcoal is given at set intervals (every 4 hours) until the patient recovers or signs of toxicity have resolved. A dose of 0.5 grams/kilogram is used. Such situations include ingestion of sustained-release

TABLE 22–6. Substances Bound to Charcoal

Acetaminophen	Imapramine	Phenothiazines
Amphetamines	Ipecac	Phenylbutazone
Arsenic	Isoniazid	Phenylpropanolamine
Atropine	Malathion	Phenytoin
Barbiturates	Mefenamic acid	Propantheline
Benzodiazepines	Mercuric chloride	Propoxyphene
Carbamazepine	Meprobamate	Quinine
Chlorpheniramine	Methaqualone	Salicylates
Chlorpromazine	Narcotics	Silver
Chloroquine	N-Acetylcysteine	Strychnine
Cocaine	Nicotine	Sulfonamides
Digoxin	Nonsteroidal antiinflammatories	Theophylline
Ethanol	Nortryptyline	Tricyclic Antidepressants
Ethchlorvynol	Paracetamol	
Glutehimide	Parathion	

preparations (Tylenol or theodur), large ingestions where a 10:1 charcoal to drug ratio is not possible with 1 dose, and drugs with large volumes of distribution (cyclic antidepressants) (Chyka, 1995; Kulig, 1987; Pond, 1986). Additionally, prolonged toxicity may benefit (Perrone, 1994). One study showed a decrease in Vancomycin half life from 33 hours to 9 hours (Kucukguclu, 1996). In cases where MD-AC will be given, an NG tube eliminates patient resistance to drinking it. Repeat doses should not include a cathartic, as will be discussed later.

Charcoal is a very porous, inert material that appears as a fine powder that results from a process where wood is burned and treated with steam and chemicals, thereby activating it. It must be mixed with liquid for consumption. Most preparations are premixed with and without sorbitol, a cathartic. A superactivated form prepared with petroleum has triple the available surface area, thus increasing its binding capacity, but problems with impurities have caused it to be unavailable in the United States. As mentioned earlier, charcoal should be administered in a quantity that approximates a 10:1 charcoal to drug ratio. Usually, 60 to 100 grams are given in an adult and 1 gram/kilogram in a child. In some cases, however, this is insufficient. Sometimes, it can be problematic to have the patient drink enough. For instance, if the patient ingests 50 Tylenol Extra-strength tablets (25 grams), 250 grams of charcoal would be required to obtain a 10:1 ratio. The problem of administering enough charcoal is worse in higher toxin quantity. A similar problem exists for any large milligram pill (ibuprofen, dolobid, theophylline).

The advantages of charcoal (Table 22–7) include its ability to bind toxin that has passed from the stomach to the intestine, its ease of use, and low cost. The entero–entero and entero–hepatic dialysis effect increases the effectiveness of charcoal by binding toxin after it has actually been absorbed into the circulation. The benefit achieved may be further enhanced by home availability where delay in coming to the hospital would not be a factor (Crokett, 1996). Home charcoal may be better than using ipecac at all, though convincing some children or adults to drink it may be more difficult than administering ipecac.

Some disadvantages include patient noncompliance due to the texture and taste. Many ways of masking the unpalatable quality have had little success (e.g., mixed in juice). It is very messy if the patient vomits, and it can be constipating (more common with MD-AC). There are reports of bowel obstruction secondary to briquette formation (Goulbourne, 1994) (usually when dosed more frequently than every 4 hours), and it can absorb an antidote, N-AC in particular (Chamberlain, 1993). Aspiration is cited as a con-

TABLE 22–7. Considerations for the Use of Activated Charcoal

Useful	1. Recent ingestion (< 1 hour): binds toxin in stomach.
	2. Late presentation (> 1 hour): binds toxin in stomach and bowel.
	3. With lavage: consider dose before and after performing lavage.
	4. Immediately effective after consumption, as opposed to delay associated with ipecac and lavage.
	5. Gastrointestinal dialysis with multi-dose regimen.
Problems	1. Not all toxins are adsorbed (iron, lithium, metals, cyanide, caustics, hydrocarbons, alcohols, organophosphates).
	2. Patient refusal to drink.
	3. Aspiration if vomiting occurs or tube is misplaced into trachea.
	4. Bowel obstruction when given too frequently.
Contraindications	1. Ileus.
	2. Caustics—may obscure damage, impeding endoscopy.
	3. Patient unable to protect airway unless protected with ETT.

cern, but it is inert and should not cause any worse pneumonitis than other substances (Harris, 1993; R. S. Hoffman 1996). Finally, charcoal does not bind everything, and in cases of single ingestions of one of these substances, charcoal may be contraindicated. Substances that do not bind to charcoal include iron, lithium, metals, cyanide, caustics, hydrocarbons, alcohols (isopropyl, ethylene glycol, methanol), and many organophosphates. Cyanide is interesting in that it may bind to charcoal somewhat, but such a small amount of the toxin is fatal that therapy must quickly go to the antidote.

Much controversy surrounds the use of charcoal in the case of an acetaminophen overdose, and some practitioners withhold it based on a concern that it may interfere with the N-AC antidote activity. Charcoal binds N-AC, thereby decreasing its bioavailability. Charcoal also binds acetaminophen, however, preventing the need for antidote in many cases. Since acetaminophen is present in many combination preparations (darvocet, percocet, cold medications), as well as being one of many other toxins sometimes ingested, withholding charcoal allows other toxins to be absorbed. Roberts (1994) interestingly points out that the dose of N-AC is standard regardless of the amount of acetaminophen ingested, because no one knows how to dose it based on quantity of toxin. Chamberlain (1993) looked at a new loading dose of 235 mg/kg after charcoal and found N-AC serum levels higher when compared with standard dosing in the absence of charcoal. This seems to show that charcoal does not significantly affect the peak serum levels. North (1981) found no effect of charcoal on N-AC levels. Spiller (1994) concluded that no increase in N-AC is needed after charcoal is given, and other investigators have had similar findings (Brent, 1993; Smilkstein, 1994). Therefore, since it is not known how to dose the N-AC for different serum acetaminophen levels and studies show no significant effect of charcoal on the antidote's effectiveness, administration of the usual dose may be given (140 mg/kg of N-AC). Additionally, charcoal should not be withheld based on an unproven concern that the N-AC won't work.

Cathartics

The logic of quickly removing toxins from the GI tract, which justifies gastric emptying, also seems to support promoting rapid movement through the bowel to evacuation per rectum. Cathartics have been used for this purpose, although no one study has proven that increasing peristalsis reduces toxin adsorption. Cathartics such as magnesium sulfate, sodium sulfate, magnesium citrate, and sorbitol act as osmotic agents, drawing water into the bowel, thereby stimulating increased movement. A study by Krenzelok (1985) showed that sorbitol is the most effective, producing a charcoal stool in less than an hour, compared with magnesium citrate at 4.2 hours and magnesium sulfate at over 9 hours. Minton (1995) looked at a simulated theophylline overdose and found that charcoal was 91% effective in preventing drug absorption at 1 hour past ingestion, 57% effective when given 6 hours post ingestion, and that adding sorbitol did not decrease drug absorption when added to charcoal. Again, benefit may exist even though it has not been demonstrated.

What is known is that sorbitol mixed with charcoal increases palatability a little, reduces the chance of constipation from charcoal, and speeds evacuation of toxin (Table 22–8). There are, however, some precautions. Repeat dosing can cause excessive fluid loss and electrolyte abnormalities, especially in children (Allerton, 1991; Caldwell, 1987; Farley, 1986). If a magnesium preparation is used, elevated serum magnesium levels may occur (Jones, 1986). Since the efficacy of a cathartic in preventing toxin adsorption is questionable, preventing constipation seems to be the only indication and 1 dose should suffice. To prevent accidental repeat dosing of a cathartic, the clinician should ensure that plain charcoal solution is available in the institution. Wax et al., (1993) found that 16% of hospitals stocked only charcoal/sorbitol preparations, and that repeat sorbitol dosing occurred in 49% of emergency departments surveyed. Reasons for repeat cathartic administration included lack of awareness of potential morbidity, no charcoal without sorbitol available, and confusion over similar packaging between charcoal with and without sorbitol. Concern about constipation is unfounded if charcoal is not given more frequently than every 4 hours. To avoid confusion, the clinician should ensure that the nursing staff is aware of this important point. Cathartics should be withheld in the presence of diarrhea, if bowel sounds are absent, or in the case of abdominal trauma.

Whole Bowel Irrigation

Like sorbitol, some believe whole bowel irrigation (WBI) accelerates passage of toxin through the bowel, thereby reducing systemic absorption of poison. Early solutions created problems with fluid absorption and electrolyte shifts. Now, products are available that have been shown to func-

TABLE 22–8. Considerations for the Use of Cathartics

Useful	1. Enhance transit of toxin through bowel. 2. Prevent constipation. 3. Improve palatability of charcoal.
Problems	1. Electrolyte and fluid disturbance if used repeatedly. 2. Abdominal cramping secondary to increased peristalsis. 3. Inadvertent repeat dosing if unaware of premixed product.
Contraindications	1. Ileus. 2. Diarrhea. 3. Obstruction. 4. Abdominal trauma.

tion without creating harmful fluid and electrolyte imbalances (Davis, 1980). Colyte and Golytely are isotonic electrolyte solutions with polyethylene glycol (PEG) that can be administered orally or by gastric tube in adults and children. This technique effectively washes the entire bowel, theoretically carrying any substances or foreign bodies out as well. As with the other methods of GI decontamination discussed, no benefit in outcome has been proven.

Nonetheless, this technique does have some utility. Many investigators support the use of WBI (Tenenbein, 1988). Many toxins are not able to be removed by lavage and emesis may be contraindicated or ineffective (sustained-release theophylline, iron, aspirin). In addition, substances such as iron or sustained-release lithium are not adsorbed by charcoal, and washing them through may limit toxicity. It is safer than repeat cathartics, since no dehydration or electrolyte abnormalities will result. Hassig (1993) found WBI to be useful in an acetaminophen overdose so large that charcoal was overwhelmed. Bernstein (1992) reported a fatal theophylline overdose where only lavage and charcoal were used. Apparently, a tablet bezoar formed that might have been washed through by whole bowel irrigation. Many studies have been done demonstrating reduced absorption of toxin, but with those toxins adsorbed by charcoal, there is not much difference. One study looking at lithium ingestion showed a 67% reduction in area under the serum concentration versus time curve (Smith, 1994). Detractors point out that washing the toxin through the bowel may just dissolve and distribute it for adsorption into the bloodstream. Also, if charcoal has absorbed much toxin, the PEG solution may displace it from the charcoal, freeing it up for systemic adsorption. Apparently, charcoal binds the irrigating solution, reducing its effectiveness. Burkhart et al., (1992) found no benefit to adding whole bowel irrigation to charcoal versus charcoal alone in sustained-release theophylline model. Roberge (1992) used WBI to clear all lead based on x-ray evidence, but serum lead levels continued to rise.

Problems must be noted in the use of this method of decontamination. This modality is labor-intensive and messy. Patients report rectal irritation, bloating, and difficulty drinking the large volumes required. Many people may vomit, placing them at risk for aspiration. Therefore, a secure airway or alert person capable of protecting the airway are important. Contraindications to the use of whole bowel irrigation include bowel obstruction, ileus, GI bleeding, and ruptured viscous.

Adults are given 1 to 2 liters/hour for 10 liters, unless known amount of foreign bodies are not yet recovered, or foreign bodies are still visible on x-ray. Children are given 500 cc/hour. Kaczorowski & Wax (1996) report 5 days of WBI in a 33-month-old boy with an iron overdose of more than 160 mg/kg. He received 44.3 liters of irrigant without adverse effect. There may be some limitations imposed by the arbitrarily accepted endpoints for terminating whole bowel irrigation. Usually, the clinician looks for clear rectal effluent or passage of all tablets or foreign bodies, if known. Scharman (1994) found that not all ingested coffee beans were passed when effluent became clear, and many more, though still not all, beans were recovered if irrigation was continued to10 liters total solution. It is hypothesized that some foreign bodies can become lodged in the folds of the large bowel, limiting effectiveness. Additional or continued irrigation may be needed. Kaczorowski & Wax (1996) found iron tablets persistently visible on x-ray after 2 days of irrigant in a 33-month-old. Scharman (1994) looked at the use of metoclopramide (Reglan) as an adjunct to whole bowel irrigation to speed up passage, but found no benefit. Metoclopramide is useful as an antiemetic in some patients who may want to vomit from toxin effects, but in higher than usual doses it may increase adverse GI effects.

In general, whole bowel irrigation must be viewed as an additional modality in the clinician's therapeutic armamentarium. It does not replace the use of lavage and charcoal, but can be useful if other methods are ineffective, if charcoal is known to be useless, or when large foreign bodies must be transported through (Table 22–9).

▶ ANTIDOTES AND TOXIDROMES

The care of the patient with a toxic exposure always includes general supportive care (ABC's, O_2, monitor, and possible venous access) and decontamination procedures

TABLE 22–9. Considerations for the Use of Whole Bowel Irrigation

Useful	1. Sustained release preparations. 2. Substances not adsorbed to charcoal (iron, lithium, lead, and other metals). 3. Massive overdose. 4. Body packers and body stuffers (heroin or cocaine packets in GI tract). 5. Dangerous foreign bodies (button batteries).
Problems	1. Tolerance of large volume of fluid (usually must use NG tube). 2. Aspiration if vomiting occurs and airway not protected. 3. Desorb toxin from charcoal or dissolve toxin, making absorption systemically more likely. 4. Messy and labor-intensive. 5. Poorly defined endpoint. 6. Rectal irritation/itching. 7. Bloating.
Contraindications	1. Bowel obstruction/ileus. 2. GI bleeding. 3. Ruptured viscous/abdominal trauma. 4. Ingestion of liquids, caustics, rapidly absorbed toxins. 5. Intravenous exposure to toxin.

TABLE 22–10. Toxicologic Syndromes (Toxidromes)

Toxin	Vital Signs	Mental Status	Symptoms	Clinical Findings	Lab Findings
Acetaminophen	Normal (early)	Normal	Anorexia, nausea, vomiting	RUQ tenderness, jaundice (late)	Abnormal LFTs
Amphetamines	Hypertension, tachycardia, tachypnea, hyperthermia	Hyperactive, agitated, toxic psychosis	Hyperalertness	Mydriasis, hyperactive bowel sounds, flush, diaphoresis	Increased CPK
Anticholinergics	Hypotension, hypertension, tachycardia, hyperthermia	Altered (agitation, lethargy to coma) hallucinations	Blurred vision	Dry mucous membranes, mydriasis, diminished bowel sounds, urinary retention	ECG abnormalities
Arsenic (acute)	Hypotension, tachycardia	Alert to coma	Abdominal pain, vomiting, diarrhea, dysphagia	Dehydration	Renal failure, abnormal abdominal radiograph; dysrhythmias
Arsenic (chronic)	Normal	Normal to encephalopathy	Abdominal pain, diarrhea	Melanosis, hyperkeratosis, sensory motor neuropathy, hair loss, Mee's lines, skin cancer	Pancytopenia, proteinuria, hematuria, abnormal LFTs
Barbiturates	Hypotension, bradypnea, hypothermia	Altered (lethargy to coma)	Slurred speech, ataxia	Dysconjugate gaze, bullae, hyporeflexia	Abnormal ABGs
Beta adrenergic antagonists	Hypotension, bradycardia	Altered (lethargy to coma)	Dizziness	Cyanosis, seizures	Hypoglycemia, ECG abnormal
Botulism	Bradypnea	Normal unless hypoxia	Blurred vision, dysphagia, sore throat, diarrhea	Ophthalmoplegia, mydriasis, ptosis, cranial nerve abnormalities	Normal
Carbamazepine	Hypotension, tachycardia, bradypnea, hypothermia	Altered (lethargy to coma)	Hallucinations, extrapyramidal movements, seizures	Mydriasis, nystagmus	ECG abnormalities
Carbon monoxide	Often normal	Altered (lethargy to coma)	Headache, dizziness, nausea, vomiting	Seizures	Elevated carboxyhemoglobin, ECG abnormalities, metabolic acidosis
Clonidine	Hypotension, hypertension, bradycardia, bradypnea	Altered (lethargy to coma)	Dizziness, confusion	Miosis	Normal
Cocaine	Hypertension, tachycardia, hyperthermia	Altered (anxiety, agitation, delirium)	Hallucinations, paranoia	Mydriasis, tremor, perforated nasal septum, diaphoresis, seizures, active bowel sounds	ECG abnormalities, increased CPK
Cyclic antidepressants	Hypotension, tachycardia, hyperthermia	Altered (lethargy to coma)	Confusion, dizziness	Mydriasis, dry mucous membranes, distended bladder, flush, seizures	Prolonged QRS complex, cardiac dysrhythmias
Digitalis	Hypotension, bradycardia	Normal to altered; visual hallucinations	Nausea, vomiting, anorexia, visual disturbances	None	Hyperkalemia, ECG abnormalities, increased digoxin level
Disulfiram/ethanol	Hypotension, tachycardia	Normal	Nausea, vomiting, headache, vertigo	Flush, diaphoresis, tender abdomen	Abnormal ECG (ventricular dysrhythmias)
Ethylene glycol	Tachypnea	Altered (lethargy to coma)	Abdominal pain	Slurred speech ataxia	Anion gap acidosis, osmolal gap, crystalluria, hypocalcemia, QTc prolongation, renal failure

(Continued)

TABLE 22–10. Toxicologic Syndromes (Toxidromes) *(Continued)*

Toxin	Vital Signs	Mental Status	Symptoms	Clinical Findings	Lab Findings
Iron	Hypotension (late), tachycardia (late)	Normal unless hypotensive, lethargy	Nausea, vomiting, diarrhea, abdominal pain, hematemesis	Tender abdomen	Hyperglycemia (child), leukocytosis (child), heme + stool/vomitus, metabolic acidosis, radiopaque material on abdominal radiograph
Isoniazid	Often normal	Normal or altered (lethargy to coma)	Nausea, vomiting	Seizures	Anion gap metabolic acidosis
Isopropyl alcohol	Hypotension, bradypnea	Altered (lethargy, irritability to coma)	Nausea, vomiting	Hyporeflexia, breath odor of acetone	Ketonemia, ketonuria, no glycosuria or acidosis
Lead	Hypertension	Altered (lethargy to coma)	Irritability, abdominal pain (colic), nausea, vomiting, constipation	Peripheral neuropathy, seizures gingival pigmentation	Anemia, basophilic stippling, radiopaque material on abdominal radiograph, proteinuria
Lithium	Hypotension (late)	Altered (lethargy to coma)	Diarrhea, tremor	Weakness, tremor, ataxia, myoclonus, seizures	Leukocytosis ECG abnormalities, renal abnormalities (Diabetes Insipidus)
Mercury	Hypotension (late)	Altered (psychiatric disturbances)	Salivation, diarrhea, abdominal pain	Stomatitis, ataxia, tremor	Proteinuria, renal failure
Methanol	Hypotension, tachypnea	Altered (lethargy to coma)	Blurred vision, blindness, abdominal pain	Hyperemic disks	Anion gap metabolic acidosis, increased osmolal gap
Opioids	Hypotension, bradycardia, bradypnea, hypothermia	Altered (lethargy to coma)	Slurred speech, ataxia	Miosis, absent bowel sounds	Abnormal ABGs
Organophosphates/ carbamates	Hypotension, bradycardia/ tachycardia, bradypnea/ tachypnea	Altered (lethargy to coma)	Diarrhea, abdominal pain, blurred vision, vomiting	Salivation,diaphoresis, lacrimation, urination, defecation, miosis, fasciculations, seizures	Depressed RBC and plasma cholinesterase activity
Phencyclidine	Hypertension, tachycardia, hyperthermia	Altered (agitation, lethargy to coma)	Hallucinations	Miosis, diaphoresis, myoclonus, blank stare, nystagmus, seizures	Myoglobinuria, leukocytosis, increased CPK
Phenothiazines	Hypotension, tachycardia, hypothermia/ hyperthermia	Altered (lethargy to coma)	Dizziness	Miosis/mydriasis, decreased bowel sounds, dystonia	Abnormal ECG, abnormal abdominal radiograph
Salicylates	Hyperthermia, tachypnea	Altered (agitation, lethargy to coma)	Tinnitus, nausea, vomiting	Diaphoresis, tender abdomen	Anion gap metabolic acidosis, respiratory alkalosis, abnormal LFTs and PT/PTT positive $Fecl_3$
Sedative-hypnotics	Hypotension bradypnea, hypothermia	Altered (lethargy to coma)	Slurred speech, ataxia	Hyporeflexia, bullae	Abnormal ABGs
Theophyline	Hypotension, tachycardia, tachypnea, hyperthermia	Altered (agitation)	Nausea, vomiting, diaphoresis	Diaphoresis, tremor, seizures, dysrhythmias	Hypokalemia, hyperglycemia, metabolic acidosis, abnormal ECG

RUQ = upper right quadrant; LFT = liver function tests; CRK = creatine phosphokinase.
From Goldfrank, L. R. et al. (1994).

appropriate to the toxin (accounting for elapsed time, quantity, identity, etc.). In some cases, the treatment may involve the administration of a specific toxin antagonist and optimal outcome could depend on the expedient administrations of the antidote. There are only a few specific antidotes that must be given soon after an exposure (i.e., cyanide, nitrites). Therefore, it behooves the clinician to become familiar with the common constellation of symptoms caused by the truly life-threatening poisons.

With many toxins, there are recognizable symptoms and findings that can clue the clinician to the identity of the offending substance. These are toxic syndromes or toxidromes and are useful only if the clinician is knowledgeable about them. Table 22-10 shows many identifiable toxidromes. It is clear that a thorough history and physical yield the greatest likelihood of successfully identifying the need for an antidote. Most often, the identity of a toxin comes from the history obtained from the patient, family, friends, or co-workers. Sometimes laboratory screens of blood and urine are useful in determining whether specific treatment is necessary (i.e., acetaminophen level, iron level, or theophylline level). Keep in mind that toxidromes are frequently distorted by multiple drug ingestions. One toxin may mask the typical signs and symptoms of another, but partial findings can give the clinician a suspicion of a particular substance's presence. Searching for the identity of an unknown toxin sometimes requires astute investigative skills that make the treatment of the poisoned patient very interesting and stimulating.

Importantly, advance awareness of the antidotes that are stocked by the hospital pharmacy will prevent surprises when the clinician needs to administer a particular antidote for a toxic exposure. Several studies have looked at availability of antidotes recommended by the American Society of Emergency Medicine for inclusion in regional toxicology centers (Chyka, 1994; Katatani, 1992; Parker, 1990; Woolf & Chrisanthus, 1997). Woolf & Chrisanthus (1997) surveyed 82 hospitals in Massachusetts and found that only 2 of 82 hospitals carried all the antidotes. Only naloxone and charcoal were carried by all the hospitals. Interestingly, 17% carried only charcoal with sorbitol, making repeat dosing inadvisable. Knowledge of available antidotes at one's institution will save time in obtaining the needed medicine if it must be obtained at another institution. In some instances, it may be more expeditious to transfer the patient to the hospital that can render appropriate care. Equally important as availability of an antidote is an adequate quantity to treat a patient. Table 22–11 shows antidotes recommended by the National Capitol Poison Center to be stocked by a poison center. Table 22–12 shows common antidotes all hospitals should stock.

Clearly, poison centers serve as a central location to stock exotic antidotes that are expensive, rarely used, and sometimes in short supply. In addition, poison centers are important in reducing overall cost to the health-care system by keeping many nontoxic exposures out of the hospital all together. Phone triage frequently allows treatment to begin at home with ipecac and prevent a need for hospitalization. Miller & Lestina (1997) note the important cost-saving function of poison centers. Additionally, the poison center is a valuable resource for the treating clinician who may need specific information about managing a poisoning. Of

TABLE 22–11. Antidotes Recommended by National Capitol Poison Center

Antidote	Action
Activated charcoal	• Adsorbs most toxins
Atropine	• Reverses cholinergic effects of organophosphates • Treats bradydysrhythmias
Calcium chloride	• Reverses calcium channel blocker overdose • Corrects low Ca^{++} secondary to ethylene glycol • Blocks muscle spasms of black widow spider bite • Corrects high magnesium, low potassium
Cyanide kit	• Binds cyanide to reverse methemoglobinemia
Dextrose	• Repletes deficiency
Ethanol	• Competes for alcohol dehydrogenase to prevent toxic metabolite (ethylene glycol and methanol poisoning)
Flumazenil[a]	• Reverses effect of benzodiazepine by competing for receptor sites in brain; may cause seizure or ventricular dysrhythmia in presence of TCA
Glucagon	• Increases myocardial cAMP to increase inotropic and chronotropic function in B-blocker O.D. • Also beneficial in calcium blocker overdose
Ipecac	• Central and gastric stimulant to produce emesis • Useful in immediate post ingestion hour if sedation not likely
Methylene Blue	• Reduces to leukomethylene blue by NADPH and methemoglobin reductase. • Reverses methemoglobinemia caused by nitrites by reduction of methemoglobin to hemoglobin by leukomethylene blue
N-Acetylcysteine[b]	• Binds toxic metabolite of acetaminophen and helps produce glutathione to detoxify toxic metabolite
Naloxone	• Directly antagonizes opiate receptors in brain
Oxygen[c]	• Supplements available oxygen to compete with carbon monoxide on hemoglobin and reverse carboxyhemoglobin
Physostigmine	• Inhibits acetylcholinesterase enzyme to increase acetylcholine in anticholinergic toxicity
Polyethylene glycol (Golytely)	• Whole bowel lavage to wash out all toxins
Thiamine hydrochloride	• Replaces B_1 deficiency common in alcoholism and other diseases causing malnutrition. • Can reverse Wernicke's encephalopathy
Vitamin K	• Treats anticoagulant toxicity (prolonged PT) by replacing cofactor • Useful in activating factors II, VII, IX, X

[a] Not for empiric use. Primary use to reverse known benzodiazepine exposures after a procedure in the emergency department.
[b] If not stocked, readily available.
[c] Hyperbaric oxygen may be necessary.

TABLE 22–12. Recommended Stock List of Antidotes and Therapeutic Agents for the Treatment of Poisonings and Overdoses[a]

Therapeutic Agent	Uses
Activated charcoal	General
Antivenin (Crotalidae), Polyvalent (Wyeth)	Crotalid snake bites
Antivenin *(Latrodectus mactans)* (MSD)	Black widow spider bites
Atropine	Bradydysrhythmias, cholinesterase inhibitors (organophosphates, physostigmine) Mushrooms: clitocybe, inocybe
Botulinal antitoxin (ABE-Trivalent)	Botulism (available from local health department or Centers for Disease Control)
Calcium chloride	Oxalates, fluoride, hydrofluoric acid, ethylene glycol, calcium channel blockers, Black widow spider bites, magnesium
Calcium gluconate	Hydrofluoric acid burns, Black widow spider bites
Cyanide kit (amyl nitrite, sodium nitrite, sodium thiosulfate)	Cyanide
Deferoxamine mesylate (Desferal)	Iron
Dextrose in water (50%), (20%)	Hypoglycemic agents, patients with altered mental status
Diazepam (Valium) or Lorazepam (Ativan)	Seizures, severe agitation, stimulants
Digoxin specific antibody fragments (Digibind)	Digoxin, digitoxin, and other cardiac glycosides
Dimercaprol (BAL, British anti-lewisite)	Arsenic, mercury, gold, lead
Dimercaptosuccinic acid (DMSA)	Lead
Diphenhydramine (Benadryl)	Extrapyramidal reactions (neuroleptics), allergic reactions
Dopamine HCl	Hypotension
Edrophonium chloride (Tensilon)	Anticholinergic agents, diagnostic test (myasthenia gravis)
Ethanol oral and parenteral dosage forms	Methyl alcohol, ethylene glycol
Ethylenediaminetetraacetic acid (Calcium disodium EDTA)	Lead, zinc, and other heavy metals
Flumazenil (Romazecon)	Benzodiazepines
Folinic acid	Methyl alcohol, methotrexate
Glucagon	Beta blockers, calcium channel blockers, oral hypoglycemics
Haloperidol (Haldol)	General (as a neuroleptic)
Ipecac, syrup of	Emetic
Magnesium sulfate (Epsom salts) or magnesium citrate	General cathartic
Magnesium sulfate injection	Digitalis, hydrofluoric acid
Methylene blue (1% solution)	Methemoglobinemia
N-acetylcysteine (Mucomyst)	Acetaminophen
Naloxone hydrochloride (Narcan)	Opioids (agonists, partial agonists/antagonists)
Nitroprusside	Antihypertensive, ergotamines
Norepinephrine (Levarterenol)	Hypotension (preferred for cyclic antidepressants), alpha blockers
Oxygen (Oxygen, hyperbaric)	Carbon monoxide, cyanide, hydrogen sulfide
d-Penicillamine	Copper, mercury, arsenic
Phenobarbital	General (as anticonvulsant, sedative)
Phenytoin injection	General (as anticonvulsant, antidysrhythmic)
Physostigmine salicylate (Antilirium)	Anticholinergic agents
Polyethylene glycol (Golytely)	General (gastric decontamination)
Pralidoxime chloride (2-PAM-chloride) (Protopam)	Acetyl cholinesterase inhibitors (organophosphates and carbamates)
Protamine sulfate injection	Heparin
Pyridoxine hydrochloride	Ethylene glycol, isoniazid, monomethylhydrazine containing mushrooms
Sodium bicarbonate (5% solution)	Ethylene glycol, methanol, salicylates, cyclic antidepressants, phenobarbital, quinidine, chlorpropamide
Sorbitol	General cathartic
Starch	Iodine
Thiamine hydrochloride	Thiamine deficiency, ethylene glycol
Vitamin K (Aquamephyton)	Oral anticoagulants

[a] Each emergency department should have all of the above agents readily available to its staff. Some of these antidotes may be stored in the pharmacy, others may be available from the Centers for Disease Control, but the precise mechanism for locating each one must be known by each staff member.

From Goldfrank, L. R. et al. (1994).

note is that the PDR cannot be used as an authority on the management of many overdoses, since incorrect information has been documented (Mullen, 1997). Unfortunately, funding for these vital components of the health-care structure remains inadequate and many poison centers are financially strapped.

▶ LABORATORY TESTING

The drug screen may serve as an important adjunct in the care of the poisoned patient or as an extraneous piece of data that only adds to the cost of care. The clinician must consider what effect a laboratory result will have on the management of the patient. Consideration should be given to first quickly developing a differential diagnosis of the most likely toxin(s) based on the history, physical examination (toxidrome), and any bedside tests that are performed (Table 22–13). At this point, selective drug screening may be done with consideration to potential impact on care. If the toxin requires more than supportive care and decontamination procedures, it is necessary to quantitate it. Obtaining the proper tests at the appropriate time maximizes the usefulness of the result.

Drug levels for salicylates and acetaminophen must be drawn at a specific time post ingestion (6 hours and 4 hours, respectively) to determine the peak plasma level and thereby provide the clinician with correct information. Since acetaminophen is a relatively asymptomatic ingestion and the blood level determination is inexpensive, every patient suspected of a suicide gesture or attempt should have this level drawn. Acetaminophen is present in combination with many OTC products so the patient may not be aware he or she ingested a toxic amount of this substance. The toxic effects of this drug are very treatable and usually preventable if detected. Unlike acetaminophen, salicylate overdose can be suspected by the presence of an anion-gapped acidosis on the electrolyte panel or by a bedside test of urine with ferric chloride, if urine can be obtained. If salicylate presence is suspected, a level can be determined at the 6-hour post-ingestion time (Sporer, 1996). Meanwhile, decontamination may prevent toxicity. Of course, there are many other reasons for acidosis (remember mudpiles) that may be considered (Table 22–14).

By familiarizing him- or herself with the standard hospital drug screen, the clinician is able to order appropriate tests in a timely manner. Most serum screens include acetaminophen, maybe salicylate, alcohol, benzodiazepine, and tricyclic antidepressants. Urine screens cover cocaine metabolites, opiates, and marijuana metabolites. Other substances must be specifically requested, especially if quantification will impact care, i.e., lithium, iron, CO, digoxin, theophylline. In addition to the specific levels, electrolytes can be used to check for acidosis (salicylates, ethylene glycol, methanol), potassium (digoxin toxicity requires monitoring K^+), or sodium (monitor in lithium toxicity). An ABG is useful to determine pH and carbon monoxide level, as well as respiratory effectiveness (opiate overdoes or other sedative). A pregnancy test should be considered if radiography may be used to follow effectiveness of decontamination. The value of a CBC is limited and rarely impacts the treatment. Coagulation studies may be considered if hepatic toxicity might occur, if there is evidence of a coagulopathy, or if the toxin has an effect on coagulation (warfarin or similar rodenticide). A liver panel is useful to follow potential hepatic toxicity.

In general, a laboratory study is useful during the time when the patient is being treated. With rare exception, obtaining studies that will not be available to assist in the management of the patient are academic. A laboratory test should confirm clinical suspicion or help determine the need for an antidote. There are some cases where broad screening may be necessary, but some selectivity is still possible. If a patient is comatose, ordering screens for toxins that can cause sedation is appropriate, while looking for cocaine or phencyclidine is not likely to change treatment. Similarly, ordering a cyanide level in a cyanotic patient with a history of cyanide exposure will not affect treatment that must be ordered quickly. The clinician should also remember the possibility of lab error if a result causes significant confusion.

TABLE 22–13. Tests for Suspected Toxins

Test	Toxin	Clue
Ferric chloride	Aspirin	Add to urine—turns purple in presence of ASA
Nitroprusside	Acetone, isopropyl alcohol, salicylism, metabolic ketoacidosis	Add to urine—turns purple in presence of ketones
Blood color	CO	Chocolate brown if CO > 15%
Wood's lamp	Ethylene glycol	Fluorescent appearance of urine due to fluorescein in antifreeze
Microscopic exam	Ethylene glycol	Appearance of calcium oxalate crystals visualized in urine
Narcan	Opiate	Response to antidote
EKG	TCA	Widened QRS complex

From Goldfrank, L. R. et al. (1994).

TABLE 22–14. Metabolic Acidosis—High Anion Gap

Methanol
Uremia
Diabetic ketoacidosis
Paraldehyde
Iron, isoniazid
Lactic acidosis (hypotension, seizures, hypoxia)
Ethylene glycol and other alcohols
Salicylates and strychnine

TABLE 22–15. Common Radio-opaque Ingestions

Chloral hydrate, cocaine condoms, calcium
Heavy metals (arsenic, lead)
Iron, iodides
Phenothiazines, psychotropics (TCA), potassium
Enteric-coated tablets, slow-release capsules

▶ IMAGING

Obtaining an x-ray of the abdomen to visualize ingested pills or foreign bodies has been variably successful. Though many substances should theoretically be radio-opaque, actual *in vivo* visualization has been very limited (Table 22–15). Substances such as calcium tablets, enteric-coated pills, and metals are variably seen and depend on many factors (type of coating, rate of dissolution, whether tablets were chewed). Also, overlying bony densities can obscure tablets and a negative x-ray does not rule out an ingestion of a particular toxin. The substance with reasonably reliable radiopacity is iron, though iron in chewable tablets will not visualize if the tablet is not intact. Also, foreign bodies may be visible, especially if metallic or large and multiple (body packer). The greatest utility of the plain film is in following the success of decontamination procedures with serial films. Other modalities such as ultrasound and CT are also limited but may be useful to follow success of decontamination if the substance is visible.

REFERENCES

Allerton, J.P., & Strom, J.A. (1991). Hypernatremia due to repeated doses of charcoal-sorbitol. *American Journal of Kidney Disease, 17,* 581.

Amitai, Y., Mitchell, A. A., McGuigan, M. A., et al. (1987). Ipecac-induced emesis and reduction of plasma concentrations of drugs following accidental overdose in children. *Pediatrics, 80,* 364.

Ashton, C. H. (1985). Benzodiazepine overdose: Are specific antagonists useful. *British Medical Journal, 290,* 805.

Atkin, S. H., Dasmahaptra, A., Jaket, A., et al. (1991). Fingerstick glucose determination in shock. *Annals of Internal Medicine, 114,* 1020.

Berg, M. J., Berlinger, W. G., Goldberg, M. J., et al. (1982). Acceleration of the body clearance of phenobarbital by oral activated charcoal. *New England Journal of Medicine, 307,* 642.

Beringer, W. G., Spector, R., Goldberg, M. J., et al. (1983). Enhancement of theophylline clearance by oral activated charcoal. *Clinical Pharmacology Therapeu, 33,* 351.

Bernstein, G., Jehle, D., Bernaski, E. & Braen, G. R. (1992). Failure of gastric emptying and charcoal administration in fatal sustained-release theophylline overdose: Pharmacobezoar formation. *Annals of Emergency Medicine, 21,* 1388–1390.

Bizovi, K. E., Aks, S. E., Paloucek, F., et al. (1996). Late increase in acetaminophen concentration after overdose of Tylenol extended relief. *Annals of Emergency Medicine, 28,* 549–551.

Blake, D. R. & Bramble, M. G. (1978). Is there excessive use of gastric lavage in the treatment of self-poisoning. *Lancet, 2,* 1362.

Bond, G. R., Requa, R. K., Krenzelok, E. P., et al. (1993). Influence of time until emesis on the efficacy of decontamination using acetaminophen as a marker in a pediatric population. *Annals of Emergency Medicine, 22,* 1403–1407.

Bond, G. R. (1995). Home use of syrup of ipecac is associated with a reduction in pediatric emergency department visits. *Annals of Emergency Medicine, 25,* 338–348.

Borowitz, J. L., Moore, P. F., Yim, G. K. W., et al. (1971) Mechanism of enhanced drug effects produced by dilution of the oral dose. *Toxicology and Applied Pharmacology, 19,* 164.

Brent, J. (1993). Are activated charcoal-N-acetylcysteine interactions of clinical significance. Editorial, *Annals of Emergency Medicine, 22,* 1859–1862.

Browning, R. G., Olson, D. W., & Steven, H. A. (1990). 50% dextrose: Antidote or toxin. *Annals of Emergency Medicine, 19,* 113.

Burke, M. (1972). Gastric lavage and emesis in the treatment of ingested poisons: A review and a clinical study of lavage in ten adults. *Resuscitation, 1,* 91.

Burkhart, K. K., Wuerz, R. C., Donovan, J. W. (1992). Whole bowel irrigation as adjunctive treatment for sustained-release theophylline overdose. *Annals of Emergency Medicine, 21,* 1316–1320.

Caldwell, J. W., Nava, A. J., & DeHaas, D. D. (1987). Hypernatremia associated with cathartics in overdose management. *Western Journal of Medicine, 147,* 593.

Candelise, L., Landi, G., Orazio, E. N., et al. (1985). Prognostic significance of hyperglycemia in acute stroke. *Archives of Neurology, 42,* 661.

Chamberlain, J. M., Gorman, R. L., Oderda, G. M., et al. (1993). Use of activated charcoal in a simulated poisoning with acetaminophen: A new loading dose for N-acetylcysteine? *Annals of Emergency Medicine, 22,* 1398–1402.

Chyka, P. A. & Conner, H. G. (1994). Availability of antidotes in rural and urban hospitals in tennessee. *American Journal of Hospital Pharmacy, 51,* 1346.

Chyka, P. A. (1995). Multiple-dose activated charcoal and enhancement of systemic drug clearance: Summary of studies in animals and human volunteers. *Journal of Toxicology, 33,* 399–405.

Chyka, P. A., Holley, J. E., et al. (1995). Correlation of drug pharmacokinetics and effectiveness of multiple-dose activated charcoal therapy. *Annals of Emergency Medicine, 25,* 356–362.

Crokett, R. Pre hospital use of activated charcoal: A pilot study. *Journal of Emergency Medicine, 14,* 335.

D'Alecy, L. G., Lundy, E. F., Barton, K. L., et al. (1986). Dextrose containing intravenous fluid impairs outcome and increases death after eight minutes of cardiac arrest and resuscitation in dogs. *Surgery, 100,* 505.

Dart, R. C. (1994). Gut decontamination review. *Audio Digest Emergency Medicine, 11,* 12.

Davis, G., Santa Ana, C., Morawski, S., et al. (1980). Development of a lavage solution associated with minimal water and electrolyte absorption or secretion. *Gastroenterology, 78,* 991.

Derlet, R. W. & Albertson, T. E. (1994). Flumazenil induces seizures and death in mixed cocaine–diazepam intoxications. *Annals of Emergency Medicine, 23,* 494–498.

Doyon, S. & Roberts, J. R. (1994). Reappraisal of the "coma cocktail": Dextrose, flumazenil, naloxone, and thiamin. *Emergency Medicine Clinics of North America, 12,* 301–316.

Farley, T. A. (1986). Severe hypernatremic dehydration after use of an activated charcoal-sorbitol suspension. *Journal of Pediatrics, 109,* 719.

Garrison, R. & Somer, E. (1995). *Nutritional desk reference* (3rd ed.). New Canaan, CT: Keats Publishing.

Goldfrank, L. R., Weisman, R. S., Flomenbaum, N. E., et al. (1994). *Goldfrank's toxicologic emergencies* (5th ed.). Norwalk, CT: Appleton & Lange.

Goldfrank, L. (1996). Poison management. *Audio Digest Emergency Medicine, 13,* 3.

Goldfrank, L., Weisman, R. S., Errich, J. K., & Lo, M. W. (1986). A dosing nomogram for continuous infusion of intravenous naloxone. *Annals of Emergency Medicine, 15,* 566.

Goulbourne, K. B. & Cisek, J. E. (1994). Small bowel obstruction secondary to activated charcoal and adhesions. *Annals of Emergency Medicine, 24,* 108–110.

Grande, G. & Ling, L. (1987). The effect of fluid volume on syrup of ipecac emesis time. *Journal of Toxicology and Clinical Toxicology, 25,* 473.

Gueye, P. N., Hoffman, J. R., Taboulet, P, et al. (1996). Empiric use of flumazenil in comatose patients: Limited applicability of criteria to define low risk. *Annals of Emergency Medicine, 27,* 730–735.

Harris, C. R. & Filandrinos, D. (1993). Accidental administration of activated charcoal into the lung: Aspiration by proxy. *Annals of Emergency Medicine, 22,* 1470–1473.

Hassig, S. R., Linscheer, W. G., Murthy, U. K., et al. (1993). Effects of PEG-electrolyte (colyte) on serum acetaminophen concentrations: A model for treatment of acetaminophen overdose. *Digestive Diseases and Sciences, 38,* 1395.

Hoffman, J. R., Schriger, D. L., & Luo, J. S. (1991). The empiric use of naloxone in patients with altered mental status: A reappraisal. *Annals of Emergency Medicine, 20,* 246.

Hoffman, J. R., Schriger, D. L., Votey, S. R., et al. (1992). The empiric use of hypertonic dextrose in patients with altered mental status: A reappraisal. *Annals of Emergency Medicine, 21,* 20.

Hoffman, R. S. (1996). Poison management. *Audio Digest and Emergency Medicine, 13,* 03.

Hoffman, R. S. (1996). Assessing the coma cocktail. *Audio Digest and Emergency Medicine, 13,* 19.

Jones, J., Heiselman, D., Dougherty, J., et al. (1986). Cathartic-induced magnesium toxicity during overdose management. *Annals of Emergency Medicine, 15,* 1214.

Kaczorowski, J. M. & Wax, P. M. (1996). Five days of whole bowel irrigation in a case of pediatric iron ingestion. *Annals of Emergency Medicine, 27,* 258–263.

Kalimo, H., Rehncrona, S., Soderfeldt, D., et al. (1981). Brain lactic acidosis and ischemic cell damage. *Journal of Cerebral Blood Flow Metabolism, 1,* 313.

Kaplan, J. L. & Marx, J. A. (1993). Effectiveness and safety of intravenous nalmefene for emergency department patients with suspected narcotic overdose: A pilot study. *Annals of Emergency Medicine, 22,* 187–190.

Katatani, M. S., Kearney, T. E., Levin, R. H., et al. (1992). Treatment of toxicologic emergencies—antidote preparedness: An evaluation of Bay Area Hospital pharmacies and impact on emergency planning. *Veterinary and Human Toxicology, 34,* 319.

Knight, K. M. & Doucet, H. J. (1987). Gastric rupture and death secondary to syrup of ipecac. *Southern Medical Journal 80,* 786.

Krenzelok, E. P. (1985). Gastrointestinal transit times of cathartics used with activated charcoal. *Clinical Pharmacology 4,* 446.

Krenzelok, E. P. (1994). Syrup of ipecac—indications, controversies, limitations. *Clinical Toxicology Forum, 6,* 2.

Kucukguclu, S., Frincok, Y., Ozkan, H., et al. (1996). Multiple-dose activated charcoal in an accidental vancomycin overdose. *Journal of Toxicology, 34,* 83–86.

Kulig, K., Bar-Or, D., Cantrill, S. V., et al. (1985). Management of acutely poisoned patients without gastric emptying. *Annals of Emergency Medicine, 14,* 562.

Kulig, K. W., Bar-Or, D., Rumack, B. H., et al. (1987). Intravenous theophylline poisoning and multiple dose charcoal in an animal model. *Annals of Emergency Medicine, 16,* 842.

Levy, G. (1982). Gastrointestinal clearance of drugs with activated charcoal. *New England Journal of Medicine, 307,* 676.

Longstreth, W. T. & Inue, T. S. (1984). High blood glucose level on hospital admission and poor neurologic recovery after cardiac arrest. *Annals of Neurology, 15,* 59.

Lukas, S. E. & Griffiths, R. R. (1982). Precipitated withdrawal by a benzodiazepine receptor antagonist (RO 15 1788) after 7 days of diazepam. *Science, 217,* 1161.

Marchant, B., Wray, R., Leach, A., et al. (1989). Flumazenil causing convulsions and ventricular tachycardia. *British Medical Journal, 299,* 860.

Mariani, P. J. & Pook, N. (1993). Gastrointestinal tract perforation with charcoal peritoneum complicating orogastric intubation and lavage. *Annals of Emergency Medicine, 22,* 606–609.

McNamara, R. M., Aaron, C. K., Gemborys, M., et al. (1989). Efficacy of charcoal cathartic versus ipecac in reducing serum acetaminophen in a simulated overdose. *Annals of Emergency Medicine, 18,* 934.

Merigian, K. S., Woodard, M., Hedges, J. R., et al. (1990). Prospective evaluation of gastric emptying in the self-poisoned patient. *American Journal of Emergency Medicine, 8,* 479.

Miller, T. R. & Lestina, D. C. (1997). Costs of poisoning in the United States and savings from poison control centers: A benefit-cost analysis. *Annals of Emergency Medicine, 29,* 239–245.

Minton, N. A. & Henry, J. A. (1995). Prevention of drug absorption in simulated theophylline overdose. *Journal of Toxicology, 33,* 43–49.

Mordel, A., Winkler, E., Almog, S., et al. (1992). Seizures after flumazenil administration in a case of combined benzodiazepine and tricyclic antidepressant overdose. *Critical Care Medicine, 20,* 1733.

Mullen, W. H., Anderson, I. B., Kim, S. Y., et al. (1997). Incorrect overdose management advice in the physicians' desk reference. *Annals of Emergency Medicine, 29,* 255–261.

Myers, R. E. & Yamaguchi, S. (1976). Effects of serum glucose concentrations on brain response to circulatory arrest. *Journal of Neuropathology and Experimental Neurology, 35,* 301.

Neuvonen, P. J., Vartiainen, M., & Tokola, O. (1983). Comparison of activated charcoal and ipecac syrup in prevention of drug absorption. *European Journal of Clinical Pharmacology, 24,* 557.

North, D. S., Peterson, R. G., & Krenzelok, E. P. Effect of activated charcoal administration on acetylcysteine serum levels in humans. *American Journal of Hospital Pharmacy, 38,* 1022.

Olson, K. R., Kearney, T. E., Dyer, J. E., et al. (1993). Seizures associated with poisoning and drug overdose. *American Journal of Emergency Medicine, 11,* 565–568.

Parker, D. P., Dart, R. C., & McNally, J. T. (1990). Critical deficiencies in the treatment of toxicologic emergencies: Antidote stocking in Arizona hospitals. *Veterinary and Human Toxicology, 32,* 376.

Perrone, J., Hoffman, R. S., & Goldfrank, L. R. (1994). Special considerations in gastrointestinal decontamination. *Emergency Medicine Clinics of North America, 12,* 285–299.

Pond, S. M. (1986). Role of repeated oral doses of activated charcoal clinical toxicology. *Medicial Toxicology, 3,* 11.

Pond, S. M. (1995). Gastric emptying in acute overdose: A prospective randomized controlled trial. *Medical Journal of Australia, 163,* 345.

Prischl, F., Donner, A., Grimm, G., et al. (1998). Value of flumazenil in benzodiazepine self-poisoning. *Medical Toxicology, 3,* 334.

Pulsinelli, W. A., Levy, D. E., Sigsbee, B., et al. (1983). Increased damage after ischemic stroke in patients with hyperglycemia with and without established diabetes mellitus. *American Journal of Medicine, 74,* 540.

Roberge, R. J. & Martin, T. G. (1992). Whole bowel irrigation in an acute oral lead intoxication. *American Journal of Medicine, 10,* 577.

Roberts, J. (1994). Acetaminophen overdose: Laboratory evaluation and gastric decontamination issues. *Emergency Medicine News, 6,* 7–10.

Robertson, W. O. (1962). Syrup of ipecac—A slow or fast emetic? *American Journal of Diseases of Children, 103,* 136.

Robertson, W. O. (1979). Syrup of ipecac associated fatality: A case report. *Veterinary and Human Toxicology, 21,* 87.

Rosen, P. & Barkin, R. (1992). *Emergency Medicine Concepts and Clinical Practice* (3rd ed.). Chicago: Mosby.

Scharman, E. J., Lembersky, R., & Krenzelok, E. P. (1994). Efficacy of whole bowel irrigation with and without metoclopramide pretreatment. *American Journal of Emergency Medicine, 12,* 302–305.

Smilkstein, M. J. (1994). A new loading dose for N-acetylcysteine: The answer is no. *Annals of Emergency Medicine, 24,* 538–539.

Smith, D. A., Leake, L., Loflin, J. R., et al. (1992). Is admission after intravenous heroin overdose necessary? *Annals of Emergency Medicine, 21,* 1326–1330.

Spiller, H. A., Krenzelok, E. P., Grande, C. A., et al. (1994). A prospective evaluation of the effect of activated charcoal before oral N-acetylcysteine in acetaminophen overdose. *Annals of Emergency Medicine, 23,* 519–523.

Spivey, W. H. (1992). Flumazenil and seizures: Analysis of 43 cases. *Clinical Therapeutics, 14,* 292.

Spivey, W. H., Roberts, J. R., & Derlet, R. W. (1993). A clinical trial of escalating doses of flumazenil for reversal of suspected benzodiazepine overdose in the emergency department. *Annuals of Emergency Medicine, 22,* 1813–1820.

Sporer, K. A. & Khayam-Bashi, H. (1996). Acetaminophen and salicylate levels in patients with suicide ingestion or altered mental status. *American Journals of Emergency Medicine, 14,* 443–446.

Tandberg, D., Liecht, E. J., & Fishbein, D. (1981). Mallory-Weiss syndrome: An unusual complication of ipecac-induced emesis. *Annals of Emergency Medicine, 10,* 521.

Tenenbein, M., Cohen, S., & Sitar, D. (1987). Efficacy of ipecac-induced emesis, orogastric lavage, and activated charcoal for acute drug overdose. *Annals of Emergency Medicine, 16,* 838.

Tenenbein, M. (1988). Whole bowel irrigation as a gastrointestinal decontamination procedure after acute poisoning. *Medical Toxicology, 3,* 77.

Vance, M. V., Selden, B. S., & Clark, R. F. (1992). Optimal patient position for transport and initial management of toxic ingestions. *Annals of Emergency Medicine, 21,* 243–246.

Votey, S. R., Bosse, G. M., Bayer, M. J., et al. (1991). Flumazenil: A new benzodiazepine antagonist. *Annals of Emergency Medicine, 20,* 181.

Wald, P., Stern, J., Weiner, B., et al. (1986). Esophageal tear following forceful removal of an impacted oral gastric lavage tube. *Annals of Emergency Medicine, 15,* 80.

Wax, P. M., Wang, R. Y., Hoffman, R. S., Mercurio, M., Howland, M., & Goldfrank, L. (1993). Prevalence of sorbitol in multidose activated charcoal regimens in emergency departments. *Annals of Emergency Medicine, 22,* 1807–1812.

Weiner, K. (1991). The effect of hematocrit on reagent strip tests for glucose. *Diabetic Medicine 8,* 172.

Weisman, R. S. (1994). Antidotes in depth: Naloxone. *In Goldfrank's Toxicologic Emergencies* (5th ed.). (pp. 784–785). Norwalk, CT: Appleton & Lange.

Welsh, F. A., Ginsberg, M. D., Rieder, B. S., et al. (1980). Deleterious effect of glucose pretreatment on recovery from diffuse cerebral ischemia in the category II regional metabolite levels. *Stroke, 11,* 355.

Wolowodiuk, O. J., McMicken, D. B., & O'Brien, P. (1984). Pneumomediastinum and retroperitoneum: An unusual complication of syrup of ipecac induced emesis. *Annals of Emergency Medicine, 13,* 1148.

Woolf, A. D. & Chrisanthus, K. (1997). On-site availability of selected antidotes: Results of a survey of Massachusetts hospitals. *American Journal of Emergency Medicine 15,* 62–66.

Wrenn, K., Rodewald, L., & Dockstader, L. (1993). Potential misuse of ipecac. *Annals of Emergency Medicine, 22,* 1408–1412.

Young, W. F. & Bivins, H. G. (1993). Evaluation of gastric emptying using radionuclides: Gastric lavage vs. ipecac-induced emesis. *Annals of Emergency Medicine, 22,* 1423–1427.

23

Preoperative Evaluation and Cardiac Risk Assessment

Catherine La Mattina Allen

The goal of preoperative evaluation is to reduce morbidity associated with the perioperative experience. Typically, internists, cardiologists, and anesthesiologists play important roles in evaluation and risk assessment of patients prior to surgery. Advanced practice nurses also evaluate patients before surgery and develop a foundation for the perioperative management plan. Risk assessment identifies those patients who may benefit from heightened perioperative surveillance. This chapter presents a general overview of surgical and anesthetic stress, discusses important elements of preoperative evaluation, examines the evolution of risk-assessment strategies, and reviews the guidelines jointly developed by the American College of Cardiology/American Heart Association Committee on Perioperative Cardiovascular Evaluation for Noncardiac Surgery.

▶ THE STRESS OF SURGERY AND ANESTHESIA

The physiologic responses to surgery are controlled by the central nervous system (CNS). Surgical stimulation activates the stress response, including catecholamine surge and increased adrenocorticotropic hormone (ACTH) and cortisol secretion. Aldosterone and antidiuretic hormone (ADH) levels rise and cause sodium and water retention and reduced urinary output. When circulating blood volume fluctuates, cardiac output is affected. Although operative stress increases insulin production, hyperglycemia prevails because of increased catecholamine, cortisol, and glucagon levels. The increased metabolic rate induces catabolism. Surgical stress is attenuated through the administration of anesthesia. Anesthetic agents decrease pain sensation, diminish the release of stress hormones and catecholamines, and directly affect cardiac and pulmonary function.

Changes in pulmonary function occur from surgical positioning, operative site, or anesthesia. Functional residual capacity (FRC) declines by approximately 20% in the supine position. Vital capacity (VC) and FRC may be reduced by 70% and 50% respectively during the immediate postoperative period after upper-abdominal surgery. Anesthesia alters oxygenation and ventilation, and can lead to hypoxemia or hypercarbia. Mucociliary function is diminished in the presence of inhalation agents which potentially increases the risk of infection. Decreases in FRC and VC are more significant in patients with morbid obesity or preexisting pulmonary disease.

Cardiovascular stress occurs during the release of catecholamines and through a direct effect of anesthetic agents or techniques. The metabolic demands of surgery increase heart rate, blood pressure, and myocardial oxygen consumption. The volatile gases decrease myocardial contractility, dilate systemic vasculature, and cause a 20 to 40% reduction in stroke volume. With accompanying blood or fluid loss, reductions in cardiac output can occur. Inadequate anesthetic depth can stress the cardiovascular system when tachycardia ensues. During surgery, the threat of myocardial ischemia exists due to potential imbalances between oxygen supply and demand (Fig. 23–1).

Surgical stress increases oxygen demand (i.e., increased heart rate or blood pressure during intubation, incision, and extubation), or decreases oxygen supply (i.e., during significant blood loss or hypoxemia).

The cardiovascular system is also affected by anesthetic choice. High doses of narcotics have little effect on myocardial contractility and are useful in patients with a compromised left ventricle. The use of narcotics more effectively blocks autonomic responses. However, the attendant respiratory and CNS depression persist into the recovery period and may require assisted ventilation. Though regional (spinal or epidural) anesthesia is more effective than general anesthesia at limiting the rise in stress hormones, it can result in arterial hypotension due to sympathetic blockade of preganglionic vasomotor efferents. As the venous capacitance system dilates, blood pooling reduces preload which impairs cardiac output.

Other intraoperative stresses, such as ocular manipulation, intraabdominal traction, carotid sinus pressure, or tracheal intubation, can increase parasympathetic activity which may result in bradyarrhythmias and hypotension. Sympathetic hyperactivity due to catecholamine release from inadequate anesthesia, hypoxia, or hypercapnea may precipitate ventricular tachyarrythmias.

Perioperative stress renders the patient hypercoagulable, increasing the risk of thrombotic complications. On the other hand, clotting may be impaired due to hypothermia or preexisting disease. The use of anticoagulants may be associated with important perioperative complications.

To summarize, perioperative stress taxes the metabolic, pulmonary, cardiovascular, central nervous, and hematologic systems in ways that can jeopardize even the most stable of patients. Patient safety is enhanced through timely, detailed preoperative evaluation. When necessary, optimization of health status can occur and the anesthesiologist can implement an anesthetic management plan designed within the context of the patient's coexistent disease.

▶ PERIOPERATIVE CONSULTATION

The term "perioperative" refers to the period immediately before, during, and after surgical intervention. The perioperative consultant evaluates the patient and recommends therapeutic interventions during these specific time intervals. The *preoperative* consultant evaluates the patient's medical condition, anticipates the effects of surgery, and recommends interventions for improvement of the patient's health status prior to operation. Internists, family practitioners, surgeons, and nurse practitioners perform preoperative evaluation. The *intraoperative* consultant assists the anesthesiologist or surgeon with the management of acute problems (e.g., cardiology consultation). The *postoperative* consultant evaluates new or preexisting problems within the context of the surgical experience. Postoperative evaluation is performed by a variety of specialists (e.g., endocrinologists, infectious disease specialists) and nurse practitioners. Anesthesiologists may be consulted for the management of postoperative pain.

The *preanesthetic* consultant is a member of the anesthesia care team and also evaluates the patient's preoperative health status. Anesthesiologists, nurse anesthetists, and nurse practitioners perform this evaluation. During the preanesthetic visit, the consultant conducts an airway evaluation, anticipates the effects of anesthesia, formulates the

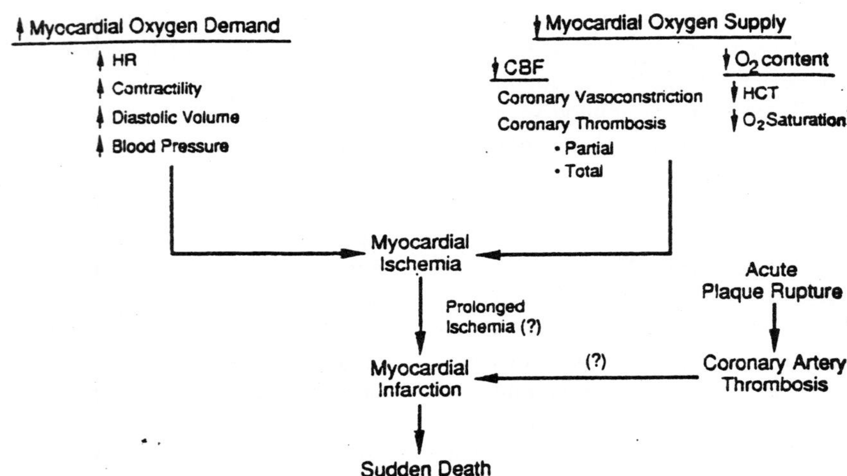

Figure 23–1. Determinants of myocardial ischemia and infarction. Intraoperative stressors can lead to an imbalance between myocardial oxygen supply and demand, resulting in ischemia or infarction. *(Used with permission from Beattie, C. & Fleisher, L. [1992].)*

anesthetic management plan within the context of the patient's medical condition, and estimates the patient's fitness for anesthesia in an attempt to minimize risk. The anesthetic management plan documents choice of anesthetic, choice of intraoperative monitors, and recommendations for airway and pain management. At this time, informed consent for anesthesia is obtained. Every patient who is expected to receive anesthesia requires a preanesthetic consultation.

▶ PREOPERATIVE EVALUATION

A formal preoperative evaluation documents all pertinent aspects of the patient's health history and concludes with a summary of the medical stability of the patient. The goal is to identify those factors that increase perioperative risk and determine whether or not the patient's medical condition can be improved. When performing the preoperative consultation, it is important to remember its audience and potential contribution towards minimizing perioperative morbidity and mortality. The surgical and anesthesia care teams use the preoperative evaluation to prepare for perioperative patient management.

These teams are often hampered by limited access to the patient's medical records, so the importance of documenting the dates and results of important prior testing (e.g., cardiovascular or pulmonary evaluations) cannot be overstated. Finally, recommendations for perioperative management should be noted with awareness of the fact that intraoperative management and anesthetic choice are the exclusive purview of the anesthesiologist.

Elements of the preoperative evaluation include assessment of medical, surgical, anesthetic, social, and family histories; documentation of medications and allergies; a review of systems; a focused physical examination; and notation of the results of preoperative testing. At the conclusion of preoperative evaluation, a complete problem list should document the stability of each medical condition.

History

The foundation of preoperative evaluation is a thorough history. The status and dates of all past and present medical conditions and recent acute illness is documented along with the outcome of each evaluation. Dates and reasons for prior hospitalizations are included. A useful way of communicating this information is through the use of a problem-oriented list that starts with the current health condition requiring surgical intervention and proceeds in reverse chronological order. Type of previous surgery and anesthesia should mention any history of surgical or anesthetic problems, such as difficult intubation. A family history of complications with anesthesia should be noted, such as malignant hyperthermia or pseudocholinesterase deficiency.

The list of medications should document recent steroid or anticoagulant use, or chemotherapy received within the preceding month. Steroids taken within six months of surgery may require stress-dose steroids for a major operation.

The documentation of allergies and specific reactions should include the presence or absence of latex sensitivity. Patients with frequent exposure to latex proteins, history of spina bifida, or multiple surgical procedures during infancy should be considered latex sensitive and appropriate precautions taken (Mendel, 1997).

The psychosocial history includes documentation of current or prior tobacco, alcohol, or drug use; status of current living situation if pertinent to postoperative care; religious preferences with surgical implication (e.g., nonacceptance of blood products); occupation; and identification of alternative medical decision-maker. When preoperative anxiety is extreme, a notation of the circumstances facilitates appropriate management.

Recording the presence or absence of a family history of cardiovascular disease assists in identifying the context of a patient's cardiac risk, along with the history, physical examination, and electrocardiogram (ECG).

For pediatric patients, the birth and developmental history documents prematurity, history of apnea (including family history of sudden infant death), or developmental delay. Postoperative apnea and bradycardia are more likely to occur in young patients with a history of premature birth. Lower respiratory tract infection typically requires the postponement of elective surgery for at least one month. When cranio–facial congenital anomaly exits, a member of the anesthesia care team should be consulted prior to the day of surgery to assess relevant intubation concerns.

For the obstetric patient, the history includes past or present complications during pregnancy and date of last menstrual period. A preanesthetic evaluation is essential for parturients so that an anesthetic management plan may be developed that is appropriate to the time of gestation. Pharmacologic agents with teratogenic potential may be contraindicated during the first trimester; for this reason, it is prudent to inquire about the possibility of pregnancy during the preoperative evaluation for women of childbearing age.

Review of Systems

The review of systems (ROS) is a methodical inquiry about symptoms that may lead to the discovery of undiagnosed medical illness. Additionally, the identification of problems with surgical or anesthetic implications enables interventions designed to maximize perioperative safety. During the system review, the clinician asks about symptoms for each major organ system. A careful review will often trigger the patient to recall medical conditions that have not been previously discussed.

The ROS begins with an inquiry of symptoms associated with neurological illness: syncope, dizziness, vision or speech changes, unexplained weakness, severe headaches, memory loss, or history of cerebrovascular insult, migraine headache, seizures, or CNS disease.

The patient is asked about pulmonary symptoms: shortness of breath at rest or with exertion, orthopnea, chronic cough or wheezes, sputum production, activity tolerance, or history of recent acute or chronic respiratory illness. When a history of chronic obstructive pulmonary disease (COPD) or asthma exists, the clinician should inquire about triggering mechanisms, use of inhalers or steroids, frequency of exacerbations, prior need for hospitalization or emergency treatment, situations requiring intubation, and tolerance of previous general anesthesia. Inquiry concerning a history of sleep apnea should be prompted during the preoperative assessment of the morbidly obese patient. Symptoms suggestive of sleep apnea include snoring and daytime somnolence. Supportive data may be obtained from a family member who has witnessed apneic episodes. With this condition, the airway can obstruct after induction of general anesthesia or during the administration of sedative anesthetics and increase the risk of hypoxia. The use of postoperative narcotics further subjects the patient to the risk of airway obstruction.

The cardiovascular review strives to determine an assessment of the functional status of this system. The clinician derives important information about cardiovascular performance through inquiry about the condition of four major aspects of cardiovascular function: vessels, valves, volts, and ventricle (the "Four Vs"). Questions concerning the "Four Vs" attempt to identify symptoms of coronary artery disease (CAD) or peripheral vascular disease (PVD), valvular heart disease, electrical instability, or congestive heart failure (CHF). Symptoms include: fatigue, palpitations, dizziness, syncope, angina, nocturnal or exertional dyspnea, claudication, swelling, or decreased exercise tolerance. The patient should be queried about a past history of myocardial infarction (MI), CHF, rheumatic fever, heart murmur, mitral valve prolapse, cardiac arrhythmia, or implantation of cardiac devices such as pacemaker or internal defibrillator. It is often helpful to ask the patient about the nature of previous cardiovascular testing or interventional procedures so that records may be obtained if necessary. When a prior history of CHF exists, severity and functional status is evaluated according to the New York Heart Association (NYHA) classification system. The Canadian Cardiovascular Society Functional Classification of Angina (CCVSA) may be used to quantify the severity of angina (Table 23–1).

During the gastrointestinal review, the patient is questioned about the following symptoms: dyspepsia, reflux, epigastric pain, or a history of peptic ulcer disease, hiatal hemia, gastroparesis, or gastroesophageal reflux disease (GERD). The presence of upper gastrointestinal disease may predispose the patient to aspiration of gastric contents during intubation. Prophylactic measures by the anesthesia care team include the administration of gastrokinetic agents or H_2-antagonists to avoid or diminish the severity of aspiration should it occur. The patient is also questioned about a prior history of hepatitis or hepatic impairment.

Patients with renal impairment should be questioned about the stability of coexisting disease. With end-stage renal disease (ESRD) related to diabetes or hypertension, the patient may have associated CAD or CHF and an investigation of symptoms pertinent to these illnesses must occur. In addition, fluid, electrolyte, and coagulation status must be determined through questioning and appropriate laboratory testing. Surgery must be coordinated with plans for dialysis.

The health history typically identifies the presence of endocrine dysfunction. A system review allows the clinician to determine the degree of control of known metabolic illness. The endocrine conditions most commonly encountered during the preoperative evaluation include thyroid disease, diabetes mellitus, morbid obesity, and adrenal insufficiency. Prior to operation, euthyroid status must be assured in patients with a history of hyperthyroidism so that the hypermetabolic changes associated with the stress of surgery are not exacerbated. The greatest surgical risks for the hyperthyroid patient are tachyarrhythmias or thyroid storm. Conversely, untreated hypothyroidism can manifest as cardiovascular or respiratory failure in the postoperative period.

For patients with diabetes mellitus, the clinician must inquire about symptoms of end-organ disease: CAD, cardiomyopathy, PVD, renal insufficiency, retinopathy, autonomic impairment, or peripheral neuropathy. Autonomic dysfunction can result in silent ischemia or gastroparesis and complicate the perioperative period with MI or aspiration.

TABLE 23–1. The New York Heart Association Classification of Heart Failure and the Canadian Cardiovascular Society Functional Classification of Angina

NYHA		CCVSA	
Class 1	No symptoms with ordinary physical activity	Class I	Ordinary physical activity does not cause angina
Class 2	Symptoms with ordinary activity; slight limitation of activity	Class II	Slight limitation with ordinary activity
Class 3	Symptoms with less than ordinary activity; marked limitation of activity	Class III	Marked limitations of ordinary activity
Class 4	Symptoms with any physical activity or even at rest	Class IV	Inability to carry on any physical activity without discomfort

Used with permission from Kurki, T. (1997).

The morbidly obese patient is at risk for sleep apnea, hypertension, left ventricular dysfunction, restrictive lung problems, gastrointestinal or hepatobiliary disease, and glucose intolerance. There is also a potential for difficult mask ventilation or intubation, aspiration, and venous access problems at the time of surgery.

Primary adrenal insufficiency caused by Addison's disease or secondary insufficiency due to exogenous glucocorticoid administration requires perioperative steroid coverage for a major operation to prevent hemodynamic instability.

An inquiry about musculoskeletal function may uncover limitations that should be known to the anesthesia care team. Specifically, arthritic conditions of the neck may limit the mobility needed to visualize the larynx during intubation and temporomandibular joint dysfunction can also challenge instrumentation of the airway. Spinal or epidural anesthesia may be problematic in patients with disorders of the spine. The pharmacologic treatment of joint conditions often requires preoperative modification and patients may be advised to stop aspirin and nonsteroidal antiinflammatory agents (NSAIDs) to minimize the risk of excessive bleeding.

The hematologic/immunologic review questions the patient about a history of anemia, prolonged bleeding, bleeding tendency, thromboembolic disease, cancer, or serious infectious illness.

The final inquiry addresses possible intubation or ventilation concerns. The patient is questioned about a history of dental, intraoral, or laryngeal disease, or prior irradiation of the head or neck.

Physical Examination

Preoperative physical examination begins with documentation of patient demographics and the recording of vital signs: age, gender, height, weight, heart rate, and blood pressure. General appearance is noted. The baseline mental status should be documented, particularly in the elderly patient, so that a basis for comparison exists if postoperative changes occur. The head and neck examination focuses on notation of the following: presence of anatomic or congenital abnormality; surgical scars; oral condition inclusive of teeth, gums, tongue, and pharynx; range of motion; presence of masses, jugular venous distention (JVD), or bruit; and evidence of tracheal deviation or thyroid abnormality. The presence of hoarseness should be noted. Anatomic features that may contribute to difficult intubation include receding mandible; small mouth opening or oropharynx; short, muscular neck; high, arched palate; protruding maxillary incisors; or a limited view of the posterior pharynx. When a suspicion of difficult intubation exists, the patient must be evaluated by a member of the anesthesia care team before the day of surgery.

The lungs are examined for adventitious sounds or wheezing and the cardiac examination includes an assessment of rhythm and notation of abnormal heart sounds, murmurs, clicks, or rubs.

The abdomen is examined for distention or masses, and the extremities are checked for pulses and the presence of edema, clubbing, or cyanosis.

Sensory impairments and gross neurologic function should be noted. Further assessment is guided by data accumulated during the history and review of systems.

Preoperative Testing

The detailed history, system review, and physical examination provide nearly all the information required to assess preoperative medical stability. Diagnostic testing should be ordered only as indicated by this information. Nevertheless, in many settings, institutional or clinical practice standards determine the nature and extent of laboratory and ancillary testing. The evidence within the literature supports a conservative approach to routine preoperative tests. A useful strategy for preoperative testing is found in Table 23–2 and Figure 23–2.

Outcome

At the conclusion of preoperative evaluation, the clinician formulates an impression of the patient's health status. The medically stable patient requires no further intervention and may proceed to surgery. When the patient's clinical condition requires additional intervention or an important abnormality is found on diagnostic testing, specific recommendations should be communicated to the surgeon and/or the anesthesiologist. Strategies for improvement of the preoperative status or the prevention of morbidity may include the prescription of pharmacologic agents. In some instances, further diagnostic testing or consultation is indicated.

With the exception of diuretics, patients are always advised to continue cardiopulmonary medications up to the time of surgery. Patients with pulmonary disease using metered dose inhalers should continue their use perioperatively. Pulmonary function may need to be maximized with bronchodilators, steroids, or antibiotics. Smoking cessation should be strongly encouraged. Lower respiratory tract infection requires the postponement of elective surgery. Asymptomatic patients with a recent upper respiratory infection may be able to safely undergo outpatient or minor elective surgery; however, there may be heightened airway reactivity, increased airway resistance, or diaphragmatic dysfunction for up to several weeks after viral infection. Patients with severe pulmonary disease may require preoperative pulmonary consultation prior to major cardio–thoracic or abdominal surgery. Pulmonary function tests should be performed before lung resection. The risk of postoperative pulmonary complications increases when the forced expiratory volume in one second (FEV_1) is less than 2 liters or the forced vital capacity (FVC) is less than 50% of the predicted value.

TABLE 23–2. Indications for Laboratory Testing

Test	Indications
Hemoglobin	Menstruating females, children less than 1 year old or with suspected sickle cell disease, history of anemia, blood dyscrasia or malignancy, congenital heart disease, chronic disease states, age greater than 60 years
WBC count	Suspected infection or immunosuppression
Platelet count	History of abnormal bleeding or bruising, liver disease, blood dyscrasias, chemotherapy, hypersplenism
Coagulation studies	History of abnormal bleeding, anticoagulant drug therapy, liver disease, malabsorption, poor nutritional status
Electrolytes, blood glucose, BUN/creatinine	Patients with hypertension, diabetes, heart disease, or disease states with the potential for fluid–electrolyte abnormalities. Patients taking digoxin, diuretics, steroids, or ACE-inhibitors
Liver function tests	Patients with liver disease, history of or exposure to hepatitis, history of alcohol or drug abuse, drug therapy with agents that may affect liver function
Pregnancy test	Patients in whom pregnancy cannot be reliably ruled out by history (some suggest all females of childbearing years)
Urinalysis	No indication in preanesthetic evaluation; surgeon may request to rule out infection before certain surgical procedures, particularly those involving prosthetic implants
Electrocardiogram	Males more than 45 years old, females more than 55 years old, history or symptoms of cardiac disease, history of hypertension, diabetes, morbid obesity, significant pulmonary disease, cocaine abuse
Chest x-ray	Patients with symptoms of pulmonary disease, airway obstruction, cardiac disease, malignancy, history of heavy smoking, age greater than 75 years
Cervical spine flexion/extension	Patients with rheumatoid arthritis or Down's syndrome

No laboratory test is indicated merely because the patient is undergoing anesthesia or surgery. Laboratory tests should be chosen according to specific indications, based on a comprehensive history and physical examination. Some guidelines are listed.
Used with permission from Everett, L. & Kallar, S. (1995).

Moderate to severe hypertension (diastolic > 110 mm Hg) may contribute to significant lability of intraoperative blood pressure which can predispose the patient to cardiac or renal morbidity. During surgery, the usual variations in heart rate and blood pressure are exaggerated in the hypertensive patient. Therefore, patients with coronary disease or left ventricular dysfunction are at risk for ischemia or heart failure. Since chronic hypertension resets autoregulation of cerebral circulation, perioperative blood pressure reductions may also induce cerebral ischemia. The patient with severe or newly diagnosed hypertension should have elective surgery postponed until initiation or reevaluation of pharmacologic therapy results in better control. Postoperative management should continue with parenteral agents when the patient is fasting.

Patients with poorly controlled cardiac disease such as unstable angina, severe valvular disease, symptomatic arrhythmia, cardiomyopathy, and decompensated CHF are at risk for perioperative MI or CHF and require cardiology consultation prior to surgery. Strategies for evaluating car-

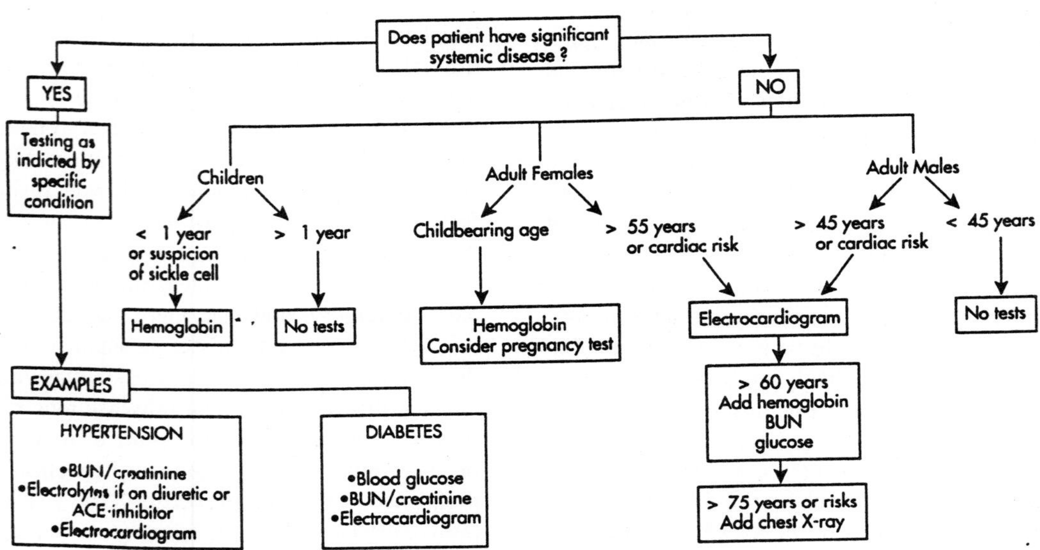

Figure 23–2. Preoperative testing algorithm. Properative testing may be ordered on disease or age criteria. *(Used with permission from Everett, L. & Kallar, S. [1995].)*

diac risk within the context of the type of proposed surgery are discussed later in this chapter. Recommendations for preoperative endocarditis prophylaxis should follow American Heart Association guidelines (Table 23–3).

Perioperative management of patients with diabetes must be individually tailored. A knowledge of preoperative glycemic control sets the stage for an appropriate management strategy. One alternative is to discontinue all types of insulin on the morning of surgery. Another approach is to give one third to one half the dose of longer-acting insulin. Blood glucose determination by fingerstick should occur within one hour of surgery with short-acting insulin coverage as needed. In circumstances of brittle control, consultation with an endocrinologist may be necessary.

Adrenal suppression is expected when patients have taken supraphysiologic doses of glucocorticoids for more than a week during the half year preceding surgery (daily administration of more than 7.5 mg prednisone or 20 mg hydrocortisone). Appropriate steroid coverage for major surgery consists of hydrocortisone 100 mg IV given one hour prior to induction of anesthesia and continued every eight hours throughout the immediate postoperative period.

To summarize, elective surgery may need to be postponed and additional consultation sought for the following clinical situations (adapted from Everett & Kallar, 1995):

- Recent myocardial infarction (< 6 months)
- Unstable angina (CCVSA Class III or IV)
- Uncontrolled systemic morbidity: hypertension (diastolic blood pressure > 110), diabetes, asthma, COPD, hepatic or renal disease
- New or symptomatic cardiac dysrhythmia
- ECG changes suggestive of ischemia or infarct
- Congestive heart failure (NYHA Class 3 or 4)
- Serious bleeding disorders
- Significant exercise intolerance
- Moderate to severe involuntary weight loss with constitutional symptoms not previously evaluated
- Syncope
- Unstable neurological disease

When the patient's medical condition is complex or not optimized, timely consultation with a member of the anesthesia care team should also be sought (Table 23–4). The Pre-Surgical Evaluation Form in use at the Allegheny University Hospitals (Pennsylvania) represents a model approach to the documentation of the patient's preoperative medical condition (Fig. 23–3).

TABLE 23–3. Endocarditis Prophylaxis Recommendations

Cardiac Conditions That Require Endocarditis Prophylaxis
- Prosthetic cardiac valves
- Previous bacterial endocarditis
- Most congenital cardiac malformations
- Rheumatic and other acquired valvular dysfunction, even after surgery
- Hypertrophic cardiomyopathy
- Mitral valve prolapse with valvular regurgitation

Surgical Procedures That Require Endocarditis Prophylaxis
- Tonsillectomy and/or adenoidectomy
- Surgical operations that involve intestinal or respiratory mucosa
- Rigid bronchoscopy
- Sclerotherapy for esophageal varices
- Esophageal dilation
- Cystoscopy
- Urethral dilation
- Urethral catheterization, if urinary tract infection is present
- Urinary tract surgery, if urinary tract infection is present
- Prostatic surgery
- Incision and drainage of infected tissue
- Dental procedures likely to cause gingival or mucosal bleeding

Procedures That May Not Require Endocarditis Prophylaxis
- Injection of local intraoral anesthetic
- Tympanostomy tube insertion
- Endotracheal intubation
- Flexible bronchoscopy
- Endoscopy
- Dental procedures not likely to induce gingival bleeding

Used with permission from Green, C. & Pandit, S. (1995). In R. Twersky (ed.). The ambulatory anesthesia handbook. *St. Louis: Mosby.*

RISK ASSESSMENT

Perioperative risk is the possibility of morbidity or mortality associated with preoperative preparation, surgery, anesthesia, and postoperative recovery. The determinants of perioperative risk are confounded by a multitude of variables that are patient-, procedure-, provider-, institution-, or anesthetic-related. The process of preoperative evaluation attempts to limit the risks associated with the surgical experience through appropriate optimization of the medical condition. However, preoperative evaluation can only be concerned with the risks that the patient himself or herself brings to surgery. The actual contribution that these risks represent in overall perioperative morbidity is not known. Murphy (1992) reported that the 1 to 2% estimate of the death rate within the first 30 days after surgery was more related to the patient's underlying disease state than to surgical or anesthetic mishap.

Anesthetic and Surgical Risk

The long history of risk measurement within the discipline of anesthesiology dates back to the 1850s when controversy focused on the relative safety of ether anesthesia (Pierce, 1990). The American Society of Anesthesiologists (ASA) has been continuously involved in the examination of anesthesia-related morbidity and, in 1941, initiated the first system for the identification of operative risk in relation to the patient's physical state (Saklad, 1941). At the time of preanesthetic evaluation, the medical condition of the patient

TABLE 23–4. Conditions for which Consultation with a Member of the Anesthesia Care Team Should Be Sought Prior to the Day of Surgery

General
Medical condition inhibiting ability to engage in normal daily activity
Medical conditions necessitating continual assistance or monitoring at home within the past 6 months
Admission within the past 2 months for acute or exacerbation of chronic condition

Cardiocirculatory
History of angina, coronary artery disease, myocardial infarction, symptomatic arrhythmias
Poorly controlled hypertension (diastolic >110, systolic >160)
History of congestive heart failure

Respiratory
Asthma or COPD requiring chronic medications, or with acute exacerbation and progression within past 6 months
History of major airway surgery or unusual airway anatomy, upper and/or lower airway tumor or obstruction
History of chronic respiratory distress requiring home ventilatory assistance or monitoring

Endocrine
Nondiet controlled diabetes (insulin or oral hypoglycemic agents)
Adrenal disorders
Active thyroid disease

Neuromuscular
History of seizure disorder or other significant CNS disease (e.g., multiple sclerosis)
History of myopathy or other muscle disorders

Hepatic
Any active hepatobiliary disease or compromise

Musculoskeletal
Kyphosis and/or scoliosis causing functional compromise
Temporomandibular joint disorder
Cervical or thoracic spine injury

Oncology
Patients receiving chemotherapy
Other oncology process with significant physiologic residual or compromise

Gastrointestinal
Massive obesity (>140% ideal body weight)
Hiatal hernia
Symptomatic gastroesophageal reflux

Used with permission from Pasternak, L.R. (1995).

was designated according to predetermined categories. The process of classifying the patient's preoperative medical status evolved over a twenty-year period and, by 1963, the ASA adopted the physical status classification system that anesthesiologists use today (Table 23–5) (American Society of Anesthesiologists, 1963). An interpretation of ASA physical status is found in Table 23–6.

The utility of the ASA classification system was documented in an important study reported by Dripps, Lamont, & Eckenoff (1961). It was found that ASA physical status predicted anesthetic morbidity and mortality. The correlation of physical status with mortality was subsequently validated by other investigators (Cohen, Duncan, & Tate, 1988; Marx, Mateo, & Orkin, 1973; Vacanti, VanHouten, & Hill, 1970). The anesthesiologist's impression of anesthetic risk is derived from the ASA physical status classification and the results of preoperative testing.

The continued evaluation of anesthesia practices and outcomes led to the ASA's formulation of intraoperative monitoring standards in 1986 which are thought to be responsible for important declines in anesthesia morbidity and mortality. Mortality rates due to anesthesia-related complications are estimated at 1:10,000 to 1:185,000; and 1:200,000 for healthier patients in ASA Class I and 2 (Hirsh, 1994; Murphy, 1992).

The precise contribution that the surgical procedure itself has on overall postoperative morbidity is difficult to quantify. Studies on postoperative mortality are confounded by patient, surgical, and anesthetic-related factors. The literature consistently confirms that the patient's underlying medical condition is the most important predictor of surgical mortality. Certain operations—such as intrathoracic, intraperitoneal, aortic, peripheral vascular, and emergency surgery—are associated with higher risk and, when serious complications occur, they are typically cardiac in nature (Abraham et al., 1991; Keenan & Boyan, 1985). As surgical technique and anesthesia safety advanced, patients with complex medical problems became more acceptable surgical risks.

Cardiovascular Risk

The leading cause of postoperative death is cardiac morbidity. Contributing factors include dysrhythmias, CHF, unstable angina, and MI (Mangano, 1990, 1991a). In Coronary Artery Surgery Study (CASS) registry patients undergoing noncardiac surgery, cardiac mortality was nearly five times greater in patients with CAD than in patients without significant CAD (2.4% versus 0.5%) (Foster, Davis, Carpenter, Abele, & Fray, 1986). In vascular surgery patients, myocardial infarction occurs in up to 15% of patients (Mangano, 1991a). The risk of postoperative MI is greater in patients with a history of infarction than in patients without previous MI (5-8% versus 0.1-0.7%), and reinfarction mortality approaches 70% (Leung, London, & Mangano, 1990; Topkins & Artusio, 1964).

Studies conducted during the 1960s and 1970s demonstrated that surgery performed within 6 months of MI was associated with significant reinfarction rates: 30% within 3 months, 15% within 3 to 6 months, and 5% after 6 months (Goldman, 1983; Kurki, 1997; Mangano, 1990). These data had been the basis for the postponement of elective surgery until 6 months following myocardial infarction. However,

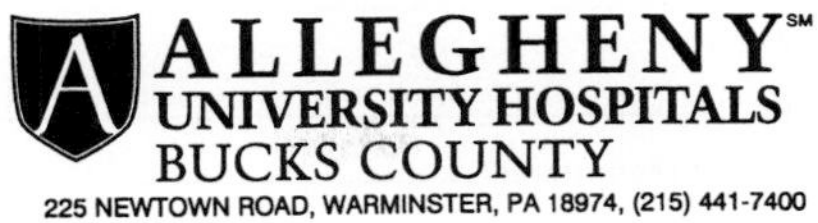

PRE-SURGICAL EVALUATION FORM

All blanks must be filled. Please record pertinent positives or indicate NL (normal) or NA (not applicable).

PATIENT STAMP

Chief Complaint / Procedure: (Reasons / indications / criteria for procedure)

Other Current Medical Problems:

Past Medical / Surgical History:

Present Medications and Allergies:

Review of Systems:

Family / Social History:

FORM #X0279BC (REV. 8/97)

(Continued on page 338)

Figure 23–3. The Pre-Surgical Evaluation Form at Allegheny University Hospitals—Bucks County. *(Used with permission.)*

in a study conducted by Rao, Jacobs, & El-Etr (1983), preoperative optimization and intensified monitoring reduced the incidence of reinfarction with surgery performed at 3 and 6 months after MI to 5.7% and 1.9%, respectively. A small study of 48 patients demonstrated no reinfarctions when surgery was performed at 3 months after MI (Wells & Kaplan, 1981). Some investigators suggest that aggressive intraoperative monitoring increases the safety of an operation, yet studies do not consistently demonstrate that intraoperative invasive monitors prevent postoperative cardiovascular complications. The decrease in reinfarction rates is more likely related to refinements in perioperative care.

After surgery, the peak incidence of MI occurs on postoperative day three. When postoperative MI does occur, a typical anginal presentation may be absent and instead, CHF, hypotension, or arrhythmia may occur.

Physical Examination: (Please check if normal, or describe abnormalities)

☐ Mental Status ______ ☐ Vital Signs ______
☐ General Appearance ______ ☐ Skin / Mucous Membranes ______
☐ HEENT ______ ☐ Heart ______
☐ Lungs ______ ☐ Lymph Nodes ______
☐ Abdomen ______ ☐ Pelvic / Rectal ______
☐ Breasts ______ ☐ Neurologic ______
☐ Extremities ______ ☐ Other ______

Laboratory / X -Ray: (Please check desired studies)

☐ CBC ☐ PT / PTT ☐ ECG
☐ SMA 6 ☐ CXR ☐ Other
☐ Urine

Impression and Plan: (Attention to status for surgery/anesthesia)

Is Patient in Optimal Medical Condition for Surgery:

☐ YES ☐ NO (If NO, please explain)

Signature: ______ **Date / Time:** ______

☐ Please check if additional information is attached

I have made positive indentification of my patient.

______ **M.D.** ______ **CRNA / RN**

Figure 23–3. *(Continued)*

Cardiac Risk Indices

By 1975, research demonstrated that many of the factors presumed to contribute to perioperative cardiac morbidity were related to the patient's medical condition and could be identified from the history and physical examination conducted preoperatively. A history of recent MI (< 6 months) or current CHF appeared to confer the greatest risk to the patient. For these reasons, the ASA physical status classification, the functional classification of heart disease by NYHA criteria, and the functional classification of angina by CCVSA criteria became useful, though limited, indices in the quantification of perioperative risk.

The cardiac risk index published by Goldman et al.

TABLE 23–5. The American Society of Anesthesiologists (ASA) Classification of Physical Status

1. A normal healthy patient.
2. A patient with a mild systemic disease.
3. A patient with a severe systemic disease that limits activity, but is not incapacitating.
4. A patient with an incapacitating systemic disease that is a constant threat to life.
5. A moribund patient not expected to survive 24 hours with or without operation.

In the event of emergency operation, precede the number with an E.

Used with permission from ASA new classification of physical status. (1963). Anesthesiology.

(1977) became the standard by which preoperative risk was measured. This study was the first prospective attempt at the prediction of cardiac risk for noncardiac surgery and included 1001 consecutive patients undergoing major surgery at the Massachusetts General Hospital between 1975 and 1976. Through multivariate analysis, nine correlates of cardiac risk were identified and weighted such that a score could be tabulated and risk assigned according to one of four categories (Table 23–7). As total point value increased, there was a statistically significant increase in cardiac morbidity and mortality among the study subjects.

The "Goldman Criteria" identified variables that were patient, surgical, and diagnostic testing related, and included data concerning history, physical exam, ECG, laboratory, and type of operation. Cardiovascular risk factors such as angina, previous MI, diabetes, hypertension, smoking, hyperlipidemia, PVD, and ECG changes indicative of ischemia or infarct were not identified as predictors of perioperative risk in Goldman's study.

The Goldman Index of Cardiac Risk was validated prospectively in a cohort of 1140 surgical patients at the Toronto General Hospital by Zeldin (1984). Although this study confirmed the reliability of the "Goldman Criteria," other investigators began to challenge the Goldman index through investigation with specific sets of surgical patients. The Goldman cardiac risk index significantly underestimated the risk of serious cardiovascular complications in an investigation of patients undergoing aortic surgery (Jeffrey, Kunsman, Cullen, & Brewster, 1983). In this study, the patients identified as the lowest risk actually represented a much higher cardiac risk when outcome data were analyzed.

Detsky et al. (1986a, 1986b) concluded that the Goldman multifactorial index omitted an important variable that reflected the severity of cardiac disease, namely angina pectoris, and proposed a modified risk index that included CCVSA criteria (Table 23–8).

The investigators also refined the variable concerning left ventricular function and excluded the variable concerning type of surgery as this was not a patient characteristic. This was the only study conducted with the modified multifactorial index on a cross section of surgical patients and its predictive validity proved to be comparable with the original Goldman index. The need for external validation of this index yet exists.

TABLE 23–6. The American Society of Anesthesiologists (ASA) Classification System[a]

ASA Class 1
No organic, physiologic, biochemical, or psychiatric disturbance
The pathologic process for which the operation is to be performed is localized and does not entail a systemic disturbance

ASA Class 2
Mild to moderate systemic disease disturbance caused either by the condition to be treated surgically or by other pathologic processes
- well-controlled hypertension
- status post-CABG without symptoms
- history of asthma
- anemia
- cigarette use
- well-controlled diabetes mellitus
- mild obesity
- age <1 year or >70 years
- pregnancy

ASA Class 3
Severe systemic disturbance or disease from whatever cause, even though it may not be possible to define the degree of disability with finality
- angina
- poorly controlled hypertension
- symptomatic respiratory disease (e.g., asthma, COPD)
- massive obesity

ASA Class 4
Indicative of the patient with severe systemic disorders that are already life-threatening, not always correctable by operation
- unstable angina
- congestive heart failure
- debilitating respiratory disease
- hepatorenal failure

ASA Class 5
The moribund patient who has little chance of survival but is submitted to operation in desperation
- Modifier: Emergency Operation (E)

[a] The preoperative medical condition of the patient may be assigned to one of five categories.
Used with permission from Pasternak, L.R. (1995).

Wong & Detsky (1992) studied the utility of the Goldman index and the modified Detsky index in the estimation of cardiac risk for patients undergoing peripheral vascular surgery. They concluded that both indices failed to identify the subset of higher risk patients likely to have significant CAD who scored low on the scales due to functional limitations imposed by their disease. In these instances, further risk stratification was recommended through the use of dipyridamole–thallium imaging.

TABLE 23–7. The Multifactorial Index of Cardiac Risk

Goldman[a]	
Variable	***Score***
Age >70 years	5
Myocardial infarction <6 months	10
ECG: nonsinus rhythm or PVCs	7
>5 PVCs anytime	7
S3 gallop or JVD	11
Aortic stenosis	3
Emergency operation	4
Intrathoracic, intraperitoneal, or aortic operation	3
Poor general status	3
Total possible score	53

[a] Goldman et al. developed a risk index for the prediction of perioperative cardiac complications. Four risk classes were identified through the assignment of weighted criteria: Class I, 0-5 points; Class II, 6-12 points; Class III, 13-25 points; Class IV, over 25 points.

Used with permission from Kurki, T. (1997).

Limitations of Risk Indices

As Wong & Detsky demonstrated, the cardiac risk indices have limited sensitivity in certain clinical situations. The lack of widespread validation of both the Goldman and Detsky scales demands caution with their use. Some also question whether the indices are effective in the identification of risk for individual versus populations of patients. Another possible shortcoming with the utilization of cardiac risk indices may actually be their prospective nature. For example, the application of the "Goldman Criteria" to a specific patient represents an estimation of cardiac risk specifically during the preoperative period. However, the patient moving through the perioperative process is subject to a multitude of risk-related variables occurring at different times. Estimates of perioperative cardiovascular risk have yet to be fully defined from intraoperative and postoperative perspectives. As simple as it may be, the ASA physical status classification remains an important standard for the identification of perioperative risk.

When history, physical exam, or type of operation suggest important cardiovascular risk, the clinician must make a determination concerning the appropriateness of nonroutine preoperative testing. In most cases, current reimbursement constraints often require cardiology consultation to implement noninvasive cardiovascular testing such as ambulatory ECG monitoring, exercise stress testing, echocardiography, or radionuclear imaging.

Finally, all of the risk indices tell us the same thing: an unstable cardiovascular status portends higher risk.

TABLE 23–8. The Modified Multifactorial Index by Detsky et al.

Detsky	
Variable	***Score***
Age >70 years	5
Myocardial infarction <6 months	10
Myocardial infarction >6 months	5
Unstable angina <3 months	10
Alveolar pulmonary edema < 1 week	10
Pulmonary edema ever in past	5
Sinus rhythm and PACs	5
Nonsinus rhythm or PVCs	5
CCVSA class III	10
CCVSA class IV	20
Critical aortic stenosis	20
Emergency operation	10
Poor general status	5
Total possible score	120

Used with permission from Kurki, (1997).

Future Directions

Twenty-five years of research on preoperative evaluation identified the utility of the history and physical examination in the estimation of perioperative risk. The focus of much of the more recent literature concerning risk assessment is on the utility of preoperative noninvasive cardiac testing, such as exercise stress testing, ambulatory ECG monitoring, or radionuclear imaging (Coley et al., 1992; Eagle et al., 1989; Fleisher et al., 1991; Mangano et al., 1991b). These tests are expected to document the severity of cardiovascular disease better than history and physical examination. Dipyridamole thallium scintigraphy has emerged as a useful way of further risk-stratifying patients unable to exercise who have been estimated at intermediate or high-risk after the collection of data by history, physical examination, and routine preoperative testing. Future studies on the utility of preoperative noninvasive cardiac testing will necessarily require the inclusion of cost-benefit and cost-effectiveness analysis.

In addition to preoperative predictors, the intraoperative and postoperative predictors of cardiovascular morbidity represent another important area of research. Mangano (1990) summarized diagnostic and therapeutic dilemmas for the three perioperative periods that best illustrate the focus of current perioperative research (Fig. 23–4).

▶ GUIDELINES FOR PERIOPERATIVE CARDIOVASCULAR EVALUATION FOR NONCARDIAC SURGERY

The collective wisdom of current preoperative assessment strategies is evident in the recently published guidelines from the American College of Cardiology (ACC) and

American Heart Association (AHA) Committee on Perioperative Cardiovascular Evaluation for Noncardiac Surgery. The guidelines provide a framework for the estimation of cardiac risk prior to noncardiac surgery. According to the guidelines, determinants of cardiac risk include severity, stability, and prior treatment of heart disease; functional capacity; age; comorbid conditions; and type of surgery. The history, physical examination, and routine ECG remain the foundation for the initial identification of important cardiovascular conditions (American College of Cardiology/American Heart Association, 1996).

The ACC/AHA guidelines include an algorithm that facilitates a stepwise approach to preoperative cardiovascular assessment and helps determine which patients are candidates for cardiac testing (Fig. 23–5). Clinical circumstances (markers) are designated as major, intermediate, or minor predictors of cardiovascular risk (Table 23–9). (Note: "Recent MI" is defined as > 7 days but less than or equal to 30 days.)

When clinical predictors are evaluated within the context of functional capacity, surgery-specific risk, and prior coronary evaluation and treatment, the best estimate of overall cardiovascular risk is possible (Table 23–10 and Table 23–11). Functional capacity is expressed in metabolic equivalent (MET) levels. Patients unable to meet a 4 MET demand are at increased perioperative risk. In addition, the higher the degree of hemodynamic stress associated with a particular surgical procedure, the greater the likelihood of adverse cardiovascular events. (Note: The guidelines define "recent coronary evaluation" to mean within the past 2 years.)

The use of the algorithm also identifies patients most likely to benefit from further noninvasive cardiac testing. Noninvasive test results may then be used by the anesthesiologist to formulate an intraoperative management plan. When coronary angiography is considered by the cardiology consultant, the risks of this invasive procedure must be weighed within the context of the risk of the proposed noncardiac surgery.

The clinician uses the ACC/AHA algorithm at the conclusion of the preoperative evaluation to determine the need for further consultation by a cardiologist. Patients with major clinical predictors of risk are referred to cardiology and elective surgery is postponed. Patients with intermediate or minor clinical predictors of risk are evaluated within the context of their individual functional capacity and expected type of surgery. Therefore, the overall estimation of risk may be high for one anticipated surgical procedure and low for another. When the need for noninvasive testing has been identified, cardiology referral is likely to be necessary.

The algorithm assists the clinician with the estimation of risk according to a unique set of conditions for the individual patient. This process represents a distinct advantage over other methods of risk assessment. With respect to elective surgery after MI, the guidelines endorse a 4- to 6-week wait (the time frame for scar formation) instead of 6 months if there is no evidence of ischemic risk by clinical symptoms or noninvasive study. Use of the algorithm facilitates treatment decisions over the entire perioperative period.

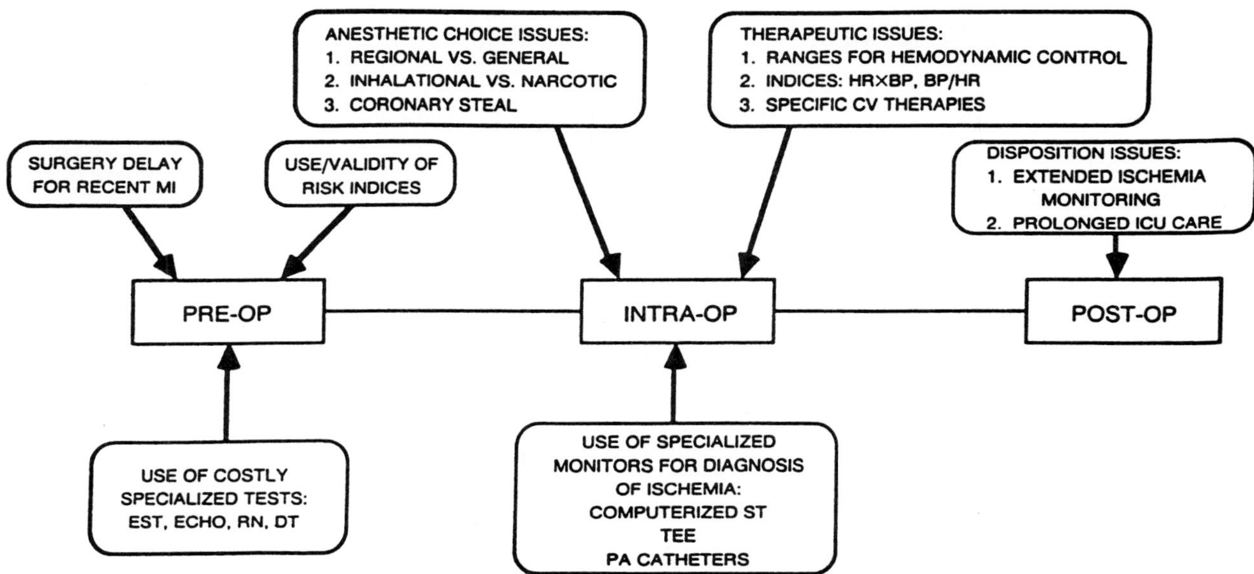

Figure 23–4. Current diagnostic and therapeutic dilemmas concerning the predictors of perioperative cardiac morbidity for the three perioperative periods. (*Used with permission from Mangano, D. 1990.* Anesthesiology.)

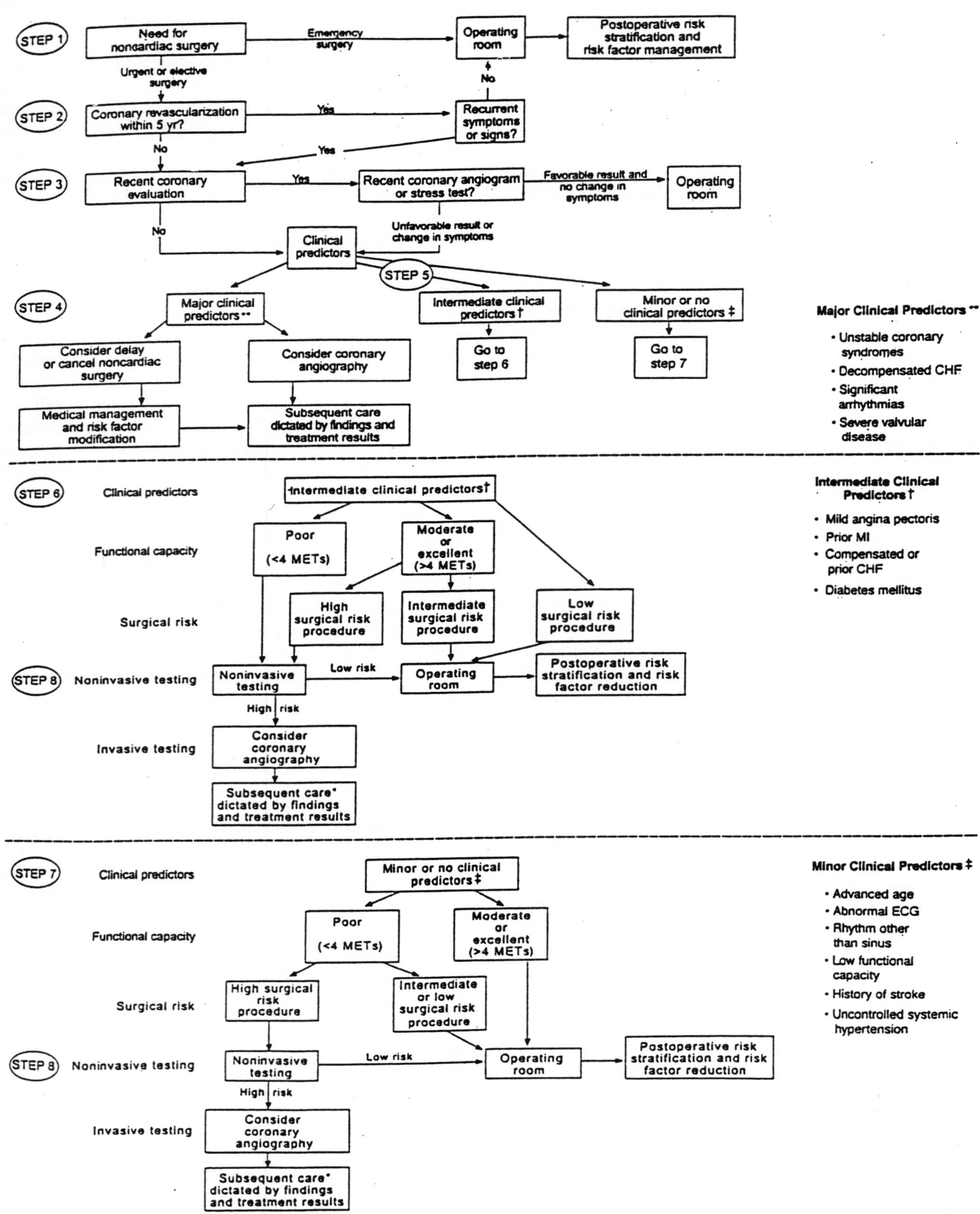

Figure 23–5. Stepwise approach to preoperative cardiac assessment.
** Subsequent care may include cancellation or delay of surgery, coronary revascularization followed by noncardiac surgery, or intensified care. (Used with permission from American College of Cardiology/American Heart Association Task Force,* Circulation, *1996.)*

TABLE 23–9. Clinical Predictors of Increased Perioperative Cardiovascular Risk

Major

Unstable coronary syndromes

- Recent myocardial infarction with evidence of important ischemic risk by clinical symptoms or noninvasive study
- Unstable or severe angina (Canadian Class III or IV)

Decompensated congestive heart failure

Significant arrhythmias

- High-grade atrioventricular block
- Symptomatic ventricular arrhythmias in the presence of underlying heart disease
- Supraventricular arrhythmias with uncontrolled ventricular rate

Severe valvular disease

Intermediate

Mild angina pectoris (Canadian Class I or II)

Prior myocardial infarction by history or pathological Q waves

Compensated or prior congestive heart failure

Diabetes mellitus

Minor

Advanced age

Abnormal ECG (left ventricular hypertrophy, left bundle branch block, ST-T abnormalities)

Rhythm other than sinus (e.g., atrial fibrillation)

Low-functional capacity (e.g., inability to climb one flight of stairs with a bag of groceries)

History of stroke

Uncontrolled systemic hypertension

Note: Recent myocardial infarction is defined as greater than 7 days but less than or equal to 1 month.

Used with permission from American College of Cardiology/American Heart Association Task Force. (1996). Guidelines for perioperative cardiovascular evaluation for noncardiac surgery. Circulation.

TABLE 23–10. Exercise Tolerance

Functional Capacity	MET Level	Daily Activities
Poor	<4 MET	Eat, dress, walk short distance slowly, light housework
Moderate	4-7 MET	Climb stairs, run short distance, walk uphill, heavy housework, doubles tennis
Excellent	>7 MET	Strenuous sports, swimming, singles tennis, skiing

Note: Patients with poor exercise tolerance are at increased perioperative risk. The level of exercise tolerance may indicate the need for preoperative cardiac testing or intraoperative invasive monitoring.

Used with permission from Mingus, M. (1997). Patients with cardiac disease for ambulatory surgery. Anesthesiology Clinics of North America.

TABLE 23–11. Cardiac Risk Stratification for Noncardiac Surgery

High

(Reported cardiac risk often >5%)

- Emergent major operations, particularly in the elderly
- Aortic and other major vascular
- Peripheral vascular
- Anticipated prolonged surgical procedures associated with large fluid shifts and/or blood loss

Intermediate

(Reported cardiac risk generally <5%)

- Carotid endarterectomy
- Head and neck
- Intraperitoneal and intrathoracic
- Orthopedic
- Prostate

Low

(Reported cardiac risk generally <1%)

- Endoscopic procedures
- Superficial procedure
- Cataract
- Breast

Note: Estimated risk includes combined incidence of cardiac death and nonfatal myocardial infarction. Low-risk procedures do not generally require further preoperative cardiac testing.

Used with permission from American College of Cardiology/American Heart Association Task Force. (1996).

Preoperative evaluation identifies the stability of the patient's medical problems and includes recommendations for strategies to improve the clinical condition when necessary. The contribution of this evaluation towards risk reduction is substantial. Most important, the preoperative evaluation assists the anesthesia care team in the formulation of a sound anesthetic plan. The patient, anesthesiologist, and surgeon are not served by documentation that simply states "patient is medically clear for surgery."

Risk-assessment tools such as the ACC/AHA algorithm for perioperative cardiovascular evaluation further enable an estimation of cardiac risk, which also facilitates patient management by the anesthesiologist and surgeon.

Adequate preoperative evaluation and patient preparation will reduce the risks of surgery, avoid unnecessary postponement or cancellation of surgery, and possibly minimize the legal risks of the perioperative management team.

REFERENCES

Abraham, S., Coles, N. A., Coley, C., Strauss, H. W., Boucher, C., & Eagle, K. (1991). Coronary risk of noncardiac surgery. *Progress in Cardiovascular Diseases, 34* (3), 205–234.

American College of Cardiology/American Heart Association Task Force. (1996). Guidelines for perioperative cardiovascular evaluation for noncardiac surgery. *Circulation, 93* (6), 1278–1317.

American Society of Anesthesiologists. (1963). New classification of physical status. *Anesthesiology, 24* (l), 111.

Cohen, D., Duncan, P., & Tate, R. (1988). Does anesthesia contribute to operative mortality? *Journal of AMA, 260* (19), 2859–2863.

Coley, C., Field, T., Abraham, S., Boucher, C., & Eagle, K. (1992). Usefulness of Dipyridamole–Thallium scanning for preoperative evaluation of cardiac risk for nonvascular surgery. *The American Journal of Cardiology, 69,* 1280–1285.

Detsky, A., Abrams, H., Forbath, N., Scott, J. G. & Hilliard, J. (1986a). Cardiac assessment for patients undergoing noncardiac surgery. *Archives of Internal Medicine, 146* (11), 2131–2134.

Detsky, A., Abrams, H., McLaughlin, J. R., Drucker, D., Sasson, Z., et al. (1986b). Predicting cardiac complications in patients undergoing non-cardiac surgery. *Journal of Internal Medicine, 1* (4), 211–219.

Dripps, R., Lamont, A., & Eckenhoff, J. (1961). The role of anesthesia in surgical mortality. *Journal of AMA, 178* (3), 261–266.

Eagle, K., Coley, C., Newell, J., Brewster, D., Darling, C., Strauss, W., et al. (1989). Combining clinical and thallium data optimizes preoperative assessment of cardiac risk before major vascular surgery. *Annals of Internal Medicine, 110* (11), 859–866.

Everett, L. & Kallar, S. (1995). Presurgical evaluation and laboratory testing. In R. Twersky (ed.). *The ambulatory anesthesia handbook* (pp. 1–34). St. Louis: Mosby.

Fleisher, L., Rosenbaum, S., Nelson, A., & Barash, P. (1991). The predictive value of preoperative silent ischemia for postoperative ischemic cardiac events in vascular and nonvascular surgery patients. *American Heart Journal, 122* (4), 980–986.

Foster, E., Davis, K., Carpenter, J., Abele, S., & Fray, D. (1986). Risk of noncardiac operation in patients with defined coronary disease: The coronary artery surgery study (CASS) registry experience. *Annals of Thoracic Surgery, 41* (l), 42–50.

Goldman, L. (1983). Cardiac risks and complications of noncardiac surgery. *Annals of Internal Medicine, 98* (4), 504–513.

Goldman, L., Caldera, D., Nussbaum, S., Southwick, F., Krogstad, D., Murray, B., et al. (1977). Multifactorial index of cardiac risk in noncardiac surgical procedures. *The New England Journal of Medicine, 297* (16), 845–850.

Hirsh, R. (1994). An approach to assessing perioperative risk. In D. Goldmann, F. Brown, & D. Guamieri, (eds.). *Perioperative Medicine* (pp. 9–13). New York: McGraw-Hill.

Jeffrey, C., Kunsman, J., Cullen, D., & Brewster, D. (1983). A prospective evaluation of cardiac risk. *Anesthesiology, 58* (5), 462–464.

Keenan, R. & Boyan, P. (1985). Cardiac arrest due to anesthesia: A study of incidence and causes. *Journal of AMA, 253* (16), 2373–2377.

Kurki, T. (1997). Preoperative assessment of patients with cardiac disease undergoing noncardiac surgery. *Anesthesiology Clinics of North America, 15* (l), 1–13.

Leung, J., London, M., & Mangano, D. (1990). Management of patients with coronary artery disease. *Seminars in Anesthesia, 9* (4), 258–269.

Mangano, D. (1990). Perioperative cardiac mobidity. *Anesthesiology, 72* (l), 153–184.

Mangano, D. (1991a). Assessment of risk for cardiac and noncardiac surgical procedures. *Anesthesiology Clinics of North America, 9* (3), 521–551.

Mangano, D., London, M., Tubau, J., Browner, W., Hollenberg, M., et al. (1991b). Dipyridamole Thallium-201 scintigraphy as a preoperative screening test: A reexamination of its predictive potential. *Circulation, 84* (2), 493–502.

Marx, G., Mateo, C., & Orkin, L. (1973). Computer analysis of postanesthetic deaths. *Anesthesiology, 39* (l), 54–58.

Mendel, H. (1997). Management of latex hypersensitivity for operating room patients and health care providers. *Contemporary Surgery, 50* (6), 325–330.

Murphy, F. (1992). Hazards of anesthesia. In D. Longnecker & F. Murphy (eds.). *Dripps Eckenhoff/Vandam—Introduction to anesthesia,* 8th ed. (pp.419–427). Philadelphia: W. B. Saunders.

Pierce, E. (1990). The development of anesthesia guidelines and standards. *Quality Review Bulletin, 16* (l), 61–64.

Rao, T., Jacobs, K., & El-Etr, A. (1983). Reinfarction following anesthesia in patients with myocardial infarction. *Anesthesiology, 59* (6), 499–505.

Saklad, M. (1941). Grading of patients for surgical procedures. *Anesthesiology, 2* (3), 281–284.

Topkins, M. & Artusio, J. (1964). Myocardial infarction and surgery. *Anesthesia and Analgesia, 43* (6), 716–720.

Vacanti, C., VanHouten, R., & Hill, R. (1970). A statistical analysis of the relationship of physical status to postoperative mortality in 68,388 cases. *Anesthesia and Analgesia, 49* (4), 564–566.

Wells, P. & Kaplan, J. (1981). Optimal management of patients with ischemic heart disease for noncardiac surgery by complementary anesthesiologist and cardiologist interaction. *American Heart Journal, 102* (6), 1029–1037.

Wong, T. & Detsky, A. (1992). Preoperative cardiac risk assessment for patients having peripheral vascular surgery. *Annals of Internal Medicine, 116* (9), 743–753.

Zeldin, R. (1984). Assessing cardiac risk in patients who undergo noncardiac surgical procedures. *The Canadian Journal of Surgery, 27* (4), 402–404.

BIBLIOGRAPHY

Beattie, C. & Fleisher, L. (1992). Ischemic heart disease. *International Anesthesiology Clinics,* 30 (1), Preface, xx.

Becker, R. & Underwood, D. (1987). Myocardial infarction in patients undergoing noncardiac surgery. *Cleveland Clinic Journal of Medicine, 54* (l), 25–28.

Carson, J. & Eisenberg, J. (1994). The preoperative screening examination. In D. Goldmann, F. Brown, & D. Guamieri (Eds.). *Perioperative medicine* (pp. 15–23). New York: McGraw-Hill.

Cassidy, J. & Marley, R. (1996). Preoperative assessment of the ambulatory patient. *Journal of PeriAnesthesia Nursing, 11* (5), 334–343.

Feigal, D. & Blaisdell, F. W. (1979). The estimation of surgical risk. *Medical Clinics of North America, 63* (6), 1131–1143.

Fleisher, L. & Eagle, K. (1996). Screening for cardiac disease in patients having noncardiac surgery. *Annals of Internal Medicine, 124* (8), 767–772.

Fleisher, L. (1997). Ischemic heart disease. *Anesthesiology Clinics of North America, 15* (l), 49–67.

Gersh, B., Rihal, C., Rooke, T., & Ballard, D. (1991). Evaluation and management of patients with both peripheral vascular and coronary artery disease. *JACC, 18* (l), 203–214.

Goldman, L. (1987). Multifactorial index of cardiac risk in noncardiac surgery: Ten-year status report. *Journal of Cardiothoracic Anesthesia, 1* (3), 237–244.

Goldman, L. (1988). Assessment of the patient with known or suspected ischaemic heart disease for non-cardiac surgery. *British Journal of Anesthesia, 61* (l), 38–43.

Goldman, L. (1994). Assessment of perioperative cardiac risk. *The New England Journal of Medicine, 330* (10), 707–709.

Goldman, L., Caldera, D., Southwick, F., Nussbaum, S., Murray, B. et al. (1978). Cardiac risk factors and complications in non-cardiac surgery. *Medicine, 57* (4), 357–370.

Goldstein, A. & Keats, A. (1970). The risk of anesthesia. *Anesthesiology, 33* (2), 130–143.

Haagenstein, R. & Steen, P.A. (1988). Perioperative myocardial infarction. *British Journal of Anesthesia, 61* (l), 24–37.

Harman, E. & Lillington, G. (1979). Pulmonary risk factors in surgery. *Medical Clinics of North America, 63* (6), 1289–1298.

Hollenberg, M., Mangano, D., Browner, W., London, M., Tubau, J., & Tateo, I. (1992). Predictors of postoperative myocardial ischemia in patients undergoing noncardiac surgery. *Journal of AMA, 268* (2), 205–209.

Khetarpal, S. (1990). Preanesthetic assessment of the patient with cardiac disease. *Anesthesiology Clinics of North America, 8* (4), 631–645.

Larsen, S., Olesen, K., Jacobsen, E., Nielsen, H., Nelsen, A., et al. (1987). Prediction of cardiac risk in non-cardiac surgery. *European Heart Journal, 8,* 179–185.

Logue, R. B. & Kaplan, J. (1982). The cardiac patient and noncardiac surgery. *Current Problems in Cardiology, 7* (2), 5–49.

Mangano, D., Browner, W., Hollenberg, M., London, M., Tubau, J., et al. (1990). Association of perioperative myocardial ischemia with cardiac morbidity and mortality in men undergoing noncardiac surgery. *The New England Journal of Medicine, 323* (26), 1781–1788.

Mingus, M. (1997). Patients with cardiac disease for ambulatory surgery. *Anesthesiology Clinics of North America, 15* (l), 171–188.

Myers, W., Davis, K., Foster, D., Maynard, C., & Kaiser, G. (1985). Surgical survival in the coronary artery surgery study (CASS) registry. *The Annals of Thoracic Surgery, 40* (3), 245–258.

Pasternak, L. R. (1995). Screening patients: Strategies and studies. In K. McGoldrick, (ed.). *Ambulatory anesthesiology: A Problem-oriented approach* (pp. 2–19). Baltimore: Williams & Wilkins.

Phillips, P. & Frost, E. (1990). Preanesthetic assessment of the ambulatory patient. *Anesthesiology Clinics of North America, 8* (4), 801–809.

Robbins, J. & Mushlin, A. (1979). Preoperative evaluation of the healthy patient. *Medical Clinics of North America, 63* (6), 1145–1156.

Rose, S., Corman, L., & Mason, D. (1979). Cardiac risk factors in patients undergoing noncardiac surgery. *Medical Clinics of North America, 63* (6), 1271–1288.

Weitz, H. & Goldman, L. (1987). Noncardiac surgery in the patient with heart disease. *Medical Clinics of North America, 71* (3), 413–432.

Yarmush, L. (1997). Noncardiac surgery in the patient with valvular heart disease. *Anesthesiology Clinics of North America, 15* (l), 69–91.

24

Trauma

Robin M. Haskell

Death and taxes, it is said, are two inevitabilities of life; trauma qualifies as a legitimate third (Walt, 1991). Injuries have a major impact on the health of Americans, causing 6% of all deaths, 8% of all hospital admissions, and 37% of all emergency department visits. Intentional and unintentional injury caused over 152,000 deaths and 9 million disabilities in 1995, with a male to female ratio of approximately 2:1 (Anderson, Kochanek, & Murphy, 1995). Trauma is the leading cause of death among people between the ages of 1 and 44, which includes their most productive years as wage-earners and parents. Because injuries disproportionately affect the young, injury mortality accounts for more potential years of life lost than all leading causes of death in the United States (National Center for Health Statistics, 1997) (Fig. 24–1).

According to the U.S. Department of Transportation, motor vehicle crashes (MVCs) are the leading cause of death among Americans between the ages of 1 and 37. The total cost of MVCs to society exceeds $150 billion annually. In 1996, MVCs accounted for 41,907 fatalities, an increase for the fourth straight year (National Center for Health Statistics, 1997).

Trauma is a multidisciplinary continuum of care, which consists of prevention, pre-hospital care, resuscitation, intensive care, convalescent care, and rehabilitation. The scope of trauma care in the hospital setting requires ex-

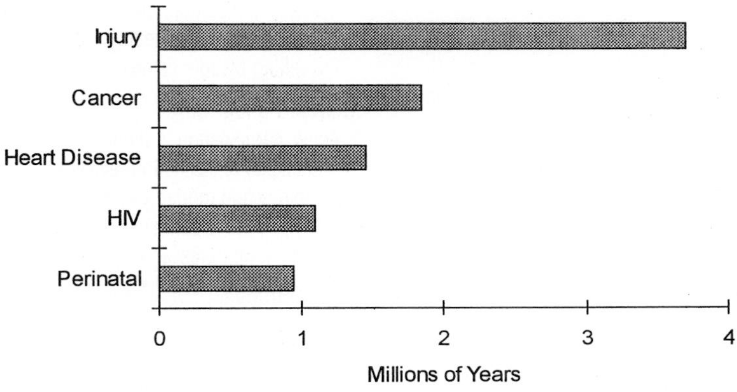

Figure 24–1. Years of potential life lost before age 65, by cause of death—United States, 1994. *(From National Center for Health Statistics System, 1996–1997, Center for Disease Control.)*

tensive knowledge of anatomy, physiology, pharmacology, and the surgical subspecialties (neurosurgery, orthopedics, plastic surgery, etc.). Trauma-care provision is labor-intensive, requiring 24-hour-a-day support from numerous hospital departments. Acute trauma care not only encompasses injury recognition and management, but also the problems of shock, infection, pulmonary support, thromboembolism, and orthopedic complications.

The trauma nurse practitioner (NP) assists with the clinical management of both inpatients and outpatients (Table 24–1). Importantly, the trauma NP provides continuity of care to patients on a surgical service staffed by rotating attending surgeons and/or house staff. Communication with consultants, nursing staff, and ancillary disciplines may be facilitated by the NP. Spisso, O'Callaghan, McKennan, & Holcroft (1990) demonstrated improved quality of care, including reduced length of stay, after the addition of NPs to the trauma team.

This chapter describes the biomechanics of injury and the essential principles of trauma care, with emphasis on those aspects most critical to the clinical practice of the trauma NP: diagnosis and management of specific injuries, injury complexes, and major complications of trauma.

▶ U.S. TRAUMA SYSTEMS

A trauma system provides trained personnel, facilities, and equipment for optimal care of the acutely injured patient, from field care through rehabilitation. A designated trauma center is a facility that has committed extensive resources to providing quality trauma care on a priority basis. Trauma center designation is provided by a recognized state or regional entity. Such designation generally requires a periodic performance-based verification process, in which the institution must demonstrate commitment, superior quality of care, and a timely response to injured patients. In addition, cost-effective resource utilization and continuous quality management are considered.

It is well established that morbidity and mortality decrease when major trauma victims are treated in trauma centers (Kilberg, Clemmer, & Claussen, 1988; Shackford, Hollingsworth-Friedlund, Cooper, & Eastman, 1986; West, Cales, & Gazzaniga, 1983; West, Trunkey, & Lim, 1979). Appropriate triage to a trauma center is accomplished by determining the actual or potential severity of a patient's injuries. Unfortunately, the assessment techniques available to prehospital personnel under field conditions are limited, and

TABLE 24–1. Components of the Trauma Nurse Practitioner Role

Direct Patient Care

Comprehensive inpatient management
- History and physical examination, as appropriate
- Primary and secondary surveys (resuscitative phase)
- Tertiary survey
- Medical diagnoses, with prescription of medical and nursing therapies
- Pharmacologic management
- Daily and incident-oriented progress notes
- Daily orders, other orders
- Laboratory test ordering and interpretation
- Radiograph ordering, interpretation with trauma surgeon or radiology consultation
- Medical specialist consultation
- Social work and clinical resource department liaison
- Patient/family education
- Communication with patients and families
- Handling nursing/ancillary staff pages
- Initiation of the evaluation and emergency management of life-threatening conditions
- Discharge physical examination
- Discharge teaching
- Discharge summaries

Outpatient care
- System-focused assessment
- History and Physical, as required
- Coordination of home services
- Communication with primary care providers
- Referral to ancillary services
- Telephone triage

Procedures
- Operating room: first assist, second assist
- Wound management, including burns
- Wound cleansing and debridement
- Suturing
- Suture removal
- Removal of superficial foreign bodies
- Surgical drain removal
- Splinting
- Cervical collar placement and removal
- Intravenous line insertion
- Pulmonary artery catheterization
- Central venous and arterial catheterization
- Chest tube insertion, management, and removal
- Gastric or intestinal feeding tube insertion
- Indwelling bladder catheterization

Indirect Patient Care
- Active participation in multidisciplinary rounds, radiology rounds
- Videotaped resuscitation review and analysis
- Morbidity and mortality conference
- Quality improvement activities
- Participation in research

Administrative
- Nursing staff education
- Consultant in trauma for nursing staff
- Critical pathway development
- Policy and procedure development
- Patient education committee representative

many potentially lethal injuries may not be apparent during the early postinjury phase. Because precise determination of injury severity is difficult at the scene, field triage guidelines serve to identify the injured patient who may benefit from trauma center care. The triage decision scheme recommended by American College of Surgeons (ACS) Committee on Trauma combines physiologic data, anatomic criteria, mechanism of injury, age, and comorbidities to provide a highly sensitive algorithm for identification of major trauma victims (Fig. 24–2).

Three levels of trauma center designation (levels I, II, and III) are defined in "Resources for the Optimal Care of the Injured Patient" (American College of Surgeons Committee on Trauma, 1989). All levels require commitment of the medical and hospital staff, an organized trauma team response, and a quality management program. Variations in

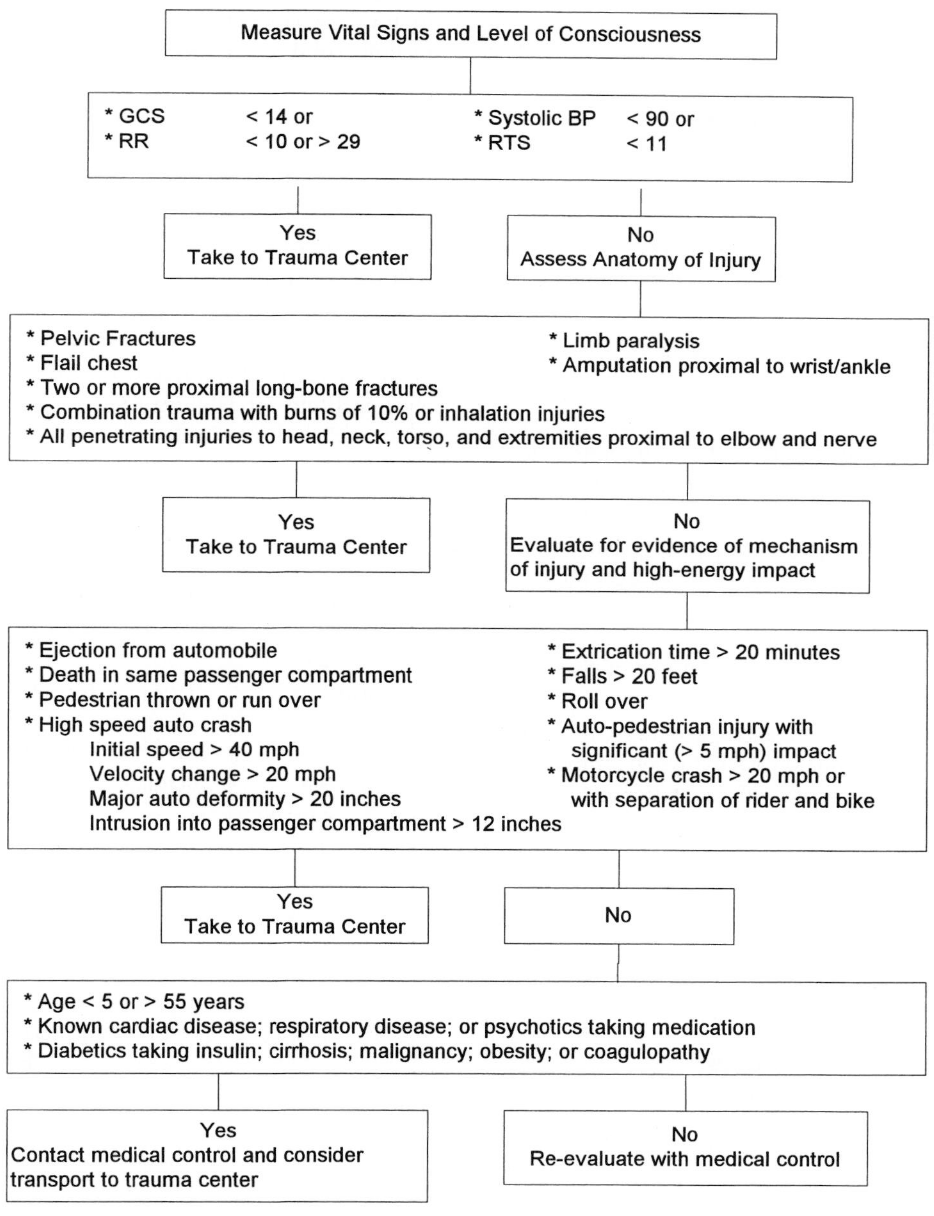

Figure 24–2. Prehospital Triage Criteria. Optimal field triage criteria should facilitate the rapid transport of patients with life-threatening injuries to verified trauma center. However, because perfect triage criteria do not exist, this triage decision scheme necessarily over-triages trauma patients so that patients needing trauma centers are transported to them in almost every case. *(Reprinted with permission from American College of Surgeons, Committee on Trauma, [1993] [p. 318].)*

requirements for medical specialist availability and equipment, such as cardiopulmonary bypass, differentiate the three levels. Level I trauma centers are obligated to support and improve trauma care through education and research.

Many trauma centers maintain a database called a trauma registry to provide epidemiologic information and demographic characteristics. Trauma registries can support quality management programs and clinical research, as well as assist in mobilizing public and political support for such projects as violence prevention and highway safety legislation.

MECHANISMS OF INJURY

Injury results from acute exposure to mechanical (e.g., crash, bullet, fall), electrical, thermal, or chemical energy, or from a lack of essential heat or oxygen. When the energy imparted causes tissue deformity greater than its recoverable limits, anatomic damage or physiologic imbalance occurs. Injuring forces are generally classified as blunt or penetrating.

Blunt Trauma

Blunt trauma is defined as an injury with no communication to the outside environment. As such, blunt mechanisms are often more life threatening because the extent of injuries is less obvious. Blunt injury typically results from MVCs, falls, assaults, and contact sports. Wounding generally occurs through compression or crushing of body parts and tissues. Internal shearing or tearing of tissue can occur by rapid deceleration, with differential movement of fixed and nonfixed parts of the body.

Victims of motor vehicle crashes actually experience three collisions. The first collision occurs when a motor vehicle impacts with another or with a stationary object. Crushing of the car in frontal or side impact may cause direct contact injuries to the driver or passengers. The second collision occurs when the occupant hits various internal parts of the car, such as the windshield, steering wheel, and dashboard. The third collision involves the impact of movable organs (brain, heart, liver, spleen, intestine) against the rigid bony structures of the body.

Protective Restraint Devices

Safety Belts. Safety belts reduce the morbidity and mortality of injury by preventing both ejection from the vehicle and impact with the vehicle interior. Safety belts are greater than 50% effective in preventing MVC fatalities (Rutledge et al., 1993). Restrained victims in MVCs have decreased hospital admission rates, number and severity of injuries, intensive care unit (ICU) days, length of stay, and hospital charges compared with unrestrained victims (Reath, Kirby, Lynch & Maull, 1989; Rutledge et al., 1993).

Paradoxically, safety belts are a direct cause of or contributing factor to many injuries in deceleration-type MVCs (Table 24–2) (Feliciano, 1996). Occupant contact with the belt during sudden deceleration may cause severe injuries, which are more likely if seat belts are positioned improperly, or if both lap and shoulder components are not used together (Sato, 1987). The shoulder belt may cause injury to the cervical spine or brachial plexus (Holbrook & Bennett, 1990), rupture of the upper abdominal organs (States, Huelke, Dance & Green, 1987), and increased incidence of injury to the chest wall and lung in the elderly (Martinez, Sharieff, & Hooper, 1994). Lap belts have been implicated in both solid and hollow visceral abdominal injury, vertebral fractures, abdominal aortic dissection, and common iliac artery transection (Appleby & Nagy, 1989; Arajarvi, Santavirta, & Tolonen, 1987; Rutledge et al., 1991).

Airbags. Airbags complement safety belts, providing an additional 12% mortality reduction for drivers who are properly restrained (Viano, 1995). The greater load distribution provided by airbags in frontal collisions enhances the protection provided by safety belts and provides substantial protection for unrestrained occupants. Airbag-only restraint of the driver is 20% effective in preventing fatality (Insurance Institute for Highway Safety, 1996). With or without safety belts, airbags reduce severity of brain injury and diminish the incidence of facial and thoracoabdominal trauma, but offer no protection from intrusion-related in-

TABLE 24–2. Injuries Related to Restraint Devices, Especially When Worn Improperly

Lap Seat Belt	
Compression	Tear or avulsion of mesentery Rupture of small bowel or colon Thrombosis of iliac artery or abdominal aorta
Hyperflexion	Chance fracture of lumbar vertebrae
Shoulder Belt	
Submarining (hyperextension and rotation)	Intimal tear or thrombosis in innominate, carotid, subclavian, or vertebral arteries Fracture or dislocation of cervical spine
Compression	Intimal tear or thrombosis in subclavian artery Fracture of ribs Pulmonary contusion Rupture of upper abdominal viscera
Airbag	
Contact	Corneal abrasions, keratitis Abrasions/contusions of the face, neck, chest Blunt cardiac injury Upper extremity soft tissue injury Upper extremity fracture
Flexion/hyperextension (unrestrained occupants)	Flexion or extension cervical fracture Thoracic fracture

Adapted with permission from Feliciano, (1996). Trauma *(3rd ed.). (p. 97).*

juries to the legs and pelvis (Burgess, Dischinger, O'Quinn, & Schmidhauser, 1995; Loo et al., 1996).

The deployment of an airbag in a crash is not without risk. Airbag inflation is accomplished by converting sodium azide to nitrogen gas, which fills a 60-liter airbag in 10 to 35 msec at a speed of up to 200 mph (Viano, 1995). Heat and aerosolized alkaline compounds are vented through holes in the back of the airbag, so that the bag begins to collapse before the occupant comes in contact with it (Smally, Binzer, Dolin, & Viano, 1992).

The significant physical and chemical forces involved in airbag deployment may cause a variety of injuries, most of which are minor. Gaseous and particulate matter emitted in the vehicle interior may cause thermal and chemical burns to the eyes and skin (Smally et al., 1992). Inhalation of airbag effluents can trigger acute bronchospasm in asthmatics (Gross et al., 1995). The high velocity of airbag inflation results in abrasions and contusions of the face and neck, and may cause blunt ocular injury. In addition, the airbag can push the head, arms, and hands, causing direct injury and secondary impact within the vehicle (Antosia et al., 1995; Blacksin, 1993).

About 1% of airbag-induced injuries are serious or fatal (Insurance Institute for Highway Safety, 1996). Risk factors include a close proximity of the front-seat occupant to the steering wheel or dashboard, and improper use of safety restraints (Lund & Ferguson, 1995). Small adults and children, who tend to sit closer to the airbag, and unbelted front-seat occupants are "slapped" or "punched" by the rigid airbag module cover or the inflating airbag (Smock & Nichols, 1995). Infants and children riding in the front seat of an airbag-equipped vehicle are at high risk of serious and fatal injury, even if properly belted or restrained in a car seat (Insurance Institute for Highway Safety, 1996).

Penetrating Trauma

Penetrating injury is produced when a foreign object (missile) dissipates energy to tissue by passing through it. Common penetrating injury mechanisms include firearms, stabbings, and impalements. Among the factors that influence the type and severity of injury are the velocity of the missile, missile mass and shape, the organs in the path of the missile, and tissue rigidity. Because of their high velocity, bullets transmit large amounts of kinetic energy to tissues and thus have a high wounding potential. Stab wounds and impalements are low velocity and therefore low energy, causing less concussive forces to tissues surrounding the path of the object (Swan & Swan, 1991).

Wounding from projectiles occurs through direct mechanisms (laceration of tissue, transfer of heat) and indirect mechanisms (compression, stretching, low-displacement shock waves, and high-displacement shear waves). Shock waves spread out behind a projectile in tissue and appear to cause no perceptible displacement of or damage to tissues. Shear waves result from medium or high velocity missiles, causing transfer of kinetic energy to surrounding tissue with compression and outward displacement. This energy transfer creates a temporary cavity along the path of the bullet (Fig. 24–3). The elasticity of the tissue determines the permanent effect of the cavity: the relative elasticity of muscle tissue results in less permanent damage, whereas permanent defects of the inelastic brain, liver, and spleen are more likely (Hinkle & Betz, 1995).

The amount of energy absorbed is determined by the density of the tissue and the frontal area of the bullet. In dense tissues, more tissue particles are put in motion away from the path of the bullet, and more energy is lost by the bullet. The most dense structures, such as bone and solid organs, create the maximum amount of energy exchange.

An increased number of tissue particles are hit by increasing the frontal area of a bullet, bullet tumble, and bullet fragmentation (Fig. 24–4). If a 0.45-caliber bullet with a cross section slightly less than 1/2 inch in diameter is flattened to a diameter of 1 inch, its frontal projection increases by 400%. Thus, four times as many tissue particles are hit, regardless of tissue density or bullet weight and velocity

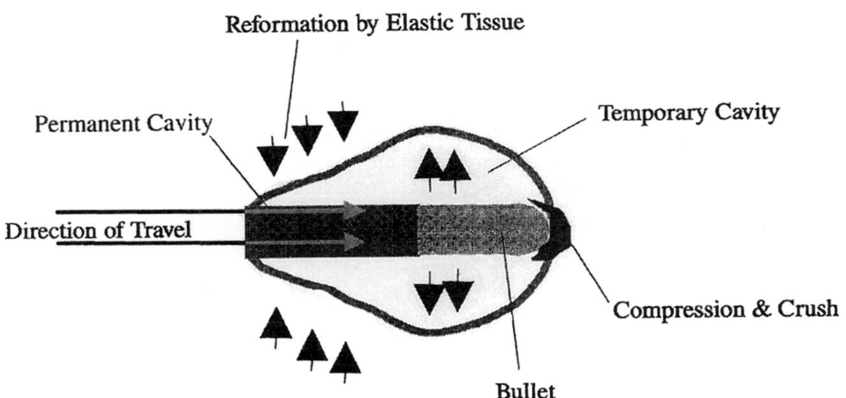

Figure 24–3. As the bullet penetrates the tissue, it crushes that part of the tissue that is directly in its pathway. The cavitation created around the pathway stretches the nearby tissue. *(Reprinted with permission from McSwain, [1996]. [p. 106].)*

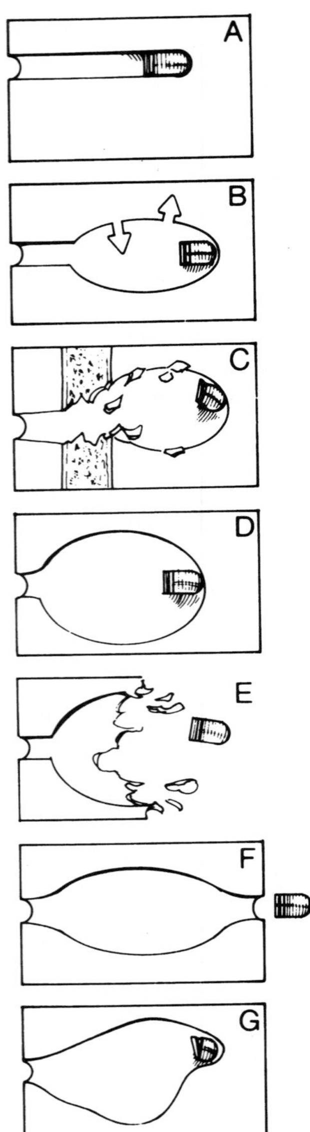

Figure 24–4. Patterns of injury in tissue secondary to variations in the ballistics of missiles and tissue characteristics. **A,** Low velocity, no cavitation, entrance, and exit small. **B,** Higher velocity, formation of cavity, arrows show direction and magnitude of acceleration of tissue. **C,** Velocity as in **(B)**, but deformation of bullet and creation of secondary missiles on penetrating bone. **D,** Very high velocity, large cavity, and small entrance. Exit may be small. **E,** Very high velocity, thin target, large and ragged exit. **F,** Velocity, caliber, and thickness of tissue such that cavitation occurs deep inside, and entrance and exit are small. **G,** Asymmetric cavitation as bullet begins to deform and tumble. *(Reprinted with permission from Cardona, Hurn, Bastnagel-Mason, Scanlon-Schilpp, & Veise-Berry (Eds.). [1988]. [p. 118].)*

(McSwain, 1996). Hollow-point bullets contain a cavity that expands on contact, causing the shell to expand and thus increasing its frontal area (Sykes, Champion, & Fouty, 1988). Similar expansion occurs with semi-jacketed or partial-jacketed bullets, and with silver-tip and exploding bullets. A missile that is tumbling on impact presents a greater frontal area, impacting more tissue particles and increasing the size of the temporary and, perhaps, permanent cavities (Feliciano, 1996). Moreover, bullet fragmentation increases frontal area as each individual fragment has a frontal area of its own (McSwain, 1996).

Factors Influencing Patterns of Injury

Similar mechanisms of injury tend to produce similar patterns of injury. Knowledge of injury mechanisms aids in the rapid diagnosis of injuries. For example: (1) the direction of impact in MVCs raises suspicion of certain types and patterns of injury (Table 24–3), and (2) unrestrained drivers in frontal impact MVCs sustain similar injuries from impact with the steering wheel, dash, and windshield (Fig. 24–5). Alterations that occur in injury patterns reflect differences in the victim's age, gender, comorbidities (including substance abuse), and individual variations in response to the energy transfer (Feliciano, 1996).

TABLE 24–3. Mechanisms of Injury and Related Suspected Injury Patterns In Automobile Accidents

Mechanisms of Injury	Suspected Injury Patterns
Frontal impact	Head or facial injury Cervical spine fracture
Bull's-eye fracture of windshield	Pneumothorax Transection of aorta (decelerating injury) Fractured spleen or liver Posterior fracture/dislocation of hip and/or knee
Bent steering wheel	Anterior flail chest
Knee imprint in dashboard	Myocardial contusion
Side impact	Contralateral neck sprain Cervical spine fracture Lateral flail chest Pneumothorax Traumatic aortic rupture Diaphragmatic rupture Fractured spleen or liver (depending on side of impact) Fractured pelvis or acetabulum
Rear impact	Cervical spine injury
Ejection from vehicle	Ejection from the vehicle precludes meaningful prediction of injury patterns, but places the patient at a greater risk from virtually all injury mechanisms. Mortality is increased significantly.
Motor vehicle–pedestrian	Head injury Thoracic and abdominal injuries Fractured lower extremities

From American College of Surgeons, Committee on Trauma, (1993). Advanced Trauma Life Support Manual *(p. 29).*

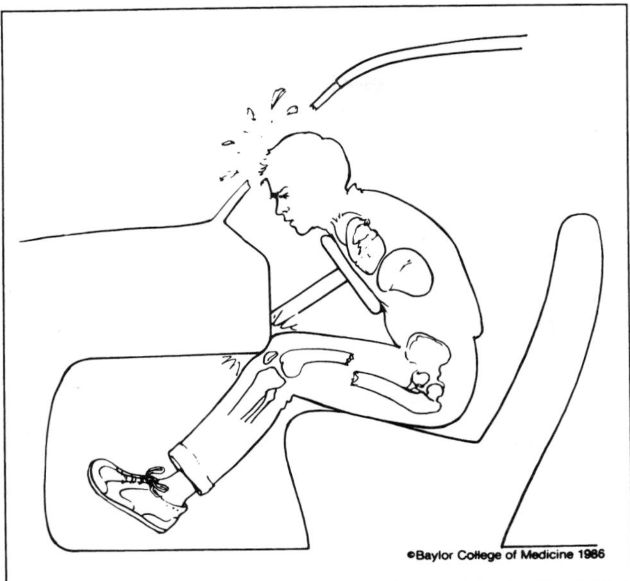

Figure 24–5. Unrestrained driver in motor vehicle accident commonly sustains injuries to the scalp, skull, face, sternum and/or ribs, heart and/or aorta, spleen and/or liver, and bones of the pelvis and lower extremities. *(Reprinted with permission from Baylor College of Medicine.)*

Certain anatomic factors also influence patterns of injury. The skeleton offers some protection to soft organs. The skull protects the brain, the ribs protect the heart and lungs, and the pelvis protects the genitourinary structures. The first and second ribs, sternum, scapula, pelvis, and femur are relatively more resistant to the deformation associated with impact trauma. Fractures of these bones provide evidence that significant kinetic energy has been transferred to the victim and that associated injuries may be present (Table 24–4) (Feliciano, 1996). Injuries from MVCs result from direct impact or from differences in deceleration between the mass of the body and its enclosed viscera. Shearing injuries subsequently occur between areas of different deceleration and at points of anatomic fixation. For example, deceleration-type crashes are a common cause of lacerations of the descending thoracic aorta at or just distal to the ligamentum arteriosum, a common point of fixation.

TABLE 24–4. The Injuries Associated with Fractures of Certain Impact-Resistant Bones in the Body

First or second ribs
Pulmonary contusion
Cranial or closed head injury
Abdominal injury
Brachial plexus contusion or disruption
Sympathetic chain injury
Ipsilateral subclavian artery tear
Great vessel injury
Sternum
Rib fractures
Pulmonary contusion
Blunt cardiac injury
Cardiac rupture
Thoracic aortic transection
Compression fractures of the thoracic spine
Scapula
Ipsilateral rib fractures
Pulmonary contusion
Ipsilateral upper extremity injury
Pelvis
Abdominal injury
Genitourinary tract disruption
Femur
Ipsilateral patella fracture
Ipsilateral knee ligamentus injury
Ipsilateral acetabular or pelvic ring fracture

▶ TRAUMA SCORING

Many indices using measures of physiologic or anatomic derangement have been developed to quantify injury severity and functional outcome. Such trauma-scoring tools can provide data for quality improvement, comparison of therapeutic modalities, evaluation of resource utilization, and collection of basic epidemiologic trauma data (Champion, Sacco, & Copes, 1996). The following are several of the more commonly used trauma indices and their applications.

Glasgow Coma Scale

The Glasgow Coma Scale (GCS) is widely used to assess level of consciousness (Table 24–5). Scores range from 3 to 15, with higher scores indicating a lesser degree of neurologic impairment. The GCS is used for prehospital triage, for determining the level of consciousness after hospital admission, for serial evaluation following severe traumatic brain injury, and for prognostication. The GCS has also been incorporated into the Trauma Score (TS) and Revised Trauma Score (RTS).

Trauma Score

The Trauma Score (TS) is based on assessment of cardiovascular status (capillary return and blood pressure), respiratory status (rate and effort), and GCS (Champion, Sacco, Carnazzo, Copes, & Fouty, 1981). Weighted values assigned to the variables are added to obtain the trauma score, which ranges from 1 (worst prognosis) to 16 (best prognosis). The trauma score is widely used to characterize the physiologic status of the injured patient in prehospital and hospital settings (Champion, Sacco, & Copes, 1996).

TABLE 24–5. Glasgow Coma Scale

Eye Opening (E)	
Spontaneous	___4
To voice	___3
To pain	___2
None	___1
Verbal Response (V)	
Oriented	___5
Confused	___4
Inappropriate words	___3
Incomprehensible sounds	___2
None	___1
Motor Response (M)	
Obeys commands	___6
Localizes pain	___5
Withdraws (pain)	___4
Flexion (pain)	___3
Extension (pain)	___2
None	___1
Total GCS Points (E + V + M)	___

Revised Trauma Score

The Revised Trauma Score (RTS) is based on the GCS, systolic blood pressure (SBP), and respiratory rate (RR), which are assigned coded values from 4 (normal) to 0 (Table 24–6) (Champion et al., 1989). The RTS is used in prehospital triage; a subnormal value for any RTS variable suggests the need for transport to a trauma center (American College of Surgeons, 1993). For evaluation of in-hospital outcome, the individual coded values are weighted and summed to yield the RTS. Scores range from 0 to 7.84; higher values are associated with better prognoses (Champion, Sacco, & Copes, 1996).

Abbreviated Injury Scale

The Abbreviated Injury Scale (AIS) is an anatomic score that characterizes injury severity by assigning a severity value to each injury listed on an established index of several hundred. The AIS ranges from 1 (minor) to 6 (nearly always fatal), and is determined for every injury sustained by an individual patient.

Injury Severity Score

The Injury Severity Score (ISS) was developed to characterize the severity of a trauma patient's injury complex. The ISS can range from 1 to 75. It is computed as the sum of the squares of the three highest AIS scores for injuries to different body regions, unless there is an AIS 6 injury, in which case an ISS of 75 is assigned. The ISS correlates with mortality (Baker, O'Neill, Haddon, & Long, 1974; Baker & O'Neill, 1976; Bull, 1975; Semmlow & Cone, 1976), but is limited in that it incorporates three injuries at most, and only the greatest AIS value from each body region. It considers injuries with the same AIS values to be of equal severity, discounting the importance of body region (Copes et al., 1988). In patients with multiple injuries within a single body region, the ISS considers only one of the injuries in that region. In patients with injuries in multiple body regions, the ISS accounts for a second, perhaps less severe injury in a second body region rather than a second, more severe injury in the first body region (Osler, Baker, & Long, 1997). Despite these limitations, the ISS is the most frequently used summary measure of anatomic injury severity (Champion, Sacco, & Copes, 1996).

TABLE 24–6. Revised Trauma Score[a]

GCS	SBP	RR	Coded Value
13–15	>89	10–29	4
9–12	76–89	>29	3
6–8	50–75	6–9	2
4–5	1–49	1–5	1
3	0	0	0

[a] RTS = 0.9368 (GCS_c) + 0.7326 (SBP_c) + 0.2908 (RR_c) where the subscript c refers to coded value.

Reprinted with permission from Champion, Sacco, & Copes, (1996). Trauma *(3rd ed.). (p. 54).*

Functional Independence Measure

The Functional Independence Measure (FIM) is a reliable and valid instrument used to document the severity of a disability as well as the outcomes of rehabilitation treatment (Christiansen, Schwartz, & Barnes, 1993). The FIM measures self-care, sphincter control, mobility, locomotion, communication, and social cognition, providing an overall score of function ranging from 18 (assistance required in all areas) to 126 (completely independent). Though not specific to trauma, the FIM is often used to determine the impact of specific acute-care and rehabilitation treatments on the functional outcome of injured patients. The FIM score of a trauma patient at discharge from an inpatient unit is a required data element in most trauma registries.

▶ INITIAL MANAGEMENT OF THE TRAUMA PATIENT

The initial management of the seriously injured patient requires rapid, systematic assessment with concurrent institution of life-saving therapy (Table 24–7). Because the most obvious injury may not be the most important one, successful resuscitation requires a deliberate and regimented team approach, with the flexibility to reset priorities based on injury identification and physiologic changes. The trauma surgeon or emergency department (ED) physician usually acts as team leader.

TABLE 24–7. Phases of Initial Management

Primary Survey (15 seconds)
- Airway with cervical spine control
  - Voice, air exchange, patency, cervical immobilization
- Breathing
  - Breath sounds, chest wall, neck veins
- Circulation
  - Mentation, skin color, pulse, capillary refill, neck veins, external bleeding
- Disability (neurologic)
  - Pupils, extremity movement, type and site, AVPU (A = alert, V = responds to verbal stimuli, P = responds only to pain, U = unresponsive)
- Expose the patient

Resuscitation
- Generic–ECG leads, pulse oximetry, IV, draw labs
- Concurrent with life-threatening injuries identified on primary survey
- Include gastric and urinary catheters, or perform with secondary survey

Secondary Survey
- Vital signs, including core temperature if patient unstable
- Head-to-toe examination (including spine)
- AMPLE history
- Imaging
- May be delayed until after operating room in unstable patient or patient in extremis

Definitive Care
- Surgery (may be in resuscitation phase)
- Splinting
- Medications (3 A's: analgesics, antibiotics, antitetanus)
- Consultants
- Transfer (ICU, surgical ward, or other facility such as regional spinal cord injury or burn center)

Tertiary Survey
- Repeat primary and secondary surveys within 24 hours for occult or missed injuries
- Creation of injury "problem" list with specific identification of physician handling each

Note: The emergency department (ED) is the portal of entry into the hospital's services, not the site of definitive care. Treatment in the ED is limited to that of life-threatening injuries only, to prevent unnecessary and hazardous delays to definitive care.

Adapted with permission from Rhodes, (1998c). The Trauma Manual *(p. 83).*

The Advanced Trauma Life Support (ATLS) course was adopted by the ACS Committee on Trauma (COT) in 1979 to provide a standardized program to train physicians in trauma care. The ATLS guidelines are accepted as the gold standard for the first hour of trauma care, whether the patient is treated in a rural general hospital or an urban Level I trauma center. Recognizing that the traditional approach used for a patient with an undiagnosed medical condition (extensive history, head-to-toe physical examination, and development of a list of differential diagnoses) does not satisfy the immediate needs of a patient with severe injuries, ATLS stresses the following tenets:

1. The greatest threat to life must be treated first.
2. The lack of a definitive diagnosis should never impede initiation of treatment.
3. A detailed history is not prerequisite to the evaluation of the acutely injured patient.
4. The mechanisms of injury suggest the degree of injury as well as specific injuries that must be confirmed or ruled out.

Primary Survey

The process of assessing and resuscitating the patient's vital functions constitutes the primary survey. The mnemonic "ABCDE" defines the ordered, prioritized evaluations and interventions recommended for all trauma resuscitations:

Airway with cervical spine control
Breathing and ventilation
Circulation with hemorrhage control
Disability (neurologic status)
Exposure (undress) with **E**nvironmental control (prevent hypothermia)

During the primary survey, identified abnormalities are treated concurrently, before proceeding to the next step in the evaluation. For example, a patient with a patent airway but no spontaneous respirations should be ventilated via mouth-to-face mask or bag–valve–face mask techniques, before circulatory evaluation. If multiple qualified personnel are present, these steps may be accomplished simultaneously, under the direction of the trauma team leader.

Airway with Cervical Spine Control

The first step in the primary survey is assessment of the patency of the airway. Airway obstruction may result from foreign bodies in the mouth, from fractures of the face, mandible, or trachea/larynx, or from bleeding. Removal of visible debris and the chin lift or jaw thrust maneuvers may clear the airway in less severely injured patients. More definitive airway control, usually endotracheal intubation, is appropriate for patients with obvious severe head injury or shock, or if there is any question about the patency of the airway. In certain patients, a surgical airway (cricothyroidotomy) may be required (Jurkovich & Carrico, 1997).

While assessing and managing the airway, care must be taken to prevent excess movement of the cervical spine. A rigid cervical collar, usually applied in the field, should remain on the patient during the primary survey. If collar removal is required for intubation, manual in-line cervical stabilization prevents inadvertent exacerbation of potential cervical spine injury. Cervical collars are left in place until cervical spine injury is excluded. *A normal neurologic examination does not rule out a cervical spine injury.* Any patient with multisystem trauma, especially with an altered level of consciousness or blunt injury above the clavicle, is assumed to have a cervical spine injury.

Breathing and Ventilation

The adequacy of gas exchange is assessed by observing chest wall movement, auscultating for breath sounds, and inspecting and palpating the chest wall for evidence of injuries that may compromise ventilation. If there is decreased respiratory drive, unequal or absent breath sounds, or an unstable chest wall, assisted ventilation is usually necessary. In cases of suspected tension pneumothorax with hemodynamic instability, needle catheter decompression of the affected hemithorax may be both diagnostic and therapeutic (Jurkovich & Carrico, 1997). Every injured patient should receive supplemental oxygen therapy (American College of Surgeons, 1993).

Circulation with Hemorrhage Control

Assessment of circulatory status includes evaluation of level of consciousness, skin color, and the quality, rate, and regularity of central and peripheral pulses. Abnormalities in circulatory status signify the need to establish two large-bore intravenous lines with rapid infusion of isotonic crystalloid. Bolus intravenous therapy may require the infusion of two to three liters to achieve an appropriate patient response (Table 24–8). Absent or transient response to two liters of crystalloid suggests ongoing hemorrhage, and an immediate need for blood transfusion and surgical intervention should be anticipated. External hemorrhage is identified and controlled using direct manual pressure (American College of Surgeons, 1993). Splinting of deformed extremities may help control bleeding from fracture sites. Hemorrhage into the thoracic or abdominal cavities, or into muscles surrounding a fracture or soft tissue injury, can account for major occult blood loss. Unreported or underestimated bleeding at the scene of the injury should also be considered in patients with signs of hypovolemia.

Disability (Neurologic Evaluation)

A brief examination to determine level of consciousness, pupillary size and reaction, and movement of extremities is necessary to identify life-threatening neurologic injuries. The GCS should also be computed in the primary survey. A decrease in the level of consciousness (LOC) may indicate cerebral hypoperfusion, decreased cerebral oxygenation, or direct cerebral injury. An alteration of LOC indicates the need for immediate reevaluation of the patient's airway, breathing, and perfusion. Alcohol or other substances may also alter LOC, but the cause should be considered of traumatic CNS origin until proven otherwise (American College of Surgeons, 1993).

Exposure/Environment Control

All garments should be cut off to facilitate thorough examination and patient assessment. After the assessment is complete, the patient should be covered with warmed blankets. Iatrogenic hypothermia can occur quickly in the emergency department but can be prevented by maintaining a warm environment and by warming intravenous fluids prior to infusion.

Monitoring

Adequate resuscitation is assessed in part by quantitative improvement in physiologic parameters. Pulse rate, blood pressure, respiratory rate, and core body temperature should be obtained as soon as possible after completing the primary survey. Electrocardiographic (ECG) monitoring is required for all trauma patients (American College of Surgeons, 1993). Dysrhythmias such as sinus tachycardia, atrial fibrillation, premature ventricular contractions, and ST segment changes may indicate blunt cardiac injury. Pulseless electrical activity (PEA) can occur with cardiac tamponade, tension pneumothorax, or profound hypovolemia. Hypoxia, hypoperfusion, and hypothermia should be suspected when bradycardia, aberrant conduction, and premature beats are present.

Pulse oximetry can be a useful adjunct, but does not measure oxygen saturation accurately in hypothermic or hypovolemic patients due to peripheral vasoconstriction. End-tidal carbon dioxide monitoring is a reliable means of confirming the position of the endotracheal tube in intubated patients, but actual values may correlate poorly with true arterial carbon dioxide levels. Arterial blood gases (ABGs) provide the most accurate measure of oxygenation and ventilation. Other monitoring devices (e.g., arterial line, pulmonary artery catheter) provide helpful information in the severely injured patient but are usually inserted in the operating room or intensive care unit.

TABLE 24–8. Responses to Initial Fluid Resuscitation[a]

	Rapid Response	Transient Response	No Response
Vital Signs	Return to normal	Transient improvement; recurrence of ↓ BP and ↑ HR	Remain abnormal
Estimated Blood Loss	Minimal (10%–20%)	Moderate and ongoing (20%–40%)	Severe (>40%)
Need for More Crystalloid	Low	High	High
Need for Blood	Low	Moderate-high	Immediate
Blood Preparation	Type and crossmatch	Type-specific	Emergency blood release
Need for Operative Intervention	Possibly	Likely	Highly likely
Surgical Consultation	Yes	Yes	Yes

[a] 2000 mL Ringer's lactate or 0.9% NaCl in adults, 20 mL/kg Ringer's lactate in children, over 10–15 minutes.

Reprinted with permission from American College of Surgeons, Committee on Trauma, (1993). Advanced Trauma Life Support Manual *(p. 88).*

Urinary and Gastric Catheters

Most severely injured patients require an indwelling urinary catheter to assess the adequacy of resuscitation. A urine specimen should be sent for laboratory analysis and toxicology screen, if indicated. Catheterization is contraindicated in patients in whom urethral transection is suspected. Signs of urethral injury include blood at the urethral meatus, scrotal or perineal hematoma, and, in males, a nonpalpable prostate on rectal examination.

A gastric tube decompresses the stomach and decreases the risk of aspiration. If a cribiform plate fracture is suspected, the tube should be inserted orally to prevent intracranial passage. Blood in the gastric aspirate may represent swallowed blood, traumatic insertion, or injury to the stomach. Gastric decompression is required prior to performing diagnostic peritoneal lavage (DPL).

Radiologic Studies

Three portable x-rays should be obtained during or immediately after the primary survey in most patients with significant blunt injury: the cross-table lateral x-ray of the cervical spine, anterior–posterior (AP) chest x-ray, and AP pelvic x-ray (Krantz, 1996). These studies should not delay or interrupt patient resuscitation. Information obtained from these x-rays may influence the early resuscitation and evaluation of the patient. Additional x-rays of the cervical spine, including the open mouth odontoid and AP views, are ultimately required for adequate radiographic evaluation (American College of Radiology, 1995). Other diagnostic studies should be directed by physical examination and mechanism of injury as the patient's condition permits. Patients with penetrating injuries need x-rays pertinent to the site(s) of the wounding and suspected missile trajectory (American College of Surgeons, 1993).

Laboratory Studies

A full battery of laboratory studies is generally not required in stable trauma patients because the results seldom alter initial management. The most useful tests are hemoglobin and hematocrit levels, which help to quantify the severity of anemia following obvious or occult hemorrhage. Recent data suggest a more selective and cost-effective tiered approach to laboratory studies in both blunt and penetrating trauma (Table 24–9) (Rhodes, 1998c).

TABLE 24–9. Suggested Laboratory Studies in Stable and Unstable Trauma Patients

Stable patients
- Hemoglobin and hematocrit
- Blood ethanol, depending upon hospital protocol
- Urine dipstick for blood
- Human chorionic gonadotropin (HCG) for women of child-bearing age

Unstable patients

All of the above, *plus:*
- Blood type and cross-match
- Arterial blood gas
- Prothrombin time, partial thromboplastin time, platelet count
- Electrocardiogram
- Selective serum metabolic tests based on patient condition and hospital protocol
    - Sodium, potassium, chloride, carbon dioxide, osmolality, blood urea nitrogen, creatinine, calcium, magnesium, amylase, lipase

Adapted with permission from Rhodes, (1998). The Trauma Manual *(p. 90).*

Secondary Survey

The secondary survey is performed following completion of the primary survey, after resuscitation has been initiated, and the patient's airway, breathing, and circulation (ABCs) have been reassessed (American College of Surgeons, 1993). The secondary survey follows the more traditional method of patient evaluation, including a complete history and head-to-toe physical examination. Additional x-rays, laboratory tests, and special studies such as computed tomographic (CT) scanning, arteriography, ultrasound, and DPL are completed during the secondary survey. An efficient secondary survey insures that delays in definitive care do not occur. If the patient requires operative intervention to correct problems with the ABCs, the secondary survey is performed postoperatively (Krantz, 1996).

History

A reliable history is often impossible to obtain from the trauma patient. Prehospital personnel and family can often furnish specific information about the patient's medical history and mechanism of injury. The mnemonic "AMPLE" provides an efficient framework for gathering the trauma patient's history (American College of Surgeons, 1993):

Allergies
Medications (current medications and immunization status, especially for tetanus)
Past illnesses and operations
Last meal
Events/**E**nvironment related to the injury

Allergic reactions can be avoided if known drug allergies are documented and communicated to the trauma team. Medications taken by the patient indicate other conditions and may affect the physiologic response to shock. Certain cardiac medications (e.g., beta blockers) can prevent a rise in pulse rate even in the setting of profound hypovolemia. Anticonvulsants or vasodilators suggest the possibility of a seizure or cardiac event as the cause of the accident. Past illnesses and operations should be considered in the context of current findings. A cardiac murmur from rheumatic heart disease has different implications than an acute murmur after trauma to the chest (Krantz, 1996). The time of last meal is important to establish in diabetic patients and in those patients who require intubation.

The events and environmental factors surrounding the injury provide valuable information that influences patient evaluation and management. Important information to obtain about MVCs includes use of safety restraints, airbag deployment, direction of impact (i.e., frontal or side), extent and type of damage to the motor vehicle, ejection from the vehicle, and the condition of the steering wheel and windshield. The medical history of patients who have fallen should include the height from which the patient fell and the type of surface on which the impact occurred. The cause of the fall, if known, has ramifications for the medical work-up, social service intervention, and injury prevention. A history of syncope or substance abuse should be sought.

Salient information regarding firearm injuries includes the velocity and caliber of the bullet, the distance from the weapon to the victim, and position of the assailant relative to the victim. In stab wounds or impalements it is important to determine the length and trajectory of the impaling object, as well as its degree of contamination.

Burn patients may have sustained associated penetrating and blunt injuries as well as exposure to hazardous materials. Specific information that may assist in the diagnosis of inhalation injury or carbon monoxide poisoning include substances burned in the fire, open or closed space, and length of exposure. Chemical fires and combustion of plastics are risk factors for serious inhalational injuries (Krantz, 1996).

Physical Examination

A thorough head-to-toe examination is critical for complete injury identification. Efficient assessment of the trauma patient can be difficult; the patient is usually examined in the supine position, altered neurologic status may interfere with patient cooperation, and immobilization devices such as cervical collars or splints may hide important abnormalities. Moreover, physiologic changes that warrant intervention interrupt the examination unless multiple practitioners are available.

All clothing, blankets, and prehospital bandages should be removed. Immobilization devices should be temporarily removed while a trauma team member maintains in-line cervical or extremity traction. Military Anti-Shock Trousers (MAST) should be removed if the patient is hemodynamically stable. The gradual deflation process begins with the abdominal compartment and proceeds distally. Air is allowed to escape slowly, while measuring blood pressure prior to deflating subsequent compartments. Once all segments have been deflated without significant change in systolic blood pressure (greater than 5 mm Hg decrease from baseline), the MAST can be safely removed.

The patient must be log-rolled while maintaining in-line cervical traction for assessment of the back of the head and neck, axillae, thoracic and lumbar spine, buttocks, rectum, and posterior extremities.

In penetrating injuries, determination of missile trajectory is critical for rapid injury identification. As soon as the primary survey is completed, wounds from penetrating objects should be inspected to determine the presence or absence of platysmal, fascial, or peritoneal penetration. The presence of such penetrations usually requires immediate operative exploration. Missile trajectory can sometimes be determined by identifying entry and exit wounds, and by palpating the direction of the wound tract.

Head. The scalp is thoroughly examined for lacerations and hematoma, which may be masked by thick hair or hair matted with blood. Occipital lacerations are frequently overlooked. If rapid suture closure of a scalp laceration was required for hemorrhage control during the primary survey, further assessment and, perhaps, reclosure can be done during the secondary survey.

The face is inspected for lacerations or contusions, and all bony prominences palpated for fracture-related deformities. Impairment of upward gaze and hypesthesia inferior to the eye suggest a "blowout" fracture of the inferior surface of the orbit. A midface fracture is likely when a gloved finger placed into the mouth can move the central incisors or palate. Acute malocclusion of the teeth indicates mandibular or maxillary fractures. Bruising around the eyes (raccoon's eyes) or behind the ears (Battle's sign) suggests a basilar skull fracture.

The eyes are examined for pupillary size and reaction, extraocular movements, visual acuity, hyphema, foreign bodies, and direct ocular trauma. Intact visual acuity of both eyes indicates that serious eye injury is unlikely. The ears are often subject to complex lacerations. A hemotympanum, disruption of the external canal, or cerebrospinal fluid leakage through the ear are diagnostic of a basilar skull fracture.

Neck. Neck evaluation involves assessment of the airway, digestive tract, vascular system, and neurologic function (Table 24–10). As previously noted, the cervical spine should be immobilized until injury has been excluded or treated. While a trauma team member maintains in-line cervical immobilization, the cervical spinous processes, trapezius muscles, and sternomastoids should be palpated for areas of tenderness or deformity. In alert, cooperative, and unintoxicated patients where there is low suspicion of cervical injury, no neck tenderness or deformity, *and* a lack of other distracting injury, active range of motion including extension, flexion, rotation, and lateral bending may be assessed. Pain or paresthesias during range of motion indicates possible injury and a rigid collar must be reapplied. Muscle tone and strength are assessed in all extremities. The sensory system is rapidly evaluated by comparing light touch on both arms and both legs. If an area of sensory loss or hypersensitivity is detected, its boundaries must be mapped out in detail. Dermatome patterns can help localize neurologic lesions (see section on spinal cord injury). A complete three-view x-ray series (open mouth odontoid, AP, and lateral views) of the cervical spine is required to exclude occult injuries or to define injury in patients with

TABLE 24–10. Clinical Signs of Injury after Neck Trauma

Respiratory Tract
- Respiratory distress
- Stridor
- Crepitus
- Hoarseness
- Dysphonia (voice change)
- Dysphagia or odynophagia
- Hemoptysis
- Pneumothorax

Neurologic
- Signs of spinal cord injury
  - Quadriparesis or quadriplegia
  - Cardiorespiratory arrest
  - Unexplained hypotension
  - Respiratory distress
- Lateralized neurologic deficit
- Cervical sensory deficits
- Cranial nerve deficits
  - Drooping of corner of mouth (VII)
  - Trapezius weakness (XI)
  - Tongue deviation (XII)
- Motor or sensory deficits of upper extremities (brachial plexus)

Vascular
- Shock
- Active external hemorrhage
- Expanding or pulsatile hematoma
- Diminished or absent carotid pulse
- Bruit
- Asymmetry of blood pressure between extremities
- Signs of hemispheric cerebrovascular compromise
  - Hemiplegia
  - Hemiparesis
  - Decreased level of consciousness
  - Aphasia
  - Monocular blindness
- Airway obstruction
- Hemothorax
- Signs of air embolus

Digestive Tract
- Dysphagia or odynophagia
- Drooling
- Hematemesis
- Crepitus
- Associated respiratory tract injury

neurologic deficits. As noted previously, the neurologic examination is normal in many cases of cervical spine injury (Krantz, 1996).

The neck should be inspected for distended neck veins, indicating cardiac tamponade or tension pneumothorax, and flat neck veins, indicating hypovolemia. Early or significant swelling of the neck suggests bleeding into a fascial plane or possible esophageal or laryngeal injury (Collincot, 1991). Wounds that penetrate the platysma, and the presence of an expanding hematoma over the carotid artery or jugular vein, warrant operative exploration (Krantz, 1996).

Palpation of the neck may reveal subcutaneous emphysema, which suggests injury to the larynx, tracheobronchial tree, esophagus, or lung (Symbus, 1996). The presence of thrills or bruits over the carotid arteries indicates the need for further evaluation with arteriography or duplex scanning (Krantz, 1996).

Thorax. Inspection of the chest involves examination for contusions, abrasions, deformity, and symmetry of expansion. Pneumothorax or splinting associated with fractured ribs may account for poor movement of one side of the chest. Discoordinate movements of the chest indicate a possible flail segment. Shortness of breath, pain, and tenderness to palpation strongly suggest the presence of soft tissue injury or fracture. Palpation of the ribs, clavicles, and scapulae may reveal tenderness, fractures, deformity, crepitus, or the presence of a flail segment. Subcutaneous emphysema, suggesting lung or tracheobronchial injury, may also be discovered on palpation. Percussion is performed to detect hyperresonance or tympany. Auscultation is important for assessment of heart sounds and reevaluation of breath sounds.

Tissue hypoxia from inadequate ventilation and oxygenation, shock, or impeded central venous return is the greatest initial threat in blunt or penetrating thoracic trauma. Immediate action is required for any hemodynamically significant pneumothorax, hemothorax, or cardiac tamponade. When signs of tension pneumothorax are present, immediate treatment requires placing a needle in the second intercostal space in the midclavicular line to decompress the hemithorax (Table 24–11). A large-bore chest tube is subsequently inserted. If a simple pneumothorax or hemothorax is suspected by clinical examination, chest tube insertion should not be delayed for a chest x-ray. Emergent treatment of an open pneumothorax (sucking chest wound) includes covering the wound with a sterile occlusive dressing taped on three sides to allow outward venting of air

TABLE 24–11. Signs of Tension Pneumothorax

- Dyspnea
- Hypotension
- Unilateral absence of breath sounds
- Distended neck veins (may be absent in hypovolemic patients)
- Hyperresonance to percussion over affected hemithorax
- Tracheal deviation toward contralateral hemithorax (late sign, not necessary to clinically confirm the diagnosis)
- Cyanosis (late sign)

from the pleural space. This must be followed immediately by chest tube insertion to avoid converting the open pneumothorax into a tension pneumothorax.

A chest x-ray should be done after chest tube insertion. Persistent pneumothorax may indicate a major airway laceration. Patients with massive hemothorax (initial chest tube drainage greater than 1500 mL or continued hemorrhage of greater than 200 mL per hour) require early transfusion and, perhaps, thoracotomy.

Cardiac tamponade occurs when blood accumulates in the pericardial sac, impeding cardiac distention during diastole (Fig. 24–6). Signs of cardiac tamponade include anxiety and Beck's triad of distended neck veins, muffled heart sounds, and hypotension. If cardiac arrest is not imminent, the patient is taken directly to the operating room. Other patients may be temporized with pericardiocentesis.

Emergency department (ED) thoracotomy is reserved for patients in extremis. This procedure is most productive in patients with life-threatening penetrating cardiac wounds, but ideal patient selection continues to be redefined (Read, Moore, & Moore, 1996). The goals of ED thoracotomy are to release pericardial tamponade, control intrathoracic or cardiac hemorrhage, and control massive air embolism or bronchopleural fistulae. It also permits open cardiac massage and temporary occlusion of the descending thoracic aorta in order to redistribute limited blood flow to the heart and brain in patients with massive intraabdominal hemorrhage.

Indications for ED thoracotomy are summarized in Table 24–12. Resuscitative thoracotomy is indicated in patients in extremis undergoing cardiopulmonary resuscitation

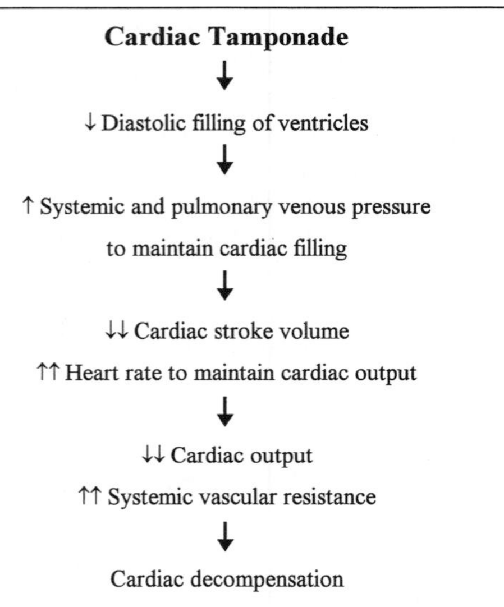

Figure 24–6. Pathophysiologic events of cardiac tamponade. *(Reprinted with permission from Kshettry & Bolman. [1994]. [p. 141.]. Copyright 1994 by W. B. Saunders.)*

TABLE 24–12. Indications for Emergency Department Thoracotomy

Clear Indications

1. "Salvageable" postinjury cardiac arrest. Patients sustaining witnessed cardiac arrest with a high likelihood of isolated intrathoracic injury, particularly penetrating cardiac wounds.
2. Severe postinjury hypotension (systolic blood pressure less than 60 mm Hg) due to:
   - Cardiac tamponade
   - Air embolism
   - Thoracic hemorrhage

Relative Indications

1. Moderate postinjury hypotension (systolic blood pressure less than 80 mm Hg) due to:
   - Potential intraabdominal aortic injury
   - Major pelvic fractures
   - Active intraabdominal hemorrhage

Adapted with permission from Read, Moore, & Moore, (1996), Trauma *(3rd ed.). (p. 196).*

following *penetrating* injury isolated to the chest. *Blunt* trauma victims in a similar condition may benefit from thoracotomy only if there is effective electrical cardiac activity (narrow–complex rhythms). Upon opening of the chest, cardiac tamponade is decompressed, hemorrhage is controlled, air is aspirated from the left ventricle, and the thoracic aorta is clamped until the patient is rapidly transported to the operating room for definitive treatment of injuries.

The chest x-ray should be carefully reviewed for acute and chronic abnormalities. Certain abnormal findings increase the likelihood of other more significant associated injuries (Table 24–13). Widening of the mediastinum (greater than 8 cm) is a hallmark of aortic injury but may be present due to obesity or supine positioning. A repeat AP chest x-ray in the upright or reverse trendelenberg position may help to exclude aortic injury in cases where the mechanism of injury does not support the diagnosis. Other radiographic signs of aortic rupture are listed in Table 24–14. Refer to the later section on chest trauma for further discussion of the diagnosis and management of aortic injury.

Abdomen. The abdomen is comprised of three basic regions: the peritoneal cavity, the retroperitoneum, and the pelvic portion (Krantz, 1996). Because the diaphragm may rise to the level of the fourth intercostal space (nipple level), blunt and penetrating trauma to the lower chest may involve the spleen, liver, or kidneys. Detecting the presence of abdominal injury is more important than searching for a specific injury to an organ or vessel. Once abdominal injury is found, a surgeon must be involved to assist with resuscitation and provide definitive care (Krantz, 1996).

Inspection of the abdomen for ecchymosis, abrasions, and penetrating injury may provide clues to underlying organ damage. Local exploration of knife wounds may help identify peritoneal penetration but do not definitively ex-

TABLE 24–13. Chest X-Ray Suggestions and Potential Associated Injuries

Abnormal Findings	Diagnoses to Consider
Any rib fracture	Pneumothorax, hemothorax
Fracture of first 3 ribs	Airway or great vessel injury
Fracture of lower ribs, 9 to 12	Abdominal injury
Two or more rib fractures in two or more places	Flail chest, pulmonary contusion
GI gas pattern in chest (loculated air)	Diaphragmatic rupture
Nasogastric tube in chest	Diaphragmatic rupture or ruptured esophagus
Air fluid level in chest	Hemothorax or diaphragmatic rupture
Sternal fracture	Blunt cardiac injury, head injury, cervical spine injury
Mediastinal hematoma	Great vessel injury, sternal fracture
Disrupted diaphragm	Abdominal visceral injury
Respiratory distress without roentgenographic findings	CNS injury, aspiration
Persistent large pneumothorax after chest tube insertion	Bronchial tear, esophageal disruption
Mediastinal air	Esophageal disruption, pneumoperitoneum, tracheal injury
Scapular fracture	Airway or great vessel injury, pulmonary contusion
Free air under diaphragm	Ruptured hollow abdominal viscus

Adapted with permission from American College of Surgeons, Committee on Trauma, (1993). Advanced Trauma Life Support Manual *(p. 133).*

clude it. Gunshot wounds should be objectively described by location and general appearance. The general contour of the abdomen should be noted.

Auscultation of the abdomen is rarely helpful in the secondary survey; the presence or absence of bowel sounds is a nonspecific finding in injured patients, although rarely auscultation may detect a bruit suggestive of vascular injury. Percussion detects localized tenderness, peritoneal irritation, and gastric distention. Abdominal distention suggests abdominal bleeding or pneumoperitoneum. Palpation identifies localized or generalized tenderness, guarding (voluntary or involuntary), rigidity, rebound tenderness, or masses. Hematuria, either gross or microscopic (detected by urine dipstick or laboratory analysis), is a marker for both renal and extrarenal abdominal injuries after blunt trauma (Knudson, McAninch, Gomez, Lee, & Stubbs, 1992).

While physical examination is the most important means of detecting the need for urgent laparotomy, several factors often confound abdominal examination in the traumatized patient. The presence of neurologic dysfunction secondary to head injury, spinal cord injury, or substance abuse poses the greatest obstacle to reliable clinical examination (Wilson, 1964). Even in alert patients, severe distracting injury, such as a fractured extremity, diminishes the reliability of abdominal examination. Pain and bleeding from associated rib or pelvic fractures may distort clinical signs of true abdominal injury. Moreover, a patient may be asymptomatic and yet have a life-threatening abdominal injury (e.g., liver laceration with contained hematoma). Patients with equivocal examination findings, an altered sensorium, or sensory impairment from a spinal cord injury need further diagnostic studies.

TABLE 24–14. Radiographic Signs of Thoracic Aortic Disruption

- Widening of the mediastinum > 8 cm
- Widening of the thoracic outlet
- Loss of aortic knob contour
- Calcium "layering" in aortic knob area
- Loss of aortico-pulmonary window
- Pleural apical cap
- Loss of paraspinal mediastinal "stripe"
- Large hemothorax
- Deviation of the trachea
- Depression of the left main stem bronchus > 140 degrees
- Deviation of the nasogastric tube from midline

No single sign reliably confirms or excludes aortic injury.

Diagnostic peritoneal lavage (DPL) is a rapid and sensitive test that can be performed in the resuscitation area and is indicated in the unstable patient requiring immediate confirmation of intraperitoneal injury (Cue, Miller, Cryer, Malangoni, & Richardson, 1990; Pachter & Hofstetter, 1981). In trauma patients, DPL is designed to identify the presence of hemoperitoneum, but it can also reveal hollow viscus injury with enteric contamination (Fabian & Croce, 1996). Once the gold standard screening test for abdominal injury, concerns about its invasiveness, oversensitivity, and nonspecificity have redefined its role in recent years. DPL is currently used for rapid screening in unstable patients and marginally stable patients with multiple injuries. Also when CT scanning results are equivocal, especially when intraperitoneal fluid is noted in the absence of solid organ injury (Fabian & Croce, 1996), DPL is a useful screening tool.

CT scanning defines specific abdominal injuries, and is especially effective in identifying solid organ and retroperitoneal injuries (Feliciano, 1991; Peitzman et al., 1986; Shuman, 1997). Patients for whom serial examination is impossible because of anesthesia, pain medication requirements, or other procedures, require CT scanning if the mechanism of injury suggests potential abdominal injury, even in the presence of a normal initial examination. CT scanning is safe, specific and noninvasive, but requires patient transport, more time and personnel, radiographic contrast, and sophisticated equipment. It should only be used in hemodynamically stable patients, and careful monitoring should be employed during the test (Feliciano, 1991).

Emergent abdominal sonography (ultrasonography) has emerged as a rapid, noninvasive, low cost, and accurate screening test for the presence of intraperitoneal fluid (Boulanger et al., 1995; Rozycki et al., 1995). Credentialed trauma surgeons can reliably detect fluid and visceral injury with dynamic "real time" images using the FAST technique (focused abdominal sonogram for trauma) (Davis, 1997; Ochsner, 1997). The major drawback of ultrasonography is its lack of specificity in defining solid organ injury, with inadequate visualization of the retroperitoneum (Fabian & Croce, 1996). In one study, 26% of patients with abdominal visceral injuries diagnosed by admission CT scan had no evidence of hemoperitoneum. Hence, dependence on hemoperitoneum as the sole criterion of visceral injury after blunt trauma results in false–negative examinations and misses significant injuries (Sherbourne, Shanmuganathan, Mirvis, Chiu, & Rodriguez, 1997).

Contrast studies may be necessary to define injuries to the urinary or gastrointestinal tract. The retrograde urethrogram, cystogram, and "one-shot" intravenous pyelogram are sometimes used for the patient with gross hematuria. These studies can be performed in the resuscitation area to detect disruption of the lower and upper genitourinary tract (Krantz, 1996). Using enterally-administered contrast, injuries to the retroperitoneal duodenum or rectum may be detected. Extravasation of contrast mandates immediate exploratory laparotomy.

Pelvis, Perineum, and Rectum. Stability of the pelvis can be determined by manually compressing the iliac crests toward midline and by rocking the pelvis with the heel of both hands. These maneuvers may increase bleeding and should be performed with care. The presence of pelvic fractures increases the likelihood of injury to the urethra or bladder.

Inspection of the external genitalia, perineum, vagina, and rectum detects lacerations, scrotal or perineal hematomas, and blood at the urethral meatus. Contraindications to insertion of a bladder catheter have been previously mentioned. During the rectal examination, sphincter tone is assessed, the prostate is palpated, and blood in the rectal canal is noted. In the absence of speculum examination, which is logistically difficult in the acute setting of trauma, digital examination may reveal blood at the introitus or a vaginal vault laceration, which indicates an open rather than a closed pelvic fracture.

If a pelvic fracture is identified on the AP x-ray of the pelvis, further films are necessary to completely characterize the fracture unless it simply involves a pubic ramus. The timing of these studies depends upon the hemodynamic stability of the patient and the presence of life-threatening injuries. The unstable patient requiring external fixation rarely needs additional x-rays. Once the patient is hemodynamically stable and other injuries have been repaired, complete radiographic and clinical characterization are necessary for the orthopedic surgeon to develop a definitive plan. Pelvic CT scanning is routinely performed in conjunction with abdominal CT scanning and is necessary to diagnose occult pelvic instability (Cryer & Johnson, 1996).

Musculoskeletal System. The extremities should be inspected for deformity, swelling, and wounds. Palpation of the extremities and passive range of motion of all joints may reveal tenderness, crepitus, and abnormal range of motion, which are clues to the presence of fractures and tendon or ligament injury. Assessment of neurovascular status is important in identifying injuries that may lead to loss of limb.

Thorough assessment of peripheral nerve function requires a cooperative patient. For each significant peripheral nerve, distal voluntary motor function and sensation must be systematically confirmed (Tables 24–15 and 24–16) (American College of Surgeons, 1993). Nerve injuries may be complete or incomplete, with some preservation of function. It is important to note that motor or sensory impairment also may be due to arterial occlusion or compartment syndrome. Peripheral nerve injury in the absence of these two conditions rarely requires emergency treatment, but immediate repair should be considered when a clean laceration is the cause of the injury (American College of Surgeons, 1993).

TABLE 24–15. Peripheral Nerve Assessment of Upper Extremities

Nerve	Motor	Sensation
Ulnar	Index finger abduction	Little finger
Median–distal	Thenar contraction with opposition	Index finger
Median–anterior interosseous	Index tip flexion	———
Musculocutaneous	Elbow flexion	Lateral forearm
Radial	Thumb extension/abduction	Dorsal web between thumb and index finger
Axillary	Deltoid contraction with shoulder abduction	Lateral shoulder

Adapted with permission from American College of Surgeons, Committee on Trauma, (1993). Advanced Trauma Life Support Manual *(p. 229).*

TABLE 24–16. Peripheral Nerve Assessment of Lower Extremities

Nerve	Motor	Sensation
Femoral	Knee extension	Anterior knee
Obturator	Hip adduction	Medial thigh
Tibial	Toe flexion	Sole of foot
Superficial Peroneal	Ankle eversion	Lateral dorsum of foot
Deep Peroneal	Ankle/toe dorsiflexion	Dorsal first to second toe web
Superior Gluteal	Hip abduction	———
Inferior Gluteal	Deltoid contraction with shoulder abduction	———

Adapted with permission from American College of Surgeons, Committee on Trauma, (1993). Advanced Trauma Life Support Manual *(p. 229).*

Abnormalities in the musculoskeletal examination require appropriate x-rays and the initiation of treatment. The x-ray studies should include the joints proximal and distal to the suspicious bone. Fractures of the spine and acetabulum usually require further definition with CT scanning. Grossly deformed limbs should be gently reduced, especially if the limb is ischemic, with peripheral pulse assessment before and after manipulation. Absence of a pulse after reduction suggests a significant vascular injury warranting exploration. Bones or joints with suspected injury should be immobilized with splints to alleviate pain, prevent further soft tissue injury (especially to nerves and vessels), and to facilitate intrahospital transportation (Harkness, Ramsey, & Harkness, 1996). Open fractures should be splinted after the wound is copiously irrigated and a sterile dressing applied. Urgent orthopedic consultation should be obtained for open fractures, and for fractures or dislocations causing limb ischemia.

Vascular System. The neck, groin, and extremities are inspected for large expanding hematomas and pallor. The carotid, brachial, radial, femoral, popliteal, dorsalis pedis, and posterior tibial arterial pulses should be palpated. The subclavian and axillary arteries can be assessed by comparing blood pressure in both arms. Decreased or absent pulses in all extremities suggests shock. Poor perfusion of one extremity with normal perfusion of the contralateral extremity suggests an arterial injury (Collincott, 1991). Skin temperature and capillary refill may also help identify local or systemic circulatory abnormalities. A continuous bruit auscultated in the area around a penetrating wound suggests an arteriovenous fistula.

Measurement of a Doppler arterial pressure index (API) can reliably and noninvasively exclude major occult arterial damage in injured extremities (Johansen, Lynch, Paun, & Copass, 1991). API is calculated by dividing the systolic arterial pressure in the injured extremity by the systolic arterial pressure in the uninjured arm. The presence of an API < 0.90 or "hard signs" of vascular injury usually warrants further study with arteriography or continued observation (Table 24–17). Arteriography is highly sensitive for significant vascular injury resulting from both penetrating injury and fractures/dislocations.

Neurologic Assessment. A complete neurologic exam is performed during the secondary survey, including the GCS score, pupillary assessment, cranial nerve evaluation, motor and sensory functions, and reflexes. The severity of brain injury can be estimated by assessing the level of consciousness, pupillary function, and lateralized weakness of the extremities. Immediate consultation with a neurosurgeon is required if there are deficiencies in these areas (Jurkovich & Carrico, 1997). Baseline findings should be carefully documented, and any abnormalities investigated with early CT scanning of the head and spine (Krantz, 1996). Sedation and neuromuscular blockade interferes with neurologic examination but may be necessary for safe, expeditious transport of the head-injured patient. Short-acting agents should be used when possible. Intracranial mass lesions (subdural or epidural hematomas), depressed skull fractures, and severe intracerebral hemorrhage identified with CT scanning or plain films require early neurosurgical consultation.

The negative influence of secondary insults (e.g., hypotension and hypoxia) on outcome from severe head in-

TABLE 24–17. Physical Signs of Arterial Injury

Hard signs
- Evidence of regional ischemia
  - Pallor
  - Pulselessness
  - Paresthesia
  - Pain
  - Paralysis
  - Poikilothermia
- Expanding or large hematoma
- Pulsatile bleeding
- Uncontrollable bleeding with direct pressure
- Bruit or thrill

Soft signs
- History of serious bleeding
- Stable, small hematoma
- Diminished distal pulses
- Adjacent nerve injury
- Fracture or dislocation in proximity to a major artery
- Anatomic proximity (≤ 1 cm) of wound to major artery

jury establishes *systemic* resuscitation as the early management priority (Chestnut et al., 1993; Fearnside, Cook, McDougall, & McNeil, 1993; Miller & Becker, 1982; Miller, Sweet, Narayan, & Becker, 1978). A single episode of hypotension (systolic BP < 90 mm Hg) in the adult with head injury increases mortality by 50% (Chestnut et al., 1993). Adequate ventilation, oxygenation, and circulatory support must be provided. When signs of transtentorial herniation or deterioration of neurologic status are present, hyperventilation should be initiated immediately to reduce intracranial hypertension. The intravenous administration of mannitol is also indicated but only under conditions of adequate volume resuscitation (Brain Trauma Foundation, 1995).

▶ MANAGEMENT OF SPECIFIC INJURIES

As trauma patients move from the ED to definitive care (OR, ICU, surgical ward, etc.), the trauma NP is responsible for ongoing injury identification and management. Comprehensive knowledge of the diagnosis and management of specific injuries and injury complexes enables the trauma NP to effectively participate in the surgical and medical care of multiply injured patients. Additionally, a variety of clinical problems encountered during rounds or identified by the nursing staff require complex diagnostic reasoning (Table 24–18). Good physical assessment skills, vigilance, astute clinical judgment, and frequent collaboration with trauma surgeons are essential components of acute trauma care.

Head Injury

Traumatic brain injury is the single most important factor in the morbidity and mortality of trauma. Approximately 2 million people per year sustain traumatic brain injuries (TBIs), with most victims between the ages of 16 and 30 years (Marion, 1998a). MVCs cause the majority of TBIs, followed by falls, blunt assaults, firearm injuries, and stabbings (Gennarelli, Champion, Copes, & Sacco, 1994). Gennarelli and associates found that patients with TBIs had three times the mortality rate, greater disability at time of discharge from the hospital, and were less likely to be discharged home than those without brain injury.

TBIs, often loosely described as head injuries, are categorized as mild, moderate, or severe depending on the degree of neurologic dysfunction at the time of initial evaluation (Marion, 1998a) (Table 24–19). Loss of consciousness is an important indicator of TBI, especially for patients with an initial GCS score of 15. Admission GCS score correlates well with outcome. Among patients with GCS score 8 or below, 41% die, and only 35% achieve any functional recovery (Pal, Brown, & Fleiszer, 1989).

Pathophysiology

Intracranial Hematomas and Contusions. Traumatic mass lesions of the brain are classified as epidural or subdural hematomas, or as intraparenchymal contusions or hematomas. Combinations of these lesions often occur (Valadka & Narayan, 1996).

The most common mass lesion due to trauma is the subdural hematoma (SDH). This lesion occurs in the potential space between the dural and arachnoid meningeal layers, and results from rupture of the small bridging veins between the cerebral cortex and venous sinuses. Clinical signs and prognosis are variable, depending on the size and location of the hematoma and the severity of injury to the underlying brain. Large subdural hematomas (> 1 cm), especially those associated with focal or global neurologic deficits, are usually managed with craniotomy and evacuation. Patients with asymptomatic SDH and GCS scores of 11 to 15 can safely be managed nonoperatively (Croce et al., 1994). Patients treated both surgically and nonsurgically require ICU observation for immediate detection of neurologic deterioration.

Epidural hematomas are caused by arterial bleeding from stripping of the dura from the skull. They are usually associated with temporal bone fractures causing laceration of the middle meningeal artery. The classic clinical course includes a lucid interval between the trauma and subsequent neurologic deterioration. Only a minority of patients with epidural hematomas present in this "classic" fashion; about one third of patients never regain consciousness, and about one third never lose it. With prompt surgical evacuation, these patients usually have a good prognosis.

Contusions represent areas of bruised tissue in which the blood–brain barrier may have lost its integrity. Intracranial hematomas and contusions occur in all areas of cerebral parenchyma but most commonly occur in the frontal and anterior temporal regions, and at the anterior base of the brain (Valadka & Narayan, 1996). Contusions may evolve into intracerebral hematomas, causing mass effect that may warrant surgical evacuation. Even small contusions and hematomas may enlarge in patients with minor head injury (Dacey, Alves, Rimel, Winn, & Jane, 1986).

Diffuse Axonal Injury. During blunt trauma to the head, linear and rotational sheer forces cause varying degrees of structural damage to axons and local axonal swelling, which over several hours culminates in separation of the axon into two segments. If axonal disconnection disrupts a significant amount of neuronal pathways, profound neurologic deficits may result. Magnetic resonance imaging (MRI) is helpful for confirmation of diffuse axonal injury (DAI), but MRI is time-consuming and does not accommodate critical care technology or allow for close patient monitoring. CT scans may show multiple small focal hemorrhagic lesions with minimal mass effect, but because CT lacks sensitivity for diagnosing DAI, it is usually a clinical

TABLE 24–18. Differential Diagnoses for Commonly Encountered Medical Problems in the Hospitalized Adult Trauma Patient

Abdominal Pain
- Abdominal wall contusion
- Incisional/postoperative
- Hollow viscus injury
- Solid organ injury
- Constipation
- Ileus
- Cholecystitis
- Pancreatitis
- Gastroduodenal ulceration
- Peritonitis
- Mesenteric ischemia or infarction

Chest Pain
- Chest-wall contusion
- Rib fracture
- Sternal fracture
- Pneumonia
- Myocardial ischemia
- Dissecting aortic aneurysm
- Pulmonary embolus
- Pneumothorax
- Anxiety

Acidosis
- *Respiratory*
  - Splinting
  - Atelectasis
  - Pneumonia
  - Pleural effusion
  - Pneumothorax
  - Oversedation
- *Metabolic*
  - Excess saline resuscitation
  - Diarrhea
  - Alcohol intoxication
  - Hyperalimentation
  - Renal tubular acidosis

Alkalosis
- *Respiratory*
  - Hypoxemia
  - Pulmonary embolus
  - Pneumonia
  - Anxiety
  - Pain
  - Fever
  - Iatrogenic (mechanical ventilation)
- *Metabolic*
  - Gastric suction
  - Vomiting
  - Exogenous steroids
  - Diuretics

Decreased Level of Consciusness
- Brain injury
- Cerebral edema
- Hydrocephalus
- Meningitis
- Fever
- Hypothermia
- Sepsis
- Oversedation
- Narcotic overdose
- Alcohol intoxication
- Hypoxia
- Pulmonary embolus
- Renal failure
- Hepatic failure
- Acid–base disturbances

Agitation
- Pain
- Anxiety
- ICU delirium
- Brain injury
- Burns
- Infection
- Fever
- Heat stroke
- Hypothermia
- Drug intoxication
- Drug withdrawal
- Adverse drug reaction
- Substance-induced psychosis
- Acid–base imbalances
- Hypoxia
- Pulmonary embolus
- Hypotension
- Shock
- Severe fecal impaction
- Renal failure
- Hypoglycemia
- Vitamin deficiencies

Anemia
- Hemorrhage
- Dilutional

Coagulopathy
- Consumptive
- Severe brain injury
- Blood loss
- Disseminated intravascular coagulation (DIC)

Fever
- *Inflammatory*
  - Trauma
  - Burns
  - Surgery
  - Deep vein thrombosis
  - Pancreatitis
  - Cholecystitis
- *Infectious*
  - Nosocomial pneumonia
  - Sinusitis
  - Urinary tract infection
  - Skin and soft tissue infections
  - Abdominal abscess
  - Device-related bacteremia
  - Osteomyelitis
  - Sepsis
- *Non-infectious*
  - CNS injury
  - Heat stroke
  - Atelectasis
  - Seizures
  - Drug reaction

Hypothermia
- *Primary*
  - Exposure
  - Immersion
- *Secondary*
  - Pharmacologic
    - Ethanol
    - Narcotics
    - Barbiturates
    - Sedatives and Hypnotics
    - Anesthesia
    - Neuromuscular blocking agents
  - Burns
  - Sepsis
  - Advanced age
  - CNS injury
  - Wernicke's encephalopathy
  - Spinal cord injury
  - Iatrogenic
    - Cold intravenous fluids
    - Patient exposure
    - Hemodialysis

Hypertension
- Pain
- Inadequate sedation
- Intracranial hypertension
- Pre-injury hypertensive conditions

Hypotension
- *Hypovolemia*
  - Blood loss
  - Third spacing of fluid
- *Relative hypovolemia*
  - Vasodilation
  - Autonomic dysfunction
- *Pump failure*
  - Blunt cardiac injury
  - Pericardial tamponade
  - Tension pneumothorax
  - Pulmonary embolus
  - Dysrhythmia
- *Inflammatory/Infectious*
  - Sepsis/septic shock
  - Systemic inflammatory response syndrome
  - Anaphylaxis
- *Medications*
  - Narcotics
  - Hypnotics and Sedatives
  - Diuretics
  - Muscle relaxants
  - Anesthetics
  - Antihypertensives

Dyspnea
- Pneumothorax
- Pleural effusion
- Pulmonary contusion
- Chest wall injury
- Pulmonary embolus
- Flail chest
- Acute respiratory distress syndrome
- Pneumonia
- Atelectasis
- Aspiration

Hypoxemia
- Atelectasis
- Pneumonia
- Splinting
- Pneumothorax
- Pleural effusion
- Pulmonary embolus
- Decreased level of consciousness

TABLE 24–19. Categories of Traumatic Brain Injury

	GCS	Clinical Hallmarks	Prognosis
Mild head injury	13–15	Brief period of loss of consciousness	Excellent prognosis Mortality < 1%
Moderate head injury	9–12	Typically confused sensorium May have focal neurologic deficits Able to follow simple commands	Good prognosis Mortality < 5%
Severe head injury	8 or less	Unable to follow commands Comatose	Significant permanent disability is likely Mortality > 40%

Adapted with permission from Marion, (1998). The Trauma Manual *(p. 242).*

diagnosis. DAI should be considered in patients whose initial CT scans show no significant pathology but who exhibit severe neurologic deficits, or in patients who remain comatose or severely disabled after evacuation of mass lesions. At present, there is no specific effective treatment for DAI (Valadka & Narayan, 1996).

Subarachnoid and Intraventricular Hemorrhage. Diffuse subarachnoid hemorrhage (SAH) is common after cranial trauma. SAH does not cause cerebral edema, but diffuse blood in the subarachnoid space predisposes patients to cerebral vasospasm, which impedes arterial blood flow and may cause tissue ischemia. Intraventricular hemorrhage is significant as an indicator of injury severity and may cause posttraumatic hydrocephalus (Valadka & Narayan, 1996).

Skull Fractures. In most cases, a skull fracture has less clinical importance than potential underlying brain contusion or clot. Since such lesions cannot be detected by plain skull x-rays, CT scanning is the diagnostic study of choice for patients with suspected skull fractures. Linear skull fractures are most common and rarely require treatment. Depressed skull fractures are usually more serious because of the increased incidence of injury to the underlying dura and brain tissue. These fractures are generally surgically elevated when the depth of depression is greater than the thickness of adjacent skull; however, this approach has not been proven to improve neurologic outcome (Marion, 1998a; Valadka & Narayan, 1996). Indications for surgical repair include evidence of cerebrospinal fluid (CSF) leak, cosmetic deformity, or contaminated bone or scalp fragments imbedded in the brain. Prophylactic anticonvulsants are often prescribed for 7 days. Broad-spectrum antibiotics are sometimes prescribed for 7 to 14 days (Marion, 1998a).

Basilar skull fractures may be associated with injury to the cranial nerves and local blood vessels. If a basilar skull fracture extends into the ethmoid bones anteriorly or petrous bones posteriorly, CSF leaks can occur through the nose or ears. The principle concern with basilar skull fractures is the risk of meningitis; however, prophylactic antibiotic administration is not recommended (Marion, 1998a). CSF leaks usually resolve spontaneously. Insertion of a lumbar drainage catheter or operative repair of the dural tear may be considered for CSF leaks that persist for more than 24 hours.

Penetrating Brain Injuries. Laceration of the scalp and fracturing of the skull occurs as a missile enters the cranium. Brain tissue damage from low-velocity mechanisms (e.g., stabbings) is relatively localized, with prognosis dependent upon trajectory. Gunshot wounds to the brain carry a high mortality rate from the extensive parenchymal destruction that results from shock waves and cavitation. Swelling of the remaining tissue may result in fatal intracranial hypertension. Injury to cerebral or dural blood vessels may cause large hematomas. Infectious complications occur locally around bone and bullet fragments, or regionally from disruption of normal anatomic barriers to the external environment. The management of gunshot wounds to the brain involves the same principles of cerebral resuscitation as for blunt TBI. Debridement of superficial entry and exit wounds is recommended, but it is not usually necessary to retrieve intracranial bullet and bone fragments. Prophylactic anticonvulsant and antibiotic therapy are usually prescribed.

Management of Intracranial Hypertension

Severe traumatic brain injury occurs from primary impact damage and from secondary injury as various inflammatory and biochemical insults evolve. Moreover, cerebral vasospasm, local vessel obstruction, and abnormalities of cerebral autoregulation threaten the adequacy of blood flow to brain tissue. Cerebral ischemia, the single most important event determining outcome after TBI, can be prevented or minimized with measures to optimize cerebral blood flow (CBF) (Rosner, Rosner, & Johnson, 1995). Prevention of secondary brain injury is of critical importance during the first 5 to 7 days after the primary insult.

In 1995, a task force of the Brain Trauma Foundation and the American Association of Neurological Surgeons developed evidence-based guidelines for the management of severe brain injury in adults. These important guidelines address key issues such as intracranial pressure monitoring and treatment, cerebral perfusion pressure management, hyperventilation, nutrition, and the use of mannitol, barbiturates, glucocorticoids, and anti-seizure medications.

Intensive care management of patients with severe TBI requires continuous monitoring of several physiologic parameters. Intracranial pressure (ICP) monitoring is indicated in patients with severe head injury (admission GCS $\leq$ 8) with an abnormal admission head CT scan (presence of hematomas, contusions, edema, or compressed basal cisterns). ICP monitoring is also appropriate in severely head-injured patients with a normal CT scan if two or more of the following are noted at admission: age over 40 years, unilateral or bilateral motor posturing, and systolic BP less than 90 mm Hg (Brain Trauma Foundation, 1995).

ICP monitoring is accomplished through the insertion of one of several devices placed in the epidural, subdural, subarachnoid, parenchymal, or ventricular locations. Ventricular pressure measurement is the most accurate and allows for therapeutic drainage of cerebrospinal fluid (CSF) in the event of intracranial hypertension. ICP monitoring complications for all devices include infection, hemorrhage, malfunction, obstruction, or malposition. Such complications are rarely a clinically significant cause of morbidity and should not deter the decision to monitor ICP. Normal ICP is between 0 and 10 mm Hg. An ICP of 10 to 20 mm Hg requires careful observation, and ICP treatment should be initiated at 20 to 25 mm Hg (Brain Trauma Foundation, 1995).

Cerebral perfusion pressure (CPP) is the greatest determinant of cerebral hemodynamic responses and effects, and is more amenable to manipulation than ICP. The injured brain is characterized by increased cerebral vascular resistance; hence, it requires CPP to be above normal before relatively "normal" levels of CBF can be attained (Rosner & Daughton, 1990). CPP is calculated by subtracting ICP from the mean blood pressure. The minimum goal for CPP is 70 mm Hg, with an average level of 85 mm Hg required for preservation of CBF. Higher CPP levels of 100 mm Hg or more may be required as defined by individual circumstances (Rosner et al., 1995). If CPP is inadequate, tissue perfusion is also inadequate and the ICP increases progressively.

CPP therapy can minimize ICP by reducing intracranial blood volume through autoregulatory vasoconstriction. CPP can be manipulated by inducing systemic hypertension without potentiating vasogenic edema and intracranial hypertension. Although CPP therapy is not isolated from that of ICP, the effects of many ICP therapies are transient, potentially toxic, and better used sparingly (Rosner et al., 1995). Interpretation and treatment of ICP based on any threshold should be corroborated by frequent clinical examination and CPP data (Brain Trauma Foundation, 1995).

Once a mainstay in the management of intracranial hypertension, prolonged hyperventilation therapy ($PaCO_2$ of 25 mm Hg or less) should be avoided due to its detrimental effect on CBF. Global CBF is typically very low after brain injury, and may be even lower in the anatomic region of tissue injury (McLaughlin & Marion, 1996). Aggressive hyperventilation reduces CBF even further, and may also cause loss of autoregulation. Muizelaar et al. (1991) found that severely head-injured patients had a significantly better outcome if they were not hyperventilated for 5 days after injury.

Mannitol is effective in lowering ICP, with limited data suggesting that intermittent doses may be more effective than continuous infusion (Brain Trauma Foundation, 1995). Mannitol also has beneficial effects on CPP, CBF, and brain metabolism. Its exact mechanisms remain unclear, but it is generally thought to have an osmotic effect at the blood–brain barrier as well as a plasma expanding effect, which reduces hematocrit, reduces blood viscosity, increases cerebral blood flow, and increases cerebral oxygen delivery. Mannitol requires an adequate CPP for its effects on ICP to be realized. It should not be given to hypovolemic patients, and serum osmolalities greater than 320 mOsm/L should be avoided.

Up to 15% of patients with severe head injury ultimately develop medically and surgically intractable intracranial hypertension with an associated mortality of 84 to 100% (Brain Trauma Foundation, 1995). In this setting, high-dose barbiturate therapy exerts cerebral protective and ICP lowering effects through suppression of cerebral metabolism, alteration in vascular tone, and inhibition of free radical-mediated lipid peroxidation. Pentobarbital is used most often, with a goal of therapy to establish serum pentobarbital levels of 3 to 4 mgm%, but literature suggests a poor correlation among serum level, therapeutic benefit, and systemic complications. The electroencephalographic (EEG) pattern of burst suppression offers a more clinically reliable form of monitoring. Burst suppression indicates near maximal reduction in cerebral metabolism and CBF (Brain Trauma Foundation, 1995).

The Guidelines for the Management of Severe Head Injury include a critical pathway which provides a framework for the management of intracranial hypertension (Fig. 24–7). Early treatment includes control of body temperature, sedation with or without neuromuscular blockade, avoidance of jugular venous outflow obstruction, elevation of the head of the bed, maintenance of adequate arterial oxygenation, and volume administration to maintain a CPP of 70 mm Hg or more. If a ventricular catheter is used for ICP monitoring, CSF drainage should be used first for ICP elevations. Bolus doses of mannitol should be given if the serum osmolality is less than 320 and the patient is not hypovolemic. Mild hyperventilation ($PaCO_2$ of 30-35 mm Hg) may be initiated.

Persistent elevation of ICP after employing these maneuvers may require "second-tier" therapy, including induced hypertensive therapy, barbiturate therapy, hyperventilation to $PaCO_2$ less than 30 mm Hg, induced hypothermia, and decompressive craniectomy. Second-tier therapies either have been proven effective in improving outcome but have significant complication rates (e.g., barbiturates) or

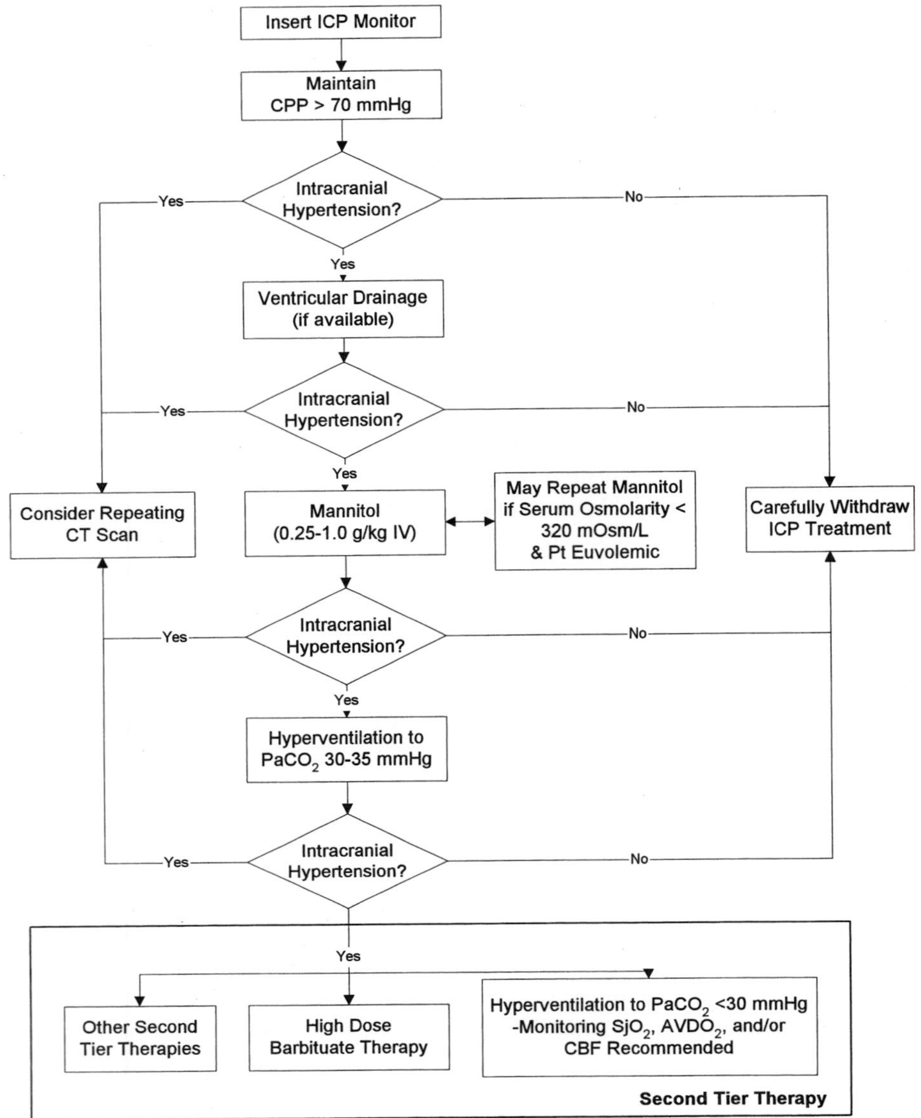

Figure 24–7. Critical pathway for treatment of intracranial hypertension in the severe head injury patient. ICP = intracranial pressure, CPP = cerebral perfusion pressure, CT = computed tomography, IV = intravenous, SjO_2 = jugular venous oxygen saturation, $AVDO_2$ = arterial-venous oxygen content difference, and CBF = cerebral blood flow. *(Reprinted with permission from* Guidelines for the management of severe head injury *[p. 13–3]. Brain Trauma Foundation, American Association of Neurological Surgeons, and Joint Section on Neurotrauma and Critical Care, 1998, Philadelphia: Lippincott-Raven. Copyright 1995.)*

appear to be effective in lowering ICP, but remain unproven in terms of the exact magnitude of their risk/benefit ratio or their influence on outcome. If available, measurement of CBF or jugular venous saturation (SjO_2) should be considered when second-tier therapies are used (Brain Trauma Foundation, 1995).

ICP elevation may signal the development of a surgical mass lesion. Consideration should be given to repeating a head CT scan when ICP cannot be controlled or when second-tier therapy is being contemplated (Brain Trauma Foundation, 1995).

Management of Mild or Moderate Head Injury

The distinction between mild and moderate head injuries is based on the initial GCS score, which reflects the severity of parenchymal injury (refer to Table 24–19) (Marion, 1998a). While most patients who are completely lucid at initial evaluation can be observed in the emergency department and safely discharged, a subset of patients are at risk for delayed posttraumatic hematomas or cerebral edema. Clinical characteristics associated with such risk include loss of consciousness associated with posttraumatic or retrograde amnesia (Duus, Boesen, Kruse, & Nielsen, 1993). Mildly head-injured patients with these characteristics should undergo a CT scan of the head (Duus, Lind, Christensen, & Nielsen, 1994; Moran, McCarthy, Uddin, & Poelstra, 1994). If CT scanning excludes intracranial pathology, these patients may be discharged, provided that a reliable adult family member can provide close observation for lethargy, disorientation, nausea and vomiting, and other signs of neurologic compromise. Patients with an abnormal CT scan, with focal neurologic deficit in the emergency department, or without a reliable family member to observe them at home should be admitted for 24-hour observation.

Patients with moderate head injury should be treated like those with severe injury. A significant portion of these decline into the latter category (Valadka & Narayan, 1996). Patients with intracranial lesions detected on initial CT scanning should be monitored closely for signs of neurologic deterioration, as contusions or hematomas may increase in size, or cause cerebral edema or hydrocephalus. In head-injured patients undergoing surgery or prolonged periods of sedation for management of other injuries, ICP monitoring can provide an alternative to physical examination for early detection of intracranial hypertension. A repeat CT scan is often performed 24 hours after initial injury, especially in elderly patients with age-related cerebral atrophy who may not manifest with neurologic deficits until significant intracranial hemorrhage or edema develops.

Postconcussive syndrome may result from mild or moderate head injuries. Symptoms may occur for weeks, months, or, rarely, years and commonly include headaches, vertigo, emotional lability, irritability, fatigue, tinnitus, sleep disturbances, and cognitive dysfunction (Levitt, Sutton, Goldman, Mikhail, & Christopher, 1994). Most patients with postconcussive syndrome experience mild intermittent symptoms and recover spontaneously within 2 to 4 weeks of injury, but for some, it can preclude return to normal life. Referral for outpatient neuropsychiatric evaluation and treatment is indicated if symptoms are debilitating or persistent for longer than 4 weeks (Barrett, Ward, Boughey, Jones, & Mychalkiw, 1994).

Upon discharge from the ED or inpatient unit, minor head-injured patients and their families should receive instructions defining signs and symptoms of neurologic deterioration (Fig. 24–8). It should be emphasized that symptoms such as headache are an expected part of recovery. Thorough description of symptoms of postconcussive syndrome with strategies for their management helps minimize phone queries or unnecessary return ED visits from overconcern about "routine" symptoms.

Injury to the Spine and Spinal Cord

Although spinal cord injury (SCI) accounts for only 1% of injury-related hospitalization, the impact of SCI on patients, families, and health-care resources is considerable (Jurkovich & Carrico, 1997). Permanent, severe disability results in loss of livelihood and psychological well-being. Once the primary injury occurs, limited surgical and pharmacologic therapies are available, and none fully reverses the initial damage. The primary objectives in the acute management of SCI are to prevent further injury by spine stabilization and by pharmacologically modulating the endogenous injury response. Such strategies may salvage a few dermatome levels and have a significant effect on functional recovery and rehabilitative potential.

SCI most commonly occurs in males (4:1 male-to-female ratio) and among persons between the ages of 15 and 30 years, but the incidence in those greater than 60 is steadily increasing. Nationally, about 50% of SCI is caused by MVCs (Marion, 1998b). Gunshot wounds to the spine are becoming more prevalent, especially in urban areas.

Injury Mechanisms

The spinal cord is normally protected by the vertebrae, which are held in alignment by strong ligaments and joints. Three columns provide stability to the spine (Fig. 24–9). Instability of the vertebral column usually results when there is injury to two of the three columns, caused by forceful flexion, hyperextension, rotation, axial loading, compression, missile penetration, or from a combination of these. Ligamentous injury can also cause spine instability and may occur without apparent bony injury (Przybylski & Marion, 1996).

Primary injury to the spinal cord occurs from displacement of bone or disk fragments, microscopic disruption of axons, and microhemorrhage. SCI in penetrating trauma occurs from direct penetration of the spinal canal or from the concussive effects of the projectile. Bullets, bullet fragments, or bone fragments often contact the spinal cord, and in many cases fragments remain inside the spinal canal (Yoshida, Garland, & Waters, 1995).

Secondary injury results from local edema and infarction due to hypoxia, or from occlusion of the anterior spinal artery or paired posterior spinal arteries. Secondary injury may also result from the release of endogenous mediators that cause progression of neuronal damage due to alterations in physiology and metabolism in the region of the direct trauma. This biochemical injury is associated with hemorrhage within the cord gray matter, release of excitatory amino acids, accumulation of endogenous opioids, free radical production, and lipid peroxidation. Ischemia may result from any of these processes and is considered the most important mechanism of secondary injury (Rhoney, Luer, Hughes, & Hatton, 1996).

The cervical spine is affected in 55% of patients with SCI, approximately 10% of whom have complete injury (Table 24–20) (Burney, Maio, Maynard, & Karunas, 1993). Between 2% and 5% of obtunded or comatose head-injured patients have a concomitant cervical spine injury (Marion, 1998b). Thoracic and lumbar spine injury accounts for 30%

Discharge Instructions for Minor Head Injury

You (or your family member) have suffered a minor head injury, also known as a concussion. A concussion causes immediate and temporary disturbances in the functioning of your brain. For example, you may not remember the events surrounding your brain injury, or you may have briefly lost consciousness.

The first 24 hours after a head injury require careful observation for signs of bruising or bleeding in the brain. There are special circumstances when an overnight hospital admission is required, but usually a friend or family member who is staying with you can safely provide this observation. If you were not admitted to the hospital after your Emergency room visit, it is important that a responsible person awakens you every 2 hours for the first 24 hours. You should sleep as you feel you need to, but someone should wake you every 2 hours to check your state of consciousness and orientation. Your family member or friend should ask you your name, address, and the date. He or she should also be alert to any unusual behavior or symptoms.

Call your doctor or return to the emergency department if any of the following symptoms occur:

1. Headache increases in intensity or is severe despite taking the pain medication in the manner that was recommended to you
2. Excessive drowsiness
3. Confusion or disorientation (cannot answer simple questions correctly or seems confused)
4. Persistent nausea and/or vomiting more than twice
5. Blood or clear fluid from the ears or nose
6. New weakness, numbness or paralysis of the arms or legs
7. Convulsions or seizures

You may now be experiencing headaches, dizziness, memory loss, or blurred/double vision. Headaches are very common after minor head injury and are an expected part of your recovery. The character, frequency and severity of the headaches vary from person to person. Patients can have headaches for a few days, a few weeks, or even several months. As time goes by your headaches should become less severe and less frequent and they should not interfere with your daily life. Your other symptoms should also resolve over time. If your dizziness, memory loss, and visual changes persist for longer than 3 days, call your doctor.

The following suggestions may help you to minimize headache discomfort for the first 3-5 days:

1. You should take the pain medication that was recommended to you by your doctor.
2. Avoid noisy, brightly lit, or crowded places.
3. Rest as much as you can and avoid strenuous activity.
4. Avoid activities that require intense concentration.

Do not take any medication for pain other than what was prescribed for you by your doctor. If the headache requires stronger medication, call your doctor as soon as possible. You should avoid taking aspirin or aspirin-containing medications. Do not drink any alcoholic beverages for one week.

It is important that you keep follow-up appointments as requested by your doctor. It is uncommon, but there may be long-term problems with your memory, vision, or cognitive abilities that your doctor can detect and treat.

Figure 24–8. Discharge instructions for patients with minor head injury.

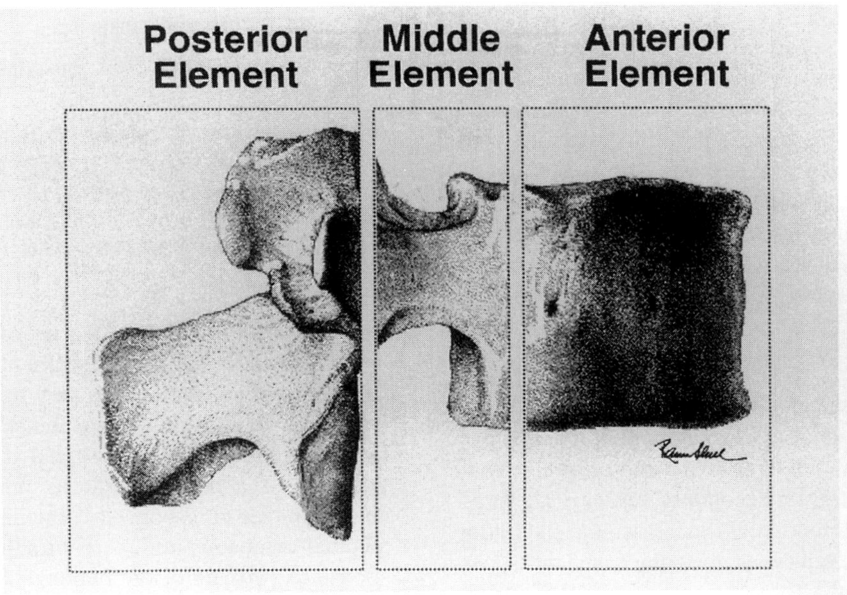

Figure 24–9. Three columns of the spine. *(Reprinted with permission from Peitzman, Rhodes, Schwab, & Yealy [Eds.]. [1998]. [p. 143].)*

TABLE 24–20. Classification, Description, and Mechanisms of Spinal Cord Injuries

Injury	Definition/Anatomic Description	Mechanism of Injury	Clinical Manifestations
Complete	A total loss of sensory and motor function in areas below the location of osseous injury to the spine with persistence for more than 48 hours Usually associated with severe vertebral fracture or disruption of vertebral alignment	Flexion with axial loading, hyperextension, compression	Quadriplegia, paraplegia, loss of voluntary and autonomic nervous function; spinal shock; minimal neurologic recovery
Incomplete			
Anterior Cord Syndrome	Loss of corticospinal and spinothalamic pathways with preservation of posterior column function	Occlusion or spasm of anterior spinal artery	Motor weakness; diminished pain and temperature sensation below level of lesion
Central Cord Syndrome	Injury to centrally located cord fibers controlling upper extremity function and voluntary bowel and bladder control	Hyperextension injury, especially with pre-existing cervical spondylosis and narrowing of canal	Loss of upper extremity strength, pain, and temperature sensation; preservation of lower extremity function Bowel/bladder control may also be lost
Brown-Sequard Syndrome	Unilateral injury to cord affecting crossed ascending spinothalamic fibers, uncrossed ascending posterior column fibers, and crossed motor pathways	Commonly penetrating injury with damage to saggital portion of spinal cord	Ipsilateral loss of motor function, vibratory and joint position sense; contralateral loss of pain and temperature sense
Conus Medullaris Lesions	Injury to the conus medullaris	Hyperflexion, compression, penetrating trauma	Bilateral, usually symmetric lower extremity deficits; disturbances of bowel and bladder function
Cauda Equina Lesions	Injury to cauda equina	Hyperflexion, compression, penetrating trauma	Asymmetrical lower extremity deficits; radicular pain; dysesthesia of the legs
Spinal Cord Contusion or Concussion	Exact pathology unknown; probably physiologic rather than anatomic disruption of cord	Acceleration/deceleration injuries of the neck especially in pre-existing spinal stenosis	Loss of neurologic function below level of injury, with spontaneous recovery within 48 hours

and 15% of the remaining SCI, respectively (Burney et al., 1993). The majority of spinal cord injuries are incomplete and, with proper care, patients may have a remarkable capacity for recovery. Persons with SCI have a greater opportunity for decreased morbidity and mortality when they are referred to a comprehensive SCI center within 72 hours of admission. Even with optimal care, mortality associated with SCI is 5.5%, ranging from 1.3% for those 30 years of age or less, to 22.7% for persons over the age of 60 (Regional Spinal Cord Injury Center of Delaware Valley, 1996).

Evaluation

Physical Examination. When the primary survey is completed, meticulous neurologic examination must be performed to identify spine tenderness and motor and sensory abnormalities (see section on secondary survey). The presence of *midline* spinous tenderness increases the likelihood of bony or ligamentous injury, as does any transient or persistent weakness, dysesthesia, or sensory loss in the extremities. If SCI is suspected, all muscle groups should be tested (Table 24–21), and their strength graded according to the motor grading scale (Table 24–22). The degree of diaphragmatic function can be assessed by measuring vital capacity. SCI below the level of the C5 nerve root does not affect diaphragmatic function; however, because the intercostal muscles and other accessory muscles of respiration are denervated by SCI, hypoventilation may occur (Chiles & Cooper, 1996).

Sensory examination should include light touch and pinprick sensation in all major dermatomes (Fig. 24–10). Key areas for assessment are outlined in Table 24–23. The identification of a sensory level on the trunk or upper extremities is virtually pathognomonic for SCI (Marion, 1998b). Vibratory sensation and proprioception should be tested in all extremities. The neurologic level of injury is defined as the most caudal segment that tests as normal or intact for both motor and sensory function.

TABLE 24–22. Motor Grading Scale

Grade	Description
5	Normal strength
4	Movement against some resistance and against gravity
3	Movement against gravity only
2	Movement only with gravity eliminated
1	Flicker or trace of contraction
0	No movement or contraction

Deep tendon reflexes, Babinski response, and sphincter tone should also be assessed if SCI is suspected. The presence of a bulbocavernosus reflex (contraction of the anal sphincter in response to pinching of the penile shaft) or an anal-cutaneous reflex (contraction of the anus in response to stroking of the perianal skin) are signs of preservation of distal function, often called *sacral sparing.* Sacral sparing suggests an incomplete spinal lesion and predicts a more favorable prognosis (Chiles & Cooper, 1996).

Radiographic Evaluation. The goals of imaging in a patient with a suspected spine injury are to assess vertebral alignment, identify fractures or ligamentous injuries, determine spine instability, and determine whether any neural structures are compressed by bone, foreign body, or soft tissue (Table 24–24).

Cervical Spine. Cervical spine radiographs may not be indicated for patients meeting the following criteria: intact mental status, sober, no distracting pain from other injuries, no spine pain and no neurologic deficit (Roberge et al., 1988; Velmahos et al., 1996). Patients who do not meet these criteria and whose mechanism of injury carries a risk

TABLE 24–21. Assessment of Motor Function According to Spinal Segment

Spinal Segment[a]	Muscle	Assessment
C1 to C4	Diaphragm	Use vital capacity and sensory level
C5, C6	Deltoid	Arm abduction
C5, **C6**	Biceps	Elbow flexion
C6, C7	Extensor carpi radialis	Wrist extension
C7, C8	Triceps	Elbow extension
C8, T1	Flexor digitorum profundus	Finger flexion, hand grasp
C8, **T1**	Hand intrinsics	Finger abduction
T2 through L1		Use sensory level
L1, **L2,** L3	Iliopsoas	Hip flexion
L2, **L3, L4**	Quadriceps	Knee extension
L4, **L5,** S1, S2	Hamstrings	Knee flexion
L4, L5	Tibialis anterior	Ankle flexion
L5, S1	Extensor hallucis longus	Great toe extension
S1, S2	Gastrocnemius	Ankle plantar flexion
S2, S3, S4	Bladder, anal sphincter	Voluntary rectal tone

[a] The predominant location of the nerve root responsible for a given muscle or mucle group is shown in bold type. The C8 nerve root exits in the foramen between C7 and T1.
Note: Motor function assessment is a useful adjunct to dermatome assessment in determining the level of spinal cord injury.

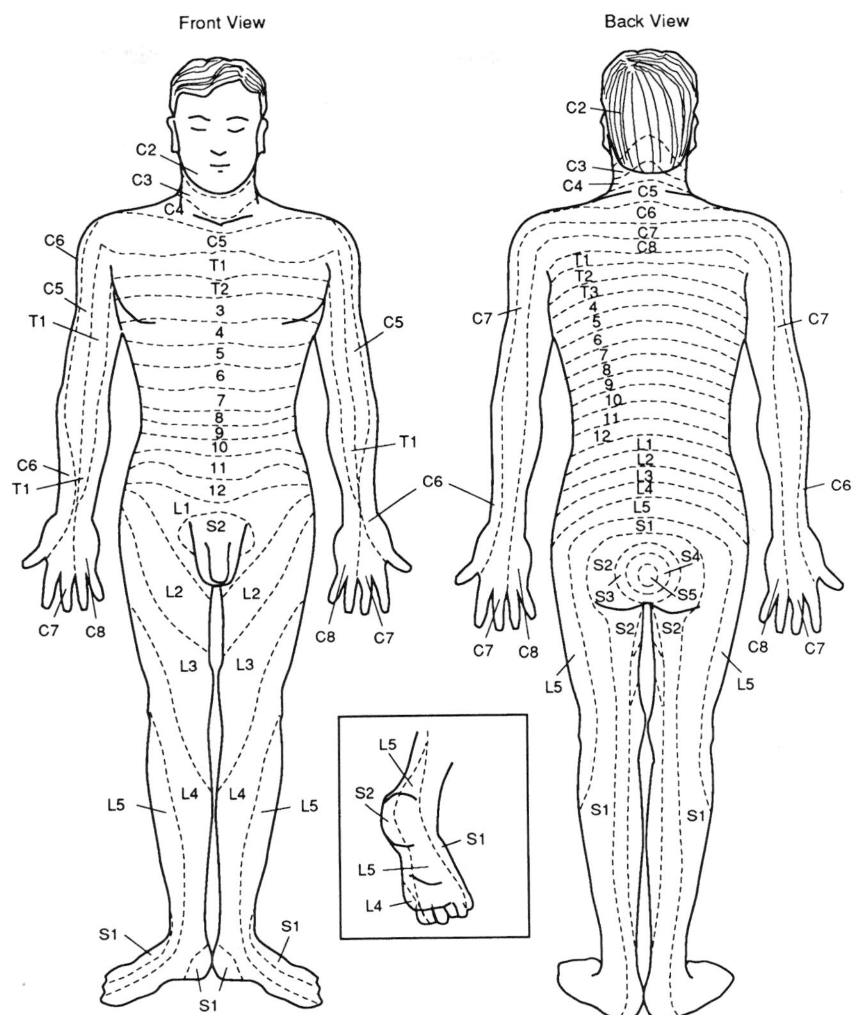

Figure 24–10. Dermatomes. *(Reprinted with permission from Cardona, Hurn, Bastnagel-Mason, Scanlon-Schilpp, & Veise-Berry [Eds.]. [1988]. [p. 427]. Copyright 1988 by W. B. Saunders.)*

of cervical spine injury should undergo radiographic evaluation of the cervical spine.

Initial c-spine radiographs include the AP, lateral, and open-mouth odontoid views. It is imperative that the lateral view include the entire cervical spine, including C7 through the top portion of T1 (Fig. 24–11). If there are suspicious areas or areas that cannot be seen on plain x-ray, axial CT scans at 3-mm intervals should be obtained, including the vertebrae above and below any areas of concern. If these images are normal, and the patient is alert and has no neck pain or distracting injuries, the cervical collar can be removed and the c-spine considered "cleared."

Patients without neurologic deficit but with cervical spine tenderness and *normal* open-mouth odontoid, AP, and lateral films should undergo flexion and extension x-rays of the cervical spine. These views identify clinically important ligament injury by detecting subluxation or distraction of cervical vertebrae as the patient actively flexes the neck forward and extends it back. Abnormal flexion or extension views warrant neurosurgical consultation and maintenance of a rigid cervical collar. If flexion and extension views show normal vertebral alignment and no vertebral distraction, the cervical collar can be removed and the c-spine considered "cleared." With bony and ligamentous injury ruled out, the patient with neck pain is diagnosed with cervical strain, commonly known as whiplash.

Immediate referral to a regional spinal cord injury center is indicated for all patients with neurologic deficits consistent with spinal cord injury. Spinal alignment must be maintained with a rigid collar, spine board, and sandbags, even if plain three-view radiographs are normal. MRI of the c-spine helps to define nonosseous injury and compression of neural structures, but MRI may not be available in certain centers or feasible in multiply injured patients.

TABLE 24–23. Assessment of Sensory Function by Spinal Segment

Spinal Segment	Sensory Area for Testing
C2	Occipital protuberance
C3	Supraclavicular fossa
C4	Top of acromioclavicular joint
C5	Lateral side of antecubital fossa
C6	Thumb
C7	Third finger
C8	Fifth finger
T1	Medial side of antecubital fossa
T2	Apex of axilla
T3	Third intercostal space
T4	Nipple line
T5 through T9	Corresponding intercostal space
T10	Umbilicus
T11	Eleventh intercostal space
T12	Inguinal ligament near femoral artery
L1	Below inguinal ligament
L2	Middle of anterior thigh
L3	Medial femoral condyle
L4	Medial malleolus
L5	Lateral calf
S2	Posterior thigh, popliteal fossa
S3	Ischial tuberosity
S4, S5	Perineum

The diagnosis of cervical spine injury in comatose or obtunded patients is difficult. Patients with a GCS score of less than 13 are unable to reliably report the presence of neck tenderness or other neurologic symptoms. Bony integrity can be evaluated with plain radiographs or CT scanning, but these static studies cannot exclude ligamentous injury. A rigid collar may be left in place until the patient regains consciousness for physical examination, but prolonged use of rigid collars and maintenance of spinal precautions increases the risk of skin breakdown and interferes with routine nursing care. Moreover, many complex facial reconstructive procedures and orthopedic procedures must be delayed until cervical spine clearance.

The use of dynamic fluoroscopy can safely and effectively evaluate ligamentous stability in obtunded patients, allowing for earlier collar removal (Davis et al., 1995). With this technique, the cervical spine is evaluated for lateral intervertebral body motion greater than 1 mm while it is passively taken through full flexion and extension. Fluoroscopy can be performed in the intensive care unit by an experienced physician or radiologist if the patient is unstable or transportation to the radiology department is not feasible.

Thoracic and Lumbar Spine. Lateral and AP views of the thoracic and lumbar spine should be obtained if there is pain in these regions or if there are motor or sensory abnormalities consistent with thoracic or lumbar dermatomal patterns. Because the presence of associated injuries or mental status impairment from head injury or intoxication reduce the reliability of clinical examination, surveillance thoracolumbar x-rays are also indicated in the following circumstances after blunt trauma: fall ≥ 10 feet (3 meters), ejection from a motor vehicle or MVC ≥ 50 mph (80 km/hr), GCS score ≤ 8, AIS scores ≥ 3, and neurologic deficit (Cooper, Dunham & Rodriguez, 1995; Frankel, Rozycki, Ochsner, Harviel, & Champion, 1994).

TABLE 24–24. Diagnostic Modalities for Evaluation of the Spine

Diagnostic Modality	Indications	Abnormality Diagnosed
Lateral cervical, lumbar or thoracic spine radiograph	Any injured patient when spine fracture is suspected	Alignment; body height; contour; cartilagenous space; soft tissue signs
Anterior–posterior (AP) spine radiograph	Follow-up to lateral spine radiograph	Spinous process; transverse processes; articular masses; vertebral bodies
Odontoid radiograph	Follow-up to lateral cervical spine radiograph	Atlanto-occipital joint; atlanto-axial joint; odontoid; lateral edge of articular masses of C1 with C2
Horizontal oblique radiograph	Normal 3-view cervical series and neck pain or neurologic deficit	Pedicle; intervertebral foramina; facet alignment; lamina
Pillar radiograph	Same as above; hyperextension injury	Posterior elements, lateral masses; lamina; limitations (visualizes C4–C7)
Flexion/extension radiographs	Same as above for cervical series; normal AP and lateral thoracic or lumbar views and back pain or neurologic deficit	Anterior subluxation; divergence of spinous or transverse processes; atlantodens interval (< 3 mm)
Computed tomography	Same as above; neurologic findings not explainable; suspicious radiograph findings; high clinical suspicion	Flexion teardrop; Jefferson; burst; lamina; hyperextension-dislocation
Magnetic resonance imaging	Same as above	Cord transection or contusion; intervertebral disk abnormality; parenchymal hemorrhagic lesions; intrinsic cord abnormality

Adapted with permission from Highland, Salciccioli, & Wilson, (1996). Management of Trauma: Pitfalls and Practice *(p. 210).*

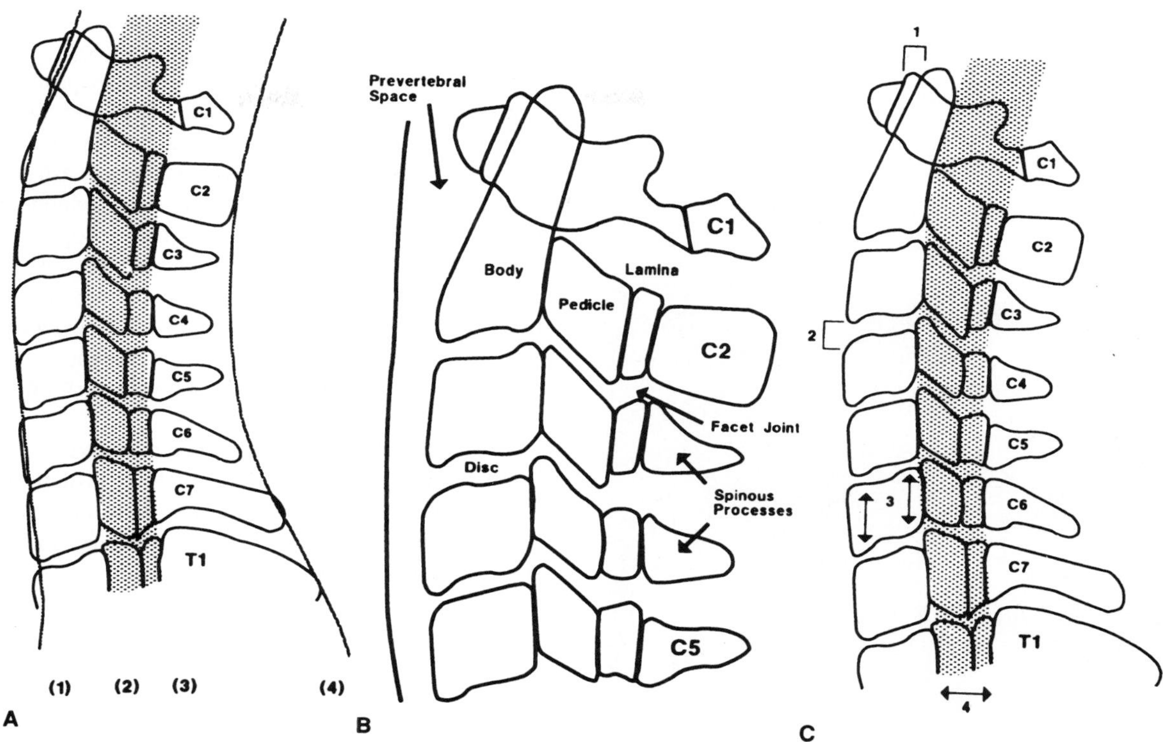

Figure 24–11. A, In evaluating the cervical spine in a lateral x-ray, one should see all seven cervical vertebrae plus the top portion of the body of T1. The alignment of the anterior portions of the vertebral bodies, the posterior vertebral bodies, the junction of the laminae with the spinous processes, and the tips of the spinous processes should all be checked carefully. **B,** When reviewing x-rays of the cervical spine, one should look closely at the various components of the prevertebral space, the alignment of the vertebral bodies, the disc spaces, the pedicles, the laminae, the facet joints, and the spinous processes. **C,** Measurements that may be helpful in evaluating a lateral x-ray of the cervical spine for injuries include: (1) atlantodental interval (normal: 2.5–3.0 mm), (2) superior vertebral body and inferior vertebral alignment (should be < 2.7 mm difference), (3) anterior to posterior bone height in a vertebral body (should be < 3 mm difference), (4) spinal canal width (should be at least 13 mm), and (5) < 5 mm prevertebral space. *(Reprinted with permission from Highland, Salciccioli, & Wilson. [1996]. [p. 210]. Copyright 1996 by Williams & Wilkins.)*

On both lateral and AP views, collapse of the vertebrae should be identified and quantified as the percentage of normal vertebral height lost. On the lateral view, alignment of the anterior and posterior borders of the vertebral bodies and the lamina should be noted. On the AP view, the distance between the pedicles at each vertebrae should be similar to the distance between the pedicles at the vertebrae above and below. If there is evidence of fracture or dislocation, or any suspicious areas, axial CT scans at 3-mm intervals should be obtained through that level, including the vertebrae above and below any areas of concern. If physical findings or mechanism of injury suggests injury but AP and lateral views are normal, flexion and extension views may be obtained. If there is a neurologic deficit consistent with SCI, MRI or CT scan and neurosurgical consultation should be obtained, or referral to a regional SCI center initiated (Marion, 1998b).

Fractures of the thoracic or lumbar vertebral bodies with less than 25% loss of height are usually stable. Unstable injuries involve more than 25% loss of vertebral body height. All spinal columns should be carefully assessed for injury—CT is often essential for determining the extent of injury, particularly to the middle column.

Management

Spinal Cord Injury. The goal of management of spinal cord injury is to reduce the resultant neurologic deficit, prevent additional loss of neurologic function, and prevent complications. Initial treatment consists of stabilizing the airway, breathing, and circulation, followed by spine stabilization.

Corticosteroid administration reduces edema and improves the functional outcome of blunt SCI patients if given within 8 hours of injury. The usual dosing strategy is an initial bolus dose of 30 mg/kg of methylprednisolone started in the emergency department, followed by a continuous infusion of 5.4 mg/kg/hour for 23 hours (Bracken et al., 1990). More recent recommendations by Bracken et al. (1997) extend the length of continuous infusion to 48 hours for patients who received the bolus dose between 3 and 8 hours after injury. There is preliminary evidence that steroid

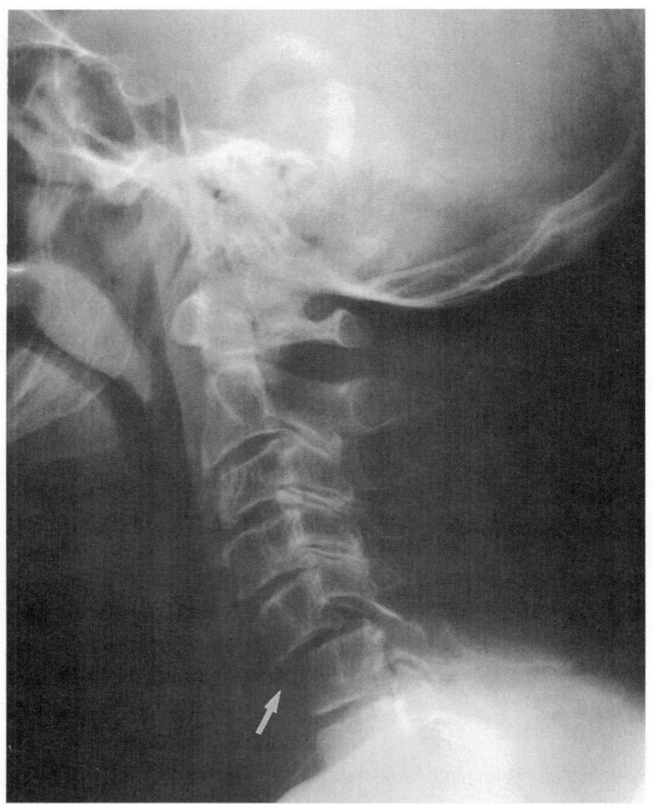

Figure 24–12. This 70-year-old patient had neck pain without neurologic deficit after a 12-step fall. Lateral cervical spine x-ray shows C5-6 subluxation, prevertebral soft-tissue swelling at the level of injury, and degenerative disc changes at multiple levels. Skull tongs with axial traction successfully reduced the injury, and surgical fixation was ultimately performed with good outcome.

administration after penetrating spinal cord injury does not significantly improve outcome (Levy et al., 1996). Other drug therapies—including antioxidants, vitamins E and C, corticosteroids, aminosteroids, opiate receptor antagonists, gangliosides, and growth factor—are being investigated for their potential role in limiting secondary injury (Rhoney, Luer, Hughes, & Hatton, 1996).

Hypotension and hypovolemia should be avoided for their potential to worsen ischemic spinal cord damage. Neurogenic shock is common in patients with complete spinal cord injuries from C1 to T6. Diminished peripheral sympathetic tone may cause vasodilatation, increased venous capacity, and profound hypotension. Associated bradycardia may help distinguish this reaction from shock due to hemorrhage, but it should never be assumed that hypotension is due to neurogenic shock until other causes (e.g., cavitary bleeding) have been excluded. Fluid resuscitation is the first-line treatment, and sometimes vasopressors may be required.

Pulmonary complications are common, especially in patients with quadriplegia. Patients with upper cervical cord injury require early intubation and mechanical ventilation, with use of positive end expiratory pressure (PEEP), suctioning, quad coughing, and bronchoscopy. All patients with SCI require an aggressive pulmonary protocol, including postural drainage, chest percussion/vibration, frequent turning, and daily assessment of pulmonary mechanics.

Nasogastric decompression prevents gastric distention and aspiration of gastric contents. Gastroduodenal ulceration is common after SCI. Stress ulcer prophylaxis is recommended and gastric pH should be closely monitored, with antacids or carafate prescribed as needed. SCI patients may lack abdominal sensation and do not develop classic peritoneal symptoms if there are unrecognized abdominal injuries or complications such as bowel perforation or peritoneal hemorrhage.

An indwelling urinary catheter should be placed during the acute phase to prevent bladder distention, provide continence, preserve upper urinary tract function, and to allow assessment of urinary output. Urinary tract infections are common in SCI patients. Intermittent catheterization, anticholinergic medications, and sphincterotomy may be employed in the recovery phase.

Decubitus ulcers develop in 32% of SCI patients and frequently occur over the bony prominences of the sacrum, heels, and ischium (Marion, 1998b). Frequent turning, optimizing nutritional status, and diligent skin care are essential.

Unstable Spine Fractures or Ligamentous Injury without Spinal Cord Injury. The management of unstable spinal column injury depends on its location, the degree of vertebral dislocation, and the presence or absence of spinal canal compromise (Marion, 1998b). When an unstable cervical spine fracture is present, but anatomic position is good, halo immobilization or surgical stabilization maintains proper alignment until healing occurs. In cases where anatomic position is significantly altered, axial traction with skull tongs helps to reduce maligned cervical vertebrae prior to operative fixation (Fig. 24–12). Some C1 and C2 fractures or cervical ligamentous injuries can be managed with a rigid external orthoses such a Miami-J collar or halo brace/vest worn for 8 to 12 weeks (Table 24–25). Many unstable lower cervical spine, thoracic, and lumbar fractures, or those associated with incomplete neurologic deficits, require surgical decompression and internal fixation. Patients with unstable injuries benefit from early operative stabilization to allow for early mobilization.

The majority of gunshot wounds to the spine are stable injuries—instability occurs when there are fractures of both pedicles or facets. The role of decompressive surgery in gunshot wounds to the spine is not clearly defined. Retained bullets rarely cause problems of delayed infection or lead toxicity, eliminating the need for prophylactic bullet removal; however, in the thoracolumbar spine, removal of bullet fragments lodged within the spinal canal has been shown to significantly improve neurologic recovery (Wa-

TABLE 24–25. Methods, Indications, Length of Therapy, and Precautions of Various Spine Immobilization Techniques

Methods	Indications	Goal of Therapy	Length of Therapy	Precautions
Cervical Spine				
Hard Cervical Collar (Short-Term) Philadelphia collar and Stif-neck collar	Prehospital immobilization Uncleared c-spine	Pre-evaluation, presumptive	< 48 hours	Ensure good collar fit Skin care Decubitus ulcers
Hard Cervical Collar (Long-Term) Miami-J collar and Aspen collar	Stable c-spine fracture Ligamentous injury	Hasten healing, diminish pain	8–12 weeks	Ensure good collar fit Worn continuously—provide second collar for washing Meticulous skin care
Soft Cervical Collar	Cervical strain, whiplash	Symptom management	Varies, dependent on symptom severity	Limit use to avoid dependence, e.g., nighttime, riding in car only
Cervical Traction				
Gardner-Wells tongs	Unstable maligned c-spine fracture, dislocation, or ligamentous injury	Cervical reduction Bridge to operative therapy	Varies	Pin site care and assessment Reposition patient every 2 hours
Halo vest	Unstable c-spine fracture, dislocation, or ligamentous injury	Definitive cervical immobilization	8–12 weeks	Pin site assessment and care Decubitus ulcers beneath vest
Four poster or Yale brace	Stable c-spine injuries or adjunct to surgery for unstable c-spine injuries	Hasten healing, diminish pain	8–12 weeks	
Thoracic or Lumbar Spine				
Hyperextension Cast and Thoraco–Lumbar Support Orthotic (Clam-Shell or Tortoise-Shell Brace)	Stable thoracic or lumbar spine column fractures; anterior compression fracture with <40% loss of height; burst fractures with no neurologic deficit, <50% vertebral body involvement, <30% canal compromise, angulation <20°	Hasten healing, diminish pain After spinal decompressive and stabilization surgery for support and comfort	8–12 weeks	Requires custom fit Meticulous skin care
Elastic Thoraco–Lumbar Supports	Minor compression fractures or transverse process fractures Lumbar strain	Symptom management	Varies, dependent on symptom severity	

ters, Adkins, Yakura, et al., 1991). A deterioration in neurologic status is the most agreed-upon indication for surgery in both blunt and penetrating injury.

Stable Spinal Injuries. Stable spine fractures or strain injuries are generally managed with external braces and symptom-relief therapies (Table 24–25). Patients generally require 24 to 48 hours of rest with antiinflammatory and analgesic medications before pain and muscle spasm are adequately controlled. Early physical therapy mitigates stiffness and hastens functional recovery.

Neck Injury

Neck injury presents a diagnostic and management challenge because of the high density of vital structures in the region. Structures at risk for injury include the trachea, esophagus, vessels, thoracic lymphatic duct, spinal column, spinal cord, thyroid gland, parathyroid glands, lower cranial nerves, brachial plexus, muscle, and soft tissue. The neck is divided into three anatomic zones (Fig. 24–13). Zone II injuries are usually vascular and are the easiest to evaluate and operatively expose, whereas exposure is difficult and diagnostic evaluation usually more extensive in zones I and III injuries.

Blunt injury to the neck occurs most commonly in MVCs, due to acceleration–deceleration forces and improper placement of the shoulder portion of three-point restraints. Significant force to the head or chest in MVCs can cause forceful flexion–extension of the neck, resulting in compression, stretching, or shearing. Other blunt mecha-

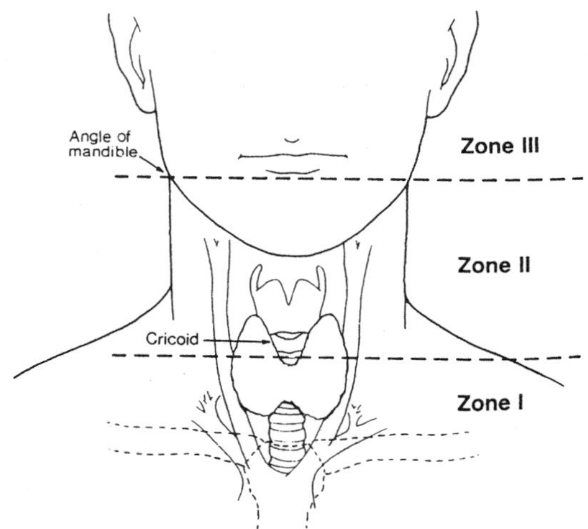

Figure 24–13. Anatomic zones of the neck. *(Reprinted with permission from Feliciano, Moore, & Mattox. [1996]. [p. 330]. Copyright 1996 by Appleton & Lange.)*

nisms of neck injury include hangings, beatings, choke holds, and sudden hyperextension as is seen when riders of motorcycles and bicycles strike the neck on unseen objects such as clotheslines. A high index of suspicion for blunt neck injury is imperative due to its often occult presentation. Failure to identify a vascular injury or cervical spine fracture can lead to devastating neurologic complications.

Penetrating injury to the neck is caused by gunshots, stabbings, and injuries by other sharp impalements. Wounding occurs through laceration and compression of tissue, as well as through the cavitary effect of high-velocity missiles. Aggressive diagnostic evaluation is indicated since it is difficult to determine the exact course of the missile through an anatomically dense area. It is often necessary to include the head, chest, and shoulder area in the evaluation process (Thal, 1996). Penetrating injuries may also occur in association with occult blunt injury to the carotid artery (Lebos & Saadia, 1994).

The history and physical examination are critical in efficient accurate diagnosis of injury to the neck. The alert patient should be questioned about pain, including its location and character, and about any difficulty breathing, swallowing, or talking. Neurologic history should include the upper extremity, especially in patients with zone I penetrating injuries. (Refer to the section on secondary survey for a complete description of physical assessment of the neck.)

The primary concern is maintenance of a patent airway. Early intubation is key, but may be complicated by associated cervical spine injury, large neck hematomas, and laryngeal trauma. Laryngeal trauma involves fracture of the thyroid cartilage, subluxation of the arytenoid cartilages, or dislocation of the cricothyroid joint. Patient complaints may include tenderness, shortness of breath, and voice change. Subcutaneous emphysema is usually noted on examination. Standard endotracheal intubation is contraindicated in the patient with a suspected or proved laryngeal fracture because of the risk of increasing the damage or creating a false passage without adequately securing the airway. If intubation is necessary, a surgical airway should be inserted below the area of injury (Thal, 1996).

Penetrating wounds should be inspected but not probed or locally explored since opening a wound tract may dislodge a clot and cause uncontrollable bleeding. If there is a potential for vascular injury, nasogastric tube insertion should be deferred until just before the induction of anesthesia in the operating room. In this way, neck bleeding induced by the gagging or retching associated with tube insertion can be rapidly controlled.

Prospective studies following *penetrating* neck trauma found that careful and repeated physical examination reliably detected significant injuries (Atteberry, Dennis, Menawat, & Frykberg, 1994; Demetriades, Charalambides, & Lakhoo, 1993). However, physical examination failed to accurately predict the presence or absence of blunt vascular neck injuries in several retrospective studies (McCormick & Burch, 1979; Sclafani, Cavaliere, Atweh, Duncan, Scalea, 1991). Approximately 50% of patients with blunt carotid injury do not have external evidence of neck injury. Most patients with such injury present with delayed focal or ischemic neurologic symptoms (Cipolle, 1998). Doppler ultrasound can be useful in screening for carotid injury in blunt-injured patients in which carotid trauma is a possibility. If the study is negative, the patient can be followed with serial neurologic examination.

Lateral and AP cervical spine x-rays, performed during the secondary survey, reveal the presence of retained fragments, soft-tissue hematomas, air column deviation or destruction, retropharyngeal thickening, and subcutaneous emphysema. Unstable patients with clear indications for surgery—such as shock, uncontrolled bleeding, or expanding hematoma—must be taken directly to the operating room. In stable patients, the type and location of injury determine the diagnostic work-up and management approach. Additional studies are often obtained, including angiography (arteriography), ultrasound, bronchoscopy, endoscopy, and contrast studies (Thal, 1996).

Arteriography is the most reliable means of identifying injuries of the carotid and vertebral arteries. It is recommended for stable patients with penetrating injuries in either zone I or zone III, or for blunt trauma if the patient has any external signs of neck injury associated with a change in the level of consciousness or lateralizing neurologic findings unexplained by CT scanning of the head. Low neck wounds (zone I) may involve superior mediastinal structures requiring thoracotomy for control and repair. High neck wounds (zone III) pose difficult problems with exposure, and defining the precise location and extent of injury may alter surgical approach. The need for angiography in zone II injuries is controversial but can be useful in allowing a selective approach to the surgical management of such injuries. It reliably rules out vascular injury, especially with soft signs of injury, allowing for nonoperative management with greater confidence. Angiography may detect unsuspected vertebral artery injury that might otherwise be undetected at the time of operation (Thal, 1996).

Patients with blunt neck injury or stable patients with penetrating injury not requiring exploration may require several diagnostic studies to rule out injury to the nonvascular structures in the neck. Laryngoscopy and bronchoscopy are used to localize or exclude injury to the hypopharynx or trachea. CT scanning is useful in confirming laryngeal fractures. Either contrast esophagography or esophagoscopy alone detects 60% of esophogeal injuries; diagnostic accuracy increases to 90% if the tests are used together (Johnson, 1998).

Management

Penetrating Neck Injury. In recent years, the age-old principle of mandatory surgical exploration of wounds that penetrated the platysma has been challenged by reports that from 46 to 89% of neck explorations may be negative for significant injury. A selective approach in stable, asymptomatic patients may be equally safe (Atteberry et al., 1994; Demetriades et al., 1993; Mansour, Moore, Moore, & Whitehill, 1991). The presence of "hard" signs or hemodynamic instability mandates surgical exploration and repair. Patients with "soft" signs such as hematoma, mild active bleeding, dyspnea, subcutaneous emphysema, hoarsenss, or dysphagia should be assessed individually, taking into account the severity of the clinical findings and the direction of the wound tract (Demetriades et al., 1993).

Intraoperative management is influenced by the type and severity of the injury, as well as by the patient's preoperative neurologic status. Injured vessels are usually repaired if the patient had no preoperative neurologic deficit.

Blunt Neck Injury. The management of blunt injury to the neck, especially vascular injury, is highly controversial. In general, localized carotid injuries in patients without neurologic deficits are surgically repaired. Carotid artery thrombosis may also be treated medically with blood pressure control and anticoagulation in selected cases. Vertebral artery injuries may be treated with repair, ligation, or balloon occlusion. Identified laryngeal or tracheal injuries are surgically repaired following evaluation of the esophagus with endoscopy and esophagography. Esophogeal perforations are usually operatively repaired; however, a small subset of patients with small injuries may be managed nonoperatively with close observation and IV antibiotics (Cipolle, 1998).

Thoracic Trauma

Chest injuries are directly responsible for approximately 25% of trauma deaths annually in the United States, contribute to an additional 25% of deaths, and cause significant long-term disability in survivors (LoCicero & Mattox, 1989). Immediate deaths are caused by great vessel injury or disruption of the heart. Early deaths (those occurring within 30 minutes to 3 hours) involve tension pneumothorax, cardiac tamponade, airway obstruction, or aspiration. Pulmonary sepsis, adult respiratory distress syndrome (ARDS), and missed injury account for the late deaths (Powell, McMahon, & Peitzman, 1998).

Chest-Wall Injury

Major chest-wall injury with fractures and disruption of musculature may allow direct injury to the underlying lungs, heart, great vessels, and upper abdominal organs. Moreover, respiration, ventilation, and oxygenation may be impaired by ineffective or paradoxical motion of a portion of the thoracic cage (Cogbill & Landercasper, 1996).

Penetrating missiles cause direct chest-wall injury through laceration and indirect injury from dissipation of kinetic energy to surrounding tissues. Although knife wounds and low-velocity handgun missiles cause more localized trauma, the extent of injuries to the chest cannot be judged by the appearance of the skin entry wound, and deep penetration should be assumed (Cogbill & Landercasper, 1996). Patients with penetrating injuries below the nipples anteriorly or inferior to the tip of the scapula posteriorly require evaluation for abdominal injury as well as thoracic injury.

Blunt forces cause chest-wall injury through direct impact, compression, and rapid deceleration in high speed MVCs and falls from heights. Direct impact can cause fractures of the ribs, sternum, or scapula with underlying pneumothorax, pulmonary contusion, or blunt cardiac injury. Compression of the chest by a heavy object may prevent respiration and markedly decrease venous return into the upper thorax, causing traumatic asphyxiation. Lateral rib fractures occur when anterior–posterior compressive forces exert indirect pressure on the rib cage (Cogbill & Landercasper, 1996).

The initial steps in the primary survey—assessment of airway and breathing—are of obvious importance in patients with chest injury. Immediate management priorities include establishment of a patent airway, initiation or support of adequate ventilation, and treatment of shock (Cogbill & Landercasper, 1996).

Specific information about the injury mechanism should be gathered in the history, including weapon characteristics and location of assailant in relation to the victim in penetrating trauma, and vehicle characteristics (type, speed, impact damage), use of restraint devices, and direction of impact in motor vehicle trauma. Important aspects of the medical history include tobacco use, prior surgeries, and medical illnesses, with emphasis on pulmonary conditions.

Refer to the section on secondary survey for discussion of physical examination of the thorax. Serial examinations are important to detect progressive changes in pulmonary function. Pneumothorax, hemothorax, and pulmonary contusion may develop or worsen several hours after injury.

In penetrating chest injury, auscultation to detect hemothorax (HTX) or pneumothorax (PTX) has been reported to have a sensitivity of 58%, specificity of 98%, and a positive predictive value of 98% (Chen, Markmann, Kauder, & Schwab, 1997). Abnormal breath sounds on auscultation indicate HTX or PTX with a fair degree of certainty, but because negative auscultation does not rule out injury, a chest x-ray is required. Conversely, this study demonstrates that abnormal breath sounds after penetrating trauma usually indicates HTX or PTX and thus can be used as a reliable indication for chest tube insertion before chest x-ray examination.

Traumatic asphyxiation is a rare syndrome that occurs following severe crushing injuries to the chest secondary to increases in intrathoracic and superior vena caval pressures. Manifestations include cyanosis of the face and neck, facial edema, petechiae, and subconjunctival hemorrhage. Occasionally, hemotympanum, epistaxis, seizures, confusion, loss of consciousness, blindness, and hematuria are seen. Associated chest-wall and intrathoracic injuries are common.

All patients with chest-wall injury should have an AP chest x-ray taken early in the evaluation. Paper clips or other radiopaque markers taped directly over entry and exit wounds may help determine missile trajectory when linked with abnormalities seen on x-ray. Systematic assessment of soft tissues, bones, pleura, lungs, mediastinum, and diaphragm identifies or provides clues for the majority of chest injuries (refer to Table 24–13). The position of bullets and foreign bodies should be noted. Clavicle fractures are usually seen on the AP view, but fractures of the ribs or sternum may not be visualized despite clinical evidence of their presence (Hunt & Schwab, 1992; Nahum, Gadd, Schneider, & Kroell, 1971). The chief purpose of chest radiography in patients with possible fractured ribs or sternum is to detect associated HTX, PTX, pulmonary contusion, and major vascular injury (Wilson & Steiger, 1996).

Flail chest is a clinical diagnosis that may or may not be confirmed radiographically (Fig. 24–14). Flail chest involves fractures of two or more ribs in two or more separate locations resulting in paradoxical motion of a chest-wall segment. Patients with flail segments are at high risk for immediate or delayed PTX, HTX, as well as pulmonary contusion. Hypoxemia results primarily from underlying pulmonary contusion, and secondarily from the increased work of breathing associated with paradoxical chest-wall motion. Morbidity and mortality are usually proportionate to the severity of the parenchymal injury rather than the chest-wall injury.

In stable patients, lateral or oblique views, tomograms, and rib films may be helpful in confirming the diagnosis of suspected bony injury. An additional AP view taken on expiration may detect small apical PTXs that are often obscured by the tangle of bones in the upper chest. Radiographic confirmation of clinically insignificant PTX may alter initial management, especially if operative procedures requiring positive pressure ventilation are planned.

A normal initial chest x-ray does not rule out signifi-

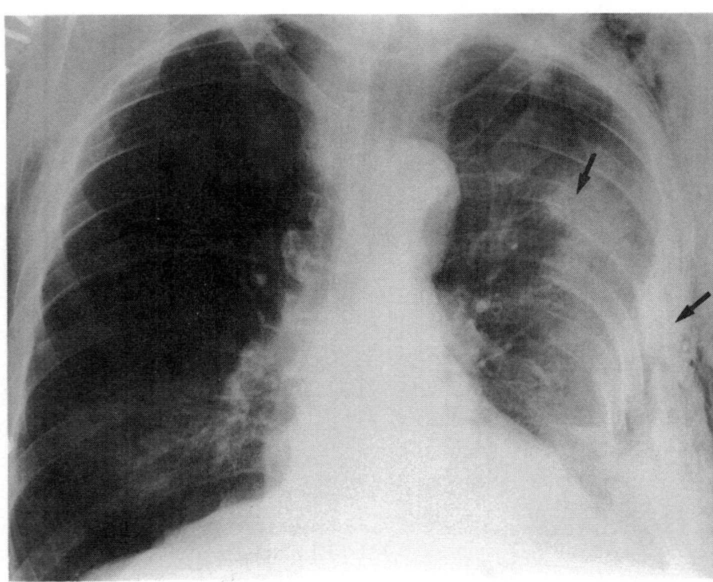

Figure 24–14. Chest x-ray of a 78-year-old male with a flail segment resulting from a fall into the corner of a table. The arrows indicate the fracture sites of three consecutive ribs. Note the associated left hemothorax, pulmonary contusion, and subcutaneous emphysema of the left lateral chest wall.

cant chest injury, as the onset of pulmonary contusion and HTX may be delayed. Serial chest x-rays are important in selected patients for identification of both delayed conditions and related pulmonary complications (Cogbill & Landercasper, 1996).

Continuous pulse oximetry and ECG monitoring are essential during the assessment and diagnostic phases. Early arterial blood gas measurements are indicated in patients with respiratory distress, suspected flail chest or pulmonary contusion, and in all elderly patients, even those with seemingly minor injuries (Cogbill & Landercasper, 1996).

Most chest-wall injuries are managed nonsurgically. The mainstay of treatment is good pain control to allow for optimal pulmonary mechanics. Nonsteroidal antiinflammatory therapy combined with intravenous or oral narcotic analgesic therapy offers the best approach to chest-wall pain control. The use of a thoracic epidural catheter for delivery of medication is a highly effective method of pain control for more severe chest-wall injuries, or for patients whose pain cannot be adequately managed using less-invasive techniques. Care must be taken to avoid oversedation of patients with chest injuries. Aggressive pulmonary toilet, including incentive spirometry, chest percussion, coughing, and deep breathing exercises, are facilitated by optimal pain control.

Intubation is used selectively. Signs of respiratory failure warranting intubation include respiratory distress, accessory muscle use, respiratory rate > 35 per minute or less than 8 per minute, $PaO_2 < 60$ mm Hg at $FiO_2 \geq 50\%$, or $PaCO_2 > 55$ mm Hg (Powell et al., 1998). Early intubation should be considered in patients with chronic pulmonary disease, cardiac disease, hemodynamic instability, the need for surgical repair of other injuries, or advanced age. Patients with flail chest should be admitted to the intensive care unit for observation.

Lung and Pleural Injury

Injury to the lung and pleura usually results from stab or gunshot wounds, or rib fractures caused by blunt forces. In penetrating thoracic injury, diagnosis is rarely a problem because clinical and radiographic manifestations usually occur within minutes to hours. Blunt injuries, on the other hand, may not be readily apparent and may not appear at their worst until 48 to 72 hours after the injury occurred (Richardson & Miller, 1996).

The most common pleural injury is a pneumothorax (PTX), which is caused by the introduction of air in the potential space between the lung parenchyma and parietal pleura. PTX occurs through several mechanisms that allow air to enter the pleural space: (1) a fractured rib penetrates the lung, (2) crush injury causes alveolar disruption, (3) deceleration injuries may tear the lung, and (4) an increase in intrathoracic pressure may cause alveolar rupture.

Tension PTX occurs when air entering the pleural space has no means to escape, allowing development of sufficient pressure to compress the lung. The lung collapses with subsequent mediastinal and tracheal shift away from the affected hemithorax. The superior and inferior vena cavas become kinked, causing impaired venous return and decreased cardiac output. Tension PTX is a clinical diagnosis—patients presenting with clinical criteria (refer to Table 24–11) require immediate needle decompression with a 12- or 14-gauge angiocatheter inserted into the second intercostal space in the midclavicular line. Radiographic confirmation is unnecessary and only delays treatment and prolongs hypotension. Needle decompression converts the tension PTX into a simple PTX; complete evacuation of the pleural space requires the insertion of a chest tube.

Thoracoscopy is currently used for diagnostic evaluation of the diaphragm, assessment of persistent hemothorax, evacuation of retained pleural clot, control of bleeding from intercostal vessels, and repair of small diaphragmatic injuries (Richardson & Miller, 1996). Thoracoscopy is also being investigated for its potential use in the evaluation of injuries to the lung, esophagus, heart, and great vessels.

The majority of injuries to the lung and pleura can be treated with tube thoracostomy. In penetrating chest trauma with hemodynamic instability, immediate operative intervention to control bleeding is paramount. Ideally, emergency operations on the chest are performed in the OR after resuscitation in the ED; however, exsanguination (≥ 1500 ml blood evacuated initially with ongoing bleeding) with hemodynamic decompensation may require ED thoracotomy (Powell et al., 1998).

Blunt Cardiac Injury

Blunt force to the chest wall may cause myocardial injury. Presentation ranges from subtle ECG changes to dysrhythmias to acute heart failure, valvular injury, or cardiac rupture and death.

Cardiac Contusion. Myocardial contusion should be suspected in patients with blunt thoracic trauma who manifest a poor cardiovascular response to their injury. Unfortunately there is no standard means by which to establish the diagnosis, except for pathologic examination at autopsy. The low severity and clinical relevance of this injury favors minimal diagnostic evaluation with treatment of cardiac abnormalities as they occur.

Symptoms are variable, with most patients reporting chest pain. The most common sign is dysrhythmia, usually sinus tachycardia (most common), premature atrial contractions, atrial fibrillation, bundle branch block, or premature ventricular contractions. Associated ECG abnormalities may include nonspecific ST segment elevation and T-wave flattening. Echocardiography, cardiac scintography, gated blood-pool scanning, and cardiac isoenzyme (CPK-MB, Troponin) analysis have not proven to be highly sensitive or specific in diagnosing cardiac contusion. Clinical outcome is not related to abnormalities in any of these tests (Ivatury, 1996).

The management of blunt cardiac injury is supportive. Patients with an abnormal admission ECG warrant telemetry monitoring for 24 to 48 hours, since almost all serious dysrhythmias occur within this time frame. Serial transthoracic echocardiography may be performed on selected patients, particularly those with prior cardiac disease or hemodynamic instability. Transesophogeal echocardiography (TEE) may be performed if the transthoracic echocardiogram is suboptimal. The impact of the information acquired from any laboratory or imaging study on clinical management decisions should be considered.

Cardiac Tamponade. Cardiac tamponade is most frequently caused by penetrating injuries but is also seen after blunt thoracic trauma. Accumulation of as little as 100 mL of blood in the pericardial sac may impair diastolic filling to the extent that shock and cyanosis develops (refer to Fig. 24–6). Beck's triad of distended neck veins, muffled heart sounds, and hypotension is present only in about one third of patients with cardiac tamponade. Two additional "classic" signs that are rarely seen include pulsus paradoxus (decrease in systolic pressure of more than 10 mm Hg during inspiration) and Kussmaul's sign (a rise in venous pressure with spontaneous inspiration). Tamponade should be suspected in patients with pulseless electrical activity or persistent hypotension in the absence of hypovolemia or tension PTX (Jurkovich & Carrico, 1997). If invasive lines are present, right and left heart pressures both rise and eventually equalize.

Pericardiocentesis is both a diagnostic and therapeutic maneuver; however, clotted hemopericardium produces a false–negative result in 15% of patients with cardiac tamponade. Echocardiography is advisable to confirm the diagnosis, but it too has a small (<5%) false–negative rate. For stable patients, subxyphoid pericardial window is the most reliable diagnostic and therapeutic procedure but takes more time and is best performed in the operating room. If pericardial blood is found, the incision can be converted to a median sternotomy for definitive cardiac repair. Immediate thoracotomy is warranted for unstable patients with suspected cardiac tamponade.

Thoracic Aortic Disruption. In cases of rapid deceleration (high-speed MVC, ejection from vehicle, or falls from great heights), the degree of external trauma may not fully predict the severity of internal injuries, and clinical suspicion of aortic injury should be heightened. Eighty-five percent of patients with aortic rupture die at the scene. If undiagnosed, 50% of the survivors suffer a ruptured aneurysm within 24 hours. Only 2% survive to develop a chronic pseudoaneurysm (Powell et al., 1998).

Prehospital personnel may verify the occurrence of hemodynamic instability or lower extremity paresis or paralysis in the field or during transport. Physical examination may reveal chest-wall contusion, palpable sternal fracture, respiratory distress, intrascapular murmur, widened pulse pressure, upper extremity hypertension, diminished or absent pulses, and hypotension. One half of patients with thoracic aortic disruption have no external signs of chest trauma. Numerous radiographic clues to the diagnosis may be found on chest x-ray, but no single sign reliably confirms or excludes aortic injury (refer to Table 24–14). The most reliable sign may be loss of the aortic knob contour (Miller, Richardson, & Thomas, 1989). It is important to obtain interval chest x-rays (at 4 to 6 hours and again at 24 hours) in patients with normal initial films if the index of suspicion for aortic injury is great (Mattox, Hirshberg, & Wall, 1996).

Aortography is the gold standard for diagnosis. A high-resolution helical chest CT scan may reveal an intimal flap or mediastinal hematoma, which are indications to perform aortography to specifically define the injury. Transesophageal echocardiogram (TEE) is useful for unstable patients in the ICU or for those requiring immediate surgery for cavitary bleeding (Minard et al., 1996). A positive TEE identifies the location of injury and expedites operative repair (Buckmaster, Kearney, Johnson, Smith, & Sapin, 1994; Kearney et al., 1993).

Management of thoracic aortic injury first requires establishing an airway, ventilation, and circulation. Identification and treatment of other life-threatening injuries must occur while arrangements are made for immediate transfer to the operating room or Level I trauma center. During transport, the risk of rupture may be reduced by minimizing contractile shear forces in the aortic wall through controlling blood pressure (SBP between 100 to 130 mm Hg) and heart rate (< 100 BPM) using a short-acting beta-agonist such as esmolol. The operative approach may involve left thoracotomy or sternotomy. Postoperative paraplegia is a rare but devastating complication resulting from prolonged aortic clamp time (> 30 minutes), or from extensive injury to intercostal arteries with disruption of flow to the anterior spinal artery (Mattox, Hirshberg, & Wall, 1996).

Injury to the Diaphragm

Injuries to the diaphragm are diagnostically challenging and surgically difficult to repair. Mortality from diaphragmatic injury ranges from 5% for penetrating injury to nearly 40% for blunt injury. Major morbidity results from acute complications such as respiratory failure, empyema, subphrenic abscesses, and hemidiaphragmatic paralysis, and from complications due to missed injury including the strangulation and perforation of herniated abdominal viscera and recurrent bowel obstruction. The incidence of diaphragmatic injuries is low, ranging from 1 to 6% of all abdominal injuries. By virtue of its anatomic location, the diaphragm is rarely injured alone. There is a 90% incidence of associated thoracic injury and a 50 to 100% incidence of associated abdominal and pelvic injury (Asensio, Demetriades, & Rod-riguez, 1996).

Penetrating injury mechanisms, the most common cause of diaphragmatic injuries, include firearm wounds and stab wounds to the thoracoabdominal region. Though the exact mechanisms of diaphragmatic injury in blunt trauma are unclear, it is postulated that abrupt increases in the pleuroperitoneal pressure gradient, which can occur with the sudden transfer of energy to the domes of the diaphragm (as in severe blunt abdominal trauma in MVCs or falls from heights), leads to diaphragmatic disruption. The left hemidiaphragm is more frequently injured than the right. In the presence of diaphragmatic laceration, perforation, or rupture, the pleuroperitoneal gradient encourages the transdiaphragmatic migration and herniation of intraabdominal viscera (Hood, 1971).

The diagnosis of diaphragmatic injury is rarely obvious and requires a high index of suspicion. Symptoms are nonspecific and may include dyspnea, orthopnea, chest pain, referred scapular pain, and abdominal pain. Physical findings may include diminished breath sounds on the affected side, bowel sounds in the hemithorax, shifting cardiac dullness, a scaphoid abdomen, and peritoneal signs.

The definitive diagnostic procedure is exploratory laparotomy with direct diaphragmatic exploration. Many patients have obvious severe associated abdominal injuries requiring laparotomy, but it is the patient without indications for laparotomy who represents the true diagnostic quandary. The initial chest x-ray may show elevation of the diaphragm, visceral herniation, irregularity of the diaphragmatic contour, and pleural fluid (Carter & Giuseffi, 1951). Occasionally a coiled nasogastric tube can be seen within the left hemithorax, which is pathognomic for ruptured left hemidiaphragm. However, only 50% of diaphragmatic ruptures can be seen on chest x-ray; in 40% the chest x-ray is abnormal but not diagnostic, and in 10% the chest x-ray is normal (Miller, Bennett, Root, Trinkle, & Grover, 1984). Diaphragmatic injury may be mimicked by HTX, PTX, gastric dilatation, atelectasis, pulmonary contusion, intraabdominal fluid, traumatic pneumatocele, or congenital eventration (Asensio et al., 1996).

DPL, ultrasonography, or CT scanning may be required for the evaluation of associated injuries, but these tests frequently miss diaphragmatic injury. Contrast studies such as upper gastrointestinal series and barium enema are useful diagnostic tools in stable patients or those with chronic abdominal visceral herniation. There is a growing body of evidence to support the use of laparoscopy or thoracoscopy, which are minimally invasive procedures with excellent diagnostic accuracy for diaphragmatic injury (Ivatury, Simon, & Stahl, 1993; Ochsner, Rozycki, Lucente, Wherry, & Champion, 1993; Salvino et al., 1993).

Primary repair of the diaphragmatic injury can almost always be accomplished through laparotomy. Perioperative intravenous antibiotics and copious irrigation are used to minimize infectious complications. Postoperative care involves pulmonary support, pain control, and early mobilization. Associated injuries usually take precedence after definitive diaphragmatic repair.

Abdominal Injury

Abdominal injury is a major cause of morbidity and mortality from both blunt and penetrating injuries. Swift diagnosis is critical but often difficult. Because physical examination is unreliable in many cases, other diagnostic modalities are employed based on the hemodynamic stability of the patient and the presence of associated injuries.

Liver

By virtue of its size and position, the liver is the most commonly injured abdominal organ after penetrating trauma and the second most commonly injured organ after blunt trauma. Many liver injuries are minor and outcomes generally good. However, the surgical and medical management of severe liver injuries can be extremely difficult. In one large series, the mortality rates for liver injuries from stab wounds, gunshot wounds, and blunt trauma were 8%, 22%, and 30%, respectively (Wilson & Walt, 1996). Most deaths occur early (within 48 hours) from shock and coagulopathy. Late mortality usually results from sepsis and multiple organ dysfunction syndrome (MODS) secondary to multiple episodes of ischemia and reperfusion.

Physical examination cannot reliably detect liver injury in the blunt-trauma patient. The diagnostic approach depends on the hemodynamic status of the patient in the ED. For stable victims of blunt trauma, CT scanning is the diagnostic study of choice (Fig. 24–15). CT can delineate the anatomic nature and severity of a liver injury as well as identify associated visceral and retroperitoneal injury. Unstable patients require DPL or ultrasound to confirm or rule out the presence of intraperitoneal fluid. Both are sensitive but not specific for liver injuries; a positive result indicates the need for immediate laparotomy.

Liver injuries are classified anatomically as grade I through grade VI, the latter indicating lethal hepatic disruption (Table 24–26). Classification should be assigned based on CT findings or direct exploration at laparotomy by an experienced trauma surgeon.

In penetrating injury, if trajectory determination suggests possible liver injury, exploratory laparotomy remains the gold standard for diagnosis and therapy. The approach to blunt trauma to the liver has evolved in recent years from one of mandatory laparotomy in all cases to more selective surgery. Nonoperative management of selected patients with all grades of liver injuries is now widely practiced (Meredith, Young, Bowling, & Roboussin, 1994; Pachter et al., 1996; Sherman et al., 1994). The advantages of nonoperative therapy include exceedingly low morbidity (5%) and mortality (0.5%) as well as improved management of associated injuries. Current data suggest that 50 to 80% of adult patients with blunt hepatic injuries are candidates for this approach, which carries a high success rate of 94% (Pachter et al., 1996).

Careful patient selection and aggressive monitoring for ongoing bleeding are key to successful nonoperative man-

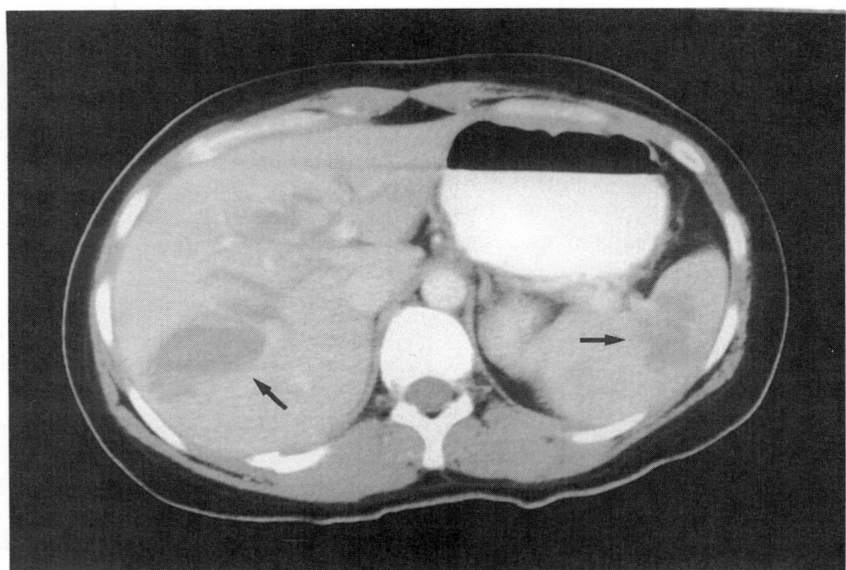

Figure 24–15. Abdominal CT scan of an unrestrained driver involved in a MVC. A grade III liver laceration *(left-hand arrow)* and grade IV splenic laceration *(right-hand arrow)* are present.

agement (Table 24–27). Patients are admitted to the ICU on bedrest, with serial examinations and hematocrits performed every 4 to 6 hours. Indications for urgent laparatomy include: (1) hemodynamic instability, (2) a greater than 2-unit red blood-cell transfusion requirement, (3) the development of peritoneal signs, and (4) a deterioration in mental status such that physical examination is no longer reliable.

If stable after 24 to 48 hours of close observation, the patient can be transferred to the ward and the diet can be advanced according to customary practice. Bedrest is maintained for 2 to 3 days to prevent hemorrhage from disruption of the protective perihepatic hematoma. Activity must be severely restricted for several days to weeks, depending on the severity of the injury. Prior to patient discharge, it is important to explicitly describe activity restrictions to the patient and family, ideally using a written template for clarity and consistency (Figure 24–16). Patients may resume normal physical activity 2 to 3 months after injury.

The need for follow-up abdominal CT scanning is controversial. Some authors support obtaining a CT within 7 to 10 days after grade IV or V injury to document healing (Pachter et al., 1996). It is also useful in young patients with active lifestyles before clearance to resume activities such as contact sports, but there is little data to support this approach. Repeat CT evaluation has proven useful in identifying complications of liver injuries such as intraperitoneal biliary leaks and subcapsular bilomas (Bynoe et al., 1992).

Operative management is required when there are clinical indications of ongoing intraabdominal hemorrhage.

TABLE 24–26. Liver Injury Scale

Grade[a]		Injury Description	AIS[b]
I	Hematoma	Subcapsular, <10% surface area	2
	Laceration	Capsular tear, <1 cm parenchymal depth	2
II	Hematoma	Subcapsular, 10–50% surface area; intraparenchymal, <10 cm in diameter	2
	Laceration	1–3 cm parenchymal depth, <10 cm in length	2
III	Hematoma	Subcapsular, >50% surface area or expanding; ruptured subcapsular or parenchymal hematoma Intraparenchymal hematoma >10 cm or expanding	3
	Laceration	>3 cm parenchymal depth	3
IV	Laceration	Parenchymal disruption involving 25–75% of hepatic lobe or 1–3 Couinaud's segments within a single lobe	4
V	Laceration	Parenchymal disruption involving >75% of hepatic lobe or >3 Couinaud's segments within a single lobe	5
	Vascular	Juxtahepatic venous injuries; i.e., retrohepatic vena cava/central major hepatic veins	5
VI	Vascular	Hepatic avulsion	6

[a] Advance one grade for multiple injuries, up to grade III.
[b] AIS = abbreviated injury scale score.
Adapted with permission from Moore et al., (1994). (p. 324).

TABLE 24–27. Guidelines for Nonoperative Management of Blunt Hepatic Trauma

1. The patient must be hemodynamically stable and have no other clinical indications for laparotomy such as peritoneal signs
2. The CT scan must be of good quality and interpreted by a physician with a sound understanding of and experience with CT in trauma. The criteria for limited liver injury must be present
3. The decision not to perform exploratory surgery must be made by a surgeon with experience in liver trauma
4. The patient must be monitored closely for bleeding or other complications by intensive care unit or floor staff who are familiar with trauma patients
5. Nonoperative management must be performed in an institution where surgery can be provided immediately, if needed. This requires not only an experienced trauma surgeon but anesthesiology, operating room, and blood bank support

Adapted with permission from Ciraulo et al., (1996). (p. 821).

The blood bank should be notified of the potential need for massive quantities of blood products. The specific method of surgical repair varies according to the severity of liver injury; most injuries are grade I or II and are repaired with electrocautery, simple suture, and topical hemostatic agents. Definitive repair of complex liver injury (grades III to V) may be accomplished with hepatotomy, resectional debridement, deep suture repair, hepatic resection, intraparenchymal balloon tamponade, and other advanced techniques. Patients should be admitted to the ICU postoperatively for close monitoring, volume resuscitation, and serial hematocrit checks. Stable patients can be allowed out of bed in 24 hours, with activity and diet progression as tolerated.

In exsanguinating patients with devastating abdominal injury, a staged procedure termed "Damage Control" has been shown to decrease mortality by interrupting the viscous cycle of hypothermia, acidosis, and coagulopathy (Hirshberg, Wall, & Mattox, 1994; Rotondo et al., 1993). Damage Control is a three-part approach including abbreviated laparotomy for hemorrhage control, ICU resuscitation, and definitive repair and reconstruction (Table 24–28). This alternative surgical approach is recommended for exsanguinating, unstable patients with multiple penetrating abdominal wounds or high blunt energy transfer.

Spleen

The spleen is the most commonly injured organ in blunt abdominal trauma. Splenic injuries are present in 30% of victims of blunt abdominal trauma and in 10% of victims of penetrating abdominal trauma. The mortality of isolated splenic injury is only about 1 to 2%; however, the majority of patients with splenic trauma have other associated abdominal injuries, increasing the mortality rate to 18 to 25%.

Physical examination is generally nonspecific in the diagnosis of splenic injury. Inspection may reveal left upper quadrant contusions, abrasions, or penetrating wounds. There may be left upper quadrant tenderness, referred left shoulder pain (Kehr's sign), or peritoneal signs (Esposito & Gamelli, 1996). Systematic palpation of the chest wall may reveal point tenderness over associated rib fractures. Twenty-five percent of patients with left lower rib fractures (ribs 9 to 12) have a splenic injury (Boone & Peitzman, 1998).

In the unstable patient, DPL or ultrasound are optimal means of rapidly diagnosing hemoperitoneum, which is often a result of splenic rupture. For stable patients, abdominal CT scanning helps delineate splenic lacerations as well as associated abdominal and lower thoracic injuries (refer to Fig. 24–15). Splenic injuries are classified anatomically as grades I to V injuries using CT findings or direct exploration at laparotomy (Table 24–29).

Until recently, splenectomy was the treatment of choice for splenic injury. Yet the spleen has important underappreciated immunologic and reticuloendothelial filtering functions. Severe sepsis after splenectomy occurs up to 200 times more frequently than in patients with normal spleens (Boone & Peitzman, 1998). This condition is called *overwhelming postsplenectomy infection* (OPSI), which occurs most frequently in children and in patients with lower respiratory infections.

Recognition of the immunologic consequences of splenectomy and CT-assisted delineation have encouraged efforts to salvage the injured spleen. Nonoperative management of splenic injuries is now commonplace. As with liver injuries, careful patient selection and aggressive monitoring for ongoing bleeding are key to successful nonoperative management (Table 24–30) (Smith, Wengrovitz, & De Long, 1992). Patients are admitted to the ICU on bedrest, with serial examinations and hematocrits performed every 4 to 6 hours. Indications for urgent laparotomy are the same as for nonoperatively managed liver injuries. The failure rate of nonoperative splenic injury management is as high as 18% (Boone & Peitzman, 1998).

Activity restriction after discharge should be enforced in accordance with the severity of the splenic rupture to minimize the risk of rebleeding from hematoma disruption (refer to Fig. 24–16). Follow-up abdominal CT scans are not routinely necessary in the absence of clinical indications (Thaemert, Cogbill, & Lambert, 1997). As with nonoperatively managed liver injuries in young patients, a CT scan performed 2 to 3 months after injury documents organ healing before clearance to return to full activities.

Patients who are hemodynamically unstable or have severe associated abdominal injuries require immediate exploratory laparotomy. The operative therapy of choice is splenorrhaphy (splenic repair) rather than splenectomy when possible. If bleeding is persistent or at least one-third of the splenic mass (necessary for immunocompetence) cannot be salvaged, attempts at splenorrhaphy are generally abandoned. Splenectomy is performed in unstable patients, patients with other life-threatening injury, patients with multiple sources for postoperative blood loss, and patients with complex grade III or grade IV/V injuries.

Discharge Instructions for Injury to the Liver, Kidney, or Spleen

Your accident or injury caused a laceration (cut) and/or bruising of your liver, kidney, or spleen. Bleeding may have occurred internally. The bleeding stops as a clot begins to form within the injured area. It is extremely important that you follow the instructions given to you by your doctors and nurses. You must limit your physical activity as instructed or you risk disrupting the clot that has formed within your injured organ. Serious internal bleeding may result.

Please check the chart below for instructions about your activity level. These instructions may change if your doctor decides it is necessary.

Date of your injury: ________	Week # __	Week # __	Week # __	Week # __	Week # _
Activities	House-bound. Remain sedentary or in bed at all times. You should only get up to go to the bathroom or to eat.	House-bound. Light household chores such as cooking, washing dishes, vacuuming.	Full activities and household chores that do not require heavy lifting. Shopping, light yard work/gardening, visiting friends, etc. is O.K.	No restriction	No restriction
Heavy Lifting* *No lifting any object weighing more than 5 lbs, or about the weight of a telephone book.	No heavy lifting	No heavy lifting	No heavy lifting	No restriction	No restriction
Traveling in a motor vehicle	You may ride in a car (but not drive) to your doctor's appointments only.	You may ride in a car (but not drive) to your doctor's appointments only.	Driving or riding within a 1 hour radius of your home.	No restriction	No restriction
Work or School	No work or school	No work or school	May return to work or school unless heavy lifting or strenuous activity is required. Discuss in detail with your doctor before returning to work or school.	No restriction	No restriction
Exercise/Sports	None permitted	None permitted	•No sports •No gym class •Light exercise is O.K. (Walking, slow treadmill or stationary bike)	No high diving, horse-back riding, and contact sports (football, karate, wrestling, lacrosse, soccer, etc.)	No restriction

Be sensible in all your activities, including sex. Unless your doctor told you otherwise, your injured organ will continue to work normally as it heals. Follow-up appointments are important and allow your doctor to advance you to the next level of activity. A CT scan of your abdomen is sometimes done to make sure that healing is complete. Please call your doctor if you have questions about what you are allowed to do.

Figure 24–16. Discharge instructions for patients with blunt injury to the liver, spleen, or kidney that was managed nonoperatively. The table must be individualized to the grade/severity of injury.

TABLE 24–28. Components of the Damage Control Procedure

	Surgical Maneuvers	Adjunctive Therapy and Studies
Part 1 Initial Laparotomy	Aortic compression Four quadrant packing Control surgical bleeding Control contamination Abdominal packing Abdominal skin closure	Actively rewarm Treat coagulopathy Consider angiography for identification and embolization of bleeding vessels
Part 2 ICU Resuscitation	Monitor intraabdominal pressure For intraabdominal hypertension, early reexploration (in operating room or at bedside if unstable)	Actively rewarm Invasive monitoring Correct volume deficits Correct coagulopathy Correct acidosis Baseline neurologic examination Sedate and paralyze Consider angiography or CT scan
Part 3 Reexploration and Reconstruction	Remove packing Reassess injuries Control surgical bleeding Reevaluate for missed injuries Debride and/or repair all injuries Consider enteral access Attempt closure of abdominal wall Consider tracheostomy	For abdominal wall/bowel edema, where fascial closure impossible: Aggressive diuresis Consider nasojejunal tube

Damage control is used in selective cases of severe abdominal injury associated with hemodynamic instability, metabolic acidosis (pH < 7.30), hypothermia (core temperature < 35° C), and coagulopathy. After initial laparotomy for contol of hemorrhage and contamination, the patient is taken to the intensive care unit (ICU) for aggressive resuscitation and active rewarming. When normal physiology has been reestablished (36–72 hours), re-laparotomy is performed for definitive repair of injuries. Angiography is an important adjunct for vascular injuries that are incompletely controlled.

Adapted with permission from Kauder, Schwab, & Rotondo, (1996). (p. 721).

Delayed splenic rupture infrequently occurs from an initially occult splenic injury following blunt abdominal trauma. Signs and symptoms of intraabdominal hemorrhage from perisplenic hematoma rupture can appear abruptly 48 hours or more after CT scanning performed during initial evaluation did not detect splenic injury. A high index of suspicion and liberal use of CT scanning are essential for diagnosis of delayed splenic rupture (Kluger et al., 1994). Management consists of volume resuscitation and urgent splenectomy.

Postoperative care involves nasogastric tube decompression of the stomach for 36 to 48 hours, early ambulation, and advancement of diet according to customary indications. Both the white blood cell count and platelet count are expected to rise after splenectomy. Postsplenectomy thrombocytosis exceeding $10^6/mm^3$ may be treated with one baby aspirin (80 mg) per day.

Splenectomy results in a lifelong risk of OPSI. The most common causative organisms include *streptococcus pneumoniae, meningococcus, haemophilus influenzae,*

TABLE 24–29. Spleen Injury Scale

	Grade[a]	Injury Description	AIS[b]
I	Hematoma	Subcapsular, <10% surface area	2
	Laceration	Capsular tear, <1 cm parenchymal depth	2
II	Hematoma	Subcapsular, 10–50% surface area; intraparenchymal, <5 cm in diameter	2
	Laceration	1–3 cm parenchymal depth which does not involve a trabecular vessel	
III	Hematoma	Subcapsular, >50% surface area or expanding; ruptured subcapsular or parenchymal hematoma Intraparenchymal hematoma >5 cm or expanding	3
	Laceration	>3 cm parenchymal depth or involving trabecular vessels	3
IV	Laceration	Laceration involving segmental or hillar vessels producing major devascularization (>25% of spleen)	4
V	Laceration	Completely shattered spleen	5
	Vascular	Hillar vascular injury which devascularizes spleen	5

[a] Advance one grade for multiple injuries, up to grade III.

[b] AIS = abbreviated injury scale score.

Adapted with permission from Moore et al., (1994). (p. 323).

TABLE 24–30. Criteria for Patient Selection for Nonoperative Management of Splenic Trauma

Age ≤ 55 years
CT scan appearance of Grade I, II or III injury
Hemodynamic stability
Absence of concomitant injuries precluding reliable abdominal assessment
Absence of other serious abdominal injuries

Reprinted with permission from Smith, Wengrovitz, & DeLong, (1992). (p. 363). Copyright 1992 by Williams and Wilkins.

staphylococcus aureus, and *escherichia coli.* All post-splenectomy patients should receive Pneumovax, *h influenzae,* and *meningococcal* vaccines within one month of operation. Asplenic adults should receive antibiotic prophylaxis before invasive procedures or with upper respiratory infections. Patients must receive explicit instructions and inform their doctors and dentists of their asplenic condition (Fig. 24–17).

Stomach

Most gastric injury results from penetrating trauma. Blunt gastric rupture is rare and creates a larger hole. Severe associated injuries are more common in blunt trauma because of the degree of force necessary to cause gastric blowout. In patients with normal gastric physiology, high intraluminal acidity renders the stomach relatively free of bacteria, so that the risk of bacterial peritonitis after perforation is low. Patients with preexisting gastric disease or those taking antacids or H2-receptor blockers have a higher risk of peritoneal contamination after full-thickness gastric injury. Undigested food contains bacteria and also increases the risk of intraabdominal infection if it is not washed out of the peritoneal cavity at time of operation.

Signs and symptoms of gastric perforation may include abdominal pain, peritoneal findings, blood in nasogastric aspirate or emesis, and free subdiaphragmatic air on chest x-ray, but none are sensitive or specific for the presence of gastric injury. Adjuncts to physical examination include DPL, CT scanning, ultrasound, and laparoscopy. DPL is highly sensitive but not specific, while CT and ultrasound have a high false–negative rate. Laparoscopy may be helpful in stable patients with penetrating wounds. Blunt-injured patients usually require exploratory laparotomy for associated injuries, which facilitates the diagnosis of gastric injury.

Most gastric injuries are treated with debridement and closure. Gastric diversion or resection is rarely necessary unless tissue destruction is extensive. Unless bacterial peritonitis develops, complications are rare and outcomes generally favorable.

Small Bowel

The small bowel is the most commonly injured organ in penetrating abdominal trauma. Blunt small bowel injuries, usually due to sudden compression by lap safety belts in high speed MVCs, are less common but not rare (Fig. 24–18). Blunt intestinal injury may also be caused by stretching and traction of the bowel at its points of fixation (Wisner, 1996). Blunt mesenteric injuries may also result in significant hemoperitoneum, small bowel devascularization, and bowel ischemia.

The presence of a Chance fracture of the lower thoracic or lumbar spine is an important indicator of a potential small bowel injury. A Chance fracture is one that is oriented longitudinally through the vertebral body and produced by a flexion–distraction mechanism, usually caused by a lap safety restraint (Wisner, 1996). Multiple solid viscus injuries, or abdominal solid viscus injury with an AIS ≥ 5, are also predictive of small bowel and other hollow viscus injury (Nance et al., 1997).

The proximal small bowel, like the stomach, contains few bacteria. However, the distal small bowel has a higher bacterial load similar to that of the colon (including anaerobes), so that injury to the distal small bowel increases the risk of bacterial peritonitis (Wisner, 1996).

The diagnosis of small bowel injury is difficult and often not made on initial presentation. Peritoneal signs may or may not be present initially, depending upon the degree of contamination and hemoperitoneum. Because CT scanning has a significant false–negative rate, serial examination is critical in patients with blunt abdominal trauma even if the initial abdominal CT was normal. Findings on CT scan suggestive of small bowel injury include fluid collections without solid viscus injury, free intraperitoneal air, bowel wall thickening, and mesenteric infiltration (Boone & Peitzman, 1998).

When physical examination is unreliable, as in patients with an altered sensorium or sensory impairment from a spinal cord injury, DPL may detect small bowel injury; however, false–negatives can occur especially if the test is performed less than 3 hours after injury. In addition to testing for red and white blood cell counts, elevated alkaline phosphatase levels in DPL effluent may prove to be diagnostic of otherwise occult blunt intestinal injuries (Jaffin et al., 1993).

Treatment of small bowel injuries requires perioperative antibiotic administration and surgical repair. The prognosis is good if diagnosis and repair occur promptly. Except in cases of extensive small bowel resection for massive injury, metabolic and nutritional complications are rare.

Pancreas

The pancreas is a retroperitoneal structure, relatively well-protected anteriorly by the upper abdominal organs and posteriorly by the thick paraspinous muscles. Consequently, pancreatic injuries occur in only 7% of patients with abdominal trauma and usually occur only with deep penetrating wounds and major blunt force trauma (Wilson, 1996). Overall, 90% of patients with pancreatic injuries have at least one associated injury (Jurkovich & Carrico, 1997). Penetrating pancreatic injuries are associated with major vascular injury, gastric rupture, liver laceration, and renal

Discharge Instructions Following Splenectomy

Your spleen was injured during your accident and had to be removed. The spleen plays a role in fighting infection in the body. There is a small chance that you may be more prone to serious infections. It is important for you to follow these instructions:

1. During your hospital stay, vaccines called **Pneumovax, Hemophilus-B,** and **Meningococcus** were given to protect you from bacteria which cause most of the infections after a spleen is removed. Keep this paper in a secure place so that you will always have a record of the vaccines you were given.

2. You may want to get a Medic-Alert™ bracelet or a card to carry in your wallet to say that your spleen has been taken out. Ask your nurse for an application.

3. If at any time you develop signs of infection, such as fever above 101 degrees, shaking chills, or serious cough, call your family doctor right away. Remind your doctor that you had your spleen removed and explain your symptoms.

4. If you visit a doctor or dentist for the first time, you should tell him/her that you have had your spleen removed so it can be noted in your medical record. Check with your family doctor periodically to see if there is any new information that you should be aware of.

Please call your Trauma Surgeon or Nurse Practitioner if you have any questions or concerns.

Figure 24–17. Discharge instructions for adult patients who have had a splenectomy following splenic trauma.

injury. The most frequent associated injuries with blunt pancreatic trauma include injuries to the duodenum, liver, spleen, kidney, colon, and major vessels. The mortality rate from pancreatic injuries can be high, usually due to hemorrhage from associated injuries. However, late deaths account for up to 40% of the overall mortality and can occur from complications such as sepsis and MODS.

A delay in diagnosis and treatment of pancreatic injury is uniformly recognized as the principle cause of morbidity and mortality after blunt pancreatic trauma (Wilson, 1996). Unfortunately there are no specific signs or symptoms for pancreatic injury and, in fact, a normal physical examination does not rule out pancreatic injury. Most isolated retroperitoneal injuries produce only mild tenderness rather than signs of frank peritonitis. Thus, injury to the pancreas must be suspected in all patients with injury to the upper abdomen.

Associated intraabdominal injuries often serve as the main indication for surgical exploration. Peritoneal signs, positive DPL, or CT findings of other serious abdominal injury indicate the need for laparotomy in patients with preoperatively unrecognized pancreatic injury. Intraoperative diagnosis depends on careful visual inspection and palpation (Jurkovich, 1996).

In patients without indications for laparotomy, serial physical examination combined with a high index of suspicion is the best means of diagnosis. Examination findings 6 to 24 hours after injury may include nonspecific abdominal pain, or pain in the mid-epigastric region or back. Eventually the patient develops peritoneal signs. DPL is not reli-

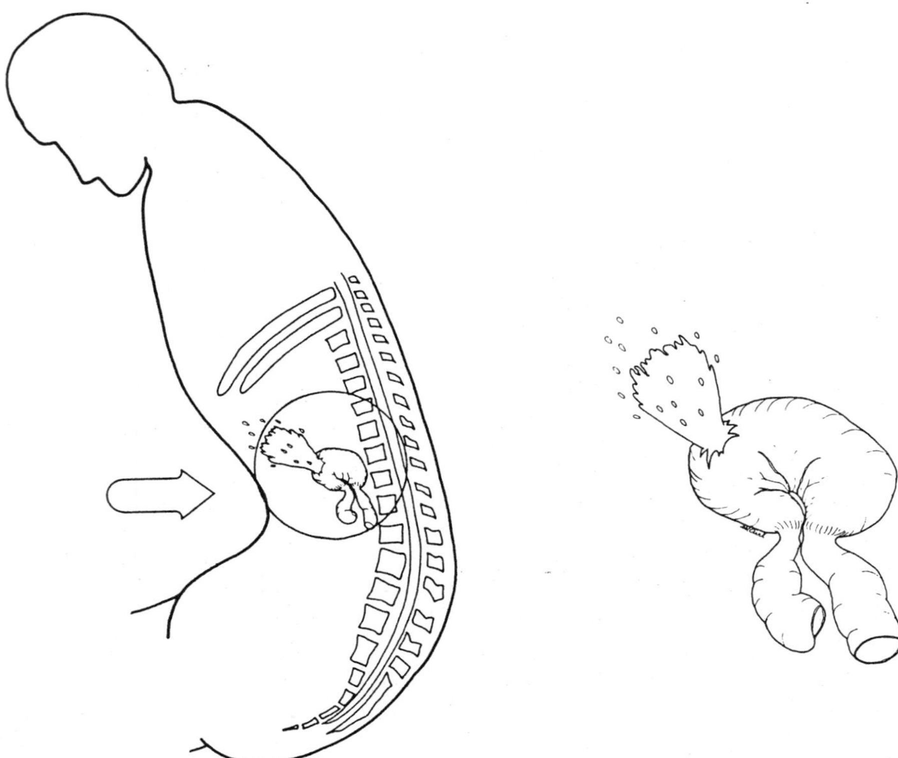

Figure 24–18. The small bowel is normally arranged in kinks and convolutions. These convolutions may become compressed by a steering wheel or seat belt, forming a closed loop under pressure. The intraluminal pressure may be high enough to cause a blowout of the bowel wall. *(Reprinted with permission from Feliciano, Moore, & Mattox (Eds.). [1996]. [p. 555]. Copyright 1998 by Appleton & Lange.)*

able in the diagnosis of retroperitoneal injuries. CT may identify peripancreatic hematomas but may not identify pancreatic lacerations early in the postinjury period (Boone & Peitzman, 1998). Serum amylase and its isoenzymes are not reliable predictors of pancreatic injury (Bouwman, Weaver, & Walt, 1984).

Surgical treatment involves hemorrhage control, debridement of devitalized tissue, preservation of maximal viable pancreatic tissue, insertion of closed suction drains for drainage of pancreatic secretions, and placement of a feeding jejunostomy for postoperative care (Boone & Peitzman, 1998). The pathogenesis of most postoperative complications, occurring in 36 to 61% of patients, is autolytic tissue destruction secondary to release of pancreatic enzymes from torn pancreatic tissue. Common complications include pancreatic fistula, intraabdominal abscess, pancreatic abscess or pseudocyst, and pancreatitis (Wilson, 1996).

Abdominal Vascular Injuries

Most abdominal vascular injuries are caused by penetrating trauma and are almost always associated with multiple intraabdominal injuries. The mortality ranges from 30 to 60%; early mortality results from exsanguination, whereas late mortality results from MODS and sepsis (Jurkovich & Carrico, 1997). Determination of trajectory is important in establishing the diagnosis. A bullet that violates the upper abdomen, posterior abdomen, or posterolateral pelvis frequently causes a vascular injury (Shapiro, 1998). Local wound exploration as well as chest and abdominal x-rays with metallic markers over wound sites can help determine trajectory. CT in the stable patient may reveal mesenteric or retroperitoneal hematoma. Patients who present early after injury with a contained hematoma may have a normal blood pressure and minimal pain.

Contrarily, a hypotensive patient with a penetrating abdominal wound is assumed to have a bleeding vascular injury and requires immediate surgical intervention. Hemorrhage control and resuscitation must occur simultaneously in the operating room. Blood transfusion should be initiated early and massive transfusion requirements should be anticipated. Every effort should be made to avoid hypothermia, including maintaining room temperature at 27°C and using warming blankets and fluid warmers (Shapiro, 1998).

Operative goals include: (1) initial hemorrhage control and damage assessment, (2) control of contamination through copious irrigation followed by repair of hollow visceral injuries, and (3) reestablishing vascular continuity with primary repair or grafting. If the patient is in extremis—hypothermic, acidotic, coagulopathic—vessel ligation or damage control are considered (see the section on liver injuries).

Genitourinary Injuries

Urinary tract injury occurs in 3 to 4% of trauma cases from blunt or penetrating trauma to the chest, abdomen, or pelvis (Wilson, Smith, & McCarroll, 1996). The kidney is the most frequently injured structure, followed by the bladder and urethra. Few genitourinary injuries are immediately life-threatening, but they are often associated with other serious injuries.

Signs and symptoms of genitourinary trauma include flank contusions, flank or abdominal pain, nausea, vomiting, and paralytic ileus. A bruit heard in the posterior midline near the first or second lumbar vertebrae may be the only indication of damage to renal vessels. Fractures of the lower ribs or lumbar vertebrae are frequently associated injuries. Hematuria suggests the presence of urologic injury and in high-risk patients is an indication for complete urologic examination, but the absence of hematuria does not rule out injury (Knudson et al., 1992).

For stable patients, CT is the diagnostic study of choice for detection of renal injury, evaluation of vascular integrity, and identification of associated injuries. If the CT scan is indeterminate, arteriography may be used to delineate renal vascular integrity and, in selected cases, to treat vascular injuries with embolization. A limited role exists for intravenous pyelography (IVP). A "one-shot IVP" (250-300 mL of high-density intravenous contrast given as a rapid bolus, followed by a single abdominal film taken 3-5 minutes after injection) helps evaluate renal function in unstable patients or when CT scanning is unavailable due to nonfunction or multiple simultaneous trauma patients (Rhodes, 1998a). The exact role of ultrasound in genitourinary trauma remains unclear, but it may be a useful clinical adjunct when intravenous contrast injection is contraindicated. Urethrography or cystography are indicated in cases of suspected urethral or bladder injury, respectively.

Renal Injury

The kidneys are among the most commonly injured organs in blunt abdominal trauma. Penetrating injury accounts for 20% of renal injuries. Renal injuries range from minor cortical contusions and lacerations to deep lacerations involving the collecting system and major vessels (Fig. 24–19). With penetrating trauma, the extent of injury is variable and cannot be estimated by the appearance of the wound or the amount of hematuria present. Since 20% of the cardiac output goes to the kidneys, blood loss from a renal pedicle injury can be massive (Wilson et al., 1996). Renal injuries are classified as grades I through V based on assessment at laparotomy or using CT findings (Table 24–31).

Grades I to III renal injuries predominate and can be managed nonoperatively in hemodynamically stable patients (Cheng, Lazan, & Stone, 1994; Evins, Thomason, & Rosenblum,1980). Surgery is indicated for unstable patients, for hilar or pedicle injuries, and for grade IV/V injuries. Hemorrhage control and renal salvage are the chief operative goals, but patient instability or major vascular damage may warrant nephrectomy.

Ureteral Injury

Most ureteral injuries are caused by penetrating injury or are iatrogenic in origin. Blunt injury is rare, usually caused by avulsion of the ureter from the renal pelvis. In addition, ureteral compression may result from retroperitoneal hematoma or entrapment in a pelvic fracture. IVP, CT scanning, and retrograde ureterography are useful diagnostic tests alone or in combination. Most ureteral injuries are treated with primary surgical repair and stenting (Rhodes, 1998a).

Bladder Injury

Bladder injuries usually result from blunt trauma and are often associated with fractures of the pelvis and long bones. The empty bladder is well protected from injury, but when it is distended with urine, it is much more easily ruptured in blunt trauma and presents a bigger target for penetrating missiles. Bladder injuries are classified as contusions or ruptures. Intraperitoneal bladder ruptures usually occur on the posterior wall as a result of blunt trauma to a full bladder, whereas extraperitoneal bladder ruptures occur on the anterior or anterolateral wall in conjunction with pelvic fractures.

A cystogram is indicated for patients with gross hematuria who also have a pelvic fracture or abdominal wall contusion. False–negative cystogram results may occur if blood clots, tissue, or peritoneal contents fill the defect. If intraperitoneal bladder rupture is seen, surgical exploration is indicated with primary bladder repair in most cases. Extraperitoneal bladder ruptures can be further delineated with CT or CT cystogram. Small extraperitoneal ruptures can be managed with bladder drainage alone, but tears with large extravasation are usually repaired.

Urethral Injury

Urethral trauma occurs most often in male victims of blunt trauma and very rarely in females. Urethral or bladder injuries are present in up to 25% of male patients with pelvic fractures (Wilson et al., 1996). Symptoms of urethral injury include pain in the perineum or lower abdomen and inability to void. Signs of urethral injury include blood at the urethral meatus, hematuria, scrotal or perineal hematoma, and, in males, a nonpalpable prostate on rectal examination. If urethral injury is suspected, a urethral catheter should not be placed until a retrograde urethrogram has excluded urethral disruption. Repeated attempts to catheterize a damaged urethra may cause further injury and prolong healing.

Many patients have associated injuries that take precedence, so that the urologist's initial efforts may be limited to placement of a suprapubic cystostomy drain. On occasion, a urologist may gently advance a urinary catheter to

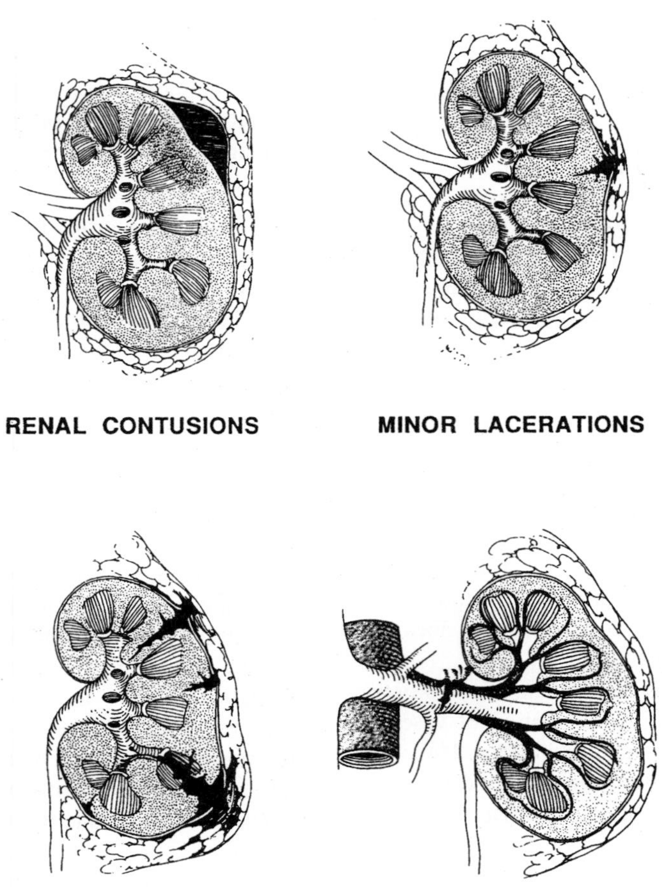

Figure 24–19. Renal injuries occurring from blunt or penetrating abdominal trauma range in severity from minor contusions and lacerations to deep parenchymal lacerations and vascular injuries. *(Reprinted with permission from Armenakas & McAninch. [1996]. [p. 681]. Copyright 1996 by Williams & Wilkins.)*

TABLE 24–31. Kidney Injury Scale

Grade[a]	Type of Injury	Description of Injury	AIS[b]
I	Contusion	Microscopic or gross hematuria, urologic studies normal	2
	Hematoma	Subcapsular, nonexpanding without parenchymal laceration	2
II	Hematoma	Nonexpanding perirenal hematoma confined to renal retroperitoneum	2
	Laceration	< 1.0 cm parenchymal depth of renal cortex without urinary extravasation	2
III	Laceration	> 1.0 cm parenchymal depth of renal cortex without collecting system rupture or urinary extravasation	3
IV	Laceration	Parenchymal laceration extending through renal cortex, medulla, and collecting system	4
	Vascular	Main renal artery or vein injury with contained hemorrhage	4
V	Laceration	Completely shattered kidney	5
	Vascular	Avulsion of renal hilum which devascularizes kidney	5

[a] Advance one grade for bilateral injuries up to grade III.
[b] AIS = abbreviated injury scale score.
Adapted with permission from Moore et al., (1989). (p. 1664). Copyright 1989 by Williams and Wilkins.

stent the urethral injury as a temporizing measure (Rhodes, 1998a). Unfortunately, the severed urethral segments are frequently distracted so that reapproximation cannot occur until associated pelvic fractures are reduced and swelling resolves. Delayed ureteroplasty or open end-to-end anastomosis are performed for definitive treatment. Long-term complications of urethral injuries include urethral stricture, impotence in male patients, and chronic urinary tract infection (Wilson et al., 1996).

Colon and Rectum

Colon injuries occur in 25% of gunshot wounds, 5% of stab wounds, and 5% of blunt injuries. Thermometer perforations, foreign bodies from sexual misadventures, and endoscopic perforations are additional causes of penetrating colon trauma. Blunt mechanisms include crushing from associated pelvic fractures and blowout from sudden compression of air-filled bowel secondary to lap safety restraints in deceleration MVCs. Rectal injuries represent up to 5% of all colon injuries. Overall mortality rates are 5 to 10% (Boone & Peitzman, 1998).

Signs and symptoms of colon injury are consistent with peritonitis; however, initially symptoms may be modest. Gross blood on rectal examination with a penetrating abdominal, pelvic, or buttock wound is pathognomonic of colorectal injury (Boone & Peitzman, 1998). Gross blood on rectal examination in patients with pelvic fractures also suggests rectal injury which may be confirmed with proctosigmoidoscopy. CT is unreliable in the detection of colorectal injuries but may help delineate associated injuries in hemodynamically stable patients.

Most colon injuries are diagnosed at laparotomy, which is indicated for patients with hemodynamic instability, peritoneal findings, anterior penetrating wounds below the fifth intercostal space, and evidence of free air or bullets below the diaphragm on x-ray (Wilson, Walt, & Dulchavsky, 1996). Current operative techniques include primary injury repair, resection and anastomosis, colostomy, and exteriorized primary repair with reoperation in 7 to 10 days (Burch, 1996). Primary repair is controversial but gaining acceptance in select patients (Table 24–32). Only partial thickness colon injuries can be cautiously observed while the patient is maintained NPO and given antibiotics.

The management of rectal injury involves fecal diversion with a sigmoid colostomy and presacral drainage with closed suction or Penrose drains. Primary repair of accessible injuries may be performed. Perioperative broad spectrum antibiotics should be administered for all colon and rectal wounds (Boone & Peitzman, 1998).

TABLE 24–32. Selection Criteria for Primary Repair of Colon Injuries

Minimal fecal spillage
Hemodynamic stability
No associated intraabdominal injuries
< 8 hour delay in diagnosis and treatment
< 1000 mL blood loss

Adapted with permission from Boone & Peitzman (1998). (p. 242).

Pelvic Fractures

Pelvic fractures typically result from vehicular trauma (occupants or pedestrians struck) and falls from heights. Fortunately, many pelvic fractures constitute rather straightforward orthopedic problems and are rarely associated with morbid sequelae. Although pelvic ring fractures account for only 3% of all fractures, the more complex pelvic injuries cause the disproportionately high mortality rate (10-50%) in these patients (Gruen, Leit, Gruen, & Peitzman, 1994). Complex pelvic ring disruptions result in severe hemorrhage from bony bleeding or disruption of the surrounding venous and arterial vessels. Such pelvic fractures are frequently associated with injuries to the abdomen, thorax, or head which contribute to morbidity and mortality. Even if the patient survives the shock and sepsis common during the acute care phase, long-term problems with pain and disability are inevitable.

The pelvic ring is comprised of the two innominate bones and the sacrum, joined anteriorly at the symphysis, and posteriorly at the sacroiliac joints by ligaments (Fig. 24–20). The innominate bones are comprised of the ilium, ischium, and pubis. Although the anterior portion of the ring is more prominent radiographically, the posterior portion is more important for structural stability and weight-bearing. In addition to bony injury, pelvic trauma often causes morbid injury to adjacent soft tissues, including nerves (pudendal, lumbar, sacral) and vessels (iliac arteries, iliac veins, and their branches).

Signs and symptoms of pelvic fractures include pelvic pain, inability to void (in cases of associated urethral disruption), pain on palpation or with attempts to flex or abduct the lower extremities, and pelvic instability. Maneuvers to assess pelvic stability must not be performed repetitively as clot disruption and exacerbation of bleeding may result. Thorough motor and sensory examination of the lower extremities and perineum (rectal tone) should be performed to evaluate for neurologic injury, particularly of the lumbosacral roots.

Inspection and palpation of the skin and soft tissue (including external genitalia) around the pelvis is important for identification of open pelvic fractures. Rectal tears indicate a contaminated pelvic fracture. Examination of females should include bimanual pelvic examination. Open pelvic fractures occur in 5% of pelvic fractures and account for 50% of the mortality (Leit & Gruen, 1998).

All patients with pelvic pain or those involved in high-energy trauma require an AP x-ray of the pelvis. If abnormalities are seen, inlet and outlet views may be obtained to determine anteroposterior and vertical displacement of the

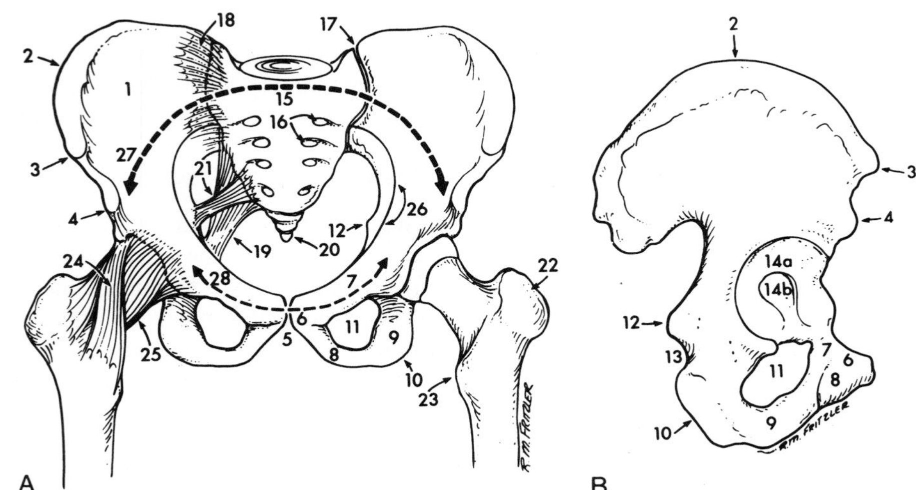

Figure 24–20. Pelvic anatomy. **A,** Anterior view of the pelvis. **B,** Lateral view of right innominate bone. 1 = iliac fossa, 2 = iliac crest, 3 = anterior superior iliac spine, 4 = anterior inferior iliac spine, 5 = symphysis pubis, 6 = body of pubis, 7 = superior ramus of pubis, 8 = inferior ramus of pubis, 9 = ramus of ischium, 10 = ischial tuberosity, 11 = obturator foramen, 12 = ischial spine, 13 = lesser sciatic notch, 14 = acetabulum (14a = articular surface, 14b = fossa), 15 = sacrum, 16 = anterior sacral foramina, 17 = sacroiliac joint, 18 = anterior sacroiliac ligament, 19 = trochanter of femur, 20 = coccyx, 21 = sacrospinous ligament, 22 = greater trochanter of femur, 23 = lesser trochanter of femur, 24 = iliofemoral ligament, 25 = pubofemoral ligament, 26 = arcuate line, 27 = posterior anterior arch. *(Reprinted with permission from Jerrard. [1993]. [p. 148]. Copyright 1993 by W. B. Saunders.)*

hemipelvis. CT scan of the pelvis should be obtained in all hemodynamically stable patients with pelvic fractures. CT provides information about the sacroiliac joint, sacrum, and iliac wing, which helps delineate the pelvic injury and determine a management plan. CT also identifies retroperitoneal hemorrhage and associated organ injury. If a urethral disruption is suspected, a retrograde urethrogram is required (see the section on urethral injury).

Numerous classification systems exist to describe the nature and stability of pelvic fractures. One such system divides fracture patterns by mechanism of injury, providing a graded likelihood of fracture-related bleeding, associated injuries, morbidity, and mortality (Table 24–33). It also serves as an aid to fracture management for the orthopedic surgeon (Cryer & Johnson, 1996).

The goals of management in patients with complex pelvic fractures include control of hemorrhage, skeletal fixation, and treatment of associated injuries. Hypotension coupled with signs or symptoms of pelvic injury suggests active bleeding from the chest or abdomen. Blood loss from pelvic fractures can be massive but is more often due to bleeding from associated injuries. Standard resuscitative measures including large-bore IV access and crystalloid/blood administration should be instituted. Chest x-ray and DPL or ultrasound help rapidly detect intrathoracic and intraperitoneal hemorrhage in unstable patients. The patient in extremis with exsanguinating hemorrhage must be taken immediately to the operating room.

Major vascular injuries require direct operative repair. If, on laparotomy, the pelvic bleeding can be controlled with pressure, the pelvis can be packed and the patient transferred for pelvic angiography and embolization (Leit & Gruen, 1998). Angiography is also an effective pre- or postoperative means of stopping hemorrhage in selected patients (Agolini et al., 1997).

Retroperitoneal bleeding from unstable pelvic fractures involves the bony surfaces near fracture sites as well as venous plexus disruption. Diastasis of the symphysis pubis (anterior widening) causes a substantial increase in the pelvic “reservoir” enabling greater hemorrhage. By using a pelvic external fixator, the innominate bones are rejoined, stabilizing clot formation and providing a splint that diminishes blood loss. A limited open reduction and internal fixation (ORIF) can also be performed acutely as part of the resuscitation laparotomy.

Definitive ORIF of anterior and posterior pelvic fractures may be performed acutely or in a delayed fashion; however, early fixation has been shown to reduce hospital stay, pain, blood loss, and long-term disability (Latenser et al., 1991). Early ORIF allows for early mobilization, which may prevent complications of immobility. Acetabular fractures are sometimes associated with pelvic fractures and can be repaired at the time of definitive pelvic ORIF.

Surgical stabilization of open fractures is performed after repeated irrigation and debridement procedures over days to weeks. Open pelvic fractures or those associated with extensive perineal soft tissue injury are selectively managed with a colostomy to divert the fecal stream.

TABLE 24–33. Classification of Pelvic Fractures

Anterior–Posterior Compression	
Type I	Disruption of the pubic symphysis with less than 2.5 cm of diastasis; no significant posterior pelvic injury
Type II	Disruption of the pubic symphysis of more than 2.5 cm with tearing of the anterior sacroiliac, sacrospinous and sacrotuberous ligaments
Type III	Complete disruption of the pubic symphysis and posterior ligament complexes, with hemiplevic displacement
Lateral Compression	
Type I	Posterior compression of the sacroiliac joint without ligament disruption; oblique pubic ramus fracture
Type II	Rupture of the posterior sacroiliac ligament; pivotal internal rotation of hemiplevis on the anterior S1 joint with a crush injury of the sacrum and an oblique pubic ramus fracture
Type III	Findings in Type II injury with evidence of an AP compression injury to the contralateral pelvis
Vertical Shear	
	Complete ligament or bony disruption of a hemiplevis associated with hemipelvic displacement

With this classification scheme, pelvic fractures ar classified according to the injuring mechanism. Frontal impact MVCs are the most common cause of anterior–posterior compression injuries. Lateral compression injuries result from lateral impact ("T-bone") MVCs or when pedestrians are struck by motor vehicles. Vertical shear injuries occcur in falls from great heights.

Reprinted with permission from Cryer & Johnson, (1996). (p. 640).

Extremity Injury

Fracture Stabilization

In patients with multiple injuries, severe deformities of the extremities are often so striking that they tend to divert much of the initial attention away from other, more serious injuries. As with all injured patients, maintaining an airway and ventilation, controlling hemorrhage, and correcting hypovolemia take priority over injured bones (Georgiadis & Wilson, 1996). Nevertheless, open fractures, classified according to the degree of overlying soft tissue injury, should receive surgical debridement and stabilization within 6 hours to minimize the risk of osteomyelitis and amputation (Trafton, 1996) (Table 24–34). Fractures and dislocations associated with neurovascular compromise also require prompt surgical attention for optimal outcome. Patterns of bone injury may be helpful in predicting associated extremity injuries not initially appreciated (Table 24–35).

Hemorrhage caused by transection or disruption of major blood vessels constitutes the only situation in which extremity injuries are immediately life threatening (Jurkovich & Carrico, 1997). However, multiple long-bone fractures have a remarkably adverse impact on morbidity and mortality following multiple trauma. Although discussion of the specific management of fractures and dislocations is beyond the scope of this chapter, the critical role of early fracture fixation in the care of the multiply injured patient deserves elucidation.

Multiple long-bone fractures often occur in patients with other serious associated injuries, creating competing priorities and difficult management decisions. In a prospective study comparing pulmonary morbidity in multiple-injured patients undergoing "early" fracture fixation (within 24 hours of injury) versus "late" fracture fixation (> 48 hours after injury), Bone et al. (1989) demonstrated decreased incidence of ARDS, fat embolism syndrome, pulmonary embolism, and pneumonia with early fixation. Numerous retrospective studies support these findings, adding that early fixation results in fewer days on mechanical ven-

TABLE 24–34. Classification of Open Fractures

Type	Wound Length	Level of Contamination	Soft-Tissue Injury	Bone Injury
I	<1 cm	Clean	Minimal	Simple, minimal comminution
II	>1 cm	Moderate	Moderate, some muscle damage	Moderate comminution
III[a]				
A	Usually >10 cm	High	Severe with crushing	Usually comminuted; soft-tissue coverage of bone possible
B	Usually >10 cm	High	Very severe loss of coverage	Bone coverage poor; usually requires soft tissue reconstructive surgery
C	Usually >10 cm	High	Very severe loss of coverage plus vascular injury requiring repair	Bone coverage poor; usually requires soft-tissue reconstructive surgery

Classification of open fractures is important because it allows comparison of treatment results and provides guidelines for management and prognosis.

[a] Segmental fractures, barnyard injuries, fractures occurring in a highly contaminated environment, shotgun wounds, or high-velocity gunshot wounds automatically result in classification as a Type III open fracture.

Adapted with permission from Chapman & Olson, (1996). (p. 309).

TABLE 24–35. Extremity X-Ray Suggestions and Potential Associated Injury

Abnormal Findings	Diagnoses to Consider
Extremity fracture	Arterial injury Nerve injury Hemorrhage with or without shock Compartment syndrome Fat embolization Anaerobic soft-tissue infection Fracture fragments within the joint Thromboembolism Joint dislocation about and below the fracture site
Femoral fracture	Acetabular or pelvic ring fracture, hip dislocation
Calcaneal fracture	Vertebral column injuries
Shoulder girdle fracture	Thoracic injuries
Soft-tissue signs without fracture	Ligamentous injuries
Multiple fractures of different ages	Abuse

Adapted with permission from American College of Surgeons, Committee on Trauma, (1993). Advanced Trauma Life Support Manual *(p. 350).*

tilation, decreased incidence of sepsis and MODS, and shorter length of stay (ICU and overall acute care) (Behrman et al., 1990). The exact mechanism of these beneficial effects is unclear, but seems related to diminished inflammatory response and an ability to mobilize the patient early. Early mobilization lessens the likelihood of venous thrombus, decubitus ulcers, and pneumonia (Jurkovich & Carrico, 1997).

Fixation of long-bone injuries should then immediately follow identification and control of life-threatening hemorrhage from associated injuries. In patients with concomitant moderate to severe head injuries, ICP monitoring provides an important intraoperative adjunct to detect intracranial hypertension in the anesthetized, unexaminable patient.

Soft-Tissue Injuries

Soft-tissue injuries, common after both blunt and penetrating trauma, range in complexity from simple bruises or lacerations to major crush injuries. Shearing and compressive forces cause most blunt soft-tissue injuries. Penetrating soft-tissue trauma results from low- or high-velocity wounds.

1. Low-velocity wounds are usually caused by stabbings and handguns. Damage to the underlying structure is generally responsible for wound morbidity (Rhodes, 1998b).
2. High-velocity gunshot wounds can create extensive soft-tissue damage, usually requiring extensive debridement and secondary closure.
3. The severity of shotgun wounding depends on distance from the assailant. A shotgun slug is a high-velocity missile at less than 2 inches. Most shotgun missiles at less than 20 feet produce a single deep complex wound, whereas those at greater than 20 feet cause multiple, less severe wounds from the wide scatter of pellets (Ordog, Wasserberger, & Balasubramaniam, 1988).

The principles of management of soft-tissue injuries include debridement of devitalized tissue, restoration of adequate blood supply, and adequate coverage of vital structures (e.g., nerves, vessels, and tendons). Because assessment of wound viability may be difficult initially, repeat examination is essential, with exploration under anesthesia if there is any question regarding the viability of muscle or underlying soft tissue. Complete debridement is the most important means of preventing infection, including tetanus and gas gangrene.

Peripheral Vascular Injury

Vascular injury must be suspected in all injured extremities. Penetrating wounds are more common and may cause direct vessel perforation, transection, or laceration (Fig. 24–21). Blunt vascular injuries occur most frequently with fractures and dislocations, and generally involve vessel contusion and intimal disruption with obstruction and thrombosis (Table 24–36). Vascular extremity injury can result in limb loss, serious disability, or death (Shackford & Rich, 1996). Poor prognostic factors include treatment delay greater than 6 to 12 hours, blunt mechanism, high-velocity missile wounds, lower extremity injury (especially the popliteal artery), atherosclerosis, and adjacent injury to nerve, vein, soft tissues, and bone.

Physical examination is critical for the diagnosis of pe-

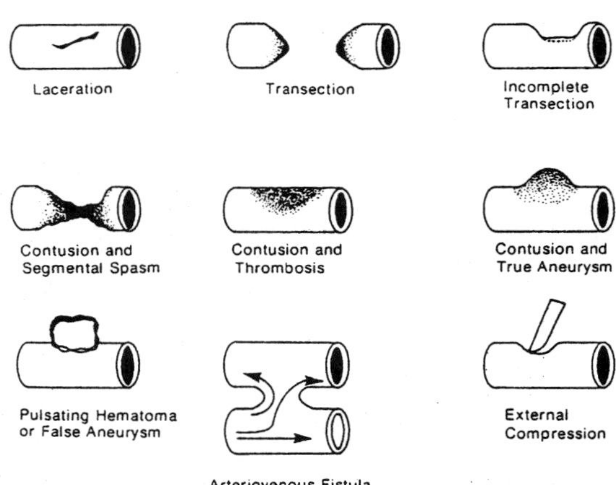

Figure 24–21. Common types of arterial injury resulting from blunt or penetrating trauma. Laceration and transection account for the vast majority of arterial injuries. Transection may be associated with avulsion of segments of the artery. External compression can be caused by displaced bone from comminuted fractures. *(Reprinted with permission from Shackford & Rich. [1996]. [p. 823]. Copyright 1996 by Appleton & Lange.)*

TABLE 24–36. Common Skeletal Injuries Associated with Vascular Injury

Skeletal Injury	Associated Vascular Injury
Clavicle fracture	Subclavian artery
Supracondylar fracture of the humerus	Brachial artery
Anterior dislocation of the shoulder	Axillary artery
Displaced fracture of the distal femur	Superficial femoral artery
Posterior knee dislocation	Popliteal vessels

ripheral vascular injury. The patient with "hard" signs of arterial injury requires immediate surgical exploration (refer to Table 24–17). More commonly, patients present with "soft" signs of injury in which the yield from routine surgical exploration is too low to justify the risks, expense, and morbidity (Jurkovich & Carrico, 1997). Patients with soft signs of injury should be evaluated with serial physical examination, noninvasive vascular studies (arterial pressure index, duplex ultrasound), or arteriography in selected patients. Arteriography is useful to exclude vascular injury (especially in patients with knee dislocations) and delineate injury prior to operation; however, performing the study should never delay revascularization in patients with limb ischemia (Gable, Allen, & Richardson, 1997). Most clinically occult intimal defects, spasm, or small pseudoaneurysms resolve spontaneously, so that arteriography in the absence of hard signs is seldom indicated.

Operative management of arterial injury involves debridement of injured vessels, thrombectomy, and grafting using polytetraflouroethylene (PTFE) or cephalic, epigastric, basilic, or saphenous veins. Venous injuries are usually found at the time of exploration for arterial injuries. Venous injuries are treated with either ligation or repair.

Early complications of peripheral vascular injury include thrombotic occlusion, venous thromboembolism, bleeding, infection, compartment syndrome, rhabdomyolysis, and amputation. Late complications include graft occlusion, infection, delayed bleeding (usually from infection), arteriovenous fistula, and pseudoaneurysm.

Mangled Extremity

When an extremity is injured to the extent that its salvageability is at question, the combined judgment of the trauma surgeon and orthopedic surgeon may lead to a decision to perform primary amputation. While every effort should be made to preserve functional and anatomic integrity, amputation and prosthesis may be more effective for a patient than a limb that is still attached but of limited use. Substantial morbidity occurs with salvage attempts (multiple surgical procedures, recurrent infection, pain, high cost, medical risks, and duration of disability and rehabilitation), and it is rare that salvage completely restores function of a severely injured limb (Trafton, 1996).

The Mangled Extremity Scoring System (MESS) is one of several scoring systems developed to help clinicians determine the benefit of early amputation versus attempts at limb salvage (Table 24–37). A limb with a MESS score of ≥ 7 suggests the need for amputation, whereas limbs with MESS < 7 may be successfully salvaged (Johansen et al., 1990). Because the MESS score has not been validated prospectively, management decisions must incorporate clinical judgment and consideration of several local and systemic variables (Table 24–38). The patient's occupation and subjective desires should also be considered.

Tetanus

Tetanus, caused by the anaerobic bacillus *Clostridium tetani,* is a preventable disease characterized by convulsive spasm of voluntary muscles and a propensity for respiratory arrest. It may occur as a complication of large or small wounds, including abrasions, lacerations, burns, and open fractures. The average incubation period is 10 days, but it can appear

TABLE 24–37. Mangled Extremity Severity Score (MESS)

Type	Characteristics	Injuries	Points
Skeletal/soft tissue	Low energy	Stab wounds, simple closed fractures, small-caliber gunshot wounds	1
	Medium energy	Open or multiple-level fractures, dislocations, moderate crush injuries	2
	High energy	Shotgun blast (close range), high velocity gunshot wounds	3
	Massive crush	Logging, railroad, oil rig accidents	4
Shock	Normal blood pressure	BP stable in field and in operating room (systolic BP > 90 mm Hg)	0
	Transiently hypotensive	BP unstable in field but responsive to intravenous fluids	1
	Prolonged hypotension	Systolic BP < 90 mm Hg in field and responsive to intravenous fluid only in the operating room	2
Ischemia (double value if ischemia > 6 hours)	None	A pulsatile limb without signs of ischemia	0
	Mild	Diminished pulses without signs of ischemia	1
	Moderate	No pulse by Doppler, sluggish capillary refill, paresthesia, diminished motor activity	2
		Pulseless, cool, paralyzed and numb without capillary refilling	3
Age	< 30 years		0
	30 to 50 years		1
	> 50 years		2

Modified with permission from Trafton, (1996). (p. 794).

TABLE 24–38. Factors Governing Limb Salvage

Fracture grade, type, level(s)
Energy imparted by wounding
Soft-tissue disruption, avulsion
Wound contamination
Delay of fracture fixation
Duration, severity of ischemia
Loss of soft tissues of the foot
Nerve disruption/division
Venous damage: repair versus ligature for venous injury
Development of compartment hypertension
Level and type of arterial injury
Delay of revascularization
Muscle viability at operation
Shock; amount of blood transfused; need for vasopressors
Wounding mechanism (blunt versus penetrating trauma)
Extent of other injuries/Injury Severity Score
Age, coexisting medical illnesses
Transport time: use of military anti-shock trousers (MAST)
Trauma center versus community hospital

Reprinted with permission from Johansen, Daines, & Howey, (1990). (p. 568). Copyright 1990 by Williams and Wilkins.

in 1 to 2 days in severely injured patients. Proper wound care and immunization are crucial for prevention. Traumatic wounds can be characterized as tetanus prone or nontetanus prone based on mechanism of injury, age of the wound, and certain wound attributes (Table 24–39). In patients with wounds, the guidelines in Table 24–39 should be used to determine if tetanus toxoid with or without tetanus immune globulin (TIG) administration is necessary.

Burns

Approximately 1% of the U.S. population incurs a burn injury each year. Of these 2 million burns, about 7500 die and 100,000 require hospitalization (Kauder, 1998). Twenty-seven percent of patients hospitalized with burns require burn center care. Burn centers provide specialized treatment for optimum care and outcome. The American Burn Association (ABA) classification of burn injuries requiring specialized care in a burn center are listed in Table 24–40. Arrangements for transfer to a burn center are made by physician-to-physician referral.

Pathophysiology

Burn injury affects virtually every organ system, and the magnitude of the pathophysiologic response is directly proportionate to the degree of cutaneous injury (McManus & Pruitt, 1996). The systemic manifestations of burn injury are generally seen in patients with greater than 20% BSA burns (Table 24–41). Mortality following burn injury increases as both age and percent BSA burned increase.

Evaluation

History. Patient history should include a thorough account of the burn event, including the source of burn (flame, liquid, chemical, steam, explosion), duration of exposure, environment in which exposure occurred (closed versus open space), smoke inhalation, and knowledge of exposure

TABLE 24–39. Wounds Characteristics and Susceptibility to Tetanus

Clinical Features	Tetanus-Prone Wounds	Non-Tetanus-Prone Wounds
Age of Wound	≥6 Hours	<6 Hours
Configuration	Stellate wound	Linear wound
Depth	≥1 cm	<1 cm
Mechanism of Injury	Missile, crush, burn, frostbite	Sharp surface (e.g., knife)
Signs of Infection	Present	Absent
Devitalized Tissue	Present	Absent
Contaminants (dirt, feces, soil, saliva)	Present	Absent
Denervated and/or ischemic tissue	Present	Absent

Guide to Tetanus Prophylaxis

History of Absorbed	Tetanus-Prone Wounds		Non-Tetanus-Prone Wounds	
Tetanus Toxoid (Doses)	*Td*[a]	*TIG*[b]	*Td*[a]	*TIG*[c]
Uncertain or < three	Yes	Yes	Yes	No
≥ Three or more[d]	No[e]	No	No[f]	No

Notes:

[a] For children less than 7 years old, diptheria and tetanus toxoids absorbed and pertussis vaccine absorbed (for pediatric use) (DPT) is recommended. Diptheria and tetanus toxoids absorbed (for pediatric use) are preferred to tetanus toxoid absorbed alone if pertussis vaccine is contraindicted. For persons 7 years or older, tetanus and diptheria toxoids absorbed (for adult use) (Td) is preferred to tetanus toxoid absorbed used.

[b] TIG = Human tetanus immune globulin.

[c] When TIG and Td are given concurrently, separate syringes and separate sites should be used.

[d] If only three doses of fluid toxoid have been received, a fourth dose of toxoid, preferably an absorbed toxoid, should be given.

[e] Yes, if more than 5 years since last dose. (More frequent boosters are not needed and can accentuate side effects).

[f] Yes, if more than 10 years since last dose.

Reprinted with permission from Rehm & Ross, (1996). (p. 779). Copyright 1996 by Williams and Wilkins.

TABLE 24–40. American Burn Association Criteria for Burn Center Referral

Age and Percent Body Surface Area Criteria
- Burns with total body surface area > 10% < 10 years of age
- Burns with total body surface area > 10% > 50 years of age
- Burns with total body surface area > 20% other ages
- Burns with total body surface area > 5% full-thickness burns

Any burns that involve the hands, feet, face, or perineum
Circumferential burns of the chest or extremities
Electric injury
Chemical injury
Significant associated injuries that have the potential of compromising the postburn course
Evidence of inhalation injury
Major preexisting diseases

Reprinted with permission from Gordon & Goodwin, (1997). (p. 239).

to toxic fumes from burning plastics or cyanide. Details regarding associated injury mechanisms (e.g., jump from window, MVC) should also be elicited. A medical and substance abuse history should also be obtained (Kauder, 1998).

Assessment. The initial management of the burn patient, including triage to a burn center, is based in part upon accurate estimation of burn depth and burned surface area. Partial-thickness burns are those in which variable amounts of the dermis may be viable (Fig. 24–22). Full-thickness burns destroy the entire thickness of the dermis and may also injure the subcutaneous fat, muscle, or bone. Each depth of burn injury has distinct physiologic characteristics (Table 24–42).

A rapid means of estimating the percentage of body surface area (BSA) burned is the "Rule of 9s," based on the fact that each anatomic region represents approximately 9% BSA or a multiple thereof (Fig. 24–23). Smaller burns (<10% BSA) or those with multiple noncontiguous burned areas are better assessed using the palm size of the patient. The size of the patient's hand is about 1% of BSA. Following initial assessment, the exact burn size and depth should be more accurately mapped using a burn diagram (Fig. 24–24). First-degree burns are generally not included in any of these calculations (Gordon & Goodwin, 1997).

The location of the burn also impacts triage to a burn center. Patients with significant burns of the face, hands, fingers, feet, toes, and perineum require specialized burn center care because of the cosmetic and functional importance of these areas.

Facial burns, singed facial hair, hoarseness, and carbonaceous sputum suggests inhalation injury. Bronchoscopy findings of airway edema and erythema assist in the diagnosis (Clark, 1992). Carbon monoxide (CO) poisoning is characterized by cherry red skin, mental status changes, hypoxemia, and acidosis. Significant amounts of CO in the blood negates the reliability of pulse oximetry.

Associated injuries often occur as people try to flee from the burning area. Chest, abdominal, and orthopedic injuries are common but may be missed due to the presence of distracting burn injury (Kauder, 1998).

TABLE 24–41. Systemic Manifestations of Burn Injury

Cardiovascular
Increased capillary permeability
Decreased cardiac output
Increased systemic vascular resistance

Pulmonary
Hyperventilation
Mild hypoxemia
Impaired chest wall expansion (circumferential chest burns)

Gastrointestinal
Paralytic ileus
Gastritis/duodenitis
Ulceration and perforation (late)

Renal
Decreased glomerular filtration rate
Sodium retention
Acute tubular necrosis

Metabolic
Increased metabolic rate
Decreased insulin levels
Increased oxygen consumption

Hematologic
Leukocytosis
Thrombocytosis (late)

Immunologic
Impaired cellular and humoral immunity
Loss of protective skin barrier

Integument
Increased insensible water loss
Increased evaporative water loss

Resuscitation

Standard resuscitation procedures apply to burn victims. All patients should receive 100% oxygen, which helps facilitate displacement of CO from the hemoglobin molecule in patients with CO poisoning. Early intubation is essential for patients with signs of airway obstruction, inhalation injury, or airway compromise from other injuries. Severe, circumferential chest-wall burns may impair adequate ventilation secondary to pain and eschar formation. Immediate chest-wall escharotomy may be necessary.

Large-bore IV access must be established and isotonic fluid therapy initiated promptly. Dextrose-containing fluids should be avoided as burn patients are frequently glucose intolerant and hyperglycemic. Osmotic diuresis resulting from hyperglycemia may manifest as polyuria. Of the numerous formulas available to estimate resuscitation fluid requirements, the Parkland formula is used most often.

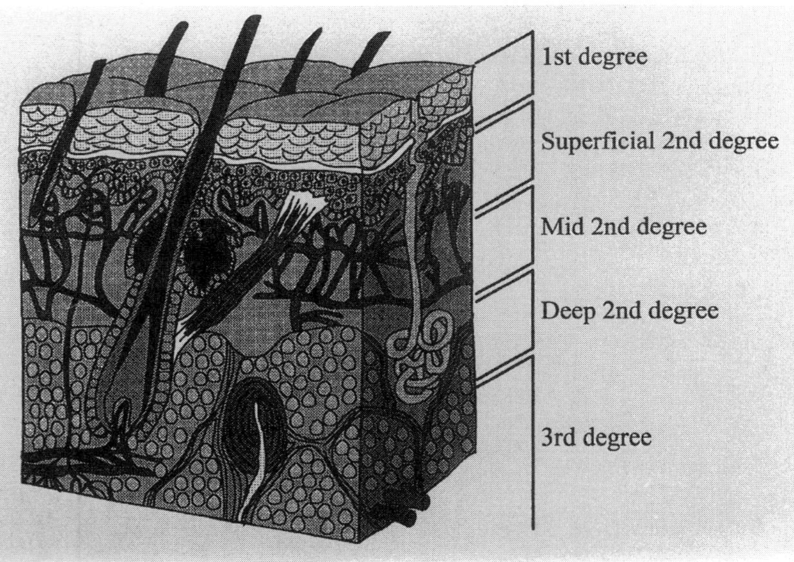

Figure 24–22. Burn wound depth. *(Reprinted with permission from Kauder. [1988]. [p. 425]. Copyright 1998 by Lippincott-Raven.)*

4 mL × body weight (kg) × % BSA burned over 24 hours
(50% of the total calculated fluid requirement
is given over the first 8 hours
and the remainder over the following 16 hours)

All formulas represent initial estimates only and require close clinical correlation with respect to urine output, mentation, blood pressure, and depth of the burn. Urine output is perhaps the most useful indicator; it should be approximately 50 mL/hour in adults. Central venous or pulmonary artery catheters should be used if the adequacy of resuscitation is in doubt.

If available, hyperbaric oxygen therapy may be an important resuscitative measure for patients with CO exposure with a history of unconsciousness or mental status changes. Hyperbaric therapy may lessen long-term or permanent neurologic sequelae.

Wound Management

The principle goals of wound care are to promote survival of remaining viable tissue, to prevent infection, and to optimize functional and aesthetic results as healing occurs. Physical and occupational therapists with training in burn-

TABLE 24–42. Physiologic Characteristics of Burn Wounds

	Superficial (First Degree)	Partial Thickness (Superficial Second Degree)	Deep Dermal Partial Thickness (Deep Second Degree)	Full Thickness (Third Degree)
Etiology	Sunburn, ultraviolet light exposure, minor flash	Brief exposure to flash flame, hot liquid spills, brief exposure to dilute chemical agents	Hot liquids or solids; flash flame, direct flame; intense radiant energy sources, chemical agents	Prolonged contact with flames, steam, chemical agents, or high voltage electrical current
Localization of cellular injury	Minimal epithelial damage	Epidermis, damage to middermal tissue plane	Entire epidermis and more dermal involvement than superficial partial thickness; hair follicles and sweat glands intact	Epidermis, dermis, and epidermal appendages; portions of subcutaneous fat; possible involvement of connective tissue, muscle and bone
Physical characteristics	Red or light red; dry or small blisters; slight erythema; exquisitely painful	Moist, bright pink or reddish color; blister formation; blanching; tactile and pain sensation intact	Pale, waxy appearance; absent blanching; usually dry; decreased pinprick sensation but pressure sensation intact	Dry, leathery, insensate, avascular, pale yellow to brown coloration, possible char; thrombosed vasculature may be visible
Healing time	7–14 days	14–21 days	Prolonged healing period >21 days; contracture formation; possible conversion to full thickness injury; hypertrophic scarring possible	Incapable of self-regeneration; requires grafting for optimal results

Reprinted with permission from Jordan & Harrington, (1997). (p. 253).

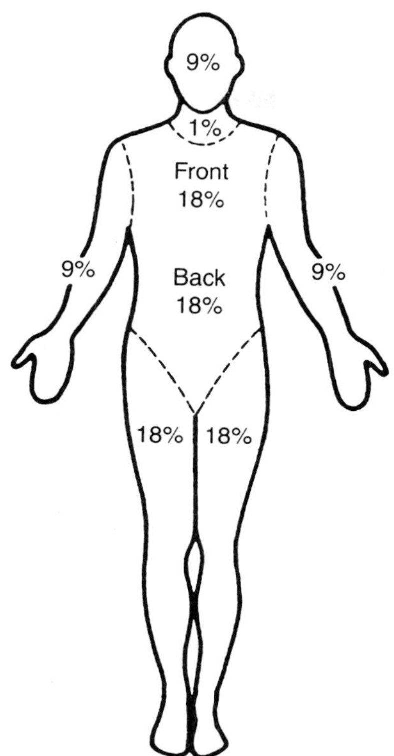

Figure 24–23. Rule of "9"s for Rapid Assessment of Percentage of Body Surface Area Burned.

wound management can provide valuable assistance in both inpatient and outpatient management.

Superficial, first-degree burns do not require special therapy. Topical or oral analgesics may be prescribed. For partial-thickness or full-thickness burn wounds, application of antimicrobial agents, meticulous wound care, and vigilant surveillance are the mainstays of initial wound management (Jordan & Harrington, 1997). Prophylactic intravenous antibiotics are not required. Three topical antimicrobial agents—Sulfamylon, Silvadene, and silver nitrate solution—demonstrate wide activity against colonizing organisms and have minimal systemic absorption and toxicity (Table 24–43). Gentamicin or Bacitracin ointment may also be used but these agents poorly penetrate eschar. Large blisters may be left intact, as they provide a sterile physiologic dressing for the burn wound. They should be debrided if they interfere with joint motion or cause pain.

The customary approach to large, deep burn wounds involves burn-wound excision and split-thickness skin grafting (Baxter, 1993). This process is often initiated following physiologic stabilization and continues at intervals until the entire burn wound is covered. Biologic dressings and synthetic materials can cover partial-thickness burns to promote healing and serve as temporary protection after burn excision when no donor sites are available for harvesting. Cadaveric allograft and porcine xenograft are commonly used biologic dressings. Biobrane and Integra are synthetic dressings with a collagen inner layer and an outer epithelial-like membrane that prevents dessication.

▶ MISSED INJURY

Missed injuries are those that are diagnosed late in the hospital course or after discharge from the trauma service. Some institutions define a missed injury relative to an arbitrary time period, such as those diagnosed beyond the first 12 or 24 hours after initial evaluation. The incidence of missed injury has been reported at 9 to 12% (Chan, Ainscow, & Sikorski, 1980; Enderson et al., 1990).

Numerous factors lead to missed injury (Table 24–44). As many as 50% of missed injuries occur in patients with altered level of consciousness, particularly head-injured or intoxicated patients (Enderson & Maull, 1991). Musculoskeletal injuries comprise approximately one half of all missed injuries; the remainder includes head, chest, abdominal, retroperitoneal, spinal, and neurovascular injury (Chan et al., 1980; Enderson & Maull, 1991).

Rare cases of missed injury are unavoidable in the complex delivery of care to multiply injured trauma patients. However, the trauma team is responsible for implementing measures to lower the risk of missed injury. A tertiary survey should be completed on all trauma patients to discover injuries that were not identified during the primary and secondary surveys. The tertiary survey is a complete head-to-toe examination performed after the patient regains consciousness or sobriety, after surgical or nonsurgical treatment has been instituted for known injuries, and before the patient is allowed to ambulate. In addition to investigating new symptoms or signs of injury, the tertiary survey provides an opportunity to compare examination findings and final radiologic study results with admission examination data (Sommers, 1995).

In addition to the tertiary survey, several routine practices help reduce the rate of missed injury: (1) suspect unidentified injuries in trauma patients with head injury or intoxication; (2) perform thorough reexaminations, temporarily holding neuromuscular blocking agents to allow for complete neurologic examination; (3) thoroughly investigate patient reports of pain, weakness, or sensory loss using radiographic studies liberally; (4) assume that postoperative hemorrhage is from a missed injury until proven otherwise; (5) actively entertain the possibility of a missed injury when a patient fails to progress as expected; (6) avoid transfer of injured inpatients to a nontrauma service for at least 24 hours; and (7) regularly review and discuss cases involving missed injury in formal peer-review sessions.

▶ COMPLICATIONS OF TRAUMA

Despite the best efforts of trauma care providers, complications of trauma do occur. Critical injuries alter tissue struc-

Burn Estimate and Diagram
Age vs Area

Initial Evaluation

Cause of Burn________________

Date of Burn________________

Time of Burn________________

Age________________

Sex________________

Weight________________

Date of Admission________________

Signature________________

Date________________

Burn Diagram

Color Code

Red - 3°
Blue - 2°

Areas	Age (y)						2°	3°	Total	Areas
	Birth–1	1–4	5–9	10–14	15	Adult				
Head	19	17	13	11	9	7				
Neck	2	2	2	2	2	2				
Ant. Trunk	13	13	13	13	13	13				
Post. Trunk	13	13	13	13	13	13				
R. Buttock	$2\frac{1}{2}$	$2\frac{1}{2}$	$2\frac{1}{2}$	$2\frac{1}{2}$	$2\frac{1}{2}$	$2\frac{1}{2}$				
L. Buttock	$2\frac{1}{2}$	$2\frac{1}{2}$	$2\frac{1}{2}$	$2\frac{1}{2}$	$2\frac{1}{2}$	$2\frac{1}{2}$				
Genitalia	1	1	1	1	1	1				
R.U. Arm	4	4	4	4	4	4				
L.U. Arm	4	4	4	4	4	4				
R.L. Arm	3	3	3	3	3	3				
L.L. Arm	3	3	3	3	3	3				
R. Hand	$2\frac{1}{2}$	$2\frac{1}{2}$	$2\frac{1}{2}$	$2\frac{1}{2}$	$2\frac{1}{2}$	$2\frac{1}{2}$				
L. Hand	$2\frac{1}{2}$	$2\frac{1}{2}$	$2\frac{1}{2}$	$2\frac{1}{2}$	$2\frac{1}{2}$	$2\frac{1}{2}$				
R. Thigh	$5\frac{1}{2}$	$6\frac{1}{2}$	8	$8\frac{1}{2}$	9	$9\frac{1}{2}$				
L. Thigh	$5\frac{1}{2}$	$6\frac{1}{2}$	8	$8\frac{1}{2}$	9	$9\frac{1}{2}$				
R. Leg	5	5	$5\frac{1}{2}$	6	$6\frac{1}{2}$	7				
L. Leg	5	5	$5\frac{1}{2}$	6	$6\frac{1}{2}$	7				
R. Foot	$3\frac{1}{2}$	$3\frac{1}{2}$	$3\frac{1}{2}$	$3\frac{1}{2}$	$3\frac{1}{2}$	$3\frac{1}{2}$				
L. Foot	$3\frac{1}{2}$	$3\frac{1}{2}$	$3\frac{1}{2}$	$3\frac{1}{2}$	$3\frac{1}{2}$	$3\frac{1}{2}$				
						Total				

Figure 24–24. Burn Diagram and Calculation Table. Based on the Lund and Browder chart, this method more accurately represents differences in body size and more accurately estimates the percent body surface area for each anatomic region. *(Reprinted with permission from Jordan & Harrington. [1997]. [p. 257]. Copyright 1997 by W. B. Saunders.)*

ture and function to the extent that complications are sometimes unavoidable. Major life-affecting decisions must be made hurriedly and often based on incomplete data, which may inevitably contribute to untoward delays in treatment (Maull, Rodriguez, & Wiles, 1996).

Shock

Shock is defined as an inadequate cardiac output resulting in cellular hypoxia. Persistent shock results in cellular dysfunction, organ failure, and death. Injured patients in shock require resuscitation using specific therapies and techniques in accordance with the cause of shock. Hypovolemic (or hemorrhagic) shock is the most common form of shock in trauma patients. Cardiogenic, obstructive, neurogenic, and septic shock states can also occur alone or in combination. Because hemorrhage is the etiology of shock in the majority of trauma patients, a major component of successful resuscitation is hemostasis, often achieved by surgical intervention (Mullins, 1996).

A priority in the initial evaluation of a trauma patient is assessment for hemorrhagic shock, which may or may not be apparent. Compensatory physiologic mechanisms (e.g., sympathetic vasoconstriction, catecholamine-mediated increases in heart rate and contractility) can mask significant hypovolemia. Cardiac output does not significantly decline until the blood volume deficit reaches between 20 to 40%, thus blood pressure alone is an inaccurate guide for estimation of blood loss. ATLS guidelines divide hemorrhagic shock into four stages based on percentage of acute volume loss (Table 24–45). Although each class is associ-

TABLE 24–43. Topical Antimicrobial Agents for Burn Wound Care

Agent	Chemistry	Method of Use	Activity	Advantages	Disadvantages
Mafenide Acetate (Sulfamylon Cream 11.2%)	Methylated sulfonamide	Topical application of drug (cream) in water miscible base applied QD or BID without dressings. Cleanse wound between applications. Apply to depth of one-sixteenth inch	Active against gram-positive and gram-negative organisms	—Penetrates through full-thickness of eschar potentiating delayed therapy —Easy application and removal, no dressings required, permits monitoring of wound appearance, and allows full joint motion —Persistent activity against pseudornonas, resistance does not develop, wide spectrum of use —Infrequent hypersensitivity, nontoxic to local tissues	—Use not compatible with dressings —Painful on application for 15–30 minutes —May cause metabolic acidosis due to biochemical breakdown into acid salt with compensatory hyperventilation and CO_2 retention
Silver Sulfadiazine (Silvadene 1%)	Silver sulfadiazine complex	Topical application of drug (cream) in water miscible base applied QD or BID without dressings. Cleanse wound between applications. Apply to depth of one-sixteenth inch	Active against gram-positive and gram-negative organisms	—Painless upon application —Convenient for outpatient use (with/without dressings) —Easy application and removal, permits easy monitoring of wound appearance and allows full joint movement (without dressings) —Wide spectrum of use	—Only partial penetration through full-thickness eschar —5%–7% incidence of hypersensitivity —Transient leukopenia reported —Potential cross sensitivity with other sulfonamides
Silver Nitrate 0.5% dressings (soaks)	Inorganic silver salt	0.5% solution in distilled water, use to dampen dressings every 2 hours, change dressing BID or TID	Effective against wide range of pathogens, including fungal elements	—No hypersensitivity reaction, painless on application —No resistant organism reported —Evaporative water and heat loss minimized with use of required dressings —Effective for use in exfoliative skin diseases	—No penetration of eschar —Labor-intensive dressing changes, difficulty in monitoring wound surfaces, and limited joint movement due to requisite dressings —Discoloration of wound renders evaluation difficult; equipment and environmental staining is permanent —Biochemical changes, particularly in children, requires close fluid and electrolyte monitoring

Reprinted with permission from Greenfield & DeFazio Quinn (Eds.), (1997). (p. 262). Copyright 1997 by W. B. Saunders Company.

ated with certain clinical signs, the distinction between classes is not always obvious, and patients may insidiously progress from one stage to another. It is jeopardous to wait until the patient fits a precise classification before initiating therapy.

Aggressive fluid resuscitation must be initiated when *early* signs of blood loss are apparent or suspected (American College of Surgeons, 1993). Two large bore intravenous catheters should be inserted for rapid administration of fluid. Hypotensive patients should receive two liters of balanced electrolyte solution. If hypotension persists and physical examination findings confirm blood loss is a principle cause of shock, a repeated fluid bolus may be indicated. No response or only transient response to the second bolus of fluid demonstrates ongoing hemorrhage. Blood transfusion should then be initiated to mitigate tissue oxygen debt and anaerobic cellular metabolism. Once life-threatening hemorrhage is identified or suspected, external bleeding should

TABLE 24–44. Factors Contributing to Missed Injuries

Factors	Possible Explanation
Hemodynamic instability	Patients who present to the emergency department in shock may require rapid evaluation and, often, emergency surgery. Injuries may be missed because of an urgency to terminate a surgical procedure to limit hypotension or hypothermia and to correct coagulopathies
Alterations in consciousness	Decreased level of consciousness from factors such as head injury or alcohol intoxication accounts for as many as half of missed injuries. When patients cannot participate in the physical examination or provide a history of the injury, hidden injuries become more difficult to identify. Intubation and mechanical ventilation are also associated with missed injuries because of the patient's inability to communicate
Errors of practitioner inexperience	Errors of practitioner inexperience occur when appropriate information is obtained during examination, but that information is misinterpreted. Examples of these errors include ignoring the significance of bruising or minimizing the importance of a lesion. A low index of suspicion by the examiner also may occur with inexperience
Radiologic errors	Radiologic errors occur when appropriate x-rays are not performed, are of inadequate quality or of the wrong view, or are incorrectly interpreted. Most commonly, errors occur when x-rays are requested, taken, and reported but the results are either not noted or are misinterpreted by the clinicians responsible for the patient's care. Particular difficulty in interpretation occurs when more than one lesion is located in the same region
Technical errors	Procedural errors in techniques such as the peritoneal lavage may contribute to the rate of missed injury. Hastily applied splints or cervical collars may obscure a less apparent injury that needs further investigation
Admission to an inappropriate service	In institutions with trauma services, admission to an inappropriate service is an unusual event. Trauma patients admitted to nonacute specialty units have a 46% rate of missed injury (Chan, Ainscow, & Sikorski, 1980)

Adapted with permission from Sommers, (1995). (p. 189). Copyright 1995 by J. B. Lippincott.

be controlled with direct pressure and the patient transported to the operating room as quickly as possible.

In patients with penetrating injury to the torso, fluid resuscitation to a normal or supranormal blood pressure before operative repair of internal injuries has been shown to increase mortality as well as increase the risk of ARDS and other complications (Bickell, et al., 1994). Increasing hydrostatic forces within injured vessels by rapid volume administration may disrupt early protective clot formation and exacerbate hemorrhage. Delaying fluid resuscitation until definitive repair of major vascular injuries has been recommended but not yet widely accepted (Mattox, Hirshberg, & Wall, 1994).

There is considerable debate regarding the optimal resuscitation endpoints following injury. Discussion of this controversy is beyond the scope of this chapter. The principle goal of volume resuscitation is to restore organ perfusion, rather than to achieve arbitrary clinical endpoints such as a target blood pressure or heart rate. Crystalloids and colloids must be used judiciously to meet *metabolic* endpoints. Lactate, base deficit, and oxygen transport variables are useful in guiding the resuscitation of trauma patients and in predicting mortality (Abramson et al., 1993; Davis et al., 1988; Durham, Neunaber, Mazuski, Shapiro, & Baue, 1996). There is preliminary evidence to suggest that gastric tonometry (measurement of gastric mucosal pH using a nasogastric catheter) may be a more direct measure of organ perfusion, with preliminary data demonstrating its superiority in predicting morbidity and mortality in trauma patients (Gutierrez & Brown, 1996; Ivatury et al., 1996).

TABLE 24–45. Classes of Hemorrhagic Shock, with Estimated Blood Loss, Based on Patient's Initial Presentation[a]

	Class I	Class II	Class III	Class IV
Pulse Rate (beats/minute)	< 100	> 100	> 120	> 140
Blood Pressure (mm Hg)	Normal	Normal	Decreased	Decreased
Pulse Pressure (mm Hg)	Normal or increased	Decreased	Decreased	Decreased
Respiratory Rate (per minute)	14–20	20–30	30–40	>35
Urine Output (mL/hour)	>30	20–30	5–15	Negligible
Mental Status	Slightly anxious	Mildly anxious	Anxious and confused	Confused, lethargic
Blood Loss (mL)	Up to 750	750–1500	1500–2000	> 2000
Blood Loss (% blood volume)	Up to 15%	15–30%	30–40%	> 40%
Fluid Replacement (3:1 rule[b])	Crystalloid	Crystalloid	Crystalloid and blood	Crystalloid and blood

[a] For a 70 kg male.

[b] Fluid replacement guidelines are based on the "three-for-one" rule. This rule derives from the empiric observation that most patients in hemorrhagic shock require as much as 300 mL of electrolyte solution for each 100 mL of blood loss. Applied blindly, these guidelines can result in excessive or inadequate fluid resuscitation. The use of bolus therapy with careful monitoring of the patient's response can help to individualize volume administration.

Adapted with permission from American College of Surgeons, Committee on Trauma, (1993). Advanced Trauma Life Support Manual *(p. 86).*

Hypothermia

Hypothermia, defined as a core body temperature less than 35°C, occurs when heat loss exceeds heat production. Hypothermia occurs in an estimated 21 to 66% of trauma patients, with direct correlation to ISS, massive fluid resuscitation, and shock (Luna et al., 1987; Steinemann, Shackford, & Davis, 1990). Primary hypothermia results from prolonged exposure or water immersion, whereas secondary hypothermia occurs as a result of dermal disruption (burns or large wounds), shock, substance abuse, or altered thermoregulation from hypothalamic injury or spinal cord injury. Iatrogenic factors contributing to the development of hypothermia in the trauma patient include the infusion of cold intravenous fluids, exposure for clinical assessment, opening of body cavities, and suppression of heat production through anesthetic agents and other medications (Haskell, Boruta, Rotondo, & Frankel, 1997).

Hypothermia causes global dysfunction of all body systems in proportion to the severity of the temperature derangement (Table 24–46). It is classified as mild, moderate, or severe depending upon core temperature readings (Table 24–47). A core temperature of 32°C or less in trauma patients has been associated with a mortality rate near 100%, even in the context of mild trauma (Jurkovich, Greiser, Luterman, & Curreri, 1987).

Prevention of further heat loss in trauma patients is critical. Warming the environment (resuscitation room, OR, or ICU) and minimizing patient exposure decreases the amount of heat lost by radiation from the skin and by evaporation from operative sites. Warm humidified oxygen should be administered. All intravenous blood products and crystalloid should be warmed prior to infusion using a fluid warmer or warming infusion device. Application of a heated blanket is indicated for high-risk patients before hypothermia ensues.

Treatment of hypothermia begins with standard resuscitation efforts, concurrent to initiation of rewarming techniques (Table 24–48). Endotracheal intubation is indicated for apnea or coma. Figure 24–25 illustrates the effects of severe hypothermia on cardiac conduction, with characteristic Osborn or "J" waves. The severe bradycardia that accompanies hypothermia may provide sufficient systemic perfusion, since hypothermia decreases metabolic requirements. Palpation of the carotid pulse for one full minute confirms pulselessness, at which time external chest compressions should be initiated. The risk of spontaneous ventricular fibrillation increases as core temperature approaches 28°C. The risk may be enhanced by physical stimuli; therefore procedures and handling of the patient should be limited when possible. Hypovolemia—caused by concomitant injuries, "cold diuresis," and capillary leak—must be treated with warmed fluids. If warmed and resuscitated, a victim of primary hypothermia may recover neurologically, even after prolonged arrest.

TABLE 24–46. Pathophysiological Effects of Hypothermia

Central Nervous System
- Decreased cerebral blood flow
- Progressive paralysis of the central nervous system
- Reduced cerebral metabolic demand

Cardiovascular
- Decreased heart rate, contractility and cardiac output
- Delayed depolarization in pacemaker tissue
- Electrocardiogram characteristics:
  - Increased PR, QRS and QT intervals
  - J wave (Osborn wave)
  - ST elevation
  - T wave inversion
- Decreased transmembrane resting potential
  - Atrial fibrillation
  - Ventricular fibrillation

Pulmonary
- Hypoventilation
- Decreased cough reflex
- Increased airway secretions (bronchorrhea)
- Paralysis of mucociliary mechanism

Gastrointestinal
- Hypomotility
- Decreased hepatic metabolism
- Decreased insulin release from the pancreas
- Stress ulceration

Renal
- Impaired renal tubular transport function causing decreased sodium and water reabsorption
- Decreased antidiuretic hormone
- Fluid shift from vascular compartment to interstitial spaces

Acid–Base Balance
- Decreased systemic carbon dioxide production
- Early respiratory alkalosis
- Eventual metabolic acidosis in severe hypothermia

Hematologic
- Shift of oxyhemoglobin dissociation curve to left causing decreased oxygen delivery to tissues
- Increased blood viscosity
- Coagulopathy due to:
  - Inhibition of the enzymatic reactions of the coagulation cascade
  - Splenic sequestration of platelets

Immunologic
- Splenic sequestration of leukocytes
- Decreased neutrophil function
- Reduced collagen deposition

Reprinted with permission from Haskell, Boruta, Rotondo, & Frankel, (1997). (p. 369).

Hypothermic patients may appear dead, but cardiopulmonary resuscitation should be initiated despite absence of vital signs. Death in a cold patient has been described as failure to revive on rewarming. If a patient has been rewarmed to 35°C or greater without return of cardiorespira-

TABLE 24–47. Signs and Symptoms of Hypothermia

Severity	Core Temperature	Signs and Symptoms
Mild	32°C to 35°C	Shivering, dysarthria, amnesia, impaired judgment, ataxia, increased blood pressure, vasoconstriction, tachycardia, bronchorrhea, tachypnea
Moderate	28°C to 32°C	No shivering, stupor, pupillary dilation, hyporeflexia, J waves, bradydysrhythmia, atrial flutter, decreased blood pressure, hypoventilation, coagulopathies
Severe	< 28°C	Coma, loss of corneal reflexes, areflexia, hypotension, apnea, J waves, metabolic acidosis, coagulopathies, ventricular fibrillation, asystole (<25°C)
Profound	< 20°C	Hypoxia, acidosis, respiratory arrest, asystole, isoelectric electroencephalogram, death

Reprinted with permission from Haskell, Boruta, Rotondo, & Frankel, (1997). (p. 370). Copyright 1997 by Lippincott.

tory function, consideration should be given to discontinuing resuscitation efforts.

Abdominal Compartment Syndrome

Abdominal compartment syndrome (ACS), also called intraabdominal hypertension, is defined as cardiovascular, respiratory, and renal impairment secondary to increased intraabdominal pressure (IAP). ACS occurs in the trauma patient from various conditions causing increased IAP or following application of pneumatic anti-shock garments (MAST trousers) (Table 24–49). Its significant morbidity manifests as MODS and sepsis, which are thought to occur when increased IAP causes a critical reduction in splanchnic perfusion. Patients with ACS have high mortality rates (42%), with death usually occurring from the underlying insult and MODS (Borst & Udekwu, 1998).

A high index of suspicion is essential for early diagnosis. Clinical manifestations of ACS are caused by profound abdominal distention in association with diaphragmatic elevation, cardiovascular dysfunction, and renal dysfunction from both direct compression of renal parenchyma and decreased renal blood flow (Table 24–50). Oliguria (in the presence of euvolemia) is often the earliest sign. ACS is often a clinical diagnosis, but in its early phase when oliguria may be the only finding, measurement of IAP is useful. IAP can be measured indirectly by measuring bladder pressure, gastric pressure, or by using a long femoral venous catheter placed in the inferior vena cava (Borst & Udekwu, 1998). The bladder method is used most often since it is simple and reliable (Table 24–51). An IAP greater than 25 mm Hg is considered diagnostic of ACS if clinical signs are present (Feliciano, Moore, & Mattox, 1996).

Once identified, ACS should be considered a surgical emergency. Decompressive laparotomy should be performed

TABLE 24–48. Warming Techniques

Warming Technique	Indications	Actions
Passive External	All stages of hypothermia Hypothermia prevention	Remove patient from cold environment Remove wet clothing Cover with warm blankets
Active External	All stages of hypothermia Presence of predisposing factors	Apply the following: Fluid-circulating heating blankets Convective air warmers Reflective blankets Heating pads and hot water bottles Radiant heat sources Warmed oxygen and inhalation gases Use of warming beds
Active Internal (Core Rewarming)	Moderate to severe hypothermia Massive volume resuscitation Hemodynamic instability	Administer heated intravenous fluids and blood products Cardiopulmonary bypass Gastric lavage Pleural lavage Peritoneal lavage Colonic and bladder irrigation Hemodialysis Continuous arterio-venous rewarming (CAVR) Open thoracotomy with myocardial/mediastinal irrigation

Selected warming techniques should be utilized prophylactically for all trauma patients at risk of hypothermia and for patients with core body temperature < 35°C.
Adapted with permission from Haskell, Boruta, Rotondo, & Frankel, (1997). (p. 377). Copyright 1997 by Lippincott.

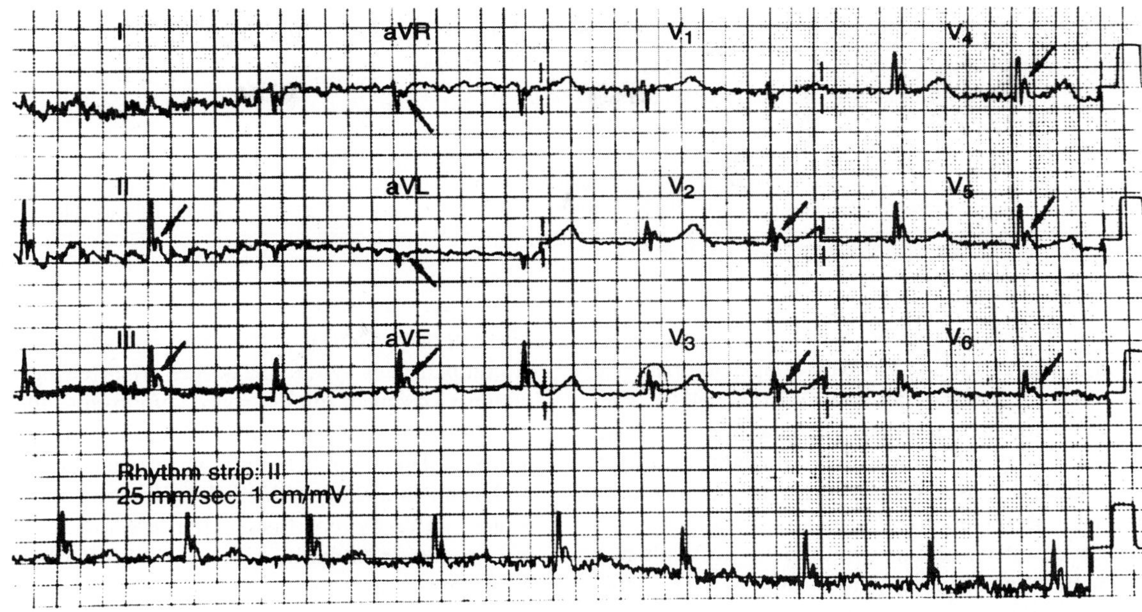

Figure 24–25. A 12-lead electrocardiogram in a 40-year-old alcoholic male with a core body temperature of 29°C from accidental exposure to cold. The tracing shows a bradycardic rhythm, prolonged QT intervals, a baseline artifact due to muscle tremors, and characteristic Osborn ("J") waves *(arrows). (Reprinted with permission from Patel & Getsos. [1994]. [p. 680]. Copyright 1994 by the Massachusetts Medical Society.)*

immediately to restore ventilation, cardiac output, and renal and splanchnic perfusion. Hemodynamic decompensation may occur after the procedure due to a sudden drop in systemic vascular resistance. Reperfusion syndrome, resulting from the release of acid and metabolites from reperfused tissues into the circulation, may cause immediate asystole. To mitigate this problem, the initial resuscitative fluid may contain mannitol and sodium bicarbonate (Borst & Udekwu, 1998). After decompression, the abdomen is temporarily closed using one of a variety of materials (e.g., mesh, plastic silo, plastic irrigation bag) (Feliciano, Moore, & Mattox, 1996).

Permanent abdominal closure is performed after metabolic abnormalities have been corrected and the intraabdominal edema is thought to have resolved. Skin grafting or delayed abdominal wall reconstruction may be required.

TABLE 24–49. Etiologies of Abdominal Compartment Syndrome in Trauma Patients

Abdominal trauma
Intraperitoneal hemorrhage
Retroperitoneal hemorrhage
Postresuscitation edema
Ileus
Bowel obstruction
Hemorrhagic pancreatitis
Pneumatic anti-shock garments (MAST trousers)
Abdominal packing
Abdominal incision closure under excessive tension

Orthopedic Complications

Fat Embolism

Fat embolism, the sudden blocking of an artery by a fat embolus or clot, is a potential complication in patients with long-bone and pelvic fractures. Fat embolism remains subclinical in most patients, but progresses to fat embolism

TABLE 24–50. Clinical Manifestations of Abdominal Compartment Syndrome

Respiratory
Decreased inspiratory tidal volumes
Increased peak airway pressures
Decreased compliance
Increased pulmonary vascular resistance
Hypoxemia
Hypercarbia
Acidosis
Cardiovascular
Increased central venous pressure (CVP)
Increased pulmonary artery wedge pressure
Increased systemic vascular resistance
Decreased cardiac output
Renal
Oliguria

TABLE 24–51. Procedure for Indirect Measurement of Intraabdominal Pressure through Bladder Pressure Measurement

1. Inject 50 to 100 mL of sterile saline in the empty bladder through an indwelling Foley catheter
2. Clamp the tubing of the urinary drainage bag just distal to the culture aspiration port
3. Connect the end of the drainage bag tubing to the indwelling Foley catheter
4. Release the clamp just enough to allow the tubing proximal to the clamp to fill with fluid from the bladder, then reapply the clamp
5. Y-connect a pressure transducer through the culture aspiration port of the tubing to the drainage bag using a 16-gauge needle
6. Determine intra-abdominal pressure from the transducer using the top of the symphysis pubis bone as the zero point with the patient supine

Adapted with permission from Peitzman, Rhodes, Schwab, & Yealy, (1998). (p. 282).

syndrome in up to 10% of patients with multiple high-risk fractures, and causes death in 10 to 20% of afflicted patients (Gossling & Pellegrini, 1982; Shier & Wilson, 1980). The etiology of fat embolism syndrome is unclear, but it is most likely an inflammatory process involving formulation of fat globules intravascularly as a result of the rapid mobilization of free fatty acids secondary to catecholamine response.

Diagnosis of fat embolism syndrome is difficult because of variable clinical presentations and because of the lack of a test that is sensitive or specific for it. The syndrome is characterized by a triad of confusion, dyspnea, and petechiae of the chest, axilla, and subconjunctival areas. Other signs may include tachypnea, chest pain, cough, tachycardia, fever, seizures, and coma. It may be difficult to distinguish the neurologic manifestations of the syndrome from those of accompanying traumatic brain injury (Table 24–52). Fat globules are present in the urine, serum, or sputum of 50% of patients with bone trauma, and, therefore, are too sensitive and nonspecific for the diagnosis of fat embolism syndrome (Benson, 1993). Thrombocytopenia and diffuse pulmonary infiltrates are often present. The clinical scenario is similar to that of pulmonary embolism, which must be investigated.

Treatment is generally supportive, with the prompt initiation of ventilatory support if respiratory failure develops. Preventive measures that may reduce the risk of fat embolism include proper splinting, adequate hydration, and early fracture reduction and fixation (Benson, 1993).

TABLE 24–52. Comparison of Clinical Manifestations of Cerebral Fat Embolism and Traumatic Brain Injury

Signs and Symptoms	Cerebral Fat Embolism	Traumatic Brain Injury
Lucid interval	18–24 hours	6–10 hours
Confusion	Severe	Moderate
Pulse rate	Rapid (140–160 beats per minute)	Slow
Respiratory rate	Rapid	Slow
Onset of coma	Rapid	Slow
Localizing signs	Usually absent	Usually present
Decerebrate rigidity	Early	Terminal

Reprinted with permission from Pelligrini, Reid, & Evarts, (1996). (p. 435).

Extremity Compartment Syndrome

A compartment syndrome occurs when elevated pressures within a confined, limited space compromise the circulation and function of tissues in that space, causing myoneural necrosis. This complication is most commonly encountered in the calf as a result of a crushing fracture or blast injury. It is also caused by reperfusion after repair of an arterial injury in an ischemic extremity. Clinical manifestations include the "P's": *pain* out of proportion to the injury, pain on *passive* muscle stretch, *paresthesias* in the distribution of nerves within a compartment, and *palpable* tenseness of the fascial boundaries of a compartment. Loss of palpable *pulse* and *paralysis* as a result of significant anoxia and necrosis are late signs (Mabee, 1993; Mabee & Bostwick, 1993).

Intracompartmental pressure measurements serve as adjuncts to serial physical examinations. In unresponsive patients or in patients with equivocal examination findings, compartment syndrome may be confirmed by elevated measurements (pressures <20 mm Hg are normal, >30 mm Hg abnormal). Compartment syndrome is considered a surgical emergency; treatment is fasciotomy of all compartments to allow restoration of adequate tissue perfusion. Fasciotomy may be done prophylactically in cases of arterial injury repair. Whenever doubt exists about the diagnosis, fasciotomy should be performed. The morbidity for fasciotomy is minimal compared with the sequelae of an undiagnosed compartment syndrome or a delay in restoring perfusion (Kane, 1998).

Rhabdomyolysis

Rhabdomyolysis is a syndrome of skeletal muscle injury or ischemia with associated local and systemic complications. Muscle injury or necrosis causes a leakage of fluid, potassium, phosphates, and myoglobin into the intravascular and intracellular spaces, where these substances affect other organs (Kane, 1998). Organ injury is compounded by intravascular depletion secondary to third spacing of fluid into the damaged muscle. Complications include acute renal failure, acid–base and electrolyte disturbances, dysrhythmias, muscle contractures, peripheral neuropathy, and disseminated intravascular coagulation (DIC).

Rhabdomyolysis is attributed to traumatic and nontraumatic causes. Traumatic causes include lower extremity fractures with crushing of soft tissues, prolonged muscular compression during unconsciousness due to drugs or anesthesia, burns, electrical shock, frostbite, surgical tourniquets, and severe muscular exertion. Direct injury to skeletal muscle results, typically accompanied by compartment syndrome. Nontraumatic causes include neuroleptic malignant syndrome, malignant hyperthermia, venom from certain insects and snakes, severe infection, and skeletal muscle toxins such as cocaine, alcohol, heroin, and theophylline. Nontraumatic causes lead to muscle ischemia or myopathy.

Diagnosis of rhabdomyolysis depends upon a high index of suspicion and several laboratory studies. Clinical findings are nonspecific and may include malaise, fever, weakness, and tenderness of involved muscles. Myoglobinuria is caused by high renal clearance of serum myoglobin and may cause rusty–brown-colored urine early after injury. Myoglobinuria may be confirmed chemically, but its absence does not exclude rhabdomyolysis. If the urine dips positive for blood but no red blood cells are seen on microscopy, myoglobinuria is likely to be present. Pigmented granular casts may also be present on urine microscopy. Creatinine phosphokinase (CPK) level is a sensitive marker of muscle injury; a fivefold increase in CPK from baseline is diagnostic for rhabdomyolysis. CPK levels rise 2 to 12 hours after injury, peak at around 1 to 2 days, and decrease by 3 to 5 days (Kane, 1998). Other associated laboratory findings include anion gap acidosis, hyperkalemia, hyperphosphatemia, hyperuricemia, hypocalcemia, and unusually low blood urea nitrogen to creatinine ratio due to creatinine release from the muscle.

Treatment of rhabdomyolysis involves volume repletion and correction of electrolyte abnormalities. Prevention of acute renal failure is critical, including intravenous fluids to maintain urine output > 100-200 cc per hour, mannitol or loop diuretics after adequate volume resuscitation is assured, and sodium bicarbonate to maintain urine pH > 5.6. Fasciotomy is performed if a compartment syndrome exists.

Embolic Complications

Deep Venous Thrombosis

Deep vein thrombosis (DVT) refers to a nonobstructing or obstructing clot in any deep venous system, including the upper extremity and the calf. DVT is a serious complication, both because of the risk of immediate death from pulmonary embolism (PE) and because of long-term disability from postphlebitic syndrome. Numerous risk factors for DVT are present in most multiply injured trauma patients (Table 24–53) (Dennis et al., 1993). Moreover, the endogenous coagulation profile is altered in multiply injured patients, causing an immediate hypercoagulable state (Engelman, Gabram, Allen, Ens, & Jacobs, 1996). If no prophylaxis is used, the incidence of DVT after major trauma ranges from 19 to 58% (Geerts et al., 1994). The actual incidence of DVT is unknown because many cases are clinically unrecognized.

TABLE 24–53. Risk Factors for Deep Vein Thrombosis after Trauma

GCS score < 8	General anesthesia
Spine fractures	Large transfusion requirements
Spinal cord injury	Age > 40 years
Femur and tibia fractures	Underlying conditions:
Complex pelvic fractures	• Obesity
Immobilized > 3 days	• Malignancy
Direct venous injury	• Hypercoagulable state
AIS ≥ 3 for chest or abdomen	• History of DVT or PE
ISS ≥ 16	• Pregnancy
Extensive soft tissue trauma	• Congestive heart failure
Presence of femoral venous catheters	• Estrogen therapy

Adapted with permission from Knudson, Lewis, Clinton, Atkinson, & Megerman, (1994). (p. 485). Copyright 1994 by Williams and Wilkins.

DVT may occur immediately after injury, within 24 to 48 hours, but it is most commonly first detected 7 to 10 days after injury. When a DVT occurs, clot formation permanently impairs venous valvular competence in the affected segment of vein. Postphlebitic syndrome—characterized by swelling, nonpitting edema, pain, and discoloration—frequently occurs in the affected extremity. Serious disability may result, especially when venous stasis ulcers develop. Proximal extremity and pelvic vein DVT carry the greatest risk of potentially lethal embolic complications.

There are numerous methods of DVT prophylaxis, and the optimal method or combination of methods continues to be investigated. The best prevention may be early ambulation. If ambulation is contraindicated, other forms of prophylaxis include elastic compression stockings, sequential pneumatic compression devices (PCDs), and low-dose anticoagulation. PCDs are indicated when access to both lower extremities is not limited by casts, splints, external fixation devices, or arterial insufficiency. Otherwise, low-dose unfractionated heparin (5000 units subcutaneous every 8 to 12 hours) or low molecular-weight heparin (30 mg subcutaneous every 12 hours) may be used (Geerts et al., 1996; Knudson, Morabito, Paiement, & Shackleford, 1996). Even though the efficacy of these methods in preventing DVT remains unclear, the morbidity associated with them is minimal, and some form of prophylaxis should be used for trauma patients at risk.

Because symptoms and signs of DVT are nonspecific and may be attributable to other conditions, DVT is a radiographic diagnosis. Over 50% of DVTs are clinically silent, and even when symptoms are present, fewer than one third have the classic syndrome of calf discomfort, edema, and Homan's sign (pain on dorsiflexion of the foot) (Geerts et al., 1994; Kudsk et al., 1989). Therefore, diagnostic studies are required when DVT is suspected, and routine screening is necessary for early detection in high-risk trauma patients.

Venography is the most accurate test for detecting DVT. However, because it is invasive, painful, expensive, and involves potentially nephrotoxic contrast injection, its use as a screening tool is limited. The routine use of venography has been largely replaced by noninvasive methods (Reilly, 1998).

Duplex ultrasonography combines flow velocity and imaging modalities to detect the presence of thrombus, abnormal venous compressibility, or venous dilatation, all of which verify DVT. It is noninvasive, painless, portable, and 99% accurate (Woolson et al., 1990). Surveillance with serial duplex sonography identifies asymptomatic DVT in 10 to 21% of trauma patients, despite adequate prophylaxis (Burns, Cohn, Frumento, Degutis, & Hammers, 1993; Napolitano, et al., 1995). Its major weakness is its limited ability to detect thrombus in pelvic veins.

CT scanning and MRI can detect DVT in abdominal and pelvic veins. Both studies are considered superior to venography in imaging such large proximal veins (Reilly, 1998). Because both techniques are expensive and require patient transport, their use as screening tools is limited. Occasionally, DVT is diagnosed incidentally when abdominal or pelvic CT scanning is performed for other purposes.

Impedance plethysmography (IPG) detects limited venous capacitance and delayed venous outflow that are suggestive of DVT. Although its overall sensitivity and specificity are close to 90%, IPG is insensitive for nonobstructing and infrapopliteal thrombi, and its sensitivity in the trauma population remains questionable (Reilly, 1998).

For patients at high risk of DVT, surveillance duplex sonography should be performed within 48 hours of admission and every 5 to 7 days thereafter, and also when symptoms or signs develop that suggest DVT. Once detected, the goals of DVT treatment include facilitation of clot lysis, prevention of clot proliferation, reduction in the risk of PE, preservation of valve function, symptom relief, and prevention of recurrence.

The principle therapy for proximal and pelvic vein DVT is anticoagulation with heparin followed by warfarin. A partial thromboplastin time (PTT) of two times normal is the goal of heparin therapy. Warfarin is started once the PTT has reached the therapeutic level; an INR between 2.0 and 3.0 is the goal of warfarin therapy. A 3- to 6-month course of anticoagulation is recommended, but severe complications (e.g., subdural hematomas, hemothorax, heparin-induced thrombocytopenia) may develop requiring termination of therapy. Older patients (age > 55) are at greater risk for such complications (Brathwaite, Mure, O'Malley, Spence, & Ross, 1993).

When anticoagulation is contraindicated, such as for patients with ongoing bleeding, closed head injury or abdominal solid viscus injury managed nonoperatively, inferior vena cava (IVC) filter insertion is recommended to prevent PE. IVC filters *do not* prevent or treat DVT, but are 98% effective in preventing the occurrence of PE from lower extremity DVT. IVC filters should also be considered for proximal iliac DVTs, recurrent DVT or PE, PE despite adequate anticoagulation, and for elderly patients (EAST Trauma Practice Guidelines, 1997).

Patients with lower extremity DVT should be placed on bedrest until therapeutic PTT has been reached. Elevation of the leg and thigh-length elastic stockings are recommended to minimize swelling and provide symptom relief.

The therapy for calf vein (distal) DVT is controversial. If left untreated, calf DVTs may propagate proximally and become a risk for embolism. Untreated calf DVTs also may resolve without complications. The treatment decision is both patient and provider dependent; if no therapy is prescribed, follow-up duplex ultrasonography is necessary to detect proximal propagation and to ensure initial thrombus resolution (Reilly, 1998).

Pulmonary Embolus

The incidence of pulmonary embolism (PE) in the overall trauma population is less than 1%, but PE tragically causes sudden death in patients who have otherwise survived their injury (Tuttle-Newhall, Rutledge, Hultman, & Fakhry, 1997). In high-risk trauma patients (refer to Table 24–53), the incidence of PE may be as high as 9% (Rogers, Shackford, Wilson, Ricci, & Morris, 1993).

As with DVT, the cornerstone of management is prevention (Reilly, 1998). Despite the routine use of DVT prophylaxis, the risk of DVT and PE in severely injured trauma patients is significant (Winchell, Hoyt, Walsh, Simons, & Eastman, 1994). Patients without documented DVT but with certain high-risk injury complexes may benefit from prophylactic IVC filters to reduce the risk of PE (Rodriguez et al., 1996). Preliminary evidence suggests that patients who cannot receive anticoagulation and have one or more of the following injury patterns may benefit from prophylactic IVC filter insertion: recent brain injury, incomplete spinal cord injury with paraplegia or quadraplegia, complex pelvic fractures with associated long-bone fractures, multiple long-bone fractures, and major eye injury (EAST Trauma Practice Guidelines, 1997). The incidence of fatal PE in these patients is greater than the risk of short-term complications from IVC filters; however, the long-term consequences of vena cava filters are unknown (Patton et al., 1996).

The diagnosis of PE in the trauma patient is difficult; many patients die too quickly to allow for diagnosis and treatment. The most common signs and symptoms of PE—tachypnea, tachycardia, and hypoxemia—are often present in patients with thoracic injuries and with comorbidities such as atelectasis, pneumonia, and myocardial ischemia. A sudden decrease in PaO_2 without explanation is suspicious for PE (Reilly, 1998). Nonspecific ECG changes may include right axis deviation, right bundle branch block, Q waves in lead I, and inverted T waves. The chest x-ray may be normal or reveal only subtle findings such as Westermark's sign (a decrease in vascular markings). If a pul-

Bone, L., Johnson, K., Weigelt, J., et al. (1989). Early versus delayed stabilization of fractures: A prospective randomized study. *Journal of Bone and Joint Surgery, 71A,* 336.

Boone, D. C. & Peitzman, A. B. (1998). Abdominal injury. In A. B. Peitzman, M. Rhodes, C. W. Schwab, & D. M. Yealy (Eds.). *The trauma manual* (pp. 226–264). Philadelphia: Lippincott-Raven.

Borst, M. J. & Udekwu, A. O. (1998). Abdominal compartment syndrome. In A. B. Peitzman, M. Rhodes, C. W. Schwab, & D. M. Yealy (Eds.), *The trauma manual* (pp. 281–283). Philadelphia: Lippincott-Raven.

Boulanger, B. R., Brenneman, F. D., McLellan, B. A., Rizoli, S. B., Culhane, J., & Hamilton, P. (1995). A prospective study of emergent abdominal sonography after blunt trauma. *Journal of Trauma, 39* (2), 325–330.

Bouwman, D. L., Weaver, D. W., & Walt, A. J. (1984). Serum amylase and its isoenzymes: A clarification of their implications in trauma. *Journal of Trauma, 24* (7), 573–578.

Bracken, M. B., Shepard, M. J., Collins, W. F., Holford, T. R., Young, W., Baskin, D. S., Eisenberg, H. M., Flamm, E., Leo-Summers, L., Maroon, J., Marshall, L. F., Perot, P. L., Piepmeier, J., Sonntag, V. K. H., Wagner, F. C., Wilberger, J. E., & Winn, H. R. (1990). A randomized, controlled trial of methylprednisolone or naloxone in the treatment of acute spinal-cord injury. *New England Journal of Medicine, 322* (20), 1405–1411.

Bracken, M. B., Shepard, M. J., Holford, T. R., Leo-Summers, L., Aldrich, E. F., Fazi, M., Fehlings, M., Herr, D. L., Hitchon, P. W., Marshall, L. F., Nockels, R. P., Pascale, V., Perot, P. L., Piepmeier, J., Sonntag, V. K. H., Wagner, F. C., Wilberger, J. E., Winn, H. R., & Young, W. (1997). Administration of methylprednisolone for 24 or 48 hours or tirilizad mesylate for 48 hours in the treatment of acute spinal cord injury. *Journal of the American Medical Association, 277* (20), 1597–1604.

Brain Trauma Foundation, American Association of Neurological Surgeons, and Joint Section on Neurotrauma and Critical Care. (1995). *Guidelines for the management of severe head injury.*

Brathwaite, C. E., Mure, A. J., O'Malley, K. F., Spence, R. K., & Ross, S. E. (1993). Complications of anticoagulation for pulmonary embolism in low risk trauma patients. *Chest, 104* (3), 718.

Buckmaster, M. J., Kearney, P. A., Johnson, S. B., Smith, M. D., & Sapin, P. M. (1994). Further experience with transesophageal echocardiography in the evaluation of thoracic aortic injury. *Journal of Trauma, 37* (6), 989–995.

Bull, J. P. (1975). The injury severity score of road traffic casualties in relation to mortality, time of death, hospital treatment time and disability. *Accident Analysis and Prevention, 7,* 249.

Burch, J. M. (1996). Injury to the colon and rectum. In D. V. Feliciano, E. E. Moore, & K. L. Mattox (Eds.), *Trauma* (3rd ed.). (pp. 595–614). Stamford, CT: Appleton & Lange.

Burgess, A. R., Dischinger, P. C., O'Quinn, T. D., & Schmidhauser, C. B. (1995). Lower extremity injuries in drivers of airbag-equipped automobiles: Clinical and crash reconstruction correlations. *Journal of Trauma, 38* (4), 509–516.

Burney, R. E., Maio, R. F., Maynard F., & Karunas, R. (1993). Incidence, characteristics, and outcome of spinal cord injury at trauma centers in North America. *Archives of Surgery, 128* (5), 596–599.

Burns, G. A., Cohn, S. M., Frumento, R. K., Degutis, L. C., & Hammers, L. (1993). Prospective ultrasound evaluation of venous thrombosis in high-risk trauma patients. *Journal of Trauma, 35*(3), 405–407.

Bynoe, R. P., Bell, R. M., Miles, W. S., Close, T. P., Ross, M. A., & Fine, J. G. (1992). Complications of non-operative management of blunt hepatic injuries. *Journal of Trauma, 32* (3), 308–315.

Cardona, V. D., Hurn, P. O., Bastnagel-Mason, P. J., Scanlon-Schilpp, A. M., & Veise-Berry, S. W. (Eds.). (1988). *Trauma nursing: From resuscitation through rehabilitation.* (p. 118). Philadelphia: W. B. Saunders.

Carter, B. N. & Giuseffi, J. (1951). Traumatic diaphragmatic hernia. *American Journal of Roentgenology, 65,* 56.

Champion, H. R., Sacco, W. J., & Copes, W.S. (1996). Trauma scoring. In D. V. Feliciano, E. E. Moore, & K. L. Mattox (Eds.), *Trauma* (3rd ed.). (pp. 53–68). Stamford, CT: Appleton & Lange.

Champion, H. R., Sacco, W. J., Carnazzo, A. J., Copes, W., & Fouty, W. J. (1981). Trauma score. *Critical Care Medicine, 9* (9), 672–676.

Champion, H. R., Sacco, W. J., Copes, W. S., Gann, D. S., Genarelli, T., & Flanagan, M. E. (1989). A revision of the trauma score. *Journal of Trauma, 29* (5), 623–629.

Chan, R. N. W., Ainscow, D., & Sikorski, J. M. (1980). Diagnostic failures in the multiple injured. *Journal of Trauma, 20* (8), 684–687.

Chapman, M. W. & Olson, S. A. (1996). Open fractures. In C. A. Rockwood, D. P. Green, R. W. Bucholz, & J. D. Heckman (Eds.), *Rockwood and Green's fractures in adults* (4th ed.). (p. 309), Philadelphia: Lippincott-Raven.

Chen, S., Markmann, J. F., Kauder, D. R., & Schwab, C. W. (1997). Hemothorax missed by auscultation in penetrating chest injury. *Journal of Trauma, 42* (1), 86–89.

Cheng, D. L., Lazan, D., & Stone, N. (1994). Conservative treatment of type III renal trauma. *Journal of Trauma, 36* (4), 491–494.

Chestnut, R. M., Marshall, L. F., Klauber, M. R., Blunt, B. A., Baldwin, N., Eisenberg, H. M., Jane, J. A., Marmarou, A., & Foulkes, M. A. (1993). The role of secondary brain injury in determining outcome from severe head injury. *Journal of Trauma, 34* (2), 216–222.

Chiles, B. W. & Cooper, P. R. (1996). Acute spinal injury. *New England Journal of Medicine, 334* (8), 514–520.

Christiansen, C. H., Schwartz, R. K., & Barnes, K. J. (1993). Self-care: Evaluation and management. In J. A. DeLisa & B. M. Gans (Eds.), *Rehabilitation medicine: Principles and practice.* (2nd ed.). (pp. 186–187). Philadelphia: J. B. Lippincott.

Cipolle, M. D. (1998). Blunt neck injury. In A. B. Peitzman, M. Rhodes, C. W. Schwab, & D. M. Yealy (Eds.), *The trauma manual* (pp. 195–198). Philadelphia: Lippincott-Raven.

Ciraulo, D. L., Nikkanen, H. E., Palter, M., Markowitz, S., Gabram, S., Cowell, V., Luk, S., & Lenworth, J. (1996). Clinical analysis of the utility of repeat computed tomographic scan before discharge in blunt hepatic injury. *Journal of Trauma, 41* (5), 821–824.

Clark, W. R. (1992). Smoke inhalation: Diagnosis and treatment. *World Journal of Surgery, 16,* 24–29.

Coben, J. H. (1998). Injury prevention/epidemiology. In A. B. Peitzman, M. Rhodes, C. W. Schwab, & D. M. Yealy (Eds.), *The trauma manual* (pp. 473–476). Philadelphia: Lippincott-Raven.

Cogbill, T. H, & Landerscaper, J. (1996). Injury to the chest wall. In D. V. Feliciano, E. E. Moore, & K. L. Mattox (Eds.), *Trauma* (3rd ed.). (pp. 355–374). Stamford, CT: Appleton & Lange.

Collincott, P. E. (1991) Initial assessment of the trauma patient. In E. E. Moore, K. L. Mattox, & D. V. Feliciano (Eds.), *Trauma* (2nd ed.). (pp. 109–125). East Norwalk, CT: Appleton & Lange.

Colohan, A. R., Pitts, L. H., & Rosegay, H. (1996). Injury to the peripheral nerves. In D. V. Feliciano, E. E. Moore & K. L. Mattox (Eds.), *Trauma* (3rd ed.). (pp. 853–864). Stamford, CT: Appleton & Lange.

Committee on Trauma, American College of Surgeons. (1993). Shock. *Advanced Trauma Life Support Manual,* pp. 75–94.

Cook, D. J., Fuller, H. D., Guyatt, G. H., Marshall, J. C., Leasa D., Hall, R., Winton, T. L., Rutledge, F., Todd, T. J., & Roy, P. (1994). Risk factors for gastrointestinal bleeding in critically ill patients. *New England Journal of Medicine, 330* (6), 377–381.

Cooper, C., Dunham, C. M., & Rodriguez, A. (1995). Falls and major injuries are risk factors for thoracolumbar fractures: Cognitive impairment and multiple injuries impede the detection of back pain and tenderness. *Journal of Trauma, 38* (5), 692–696.

Copes, W. S., Champion, H. R., Sacco, W. J., Lawnick, M. M., Keast, S. L., & Bain, L. W. (1988). The injury severity score revisited. *Journal of Trauma, 28* (1), 69–77.

Croce, M. A., Dent, D. L., Menke, P. G., Robertson, J. T., Hinson, M. S., Young, B. H., Donovan, T. B., Pritchard, F. E., Minard, G., Kudsk, K. A., & Fabian, T. C. (1994). Acute subdural hematoma: Nonsurgical management of selected patients. *Journal of Trauma, 36* (6), 820–827.

Cryer, H. G. & Johnson, E. E. (1996). Pelvic fractures. In D. V. Feliciano, E. E. Moore, & K. L. Mattox (Eds.), *Trauma* (3rd ed.). (pp. 635–660). Stamford, CT: Appleton & Lange.

Cue, J. I., Miller, F. B., Cryer, H. M., Malangoni, M. A., & Richardson, J. D. (1990). A prospective, randomized comparison between open and closed peritoneal lavage techniques. *Journal of Trauma, 30* (7), 880–883.

Dacey, R. G., Alves, W. M., Rimel, R. W., Winn, H. R., & Jane, J. A. (1986). Neurosurgical complications after apparently minor head injury—Assessment of risk in a series of 610 patients. *Journal of Neurosurgery, 65* (2), 203–210.

Davis, F. E. (1997). The evolution of ultrasound as a diagnostic modality for evaluation of the abdomen in blunt-injured patients. *Trauma Quarterly, 13* (2), 155–171.

Davis, J. W., Parks, S. N., Detlefs, C. L., Williams, G. G., Williams, J. L., & Smith, R. W. (1995). Clearing the cervical spine in obtunded patients: The use of dynamic fluoroscopy. *Journal of Trauma, 39* (3), 435–438.

Davis, J. W., Parks, S. N., Kaups, K. L., Gladen, H. E., & O'Donnell-Nicol, S. (1996). Admission base deficit predicts transfusion requirements and risk of complications. *Journal of Trauma, 41* (5), 769–774.

Davis, J. W., Shackford, S. R., Mackersie, R. C., & Hoyt, D. B. (1988). Base deficit as a guide to volume resuscitation. *Journal of Trauma, 28* (10), 1464–1467.

Demetriades, D., Charalambides, D., & Lakhoo, M. (1993). Physical examination and selective conservative management in patients with penetrating injuries of the neck. *British Journal of Surgery, 80,* 1534–1536.

Dennis, J. W., Jagger, C., Butcher, L., Menawat, S. S., Neel, M., & Frykberg, E. R. (1993). Reassessing the role of arteriograms in the management of posterior knee dislocations. *Journal of Trauma, 35* (5), 692–697.

Dennis, J. W., Menawat, S., Von Thron, J., Fallon, W. F., Vinsant, G. O., Laneve, L. M., Jagger, C., & Frykberg, E. R. (1993). Efficacy of deep venous thrombosis prophylaxis in trauma patients and identification of high-risk groups. *Journal of Trauma, 35* (1), 132–139.

Durham, R. M., Neunaber, K., Mazuski, J. E., Shapiro, M. J., & Baue, A. E. (1996). The use of oxygen consumption and delivery as endpoints for resuscitation in critically ill patients. *Journal of Trauma, 41* (1), 32–40.

Duus, B. R., Boesen, T., Kruse, K. V., & Nielsen, K. B. (1993). Prognostic signs in the evaluation of patients with minor head injury. *British Journal of Surgery, 80* (8), 988–991.

Duus, B. R., Lind, B., Christensen, H., & Nielsen, O. A. (1994). The role of neuroimaging in the initial management of patients with minor head injury. *Annals of Emergency Medicine, 23* (6), 1279–1283.

Eastern Association for the Surgery of Trauma (EAST). (1997). The role of the vena cava filter in the prophylaxis and treatment of PE. From the World Wide Web: www.east.org.

Enderson, B. L & Maull, K. I. (1991). Missed injuries: The trauma surgeon's nemesis. *Surgical Clinics of North America, 71,* 399–418.

Enderson, B. L., Reath, D. B., Meadors, J., Dallas, W., DeBoo, J., & Maull, K. I. (1990). The tertiary trauma survey: A prospective study of missed injury. *Journal of Trauma, 30* (6), 666–669.

Engelman, D. T., Gabram, S. G. A., Allen, L., Ens, G. E., & Jacobs, L. M. (1996). Hypergoagulability following multiple trauma. *World Journal of Surgery, 20* (1), 5–10.

Esposito, T. J. & Gamelli, R. L. (1996). Injury to the spleen. In D. V. Feliciano, E. E. Moore & K. L. Mattox (Eds.), *Trauma* (3rd ed.). (pp. 525–550). Stamford, CT: Appleton & Lange.

Evins, S. C., Thomason, W. B., & Rosenblum R. (1980). Nonoperative management of severe renal lacerations. *Journal of Urology, 123,* 247.

Fabian, T. C. & Croce, M. A. (1996). Abdominal trauma, including indications for celiotomy. In D. V. Feliciano, E. E. Moore, & K. L. Mattox (Eds.), *Trauma* (3rd ed.). (pp. 441–486). Stamford, CT: Appleton & Lange.

Fearnside, M. R., Cook, R. J., McDougall, P., & McNeil, R. J. (1993). The Westmead Head Injury Project outcome in severe head injury. A comparative analysis of prehospital, clinical, and CT variables. *British Journal of Neurosurgery, 7* (3), 267–279.

Feliciano, D. V. (1991). Diagnostic modalities in abdominal trauma. Peritoneal lavage, ultrasonography, computerized tomography scanning, and arteriography. *Surgical Clinics of North America, 71* (2), 241–256.

Feliciano, D. V. (1996). Patterns of Injury. In D. V. Feliciano, E. E. Moore, & K. L. Mattox (Eds.), *Trauma* (3rd ed.). (pp. 85–104). Stamford, CT: Appleton & Lange.

Feliciano, D. V., Moore, E. E., & Mattox, K. L. (1996). Damage control and alternate wound closures in abdominal trauma. In D. V. Feliciano, E. E. Moore, & K. L. Mattox (Eds.), *Trauma* (3rd ed.). (pp. 717–732). Stamford, CT: Appleton & Lange.

Frankel, H. L., Rozycki, G. S., Ochsner, G., Harviel, J. D., & Champion, H.R. (1994). Indications for obtaining surveillance thoracic and lumbar spine radiographs. *Journal of Trauma, 37* (4), 673–676.

Gable, D. R., Allen, J. W., & Richardson, J. D. (1997). Blunt popliteal artery injury: Is physical examination alone enough for evaluation? *Journal of Trauma, 43* (3), 541–544.

Geerts, W. H., Code, K. I., Jay, R. M., Chan, E., & Szalai, J. P. (1994). A prospective study of venous thromboembolism after major trauma. *New England Journal of Medicine, 331* (24), 1601–1606.

Geerts, W. H., Jay, R. M., Code, K. I., Chen, E., Szalai, J. P., Saibil, E. A., & Hamilton, P. A. (1996). A comparison of low-dose heparin with low-molecular weight heparin as prophylaxis against venous thromboembolism after major trauma. *New England Journal of Medicine, 335* (10), 701–707.

Gennarelli, T. A., Champion, H. R., Copes, W. S., & Sacco, W. J. (1994). Comparison of mortality, morbidity, and severity of 59,713 head injured patients with 114,447 patients with extracranial injuries. *Journal of Trauma, 37* (6), 962–968.

Georgiadis, G. M. & Wilson, R. F. (1996). Musculoskeletal trauma. In R. F. Wilson & A. J. Walt (Eds.), *Management of trauma: Pitfalls and practice* (2nd ed.). (pp. 643–671). Baltimore: Williams & Wilkens.

Gordon, M. & Goodwin, C. W. (1997). Initial assessment, management, and stabilization. *Nursing Clinics of North America, 32,* 237–249.

Gossling, J. R. & Pellegrini, V. D. (1982). Fat embolism syndrome: A review of the pathophysiology and physiologic basis of treatment. *Clinical Orthopedics, 165,* 68–82.

Greenfield, E. & Jordan B. (1996). Advances in burn wound care. *Critical Care Nursing Clinics of North America, 8* (2), 203–215.

Greenfield E. & McManus, A. T. (1997). Infectious complications: Prevention and strategies for their control. *Nursing Clinics of North America, 32,* 297–309.

Greenfield, E. & Quinn, D. M. DeFazio (Eds.). (1997). *The nursing clinics of North America.* (p. 262). Philadelphia: W. B. Saunders.

Gross, K. B., Koets, M. H., D'Arcy, J. B., Chan, T. L., Wooley, R. G., & Basha, M. A. (1995). Mechanism of induction of asthmatic attacks initiated by the inhalation of particles generated by airbag system deployment. *Journal of Trauma, 38* (4), 521–527.

Gruen, G. S., Leit, M. E., Gruen, R. J., & Peitzman, A. B. (1994). The acute management of hemodynamically unstable multiple trauma patients with pelvic ring fractures. *Journal of Trauma, 36* (5), 706–711.

Gutierrez, G. & Brown, S. D. (1996). Gastrointestinal tonometry: A monitor of regional dysoxia. *New Horizons, 4,* 413.

Harkness, J. W., Ramsey, W. C., & Harkness, J. W. (1996). Principles of fractures and dislocations. In C. A. Rockwood, D. P. Green, R. W. Bucholz, & J. D. Heckman (Eds.), *Fractures in adults* (4th ed.). (pp. 3–120). Philadelphia: Lippincott-Raven.

Haskell, R. M., Boruta, B., Rotondo, M. F., & Frankel, H. L. (1997). Hypothermia. *AACN Clinical Issues: Advanced Practice in Acute and Critical Care, 8* (3), 368–382.

Highland, T., Salcieeioli, G., & Wilson, R. F. (1996). In R. F. Wilson & A. J. Walt (Eds.), Management of trauma: Pitfalls and practice (2nd ed.). (p. 210). Baltimore: Williams & Wilkens.

Highway Loss Data Institute. (1996). Addressing the risks from airbag inflation for infants, children, and short drivers. In K. Stewart (Ed.), *Insurance institute for highway safety advisory.* Arlington, VA.

Hinkle, J. & Betz, S. (1995). Gunshot injuries. *AACN Clinical Issues, 6* (2), 175–186.

Hirshberg, A., Wall, M. J., & Mattox, K. L (1994). Planned reoperation for trauma: A two year experience with 124 patients. *Journal of Trauma, 37* (3), 365–369.

Holbrook, J. L. & Bennett, J. B. (1990). Brachial plexus injury associated with chest restraint seatbelts: Case report. *Journal of Trauma, 30* (11), 1413–1414.

Hood, R. M. (1971). Traumatic diaphragmatic hernia. *Annals of Thoracic Surgery, 12,* 311.

Huelke, D. F., Moore, J. L., Compton, T. W., Samuels, J., & Levine, R. S. (1995). Upper extremity injuries related to airbag deployments. *Journal of Trauma, 38* (4), 482–488.

Hunt, D. M. & Schwab, F. J. (1992). Chest trauma. In P. Rosen (Ed.), *Diagnostic radiology in emergency medicine* (p. 77). St. Louis: Mosby.

Insurance Institute for Highway Safety. (1996). *Status Report, 30* (3).

Ivatury, R. R. (1996). Injury to the heart. In D. V. Feliciano, E. E. Moore, & K. L. Mattox (Eds.), *Trauma* (3rd ed.). (pp. 409–422). Stamford, CT: Appleton & Lange.

Ivatury, R. R., Simon, R. J., Islam, S., et al. (1996). A prospective randomized study of end points of resuscitation after major trauma: Global oxygen transport indices versus organ-specific gastric mucosal pH. *Journal of the American College of Surgery, 183,* 145.

Ivatury, R. R., Simon, R. J., Stahl, W. M. (1993). A critical evaluation of laparoscopy in penetrating abdominal trauma. *Journal of Trauma, 34* (6), 822–827.

Jaffin, J. H., Ochsner, M. G., Cole, F. J., Rozycki, G. S., Kass, M., & Champion, H. R. (1993). Alkaline phosphatase levels in diagnostic peritoneal lavage fluid as a predictor of hollow visceral injury. *Journal of Trauma, 34* (6), 829.

Jerrard, D. A. (1993). *Emergency medicine clinics of North America, (11),* p. 148. Philadelphia: W. B. Saunders.

Johansen, K., Daines, M., Howey, T., et al. (1990). Objective criteria accurately predict amputation following lower extremity trauma. *Journal of Trauma, 30,* 568.

Johansen, K., Lynch, K., Paun, M., & Copass, M. (1991). Non-invasive vascular tests reliably exclude occult arterial trauma in injured extremities. *Journal of Trauma, 31* (4), 515.

Johnson, M. L. (1998). Penetrating neck trauma. In A. B. Peitzman, M. Rhodes, C. W. Schwab, & D. M. Yealy (Eds.), *The trauma manual* (pp. 187–194). Philadelphia: Lippincott-Raven.

Jordan, B. S. & Harrington, D. T. (1997). Management of the burn wound. *Nursing Clinics of North America, 32,* 251–273.

Jurkovich, G. J. (1996). Injury to the duodenum and pancreas. In D. V. Feliciano, E. E. Moore, & K. L. Mattox (Eds.), *Trauma* (3rd ed.). (pp. 573–594). Stamford, CT: Appleton & Lange.

Jurkovich, G. J. & Carrico, C. J. (1997). Management of the acutely injured patient. In D. C. Sabiston & H.K. Lyerly (Eds.), *Textbook of surgery* (15th ed.). (pp. 296–339). Philadelphia: W. B. Saunders.

Jurkovich, G. J., Greiser, W. B., Luterman, A., & Curreri, P. W. (1987). Hypothermia in trauma victims: An ominous predictor of survival. *Journal of Trauma, 27* (9), 1019–1021, 1027.

Kane, J. M. (1998). Compartment syndrome. In A. B. Peitzman, M. Rhodes, C. W. Schwab, & D. M. Yealy (Eds.), *The trauma manual* (pp. 331–334). Philadelphia: Lippincott-Raven.

Kauder, D. R. (1998). Burns/inhalational injury. In A. B. Peitzman, M. Rhodes, C. W. Schwab, & D. M. Yealy (Eds.), *The trauma manual* (pp. 423–430). Philadelphia: Lippincott-Raven.

Kauder, D. R., Schwab, C. W., & Rotondo, M. F. (1996). In R. R. Ivatury & C. G. Cayten (Eds.), The textbook of penetrating trauma. (p. 721). Baltimore: Williams & Wilkins.

Kearney, P. A., Smith, D. W., Johnson, S. B., Barker, D. E., Smith, M. D., & Sapin, P. M. (1993). Use of transesophogeal echocardiography in the evaluation of traumatic aortic injury. *Journal of Trauma, 34* (5), 696.

Kellerman, A. L. & Todd, K. H. (1996). Prevention. In D. V. Feliciano, E. E. Moore & K. L. Mattox (Eds.), *Trauma* (3rd Ed., pp. 31–40). Stamford, CT: Appleton & Lange.

Kennedy, F., Gonzalez, P., Dang, C., Fleming, A. & Sterling-Scott, R. (1993). The Glasgow coma scale and prognosis in gunshot wounds to the brain. *Journal of Trauma, 35* (1), 75–77.

Kilberg, L., Clemmer, T. P. & Claussen, J. (1988). Effectiveness of implementing a trauma triage system on outcome: A prospective evaluation. *Journal of Trauma, 10* ( ), 1493.

Kluger, Y., Paul, D. B., Raves, J. J., Fonda, M., Young, J. C., Townsend, R. N., & Diamond, D. L. (1994). Delayed rupture of the spleen—Myths, facts, and their importance: Case reports and literature review. *Journal of Trauma, 36* (4), 568–571.

Knudson, M. M., Lewis, F. R., Clinton, A., Atkinson, K., & Megerman, J. (1994). Prevention of venous thromboembolism in trauma patients. *Journal of Trauma, 37* (3), 480–487.

Knudson, M. M., McAninch, J. W., Gomez, R., Lee, P., & Stubbs, H. A. (1992). Hematuria as a predictor of abdominal injury after blunt trauma. *American Journal of Surgery, 164,* 482–486.

Knudson, M. M., Morabito, D., Paiement, G. D., & Shackleford, S. (1996). Use of low molecular weight heparin in preventing thromboembolism in trauma patients. *Journal of Trauma, 41* (3), 446–459.

Krantz, B. E. (1996). Initial assessment. In D. V. Feliciano, E. E. Moore & K. L. Mattox (Eds.), *Trauma* (3rd ed.). (pp. 123–140). Stamford, CT: Appleton & Lange.

Kshettry, V. R. & Bolman, R. M. (1994). Chest trauma. *Clinics in Chest Medicine, 15* (1), 137–146.

Kudsk, K. A., Fabian, T. C., Baum, S., et al. (1989). Silent deep vein thrombosis in immobilized trauma patients. *American Journal of Surgery, 158,* 515.

Kuhlmann, R. S. & Cruikshank, D. P. (1994). Maternal trauma during pregnancy. *Clinical Obstetrics and Gynecology, 37* (2), 274–293.

Latenser, B. A., Gentilello, L. M., Tarver, A. A., Thalgott, J. S., & Batdorf, J. W. (1991). Improved outcome with early fixation of skeletally unstable pelvic fractures. *Journal of Trauma, 31* (1), 28–31.

Lebos, M. R. & Saadia, R. (1994). The overlooked blunt component in penetrating neck injuries: Three case reports. *Journal of Trauma, 36* (3), 410–411.

Leit, M. E. & Gruen, G. S. (1998). Pelvic fractures. In A. B. Peitzman, M. Rhodes, C. W. Schwab, & D. M. Yealy (Eds.), *The trauma manual.* (pp. 307–314). Philadelphia: Lippincott-Raven.

Levitt, M. A., Sutton, M., Goldman, J., Mikhail, M., & Christopher, T. (1994). Cognitive dysfunction in patients suffering minor head trauma. *American Journal of Emergency Medicine, 12* (2), 172–175.

Levy, M. L., Gans, W., Wijesinghe, H. S., SooHoo, W. E., Adkins, R. H., & Stillerman, C. B. (1996). Use of methylprednisolone as an adjunct in the management of patients with penetrating spinal cord injury: Outcome analysis. *Neurosurgery, 39* (6), 1141–1148.

LoCicero III, J. & Mattox, K. L. (1989). Epidemiology of chest trauma. *Surgical Clinics of North America, 69,* 15.

Loo, G. T., Siegel, J. H., Dischinger, P. C., Rixen, D., Burgess, A. R., Addis, M. D., O'Quinn, T., McCammon, L., Schmidhauser, C. B., Marsh, P., Hodge, P. A., & Bents, F. (1996). Airbag protection versus compartment intrusion effect determines the pattern of injuries in multiple trauma motor vehicle crashes. *Journal of Trauma, 41* (6), 935–951.

Luna, G. K., Maier, R. V., Paulin, A. G., Anardi, D., Copass, M. K., & Oreskovich, M. (1987). Incidence and effect of hypothermia in seriously injured patients. *Journal of Trauma, 27,* 1014–1018.

Lund, A. K. & Ferguson, S. A. (1995). Driver fatalities in 1985-1993 cars with airbags. *Journal of Trauma, 38* (4), 469–475.

Mabee, J. R. (1993). Compartment syndrome: a complication of acute extremity trauma. *Journal of Emergency Medicine, 12* (5), 651–656.

Mabee, J. R. & Bostwick, T. L. (1993). Pathophysiology and mechanisms of compartment syndrome. *Orthopaedic Review, Feb,* 175–181.

Maier, R. V., Mitchell, D., & Gentilello, L. (1994). Optimal therapy for stress gastritis. *Annals of Surgery, 220,* 353–360.

Mansour, M. A., Moore, E. E., Moore, F. A., & Whitehill, T. A. (1991). Validating the selective management of penetrating neck trauma. *American Journal of Surgery, 162* (6), 517–521.

Marion, D. W. (1998a). Head injury. In A. B. Peitzman, M. Rhodes, C. W. Schwab, & D. M. Yealy (Eds.), *The trauma manual.* (pp. 134–141). Philadelphia: Lippincott-Raven.

Marion, D. W. (1998b). Injuries of the spinal cord and spinal column. In A. B. Peitzman, M. Rhodes, C. W. Schwab, & D. M. Yealy (Eds.), *The trauma manual.* (pp. 142–155). Philadelphia: Lippincott-Raven.

Martinez, R., Sharieff, G., & Hooper, J. (1994). Three-point restraints as a risk factor for chest injury in the elderly. *Journal of Trauma, 37* (6), 980–984.

Mattox, K. L. & Wall Jr., M. J. (1996). Injury to the great thoracic vessels. In D. V. Feliciano, E. E. Moore, & K. L. Mattox (Eds.), *Trauma* (3rd ed.). (pp. 423–440). Stamford, CT: Appleton & Lange.

Mattox, K. L., Hirshberg, A., & Wall, M. J. (1996). Alternate approaches to resuscitation. In R. R. Ivatury & C.G. Cayten (Eds.), *Textbook of penetrating trauma.* (p. 195). Baltimore: Williams & Wilkins.

Maull, K. I., Rodriguez, A., & Wiles, C. E. (1996). Preface. In K. I. Maull, A. Rodriguez, & C. E. Wiles (Eds.), *Complications in trauma and critical care.* (p. xiii). Philadelphia: W. B. Saunders.

McCormick, T. M. & Burch, B. H. (1979). Routine angiographic evaluation of neck and extremity injuries. *Journal of Trauma, 19* (5), 384.

McLaughlin, M. R. & Marion, D. W. (1996). Cerebral blood flow and vasoresponsivity within and around cerebral contusions. *Journal of Neurosurgery, 85* (5), 871–876.

McManus, W. F. & Pruitt Jr., B. A. (1996). Thermal injuries. In D. V. Feliciano, E. E. Moore, & K. L. Mattox (Eds.), *Trauma* (3rd ed.). (pp. 937–950). Stamford, CT: Appleton & Lange.

McSwain, N. E. (1996). Ballistics. In R. R. Ivatury & C. G. Cayten (Eds.), *The textbook of penetrating trauma.* (pp. 105–120). Baltimore: Williams and Wilkins.

Meredith, J. W., Young, J. S., Bowling, J., & Roboussin, D.

(1994). Nonoperative management of blunt hepatic trauma; The exception or the rule? *Journal of Trauma, 36* (4), 529–535.

Miller, F. B., Richardson, J. D., & Thomas, H. A. (1989). Role of CT in the diagnosis of major arterial injury after blunt thoracic trauma. *Surgery, 106,* 596.

Miller, J. D. & Becker, D. P. (1982). Secondary insults to the injured brain. *Journal of the Royal College of Surgery, 27,* 292–298.

Miller, J. D., Sweet, R. C., Narayan, R., & Becker, D. P. (1978). Early insults to the injured brain. *Journal of the American Medical Association, 240* (5), 439–442.

Miller, L., Bennett, E. V., Root, H. D., Trinkle, J. K., & Grover, F. L. (1984). Management of penetrating and blunt diaphragmatic injury. *Journal of Trauma, 24* (5), 403–409.

Minard, G., Schurr, M. J., Croce, M. A., Gavant, M. L., Kudsk, K. A., Taylor, M. J., Pritchard, F. E., & Fabian, T. C. (1996). A prospective analysis of transesophageal echocardiography in the diagnosis of traumatic disruption of the aorta. *Journal of Trauma, 40* (2), 225–230.

Moore, E. E., Cogbill, T. H., Jurkovich, G. J., Shackford, S. R., Malangoni, M. A., & Champion, H. R. (1989). Organ injury scaling: Spleen, liver, and kidney. *Journal of Trauma, 29* (12), 1664.

Moore, E. E., Cogbill, T. H., Jurkovich, G. J., Shackford, S. R., Malangoni, M. A., & Champion, H. R. (1994). Organ injury scaling: Spleen and liver (1994 revision). *Journal of Trauma, 38* (3), 323–324.

Moore, E. E., Mattox, K. L., & Feliciano, D. V. (Eds.). (1991). *Trauma,* (2nd ed.). (p. 90). Norwalk, CT: Appleton & Lange.

Moran, S. G., McCarthy, M. C., Uddin, D. E., & Poelstra, R. J. (1994). Predictors of positive CT scans in the trauma patient with minor head injury. *American Surgeon, 60* (7), 533–535.

Morris Jr., J. A., Limbird, T. J., & MacKenzie, E. (1996). Rehabilitation of the trauma patient. In D. V. Feliciano, E. E. Moore & K. L. Mattox (Eds.), *Trauma* (3rd ed.). (pp. 1013–1022). Stamford, CT: Appleton & Lange.

Muizelaar, J. P., Marmarou, A., Ward, J. D., Kontos, H. A., Choi, S. C., Becker, D. P., Gruemer, H., & Young, H. F. (1991). Adverse effects of prolonged hyperventilation in patients with severe head injury. *Journal of Neurosurgery, 75* (5), 731–739.

Mullins, R. J. (1996). Management of shock. In D. V. Feliciano, E. E. Moore, & K. L. Mattox (Eds.), *Trauma* (3rd ed.). (pp. 159–180). Stamford, CT: Appleton & Lange.

Nahum, A. M., Gadd, C. W., Schneider, D. C., & Kroell, C. K. (1971). The biomechanical basis for chest impact protection: I. Force-deflection characteristics of the thorax. *Journal of Trauma, 11* (10), 874–882.

Nance, M. L., Peden, G. W., Shapiro, M. B., Kauder, D. K., Rotondo, M. F., & Schwab, C. W. (1997). Solid viscus injury predicts major hollow viscus injury in blunt abdominal trauma. *Journal of Trauma, 43* (4), 618–623.

Napolitano, L. M., Garlapati, V. S., Heard, S. O., Silva, W. E., Cutler, B. S., O'Neill, A. M., Anderson, F. A., & Wheeler, H. B. (1995). Asymptomatic deep venous thrombosis in the trauma patient: Is an aggressive screening protocol justified? *Journal of Trauma, 39* (4), 651–659.

National Center for Health Statistics. (1997). Health, United States, 1996–1997 and injury chartbook.

Ochsner, M. G. (1997). The basic abdominal ultrasound exam for the presence of fluid in the abdomen. *Trauma Quarterly, 13* (2), 173–189.

Ochsner, M. G., Rozycki, G. S., Lucente, F., Wherry, D. C., & Champion, H. R. (1993). Prospective evaluation of thoracoscopy for diagnosing diaphragmatic injury in thoracoabdominal trauma: A preliminary report. *Journal of Trauma, 34* (5), 704–710.

Ordog, G. J., Balasubramanium, S., Wasserberger, J., Kram, H., Bishop, M., & Shoemaker, W. (1994). Extremity gunshot wounds: Part one—Identification and treatment of patients at high risk of vascular injury. *Journal of Trauma, 36* (3), 358–368.

Ordog, G. J., Wasserberger, J., & Balasubramaniam, S. (1988). Shotgun wound ballistics. *Journal of Trauma, 28* (5), 624–631.

Osler, T., Baker, S. P., & Long, W. (1997). A modification of the injury severity score that both improves accuracy and simplifies scoring. *Journal of Trauma, 43* (6), 922–926.

Pachter, H. L. & Hofstetter, S. R. (1981). Open and percutaneous paracentesis and lavage for abdominal trauma. *Archives of Surgery, 116* (3), 318.

Pachter, H. L., Knudson, M. M., Esrig, B., Ross, S., Hoyt, D., Cogbill, T., Sherman, H., Scalea, T., Harrison, P., Shackford, S., Ochsner, G. & Mucha, P. (1996). Status of nonoperative management of blunt hepatic injuries in 1995: A multicenter experience with 404 patients. *Journal of Trauma, 40* (1), 31–34.

Pachter, H. L., Liang, H. G. & Hofstetter, S. R. (1996). Liver and biliary tract trauma. In D. V. Feliciano, E. E. Moore & K. L. Mattox (Eds.), *Trauma* (3rd Ed.), (pp. 487–524). Stamford, CT: Appleton & Lange.

Pal, J., Brown, R. & Fleiszer, D. (1989). The value of the Glasgow coma scale and injury severity score: Predicting outcome in multiple patients with head injury. *Journal of Trauma, 29* (6), 746–748.

Patel, A. & Getsos, J. (1994). Osborn waves of hypothermia. *New England Journal of Medicine, 330,* p. 680.

Patton, J. H., Fabian, T. C., Croce, M. A., Minard, G., Pritchard, F. E. & Kudsk, K. A. (1996). Prophylactic Greenfield filters: acute complications and long-term follow-up. *Journal of Trauma, 41* (2), 231–237.

Peitzman, A. B., Makaroun, M. S., Slasky, B. S., & Ritter, P. (1986). Prospective study of computed tomography in initial management of blunt abdominal trauma. *Journal of Trauma, 26* (7), 585–592.

Peitzman, A. B., Rhodes, M., Schwab, C. W., & Yealy, D. M. (Eds). (1998). *The trauma manual,* (p. 143). Philadelphia: Lippencott-Raven.

Peterson, N. E. (1996). Genitourinary trauma. In D. V. Feliciano, E. E. Moore & K. L. Mattox (Eds.), *Trauma* (3rd ed.). (pp. 661–694). Stamford, CT: Appleton & Lange.

Powell, M. A., McMahon, D., & Peitzman, A. B. (1998). Thoracic injury. In A. B. Peitzman, M. Rhodes, C. W. Schwab, & D. M. Yealy (Eds.), *The trauma manual.* (pp. 187–194). Philadelphia: Lippincott-Raven.

Przybylski, G. & Marion, D. W. (1996). Injury to the vertebrae and spinal cord. In D. V. Feliciano, E. E. Moore, & K. L. Mattox (Eds.), *Trauma* (3rd ed.). (pp. 307–328). Stamford, CT: Appleton & Lange.

Read, R. A., Moore, E. E., & Moore, J. B. (1996). Emergency department thoracotomy. In D. V. Feliciano, E. E. Moore, & K. L. Mattox (Eds.), *Trauma* (3rd ed.). (pp. 193–206). Stamford, CT: Appleton & Lange.

Reath, D.B., Kirby, J., Lynch, M., & Maull, K. I. (1989). Injury and cost comparison of restrained and unrestrained motor vehicle crash victims. *Journal of Trauma 29,* (8), 1173–1176.

Regional Spinal Cord Injury Center of Delaware Valley. (1996). Spinal cord injury facts. Philadelphia: Thomas Jefferson University.

Reilly, P. M. (1998). Deep vein thrombosis/prophylaxis. In A. B. Peitzman, M. Rhodes, C. W. Schwab, & D. M. Yealy (Eds.), *The trauma manual.* (pp. 466–472). Philadelphia: Lippincott-Raven.

Rhodes, M. (1998a). Genitourinary injuries. In A. B. Peitzman, M. Rhodes, C. W. Schwab, & D. M. Yealy (Eds.), *The trauma manual.* (pp. 285–292). Philadelphia: Lippincott-Raven.

Rhodes, M. (1998b). Soft-tissue injuries. In A. B. Peitzman, M. Rhodes, C. W. Schwab, & D. M. Yealy (Eds.), *The trauma manual.* (pp. 348–350). Philadelphia: Lippincott-Raven.

Rhodes, M. (1998c). Trauma resuscitation. In A. B. Peitzman, M. Rhodes, C. W. Schwab, & D. M. Yealy (Eds.), *The trauma manual.* (pp. 82–90). Philadelphia: Lippincott-Raven.

Rhoney, D. H., Luer, M. S., Hughes, M., & Hatton, J. (1996). New pharmacologic approaches to acute spinal cord injury. *Pharmacotherapy, 16* (3), 382–392.

Rehm, C.C. & Ross, S.E. (1996). Extremities: Soft tissue. In R. R. Ivatury D. C. G. Cayten (Eds.). Textbook of penetrating trauma. (p. 779). Baltimore: Williams and Wilkins.

Richardson, J. D. & Miller F. B. (1996). Injury to the lung and pleura. In D. V. Feliciano, E. E. Moore, & K. L. Mattox (Eds.), *Trauma* (3rd ed.). (pp. 387–408). Stamford, CT: Appleton & Lange.

Roberge, J. R., Wears, R. C., Kelly, M., Evans, T. C., Kenny, M. A., Daffner, R. D., Kreman, R., Murray, B. S., & Cottington, E. C. (1988). Selective application of cervical spine radiography in alert victims of blunt trauma: A prospective study. *Journal of Trauma, 28* (6), 784–793.

Rodriguez, J. L., Lopez, J. M., Proctor, M. C., Conley, J. L., Gerndt, S. J., Marx, M. V., Taheri, P. A., & Greenfield, L. J. (1996). Early placement of prophylactic vena caval filters in injured patients at high risk for pulmonary embolism. *Journal of Trauma, 40* (5), 797–804.

Rogers, F. B., Shackford, S. R., Wilson, J., Ricci, M. A., & Morris, C. S. (1993). Prophylactic vena cava filter insertion in severely injured trauma patients: Indications and preliminary results. *Journal of Trauma, 35* (4), 637–642.

Rosner, M. J. & Daughton, S. (1990). Cerebral perfusion pressure management in head injury. *Journal of Trauma, 30* (8), 933–941.

Rosner, M. J., Rosner, S. D., & Johnson, A. H. (1995). Cerebral perfusion pressure: Management protocol and clinical results. *Journal of Neurosurgery, 83* (6), 949–962.

Rotondo, M. F., Schwab, C. W., McGonigal, M. D., Phillips, G. R., Fruchterman, T. M., Kauder, D. K., Latenser, B. A., & Angood, P. A. (1993). 'Damage Control': An approach for improved survival in exsanguinating penetrating abdominal injury. *Journal of Trauma, 35* (3), 375–383.

Rozycki, G. S., Ochsner, G., Schmidt, J. A., Frankel, H. L., Davis, T. P., Wang, D., & Champion, H. R. (1995). A prospective study of surgeon-performed ultrasound as the primary adjuvant modality for injured patient assessment. *Journal of Trauma, 39* (3), 492–500.

Rutledge, R., Lalor, A., Oller, D., Hansen, A., Thomasen, M., Meredith, W., Foil, B., & Baker, C. (1993). The cost of not wearing seat belts. A comparison of outcome in 3396 patients. *Annals of Surgery, 217* (2), 122–127.

Rutledge, R., Thomason, M., Oller, D., Meredith, W., Moylan, J., Clancy, T., Cunningham, P., & Baker, C. (1991). The spectrum of abdominal injuries associated with the use of seat belts. *Journal of Trauma, 31* (6), 820–826.

Salvino, C. K., Esposito, T. J., Marshall, W. J., Dries, D. J., Morris, R. C., & Gamelli, R. L. (1993). The role of diagnostic laparoscopy in the management of trauma patients: A preliminary assessment. *Journal of Trauma, 34* (4), 506–515.

Sastry, S. M., Copeland, R. A., Mezghebe, H., & Siram, S. M. (1995). Retinal hemorrhage secondary airbag-related ocular trauma. *Journal of Trauma, 38* (4), 582.

Sato, T. B. (1987). Effects of seat belts and injuries resulting from improper use. *Journal of Trauma, 27* (7), 754–758.

Sclafani, S. J. A., Cavaliere, G., Atweh, N., Duncan, A. O., & Scalea, T. (1991). The role of angiography in penetrating neck trauma. *Journal of Trauma, 31* (4), 557–563.

Semmlow, J. L. & Cone, R. (1976). Application of the injury severity score: An independent correlation. *Health Service Research, 11* (1), 45–52.

Shackford, S. R. & Rich, N. M. (1996). Peripheral vascular injury. In D. V. Feliciano, E. E. Moore, & K. L. Mattox (Eds.), *Trauma* (3rd ed.). (pp. 819–852). Stamford, CT: Appleton & Lange.

Shackford, S. R., Hollingsworth-Friedlund, P., Cooper, G. F., & Eastman, A. B. (1986). The effect of regionalization on quality of trauma care as assessed by concurrent audit prior to and after institution of a trauma system: A preliminary report. *Journal of Trauma, 26* (9), 812–820.

Shapiro, M. B. (1998). Abdominal vascular injury. In A. B. Peitzman, M. Rhodes, C. W. Schwab, & D. M. Yealy (Eds.), *The Trauma Manual.* (pp. 265–274). Philadelphia: Lippincott-Raven.

Sherbourne, C. D., Shanmuganathan, K., Mirvis, S. E., Chiu, W. C., & Rodriguez, A. (1997). Visceral injury without hemoperitoneum: A limitation of screening abdominal sonography for trauma. *Emergency Radiology, 4* (6), 349–354.

Sherman, H. F., Savage, B. A., Jones, L. M., Barrette, R. R., Latenser, B. A., Varcelotti, J. R., McAuley, C. E., Jones, R. T., & Myers, A. H. (1994). Nonoperative management of blunt hepatic injuries: Safe at any grade? *Journal of Trauma, 37* (4), 616–621.

Shier, M. R. & Wilson, R. F. (1980). Fat embolism syndrome: traumatic coagulopathy with respiratory distress. *Surgery Annals, 12,* 139–168.

Shuman, W. P. (1997). CT of blunt abdominal trauma in adults. *Radiology, 205,* 297–306.

Simons, R. K., Hoyt, D. B., Winchell, R. J., Holbrook, T., & Eastman, A. B. (1995). A risk analysis of stress ulceration after trauma. *Journal of Trauma, 39* (2), 289–294.

Smally, A. J., Binzer, A., Dolin, S., & Viano, D. (1992). Alkaline chemical keratitis: Eye injury from airbags. *Annals of Emergency Medicine, 21* (11), 1400–1402.

Smith, J. S., Wengrovitz, M. A., & DeLong, B. S. (1992). Prospective validation of criteria, including age, for safe, nonsurgical management of the ruptured spleen. *Journal of Trauma, 33* (3), 363–369.

Smock, W. S. & Nichols, G. R. (1995). Airbag module cover injuries. *Journal of Trauma, 38* (4), 489–493.

Sommers, M. S. (1995). Missed injuries: a case of trauma hide and seek. *AACN Clinical Issues: Advanced Practice in Acute and Critical Care, 6* (2), 187–195.

Spisso, J., O'Callaghan, C., McKennan, M., & Holcroft, J. W. (1990). Improved quality of care and reduction of housestaff workload using trauma nurse practitioners. *Journal of Trauma, 30* (5), 660–665.

States, J. D., Huelke, D. F., Dance, M., & Green, R. N. (1987). Fatal injuries caused by underarm use of shoulder belts. *Journal of Trauma, 27* (7), 740–745.

Steinemann, S., Shackford, S. R., & Davis, J. W. (1990). Implications of admission hypothermia in trauma patients. *Journal of Trauma, 30* (2), 200–202.

Swan, K. G. & Swan, R. C. (1991). Principles of ballistics applicable to the treatment of gunshot wounds. *Surgical Clinics of North America, 71* (2), 221–239.

Sykes, L. N., Champion, H. R., & Fouty, W. J. (1988). Dum-dums, hollow-points, and devastators: Techniques designed to increase wounding potential of bullets. *Journal of Trauma, 28* (5), 618–623.

Symbus, P. N. (1996). Injury to the esophagus, trachea, and bronchus. In D. V. Feliciano, E. E. Moore & K. L. Mattox (Eds.), *Trauma* (3rd ed.). (pp. 375–386). Stamford, CT: Appleton & Lange.

Thaemert, B. C., Cogbill, T. H., & Lambert, P. L. (1997). Nonoperative management of splenic injury: Are follow-up computed tomographic scans of any value? *Journal of Trauma, 43* (5), 748–751.

Thal, E. R. (1996). Injury to the neck. In D. V. Feliciano, E. E. Moore, & K. L. Mattox (Eds.), *Trauma* (3rd Ed.). (pp. 329–344). Stamford, CT: Appleton & Lange.

Trafton, P. G. (1996). Lower extremity fractures and dislocations. In D. V. Feliciano, E. E. Moore & K. L. Mattox (Eds.), *Trauma* (3rd ed.). (pp. 791–818). Stamford, CT: Appleton & Lange.

Tuttle-Newhall, J. E., Rutledge, R., Hultman, C. S., & Fakhry, S. M. (1997). Statewide, population-based, time-series analysis of the frequency and outcome of pulmonary embolus in 318,554 trauma patients. *Journal of Trauma, 42* (1), 90–99.

Valadka, A. B. & Narayan, R. K. (1996). In D. V. Feliciano, E. E. Moore & K. L. Mattox (Eds.), *Trauma* (3rd ed.). (pp. 267–278). Stamford, CT: Appleton & Lange.

Velmahos, G. C., Theodorou, D., Tatevossian, R., Belzberg, H., Cornwell, E. E., Berne, T. V., Asensio, J. A., & Demetriades, D. (1996). Radiographic cervical spine evaluation in the alert asymptomatic blunt trauma victim: Much ado about nothing? *Journal of Trauma, 40* (5), 768–774.

Viano, D. C. (1995). Restraint effectiveness, availability and use in fatal crashes: Implications to injury control. *Journal of Trauma, 38* (4), 538–545.

Walt, A. J. (1991). Foreword to E. E. Moore, K. L. Mattox, & D. V. Feliciano (Eds.), *Trauma* (2nd ed.). (pp xvii–xviii). Norwalk, CT: Appleton & Lange.

Waters, R. L., Adkins, R. H., Yakura, J. et al. (1991). Profiles of spinal cord injury and recovery after gunshot injury. *Clinical Orthopedics, 267,* 14–21.

West, J. G., Cales, R. H., & Gazzaniga, A. G. (1983). Impact of regionalization: The Orange County experience. *Archives of Surgery, 118* (6), 740–744.

West, J. G., Trunkey, D. D., & Lim, R. C. (1979). Systems of trauma care: A study of two counties. *Archives of Surgery, 114* (4), 455–460.

Wilson, C. B. (1964). Unrecognized abdominal trauma in patients with head injuries. *Annals of Surgery, 161,* 608–613.

Wilson, R. F. (1996). Injury to the pancreas and duodenum. In R. F. Wilson & A. J. Walt (Eds.), *Management of Trauma: Pitfalls and Practice* (2nd ed.). (pp. 510–533). Baltimore: Williams & Wilkins.

Wilson, R. F. & Steiger, Z. (1996). Thoracic trauma: Chest wall and lung. In R. F. Wilson & A. J. Walt (Eds.), *Management of trauma: Pitfalls and practice* (2nd ed.). (pp. 314–342). Baltimore: Williams & Wilkins.

Wilson, R. F. & Walt, A. J. (1996). Injuries to the liver and biliary tract. In R. F. Wilson & A. J. Walt (Eds.), *Management of trauma: Pitfalls and practice* (2nd ed.). (pp. 449–472). Baltimore: Williams & Wilkins.

Wilson, R. F., Smith, J. B., & McCarroll, K. A. (1996). Trauma to the urinary tract. In R. F. Wilson & A. J. Walt (Eds.), *Management of trauma: Pitfalls and practice* (2nd ed.). (pp. 600–620). Baltimore: Williams & Wilkins.

Wilson, R. F., Walt, A. J., & Dulchavsky, S. (1996). Injuries to the colon and rectum. In R. F. Wilson & A. J. Walt (Eds.), *Management of trauma: Pitfalls and practice* (2nd ed.). (pp. 534–553). Baltimore: Williams & Wilkins.

Winchell, R. J., Hoyt, D. B., Walsh, J. C., Simons, R. K., & Eastman, A. B. (1994). Risk factors associated with pulmonary embolism despite routine prophylaxis: implications for improved protection. *Journal of Trauma, 37* (4), 600–606.

Wisner, D. H. (1996). Injury to the stomach and small bowel. In D. V. Feliciano, E. E. Moore & K. L. Mattox (Eds.), *Trauma* (3rd ed.). (pp. 551–572). Stamford, CT: Appleton & Lange.

Woodring, J. H. & Lee, C. (1993). Limitations of cervical radiography in the evaluation of acute cervical trauma. *Journal of Trauma, 34* (1), 32–39.

Woolson, S. T., McCrory, D. W., Walter, J. F., Maloney, W. J., Watt, J. M., & Cahill, P. D. (1990). B-mode ultrasound scanning in the detection of proximal venous thrombosis after total hip replacement. *Journal of Bone and Joint Surgery, 72* (7), 983–987.

Yoshida, G. M., Garland, D., & Waters, R. L. (1995). Gunshot wounds to the spine. *Orthopedic Clinics of North America, 26* (1), 109–116.

25

Plastic and Reconstructive Surgery

Janet Bienkowski

▶ HISTORY OF PLASTIC AND RECONSTRUCTIVE SURGERY

The roots of reconstructive surgery dates back at least 2500 years according to records that describe nasal and earlobe reconstruction (Bhishagratna, 1916). The term *plastic* comes from the Greek word *plastikos* meaning "fit for molding." Throughout the history of surgery, plastic (constructive) and reconstructive surgical techniques were developed in conjunction with general surgery. These procedures did not become a separate branch of surgery until after World War I, when instructional seminars for plastic surgery of the face were held. After World War II, reconstructive plastic surgery established itself through tissue transplantation, hand surgery, and limb replantation.

Definition

Plastic and reconstructive surgery includes reconstruction and aesthetics for all parts of the body. This includes subspecialities of microsurgery, peripheral nerve surgery, craniofacial and hand surgery, burns, and cosmetics. This chapter addresses the reconstructive aspects of plastic surgery.

Role of the Nurse Practitioner

The role of the nurse practitioner in plastic and reconstructive surgery is diverse. The nurse practitioner is often introduced to the patient at the initial consult. The presurgical history and physical is performed, at which time any further questions regarding the surgery are answered and pre- and postoperative instructions are given. A knowledge of the surgical procedures is essential. The plastic surgery nurse practitioner should have a surgical nursing background that encompasses management of surgical wounds and drains.

The role can include assisting in surgery, in hospital rounds, and discharge of the patient, including drain removal and postoperative follow-up. This allows for total continuity of patient care. Clinical techniques may include minor suturing, performing punch biopsies, suture removal and drainage of seromas and minor wound debridements, and placement and removal of splints and casts. These techniques are learned through various conference offerings of suturing and cast placement and removal workshops, and clinical experience.

▶ PSYCHOSOCIAL ASPECTS OF RECONSTRUCTIVE SURGERY

Body image represents a person's perception of his or her body as well as the emotional significance ascribed to various body parts ([Dhillon et al., 1982] in Bronheim, Strain & Biller, 1991). It is a complex phenomenon that evolves throughout one's life at a preconscious level. It is the result of input from a person's formative psychological development and from stimuli from one's environment. It is a synthesis of one's past and present.

Body image begins to be formed during infancy and has a strong link to a child's interaction with his or her environment and family members. According to social developmental psychologists, children develop levels of attachment with parents or caregivers depending on how well a child's needs are met during infancy and early childhood (Bretherton, 1997). This theory of attachment helps to explain how a child organizes his or her emotional experiences. For example, a positive, securely attached child has the capacity to admit to normal imperfections within him- or herself and reveal both strong and weak points of the self. Conversely, for children experiencing weak attachment to their parents, an overwhelming change and/or disfigurement in the body can superimpose on earlier experiences of bodily changes that were painful or conflict-ridden.

Children learn a great deal of interpersonal behavior and problem-solving strategies from within the family context. Early insecure patterns of attachment and deficits in problem-solving strategies can lead to deficits in social and cognitive abilities that can have a significant effect on future coping skills. One major factor in coping with body disfigurement—whether congenital or acquired—is the protective function of perceived social support from family, teacher, classmate, and friends. This experience greatly helps in advocating a healthy adaptation to a person's injury or handicap (Wallander, 1988).

Societal stimuli can also affect a person's body image. The psychosocial effects of physical attractiveness may have a strong influence on social development and behavior. Physical attractiveness can influence people's expectations about personality, likability, behavior, and future performance. People often view others with anomalies differently. Our social construct is imbued with the image of the perfect body. According to media messages, if we are one of the beautiful people, we will get the "man of our dreams," the perfect job, and whatever else our heart desires. Villains are portrayed as ugly (wicked witches) or old and haggard, and handicapped characters are portrayed as social outcasts. In light of these societal views on physical attractiveness, an altered body image may cause a patient to experience disturbing personal and social adjustments.

Coping with a changed body image can be a crucial issue. One must deal not only with the original disfigurement, but also with the resultant scars at reconstruction. The psychological impact on patients who are surgically treated with muscle flaps and skin grafts and who have disfiguring scars to their body, face, and neck often results in overall distress, including social isolation, decreased self esteem and sexual attractiveness, and fear of rejection and abandonment (Gamba et al., 1992). Breast cancer patients have to cope with not only their disease and fear of death, but also decreased femininity. The chronic stress produced by being diagnosed with cancer, fear of recurrence, and constant need to cope and act normal and healthy may impair their long-term coping skills. (Rappaport et al., 1993). Patients who have survived head and neck cancer reported decreased sexuality with their partners and decreased social interaction with friends due to the resultant deformity. They were noted to feel increasing distress and anxiety from their decreased sense of the familiar self up to 11 years after diagnosis and treatment (Bjordal & Kaasa, 1995).

The psychosocial impact on these patients needs to be addressed preoperatively. Patterns of coping with past stresses, the presence of psychiatric disorders and addictive behaviors, and an appraisal of the patient's support system needs to be identified so potential difficulties can be identified and addressed before surgery. This type of intervention is imperative at the initial consult. Nursing personnel and psychiatric consults can help foster a patient's emotional support and lead to exploration of his or her fears and thoughts. Other treatment options can be recommended if necessary. Referral to support groups with counselors trained in the management of cancer patients can be effective in reducing anxiety and depression (Fallowfield & Baum, 1986). Organizations such as Reach to Recovery for mastectomy patients can be contacted. It is composed of women who have undergone breast cancer treatment as well as reconstruction and can provide patients with empathy and emotional support. Social workers can ensure help with finances or homemaking assistance where needed. Follow-up visits at yearly intervals should be scheduled to see how these patients are coping with the physical and emotional responses to plastic and reconstructive surgery. Further studies are needed to determine the ability of these patients to cope long term.

▶ PREOPERATIVE ASSESSMENT

Patients undergo a preoperative history and physical. Those with diabetes, severe pulmonary disease, emphysema, COPD, or a cardiac history often need surgical clearance from their primary-care provider or medical specialist.

Laboratory results are reviewed prior to surgery. EKG abnormalities need to be reviewed by a cardiologist. Albumin and prealbumin levels should be determined in malnourished or anorexic patients. An albumin level <3.5 is deleterious to wound healing and should be corrected before proceeding with surgery. Protein building blocks are needed to heal wounds as amino acids are necessary for wound remodeling and tensile tissue strength. Proper nutritional teaching is essential and a nutritional consult may be helpful.

Patients who smoke are counseled on the deleterious effects of smoking. In addition to worsening the risk of perioperative pneumonia, smoking can increase platelet aggregation resulting in blood clots (Nolan et al., 1985). Nicotine constricts blood vessels thereby decreasing blood flow to the operative site (Van Adrichem et al., 1992). The carbon monoxide in cigarette smoke competes with the hemoglobin molecule, reducing the amount of oxygen that reaches the wound (Sherwin & Gastwirth, 1987). Patients should stop smoking at least 2 weeks prior to surgery; however, the effects of smoking on wound healing persist up to years after quitting. If a patient is seen for preoperative assessment a few days before the procedure, he or she is advised to stop smoking immediately, and is taught how to use an incentive spirometer to maintain sufficient lung expansion pre- and postoperatively.

Any further questions regarding the surgery are answered at this time. These questions may concern length of the surgical procedure, potential complications relating to the intervention, and level of postoperative care required in order to maintain maximal functioning.

▶ RECONSTRUCTIVE TECHNIQUES

Among the most common reconstructive procedures are those related to wound closure, breast reconstruction, craniofacial deformities, and hand reconstruction. Risk factors, surgical procedures, and postoperative care for each of these techniques are discussed.

Wound Closure

Wound preparation prior to suturing includes obtaining hemostasis through gentle continuous pressure. The periphery of the wound is disinfected with betadine or phisohex. These substances should be avoided in the depth of the wound as they can cause damage to the deep tissues. After adequate local anesthesia, the depth of the wound should be irrigated prior to suturing to remove any contaminants. This may be accomplished by using an 18 to 20 gauge plastic angiocath needle attached to a 30-cc syringe and copious amounts of saline to reduce bacterial contamination, dirt, and debris. Any gravel, glass, and so on should be removed prior to closure. Excision or debridement of devitalized or nonviable tissue is accomplished with a #3 knife handle and a 15 blade (Fig. 25–1).

Closure of clean open wounds involves assessment of tissue loss. Wounds without tissue loss can be allowed to close secondarily or closed primarily using layered closure to avoid any tension on the final skin repair. Wounds may also be covered with flaps or skin grafts.

If the wound edges are macerated (such as occurs with blunt trauma), it is often necessary to trim the edges. A fine-point cautery tip may be used to control bleeding. Never cauterize the skin edge as this can lead to tissue necrosis.

Tetanus Prophylaxis

The administration of tetanus prophylaxis is recommended within 5 years if the wound is deep or contaminated and within 10 years if the wound is clean and minor. The recommended preparation is the Td preparation, which includes both tetanus and diphtheria toxoid (Lutwick, 1996).

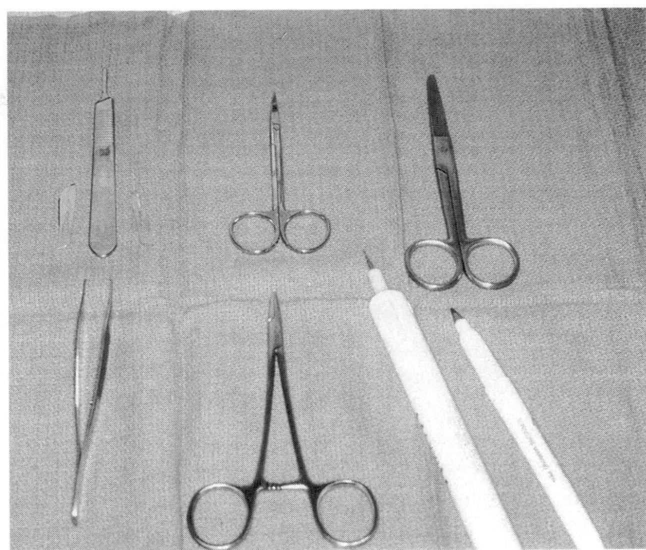

Figure 25–1. Instruments used for suturing. *Top left to right:* #10 blade, #3 knife handle, #15 blade, Steven's scissors, utility scissors. *Bottom left to right:* Adson fine-toothed forcep, Webster needle holder, disposable cautery, marking pen.

Anesthesia

The most common choice of anesthesia for simple wound closure is local. A common solution for local infiltration is 1% lidocaine (Xylocaine HCL) in a 1:100,000 solution with epinephrine. Epinephrine provides hemostasis through vasoconstriction. If a person has a known cardiac or hypertensive history, avoid use of epinephrine. It is important to use plain lidocaine without epinephrine when injecting into fingers or toes, due to risk of ischemia from digital artery spasm. Sodium bicarbonate (8.4%) may be added to the lidocaine to decrease pain on injection and hasten the anesthesia. The two components should be combined just prior to injection, to avoid precipitation of the components. The ratio of bicarbonate to lidocaine with or without epinephrine is 1:5.

Always aspirate prior to injection to avoid infiltration in surrounding vessels. The anesthetic should be administered subcutaneously initially on one side, parallel to the wound edge, using a 27-gauge, 1-inch needle. Initial injection with a small needle causes less pain. Once an anesthetized area is achieved, a 25-gauge, 1½-inch needle can be used. Progress with injections, always injecting into an anesthetized area parallel to the wound edges until all sides of the wounds are infiltrated.

Maximum allowable single dose for lidocaine without epinephrine is 4.5 mg/kg (approximately 30 ml per 70-kg adult) and 7 mg/kg (approximately 50 ml per adult) for 1%

lidocaine with epinephrine. A small laceration usually requires about 3 to 6 ml of the lidocaine solution. Lidocaine with epinephrine's duration of action is about 60 to 240 minutes. Lidocaine without epinephrine lasts about 30 to 120 minutes. If a patient has allergies to the preservatives in local anesthetics, use preservative-free anesthetics.

Suturing

Suture Materials

There are many types of suture materials to choose from, depending on the characteristics of the wound. Suture material is marketed as monofilament or braided (multifilament) according to the number of strands of which they are made. Monofilament sutures are made of a single strand of material, whereas multifilament sutures contain many strands braided together. Sutures are also marketed as nonabsorbable or absorbable.

Nonabsorbable. The most frequently used nonabsorbable sutures are silk and synthetic materials such as monofilament nylon (Ethilon, Dermalon), polypropylene (Prolene), or polybutester (Novafil). Braided sutures have the potential for capillarity, an ability to carry fluid along any of its strands, including infected tissue fluid. For this reason, braided sutures have fallen into disfavor, unless removed within 5 days, so are used less often. Nonabsorbable sutures cannot be digested by body enzymes or hydrolyzed by tissue fluids. Synthetic fibers such as nylon, polyester, or polyethylene cause less tissue irritation and have a higher tensile strength than the natural fibers of silk. Nonabsorbable sutures that are used on exposed tissue, such as the eye or skin, must be removed.

Absorbable. Synthetic absorbable sutures are made of polymers of polyglycolic acid. Plain gut is made from the submucosa of sheep or beef intestine. They are digested by body enzymes or hydrolyzed by tissue fluids within 5 days. Plain surgical gut and chromic gut, which is surgical gut treated in a chromiun salt, are digested by body enzymes that results in varying degrees of inflammatory reaction. Gut sutures provide only minimal support so are used on tissues that heal very rapidly. They are not recommended for surface sutures because they can lead to strong reactions and inflammation. Synthetic absorbable sutures, such as Maxon, Dexon, vicryl, and PDS, are absorbed by hydrolysis in which water combines with a salt to form an acid and a base, thus causing very little tissue reaction. Absorption occurs over 3 to 6 months.

Suture Diameter

Suture diameter ranges from a heavy size 0 to a very fine size 11-0. Thickness decreases as the suture size increases; therefore, tensile strength decreases as suture diameter decreases. The thickness of the suture material is determined by the location on the body, using smaller sutures for the face and larger sutures for the trunk and extremities.

Suture Needles

Surgical needles have either a straight or curved shaft. The most frequently used in plastic surgery is the curved. The curvature may be 1/4, 3/8, 1/2, or 5/8 circle. The 1/2 and 3/8 circles are the most common skin closure needles. The needle point most commonly used in plastic surgery for skin suturing is the cutting needle. In tissues that offer only slight resistance, such as the oral cavity, muscle fascia, or peritoneum, use of a tapered needle is usual. Plastic surgery needles are less traumatic and are recommended for wound repair. They are identified by the letter P or PS appearing next to the needle size on the package (Fig. 25–2). A P1 is smaller than a P3 needle, and both are commonly used.

Placement of Sutures

The most important aspect of suturing is to be certain that all dermal layers meet at the same level. A bite is the amount of tissue taken when the needle is set into the skin. If a superficial bite is taken on one side of the wound and a deep bite on the other side, the wound edges will not meet correctly. Because wounds tend to invert or indent after wound contraction, it is important to evert or slightly raise the wound edges above the normal skin plane, as wounds will flatten over time with healing (Fig. 25–3).

To achieve wound edge eversion, the needle point should enter the epidermis and dermis at a 90-degree angle before it curves around the tissue.

When lifting the wound edge up for suture application, the tissue should not be crushed between the dermis and epidermis as this can damage the tissue, leading to tissue necrosis. The skin edge should be retracted gently prior to suture needle placement (Fig. 25–4).

One also needs to be familiar with the tension component of the wound. Tension is a force that produces elongation or extension (American Heritage Dictionary, 1993). All body structures have a natural tension inherent to that particular area, for example, tension over a joint is greater than tension on the top of the scalp. Inflammation and swelling place increased tension on a wound. If a suture is placed too near the closure, it will possibly tear. When the swelling decreases, the tear leaves a wider unsightlier scar. The suture should be placed so that most of the tension is deeper in the dermis where the possibility of tears and scars is decreased. Sutures should, therefore, be placed *parallel* to lines of tension rather than *against* them. Table 25–1 gives the length of time sutures should remain in place for both adults and children.

Interrupted Suture

Interrupted sutures are single sutures separately placed and tied individually with the wound edges in an everted position. This is a secure suture in that if one of the sutures breaks, the wound edges remain intact with the rest of the sutures. Every other suture can be removed if necessary. Sutures should be placed closer together and closer to the

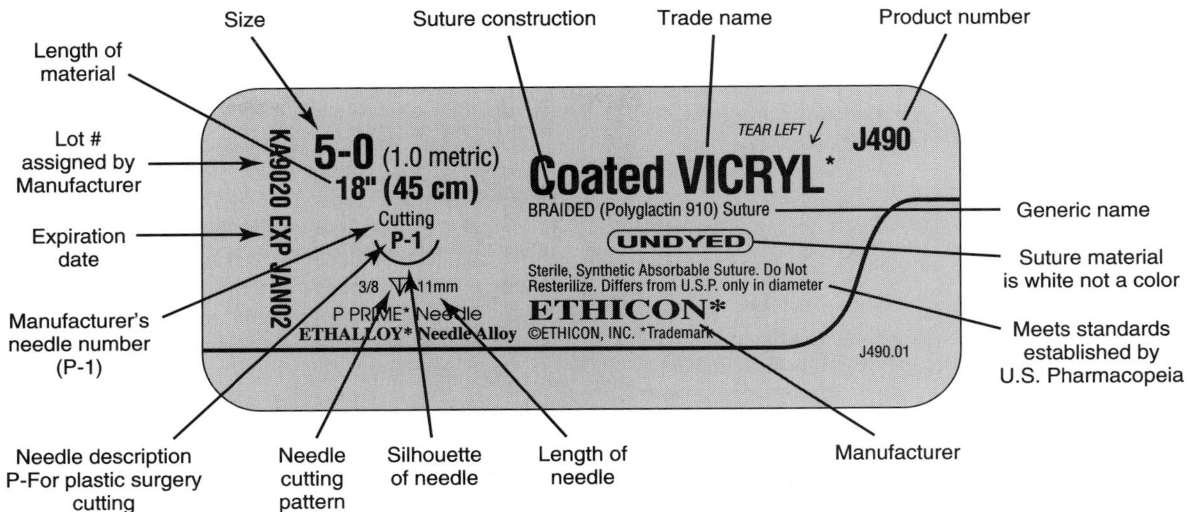

Figure 25–2. The suture package contains the following information.

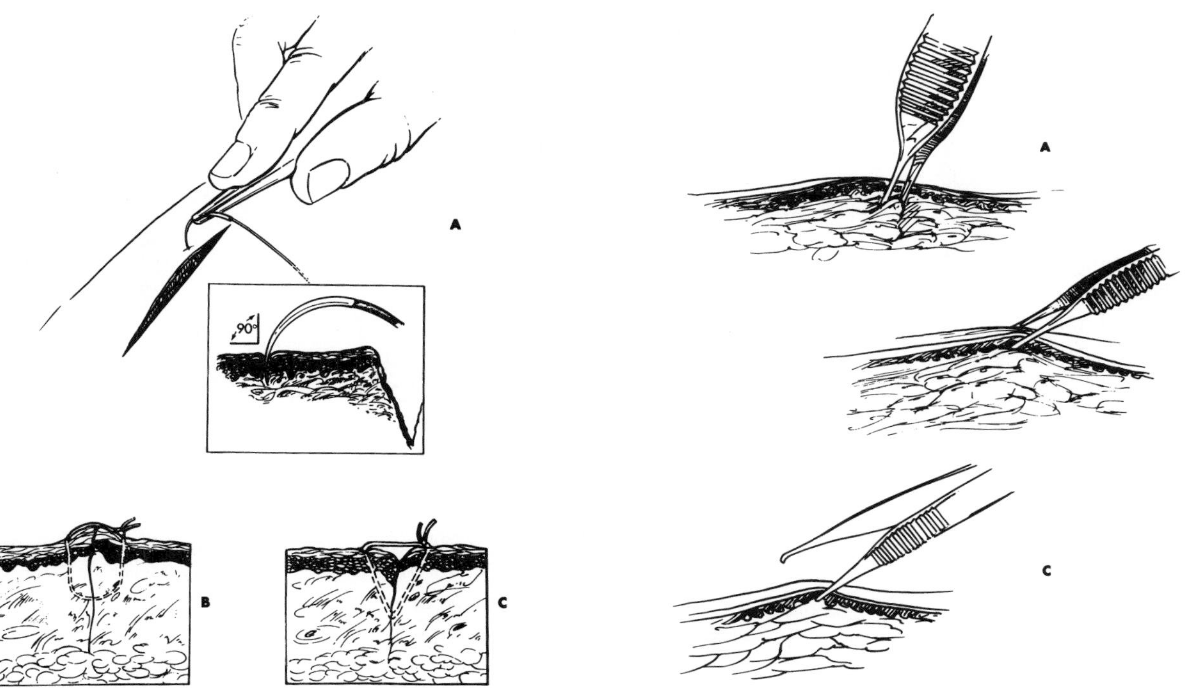

Figure 25–3. Wound edge eversion. **A,** The suture needle is placed at a 90 degree angle to the skin and epidermis. **B,** For proper wound edge eversion, the suture should have a squared or jar configuration when curving around the tissue to exit the other side. **C,** Angling the suture in a wedge shape toward the center of the wound can lead to wound edge inversion with scar depression. *(Used with permission from A. T. Trott, [1977]. [p. 145].)*

Figure 25–4. Tissue handling. **A,** Tissue should be grasped gently by the subcutaneous tissue. **B,** Grasping the dermis and epidermis with the tips of the forcep can lead to compression and damage to the dermis. **C,** Retraction or anchoring of the tissue for needle placement can be accomplished by using one edge of the toothed forcep at the dermal edge. *(Used with permission from A. T. Trott, [p. 107]).*

TABLE 25–1. Length of Time Sutures Should Remain in Place

	Adult (days)	Children (days)
Face	3–5	3–4
Scalp	6–7	5–6
Trunk	7–10	6–8
Arm (not joints)	7–10	5–9
Leg (not joints)	8–10	6–8
Joint extensor surface	8–14	7–12
Joint flexor surface	8–10	7–12
Dorsum of hand	7–9	5–7
Palm	7–12	7–10
Sole of foot	7–12	7–10

wound edge approximately 3 mm on the face and approximately 4 mm elsewhere to reduce tension on the wound (Fig. 25–5). All knots are placed evenly on the same side of the wound.

Running Suture

A running suture can be used on any wound with minimal tension. It is similar to an interrupted suture, except that the suture material is not cut and tied with each succeeding stitch. After the initial suture and knot is placed, the next bite is made at a 45-degree angle to the wound direction starting at the original knot. The primary benefit of the running suture is speed. The main drawback is if the suture breaks anywhere along its length, the whole suture line can unravel. Wound edge eversion may be difficult to achieve with this method.

Vertical Mattress Suture

This suture involves placing a double line of suture material across the wound. Skin is entered and exited twice, with the two lines of suture lying one above the other. The needle is brought through the skin, taking a large bite, to an equal distance on the opposite side of the wound. The needle then enters the skin on the same plane and same side as where it just exited to take a small bite into the epidermal–dermal edge through an equal distance to the other side (Fig. 25–6). It is useful in single layer closures of wounds under great tension. The disadvantages of this type of suture is that it is time consuming and results in a double suture track.

Horizontal Mattress Suture

In a horizontal mattress suture, two lines of suture lie parallel to one another in a horizontal plane. The needle is brought through the skin to the opposite side of the wound. The next needle is placed about 0.5 cm adjacent or next to where the needle just exited. It is again brought through the skin to the opposite side where the original needle entered approximately 1/2 cm from the original entry (Fig. 25–7). It takes the place of two simple ties to repair a small laceration, saving time. This method is less likely to rip through the skin, and therefore the technique is useful in areas

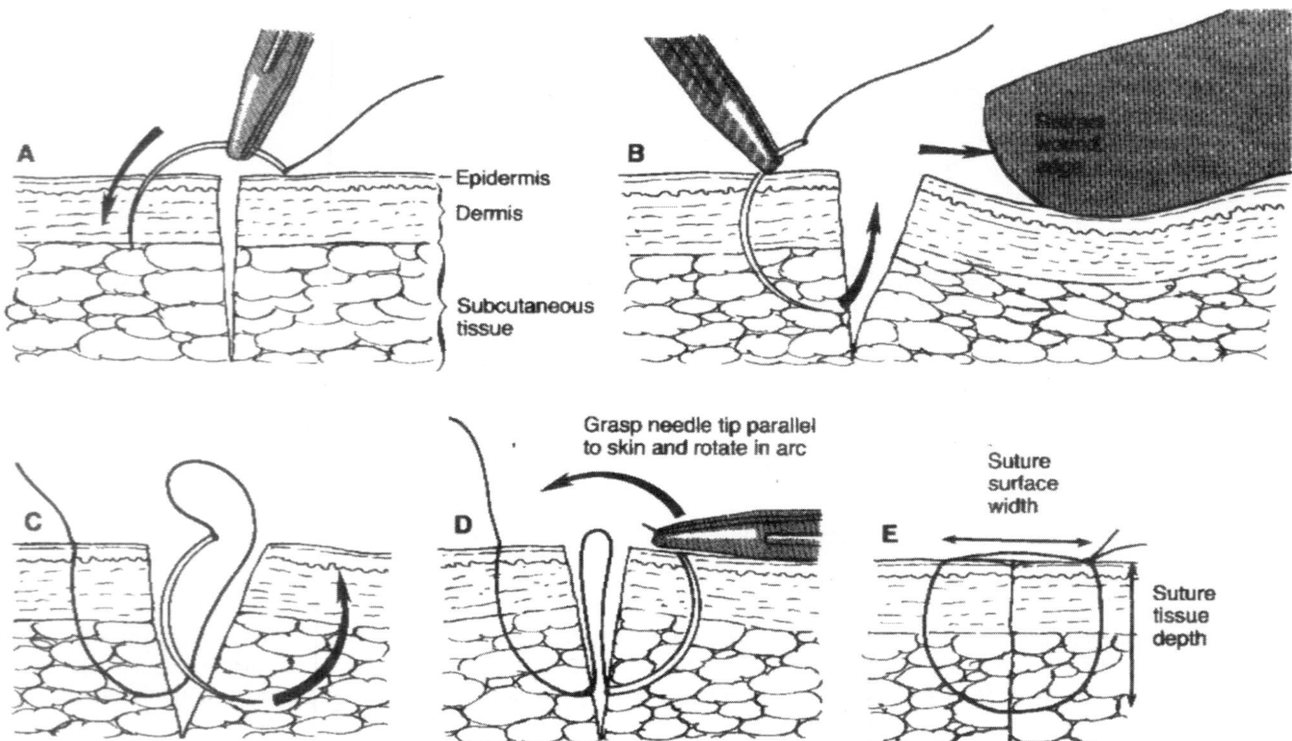

Figure 25–5. Simple interrupted suture. Each suture is tied after passing through each side equivocally being careful to evert the wound edge. All knots are placed on the same side.

where the skin is atrophic, such as the lower leg in elderly patients or at the scalp–skin junction.

Pullout Subcuticular Suture

Plastic surgeons often use the pullout subcuticular suture, which consists of a running buried stitch that is placed just below the dermal–epidermal junction. The skin is entered through the epidermis about 2 to 4 mm from one end of the wound, emerging in the dermis at the apex or top of the

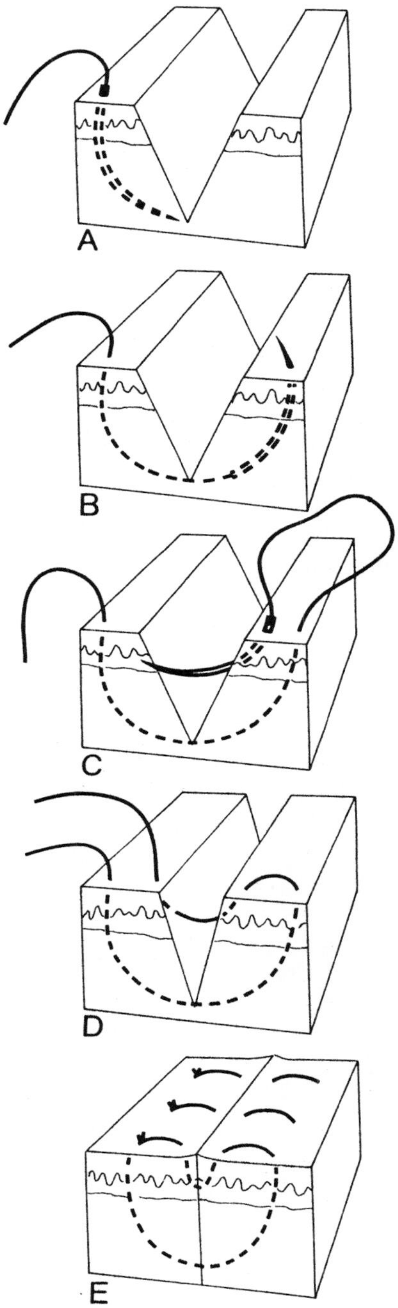

Figure 25–6. Vertical mattress suture. **A,** The needle enters the skin at a 90 degree angle. **B,** It is brought through to the opposite side of the wound and exits an equal distance from the wound edge as it entered on the other side. **C,** The needle reenters the skin on the same side and same plane as where it just exited, **D,** taking a smaller bite into the epidermal edge through to the other side, exiting an equal distance from the wound edge to where it entered on the opposite side. **E.** A knot is tied and all knots are placed evenly on the same side of the wound.

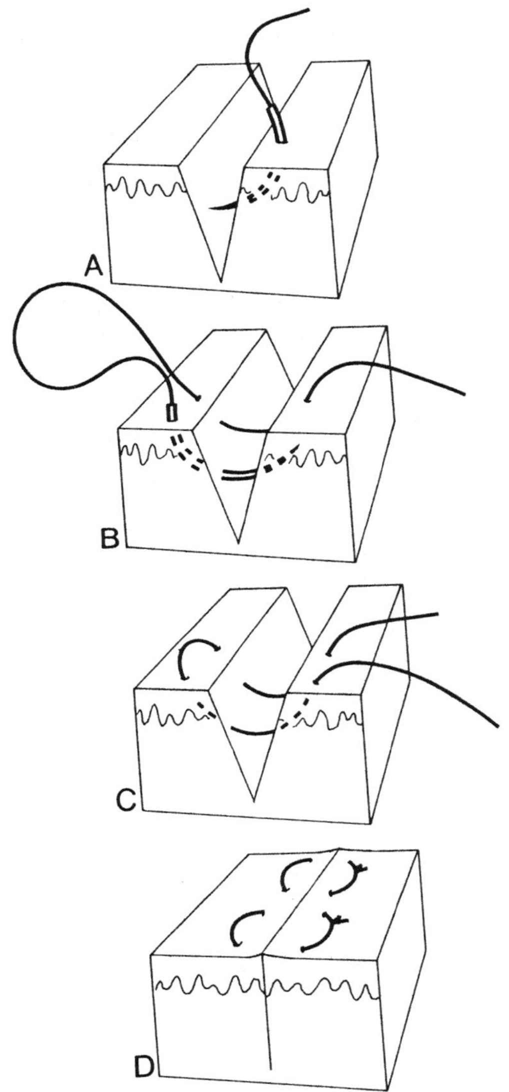

Figure 25–7. Horizontal mattress suture. **A,** The needle is placed 0.5-1 cm away from the wound edge at a 90 degree angle. **B,** The needle is brought out to the opposite side, the same distance from the wound edge that it entered. The needle is then placed about 0.5 cm next to where it just exited. **C,** It is again brought through the skin at a 90 degree angle to the opposite side parallel to the initial suture and exits where the initial suture started on the oposite side. **D,** Care should be made to enter and exit the wound at the same depth on each bite to prevent buckling.

wound. The suture is then passed to the alternate side directly across or slightly behind the exit point of the previous stitch throughout the plane of the dermis to a depth of about 2 to 3 mm into the dermis. Each bite should be a mirror image of the previous one. When completed, the suture is brought out through the dermis, exiting the skin. A tail is left on both sides of the wound and taped into place using steri strips. The steri strips may be placed along the wound edge's length (Fig. 25–8). The patient needs to be instructed not to pull on or cut the end sutures if the steri strips become loose; they could potentially remove the whole suture if they pull it through or lose the suture if both ends are cut. The pullout subcuticular stitch avoids the problem of suture marks. It is useful in approximating sutures if tension is present and a widened scar is feared such as in areas of the arms, legs, or back. It can be left in for a much longer period of time in high tension areas without fear of suture track marks. It is best suited for straight lacerations. It is, however, a harder stitch to learn and takes more time to perform than simple running sutures.

Z-Plasties. Z-plasties change the direction of the scar so it is more in line with natural creases. The scar's appearance is improved by changing its direction. This is useful in areas where scars limit movement, such as in areas over joints or the axilla or neck. Tissue is transposed, lengthened, and rearranged. The resulting scar tissue is shaped like a Z (Fig. 25–9).

V-Y Advancement Flaps. A V-shaped incision is made through the skin, the skin on the other side of the V is advanced in the direction of the apex of the V, and the incision is closed as a Y. The dermis and subcutaneous tissue are raised. This technique helps to lengthen structures such as correction of lip notching.

Grafts and Flaps

Any tissue can be transferred as a flap or a graft. These include tendons, bones, cartilage, fascia, dermis, muscles, nerves, and vessels. Fat can also be transferred as a graft, but the long-term results are questionable as fat breaks down and scars over. Grafts don't have a blood supply initially reestablished. The diffusion of gases and nutrients from the underlying bed develops perfusion after a few days. Reconstruction of flaps may involve transposition of

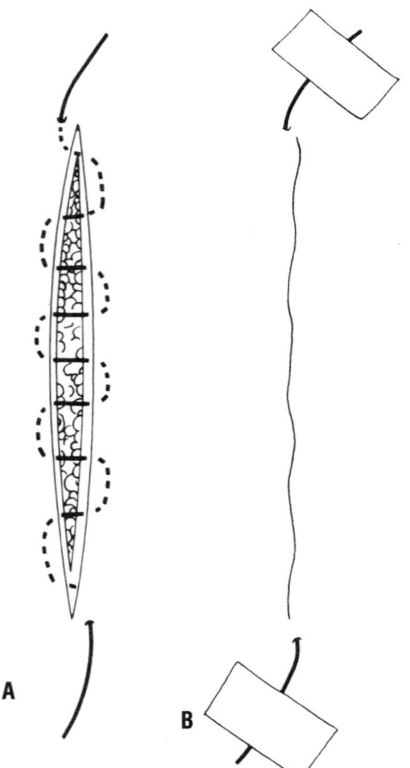

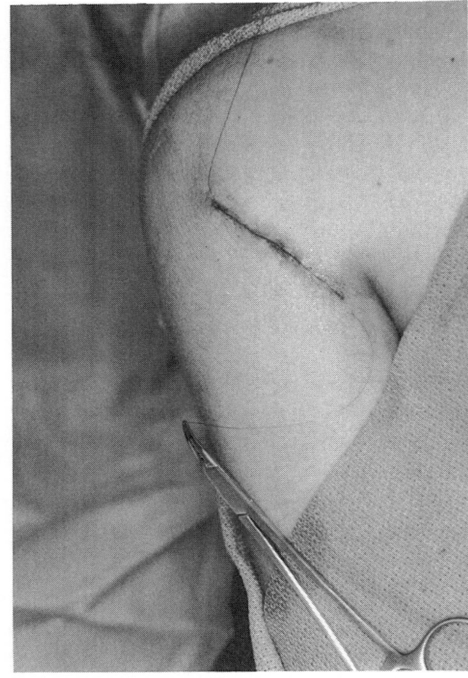

Figure 25–8. Pullout subcuticular. **A,** The skin is entered through the epidermis about 2 to 4 mm above one end of the wound then exits in the subcuticular plane at the top of the wound. The suture is then passed to the opposite side directly across or slightly behind the exit point of the previous stitch to a depth of about 2 to 3 mm into the dermis. Each corresponding stitch should mimic the one before it. When completed, the suture is brought out through the dermis exiting the skin. **B,** A tail is left on both sides of the wound and taped in place using steri strips. **C,** The strips may be placed along the wound edges length.

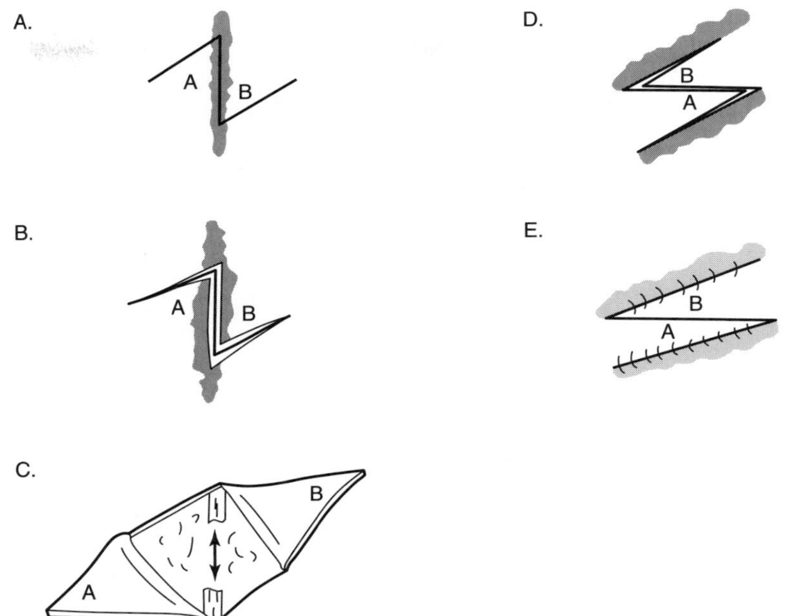

Figure 25–9. Z-plasty. **A,** Three lines of equal length are drawn (if the incisions are not the same length, puckering of the flaps can occur), the vertical line is drawn along the vertical scar line. The lines are then cut at a 60 degree angle. You end up with angle A and angle B. **B,** Both flaps are then undermined (the dermal layers are raised). **C,** The deeper portion of the scar is released. **D,** The triangular flaps are transpositioned B goes atop A. **E,** The wound edges are then sutured. The scar is lengthened and has a new Z shape.

tissues attached at one site onto an open wound bed, which eventually develops its own perfusion, or transfer of tissue from one site to another in which the flap's blood supply is severed at the donor site and reestablished at the receipient site by microsurgery.

Skin Grafts

Skin grafts are classified as either split thickness (which involves the epidermis and only part of the dermis) or full thickness (which involves the epidermis and the whole dermis) (Fig. 25–10). For both types of grafts, the recipient bed should be free of infection and well perfused. Skin grafts can be taken from any body part. They are usually harvested from hidden areas such as the upper thigh or buttock, as they leave a significant scar. Areas of the lateral neck, postauricular area, or supraclavicular area are used as a donor site when skin grafting the face.

Skin grafts can be harvested by using a free-hand knife or by using a dermatome. There are several types of dermatomes, including air- or electric-powered models (Fig. 25–11). The width of the graft is determined by the width setting on the dermatome. The donor site is first cleaned with a surgical solution. If betadine is used, it must be washed off to prevent the dermatome from sticking to the skin. Mineral oil is applied to the donor site to expedite graft cutting. The dermatome is laid flat on the skin and is moved across the skin surface with a gentle downward pressure.

Skin grafts can be meshed using a skin graft mesher. This procedure is used when there is an insufficient amount of skin available to be harvested as a graft for use with large burns or to expand the surface area. The holes created from meshing allow for drainage of blood and serum (Fig. 25–12). Split-thickness skin grafts are either sutured or stapled to the recipient site.

Full-thickness skin grafts are ordinarily cut using a scalpel; a dermatome can be used. The grafts are usually small. A pattern of the defect is outlined on the donor site

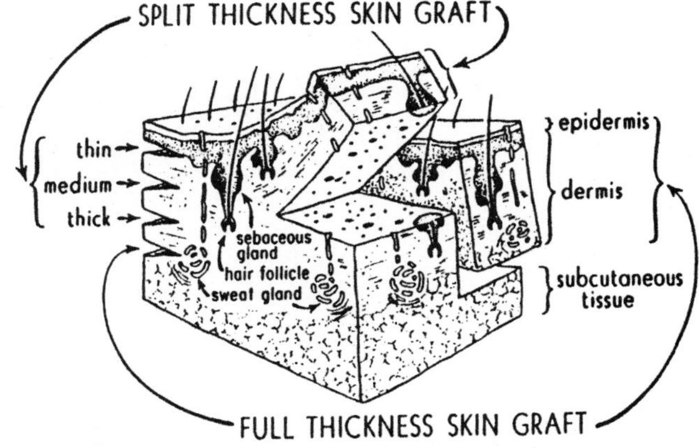

Figure 25–10. Skin grafts. A split thickness graft includes: epidermis and part of the dermis. Thickness may be thin to thick. A contraction at the recipient site is less with a thicker graft. A thinner graft has a better survival rate. A full thickness graft includes the epidermis and all the dermis. It is slower to vascularize than a split thickness graft. Capillary blood vessels begin to grow at the recipient site within 48 to 72 hours giving the graft new circulation.

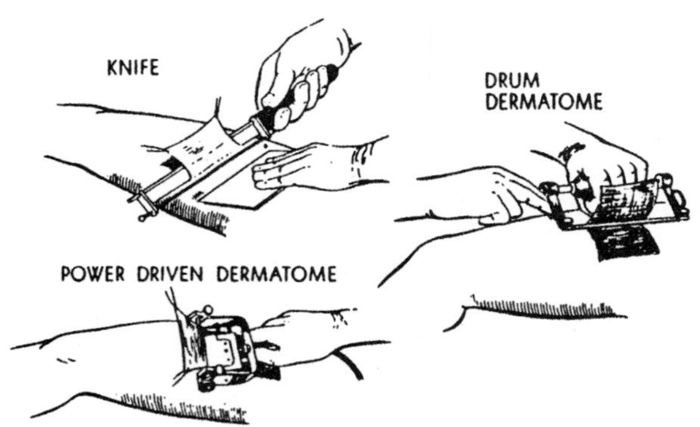

Figure 25–11. Dermatome. There are several types: *Top left:* A free hand knife. *Top right:* A drum dermatome and *bottom left* is a power driven dermatome. The type of blade and thickness of the graft is determined by the surgeon.

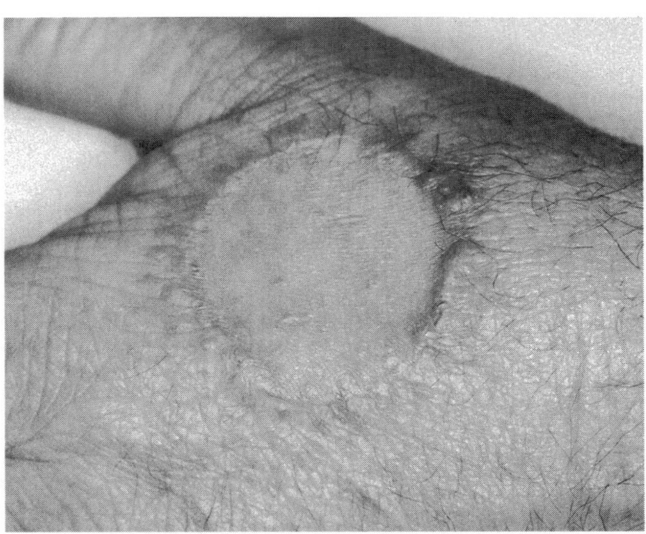

Figure 25–13. A full-thickness graft is good for smaller areas such as the hand. It can be sutured or stapled in place.

before cutting and transplanting to the recipient site. Full-thickness skin grafts are sutured in place, and the donor site is closed primarily (Fig. 25–13).

Skin grafts need to adhere well to their grafted site to allow for growth of new blood vessels. A pressure dressing is used to promote graft adherence and to prevent graft shearing from a loose dressing. It is composed of an inner layer of a nonstick bacteriostatic (prevents bacteria from entering the site) material such as a petrolatum gauze with bismuth (Xeroform gauze) or an oil emulsion dressing—on which a compacted layer of sterile fluffed gauze, a gauze roll, and an ACE wrap—is applied. In areas where a pressure dressing cannot be applied to a full-thickness and split-thickness graft, such as the face or chest, tie-over dressings can be used. These bulky dressings are composed of a Xeroform gauze outer layer with inner layers of cotton sheeting that are sutured and tied over the site (Fig. 25–14). Tie-over dressings are usually left on for approximately 5 to 7 days. Non–tie-over dressings are maintained for a period of about 4 to 7 days to allow for the new blood supply to form.

Skin grafts are initially pale when first applied, but start to regain a pink color with the growth of new circulation. Great care is taken when removing the postoperative dressing so as not to dislodge the graft.

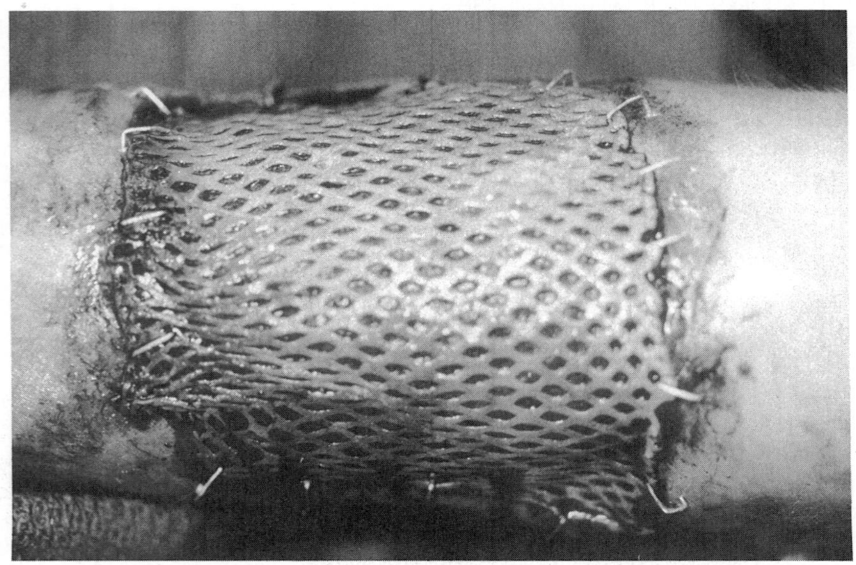

Figure 25–12. A meshed skin graft. This is a split thickness graft. The holes in the mesh allow for serous drainage as well as for coverage of larger surface areas.

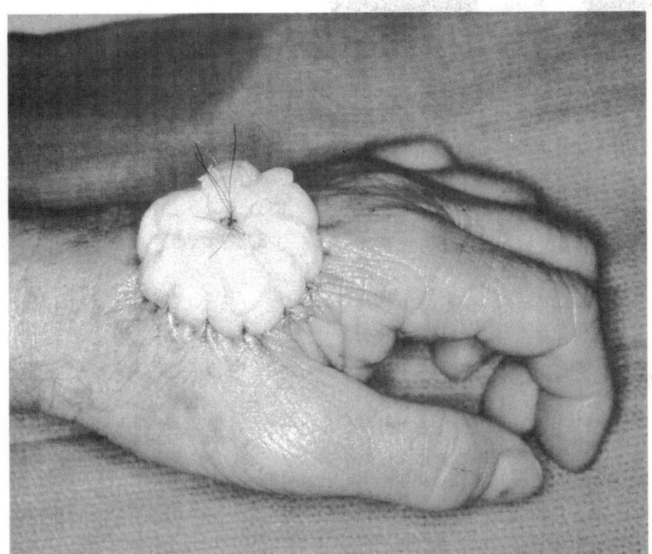

Figure 25–14. A tie over dressing is composed of a nonstick petroleum gauze with bismuth on which layers of compacted sterile gauze is placed. It is then sutured to the circumference of the skin graft in a circular manner with all the ties at the center.

The donor site of a split-thickness graft is usually covered with a Xeroform gauze and a sterile gauze dressing over it. The sterile gauze is removed the first postoperative day, leaving the Xeroform gauze in place to allow for epithelial growth. Patients are instructed to leave the donor site open to air to allow for quicker healing. A heat lamp on a very low setting may also be used to speed drying. The donor site where a full-thickness graft was taken has a primary suture line that is covered with a Xeroform gauze and a dry sterile dressing. This dressing is usually removed the first or second postoperative day and changed daily thereafter until the site is healed.

Flaps

Flaps are classified as either local or distant. Any type of tissue including skin, fascia, muscle, bone, or nerves may be transferred from one site to another with its vascular supply intact. Local flaps use tissue in close proximity to the wound site. They can be advanced forward, rotated sideways, or transferred close to the recipient site. Distant flaps involve harvesting tissue from a donor site and temporarily attaching it to the wound bed. It is then released after new tissue has formed. A distant flap may be in the form of a free tissue transfer where the blood supply is severed at the donor site and reestablished at the recipient site by microsurgical means (Fig. 25–15).

Complex wounds involving the head and neck may require reconstruction with flaps composed of skin, muscle, and bone. The type of flap used in this process is based on the degree of tissue loss, achievement of optimal function, and on individual patient's needs and goals.

A

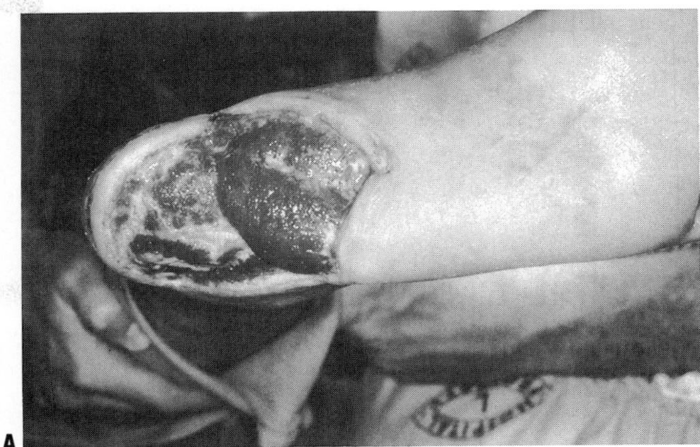

B

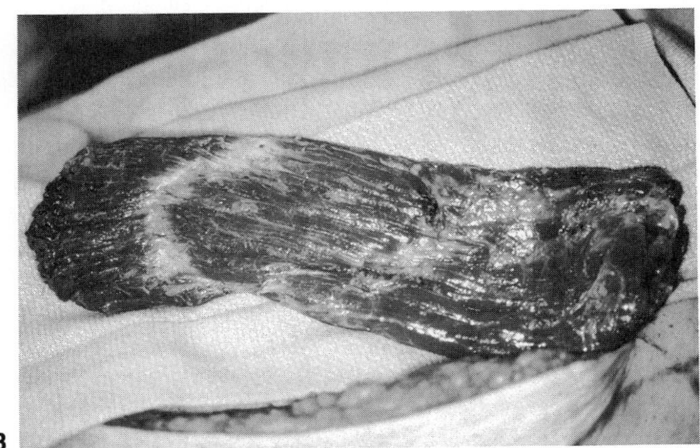

C

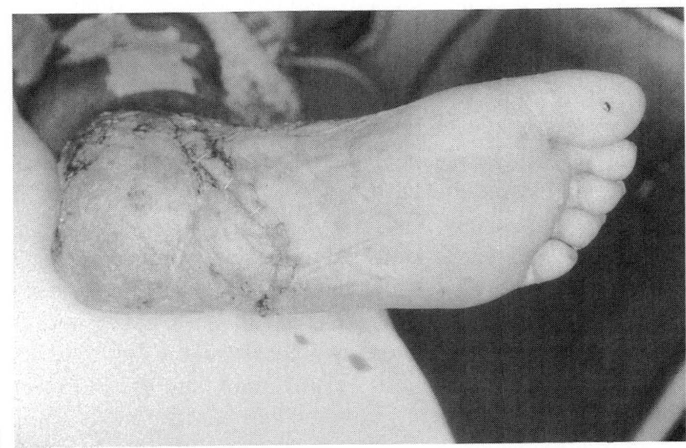

Figure 25–15. Muscle flap. **A,** A large open wound on plantar surface of a foot. **B,** The rectus muscle is harvested from the abdomen. **C,** The rectus muscle covers the foot defect and is covered with a skin graft and stapled in place.

Postoperatively, patients who receive flaps are placed on a low air loss or fluidized air beds with a capillary closure pressure between 12 to 25 mm Hg. The pressure within the capillary circulation is approximately 28 to 32 mm Hg in a healthy adult. This pressure may be lower in certain disease states. Any external or internal force of greater than 32 mm Hg applied to a bony prominence for prolonged periods can produce a capillary shutdown from inadequate capillary blood flow, and decrease cellular metabolic exchanges, thereby causing tissue hypoxia and necrosis. Low air loss or fluidized air beds help keep the flap's capillary circulation intact. Some surgeons may prefer to place patients with ischial, sacral, or trochanteric flaps who are able to move on a fluidized air bed so as to decrease movement and shearing of the flap.

Free flaps are monitored very closely for the first 48 to 72 hours. This is a critical time when clotting of the reanastomosed vessels can occur. Patients are therefore placed in an intensive care unit or closely monitored unit where the flaps can be monitored every hour. Flaps can fail from infection, arteriosclerosis, anastomotic thrombosis, hypotension, kinking of the flap's pedicle or blood supply, malnutrition, or compression (Kerrigan, 1983). The flap is observed for color, warmth, capillary blanching and refill, and bleeding from stab wounds. Color observation can depend on the donor site. If a flap is transferred from a nontanned area to a tanned area, it can be mistaken for being underperfused. Flaps generally look pale pink or pink. Increased redness can indicate venous congestion. A purple or blue color can be an indicator of severe ischemia or venous failure (Acland, 1981).

Capillary blanching and refill to assess perfusion is checked using gentle pressure on the flap. Another method to test perfusion is to stab the flap with an 18-gauge needle to make it bleed. Vascular patency can be monitored through flap temperature. Flap temperature may be monitored and compared with a control site by using specifically designed machines. A difference of three degrees between the flap temperature and the control site is considered significant and may indicate decreased patency (May & Halls, 1985). This is monitored every hour for the first 48 to 72 hours postoperatively.

Because a decrease in body core temperature can lead to vasoconstriction and decreased blood flow, a patient's room temperature is kept at 72°F or higher. A heat shield is often used over the extremity flaps to keep them warm. Some surgeons have all intravenous fluids warmed. Dopplers are also used to moniter flap blood flow. An area of arterial reanastomosis is marked on the flap and the pulse is checked for audibility every hour.

A combination of all the previous procedures may be performed to test flap circulation. In addition, blood pressure is also monitored since hypertension and hypotension can induce decreased perfusion to the flap or rupture the anastomosis. Input and outputs are monitored every hour for the first 24 hours. Hypotension is usually treated with fluid boluses instead of vasopressor agents, which can increase peripheral vascular resistance and thereby decrease blood flow to the flap. Hypertension can often be regulated by analgesic preparations and other measures. Hypertensive medications are used if pain control fails to lower the blood pressure.

Output from drains placed in the operating room is recorded every shift. If a flap is placed on a joint surface or on a lower extremity, immobilization is necessary to prevent shearing of the graft or flap. Patients with below-the-waist grafts or flaps are generally kept on complete bed rest for a period of at least one week. If a lower extremity flap or graft is performed, the patient may be out of bed after four or five days with the leg elevated at all times for another week and then is gradually allowed intermittent leg dependency. This intervention prevents venous congestion and flap or graft loss. Physical therapy usually works with the patients to teach transfers or intermittent leg dependency.

Patients with greater trochanter, ischial or, sacral myocutaneous flaps are usually kept on low air loss or fluidized air beds for a period of 10 days to 2 weeks. After discharge, the patient will need to use a specialized bed to keep the capillary pressures low until the flap is well healed. If a patient has had frequent pressure ulcers, an arrangement is made to have a low air loss lay-over mattress placed permanently on the patient's bed at home to prevent further breakdown. Patients are also instructed on factors that may promote impaired healing, such as smoking, malnutrition, or infrequent turning while lying in bed.

Tissue Expansion

Normal skin and subcutaneous tissue have the physiologic capacity to stretch and reproduce. Tissue cells and the connective tissue between the cells yield to pressure placed upon them by stretching to reduce the tension placed on them. This is well noted in pregnancy, weight gain, and skin tumor growth. Tissue expansion surgically enhances this normal biologic process by increasing tissue surface area (Austad & Pasyk, 1987). Tissue expansion is usually carried out as a secondary reconstructive procedure to improve scar appearance such as occurs with burns; to cover defects resulting from trauma, radiation, surgical, or infective processes; or to increase skin surface area such as in expansion of the chest wall skin after a mastectomy to allow for implant placement. Tissue expansion was first successfully used in the 1970s for breast tissue expansion after mastectomy.

In discussing the implications of this procedure, patients are informed that the expansion may take several months. At least two operations are needed: one for placement of the expander and another for removal of the expander and excision of the defect. Patients are also informed of the temporary deformity to their body while the expander is in place. If an infection develops within the site, or if the expander ruptures, the expander must be removed and either immediately replaced in the case of a rupture or reinserted after the infection clears. Either way, an additional surgical procedure would have to be performed.

Tissue expanders are selected according to the shape

and size of the defect. They are made of a silicone shell and come in a variety of shapes and sizes. Many types have remote filling ports, a mechanism that decreases the risk of inadvertent implant puncture during inflation. Others types of expanders have internal filling ports that contain a metal insert to denote the port area, a component that is detected with a magnet. Tissue expanders are usually placed under the skin and subcutaneous tissue. Expanders that feature remote ports are usually placed in areas where they are easy to palpate and remove. The connector tube that joins the filling port to the expander should not be placed over a joint, since sudden movement may dislodge the tube and rupture the implant.

When the implant is first surgically placed, it is filled with only a small amount of saline to prevent excessive tension on the suture line. Inflations are usually started approximately 2 weeks after initial placement to allow for the suture line to heal sufficiently. Expanders are inflated on an individualized basis according to the anatomical location and patient comfort. Saline is injected into the port with a 23-gauge or smaller needle until there is blanching of the overlying skin or patient discomfort. Expansion occurs until adequate soft tissue can be obtained to cover the defect. The expander is then removed, the defect is corrected, and a primary closure is performed.

▶ BREAST RECONSTRUCTION

Breast reconstruction is performed to correct breast deformities resulting from mastectomies, bilateral hypoplasia or unilateral hypoplasia from radiation injury, trauma, or Poland's syndrome (Fig. 25–16). Poland's syndrome can occur in varying degrees and may involve not only maldevelopment or absence of the breast and nipple but may also include absence of part or all of the pectoralis major muscle, deficiency or absence of the subcutaneous fat and axillary hair, abnormalities of costal cartilages and anterior ribs, and various abnormalities of the upper extremities including shortening and syndactyly (Hester & Bostwick, 1982).

Breast deformities—whether congenital or surgically induced—can evoke distressing feelings regarding body image and psychological well being. Breast reconstruction is a matter of choice and every woman who has a congenital deformity or who considers a mastectomy should be given the information necessary to make that choice. Some women choose not to undergo reconstruction because of the fear of both the risks involved with this surgery and multiple operations. Other women are reluctant to pursue this treatment because they feel they are too old, or their family or significant others do not support the decision to have extensive surgery. Women with young children fear that reconstruction will put too much of a financial burden on the family. They worry whether they can afford to be out of work for a long period of time and if their insurance carriers will cover the cost of reconstruction. Others fear implant placement and/or rejection of the implant. Others reflect that if the cancer recurs, it would not be easily detected because of the reconstruction.

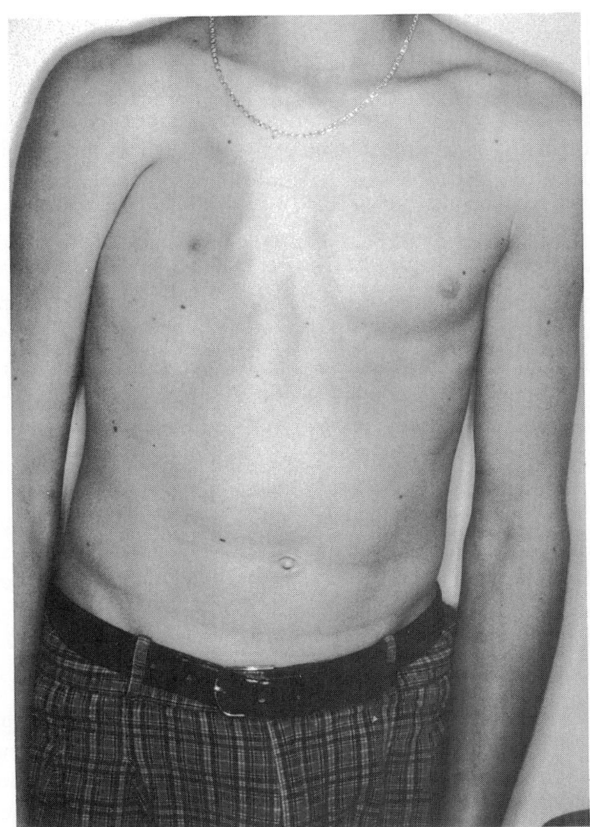

Figure 25–16. Poland syndrome. There is an absence of the pectoralis muscle and breast tissue on the right chest wall.

Breast reconstruction should be viewed as a part of cancer rehabilitation, *not* cosmetic surgery. Breast cancer patients are now given the option at the time of diagnosis whether to undergo immediate reconstruction after mastectomy. In general, patients who have undergone breast reconstruction—whether immediate or delayed—are satisfied with the end result. Several studies from the National Survey on Breast Cancer (1991) demonstrate breast reconstruction helps women experience a greater sense of psychological well being and a sense of physical comfort by improving their body image and sense of femininity.

Treating women with breast cancer requires a team approach that includes the general surgeon, medical oncologist, radiation oncologist, plastic surgeon, family physician, pathologist, nurses, psychiatrists, social workers, and physical therapists.

During the consult between the patient and the plastic surgeon, all of the treatment options related to breast reconstruction are outlined. They are tailored to meet the patient's expectations of breast appearance and symmetry incorporating the patient's physiological make-up. The patient then decides whether or not she wants to have immediate or delayed reconstruction. Reconstruction is a process with many stages and usually involves a commitment for several months to a year. Several operations are performed depending on the method of reconstruction. If the opposite breast is ptotic, a breast reduction or a mastopexy to lift the breast to match the reconstruction is also performed. The areola and nipple reconstruction are all performed separately. Adjuvent chemotherapy or radiation is not a contraindication to immediate reconstruction. Patients may begin their chemotherapy at the scheduled time postoperatively. If patients choose to delay their reconstruction, plastic surgeons recommend waiting at least one month after chemotherapy ends.

Breast reconstruction options are decided by the patient and the plastic surgeon. Not all patients are good candidates for all methods of reconstruction; therefore, patient selection is an important aspect in breast reconstruction.

Breast Implants

There are many techniques available for breast reconstruction. The simplest procedure is placement of a saline breast implant beneath the pectoralis muscle. Silicone breast implants were banned by the FDA in 1992 and are no longer placed unless one is part of a study. After a mastectomy, there is usually a significant loss of tissue. Immediate placement of a breast implant may not allow for skin closure if there is inadequate tissue. Placement of an implant immediately postmastectomy can create tension in a taut skin envelope leading to tissue necrosis. An anatomic tissue expander is placed under the pectoralis muscle and inflated over a period of several weeks or months to expand the chest tissue to allow for implant placement. The implant allows a good match of color and skin texture between the reconstructed and the other breast. The operating time and hospitalization for this method is much less than that of other procedures. If an implant is inserted as part of a delayed reconstruction, it can be done as outpatient surgery, a procedure that takes approximately 1 hour. If done as an immediate reconstruction, patients can go home when they have recovered from the mastectomy. With this method, women are able to return to work and get on with their lives sooner than with the other procedures. Since the implant is placed submuscularly, any local recurrences of the breast cancer are not covered by the implant.

Patient Selection

The patient who is to undergo an implant without a flap reconstruction needs an intact pectoralis muscle and an anterior axillary fold. It is not the preferred method when the opposite breast is large and pendulous; when the chest wall skin is tight, extremely thin, or has been irradiated; or there is not enough tissue available to close the mastectomy scar.

Risk Factors

The risks involved with tissue expansion and implant placement following a mastectomy include infection, failure of the expander device, or failure of the implant. These conditions require immediate surgical removal, additional healing time, and placement of another expander/implant at a later date.

After a mastectomy, the chest tissue is thin. Necrosis of the skin flap can occur with tissue expansion and needs to be closely monitored. Nerve compression from the expansion may occur in the ipsilateral arm and cause pain and numbness. Removal of some of the fluid usually relieves these symptoms (D'Angelo & Gorrell, 1989).

Risks associated with saline implant placement postmastectomy include capsular contracture. The risk of capsular contracture is greater when just an implant is used without extra muscle coverage. An implant that comes in contact with skin dermis has a higher reactivity rate to form a fibrous capsule. A grade 3 or 4 capsule causes the implant to shift, giving an unsightly appearance and becoming hard and painful. Surgical excision of the fibrous capsule and replacement of the implant is then necessary.

Since the chest tissue is thin, wrinkling of the implant—noticeable on the chest wall—is increased.

Surgical Procedure

Reconstruction with insertion of an implant is done through the mastectomy scar without a second incision and scar. After tissue expansion is complete, the expander is removed and the deflated implant is inserted under the pectoralis muscle with the fill tube intact. Saline is then placed in the implant according to manufacturer's directions and the fill tube is then removed. The opening is primarily closed with sutures. A drain is placed to prevent hematoma formation and removed prior to discharge from the hospital.

Breast Reconstruction with a TRAM Flap

The lower abdominal skin, fat, and rectus muscle provide a generous amount of tissue for a patient who wants a breast reconstruction without use of an implant and wants a reduction of her extra lower abdominal tissue. The transverse rectus abdominus musculocutaneous (TRAM) flap is well suited to this specific indication.

Patient Selection

This procedure requires a select patient population. Women who are not good candidates for this procedure are those with conditions such as cardiac disease, pulmonary diseases, diabetes mellitus, or collagen vascular diseases. All of these disease processes can compromise the microcirculation and oxygen delivery to the flap. Abdominal scars also need to be taken into consideration when considering use of the TRAM flap.

After menopause, blood flow to the lower abdomen

decreases. Older patients must therefore be in excellent health, of normal weight, and without systemic disease that could affect the microcirculation.

Obese patients with weights greater than 25% of ideal body weight are also not good candidates because the fat of the obese patient is poorly vascularized, requiring greater microcirculation leading to a greater risk of development of fat necrosis. The thickness of the abdominal wall affects the breast thickness and projection; therefore, a very thin women with a flat abdomen is also not a good candidate as there is not enough tissue to create an asethetic breast with a small amount of ptosis to hide the inframammary crease.

Heavy long-term cigarette smokers often have permanent damage to their microcirculation which could compromise the flap, so they are not good candidates for a TRAM flap. Women with radiation to the abdomen or mediastinum or surgical division of the superior epigastric artery, which is used as the blood supply for the TRAM flap, are also not candidates for this procedure. Those with a previous psychiatric instability may not be suited for this procedure, as the recuperation period is longer and more intensive than with other reconstructive methods.

Risk Factors

Potential risks from this procedure include bleeding, infection, scarring, and tissue necrosis.

Fat necrosis or a thickening in the fat portion of the flap can mimic a breast mass. Breast cancer is not known to recur in the abdominal wall fat, but can occur in the chest wall skin, musculofascia, or axilla. There is no evidence to suggest that breast reconstruction increases the risk of local recurrence (Sadove & Scherl, 1992). Breast cancer patients are closely monitored by their oncologist for any recurrences.

Other risks to TRAM flap surgery include loss of part or all of the flap due to thrombosis of the vessels. Deep vein thrombosis (DVT) can occur due to the length of the operation and prolonged bed rest.

A hematoma or a seroma can develop as a result of TRAM flap surgery. Patients are advised to avoid taking aspirin or aspirin-containing products as well as ibuprofen products at least one week prior to surgery to decrease risk of bleeding.

An abdominal wall hernia may also develop as a result of this procedure. To compensate for this factor, the wall is usually reinforced with a prolene mesh to prevent protrusion of intraabdominal contents. The abdominal wall fascia and part of the rectus sheath are preserved to maintain abdominal wall strength. Most patients report no long-term limitations with routine activities. Some have problems doing situps, but can be taught to strengthen the external oblique muscle to help with this activity.

Surgical Procedure

The operation takes approximately 4 to 8 hours or longer if additional procedures are performed. The patient's abdomen and chest are marked the day before or day of surgery to outline the site from which the flap will be taken (Fig. 25–17). Zones I through IV are marked on the abdomen. Zone I is usually on the same side as the pedicle or main blood supply. Zone II is adjacent to it. Zone III is at the end of the same side as the rectus muscle that is to be used as the flap and Zone IV is on the opposite side where only skin and underlying fat are taken. Many surgeons often discard Zone IV because this area may have inadequate blood supply and may cause prolonged hardening of the necrotic fat.

To begin this procedure, the abdomen is incised along the preoperative markings down to the outer layer of rectus fascia. The inner layer of fascia is preserved for abdominal wall strength. The skin and subcutaneous tissue is then dissected laterally to medially. The umbilicus is incised and left intact for closure at the end. The rectus abdominus muscle is then elevated out of the rectus sheath up to the

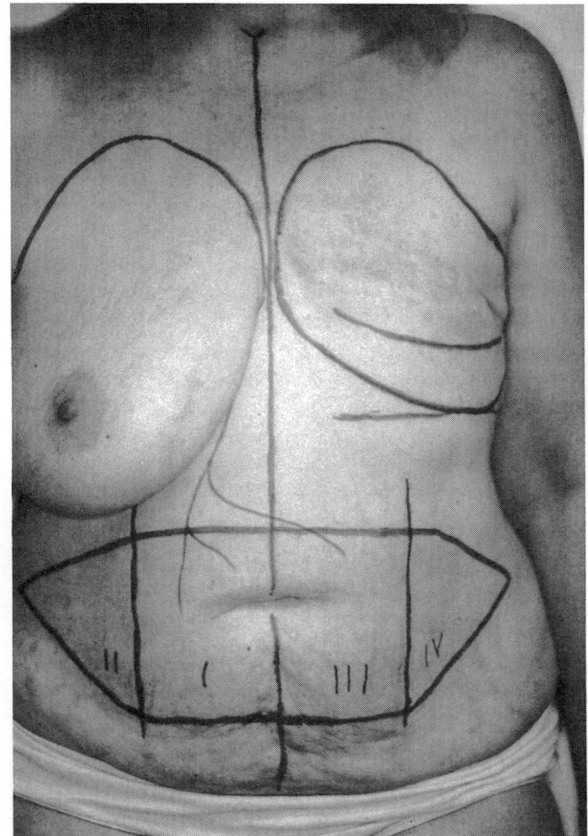

Figure 25–17. TRAM flap markings. Lines are drawn on the patient the day before or the day of surgery to guide with incisions and placement of the flap. The abdominal zones are drawn. When using a contralateral muscle flap, zones 1 and 2 have the best blood supply as that is the side where the muscle will be taken from. Zones 3 and 4 are skin and subcutaneous tissue with zone 4 being the most distal part of the flap with the least blood supply.

costal margin, tunneled (Fig. 25–18), and transposed gently—making sure there is no constriction or twisting of the pedicle—to fit into the breast region. Blood pressure and body temperature are frequently checked from this time on. A Doppler is used to determine blood flow.

Next, the abdominal posterior sheath is plicated or tucked towards midline to reinforce the abdominal wall. A mesh is used on the lower abdomen for further reinforcement. The abdomen is sutured and the umbilicus is recreated through the outer skin. The flap is then placed to pro-

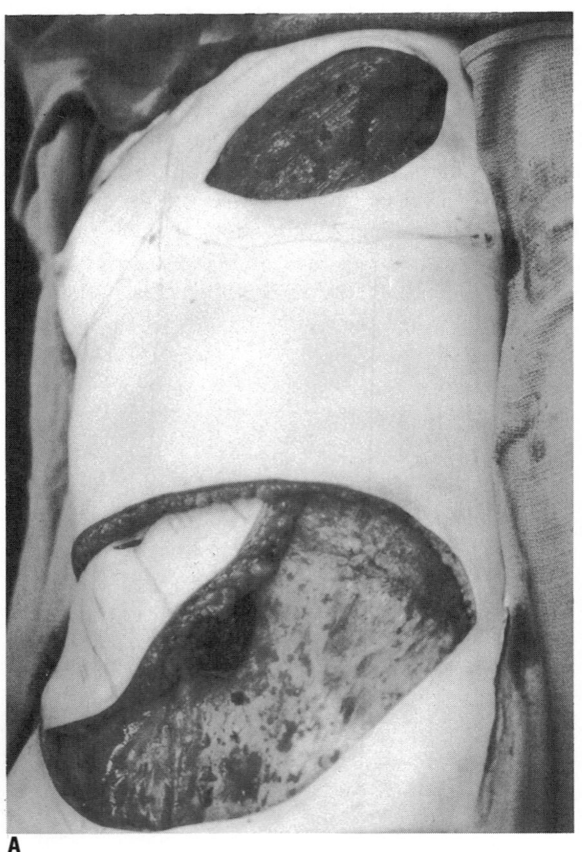

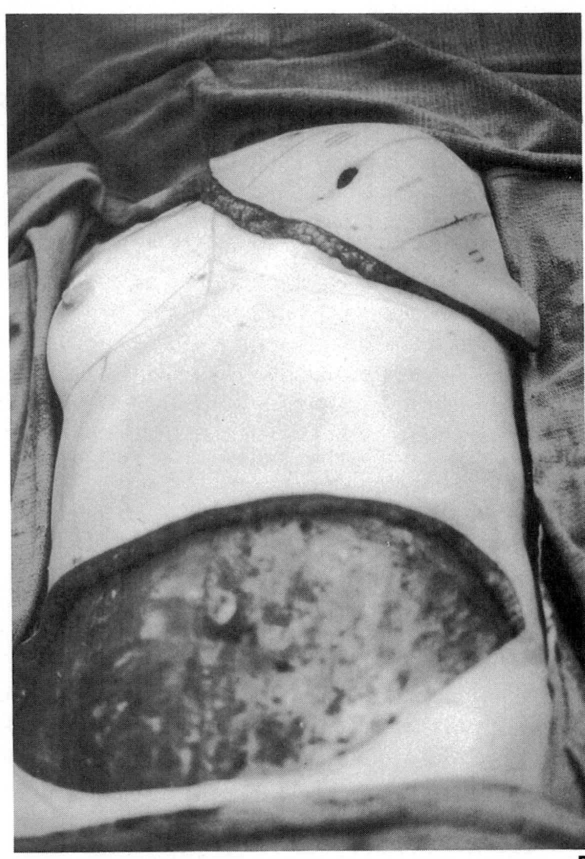

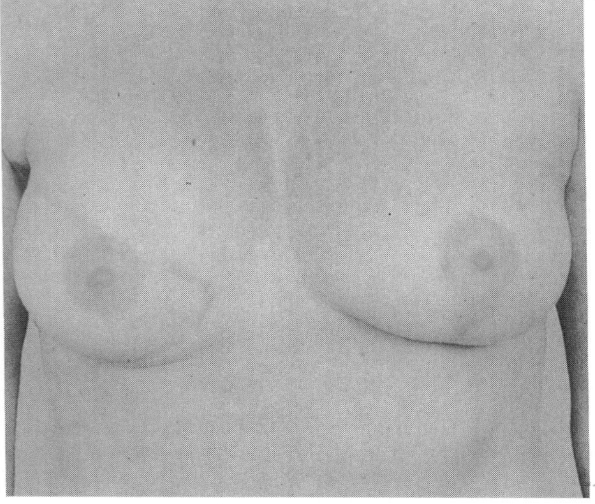

Figure 25–18. TRAM flap. **A,** The abdominal flap is harvested and tunneled under the chest wall. **B,** The flap is placed at the recipient site. The abdomen is sutured first then the flap is formed and sutured in place. Drains are placed in the abdomen and breast prior to suturing. **C,** Postop view after reduction of the opposite breast, and nipple and areola placement.

vide symmetry with the other breast and sutured closed. The TRAM breast is reconstructed slightly larger because the rectus muscle atrophies and there is some development of perioperative edema which subsides after a few months.

Drains are placed on the lateral chest wall of the flap site and along the abdominal wall. A light dressing of Xeroform strips along the suture lines followed by a sterile dressing are applied along the abdomen and breast. The TRAM flap has a light covering to allow close monitoring for the first 48 to 72 hours. Sequential compression stockings are applied during surgery and are worn until the patient is discharged.

Postoperative Care

The patient is transferred in a semi-Fowler's or jack-knife position with head and legs elevated to keep pressure off the flap's pedicle. The patient remains this way while in bed. When out of bed to a chair, usually after 48 hours, the feet are elevated while in a chair with knees bent to reduce strain on the flap. The flap is monitored every hour for 48 hours, assessing the flap's color temperature and capillary refill. Sequential compression stockings are kept on the patient while in bed to prevent DVT. The drains are emptied every shift and are removed when output is less than 30 ml per 24 hours (Cohen, 1994). If output is not less than 30 ml per 24 hours, the patient is instructed in wound and drain care. During hospitalization, mastectomy patients are put in contact with a Reach for Recovery representative. Length of hospitalization is usually 4 to 6 days.

After discharge, patients are instructed not to straighten up completely for at least 10 days. Sutures are removed about two weeks after surgery. Patients may not drive for approximately 6 weeks and are to avoid lifting anything heavier than a loaf of bread for 3 to 4 weeks, and avoid lifting objects heavier than 10 pounds for 8 to 12 weeks. It often takes 6 to 12 weeks before patients regain their strength and resume preoperative activities. Patients usually experience a discomforting pulling sensation in the abdomen for several weeks after the surgery when trying to stand upright.

Reconstruction with a Latissimus Dorsi Flap

A latissimus dorsi flap is used when there is insufficient tissue to place an implant and additional fullness is required to create a more symmetrical result. The latissimus dorsi is the largest muscle in the body. It extends from the lower thoracic spine to the iliac crest and can cover an area 15 cm by 12 cm (McCraw & Maxwell, 1988). The latissimus muscle is a hearty muscle as the thoracodorsal artery that supplies the muscle is not affected by atherosclerosis as are other arteries. It can be used to cover the chest wall when the pectoralis major is removed in a radical mastectomy or if the muscle is denervated. The flap consists of an island of skin, fat, and muscle. The latissimus dorsi gets its blood supply from the thoracodorsal artery and vein in the posterior axillary line. In patients who are having delayed surgery, it is imperative to obtain the operative report from their mastectomy to note if this artery or the thoracodorsal nerve was cut. If the nerve is cut, the muscle significantly atrophies. If the thoracodorsal artery is cut, the flap may not survive.

Patient Selection

As previously mentioned, the latissimus dorsi flap has excellent survival rates. There are few contraindications for patient selection. Those that are relevant include any woman who has had extensive radiation to the axilla or a thoracotomy excision in the area of the flap, as both could result in decreased blood supply to the flap. If a patient has had the thoracodorsal artery or nerve cut, she may not be a canididate for this reconstruction.

Risk Factors

With the latissimus dorsi flap, a rather large diagonal incision is created across the back. It usually can be concealed by undergarments or a bathing suit. There is a notable difference in skin color and texture between the reconstructed breast and back.

Loss of muscle function is a concern to many patients who undergo this procedure. The latissimus dorsi adducts, medially rotates and extends the shoulder. Weakness may be noted when pushing up from a chair or in cross country skiing or in climbing activities. Most patients have no significant functional loss (Laitung & Peck, 1985). When using a latissimus flap, an implant needs to be placed at the site, as the latissimus is a very thin flat muscle that doesn't give sufficient breast projection. The risks of using a saline implant are the same as noted in saline implant reconstruction. The risk of capsular contracture are less when using muscle coverage, so this is an advantage.

Breast cancer does not spread to the back or back scar. If the cancer recurs, it would be in the chest wall tissue, the mastectomy scar area, or on the musculofascia of the chest wall.

Seroma formation is a common complication with this surgery (Strombeck & Rosato, 1986) since a large surface area is initially created between the dissected flap and the chest wall. Drains are left in until there is less than 30 cc of drainage per 24 hours. If seroma formation continues after the drains are taken out, then the fluid is aspirated with a needle and a 60-cc syringe.

The area in which the latissimus dorsi flap is used is insensate so there is little discomfort for the patient. If an infection at the site ensues, the implant may have to be removed to allow the infection to clear, after which time it can be replaced. There is a possibility of partial loss of the flap, but this occurs in less than 2% of patients (Bostwick, 1989). If done as an immediate procedure, tissue necrosis from the mastectomy dissection can occur with some tissue sloughing.

Surgical Procedure

With latissimus dorsi flap reconstruction, the patient is marked either the day before or the day of surgery (Fig. 25–19). The patient is placed in a lateral position in the operating room to harvest the latissimus muscle. The skin island that will replace the amount of skin loss is incised to the subcutaneous tissue and the skin is lifted from the latissimus to the margins of the muscle excision. After the muscle is dissected from its lower rib origin, the flap is elevated and rotated either under the axilla or straight across through an axillary incision. A drain is placed and the back incision line is closed.

The patient is then placed in a supine position and the latissimus muscle is sutured to the pectoralis major muscle and the skin just above the inframammary crease. An opening is left for placement of the tissue expander or implant at this time. A drain is inserted and the area is closed with sutures; Xeroform gauze and a dry sterile dressing are then applied.

Postoperative Care

The patient is often put on a low air loss bed to prevent pressure on the blood supply to the flap. The patient is positioned with the surgical side up and the affected arm is elevated to heart level to avoid pressure on the flap and pedicle. The patient is also instructed not to abduct her elbow for the first 24 to 72 hours. The flap is closely monitored for the first 48 hours. Sequential compression stockings are worn while in bed to prevent thrombosis. Patients are expected to be out of bed the following postoperative day. Patients are discharged home after 3 to 5 days. They are instructed on how to care for their drains and are told to limit arm movement, as this increases seroma formation. Patients may not lift anything heavier than a loaf of bread for a period of 4 to 6 weeks and may return to work at that time.

The Contralateral Breast

On initial consultation for reconstruction, the contralateral breast is discussed. One consideration in breast reconstruction is to provide symmetry between the reconstructed and original breast. This can be accomplished through breast reduction if the contralateral breast is large and ptotic or through a mastopexy if the size of the contralateral breast matches but there is ptosis. Augmentation with an implant may also be another option.

Breast Reduction of the Opposite Breast

If the opposite breast is large and ptotic, it may need to be reduced to provide symmetry.

Breast reduction or mammoplasty involves uplift of the breast with significant dissection of breast mass and volume. This is performed usually 3 to 6 months after the initial reconstruction. A mammography is recommended prior to any breast reduction surgery. If there are any suspicious areas, the patient's general surgeon and oncologist are notified.

Risk Factors. The surgical risks associated with breast reduction include bleeding, infection, and scarring. Vertical and horizontal scars are created by this surgery. There is also the possiblity of tissue necrosis, hematoma, asymmetry, possible loss of nipple sensation, inability to lactate, possible loss of the nipple, and loss of nipple pigmentation. When breasts are very large and ptotic, the nipple is removed and placed as a free graft on the breast with a tie-over dressing. This greatly increases the risk of depigmentation.

Surgical Procedure. The breast to be reduced is marked the day before or day of surgery. The tissue is incised, lifted, and resected. The nipple is either placed as a free graft or placed along its pedicle or blood supply in a superior position. If the areola nipple complex has to be lifted more than six inches to its new site, the blood supply may not be adequate, so a free nipple graft technique is typically used. The desired amount of breast tissue is removed. The nipple and areola are positioned and sutured in place, and horizontal and vertical openings are closed with a dou-

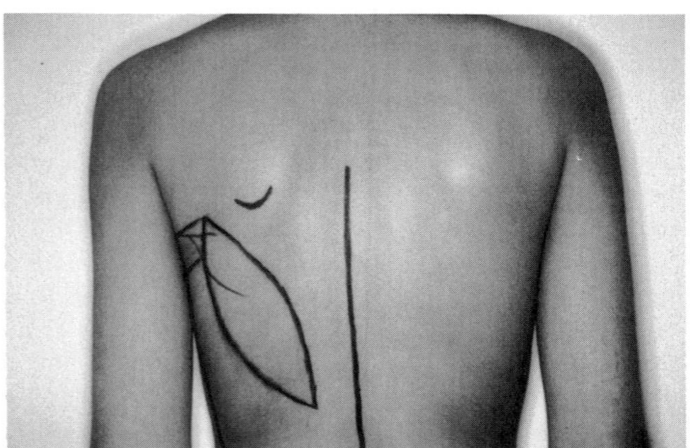

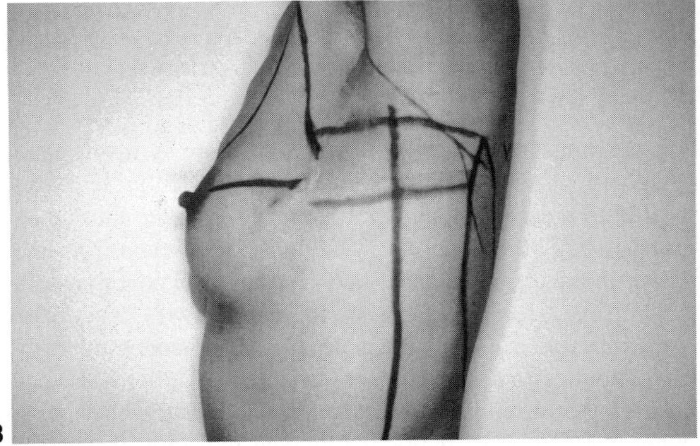

Figure 25–19. Latissimus dorsi flap preop markings. **A,** Back markings showing where the island of skin and muscle will be taken from. The patient will end up with a vertical scar the length of the flap. **B,** This shows where the flap is tunneled under to the front of the chest wall.

ble layer closure with a buried dermal and running suture. A drain may or may not be used, depending on the surgeon's preference. If one is placed in the breast, it is removed prior to discharge from the hospital. Adhesive (steri) strips are placed to further reinforce the closure. A grease-impregnated gauze (Xeroform) and a dry sterile dressing with a snug ACE bandage are wrapped over the chest.

Postoperative Care. The patient is usually kept overnight to monitor the nipple and areola for appropriate blanching and to monitor for hematoma formation. If areola–nipple viability decreases as noted by a purplish hue, the patient would have to be brought back to the operating room for removal of the areola/nipple complex which is then replaced as a full-thickness free skin graft. The patient is usually discharged the next day. The discharge dressing is according to surgeon preference which is either a snug bandage with an ACE wrap, or a noncommercial brassiere without underwire to be worn continually for 6 weeks. Patients are instructed to sleep prone for a period of several weeks. They are not to lift anything heavier than 2 pounds for 4 weeks.

Mastopexy

A mastopexy is performed if there is close symmetry to the reconstructed breast, but ptosis is present. It resuspends and reshapes an elongated and lax breast.

Risk Factors. The risks are the same as for reduction mammoplasty except the loss of pigmentation is greatly reduced. The nipple is not usually taken as a free graft, just raised on a pedicle. The risks include bleeding, infection, scarring, possible hematoma, tissue necrosis, loss of nipple sensation, possible inability to lactate, and a small possibility of loss of pigmentation. Patients are counseled that an unnatural flatness of the inferior (lower) breast and downward point of the nipple usually corrects themselves within the first few months after surgery.

Surgical Procedure. The surgical procedure is the same as for a reduction, except with little or no reduction of tissue. A drain is rarely placed. If a patient prefers more upper breast projection, then an implant is placed at the same time. This is discussed with the patient at a preoperative visit.

Postoperative Care. The postoperative care is the same as for the breast reduction except that this procedure is usually done as an outpatient procedure. The patient goes home the same day and follows up within a week.

Nipple–Areola Reconstruction

Creating the areola and nipple are the final stages of reconstruction, in order to form a more natural-looking breast. This is performed 3 to 9 months after the initial reconstruction, depending on the type of the original reconstruction and what needed to be performed on the contralateral breast. The surgery is delayed until the reconstructed breast has softened from the postoperative swelling. The delay is also dependent on how well the patient tolerated chemotherapy and/or radiation. It is usually preferable to reconstruct the nipple prior to radiation therapy to increase areola–nipple viability, but this is not a contraindication.

Risk Factors

The risk factors for nipple and areola reconstruction are very minimal. This is a minor procedure performed under local anesthesia and as an ambulatory surgery. The usual surgical risks such as bleeding infection and scarring are included. There is a possibility of loss of part or all of the graft or the flap.

Surgical Procedure

There are various options for recreating the areola and nipple. The areola can be tattooed. This does not produce an areolar projection. Tissue from the upper inner thigh has a texture similar to a natural areola. It is taken as a full-thickness skin graft, and is usually done as a separate procedure. A tie-over dressing is placed over the recipient site. A grease-impregnated gauze (Xeroform) is placed over the donor suture site, which is closed primarily with sutures. If a patient has a very large areola on the opposite side and requires a reduction or a mastopexy, part of the areola can be used at the same time or placed as a free graft on the upper thigh for future use.

To create a nipple, one can use the opposite nipple which has good color and texture match. The patient, however, needs to have a nipple on the opposite side that is large and has a good projection. There are also various cutaneous flaps utilizing local tissue at the site of the nipple reconstruction. A common flap is the skate flap in which an areola circle is drawn and the upper third of skin within the circle is deepithelialized. The subcutaneous tissue is lifted up and the wings of the skate are wrapped around the subcutaneous tissue to form a mound (Fig. 25–20). The mound is made much larger than the opposite nipple because there is approximately 50% shrinkage after a few months. The nipple is sutured vertically and the areola graft is sutured circumferentially. There are many variations on the various flaps, but they all have projection as their main goal. If a patient does not want to go through creation of a nipple, there are polyester nipple buds of various sizes that can be sewn into bras and bathing suits.

Postoperative Care

The patient is discharged the same day of surgery. The dressings are left dry and intact until a follow-up visit within 1 week. The patient is instructed not to shower and not to sleep prone for several weeks.

▶ CRANIOFACIAL DEFORMITIES

Craniofacial deformities include all deformities of the cranium and face. The anomalies are often complex and may

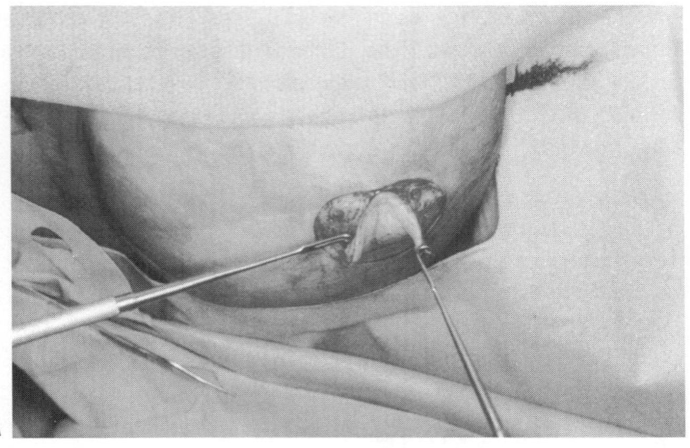

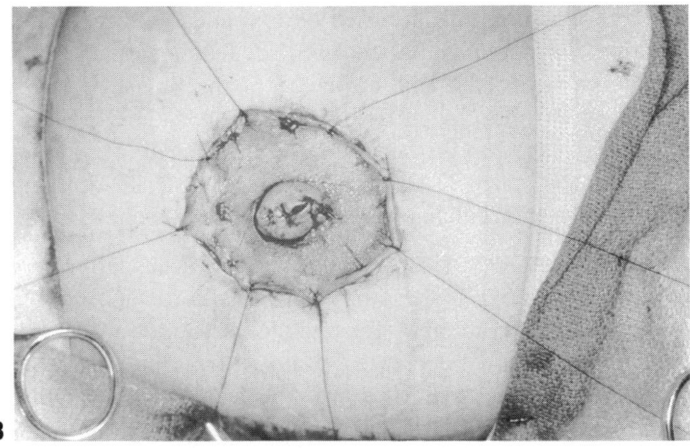

Figure 25–20. Areola/nipple reconstruction. **A,** The skate flap. A circle is drawn and the upper and lower third of the skin is deepithelialized. The tissue is lifted and the wings of the skate are wrapped around the subcutaneous tissue to form a mound. **B,** The areola is obtained from a full thickness skin graft usually from the inner upper thigh and placed around the nipple. The nipple is sutured vertically and the areola is sutured circumferentially.

involve the neurocranium, eye, mouth, and facial bones. Their management, therefore, requires a team approach that includes plastic surgeons, pediatricians, neurologists, neurosurgeons, opthalmologists, otolaryngologists, oral surgeons, speech pathologists, social workers, psyschiatrists, psychologists, and geneticists.

There are various types of craniofacial deformities from mild to severe. There are plastic surgeons who specialize in performing the reconstructions for moderate to severe craniofacial deformities. For the purpose of this chapter, only cleft palate and lip repair will be discussed, as these types of deformity are more commonly seen.

Clefts

Clefts result from the nonunion of soft tissue or bone. They are a result of failure of suture formation and occur in the soft palate, hard palate, lip, or nose. They can be unilateral or bilateral.

The palate is divided into the primary and secondary palate (Fig. 25–21). The primary palate consists of the columella, which is the soft tissue connecting the nasal tip to the upper lip, the upper lip, the four incisors, and a small triangle of hard palate (known as the premaxilla or central maxillary alveolus). The alveolar process is part of the maxilla that contains the tooth sockets. The secondary palate contains the rest of the hard palate and soft palate.

Clefts can be complete or incomplete. A complete primary cleft extends from the nose through the vermillion border (the junction of the pinkish red area of the lips with the surrounding skin). An incomplete cleft has some union of skin beneath the nares. A complete cleft of the secondary palate extends from the uvula to the incisive foramen. An incomplete cleft of the secondary palate stops before the incisive foramen (Fig. 25–22).

Cleft Palate

A cleft palate is repaired to separate the nasal cavity from the oropharynx to eliminate nasal regurgitation of liquids and solids. It also improves middle ear ventilation and speech. Appropriate timing of the repair is necessary to prevent decreased growth of the anteroposterior maxilla. The

B. Cleft palate

1. Normal palate anatomy

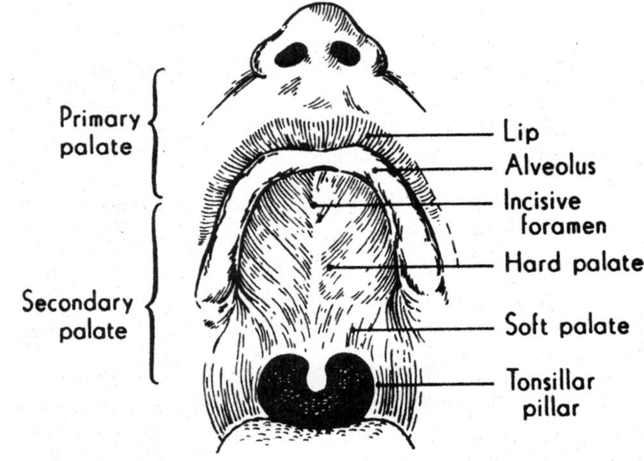

2. Classification
a. Types of clefts

Figure 25–21. Cleft palate anatomy. The primary palate consists of the soft tissue connecting the nasal tip to the upperlip; the alveolus which is part of the maxilla that contains the tooth sockets and a small triangle of the hard palate. The secondary palate contains the rest of the hard palate, the soft palate, and the tonsillar pillar.

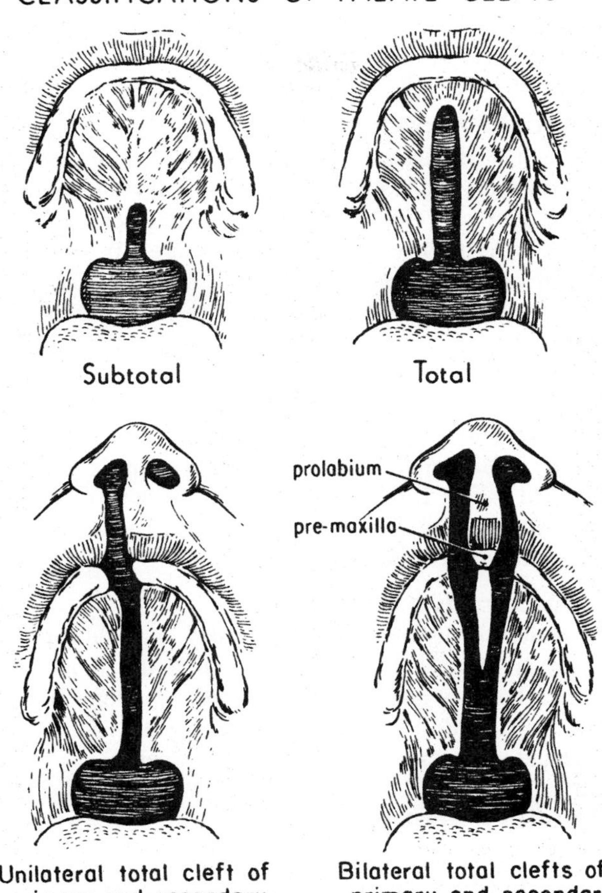

Figure 25–22. Classifications of cleft palates. *Top left:* A subtotal cleft of the secondary palate stops before the incisive foramen. *Top right:* A complete or total cleft of the secondary palate. *Bottom left:* A unilateral cleft of the primary and secondary palates. *Bottom right:* Bilateral complete cleft of the lip and palate.

soft palate is closed at about 6 to 8 months of age and the hard palate is repaired at approximately 18 months of age. Myringotomy tubes may be placed at this time.

Infants often tire easily during feeding, and may experience a failure to thrive. They need to be followed very carefully for weight gain. When bottle feeding, parents need to be instructed to make larger crosscuts in the nipple to allow for more flow. Infants should be fed at a 45-degree angle so that less milk escapes into the nasal passages. These infants ingest a large amount of air with the milk and need to be burped more often. Sour or acid foods should be avoided so as to prevent irritation of the nose while the cleft is still open.

Risk Factors

Surgical correction of cleft palate can result in bleeding/hemorrhage that can be life threatening if clotted blood becomes lodged on the vocal cords causing respiratory obstruction. There can be suture-line dehiscence and development of an oronasal fistula between the palate and nose. In addition, velopharyngeal incompetence, an inability to close the sphincter between the oral and nasal cavities that results in hypernasal speech, can also be associated with these procedures.

Surgical Procedure

There are various methods of cleft palate repair. Surgeons have their preference for closure, which all involve the use of local flaps with either V-Y advancement flaps or Z-plasties to close the defect. A tongue suture is placed to prevent tongue movement, impeding the infant/child from irritating the suture line with his or her tongue.

Postoperative Care

The patient is usually positioned supine with the head elevated or crib mattress in a slight reverse trendelenburg position to reduce swelling. The tongue suture is removed in 24 to 48 hours. Liquid feeding may be initiated but most babies refuse feeding for the first 48 hours. IV supplementation is required. Arm restraints are placed for 2 weeks and worn at all times except for bathing. Bottle feeding is usually delayed for 2 weeks after surgery. The parents are instructed to keep the baby on only liquidy soft baby food from the edge of a cup or through a syringe and a soft red tube feeder during this period. No foreign objects are allowed near the mouth during this postoperative period. After 3 to 6 months of palate closure, parents are encouraged to have the child suck with straws.

Following the cleft palate repair, the patient continues to see the various members of the cleft palate team for evaluation and continued therapy.

Cleft Lip

Cleft lips are repaired when the child weighs at least 10 to 14 pounds, which is about 3 months of age, to ensure an adequate amount of tissue with which to work. This time frame varies as some surgeons will repair these deformities earlier.

Risk Factors

Risk factors for cleft lip repair include hypertrophic or widened scars, residual asymmetry, excessive lip shortening, redundancy of the vermilion, tissue deficit in the vermilion (a whistle deformity), or malalignment. The alar deformity is expected until definitive nasal surgery is performed. Wound dehiscence is unusual, but may occur from direct trauma.

Surgical Procedure

Closure of the cleft lip involves use of various flaps. It is usually repaired with a sutured closure of the muscle and skin; the technique is surgeon specific. The goal of a cleft lip repair is to join the cleft edges along the natural lip line, creating symmetry without loss of the natural border (Fig. 25–23).

Postoperative Care

Elbow/arm restraints are placed to prevent fingers or objects from interfering with the surgical repair, and are worn continuously for a period of 2 to 3 weeks except for bathing. Soft liquidy foods using a cup or syringe and a red tube are used to feed the infant/child for a period of 3 weeks. Parents are instructed to apply antibiotic ointment to the suture line with a cotton-tipped applicator twice daily.

These patients continue to follow up with the cleft palate/lip team. Further reconstruction is often necessary in the preschooler and adolescent stages because residual lip and nose deformities may affect psychosocial growth at this time. In the preschooler stage, the alar is reconstructed and orthodontic repairs—such as straightening rotated teeth or replacing missing teeth—are implemented. Impaired hearing and speech difficulties are also addressed at this time. In adolescence, septal repair and osteotomies (breaking of the nasal bone to narrow it) are done when the nose has fully matured and no further growth is expected.

TRAUMATIC FACIAL FRACTURES

Facial fractures can occur to pedestrians hit by cars, from motor vehicle accidents, or blows to the face from fists, objects, or gunshot wounds.

Nasal Fractures

Nasal fractures are the most common facial fractures. Most are minor with little or no displacement.

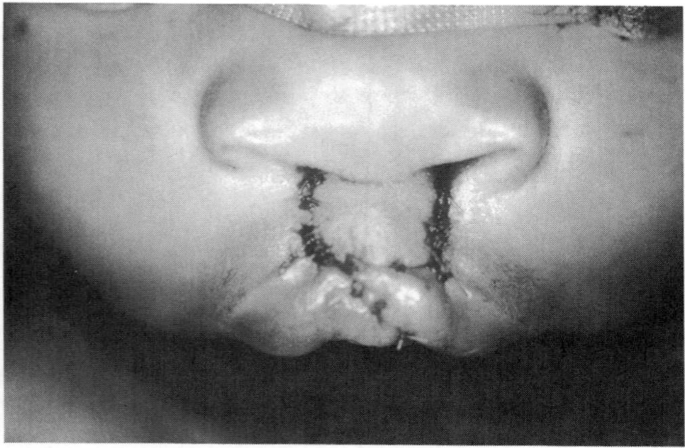

Figure 25–23. Cleft lip repair. The cleft edges are joined along the natural lip line to create symmetry without loss of the natural border.

Risk Factors

The possible risks for repair of nasal fractures is severe bleeding, late nasal deformity, and septal deviation which may require addition surgery.

Surgical Procedure

The method of surgical intervention selected for displaced nasal fractures is a closed reduction, whereby the bones are manipulated with either a #3 knife handle or padded Kelly forceps or Asch forceps and digital pressure. The fracture is reduced when the bones are back in midline. Steri strips and adhesive tape are then applied to the bridge of the nose to prevent edges of the splint from damaging the skin. The splint is applied over the tape and is removed after one week. If a laceration accompanies the fracture, the fracture is reduced through the open wound designating an open reduction. The laceration is sutured and a splint is placed as described earlier. If there is collapse of the bone in a downward manner, then a combination of nasal packing and external splinting as described is used.

Postoperative Care

The patient is discharged the same day as the repair. The patient is instructed to sneeze through the mouth, not through the nose, and not blow the nose for at least 10 to 14 days. Any nasal discharge can be very gently patted. The splint and any packing are removed in 1 week.

Maxillary Fractures

The maxilla forms a portion of the orbit nasal fossa, oral cavity, and palate. In 1901, LeFort determined the areas of structural weaknesses in the facial bones (Fig. 25–24), which are confirmed by a CT scan and radiologic views:

LeFort I: Transverse fracture that involves the alveolar process and the roof of the mouth to the floor of the nose.
LeFort II: Pyrimidal-shaped fracture that begins at the apices of the teeth and across the nasal bones and inferior and medial orbit.
LeFort III: Fracture that extends along the zygomatic frontal suture line and meets in the midline along the nasofrontal suture line.

Risk Factors

The risks involved with repair of maxillary fractures include pain, hemorrhage, nasal airway obstruction from edema, nonunion of the fracture, CSF rhinorrhea or meningitis, blindness/double vision from a displaced bone fragment severing or compressing the optic nerve, lacrimal obstruction, extraocular muscle imbalances, malocclusion, periorbital edema, enopthalmos (recession of eyeball into the socket), hypoasthesia of the infraorbital nerve devitalization of the teeth, and malocclusion of the teeth.

Surgical Procedure

Treatment of LeFort fractures consists of an open reduction through a buccal sulcus incision (mouth) for lower maxil-

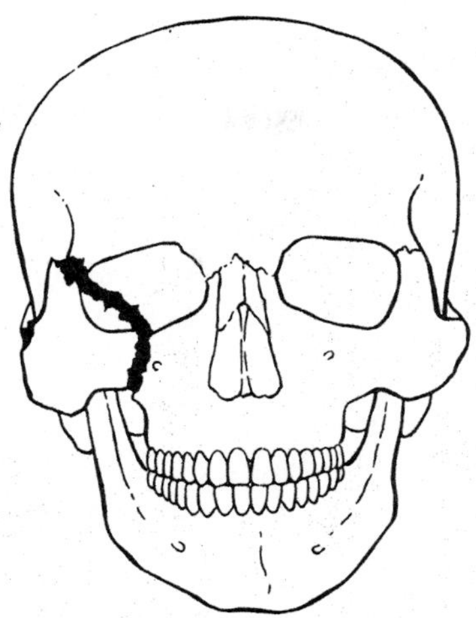

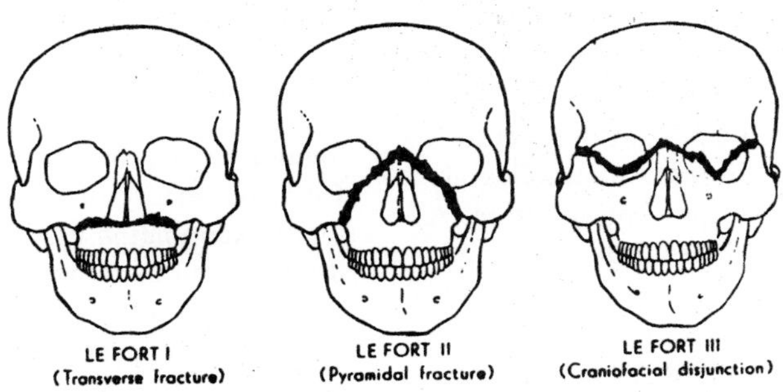

Figure 25–24. LeFort fractures. *Bottom left:* LeFort I—transverse fracture that involves the alveolar process, roof of the mouth, and floor of the nose. *Middle:* LeFort II—starts at the apices of the teeth and crosses the nasal bones and inferior and medial orbit. *Bottom right:* LeFort III—extends along the zygomatic frontal suture line and meets in the middle along the nasofrontal suture line.

lary fractures or through coronal or eyelid incisions for higher level maxillary fractures. Fractures are reduced with interfragmentary wiring or plate fixation using titanium screws. Stainless steel should not be used as a permanent implant as it may cause erosion, tonicity, and hypersensitivity in maxillofacial fixation (Haug, 1996). In complex fractures, bone grafts may be needed if the structural supports cannot be reconstructed using suspension wires.

Zygomatic Fractures

The zygoma joins the frontal bone superiorly and the maxilla in the medial orbit. It forms the lateral wall and a large portion of the lateral floor of the orbit. It also joins with the temporal bone adjacent to the ear.

These fractures are manifested by cheek and eyelid edema, depression of the cheek bone, circumoral and periorbital ecchymosis (raccoon eyes), unilateral nosebleed, and anesthesia or hyperesthia of the zygomatic area.

Risk Factors

The risks involved with surgical management include bleeding, maxillary sinus infection, double vision, malfunction of the extraocular movements of the eyes, blindness, and malunion of the fracture.

Surgical Procedure

Surgery consists of an open reduction through either the buccal vestibule, the lateral third of the eyebrow, infraorbital region, or temporal region. The bones are repaired with wires or titanium miniplates/screws and/or a bone graft depending on the severity of the break.

Mandibular Fractures

Mandibular fractures are manifested by malocclusion, inability to open the mouth, swelling, ecchymosis, jaw and muscle spasms, and numbness to the lower lip. They are classified according to the fracture's location, condition of the teeth, and direction of the teeth.

Risk Factors

The risks involved with surgical management include hemorrhage, airway obstruction in greatly displaced fractures due to tongue and edemic tissues of the floor of the mouth falling back to occlude the pharynx, nonunion, malocclusion, infection, osteomylitis, nutritional defects, and anklylosis of the TMJ joint.

Surgical Procedure

Mandibular fractures can be repaired either with closed reduction and fixation with wires and arch bars; with open reduction and internal fixation with plates and screws; or with wires for a displaced fracture.

Postoperative Care

Patients with fractures of the maxilla or zygoma requiring internal fixation with plates and screws are monitored for the first 24 to 48 hours for diplopia (double vision), blurred vision, and impaired extraocular movements. If reduced blinking is noted, liquid tears may be ordered. Postoperative edema often increases for the first 12 to 24 hours. Ice is applied gently to the face (not directly to the skin) and the head is elevated postoperatively to decrease edema.

If the patient has intermaxillary fixation, which varies according to the type and severity of the fracture, the jaw is wired shut. Suction equipment and wire cutters are at the patient's bedside at all times. Antiemetics are usually prescribed postoperatively to prevent vomiting. A nasogastric tube may or may not be present. If vomiting is imminent, the wires are cut at once at the wire loops noted inside the cheek. The wires (intermaxillary fixation) are usually maintained for a period of 4 to 8 weeks, depending on the degree of displacement for the fracture. The patient is instructed to carry a wire cutter at all times and know which wires to cut if in a situation where vomiting is imminent. If this happens, the surgeon should be notified immediately.

If the patient's airway cannot be maintained after surgery, a nasopharyngeal airway may be needed. The patient is suctioned through this airway p.r.n. If bleeding is present, breath sounds and airway patency are assessed every two hours. A tracheostomy set should be immediately available. Assess for signs of hypoxia, such as tachypnea, tachycardia, and restlessness.

When the patient is tolerating oral fluids while clamping the nasogastric tube, the tube may be removed. Patients may drink from a glass or use a catheter and a syringe to ingest a thoroughly strained formula. Straws need to be avoided for the first 7 to 14 days as this can stimulate bleeding. Patients need supplemental liquid nutrition as well as nutritional services for dietary counseling. Patients need to maintain a balanced dietary mix of protein, carbohydrates, and fats to maintain enough calories. When discharged home, patients may use blenderized food from all food groups but without particles that could get lodged in the wiring and increase postoperative infection. Patients should avoid alcoholic and carbonated beverages, as they may fizz or foam in the back of the throat and cause airway problems (Steur, 1991).

Patients are taught to irrigate the inside of the mouth with water or a mouthwash, according to the surgeon's preference, using a syringe and red rubber catheter or any low-pressure water device after every meal and at bedtime as long as the wires are in place.

Pieces of paraffin wax can be placed on the open ends of the wires if they irritate buccal surfaces.

▶ HAND SURGERY

Hand surgery encompasses injuries involving fractures; dislocations; amputations; replantations; tendon, nerve, and nail injuries; infections; and soft-tissue coverage. It also includes congenital disorders, osteo and rheumatoid arthritis, burns, tenosynovitis, vascular disorders, and Dupuytren's contractures. This section will cover the surgical aspect of tendon injuries, replantations, tenosynovitis, Dupuytren's contractures, and carpal tunnel syndrome.

Tendon Injuries

Tendon injuries of the hand are noted on initial evaluation from the history of the mechanism of the injury and thorough examination of motor function and strength of each digit as well as radiographic views. Uncomplicated tendon lacerations should be repaired within 7 to 10 days after injury. Tendon lacerations associated with compound fractures, vascular injuries, and/or devitalized tissue should be repaired immediately. The goal of tendon repair is to restore maximum function. To achieve maximal function, it is necessary to have a well-aligned bony structure with good skin coverage as well as a sufficient blood and nerve supply. Tendon injuries may involve the extensor tendons, which extend the hand and wrist, and/or the flexor tendons, which flex the hand and wrist.

Extensor Tendons. Extensor tendon injuries at or near its insertion on the distal phalanx (mallet finger), do not usually separate widely when lacerated or avulsed and may be treated by splinting. Splinting of the distal interphalangeal joint in hyperextension should be done as soon after injury as possible. Even closed injuries greater than one month can be splinted (Patel, Shekhar et al., 1986). A metal splint can be taped in place for a period of 6 weeks. The degree of extension for splinting can be obtained by observing the digit for the degree of extension at which the digital dorsal skin blanches prior to placing the splint. The amount of hyperextension in the splint should not exceed this point (Ryan & Mullins, 1987). The splint is worn continuously and removed only when very soiled. When the splint is replaced, the distal phalanx is continuously maintained in extension on a table top while the new splint is placed and taped. After 6 weeks, the patient may begin guarded flexion exercise. If any lag is noted, the splint is placed for another 2 weeks.

Injury to the extensor tendon over the proximal interphalangeal joint may result in a boutonnière deformity. This also may be treated with splinting for 4 to 6 weeks. The distal interphalangeal joint is left free for active flexion. If there is a long delay between injury and initial presentation, avulsion of the bone fragment from the base of the middle phalanx, or dislocation of the proximal interphalangeal joint, then surgical repair is indicated.

Tendons lacerated over the metacarpal joints are repaired surgically.

Flexor Tendons. The flexor tendons located on the palmar surface of the hand have a double-walled hollow tube or sheath for each finger that immerse the tendons with synovial fluid. A fibrous band or retinaculum overlies the tendon sheath, which extends from the neck of the metacarpals and ends at the distal phalanx. It consists of several pulleys that crisscross and surround the flexor tendon. The annular or circular pulleys prevent the tendons from bowstringing during finger flexion.

Risk Factors

The risk factors involved with surgical management include bleeding, infection, scarring, need for surgery later to cut scar tissue adhesions if scarring decreases function, stiffness from postoperative splinting, loss of grip strength due to immobilization of the hand, need for hand therapy, rupture of tendon repair, possible injury to blood vessel and nerves, and possible tissue necrosis.

Surgical Procedure

Tendons are repaired using magnification either through the microscope or by using magnification loops. The incision to repair a tendon is often extended proximally to the laceration, as the proximal end of the lacerated tendon usually retracts. Once the two ends of the tendon are located, they are sutured together using surgeon-specific techniques. The wound is then irrigated and, when hemostasis is achieved, the wound is closed with nonabsorbable nylon sutures that are removed in 10 to 14 days. If there is loss of tendon tissue, such that the two ends cannot be joined, then a tendon graft or transfer may be indicated.

Postoperative Care

Careful padding of the hand in the web spaces between the fingers should be done before applying the rest of the bandage. This action evenly distributes pressure and helps to prevent moisture buildup, thereby preventing skin irritation. Failure to pad the palm and dorsum can cause unnecessary pressure on the radial and ulnar sides of the hand. The hand is placed in a plaster cast and immobilized for a period of 3 to 6 weeks if the extensor tendon is repaired. Patients are then referred to hand therapy for passive extension and active flexion exercises. It is preferable to have a certified hand therapist conduct these sessions. Adhesions are less of a problem with extensor tendons than with flexor tendons.

If the repair is a flexor tendon, a sterile dressing is applied and a dorsal plaster splint extending from beyond the fingertips to the proximal forearm is applied to keep the metacarpal phalangeal joints in 60-degree flexion. Hand therapy is started within a few days to prevent adhesion formation that can impair movement of the flexor tendons through the pulleys. A rubber-band splint is made for the patient by the hand therapist to allow active extension followed by passive flexion. Early protected mobilization improves the strength of the repair and minimizes adhesions. Patients are counseled about the importance of compliance in following the therapy to regain function. They are also told that they cannot be too aggressive as this may rupture the tendon repair.

The fingertips are usually exposed to assess the vascularity of the hand. Color, temperature, and capillary refill are noted for the first 24 to 48 hours postoperatively if the patient is an inpatient. If the patient is discharged the same day, he or she is instructed to assess the fingertips for color and temperature changes as well as increased swelling. The patient is also instructed to keep the hand elevated above the level of the heart at all times to decrease swelling and pain; a sling is provided for this. While sitting or lying at home, the patient can keep the hand propped up on pillows.

Digit Replantations

In the event of the amputation of a digit, it may be replanted if the digit is wrapped in ice immediately after the injury and is not crushed. Revascularization of incomplete amputations may also be performed if there is not extensive injury to the afflicted limb. Replantations of avulsed thumbs have an unpredictable survival rate. Therefore, tendon and nerve reconstructions on the thumb are usually carried out as a secondary procedure about 6 weeks after the vessels are repaired.

Risk Factors

These include bleeding, infection, scarring, arterial or venous insufficiency, failure of replantation, amputation, nonunion, angulation, and malrotation of the replanted finger bone.

Surgical Procedure

The pneumatic tourniquet is applied to the affected extremity and is let down for 15 minutes after 2 hours to allow for clearing of metabolic cellular wastes accumulated during inflation from lack of blood flow. The bones are fixated with interosseous pins, wires, or plates. The arteries and veins are then repaired microscopically. If nerves or vessels are exposed, a skin graft is applied. The postoperative dressing provides immobilization without constriction allowing the finger to be exposed for observation.

Postoperative Care

After replantation of a digit, antithrombotic medications are usually begun. This often includes 600 mg of aspirin twice daily for 3 weeks. In addition, IV low molecular-weight dextran in 500 ml of glucose is given over 8 hours for the first 5 days. Postoperative monitoring of the circulation with cutaneous temperature probes and observation as to color, temperature, and capillary refill is important. A very rapid refill may represent venous congestion. A very slow refill or blanching may indicate arterial insufficiency. Vascular occlusion commonly occurs during the first 2 to 3 postoperative days. The hand is kept warm with some type of warming hood or blanket to prevent vasospasms; it is also kept elevated to prevent congestion and minimize edema. Patients are instructed at discharge to monitor the color and temperature of the finger and are told to call the surgeon immediately if there are any changes. Hand therapy for progressive range of motion is started at approximately 4 weeks postoperative.

Tenosynovitis

Tendons of a musculotendonous unit pass through tunnels or canals in various locations of the upper extremity. Movement of the hand in these areas produces movement of the tendons through the tunnels. When the synovium, which is a fluid-filled membrane, becomes inflammed, movement through these tunnels becomes painful. The areas most frequently involved are the abductor pollicis longus tendon in the first dorsal compartment in de Quervain's disease and the digital flexors (trigger fingers). In de Quervain's tenosynovitis, the first dorsal compartment located in front of the radius is where tenderness is localized. Acute pain on any movement of the thumb is the primary symptom. It can radiate into the forearm. The Finkelstein test, in which the patient is asked to grasp the thumb firmly in the palm of his or her hand and the examiner deviates the hand in an ulnar direction, helps to confirm the diagnosis. The opposite hand is also tested. If injection with steroids and splinting over a period of 6 weeks fails to relieve the symptoms, then surgical release is performed.

Flexor tenosynovitis usually presents with a painful arresting–locking motion of the finger when attempts are made to straighten the finger from a flexed position. Triggering occurs from the formation of a nodule on the tendon which jams in the tunnel on attempts to straighten the finger. The nodule can be felt by placing one's finger over the region of the palmar crease at the base of the involved finger. The examiner may feel a small nodule passing beneath his or her fingers. Trigger finger may occur in diabetic and rheumatoid patients, but frequently the etiology is unknown. If steroid injections do not provide lasting relief for the pain, then surgery is performed.

Risk Factors

The risks involved with this surgery include bleeding, infection, scarring, stiffness from splinting, possible loss of grip strength, possible injury to blood vessels/nerves, possible neuroma, and possible need for hand therapy.

Surgical Procedure

A pneumatic arm tourniquet and local anesthesia are generally used. The skin and subcutaneous tissue are incised, taking care to protect nerves and blood vessels. In trigger finger, a scalpel is used to divide the A1 pulley longitudinally to relieve triggering. If awake, the patient is asked to actively move his or her finger to make certain that the triggering and locking has ceased. In deQuervain's tenosynovitis, the first annular ligament is dissected or divided longitudinally with a scalpel. The patient is asked to move his or her thumb to confirm good movement without entrapment.

Postoperative Care

Padding is placed in the web spaces between each finger; the hand and operative site are also well padded. A compression dressing is placed over the operative site, and the thumb is immobilized after repair of the first compartment to minimize pain. A splint is placed with the fingers exposed to allow for observation of color and temperature of the digits. The patient is to keep the hand elevated above the level of the heart to decrease swelling for the first several postoperative days. Approximately 6 to 7 days postoperatively, the bulky splint is removed and the hand is placed in a smaller splint covering only the first compartment with gauze padding to protect the suture lines. The patient may perform very gentle range-of-motion exercises with his or her fingers, but may not use the hand for lifting or performing repetitive motion. The sutures are removed the following week and the patient may begin using the hand for very limited movements, such as writing or using the computer for no longer than 15 minutes at a time, resting for 20 minutes in between. Lifting is prohibited for another 2 weeks; then lifting may be gradually incorporated over the next several weeks.

Dupuytren's Disease

The first sign of the disease is a painful nodule made up of fibroblasts in the distal palmar crease in the area of the base of the finger, frequently the ring small or middle fingers. This nodule may progress to development of bands that produce the Dupuytren's contracture of the flexor tendons in the afflicted digit (Fig. 25–25). The nodule may either remain for years and never advance or pro-gress slowly or rapidly to a flexion joint contracture. The disease is attributed to an inherited autosomal dominant trait.

The goal of surgery is to improve function to the hand. The use of steroids or splinting have not been found of value to prevent contracture. Surgery is indicated when there is a digital flexion contracture of the metacarpal joint or proximal interphalangeal joint.

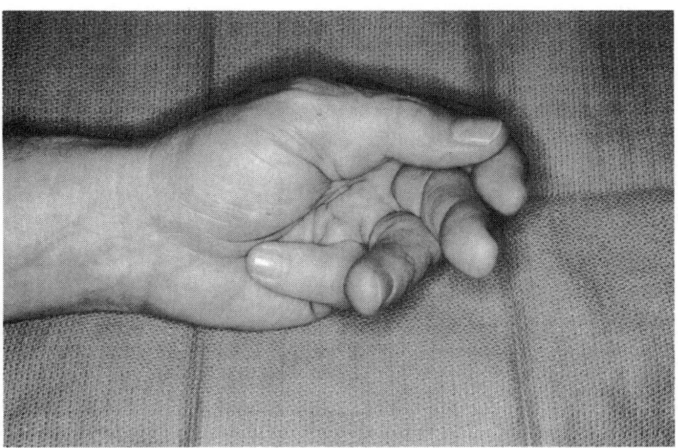

Figure 25–25. Dupuytren's contracture. A severe flexion contracture of the fourth and fifth finger with moderate contracture of the second and third. This patient lost function of his hand with all the contractures. He had this for many years and progressively worsened over time.

Risk Factors

The risks involved with the surgery are bleeding, infection, scarring, possible tissue necrosis, stiffness from splinting, need for hand therapy, recurrence of the disease, scar adhesion limiting function, failure to regain full extension, and possible injury to blood vessels and nerves.

Surgical Procedure

An incision is made in the palm and a fasciectomy is performed to excise the nodule and pretendinous bands.

Postoperative Care

Padding is placed in the web spaces between each finger, and the hand and operative site are well padded. A splint is placed and removed approximately 1 week after surgery. Active exercises and dynamic splinting by a certified hand therapist are initiated days after surgery. The sutures are removed two weeks postoperatively, and the patient continues to receive hand therapy for severals weeks to prevent flexion contractions.

Carpal Tunnel Syndrome

The most frequent peripheral nerve compression is at the median nerve at the carpal tunnel. There are ten structures that pass through this tunnel: the median nerve and nine flexor tendons. The carpal tunnel is inelastic and unable to accommodate any change in volume through the tunnel. Factors involved in carpal tunnel syndrome are any inflammatory conditions or nonspecific tenosynovitis; alterations in fluid balance from pregnancy, hypothyroidism, menopause, renal failure, and obesity; and external forces, such as vibrations, direct pressure, fractures of the forearm or wrist, or tumors.

The most frequent complaint is numbness and tingling in the region of the median nerve distribution. The digits most involved are the middle and index fingers. Pain is also noted at the wrist, often radiating to the forearm. These symptoms often awaken the patient at night. Weakness in grip strength with patient complaints of frequent dropping of objects is also noted.

Examination includes the Phalens test, in which the wrist is flexed, and Tinels sign, in which tapping over the carpal tunnel at the wrist produces numbness and tingling over the median nerve distribution. Examination for muscle wasting at the thenar prominance is performed by comparing both hands. Electrical conduction studies are performed to note if there is a slowing of nerve conduction through this area. If splinting and use of nonsteroidal antiinflammatories for 6 weeks or longer fail to improve symptoms, or if thenar muscle wasting and decreased sensation (which are advanced signs of neuropathy) are evident, then surgery is indicated. Injection into the carpal tunnel is suggested when the entrapment is temporary, such as in pregnancy. A few weeks after pregnancy, symptoms usually subside. Injecting into the carpal tunnel carries a risk of injuring the median nerve.

Risk Factors

The risk factors involved include bleeding, infection, scarring, stiffness from splinting, possible need for hand therapy, possible injury to blood vessels and nerves, failure to relieve symptoms, and loss of grip strength.

Surgical Procedure

A longitudinal incision following the crease of the palm is made over the carpal tunnel area and the carpal ligament is divided longitudinally along its ulnar border. The wrist is closed with nonabsorbable sutures. Endoscopic carpal tunnel release may also be performed. Outcomes are similar between the two techniques, with scar tenderness the only significant factor.

Postoperative Care

Padding is placed in the web spaces of each finger, and the hand and operative site are well padded. A plaster splint is then placed over the bulky dressing. The patient is instructed to keep the arm elevated above the level of the heart to reduce swelling. In approximately 1 week the bulky splint is removed and a wrist splint is placed with a gauze dressing over the operative site. The patient is instructed to remove the splint several times per day, performing very gentle range-of-motion exercises of the fingers and wrist. The sutures are removed the following week and the patient is instructed to use the splint at night over the next 2 weeks. Limited repetitive hand movements such as typing are limited to 15 minutes with 20-minute rest periods in between for a period of 2 weeks. Heavy lifting of objects greater than a pound are discouraged for a period of 6 weeks postoperatively and then gradually after that. Swelling over the thenar and hypothenar prominence (pillar pain) usually persists for 12 to 16 weeks after surgery. Constant use of the hand without rest and gripping will aggravate the pain. Maximum grip strength returns in about 6 months.

REFERENCES

Acland, R. D. (1981). Discussion on experiences in monitoring the circulation in free-flap transfer. *Plastic and Reconstructive Surgery, 68,* 554.

Allen, J. G., Kelly, K. A., & Glodich, A. (1997). A psychoeducational program for patients with trauma-related disorders. *Bulletin of the Menninger Clinic, 61* (2), 222–239.

Ainslie, N. B. & Ojeda-Fournier, H. (1996). Creating a nipple–areola reconstruction. *Plastic Surgical Nursing, 16* (3), 156–165.

American Heritage College Dictionary, 3rd ed. (1993). New York: Houghton Mifflin.

Austad, E. D. & Pasyk, K. A. (1987). Origin of expanded tissue. *Clinics of Plastic Surgery, 14* (3), 431–433.

Bartfield, J. M. et al. (1995). The effects of warming and buffering on pain of infiltration of lidocaine. *Academic Emergency Medicine, 2,* 254–258.

Bartkiw, T. P., Fynn, B. R., & Brown, D. H. (1995). Diagnosis and management of nasal fractures. *International Journal of Trauma Nursing, 1* (1), 11–18.

Beasley M. E. (1994). The pedicled TRAM as preference for immediate autogenous tissue breast reconstruction. *Clinics in Plastic Surgery, 21,* 191–205.

Bhishagratna, K. K. (1916). An English translation of the Sushruta samhita based on original Sanskrit text. (3 vols.). Calcutta: Bose, p. 107.

Bjordal, K. & Kaasa, S. (1995). Psychological distress in head and neck cancer patients 7-11 years after curative treatment. *British Journal of Cancer, 71,* 592–597.

Bradbury, E. T. & Hewison, J. (1994). Early parental adjustment to visible congenital disfigurement. *Child Care, Health and Development, 20,* 251–266.

Bretherton, I. (1997). Bowlby's legacy to developmental psychology. *Child Psychiatry and Human Development, 28* (1), 33–43.

Bronheim, H., Strain, J. J. & Biller, H. F. (1991). Psychiatric aspects of head and neck surgery—Part II: Body image and psychiatric intervention. *General Hospital Psychiatry, 13,* 225–232.

Brown, R. A., Gelberman, R. H., Seiler, J. G. et al. (1993). Carpal tunnel release. A prospective randomized assessment of open and endoscopic methods. *Journal of Bone and Joint Surgery, 75A,* 1265–1274.

Brzezienski, M. A. & Schneider, L. H. (1995). Extensor tendon injuries at the distal interphalangeal joint. *Hand Clinics, 11* (3), 373–386.

Calloway, D. M. et. al. (1992). Changing concepts and controversies in the management of mandibular fractures. *Clinics in Plastic Surgery, 19* (1), 59–69.

Chisholm, C. D. & Howell, J. M. (1992). Soft tissue emergencies. Wound evaluation and cleansing. *Emergency Medicine Clinics of North America, 10* (4), 665–672.

Clayton, B. & Waller, A. L. (1996). The TRAM flap in breast reconstruction. *Plastic Surgical Nursing, 16* (3), 133–138.

Cohen, M. (1994). Mastery of plastic and reconstructive surgery. (vol 2), pp. 1324–1335. Boston: Little Brown.

Coons, M. S. & Green, S. M. (1995). Boutonnière deformity. *Hand Clinics, 11* (3), 387–402.

D'Angelo, T. M. & Gorrell, C. R. (1989). Breast reconstruction using tissue expanders. *Oncology Nursing Forum, 16* (1), 23–26.

Elliot, F. L. & Hartrampf, C. R. (1983). Tailoring of the new breast using the transverse abdominal island flap. *Plastic and Reconstructive Surgery, 72* (6), 887–893.

Enich, R. F. et al. (1988). Principles of emergency wound management. *Annals of Emergency Medicine, 17,* 1284–1302.

Fallowfield, L. J. & Baum, M. (1986). Psychological welfare of patients with breast cancer. *Journal of the Royal Society of Medicine, 79,* 165–169.

Fariss, B. L. et al. (1987). Anesthetic properties of bupivicaine and lidocaine for infiltration anesthesia. *Journal of Emergency Medicine, 5,* 275–282.

Gamba, A. et. al. (1992). Psychosocial adjustment of patients surgically treated for head and neck cancer. *Head and Neck, 14,* 218–223.

Haug, R. H. (1996). Retention of asymptomatic bone plates used for orthognathic surgery and facial fractures. *Journal of Oral and Maxillofacial Surgery, 54* (5), 611–617.

Hester, Jr., T. R. & Bostwick III, J. (1982). Poland's syndrome: Correction with latissimus muscle transposition. *Plastic and Reconstructive Surgery, 2,* 226–233.

Hinojosa, R. J. & Layman, A. S. (1996). Breast reconstruction through tissue expansion. *Plastic Surgical Nursing, 16* (3), 139–145.

Hobar, P. C. (1992). Methods of rigid fixations. *Clinics in Plastic Surgery, 19* (1), 31–39.

Holmes, J. D. (1989). Capsular contracture after breast reconstruction with tissue expansion. *British Journal of Plastic Surgery, 42* (5), 591–594.

Ingari, J. V. & Pederson, W. C. (1997). Update on tendon repair. *Clinics in Plastic Surgery, 24* (1), 161–171.

Jurkiewicz, M. J. et al. (1990). *Plastic Surgery Principles and Practice* (Vols. One and Two). St. Louis: Mosby.

Kerrigan, C. L. (1983). Skin flap failure: Pathophysiology. *Plastic and Reconstructive Surgery, 72,* 766.

Krueckeberg, S. M. & Kapp-Simon, K. A. (1993). Effect of parental factors on social skills of preschool children with craniofacial anomalies. *Cleft Palate–Craniofacial Journal, 30* (5), 490–496.

Laitung, K. G. & Peck, F. (1985). Shoulder function following the loss of the latissimus dorsi muscle. *British Journal of Plastic Surgery, 38,* 375–379.

Lewis, M. B. (1993). Unilateral cleft lip repair Z plasty. *Clinics in Plastic Surgery, 20* (4), 647–657.

Little, J. (1984). Nipple–areola reconstruction. *Clinics in Plastic Surgery, 11,* 351.

Luce, E. A. (1992). Developing concepts and treatment of complex maxillary fractures. *Clinics in Plastic Surgery, 19,* 125–131.

Lutwick, L. E. (1996). Postexposure prophylaxis. *Infectious Disease Clinics of North America, 10* (4), 899–915.

Markovchick, V. (1992). Suture materials and mechanical aftercare. *Emergency Medicine Clinics of North America, 10* (4), 673–689.

Marks, M. R., & Gunther, S. F. (1989) Efficacy of cortisol injection in treatment of trigger fingers and thumb. *Journal of Hand Surgery, 14,* 722–727.

May, J. W. & Halls, M. J. (1985). Thermocouple probe monitoring for free tissue transfer replantation and revascularization procedures. *Plastic and Reconstructive Surgery, 12* (2), 197–207.

McCarthy, J. G. (1990). Plastic surgery, vol 1. General Principles. p. 2. Philadelphia: W. B. Saunders.

McCraw, J. B. & Maxwell, G. P. (1988). Early and late capsular "deformation" as a cause of unsatisfactory results in the latissimus dorsi flap for breast reconstruction. *Clinics in Plastic Surgery, 15* (4), 717–726.

McCraw, J. B. et. al. (1994). The autogenous latissimus breast reconstruction. *Clinics in Plastic Surgery, 21* (2), 279–296.

Merle, M. & Dautel, G. (1991). Vascularized nerve grafts. *Journal of Hand Surgery, 16,* 483–488.

Mizgala, C. A. et al. (1994). Abdominal function after pedicled TRAM flap surgery. *Clinics in Plastic Surgery, 21* (2), 255–272.

Moy, R. L., Waldman, B., & Hein, D. W. (1992). A review of sutures and suturing techniques. *Journal of Dermatologic Surgery and Oncology, 18* (9), 785–795.

Nelles, W. B. et al. (1991). Social supports and breast cancer: A review. *Journal of Psychosocial Oncology, 9* (1), 21–34.

Netscher, D. T. & Clamon, J. (1994). Smoking: Adverse effects on outcomes for plastic surgical patients. *Plastic Surgical Nursing, 14* (4), 205–210.

Ngu Yen, P. N. & Sullivan, P. K. (1993). *Clinics in Plastic Surgery, 20* (4), 671–681.

Nolan, J. et al. (1985). The acute effects of cigarette smoking exposure on experimental skin flaps. *Plastic and Reconstructive Surgery, 75,* 544–549.

Nordstrom, R. A. & Nordstrom, R. M. (1986). Absorbable versus nonabsorbable sutures to prevent postoperative stretching of wound area. *Plastic and Reconstructive Surgery, 78* (2), 186–190.

Orlinsky, M. et al. (1992). Pain comparison of unbuffered versus buffered lidocaine in local wound infiltration. *Journal of Emergency Medicine, 10,* 411–415.

Patel, M. R., Shekhar, S. et al. (1986). Conservative management of chronic mallet finger. *Journal of Hand Surgery, 11A,* 570–573.

Rappaport, Y. et al. (1993). Psychosocial problems in head-and-neck cancer patients and their change with time since diagnosis. *Annals of Oncology, 4* (1), 69–73.

Rockwell, W. B. & Lister, G. D. (1993). Soft tissue reconstruction. Coverage of hand injuries. *Orthopedic Clinics of North America, 24* (3), 411–424.

Rowland, J. et al. (1993). Psychological response to breast reconstruction. *Psychosomatics, 34* (3), 241–250.

Rutter M. (1995). Clinical implications of attachment concepts: Retrospect and prospect. *Journal of Child Psychology & Psychiatry & Allied Disciplines, 36* (4), 549–571.

Ryan, G. M. & Mullins, P. T. (1987). Skin necrosis complicating mallet finger splinting and vascularity of the DIP joint overlying skin. *Journal of Hand Surgery, 12A,* 548–552.

Saber, S. K. (1991). Nutritional management of intermaxillary fixation patients. *Advancing Clinical Care, 6* (5), 24–25.

Sadove, R. C. & Scherl, E. R. (1992). Immediate breast reconstruction at the time of mastectomy for breast cancer. *Journal of Kentucky Medical Association, 90* (5), 225–231.

Schain, W. S. et al. (1985). The sooner the better: A study of psychological factors in women undergoing immediate versus delayed breast reconstruction. *American Journal of Psychiatry, 142,* 40–46.

Schover, L. R. (1991). The impact of breast cancer on sexuality, body image and intimate relationships. *Cancer, 41,* 112–120.

Seckel, B. R. & Hyland, W. T. (1985). Soft-tissue expander for delayed and immediate breast reconstruction. *Surgical Clinics of North America, 65* (2), 383–391.

Sherwin, M. A. & Gastwirth, C. M. (1987). Detrimental effects of cigarette smoking on lower extremity wound healing. *Journal of Foot Surgery, 29,* 84–87.

Spear, S. L. & Arias, J. (1995). Long term experience with nipple–areola tattooing. *Annals of Plastic Surgery, 35* (3), 232–236.

Spencer, K. W. (1996). Using the latissimus dorsi flap for breast reconstruction. *Plastic Surgical Nursing, 16* (3), 147–155.

Steinberg, D. R. (1992). Acute flexor tendon injuries. *Orthopedic Clinics of North America, 23,* 125–141.

Steur, K. (1991). Facial fractures: Diagnosis to discharge. *AORN Journal, 54* (4), 773–787.

Strickland, J. W. & Leibovic, S. J. (1991). Anatomy and pathogenesis of the digital cords and nodules. *Hand Clinics,* 645–657.

Strombeck, J. O. & Rosato, F. E. (1986). *Surgery of the breast: Diagnosis and treatment,* pp. 256–261. New York: Thieme Inc.

Summers B. K. & Siegle, R. J. (1993). Facial cutaneous reconstructive surgery: General aesthetic principles. *Journal of the American Academy of Dermatology, 29* (5), Part 1, 669–683.

Tobiasen, J. M. (1993). Combined effects of severity of cleft impairment and facial attractiveness on social perception: An experimental study. *Cleft Palate–Craniofacial Journal, 30* (1), 82–86.

Trott, A. T. (1997). *Wounds and Lacerations. Emergency Care and Closure.* St. Louis: Mosby.

Valanis, B. & Rumpler, C. (1985). Helping women to choose breast cancer treatment alternatives. *Cancer Nursing, 8* (3), 167–175.

Van Adrichem, L. N. A., Hovius, S. E. R., van Strik, R., & van der Meulem, J. C. (1992). The acute effects of cigarette smoking on microcirculation of the replanted digit. *Journal of Hand Surgery, 17A,* 230–234.

Van der Meulen, J. C. (1992). Columellar elongation in bilateral cleft lip repair: Early results. *Plastic and Reconstructive Surgery, 89* (6), 1060–1067.

Wallander, J. L. et. al. (1988). Children with chronic physical disorders: Maternal reports of their psychological adjustment. *Journal of Pediatric Psychology, 13,* 197–212.

Watt-Watson, J. & Graydon, J. (1995). Impact of surgery on head and neck cancer patients and their caregivers. *Nursing Clinics of North America, 30* (4), 659–670.

Wong, N. L. (1993). Review of continuous sutures on dermatologic surgery. *Journal of Dermatologic Surgery and Oncology, 19,* 923–931.

Wood, M. B. (1992). Finger and hand replantation. *Hand Clinics, 8* (3), 397–408.

Wyrick, J. D. & Stern, P. J. (1992). Secondary nerve reconstruction. *Hand Clinics, 8,* 587–597.

26

Cancer Treatment

Kim Marie Falk

It is expected that approximately 1,228,600 people in the United States will be diagnosed with cancer in 1998. This does not include cancer *in situ,* except urinary bladder. This figure also does not include basal- and squamous-cell skin cancers, of which approximately one million are predicted in 1998. The number of those expected to die from cancer this same year is about 564,800 Americans (Landis, Murray, Bolden, & Wingo, 1998), making cancer the second leading cause of death in the United States. It is also estimated that about 7.4 million Americans have a history of cancer. This figure includes survivors with no current indication of cancer and those who do have evidence of the disease, including patients receiving treatment (American Cancer Society, 1997). Thus, it is reasonable to expect that most acute care nurse practitioners (ACNPs) will encounter people in their practice whom have been or will be diagnosed with cancer, including patients who underwent, are currently undergoing, or will undergo cancer treatment.

Because cancer includes numerous distinct diseases, largely due to the multitudinous number of possible sites of origin in the human body, cancer treatment encompasses a wide variety of disease processes and specific treatment modalities. This chapter primarily focuses on the modalities of cancer treatment in general. Additional information on specific types of cancers can be found in other chapters.

▶ PATHOPHYSIOLOGY

Many advances have been made in the field of oncology, including expanded knowledge related to the biological basis of cancer. It has been observed that genes involved in controlling the growth and development in a normal cell undergo a series of mutations that eventually cause subsequent cells to become cancer cells. Thus, cancer is a genetic disease (Calzone, 1997). The genetic basis for this transformation of normal cell to cancer cell can be understood through a comparison of normal cellular growth and cancer cell growth.

Cellular Growth

In normal cellular growth, cells replicate through a process known as the cell cycle. The cell cycle consists of four active stages: G1-interphase, S-DNA synthesis, G2-intermediate phase, and M-mitosis. Cells that are not replicating are in a fifth phase known as the G0 or resting phase. For a cell to replicate, it must leave the G0 phase and enter the cell cycle. Thus, a specific stimulation must occur to induce a cell to leave the G0 phase and enter the cell cycle. After a cell goes through a number of cycles of division and growth is no longer needed, the need to grow is repressed (Bullock, 1996).

It is known that cancer cells also grow and replicate through the same cell cycle as a normal cell. However, as a result of genetic mutations, cancer cells continue to replicate even when the need for growth no longer exists. One reason why this happens is attributed to a loss of contact inhibition (Bullock, 1996; Gallucci, 1991; Pfeifer, 1994a).

Contact inhibition, also called density-dependent growth control, refers to a property of normal cells in a culture medium; they stop replicating when the bottom of the Petri dish has been covered. Normal cells in the body also exhibit this property. Additionally, normal cells adhere to each other, forming tight junctions with other cells of their kind (Bullock, 1996; Gallucci, 1991; Pfeifer, 1994a).

Cancer cells, however, do not have contact inhibition; they continue to replicate, crowding on top of each other and forming multiple layers. Cancer cells also have decreased adhesiveness, thus enabling them to be more mobile. It is this loss of contact inhibition and decreased adhesiveness that contribute to cancer cells' loss of proliferative control. Unhindered proliferation is a hallmark property of cancer cells (Bullock, 1996; Gallucci, 1991; Pfeifer, 1994a).

Another classic property demonstrated by cancer cells is anaplasia, or loss of cellular differentiation. When normal cells grow and develop they become specialized through a process called differentiation. Differentiated cells are mature cells that have specific functions, depending on their tissue types. There are many types of differentiated cells within the body and they differ from one another both physically and functionally. Cells are considered well differentiated when they look and act like their cell of origin (Bullock, 1996; Gallucci, 1991; Pfeifer, 1994a).

But cancer cells do not resemble their cells of origin and are classified as poorly differentiated cells (Bullock, 1996; Gallucci, 1991; Pfeifer, 1994a). In fact, as cancer cells continue to replicate, they lose more of their differentiation. Cancer cells can become so poorly differentiated that a clinician may not be able to determine the original site of cancer.

When a normal cell undergoes these characteristic changes of malignancy, carcinogenesis has occurred. Therefore, the process through which normal cells lose their ability to stop replicating, become poorly differentiated, and thus become cancerous is termed carcinogenesis (Bullock, 1996; Gallucci, 1991; Pfeifer, 1994a).

TABLE 26–1. A Comparison of Benign and Malignant Neoplasms

Benign	Malignant
Similar to cell of origin	Dissimilar from cell of origin
Edges move outward smoothly (encapsulated)	Edges move outward irregularly
Compresses	Invades
Slow growth rate	Rapid to very rapid growth rate
Slight vascularity	Moderate to marked vascularity
Seldom recur after removal	Frequently recur after removal
Necrosis and ulceration unusual	Necrosis and ulceration common
Systemic effects unusual unless it is a secreting endocrine neoplasm	Systemic effects common

Reprinted with permission from Bullock (1996).

Development of a Malignancy

Cancers can be broadly classified as hematologic or solid tumor malignancies. Cancers of the hematologic system (e.g., leukemia, multiple myeloma, lymphoma) are characterized by abnormalities of bone marrow and lymphoid tissue. In the case of solid malignancies, carcinogenesis leads to the development of an abnormal growth, referred to as a neoplasm. Certainly not all tumors are malignant; many tumors are benign. Table 26–1 highlights the differences between benign and malignant tumors.

The possibility that a malignancy develops is dependent on many factors. Some of the major factors include a three-stage theory of carcinogenesis and the presence of regulatory genes.

Three-Stage Theory of Carcinogenesis

The three-stage theory of carcinogenesis evolved from Berenblum's two-stage theory, proposed in 1947. Berenblum's theory suggested that cancer occurred as a result of two distinct events: initiation and promotion. The three-stage theory that developed from this consists of three distinct phases: initiation, promotion, and progression (Pfeifer, 1994a).

Initiation involves a carcinogenic insult to a cell's deoxyribonucleic acid (DNA). The damaged gene is affected in one of three ways. First, the gene may undergo repair and no cancer results. Second, the gene may suffer permanent changes but no cancer results at the time, or third, the gene causes carcinogenesis. This last scenario occurs when the initiator is a complete carcinogen. Complete carcinogens are capable of producing cancer on their own because they possess both initiating and promoting properties (Pfeifer, 1994a).

The second stage, promotion, occurs when the gene encounters a cocarcinogen. Cocarcinogens are promoting agents that increase the activity of carcinogens. The resultant damage to the cell is either irreversible or reversible. Fortunately, DNA damage may be reversible in the presence of certain cancer-reversing agents. However, if a cell proceeds to the final stage, morphologic changes occur within the cell that ultimately lead to irreversible malignant responses (Bullock, 1996; Pfeifer, 1994a).

Regulatory Genes

Several types of regulatory genes associated with cancer development have been identified and named, including oncogenes and tumor suppressor genes. Oncogenes are genes that, when activated, cause a cell to undergo malignant transformation. Similarly, when tumor suppressor genes are inactivated, malignant cellular growth is promoted (Bullock, 1996; Calzone, 1997).

The Spread of Cancer

Cancer treatment is largely influenced by the ability of cancer cells to spread. The two primary ways that cancer cells spread is through direct invasion and metastasis. Direct invasion occurs when cancer cells extend beyond the primary site and thus destroy adjacent tissues. This direct spread is often the first step toward metastases (Bullock, 1996; Hubbard & Liotta, 1991; Pfeifer, 1994a).

Metastasis is the ability of cancer cells to migrate from their site of origin and establish growth at distant sites. An overwhelming majority of patients with cancer die from metastatic disease; therefore, one of the underlying principles of cancer treatment is aimed at preventing or eliminating cancer metastasis.

Etiology

The etiology of cancer is thought to be multifactorial with heredity, environmental components, and personal factors all interacting to produce malignancy. While the number of cancers thought to be associated with an inherited predisposition is low, research in this area has been instrumental in furthering an understanding of the pathophysiology of cancer in general (Calzone, 1997). Table 26–2 lists common hereditary cancer syndromes and their clinical manifestations.

Many environmental components are associated with the development of cancer. The American Cancer Society (1997) estimates that more than half of all cancer cases are caused by the environment, most of which result from lifestyle choices. Examples of known environmental carcinogens include polycyclic aromatic hydrocarbons and nitrosamines found in tobacco smoke; asbestos; benzene; polyvinyl chloride, used in manufacturing plastics; ultraviolet, high-frequency, and ionizing radiation; certain insecticide ingredients such as naphthalene and 2-acetylaminofluorene; arsenic; aflatoxin B, a mold found on some nuts, fruits, and grains; and diethylstilbestrol, used in the 1950s to prevent spontaneous abortion (American Cancer Society, 1997; Bullock, 1992, 1996; Meili, 1994; Mettlin & Mirand, 1991).

Another environmental component associated with the development of cancer in humans is viruses. These viruses, labeled oncogenic viruses, are selective, thus infecting only specific tissues. Knowledge about oncogenic viruses and their direct link to cancer is limited, though various specific viruses have been identified (Bullock, 1996; Pfeifer, 1994a). Table 26–3 lists several oncogenic viruses and their associated cancers.

Personal factors that contribute to the development of cancer include diet, sexual practices, and reproductive history. A low-fiber, high-fat diet has been implicated in colon cancer. Other cancers associated with a high-fat diet include breast, uterine, prostate, and ovarian cancer. Additionally, alcohol consumption is linked with cancer of the mouth, pharynx, larynx, esophagus, stomach, liver, breast, and pancreas (Bullock, 1996; Meili, 1994).

Multiple partners and early age at first intercourse are both examples of sexual practices that are related to the de-

TABLE 26–2. Common Hereditary Cancer Syndromes and Associated Cancer Susceptibility Genes

Syndrome/Condition	Clinical Manifestations
Ataxia-Telangiectasia	Cerebral ataxia, oculocutaneous telangiectasias, radiation hypersensitivity, leukemia, lymphoma, breast cancer, and other solid tumors
Beckwith-Wiedemann Syndrome	Wilms' tumor, adrenal carcinomas, hepatoblastomas
Breast/Ovarian Cancer Syndrome	Breast cancer, ovarian cancer, prostate cancer, colon cancer Breast cancer (male and female), ovarian cancer
Cowden's Disease	Multiple mucocutaneous lesions, vitiligo, angiomas, benign proliferative disease of multiple organ systems, breast cancer, thyroid cancer, colonic neoplasms
Familial Adenomatous Polyposis (Gardner Syndrome)	Colon polyposis (adenomas), desmoid tumors, osteomas, thyroid cancer, hepatoblastoma
Fanconi Anemia	Leukemia, esophageal cancer, hepatoma
Gorlin Syndrome	Basal cell carcinoma, brain tumors, ovarian cancer
Hereditary Nonpolyposis Colorectal Cancer (Lynch Syndromes)	Gastrointestinal (GI) cancers, endometrial cancer, ovarian cancer, ureteral cancer
Li-Fraumeni Syndrome	Breast cancer, sarcoma, brain tumors, leukemia, adrenocortical carcinoma
Melanoma	Melanoma
Muir-Torre Syndrome	GI and genitourinary cancers, skin cancer, breast cancer, benign breast tumors
Multiple Endocrine Neoplasia Type I	Pancreatic cancer, pituitary adenomas
Multiple Endocrine Neoplasia Type II	Thyroid cancer, pheochromocytomas
Neurofibromatosis	Neurofibromatosis, pheochromocytomas, optic gliomas
Peutz-Jeghers Syndrome	Abnormal melanin deposits, GI polyposis, GI cancer, breast cancer, uterine cancer, ovarian cancer, testicular cancer
Prostate Cancer	Prostate cancer
Retinoblastoma	Retinoblastoma, osteosarcoma
Von Hippel-Lindau Syndrome	Hemangioblastoma, renal cell cancer, pheochromocytomas
Wilms' Tumor	Wilms' Tumor
Xeroderma Pigmentosum	Skin cancer, melanoma, leukemia

Adapted with permission from Calzone (1997).

TABLE 26–3. Viruses and Their Associated Cancers

Virus	Associated Cancers
Cytomegalovirus	Kaposi's sarcoma
Epstein–Barr virus	Burkitt's lymphoma Nasopharyngeal carcinoma
Hepatitis B group	Liver cancer
Herpes simplex type 2 (HSV-2)	Cervical cancer
Human papilloma virus (HPV)	Cervical cancer, cancer of the vulva, anogenital cancers, penile cancer
Human T-cell lymphotropic virus, type 1 (HTLV-1)	Adult T-cell leukemia

Adapted with permission from Otto (1997) and Frank-Stromborg (1991).

velopment of cervical cancer. Conversely, cervical cancer is rare among women who are not sexually active. In males, cancer of the penis is rare in circumcised males (Bullock, 1996; Frank-Stromborg, 1991; Mettlin & Mirand, 1991).

Reproductive history plays a role in breast cancer development. Women who are nulliparous or who have their first full-term pregnancy after the age of 30 have a higher rate of breast cancer (Frank-Stromborg, 1991; Mettlin & Mirand, 1991). Induced abortions, particularly a first pregnancy in a very young woman, may also increase a woman's risk for breast cancer (Canty, 1997).

▶ HISTORY, PHYSICAL FINDINGS, AND DIAGNOSTIC STUDIES

One of the primary goals of assessment for any disease is early detection. For cancer, early detection is especially crucial. Treatment is most successful for cancers treated in the early stage and the very early stage (cancer *in situ*). Therefore, it is important for ACNPs to be familiar with the American Cancer Society's recommendations for early detection of cancer in asymptomatic people. Current recommendations for breast, cervical, colorectal, ovarian, and prostate checkups are presented in Table 26–4.

As discussed in Chapter 12, all patients initially deserve a comprehensive health history and a thorough physical exam. When cancer is a suspected diagnosis or when the patient has a history of cancer, the ACNP should include specific content in the history to assist him or her in a thorough assessment. This section presents certain areas the ACNP should explore for the patient he or she suspects has cancer and for the patient who has a history of cancer.

Comprehensive Health History

Chief Complaint

Beginning with the patient's chief complaint can initially sensitize the ACNP to the possibility of cancer. However, because of the great diversity in types of cancers, the numerous possible sites of origin, and the fact that patients present in various stages of the disease, there is no typical presenting chief complaint for all cancers. Nonetheless, common complaints for patients with cancer in general include significant weight loss, the presence of a new mass, pain, unusual bleeding (e.g., rectal or vaginal), persistent cough, fatigue, and general malaise. While most of these signs and symptoms are too general to help the ACNP focus on the particular type of cancer suspected, they can be an important starting point to help guide the rest of the health history. However, some complaints, like rectal bleeding and pain at a particular location, direct the ACNP to specific body systems that may be the site of origin or sites of metastases.

TABLE 26–4. Selected Cancer Screening Recommendations for Asymptomatic Patients

Cancer	Screening Recommendation
Breast	For women Age 20–39: clinical breast examination (CBE) every 3 years, monthly breast self exam (BSE) Age 40+: annual mammography, annual CBE, monthly BSE
Cervical	Age 18 (or age when become sexually active, if earlier): annual Pap test and pelvic exam (Pap test: after 3 consecutive satisfactory normal, annual Pap tests may be performed less frequently)
Colorectal	Age 50+: annual fecal occult blood test plus flexible sigmoidoscopy every 5 years OR colonoscopy and digital rectal exam every 10 years OR double contrast barium enema and digital rectal exam every 5–10 years
Ovarian	Age 18–40: pelvic examination every 1–3 years Age 41+: annual pelvic examination
Prostate	Age 50: discuss with health-care provider about beginning annual prostate-specific antigen and digital rectal examination

Compiled from data from the American Cancer Society (1997).

Risk Factors

Once the ACNP has elicited the patient's chief complaint, an assessment for cancer risks should follow. The data that a patient supplies from questions concerning cancer risk factors can provide additional support of a suspected cancer and possibly further focus the history and physical exam. Questions should focus on the patient's histories and include the following areas: family, social, and personal health.

Family History

A family history should include information about family members who presently have or had cancer and specifically what type. Because the general public often has avoided the term "cancer," the ACNP should also question the patient about "tumors" or "growths" of family members (Olsen & Frank-Stromborg, 1991).

While it is true that only a small percentage of cancers are thought to be caused from an inherited predisposition, there are families that demonstrate an unusually high incidence of certain cancers. Characteristics shared by these families include an early age of onset of cancer, an increased frequency of multiple primary malignancies, and a tendency for the same type of neoplasm or histologic type to develop in one or multiple sites (Calzone, 1997; Frank-Stromborg, 1991).

Social History

A social history has many elements including drug and alcohol use, sexual habits, occupational factors, leisure-time activities, and places of residence. The patient should be asked if he or she currently uses or has ever used in the past tobacco, alcohol, or illicit drugs. If the patient provides a positive response to using any of these substances, further questioning should clarify the specific substances, length of use, amount, and complications from use (Olsen & Frank-Stromborg, 1991).

Cigarette smoking is a significant risk factor; it is the single most important source of preventable morbidity and premature mortality. It is associated with many cancers including mouth, pharynx, larynx, lung, esophagus, pancreas, cervix, kidney, and bladder (Frank-Stromborg, 1991; Gullatte, 1994). As mentioned earlier, alcohol has also been linked to numerous cancers. Additionally, the additive effects of both tobacco use and alcohol consumption make them greater risk factors when combined. It is supposed that alcohol's direct damage to epithelial tissues or its ability to increase the delivery of smoke-derived chemicals makes this synergistic effect possible (Meili, 1994).

A sexual history is very important, considering that a direct relationship exists between sexual lifestyles and practices and genital cancers. Questions concerning sexual habits should include the age of first intercourse, number of sexual partners, type of protection used, history of sexually transmitted diseases (STDs), and, for women, past Papanicolaou results. As mentioned earlier, multiple sexual partners and early age of first intercourse are risk factors for cervical development. Additional risk factors for cervical cancer include a high rate of STDs and exposure to high-risk sexual partners (Frank-Stromborg, 1991; Gullatte, 1994).

Assessment of occupational risk factors should include areas of employment, work materials, work locations, known carcinogenic exposures, and safety procedures implemented by the patient. Table 26–5 presents a comprehensive list of occupations carrying an increased risk of cancer, sites of cancer, and causative agents (Frank-Stromborg, 1991; Olsen & Frank-Stromborg, 1991).

Questions concerning leisure-time activities should focus on possible exposure to carcinogenic materials the patient may have either encountered exclusively outside of the work place or exposure in addition to that at the work site. For some patients, it is possible that valuable information pertaining to possible exposure to chemical or physical carcinogens may be only obtained if the ACNP explores this domain. People who engage in artistic or craft projects as a leisure activity may unknowingly become exposed to carcinogens from the products they use to create their work and the materials to clean their supplies.

A residential history should include questions about former, as well as, current habitats. Exposure to potentially carcinogenic substances from the actual dwelling place (e.g., lead paint or asbestos) and the area of the habitat (e.g., polycyclic hydrocarbons from industrialization) should be assessed. Table 26–5 includes many environmental carcinogens.

Personal History

Finally, a health history for a patient with suspected cancer includes a past personal health history. Olsen & Frank-Stromborg (1991) suggest that ideally the following information be obtained: all prior acute and chronic illnesses and their treatments; past x-ray treatments, including treatments for acne, swollen tonsils, and enlarged thymus (a practice abandoned in the 1950s); maternal use of diethylstilbestrol (DES); blood transfusions; past surgeries; all prior medications (including birth control pills); vitamins and over-the-counter drugs; relevant dietary practices and, if appropriate, a history of obesity; reproductive history, including menses and menopause history.

Additionally, it is important to consider the age of the patient. Since a person's lifetime risk of developing cancer increases as he or she ages, the ACNP should consider all middle age and older adults at risk for developing cancer (American Cancer Society, 1997).

Physical Exam

Some of the major sites of cancer incidence and cancer deaths, presented in Figures 26–1 and 26–2, include breast, prostate, lung, and colon and rectum (Landis et al., 1998). Each of these sites has typical presenting signs and symptoms of which the ACNP should be aware.

Breast Cancer

Breast cancer most often presents as a lump or thickening in the breast. However, not all breast lumps are malignant; in fact 75% to 80% are benign. Other possible presenting symptoms include nipple discharge, nipple retraction, scaling of the skin around the nipple, dimpling, and skin inflammation. In addition, the skin may become roughened, resembling the skin of an orange, termed "peau d'orange." Unfortunately, this condition and the previously mentioned symptoms, other than breast lump, are often indicative of an advanced stage of cancer (Knobf, 1991).

Prostate Cancer

In its early stages, the patient with prostate cancer often has no discernible signs or symptoms. However, on rectal

(Text continued on p. 459)

TABLE 26–5. Occupations Carrying an Increased Risk of Cancer

Industry	Occupation	Site	Reported or Suspected Causative Agent
(a) Occupations recognized to present an increased risk of cancer, causally related to the occupation			
Agriculture, forestry, and fishing	Vineyard workers using arsenical insecticides	Lung, skin	Arsenic
Extractive	Arsenic mining	Lung, skin	Arsenic
	Iron-ore mining	Lung	Causative agent not identified
	Asbestos mining	Lung, pleural and peritoneal mesothelioma	Asbestos
	Uranium mining	Lung	Radon
Asbestos production industry	Insulated material production (pipes, sheeting, textile, clothes, masks, asbestos cement manufacts)	Lung, pleural and peritoneal mesothelioma	Asbestos
Petroleum industry	Wax pressmen	Scrotum	Polycyclic hydrocarbons
Metal industry	Copper smelting	Lung	Arsenic
	Chromate producing	Lung	Chromium
	Chromium plating	Lung	Chromium
	Ferrochromium producing	Lung	Chromium
	Steel production	Lung	Benzo(a)pyrene
	Nickel refining	Nasal sinuses, lung	Nickel
Shipbuilding, motor vehicles, and transport	Shipyard and dockyard workers	Lung, pleural and peritoneal mesothelioma	Asbestos
Chemical industry	BCME and CMME products and users	Lung (oat cell carcinoma)	BCME, CMME
	Vinyl chloride producers	Liver angiosarcoma	Vinyl chloride monomer
	Isopropyl alcohol manufacturing (strong acid process) workers	Paranasal sinuses	Causative agent not identified
	Pigment chromate producing	Lung	Chromium
	Dye manufacturers and users	Bladder	Benzidine, 2-naphthylamine, 4-aminodiphenyl
	Auramine manufacture	Bladder	Auramine (together with the other aromatic amines used in the process)
Pesticides and herbicides production industry	Arsenical insecticide production and packaging	Lung	Arsenic
Gas industry	Coke plant workers	Lung	Benzo(a)pyrene
	Gas workers	Lung, bladder, scrotum	Coal carbonization products, β-naphthylamine
	Gas-retort house workers	Bladder	α/β-naphthylamine
Rubber industry	Rubber manufacture	Lymphatic and hematopoietic system (leukemia)	Benzene
		Bladder	Aromatic amines
	Calendering, tire curing, tire building	Lymphatic and hematopoietic system (leukemia)	Benzene
	Millers, mixers	Bladder	Aromatic amines
	Synthetic latex producers, tire curing, calendar operatives, reclaimers, cable makers	Bladder	Aromatic amines
Construction industry	Insulators and pipe coverers	Lung, pleural, and peritoneal mesothelioma	Asbestos
Leather industry	Boot and shoe manufacturers, repairers	Nose, marrow (leukemia)	Leather dust, benzene
Wood pulp and paper industry	Furniture and cabinet makers	Nose (adenocarcinoma)	Wood dust
Other	Roofers, asphalt workers	Lung	BAP
(b) Occupations reported to present an increased risk of cancer but for which the assessment of the causal relation with the occupation is not definitive			
Agriculture, forestry, and fishing	Fishermen	Skin, lip	Pitch, ultraviolet radiation
	Farmers	Lymphatic and hematopoietic system (leukemia, lymphoma)	Undefined

TABLE 26–5. Occupations Carrying an Increased Risk of Cancer *(Continued)*

Industry	Occupation	Site	Reported or Suspected Causative Agent
	Basal bark sprayers	Lymphatic and hematopoietic system (lymphoma), soft tissue sarcomas	Phenoxyacetic acids, chlorophenols (presumably contaminated with PCDF, PCDD, and polychlorinated benzodioxins)
	Railway embankment sprayers	Lymphatic and hematopoietic system (lymphoma), lung cancer	Phenoxyacetic acids, amitrol, monuron, durion
	Pesticide appliers	Lung	Hexachlorocyclohexane combined and other pesticides
Extractive	Zinc-lead mining	Lung	Radiation
	Coal	Stomach	Coal dust
	Talc	Lung, pleura	Talc (contaminated with asbestos?)
Asbestos production industry	Insulation material production (pipes, sheeting, textiles, clothes, masks, asbestos cement manufacts)	Larynx, gastrointestinal tract	Asbestos
Petroleum industry	Oil refining	Esophagus, stomach, lung	Polycyclic hydrocarbons
	Boilermakers, painters, welders, oilfield workers	Lung	Polycyclic hydrocarbons
	Petrochemical plant workers	Brain, stomach	Polycyclic hydrocarbons
	Petroleum refining	Marrow (leukemia)	Benzene
Metal industry	Aluminium production	Lung	Benzo(a)pyrene
	Beryllium refining	Lung	Beryllium
	Smelters	Respiratory and digestive system	Lead
	Nickel refining	Larynx	Nickel
	Battery plant workers, cadmium alloy producers, electroplating workers	Prostate, kidney	Cadmium
	Cadmium smelters	Prostate, lung	Cadmium
Shipbuilding, motor vehicles, and transport	Filling station, bus and truck drivers, operators of excavating machines	Marrow (leukemia)	Petroleum products and combustion residues containing benzene
	Haulers	Lung	Polycyclic aromatic hydrocarbons
	Shipyard and dockyard workers	Larynx, digestive system	Asbestos
Chemical industry	Acrylonitrile production	Lung, colon	Acrylonitrile
	Vinylidene chloride producers	Lung	Vinylidene chloride (mixed exposure to VC and acrylonitrile)
	Isopropyl alcohol manufacturing (strong acid process) workers	Larynx	Undefined
	Polychloroprene producers	Lung	Chloroprene
	Dimethylsulfate producers	Lung	Dimethylsulfate
	Epichlorohydrin producers	Lung, lymphatic and hematopoietic system (leukemia)	Epichlorohydrin
	Ethylene oxide producers	Lymphatic and hematopoietic system (leukemia), stomach	Ethylene oxide
	Ethylene dibromide producers	Digestive system	Ethylene dibromide
	Flame retardant and plasticizer users	Skin (melanoma)	Polychlorinated biphenyls
	Styrene and polystyrene producers	Lymphatic and hematopoietic system (leukemia)	Styrene
	Ortho- and *para*-toluidine producers	Bladder	*Ortho/para*-toluidine
	Benzoylchloride producers	Lung	Benzoylchloride
	Magenta producers	Bladder	Aniline, *o*-toluidine

(Continued)

TABLE 26–5. Occupations Carrying an Increased Risk of Cancer *(Continued)*

Industry	Occupation	Site	Reported or Suspected Causative Agent
Pesticides and herbicides production industry	Tetrachlorodibenzodioxin producers and those exposed after accidents	Lung, stomach	DCDD and TCDD dichlorodibenzodioxin, trichlorodibenzodioxin
Rubber industry	Rubber manufacturing	Lymphopoietic system, stomach, brain, pancreas	Undefined
	Processors, composers, cementing synthetic plant	Stomach	Undefined
	General service	Lymphatic and hematopoietic system (leukemia), lymphatic and hemopoietic tissue	Undefined
	Synthetic latex producers and tire curing	Lung	Undefined
	Calender operatives and reclaimers	Prostate, lung	Undefined
	Compounding, mixing, and calendering	Prostate	Undefined
	Styrene butadiene rubber producers	Lymphatic and hematopoietic system (lymphomas)	Styrene
	Pliofilm producers	Lymphatic and hematopoietic system (leukemia)	Benzene
	Rubber compounding, extruding, milling	Stomach	Undefined
	Tire assembly	Skin	Mineral extender oil
		Brain	Undefined
Construction industry	Insulators and pipe coverers	Larynx, gastrointestinal tract	Asbestos
Printing industry	Rotogravure workers, binders	Marrow (leukemia)	Benzene
	Printing pressmen	Buccal cavity, rectum, pancreas, lung, prostate, kidney	Oil mist, solvents, dyes, cadmium, lead
	Newspaper pressmen	Buccal cavity	Oil mist, solvents, dyes, cadmium, lead
	Commercial pressmen	Pancreas, rectum	Oil mist, solvents, dyes, cadmium, lead
	Compositors	Multiple myeloma	Solvents
	Machine room workers	Lung	Oil mist
Leather industry	Tanners and processors	Bladder, nasal, lung	Leather dust, other chemicals, chromium
	Leather workers, unspecified	Nose, larynx, lung, bladder, lymphatic and hematopoietic system (lymphomas)	Undefined
	Boot and shoe manufacturers and repairers	Buccal cavity	Undefined
	Other leather goods manufacturers	Marrow (leukemia)	Benzene
Textile industry	Cotton and wool workers	Mouth, pharynx	Cotton and wool dust
Wood pulp and paper industry	Lumbermen and sawmill workers	Nose, Hodgkin's lymphoma	Wood dust, chlorophenols
	Pulp and papermill workers	Lymphopoietic tissue	Undefined
	Carpenters, joiners	Nose, Hodgkin's lymphomas	Wood dust, solvents
	Wood workers, unspecified		Undefined
Other	Radium dial workers	Breast	Radon
	Laundry and dry cleaners	Lung, skin, cervix uteri	Tritetrachloroethylene and carbon tetrachloride
	Roofers, asphalt workers	Mouth, pharynx, larynx, esophagus, stomach	Benzo(a)pyrene, other pitch volatile agents

Reprinted with permission from Simonato & Saracci (1983).

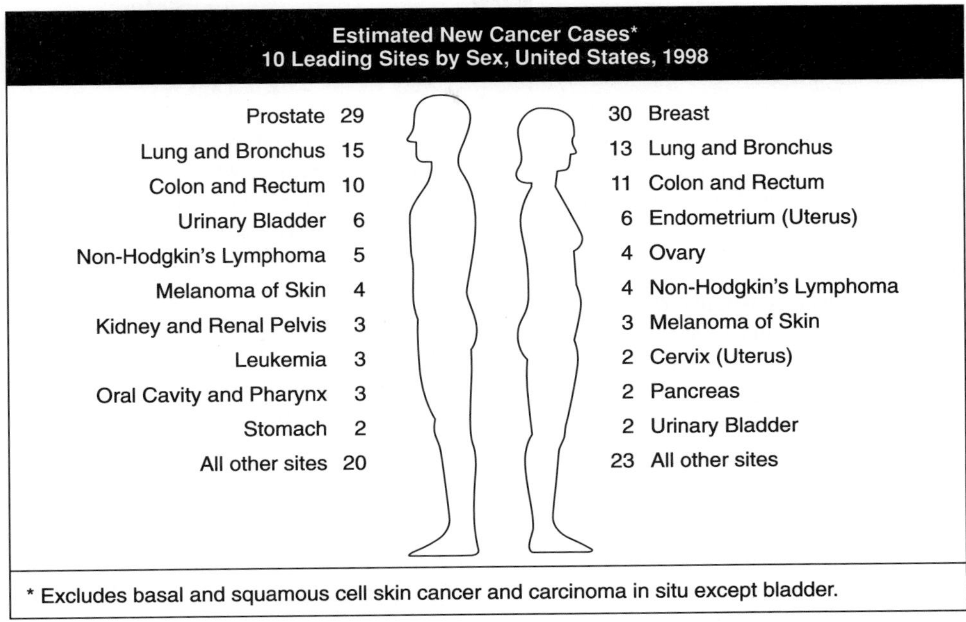

Figure 26–1. Estimated new cancer cases—ten leading sites by sex, United States, 1988. *(From Landis, Murray, Bolden, & Wingo [1998].)*

exam, a clinician may detect a prostate that feels firm, perhaps with sharp edges, unlike the normal rubbery feel of a noncancerous prostate. Late-stage prostate cancer can cause urinary complications such as frequency, dysuria, and obstruction (Lind & Irwin, 1991).

Lung Cancer

Lung cancer has diverse clinical manifestations due to the many possible sites of origin within the respiratory system. Additionally, lung cancer typically presents in the metastatic stage. It is likely that a patient may be asymptomatic and

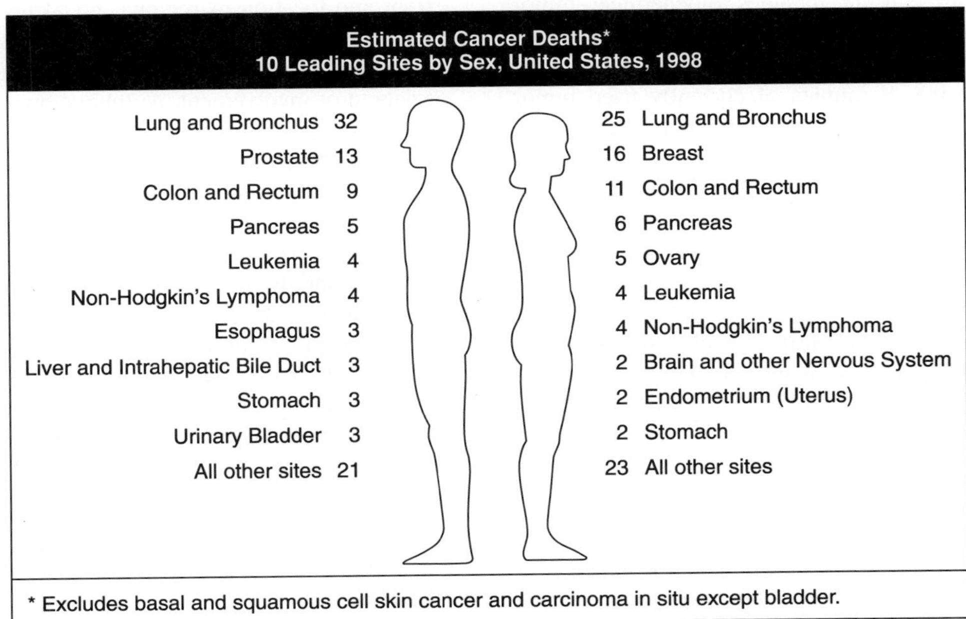

Figure 26–2. Estimated cancer deaths—ten leading sites by sex, United States, 1988. *(From Landis, Murray, Bolden, & Wingo [1998].)*

that the cancer is first detected on chest x-ray. Chest x-rays may reveal pneumonia, atelectasis, or perhaps a pleural effusion. Some other common presenting signs and symptoms are cough, hoarseness, dyspnea, and hemoptysis. Since smoking is associated with lung cancer and many smokers typically have a cough, it is important for the ACNP to assess for a change in cough with an increase in sputum production (Lindsey, 1991).

Colon Cancer

A patient with colorectal cancer is usually older than 50. Colorectal cancer in younger patients is associated with a history of familial polyposis or ulcerative colitis. Typically, patients with colorectal cancer present with abdominal pain, rectal bleeding, and a change in stool manifesting as either diarrhea or constipation. Hemoccult tests should be used to verify blood in stool. Laboratory results may reveal anemia. Unfortunately, sometimes the patient presents with either obstruction or perforation of the bowel, two problems associated with a poor prognosis (Ehlke, 1991).

Specific Cancer and Cancer in General

Table 26–6 lists appropriate physical examination and diagnostic testing for most of the major cancers including cervical, endometrial, vaginal, ovarian, breast, stomach, liver, lung, colorectal, skin, thyroid, testicular, prostate, bladder, and even cancer in general.

Diagnostic Testing

In addition to the diagnostic tests listed in Table 26–6, additional diagnostic testing for patients with suspected cancer includes laboratory studies. Besides the standard battery of tests (e.g., complete blood count), laboratory blood work useful in detecting cancers includes biochemical tumor markers. Tumor markers are substances released by either tumor cells or in response to the tumor and can be detected in the blood or urine. Examples of currently used tumor markers include carcinoembryonic antigen (CEA), alpha-fetoprotein (AFP), prostate-specific antigen (PSA), beta human chorionic gonadotropin (BHCG), and CA-125. Elevations in these values can indicate the presence or recurrence of certain cancers. However, many of these markers can also be elevated in the presence of other diseases. Therefore, most are not used as screening tests for the general public. Nonetheless, they have proven useful in monitoring the course of cancers, as well as the effectiveness of treatments (Alexander, 1994; Brock et al., 1993; Higgins, 1996; Schindler, 1991). Table 26–7 lists some of the commonly used tumor markers.

The Patient with a History of Cancer

Patients who have previously been treated for cancer deserve special consideration. This includes any patient with a history of childhood or adult cancers. Specific considerations can be grouped into two categories: patients in remission and survivors. The difference between a patient in remission and a survivor is a subtle distinction. In the past, clinicians considered a specific amount of time (e.g., five years or ten years) with a cancer-free period as cure. However, with more successful cancer treatments, patients are living longer and maintaining longer cancer-free periods. This is one reason why ACNPs should give special consideration to any patient with a history of cancer.

Patients who are long-term survivors of childhood cancer comprise a significant subset of survivors. Like all cancer survivors, they owe their success to improvements in both multimodal therapy and supportive care. A child diagnosed in the 1960s with leukemia had a 1% chance of being disease free in five years. However, a child who is diagnosed with cancer today has a 70% chance of becoming a long-term survivor (Hobbie, 1997).

An important issue to consider when you encounter survivors of cancer is the late effects of treatment modalities, particularly chemotherapy and radiation therapy. Table 26–8 lists late effects from chemotherapy and radiation that occur to the major body systems, the causative agents, and known threshold doses.

▶ STAGING

Staging of cancer, performed at the time of diagnosis, is primarily done to establish the extent of the disease. Unfortunately, there are many different types of classifications used for staging cancers. Furthermore, some cancers can be classified using several different systems, depending on the clinician's preference. However, the most common staging classification involves the use of the acronym TNM, where the T stands for tumor size, extent, or depth, the N for the extent and location of regional nodal involvement, and the M for absence or presence of distant metastases. Each area is assigned a number, corresponding to the size of the tumor or degree of involvement. Numbers range from 0 to 4, with the best prognosis associated with a 0. Table 26–9 displays a general TNM classification and Table 26–10 shows all the possible TNM classifications for lung cancer.

Once a patient's cancer has been staged, the clinician can estimate patient prognosis and, most important, determine appropriate therapy. What may be most beneficial for early-stage cancers can be ineffective for late-stage cancers. In addition, most of the research related to the treatment and cure of cancer uses staging as a framework. Variables within therapies and combinations of therapies are altered in an attempt to find the best treatment for a specific cancer at a certain stage.

▶ TREATMENT

Goals

The ultimate goal of cancer treatment is to cure the patient with minimal functional and structural impairment to the physical body. This is a realistic goal for many cancers,

(Text continued on p. 464)

TABLE 26–6. Cancer Detection: Physical Examination and Diagnostic Testing

Site	Physical Examination	Diagnostic Testing
Cervical Cancer ("ACS modified guideline," 1987; Perez, Knapp, Disaia, & Young, 1985; Smith, Clarke-Pearson, & Creasman, 1985).	**Vagina:** Evaluate consistency of cervix, check for presence of papilloma, Bartholin's cysts, unusual vaginal discharge and tissue friability; evaluate depth of vaginal fornices; check size, position, and mobility of uterus; evaluate color, discharge, and presence of any lesions **Rectum:** Evaluate elasticity and softness of parametrium; evaluate Douglas' pouch (retrouterine pouch)—normally not palpable; evaluate consistency and shape of cervix; evaluate size, position, and mobility of uterus	**Papanicolaou smear:** Cytologic examination of exfoliated cervical cells; sample taken from transition zone, ectocervix, and endocervix **Colposcopy:** The vagina and cervix are washed with acetic acid to highlight abnormal tissue and then examined with magnifying instrument; colposcopy is done following an abnormal Papanicolaou smear or the presence of cervical lesions; a directed biopsy may be done if abnormal tissue is found **Conization:** A cone-shaped excision is made of the abnormal areas of the cervix **Biopsy:** In the presence of gross lesions, multiple punch biopsies are taken
Endometrial Cancer	**Vagina:** Palpate vagina, sub-uretheral areas, and meatus to detect metastases **Rectum:** Palpate cul-de-sac of Douglas, noting consistency and thickening; palpate rectum for extension of neoplasm	**Endometrial biopsy:** Use a Novack curette or less widely used Gravlee jet washer to obtain specimens **Suction curettage:** Tissue is obtained from endometrial cavity **Fractional dilatation and curettage (D & C):** This is done if endometrial pathology is suspected
Vaginal Cancer	**Inspect** vulva and palpate vagina, noting areas of induration; note vaginal bands and cervical structural changes; rotate speculum to visualize entire vagina (vividly red focal areas should arouse suspicion)	**Colposcopy:** Colposcopy is used for directed biopsies of abnormal sites in the vagina
Ovarian Cancer (Khan, Slack, & Cosgrove, 1985; Sargris, 1983; Young, Knapp, Fules, & Disaia, 1985)	**Inspect** for skin signs of abdominal distention, contour for distention, masses (generalized or symmetrical or asymmetrical), bulging flanks **Palpate** for masses and tenderness **Percussion:** Solid tumor is dull to percussion and fluid wave will be dull to percussion **Bimanual pelvic examination:** Palpate adenexa for masses; any enlargement in a premenarchal or postmenopausal woman should be evaluated; solid, bilateral, or fixed masses greater than 10 cm should raise suspicion of malignancy; palpate cul-de-sac via rectovaginal examination (nodularity in cul-de-sac is suspect)	**Ultrasound:** Used in prestaging assessment of suspected ovarian cancer and preoperatively to assess degree of tumor extension in pelvic, abdominal, and retroperitoneal regions; high level of accuracy in detecting tumors **Lymphangiography:** For prestaging evaluation of women known or suspected to have ovarian cancer **Computed tomography:** Computed tomography (CT) provides additional diagnostic and staging information
Breast Cancer (Carlile & Hadaway, 1985; Paulus, 1987)	**Inspection:** Sitting with arms at the side, sitting with arms elevated, sitting with pectoral muscle contraction, sitting bending forward **Palpation:** Inspect breasts with patient in sitting and supine positions with superficial palpation for thickening and temperature changes, and with deeper palpation for lesions; palpate with patient in sitting position for women with pendulous breasts and women with present or past complaints of breast masses; supine: have women lie in left and right lateral decubitus positions to check for lesions between ribs **Examine** nipples for discharge and fix discharge for cytologic examination	**Film-screen mammography or xeromammography:** These methods detect noninvasive or invasive cancers smaller than 0.5 cm **Galactography:** Used in evaluation of nipple discharge; detects papillomas; water-soluble contrast medium is injected into duct **Pneumocystography:** Mammography is performed after removal of fluid and introduction of air into a breast cyst; this is definitive in the detection of intracystic tumors
Stomach Cancer (Macdonald, Cohn, & Gwnderson, 1985; Thompson, 1985)	**Abdominal examination:** Inspect contour for ascites, peristaltic waves (which move from left to right), pallor of mucous membranes indicating anemia, jaundice **Palpate abdomen:** Check painless mass in	**Double-contrast barium studies:** Reported to miss 8 to 10% of gastric cancers; combination of air and barium enables radiologist to better visualize colonic mucosa **Fiberoptic endoscopy:** Supplemented by biopsy and cytology techniques, this is judged to be superior to

(Continued)

TABLE 26–6. Cancer Detection: Physical Examination and Diagnostic Testing *(Continued)*

Site	Physical Examination	Diagnostic Testing
	epigastrium (cancer of stomach is palpable to left of midline). Nodular liver may indicate metastasis to liver; ovarian mass (Krukenberg tumors) may indicate metastasis to ovaries; check for umbilical metastasis **Percussion of abdomen:** Check for dullness, ascites, fluid wave, shifting dullness, puddle test done for small amounts of fluid in the abdomen; palpate nodes in supraclavicular region (Virchow's node is usually on the left) and axillary region **Rectal examination:** Palpate cul-de-sac for metastasis **Skin:** Inspect skin for acanthosis nigricans (suggests cancer of the stomach). Acanthosis nigricans is brown to black pigmentation of the skin	barium examination; sensitivity reported to be 100% and specificity is 99% **Gastric biopsy:** Take specimens from suspected lesions or ulcers; diagnostic accuracy as high as 96% **Cytology:** Obtain specimens of gastric walls using brushing technique, gastric washings, or endoscopic jet wash technique. Accuracy rates are reported to be over 90%
Liver Cancer (Cody, Macdonald, & Gunderson, 1985)	**Abdomen:** Inspect for masses, signs of portal hypertension, jaundice; palpate liver—note tenderness and surface consistency (hard, nodular, irregular masses or masses adjacent to the liver are suspicious for cancer); percuss liver borders, fist percussion of liver for tenderness, percuss for fluid; palpate extremities for edema **Respiratory tract:** Impairment of air entry in right basal segments may be heard in cancer of the liver; check for restriction of diaphragmatic movement on the right side with a friction rub in cancer of the liver **Skin:** Inspect for signs suggesting cirrhosis—e.g., spider angiomas, palmar erythemia, gynecomastia in males, sparse axillary, pubic, and pectoral hair in men	**Serum alkaline phosphatase:** This enzyme is elevated in 70 to 80% of patients with hepatic metastases **Alpha-fetoprotein (AFP) assay:** This is useful in diagnosis and follow-up of people with hepatocellular carcinoma; AFP strongly associated with hepatocellular carcinoma; reports suggest that 75 to 90% of people with primary hepatic cancer have levels above the normal values of 20 to 40 ng/ml **Posteroanterior and lateral chest x-ray films:** These depict the shape of diaphragm **Radionuclide liver scanning:** This demonstrates whether the liver has an abnormality consistent with hepatoma. **Biopsy:** Biopsy may be considered to establish a tissue diagnosis
Lung Cancer (Grant, 1985; Menna, Higgins, & Glatstein, 1985)	**Palpation:** Palpate supraclavicular region for lymphadenopathy; palpate liver for nodularity, indicating metastatic spread **Wheeze:** Any unilateral wheeze merits further evaluation	**PA (posteroanterior) chest x-ray film:** PA and lateral films should be obtained if a lesion is seen on PA film; conventional and computed tomography also are done in presence of peripheral opacity **Cytology:** Examination of 3-day pooled sputum has identified cancer in persons with normal chest radiographs **Flexible fiberoptic bronchoscopy:** This technique provides a visual examination of the interior of the bronchi and, when used with bronchial washings, the combined technique gives an overall accuracy of 79% with a false-positive rate of 0.8% **Transthoracic fine needle aspiration biopsy:** This new procedure is done under fluoroscopic guidance and can diagnose intrapulmonary and solitary pulmonary nodules; research shows low false-positive and false-negative results
Colorectal Cancer (Boyle, Michatek, Bersani, Nemoto, & Mettlin, 1981; Sugarbaker, Gunderson, & Wittes, 1985; Thompson, 1987)	**Rectum:** Palpate entire circumference of anorectal segment for masses and ask patient to strain while examining, palpate Blumer's rectal shelf, check for occult blood in stool **Abdomen:** Inspect contour for distention or masses, use light palpation for subcutaneous nodules or signs of metastatic cancer (enlarged nodular liver, bilateral ovarian tumors, umbilical metastases); percuss for ascites, distention, or areas of dullness indicating masses	**Fecal occult blood testing:** The patient collects stool samples for 3 days using Hemoccult slides; these slides are designed to detect blood in the stool when a chemical is applied **Barium enema x-ray studies:** Barium plus air contrast is recommended over single-contrast technique because the latter can miss up to 40% of polypoid lesions and 20% of carcinomas; reports suggest that barium and air contrast technique can detect 92% of cancers **Proctosigmoidoscopy:** This technique finds lesions low in rectum; approximately 55% of colon cancers occur within 25 cm of anal verge

TABLE 26–6. Cancer Detection: Physical Examination and Diagnostic Testing *(Continued)*

Site	Physical Examination	Diagnostic Testing
		Flexible sigmoidoscopy: Physician can see 50 to 60 cm of colon, and biopsy and polyp removal can be performed. Nearly two thirds of cancers seen with this instrument **Colonoscopy:** If barium enema shows lesions, additional lesions are often found at colonoscopy; can provide specimens for cytologic examination (biopsy, brushing, or washing); polypectomy can also be done; entire colon can be visualized
Skin Cancer (Finley, 1986)	**Inspection:** Entire skin. Note size, shape, color, surface, location, sensations, and surrounding skin of any lesions; note development of any itchiness or irritation. **Malignant melanoma:** inspect back above the waist; head, scalp, and neck; finger and toe webs and soles of feet in deeply pigmented people; the skin between the border of mucous membranes and body orifices; fingernails. Any pigmented nevus that grows rapidly, ulcerates, bleeds or becomes infected should be considered a possible melanoma. Persons with dysplastic nevus syndrome and high-risk characteristics should be examined routinely	**Biopsy:** Definitive diagnosis can be made
Thyroid Cancer (Brennan & Macdonald, 1985)	**Inspect:** Inspect neck, especially on swallowing, for mass or asymmetry; palpate cervical lymph nodes, salivary glands, and thyroid gland, (noting size, contour, symmetry, consistency); masses should be evaluated for firmness, fixation irregularity, or pain; indirect laryngoscopy should be done	**Biopsy:** Biopsy of the thyroid nodule is the only unequivocal diagnostic tool; percutaneous needle biopsy can provide tissue for histologic analysis; fine-needle aspiration is used to obtain tissue for cytologic examination **Ultrasonography:** Ultrasonography is used to distinguish benign from malignant thyroid lesions **Thyroid scintigram:** This is useful in demonstrating size, shape, and position of lesions detected clinically; with both ultrasound and radionuclide methods, tumors of 0.5 cm can be detected
Testicular Cancer (Einhorn, Donohue, Peckham, Williams, & Loehrer, 1985; Hogan, 1983)	**Palpation:** Palpate the scrotum and testicles with both hands while patient stands; note size, shape, consistency, tenderness, and weight of testicles; weight differential between testicles is a clue to malignancy—tumor will feel weighty Testicle feels neither hard nor soft—it has a somewhat rubbery consistency; surface should be smooth and free of lumps except for the ductus deferens; common sitesfor tumors are on the testicular anterior and lateral surfaces; check for hydrocele **Transillumination:** When scrotum is transilluminated, tumors do not permit passage of light, but cysts do; palpate abdomen to check for retroperitoneal lymph node involvement; metastatic nodes usually lie at the level of, or slightly caudal to, the umbilicus; palpate supraclavicular node area for evidence of metastasis	**Ultrasonography:** This technique is reported to distinguish a solid mass from a cystic mass and to be able to show whether the mass involves testis or epididymis or both **Serum markers (AFP and beta-human chorionic gonadotropin):** When measured together one or the other will be positive 85% of the time in men with testicular cancer; not sufficiently sensitive to be relied on alone and not used in early detection Definitive diagnosis is by removal of testes and pathologic analysis
Prostate Cancer ("New prostate cancer detection group," 1987; Perez, Fair, Ihde, & Labrie, 1985)	**Rectal examination:** With patient in knee-chest position, evaluate anal sphincter (which is relaxed in prostate cancer); when palpating prostate, note size, median furrow, surface, shape, consistency, mobility, and sensitivity; cancer is usually a nontender, palpable hard nodule on posterior surface; palpable lymph nodes in groin and	**Digital rectal examination:** Earliest stage detectable by rectal examination is Stage B disease; however, digital rectal examination is judged to be the best method of early detection **Needle biopsy:** Needle biopsy is the standard method to diagnose tumor in United States; aspiration biopsy is the preferred method in Europe

(Continued)

TABLE 26–6. Cancer Detection: Physical Examination and Diagnostic Testing *(Continued)*

Site	Physical Examination	Diagnostic Testing
	supraclavicular region suggest metastasis	**Transrectal Ultrasonography:** This method currently is in testing state to assess its value in early detection; it is useful in detecting tumor invasion through the prostatic capsule (anteriorly)
Bladder Cancer (Cetrin, 1983; Richie, Shipley, & Yagoda, 1985)	Tumor may be palpated suprapubically; bladder can be best felt by rectal or vaginal palpation under anesthesia	**Urinary cytology:** This test may lead to presumptive diagnosis of bladder cancer **Cytoscopy:** Cytoscopic examination and transurethral biopsy confirm the diagnosis **Ultrasonography:** This technique is used in staging to assess invasion of the bladder wall by cancer
Detection of Cancer in General (Van Der Werf, 1987)		**Water-suppressed nuclear magnetic resonance (NMR) spectroscopy:** Blood test should be done when lipoprotein widths are measured. Differences will be noted between persons with benign and malignant tumors, and in persons with tumors and without tumors. This method is in the investigative stage

Reprinted with permission from Olsen & Frank-Stromborg (1991).

particularly when diagnosed in the early stages. Five-year survival rates vary greatly among the types of cancer, ranging from 4% for pancreatic cancer diagnosed at all stages to 99% for localized prostate cancer. These figures exclude cancer *in situ,* which are early-stage cancers, and basal- and squamous-cell skin cancers, which typically have higher survival rates than invasive cancer (American Cancer Society, 1997). Other possible goals for cancer treatment in general include induction of remission, prolonging a remission, and maintaining or restoring a patient to his or her optimal quality of life.

Modalities

The treatment modalities for cancer include surgery, radiation, chemotherapy, hormones, immunotherapy, and bone marrow transplantation. The type of treatment a patient receives is dependent on the type of cancer, its stage, its location, and the patient's functional status. The type of cancer does not change throughout treatment; metastatic cancer is still the same type of cancer as it was at diagnosis, just in a different location. However, the cancer stage, its location, and the patient's functional status can, and often does, change throughout the whole cancer experience. Therefore,

TABLE 26–7. Commonly Used Tumor Markers

Marker	Elevations may indicate	Useful for
CEA (carcinoembryonic antigen)	Breast, colorectal, and lung cancers	Monitoring or management of patients with known disease
PSA (prostate-specific antigen)	Prostate cancer, benign prostate enlargement	Prostate cancer screening when combined with rectal examination; monitoring response to treatment and recurrence
HCG (human chorionic gonadotropin)	Germ cell tumors (testicular, certain types of ovarian, others), pregnancy	Differentiation of germ cell tumors
AFP (α-fetoprotein)	Germ cell tumors, liver cancer, benign liver disease, pregnancy	Differentiation of germ cell tumors
CA-125 (antigen)	Ovarian, colorectal, and gastric cancers	Monitoring response to treatment
CA-15-3 (two antigens)	Metastatic or recurrent breast cancer	Monitoring recurrence of disease
CA-19-9 (antigens)	Pancreatic, colorectal, and gastric cancers; inflammatory bowel and biliary disease	Monitoring response to treatment
CA-72-4 (antigens)	Ovarian, colorectal, and gastric cancers	Detection of primary disease and monitoring of treatment progress
CA-242	Pancreatic cancer	Monitoring disease progress when combined with CA-19-9

From Otto (1997).

TABLE 26–8. Late Effects of Chemotherapy and Radiation Therapy

Organ System	Agent	Mechanism of Injury	Effect	Threshold Dose	Comments
Heart	Doxorubicin (Adriamycin)	Cytotoxic to cardiomyocytes via direct cell damage to myocyte with resultant loss of contractile component	Congestive heart failure	550 mg/m^2	300–350 mg/m^2 when used with radiation
	Radiation	Mycocardial capillary endothelial cell injury that produces myocardial fibrosis with exudate; no damage to myocytes	Myocardial fibrosis (may occur 5–10 years after radiation when doxorubicin given)	45–50 Gy	—
Lungs	Bleomycin	Changes in nucleus in alveolar cells	Alveolitis; parenchymal fibrosis; interstitial changes	400–500 U	When combined with radiation, dose response is increased
	Radiation	Ablation of alveolar cells and release of surfactant; injury to lung vasculature	Arterial hypoxia; decreased blood flow; acute pneumonitis	>6.0 Gy	
Kidney	Cisplatin	Acute tubular necrosis and atrophy due to changes in renal tubular cell	Renal failure due to tubular damage	—	Added and enhanced problems occur
	Radiation	Changes in the arteriolar glomerular area	Nephritis due to microvascular damage	5–20 Gy	10 Gy when used with chemotherapy
Liver	Methotrexate 6-Mercaptopurine Doxorubicin (Adriamycin)	Direct effect on hepatocytes	Hepatocellular necrosis and fat replacement	—	—
Skin	Doxorubicin (Adriamycin) Actinomycin D Carmustine	—	Enhancement or "recall" of previous radiation skin reactions when chemotherapy is given	—	—
Central nervous system	Methotrexate (intrathecal and intravenous)	Contacts white matter; damage to vascular choroid plexus; alters drug clearance	Leukoencephalopathy	—	—
	Brain irradiation	Alters capillary permeability of blood-brain barrier	Leukoencephalopathy	—	—
Gastrointestinal (major dose-limiting organ in acute reaction)	5-Fluorouracil	*Acute* mucosal loss	Stomatitis; enteritis; ulceration	—	Late effects occur only with addition of radiation therapy
	Radiation	*Acute* mucosal loss Late progressive endarteritis	 Ulceration and infarction necrosis of vessels resulting in fistulae and perforation; slow fibrosis and stricture of bowel	— —	—
Bone marrow (major dose-limiting organ in acute reaction)	Chemotherapy	*Acute* suppression of cycling stem cells	Leukopenia, thrombocytopenia, gradual anemia	—	—
	Radiation	*Acute* suppression of resting cells 10–15% irradiated marrow ablated at doses <30.0 Gy	Gradual with time		Recovery of bone marrow suppressed when combined treatment given simultaneously

(Continued)

TABLE 26–8. Late Effects of Chemotherapy and Radiation Therapy *(Continued)*

Organ System	Agent	Mechanism of Injury	Effect	Threshold Dose	Comments
		25–50% irradiated marrow ablated at doses >30.0 Gy 50–75% irradiated marrow ablated but responds quickly due to increased sensitivity to total volume ablated (new islands of hematopoiesis become active; protected marrow compensates with overproduction)			

Reprinted with permission from Scofield, Liebman, & Popkin (1991).

while there is a limited number of treatment modalities, each patient's experience with cancer treatment is a unique and diverse encounter.

Surgery. Patients receive surgery for cancer at all stages of the disease process. The reasons patients receive surgery are numerous and include diagnosis, staging, prevention, cure, palliation, reconstruction, cytoreduction, resection of metastases, supportive care, and following complications from other treatment modalities (Havard & Topping, 1991).

Often, a suspected cancer diagnosis is confirmed through surgical biopsy of the suspicious tissue and subsequent examination of the specimen. Possible biopsy techniques include exfoliative, needle, incisional, excisional, and endoscopic. An exfoliative biopsy is obtained by scraping cells from the suspected tissue, as in a Papanicolaou test. A needle biopsy involves aspiration of fluid or tissue through a needle, usually inserted after local anesthesia. Done under local or general anesthesia, an incisional biopsy is the removal of a small section of tissue. Punch or shave biopsies are specific types of incisional biopsies. An excisional biopsy includes complete removal of the tumor with little or no margin of surrounding tissue. When the suspected tissue is not in an easily accessible site, a scope is used so that a tissue sample may be obtained. Common endoscopic biopsies include the use of a laryngoscope, cystoscope, and bronchoscope (Havard & Topping, 1991).

The staging of cancer most often involves surgery. Surgical staging techniques include open incisional procedures as well as laparoscopic techniques. Laparoscopic techniques are becoming the preferred method of staging for many cancers. Among the many benefits of laparoscopy are that it is less invasive than open incision, potentially allowing a shorter recovery time, shorter hospitalization, and reduced medical costs (Ramshaw, 1997).

In a small number of cases, patients may elect to have

TABLE 26–9. General TNM Definitions

T	Primary tumor	Size, extent, depth of primary tumor
	TX	Primary tumor cannot be assessed
	T0	No evidence of primary tumor
	Tis	*In situ*
	T1–T4	Increasing size or extent of primary tumor
N	Nodal metastasis	Extent and location of involved regional lymph nodes
	NX	Regional lymph nodes cannot be assessed
	N0	No regional lymph node metastasis
	N1–N3	Increasing numbers and size of involved regional lymph nodes
M	Metastasis	Absence or presence of distant spread of disease
	MX	Distant disease cannot be assessed
	M0	No distant spread of disease
	M1	Distant spread of disease

Reprinted with permission from Alexander (1994).

TABLE 26–10. An Example of TNM Staging: Lung Guidelines

Stage	Lung
Occult	**TX-N0-M0** TX: primary proven only by cells (sputum)
0	**Tis-N0-M0** Tis: carcinoma *in situ*
I	**T1 or T2-N0-M0** T1: tumor ≤ 3 cm T2: >3 cm and/or involving main bronchus or pleura
II	**T1 or T2-N1-M0** N1: peribronchial or hilar lymph node metastasis; same side as tumor
IIIA	**T1 or T2-N2-M0** T3-any N-M0 N2: mediastinal or subclavian nodes; same side T3: tumor invades chest wall, diaphragm, mediastinal pleura, pericardium
IIIB	**Any T-N3-M0** **T4-any N-M0** N3: metastasis in lymph nodes opposite side T4: invades other organs (heart, mediastinum, etc.) or pleural effusion
IV	**Any T, any N, M1** M1: distant metastasis

Reprinted with permission from Alexander (1994).

prophylactic surgery. These patients usually have a precancerous condition or a high familial risk for a particular type of cancer. Examples of surgery done for prevention of cancer include a colectomy for familial polyposis coli, orchiopexy for cryptorchidism, oophrectomy for familial ovarian cancer, and mastectomy for familial breast cancer (Havard & Topping, 1991).

Surgery is the dominant treatment method for those patients with cancer who achieve a cure. The surgical procedure can be either a local excision or a wide excision, also called *en bloc* dissection. For a local excision the malignant tumor is removed with a small margin of normal tissue. For a wide excision the tumor, regional lymph nodes, lymphatic channels, and adjoining structures are all removed. Examples of cancers whose primary method of cure is surgical include skin cancers (with the exception of melanoma), early rectal and colon cancers, early breast cancer, early cervical cancer, and differentiated thyroid cancer (Havard & Topping, 1991; Pfeifer, 1994a).

When cure is not a realistic expectation, surgery can still be used as a treatment option for palliative reasons. Indications for palliative surgery include relief from symptoms and improvement in function. Examples of palliative surgical procedures include treatment for oncologic emergencies, bone stabilization, and sympathectomy for pain (Havard & Topping, 1991; Pfeifer, 1994a).

Reconstructive surgery is often necessary after radical surgical resections have occurred. Creation of an ileostomy, urostomy, or colostomy is an example of possible necessary reconstructive surgical procedures associated with cancer treatment (Havard & Topping, 1991). Chapter 25 discusses reconstructive surgery in more detail.

Cytoreductive surgery, also called debulking, is undertaken with the intent to reduce tumor mass to a level that is more manageable for the other treatment modalities. It is thought that the residual tumor volume will be more susceptible to postoperative chemotherapy or radiation (Havard & Topping, 1991; Martin & Braly, 1991).

Metastases may be resected if they are isolated, if the goal of treatment is curative, for palliation, or if the original site of cancer is controlled. Areas of metastases that have been successfully resected include bone, lung, liver, and brain (Havard & Topping, 1991).

In some instances surgery may be indicated for treatment of oncologic emergencies. However, the decision to surgically intervene during an oncologic emergency is controversial because sometimes the outcome results in a poorer quality of life for the patient. Those emergencies needing surgical intervention include airway obstruction, perforations, and spinal cord compression (Havard & Topping, 1991).

Surgical techniques for cancer treatment are also used in a supportive role. Placement of a gastrostomy or jejunostomy tube to aid in nutrition, radioactive implants for radiation therapy, and placement of vascular access devices to aid in delivery of chemotherapy are all examples of supportive surgical measures (Havard & Topping, 1991).

Unfortunately, sometimes radiation therapy and chemotherapy cause complications that need to be surgically treated. Both therapies infrequently have the potential to cause new malignancies, which may require surgical resection. Additionally, radiation therapy is associated with other possible complications that may need surgical intervention including skin necrosis, fistula development, muscle contraction or stricture, and bone fracture. Potential complications from chemotherapy that may require surgical intervention include tissue necrosis from extravasation and intestinal inflammation and perforation. Surgical procedures to repair these complications can include excision, grafting, resection, dilatation, stent insertion, debridement, fixation, and possibly amputation (Havard & Topping, 1991).

Radiation Therapy. Radiation as a treatment modality involves the use of high energy, ionizing rays. The aim of radiation therapy is to deliver a precise dose of radiation to the specific area of carcinogenic tissue so that the cells are either killed or can no longer reproduce, while sparing the surrounding healthy tissues. Realistically, some healthy tissues also receive radiation; but radiation is delivered in such a way as to minimize healthy tissue exposure. The exception to this is total body irradiation used before bone marrow transplantation or hemibody treatment for extensive bone metastases (Hilderley & Dow, 1991; Iwamoto, 1994).

Radiation can be delivered as either teletherapy or brachytherapy. Teletherapy is given through the use of a machine, such as a linear accelerator, while brachytherapy involves insertion of a radiation source near the carcinogenic tumor. Thus, the primary difference between the therapies involves the use of radiation from an external versus an internal source (Hilderley & Dow, 1991).

Patients can receive radiation therapy at any stage of the disease process and for a variety of reasons including cure, control of local disease, adjuvant therapy, and palliation. Prostate cancer and early stage Hodgkin's disease are two examples of cancer that are curable through the use of radiation (Hilderley & Dow, 1991; Iwamoto, 1994).

Radiation is used locally to control the growth and spread of malignancies. Examples of radiation therapy used for local control include head and neck cancers and cancer of the breast (Hilderley & Dow, 1991; Iwamoto, 1994).

Radiation is also frequently used as an adjunct to chemotherapy and surgery. The concept of adjuvant therapy is an important one in cancer treatment and discussed more fully in the section on multimodal therapy. The goal of adjuvant radiation therapy is dependent on the primary site of cancer and the site receiving the radiation; however, in general, adjuvant radiation therapy aims to eliminate microscopic disease beyond surgical tumor margins, reduce tumor bulk, and decrease the need for further surgical procedures.

Additionally, radiation therapy that is used as an adjunct chemotherapy can facilitate transfer of chemotherapeutic agents across the blood–brain barrier, a difficult area for most chemotherapeutic agents to reach. When chemotherapy is used for this purpose, it acts as a radiosensitizer. Radiosensitizers are substances that are administered concurrently with radiation therapy to increase tumor response. Chemotherapeutic agents used as radiosensitizers include cisplatin, 5-fluorouracil, bleomycin, and mitomycin. Other radiosensitizers include etanidazole, fluosol DA, metronidazole, SR2508, and Ro-03-8799 (Hilderley & Dow, 1991; Iwamoto, 1994, Wilkes, Ingwersen, & Burke, 1997).

Another frequent use for radiation in the treatment of cancer is palliation. Common signs and symptoms that necessitate the use of radiation for relief include pain, loss of mobility, bleeding, and pressure. Pain, particularly when in the bones, has been effectively managed through radiation (Hilderley & Dow, 1991; Iwamoto, 1994).

Chemotherapy. Many cancers benefit from antineoplastic drug therapy, frequently referred to as chemotherapy. They are rarely used as single agents because combination therapy is more effective with longer disease-free intervals, has less toxic effects, and produces less drug resistance than single agents. Additionally, greater cell kill can be achieved (Walter-Coleman, 1996). Standard combinations exist for most cancers.

Chemotherapy is delivered by a variety of routes including po, SC, IM, IV (bolus, piggyback, or continuous infusion), topical, intrathecal, intraperitoneal, intracavity, intraarterial, and intralesional. Special precautions are needed when delivering chemotherapy because studies have shown that many antineoplastic drugs are teratogenic, mutagenic, and carcinogenic. The Occupational Safety and Health Administration (OSHA) has developed guidelines for the safe administration of all hazardous drugs, including antineoplastics. The guidelines recommend that specific education and training be provided for all staff involved in handling cytotoxic drugs (Mahon et al., 1994; Walter-Coleman, 1996; Wilkes et al., 1997). Many institutions provide special training for those health-care personnel who are required to administer chemotherapy.

Chemotherapeutic drugs used in the treatment of cancer interfere with cell division and are either cytostatic or cytocidal. They may be classified by several different methods including the point in the cell cycle at which they exert their effect or by their mechanism of action, derivation, and chemical structure. If categorized by the former method, chemotherapeutic drugs are either cell-cycle specific or cell-cycle nonspecific. Drugs that are cell-cycle specific primarily destroy cells that are dividing—those cells in G1, S, G2, and M phase. Cell-cycle nonspecific drugs are most toxic to cells in the resting, or G0, phase. The most common classification system uses the chemical properties of the drugs. Using this system, there are five main categories: alkylating agents, plant alkaloids, antimetabolities, antibiotics, and miscellaneous (Guy, 1991; Walter-Coleman, 1996; Wilkes et al., 1997).

The alkylating agents are cell-cycle nonspecific and work by substituting an alkyl group for a hydrogen atom, thus causing abnormal breaks and cross-linking of DNA strands. The inability of the DNA strands to separate during DNA replication leads to cell death. The alkylating agents can be further classified into mustard derivatives, ethylenimines, alkyl sulfonamides, triazenes, nitrosoureas, and metal salts (Guy, 1991; Wilkes et al., 1997).

The plant alkaloids, derived from foliage, are cell-cycle specific for the G1 and S phases. Their mechanisms of action involve crystallization or destabilization of the microtubules or inhibition of the mitosis phase. The drugs extracted from the periwinkle plant are called vinca alkaloids, those derived from the May apple plant are called podophyllotoxins, and those derived from the yew tree bark are called taxanes (Guy, 1991; Walter-Coleman, 1996; Wilkes et al., 1997).

The antimetabolities are cell-cycle specific in the S phase and "interfere with DNA and RNA synthesis by acting as false metabolites which are incorporated into the DNA strand, or block essential enzymes, so that DNA synthesis is prevented" (Wilkes et al., 1997, p.14). Antimetabolities can be further classified into folic acid antagonists, pyrimidine antagonists, or purine antagonists.

The antineoplastic antibiotics are derived from a species of soil fungus and are cell-cycle nonspecific. They incorporate a variety of mechanisms to disrupt cell division, including interference with protein and RNA synthesis, thus causing cell death. They can be further classified into anthracyclines, chromomycins, or miscellaneous (Guy, 1991; Wilkes et al., 1997).

The miscellaneous category encompasses the remaining chemotherapeutic drugs in current clinical practice whose mechanisms of action are poorly understood or unique (Guy, 1991). Specific drugs in this category include L-asparaginase and procarbazine.

There are a large number of chemotherapeutic drugs currently in use; Table 26–11 lists some of the more common ones.

Like radiation therapy, patients receive chemotherapy for a variety of reasons. Chemotherapy can be the primary method of treatment aimed at curing the patient or it can be given adjuvantly. Testicular cancer and acute lymphocytic leukemia are primarily cured through chemotherapy (Guy, 1991). Adjuvant use is discussed under the section of multimodal therapy.

Hormonal Therapy. Many cancers arise from hormonally active tumors and thus are hormonally sensitive. "Antineoplastic hormonal manipulations include obliterating host production of the required hormone; blocking the

TABLE 26–11. Classification of Some Commonly Used Antineoplastic Drugs

Alkylating Agents	Plant Alkaloids	Antimetabolites	Antibiotics	Miscellaneous
Busulfan	Docetaxel	Cytosine-arabinoside	Bleomycin	L-asparaginase
Carmustine	Etoposide	5-Fluorouracil	Dactinomycin	Procarbazine
Cisplatin	Paclitaxel	Hydroxyurea	Daunorubicin	
Cyclophosphamide	Teniposide	Methotrexate	Doxorubicin	
Dacarbazine	Vinblastine		Mithramycin	
Ifosfamide	Vincristine		Mitomycin C	
Lomustine			Mitoxantrone	
Mechlorethamine			Plicamycin	
Streptozocin				
Triethylene-thiophosphoramide				

Data compiled from Guy (1991), Wilkes, Ingwersen, & Burke (1997).

hormone receptors with competing agents; and substituting chemically similar agents for the active hormone, which cannot be used by the tumor cell" (Guy, 1991, p. 287). Currently, cancers that use hormones for treatment include breast, ovarian, endometrial, renal, and prostate. Additionally, hematologic malignancies benefit from adrenocorticosteroids, which have demonstrated direct antineoplastic effects.

Besides the adrenocorticosteroids, other hormone classifications include steroids, steroid blockers, androgens, antiandrogens, estrogens, antiestrogens, progestins, aromatase inhibiters, and luteinizing hormone-releasing hormone (LHRH) blockers (Guy, 1991; Wasaff, 1997; Wilkes et al., 1997).

Hormone therapy is often used in the treatment of metastatic breast cancer, allowing for an increased understanding of its role in cancer treatment. In breast cancer tumors that are estrogen receptor positive, antiestrogens act by binding to estrogen receptors. This action blocks estrogen from binding to the receptors, thus making these receptors inactive. Specific drug names of some estrogens are diethylstilbestrol, ethinyl estradiol, conjugated equine estrogen, and chorotrianisene. Tamoxifen is an example of an antiestrogen (Wasaff, 1997; Wilkes et al., 1997).

Also in the case of breast cancer, aromatase inhibiters suppress the enzyme involved in estrogen production, thus causing a decrease in serum estrogen in postmenopausal women. Aromatase inhibiters are either steroidal or nonsteroidal and either selective or non-selective, depending on their affinity for the aromatase enzyme. Drugs that are aromatase inhibiters include amino-glutethimide, formestane, exemestane, and anastrozole (Wasaff, 1997).

Though in use for many years, the mechanism of action of the androgens is unclear but, in research, progestins compete for both progestin and androgen receptor sites. Examples of androgens include testosterone, obfluoxymesterone, and obtestolactone, while bicalutamide and flutamide are antiandrogens. Megestrol acetate and medroxyprogesterone are examples of progestin drugs. LHRH blockers inhibit pituitary gonadotropin secretion and include the drugs leuprolide and goserelin (Guy, 1991; Wasaff, 1997; Wilson, Shannon & Stang, 1998).

Immunotherapy. Immmunotherapy, also called biotherapy, involves the use of agents called biologic response modifiers (BRMs). BRMs are naturally found in the body's immune system; they alter the body's immune response either through stimulation, restoration, augmentation, or modulation. Additionally, some BRMs have direct antitumor properties. Because gastric enzymes destroy BRMs, routes of administration are always parenteral including topical, intralesional, SC, IM, and IV (Schindler, 1991; Wilkes et al., 1997).

Because BRMs are found in the body's immune system they can be obtained through living sources; however, they are also synthesized in the laboratory. BRMs that have been made in the laboratory through recombinant DNA have a lower case "r" in front of them, e.g., r-IL-2 (Schindler, 1991; Wilkes et al., 1997). This may be an important aspect for the ACNP to know because those patients who object to blood products may be willing to receive recombinant BRMs.

At this time, most BRMs are investigational; however, several have demonstrated highly desirable properties and others are fulfilling much needed functions. Additionally, recent technology has created fused BRMs, potentially allowing for a synergistic effect (Wilkes et al., 1997).

BRMs are further classified into cytokines or monoclonal antibodies (MoAbs). Cytokines are substances released from activated lymphocytes. Specific cytokines currently in use include colony stimulating factors (CSFs), interferons (IFNs), interleukins (ILs), and tumor necrosis factor (TNF).

The CSFs are glycoproteins and include granulocyte colony stimulating factor (G-CSF), macrophage colony stimulating factor (M-CSF), granulocyte–macrophage colony stimulating factor (GM–CSF), and erythropoietin (EPO). As indicated by their name, CSFs stimulate the differentiation of particular blood cells. CSFs are used to combat a common side effect of chemotherapeutic drugs: myelosuppression. G-CSF accelerates the recovery of neutraphil counts, M-CSF affects macrophages, GM–CSF regulates the growth of all granulocytes and stimulates monocytes and macrophages, and EPO stimulates erythrocyte production and differentiation (Farrell, 1996; Wilkes et al., 1997).

Two types of IFNs include alpha and beta, with numerous alpha subtypes. IFNs have antiviral, antiproliferative, and immunomodulatory effects. Alpha interferon was the first BRM to be approved by the Food and Drug Administration and is currently indicated for hairy-cell leukemia and AIDS-related Kaposi's sarcoma (Farrell, 1996; Wilkes et al., 1997).

The ILs exert their effects on the T lymphocytes including stimulation of T-lymphocyte proliferation, enhanced killer T-cell activity, and proliferation of cytotoxic T cells. The ILs are also capable of stimulating other cytokines. IL-2 is currently indicated for metastatic renal cell carcinoma. Other ILs, e.g., IL-1 and IL-4, are still investigational (Farrell, 1996; Wilkes et al., 1997).

TNF is produced by activated macrophages, may be cytostatic in the G2 stage, and may also cause injury to a tumor's capillaries, causing tumor cells to hemorrhage and necrose. TNF also activates other immune cells. The use of TNF in cancer treatment is still investigational (Wilkes et al., 1997).

MoAbs "are identical antibodies made by the many descendants (clones) of a single plasma cell. Typically, the target antigen is injected into a mouse, then antibody-producing plasma cells are 'harvested' from the mouse. The mouse plasma cell is fused with a long-lived laboratory-grown plasma cell, within a single-cell membrane. The fused cells, or hybrids, are then cloned. Over a long period of time, clones secrete the made-to-order monoclonal (single clone) antibodies" (Schindler, 1992, pp. 22–23). Figure 26–3 depicts monoclonal antibody production.

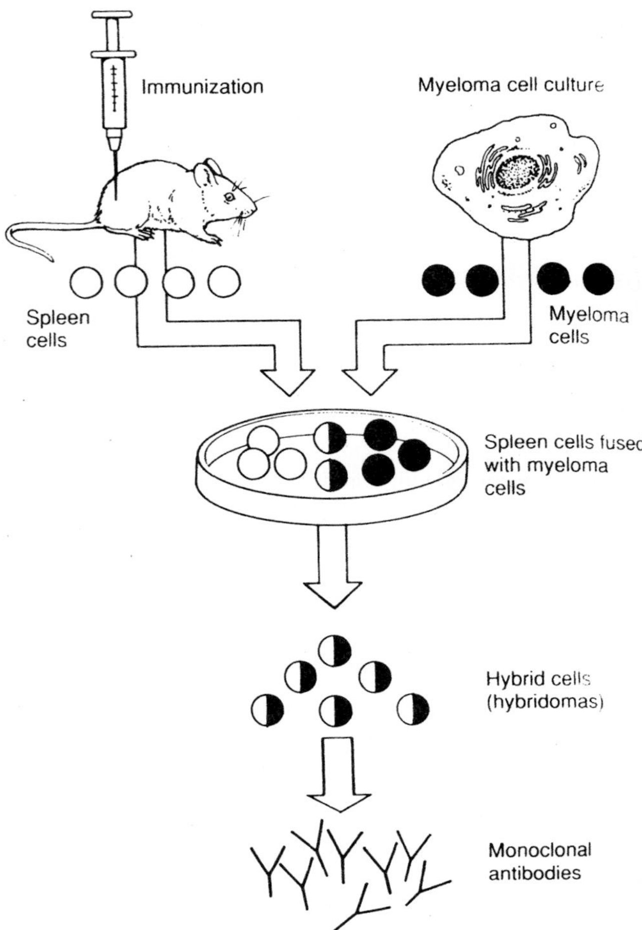

Figure 26–3. Monoclonal antibody production. *(From Rieger [1994].)*

MoAbs selectively bind to tumor cell surfaces and could provide the most tumor-specific therapy for cancer. Additionally, MoAbs may be conjugated to radioisotopes, chemotherapeutic drugs, or toxins. Thus, conjugated MoAbs can deliver cytotoxic agents directly to tumor cells (Karius & Marriott, 1997). MoAbs have already undergone numerous clinical trials but most remain largely investigational. However, in late 1997 the Food and Drug Administration approved the first monoclonal antibody for clinical use: rituximab. Initial clinical trials established rituximab as safe and effective for treatment of relapsed or refractory low-grade or follicular CD20+, B-cell non-Hodgkin's lymphoma (Cabanillas, Maloney, Link & Jonas, 1998; Grillo-Lopez & Fyfe, 1997).

Bone Marrow Transplant. Bone marrow transplant (BMT) involves the replacement of diseased or damaged bone marrow with healthy bone marrow. There are two main types of BMT: autologous and allogeneic. Autologous BMT occurs when a patient uses his or her own bone marrow. In allogeneic BMT a patient receives the bone marrow of someone other than him- or herself. Table 26–12 lists current diseases treated with BMT.

Allogenic BMTs can be further classified into syngeneic, related, or unrelated. When the donor is the patient's identical twin, this is a syngeneic BMT. A related allogenic BMT is when the donor is related to the recipient, usually a sibling. An unrelated allogenic BMT is from an unrelated donor, one who is either a human leukocyte antigen (HLA) match or only a partial HLA match. HLA-matched donors are often obtained through The National Marrow Donor Registry Program. This registry, created in 1987, contains over 600,000 individuals who have had tissue typing and are willing to be BMT donors. HLA matching is an important concept because the more matched the donor's marrow is to the recipient, the less chance there is for graft rejection and other possible side effects, particularly graft versus host disease (Cook, 1996; Moore & Szekley, 1994; Poliquin, 1997).

TABLE 26–12. Diseases Treated with Bone Marrow Transplantation

Malignant	Nonmalignant
Leukemia (acute and chronic, lymphocytic and myelogenous)	Myelodysplastic syndrome
Hodgkin's lymphoma	Myelofibrosis
Non-Hodgkin's lymphoma	Aplastic anemia
Burkitt's lymphoma	Thalassemia
Multiple myeloma	Severe combined immunodeficiency syndrome
Breast cancer	Mucopolysacharoidosis
Testicular cancer	Lipid storage disease
Lung cancer	Osteopetrosis
Neuroblastoma	Paroxysmal nocturnal hemoglobinuria
Ewing's sarcoma	
Wilms' tumor	
Rhabdomyosarcoma	
Melanoma	

Data compiled from Moore & Szekley (1994), Poliquin (1997), Shivnan, Shelton, & Onners (1996).

TABLE 26–13. Malignant Diseases Treated with PBSC Transplantation

Acute myelogenous leukemia
Chronic myelogenous leukemia
Hodgkin's lymphoma
Non-Hodgkin's lymphoma
Multiple myeloma
Sarcoma
Neuroblastoma
Brain tumors
Breast cancer
Testicular cancer
Ovarian cancer
Small cell lung cancer
Wilms' tumor

Data from Moore & Szekley (1994), Wujcik (1997).

BMT is an aggressive treatment that requires both the donor and the recipient to undergo procedures. For allogeneic BMT, the donor must have his or her marrow harvested, a procedure usually performed in the operating room that lasts several hours. The recipient must undergo a demanding pre-BMT chemotherapy regimen and sometimes total body radiation before receiving the donor's bone marrow. Intravenous infusion of bone marrow usually takes place in the recipient's room. In the case of autologous BMT the procedure is similar except that the patient must be in remission and recovered from other treatments before harvesting. Also, more volume may be needed during harvesting due to purging. Purging, through the use of chemotherapy or MoAbs, is done to rid the bone marrow of possible occult cancer cells (Moore & Szekley, 1994; Poliquin, 1997).

Another type of marrow transplant, one that uses peripherally circulating functional hematopoietic stem cells, is called peripheral blood stem cell (PBSC) transplant. Like BMT, PBSC transplantation can be autologous or allogeneic; however, most PBSC transplants are autologous. Table 26–13 lists current malignant diseases treated with PBSC transplantation.

Transplantation of PBSCs entails the collection of blood cells through a process called aspheresis. Aspheresis extracts the blood cells from peripherally circulating blood, separates the various components, retains the peripheral stem cells, and returns the remaining blood back to the patient. The collected stem cells are transplanted at a later date. The main advantages of PBSC transplant are that it is often an outpatient procedure, less intensive, and less expensive with a shorter recuperation period than BMT. However, the reinfusion of stem cells is similar to bone marrow (Moore & Szekley, 1994; Poliquin, 1997). Table 26–14 displays types of transplantations.

Side Effects

The ACNP should be familiar with both acute and long-term side effects of surgery, radiation therapy, chemotherapy, hormonal therapy, immunotherapy, and bone marrow transplant. Familiarity with expected side effects and effective treatments for resolution of, or relief from, such side effects aid the ACNP in competent management of patients with cancer. This section introduces the ACNP to the major side effects associated with cancer treatment. Procedures and therapies for resolution and relief of side effects can be found in other chapters of the book.

Surgery. As expected, many of the side effects of surgery correlate with the area that received the surgical operation; however, surgical treatment for cancer in general is associated with skin impairment and fatigue. Additionally,

TABLE 26–14. Types of Transplantations

Type of Transplantation	Source of Bone Marrow/Stem Cells
Autologous bone marrow	• Patient (self)
Allogeneic bone marrow	
• Related	• Human leukocyte antigen-matched (HLA-matched) family member, usually a sibling
• Syngeneic	• Patient's identical twin (HLA identical)
• Unrelated	• HLA-matched nonfamily member
• Mismatched	• Partially HLA-matched family or nonfamily member
Peripheral blood stem cell	
• Autologous	• Patient (self)
• Allogeneic	• HLA-matched family or nonfamily member

From Poliquin (1997).

when surgery has resulted in the loss of a body part (e.g., breast or leg), many patients experience a change in body image. Skin impairment and disruption in body image are discussed previously in Chapter 25. Fatigue is a significant experience for all patients undergoing treatment for cancer, no matter the modality, and is discussed here.

Fatigue is a common postoperative experience; however, very little research has been done to examine the exact correlation and causes. Winningham et al. (1994), in a comprehensive article concerning fatigue and the cancer experience, reviewed several studies that analyzed physiologic and psychosocial factors and their relevance to surgery and fatigue. Most of the study results have limited application because of small sample sizes, incomplete information on research methods, and lack of replication. Additionally, only one study involved patients with cancer. The reviewers conclude that while postoperative fatigue is a problem that improves with time, it is not well understood.

Patients who receive radiation therapy frequently experience some degree of fatigue. It has been noted that as radiation therapy progresses over time, more fatigue is experienced (Irvine, Vincent, Graydon, Bubela, & Thompson, 1994). After reviewing research findings on radiation therapy and fatigue, Winningham et al. (1994) conclude that the etiologic factors and correlates of fatigue for radiation therapy have not been identified.

Studies have also demonstrated that 80% to 96% of patients receiving chemotherapy experience fatigue (Blesch et al., 1991; Nail, Jones, Greene, Schipper, & Jensen, 1991). Reviewing studies on fatigue and chemotherapy, Winningham et al. (1994) noted that both psychological and physiological responses were cited as contributing factors. Also, fatigue patterns varied depending on disease type, size, duration, magnitude, and specific chemotherapeutic drugs used. Furthermore, fatigue was usually reported in the first 3 to 4 days following chemotherapy administration, became more noticeable 6 to 7 days later, and faded until the next treatment.

The relationship between biotherapy and fatigue is well established; fatigue is often a dose-limiting toxicity. The major side effect of biotherapy, a flu-like syndrome, includes fatigue (Winningham et al., 1994).

Radiation Therapy. Common side effects of radiation therapy include alopecia; mucositis; nausea, vomiting, and diarrhea; bone marrow depression; skin reactions; and fatigue. The manifestation of radiation side effects is often site and dose dependent.

Alopecia, or hair loss, is associated with radiation to the head. Hair loss may be regional (at the location of the treatment site) and may also occur directly opposite the site, where the x-rays exit. Only with large doses, as in treatment for brain tumors, is alopecia likely to be permanent (Iwamoto, 1994).

Mucositis is inflammation of the mucous membranes and can occur in the respiratory, digestive, and genitourinary tracts. Inflammation of the oral cavity (stomatitis) and inflammation of the esophagus (esophagitis) may occur after receiving radiation to the head, neck, and chest. The tissues may become erythematous or whitish, edematous, and are usually very sensitive (Hilderley & Dow, 1991; Iwamoto, 1994).

Nausea, vomiting, and diarrhea are associated with radiation to the abdomen and pelvis. These symptoms occur due to the effects of radiation on the intestines. The mucosa of the intestinal lining becomes slick causing stool to move quickly through the intestines. In addition the bowel lining may atrophy, causing decreased fluid resorption and malabsorption of bile salts. Symptoms often occur within 6 hours after treatment and may last for 3 to 6 hours. The patient may experience diarrhea throughout the course of treatment, resolving several weeks after completion (Bisanz, 1997; Hilderley & Dow, 1991; Iwamoto, 1994).

Bone marrow depression occurs when sites with large amounts of active bone marrow are irradiated. These sites include the skull, sternum, ribs, pelvis, and spine. Bone marrow depression is not often an acute reaction so blood counts must be routinely followed (Iwamoto, 1994).

Skin reactions occur because radiation must enter and exit the body through the skin. An expected and normal side effect, erythema begins to develop 2 weeks into treatment. In some cases the erythema progresses to dry, flaky skin and then moist desquamation. Healing usually occurs several weeks after radiation treatments have ceased (Hilderley & Dow, 1991; Iwamoto, 1994).

Long-term skin changes may include increased pigmentation and radiation recall. Radiation recall develops when skin that has received radiation in the past is exposed to sunlight. The amount of sunlight exposure needed to induce radiation recall varies for each patient and is dependent on the total amount of radiation received and the patient's own pigmentation. Radiation recall can also occur with the administration of certain chemotherapeutic agents. Areas that sustain changes from previous radiation again demonstrate alterations when certain chemotherapeutic agents are delivered.

Chemotherapy. Due to the systemic nature of treatment, the expected side effects of chemotherapy are numerous. Many side effects occur at standard doses while others more often occur when the drug is given in high-dose or long-term therapy. This chapter lists the main side effects associated with chemotherapy by grouping them under body systems: neurological; cardiac; pulmonary; gastrointestinal; renal; hematologic; immunologic; and skin, nails, and hair. Additionally, specific drugs that induce these side effects are also given.

Neurological. Neurological changes include central nervous system disturbances that range from mild confusion, dizziness, and somnolence to hallucinations and seizures.

These side effects are often dose related, higher doses causing more incidence, and usually not permanent. Some agents associated with central nervous system changes include methotrexate, ifosfamide, procarbazine, busulfan, and mitotane (an antihormone) (McCoy-Adabody & Borger, 1996; Wilkes et al., 1997).

Peripheral nervous system changes include paresthesias and peripheral neuropathy, due to myelin sheath destruction. Some agents associated with peripheral side effects include cisplatin, paclitaxel, docetaxel, procarbazine, vinblastine, and vincristine (McCoy-Adabody & Borger, 1996; Wilkes et al., 1997).

Cardiac. The most significant side effect to the cardiac system is caused by the anthracyclines, which are cardiotoxic. They cause direct damage to the myocardium resulting in left ventricular hypertrophy and clinical cardiomyopathy. Complications can include congestive heart failure, dysrhythmias, and ischemic changes. In the past patients were dose limited by this side effect; however, with the addition of the cardioprotective drug dexrazoxane, patients can receive higher doses of the anthracyclines without increasing damage to the heart. Besides the anthracyclines (e.g., daunorubicin, doxorubicin) other chemotherapeutic drugs that cause cardiac changes include mitoxantrone, cyclophosphamide, and paclitaxel (McCoy-Adabody & Borger, 1996; Wilkes et al., 1997).

Pulmonary. Pulmonary complications include pneumonitis, fibrosis, and noncardiogenic pulmonary edema. The most common of these toxicities is pneumonitis and the subsequent development of fibrosis. These side effects can be acute or develop over several weeks after chemotherapy administration. Those most at risk for pulmonary complications include concomitant or previous chest radiation, older age, cumulative drug dosage, vital organ function, and preexisting lung disease. Drugs associated with pulmonary side effects include bleomycin, carmustine, and methotrexate (McCoy-Adabody & Borger, 1996; Wilkes et al., 1997).

Another potential complication, bleomycin pulmonary toxicity is unique because it causes permanent structural changes in the alveoli. Consequently, when the cells that line the alveoli encounter oxygen, they secrete substances that the immune system perceives as foreign. This precipitates a rejection response. Therefore, once a patient has received bleomycin, he or she should be given only low concentrations of oxygen (30–40%) during anesthesia (McCoy-Adabody & Borger, 1996).

Gastrointestinal. Because its cells are rapidly dividing, the GI tract is one of the three main body systems that most often manifests chemotherapeutic side effects. The five main insults are nausea and vomiting; constipation; diarrhea; mucositis and stomatitis; and anorexia.

Many chemotherapeutic drugs cause nausea and vomiting; however, only a limited few have a high emetogenic potential. Table 26–15 lists the chemotherapy drugs associated with a very high, high, and moderate emetogenic potential.

Other potential GI side effects of chemotherapy are constipation and diarrhea. The vinca alkaloids (e.g., vincristine, vinblastine) are most often the chemotherapy drugs associated with constipation. The chemotherapy drugs associated with diarrhea include 5-fluorouracil, methotrexate, dactinomycin, doxorubicin, daunorubicin, docetaxel, leucovorin (a vitamin in the folate group), and streptozocin (Anastasia & Blevins, 1997; Bisanz, 1997).

With chemotherapy treatment, mucositis can exist throughout the GI tract, from the mouth to the anus. In addition to being very painful, mucositis is a great threat to the patient with cancer because it predisposes him or her to anorexia. Mucositis of the GI tract is caused by bleomycin, docetaxel, 5-fluorouracil, and doxorubicin (Anastasia & Blevins, 1997).

All of the aforementioned GI disturbances can lead to anorexia. In addition, anorexia may also be caused from an altered sense of taste associated with the metal-based drugs. The chemotherapy drugs associated with anorexia include cisplatin, dactinomycin, and doxorubicin (Wilkes et al., 1997).

Renal. Renal damage from chemotherapeutic drugs includes altered kidney filtration and hemorrhagic cystitis. Altered kidney filtration function may result in azotemia, increased blood urea nitrogen, increased creatinine, decreased creatinine clearance, and electrolyte imbalances. Cisplatin, methotrexate, and streptozocin cause the most significant nephrotoxic damage (McCoy-Adabody & Borger, 1996).

Two particular chemotherapeutic drugs—cyclophosphamide and ifosfamide—are associated with hemorrhagic cystitis. Hemorrhagic cystitis is an irritation of the bladder that causes hematuria. Therefore, when cyclophosphomide and ifosfamide are given intravenously, they are administered concomitantly with a bladder protectant, such as mesna, to prevent hemorrhagic cystitis.

TABLE 26–15. Chemotherapeutic Drugs with Very High, High, and Moderate Emetogenic Potential

Very High (>90%)	High (60–90%)	Moderate (30–60%)
Cisplatin	Carmustine	Carboplatin
Dacarbazine	Cyclophosphamide	Daunorubicin
Mechlorethamine	Dactinomycin	Doxorubicin
Streptozocin	Lomustine	5-Fluorouracil
	Plicamycin	Ifosfamide
	Procarbazine	L-Asparaginase
		Mitomycin-C
		Mitoxantrone

Compiled from Goodman (1997), Wilkes, Ingwersen, & Burke (1997).

Hematologic. Because its cells are rapidly dividing, bone marrow is another one of the three main areas that most often manifests chemotherapeutic side effects. Bone marrow depression is often an expected hematologic side effect of most chemotherapeutic drugs. Bone marrow depression includes neutrapenia, anemia, and thrombocytopenia and is collectively termed myelosuppression.

Neutrapenia is low white blood cell count. When the white blood cell count reaches its lowest point (the nadir) is when the patient is at the greatest risk for infection. The length of time before a patient reaches his or her nadir is dependent on the specific drugs the patient has received and his or her own individual response to the drugs. However, on average, most chemotherapeutic drugs nadir at 7 to 10 days after the beginning of treatment (Anastasia & Blevins, 1997).

An important indicator of infection is fever. Therefore, most oncology centers have established guidelines for when a patient should report a temperature elevation, commonly any reading 100.5°F or above. Obtaining a complete blood count with differential is necessary to confirm suspected neutrapenia. A patient with an absolute neutrophil count less than 500/mm^3 is most often considered neutropenic (Anastasia & Blevins, 1997; Brandt, 1990).

Like neutrapenia, anemia can be confirmed by obtaining a complete blood count. The most effective drug intervention to combat anemia is the colony stimulating factor erythropoietin. Anemia is further discussed in Chapter 46.

Thrombocytopenia can be confirmed through obtaining a platelet count, with normal considered to be 150,000 to 300,000. Risk for hemorrhage exists at under 50,000, with severe risk at under 20,000.

The chemotherapeutic drugs associated with severe and dose-limiting myelosuppression include busulfan, dacarbazine, doxorubicin, carmustine, lomustine, mechlorethamine, mitomycin C, and vinblastine (Haeuber & Spross, 1991; Wilkes et al., 1997).

Fortunately, once identified, myelosuppression can usually be reversed through the use of the previously mentioned CSFs. Thus, with the development of CSFs the impact of myelosuppression on the patient's course of therapy has been greatly reduced.

Immunologic. The potential for a hypersensitivity reaction to chemotherapy is relatively common. However, premedication with steroids, antihistamines, and nonsteroidal antiinflammatory medications are standard therapy for those drugs that have been associated with hypersensitivity. Hypersensitivity reactions range from flushing, pruritis, rash, dyspnea, and hypotension to anaphylactic reactions with severe bronchospasm, severe hypotension, diffuse urticaria, and angioedema. The chemotherapeutic drugs associated with hypersensitivity reactions include bleomycin (lymphoma patients), cisplatin, docetaxel, L-asparaginase, paclitaxel, and teniposide (McCoy-Adabody & Borger, 1996; Wilkes et al., 1997).

Skin, Nails, and Hair. Changes in the skin from chemotherapy include vein streaking, keratosis, hyperpigmentation, peeling, and extravasation. Other than extravasation, most are expected and resolve over time: vein streaking and hyperpigmentation usually fade and peeling is temporary. The drugs associated with skin changes include bleomycin, cyclophasphamide, dactinomycin, daunorubicin, docetaxel, and doxorubicin (Wilkes et al., 1997).

Nail changes can include hypopigmentation or hyperpigmentation and onycholysis. These changes are not usually permanent and regrowth with normal color restoration is typical. Chemotherapeutic agents associated with nail changes include daunorubicin, docetaxel, and 5-flourouracil (Wilkes et al., 1997).

Extravasation is a serious side effect that may be caused by inadvertent instillation of vesicant chemotherapeutic drugs into the tissues instead of the vein. Because vesicant drugs are toxic to subcutaneous tissue, the resulting damage of extravasations ranges from erythema, edema, skin discoloration, and blistering to ulceration, soft tissue necrosis, and tendon necrosis. Permanent damage to the limb resulting in disfigurement and loss of function is a possible outcome (Boyle & Engelking, 1995).

While some initial damage from an extravasation is often readily apparent, extravasations can progressively worsen over a period of days. Ulceration is thought to be an insidious development; damage can begin internally and extend to the skin surface (Boyle & Engelking, 1995; Davis, DeSantis, & Klemm, 1995).

Another category of chemotherapeutic drugs similar to vesicants is irritants. Irritants are drugs that are able to produce pain at the site of injection and along the vein when instilled intravenously. However, these drugs generally do not cause tissue necrosis (Boyle & Engelking, 1995).

While the majority of chemotherapeutic drugs are neither vesicants nor irritants, it is imperative that clinicians have knowledge of these properties and how to administer these types of drugs beforehand. Table 26–16 lists vesicant and irritant chemotherapeutic drugs.

Because its cells are rapidly dividing, hair is the third of the three main areas most often effected by chemotherapy. Alopecia occurs with the following drugs: bleomycin, cyclophosphamide, dacarbazine, dactinomycin, daunorubicin, docetaxel, doxorubicin, mitomycin, and paclitaxel. Hair loss is not usually permanent; regrowth usually begins a few months after treatment when the drug is finished (Wilkes et al., 1997). Table 26–17 summarizes common organ system toxicities of antineoplastics.

Hormonal Therapy. Two side effects common to all hormonal drugs used in cancer treatment are fluid retention and sexual changes (Greifzu, 1996). Side effects are also dependent on the type of cancer being treated and the gender of the patient.

TABLE 26–16. Chemotherapeutic Vesicants and Irritants

Vesicants	Irritants
Dactinomycin	Bleomycin
Daunorubicin	Carmustine
Doxorubicin	Cisplatin
Mechlorethamine	Dacarbazine
Mithramycin	Etoposide
Mitomycin C	5-Fluorouracil
Vinblastine	Mitoxantrone
Vincristine	Paclitaxel
	Plicamycin
	Streptozocin
	Teniposide

Data from Boyle & Engelking (1995), Wilkes, Ingwersen, & Burke (1997).

The side effects from steroids are well documented and include increased gastric hydrochloric acid secretion, decreased secretion of gastric mucus, sodium and water retention, and emotional lability. Long-term steroid use additionally can cause suppression of the normal renal function, Cushingoid state, glaucoma, and the development of cataracts (Wilkes et al., 1997).

Females who take androgens for more than 3 months often experience masculinization. Signs and symptoms of masculinization include increased libido, excessive body hair growth, clitoral hypertrophy, and deeping of voice. Men on androgens may experience priapism and reduced ejaculatory volume. Additional side effects include sodium and water retention. Antiandrogens may cause gynecomastia, hot flashes, and breast tenderness (Wilkes et al., 1997).

TABLE 26–17. Common Organ System Toxicities of Antineoplastics*

Organ System	Toxicity	Class of Agent					
		AA	PA	A	AM	M	H
Gastrointestinal (Coons, Leventhal, Love, & Larson, 1987; Conrad, 1986; Dorr & Fritz, 1980; Mitchell & Schein, 1982)	Nausea, vomiting (Duigon, 1986; Needleman, 1987; Sallan & Cronin, 1985; See-Lasley & Ignoffo; 1981)	1–4	1–2	3	2	3–4	1
	Diarrhea	1	1	1	2–3	1	1
	Constipation	1	2	1	1	1	1
	Mucositis	1–2	1	2	3–4	1	1
Hepatotoxicity	↑ LFT results	1	1	1	2	1	1
	Cholestatic jaundice	1	1	2	2	1	1
	Hepatitis	1	1	1	2	1	1
Bone marrow (Grant Medical Center, 1987; Hoagland, 1982)	Leukopenia	4	4	4	4	1–4	1
	Thrombocytopenia	2–3	1–4	2–3	2	1–4	1
Cutaneous (Doll & Weiss, 1985; Duagin, 1982; Lovejoy, 1979; Parker, 1987; Weiss, 1982)	Rash	1	1	2–3	2–3	2–3	1
	Nail changes	1	1	1–2	2	1	1
	Hyperpigmentation	1	1	1–2	1–3	1	1
	Radiation recall	1	1	2	2	1	1
	Alopecia (Dean, Salmon, & Griffith, 1979; O'Brian, Zelson, Schwartz, & Pearson, 1970; Parker, 1987; Seipp, 1985)	1–4	1	1–4	1–4	1	1
Pulmonary (Buzdar et al., 1980; Ginsberg & Comis, 1982; Wickham, 1986)	Allergic pneumonitis	1	1	1	2	2	1
	Pulmonary fibrosis	1–2	1	1–2	1	1	1
Genitourinary (Lydon, 1986; Schilsky, 1982; Verway et al., 1984)	Kidney (Schilsky, 1982)	2–4	1	1	2	1	1
	Bladder	1	1	1	1	1	1
Cardiac (Kaszyk, 1986; Myers et al., 1983; Unverferth et al., 1981; Von Hoff, Rosenczweiz & Piccart, 1982)	Myocardial damage	1	1	2	1	1	1
	Electrocardiographic changes	1	1	2	1	1	1
Neurologic (Conrad, 1986; Holden & Felde, 1987; Kaplan & Wiernik, 1982; Lopez & Agrwal, 1984)	Central nervous system	1	1	1	2	2	1
	Peripheral nerves	1	2	1	2	1	1
Reproductive (Chapman, 1982; Grant Medical Center, 1987)	Gondal function	2–3	?	1–3	?	1–2	1–4

* Based on reported incidence and the likelihood of occurrence in general medical oncology practice.
↑, increased; LFT, liver function test; AA, alkylating agents; PA, plant alkaloids; A, antibiotics; AM, antimetabolites; M, miscellaneous; H, hormones.
1, Rare; incidence range, 0–19%.
2, Occasional; incidence range, 20–49%.
3, Common; incidence range, 50–75%.
4, Frequent; incidence range, greater than 75%.
?, Requires further definition.
When ranges are given, there is marked variability among drugs, doses, and routes.
Reprinted with permission from Guy (1991).

The use of estrogens in the postmenopausal female can lead to breast engorgement and tenderness. Additionally, women may experience uterine prolapse and urinary incontinence. Males taking estrogens usually undergo voice change, gynecomastia, loss of libido, and impotence during therapy. These side effects disappear after drug cessation (Wilkes et al., 1997).

One of the most commonly used antiestrogen is the drug tamoxifen. For females, tamoxifen may worsen or induce menopause with side effects including menstrual irregularities, hot flashes, weight gain, and vaginal dryness. Other possible side effects include nausea, vomiting and vaginal discharge. Patients on tamoxifen with skin or bone metastases have also developed a flare reaction characterized by erythema, pruritis, bone pain, hypercalcemia, and transient tumor growth. Even though tamoxifen is an antiestrogen, estrogen-like properties have been noted with effects on bone, endometrium, and serum lipid levels (Wasaff, 1997; Wilkes et al., 1997).

Progestins can cause hypertension, fluid retention, weight gain, and thromboembolisms. Aromatase inhibitors can cause hot flashes, vaginal dryness, asthenia, nausea, anorexia, and headache (Wasaff, 1997).

Immunotherapy. As expected, the side effects of BRMs vary according to the specific drug, dosage, and length of treatment; however, the most common side effect of the BRMs is a flu-like reaction. The patient may experience fever, malaise, fatigue, headache, chills, rigors, rash, arthralgias, myalgias, nausea, vomiting, and anorexia. Additionally, the patient may have erythema at the injection site. In most cases these side effects lessen as therapy continues and disappear within a month after the drug is discontinued (Caliendo, Joyce, & Altmiller, 1993; McCoy-Adabody & Borger, 1996; Wilkes et al., 1997).

Bone Marrow Transplant. Because bone marrow cells take 12 to 28 days before beginning engraftment, a bone marrow recipient is closely monitored for several weeks. Additionally, a BMT recipient's immune system does not fully recover before 6 months and may take up to 2 years, so follow-up care is a long-term process. The patient may manifest side effects all during this time period. During the infusion phase of BMT, the patient may experience any of the following side effects: fever, chills, shortness of breath, chest pain, bradycardia or tachycardia, hypotension or hypertension, nausea and vomiting, abdominal pain, rash, facial flushing, and anxiety (Poliquin, 1997; Wujcik, 1997).

For 24 to 48 hours after reinfusion, the recipient's urine may be pink or blood tinged. Other acute side effects that may be experienced include bleeding, infection, nausea and vomiting, acute renal failure, hemorrhagic cystitis, veno–occlusive disease, radiation recall, and delayed or failed engraftment (Poliquin, 1997).

BMT can cause long-term side effects as well. Potential long-term side effects include pulmonary damage, endocrine dysfunction, secondary malignancy, infection, and neurotoxicity (Poliquin, 1997).

A potential side effect of BMT and PRBC transplantation is graft versus host disease (GVHD). GVHD may be acute or chronic and is one of the most serious side effects of transplantations. GVHD occurs when the recipient's body is attacked by the T lymphocytes from the donor's marrow. Acute GVHD develops within 3 months and primarily affects the skin, liver, and gastrointestinal system. Rash, jaundice, liver disease, and diarrhea characterize acute GVHD. Chronic GVHD may develop several months or up to 3 years after transplantation and it mainly affects the skin, eyes, gastrointestinal tract, oral mucosa, vaginal mucosa, sinuses, and serosal surfaces. Chronic GVHD results in fibrosis of the cutaneous and subcutaneous tissues, photosensitivity, dry mucus membranes with atrophy and secretory gland destruction possible, hair loss, weight loss, and frequent infections. Because GVHD may be serious enough to cause death, most BMT patients receive immunosuppressive drug therapy after reinfusion (Cook, 1996; DeMeyer, Fletcher, & Buchsel, 1997).

During apheresis of PBSC transplantation, patients may experience hypocalcemia (due to the anticoagulant—sodium citrate—mixed with the blood) and hypovolemia. Additional risks, though rare, include allergic reaction, air embolism, syncope, and cardiac arrest. During and immediately after marrow return, potential side effects include erythema, headache, dyspnea, chest tightness, nausea, vomiting, tachycardia, hypertension, arrythmias, hematuria, hemaglobinuria, increased serum bilirubin, and increased serum creatinine. Fortunately, these side effects are usually short term and spontaneously subside within 24 hours. Like BMT, PBSC transplantation may result in delayed or failed engraftment (Hooper & Santas, 1993; Shivnan et al., 1996; Walker, Roethke, & Martin, 1994).

Multimodal Therapy

While each modality can be used as the sole treatment for a patient, most cancers are treated with a combination of modalities, termed multimodal therapy. The goals of multimodal therapy include the desire to improve therapeutic outcomes through improving response rates, inducing remissions and creating longer remission periods, and reducing toxicities (Scofield, Liebman, & Popkin, 1991).

Multimodal therapy usually consists of one primary treatment method and either one or more other treatment methods. The term given to therapy that is used in addition to the primary method of treatment is adjuvant therapy. Adjuvant therapy is given to enhance the body's overall response to therapy. Studies have demonstrated definite improvement in survival rates through the use of adjuvant therapy (Scofield et al., 1991). Traditionally, adjuvant therapy was given after the primary treatment; however, it can also be given prior to the primary treatment modality and is thus termed neoadjuvant.

As with all therapy, the risks of toxicities and side effects must be weighed against the potential outcomes of treatment. The use of multimodal therapy carries with it the risk of increased toxicity and the potential for more side effects due to the combination of therapies (Scofield et al., 1991).

▶ EMERGENCIES

Many cancer patients are at risk for oncologic emergencies. Sometimes a patient's first indication of cancer may be a medical emergency. Additionally, a patient who has been successfully free from cancer for a time period may suddenly experience an oncologic emergency as the first sign of recurrence (Miaskowski, 1991).

Emergencies commonly seen in patients with cancer can be categorized into three areas: obstructive, metabolic, and infiltrative. The obstructive emergencies include superior vena cava syndrome and intestinal obstruction. The metabolic emergencies are syndrome of inappropriate antidiuretic hormone secretion (SIADH), hypercalcemia, septic shock, disseminated intravascular coagulation (DIC), and tumor lysis syndrome. Cardiac tamponade, spinal cord compression, and carotid artery rupture are all considered infiltrative emergencies (Miaskowski, 1991). With the exception of tumor lysis syndrome, all these conditions can also occur in patients who do not have cancer; therefore, only tumor lysis syndrome is discussed.

Tumor lysis syndrome is a metabolic emergency most often associated with patients who have a large tumor cell burden that is rapidly proliferating (e.g., acute leukemia, non-Hodgkin's lymphoma). Cells undergoing rapid proliferation are very sensitive to cytotoxic therapy and, thus, tumor lysis syndrome most often occurs after cytotoxic therapy. Such therapy includes corticosteroids, chemotherapy, BRMs, and radiation (Anderson & Holmes, 1993; Robison, 1997).

This lysing of numerous cells causes intracellular contents to be released into extracellular fluid. If extracellular circulation cannot properly adjust to this influx, the patient may develop hyperurecemia, hyperphosphatemia, hyperkalemia, hypocalcemia, and metabolic acidosis. These biochemical alterations can lead to acute renal failure or cardiac dysrhythmias and, if unchecked, eventually death (Anderson & Holmes, 1993; Robison, 1997).

Patients usually manifest signs and symptoms of tumor lysis syndrome within 24 to 48 hours after initiating chemotherapy administration. The resolution may take up to 7 days posttreatment; however, the initial crisis must be managed immediately (Anderson & Holmes, 1993).

▶ PSYCHOSOCIAL CONCERNS

Like most diseases, cancer affects the whole person. Beyond insults to the physical body, patients can experience mental, emotional, and spiritual crises. And, in addition to patients' concerns, the ACNP should be aware that cancer also affects patients' families and significant others as well. Therefore, support must be directed to both patients and their significant others. Psychosocial concerns of patients with cancer and their significant others are numerous and beyond the scope of this chapter. Chapter 54 provides more detailed information about the management of psychosocial concerns.

▶ RESOURCES

Fortunately, there are many resources for patients with cancer and their families. Resources can be found nationwide as well as within communities. Many regions have chapters of national organizations within or nearby the area. The following is a partial list of national resources obtained from *Oncology Nursing Forum* (1997).

1. The address for the national home office of the

   American Cancer Society, Inc. (ACS) is
   1599 Clifton Road, NE
   Atlanta, GA 30329-4251
   404-329-7623 (patient services)
   800-ACS-2345 (cancer information)

   There are, however, chartered divisions for each state, the District of Columbia, and Puerto Rico with their own addresses. Additionally, there are many local chapters in each state.

   Some of the programs and services offered by the ACS include Reach to Recovery, Road to Recovery, Look Good . . . Feel Better, I Can Cope, Resource Information & Guidance, Man to Man, International Association of Laryngectomees, Ostomy Rehabilitation Program, housing, and home-care equipment.

2. The **Cancer Conquerors Foundation,** founded by a lung cancer survivor, is committed to teaching patients and families how to cope with cancer through education and support. Its telephone number is 800-238-6479.

3. The **Cancer Information Service (CIS)** is a program of the National Cancer Institute that gives accurate, personalized answers to cancer-related questions from patients, their families, health-care professionals, and the general public.

   Cancer Information Service (CIS)
   National Cancer Institute
   31 Center Drive MSC 2580
   Building 31, Room 10A16
   Bethesda, MD 20892-2580
   800-4-CANCER

4. The **Candlelighters Childhood Cancer Foundation** is an international organization that also has local chapters. The foundation serves parents who have or have had children with cancer, survivors of childhood cancer, and professionals. The foundation provides information, resource referrals, and support groups.

   Candlelighters Childhood Cancer Foundation
   7910 Woodmont Avenue, Suite 460
   Bethesda, MD 20814-3015
   800-366-CCCF

5. The **Gynecologic Cancer Foundation** aims to educate both the medical community and the general public about current trends and techniques in gynecologic cancers. The foundation assists in education, research efforts, and the reporting of findings related to gynecologic cancer.

   Gynecologic Cancer Foundation
   401 North Michigan Avenue
   Chicago, IL 60611
   312-644-6610

6. The **Leukemia Society of America, Inc.** has 57 local chapters that provide services to patients and families with leukemia and its related diseases (lymphoma and multiple myeloma). Services provided include support groups, educational materials, and financial assistance. The home office is

   Leukemia Society of America, Inc.
   600 Third Avenue
   New York, NY 10016
   800-955-4LSA

7. The **National Black Leadership Initiative on Cancer (NBLIC)** is a program of the National Cancer Institute aimed at reducing cancer incidence and mortality rates and increasing survival rates among black Americans. The NBLIC is a community-based program.

   National Black Leadership Initiative on Cancer (NBLIC)
   6130 Executive Boulevard (EPN-240)
   Bethesda, MD 20892
   301-496-8589

8. The **National Brain Tumor Foundation (NBTF)** provides information and resources to patients with brain tumors and their families. In addition to conferences, the foundation offers assistance through a one-on-one telephone support line.

   National Brain Tumor Foundation (NBTF)
   785 Market Street, Suite 1600
   San Francisco, CA 94130
   800-934-CURE

9. The focus of the **National Breast Cancer Coalition** is to end breast cancer through action and advocacy.

   National Breast Cancer Coalition
   1707 L Street NW, Suite 1060
   Washington, DC 20036
   202-296-7477

10. The **National Coalition for Cancer Survivorship (NCCS)** represents cancer survivors from all types of cancers and provides assistance through linking them with appropriate services and supports.

    National Coalition for Cancer Survivorship (NCCS)
    1010 Wayne Avenue, Suite 505
    Silver Spring, MD 20910
    301-650-8868

11. **En Accion: National Hispanic Leadership Initiative on Cancer** aims to develop programs to reduce cancer risk factors for all Hispanic/Latino people.

    National Hispanic Leadership Initiative on Cancer
    En Accion Coordinating Center
    South Texas Health Research Center
    The University of Texas Health Sciences Center at San Antonio
    7703 Floyd Curl Drive
    San Antonio, TX 78284-7791
    210-614-4496

12. The **National Hospice Organization (NHO)** is a nonprofit organization that supports the needs of people who are terminally ill through the promotion of hospice care. The organization provides education, training, and technical assistance to terminally ill people and their families.

    National Hospice Organization (NHO)
    1901 North Moore Street, Suite 901
    Arlington, VA 22209
    800-658-8898 (Hospice Helpline)

13. The **Oncology Nursing Society (ONS)** is a professional nursing organization that provides support to oncology nurses. The aim of the society is to promote the highest professional standards of oncology nursing.

    Oncology Nursing Society (ONS)
    501 Holiday Drive
    Pittsburgh, PA 15220-2749
    412-921-7373

14. The **Physician Data Query (PDQ)**, updated monthly, provides access to the most current can-

cer treatment information available. Information is beneficial for clinicians and can also be useful for patient teaching.

Physician Data Query (PDQ)
National Cancer Institute's (NCI) Computerized Database
9030 Old Georgetown Road
Bethesda, MD 20814-1519
800-345-3300 (health-care professionals)
800-4-CANCER (patients)

15. The **Skin Cancer Foundation** supports research and provides patient education materials related to skin cancer.

The Skin Cancer Foundation
245 Fifth Avenue, Suite 2402
New York, NY 10016
212-725-5176

16. **The Wellness Community** has various national locations that provide free psychosocial and educational support.

The Wellness Community
2716 Ocean Park Boulevard, Suite 1040
Santa Monica, CA 90405
310-314-2555

Many people within the health-care system today are patients with cancer. Most of these patients have experienced, or are experiencing, treatment for their cancer. While this treatment is usually done at specialized treatment centers under the direction of clinicians with specific training in oncology, many ACNPs still have contact with a large percentage of patients with cancer. Because these patients have special needs, it is imperative that ACNPs remain cognizant of the main issues regarding their care.

REFERENCES

Alexander, J. (1994). Diagnosis and staging. In S. E. Otto (Ed.), *Oncology nursing* (2nd ed.). (pp. 47–56). St. Louis: Mosby.

American Cancer Society, Inc. (1997). *Cancer facts & figures—1997* (97–300M-No. 5008.97). Atlanta: ACS.

Anastasia, P. J. & Blevins, M. C. (1997). Outpatient chemotherapy: Telephone triage for symptom management. *Oncology Nursing Forum, 24 (Suppl),* 13–22.

Anderson, B. & Holmes, W. (1993). Altered mental status: An algorithm for assessment of delirium in the cancer patient. *Current Issues in Cancer Nursing Practices Updates, 2* (5), 1–10.

Bisanz, A. (1997). Managing bowel elimination problems in patients with cancer. *Oncology Nursing Forum, 24,* 679–686.

Blesch, K. S., Paice, J. A., Wickham, R., Harte, N., Schnoor, D. K., Purl, S., Rehwalt, M., Kopp, P. L., Manson, S., Coveny, S. B., McHale, M., & Cahill, M. (1991). Correlates of fatigue in people with breast or lung cancer. *Oncology Nursing Forum, 18,* 81–87.

Boyle, D. M. & Engelking, C. (1995). Vesicant extravasation: Myths and realities. *Oncology Nursing Forum, 22,* 57–67.

Brandt, B. (1990). Nursing protocol for the patient with neutrapenia. *Oncology Nursing Forum, 17 (Suppl),* 9–15.

Brock, D., Fox, S., Gosling, G., Haney, L., Kneebone, P., Nagy, C., & Qualtza, B. (1993). Testicular cancer. *Seminars in Oncology Nursing, 9,* 224–236.

Bullock, B. L. (1992). Benign and malignant neoplasia. In B. L. Bullock & P. P. Rosendahl (Eds.), *Pathophysiology: Adaptations and alterations in function.* (3rd ed.). (pp. 349–366). Philadelphia: J. B. Lippincott.

Bullock, B. L. (1996). Neoplasia. In B. L. Bullock (Ed.) *Pathophysiology: Adaptations and alterations in function.* (4th ed.). (pp. 44–63). Philadelphia: J. B. Lippincott.

Cabanillas, F., Maloney, D., Link, B., & Jonas, C. (1998, January). Monoclonal antibody therapy in lymphoma: Introduction to Rituxan. Teleconference presented by Medical Programs Incorporated.

Caliendo, G., Joyce, D., & Altmiller, M. C. (1993). Nursing guidelines and discharge planning for patients receiving recombinant Interleukin-2. *Seminars in Oncology Nursing, 9 (Suppl 1),* 25–31.

Calzone, K. A. (1997). Genetic predisposition testing: Clinical implications for oncology nursing. *Oncology Nursing Forum, 24,* 712–718.

Canty, L. (1997). Breast cancer risk: Protective effects of an early first full-term pregnancy versus increased risk of induced abortion. *Oncology Nursing Forum, 24,* 1025–1031.

Cook, A. R. (Ed.) (1996). *The New Cancer Sourcebook.* Detroit: Omnigraphics, Inc.

Davis, M. E., DeSantis, D., & Klemm, K. (1995). A flow sheet for follow-up after chemotherapy extravasation. *Oncology Nursing Forum, 22,* 979–981.

DeMeyer, E. S., Fletcher, M. A., & Buchsel, P. C. (1997). Management of dermatologic complications of chronic graft versus host disease: A case study. *Clinical Journal of Oncology Nursing, 1,* 95–104.

Ehlke, G. (1991). Gastrointestinal cancers. In S. B. Baird, R. McCorkle, & M. Grant (Eds.), *Cancer nursing: A comprehensive textbook* (pp. 485–501). Philadelphia: W. B. Saunders.

Farrell, M. M. (1996). Biotherapy and the oncology nurse. *Seminars in Oncology Nursing, 12,* 82–88.

Frank-Stromborg, M. (1991). Evaluating cancer risk. In S. B. Baird, R. McCorkle, & M. Grant (Eds.), *Cancer nursing: A comprehensive textbook* (pp. 155–189). Philadelphia: W. B. Saunders.

Gallucci, B. B. (1991). Cancer biology: Molecular and cellular aspects. In S. B. Baird, R. McCorkle, & M. Grant (Eds.), *Cancer nursing: A comprehensive textbook* (pp. 115–129). Philadelphia: W. B. Saunders.

Goodman, M. (1997). Risk factors and antiemetic management of chemotherapy-induced nausea and vomiting. *Oncology Nursing Forum, 24* (7) (Suppl), 20–32.

Greifzu, S. (1996). Chemo quick guide hormonal agents. *RN, 59* (5), 41–42.

Grillo-Lopez, A. J. & Fyfe, G. (1997). Rituxan. G71416-RO.

Gullatte, M. M. (1994). Prevention, screening, and detection. In S. E. Otto (Ed.), *Oncology nursing* (2nd ed.). (pp. 29–46). St. Louis: Mosby.

Guy, J. L. (1991). Medical oncology—The agents. In S. B. Baird, R. McCorkle, & M. Grant (Eds.), *Cancer nursing: A comprehensive textbook* (pp. 266–290). Philadelphia: W. B. Saunders.

Haeuber, D. & Spross, J. A. (1991). Alterations in protective mechanisms: Hematopoiesis and bone marrow depression. In S. B. Baird, R. McCorkle, & M. Grant (Eds.), *Cancer nursing: A comprehensive textbook* (pp. 759–781). Philadelphia: W. B. Saunders.

Havard, C. P. & Topping, A. E. (1991). Surgical oncology. In S. B. Baird, R. McCorkle, & M. Grant (Eds.), *Cancer nursing: A comprehensive textbook* (pp. 235–245). Philadelphia: W. B. Saunders.

Higgins, C. (1996). Use of tumour markers in cancer diagnosis and treatment. *Nursing Times, 92* (16), 36–37.

Hilderley, L. J. & Dow, K. H. (1991). Radiation oncology. In S. B. Baird, R. McCorkle, & M. Grant (Eds.), *Cancer nursing: A comprehensive textbook* (pp. 246–265). Philadelphia: W. B. Saunders.

Hobbie, W. (1997, October). *PACONS News.* Available from Philadelphia Area Chapter Oncology Nursing Society, 44 Dawn Road, Levittown, PA 19056.

Hooper, P. J. & Santas, E. J. (1993). Peripheral blood stem cell transplantation. *Oncology Nursing Forum, 20,* 1215–1221.

Hubbard, S. M. & Liotta, L. A. (1991). The biology of metastases. In S. B. Baird, R. McCorkle, & M. Grant (Eds.), *Cancer nursing: A comprehensive textbook* (pp. 130–142). Philadelphia: W. B. Saunders.

Irvine, D., Vincent, L., Graydon, J. E., Bubela, N., & Thompson, L. (1994). The prevalence and correlates of fatigue in patients receiving treatment with chemotherapy and radiotherapy: A comparison with the fatigue experienced by healthy individuals. *Cancer Nursing, 17,* 367–378.

Iwamoto, R. (1994). Radiation therapy. In S. E. Otto (Ed.), *Oncology nursing* (2nd ed.). (pp. 467–492). St. Louis: Mosby.

Karius, D. & Marriott, M. A. (1997). Immunologic advances in monoclonal antibody therapy: Implications for oncology nursing. *Oncology Nursing Forum, 24,* 483–504.

Knobf, M. T. (1991). Breast cancer. In S. B. Baird, R. McCorkle, & M. Grant (Eds.), *Cancer nursing: A comprehensive textbook* (pp. 425–451). Philadelphia: W. B. Saunders.

Landis, S. H., Murray, T., Bolden, S., & Wingo, P. A. (1998). Cancer statistics, 1998. *CA A Cancer Journal for Clinicians, 48,* 6–29.

Lind, J. & Irwin, R. J. (1991). Genitourinary cancers. In S. B. Baird, R. McCorkle, & M. Grant (Eds.), *Cancer nursing: A comprehensive textbook* (pp. 466–484). Philadelphia: W. B. Saunders.

Lindsey, A. M. (1991). Lung cancer. In S. B. Baird, R. McCorkle, & M. Grant (Eds.), *Cancer nursing: A comprehensive textbook* (pp. 452–465). Philadelphia: W. B. Saunders.

Mahon, S. M., Casperson, D. S., Yackzan, S., Goodner, S., Hasse, B., Hawkins, J., Parham, J., Rimkus, C., Schlomer, M., & Witcher, V. (1994). Safe handling practices of cytotoxic drugs: The results of a chapter survey. *Oncology Nursing Forum, 22,* 1157–1165.

Martin, L. K. & Braly, G. (1991). Gynecologic cancers. In S. B. Baird, R. McCorkle, & M. Grant (Eds.), *Cancer nursing: A comprehensive textbook* (pp. 502–535). Philadelphia: W. B. Saunders.

McCoy-Adabody, A. M. & Borger, D. L. (1996). Selected critical care complications of cancer therapy. *AACN Clinical Issues, 7,* 26–36.

Meili, L. (1994). Epidemiology. In S. E. Otto (Ed.), *Oncology nursing* (2nd ed.). (pp. 20–28). St. Louis: Mosby.

Mettlin, C. & Mirand, A. L. (1991). The causes of cancer. In S. B. Baird, R. McCorkle, & M. Grant (Eds.), *Cancer nursing: A comprehensive textbook* (pp. 104–114). Philadelphia: W. B. Saunders.

Miaskowski, C. (1991). Oncologic emergencies. In S. B. Baird, R. McCorkle, & M. Grant (Eds.), *Cancer nursing: A comprehensive textbook* (pp. 885–893). Philadelphia: W. B. Saunders.

Moore, J. G. & Szekley, S. (1994). Bone marrow transplantation. In S. E. Otto (Ed.), *Oncology Nursing* (2nd ed.). (pp. 561–584). St. Louis: Mosby.

Nail, L. M., Jones, L. S., Greene, D., Schipper, D. L., & Jensen, R. (1991). Use and perceived efficacy of self-care activities in patients receiving chemotherapy. *Oncology Nursing Forum, 18,* 883–887.

Olsen, S. J. & Frank-Stromborg, M. (1991). Cancer screening and early detection. In S. B. Baird, R. McCorkle, & M. Grant (Eds.), *Cancer nursing: A comprehensive textbook* (pp. 190–218). Philadelphia: W. B. Saunders.

Oncology Nursing Society. (1997). Cancer resources in the United States. *Oncology Nursing Forum, 24,* 1607–1620.

Otto, S. E. (1997). *Oncology Nursing.* (3rd ed.). St Louis: Mosby.

Pfeifer, K. A. (1994a). Pathophysiology. In S. E. Otto (Ed.), *Oncology nursing* (2nd ed.). (pp. 3–19). St. Louis: Mosby.

Pfeifer, K. A. (1994b). Surgery. In S. E. Otto (Ed.), *Oncology nursing* (2nd ed.). (pp. 443–466). St. Louis: Mosby.

Poliquin, C. M. (1997). Overview of bone marrow and peripheral blood stem cell transplantation. *Clinical Journal of Oncology Nursing, 1,* 11–17.

Ramshaw, B. J. (1997). Laparoscopic surgery for cancer patients. *CA A Cancer Journal for Clinicians, 47,* 327–350.

Robison, J. (1997). Tumor lysis syndrome. In C. C. Chernecky & B. J. Berger (Eds.), *Advanced and Critical Care Oncology Nursing* (pp. 637–659). Philadelphia: W. B. Saunders.

Schindler, L. W. (1991). *Understanding the immune system.* (NIH Publication No. 92-529). Washington, DC: U.S. Government Printing Office.

Schindler, L. W. (1992). *The immune system—How it works.* (NIH Publication No. 92-3229). Washington, DC: U.S. Government Printing Office.

Scofield, R. P., Liebman, M. C., & Popkin, J. D. (1991). Multimodal therapy. In S. B. Baird, R. McCorkle, & M. Grant (Eds.), *Cancer nursing: A comprehensive textbook* (pp. 344–354). Philadelphia: W. B. Saunders.

Shivnan, J., Shelton, B. K., & Onners, B. K. (1996). Bone marrow transplantation: Issues for critical care nurses. *AACN Clinical Issues, 7,* 95–108.

Simonato, L. & Saracci, R. (1983). Cancer: Occupational *Encyclopedia of occupational health and safety* (3rd rev. ed.). Geneva: International Labor Organisation.

Walker, F., Roethke, S. K., & Martin, G. (1994). An overview of the rationale, process, and nursing implications of peripheral blood stem cell transplantation. *Cancer Nursing, 17,* 141–148.

Walter-Coleman, S. (1996). Oncologic pharmacology: Selected topics for critical care nurses. *AACN Clinical Issues, 7,* 46–64.

Wasaff, B. (1997). Current status of hormonal treatments for metastatic breast cancer in postmenopausal women. *Oncology Nursing Forum, 24,* 1515–1520.

Wilkes, G. M., Ingwersen, K., & Burke, M. B. (1997). *1997–1998 Oncology nursing drug handbook.* Sudbury, MA: Jones and Bartlett.

Wilson, B. A., Shannon, M. T., & Stang, C. L. (1998). *Nurses Drug Guide.* Stamford, CT: Appleton & Lange.

Winningham, M. L., Nail, L. M., Burke, M. B., Brophy, L., Cimprich, B., Jones, L. S., Pickard-Holley, S., Rhodes, V., St. Pierre, B., Beck, S., Glass, E. C., Mock, V. L., Mooney, K. H., & Piper, B. (1994). Fatigue and the cancer experience: The state of the knowledge. *Oncology Nursing Forum, 21,* 23–36.

Wujcik, D. (1997). Autologous bone marrow and blood cell transplantations. In S. C. Groenwald, M. H. Frogge, M. Goodman, & C. H. Yarbro (Eds.), *Cancer nursing: Principles and practice* (pp. 507–526). Sudbury, MA: Jones and Bartlett.

27

Organ Donation and Transplantation

Verdi J. DiSesa

Solid organ transplantation has become effective therapy for end-stage failure of the heart, lungs, liver, kidneys, and pancreas. Small bowel transplantation, while still experimental, may one day join these other procedures in the therapy of patients with otherwise untreatable disease. The first successful transplantation of a solid organ from one human to another was accomplished in 1954 when Joseph Murray of the Peter Bent Brigham Hospital in Boston took a kidney from a healthy man and transplanted it into his twin brother who suffered from terminal uremia due to glomerulonephritis (Merrill, 1956). Since that time, of course, the sciences of immunology and surgical therapy have progressed to the extent that transplantation of a variety of organs between completely unrelated individuals can be accomplished successfully.

Over this period of time, the complexity of the logistics of organ transplantation has increased as well. Most organ donors are identified at hospitals distant from the hospital in which the recipient is cared for. In addition, the success of transplantation has so increased the demand for organs that a rational system for organ allocation has had to be devised. These realities have led to the establishment of a detailed national infra-structure to support the procurement and allocation of organs for transplantation.

This chapter examines several important aspects of solid organ transplantation as it is presently practiced in the United States. General comments about organ supply and demand, the coordination of organ procurement, and immunologic considerations in organ transplantation introduce more detailed discussions of these factors in heart, lung, liver, kidney, and pancreas transplantation. The goal is to provide useful information of a general nature, not to explore the minute complexities of the broad field of organ grafting.

▶ ORGAN DEMAND AND SUPPLY

The number of organ transplants done depends completely on the supply of usable donor organs (Council on Ethical and Judicial Affairs, AMA, 1994; Hauptman, 1997). The growth in success of organ transplantation as treatment for patients with otherwise untreatable disease has led to acceleration of the demand for organs that far outweighs the supply. For example, it is estimated that as many as 40,000 to 60,000 Americans annually could benefit from heart transplantation. However, in this country, only about 2500 are performed annually. Even the most optimistic estimates of the total theoretical number of available transplantable hearts—less than 10,000—could never meet this demand (Randall, 1991).

This section discusses the indications for transplantation, recipient evaluation and selection, and the development of the waiting list for organ recipients. The discussion also covers how the supply of organs for transplantation is determined and how organs for transplantation are allocated through the national network of organ procurement organizations that is coordinated by the United Network for Organ Sharing (UNOS). The discussion concentrates on procurement of organs from cadavers, usually individuals who are brain dead but with intact circulation (beating-heart cadavers). While living related transplantation is practiced in kidney transplantation, and reduced volume liver and lung transplants have been performed using living donors, all pancreas and heart transplants must rely on cadaver donors.

Demand

As noted, the demand for cadaver organs far exceeds the supply, and probably always will. Because transplantable organs are a scarce resource, relatively stringent criteria have been developed that guide the selection of recipients for organ grafts. In general, organ transplant recipients have end-stage organ failure that is not amenable to other, more conventional forms of medical or surgical therapy. Recipients should be free of irreversible, untreatable other organ failure or be considered candidates for multiple organ grafting. Because of the dangers of the required immunosuppression, recipients should not have recent or partially treated malignancies, and should be free of infection.

These general criteria apply to recipients of organs of all types. The evaluation of the potential organ transplant recipient, therefore, requires a careful history and physical examination and appropriate laboratory, radiographic, and other tests to fully evaluate the patient's general health and to define the extent and severity of target organ failure. In addition, potential recipients undergo a battery of serologic tests to assess previous exposures to infectious agents such as hepatitis, cytomegalovirus (CMV), toxoplasmosis, and HIV. Only the latter is always a contraindication to organ transplantation, again because of the fear that treatment with immunosuppressive drugs might precipitate or exacerbate the acquired immunodeficiency syndrome (AIDS).

In addition, patients are evaluated for psychological stability and the extent to which they have a network of "supports" to assist them both during the waiting time before transplantation and during the recovery and maintenance phases after. This evaluation is done not to discriminate against individuals with a history of psychiatric or social problems but to identify them in the hopes of setting up a system of supports so that the potential organ transplant recipient can undergo the procedure and the complex posttransplant follow-up successfully. This not only makes sense from the standpoint of the individual patient, but as prudent management of a scarce resource, the transplantable organ graft. Therefore, potential recipients undergo a psychological evaluation and counseling with their significant others so that problem areas including smoking, substance abuse, or other difficulties can be addressed. As noted, these activities do not necessarily rule out transplantation as therapy for an individual, but identify areas in which intensive pretransplant therapy is needed.

The final area investigated prior to transplantation in all recipients is the state of the patient's medical insurance. Again, this is done not in an attempt to discriminate, but so that potential problems can be avoided. Transplantation is expensive therapy, both for the operation itself, and especially during the posttransplant period. Patients, by definition, are terminally ill, and therefore often have complicated postoperative recoveries. More important, posttransplant outpatient follow-up is critical, as is scrupulous administration of the required immunosuppressive drugs. This takes time and money. If a patient cannot adhere to this regimen or cannot afford it, the quality of the result of transplantation is compromised with potential loss of the organ and possibly the death of the patient. Therefore, careful pretransplant attention to these details is crucial. This is less of an issue in renal transplantation since, by law, all patients with renal failure in the United States have their medical care paid for under the End-Stage Renal Disease Program. The comprehensive scope of this program has not been duplicated for other organ grafts, although patients covered by Medicare have their transplants paid for by this program.

Indications, Evaluation, Exclusions

Heart. During a representative month in 1997, there were 3811 patients listed by UNOS and awaiting heart transplantation in the United States (*The UNOS Bulletin,* 1997). This represents the typical "instantaneous" demand for hearts according to present practice patterns. As in all organ transplantation, the underlying principal indication for heart transplantation is end-stage heart disease not amenable to other medical or surgical therapy (Baumgartner, 1979) (Table 27–1). The most common specific indication for heart transplantation is contractile failure of the myocardium producing congestive heart failure, which accounts for the vast majority (90% or better) of patients. About half of these patients have end-stage heart failure due to coronary artery disease and the other half due to idiopathic or, in a few cases, postviral myocarditis cardiomyopathy. The remainder of patients with heart failure have underlying valvular or congenital heart disease, while a few have postpartum cardiomyopathy or other rare conditions.

TABLE 27–1. Indications for Heart Transplantation

Congestive Cardiomyopathy
- Idiopathic
- Ischemic (Coronary Artery Disease)
- Post-viral
- Post-partum
- Secondary to
  - Valvular heart disease
  - Congenital heart disease

Intractable Angina
Intractable Arrhythmias

A much smaller number of patients have preserved contractile function but undergo heart transplantation for intractable and untreatable angina pectoris or ventricular arrhythmias.

All candidates for heart transplantation undergo the complete evaluation outlined above. In addition, echocardiography is an important test to confirm the diagnosis and to assess cardiac function. Left-heart catheterization with coronary angiography is often done in patients with ischemic heart disease to make certain that the patient does not have coronary anatomy suitable for angioplasty or coronary bypass surgery. In cases in which coronary anatomy is suitable for revascularization, a careful examination for reversible myocardial dysfunction is performed. This often involves thallium or positron emission tomographic (PET) scanning to detect the presence of viable, but "hibernating," hypocontractile muscle. This is a controversial and complicated topic.

Two important evaluative tools specific for candidates for heart transplantation include the right-heart catheterization and the exercise test with oxygen uptake. Right-heart catheterization with measurement of pulmonary artery pressures and resistance is mandatory prior to listing for heart transplantation. In heart failure, elevated left-heart filling pressures are common due to decompensation of the left ventricle. Increases in left-sided pressures lead to reflex increases in pulmonary artery pressures that rise gradually over time. The native right ventricle can adapt to these pressure increases if they occur gradually. It is important, however, to document pretransplant that these pressures are neither too high nor irreversible. That is because the transplanted normal donor heart has a right ventricle that has not adapted to pumping against increased pulmonary arterial pressure. When the donor heart is placed in a recipient with elevated pulmonary pressures that do not fall immediately, the new right ventricle may be unable to handle an excessive pressure load. In fact, acute right-heart failure is a recognized complication of heart transplantation. Therefore, in most cases, patients whose pulmonary artery systolic pressure *irreversibly* exceeds 70 mm Hg, or whose transpulmonary gradient (difference between mean PA pressure and wedge pressure) *irreversibly* exceeds 15 mm Hg, or whose pulmonary vascular resistance *irreversibly* exceeds 4 Wood units, cannot be considered for heart transplantation.

Precise measurement of exercise capacity is also an important evaluative tool for prospective heart transplant recipients. An exercise test with graded levels of exertion provides a relatively quantitative and objective assessment of the extent of the patient's cardiac disability. When combined with O_2 uptake, this test also provides important prognostic information. An O_2 uptake during exercise of less than 14 ml/min, in addition to signifying severe functional impairment, has been associated with excess mortality in patients with severe heart failure. Therefore, patients with appropriate indications and this level of physiologic derangement are usually listed for heart transplantation, whereas primary medical management may be attempted in patients with similar subjective symptoms but higher O_2 uptake measurements with exercise.

The contraindications and exclusions specific for heart transplantation follow from the above discussions. Patients with irreversible pulmonary hypertension are usually excluded from evaluation for cardiac transplantation because of the excessive risks of postoperative right-heart failure. In the past, these patients might have been considered candidates for simultaneous heart and lung transplantation. For several reasons, this is rarely the practice today. The primary reason is the absolute paucity of suitable heart–lung donors and the overwhelming demand for hearts for isolated heart transplantation and lungs for isolated lung transplantation. A heart–lung block can provide organs to help three patients (one heart and two lung recipients); therefore, the argument has been made that this scarce resource should be used in this way. Second, since severe heart failure that causes severe pulmonary hypertension occurs by definition in patients who are very ill, the results of heart–lung transplantation are not so good. Finally, heart–lung transplantation has fallen out of favor except in extremely rare circumstances both because the results in general have been of lower quality than hoped and many disease states that were thought initially to require simultaneous heart–lung transplantation can be managed successfully with lung transplantation alone.

Heart transplantation may not be indicated in patients with significant heart failure but preserved exercise capacity and O_2 uptake. These patients may be managed successfully with medications. Many of these patients, of course, have subsequent progression of dysfunction and end up as candidates for heart transplantation.

Lung. In 1 month in 1997, UNOS records showed 2407 patients awaiting lung transplantation (*The UNOS Bulletin,* 1997). Candidates for pulmonary transplantation have irreversible end-stage lung disease (Egan, 1989) (Table 27–2). Although life expectancy is difficult to predict in patients with severe pulmonary impairment, patients referred for lung transplantation in general have a life expectancy of less than 1 year.

TABLE 27–2. Indications for Lung Transplantation

Obstructive Lung Disease
Emphysema
Chronic bronchitis including cystic fibrosis
α_1-antitrypsin deficiency
Restrictive Lung Disease
Pulmonary Vascular Disease
Primary pulmonary hypertension
Eisenmenger's syndrome (congenital left to right shunts)

End-stage pulmonary pathology is usually either primarily obstructive or restrictive, although mixed forms exist. Patients with obstructive lung disease usually have emphysema that may be bullous or nonbullous. The most common causes of this form of severe obstructive lung disease are smoking or congenital deficiency of α_1-antitrypsin protease. Patients with the latter usually have bullous disease concentrated in the lung bases.

Patients with chronic infectious pulmonary disorders may also present with obstructive disease. Severe end-stage chronic bronchitis can lead to pulmonary dysfunction severe enough to require lung replacement. Patients with cystic fibrosis and chronic pulmonary infections present with this sort of obstructive pulmonary pathology. While many patients with noninfected lung pathology can be managed successfully with single-lung transplantation, patients with chronic infection such as those with cystic fibrosis must be managed with bilateral transplantation. This is because of the risk in single-lung transplantation that the transplanted lung will be infected by the remaining diseased lung, especially in the presence of immunosuppression.

Restrictive lung disease may also be severe enough to require lung replacement. Most of these patients have idiopathic pulmonary fibrosis. While this pathology may have several etiologies, when it has reached end-stage, the functional and pathological manifestations are similar and no therapy short of lung transplantation is effective. Patients with these forms of severe obstructive and restrictive lung disease often have secondary pulmonary hypertension and enlargement of the right ventricle. In the early days of lung transplantation, it was feared that this right ventricular dysfunction might be permanent and require cardiac replacement as well. The observation has been, however, that in most cases the right ventricular and pulmonary vascular changes secondary to primary lung disease reverse with single- or double-lung transplantation (Kramer, 1994). Only in patients with these lung pathologies and irreversible left ventricular dysfunction is heart and lung transplantation considered.

Pulmonary vascular disease is a separate entity that can be managed with single- or double-lung transplantation. Despite the fact that this is a diffuse process, in some cases it can be managed with single-lung transplantation since the normal pulmonary vascular bed, even of one lung, is so capacious. Patients with end-stage pulmonary vascular disease may have primary pulmonary hypertension. The etiology of this disease is unknown. A smaller subset of patients have end-stage pulmonary vascular changes due to a cardiovascular defect that causes shunting of blood from left to right. When this process is chronic and severe, irreversible pulmonary vascular changes can occur leading to pulmonary hypertension and reversal of the shunt to right to left (called Eisenmenger's Syndrome). In the past, some of these patients were referred for heart and lung transplantation. However, presently, when these patients have a correctable cardiovascular defect, such as a ventricular septal defect (VSD) or patent ductus arteriosus (PDA), they can be managed with single-lung transplantation combined with repair of the defect. As a result of this observation and the one noted above, and because of the limited donor supply, today combined heart and lung transplantation is performed rarely and only in patients with both end-stage irreversible cardiac and pulmonary processes.

The general indications for lung transplantation are similar to those noted above for heart transplantation. Patients usually have end-stage lung disease with limited life expectancy. They should have no other irreversible systemic disease or contraindication to immunosuppression. In general, patients with severe lung disease who require support on a ventilator are excluded from lung transplantation since the rates of morbidity and mortality in these patients are excessive. Candidates for lung transplantation must be free of significant psychiatric disorder and able to comply with the complex medical and rehabilitative regimens required before and after lung transplantation. Pretransplantation pulmonary rehabilitation is particularly important in patients awaiting lung transplantation, especially when obstructive lung disease is the underlying disorder.

Evaluation of the lung transplantation candidate is similar to that for cardiac transplantation. A complete history, physical, and basic laboratory examination are performed. Obviously, the chest x-ray and pulmonary function studies are keys to making the diagnosis of lung disease and assessing its severity. One evaluation that has proven extremely useful in evaluating patients for lung transplantation is the 6-minute walk. This test measures global functional capacity by quantifying the distance in feet that a patient is able to walk in 6 minutes. The patient may proceed at his or her own pace and rest as often as needed. Very low 6-minute walk distances such as 400 to 500 feet suggest that the lung disease is severe enough to warrant transplantation.

Some patients with obstructive lung disease referred for lung transplantation may be candidates for volume reduction surgery. In this procedure, the most diseased, usually apical, segments of the emphysematous lung are resected. Many of these patients have remarkable subjective and objective improvements in pulmonary function including better 6-minute walk distances. This procedure, of course, does not reverse the underlying lung disease. Therefore, some of these patients may ultimately need lung replacement with transplantation.

Liver. The waiting list for liver transplantation during April of 1997 included 8211 patients (*The UNOS Bulletin,* 1997). As with heart and lung transplantation, the primary indication for liver transplantation is end-stage liver disease with life expectancy of one year or less (Starzl, 1990) (Table 27–3). End-stage liver disease may be the consequence of a variety of pathological processes. The patient's

TABLE 27–3. Indications for Liver Transplantation

Cirrhosis
Alcoholic (Laennec's)
Cryptogenic
Primary biliary
Hepatitis
Fulminant Hepatic Failure
Primary Sclerosing Cholangitis
Biliary Atresia
Inborn Errors of Metabolism
Neoplasm
Budd–Chiari Syndrome

history and, in some cases, liver biopsy may determine the reason that the patient's liver function is minimal and with no chance of recovery. While the history may suggest the diagnosis, the biopsy is important in making the determination that the liver dysfunction is irreversible.

Equally as important as making the diagnosis of end-stage liver disease is the determination of when is the appropriate time to proceed to liver transplantation. The rate of progression of liver disease to ultimate complete failure and patient death is variable. Certain clinical conditions, however, have been associated by experience with an increased risk of death within 6 months. These include rapidly deepening jaundice, ascites that does not respond to diuretic therapy, spontaneous hepatic encephalopathy, recurrent sepsis including spontaneous bacterial peritonitis, recurrent bleeding from varices, and prolongation of the prothrombin time (PT) to over 8 seconds above control despite adequate therapy with vitamin K.

Other, more subjective, symptoms may contribute to the decision to proceed with liver transplantation. These include severe fatigue interfering with most activities of daily living and intractable pruritis. Another situation in which liver transplantation may be recommended is acute fulminant hepatic failure. Patients with this condition can progress from good health to hepatic encephalopathy very rapidly. While recovery can occur, it is rare, and timely transplantation may be life-saving. The rate of neurologic deterioration in these patients is often used as an indication for transplantation along with documentation of severe hepatic insufficiency.

A number of specific conditions can lead to liver failure severe enough to require transplantation. The most common is cirrhosis, accounting for nearly half of patients undergoing primary liver transplantation. Alcoholic cirrhosis is most common although indications also include primary biliary cirrhosis and cryptogenic cirrhosis. Chronic hepatitis, fulminant hepatic failure, primary sclerosis cholangitis, biliary atresia, inborn errors of metabolism, neoplasm, and other less common ailments constitute the other diagnostic groups, although each of these accounts for less than 10% of the total liver transplant patient population.

As in all of organ transplantation, the number of absolute contraindications to liver transplantation is relatively small. Patients who for cardiovascular or pulmonary reasons cannot tolerate the major operative procedure are not considered for transplantation. Similarly, recent intracranial hemorrhage, irreversible neurologic impairment, HIV infection, ongoing bacterial infection, hypotension requiring pressor agents, and active substance abuse are considered absolute contraindications to transplantation. Insulin-dependent diabetes and thrombosis of the portal vein, once thought to preclude liver transplantation, are no longer absolute contraindications to the procedure. Renal insufficiency may improve after liver transplantation, or if the condition is irreversible, simultaneous kidney transplantation may be performed. Older patients, including those over 70 years old, may be considered for transplantation since it is the physiologic age of the patient that affects the results of this (or any transplant) procedure more than the patient's chronologic age.

Kidney. There were 35,730 potential recipients waiting for cadaver kidneys on UNOS's transplant waiting list in a single month of 1996 (*The UNOS Bulletin,* 1997). The indication for kidney transplantation is the presence of end-stage renal disease (Table 27–4). While most patients undergoing kidney transplantation are undergoing dialysis at the time of the procedure, in certain cases the patient may receive an organ graft before dialysis is required. This determination is based mostly on logistical considerations. The causes of end-stage renal disease include hypertension, diabetes, glomerulonephritis, chronic upper urinary tract infection, obstructive disorders, and other less common vascular and inflammatory conditions.

The evaluation of a patient being considered for kidney transplantation is similar to that already described for other organs. Patients undergo a complete history, physical examination, and series of blood studies and other tests designed to uncover conditions that would be a contraindication to kidney transplantation. Absolute contraindications include systemic malignancy, active infection, HIV infection, and psychological or social problems that preclude un-

TABLE 27–4. Indications for Kidney Transplantation

Diabetic Nephropathy
Chronic Pyelonephritis
Glomerulonephritis
Hypertension
Lupus Nephritis
Nephrotic Syndrome
Obstructive Uropathies
Congenital
Acquired
Polycystic Kidney Disease
Amyloidosis

derstanding of the procedure or compliance with the postoperative medical regimen required. Patients must have adequate cardiovascular and pulmonary function to withstand the transplant operation. However, kidney transplantation, in general, is less rigorous surgery than the hepatic transplant operation.

Pancreas. In April of 1997, 346 patients were listed for pancreas transplants and 1421 for combined kidney–pancreas transplants according to UNOS records (*The UNOS Bulletin,* 1997). All patients undergoing pancreatic transplantation have diabetes mellitus (Sutherland, 1989). This operation is applied to three groups of patients all of whom have insulin-dependent diabetes. The first group is patients who already have a functioning renal allograft. The second group constitutes diabetic patients with uremia who undergo simultaneous kidney and pancreas transplantation. The third group is patients with diabetes but without renal failure who undergo pancreatic transplantation to treat nonuremic complications of the disease (Barbosa, 1994).

Pancreatic transplantation is a relatively new procedure the way it is currently practiced. Therefore, the specific selection criteria may be somewhat more stringent than with other transplantation procedures. Patients should be between the ages of 18 and 50 years and have insulin-dependent diabetes as documented by absence of circulating C-peptide. They should either have preserved renal function with microalbuminuria and a creatinine clearance of more than 60 to 70 ml/min or be candidates for the combined kidney–pancreas procedure with impaired renal function (creatinine clearance less than 60 ml/min). Patients considered for pancreas transplantation may also have autonomic neuropathy, retinopathy, and labile diabetes, but these conditions are not usually independent inclusion criteria. As noted above, patients must have sufficient cardio–pulmonary reserve and psychological fitness to understand the procedure and adhere to the postoperative medical treatment plan.

There are advantages to simultaneous pancreas–kidney transplantation. These include the recipient's exposure to only one set of transplant antigens from the single donor, the immunosuppressive effects of uremia that appear to improve the early immunologic results of the combined transplant operation, and a single anesthetic exposure. In addition, it is possible to monitor rejection of the pancreatic graft by monitoring the function of the simultaneous kidney graft. Patients without a prior kidney graft, furthermore, obviously undergo the pancreas transplant procedure not already taking immunosuppressive drugs. Finally, the transplanted kidney of the recipient of a pancreas–kidney transplant may be protected from the late complications of diabetes by the functioning pancreatic graft.

The selection process is most rigorous for the candidate without either a functioning kidney graft or uremic complications of diabetes. In these patients, the risks of surgery and chronic immunosuppression must be compared to the benefits of restoration of normal pancreatic function. These patients, however, may derive the most benefit from the procedure and avoid the irreversible complications of diabetes. The judgment must be made that the risks of surgery and immunosuppression are less than the risk of the patient developing irreversible secondary complications of diabetes.

The contraindications for pancreatic transplantation are identical to those discussed for kidney and other organ transplants, although the criteria are somewhat more rigid as noted. The patient must not have irreversible other organ failure, active malignancy or infection, including from HIV, and must have the ability to adhere to a complex medical regimen.

Supply

Organ Allocation System

United Network for Organ Sharing. In 1984, the United States Congress enacted legislation mandating the establishment of principles and regulations for the equitable distribution of cadaver organs for transplantation. The contract for administration of the system for organ procurement and distribution was awarded to the United Network for Organ Sharing (UNOS). UNOS, which is headquartered in Richmond, Virginia, was established and is run by health-care professionals and lay people with interests and expertise in organ transplantation (Pierce, 1996).

UNOS has promulgated standards for its members that include transplanting hospitals, transplanting surgeons and physicians, tissue-typing laboratories, and organ procurement organizations (OPOs). UNOS also devised a system, which undergoes periodic modification, that is used to stratify priority of patients waiting on transplant waiting lists and to distribute organs nationally that are procured by an OPO in a specific geographic area but for whatever reason cannot be used for a patient in that region.

While UNOS has standards and regulations, these policies do not, in general, have the force of law. Since UNOS is a federal contractor, for its policies to be legally enforceable they would have to satisfy the government's requirements for publication in the Federal Register, commentary, and modification. As it is, UNOS policies are circulated for comment to the transplantation and interested lay community prior to enactment. The additional federal publication requirements would make the process of policy development so cumbersome that the system would likely come to a halt. However, since UNOS is supported so heavily by the transplant community, voluntary adherence to its policies and guidelines is nearly universal.

In addition to setting standards and developing policies, UNOS keeps an updated list of all patients awaiting transplantation and a record of all organ grafts performed in the United States. It issues periodic reports of transplantation activity and responds to issues relating to the equity and morality of transplantation as these arise. As noted, when an organ cannot be used in a local area, UNOS coordinates the timely and equitable sharing of that organ among the nation's transplant centers. For this reason and to simplify some administrative issues, UNOS has divided the country into eleven regions of roughly equal total population (Fig. 27–1). Policy making may vary somewhat from region to region but must be approved by the appropriate UNOS committee. When inter-OPO sharing takes place, other OPOs in the region usually have first priority for the organ.

Local Organ Procurement Organization (OPO). The local OPO has the primary responsibility for identification of potential donors, obtaining consent for donation from relatives, pretransplant management of the donor's medical conditions, and allocation to local transplant centers. Each transplant center is affiliated with a local OPO that is the contact point for distribution of donor organs. There must be at least one tissue-typing laboratory available to the OPO, but in some regions there are several. Each OPO keeps a prioritized list of patients waiting for transplantation. The waiting lists for different organs are kept separately. For example, a patient awaiting a heart transplant waits on a list separate from the list of patients awaiting liver transplantation. In cases of multiple organ grafts, patients are prioritized according to the highest priority organ (Blanche, 1994b).

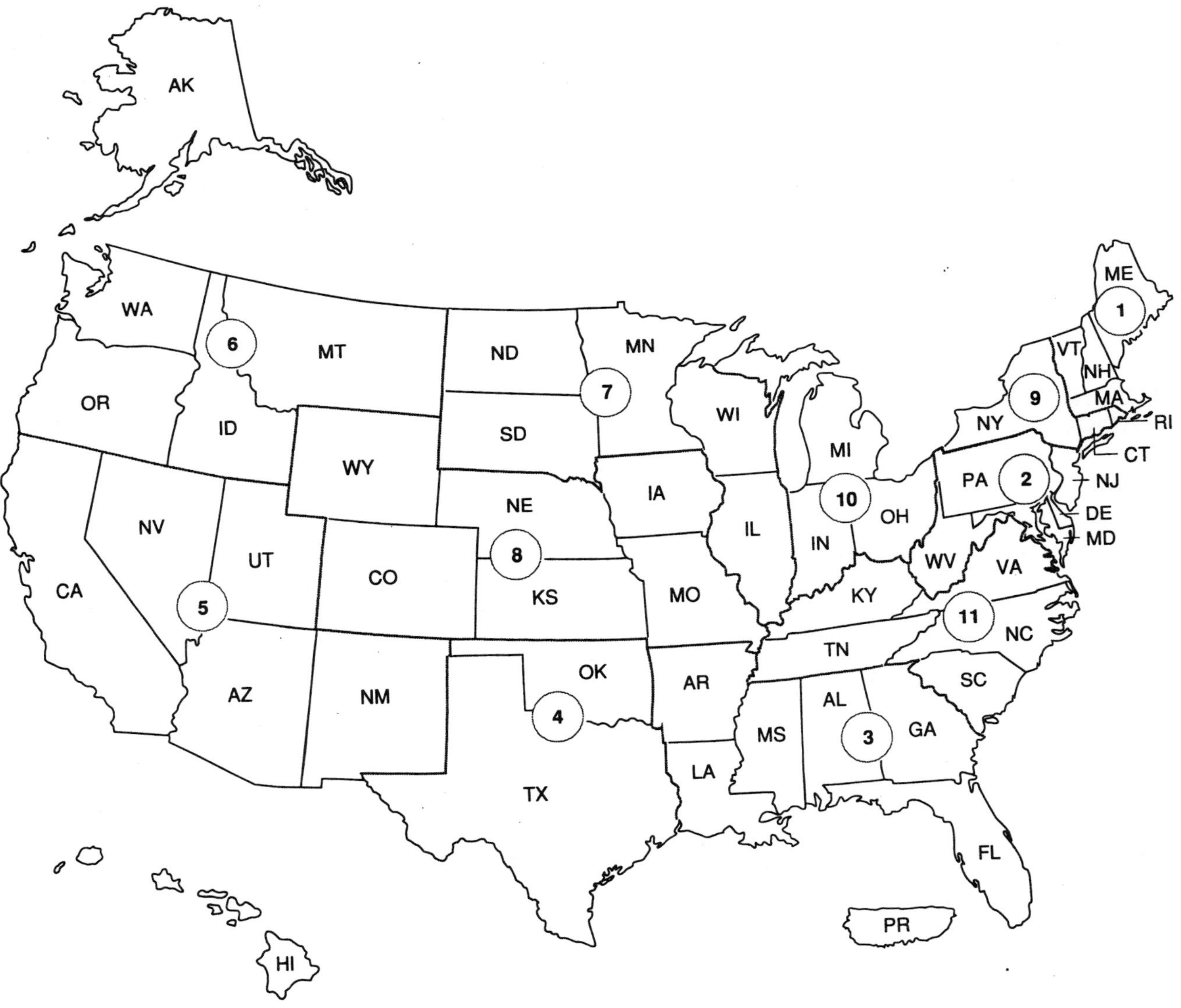

Figure 27–1. The eleven regions as defined by UNOS. The population contained in each region is intended to be approximately equal but obviously, the geographic size of the regions varies greatly. *(Reproduced with permission from Bromberg et al. [1997], illustrations by Holly R. Fischer, MFA.)*

The schemes for assigning patient priority vary from organ to organ and are modified from time to time. For example, hearts are allocated according to clinical status (1 or 2) and waiting time. No pretransplant tissue typing is done. In kidney transplantation, priority is assigned not only on the basis of waiting time but according to the degree of donor–recipient tissue matching (Cho, 1994). In human transplantation, six histocompatibility antigens (HLA antigens) are usually typed. Recipients with "six antigen matches" with a particular donor receive priority for a kidney from that donor. Other allocation procedures exist for distribution of lungs, livers, and pancreata.

Historical Procurements. In 1996, a total of 16,801 transplantations using organs from cadaveric donors were performed in the United States under the auspices of UNOS (*The UNOS Bulletin,* 1997). For comparison, during this time interval 3459 living donors contributed organs (predominately kidneys) for transplantation. The total of cadaveric organs included 2340 hearts, 795 lungs, 39 heart–lungs, 4012 livers, 8560 kidneys, and 1012 pancreata. While over the last 10 years the numbers of donations of all types of organs have increased significantly, the rate of rise in donations of hearts, livers, and kidneys recently is less steep. The rates of donation of lungs and pancreata are increasing more rapidly, reflecting the progressively widening application of transplantation of these organs in recent years.

▶ COORDINATION OF ORGAN PROCUREMENT

Logistics

The logistics of procurement of organs for transplantation from cadaveric donors are coordinated by the local OPO. When a donor, or potential donor is identified, usually in a hospital intensive care unit, coordinators from the local OPO are contacted. These coordinators are trained experts not only in the allocation of organs for transplantation, but more important in ways to approach the family of the donor about organ donation, and in the maintenance of the donor in a stable condition prior to procurement (Soifer, 1989).

The issues surrounding the approach to the donor family are naturally sensitive but also critical to gaining access to the maximum number of transplantable organs. While brain death must be established prior to organ procurement, discussions about donation can begin even before brain death is declared formally. It is preferable to have coordinators from the local OPO available as these discussions are initiated. Many times a donor's family hesitates to give consent based on misinformation or a misunderstanding to which the OPO professional can respond effectively (Darby, 1989).

In addition, the tests done to establish the viability and transplantability of the potential donor's organs can begin when it is anticipated that the patient will become an organ donor (Emery, 1986). The OPO coordinator oversees the performance of this evaluation and insures not only that the appropriate tests are done but that the interests and rights of the donor and the donor family are protected during this process. Primarily, no organ donation can take place until brain death has been declared. Recently, there has been some publicity regarding organ procurement from terminally ill but not brain dead donors who at the family's request are withdrawn from life support (D'Allessandro, 1995). These "non-heart beating" cadaver donors are relatively infrequent and will not be discussed further.

The declaration of brain death is performed by a neurologist or neurosurgeon not involved in the transplant process. Brain death is determined according to standard criteria (Angstwurm, 1984). It is the responsibility of the OPO coordinator and of each organ procurement team to make certain that there is adequate documentation that these criteria have been met. As noted, the OPO coordinator also assures that the appropriate tests are done to assess the suitability of organs for transplantation and to determine the presence of medical conditions in the donor (infection, cancer, etc.) that would preclude organ donation.

When brain death is declared or anticipated and the other evaluations are underway or complete, the OPO coordinator contacts the various organ transplant surgical teams according to the priority schema and waiting lists in the OPO cachement area. Each team, in recipient priority order, is offered the appropriate organ for that patient. Offers are made until the organ is accepted by a team for a specific patient. Transplant teams cannot jump the queue in favor of one of their patients with lower priority. In other words, if a transplant team has patients who are first and third on the waiting list, it cannot preferentially transplant the number three patient unless the transplant team caring for patient number two declines to use the organ or can be convinced to defer in favor of patient three. If no local transplant team can use the organ, it is offered nationally through UNOS and according to the UNOS priority schemes for each organ.

When all transplantable organs have been placed with specific transplant teams, the OPO coordinator arranges appropriate transportation for the several surgical teams that will procure the organs. The specifics of the travel arrangements depend on the distances involved and the length of time that an organ can be maintained and stored prior to implantation. The shortest allowable waiting times are for hearts (4-6 hours), the longest for kidneys (48-72 hours), with the safe storage times for the other organs intermediate between these extremes. Typically, surgical transplant teams are transported by ambulance, helicopter, propeller or jet airplane, or some combination of these.

Not only does the OPO coordinator arrange transportation for the transplant teams, but he or she also must arrange operating room time at the donor hospital and communicate these timing issues to the transplant teams. The recipient operations are obviously dependent for their timing on the timing of the procurement procedures. This is especially important for heart transplantation since the safe storage times are relatively short and the number of distant procurements has increased as the demand for donors has increased. In general, the implanting team is also the procurement team for heart, lung, liver, and pancreas transplantation. The practice in kidney transplantation is for a local transplant surgeon to do the procurement, even if the allocation scheme does not give his or her patients access to the specific donor's kidneys.

Finally, the local OPO is in charge of billing the various transplant centers for the costs of organ procurement. Of course, these charges are subsequently billed to the recipient's insurance carrier. The actual charges are computed by the OPO by adding the total costs, on a yearly basis, assignable to procurement of each type of organ (with some assignment of shared expenses) and dividing by the numbers of each organ procured. This charge is adjusted annually.

Operative Details

When an organ donor is identified, the operations to procure the various organs happen simultaneously and are coordinated, as noted, by the local OPO. This is true even if one or more of the procurement teams is from out of the region. In addition to coordinating the timing of the donor and recipient operations, the sequence of organ procurements in an individual donor is important. This is because of the obvious fact that the various organs all help sustain the physiologic milieu that is necessary to maintain their viability and suitability for transplantation.

Procurement of the heart, lungs, liver, pancreas, and kidneys is accomplished in the operating room with the donor monitored and supported by a team of anesthetists. Since the patient is brain dead, no anesthetic agent is required. An incision is made from the sternal notch to the pubis and a median sternotomy performed. This incision provides facile access to the intrathoracic and intraabdominal organs (Fig. 27–2).

The usual sequence is to do a physical examination and preliminary dissection of the heart and lungs early in the procurement operation (Fig. 27–3). This is important since coordination with the recipient operation is most critical with these organs and since removal of the heart and lungs cannot be performed until the abdominal organs are ready to be removed and cannulated for perfusion prior to storage. Also, the operations to remove the heart and lungs are relatively simpler and less time consuming.

The liver, kidney, and pancreas teams—which may be all the same surgeons—then examine and dissect out the vascular supply of these intraabdominal organs. The liver and pancreas dissections are the most complex and time consuming (Fig. 27–4). The blood supply of the liver includes not only the hepatic arteries and veins but also the portal system. Arterial variability is common and must be recognized. Similarly, the pancreatic dissection is complicated by vascular variability and the complex relationships among the pancreas, the pancreatic duct, and surrounding organs like the duodenum and the spleen. Finally, anomalies of the renal arterial supply must be recognized so as not to damage the kidneys during harvesting (Fig. 27–5).

Depending on the donor's anatomy and the experience of the procurement team, dissection of the abdominal organs can take from 45 minutes to two or more hours. During this period, the donor must be monitored closely and appropriate fluid resuscitation and pharmacologic support given by the anesthetist. Preservation of the organs for transplantation, which actually begins once the donor is identified, must continue in the operating room if organs of optimal condition are to be procured.

Once the intrathoracic and intraabdominal dissections are completed, the donor is heparinized and perfusion cannulas placed in the thoracic aorta, the pulmonary artery, the abdominal aorta, and the portal vein (Fig. 27–6). The venous return to the heart is ligated and the ascending aorta clamped, effectively ending the circulation. Cold preservation solution is perfused into each organ via the perfusion cannulae while each organ is cooled further by the topical application of iced slush saline solution.

Organ Preservation and Transport

The removal, storage, transportation, and implantation of solid organs from cadaveric donors requires a means to preserve the organs so that they can perform their physiologic functions when implanted in the recipient (Belzer, 1988). The injury sustained by an organ that is removed for transplantation is primarily one of ischemia and reperfusion. In transplantation, ischemia is classified as cold or warm. Cold ischemia refers to that period of time during which the organ is deprived of blood, but kept in a cold environment. Warm ischemia occurs predominantly during the implantation operation. Secondarily, the solutions used to preserve and cool organs, and hypothermia itself, may contribute to reversible damage. Finally, reestablishment of blood flow to the organ, reperfusion, can induce injury itself mediated by oxygen free radicals, cytokines, and nitric oxide.

The integrity of an organ depends on the integrity of the cells that make up that organ and perform the biochemical and mechanical functions of the organ. During organ storage, physiologic events can affect the structural integrity, ionic composition, and energy systems of the cells of the organ. To minimize ischemic damage to the cells and these energy-requiring attributes, reduction of the metabolic energy demands of the cells is the underlying principle of organ preservation. The primary way this is achieved is

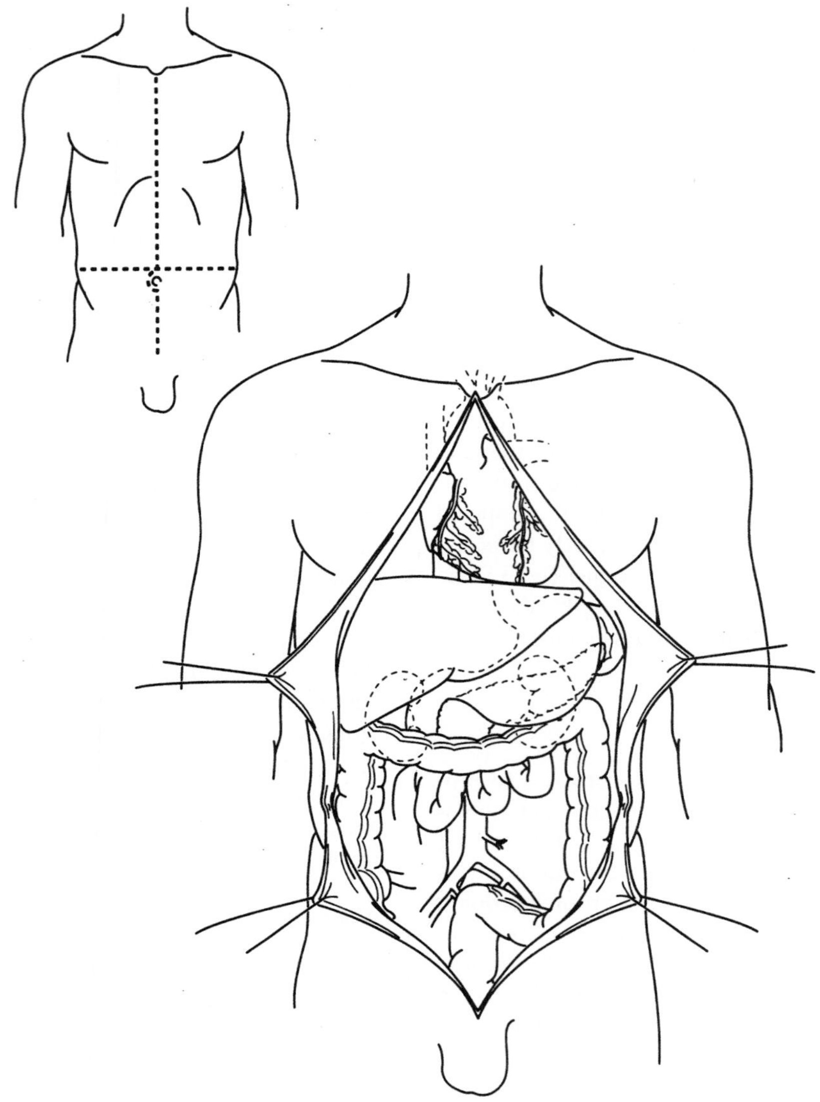

Figure 27–2. The incision for multiple organ procurement is made from sternal notch to pubis. A median sternotomy is performed. As noted in the smaller inset, transverse abdominal incisions may be added to facilitate exposure. *(Reproduced with permission from Bromberg et al. [1997], illustrations by Holly R. Fischer, MFA.)*

through reduction of temperature, since hypothermia is among the most reliable ways to reduce the energy requirements of complex organ systems. Hypothermia is used as a component of the strategy for preservation of heart, lungs, liver, kidney, and pancreas.

Until recently, the most commonly used preservation solutions were crystalloid formulations that mimicked intracellular ionic complications. These hypertonic solutions, like the Euro–Collins solution (Table 27–5), were designed to cool the organ and reduce cellular swelling. Preservation times for organs other than the kidney were relatively short using such solutions. Transplant investigators at the University of Wisconsin developed a preservation solution (UW Solution) that dramatically increased the safe cold ischemic times for liver and pancreas storage (D'Allessandro, 1990) (Table 27–6).

UW Solution uses lactobionate, raffinose, hydroxyethyl starch, and other ingredients designed to provide energy precursors, acid buffering capacity, and antioxidant capability. Using UW Solution, liver and pancreas can be stored for more than 24 hours with reliable and predictable return of function upon reperfusion (Todo, 1989). It is not clear that UW Solution has altered the safe interval for kidney storage. With conventional solutions like Euro–Collins, kidneys have been stored and reimplanted after 48 to 72 hours with return of function. UW Solution appears not to alter this interval significantly. Neither does the continuous perfusion of kidneys that is practiced in some centers

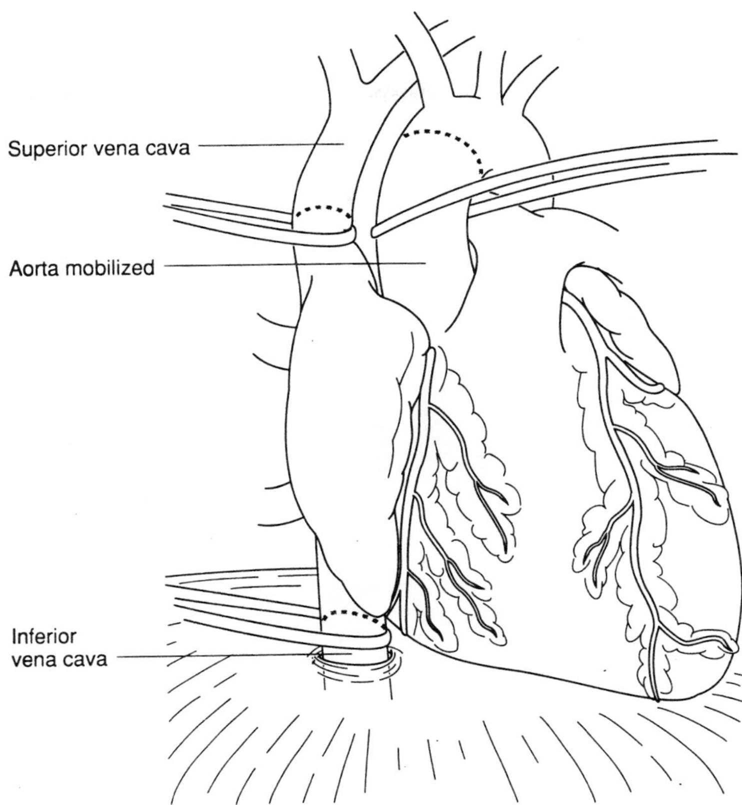

Figure 27–3. The projected resection lines for the aorta and venae cavae are depicted. The pulmonary artery is divided proximal to the bifurcation if the lungs are to be procured. *(Reproduced with permission from Bromberg et al. [1997], illustrations by Holly R. Fischer, MFA.)*

(Merion, 1990). The safe perfusion interval is identical. It must be acknowledged, however, that occasionally kidneys stored cold or perfused do not function immediately, forcing the patient to remain on dialysis until transplant function returns.

In heart transplantation, UW Solution is used with added concentrations of potassium. While the specific ingredients of UW Solution may contribute to cardiac preservation, cold and the diastolic arrest that hyperkalemia induces are probably most important for reducing the metabolic rate and therefore ischemic damage to the heart during storage and transport. Possibly because the heart must be able to perform mechanical, as opposed to biochemical, work immediately, safe ischemia times with UW Solution are similar to the 4 to 6 hours achievable with conventional solutions. No practical means of continuous heart perfusion have been devised to lengthen this interval.

Typically, lungs are preserved with a Euro–Collins intracellular-type cold preservation solution (Haverich, 1985). The administration of the preservation solution is often preceded by injection of a prostaglandin to dilate the pulmonary arterial bed and insure complete distribution of the cold preservation solution. Safe ischemia times range from 4 to 8 hours using these techniques for lung preservation.

Recipient Issues

Within the limits determined by the safe organ preservation times noted above, the recipient operation takes place coordinated with the donor procedure. In heart and lung transplantation, the organs must be implanted within a relatively few hours. Cold ischemia times can be significantly longer with liver, kidney, and pancreas transplantation. This has implications beyond the logistics of surgery, since in kidney transplantation, for example, the extended time interval allows time for histocompatibility typing of the donor and matching with the recipient.

Heart, lung, and liver transplantation is generally done orthotopically, that is, the organs are implanted in the usual anatomic positions after removal of the native organ. In heart transplantation, this requires anastomosis of the aorta, pulmonary artery, and the left and right atria. In general, the left and right atria are anastomosed as two single connections, although recently some centers have taken to doing separate anastomoses of the venae cavae and the left and right pulmonary veins (Blanche, 1994a). The lung connections are the pulmonary artery, the pulmonary veins—done as a single patch—and the bronchus. The integrity of the bronchial anastomosis is crucial since the complications of bronchial dehiscence can be devastating, especially in the

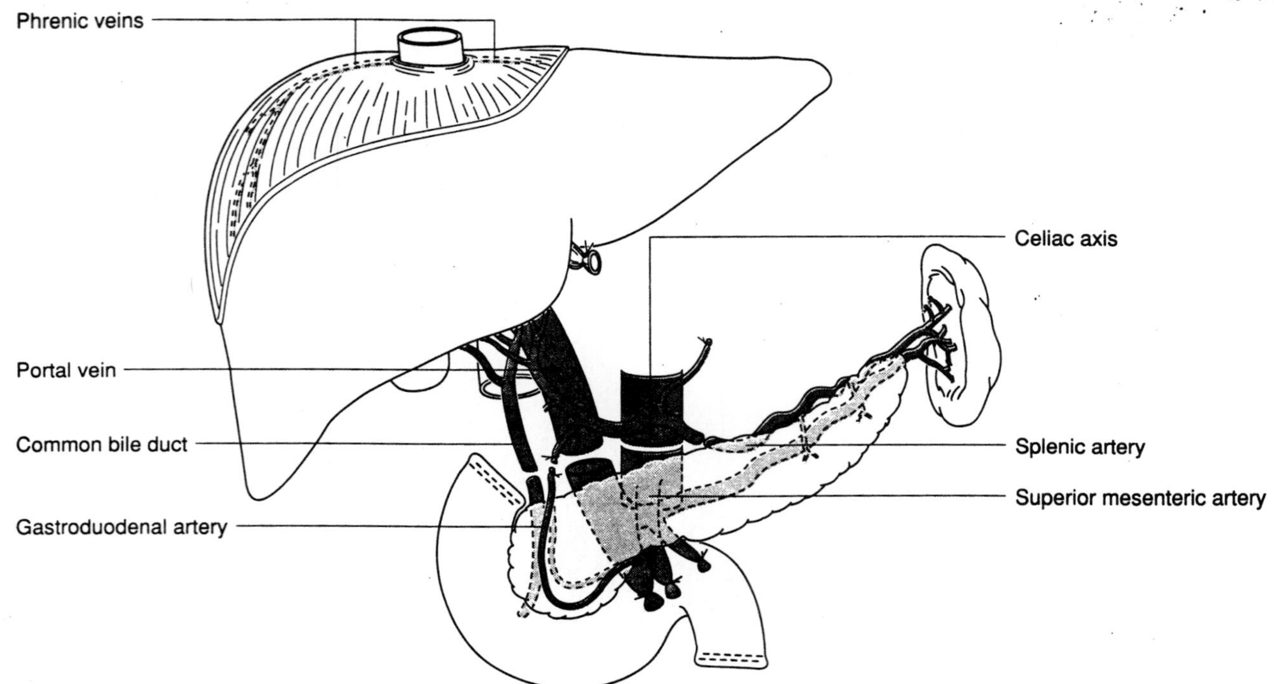

Figure 27–4. The liver and the pancreas are removed from the donor together and separated as a bench procedure. The various branches of the aorta and celiac axis must be divided and apportioned so as to insure adequate perfusion of both organs. *(Reproduced with permission from Bromberg et al. [1997], illustrations by Holly R. Fischer, MFA.)*

presence of immune suppression. Some surgeons wrap the bronchial anastomosis with omentum to try to enhance its blood supply and reduce the likelihood and complications of dehiscence.

Liver implantation requires reestablishment of the hepatic arterial and venous connections and that of the portal vein. Because of the complexity of the anatomy, the frequency of previous procedures in hepatic transplant candidates, and in many cases the presence of portal venous collaterals, the liver transplant procedure is one of the most difficult and potential bloody of the transplant operations. Using modern techniques, however, the rate of complications has been reduced, especially the requirement for transfusion which sometimes exceeded 100 units of blood

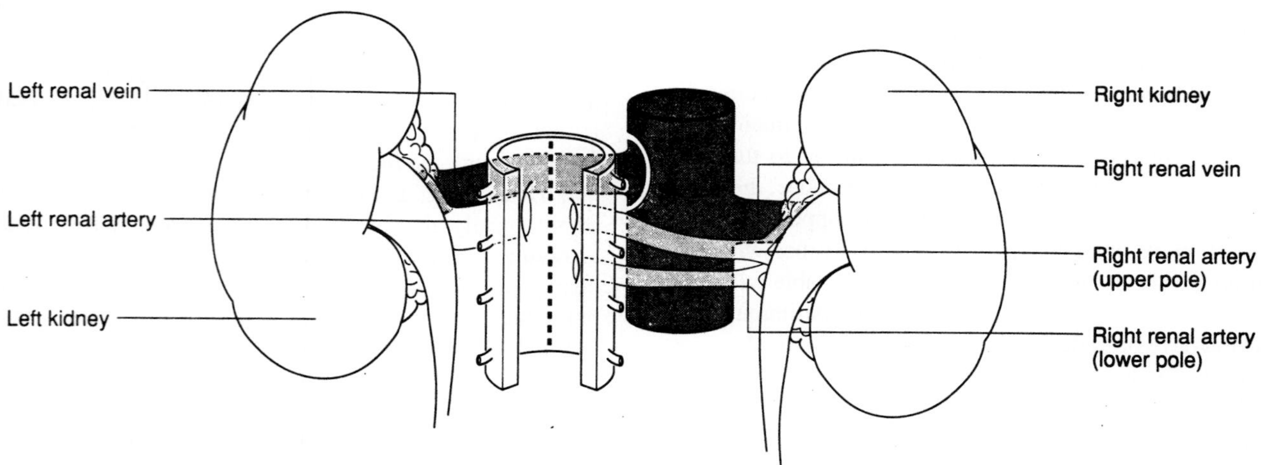

Figure 27–5. The kidneys are removed also as a single block. Division of the arterial and venous supply to each kidney is done as a bench procedure. Dissection in the hilum of each kidney is avoided to minimize the chance of damaging the vascular structures. *(Reproduced with permission from Bromberg et al. [1997], illustrations by Holly R. Fischer, MFA.)*

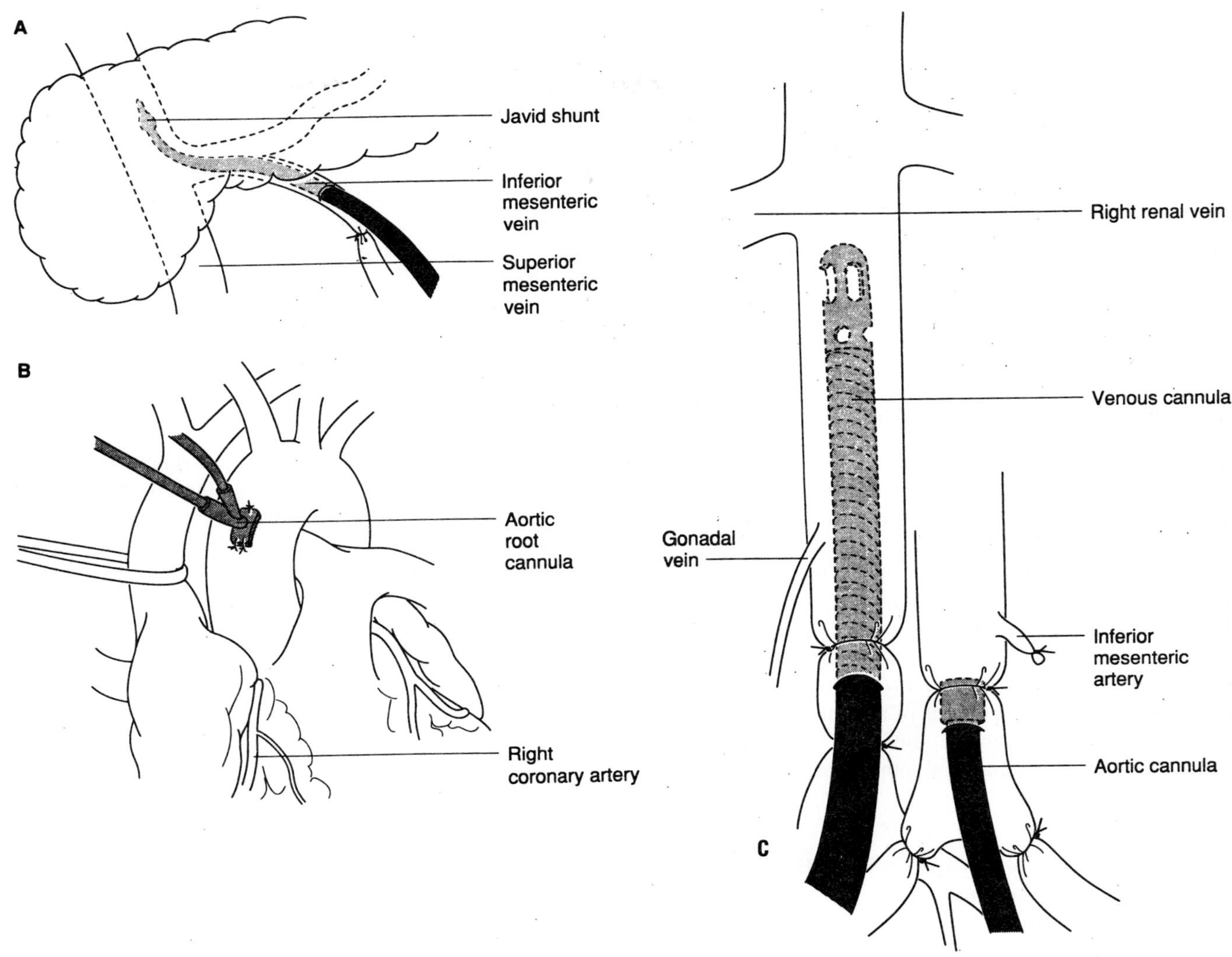

Figure 27–6. The placement of perfusion catheters prior to organ removal. **A,** The portal venous cannula is placed via the inferior mesenteric vein. **B,** A cardioplegia cannula is placed in the aortic root. The lung perfusion cannula positioned in the main pulmonary artery is not depicted in this drawing. **C,** The liver, pancreas, and kidneys are perfused via a cannula in the abdominal aorta. The inferior vena caval cannula is for drainage during perfusion. *(Reproduced with permission from Bromberg et al. [1997], illustrations by Holly R. Fischer, MFA.)*

per case. A cell-saver may be used during the liver transplantation procedure.

The kidney and pancreas are implanted heterotopically in the iliac fossa in the groin. The arterial and venous connections for these organs are based on the iliac vessels. Both the kidney and pancreas also establish connections with the uri-

TABLE 27–5. Composition of Euro-Collins Solution

Component	Concentration (per Liter)
KH_2PO_4	2.05 gm
K_2HPO_4	7.4 gm
KCl	1.12 gm
$NaHCO_3$	0.84 gm
Glucose	35 gm

TABLE 27–6. Composition of University of Wisconsin (UW) Solution

Component	Concentration (per Liter)
K-lactobionate	100 mmol
K_2HPO_4	25 mmol
$MgSO_4$	5 mmol
Raffinose	30 mmol
Adenosine	5 mmol
Glutathione	3 mmol
Insulin	100 IU
Penicillin	40 IU
Dexamethasone	8 mg
Allopurinol	1 mmol
Hydroxyethyl starch	50 gm

nary bladder. Naturally, the ureter is implanted in the bladder. In addition, the pancreatic duct is connected to the bladder by leaving the pancreas attached to a segment of duodenum that includes the opening of the duct. This pancreatico–duodenocystostomy allows drainage of the exocrine pancreatic secretions into the bladder (Nghiem, 1986). This not only provides a convenient way to drain the duct, but also provides a portal to examine the pancreas for rejection since analysis of ductal effluent in the urine can provide evidence of pancreatic injury associated with rejection.

▶ IMMUNOLOGIC CONSIDERATIONS

Matching Donor and Recipient

Although there is a fair degree of variability, some degree of matching of donor and recipient occurs in heart, lung, liver, kidney, and pancreas transplantation. Donor and recipient must be ABO blood-type compatible. While there have been occasional examples of organs from ABO incompatible donors accepted in transplant recipients, this should be avoided since there is the risk of rapid, hyperacute rejection and destruction of the transplanted organ. Presumably this is mediated by antibodies in the recipient that react with blood cell or other proteins of the donor. Requirements for HLA (human leukocyte antigen) histocompatibility matching, size matching, and other considerations vary with individual organs.

Heart

In addition to ABO blood-type compatibility, heart donor and recipient must be of more or less the same size. This is because the heart must be large enough to support the circulation of the recipient, but not so large that it cannot fit in the pericardial cavity without undue compression and compromise of function. In practical terms, since most heart transplant recipients have dilated myopathies, over sizing is rarely an issue. On the other hand, considerable thought is given to making sure that the heart is large enough. This is particularly important when the recipient has significant pulmonary hypertension since the right ventricle must have the capacity to support the pressures in the pulmonary circuit. Nonetheless, hearts from donors who weigh half of the weight of the recipient have been used successfully in carefully selected circumstances. A closer weight match, such that the donor is no more than 10% to 25% below the recipient weight, is the more usual practice.

The human histocompatiblity antigens are termed HLA (for human leukocyte antigen) antigens. In heart transplantation, prospective matching for the six routinely typed antigens is not done. However, retrospective data suggest that fortuitous matching is associated with a better outcome (Opelz & Wujciak 1994). The number of donors, the short preservation times, and the resultant logistical difficulties presently preclude HLA matching in heart transplantation.

All patients waiting for a heart transplant undergo screening for preformed antibodies against a panel of likely donor antigens (PRA, or panel reactive antibodies). Patients with high levels of reactivity (20-100% of antigens tested) usually undergo a lymphocyte crossmatch with donor cells prior to accepting a specific donor heart. In this test, serum from the recipient is mixed with lymphocytes from the donor to detect the presence of donor-directed antibodies that might destroy the graft hyperacutely.

ABO compatible donors of appropriate size are allocated to heart recipients based on their medical acuity and time waiting for transplantation. If needed, a lymphocyte crossmatch is done prior to assigning the organ to a specific recipient.

Lung

Size matching is important in lung transplantation as well since the lung must fit properly in the pleural cavity to function optimally. Size matching is done on the basis of chest x-ray measurements of the thorax rather than by patient weight. As in heart transplantation, HLA matching is not done but a lymphocyte crossmatch may be required. Assignment of lungs is prioritized by clinical status and waiting time.

Liver

Size matching is much less critical in liver transplantation but the donor and recipient should be of roughly the same size for anatomic reasons and to insure adequate metabolic capacity. HLA matching is not done and recipients waiting are prioritized by clinical status and waiting time.

Kidney

Size matching is nearly irrelevant in kidney transplantation. However, when pediatric kidneys are to be used in an adult, both kidneys on an aortic pedicle may be used for one patient. HLA matching does determine kidney distribution in most regions. Recipients who share six HLA antigens with a specific donor are given preference for kidneys from that donor with fairly complex organ payback schemes between OPOs. For example, if an organ is exported from one OPO to another because of matching criteria, the recipient OPO owes the exporting OPO a "payback" kidney. Clinical status and waiting time also play roles in kidney allocation.

Pancreas

HLA matching directs organ allocation in pancreatic transplantation only when the pancreas is transplanted simultaneously with a kidney that is assigned based on a six-antigen match. Size is not an important consideration and priority for isolated pancreas transplantation is on the basis of time waiting.

Managing Rejection

Even with HLA matching, all transplant recipients must take immunosuppressive medications to prevent their immune systems from attacking and destroying the transplanted organ. Immune suppression is based on combination therapy with multiple agents. Adequate levels of immune suppression must be achieved to prevent the immune response from damaging the graft. At the same time, immune suppression must not be too intense lest the patient become susceptible to opportunistic infection (Brooks, 1986; Flint, 1994; Flume, 1994; Hughes, 1987; Rubin, 1990; Saliba, 1989). As it is, patients do suffer both infectious complications and episodes of acute rejection so the therapeutic margin for immunosuppressive drugs is very narrow. Acute rejection is treated with a short course of heavily intensified immune suppression.

Maintenance Immunosuppression

Maintenance immunosuppression for heart, lung, liver, kidney, and pancreas is achieved with a combination of steroids, cyclosporine, and azathioprine (Olivari, 1990; Opelz, 1994). Steroids have been a component of transplant immune suppression from the earliest days of transplantation. The immune suppressive actions of prednisone are nonspecific. Because its administration can retard healing, prednisone is usually withheld from lung transplant recipients for approximately 1 week following transplantation to allow for bronchial healing (Lima, 1981). Steroids are usually given initially in high dosages (1 mg/kg), then tapered to 0.05 to 0.1 mg/kg for long-term maintenance. Some patients can be withdrawn from steroids completely. Steroid complications include hypertension, glucose intolerance, obesity, wound-healing problems, and personality changes (Table 27–7).

Cyclosporine was introduced in 1980 and has been a cornerstone of transplant immune therapy since then (Burke, 1994; Ferguson, 1985). Cyclosporine can be given orally or IV but the usual route is oral. Its immune effects are not donor specific since it appears to act through nonspecific cellular signaling mechanisms including interleukin-2 (IL-2) (Kimball, 1993). Cyclosporine dosing is determined by blood level and adjusted for the patient's creatinine since the drug is quite nephrotoxic. Early blood levels of 200-300 ng/mL are sought with longer term maintenance levels of 100-200 ng/mL. Cyclosporine's toxicities include renal insufficiency, hypertension, hirsutism, tremor, and seizures (refer to Table 27–7).

TABLE 27–7. Nonimmunologic Complications of Immunosuppressive Drugs

Steroids
Obesity
Glucose intolerance
Hypertension
Wound-healing problems
Personality changes
Azathioprine
Bone marrow suppression
Cholestatic jaundice
Cyclosporine
Hypertension
Renal failure
Tremor
Hirsutism
Seizures

Azathioprine (Imuran) is one of the oldest synthetic drugs used for transplant immunosuppression having been introduced to clinical use in 1962. After the introduction of cyclosporine, the use of azathioprine decreased but subsequent experience has demonstrated that triple drug therapy is superior to regimens that do not include azathioprine (Montagnino, 1994). The actions of this drug are nonspecific since it works by preventing the proliferation of actively dividing cells. Its dosage is 2 mg/kg. White blood cell counts are monitored and the dose of azathioprine reduced or the drug held when the count falls below 4000 per mm^3. Toxicities include marrow suppression, as noted, and cholestasis (refer to Table 27–7).

Many transplant centers include a so-called "induction" regimen early after implantation of the organ (Costanzo-Nordin, 1990). In addition to higher doses of prednisone and cyclosporine, an antibody preparation against human lymphocytes may be used for 7 to 10 days. The most commonly used agents are ATGAM, a polyclonal antilymphocyte preparation of horse antibodies and OKT3, a murine (made in mice) monoclonal antilymphocyte. These agents have the potential to produce a severe systemic inflammatory response on first exposure and as foreign proteins can induce a host immune response that limits their subsequent effectiveness. Since these are some of the more powerful agents used to treat episodes of acute rejection, some centers prefer to defer their use until therapy of acute rejection is required.

Acute Rejection

All transplanted organs may be subject to episodes of acute rejection although in liver transplantation this is fairly rare. Acute rejection, when it is severe enough, can lead to the temporary or even permanent loss of function of the transplanted organ. Obviously, detection and treatment of rejection before this occurs is important. In fact, an effort is made to detect and treat rejection before it causes even mild loss of organ function.

The way rejection is diagnosed varies from organ to organ. Histologically, however, most episodes of acute rejection are characterized by infiltration of lymphocytes and destruction of organ cells. In severe cases, damage to blood vessels causes intraparenchymal hemorrhage. Some rejection episodes have relatively sparse cellular infiltrates. These episodes may be caused primarily by antidonor antibodies that destroy the graft directly and through activation of complement and other chemical agents.

Transvenous endomyocardial biopsy is used to monitor for and diagnose rejection in heart transplantation (Imakita, 1986). Indirect, noninvasive means have not proven to be reliable. The diagnosis of lung rejection can be more difficult. Patients may have fever and a new pulmonary infiltrate but in these circumstances rejection must be distinguished from infection. Pulmonary lavage has been tried as a means to detect inflammatory cells indicative of rejection but this method is not uniformly reliable. Transbronchial biopsy is used increasingly and ultimately may be the preferred diagnostic method in lung transplantation.

Biopsy is not used routinely to diagnose rejection in liver, kidney, and pancreas transplantation. As noted, acute rejection is less common in liver transplantation. Blood tests that measure function of these organs or that are measures of parenchymal cellular damage are used as indications for percutaneous needle biopsy of the liver or kidney. In liver transplantation, therefore, serum bilirubin and liver enzymes may be followed as well as synthetic hepatic function as measured by clotting studies (prothrombin time, etc.). In kidney transplantation, renal function as measured by serum creatinine and urine output are the key measures of function that deteriorate when rejection occurs. As noted, a definitive diagnosis of acute rejection can be made by percutaneous needle biopsy.

The transplanted pancreas cannot be biopsied easily. The signs of acute pancreatic rejection are similar to and must be distinguished from those of graft thrombosis and pancreatitis. A rise in serum glucose is a relatively late manifestation of rejection as 90% of the islet cell mass must be destroyed before hyperglycemia occurs. Urinary amylase is a useful way to monitor the exocrine function of the pancreas and therefore detect rejection. A fall of 30% to 50% in the level of urinary amylase—which by week 2 following transplantation can be expected to reach 30,000 IU/Liter—appears to be a good indicator of pancreatic rejection. The pancreas also excretes bicarbonate. Urine pH should be above 7 after pancreas transplantation with duct implantation in the bladder. Early rejection may cause a fall in urine pH.

The treatment of acute rejection of any transplanted organ is a short course of intensified immunosuppression. This most commonly takes the form of a bolus of steroids, such as solumedrol 1 gm intravenously daily for three days. Persistent or severe rejection may be treated also with a course of antilymphocyte globulin such as ATGAM or OKT3 (Tesi, 1993). Refractory rejection has led some groups to put patients on such newer agents as tacrolimus (FK-506), rapamycin, or mycophenolate mofetil (European FK506 Multicentre Study Group, 1994; Griffith, 1994; Jordan, 1994). Some of these agents are also being tried in routine maintenance regimens. In some cases, less conventional agents like cyclophosphamide, methotrexate, or vincristine have been used when rejection does not respond to conventional therapy (Costanzo-Nordin, 1988).

Chronic Rejection

In addition to acute rejection, all transplant recipients are susceptible to chronic rejection. While presumably this also has an immune etiology, the histologic and functional features of chronic rejection are different from acute rejection. In all cases, however, chronic rejection seems to be marked by a proliferative–obliterative process. In hearts, chronic rejection is marked by graft coronary artery disease (Crisp, 1994; Gao, 1989). This process leads to diffuse myointimal hyperplasia of the coronary arteries. When this process is severe, myocardial ischemia results. Because of the diffuse nature of this process, it is rarely amenable to usual means of revascularization like angioplasty or bypass surgery.

Similarly, transplanted lungs are susceptible to a chronic process called obliterative bronchiolitis (Novick, 1994). This proliferative process affects the bronchioles rather than blood vessels but has equally dire prognostic implications for the lung graft. The liver is susceptible to obliterative bile duct changes (Backman, 1993) and the kidney may suffer a proliferative glomerulopathy that destroys glomerular function (Almond, 1993). The etiology of these processes is not well understood and therefore effective therapy is not available. Development of these manifestations of chronic rejection does not seem to depend on the frequency or severity of prior episodes of acute rejection. Nor can they be controlled with immunosuppressive drugs.

Results

In addition to the limitations that chronic immune processes put on the results of organ transplantation, transplant recipients are susceptible to long-term complications of immunosuppression. Some of these, including infection, which is less common late when the intensity of immune suppression is less, have been noted. Another consequence of long-term immune suppression is malignancy, particularly lymphoproliferative disorders (Penn, 1993; Penn & First, 1986; Ritter, 1994; Swinnen, 1990). These are difficult to treat, requiring diminution of the level of immune suppression and sometimes chemotherapy. Acute rejection of the graft is clearly a risk in these circumstances.

Despite these limitations, the results of modern organ transplantation are in general quite spectacular (Bromberg, 1997). In heart transplantation, 1-year survivals are over 90% in many centers, with 5-year survival over 70%. The results of lung transplantation are not yet this good. Overall 1-year survival is about 70%. This drops to 63% at 2 years and 46% at 5 years. Patients with emphysema have the best survival rates whereas those with pulmonary hypertension appear to have the worst. In most centers doing liver transplantation, patient survival rates for 1 and 5 years are 75% and 65%, respectively. Interestingly, an important determinant of patient survival after liver transplantation is the condition of the patient at the time of transplantation. The survival rate for patients taken to surgery directly from the intensive care unit is 42%, compared with 84% in patients not sick enough to require ICU care. In cadaveric renal transplantation, 1-year kidney survival is 90% or better, with graft survival 80% at 5 years, and nearly that good at 8 years. For recipients of pancreas transplants, 1- and 5-year patient survivals are about 90% and 80%, and graft survivals at these intervals are approximately 75% and 60%.

REFERENCES

Almond, P. S., Matas, A., Gillingham, K., et al. (1993). Risk factors for chronic rejection in renal allograft recipients. *Transplantation, 55,* 752–757.

Angstwurm, H. & Einhaupt, K. (1984). Organ donors and brain death diagnosis: Experiences in the diagnosis and documentation of brain death. *Transplant Proceeding, 16,* 95–97.

Backman, L. K., Gibbs, J., Levy, M., et al. (1993). Causes of late graft loss after liver transplantation. *Transplantation, 55,* 1078–1082.

Barbosa, J., Steffes, M. W., Sutherland, D. E. R., Connett, J. D., Rao, K. V., & Mauer, S. M. (1994). Effect of glycemic control on early diabetic renal lesions: A 5-year randomized controlled trial of insulin-dependent diabetic kidney transplant recipients. *JAMA, 272,* 600–606.

Baumgartner, W. A., Reitz, B. A., Oyer, P. E., et al. (1979). Cardiac homotransplantation. *Current Problems in Surgery, 16,* 1–61.

Belzer, F. O. & Southard, J. H. (1988). Principles of solid-organ preservation by cold storage. *Transplantation, 45,* 673–676.

Blanche, C., Valenza, M., Czer, L. S. C., et al. (1994a). Orthotopic heart transplantation with bicaval and pulmonary venous anastomoses. *Annals of Thoracic Surgery, 58,* 1505–1509.

Blanche, C., Valenza, M., Czer, L. S. C., et al. (1994b). Combined heart and kidney transplantation with allografts from the same donor. *Annals of Thoracic Surgery, 58,* 1135–1138.

Bromberg, J. S., Punch, J. D., Merion, R. M., et al. (1997). Transplantation and immunology. In L. J. Greenfield, M. Mulholland, K. T. Oldham, G. B. Zelenock, K. D. Lillemoe (Eds.), *Surgery: Scientific Principles and Practice* (pp. 527–632). Philadelphia: Lippincott-Raven.

Brooks, R. G. & Remington, J. S. (1986). Transplant-related infections. In J. V. Bennet & P. S. Brachman (Eds.). *Hospital Infections (2nd ed.).* (pp. 561–618). Boston: Little, Brown.

Burke, Jr., J. R., Pirsch, J. D., Ramos, E. L., et al. (1994). Long-term efficacy and safety of cyclosporine in renal transplant recipients. *New England Journal of Medicine, 331,* 358–363.

Cho, Y. W., Cecka, J. M., & Terasaki, P. I. (1994). HLA matching effect: Better survival rates and graft quality. In P. I. Terasaki & J. M. Cecka (Eds.), *Clinical Transplants 1994* (pp. 435–449). Los Angeles: UCLA Tissue Typing Laboratory.

Costanzo-Nordin, M. R., Grusk, B. B., Silver, M. A., et al. (1988). Reversal of recalcitrant cardiac allograft rejection with methotrexate. *Circulation, 78* (Suppl III), 47–57.

Costanzo-Nordin, M. R., O'Sullivan, J., Johnson, M. R., et al. (1990). Prospective randomized trial of OKT3 versus horse antithymocyte globulin-based immunosuppressive prophylaxis in heart transplantation. *Journal of Heart and Lung Transplantation 9,* 306–315.

Council on Ethical and Judicial Affairs, American Medical Association (1994). Strategies for cadaveric organ procurement. *JAMA, 272,* 809–812.

Crisp, S. J., Dunn, M. J., Rose, J. S., Barber, J., & Yacoub, M. H. (1994). Antiendothelial antibodies after heart transplantation: The accelerating factor in transplant-associated coronary artery disease? *Journal of Heart and Lung Transplantation, 13,* 81–92.

D'Allessandro, A. M., Hoffmann, R. M., Knechtle, S. J., et al. (1995). Successful extra-renal transplantation from non-heart beating donors. *Transplantation, 59,* 977–982

D'Allessandro, A. M., Sollinger, H. W., Hoffmann, R. M., et al. (1990). Experience with Belzer UW cold storage solution in simultaneous pancreas–kidney transplantation. *Transplant Proceedings, 22,* 532–534.

Darby, J. M., Stein, K., Grevnik, A., & Stuart, S. A. (1989). Approach to management of the heartbeating "brain dead" organ donor. *JAMA, 261,* 2222–2228.

Egan, T. M, Kaiser, L. R., & Cooper, J. D. (1989). Lung transplantation. *Current Problems in Surgery, 10,* 681–751.

Emery, R. W., Cork, R. C., Levinson, M. M., et al. (1986). The cardiac donor: A six-year experience. *Annals of Thoracic Surgery, 41,* 356–362.

European FK506 Multicentre Liver Study Group (1994). Randomised trial comparing Tacrolimus (FK506) and Cyclosporin in prevention of liver allograft rejection. *Lancet, 344,* 423–428.

Ferguson, R. M. & Sommer, B. G. (1985). Cyclosporine (CsA) in renal transplantation: A single institution experience. *American Journal of Kidney Diseases, 5,* 296–306.

Flint, A. & Frank, T. S. (1994). Cytomegalovirus detection in lung transplant biopsy samples by polymerase chain reaction. *Journal of Heart and Lung Transplantation, 13,* 38–42.

Flume, P. A., Egan, T. M., Paradowski, L. J., Detterbeck, F. C., Thompson, J. T., & Yankaskas, J. R. (1994). Infectious complications of lung transplantation: Impact of cystic fibrosis. *American Journal of Respiratory and Critical Care Medicine, 149,* 1601–1607.

Gao, S. Z., Schroeder, J. S., Alderman, E. L., et al. (1989). Prevalence of accelerated coronary artery disease in heart transplant survivors. *Circulation, 80* (Suppl III), III 100–105.

Griffith, B. P., Bando, K., Hardesty, R. L., et al. (1994). A prospective randomized trial of FK506 versus cyclosporine after human pulmonary transplantation. *Transplantation, 57,* 848–851.

Hauptman, P. J. & O'Connor, K. J. (1997). Procurement and allocation of solid organs for transplantation. *New England Journal of Medicine, 336* (6), 422–431.

Haverich, A., Scott, W. C., & Jamieson, S. W. (1985). Twenty years of lung preservation: A review. *Journal of Heart and Lung Transplantation, 4,* 234–240.

Hughes, W. T., Rivera, G. K., Shell, M. J., Thornton, D., & Lott, L. (1987). Successful intermittent chemoprophylaxis for *Pneumocyctis carinii* pneumonitis. *New England Journal of Medicine, 316,* 1627–1632.

Imakita, M., Tazelaar, H. D., & Billingham, M. E. (1986). Heart allograft rejection under varying immunosuppressive protocols as evaluated by endomyocardial biopsy. *Journal of Heart and Lung Transplantation, 5,* 279–285.

Jordan, M. D., Shapiro, R., Vivas, C. A., et al. (1994). FK506 "rescue" for resistant rejection of renal allografts under primary cyclosporine immunosuppression. *Transplantation, 57,* 860–865.

Kimball, P. M., Kerman, R. K., Van Buren, C. T., Lewis, R. M., Katz, S., & Kahan, B. D. (1993). Cyclosporine and Rapamycin affect protein kinase C induction of the intracellular activation signal, activator of DNA replication. *Transplantation, 55,* 1128–1132.

Kramer, M. R., Valentine, H. A., Marshall, S. E., Starnes, V. A., & Theodore, J. (1994). Recovery of the right ventricle after single-lung transplantation in pulmonary hypertension. *American Journal of Cardiology, 73,* 494–500.

Lima, O., Goldberg, M., Peters, W. S., et al. (1981). Effects of methylprednisolone and azathioprine on bronchial healing following lung transplantation. *Journal of Thoracic and Cardiovascular Surgery, 83,* 211–215.

Merion, R. M., Oh, H. K., Port, F. K., et al. (1990). A prospective randomized trial of cold-storage versus machine-perfusion preservation in cadaveric renal transplantation. *Transplantation, 50,* 230–233.

Merrill, J. P., Murray, J. E., Harrison, J. H., & Guild, W. R. (1956). Successful homotransplantation of the human kidney between identical twins. *JAMA, 160,* 277–282.

Montagnino, G., Tarantino, A., Banfi, G., Aroldi, A., Cesana, B., & Ponticelli, C. (1994). A randomized trial comparing triple-drug and double-drug therapy in renal transplantation: Analysis at 7 years. *Transplantation, 58,* 149–154.

Nghiem, D. D., Beutel, W. D., & Corry, R. J. (1986). Duodenocystostomy for exocrine pancreatic drainage in total pancreatic transplantation: A preliminary report. *Transplant Proceedings, 18,* 1874–1876.

Novick, R. J., Andreassian, B. Schafers, H. J., et al. (1994). Pulmonary retransplantation for obliterative bronchiolitis: Intermediate-term results of a North American–European series. *Journal of Thoracic Cardiovascular Surgery, 107,* 755–763.

Olivari, M. R., Kubo, S. H., Braulin, E. A., Bolman, R. M., & Ring, W. S. (1990). Five-year experience with triple-drug immunosuppressive therapy in cardiac transplantation. *Circulation, 82,* 276–280.

Opelz, G. (1994). Effect of the maintenance immunosuppressive drug regimen on kidney transplant outcome. *Transplantation, 58,* 443–436.

Opelz, G. & Wujciak, T. (1994). The influence of HLA compatibility on graft survival after heart transplantation. *New England Journal of Medicine, 330,* 816–819.

Penn, I. (1993). The effect of immunosuppression on pre-existing cancers. *Transplantation, 55,* 742–747.

Penn, I. & First, M. R. (1986). Development and incidence of cancer following cyclosporine therapy. *Transplant Proceedings, 18* (2 suppl 1), 210–215.

Pierce, G. A., Graham, W. K., Kauffman, H. M. Jr., & Wolf, J. S. (1996). The United Network for Organ Sharing: 1984-1994. *Transplant Proceedings, 28,* 12–15.

Randall, T. (1991). Too few human organs for transplantation, too many in need . . . and the gap widens. *JAMA, 265,* 1223–1227.

Ritter, J. H. & Wick, M. R. (1994). Posttransplant lymphoproliferative disorders: Immunohistologic differential diagnosis with severe allograft rejection. *International Journal of Surgical Pathology, 2,* 105–116.

Rubin, R. H. (1990). Impact of cytomegalovirus infection on organ transplant recipients. *Review of Infectious Diseases, 12* (Suppl), S754–766.

Saliba, F., Ephraim, R., Mathieu, D. et al. (1994). Risk factors for bacterial infection after liver transplantation. *Transplant Proceedings, 26,* 266.

Soifer, B. E. & Gelb, A. W. (1989). The multiple organ donor: Identification and management. *Annals of Internal Medicine, 110,* 814–823.

Starzl T. & Demetrius, A. (1990). Liver transplantation: A 31-year perspective. *Current Problems of Surgery, 27,* 49–116.

Sutherland, D. E. R., Dunn, D. L., Goetz, F. C., et al. (1989). A 10-year experience with 290 pancreas transplants at a single institution. *Annals of Surgery, 210,* 274–285.

Swinnen, L. J., Costanzo-Nordin, M. R., Fisher, S. G., et al. (1990). Increase incidence of lymphoproliferative disorder after immunosuppression with the monoclonal antibody OKT3 in cardiac transplant recipients. *New England Journal of Medicine, 323,* 1723–1728.

Tesi, R. J., Elkhammas, E. A., Henry, M. L., et al. (1993). OKT3 for primary therapy of first rejection episode in kidney transplants. *Transplantation, 55,* 1023–1029.

The UNOS Bulletin, 2 (1997).

Todo, S., Nery, J., Yanaga, K., et al. (1989). Extended preservation of human liver grafts with UW solution. *JAMA, 261,* 711–714.

28

Rehabilitation

Judi Kuric

Rehabilitation has traditionally been thought of as health care provided to neurologically injured patients (stroke, head injury, spinal cord injury) in a specialized setting. By definition, rehabilitation helps patients affected by disability, chronic illness, and aging adapt to a changed lifestyle, attain the highest possible level of functional ability, and maintain optimal health (Hartmann & Cordis, 1997). The continual changes in the health-care delivery system have facilitated the growth of rehabilitation concepts used by nearly every health-care professional in all settings.

The major goals of rehabilitation are to improve function, promote independence and life satisfaction, and preserve self esteem (Brummel-Smith, 1990). These goals are accomplished by the management of complex medical issues, consultation with specialists, ongoing patient and family education, improving function for maximal independence, and establishment of plans of care to maintain optimal wellness (Hartmann & Cordis, 1997). Improving function means maximizing the person's abilities to live in the least restrictive and most desirable environment. This is accomplished by preventing complications, modifying the effects of disability, and increasing independence (Sayles, 1981).

The diverse and encompassing needs of each patient require an interdisciplinary treatment team to assist each patient in achieving his or her highest functional level. In rehabilitation, the patient is considered to be the most important member of the team. This participation in the planning and execution of goals and activities is essential. Other professionals participating on the treatment team are determined by the patient's needs, facility or program, and reimbursement.

Rehabilitation begins the moment a person seeks health care. The provider is focused on the diagnosis and treatment of the primary condition and preventing further complications. In the acute care setting, the primary problems are often life threatening and multisystem in nature. The treatment plan is aimed at preventing complications critical to the long-term outcome of the patient. For example, early intervention in the patient with a severe head injury focuses on the control of intracranial pressure via pressure monitoring, osmotic diuretics, hyperventilation, and drug-induced coma. While these interventions are primarily aimed at patient survival, they also are directed at prevention of secondary complications and further neurologic deterioration. This patient's long-term function will be influenced by these aggressive efforts at prevention of secondary injury and other complications.

▶ ASSESSING THE POTENTIAL FOR REHABILITATION

"Rehabilitation potential" is the unrealized power to improve function that exists within a person that can eventually become realized. Some diagnoses such as stroke, head injury, and spinal cord injury lend themselves to automatic rehabilitation referrals due to the nature and lasting effects of these injuries. Patients with deficits in their abilities to manage their disease, provide for their own self care, or manage their environment may also benefit from rehab services. Table 28–1 lists some diagnoses with which patients may benefit from rehabilitation.

Activities of daily living (ADLs) are activities that must be accomplished for a patient to assume responsibility for his or her own needs and to participate in society. A patient's ability to accomplish these activities can be done through independent performance or verbal direction to a caregiver. Independence can be measured by the degree of responsibility assumed by the patient for these ADLs as necessary for successful function at home, at work, and in social situations.

Three areas of ADLs focus on different aspects of function:

1. **Personal/physical—**Deficits in personal care and health can be conceptualized using Gordon's Functional Health Patterns (1991).
   - Health Perception/Health Management—improve the patient's (and/or caregivers) knowledge level and/or modify health-related behaviors
   - Nutritional/Metabolic—impaired swallowing, risk for changes in skin integrity, inability to manage complications
   - Elimination—incontinence, retention, or ineffective patterns of bowel and bladder function; high risk or presence of infection
   - Activity/Exercise—paralysis, safety issues, orthostatic hypotension, generalized weakness and/or muscle wasting, poor endurance; inability to perform activities including bathing, toileting, grooming, eating, oral hygiene, dressing, mobility
   - Cognitive/Perceptual—problems with orientation, poor concentration or judgment, confusion, difficulty with problem solving, decreased memory, poor attention span, visual field deficits
   - Self-Perception/Self Concept—body image (visual neglect), changes in body image/self esteem
   - Coping/Stress/Tolerance—coping patterns, delayed or ineffective in reducing or managing stressful responses, depression
   - Communication Deficits—aphasias (fluent and non-fluent), hearing deficit or loss, inappropriate communication patterns
   - Sexual—physiologic dysfunction
   - Role/Relationship—changes in personal, vocational, or social roles and abilities
2. **Instrumental—**Management of the telephone, shopping, transportation, mobility outside the home
3. **Occupational/role activities—**Management of homemaking, parenting, spousal roles, vocational activities

TABLE 28–1. Common Diagnoses Seen in Rehabilitation

AIDS
ALS
Amputation
Brain Injury
Burns
COPD
CVA
Guillian-Barré Syndrome
Joint Replacement
Multiple Sclerosis
Oncology
Spinal Cord Injury

Patients with any of the deficits described above should be evaluated by a rehabilitation professional to determine their rehab potential. A patient's rehab potential is influenced by the likelihood to increase his or her independence, increase his or her knowledge level, reach a set of mutually agreeable goals, and/or improve the quality of life for that patient. The extent of services will be influenced by the patient's physical limitations, caregiver support, financial resources, and motivation.

For example, following an acute hospitalization for pneumonia, an AIDS patient may benefit from a short inpatient rehab stay to improve endurance, enhance energy conservation, provide caregiver education, and modify the living environment. Achieving these goals would allow this patient to remain in his or her own home in lieu of placement in an extended-care facility. On the other hand, a similar patient without caregiver support or lack of desire to meet these goals would probably not be considered an inpatient rehab candidate.

▶ PLANNING AND IMPLEMENTATION

During the early phases of acute illness or injury, prevention of secondary complications is essential in achieving positive long-term outcome of the patient. Early consultation with a physiatrist (within 24 hours of admission) and initiation of physical and occupational therapy services is recommended. It is common for health-care providers to delay consultation with rehabilitation professionals initially until it is determined if the patient is going to survive his or her initial insult. Early consultation and intervention maximize the rehab process and improve the patient's outcomes.

Early implementation of rehabilitation should include these interventions:

- Health Perception/Health Management—initiation of patient/family education, reinforcement of education, elimination of misconceptions and unfounded fears; involve patient/family in planning rehab program
- Nutritional/Metabolic—aggressive prevention of skin breakdown; early nutritional supplementation; prevention of complications

- Elimination—prevention of infections; early initiation of bladder management (Table 28–2) and bowel management programs (Tables 28–3 and 28–4)
- Activity/Exercise—range-of-motion exercises; maintenance/improvement of muscle strength, early mobilization, increasing sitting tolerance; aggressive respiratory support and hygiene; prevention of thrombic events; prevention of secondary complications
- Cognitive/Perceptual—early assessment of cognitive function; incorporation of compensatory techniques in care and education
- Self-Perception/Self Concept—environmental management (visual neglect); emotional support for physical adaptations
- Role/Relationship—support for the patient, family, and significant others
- Sexuality/Reproductive—education; elimination of fears and myths
- Coping/Stress/Tolerance—support of patient/family coping patterns; early family involvement in care
- Value-Belief—support of patient/family spirituality

TRANSITION TO THE REHAB SETTING

There is a diverse range of inpatient rehabilitation settings available. Each of these settings provides varying services that can be beneficial to the same patient at different points in his or her rehabilitation process. The patient's most immediate goals and physical status will dictate the most appropriate setting and need for transfer to other settings.

Long-term acute care hospitals (LTAH) provide care to a medically stable patient with a high level of acuity. Patents who require medical ventilation, vasoactive medications, dialysis, or other acute physiologic support are candidates for this setting. The advantages to this setting is the higher staffing ratio for the more acute patient without the restriction on length of stays and diagnosis-related groups (DRGs).

Comprehensive inpatient rehabilitation settings have the broadest range of services available. They are required by Council on Accreditation of Rehabilitation Facilities (CARF) to use an interdisciplinary treatment team that includes a physician who specializes in rehabilitation, rehab nursing, physical therapist, occupational therapist, speech–language pathologist, social worker/discharge planner, psychologist, and therapeutic recreation therapist. These professionals are the core team members. Other professionals must also be available for consultation to meet the patient's needs; for example, a plastic surgeon for a burn patient or pulmonologist for ventilator management.

Subacute units are designed for patients who do not require or cannot tolerate the full range of services provided by a comprehensive program. These programs may also be limited by the amount and type of therapy provided. A comatose patient or an oncology patient undergoing chemotherapy are examples of patients requiring care and support within a rehab framework but probably not appropriate for a comprehensive program.

A rising trend in the rehabilitation arena is the increase in outpatient rehabilitation programs. These programs can be compared with home infusion programs. The patient returns home with assistance and receives intense rehabilitation from professionals coming to the home. Home-based rehabilitation has proven effective for patients with a variety of diagnoses. Work-hardening programs are for patients who need additional therapy, increasing strength/endurance, or compensatory techniques to return to their vocational setting.

Facilities and treatment programs will usually assess the patient to determine his or her appropriateness for the particular facility or program. The factors in this decision usually include the patient's physical condition, goals, potential to reach rehab goals, caregiver support, financial resources, and patient/caregiver preferences. Other potential discharge locations include an extended-care facility, home with inclusion

TABLE 28–2. Initiating a Bladder Management Program

1. Discontinue indwelling catheter when urine volume is less than 600 cc every 4 hours
2. For urinary retention, use intermittent catheterization every 4 to 6 hours. Urine volumes should be 600 cc or less
3. For urinary incontinence, use external collection devices, timed voiding, absorbent padding with frequent skin care

TABLE 28–3. Initiating a Bowel Management Program

Goal: Elimination of soft, formed stool every 1 to 3 days.
Initiate an individualized program based on the following components
- Empty lower bowel, an enema may be necessary
- Establish a time of day based on patient's pre-admission pattern
- Diet high in roughage
- Increased fluid intake if not contraindicated
- Administer medications as indicated
- A sitting position is encouraged
- Insert suppository or use digital stimulation
- Repeat every day at the same established time

TABLE 28–4. Common Bowel Medications

Bulk formers—e.g., Metamucil 15 ml daily
Stool softeners—e.g., docusate sodium 100 mg TID
Mild laxatives—e.g., Milk of Magnesia 30 ml daily
Suppositories—glycerin or dulcolax as needed

in a day treatment or home therapy program, group homes, work tolerance settings, supervised living, behavior management programs, or residential treatment facilities.

A positive transition to any rehabilitation setting is facilitated by familiarity of the new setting, ongoing education, and psycho–social support of the patient and family. Always encourage family members to visit the facility (or program) and share information with the patient. The nurse or other health professional who assesses the patient is an excellent source of information and support, and many times can make recommendations for treatment until transfer arrangements can be arranged. These interventions decrease the patient's anxiety and support his or her coping and adaptation to the new setting.

Fear, frustration, loneliness, and anxiety are all common in a patient moving to another health-care setting. These emotions are not only uncomfortable but can also interfere with rehabilitation goal attainment (Nypervar et al., 1996). Patient/family education, and facilitation of control and decision-making activities, support a more positive transition and enhance the early rehabilitation period.

With medical and pharmacological advances, more patients are surviving catastrophic injuries and illnesses. Rehabilitation is useful to a wide variety of patients in order to increase individual self-care abilities, reach their maximal functional level, and improve their ability to function within society. Shorter lengths of stay in the acute care setting and increased acuity mean an increase in the number of patients who should be considered for rehabilitation. No particular diagnosis or functional limitation should determine a patient eligible or ineligible for rehabilitation. Each patient should be evaluated based on his or her deficits, functional needs and abilities, and other resources to determine the patient's rehabilitation needs and the mechanism to best meet those needs.

REFERENCES

Bronstein, J. S., Popovich, J., & Steward-Amidei, C. (1991). *Promoting stroke recovery: A research-based approach for nurses.* St. Louis: Mosby.

Brummel-Smith, K. (1990). *Introduction to rehabilitation.* In B. Kemp, K. Brummel-Smith, & J. W. Ramsdell (Eds.), *Geriatric Rehabilitation.* Austin, TX: Pro-Ed.

Gordon, M. (1991). *Manual of nursing diagnosis, 1991–1992.* St. Louis: Mosby.

Hartmann, J. & Cordis, A. (1997). The association of rehabilitation nurses. *Rehabilitation Management, 10* (6), 13–16.

Hickey, J. V. (1996). Rehabilitation of neuroscience patients. In J. V. Hickey, *The clinical practice of neurological and neurosurgical nursing* (4th ed.). Philadelphia: Lippincott.

Hoeman, S. P. (Ed.). (1996). *Rehabilitation nursing: Process and application.* St. Louis: Mosby.

Johnson, K. M. M. (Ed.). (1997). *Advanced practice nursing in rehabilitation: A core curriculum.* Glenview, IL: The Rehabilitation Nursing Foundation.

McCourt, A. E. (Ed.). (1993). *The Speciality Practice of Rehabilitation Nursing: A Core Curriculum* (3rd ed.). Glenview, IL: The Rehabilitation Nursing Foundation.

Nypaver, J. M., Titus, M., & Brugler, C. J. (1996). Patient transfer to rehabilitation: Just another move? *Rehabilitation Nursing, 21* (2), 94–97.

Patterson, T. (1994). Rehabilitation. In E. Barker (Ed.), *Neuroscience Nursing.* St. Louis: Mosby.

Sayles, S. M. (Ed.). (1981). *Rehabilitation nursing: concepts and practice: A core curriculum.* Evanston, IL: Rehabilitation Nursing Institute.

Zedjlik, C. (1992). *Management of spinal cord injury* (2nd ed.). Boston: Jones and Barlett.

IV

Approach to the Patient with an Acute Illness

29

Lipid Problems

Hugh Lipshutz

Despite a recent decline in mortality, coronary artery disease (CAD) remains the major cause of death in the United States. Surprising to many patients, this remains true today in both male and female populations. Concomitant with the growth of the managed care industry in this country, we have witnessed an increased emphasis on primary prevention. Remarkably, this has occurred in both the medical and lay communities.

The decline in the CAD mortality in this country is almost certainly multifactorial, and is not totally understood. A large portion of the mortality reduction, however, is likely attributable to changes in lifestyle associated with risk-factor modification.

Risk factors are those factors present in a patient or population that have been shown to be associated with an increased prevalence of morbidity and mortality due to coronary artery disease. One of the largest and best known trials, the Framingham Study, was the first to describe both primary and secondary risk factors for CAD. Primary risk factors identified to date include hypercholesterolemia, tobacco use, hypertension, sedentary lifestyle, obesity, family history of cardiovascular disease, Type A personality, and diabetes mellitus.

The role of lipids and cholesterol in the development of coronary artery disease and the pathophysiology of acute myocardial syndromes (infarction and unstable angina) have recently garnered much attention. We are in the midst of the cholesterol revolution, with increased public awareness leading to lifestyle and other changes resulting in lowered levels of plasma lipids. We have also recently seen the introduction of a new pharmacologic class of drugs, the HMG–CoA reductase inhibitors, capable of dramatically lowering plasma lipid levels and affecting cardiovascular morbidity and mortality profoundly.

This chapter examines lipid problems. A brief overview of normal anatomy and physiology is provided, followed by a review of the pathophysiology of hyperlipidemia. Pertinent findings of the history and physical examination are reviewed, along with pertinent laboratory findings. The management and follow-up of hypercholesterolemic patients are covered extensively.

▶ SERUM LIPIDS AND LIPOPROTEINS

The major plasma lipids include cholesterol, triglyceride, phospholipid, and cholesterol ester. Lipids by definition are not water soluble and therefore cannot circulate in free form in the blood. Lipids, therefore, circulate as macromolecular complexes known as lipoproteins. Lipoproteins consist of a hydrophobic fatty core surrounded by a hydrophilic surface. Specific proteins known as apolipoproteins bind to the outer membrane of the molecule.

The hydrophobic core of a typical lipoprotein particle consists largely of triglyceride and cholesterol ester. The surrounding hydrophilic layer consists of primarily phospholipid and some free cholesterol, as well as the apolipoproteins, that are bound to the outer layer of the molecule. The apolipoproteins primarily determine the metabolic actions of the lipoprotein molecule.

The two apolipoprotein molecules of clinical interest are apolipoprotein A-1 (apoA-1) and apolipoprotein B-100 (apoB-100). ApoA-1 is the primary surface protein component of HDL particles. ApoA-1 is responsible for the metabolic effects of HDL-C through its activation of the enzyme lecithin cholesterol acyl transferase (LCAT). ApoB-100 is the major surface protein component of LDL particles and is responsible for recognition and binding at the LDL receptor site.

There are four major classes of lipoproteins: chylomicrons, very-low density lipoproteins (VLDL), low-density lipoproteins (LDL), and high-density lipoproteins (HDL). These are classified by ultracentrifugation according to density.

Chylomicrons are the largest of the lipoprotein particles. Their core consists mainly of triglycerides. Chylomicrons are formed in the intestinal epithelium and are derived almost exclusively from dietary fat. Chylomicrons appear early after ingestion of a fatty meal, and circulate for approximately 12 to 14 hours. They are cleared by the enzyme lipoprotein lipase located in the capillary endothelial wall. Their function is to transport dietary fat from the gut to peripheral sites for further metabolism.

VLDL particles are manufactured in the liver. Their core also consists of triglycerides, in this case synthesized by the liver from plasma glucose and free fatty acids. VLDL particles are also broken down by lipoprotein lipase, in this case to an intermediate particle known as intermediate-density lipoprotein (IDL). IDL is eventually either directly taken up into the liver or metabolized to LDL.

Low-density lipoprotein (LDL) is the major cholesterol-containing lipoprotein. LDL particles are formed mainly by breakdown of IDL. Apolipoprotein B-100 is the major apolipoprotein present in LDL. LDL is metabolized in the liver, after binding to specific LDL receptors.

High-density lipoprotein (HDL) is manufactured by both liver and intestine, and is also derived from peripheral catabolism of chylomicrons and VLDL. HDL plays a role in the transfer of cholesterol, removing it from the peripheral tissue.

▶ DYSLIPIDEMIA

As noted earlier, LDL, the major cholesterol carrying lipoprotein, is metabolized in the liver after binding to an LDL receptor. This LDL receptor is found in reduced numbers in patients with a diet high in saturated fat and cholesterol. Decreased numbers of hepatic LDL receptors in turn lead to elevated circulating levels of LDL. Circulating LDL may then be oxidized to a form that is readily taken up by macrophages, resulting in the formation of foam cells. Early atherosclerotic lesions or fatty streaks consist primarily of foam cells and lipid-filled smooth muscle cells. LDL is the major lipoprotein found in these atherosclerotic lesions.

HDL particles may protect against the development of atherosclerosis through a process known as reverse cholesterol transport. Cholesterol is taken up at the peripheral cell and transported back to the liver where it is metabolized. In general, therefore, HDL levels are inversely related to the risk of developing atherosclerosis.

HDL levels are largely genetically predetermined and are difficult to modify even in the diseased state. Factors that tend to increase levels of HDL include exercise and moderate ingestion of alcohol. There are at least two subtypes of HDL: HDL2 and HDL3. Both subtypes appear to confer protection against the development of atherosclerosis.

History and Physical Exam

Often overlooked in the field of hyperlipidemia are the roles of the history taking and physical examination. In this era of cost containment and managed care, the relative cost effectiveness of the office visit increases in importance. Treatment of hyperlipidemia in any given patient requires an understanding of that patient's risk of atherosclerosis. Special attention should be given to any documented history of atherosclerosis such as previous history of myocardial infarction, angina pectoris, cerebrovascular accident or transient ischemic attack, as well as peripheral vascular disease. Risk factors for coronary disease, including a history of hypertension, cigarette smoking, diabetes, or a family history of coronary artery disease, should be carefully assessed.

The physical examination should include a thorough search for signs of hyperlipidemia, including the presence of xanthalasma or corneal arcus. Signs of vascular disease such as the presence of carotid, abdominal, or femoral bruits should be noted. Carotid, brachial, radial, femoral, popliteal, as well as dorsalis pedis and posterior tibial pulses should be assessed.

Laboratory and Diagnostic Tests

No clinical evaluation for hyperlipidemia is complete without an assessment of serum lipid levels. In a perfect world, all patients should have knowledge of values for total cholesterol as well as HDL-C, LDL-C, and triglyceride levels. Unfortunately, recommendations for lipid testing must take into account the cost effectiveness of such testing.

In the United States, an expert panel convened by the National Heart Lung and Blood Institute offers pertinent guidance. Published in 1993, the Summary of the Second Report of the National Expert Panel on Detection, Evaluation, and Treatment of High Blood Cholesterol in Adults (NCEP II) presents the panel's updated recommendations for cholesterol management in adults.

The NCEP II report calls for measurement of total serum cholesterol (TC) in all adults 20 years of age and older at least once every 5 years. This measurement may be made in the nonfasting state, and should include an HDL level at the time of initial screening. Those with a high blood cholesterol, defined as a TC > 240 mg/dL, should undergo a fasting lipoprotein analysis. The initial screening exam may be performed in the nonfasting state because NCEP guidelines for the management of healthy adults without overt coronary artery disease are based on levels of total cholesterol and HDL cholesterol. In comparison with the fasting state, nonfasting lipid levels are remarkable mainly for an elevation in the serum triglyceride level. As discussed later, this will also lead to a spuriously low LDL cholesterol calculation. Since neither the LDL-C nor the TG levels are considered in the NCEP II guidelines, this initial screening exam need not be performed in the fasting state.

NCEP II defines a desirable TC as <200 mg/dL, a borderline high TC as 200 to 239 mg/dL, and a high blood cholesterol as >240 mg/dL. Coronary heart disease risk factors are summarized in Table 29–1. Negative risk factors include an HDL cholesterol greater than or equal to 60 mg/dL.

Primary prevention of coronary artery disease refers to recommendations designed to prevent the development of atherosclerosis in those patients without overt clinical evidence of coronary disease at the time of presentation. NCEP II guidelines for primary prevention are as follows.

Patients who have both a desirable TC and an HDL > 35 mg/dL are recommended to have a repeat TC and HDL study in 5 years. General education regarding risk-factor modification including exercise and diet should be given to all patients. Those patients with a desirable TC and HDL<35 mg/dL should be reevaluated in 1 to 2 years.

Patients with a borderline–high TC (200-239 mg/dL) as well as a low HDL (<35 mg/dL) and two or more CHD risk factors should undergo a fasting lipid profile. Other patients with a borderline–high TC level should be reevaluated in 1 to 2 years. Those patients with a high TC level (>240 mg/dL) should also undergo a fasting lipid profile. The studies should be performed after fasting between 9 and 12 hours.

Recommendations regarding cholesterol screening for primary prevention were formulated with implications for the entire population in mind. Limiting costs as well as the desirability of measuring lipids in the nonfasting state factored heavily in the decision to limit lipid testing in the manner described. For the individual practitioner and for the individual patient, however, it is often useful to know exactly what the LDL cholesterol is at baseline. Most practitioners in the United States, therefore, go beyond the NCEP guidelines and perform a fasting lipoprotein analysis to have data on total cholesterol, LDL-C, HDL-C, and triglycerides.

Progress in the science of lipid measurement has also begun to factor into clinical practice. Traditionally, TC, HDL, and triglycerides are measured in the fasting state. LDL-C is then calculated by the formula

$$\text{LDL} = (\text{TC} - \text{HDL}) - \left(\frac{\text{TG}}{5}\right)$$

The recent introduction of a relatively simple assay for the direct measurement of LDL-C has made it possible to obtain a screening lipid panel in the nonfasting state. As previously noted, TC and HDL-C may be measured in the nonfasting state; it is the wide swings in triglyceride levels associated with eating that formerly made it impossible to calculate the LDL-C in the absence of a fast. Although in the nonfasting state triglyceride levels may be artificially high, this does not affect the measurement of the direct LDL-C. Accurate determinations of TC, HDL-C, and LDL-C can therefore be made without the need for a 12- to 14-hour fast. As in all aspects of modern medicine, whether this approach eventually evolves into standard practice will have as much to do with the cost to society of measuring direct LDL-C as it will with the excellence and convenience of the medical care rendered.

For secondary prevention, that is, treatment of those adults with clinical evidence of coronary heart disease, NCEP II recommends measurement of a baseline lipoprotein panel in all patients. Subsequent recommendations regarding treatment are then made by way of LDL-C levels. For those patients with evidence of coronary artery disease (CAD), the desirable LDL-C level is less than 100 mg/dL. In those patients with desirable LDL-C levels, instructions regarding diet and physical activity should be routinely given and the fasting lipoprotein panel should be repeated annually. Cholesterol-lowering therapy should be instituted for those patients with LDL-C >100 mg/dL. These recommendations are summarized in Figure 29–1.

Patients with hyperlipidemia may be classified based on the type of lipid present in increased levels. Type I hyperlipoproteinemia is characterized by marked elevations in serum TG levels. Primary Type I hyperlipoproteinemia is not felt to be associated with increased risk of cardiovascular mortality. Diabetes mellitus as well as pancreatitis may lead to elevated serum TG levels.

Type II hyperlipoproteinemia is associated with elevated LDL cholesterol levels. Type IIa, or familial hypercholesterolemia, is characterized by elevated TC and LDL-C levels. Homozygotes for this condition have TC levels of 600 to 1200 mg/dL and typically exhibit signs of premature atherosclerosis in early childhood. Heterozygotes typically have TC levels of 300 to 500 mg/dL, and also exhibit pre-

TABLE 29–1. Risk Factors for Coronary Artery Disease

1. Age (men greater than or equal to 45, women greater than or equal to 55 or premature menopause without estrogen replacement therapy)
2. Family history of premature coronary heart disease
3. Smoking
4. Hypertension
5. HDL cholesterol <35 mg/dL
6. Diabetes mellitus

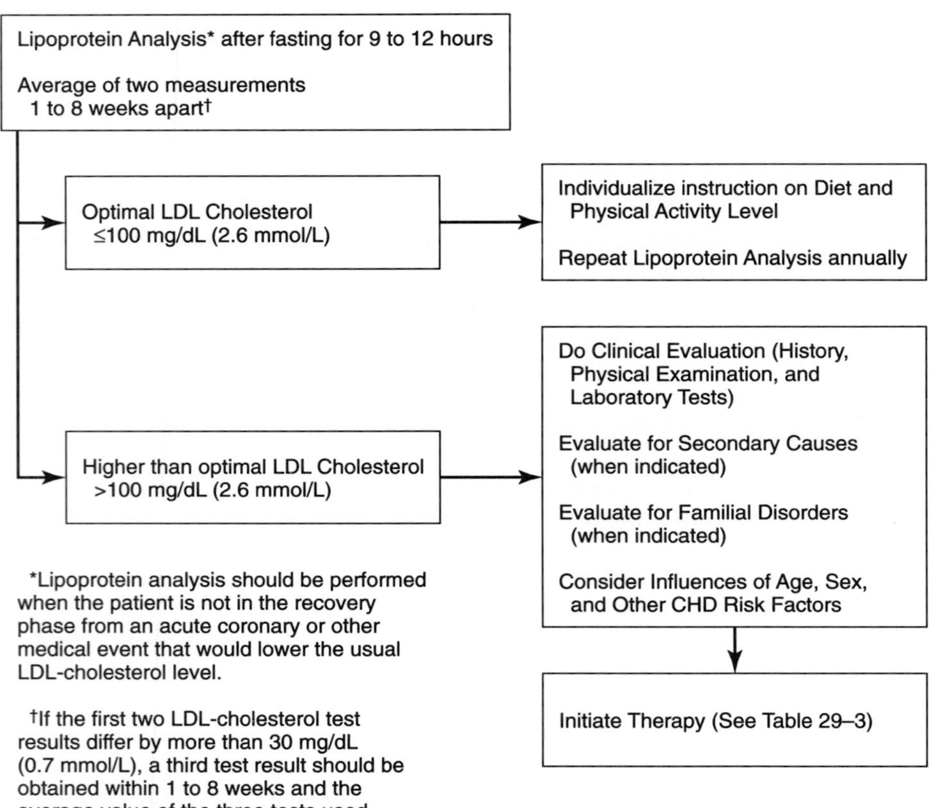

Figure 29–1. National cholesterol education panel recommendations for secondary prevention of coronary artery disease. Classification is based on low-density lipoprotein (LDL) cholesterol level. *(Adapted from Expert Panel on Detection, Evaluation and Treatment of High Blood Cholesterol in Adults [1993].)*

mature atherosclerosis, often manifested by myocardial infarction in the 40 through 50 age range. Type IIb, or polygenic hypercholesterolemia, is also associated with elevated levels of triglycerides. This is the most common cause of an elevated TC level; both forms are associated with premature atherosclerosis.

Type III hyperlipoproteinemia, or broad beta disease, is characterized by premature atherosclerosis in a patient in his or her 20s. Patients exhibit markedly elevated TC and TG levels due to incomplete breakdown of chylomicrons and VLDL.

Type IV hyperlipoproteinemia, or familial hypertriglyceridemia, is associated with overproduction of VLDL and TG by the liver. Premature atherosclerosis is not usually present in this group of patients with normal levels of LDL-C.

Type V hyperlipoproteinemia, or mixed hypertriglyceridemia, is characterized by elevated levels of VLDL and chylomicrons, with normal LDL-C levels. Familial forms are often associated with diabetes mellitus and hyperuricemia.

Management of Hyperlipidemia

Interventional Studies

The NCEP II guidelines, while remaining somewhat controversial, especially regarding recommendations concerning screening in asymptomatic adults, do provide a framework for the evaluation and treatment of adults with hyperlipidemia. This expert panel reviewed numerous studies, both observational and interventional, before issuing their recommendations. While a thorough review of the pertinent literature is beyond the scope of this chapter, and in fact the pace of research renders any such review out of date at the time of publication, the rational treatment of adults with hyperlipidemia requires at least an appreciation of the landmark studies in the field.

As of 1998, well-defined clinical studies have demonstrated without doubt that lowering total serum cholesterol levels reduces morbidity and mortality associated with CAD in those patients with established CAD. The Multiple Risk Factor Intervention Trial (MRFIT) (Stamler, Wentworth, & Neaton, 1986), demonstrated the positive association between total cholesterol levels and CAD mortality in 350,000 men screened as part of the study.

Early interventional studies such as POSCH (Program on the Surgical Control of the Hyperlipidemias) (Buchwald, Varco, Matts, et al., 1990), CLAS (Cholesterol Lowering Atherosclerosis Study) (Blankenhorn, Nessim, & Johnson, 1987), and FATS (Familial Atherosclerosis Treatment Study) (Brown, Albers, Fisher, et al., 1990), provided evidence for a trend towards decreased cardiovascular morbidity and mortality associated with lowering of serum cholesterol levels in patients with known CAD. (They also reaffirmed the now-inviolate rule of clinical research, that a study is only as good as its acronym is clever.)

Perhaps the strongest evidence that lowering of cholesterol levels can improve not only cardiovascular morbidity and mortality, but also lower all-cause mortality in patients with CAD is provided by the Scandinavian Simvastatin Survival Study (4S) (1994). This often-quoted study involved the multicenter randomization of 4444 men and women with established CAD. Patients at baseline had TC levels of between 210 and 310 mg/dL and TG levels of 220 mg/dL or less after being placed on low-fat, low-cholesterol diets. Simvastatin dosage was titrated to achieve a total cholesterol of less than 200 mg/dL. Patients were studied for a median of 5.4 years.

Drug therapy in the 4S trial resulted in a reduction of TC by 25%, LDL-C by 35%, and TG by 10%. HDL-C increased by 8%. The 4S Study was a mortality study, designed to have statistical power to examine the effect of lipid lowering on total mortality. The results were highly significant, with the treatment group showing a 30% decrease in total mortality in comparison with the placebo group. Even more impressive reductions were observed in coronary mortality (42%) and in the combined endpoint of coronary death, nonfatal MI, and resuscitated sudden cardiac death. The legacy of this study is such that it is now considered unethical to again conduct a placebo–control study of lipid lowering for secondary prevention of coronary heart disease.

In view of the overall lower event rates, it has proven to be more difficult to definitively demonstrate the value of primary prevention in ischemic heart disease. Given that at baseline the populations in these studies do not have clinical evidence of overt CAD, the study endpoints are often the development of a serious cardiovascular event rather than cardiac death or all cause mortality.

A landmark primary prevention study is the Lipid Research Clinics Coronary Primary Prevention Trial (LRC–CPPT) (1984). This study involved the randomization of nearly 4000 men with total cholesterol of greater than 265 mg/dL and LDL-C greater than 190 mg/dL to the bile acid sequestrant cholestyramine versus placebo. Patients were followed for a mean of 7.4 years. TC decreased by 13% (versus 5% in the placebo group) and LDL-C decreased by 20% (versus 8% in the placebo group.) The primary endpoint, combined CAD death and nonfatal MI, was reduced significantly (20%) in the cholestyramine group. Reduction in total mortality in this study, however, was not statistically significant.

The next landmark study in primary prevention was the Helsinki Heart Study (Huttunen, Manninen, Manttari, et al., 1991). This study involved the randomization of approximately 4000 men with hypercholesterolemia or hypertriglyceridemia to treatment with gemfibrozil versus placebo. Patients were studied for a mean of 5 years. Drug therapy resulted in reduction of TC by 10%, LDL-C by 11%, and TG by 35%. HDL-C increased by 11%. The primary endpoint, combined cardiac death plus fatal and nonfatal MIs, was significantly reduced by 34%. Despite significant reduction in CAD mortality, total mortality was observed to trend higher in the gemfibrozil group, secondary to an observed increase in noncardiovascular deaths due to accidents, violence and suicide, as well as intracerebral bleeds.

The value of lipid lowering in primary prevention was effectively demonstrated in the West of Scotland Primary Prevention Study (WOSCOPS) (Shepherd, Cobbe, Ford, et al., 1995). In this study, approximately 6500 men with elevated LDL-C but no evidence of prior myocardial infarction were randomized to pravastatin 40 mg or placebo. The mean follow-up was 4.9 years. The primary endpoint was cardiovascular death or myocardial infarction. This endpoint was reduced by 31% in the pravastatin group compared with the placebo group, a statistically significant result. There was a trend towards decrease in all cause mortality in the treatment group, but this result failed to achieve statistical significance.

Secondary Prevention

NCEP recommendations regarding diet and drug therapy for secondary prevention of CAD are summarized in Table 29–2. All CAD patients with LDL-C >100 mg/dL should be

TABLE 29–2. Treatment Decisions Based on LDL Cholesterol Level[a]

Patient Category	Initiation Level	LDL Goal
	Dietary Therapy	
Without CHD and with fewer than two risk factors	≥160 mg/dL (4.1 mmol/L)	<160 mg/dL (4.1 mmol/L)
Without CHD and with two or more risk factors	≥130 mg/dL (3.4 mmol/L)	<130 mg/dL (3.4 mmol/L)
With CHD	>100 mg/dL (2.6 mmol/L)	≤100 mg/dL (2.6 mmol/L)
	Drug Treatment	
Without CHD and with fewer than two risk factors	≥190 mg/dL (4.9 mmol/L)	<160 mg/dL (4.1 mmol/L)
Without CHD and with two or more risk factors	≥160 mg/dL (4.1 mmol/L)	<130 mg/dL (3.4 mmol/L)
With CHD	≥130 mg/dL (3.4 mmol/L)	≤100 mg/dL (2.6 mmol/L)

[a] LDL indicates low-density lipoprotein; and CHD, coronary heart disease.

placed on a Step I diet. In reality, all Americans interested in maintaining cardiovascular health should be placed on a Step I diet. This diet limits intake of saturated fats to 8% to 10% of total calories, with 30% or less of total calories from fat and less than 300 mg of cholesterol daily. If patients are already following a Step I diet, they should be instructed on adherence to a Step II diet, which provides progressive reduction in intake of saturated fats and cholesterol. This diet further limits intake of saturated fats to 7% of total calories, and intake of cholesterol to 200 mg/day. Weight loss should also be counseled as appropriate. Effective dietary counseling, especially use of a Step II Diet, often requires the services of a registered dietician. Unfortunately, these services are often not covered under health insurance policies and dietary instruction often falls to the province of the specialist as well as the primary care provider. Advanced practice nurses are particularly suited to provide this service for patients.

NCEP II guidelines recommend institution of drug therapy for secondary prevention in those patients with LDL-C >130 mg/dL while on dietary therapy. In practice, given the often modest effects dietary therapy achieves in the long-term LDL-C levels, as well as the availability of safe and effective drugs to lower LDL-C, drug therapy is often instituted concomitantly with dietary therapy, and often is prescribed for patients with LDL-C levels of between 100 and 130 mg/dL.

Primary Prevention

For primary prevention of CAD in adults, NCEP II recommendations are summarized in Figure 29–2. As previously described, initial classification is based on total cholesterol and HDL-C. Those patients with a total cholesterol of > 240 mg/dL, a borderline high TC level of 200 to 239 mg/dL, and two or more risk factors for CAD, as well as any TC level with an HDL < 35 mg/dL should have a fasting lipoprotein panel performed. As in secondary prevention, recommendations are then based on the LDL-C level.

Figure 29–3 summarizes treatment recommendations based on LDL-C for primary prevention in adults without evidence of CAD. In this group, the desirable range for LDL-C is liberalized to include levels up to 130 mg/dL. Patients in this group are provided counseling regarding diet and exercise. Those patients with borderline–high LDL-C levels (130-159 mg/dL) and fewer than two additional risk factors are placed on a Step I diet and should be reevaluated annually. Patients with borderline–high LDL-C levels as well as two or more additional risk factors should be placed on drug therapy, as should those patients with high-risk LDL-C levels (> 160 mg/dL).

Drug Therapy for Treatment of Hyperlipidemia

Concurrent with the demonstration that lowering of serum cholesterol levels is associated with decreased cardiovascular events in patients both with and without overt coronary artery disease, we have witnessed the development of many safe and effective drugs for achieving this goal. The availability of these agents provides the tools to affect a fundamental change in the natural history of coronary artery disease. Although underused and under appreciated, these drugs have the potential to reduce morbidity and mortality in a way that no new drug has done since the introduction of penicillin earlier in this century. The following briefly reviews the various classes of drugs and their indications and potential uses. Table 29–3 summarizes the effects of the lipid-lowering agents.

Bile–Acid Sequestrants. Among the earliest available agents for the treatment of hypercholesterolemia are the bile–acid sequestrants. Two agents are clinically available for use in the United States: cholestyramine and colestipol. Each of these drugs is available in a powdered resin form. They exert their lipid-lowering action by binding to bile acids in the gut, preventing their absorption and leading to loss in the feces. The increased fecal loss of bile acids with resin therapy leads to a compensatory increase in the conversion of cholesterol to bile acids.

Bile–acid resins are administered as powders, dissolved in water or orange juice. Attempts to increase palatability of these drugs have included dosing in the form of a capsule as well as a solid bar. Use of cholestyramine (4-16 gm/day) and colestipol (5-20 gm/day) may result in reduction of LDL-C levels between 15 to 30%. Because these drugs are not systemically absorbed, side effects are limited to those caused by transit of the resins through the GI system, including nausea, constipation, and bloating. The drugs are considered unpalatable by many patients, and this often limits patient compliance. The resins must also be administered with caution, as they are prone to bind to and decrease absorption of other drugs taken at the same time. Patients should be cautioned to take all other medications at least one hour before or two hours after taking a bile–acid sequestrant.

In the past bile–acid sequestrants were often used as first-line therapy for patients with elevated LDL-C levels. The availability of the statins has largely relegated the resins to use as second-line agents, used in combination with statins when monotherapy fails to achieve reduction in LDL-C to target levels.

Niacin (Nicotinic Acid). Another drug that has been available for some time for the treatment of hypercholesterolemia is niacin. Niacin works by decreasing plasma levels of free fatty acids and by decreasing hepatic VLDL synthesis. The drug is available both as a short-acting preparation, dosed at 1 to 6 gms/day, and also as a sustained-release preparation. Niacin is typically capable of lowering LDL-C by 10 to 25%, and increasing HDL-C by 15 to 35%.

As with the bile–acid sequestrants, the use of niacin is often limited by unacceptable side effects. Flushing is seen in virtually all patients, and the dosage of niacin must be

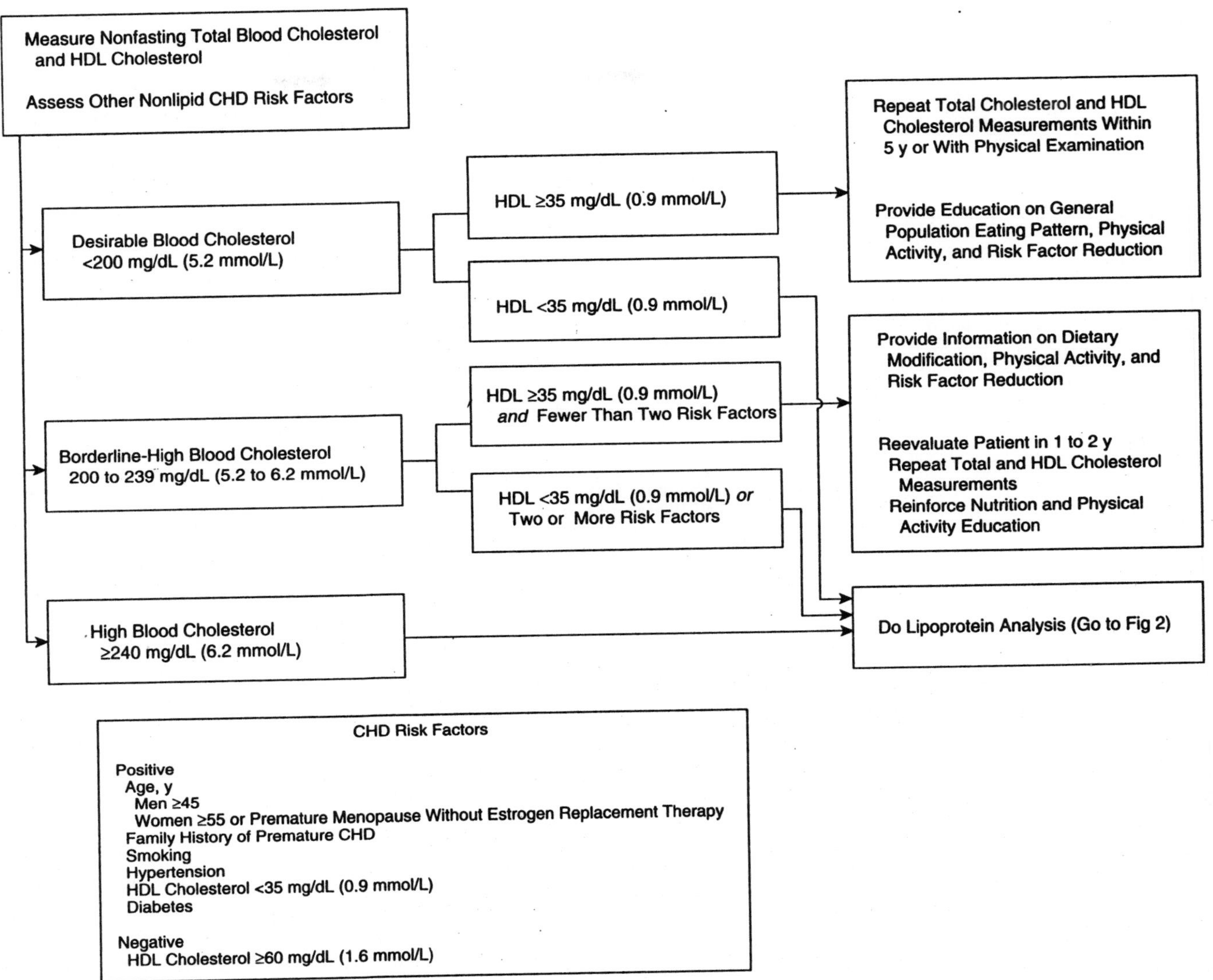

Figure 29–2. Risk factors for coronary artery disease. Initial classification is based on total cholesterol and high-density lipoprotein (HDL) cholosterol levels. *(Adapted from Expert Panel on Detection, Evaluation and Treatment of High Blood Cholesterol in Adults [1993].)*

gradually increased to avoid intolerable flushing. This side effect may be somewhat attenuated by pretreatment with aspirin. Use of the sustained-action niacin preparations has historically been associated with decreased flushing, though at the expense of increased liver toxicity. A newly released long-acting niacin preparation (Niaspan) may now potentially avoid this increased incidence of liver toxicity.

Patients treated with niacin require careful follow-up including periodic assessment of liver transaminase levels. Increase in transaminase levels to more than three times normal range requires discontinuation of therapy. Use of niacin along with the HMG–CoA reductase drugs is associated with an increased incidence of myositis, and should, in general, be avoided.

Fibric-Acid Derivatives. The fibric–acid derivatives have a complex mechanism of action that is not completely understood. Two agents are available for clinical use in the United States: gemfibrozil and clofibrate. They function by decreasing hepatic production of VLDL and by increasing activity of the enzyme lipoprotein lipase. The result is a decrease in TG levels of 20 to 50% as well as an increased HDL-C of 10 to 15%. LDL-C typically decreases by 10 to 15%, but this response is highly variable. These drugs also result in decreased levels of small dense LDL particles that may therefore lead to production of a less atherogenic LDL particle.

In the United States, the most often used fibric–acid derivative is gemfibrozil, dosed at 600 mg twice daily. The

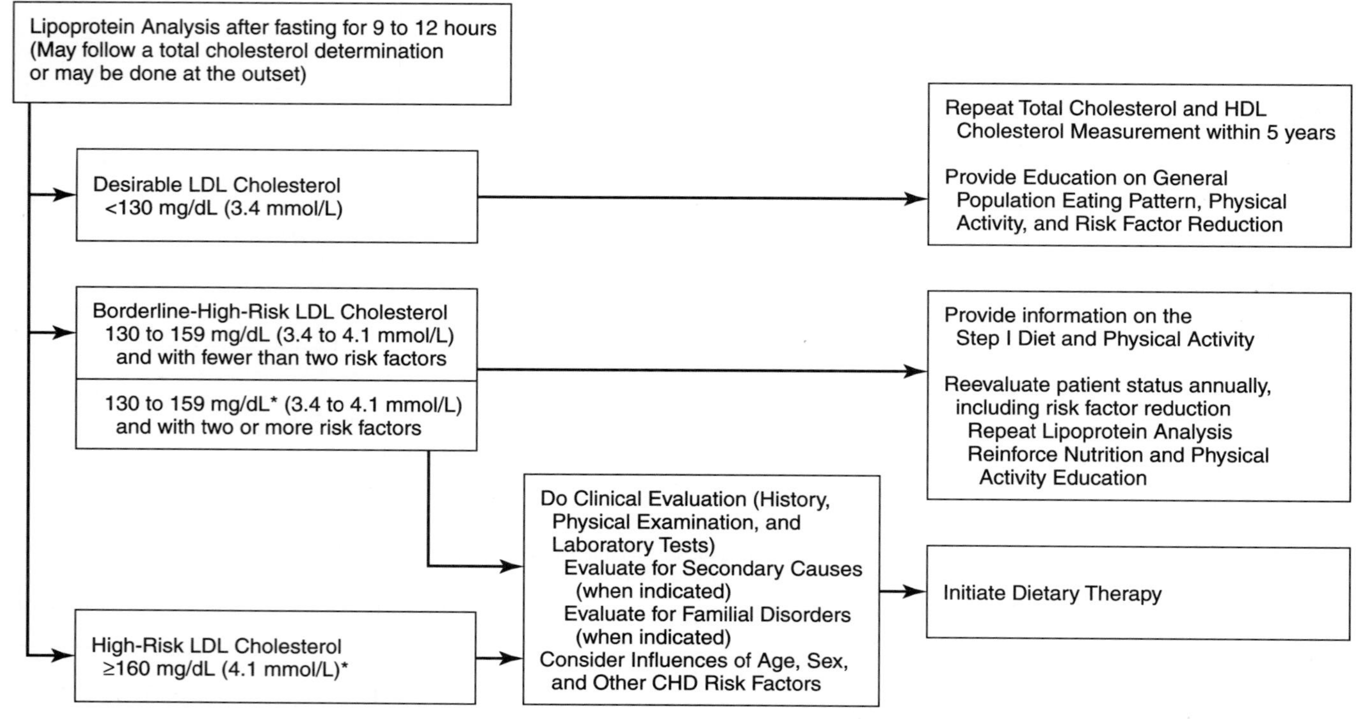

Figure 29–3. National cholesterol education panel recommendations for primary prevention of coronary artery disease. Subsequent classification is based on low-density lipoprotein (LDL) cholesterol level. *(Adapted from Expert Panel on Detection, Evaluation and Treatment of High Blood Cholesterol in Adults [1993].)*

drugs are most useful in those patients with elevated triglyceride levels and low HDL-C levels, in association with normal to modest elevations in LDL-C and TC levels. Side effects are generally mild and gemfibrozil is generally well tolerated. Once again, mild GI symptoms predominate. As with niacin, administration of gemfibrozil in conjunction with the statins results in an increased incidence of myositis. Although this combination of drugs is often effective in treating patients with severe hyperlipidemia, it should be done only with extreme caution.

Probucol. The mechanism of action of probucol is not well understood. At dosages of 1 gm/day, LDL-C decreases by 5 to 15%. The HDL-C decreases by 20 to 30%, however, and is of concern because of the known cardioprotective effects of HDL-C. For this reason probucol is not often used in the United States. Interestingly, probucol is chemically related to agents that are potent antioxidants, and there is interest in the possibility that probucol may inhibit the oxidation of LDL particles.

HMG–CoA Reductase Inhibitors. As previously noted, the introduction into clinical practice of the HMG–CoA reductase inhibitors is truly one of the major advances in modern medicine. Also referred to as the statins, these drugs inhibit the enzyme HMG–CoA reductase, which is the rate-limiting step in the body's production of cholesterol. This results in upregulation of LDL receptors and increased peripheral clearance of lipoproteins. The net effect is lower LDL-C levels.

TABLE 29–3. Relative Effects of Lipid-Lowering Agents on Blood Lipids

	Total Cholesterol	HDL-C	LDL-C	Triglycerides
Bile–Acid Sequestrants	↓		↓	
Niacin		↑↑	↓	↓↓
Fibric–Acid Derivatives		↑		↓↓
Probucol	↓	↓↓	↓	
HMG–CoA Reductase Inhibitors	↓↓	↑	↓↓	↓

There are currently six agents available in the United States. Despite some controversial data to the contrary, most experts believe that the drugs have a similar mechanism of action and differ only in their relative potency. Fluvastatin (20-40 mg/day), lovastatin (10-80 mg/day), simvastatin (5-40 mg/day), atorvastatin (5-40 mg/day), and cerivastatin (0.2 or 0.3 mg/day) are effective at reducing LDL-C by 20 to 40% and increasing HDL-C by 5 to 15%. In general, there is a linear relationship between dose and LDL-C reduction. It is useful to consider these drugs similar in efficacy albeit at different dosages. In general, 5 mg of atorvastatin is similar to 10 mg of simvastatin, 20 mg of lovastatin and pravastatin, and 40 mg of fluvastatin. Each subsequent stepwise increase in dosage may be expected to further decrease LDL-C by an additional 7%, as shown in Table 29–4. The most dramatic reductions in LDL-C may be achieved with atorvastatin 40 mg or with simvastatin 80 mg (a dose that is not approved by the FDA, but that many experts in the field believe may be safe). Atorvastatin is somewhat more effective at lowering TG levels than the other agents.

Although other mechanisms of action for the statin drugs have been proposed, such as inhibition of plasminogen activator inhibitor-1 (PAI-1), there is no evidence to clearly suggest that any one statin has a novel mechanism of action compared with the others. Many lipid experts advocate determination of the percent reduction in LDL-C needed to reach goal (depending on the clinical situation), and then instituting therapy with one of the previous drugs at a dose sufficient to achieve that target.

Statin drugs represent a huge advance in lipid-lowering therapy not only because of their marked efficacy, but also because they are remarkably well tolerated. Side effects commonly seen include GI upset and headache. Myositis is rare, but may be increased if used concomitantly with niacin, gemfibrozil, erythromycin, or cyclosporin. Elevated transaminase levels are common but do not often require discontinuation of therapy. Most cases occur early in therapy and current recommendations call for screening transaminase levels at 6 weeks and 12 weeks after institution of therapy, and periodically thereafter. The FDA recommends semi-annual screening for patients on simvastatin, and somewhat more frequent testing for patients on the other drugs. Statin therapy should be discontinued if transaminase levels rise to three times control levels.

TABLE 29–4. Approximate Equivalent Doses of HMG–CoA Reductase Inhibitors

% Reduction LDL-C	Drug
27	Lipitor 5 mg (atorvastatin) Zocor 10 mg (simvastatin) Pravachol 20 mg (pravastatin) Mevacor 20 mg (lovastatin) Leschol 80 mg (fluvastatin)
34	Lipitor 10 mg Zocor 20 mg Pravachol 40 mg Mevacor 40 mg
41	Lipitor 20 mg Zocor 40 mg
48	Lipitor 40 mg

The efficacy and safety of the statin drugs have led many clinicians to rely heavily on these agents in the treatment of hypercholesterolemia. They are often used as first-line monotherapy for both primary and secondary prevention, although in a young patient being treated for primary prevention, consideration should be give to use of the non-systemically absorbed bile–acid sequestrants.

HOMOCYSTEINE AND CORONARY ARTERY DISEASE

Recent studies have demonstrated a strong association between elevated plasma levels of homocysteine and the development of atherosclerosis. Homocystinuria is a rare inherited metabolic disorder resulting from deficiency in the enzyme cystathionine B-synthase, which causes patients to have high levels of homocysteine in the blood (hyperhomocysteinemia) as well as to spill homocysteine into the urine (homocystinuria.) These patients present with visual disturbances secondary to lens dislocation and glaucoma, mental retardation, and severe atherosclerosis and thromboembolic venous disease. The disorder is inherited via an autosomal recessive mechanism. It is believed that the high levels of homocysteine in the bloodstream results in a direct toxic effect on the vascular endothelium, as well as the induction of a hypercoaguable state.

Heterozygotes for the gene have elevated blood homocysteine levels but not high enough to result in spillage into the urine. This condition is relatively common, estimated at 1 in 100 in the general population. Other conditions associated with hyperhomocysteinemia include other (and more common) genetic mutations, folic acid deficiency, as well as vitamin B_6 and B_{12} deficiency. Patients with renal insufficiency also exhibit hyperhomocysteinemia.

Many studies have demonstrated that elevated blood homocysteine levels are at least as important a risk factor in the development of atherosclerosis as is elevated cholesterol. Many studies have demonstrated the prevalence of elevated homocysteine levels at 20 to 30% in patients with vascular disease, while only weighing in at 2% in the control group.

Unlike hypercholesterolemia, hyperhomocysteinemia may be treated safely, effectively, and inexpensively. Most experts advocate the use of folic acid to reduce homocysteine levels. This drug causes remethylation of homocysteine, and may result in up to a 40 to 50% reduction with therapy. Doses in the 1 to 2 mg/day range are generally recommended, with higher doses needed in patients with renal insufficiency.

In 1998, it is generally recommended to measure homocysteine levels in patients presenting with atherosclerotic disease in the absence of other risk factors, especially if a family history of atherosclerosis is present. Patients with hyperhomocysteinemia may then be treated with folic acid.

The issue of homocysteine as a risk factor remains unresolved at this time. Measurement of homocysteine levels only in those patients without other risk factors for vascular disease ignores the possible contribution of hyperhomocysteinemia in those patients who do have additional risk factors for CAD. In addition, homocysteine levels are often difficult to measure reliably in the clinical setting, and with a treatment as inexpensive and seemingly as innocuous as folic-acid supplementation, it is tempting to treat all patients presenting with vascular disease or with a strong family history of atherosclerosis with folic acid. Large-scale interventional studies will be needed to further define the role of folic-acid supplementation in the treatment of coronary artery disease.

▶ ELEVATED LIPOPROTEIN (A)

Lipoprotein (a), abbreviated Lp(a), has been shown preliminarily to be an independent risk factor for the development of atherosclerosis. Structurally, Lp(a) is closely related to LDL-C. The mechanism by which Lp(a) is associated with the development of atherosclerosis is not yet well understood.

Unlike in the case with homocysteine, there is no inexpensive safe and available treatment for patients with elevated levels of Lp(a). Although niacin and estrogen may be effective in lowering Lp(a) levels, there are as yet no convincing studies demonstrating that lowering Lp(a) levels results in a decrease in cardiovascular morbidity or mortality. Routine measurement of Lp(a) levels are therefore not routinely recommended, although they are often considered in patients with strong family histories of premature atherosclerosis or in patients presenting with vascular disease and no other definable risk factors. Treatment for now, however, is limited to aggressive risk factor modification (for the standard cardiac risk factors) including aggressive optimization of serum lipid levels.

Unfortunately, despite the overwhelming evidence that lowering of elevated serum cholesterol levels results in decreased cardiovascular and all-cause mortality, as well as the ready availability of safe and effective agents to achieve these goals, most patients with coronary artery disease never achieve a desirable serum lipid level. Causes for this failure are many and varied, including the expense of the medications, the unwillingness of many patients to commit to a lifetime of drug and dietary therapy, a preoccupation with potential drug side effects, and difficulties arising from reduced access to cardiovascular specialists within the managed care setting.

Patients must be convinced to become their own advocate, and education is the key. Many patients who balk at spending several dollars a day to pay for statin drugs will readily spend at least that much on a daily basis for cigarettes. With proper education, hopefully more patients can be made aware of the miraculous new tools available to reduce the progression of coronary atherosclerosis and can become partners with their health-care providers in this endeavor.

REFERENCES

Blankenhorn, D.H., Nessim, S.A., & Johnson, R.L. (1987). Beneficial effects of combined colestipol-niacin therapy on coronary atherosclerosis and coronary venous bypass grafts. *Journal of the American Medical Association, 257* (23), 3233–3240.

Brown, G., Albers, J.J., Fisher, L.D., et al. (1990). Regression of coronary artery disease as a result of intensive lipid-lowering therapy in men with high levels of apolipoprotein B. *New England Journal of Medicine, 323* (19), 1289–1298.

Buchwald, H., Varco, R.L., Matts, J.P., et al. (1990). Effect of partial ileal bypass surgery on mortality and morbidity from coronary heart disease in patients with hypercholesterolemia. Report of the Program on the Surgical Control of the Hyperlipidemias. *New England Journal of Medicine, 323* (14), 946–955.

Expert Panel on Detection, Evaluation and Treatment of High Blood Cholesterol in Adults. (1993). Summary of the second report of the National Cholesterol Education Program (NCEP) Expert Panel on Detection, Evaluation and Treatment of High Blood Cholesterol in Adults. (Adult Treatment Panel II). *Journal of the American Medical Association, 269* (23), 3015–3023.

Huttunen, J.K., Manninen, V., Manttari, M., Koskinen, P., Romo, M., Tenkanen, L., Heinonen, O.P., & Frick, M.H. (1991). The Helsinki Heart Study: Central finding and clinical implications. *Annals of Medicine, 23* (2), 155–159.

Lipid Research Clinics Program. (1984). The Lipid Research Clinics Coronary Primary Prevention Trials results. I. Reduction in incidence of coronary heart disease. *Journal of the American Medical Association, 251* (3), 365–374.

Scandinavian Simvastatin Survival Study Group. (1994). Randomized trial of cholesterol lowering in 4444 patients with coronary heart disease: The Scandinavian Simvastatin Survival Study (4S). *Lancet, 344* (8934), 1383–1389.

Shepherd, J., Cobbe, S.M., Ford, I., Isles, C.G., Lorimer, A.R., McFarlane, P.W., McKillop, J.H., & Packard, C.J. (1995). Prevention of coronary heart disease with pravastatin in men with hypercholesterolemia. West of Scotland Coronary Prevention Study Group. *New England Journal of Medicine, 333* (20), 1301–1307.

Stamler, J., Wentworth, D., & Nelson, J.D. (1986). Is relationship between serum cholesterol and risk of premature death from coronary artery disease continuous and graded? Findings in 356,222 primary screenees of the Multiple Risk Factor Intervention Trail (MRFIT). *Journal of the American Medical Association, 256* (20), 2823–2828.

30

Hypertension

Catherine Congdon

Hypertension is one of the most significant public health concerns in the United States. Hypertension is a major modifiable risk factor for cardiovascular disease that, if left untreated, can result in cerebrovascular, cardiac, peripheral vascular, and renal disease. Between 50 and 62 million Americans, age 6 and older, have high blood pressure.

The National High Blood Pressure Education Program (NHBPEP) has succeeded in increasing awareness, prevention, treatment, and control of hypertension. The percentage of Americans who were aware of having high blood pressure increased from 51% in the 1976–1980 National Health and Nutrition Examination Survey (NHANES II) to 73% in the 1988–1991 survey (NHANES III, phase 1). During the same period, treatment increased from 31% to 55%, and the percentage of those persons with high blood pressure that were controlled (less than 140/90) increased from 10% in NHANES II to 29% in NHANES III, phase 1. These changes dramatically reduced morbidity and mortality rates attributable to hypertension.

Heart disease and stroke remain the first and third leading causes of death in the United States and have become tremendous financial and social burdens on Americans (JNC VI, 1997). Mortality figures for high blood pressure are deceiving because, for many, the cause of death is disguised as heart attack or stroke, that was caused, at least in part, by hypertension. The incidence of undiagnosed and/or untreated cases of high blood pressure has significantly decreased with both private and governmental educational programs (Williams, 1994).

PUBLIC HEALTH CHALLENGE OF HYPERTENSION

The Joint National Committee outlines major public health challenges for the prevention and treatment of hypertension. These challenges are:

1. Prevent the rise of blood pressure with age.
2. Decrease the prevalence of hypertension.
3. Increase hypertension awareness and detection; many adult Americans are unaware of their diagnosis of high blood pressure.
4. Improve control of hypertension to below 140/90 mm Hg.
5. Reduce the risk for cardiovascular disease.
6. Increase recognition of the importance of controlled isolated systolic hypertension.
7. Improve recognition of the importance of high–normal blood pressure. The role that high–normal blood pressure has on the development of hypertension and target organ damage is unappreciated.
8. Reduce ethnic, socioeconomic, and regional variations in hypertension.
9. Improve universal access to treatment.
10. Enhance community programs.

The NHBPEP has developed many community-based activities designed to promote prevention, increase awareness, screen for elevated blood pressure and cardiovascular risk factors, improve therapy compliance, and reduce morbidity and mortality. More information on community programs and activities can be obtained from the National Heart, Lung, and Blood Institute (NHLBI) publications.

▶ CLASSIFICATION, DETECTION, AND CONFIRMATION

According to The Sixth Report of the Joint National Committee on Detection, Evaluation, and Treatment of High Blood Pressure (JNC VI, 1997), the definition of hypertension requires the minimum average levels of systolic blood pressure (SBP) greater than or equal to 140 mm Hg and a diastolic pressure (DBP) of 90 mm Hg or more, or current therapy with antihypertensive medication. The objective of identifying and treating high blood pressure is to reduce the risk of cardiovascular complications and associated morbidity and mortality.

To identify high-risk individuals and to provide guidelines for therapy, a classification system of adult blood pressure has been provided by the JNC VI. This classification is for adults age 18 and older who are not taking antihypertensive drugs and who are not acutely ill (Table 30–1). Any diagnosis and classification of hypertension should be based on the average of two or more blood pressure readings, taken over several weeks, after an initial screening visit. When SBP and DBP fall into different categories, the higher category should be chosen to classify the individual's blood pressure. The classification system now combines stages 3 and 4 because of the infrequency of stage 4 hypertension (JNC VI, 1997). The designations of "mild," "moderate," and "severe" hypertension are discouraged to avoid the misconception that some cases of hypertension are not significant health risks. High–normal blood pressure is included as a separate category because persons with SBP and/or DBP in these ranges are at increased risk of developing definite hypertension and of experiencing fatal and nonfatal complications, when compared with people with normal blood pressures.

TABLE 30–1. Classification of Blood Pressure for Adults Age 18 and Older[a]

Category	Systolic (mm Hg)		Diastolic (mm Hg)
Optimal[b]	<120	and	<80
Normal	<130	and	<85
High-normal	130–139	or	85–89
Hypertension[c]			
Stage 1	140–159	or	90–99
Stage 2	160–179	or	100–109
Stage 3	≥180	or	≥110

[a] Not taking antihypertensive drugs and not acutely ill. When systolic and diastolic blood pressures fall into different categories, the higher category should be selected to classify the individual's blood pressure status. For example, 160/92 mm Hg should be classified as stage 2 hypertension, and 174/120 mm Hg should be classified as stage 3 hypertension. Isolated systolic hypertension is defined as SBP of 140 mm Hg or greater and DBP below 90 mm Hg and staged appropriately (e.g., 170/82 mm Hg is defined as stage 2 isolated systolic hypertension). In addition to classifying stages of hypertension on the basis of average blood pressure levels, clinicians should specify presence or absence of target organ disease and additional risk factors. This specificity is important for risk classification and treatment (see Table 30–5).

[b] Optimal blood pressure with respect to cardiovascular risk is below 120/80 mm Hg. However, unusually low readings should be evaluated for clinical significance.

[c] Based on the average of two or more readings taken at each of two or more visits after an initial screening.

From the Joint National Committee on Detection, Evaluation, and Treatment of High Blood Pressure. (1997).

Follow-Up Recommendations

The following recommendations and follow-up scheduling should be modified according to reliable information about past blood pressure measurements, other cardiovascular risk factors, or target organ disease. An initial blood pressure reading that is normal or SBP < 130 and DBP < 85 should be rechecked in two years. High–normal readings (SBP 130-139 or DBP 85-89 mm Hg) should be rechecked in one year. Stage 1 hypertension or readings of SBP 140-159 and/or DBP 90-99 should be confirmed in two months. Stage 2 (SBP 160-179 or DBP 100-109) should be reevaluated or treated within one month. Stage 3 (SBP ≥ 180 or DBP ≥ 110) should be reevaluated or treated immediately or within one week depending on clinical situation (JNC VI, 1997).

Self-Measurement of Blood Pressure

Valuable information can be obtained from blood pressure measurements obtained outside the health-care practitioner's office. Advantages include: (1) distinguishing sustained hypertension from white coat hypertension; (2) monitoring response to antihypertensive therapy; (3) improving patient adherence to therapy and giving them a more active role in their care; and (4) potential cost reduction. Mercury sphygmomanometer is not practical for home use. Therefore, validated electronic devices or aneroid sphygmomanometers are recommended if accurate under standardized testing. Finger monitors are not recommended. The patient's device should be periodically compared with auscultatory readings obtained with a mercury device.

Ambulatory Blood Pressure Monitoring

Between 20% and 30% of patients with clinically diagnosed hypertension have normal blood pressure readings during automated ambulatory 24-hour blood pressure monitoring. Commercial monitors are available for accurate ambulatory blood pressure monitoring. These monitors are usually programmed for readings every 15 to 30 minutes throughout the day and night while patients go about their normal daily routine. The readings can be downloaded onto a personal computer for analysis (JNC VI, 1997). Ambulatory blood pressure monitoring is most clinically useful in those patients with white coat hypertension, in those patients with drug therapy resistance, hypotensive symptoms with medications, episodic hypertension, and autonomic dysfunction (JNC VI, 1997). The expense and relative inaccessibility of ambulatory blood pressure monitors, however, make the devices largely impractical clinically.

▶ HISTORY AND PHYSICAL FINDINGS

Clinical Evaluation

According to Kaplan (1998) and Williams (1994), the initial history, physical examination, and clinical work-up for the patient with hypertension should be directed toward three goals.

1. Firmly establish the diagnosis and distinguish between primary and secondary hypertension, specifically looking for secondary causes.
2. Determine the presence or absence of target-organ damage and cardiovascular disease, and the impact the hypertension has had on target organs.
3. Evaluate the patient's overall risk factors for the development of cardiovascular disease or concomitant disorders that may outline prognosis and treatment guidelines.

Data for evaluation should be obtained through medical history, physical examination, laboratory testing, and other diagnostic procedures (JNC VI, 1997). Table 30–2 lists the necessary components of the medical history.

Signs and Symptoms

Hypertension is asymptomatic in the vast majority of patients and is often undetected until years after the onset of the disease when symptoms of target-organ damage occur. Williams (1994) reports that when symptoms bring patients to the health-care provider, they fall into one or more of three categories: (1) The elevated blood pressure itself, (2) hypertensive vascular disease, or (3) the underlying disease of secondary hypertension.

The most common symptom reported by patients is headache. Kaplan (1998) reports that the majority of those patients who complain of headache are already aware of their diagnosis. The headache is often related to the anxiety over the diagnosis and its implications. Other symptoms sometimes reported by hypertensives are dizziness and lightheadedness, band-like headache, fatigue, palpitations, and chest discomfort. Chest discomfort is common among patients with hypertension and is often related to recurrent hyperventilation, occurring in conjunction with anxiety. That most symptoms, especially headache, are related to anxiety rather than blood pressure, is supported by the fact that headache among newly diagnosed hypertensives has little variation with respect to the blood pressure (Kaplan, 1998).

Headache, however, is more commonly characteristic of severe hypertension. The headache is most commonly localized to the occipital area, present upon awakening in the morning, may or may not throb, and often subsides after several hours without analgesics. Other complaints include dizziness, fatigue, palpitations, and impotence. The symptoms are usually related to hypertensive vascular disease or the underlying disease in secondary hypertension. For example, the symptoms related to vascular disease include epistaxis, hematuria, blurred vision secondary to reti-

TABLE 30–2. Components of the Medical History for Hypertension

Any known duration and levels of elevated blood pressure
Any prior treatment; results and/or side effects of previously used antihypertensive medications
Current and past history of all prescribed or self-prescribed medications, over-the-counter medications, herbal remedies, and illicit drugs in order to uncover any agents that may cause hypertension (i.e., oral contraceptives, sympathomimetics, etc.)
Patient history or current symptoms of target organ dysfunction; syptoms of cardiovascular disease, cerebrovascular disease, peripheral vascular disease, renal disease, diabetes mellitus; dyslipidemia; gout, or sexual dysfunction
Family history (first-degree relatives: siblings, parents, children, aunts, uncles) of high blood pressure, premature cardiovascular heart disease, CVA, diabetes, dyslipidemia, or renal disease
Symptoms suggesting secondary causes of hypertension (i.e., hirsutism, easy bruising, tachycardia, palpitations, weight gain, sweats, weakness, muscle cramps, or flank pain)
Symptoms of target organ damage (i.e., headache, transient weakness or blindness, chest pain, shortness of breath, syncope, intermittent claudication)
Presence of other risk factors: elevated cholesterol, diabetes mellitus, smoking or other tobacco history, and physical inactivity
History of recent changes in weight, recreational physical activities, regular physical exercise
Alcohol use
Dietary assessment including intake of sodium, cholesterol, saturated fat, and caffeine
Features of sleep apnea: headaches in early morning and daytime somnolence, snoring, irregular sleep patterns
Psychosocial status and enviromental factors that may contribute to hypertension and its control (i.e., family situation and employment status with working conditions, educational level and the degree of knowledge about hypertension, the willingness to make necessary changes in lifestyle and to follow a treatment regimen)
Sexual dysfunction: sexual function is an important area overlooked in the history-taking until after antihypertensive therapy is initiated; according to Kaplan (1998), impotence, which is most often credited to antihypertensive medications, may be present in as many as one-third of untreated hypertensive men and is most likely related to an underlying vascular disease

nal ischemia, weakness or dizziness from TIAs, angina, and dyspnea due to cardiac disease (Williams, 1994). Labile hypertension with headache, palpitations, pallor, and sweating suggests pheochromocytoma. It should also be noted that many obese hypertensive patients have sleep apnea and their early-morning headache may be due to nocturnal hypoxia in addition to the hypertension (Kaplan, 1998).

Physical Examination

The physical exam in the hypertensive patient should include a search for evidence of end-organ damage. Those patients with a blood pressure that is resistant to medical therapy, who have malignant hypertension, or who have a sudden onset of hypertension should have a thorough investigation for a secondary etiology.

Establishing the diagnosis with proper technique is essential. The initial physical examination should include:

1. Multiple blood pressure measurements (two or more) separated by two minutes with the patient lying supine or sitting comfortably with arms supported, and then again after standing for at least two minutes. The cuff should be level with the heart. If arm circumference exceeds 33 cm, a large cuff should be used (Kaplan, 1998).
2. Blood pressure measurement in both arms. If values are different, the higher value should be used.
3. Thigh blood pressure readings: To avoid falsely elevated readings, a large cuff should be used. The patient should lie prone with leg bent and supported. Listen over the popliteal fossa. This should be done for every young patient diagnosed with hypertension because coarctation of the aorta is more common in this population. The systolic blood pressure is usually slightly higher and diastolic blood pressure a little lower in this area compared with the arm.

Elderly patients who have rigid, calcified arteries may have falsely elevated blood pressure readings (pseudohypertension) because of difficulty in collapsing the brachial artery. This should be suspected in those patients whose vessels feel rigid and have few signs of vascular damage that occur with hypertension. These patients also experience postural symptoms with modest blood pressure reduction. If pseudohypertension is suspected, an automatic oscilometric machine or a finger blood pressure device should be used. Rarely, intraarterial measurement is necessary (Kaplan, 1998).

Examine the neck for carotid bruits, distended neck veins, and an enlarged thyroid gland. Palpation and auscultation of carotid arteries may reveal evidence of stenosis or occlusion. Carotid artery stenosis may be a manifestation of hypertensive vascular disease (Williams, 1994).

Observe for hypertensive retinopathy. Characteristic ocular findings of hypertensive retinopathy include arteriolar narrowing, focal arteriolar constriction, arteriovenous nicking, flame hemorrhages, hard exudates, and papilledema (Graettinger, 1995). Hypertensive retinopathy is caused by damage to endothelial lining of the capillaries, transudation of proteins from infarcted nerve fibers, and obstruction of venous outflow from the optic disc, causing papilledema. The hallmarks of papilledema are loss of venous pulsation, hyperemia of the disks, blurred disk margins, and pronounced physiologic cupping, which can be seen with the ophthalmoscope. Flame-shaped hemorrhages occur with a breakdown in the blood–retinal barrier. Sclerosis of the small retinal arterioles will lead to areas of infarction that become evident as round to oval white patches with soft borders, referred to as "cotton-wool" patches (Ramachandran & Frank, 1993). According to Kaplan (1998), in clinical practice other than ophthamology, fundoscopic findings are of limited value, with only a 60% predictive value, positive or negative. Any newly diagnosed hypertensive should have a fundoscopic examination and if malignant changes are found, further evaluation and more aggressive therapy should be implemented. Any hypertensive patient with diabetes should have a thorough ophthalmologic exam annually to monitor for diabetic retinopathy, which is treatable.

According to Shub (1993), hypertensive heart disease can be detected by physical examination and noninvasive testing. The detection of left ventricular hypertrophy (LVH) is of critical importance in the hypertensive patient because of its prognostic implications. Examination of the patient should include observation for precordial heave and palpation of the cardiac apex for the apical impulse. Also, abnormalities in rate and rhythm and the presence of clicks, murmurs, and third (S_3) and fourth (S_4) heart sounds should be noted.

The left ventricular hypertrophy that occurs with hypertension causes an increased resistance to ventricular filling during atrial contraction. This resistance or diastolic noncompliance of the ventricle causes the left-sided S_4 that can be auscultated when the bell of the stethoscope is placed lightly over the PMI or the lower left sternal border. It is louder on expiration. According to Shub (1993), between 50 and 70% of hypertensive patients have an S_4, especially if LVH is present or if the patient is elderly. A sustained impulse that is diffuse and forceful is a strong indicator of LVH. If the impulse is displaced laterally, left ventricular dilation with systolic dysfunction could present (Shub, 1993).

The practitioner should examine the lungs for rales that could be due to diastolic failure. Evidence of bronchospasm, such as wheezing, should be noted so that appropriate medications can be chosen.

The abdomen should be auscultated for bruits, possibly originating from stenotic renal arteries. Bruits from narrowing renal arteries are high pitched, often intermittent, frequently having a diastolic component or may be continuous. These bruits are heard best in the midepigastrium, just to the right or left of midline radiating toward one or both of the upper quadrants. Benign epigastric bruits radiate vertically but not laterally (Hall, Wollam, & Tuttle, 1994). Renal bruits are present in approximately 60% of patients with renal artery stenosis due to fibrous dysplasia (Hall et al., 1994) and in 40 to 50% of those with significant stenosis from arteriosclerosis (Williams, 1994). The abdomen should be examined and palpated for an abnormal abdominal pulsation of a possible aortic aneurysm. Abdominal or flank masses palpable may be enlarged kidneys of polycystic renal disease. Truncal obesity with purple striae suggests Cushing's syndrome, a secondary cause for hypertension.

The extremities should be examined for diminished or absent peripheral arterial pulsations, femoral bruits, and edema. The femoral pulses should be palpated simultaneously with the radial artery pulse and compared for diminished or delayed pulsation. Delayed or absent femoral arterial pulses and decreased blood pressure in lower extremities may indicate coarctation of the aorta. In the patient who is diagnosed before the age of 30, arterial pressure in the lower extremities should be measured at least once (Kaplan, 1998). Femoral bruits suggest obstruction of vasculature, most likely secondary to atherosclerosis.

A thorough neurological assessment should be performed. A complete neurovascular evaluation is indicated for all hypertensive patients who have painless vision loss in one eye. Possible neurovascular complications include hypertensive encephalopathy, retinal ischemia or infarction, anterior ischemic optic neuropathy, transient focal cerebral ischemia, cerebral infarction, and intracerebral hemorrhage.

Laboratory and Diagnostic Tests

Initial Laboratory Evaluation

Routine laboratory tests are recommended before initiating therapy to determine the presence of target-organ damage and other risk factors. Standard testing should be done to rule out any cases of secondary hypertension or important associated conditions. The standard baseline testing is shown in Table 30–3.

Many of these standard tests do not reveal much information in early, uncomplicated phases of essential hypertension, but are useful as baseline measurements. Occasionally, they identify patients with concomitant problems or evidence of target-organ damage.

Additional Testing for Target-Organ Damage

Additional diagnostic procedures may be indicated to determine the etiology of the hypertension or to determine the presence of any target-organ damage. The following instances may require further testing:

1. Initial history, physical, severity of the blood pressure readings, or screening laboratory data suggest further investigation.
2. Blood pressures responding poorly to pharmacologic treatment.
3. Previously well-controlled blood pressure that begins to increase.
4. Stage 3 hypertension.
5. Sudden onset of hypertension.

Although hypertensive patients have CAD more commonly than nonhypertensives, defects in myocardial perfusion may occur without obstructive coronary artery disease. Microvascular hypertensive disease without obstructive coronary artery disease may occur, increasing positive exercise stress tests. Symptoms of myocardial ischemia may occur because of increased myocardial oxygen demand, limited coronary reserve from ventricular hypertrophy, or greater systolic wall stress.

Unless the hypertension is accelerated, with resultant encephalopathy, neurological symptoms related to the hypertension may not occur. If symptoms of cerebral ischemia occur in the presence of a carotid bruit, a carotid ultrasound is indicated. Severe headache, nausea and vomiting, visual

TABLE 30–3. Baseline Laboratory and Diagnostic Tests for Patients with Essential Hypertension

Complete blood cell count	Hemoglobin and hematocrit
BUN/Creatinine	Reveals renal compromise. Hyperuricemia is found in half of untreated hypertensives, possibly indicating underlying nephrosclerosis. Gout and kidney stones are more common in hypertensives secondary to the increased urinary calcium excretion
Serum potassium	Should be known before initiating diuretic therapy. Also, hypokalemia is a indicator for primary aldosteronism
Serum calcium	Hypercalcemia may be indicative of hyperparathyroidism
Serum lipid profile	Hypertriglyceridemia and hypercholesterolemia (even more threatening) are found twice as often in untreated hypertensives as in normotensives, and the prevelance increases as the blood pressure level rises. This association is felt to be related to the relationship among upper body obesity, hyperlipidemia, glucose intolerance, and hypertension related to hyperinsulinemia (Kaplan, 1998)
Fasting glucose	Screens for diabetes
Urinanalysis	Red cell casts always indicate glomerular inflammation; proteinuria
EKG	All hypertensives should have a baseline EKG. LVH can be detected on EKG, though this is not so sensitive and is less specific than echocardiogram, especially in blacks. The EKG will detect ischemia and rhythm disturbances

disturbances, transient focal neurological signs and symptoms, altered level of consciousness (confusion, drowsiness, stupor, or coma), and seizures are all characteristic of hypertensive encephalopathy. Three or more of the symptoms are diagnostic of hypertensive encephalopathy. CT scan should be performed to rule out subarachnoid hemorrhage, cerebral infarction, or intracerebral hemorrhage.

Nocturia is usually the first symptom of renal involvement with hyperuricemia and microalbuminuria being the most common identifiable markers of nephrosclerosis, secondary to hypertension. Proteinuria is rare, but can indicate progression to nephrotic stage, which is followed by an elevated creatinine. A creatinine clearance and a 24-hour urine for quantitative protein should be done in all patients with proteinuria (Kaplan, 1998; Moore, 1993).

Hypertension is a contributing risk factor for aortic aneurysm. Careful examination and palpation of the abdomen are necessary, especially in thin, elderly hypertensive males, who have evidence of vascular disease elsewhere. If aneurysm is suspected, ultrasound is necessary for proper diagnosis.

Additional optional tests that may be beneficial include uric acid, fasting triglycerides, low-density lipoprotein (LDL) cholesterol, glycosolated hemoglobin, and thyroid-stimulating hormone.

TABLE 30–4. Components of Cardiovascular Risk Stratification in Patients with Hypertension[a]

Major Risk Factors
- Smoking
- Dyslipidemia
- Diabetes mellitus
- Age older than 60 years
- Sex (men and postmenopausal women)
- Family history of cardiovascular disease: women under age 65 or men under age 55

Target Organ Damage/Clinical Cardiovascular Disease
- Heart diseases
  - Left ventricular hypertrophy
  - Angina/prior myocardial infarction
  - Prior coronary revascularization
  - Heart failure
- Stroke or transient ischemic attach
- Nephropathy
- Peripheral arterial disease
- Retinopathy

[a] See Table 30–5.
From the Joint National Committee on Detection, Evaluation, and Treatment of High Blood Pressure. (1997).

▶ RISK STRATIFICATION

Cardiovascular risk of patients with hypertension is noted by the level of blood pressure and the presence or absence of target organ damage or other risk factors (Table 30–4). During the routine evaluation of patients with hypertension, it should be determined if these risk factors are present. If present, these risk factors modify the patient's risk for subsequent cardiovascular disease. Based on the initial assessment of risk factors, presence of target-organ damage, and level of blood pressure, the patient is risk-stratified (Table 30–5).

Risk Group A

This group is made up of those patients who have either high–normal blood pressure or have stage 1, 2, or 3 hypertension without clinical evidence of cardiovascular disease, target-organ damage, or other risk factors. In this group, those patients who have stage 1 hypertension may be managed with lifestyle modifications for up to 1 year with frequent blood pressure monitoring. Those patients with stage

TABLE 30–5. Risk Stratification and Treatment[a]

Blood Pressure Stages (mm Hg)	Risk Group A (No Risk Factors No TOD/CCD)[b]	Risk Group B (At Least 1 Risk Factor, Not Including Diabetes; No TOC/CCD)	Risk Group C (TOD/CCD and/or Diabetes, with or Without Other Risk Factors)
High-normal (130–139/85–89)	Lifestyle modification	Lifestyle modification	Drug therapy[d]
Stage 1 (140–159/90–99)	Lifestyle modification (up to 12 months)	Lifestyle modification[c] (up to 6 months)	Drug therapy
Stages 2 and 3 (≥160/≥100)	Drug therapy	Drug therapy	Drug therapy

For example, a patient with diabetes and a blood pressure of 142/94 mm Hg plus left ventricular hypertrophy should be classified as having stage 1 hypertension with target organ disease (left ventricular hypertrophy) and with another major risk factor (diabetes). This patient would be categorized as Stage 1, Risk Group C, and recommended for immediate initiation of pharmacologic treatment.

[a] Lifestyle modification should be adjunctive therapy for all patients recommended for pharmacologic therapy.
[b] TOD/CCD indicates target organ disease/clinical cardiovascular disease (see Table 30–4).
[c] For patients with multiple risk factors, clinicians should consider drugs as initial therapy plus lifestyle modifications.
[d] For those with heart failure, renal insufficiency, or diabetes.
From the Joint National Committee on Detection, Evaluation, and Treatment of High Blood Pressure. (1997).

2 or 3 hypertension should have antihypertensive medications initiated (JNC VI, 1997).

Risk Group B

Patients in this group also have no clinical cardiovascular disease or target-organ involvement, but do have one or more of the following major risk factors (*excluding* diabetes mellitus): smoking, dyslipidemia, >60 years old, male or postmenopausal female, family history of premature heart disease (men < 55 years; women < 65 years). Lifestyle modification can be used for those with high–normal blood pressure readings (SBP 130-139, DBP 85-89). Those patients with stage 1 hypertension (SBP 140-159, DBP 90-99) can use a trial of lifestyle modification for 6 months unless multiple-risk factors are present, then antihypertensive drugs should be considered as initial therapy in conjunction with lifestyle modifications.

Risk Group C

These patients have diagnosed cardiovascular disease and target-organ damage and/or diabetes mellitus. It is recommended (JNC VI, 1997) that patients with high–normal blood pressure and either renal insufficiency, heart failure, or diabetes mellitus be considered for immediate drug therapy. Lifestyle modifications should always be used as adjunctive therapy with pharmacologic treatment.

▶ PRIMARY (ESSENTIAL) HYPERTENSION

Approximately 95% of all hypertension cases have no identifiable cause. The condition occurs in 10 to 15% of white adults and 20 to 30% of black adults in the United States. The onset of essential hypertension is usually between ages 25 and 55 and is uncommon before age 20 (Massie, 1995). The pathogenesis of essential hypertension is multifactorial.

Pathogenesis

Currently, no single cause for primary hypertension has been identified. There is ongoing research to uncover possible biochemical or physiologic markers to identify people who have a genetic predisposition to high blood pressure.

The major hemodynamic alteration in hypertension is increased vascular resistance, an increase in the tonicity of vascular smooth muscle in both the arterioles and the venules. The total body venous capacity is reduced, resulting in increased afterload often leading to left ventricular hypertrophy (LVH). During the early stages of hypertension, venoconstriction redistributes volume to the cardiopulmonary circulation from the periphery. As the disease progresses, the vasoconstriction is more intense and the intravascular volume contracts progressively, leading to a diminished right atrial venous return and normalization of the cardiac output. As left ventricular hypertrophy manifests itself, there is dysfunction of the left ventricle and resting cardiac output is diminished.

Excess Sodium Intake

Researchers do not agree on the significance of sodium in hypertension. In cultures that have low dietary intake of sodium, the incidence of hypertension is low. In societies that have a dietary intake many times the daily sodium requirements, approximately 25 to 30% develop hypertension (Treadway, 1995). This is presumably related to an additional inherited defect in the ability of the kidney to excrete excess sodium. A high-sodium intake may activate a number of pressor responses. The increased intravascular volume and subsequent elevated preload related to excess sodium intake or abnormal retention of sodium increases cardiac output (Porsche, 1995) and raises free intracellular calcium and plasma catecholamines. This, in turn, heightens vascular tone and elevates blood pressure. Additionally, insulin resistance is worsened and there is a paradoxical rise in atrial natriuretic peptide (Kaplan, 1998; Treadway, 1995). Kaplan (1998) outlines several possible mechanisms responsible for sodium sensitivity.

A defect in sodium excretion from the kidneys as evidenced by higher rates of glomerular filtration and proximal sodium reabsorption, may be responsible for hypertension in some cases. Defective sodium excretion may translate into an exaggerated suppression of intrarenal renin release and a contradictory decrease in secretion of atrial natriuretic peptide. Another theory is that sodium sensitivity may be related to an elevated level of sympathetic nervous system activity and a greater pressor effect than normal.

As with other possible mechanisms for essential hypertension, there are multiple avenues that can influence renal sodium retention. Normally, when blood pressure rises there is an increase in renal excretion of sodium and water, in an attempt to normalize fluid volume and blood pressure. This is known as pressure-natriuresis. In patients with essential hypertension, the normal pressure-natriuresis curve is reset, preventing the normalization of blood pressure. An alteration in the renal function responsible for resetting the pressure-natriuresis curve is hypothesized to be inherited (Kaplan, 1998).

One hypothesis on the renal contribution to hypertension is based on a subset of ischemic nephrons, from arteriolar vasoconstriction or lumenal narrowing, with impaired sodium excretion. Renin secretion from these nephrons is elevated, interfering with overall blood pressure homeostasis. It has also been suggested that a loss in nephron number with age or a reduced filtration surface area per glomerulus limits sodium excretion (Kaplan, 1998; Porsche, 1995).

Renin–Angiotensin System

Renin is secreted by the juxtaglomerular cells in response to a number of stimuli, including decreased renal perfusion, decreased intravascular volume, increased circulating catecholamines, increased sympathetic nervous system activity, and hypokalemia. It is thought that renin may play a critical role in the pathogenesis of most hypertension, both as a direct pressor and as a growth promotor (Kaplan, 1992a, 1995).

All functions of renin are mediated through angiotensin II synthesis. Renin acts on the protein, angiotensinogen, to release angiotensin, which is converted in the lung to angiotensin II by angiotensin converting enzyme (ACE). This system is the primary stimulus for the secretion of aldosterone and intercedes for the mineralcorticoid response to sodium intake and volume loads. When sodium intake is low or plasma volume shrinks, there is an increase in renin–angiotensin II, which stimulates the secretion of aldosterone. The result of aldosterone is renal retention of sodium and water. Although this system plays an important role in the regulation of blood pressure, its importance in the pathogenesis of primary hypertension is debated.

Many patients with primary hypertension have lower plasma renin activity (PRA) than do normotensives of the same age and sex. The majority of these patients, however, have normal levels of plasma renin. Because low renin levels are expected in primary hypertension, the surprising presence of normal or high levels in most patients has generated a search for an explanation. Kaplan (1998) points out two explanations for this unexpected finding: (1) the possibility of nephron heterogeneity with a group of ischemic nephrons, contributing to excess renin, and (2) the possibility that an increased sympathetic drive is responsible.

Renin production is inversely proportional to effective blood volume. For example, anything that increases blood volume suppresses renin, and anything that decreases blood volume increases renin. With sodium restriction, aldosterone secretion is enhanced and vascular responses and renal blood flow are reduced to retain sodium. With increased dietary sodium, the adrenal response is restricted and vascular responses are enhanced, especially within the renal circulation, promoting sodium excretion.

It is believed that some patients with primary hypertension abnormally regulate, and have fixed levels of, angiotensin II (A-II) in the adrenal tissues. The A-II, it is theorized, does not increase aldosterone secretion when sodium is restricted. Also, renal blood flow does not increase with sodium loading. This hypothesis was supported when both adrenal and renal defects were corrected with suppression of A-II by administering ACE inhibitors (Kaplan, 1998).

Sympathetic Nervous System Response

The cardiovascular system is abundantly innervated by fibers of the autonomic nervous system. The sympathetic nervous system (SNS), along with the parasympathetic nervous system, make up the autonomic nervous system and have opposite effects and operate jointly to effect changes in the heart rate. When the SNS is stimulated, it is coupled with inhibition of the parasympathetic nervous system, and vice versa. This mutual action increases the accuracy of neural regulation by the autonomic nervous system.

Stimulation of the SNS causes release of epinephrine and norepinephrine. These catecholamines cause acceleration of heart rate and AV nodal conduction and increase the force of myocardial contraction, both of which are components of the adrenergic response. When the alpha-receptors in the vasculature are stimulated by the SNS, vasoconstriction results. Alpha$_1$-adrenergic receptors are located in the heart, smooth muscle, vas deferens, and the brain. Many alpha$_2$-adrenergic receptors are autoreceptors that synthesize norepinephrine. Alpha$_2$-receptors are presynaptic receptors that, when activated, inhibit further norepinephrine release. Activation of alpha$_2$-receptors in the brain reduces systemic sympathetic outflow. Blocking these receptors facilitates release of norepinephrine from sympathetic nerve endings.

Activation of beta$_1$-receptors stimulates heart rate and force of contraction, lipolysis of fat cells, and secretion of renin from the kidneys. Stimulation of the beta$_2$-adrenergic receptors relax smooth muscle in the bronchi, vasculature, uterus, gut, and bladder.

Repeated stimulation of both alpha and beta-adrenergic receptors leads to a decreased response to further stimulation, from desensitization following prolonged exposure (Berecek & Wyss, 1993). Cardiac output and arterial blood pressure can be increased by stimulation of the SNS and inhibition of the parasympathetic nervous system, resulting in vasoconstriction, increased heart rate, and force of myocardial contraction. On the other hand, an elevation in blood pressure causes the opposite.

There is evidence that increased SNS activity plays a role in early hypertension and in normotensive offspring of hypertensive parents. In addition, there is evidence that an excess of renin–angiotensin activity could interact with the SNS to mediate most of its effects. In addition, stress can directly activate the SNS and overactivity of the SNS can interact with a high-sodium intake, the renin–angiotensin system, and insulin resistance (Kaplan, 1998).

Baroreceptor Dysfunction. Baroreceptors of the SNS have a role in hypertension. The sinoaortic (high pressure) and cardiopulmonary (low pressure) baroreceptors are reflexes that when activated by a rise in blood pressure or central venous pressure normally reduce heart rate and lower blood pressure by vagal stimulation (i.e., inhibition of the SNS).

There are two major neural mechanisms responsible for the regulation of blood pressure. The high-pressure baroreceptors located in the aortic arch and carotid sinuses are sensitive to stretch of the vessel wall caused by a rise in the arterial blood pressure or central venous pressure. The elevation of blood pressure activates these receptors, stimulating the cardioregulatory center to inhibit SNS activity, reducing heart rate and blood pressure by vagal stimulation. Their firing rate is directly related to the level of arterial pressure (Carleton, 1992; Kaplan, 1998). During sustained hypertension, these reflexes are reset rapidly so when the blood pressure rises, the subsequent decreased heart rate is less dramatic (Kaplan, 1998). The low-pressure cardiopulmonary baroreceptors located predominately in the ventricles, but also in the atria and the venoatrial junctions, discharge during systole. Their firing rate is directly related to the force of myocardial contraction and the cardiac filling pressures.

Excitation of these two sets of receptors cause inhibition of sympathetic neural outflow to the heart and vasculature, causing a reduction in arterial blood pressure and vascular resistance. Also, stimulation of the receptors causes an increased parasympathetic neural outflow to the heart. This results in slowing of the sinus node, reducing the speed of conduction through the atrioventricular node (Rea, 1993), and decreased force of contraction of the atria and, perhaps, the ventricle (Carleton, 1992).

Normally, when arterial and cardiac filling pressures are reduced, the discharge of these receptors declines, sympathetic neural outflow increases leading to elevated vascular resistance, and parasympathetic outflow decreases resulting in tachycardia. The opposite is also true. These negative feedback loops are the major reflex mechanisms that regulate arterial blood pressure (Rea, 1993).

Abnormalities of the nervous system's reflex mechanisms for blood pressure regulation were once thought to explain the pathogenesis of hypertension. Now, it is believed that the state of hypertension itself can also cause secondary irregularities of reflex blood pressure control. Also, baroreceptor abnormalities may promote the persistence of hypertension (Rea, 1993).

The Role of Epinephrine. Intermittent stress can be translated into sustained hypertension. When epinephrine is secreted from the adrenomedulla, blood pressure effects can be longer and more intense, when compared with the short "fight or flight" response. Levels of epinephrine similar to those reached during stress maintain an elevated blood pressure for awhile after the initial response. It is felt that some of the epinephrine enters the sympathetic nerve endings and is rereleased during subsequent sympathetic nerve stimulation. In addition, this epinephrine acts on the presynaptic beta$_2$-receptor to facilitate additional norepinephrine release. Therefore, intermittently secreted epinephrine from the adrenal medulla may provoke a sustained increase in neuronal release of both epinephrine and norepinephrine, causing vasoconstriction and an incessant blood pressure elevation (Kaplan, 1998; Goldstein, 1993).

Stress Exposure. It is not just the level of stress that influences hypertension, but also how the person responds to stress. According to Kaplan (1998), there is greater cardiovascular and sympathetic nervous system reaction to various stresses in hypertensive patients and those with normal blood pressures who are at increased risk for developing hypertension. Stress causes more frequent and intense catecholamine release from the adrenal medulla, leading to increased SNS overactivity, vasoconstriction, increased force of myocardial contraction, increased renin–angiotensin release, and subsequent structural hypertrophy. Excess of renin–angiotensin can also increase SNS activity (Kaplan, 1998; Porsche, 1995). It has been hypothesized that repeated exposures to stressors can cause a persistant rise in blood pressure in hyperreactive patients.

Ion Transport Alterations

There is some evidence that hypertensive patients have cell membrane abnormalities, allowing abnormal intracellular ion exchange that promotes contraction and growth (Kaplan, 1998). This may be secondary to an acquired inhibition of the sodium pump, leading to increased intracellular calcium, subsequently increasing vascular tone and contraction, leaving an increased vascular resistance (Porsche, 1995).

Endothelial Dysfunction

One of the most potent substances, nitric oxide (NO), is released from the endothelial lining of the vessels and acts as the primary endogenous vasodilator. Patients with essential hypertension have diminished production of NO throughout their bodies. Decreased NO release may play a role in the pathogenesis of hypertension, in addition to hypercholesterolimia, diabetes, smoking, and physical inactivity.

Long-acting NO agonists are not yet available for the treatment of hypertension. Medications available today that influence NO are nitroglycerine, for the treatment of angina, and nitroprusside for hypertensive emergencies (Kaplan, 1998).

Obesity

Obesity affects more than one-third of adults in the United States. Obese individuals have higher cardiac outputs, stroke volume, and circulating blood volume with a lower peripheral resistance compared with nonobese patients. The increased body mass is most likely the sole reason for the higher cardiac output and subsequent rise in blood pressure. Truncal obesity is associated with higher incidence of morbidity and mortality.

Virtually all obese people are insulin resistant, which is also associated with increased incidence of hypertension. Addtionally, Kaplan (1998) points out that there is increased sympathetic activity with obesity-induced hyperinsulinemia and increased calorie intake. The normal skeletal muscle and peripheral vascular vasodilation that normally occur with insulin are decreased in the obese population. This results in decreased tissue perfusion and insulin levels, contributing to impaired glucose tolerance and the development of hypertension.

Contributing Factors

Alcohol. Excessive alcohol intake can be blamed for approximately 10% of hypertensive cases in men. Episodic drinkers have less incidence of hypertension than those who drink daily. Alcohol has a pressor effect that may arise from: increased SNS activity; cell membrane dysfunction, allowing increased calcium into the cell and magnesium to leave the cell; increased insulin resistance and hyperinsulinemia; and increased cortisol secretion in heavy drinkers (Kaplan, 1998; Klatsky, 1993). There may be alterations in baroreflex activity, and, in addition to the link between hypertension and alcohol, there is also a relationship between heavy alcohol consumption and cardiac arrhythmias, cardiomyopathy, and hemorrhagic stroke (Klatsky, 1993). Heavy alcohol consumption should always be considered a possible hypertensive risk factor.

Tobacco and Caffeine. Nicotine in cigarette smoke can raise blood pressure acutely, even in long-time smokers. This is most likely related to nicotine-induced release of norepinephrine from adrenergic nerve endings. Cigars (if inhaled) and smokeless tobacco produce the same pressor response. Nicotine patches do not appear to have the same effect on blood pressure. Because no tolerance develops to the nicotine, the blood pressure remains elevated as long as the person smokes. The effects are transient so they may not be observed during an office visit or random blood pressure check. Other adverse effects contributing to nicotine's role in hypertension include increased insulin resistance and a decrease in endothelium-dependent relaxation (Kaplan, 1998).

Caffeine is also associated with hypertensive responses. Tolerance develops to the pressor effects of caffeine, though it is reacquired within a few hours.

Physical Inactivity. Many cross-sectional and prospective observational trials have shown the benefits of regular, vigorous physical exercise. Physical fitness is associated with lower blood pressure levels and prevalence of hypertension. The most beneficial forms of exercise are aerobic or endurance training such as walking, rowing, jogging, biking, swimming, stair climbing, and cross-country skiing. These forms of exercise use the large muscle groups in a repetitive manner to increase heart rate in the target range for a prolonged period of time (Cushman, 1993).

Minerals. Decreased levels of potassium have been noted in the skeletal muscle of untreated hypertensive patients. Potassium supplementation or a diet higher in potassium and lower in sodium may lower blood pressure (Moser, 1997). Serum magnesium levels are normal in hypertensives, although there is an inverse effect of magnesium intake on blood pressure. This is evidenced by clinical trials and a decline in blood pressure with intravenous magnesium salt for the treatment of preeclampsia (Kaplan, 1998; Kuller, 1993).

Genetic Factors. Blood pressure levels have been shown to correlate among family members, with a stronger contribution from the father than from the mother (Kaplan, 1998). This has been attributed to a common genetic link, shared environment, or lifestyle habits. Hypertension does not follow the traditional rules of inheritance seen with a single gene locus. According to the JNC VI (1997), high blood pressure is polygenic and multifactorial—the interaction of several genes and the environment are significant. It is clear that heredity plays a role, but there are no specific gene markers available at this time. The genes that have been suggested to play a role in hypertension are those that affect the renin–angiotensin–aldosterone system, the kalcikrein–kinin system, and the SNS (JNC VI, 1997). Normotensive offspring with a family history of hypertension have been noted to have thicker LV walls and alterations in diastolic filling when compared with control subjects (Graettinger, 1995). Children with one or more parents with hypertension tend to have higher blood pressures.

Ethnic and Socioeconomic Factors. Blacks have an earlier onset and greater prevalence of hypertension when compared with caucasians, Asians, and Native Americans of all ages. Hypertension is present in > 40% of black men 50 years old or greater, compared with 27% in white males. Stage 3 hypertension (DBP ≥ 110) is five times more common in black men than white men, and seven times more common in black women than white women. In all ethnic groups, the less educated have a higher prevalence of hypertension than more educated individuals. This is especially true in the lower socioeconomic groups (Graettinger, 1995).

Environmental Factors. Environment also plays some role in hypertension. There is a significant correlation between blood pressures of spouses, but there is no recognizable explanation. Environmental effects are most clearly shown between populations, not between individuals. However, within populations it is difficult to determine significant relationships between environmental factors and blood pressure. At this time it is unclear the role environment has on blood pressure, and it is likely that blood pressure differences among populations are determined genetically.

Complications of Primary Hypertension

The pathogenesis of hypertension involves structural changes of the resistant vasculature leading to hypertrophy and remodeling. These changes are also closely involved in arteriosclerosis of small vessels and are responsible for the majority of target-organ damage seen with longstanding hypertension. In addition, high pressures accelerate large-vessel atherosclerosis (Kaplan, 1998). The higher the degree of blood pressure elevation, the greater the chances of developing various cardiovascular complications from acceleration of atherosclerosis.

Vascular disease from hypertension involves three interrelated mechanisms:

1. Pulsatile flow: High arterial pressures and changes in pressure waves are destructive on the arteries

leading to fracture of elastic fibers, dilation, thinning, and eventual rupture of the arterial wall (O'Rourke, 1993).

2. Endothelial cell dysfunction: The endothelial cells lining the vessels are both a victim of and a contributor to the vascular damage that is caused by hypertension. In addition to serving as a lining to the vessel, the endothelial cells contain substances that relax and constrict the underlying smooth muscle. The two most active substances contained in these cells are endothelium-derived relaxing factor (EDRF) characterized as nitric oxide, and the endolithins, which are long-acting vasoconstrictors. These along with other endothelium-derived factors may have a significant role in the development of hypertension and the eventual vascular damage. Their production may be modified by lipoproteins, strengthening the relationship among hyperlipidemia, hypertension, and arterial dysfunction (Kaplan, 1992a).
3. Smooth muscle hypertrophy: Vascular smooth muscle hypertrophy is a mechanism responsible for the initiation and persistence of hypertension.

These three interrelated mechanisms are responsible for the consequences of longstanding hypertension that lead to target-organ damage described in the following section.

Target-Organ Involvement

The organs that suffer the devastating effects of hypertension are the heart, brain, kidneys, and blood vessels.

Hypertensive Heart Disease. Cardiac complications are the major causes of morbidity and mortality in primary hypertension. Hypertensive patients have twice the risk for developing symptomatic coronary artery disease, including myocardial infarction and sudden death, and triple the risk for developing congestive heart failure. This increased risk is the result of hypertrophic changes that occur to the left ventricle from the increased afterload imposed by the hypertension, and accelerated atherosclerotic changes within the coronary arteries (Kaplan, 1992a, 1998).

Left Ventricular Hypertrophy. Left ventricular hypertrophy (LVH) is a major independent risk resulting from hypertension and the most common cardiac complication of hypertension. Approximately 5–10% of chronic hypertensives have electrocardiographic evidence of LVH; up to 50% of chronic hypertensives meet echocardiographic criteria for LVH (Kaplan, 1998; Massie, 1995). With increased arterial blood pressure and peripheral vascular resistance, there is an increase in left ventricular wall thickness and mass size resulting from progressive overload and increased stress on the ventricle. There are increased functional and biological responses of the cardiac myocytes to increased protein synthesis and cellular hypertrophy (Frolich, 1994). Diastolic dysfunction is one of the earliest changes related to the development of LVH, manifested by slow diastolic filling. According to Kaplan (1992a), those with minimally increased left ventricular muscle mass may have hyperdynamic contractility reflecting an increased inotropic state with a high percentage of muscle fiber shortening and increased wall stress. If the blood pressure and afterload are not reduced, cardiac failure ensues. Specific associations have been noted between LVH and myocardial ischemia, carotid artery disease, retinopathy, and renal damage. The increased risk for sudden death is most likely related to ventricular ectopy seen with LVH. Hypertensive LVH regresses with therapy, and should be managed aggressively.

Congestive Heart Failure. According to Kaplan (1998), the majority of episodes of congestive heart failure (CHF) in hypertensive patients are associated with dilated cardiomyopathy and a reduced ejection fraction. However, approximately 40% of the cases of CHF are associated with normal systolic function and impaired diastolic function secondary to LVH, fibrosis, myocardial ischemia, and increased afterload.

Coronary Artery Disease. Hypertension is an important risk factor for coronary artery disease (CAD). Mortality from CAD increases with the elevation of blood pressure and incidence of myocardial infarction (MI) greatly increases in the presence of hypertension. Myocardial ischemia results from hypertension when there is an increased demand and decreased supply to the heart. Hypertension increases atherosclerosis of the coronary arteries, increases the resistance in the coronary microvasculature, impairs endothelium-dependent vasodilation, and limits coronary reserve (Kaplan, 1998). Atherosclerotic complications are the most common cause of death in those patients with hypertension (Graettinger, 1995). According to the Framingham Cohort study, the prevalence of silent myocardial infarction was substantially increased in those patients with hypertension. These patients are also at risk for sudden death. (Kaplan, 1992a).

Peripheral Vascular Disease. Changes in the elasticity of the vessels are manifest early in the course of hypertension as arterial compliance is reduced from the elevated blood pressure and increased resistance. Symptomatic peripheral vascular disease (PVD), manifested by intermittent claudication, presents an increased risk for subsequent cardiovascular mortality.

Also, the majority of patients with aortic dissection have hypertension. Dissection most likely results from a combination of wall stress from high pulsatile pressures and accelerated atherosclerosis. The higher the pressure, the greater chance of dissection.

Cerebrovascular Disease. Hypertension is the major cause of stroke and is the most important modifiable risk factor for ischemic stroke, intracerebral hemorrhage, and transient ischemic attack (TIA). Approximately 80% of strokes in hypertensive patients are secondary to ischemic events, caused by either thrombosis or embolism; 10 to 15% are secondary to intraparenchymal hemorrhage; 5% secondary to subarachnoid hemorrhage; and 5 to 15% are related to an unknown etiology. Cerebrovascular complications correlate more with systolic blood pressure than with diastolic pressure. Elderly hypertensives often have silent cerebrovascular disease leading to brain atrophy and vascular dementia. One third of middle-aged hypertensives have regional and global reductions in cerebral blood flow and are neurologically asymptomatic (Kaplan, 1998).

Renal Disease. Renal impairment is both structural and functional in hypertensive patients, even those with mild elevation of blood pressure. Hypertensive nephrosclerosis is the hyalinization and sclerosis of the wall of the afferent arterioles. Renal involvement is usually asymptomatic except for complaints of nocturia secondary to the inability to concentrate urine. The first objective finding is microalbuminuria secondary to impaired intrarenal vasodilatory response. Heavy proteinuria advancing to the nephrotic range can occur. Investigators do not agree on the relationship between hypertension and renal disease. Only a small minority of hypertensives develop progressive renal disease (Kaplan, 1998). Hypertension plays a hand in accelerating the course of other types of renal disease, such as diabetic nephropathy (Massie, 1995). It is agreed that it is more prevalent among diabetics and blacks.

Retinal Changes. Vascular changes of the fundus reflect both hypertensive and arteriosclerotic retinopathy. Initially there is narrowing of the arteriolar lumen (Grade 1) and then sclerosis of the arteriolar wall evident by arteriovenous nicking (Grade 2). Persistent hypertension induces rupture of small vessels, seen as hemorrhages or exudates (Grade 3). Eventually there is papilledema (Grade 4) (Kaplan, 1992a).

Primary Prevention

According to JNC VI (1997) the goal of prevention and management of hypertension is to reduce morbidity and mortality by being as unintrusive as possible. Prevention of disease needs to be recognized as being just as important if not more important than active treatment for established hypertension. Primary prevention gives us the opportunity to interrupt and stop the continuous and costly cycle of managing hypertension and treating its complications. The JNC VI recommends a nationwide approach to prevent blood pressure rise with age and to reduce overall blood pressure levels. In turn, this will improve overall cardiovascular morbidity and mortality as much as, or more than, treating only those with an established diagnosis of hypertension. This approach to prevention is based on lifestyle modifications that have been shown to prevent or delay the expected rise in blood pressure in susceptible people (JNC VI, 1997). Lifestyle modifications, discussed later, could have a greater impact on disease prevention than on treatment of established hypertension, and should be recommended to everyone.

The "J-curve phenomenon" results when blood pressures of large groups of people are plotted on a graph against cardiovascular mortality. This curve illustrates that those with higher blood pressure, closer to the top of the curve, are more likely to die from cardiovascular disease. The curve also shows that those at the lower end (those with very low blood pressures) have increased mortality from cardiovascular disease, too. This accounts for the J shape. The J-curve hypothesis suggests that lowering DBP too much increases the risk for coronary events, presumably due to a lower diastolic perfusion pressure in the coronary circulation. This phenomenon may be more relevant in patients with hypertension and coexisting coronary artery disease and those with a pulse pressure of greater than 60 mm Hg (JNC VI, 1997). Most evidence, however, indicates that the group at the bottom of the curve (with the very low blood pressures) tends to differ from the general population in other ways that may contribute to the higher mortality rates. Data supports a progressive reduction in both cerebrovascular disease and renal disease with even greater reductions in blood pressure. The JNC states that all available data supports the value of the reduction of DBP and SBP at all ages to the levels achieved in clinical trials (DBP to < 90 mm Hg and SBP to < 140 mm Hg) in those patients with isolated systolic hypertension. In these clinical trials there was no increase in cardiovascular morbidity and mortality with further reductions of DBP.

▶ MANAGEMENT

The goal for treatment of hypertension is to prevent morbidity and mortality associated with high blood pressure in a way that the patient will be most compliant. The practitioner should first strive to achieve and maintain arterial blood pressures below 140 mm Hg systolic and 90 mm Hg diastolic. This goal for therapy can be achieved by using lifestyle modifications solely, or as an adjunct to medications.

Nonpharmacologic Therapy

Nonpharmacologic therapy—also known as lifestyle modifications—should be standard practice for all hypertensive patients and should be adjunctive therapy for all patients treated pharmacologically. According to the JNC, these lifestyle modifications have been shown to lower blood pressure to a safe level in most patients, especially those with blood pressures that are minimally elevated, and reduce other cardiovascular risk factors at little cost and low risks. Even minimally elevated pressures have been associated with increased risk for premature cardiovascular disease (CVD). All patients should be encouraged to adopt these lifestyle modifications, especially if they have risk factors for premature CVD, such as high cholesterol or diabetes. For others, this nondrug therapy may not be enough, but it may contribute to reducing the amount of medication necessary to manage their condition.

Weight Reduction

The JNC VI (1997) outlines that a body mass index (weight in kilograms divided by height in meters squared) of 27 or greater is closely correlated with an increased blood pressure. People who carry their body fat in the upper part of the body (visceral or abdominal) and have a waist circumference of 34 inches (85 cm) or greater in women, or 39 inches (98 cm) or greater in men, are at increased risk for high blood pressure, dyslipidemia, diabetes, and fatalities from coronary artery disease. A weight reduction of at least 10 pounds can reduce blood pressure in a large percentage of the overweight, hypertensive population. In overweight patients taking antihypertensive medications, weight reduction can enhance the effectiveness of these agents and reduce cardiovascular risk factors. All hypertensive patients who are overweight should be encouraged to participate in a nutritional program of instruction and calorie restriction along with increased physical activity.

Dietary Approaches

The JNC VI (1997) recommends a diet rich in fresh fruits, vegetables, low-fat dairy products, and foods low in saturated and total fat. A diet low in cholesterol and high in fiber, potassium, calcium, and magnesium, with moderate intake of protein and based on 2000 calories per day is recommended. The DASH (Dietary Approaches to Stop Hypertension) eating plan is from the DASH clinical trial funded by the NHLBI and was found to lower blood pressure. Figure 30–1 contains the DASH diet and sample menu.

Dyslipidemia is a major risk factor for coronary artery disease. Therefore, dietary restriction of fats and possible lipid-lowering agents are an important addition to antihypertensive therapy. Omega-3 fatty acids in large quantities may lower blood pressure, though some abdominal discomfort has been reported with its use.

Physical Activity

Those who live a sedentary lifestyle have a 20 to 50% increased risk of developing hypertensive disease when compared with their more active peers. It is suggested that 30 to 45 minutes/day, 5 to 6 days/week of moderately intense physical activity (i.e., brisk walking) will lower blood pressure. Any patient with cardiac or other serious health conditions may need a stress test or referral to a specialist before beginning an exercise program. A medically supervised exercise program is ideal for these patients.

Relaxation and Biofeedback

There is conflicting data on the role of stress-management techniques in the control of blood pressure. Anxiety and pressures from job or family may be involved in the development of high blood pressure. There have been many attempts to lower blood pressure with various stress-relieving techniques such as meditation, yoga, and biofeedback. These techniques have shown transient reduction in blood pressure; however, there is no conclusive evidence to support their long-term effectiveness in the majority of the hypertensive population. These techniques may be attempted because there may be additional benefits of reducing coronary risk beyond the effect on blood pressure.

Drug Therapy

The decision to begin a patient on a medication requires careful consideration of several factors: severity of the blood pressure elevation, presence of target-organ disease and/or cardiovascular disease, and the presence of other risk factors (JNC VI, 1997) (Fig. 30–2). Overall cardiovascular morbidity and mortality have been reduced by lowering blood pressure with pharmacological therapy (JNC VI, 1997), especially through a decrease in stroke mortality (Kaplan & Opie, 1997). In addition to a decreased mortality from stroke, mortality has been decreased from all causes and protection has been demonstrated for coronary events, heart failure, renal disease progression, and progression to a more severe form of hypertension. This is true among all patients in the adult population regardless of sex, age, race, blood pressure, and socioeconomic status (JNC VI, 1997).

General Guidelines

After careful consideration of the recommendations for risk stratification and treatment put forth by the Joint National Committee, the decision may be made to initiate antihypertensive medications. The initial drug of choice should be given at low dose and titrated up depending on the individual patient's needs, age, and response. The treatment should provide 24-hour effectiveness at once-daily dosing with at least 50% of peak effect to occur at the end of the 24-hour period (JNC VI, 1997). Refer to Tables 30–5 and 30–6 for a listing of oral antihypertensive agents.

Benefits of Long-Acting Formulations Over Short-Acting

1. Compliance is better with once-daily dosing.
2. May be cost effective in many situations because of less pills being used.
3. There is a consistent release/level of medication in the bloodstream to provide a constant coverage; control of blood pressure should be smooth and not intermittent.
4. Protection against risk of sudden death, cardiac event, and stroke that occurs with an abrupt rise in blood pressure after arising from sleep in the morning.

(Text continued on p. 533)

National Institutes of Health

The DASH Diet

This eating plan is from the "Dietary Approaches to Stop Hypertension" (DASH) clinical study. The research was funded by the National Heart, Lung, and Blood Institute (NHLBI), with additional support by the National Center for Research Resources and the Office of Research on Minority Health, all units of the National Institutes of Health. The final results of the DASH study appear in the April 17, 1997, issue of the *New England Journal of Medicine*. The results show that the DASH "combination diet" lowered blood pressure and, so, may help prevent and control high blood pressure.

The "combination diet" is rich in fruits, vegetables, and low-fat dairy foods and low in saturated and total fat. It also is low in cholesterol; high in dietary fiber, potassium, calcium, and magnesium; and moderately high in protein.

The DASH eating plan shown below is based on 2,000 calories a day. Depending on your caloric needs, your number of daily servings in a food group may vary from those listed.

Food Group	Daily Servings	Serving Sizes	Examples and Notes	Significance of Each Food Group to the DASH Diet Pattern
Grains and grain products	7-8	1 slice bread 1/2 C dry cereal 1/2 C cooked rice, pasta, or cereal	whole wheat bread, English muffin, pita bread, bagel, cereals, grits, oatmeal	major sources of energy and fiber
Vegetables	4-5	1 C raw leafy vegetable 1/2 C cooked vegetable 6 oz vegetable juice	tomatoes, potatoes, carrots, peas, squash, broccoli, turnip greens, collards, kale, spinach, artichokes, beans, sweet potatoes	rich sources of potassium, magnesium, and fiber
Fruits	4-5	6 oz fruit juice 1 medium fruit 1/4 C dried fruit 1/4 C fresh, frozen, or canned fruit	apricots, bananas, dates, grapes, oranges, orange juice, grapefruit, grapefruit juice, mangoes, melons, peaches, pineapples, prunes, raisins, strawberries, tangerines	important sources of potassium, magnesium, and fiber
Low-fat or nonfat dairy foods	2-3	8 oz milk 1 C yogurt 1.5 oz cheese	skim or 1% milk, skim or low-fat buttermilk, nonfat or low-fat yogurt, part-skim mozzarella cheese, nonfat cheese	major sources of calcium and protein
Meats, poultry, and fish	2 or less	3 oz cooked meats, poultry, or fish	select only lean; trim away visible fats; broil, roast, or boil, instead of frying; remove skin from poultry	rich sources of protein and magnesium
Nuts, seeds, and legumes	4-5 per week	1.5 oz or 1/3 C nuts 1/2 oz or 2 Tbsp seeds 1/2 C cooked legumes	almonds, filberts, mixed nuts, peanuts, walnuts, sunflower seeds, kidney beans, lentils	rich sources of energy, magnesium, potassium, protein, and fiber

Figure 30–1. The DASH diet.

National Institutes of Health

The DASH Diet • Sample Menu • based on 2,000 calories/day

Food	Amount	Servings Provided
Breakfast		
orange juice	6 oz	1 fruit
1% low-fat milk	8 oz (1 C)	1 dairy
corn flakes (with 1 tsp sugar)	1 C	2 grains
banana	1 medium	1 fruit
whole wheat bread (with 1 Tbsp jelly)	1 slice	1 grain
soft margarine	1 tsp	1 fat
Lunch		
chicken salad	3/4 C	1 poultry
pita bread	1/2, large	1 grain
raw vegetable medley:		
carrot and celery sticks	3-4 sticks each	
radishes	2	1 vegetable
loose-leaf lettuce	2 leaves	
part-skim mozzarella cheese	1.5 slice (1.5 oz)	1 dairy
1% low-fat milk	8 oz (1 C)	1 dairy
fruit cocktail in light syrup	1/2 C	1 fruit
Dinner		
herbed baked cod	3 oz	1 fish
scallion rice	1 C	2 grains
steamed broccoli	1/2 C	1 vegetable
stewed tomatoes	1/2 C	1 vegetable
spinach salad:		
raw spinach	1/2 C	
cherry tomatoes	2	1 vegetable
cucumber	2 slices	
light Italian salad dressing	1 Tbsp	1/2 fat
whole wheat dinner roll	1 small	1 grain
soft margarine	1 tsp	1 fat
melon balls	1/2 C	1 fruit
Snacks		
dried apricots	1 oz (1/4 C)	1 fruit
mini-pretzels	1 oz (3/4 C)	1 grain
mixed nuts	1.5 oz (1/3 C)	1 nuts
diet ginger ale	12 oz	0

Total number of servings in 2,000 calories/day menu:

Food Group	*Servings*
Grains	= 8
Vegetables	= 4
Fruits	= 5
Dairy Foods	= 3
Meats, Poultry, and Fish	= 2
Nuts, Seeds, and Legumes	= 1
Fats and Oils	= 2.5

Tips on Eating the DASH Way

- Start small. Make gradual changes in your eating habits.
- Center your meal around carbohydrates, such as pasta, rice, beans, or vegetables
- Treat meat as one part of the whole meal, instead of the focus.
- Use fruits or low-fat, low-calorie foods such as sugar-free gelatin for desserts and snacks.

REMEMBER! If you use the DASH diet to help prevent or control high blood pressure, make it part of a lifestyle that includes choosing foods lower in salt and sodium, keeping a healthy weight, being physically active, and, if you drink alcohol, doing so in moderation.

To learn more about high blood pressure, call 1-800-575-WELL or visit the NHLBI Web site at http://www.nhlbi.nih.gov/nhlbi/nhlbi.htm. DASH is also online at http.//dash.bwh.harvard.edu.

Figure 30–1. *(Continued)*

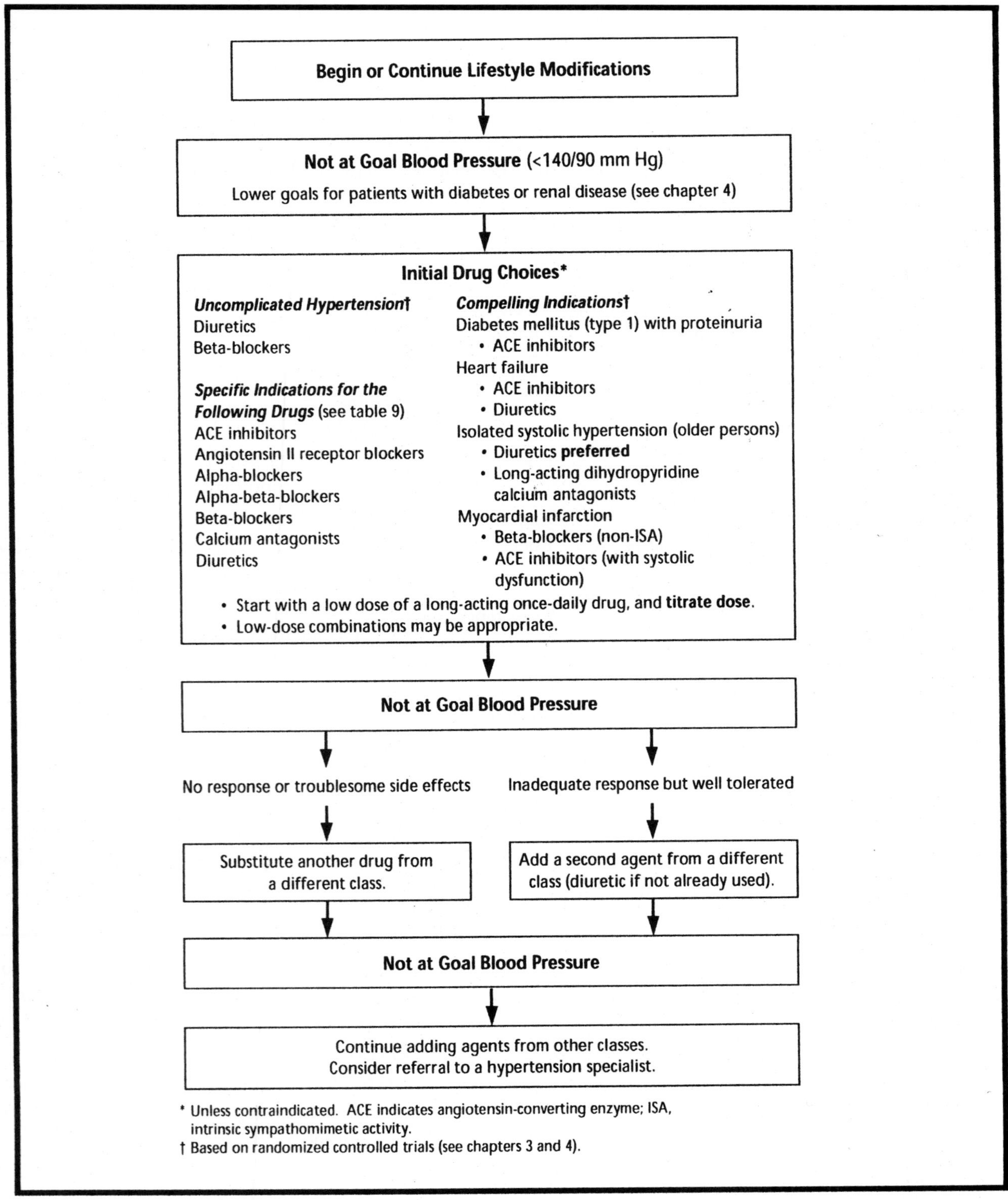

Figure 30–2. Algorithm for the treatment of hypertension. *(From the Joint National Committee on Detection, Evaluation, and Treatment of High Blood Pressure [1997].)*

TABLE 30–6. Considerations in Selecting Pharmacological Therapy

Demographics	Hypertension in African-Americans is generally more responsive to diuretics and calcium antagonists than beta blockers or ACE inhibitors
Concomitant illnesses	Antihypertensive medications can either improve or adversely effect some diseases. It is best to choose an agent that complements the treatment regimen
Quality of life	Most agents recommended for initial therapy maintain or improve quality of life, despite some adverse effects
Cost	The cost of therapy is often a barrier to adequate blood pressure control and compliance. Medication expenses may be reduced by using combination agents and generic formulations. Patients should be instructed to do price comparison at different sources
Drug Interactions	
Physiological and biochemical measurements	In certain circumstances heart rate, body weight, and hemodynamic measurements are helpful in choosing specific agents.

5. Many patients miss at least one dose of medication each week and, for this reason, agents with duration of action of greater than 24 hours are beneficial.

Initial Therapy and Special Considerations. Table 30–6 lists considerations for selecting initial therapy.

Therapy for uncomplicated stages I and II hypertension should be initiated with the lowest dosages of medications to prevent adverse effects associated with too dramatic a reduction in blood pressure. If there is not an adequate response from the initial agent after one to two months, the next dosage level should be prescribed. If there is still no adequate response from the initial agent once full dose is reached, it is recommended that a second agent be added. Or, if adverse effects exist, the medication can be substituted with an agent from another class. Addition of a low-dose thiazide diuretic is an ideal second step because it generally enhances the effects of other agents. The initial agent can be reduced if the second agent achieves satisfactory results (JNC VI, 1997). Before progressing to the next treatment step in unresponsive patients, the practitioner should always evaluate reasons for lack of responsiveness to therapy.

High-Risk Patients. Modifications to the general approach of treating hypertension may need to be implemented for those patients with stage 3 hypertension, those in risk group C, or those patients who are at greater risk for coronary event or stroke. Drug therapy should be initiated without delay. Two or more agents are often necessary if responsiveness to single drug therapy is inadequate. Patients with an average SBP of 200 mm Hg or higher and an average DBP of 120 mm Hg or higher require more immediate attention and hospitalization if there is symptomatic target-organ damage (JNC VI, 1997).

Step-Down Therapy. According to the JNC, once blood pressure has been adequately controlled for at least one year, it is appropriate to attempt to decrease the dosage and number of antihypertensive drugs. The reduction should progress in a slow and deliberate manner. Patients who are instituting lifestyle modifications are more successful with step-down therapy. Follow-up visits should be scheduled to closely follow blood pressure, which usually rises again to hypertensive levels several months or years after treatment has been discontinued, particularly in those patients who do not continuously follow lifestyle modifications.

Thiazide Diuretics

The diuretic as first-step care approach has been studied in the majority of large therapeutic trials in the United States. To be effective, the diuretic chosen must provide enough natriuresis to decrease blood volume. A persistent volume reduction, with continued diuretic use, is required to have a consistent lowering of blood pressure. Therefore, a long-acting thiazide diuretic is often chosen to treat hypertension (Opie, Kaplan, & Poole-Wilson, 1997).

The traditional role of standard or high doses of diuretics as first-line therapy in mild hypertension is challenged more often because of the metabolic side effects. The metabolic side effects of diuretics should be monitored. By administering lower doses of diuretics, especially in special populations (i.e., elderly, obese, and blacks) these side effects are minimized. Because low-dose diuretics given over long periods of time result in few changes in blood lipids, glucose, and electrolytes, the JNC recommend that diuretics and beta blockers be instituted in first-line therapy for hypertension.

Treatment of hypertension is usually initiated with thiazide-type diuretics (Table 30–7). If renal function is severely impaired (creatinine >2.5), a loop diuretic is needed. A potassium-sparing diuretic may be given in combination with the diuretic to decrease the incidence of hypokalemia.

Thiazide diuretics remain the most commonly used drugs for the treatment of hypertension. Thiazide diuretics inhibit sodium and chloride reabsorption in the early portion of the distal convoluted tubule (Kaplan, 1998; Treadway, 1995). Sodium and water excretion increases causing decreased plasma volume, intracellular sodium, and peripheral resistance. However, thiazide diuretics are only moderately effective in that the maximum excretion of filtered sodium is only 5 to 8% and nearly 90% of filtered sodium is reabsorbed before reaching the distal convoluted tubule.

TABLE 30–7. Combination Drugs for Hypertension

Drug	Trade Name
Beta–adrenergic blockers and diuretics	
Atenolol, 50 or 100 mg/chlorthalidone, 25 mg	Tenoretic
Bisoprolol fumarate, 2.5, 5, or 10 mg/hydrochlorothiazide, 6.25 mg	Ziac[a]
Metoprolol tartrate, 50 or 100 mg/hydrochlorothiazide, 25 or 50 mg	Lopressor HCT
Nadolol, 40 or 80 mg/bendroflumethiazide, 5 mg	Corzide
Propranolol hydrochloride, 40 or 80 mg/hydrochlorothiazide, 25 mg	Inderide
Propranolol hydrochloride (extended release), 80, 120, or 160 mg/hydrochlorothiazide, 50 mg	Inderide LA
Timolol maleate, 10 mg/hydrochlorothiazide, 25 mg	Timolide
ACE inhibitors and diuretics	
Benazepril hydrochloride, 5, 10, or 20 mg/hydrochlorothiazide, 6.25, 12.5, or 25 mg	Lotensin HCT
Captopril, 25 or 50 mg/hydrochlorothiazide, 15 or 25 mg	Capozide[a]
Enalapril maleate, 5 or 10 mg/hydrochlorothiazide, 12.5 or 25 mg	Vaseretic
Lisinopril, 10 or 20 mg/hydrochlorothiazide, 12.5 or 25 mg	Prinzide, Zestoretic
Angiotensin II receptor antagonists and diuretics	
Losartan potassium, 50 mg/hydrochlorothiazide, 12.5 mg	Hyzaar
Calcium antagonists and ACE inhibitors	
Amlodipine besylate, 2.5 or 5 mg/benazepril hydrochloride, 10 or 20 mg	Lotrel
Diltiazem hydrochloride, 180 mg/enalapril maleate, 5 mg	Teczem
Verapamil hydrochloride (extended release), 189 or 240 mg/trandolapril, 1, 2, or 4 mg	Tarka
Felodipine, 5 mg/enalapril maleate, 5 mg	Lexxel
Other combinations	
Triamterene, 37.5, 50, or 75 mg/hydrochlorothiazide, 25 or 50 mg	Dyazide, Maxide
Spironolactone, 25 or 50 mg/hydrochlorothiazide, 25 or 50 mg	Aldactazide
Amiloride hydrochloride, 5 mg/hydrochlorothiazide, 50 mg	Moduretic
Guanethidine monosulfate, 10 mg/hydrochlorothiazide, 25 mg	Esimil
Hydralazine hydrochloride, 25, 50, or 100 mg/hydrochlorothiazide, 25 or 50 mg	Apresazide
Methyldopa, 250 or 500 mg/hydrochlorothiazide, 15, 25, 30, or 50 mg	Aldoril
Reserpine, 0.125 mg/hydrochlorothiazide, 25 or 50 mg	Hydropres
Reserpine, 0.10 mg/hydralazine hydrochloride, 25 mg/hydrochlorothiazide, 15 mg	Ser-Ap-Es
Clonidine hydrochloride, 0.1, 0.2, or 0.3 mg/chlorthalidone, 15 mg	Combipres
Methyldopa, 250 mg/chlorothiazide, 150 or 250 mg	Aldochlor
Reserpine, 0.125 or 0.25 mg/chlorthalidone, 25 or 50 mg	Demi-Regroton
Reserpine, 0.125 or 0.25 mg/chlorothiazide, 250 or 500 mg	Diupres
Prazosin hydrochloride, 1, 2, or 5 mg/polythiazide, 0.5 mg	Minizide

[a] Approved for initial therapy.
(From the Joint National Committee on Detection, Evaluation, and Treatment of High Blood Pressure [1997].)

Potassium excretion is also increased. The decreased plasma volume activates the renin–angiotensin–aldosterone system to limit the extent of volume depletion. According to Kaplan (1998), counterregulatory mechanisms rapidly reestablish a constant state so that sodium intake and excretion are balanced within 3 to 9 days in the presence of decreased body fluid volume. With continued use, the blood volume and cardiac output normalize while peripheral vascular resistance decreases. The mechanism for the lowered peripheral vascular resistance is unknown. Potential mechanisms for the reduction of vascular resistance by small but persistent reduction in sodium include a decrease in interstitial volume, a fall in smooth muscle sodium concentration, and a change in association and response of receptors on the surface of cells to vasoconstrictor hormones (Oates, 1996).

The degree of blood pressure response depends on the individual's ability to initiate counterregulatory responses to the lowered blood pressure and plasma volume. Increased secretion of renin and aldosterone retard the continued sodium diuresis. Both renin-induced vasoconstriction and aldosterone-induced sodium retention inhibit continued reduction of body fluids and progressive fall in blood pressure while therapy continues (Kaplan, 1992b, 1998). Those who initially have low, suppressed plasma renin levels and have a weak renin response after diuretics are begun, have been shown to be more diuretic responsive (Kaplan, 1998).

Dosage. When a thiazide diuretic is used as monotherapy, it should be administered in low doses. Most patients with mild to moderate hypertension and serum creatinine concentrations below 2.0mg/dL will respond to lower doses. Lower levels of hydrochlorothiazide (HCTZ) 12.5

mg are equally as effective as 25 mg in most uncomplicated hypertensives within several weeks of initiation. This is especially true if used in combination with beta blockers or ACE inhibitors. The advantage of low-dose HCTZ (or its equivalent) is that the adverse metabolic and lipid effects are minimized while maintaining the antihypertensive potency. The response rate to thiazide monotherapy is variable and depends on the degree of blood pressure elevation, age, race, renal function, sodium ingestion, and intensity of counterregulatory renin–aldosterone response of the patient (Kaplan, 1992b). By increasing HCTZ, for example, past 25 mg/day, risks of side effects increase, making combination therapy favorable (Opie, Kaplan & Poole-Wilson, 1997).

The thiazide-class of drugs has the same pharmacologial effects and, therefore, is interchangeable with appropriate adjustment of dosage. The majority, including HCTZ, have an intermediate duration of action (6-12 hours). Preference is given to those compounds proven to be effective in low doses, such as HCTZ, bendrofluazide, cyclopenthiazide, and chlorthelidone (Opie, Kaplan, & Poole-Wilson, 1997).

Side Effects. The degree of hypokalemia is dose dependent. Diuretic-induced hypokalemia is exaggerated by increased amounts of sodium intake and those with depleted potassium stores, including older adults. Most of the adverse reactions from diuretic-induced hypokalemia occur with marked potassium depletion. Digitalis toxicity may occur with mild hypokalemia possibly because the sodium/potassium/ATPase pump is inhibited with both digitalis and hypokalemia, disturbing the normal electrolyte balance and membrane potential within the cells (Kaplan, 1998).

Diuretic-induced hypokalemia is a potentially lethal side effect that can lead to ventricular arrhythmias and sudden death. Proper monitoring of potassium levels is important. Although it occurs more frequently in those patients taking loop diuretics, hypomagnesemia may also occur with thiazide diuretic use.

With chronic use of thiazide diuretics there is a slight, asymptomatic fall in serum sodium. Rarely there is severe symptomatic hyponatremia following initiation of the diuretic therapy. Hyperuricemia also increases with thiazide diuretic use and may precipitate gout or kidney stones.

Higher doses of diuretics raise total serum cholesterol, LDL cholesterol, and triglyceride levels with little effect on HDL levels. There can be an increase in cholesterol of 15 to 20 mg/dL mostly in the LDL and an increase in triglyceride concentration, sometimes even at low doses (Opie, Kaplan, & Poole-Wilson, 1997). This rise in serum cholesterol and triglyceride concentrations usually occurs within the first 3 to 12 months of therapy (Moser, 1997).

The degree of glucose intolerance due to thiazide diuretics is usually mild. But, because of the possible relationship between insulin resistance and the development of hypertension, this is an undesirable effect.

Sexual dysfunction is a side effect seen more often with diuretics than with any other drug. It is most often seen in men, but can occur in women in the form of decreased libido and orgasmic delay. The symptoms may be diminished by decreasing the dose, alternating days of therapy, and omitting the drug for two to three days at a time. The symptoms may disappear when the diuretic is stopped. However, many patients will not experience improvement in their symptoms, possibly because a high percentage of patients have symptoms of sexual dysfunction prior to starting on diuretic therapy (Moser, 1997).

Drug Interactions. Thiazide diuretics may diminish the effects of anticoagulants, agents used for the treatment of gout, sulfonylureas, and insulin. Increased effects may be seen when thiazides are used with digitalis, anesthetics, diazoxide, lithium, loop diuretics, and vitamin D. Nonsteroidal antiinflammatory drugs (NSAIDs) may reduce the effectiveness of thiazide diuretics.

Loop Diuretics

Loop diuretics are usually needed in the treatment of hypertensive patients with renal failure and a creatinine exceeding 2.0. Loop diuretics block chloride reabsorption by inhibiting the sodium/potassium/chloride cotransport system within the lining of the thick ascending limb of the loop of Henle. This is where 35 to 45% of filtered sodium is reabsorbed. Loop diuretics are more potent with a more rapid onset when compared with thiazide diuretics. However, they are no more effective in lowering blood pressure and do not cause less side effects than thiazide diuretics (Kaplan, 1998). The site of action is reached intraluminally; they must enter the tubular fluid to be effective. Chloride, sodium, and potassium ions stay inside the lumen and are wasted in the urine with the possible side effects of hyponatremia, hypochloremia, hypokalemia, and alkalosis (Opie, Kaplan, & Poole-Wilson, 1997). When blood flow to the kidneys is reduced, larger doses are needed. Organic acids and drugs such as Probenecid may compete for entry into the tubule.

Dosing. Loop diuretics must be given two to three times each day to maintain reduced plasma volume that is necessary for lowering blood pressure with diuretic therapy. The short duration of furosemide (Lasix) (less than six hours for oral dose) does not maintain this decreased body fluid volume, sodium is retained, and the 24-hour fluid balance is not effectively altered. Twice-daily dosing of low-dose furosemide can be effective as monotherapy or combined with other agents. If twice-daily dosing is used, the first dose should be given early in the morning and the second dose given in midafternoon or early evening, so diuretic action occurs at the time of sodium intake and to avoid nocturia. If patients are not responsive to thiazide diuretics, then furosemide will probably not work unless the problem is a low GFR. In severe hypertension, IV furosemide is occasionally used for rapid antihypertensive effect, especially if fluid overload is present (Opie, Kaplan, & Poole-Wilson, 1997).

Bumetanide (Bumex) is 40 times more potent than furosemide, but has similar actions when given in equipotent doses.

The longer acting torsemide (Demadex) has been well studied and may provide a sustained antihypertensive effect with once-daily dosing (Kaplan, 1995; Opie, Kaplan, & Poole-Wilson, 1997). Torsemide differs from other diuretics in that it is mainly metabolized by the liver; only 20% is eliminated unchanged in the urine, giving it a longer duration of action.

Ethacrinic acid (Edecrin), also a loop diuretic, has greater side effects of ototoxicity and is rarely used.

Side Effects. Loop diuretics may cause fewer metabolic side effects than their longer acting counterparts because of their shorter duration of action. Side effects of loop diuretics are similar to the thiazide diuretics. The hyperlipidemic effect occurs from immediate rise in serum lipid levels from hemoconcentration following their administration. Reversible dose-related ototoxicity is seen with furosemide and can be avoided by not infusing it at rates greater than 4 mg/min (Opie, Kaplan, & Poole-Wilson, 1997).

Other Thiazide-like Diuretics

Metolazone (Zaroxylyn) also belongs to the thiazide diuretic category, but the difference is that it is effective in those patients with reduced renal function. The duration of action is up to 24 hours and when combined with loop diuretics can cause profound diuresis, with risk of volume depletion and hypokalemia. This combination, however, is used in patients with renal and heart failure. The side effects are similar to that of other thiazide diuretics (Opie, Kaplan, & Poole-Wilson, 1997).

Indapamide (Lozol) is also a thiazide-type diuretic with a half life of 14 to 16 hours. The initial dose is usually 1.25 mg daily for 4 weeks and increased to 2.5 mg daily. At these low doses, blood pressure is lowered, possibly from vasodilation. At higher doses of 2.5 to 5 mg daily, diuresis is achieved. Hypokalemia is slightly more frequent with indapamide than with HCTZ. Doses of 2.5 mg of indapamide seem to be better at provoking regression of left ventricular hypertrophy than does HCTZ 25 mg. Indapamide is thought, by many, to be the diuretic of choice for diabetics because of its ability to reduce microalbuminuria. However, there are no good comparison studies with other low-dose thiazide diuretics.

Potassium-Sparing Diuretics

The site of action is the distal tubule to prevent potassium loss. There are three potassium-sparing agents available. One is aldactone (Spironolactone), which is an aldosterone antagonist. The other two agents (Amiloride and Triamterene) act as direct inhibitors of tubular secretion. These agents are helpful in reducing thiazide-induced potassium wasting and in treating hyperaldosteronism. However, progressive hypokalemia may still occur with their use. Used alone, they are relatively weak antihypertensives. Caution should be taken with patients who have renal insufficiency because of their decreased ability to excrete potassium (Kaplan, 1995, 1998).

The most commonly reported side effects are nausea, flatulence, and skin rash. Hyperkalemia also occurs and is the most serious side effect.

Combination Agents with Diuretics

Diuretics may add to the effectiveness of all other types of antihypertensives, except the dihydropyridine calcium channel blockers. An adequate blood pressure reduction can be obtained with low doses of thiazide diuretics (6.25 mg) when added to low doses of a second agent. A logical combination is the low-dose thiazide diuretic with an ACE inhibitor. Thiazide diuretics increase renin levels and ACE inhibitors decrease metabolic side effects of thiazides (Opie, Kaplan, & Poole-Wilson, 1997). Ziac (bisoprolol and HCTZ) and Capozide (captopril and HCTZ) have been approved by the JNC VI for first-line therapy (refer to Table 30–7).

Beta Blockers

Beta blockade is recommended as an alternative to diuretics for initial therapy in the treatment of hypertension. Beta blockers are especially suitable for patients with angina pectoris or postmyocardial infarction.

Mechanism of Action. There is no consensus on the antihypertensive mechanisms of beta blockers. The following proposed mechanisms most likely contribute either partially or completely: (1) reduction in cardiac output and heart rate; (2) inhibition of renin release; (3) reduction in venous return and plasma volume; (4) reduction in peripheral vascular resistance (Kaplan & Opie, 1997); (5) resetting baroreceptor levels; (6) reduction in norepinephrine release from neurons; and (7) prevention of pressor response to catecholamines with exercise and stress (Frishman, 1993; Massie, 1995).

Differences Among Beta Blockers. The various beta–adrenergic blockers differ in terms of the presence or absence of intrinsic sympathomimetic activity (ISA), membrane-stabilizing activity (MSA), $beta_1$ selectivity, presence of alpha–adrenergic blocking activity, lipid solubilities, and relative potencies and duration of action (Frishman, 1993; Kaplan, 1995). All beta blockers are similar in their antihypertensive capabilities, regardless of these potential differences. The side effects differ, however, and all agents are nonselective at higher doses (Table 30–8).

Beta blockers are especially useful in those patients with angina pectoris, hypertrophic cardiomyopathy with diastolic dysfunction (Swartz & Moore, 1996), vascular

TABLE 30–8. Differences Among Beta Blockers

	Physiologic Effects	Examples
Intrinsic sympathomimetic activity (ISA)	Lower blood pressure with minimal effect cardiac output; less bradycardia	pindolol, carteolol, penbutolol, acebutolol
Membrane stabilizing activity	Membrane-stabilizing effect on action potential of the heart	
Beta-1 selectivity	Selectively block cardiac beta-1 receptors and have less effect on bronchial beta-2 receptors	esmolol, atenolol, metoprolol, bisoprolol, acebutolol
Alpha–adrenergic activity	Direct vasodilatory effect; less vasoconstriction	labetolol and carvedilol
Lipid-solubility	Poorly lipid-soluble agents do not cross the blood–brain barrier so readily, and may have less neurologic effects	acebutolol, atenolol

headaches, and somatic manifestations of anxiety (Massie, 1995). Beta blockers have also been shown to prevent fatal and nonfatal cardiac events in patients with previous history of myocardial infarction (Massie, 1995; Swartz & Moore, 1996) and they negate the reflex tachycardia caused by vasodilators like hydralazine and alpha–adrenergic blockers.

Beta blockers should not be used in patients with chronic obstructive pulmonary disease, heart block of greater than first degree, and sick sinus syndrome. Caution should be taken when given to patients with diabetes and hyperlipidemia. In those patients with noninsulin diabetes mellitis, beta blockers may worsen glucose intolerance and may mask symptoms of insulin-induced hypoglycemia. Beta blockers should not be discontinued suddenly in those patients with known ishcemic heart disease. For patients with Raynaud's phenomenon, beta blockers can be harmful, although beta blockade (as well as ACE inhibitors) improves microalbuminemia and hypertension. In hypertensive patients with diabetic nephropathy, these agents should be used with caution, or avoided, except in the presence of angina or postinfarct states (Opie, Poole-Wilson, et al., 1997).

Side Effects. Three major mechanisms producing adverse reactions to beta blockade are smooth muscle spasm (bronchospasm and cold extremities), exaggeration of cardiac effects (i.e., bradycardia, heart block), and central nervous system infiltration, causing insomnia and depression.

Beta blockers without ISA can cause asymptomatic bradycardia. The maximal heart rate is lowered approximately 20% with the use of beta blockers. Often patients notice decreased exercise tolerance and easy fatigability, which also noted less in agents with ISA. Rate of atrioventricular (A-V) conduction slows and may worsen heart block, exacerbate left ventricular dysfunction, and decrease cardiac output.

Bronchospasm can occur. $Beta_1$ selective agents cause less bronchial constriction at lower doses, but at higher doses they are similar to $beta_2$ nonselective agents.

Fatigue is a common side effect. Lipid-soluble beta blockers, which cross the blood–brain barrier, cause more central nervous system disturbances such as nightmares, hallucinations, confusion, lethargy, and depression (Graettinger, 1995; Kaplan, 1995).

Beta blockers should be used with caution in insulin-dependent diabetics. The response to hypoglycemia is dependent on catecholamine stimulation of glucose synthesis and release, especially in these patients who cannot secrete glucagon. Insulin induced hypoglycemia may be prolonged and more severe when using a beta blocker. The symptoms of hypoglycemia (i.e., tremors, tachycardia, hunger) are masked. Sweating is not affected, however, and patients should be educated as to the significance of sweating as a warning sign of a hypoglycemic event (Frishman, 1993; Kaplan, 1995).

Beta blockers may elevate plasma triglyceride levels and reduce high-density lipoproteins (HDL) cholesterol levels. This is seen to a lesser extent with those agents that have high ISA. According to Kaplan (1995), triglyceride levels rise an average of 30% with use of most beta blockers, which might explain why these agents have failed to reduce the incidence of coronary artery disease in controlled clinical trials. However, beta blockers without ISA are the only agents shown to decrease the incidences of sudden death, overall mortality rate, and recurrent myocardial infarction (MI) in patients with a history of previous MI. However, they do not protect against a first heart attack. Beta blockers with ISA have no negative influence on plasma lipid levels, but do not possess the ability to protect patients against recurrent MIs.

According to Kaplan (1995), with most beta blockers, except nadolol, there has been a 10 to 20% decline in renal blood flow and GFR, possibly secondary to renal vasoconstriction.

Nasal congestion and impotence are other potential side effects of beta-blocker therapy. Package inserts report a 1% incidence of impotence, but Opie, Sonnenblick et al. (1997) report that erectile dysfunction may be as high as 11% when compared with 26% in patients taking diuretics and 3% taking placebo. A change to a vasodilatory beta blocker or to a combination agent such as Ziac, which has low doses of the beta blocker and a diuretic, may be helpful.

Special Considerations. Combinations of diltiazem or verapamil with beta blockers may have additional sinoatrial and atrioventricular node depressant and negative inotropic effects. Combinations of beta blockers and reserpine may induce profound bradycardia and syncope. Phenylpropanolamine, pseudoephedrine, ephedrine, and epinephrine can cause elevations in blood pressure secondary to unopposed alpha-receptor induced vasoconstriction (Frishman, 1993).

Beta blockade is as effective in older adults as in younger patients, especially in the white population. Despite this fact, American health-care providers are prescribing ACE inhibitors and calcium antagonist more frequently for the control of elderly hypertensives (Opie, Sonnenblick, et al., 1997).

In a study comparing six antihypertensive agents with placebo, Materson, et al. (1993) showed that atenolol was only minimally more effective than placebo, with the ACE inhibitor captopril being less effective than placebo. Diltiazem was the most effective. In black hypertensives (< 60 years old), atenolol was the second most effective agent after diltiazem and was more effective than HCTZ.

Other Beta Blockers. Table 30–9 lists several new oral beta blockers and esmolol, a short-acting IV beta blocker.

Alpha-Adrenergic Blockers

Alpha blockers are a class of antihypertensive agents that can be used as monotherapy for the initial treatment of mild to moderate hypertension. Tachyphylaxis may occur with long-term use and side effects are common. For more advanced forms of hypertension, alpha–adrenergic blockers can be combined with other agents. The most commonly used alpha blockers are the selective agents that block postsynaptic $alpha_1$ adrenergic receptors. These agents lower blood pressure by blocking the uptake of catecholamines, thereby relaxing vascular smooth muscle, leading to vasodilation and decreased peripheral vascular resistance (PVR) without major changes in cardiac output. This is probably secondary to decreased venous return (preload) and a small amount of reflex sympathetic stimulation from vasodilation.

The advantages of $alpha_1$ blockers are the lower incidence of metabolic and lipid side effects. Selective $alpha_1$ adrenergic blockers decrease insulin resistance and have a favorable effect on glucose metabolism. Tolerance often develops with long-term therapy secondary to fluid retention, requiring higher doses and additional diuretics. Alpha blockers are especially chosen in those patients with dyslipidemia, diabetes, or men with benign prostatic hypertrophy. Unlike beta blockers and diuretics, alpha blockers increase HDL cholesterol levels while reducing total cholesterol levels. The LDL cholesterol-lowering effect of Doxazosin is similar to a dose of 10 mg of Lovastatin (Graettinger, 1995).

Efficacy and Dosage. These agents are effective in lowering blood pressure equivalent overall to diuretics, beta blockers, ACE inhibitors, and calcium channel blockers. They are equally as effective in blacks as in nonblack patients and in older adults. Prazosin is effective in more severe cases of hypertension and with patients who have congestive heart failure. Lower doses should be used because excessive hypotension is more prevalent with these agents, especially if compared with a diuretic. To avoid first-dose hypotension, stop the diuretic two days before starting, or give only 1 mg of the drug. The patient should be educated to the possibility of postural symptoms. These are often given before bedtime for this reason. Dosage should be slowly increased to a maximum of 20 mg/day. Prazosin is 2 to 3 times daily dosing, while doxazosin/terazosin is once-daily dosing.

Side Effects. The most serious potential effects are profound hypotension and syncope with the initial dose, though these effects rarely occur. It is, therefore, recommended that the first dose be given before bedtime. These effects may be less severe with Doxazosin because the onset of action is gradual. When combined with calcium antagonists, exaggerated hypotension may occur because the

TABLE 30–9. New Oral Beta Blockers and Esmolol

Betaxolol (Kerlone)	Long-acting lipid-soluble cardioselective beta blocker now available for the treatment of hypertension (oral dose is 10-40 mg daily)
Bisoprolol (Emcor, Monocor, Zebeta)	Cardioselective agent ($beta_1$) thought to be more selective than atenolol, licensed for the treatment of hypertension in the United States (oral dose 2.5 mg to 20 mg daily; average dose is 10 mg which has similar antihypertensive effects as 100 mg atenolol)
Carteolol (Cartrol)	Nonselective beta blocker with low lipid solubility and a half life similar to atenolol and licensed for the treatment of hypertension in the United States. The initial dose is 2.5 mg daily and can be increased to a maximum of 10 mg daily. It is excreted primarily through the kidneys
Carvedilol (Coreg)	This is a newer nonselective beta blocker/$alpha_1$-blocker that is similar to labetolol with alpha-mediated vasodilatory capacity and a longer half life. Carvedilol is contraindicated in decompensated class IV NYHA heart failure that requires intravenous inotropic therapy
Penbutolol (Levatol)	Nonselective and highly lipid soluble. The dose is 20 mg daily for the treatment of mild to moderate hypertension
Esmolol (Brevibloc)	Intravenous agent with a half life of 9 minutes. It is indicated for the treatment of perioperative hypertension and supraventricular tachycardias (SVT). For hypertension, give 80 mg (1mg/kg) over 30 seconds and infuse at 150 to 300 ug/kg/min if needed

From Opie, Sonnenblick, Frishman, & Thadani (1997).

combination eliminates two of three major vasoconstrictive mechanisms; therefore, this combination could be beneficial, but must be used with caution (Kaplan & Opie, 1997; Massie, 1995).

Nonselective alpha blockers, phentolamine (Regitine), and phenoxybenzomine (Dibenzyline) are used almost exclusively for the medical treatment of pheochromocytoma. They are effective in acutely lowering blood pressure, but the effects are neutralized by coexisting elevations in cardiac output; side effects are annoying and frequent. These agents combine well with beta blockers and diuretics.

Headache, drowsiness, dizziness, weakness, and fatigue are all most likely related to the drop in blood pressure. For most patients, these side effects decrease with ongoing therapy.

Because they do not affect exercise tolerance as beta blockers sometimes do, selective alpha$_1$ receptor blockers are particularly well-suited to young patients who are physically active (Kaplan, 1995). Also, alpha$_1$ blockers relax the prosthetic muscle tone, relieving obstructive symptoms of benign prostatic hypertrophy. These agents are often initial treatment for the elderly hypertensive male with prostatism (Kaplan, 1995).

Peripheral Alpha Blockers

Reserpine, guanethidine, and guanedrel inhibit the release of norepinephrine from the peripheral adrenergic neurons. Guanethidine and guanedril are rarely used and are usually reserved for refractory hypertension. Reserpine acts upon peripheral neuronal sites as well as the central nervous system. These agents were among the first used to treat high blood pressure, but are much less used now that other agents have become available.

Reserpine blocks norepinephrine transport into its storage vesicles in the adrenergic nerve endings so that less of the neurotransmitter is available when the nerves are stimulated. The result is decreased sympathetic tone and a subsequent lower peripheral vascular resistance. As a result of catecholamine depletion in the heart, there is a reduced cardiac output and a slight bradycardia. Although the peripheral effects dominate, the drug does enter the brain depleting central catecholamine stores as well. This most likely accounts for the depression and sedative effects of the drug (Kaplan, 1995, 1998).

Small doses are effective. If used in combination with a diuretic, 0.05 mg/day, they may be adequate and as effective as larger doses, but with fewer side effects. Although in 1974 there were claims regarding the possible risk of breast cancer associated with reserpine, these claims have not been substantiated. When cost is crucial, reserpine in addition to a diuretic, is the most inexpensive combination.

Central Alpha Agonists

Central agonists act as alpha$_2$-receptor agonists, primarily on vasomotor centers in the brain, resulting in a decreased outflow of sympathetic impulses, and is reflected in lower levels of norepinephrine (Kaplan, 1998; Malseed, Goldstein & Balkon, 1995). With these agents, there is a decreased ability of the baroreceptor reflex to compensate for the lower blood pressure, accounting for a moderate reduction in pulse rate, cardiac output, and PVR. There is also a fall in plasma renin activity (Kaplan, 1998).

Efficacy and Dosage. The onset of action for all of these drugs is 30 to 60 minutes with maximal effect seen 1 to 3 hours after an oral dose; duration of action is 6 to 8 hours. Plasma half life ranges from 6 to 24 hours for clonidine with a mean of 12 hours; 12 to 24 hours for guanfacine; and 4 to 6 hours for guansbenz (Hoffman & Lefkowitz, 1996; Perry, 1993). With Methldopa, peak levels occur in 2 to 3 hours, but maximal effect may not occur until 4 to 6 hours later. Although this drug has a rapid absorption rate and short half life, the duration may last for 24 hours even though elimination half life is 2 hours, which is prolonged to 4 to 6 hours in patients with renal failure (Oates, 1996).

Methyldopa. Prior to the advent of beta blockers in the late 1970s, methyldopa (Aldomet) was the most popular drug used in the treatment of hypertension. This drug acts like the other central adrenergic inhibitors. For patients with renal insufficiency, the dose should be halved. Metabolism and absorption of the drug may be slowed if taken with drugs containing sulfate, i.e., ferrous sulfate, resulting in a decreased antihypertensive effect (Kaplan, 1998). Methyldopa, given as monotherapy, is the treatment of choice for managing hypertension associated with preeclampsia and hypertension during pregnancy; little of the drug is transferred to the fetus.

Side effects of methyldopa and all other central alpha agonists include sedation, headache, dry mouth, drowsiness, constipation, and fatigue. Methyldopa, however, causes a number of autoimmune disorders, such as positive direct Coomb's test in as many as 25%; hemolytic anemia is rare; abnormal liver function tests in approximately 8%; severe hepatic necrosis in a few; positive antinuclear antibody results in 10%; lupus erythematosis; and fevers. According to Kaplan (1998), these effects may be related to inhibition of suppressor T cells and an unregulated production of autoantibodies by the B cells. These effects are not seen with other central agonists, which are equal in effectiveness. Other side effects include: myocarditis, bradycardia, edema, pardoxical pressor response with intravenous use, dizziness, parasthesias, Parkinson-like symptoms, psychosis, and choreoathetoid movements. Contraindications to using methyldopa include: active liver disease, depression, and pheochromocytoma. Drug interactions with methyldopa include tricyclic antidepressants, barbituates, phenothiazines, haloperidol, monoamine oxidase inhibitors, lithium, and L-dopa (Khan, 1995).

Clonidine. Clonidine acts at the same central sites as methyldopa and has similar effectiveness in treating hypertension, but does not share the same serious autoimmune and inflammatory side effects. Clonidine has been used to prevent reflex overactivity of the sympathetic nervous system that is seen with direct vasodilator therapy, and is also used as a screening tool for pheochromocytoma.

Renal blood flow and GFR are maintained with use of clonidine. Approximately 50% of the administered dose can be recovered unchanged in the urine; therefore, a dose reduction is required for patients with renal failure (Hoffman & Lefkowitz, 1996; Khan, 1995; Perry, 1993). The drug is not eliminated during dialysis. Patients may be given most or the entire dose at bedtime to alleviate some of the sedative side effects.

Clonidine has been useful in the management of accelerated hypertension with an initial 0.1 mg to 0.2 mg dose followed by 0.05 to 0.1 mg dose per hour. A transdermal patch has become more popular because of smoother blood pressure control continuously over 7 days. This preparation causes fewer side effects but may cause skin irritation. This drug should not be used in poorly compliant patients. The patient must be warned against discontinuing therapy suddenly. If therapy is discontinued abruptly (oral or transdermal), rebound hypertension (or above prior blood pressure levels), tachycardia, agitation, and sweating may occur. If these symptoms occur, the drug should be restarted, or if needed, administration of both an alpha and beta–adrenergic inhibitor (i.e., labetolol) should be given (Kaplan, 1998).

Because clonidine causes fluid retention, it should be used in combination with a diuretic. The most common side effects include dry mouth and sedation. The sedative effect is increased by the use of alcohol, barbiturates, benzodiazepines, and other tranquilizers. The antihypertensive effect may be diminished by concomitant use of tricyclic antidepressants and tranquilizers. The autoimmune, hepatic, and hematologic side effects of methyldopa are not seen with clonidine. There have been a few cases of severe bradycardia with use of clonidine related to depression of the sinoatrial and atrioventricular nodes (Kaplan, 1998).

Gaunabenz (Wytensin). This drug is very similar to clonidine, but has a few beneficial differences. It has been shown to decrease total serum cholesterol levels by 5 to 10%. Also, because of a natriuresis that occurs with this drug, a diuretic may not be needed. Side effects are similar to the other central alpha agonists.

Guanfacine (Tenex). This drug is also similar to clonidine but appears to enter the brain at a slower rate and maintain its antihypertensive effect longer. Main side effects are sedation and dry mouth (Kaplan, 1998).

Combined Alpha and Beta Receptor Blockers

Combined receptor antagonists (i.e., labetolol and carvedilol) have both alpha and beta receptor activity with many similar side effects to nonselective beta blockers. Labetolol is a nonselective beta blocker and is highly selective for alpha$_1$ receptors. The alpha-to-beta blocking action has a ratio of 1:4. Carvedilol differs from labetolol in that it has a lesser degree of alpha blocking action, causing less vasodilatory effect. In higher concentrations, carvedilol acts as a calcium channel blocker. Additionally, carvedilol acts as a free-radical scavenger, preventing lipid oxidation and resultant injury to the cells of the endothelium (Kaplan, 1998).

These drugs are effective when given twice daily. Orthostatic hypotension is the most commonly reported side effect for both labetolol and carvedilol, and is usually seen with initial therapy and with larger doses. With labetolol, scalp itching, ejaculatory failure, bronchospasm, elevated ANA, and elevated antimitochondrial antibodies have been reported. The most serious side effect with labetolol, although rare, is hepatotoxicity. Appropriate testing for liver dysfunction should be done (Kaplan, 1998).

Angiotensin-Converting Enzyme Inhibitors

Angiotensin-converting enzyme (ACE) inhibitors are recognized as one of several agents for first-choice therapy for many patients with hypertension. They are popular because of minimal side effects and contraindications, flat dose response curve, and many agents have once-daily dosing. These agents are preferred for patients with type 1 diabetes mellitus, heart failure, and postmyocardial infarction with systolic dysfunction (JNC VI, 1997). ACE inhibitors are particularly useful in diabetic patients with proteinuria or evidence of renal insufficiency because they slow the development of glomerulopathy (Oates, 1996).

In mild to moderate hypertension, ACE inhibitors can be used as monotherapy or in conjunction with other agents. There have been varying degrees of responsiveness to monotherapy with these agents (from less than 50% to 75%). This is related to an inconsistent intake of sodium in their diet and differences in white and black patients (Kaplan & Opie, 1997). The ACE inhibitors appear to be less effective in blacks and older adults and most effective in younger white patients.

Mechanism of Action. Angiotensin converting enzyme (ACE), which is available in vascular beds throughout the body, is responsible for the conversion of inactive angiotensin I (A-I) to angiotensin II (A-II), the potent vasoconstrictor and stimulator of aldosterone secretion. A-I originates in the liver from angiotensinogen, under the influence of the enzyme renin, which is formed in the renal juxtaglomerular cells. Renin is released when there is a decreased blood flow to the kidneys secondary to low blood pressure, sodium depletion or diuresis, or beta–adrenergic stimulation (Opie, Poole-Wilson, et al., 1997). This renin release leads to the cycle of converting A-I to A-II leading to vasoconstriction, aldosterone secretion, and subsequent sodium and water retention.

ACE is also responsible for inactivating the hormone bradykinin, which is responsible for vasodilation. ACE inhibition results in the suppression of A-II and the stimulation of bradykinin leading to vasodilation, decreased PVR, and lowering of systemic blood pressure (Gavras, 1993; Kaplan, 1995). There is preferential vasodilation in the organs sensitive to the effects of the angiotensin and bradykinin, such as the kidneys, brain, adrenal glands, and the heart. As a result, there is increased blood flow to these organs helping to maintain adequate perfusion to these organs.

ACE inhibitors inhibit ACE by attaching to its binding sites. These agents block the synthesis of A-II, vasoconstriction is overcome, and blood pressure lowers. Renin release and aldosterone synthesis from A-II is inhibited, leading to decreased sodium retention and potassium wastage (Kaplan, 1995; Opie, Poole-Wilson, et al., 1997). According to Opie, Poole-Wilson, et al. (1997), aldosterone formation does not continue to be fully inhibited with prolonged use of ACE inhibitors, which does not jeopardize their antihypertensive effectiveness; however, it could adversely effect the prolonged benefits of these agents in patients with heart failure.

Advantages of ACE Inhibitors. ACE inhibitors also improve the compliance of large vessels, contributing to the reduction of systolic pressure. In the uncomplicated hypertensive this effect may not be noticeable, though stroke volume and cardiac output may increase slightly. There is improvement in patients with left ventricular systolic dysfunction (ranging from modest and asymptomatic to severe impairment of function) by altered remodeling and sustained reduction in preload and afterload. There has been a greater regression of left ventricular hypertrophy in patients receiving ACE inhibitors than with any other class of drug.

ACE inhibitors enhance the favorable effects of diuretics because the normal aldosterone response to sodium loss and aldosterone's natural propensity to oppose diuretic-induced natriuresis is diminished with their use. The kidneys may be protected by the vasodilation of the efferent arterioles that occurs from decreased amounts of A-II. This increases renal blood flow and decreases intraglomerular pressure, providing the kidneys with protection in those patients who are susceptible to damage from glomerular hypertension. Additionally, ACE inhibitors have been shown to improve insulin sensitivity and lower plasma insulin levels (Kaplan, 1994; Opie, Poole-Wilson, et al., 1997).

ACE inhibitors improve walking distance in hypertensive patients with intermittent claudication. Caution should be taken in these and all patients with advanced atherosclerosis because of their increased prevalence of renovascular disease (Kaplan, 1998).

Differences Among ACE Inhibitors. In most obvious ways all ACE inhibitors are very much alike. There is no compelling reason to favor one ACE inhibitor over another. Most of these agents have the same indications, side effects, and contraindications. These agents are categorized among three chemically different classes: sulfhydryl, carboxyl, and phosphoryl. Their different class influences their tissue distribution and routes of elimination. Most ACE inhibitors are ester-containing prodrugs that are more lipid-soluble so that they are more quickly and completely absorbed. The exception is lisinopril, which is not a prodrug, is not metabolized by the liver, and is water-soluble, excreted unchanged by the kidneys. These agents differ with regards to potency, absorption, plasma half-life, tissue distribution, and mechanisms of elimination. Most ACE inhibitors, except for fosinopril and spirapril, are eliminated through the kidneys. Fosinopril (Monopril) has a balanced route of elimination and as renal function declines, increasingly more of the drug is eliminated through the liver; therefore, no decrease in dose should be necessary in the presence of renal failure. With all other ACE inhibitors that are cleared through the kidneys, impaired renal function will significantly decrease the plasma clearance requiring a reduction in dose (Jackson & Garrison, 1996; Kaplan, 1998). There was a quality-of-life study that compared ACE inhibitors and found that captopril conferred an enhanced sense of well being over all the others. The reason for this is unknown although some have raised the question of it having a beneficial central effect (Treadway, 1995).

Class Side Effects of ACE Inhibitors. ACE inhibitors have undesirable reactions that are often noted as class side effects that are related to the mechanism of action of this particular class of drug, as opposed to individual reaction to a specific drug, and is likely to occur with every ACE inhibitor.

Occurring in approximately 5 to 20% of users, cough is the most common side effect of ACE inhibitors. This is usually not reported initially and could begin months after starting the drug. The cough is described as a dry, hacking, and nonproductive cough that is often intolerable by many patients, and is more common in white women. It is most likely related to the increased formation of bradykinin and prostaglandins, arising from the inhibition of the ACE. Relief may be obtained by adding nonsteroidal antiinflammatory (NSAIDs) agents, though this may lead to a diminished antihypertensive effect (Kaplan, 1998; Opie, Poole-Wilson, et al., 1997). Also, it has been observed that the combination of low-dose ACE inhibitor and a calcium antagonist, nifedipine, lessens cough for unknown reasons (Opie, Poole-Wilson, et al., 1997). Sodium cromoglycate may also be helpful or a change to an angiotensin II receptor antagonist would be beneficial (Kaplan, 1998).

There is an immediate drop in mean arterial pressure of greater than 30% in many patients. Many patients do well with systolic blood pressures of 80 to 90 mm Hg. If orthostatic symptoms occur, dose reduction or discontinuation of the ACE inhibitor may be necessary.

In the presence of volume depletion, there is an increase in A-II to compensate and maintain homeostasis. This response is blunted with ACE inhibitor therapy and there have been a few isolated cases of marked hypotension with prerenal azotemia in these patients who are experiencing volume depletion (i.e., gastrointestinal fluid loss) (Kaplan, 1998).

Elevated plasma potassium levels may occur because there is decreased potassium excretion and sodium retention, arising from aldosterone inhibition with use of ACE inhibitors. This is true especially in patients with renal insufficiency or those receiving potassium-sparing diuretics. Any potassium supplementation should stop when ACE inhibition therapy is initiated.

In most patients there is no significant change in GFR following the administration of an ACE inhibitor. Hypotension can precipitate reversible renal failure. Angiotensin II assists in maintaining adequate glomerular filtration when perfusion to the kidney is low by constricting the efferent arteriole. It is rare, but irreversible renal failure has occurred in those patients with bilateral renal artery stenosis, or renal artery stenosis of a solitary remaining kidney, because of the inhibition of ACE resulting in a substantial decrease in the GFR. In unilateral renal artery stenosis where there is decreased perfusion pressures in the renal arteries leading to increased production of renin, ACE inhibitors may cause excessive hypotensive responses with associated oliguria and/or azotemia (Jackson & Garrison, 1996). A low first-test dose is required with frequent blood pressure monitoring. A mild yet stable increase in serum creatinine does not preclude its use.

Angioedema is rare (approximately 0.1%), but is unpredictable and life-threatening. The reaction typically occurs within hours, but could present after prolonged use. It is possibly related to the formation of bradykinin. Immediate administration of subcutaneous epinephrine is the treatment.

All ACE inhibitors cause fetal injury and death, especially in second and third trimesters. Other side effects of ACE inhibitors include rash (macculopapular, pruritic eruptions appear within the first few weeks of therapy), severe erythema and/or eczema taste disturbance, fever, blood dyscrasias (ranging from granulopenia to pancytopenia), and pancreatitis (rare).

Combination Therapy with ACE Inhibitors. ACE inhibitors are frequently combined with thiazide diuretics to provide additional hypotensive effects and limit metabolic side effects when used in low doses. This combination is beneficial because diuretics increase renin, the effects that are opposed by ACE inhibitors. The ideal thiazide dose, when used in combination, should not exceed 12.5 mg of hydrochlorothiazide. No greater antihypertensive effect is achieved with higher doses. When combined with potassium-retaining diuretics (i.e., Dyazide, Moduretic, Maxzide, spironolactone), there is an increased risk of hyperkalemia because ACE inhibitors decrease aldosterone secretion and retain potassium (Opie, Kaplan, & Poole-Wilson, 1997). The combination agent Capozide, which is a combination of Captopril and HCTZ, is now approved for initial therapy by the JNC VI.

The combination of ACE inhibitors and beta blockers is used frequently in hypertension because they have been shown to have additive antihypertensive effects, even though they both have antirenin properties.

ACE inhibitors and calcium channel blockers are being used together more frequently because they both work on the renin–angiotensin system and the increased peripheral vascular resistance found in hypertension. ACE inhibitors provide balance to the counterregulation that occurs with the powerful vasodilation of calcium channel blockers.

Angiotensin II Receptor Antagonists

The angiotensin II receptor has been found to have at least two major subtypes: type I (AT_1) receptor negotiates all of the physiologic roles of A-II, and the AT_2 receptors may be involved in the trophic changes of A-II on the vasculature. Agents that selectively block AT_1 receptors are now being used in the treatment of hypertension.

These agents work by blocking the vasoconstrictor and aldosterone-secreting effects of angiotensin II by displacing A-II from its specific AT_1 receptor. By preventing the effects of A-II, such as vasoconstriction and aldosterone secretion, smooth muscle is relaxed promoting vasodilation; and sodium and water excretion is increased reducing plasma volume. By avoiding the independent pathways for the synthesis of A-II, disadvantages of ACE inhibition are avoided. By directly blocking the A-II receptor sites, the conversion from A-I to A-II and the ACE-mediated breakdown of bradykinin and substance P are avoided. By blocking the AT_1 receptor, the negative feedback system of A-II on the secretion of renin is eliminated. The increases in plasma renin levels and circulating A-II that result do not overpower the effects of these agents on blood pressure. The major differences between A-II-receptor blockers and ACE inhibitors is the absence of elevated kinin levels that may be responsible for some of the advantages of ACE inhibitors and many of the disadvantages. In comparison, their antihypertensive effects show little differences. A-II-receptor blockers have no incidence of cough; however, angioedema has been reported with losartan.

Losartan (Cozaar) is rapidly absorbed with a peak plasma level reached in 1 hour. It is a potent AT_1 receptor antagonist, but has a short half life of approximately 2 hours. The once-daily dosing with this drug is effective because approximately 14% of an oral dose of losartan is converted to a metabolite, that is, a AT_1 receptor antagonist, which is at least 10 to 40 times more potent than losartan itself, and has a much longer half life (6-9 hours). Approximately 4% to 7% of a losartan dose is unchanged in the urine. Dosing should be reduced in those patients with liver impairment. Neither losartan, nor its metabolite, cross the blood–brain barrier. A 50-mg dose is effective in most patients; a lower dose in most patients is ineffective. However, some patients find that 25 mg twice a day gives a more steady 24-hour antihypertensive response (Jackson & Garrison, 1996).

Other A-II-receptor blockers approved for use in the treatment of hypertension are valsartan (Diovan) and irbesartan (Avapro).

The role of A-II receptor antagonists in left ventricular systolic dysfunction and renal impairment is not yet known. As results of clinical trials become available, most likely the clinical indications for A-II blockers will expand (Jackson & Garrison, 1996).

According to the JNC (1997) because there are no data that document long-term cardiac and renal protection in patients with these conditions, A-II-receptor blockers should be used when ACE inhibition is preferred, but not tolerated.

Vasodilators

Because hypertension is characterized by increased peripheral vascular resistance, directly relaxing the vessels is beneficial in the management of high blood pressure. Direct vasodilators enter the vascular smooth muscle, primarily arteriolar, and cause peripheral vasodilation. Unfortunately, the effectiveness of direct vasodilators, such as hydralazine and minoxidil, is blunted by reflex sympathetic responses to vasodilation (i.e., tachycardia). These drugs work in contrast to other vasodilators that work indirectly by preventing hormonal vasoconstrictor mechanisms (ACE inhibitors) or calcium channel blockers that inhibit vasoconstriction by preventing calcium entry into the cells.

When these direct-acting vasodilators are used alone, the arterioles dilate with a resultant drop in blood pressure causing a baroreceptor-mediated sympathetic response. This sympathetic response causes a release in both renin and catecholamines, stimulating reflex tachycardia, constriction of veins, an increased cardiac output, and myocardial oxygen demand, which could be deleterious to patients with coronary artery disease. In addition, the drop in blood pressure can cause renal retention of sodium and subsequent plasma volume expansion. These agents are usually given in combination with diuretics and beta blockers (Kaplan, 1995, 1998; Massie, 1995; Ram & Featherston, 1993). Hydralazine has often been chosen as the third drug in treating hypertension not responsive to diuretics and beta blockers. By using this combination of drugs, the various compensatory responses and side effects are reduced.

Hydralazine. Hydralazine along with minoxidil is used infrequently because of their activation of the sympathetic nervous system. Hydralazine's use did increase when a rationale for triple therapy in hypertension was demonstrated. However, with the advent of newer vasodilating drugs that block sympathetic activity, they are still used infrequently. Peak concentration can be reached within 1 hour. The half life is 1 to 3 hours, although the duration of the hypotensive effect can last up to 12 hours (Oates, 1996). This is probably because hydralazine is so eagerly taken up by the arterial walls. An oral dose of 75 to 100 mg of hydralazine is equipotent to 10 to 25 mg given parenterally (Ram & Featherston, 1993).

Side effects such as fluid retention may occur, secondary to renin release making diuretic therapy necessary. The direct inotropic effect and tachycardia make hydralazine contraindicated in those patients with angina pectoris who are not on beta blockers. The baroreceptor-mediated sympathetic response causing increased oxygen demand can lead to myocardial ischemia. This is also true because hydralazine does not dilate the epicardial coronary arteries, creating a "steal" of blood flow away from the ishemic area with arteriolar dilation (Oates, 1996). In congestive heart failure, however, reflex tachycardia is rare, perhaps because reflex arcs are blunted (Opie, Poole-Wilson, et al., 1997).

Drug-induced lupus syndrome is rare with doses below 200 mg per day or with total doses below 100 gm. The syndrome usually occurs after 6 months or longer of continuous therapy. The incidence is four times greater in women than in men and seen more commonly in whites than in African-Americans. Patients on prolonged therapy should be checked for antinuclear factors. The drug need not be discontinued with positive antinuclear antibody results, unless the patient presents with clinical features of the syndrome, i.e., arthralgias, arthritis, and fever. Pleuritis and pericarditis may occur. If symptoms persist after discontinuation of the drug, corticosteroids may be necessary. Polyneuropathy may occur and is usually responsive to pyridoxine (Oates, 1996; Opie, Poole-Wilson, et al., 1997).

Hydralazine can lower LDL and raise HDL cholesterol levels. The same beneficial effects have been noted with minoxidil.

Minoxidil. Minoxidil is a more potent vasodilator than hydralazine and its use is usually reserved for patients with severe hypertension that is refractory to other drugs, especially when associated with renal insufficiency (Kaplan, 1995, 1998).

The mechanism of action with minoxidil is slightly different in that the smooth muscle relaxation and arteriolar vasodilation are achieved by modulating potassium channels in vascular smooth muscle, which is apparently unique among vasodilators (Kaplan, 1998). Venodilation does not occur; therefore, postural hypotension is avoided (Ram & Featherston, 1993).

When used in combination with diuretics and adrenergic inhibitors, minoxidil will control blood pressure in the majority of patients who were previously resistant to other drug regimens. It can be administered with daily doses ranging from 2.5 mg to 80 mg.

The most common side effect found in 80% of patients is hypertrichosis, which initially begins with fine hair on the face and then with coarse hair increasing all over the body. This effect is thought to be related to activation of potassium channel activation, and not hormonal changes (Oates, 1996). This can be treated with depilatory agents.

Topical minoxidil (Rogaine) is now marketed for the treatment of male pattern baldness. Some of the topical ointment is absorbed and can cause significant cardiovascular effects in some individuals (Kaplan, 1998; Oates, 1996).

Because minoxidil is more potent and longer lasting than hydralazine, the cardiac sympathetic compensatory responses to direct arteriolar vasodilation are greater, making larger doses of diuretics and beta adrenergic blockers necessary (Kaplan, 1998).

The increased cardiac output that is seen with minoxidil has adverse effects on patients with left ventricular hypertrophy and poor diastolic function. The noncompliant ventricle cannot tolerate the increased volume loads, with resulting increase in left ventricular filling pressures. Cardiac failure and increased pulmonary pressures can be prevented by administering adequate amounts of diuretic therapy.

Pericardial effusion is not an uncommon finding in those patients treated with minoxidil, even in those patients with normal cardiovascular and renal function. Flattened and inverted T waves can be found on the electrocardiogram of these patients. These changes are not ischemic in nature and can be found with other drugs that activate potassium channels. Other drugs that activate potassium channels, such as pinacidil not available in the United States, accelerates myocardial repolarization, shortens refractory period, and lowers the ventricular fibrillation threshold. The effect of minoxidil on ischemic ventricular fibrillation threshold and refractory period has not been studied (Oates, 1996).

Calcium Channel Blockers

Calcium channel blockers are among the most frequently used agents for the treatment of hypertension. All calcium channel blockers lower blood pressure by relaxing arteriolar smooth muscle and thereby decreasing peripheral vascular resistance. This is done by interfering with calcium entry into the vascular smooth muscle and reducing intracellular calcium, vascular tone, and contractility. The peripheral vasodilatation is associated with less reflex tachycardia and fluid retention than is seen with other vasodilators.

Calcium channel blockers facilitate natriuresis, most likely related to the vasodilation of the renal vascular beds, diminished sodium reabsorption in the renal tubules, and interference with the secretion of aldosterone (Kaplan, 1992b; Weir, 1993). This may forestall the need for concurrent use of diuretics. Dihydropyridines are less likely to adversely effect cardiac function in those patients with left ventricular systolic dysfunction when compared with nondihydropyridines.

Calcium channel blockers have been divided into three different categories according to their structural properties: verapamil, dihydropyridines (nifedipine, felodipine, nicardipine, amlodipine, and isradipine), and diltiazem. The dihydropyridines differ from verapamil and diltiazem in that they have the greatest vasodilatory action with very little effect on the myocardium, whereas verapamil—and to a lesser extent diltiazem—slow atrioventricular conduction and depress contractility. As a consequence to the vasodilatation and subsequent decrease in peripheral vascular resistance, the dihydropyridines produce a baroreceptor-mediated sympathetic discharge causing an initial mild to moderate reflex tachycardia. With verapamil and diltiazem, there is minimal or no adrenergic stimulation on the sinoatrial node because of their direct negative chronotropic effect. For patients with a faster heart rate or atrial fibrillation, agents such as verapamil and diltiazem may be preferred, whereas those patients with bradycardia or heart block are generally better served by the dihydropyridines (Opie, Frishman, & Thadani, 1997).

Immediate-release nifedipine has been known to precipitate ischemic events and—in large doses—to increase coronary mortality in those patients with a previous history of myocardial infarction. There is inconsistent data regarding adverse effects of short-acting formulations of nifedipine, diltiazem, and verapamil. There are studies currently in progress evaluating long-acting formulations of calcium antagonists approved for the treatment of hypertension.

Table 30–10 includes a listing of selected drug interactions emphasized by the JNC VI.

▶ CONSIDERATIONS FOR SPECIAL POPULATIONS

Table 30–11 contains considerations for individualizing antihypertensive drug therapy.

Ethnic Groups

Black patients seem to have a better response to monotherapy with a diuretic, calcium channel blocker, or an alpha blocker, than they do with beta blockers and ACE inhibitors (Kaplan, 1998). In elderly blacks, a beta blocker and an ACE inhibitor were only slightly better than placebo; however, younger blacks respond well to beta blockers (Kaplan & Opie, 1997). This may be because black patients tend to have lower renin levels than whites (Kaplan, 1998; Kaplan & Opie, 1997). Overall, response to beta blockers and ACE inhibitors in this population is improved with the addition of a diuretic, most likely because renin is increased with the diuretic therapy. Adequate blood pressure control often requires combination therapy with a diuretic more often in the black population (Kaplan, 1998).

TABLE 30–10. Selected Drug Interactions with Antihypertensive Therapy[a]

Class of Agent	Increase Efficacy	Decrease Efficacy	Effect on Other Drugs
Diuretics	• Diuretics that act at different sites in the nephron (e.g., furosemide + thiazides)	• Resin-binding agents • NSAIDs • Steroids	• Diuretics raise serum lithium levels • Potassium-sparing agents may exacerbate hyperkalemia due to ACE inhibitors
Beta-blockers	• Cimetidine (hepatically metabolized beta-blockers) • Quinidine (hepatically metabolized beta-blockers) • Food (hepatically metabolized beta-blockers)	• NSAIDs • Withdrawal of clonidine • Agents that induce hepatic enzymes, including rifampin and phenobarbital	• Propranolol hydrochloride induces hepatic enzymes to increase clearance of drugs with similar metabolic pathways • Beta-blockers may mask and prolong insulin-induced hypoglycemia • Heart block may occur with nondihydropyridine calcium antagonists • Sympathomimetics cause unopposed alpha-adrenoceptor-mediated vasoconstriction • Beta-blockers increase angina-inducing potential of cocaine
ACE inhibitors	• Chlorpromazine or clozapine	• NSAIDs • Antacids • Food decreases absorption (moexipril)	• ACE inhibitors may raise serum lithium levels • ACE inhibitors may exacerbate hyperkalemic effect of potassium-sparing diuretics
Calcium antagonists	• Grapefruit juice (some dihydropyridines) • Cimetidine or ranitidine (hepatically metabolized calcium antagonists)	• Agents that induce hepatic enzymes, including rifampin and phenobarbital	• Cyclosporine levels increase[b] with diltiazem hydrochloride, verapamil hydrochloride, mibefradil dihydrochloride, or nicardipine hydrochloride (but not felodipine, isradipine, or nifedipine) • Nondihydropyridines increase levels of other drugs metabolized by the same hepatic enzyme system, including digoxin, quinidine, sulfonylureas, and theophylline • Verapamil hydrochloride may lower serum lithium levels
Alpha-blockers			• Prazosin may decrease clearance of verapamil hydrochloride
Central alpha$_2$-agonists and peripheral neuronal blockers		• Tricyclic antidepressants (and probably phenothiazines) • Monoamine oxidase inhibitors • Sympathomimetics or phenothiazines antagonize guanethidine monosulfate or guanadrel sulfate • Iron salts may reduce methyldopa absorption	• Methyldopa may increase serum lithium levels • Severity of clonidine hydrochloride withdrawal may be increased by beta-blockers • Many agents used in anesthesia are potentiated by clonidine hydrochloride

[a] See *Physicians' Desk Reference* (51st edition) and *Cardiovascular Pharmacotherapeutics* (New York: McGraw Hill), 1997. NSAIDs indicate nonsteroidal anti-inflammatory drugs; ACE, angiotensin-converting enzyme.

[b] This is a clinically and economically beneficial drug–drug interaction because it both retards progression of accelerated atherosclerosis in heart transplant recipients and reduces the required daily dose of cyclosporine.

(From the Joint National Committee on Detection, Evaluation, and Treatment of High Blood Pressure [1997].)

A higher percentage of blacks and Asians report ACE inhibitor-related cough (Kaplan, 1998). There is no strong evidence that Hispanics, Asians, or other ethnic groups respond to antihypertensive agents differently from whites.

Older Adults

Hypertension is very common in older adults. According to the JNC VI (1997), among Americans age 60 and older, elevated blood pressure was found in 60% of nonHispanic whites, 71% of nonHispanic African-Americans, and 61% of Mexican-Americans. SBP is a stronger predictor than DBP for deleterious events in older adults (i.e., stroke, heart failure, cardiac event, renal disease, and all-cause mortality). Recently, more attention has been paid to an elevated pulse pressure, which indicates reduced vascular compliance in the large vessels. This may be an even more important marker of increased cardiovascular risk than either SBP or DBP alone.

TABLE 30–11. Considerations for Individualizing Antihypertensive Drug Therapy[a]

Indication	Drug Therapy
Compelling Indications Unless Contraindicated	
Diabetes mellitus (type 1) with proteinuria	ACE I
Heart failure	ACE I, diuretics
Isolated systolic hypertension (older patients)	Diuretics (preferred), CA (long-acting DHP)
Myocardial infarction	Beta-blockers (non-ISA), ACE I (with systolic dysfunction)
May Have Favorable Effects on Comorbid Conditions[b]	
Angina	Beta-blockers, CA
Atrial tachycardia and fibrillation	Beta-blockers, CA (non-DHP)
Cyclosporine-induced hypertension (caution with the dose of cyclosporine)	CA
Diabetes mellitus (types 1 and 2) with proteinuria	ACE I (preferred), CA
Diabetes mellitus (type 2)	Low-dose diuretics
Dyslipidemia	Alpha-blockers
Essential tremor	Beta-blockers (non-CS)
Heart failure	Carvedilol, losartan potassium
Hyperthyroidism	Beta-blockers
Migraine	Beta-blockers (non-CS), CA (non-DHP)
Myocardial infarction	Diltiazem hydrochloride, verapamil hydrochloride
Osteoporosis	Thiazides
Preoperative hypertension	Beta-blockers
Prostatism (BPH)	Alpha-blockers
Renal insufficiency (caution in renovascular hypertension and creatinine ≥265.2 mmol/L [3 mg/dL])	ACE I
May Have Unfavorable Effects on Comorbid Conditions[b,c]	
Bronchospastic disease	Beta-blockers[d]
Depression	Beta-blockers, central alpha-agonists, reserpine[d]
Diabetes mellitus (types 1 and 2)	Beta-blockers, high-dose diuretics
Dyslipidemia	Beta-blockers (non-ISA), diuretics (high-dose)
Gout	Diuretics
2° or 3° heart block	Beta-blockers,[d] CA (non-DHP)[d]
Heart failure	Beta-blockers (except carvedilol, CA (except amlodipine besylate, felodipine)
Liver disease	Labetalol hydrochloride, methyldopa[d]
Peripheral vascular disease	Beta-blockers
Pregnancy	ACE I,[d] angiotensin II receptor blockers[d]
Renal insufficiency	Potassium-sparing agents
Renovascular disease	ACE I, angiotensin II receptor blockers

[a] For references, see chapter 4, *Physicians' Desk Reference* (51st edition), and Kaplan, N. M. & Gifford, R. W. Jr. (1996). Choice of initial therapy for hypertension. *JAMA, 275:* 1577–1580. ACE I indicates angiotensin-converting enzyme inhibitors; BPH, benign prostatic hyperplasia; CA, calcium antagonists; DHP, dihydropyridine; ISA, intrinsic sympathomimetic activity; MI, myocardial infarction; and non-CS, noncardioselective.
[b] Conditions and drugs are listed in alphabetical order.
[c] These drugs may be used with special monitoring unless contraindicated.
[d] Contraindicated.
(From the Joint National Committee on Detection, Evaluation, and Treatment of High Blood Pressure [1997].)

The choice of antihypertensive therapy should be based on concurrent illnesses and treatments. Therapy should be individualized rather than using a stepped-care approach. Low-dose diuretics remain the first choice for the treatment of uncomplicated hypertension in older adults. The starting dose in the older patient should be approximately half of that used in younger patients. Thiazide diuretics or beta blockers in combination with thiazide diuretics are recommended because they have been shown in randomized controlled trials to reduce morbidity and mortality rates in the older adults with hypertension. Comparatively, diuretics are preferred over beta blockers. Although ACE inhibitors, calcium channel blockers, and alpha blockers have not been studied in controlled trials in older adults, long-acting dihydropyridine calcium channel blockers are acceptable alternatives to diuretics, especially when diuretics or beta blockers are contraindicated.

Because older adults have sluggish baroreceptor and SNS responses, therapy should be gradual and cautious. Medications that exaggerate postural hypotension (peripheral adrenergic blockers, alpha blockers, and high-dose diuretics) or those that cause cognitive impairment (central alpha$_2$-agonists) should be avoided or used with caution (JNC VI, 1997; Kaplan, 1998).

Cerebrovascular Disease

Immediately following an ischemic cerebral infarction, it is safe to withhold treatment, unless the blood pressure is very high. Following the onset of a stroke, the blood pressure may rise considerably, and then fall prematurely if potent antihypertensive agents are used. Medications should be held until the patient has been stabilized. The goal should be to lower blood pressure gradually to avoid orthostatic hypotension. Patients with acute ischemic stroke who are treated with fibrinolytic agents require careful blood pressure monitoring, especially over the first 24 hours of starting treatment (JNC VI, 1997). According to Kaplan (1998), antihypertensive agents should be withheld unless the mean arterial blood pressure is greater than 130 mm Hg or the SBP is greater than 220 mm Hg. Additionally, Kaplan (1998) states that for patients with an acute thrombotic stroke, a blood pressure of 185/110 (pretreatment) is a contraindication for thrombolytic therapy.

Peripheral Vascular Disease

Beta blockers with ISA and cardioselectivity, and combination alpha–beta blockers aggravate intermittent claudication. ACE inhibitors, calcium channel blockers, and alpha blockers are better choices because of the vasodilation they provide (Kaplan, 1998).

Coexisting Coronary Artery Disease

These patients are at increased risk for cardiovascular morbidity and mortality. Rapid lowering of blood pressure below the target range should be avoided, especially when it causes reflex tachycardia and sympathetic nervous system activation. Blood pressure should be lowered gradually to the usual target range (140/90 mm Hg), or lower if angina continues.

Following myocardial infarction (MI), beta blockers such as metoprolol or atenolol that do not have intrinsic sympathomimetic activity (ISA) should be used because they decrease the risk for a recurrent heart attack or sudden cardiac death. ACE inhibitors are also beneficial following a MI, especially in the presence of left ventricular dysfunction. ACE inhibitors prevent subsequent heart failure, remodeling, and mortality. If beta blockers are contraindicated, verapamil or diltiazem may be used because they have been shown to reduce cardiac events and mortality following a non–Q-wave MI and following a MI where the left ventricular function is preserved (JNC VI, 1997).

Left Ventricular Hypertrophy

Left ventricular hypertrophy (LVH) is a major independent risk factor for sudden cardiac death, myocardial infarction, stroke, and other cardiovascular events that increase morbidity and mortality. According to the JNC VI (1997), most antihypertensive agents, except direct-acting vasodilators, along with weight reduction and modifications in dietary salt intake can reduce increased left ventricular mass and wall thickness.

Congestive Heart Failure

Hypertension is a major cause of left ventricular heart failure, whether due to systolic or diastolic dysfunction. Following MI, ACE inhibitor therapy prevents subsequent heart failure, reducing related morbidity and mortality. When ACE inhibitors are not well tolerated or are contraindicated, the vasodilator combination of hydralazine and isosorbide is appropriate in systolic dysfunction. The combination alpha–beta blocker Carvedilol used with ACE inhibitors is also effective.

When a calcium channel blocker is indicated, amlodipine has been found to be safe and effective, especially in those patients with nonischemic heart failure. Calcium channel blockers that are short acting and slow the heart rate (i.e., diltiazem) should be avoided in those patients with systolic dysfuntion.

Diabetes Mellitus

The most important need for the control of both hypertension and diabetes in type II diabetics is weight reduction. Weight loss through diet and exercise improves insulin resistance. Even without weight loss, exercise improves insulin sensitivity. ACE inhibitors, alpha blockers, calcium channel blockers, and diuretics in low doses are preferred because of less adverse effects on lipid profiles, renal function, and improved glucose tolerance and insulin sensitivity. Beta blockers should be used cautiously because of their adverse effects on peripheral blood flow, prolonged hypoglycemia, and masking of hypoglycemic symptoms. However, when diabetic patients are treated with beta blockers and diuretics, they experience similar or greater reduction of cardiovascular events compared with persons without diabetes. ACE inhibitors are preferred for patients with diabetic nephropathy; if contraindicated, A-II receptor blockers may be beneficial (JNC VI, 1997).

Dyslipidemia

Hypertensive patients should have a lipid profile done before instituting antihypertensive therapy. If hypercholesterolemia is present, diet and medication should be started to help control lipid levels. Patients must be instructed to increase physical activity and decrease dietary saturated fat, cholesterol, sodium chloride, and alcohol. The two most commonly used medications (beta blockers and diuretics) for the treatment of hypertension may induce dyslipidemia. In high doses, thiazide diuretics and loop diuretics induce elevations in total cholesterol, LDL cholesterol, and triglycerides. Dietary changes can reduce or eliminate these effects. Lower doses of thiazide diuretics have no effect on cholesterol levels. Beta blockers may increase levels of triglycerides temporarily and lower HDL levels. Nonetheless, beta blockers have been found to reduce the rate of sudden death, recurrent MI, and overall mortality.

Alpha blockers may reduce serum cholesterol levels significantly and increase HDL levels. ACE inhibitors, A-II receptor blockers, calcium channel blockers, and central adrenergic atagonists have no effect on lipid profiles. Many clinical trials have provided evidence that aggressive lipid lowering with statin drugs provides both primary and secondary protection against coronary disease. Lifestyle modifications and lipid-lowering agents should be initiated to reach appropriate goals in those patients with hypertension and hyperlipidemia (JNC VI, 1997; Kaplan, 1998).

Patients with Bronchial Asthma and Chronic Obstructive Pulmonary Disease

Beta blockers and combination alpha–beta blockers should be avoided in those patients with asthma or chronic lung disease because of their ability to exacerbate these conditions. Also, topical ophthalmic solutions that contain beta blockers (timolol) may worsen asthma. ACE inhibitors are a safe alternative; however, if a dry cough develops, A-II receptor blockers can be used.

Many over-the-counter cold and asthma formulations contain sympathomimetic agents that raise blood pressure, but may be safe if taken in limited amounts. Cromylyn sodium, ipratropium bromide, or inhaled corticosteroids can be used safely in hypertensive patients (JNC VI, 1997).

Patients Undergoing Surgery

Blood pressure exceeding 180/110 mm Hg is associated with higher risk for perioperative ishemic events. If possible, blood pressure should be controlled before proceeding with surgery. The perioperative risk for all patients, especially hypertensive patients, is partly related to the adrenergic stimulation that occurs before, during, and after surgery. Patients who are not already on a medication regimen may benefit from cardioselective beta blockade before and after surgery.

Patients should be instructed to continue their antihypertensive regimen right up to the time of surgery, and should be restarted as soon as possible postoperatively. Intravenous therapy with diuretics, adrenergic inhibitors, vasodilators, ACE inhibitors, or transdermal clonidine is recommended until the patient can resume oral intake; this will prevent rebound hypertension that can occur with abrupt discontinuation of some adrenergic-blocking agents. Calcium channel blockers have been associated with increased surgical bleeding in two studies; therefore, caution should be exercised with their use. Intraoperative blood pressure control can be obtained with intravenous labetolol, nitroprusside, nicardipine, or esmolol (JNC VI, 1997; Kaplan, 1998).

Considerations for Adherence to Therapy

The lack of adequate control in greater than two-thirds of hypertensive patients is, in part, related to poor adherence to antihypertensive therapy. Patients should be well-informed and active participants in their care. Achieving and maintaining adequate blood pressure control requires continued encouragement, ongoing lifestyle modifications, and medication adjustment. Most patients should have follow-up visits within 1 to 2 months after initiation of drug therapy to evaluate effectiveness, adherence, and possible side effects. Once blood pressure is stabilized, there should be follow up at 3 to 6 month intervals. The JNC lists several approaches that may improve adherence to therapy (Table 30–12).

▶ RESISTANT HYPERTENSION

Blood pressure that cannot be lowered below 140/90 mm Hg despite adherence to an appropriate triple-drug regimen (including a diuretic) at near maximal doses is resistant. In older adults who have isolated systolic hypertension, resistance is the failure of an adequate triple-drug regimen to reduce SBP to below 160 mm Hg. One of the most common causes of true resistance is volume overload secondary to inadequate diuretic therapy. Table 30–13 lists additional causes of inadequate responsiveness to antihypertensive therapy.

The search for secondary causes should be more aggressive in the patient who is younger and/or has the higher blood pressure. Sudden onset of high blood pressure at an early age, especially when refractory to treatment and with

TABLE 30–12. General Guidelines to Improve Patient Adherence to Antihypertensive Therapy

- Be aware of signs of patient nonadherence to antihypertensive therapy
- Establish the goal of therapy: to reduce blood pressure to nonhypertensive levels with minimal or no adverse effects
- Educate patients about the disease, and involve them and their families in its treatment. Have them measure blood pressure at home
- Maintain contact with patients; consider telecommunication
- Keep care inexpensive and simple
- Encourage lifestyle modifications
- Integrate pill-taking into routine activities of daily living
- Prescribe medications according to pharmacologic principles, favoring long-acting formulations
- Be willing to stop unsuccessful therapy and try a different approach
- Anticipate adverse effects, and adjust therapy to prevent, minimize, or ameliorate side effects
- Continue to add effective and tolerated drugs, stepwise, in sufficient doses to achieve the goal of therapy
- Encourage a positive attitude about achieving therapeutic goals
- Consider using nurse case management

(From the Joint National Committee on Detection, Evaluation, and Treatment of High Blood Pressure [1997].)

TABLE 30–13. Causes of Inadequate Responsiveness to Therapy

Pseudoresistance
- "White-coat hypertension" or office elevations
- Pseudohypertension in older patients
- Use of regular cuff on very obese arm

Nonadherence to therapy

Volume overload
- Excess salt intake
- Progressive renal damage (nephrosclerosis)
- Fluid retention from reduction of blood pressure
- Inadequate diuretic therapy

Drug-related causes
- Doses too low
- Wrong type of diuretic
- Inappropriate combinations
- Rapid inactivation (e.g., hydralazine)
- Drug actions and interactions
  - Sympathomimetics
  - Nasal decongestants
  - Appetite suppressants
  - Cocaine and other illicit drugs
  - Caffeine
  - Oral contraceptives
  - Adrenal steroids
  - Licorice (as may be found in chewing tobacco)
  - Cyclosporine, tacrolimus
  - Erythropoietin
  - Antidepressants
  - Nonsteroidal anti-inflammatory drugs

Associated conditions
- Smoking
- Increasing obesity
- Sleep apnea
- Insulin resistance/hyperinsulinemia
- Ethanol intake of more than 1 oz (30 mL) per day
- Anxiety-induced hyperventilation or panic attacks
- Chronic pain
- Intense vasoconstriction (arteritis)
- Organic brain syndrome (e.g., memory deficit)

Identifiable causes of hypertension
- (see Resistant Hypertension)

(From the Joint National Committee on Detection, Evaluation, and Treatment of High Blood Pressure [1997].)

no family history, suggests a secondary cause (Treadway, 1995). Overall cardiovascular risk profile should be evaluated in the middle-aged and elderly population with hypertension because of their greater susceptibility to sudden deleterious adverse events.

The prevalence of secondary hypertension is estimated at 5%. Because the underlying condition in secondary hypertension is generally treatable either surgically or medically, it is essential to differentiate it from primary hypertension. Secondary hypertension has a definable etiology, occurs within a wide age range, often is abrupt in onset with severe consequences, and family history is often negative.

Renal Parenchymal Diseases

Renal parenchymal diseases (RPDs) include cystic renal disease, glomerular disease, interstitial nephritis, nephrosclerosis, and end-stage renal disease, and are almost always associated with impaired renal function (Moore, 1993). RPDs are responsible for approximately half of all secondary cases of hypertension. Hypertension is very common in all forms of RPD and, when hypertension is present, it always accelerates the loss of renal function. Hypertension may result from any form of renal disease that decreases the number of functioning nephrons, leading to sodium and water retention. It is a cyclical situation where the kidney is both the victim and the culprit. This cycle can be broken with adequate antihypertensive therapy (JNC VI, 1997; Kaplan, 1998).

It is essential to detect hypertensive renal damage early. Small increases in the serum creatinine reflect significant losses in the glomerular filtration rate. Work-up should include urinalysis to detect proteinuria or hematuria and possibly renal ultrasound to rule out lower tract obstruction, polycystic kidney disease, and to evaluate the size of the kidney. A 24-hour urine for quatitative protein should be done in all patients with proteinuria (Moore, 1993).

Blood pressure should be controlled to 130/85 mm Hg or lower (127/85 mm Hg) in patients with proteinuria greater than 1 gram/24 hours. The most significant step in slowing progressive renal failure is to lower blood pressure. Unless contraindicated, patients with type 1 diabetic nephropathy, proteinuria of greater than 1 gram/24 hours, or chronic renal insufficiency should receive treatment with ACE inhibitors. Often a diuretic is used in addition to the ACE inhibitor. In patients with a creatinine of 3 mg/dL or greater, ACE inhibition should be used with extreme caution or stopped (JNC VI, 1997). In addition to the control of blood pressure, decreasing dietary intake of protein, control of hyperlipidemia, and restriction of phosphorus may also be helpful (Kaplan, 1998).

During the initial 3 months of antihypertensive therapy as blood pressure is being controlled, there may be a temporary decrease in the glomerular filtration rate. If euvolemic patients have a creatinine increase of 1 mg/dL above baseline, creatinine and potassium levels should be repeated within several days. If they remain elevated, a diagnosis of renal artery stenosis should be considered and ACE inhibitors or A-II-receptor blockers should be discontinued because they can reduce renal blood flow in patients with bilateral renal artery stenosis or renal artery stenosis to a solitary kidney.

Usually large doses of loop diuretics are needed in advanced renal insufficiency. Thiazide diuretics alone are not effective. Combining a long-acting thiazide diuretic (i.e., metazolone) with a loop diuretic, however, works well in patients who are resistant to loop diuretics alone. Potassium-sparing diuretics should not be used in patients with renal insufficiency.

According to Kaplan (1998), ACE inhibitors lower blood pressure, decrease proteinuria, and slow the loss of renal function. However, it is not clear whether ACE inhibitors are better than conventional antihypertensive agents. The excretion of ACE inhibitors is reduced in ESRD requiring a lower dose of the drug except with fisonopril, which is excreted by the liver. Calcium channel blockers have been found to provide equal protection to the kidney as ACE inhibitors. The combination of an ACE inhibitor with a calcium channel blocker may be more effective than either one used alone.

There is limited data documenting the ability of antihypertensive therapy to slow the progression of nondiabetic renal insufficiency. Use of diuretics and other antihypertensive agents may cause reduction in blood pressure that translates into reduction of renal perfusion and glomerular filtration rate. Unless the patient is believed to be hypovolemic or there is drug-related nephrotoxicity, it is best to proceed with controlling the blood pressure despite elevations in serum creatinine. In the end, renal function may be preserved by firm control of the blood pressure (Kaplan, 1998).

Renovascular Hypertension

Renovascular disease is one of the more common causes of potentially correctable secondary hypertension. Renovascular hypertension (RVHT) has been reported to affect as little as 1% of the unselected hypertensive population to as many as 30% of the patients referred to specialists (Kaplan, 1998; Nally, 1993). RVHT is more common in women than men under the age of 40, is less common in black patients with hypertension (Hall et al., 1994), and is less common in diabetics, even though they have a higher incidence of renovascular disease (Kaplan, 1998).

RVHT refers to hypertension that is caused by renal hypoperfusion. The hypoperfusion caused by renovascular disease, usually renal artery stenosis (Nally, 1993), may or may not cause hypertension; renovascular disease is much more common than RVHT (Kaplan, 1998). Hemodynamically significant renal artery stenosis is most often associated with stage 3 or resistant hypertension, and, when bilateral renal artery stenosis is present, it can lead to ishcemic nephropathy (JNC VI, 1997).

The hallmark of RVHT is the overproduction of renin by a kidney that is hypoperfused, which results in an increase in blood pressure secondary to an elevation of total peripheral resistance and sodium retention.

Types of Renal Artery Stenosis

Fibrous dysplasia accounts for 30% of renal vascular disease (Massie, 1995) occurring in younger women before age 35 (Hall et al., 1994), and is usually unilateral initially, but can occur in both renal arteries. This is a process that can involve multiple vessels arising from the aorta, including the carotid and celiac arteries (Kaplan, 1998). An epigastric bruit is heard in approximately 60 percent of patients. When combined with the presence of hypertension of less than 3 years, a systolic–diastolic bruit is predictive of a favorable response to surgery in patients with fibrous dysplasia (Hall et al., 1994). Fibroplastic disease involves mostly the distal two-thirds and branches of the renal arteries. All nonatherosclerotic lesions involve all layers of the renal artery; the most common is medial fibroplasia. Cigarette smoking was found to be a common denominator in many patients with fibromuscular dysplasia (Kaplan, 1992).

Atherosclerotic renovascular disease accounts for the majority of patients with renovascular hypertension and occurs predominantly in men over the age of 45. Specifically, renal artery stenosis (RAS) is the most common curable cause of hypertension, though it occurs in only approximately 3% of the population with hypertension (Hall et al., 1994). These patients have higher systolic pressures and vascular disease elsewhere. Abdominal bruits are found less often than in fibrous dysplasia because other abdominal vessels undergoing the same atherosclerotic changes may generate bruits (Hall et al., 1994). Atherosclerotic disease affects the proximal third of the main renal artery (Kaplan, 1992a). Approximately one third of patients with renovascular disease from atherosclerotic changes have bilateral lesions at the time of diagnosis. Their disease tends to progress if the stenoses is not relieved, even if the hypertension has been adequately managed (Kaplan, 1998). Diabetes mellitus has been found to be more prevalent in these patients and should alert the clinician to the possibility of renal artery stenosis.

History and Physical Findings

A complete and accurate medical history and physical examination is of extreme importance in determining clinical clues that may suggest RVHT as well as recognizing target-organ damage from the hypertension. Clinical clues to RVHT are listed in Table 30–14.

Diagnosis

There is no ideal "screening" test for RVHT. All screening tests are nonspecific and run the risk of high false–positives. Isoptic renography and plasma renin measurements after oral captopril challenge may be sensible initial tests in those patients with appropriate clinical presentation, and followed by renal arteriography. When the suspicion is moderate to low for renal vascular disease, captopril renography is the best noninvasive diagnostic test. The radioisotope renography is performed before and after administration of an angiotensin-converting enzyme inhibitor. This test estimates renal perfusion and function. In an affected kidney, captopril reduces the angiotensin II-mediated vasoconstriction of the efferent arteriole, lowering the glomerular filtration rate. This reduction in GFR occurs in the kidney distal to the stenosis and can be evaluated noninvasively with renogram (Massie, 1995; Nally, 1993). If both kidneys are equally affected, it may be difficult to diagnose bilateral disease.

TABLE 30–14. Clinical Suggestions of Renovascular Hypertension

Abrupt onset of hypertension before age 30 or after age 55 or uncontrolled hypertension in a patient who previously had well-controlled blood pressure
Diastolic blood pressure > 120 mm Hg
Hypertension not responding to triple-drug therapy
Accelerated/malignant hypertension with evidence of grade III or IV retinopathy (hemorrhages, exudates, papilledema)
Hypertension with evidence of arteriosclerotic disease elsewhere (carotid, coronary, and peripheral vascular disease)
Epigastric bruit—especially high-pitched, both systolic and diastolic, and radiates laterally—strongly suggests functionally significant renal arterial stenosis (heard in 46% of those with RVHT and only 9% of those with essential hypertension); benign epigastric bruits radiate vertically, not laterally
Sudden worsening of renal function in the hypertensive patient
Azotemia induced by ACE inhibitor or A-II-receptor blocker therapy
Recurrent (flash) pulmonary edema

From: Nally (1993), Hall et al. (1994), Kaplan (1998), JNC VI (1997).

Duplex Doppler-flow studies and magnetic resonance angiography may be used as noninvasive screening tests. Three-dimensional images can be obtained with a spiral-computed tomography. This study, however, requires intravenous radioconstrast dye. Absolute diagnosis requires renal angiography, which involves some risk, including atheroembolism or acute renal failure from the contrast dye (JNC VI, 1997).

Angiography remains the gold standard in the diagnosis of RAS and is recommended as the definitive test when renovascular hypertension is strongly suspected, but should never be used as a screening test. The downside is that the test is expensive, invasive, and potentially nephrotoxic. According to Nally (1993), the angiogram should be used to: determine presence, location and extent of RAS; differentiate between athersclerosis and fibromuscular dysplasia; determine kidney size and function; and, assess collateral circulation.

Management

Percutaneous transluminal renal angioplasty (PTRA) has given excellent results to patients, especially younger patients with fibromuscular dysplasia, as opposed to atherosclerosis. The results have been comparable to surgical revascularization. Patients who have atherosclerotic renal artery stenosis that is focal, unilateral, nonostial, and without evidence of atherosclerosis elsewhere, should be managed the same as patients with fibromuscular dysplasia. Renal artery stenting is being performed along with the PTRS to avoid the spontaneous elastic recoil and recurrent stenosis that can occur following PTRA (JNC VI, 1997).

Surgery is indicated for those patients whose blood pressure is not well controlled or whose renal function worsens with medical therapy. Also, surgery may be necessary when the patient does not respond to angioplasty.

Renin-Secreting Tumors

Renin-secreting tumors are not common, but the practitioner should be aware of the possibility of their occurrence. These tumors are small and are made up of juxtaglomerular cells that make renin. These patients have hypertension with high renin levels from one kidney. They mostly are found in young patients, with very high prorenin and renin levels in the peripheral blood. Secondary aldosteronism may manifest with hypokalemia. CT scan should be performed to identify the tumor. Removal of the tumor reverses the problem. If surgery is not an option, the hypertension should be managed with ACE inhibitors or calcium channel blockers (Kaplan, 1998).

Coarctation of the Aorta

The lumen of the aorta can be constricted at any level of the thoracic or abdominal aorta; however, it most often occurs just beyond the origin of the left subclavian artery, or distal to the insertion of the ligamentum arteriosum. This lesion accounts for 7% of all congenital heart disease and presents in either infantile or adult form, differing in clinical features.

According to Kaplan (1998), patients who are born with less severe postductal lesions may have no clinical presentation during childhood. There is almost always premature cardiovascular disease with the mean age of death at 34 years. Because of obstruction of blood flow, blood pressure is elevated in the aorta and its branches proximal to the coarctation, and decreased distally. Collateral circulation develops through the intercostal arteries and branches of the subclavian arteries (Massie, 1995).

History and Physical Findings

Adults and children are usually asymptomatic, presenting with hypertension. With minimal constriction, symptoms may not appear until late in life. The classic physical findings are absent or weak femoral pulses, harsh systolic murmur heard in the back, and systolic blood pressure higher in upper extremities than lower extremities; diastolic pressures are similar.

Laboratory and Diagnostic Tests

ECG shows left ventricular hypertrophy or strain. Chest x-ray shows rib notching or scalloping secondary to enlarged collateral intercostal arteries, dilation of the left subclavian artery, dilation of the aorta above and below the area of constriction, and left ventricular enlargement.

The lesion may be detected by two-dimensional echocardiography and confirmed by aortography. The gradient across the lesion can be measured by catheterization and aortogram, but are not always necessary (Kaplan, 1992a, 1998; Massie, 1995).

Management

Surgical mortality rate from resection of the coarcted site is 1% to 4%. Because the risks of the disease are so high, all coarctations in patients up to age 20 years should be resected. In those patients under 40 years of age, the patient should undergo surgery if the hypertension is refractory or if significant left ventricular hypertrophy exists. The surgical mortality rises dramatically in patients over 50 and is thought to be of little value. Immediately after surgical repair, there may be a paradoxical rise in blood pressure that is transient and most likely related to both renin–angiotensin and sympathetic nervous system overactivity (Kaplan, 1998; Massie, 1995). Balloon angioplasty has also been performed successfully and may soon become the treatment of choice.

Prognosis

Most untreated patients with adult form of coarctation die before the age of 40 from complications of hypertension, rupture of the aorta, infective endarteritis, or cerebral hemorrhage. Aortic dissection occurs more frequently in coarctation.

As many as 70% of patients who undergo surgical repair have recurrence or persistence of hypertension. Other risks include recurrence of coarctation and arterial aneurysms in various sites (Kaplan, 1998).

Primary Aldosteronism

Primary aldosteronism is a syndrome resulting from excess secretion of aldosterone from the adrenal cortex. The etiology is usually a solitary unilateral adenoma (Conn's syndrome), but could be related to bilateral cortical hyperplasia. Most aldosteronism is related to an increase in renin–angiotensin activity. There are various forms of *secondary aldosteronism* that can be caused by any clinical condition that affects renin levels (e.g., conditions that cause decreased fluid volume, decreased renal perfusion pressure, sympathetic activation, renin-secreting tumors, etc.). The ability to measure plasma renin activity (PRA) has been instrumental in differentiating between primary and secondary aldosteronism because the PRA is elevated in secondary aldosteronism and suppressed in primary aldosteronism (Kaplan, 1998).

The hypertension is related to an increased peripheral resistance, an expanded plasma volume, and an increased total body sodium content.

The majority of the people with the *primary aldosteronism* are between the ages of 30 and 50, although rarely cases are detected in patients between ages 3 and 75 (Kaplan, 1998) and is more common in females (Fitzgerald, 1995). The classic features of the disease are shown in Table 30–15.

The diagnosis of primary aldosteronism is confirmed by plasma or 24-hour urine levels of aldosterone that increase proportionately to sodium intake and excretion and that fail to suppress normally with volume expansion (Hall et al., 1994). Once the diagnosis of adrenal adenoma has been made, it can be located on CT scan or MRI of the adrenals. If not seen on CT scan, adrenal venous sampling or adrenal scintigraphy should be obtained (Fitzgerald, 1995; Kaplan, 1998).

If the diagnosis of adenoma is made, surgery should be done. If the diagnosis is bilateral hyperplasia, medical therapy with spironolactone is indicated. Bilateral adrenalectomy corrects the hypokalemia but not the hypertension and is not recommended.

TABLE 30–15. Classic Features of Primary Aldosteronism

Hypertension (some patients only have diastolic hypertension)
Hypokalemia with excessive urinary potassium excretion
Polyuria
Polydipsia
Muscular weakness (at times periodic paralysis)
Hypernatremia
Headache
Metabolic alkalosis
Elevated plasma and urine aldosterone levels
Low plasma renin levels

From Fitzgerald (1995), Kaplan (1998).

Pheochromocytoma

Pheochromocytoma is a rare tumor that can occur at any age. This tumor is made up of chromaffin cells (Sheps, 1993) that have the capacity to synthesize and store catecholamines (Kaplan, 1998). The chromaffin cells arise from the cells of the neural crest that contribute to the central nervous system and sympathetic ganglia (Sheps, 1993). Neuroblastomas, ganglioneuromas, and pheochromocytomas may develop from these tissues. A pheochromocytoma may be located in either or both adrenals or anywhere along the sympathetic nervous system chain. It is rare but possible that extraadrenal chromaffin tissue may be located anywhere from the brain to the gonads, including heart and bladder walls. Most tumors are within the abdomen, though rarely they occur within the chest and neck (Sheps, 1993). Functioning tumors arising outside the adrenal medulla are referred to as extraadrenal pheochromocytomas and nonsecreting extraadrenal tumors are known as paragangliomas. As many as 10 to15% of pheochromocytomas in adults are extraadrenal (Fitzgerald, 1995; Kaplan, 1994). Ninety percent of pheochromocytomas arise in the adrenal medulla. Solitary lesions are more common on the right. Approximately 5% of occurrences are bilateral, and 10% of tumors are extraadrenal and solitary. About 10% of tumors recur

(Sheps, 1993). Incidence of malignancy may range from 3% to 14% because of the difficulty to diagnosis. To diagnose malignancy, tumor cells must be found in sites where chromaffin tissue does not normally exist (i.e., lymph nodes, liver, bone, muscle, and lungs) (Sheps, 1993).

The chromaffin cells synthesize catecholamines from the dietary amino acid tyrosine. Norepinephrine is the end-product, except in the adrenal medulla where the majority of the norepinephrine is converted into epinephrine, but a few, usually small in size, secrete only norepinephrine. Conversely, except for a rare few, extraadrenal pheochromocytomas do not secrete epinephrine (Kaplan, 1992a).

History and Physical Findings

Because of the increased secretion of epinephrine and norepinephrine by these tumors, there is excessive adrenergic receptor stimulation which translates into peripheral vasoconstriction and cardiac stimulation (Williams, 1994). The patient initially presents with complaints of severe headache, profuse sweating, and/or palpitations. The symptoms are usually episodic with the onset being sudden and the peak severity being reached within a few minutes. In approximately 50% of the patients, the duration of the episode is less than 15 minutes and usually lasts less than an hour in most patients. The attacks are usually brought on by exercise, bending over, urination, defecation, pressure on the abdomen, induction of anesthesia, or injection of drugs (i.e., histamine, glucagon, droperidol, tyramine, metoclopramide, cytotoxic drugs, tricyclic antidepressants, or phenothiazines) (Sheps, 1993). The hypertension is often difficult to control and unusually labile, which is often the first clue to the health-care practitioner. Other clinical clues to the diagnosis are listed in Table 30–16.

Dramatic fluctuations may be missed and the hypertension may only appear with an episode or may be persistent (Kaplan, 1992a). The symptoms may be attributed to psychoneurosis by practitioners, representing menopausal hot flashes or anxiety-induced hypertension. If the diagnosis is missed, severe complications may arise from exceedingly high blood pressure and damage to the heart by catecholamines. Stroke, hypertensive crisis with encephalopathy, and retinal hemorrhage may occur because these abrupt elevations in blood pressure damage the vessels that are not conditioned as would be in a chronicly hypertensive patient.

TABLE 30–16. Diagnostic Findings in Pheochromocytoma

Inappropriate sinus tachycardia
Exaggerated orthostatic blood pressure changes
Postural tachycardia
Mild elevation of basal body temperature
Vasomotor changes (i.e., facial pallor)
Precordial or abdominal pain
Suprarenal or midline abdominal mass on physical examination
Recurrent arrhythmias
Increased nervousness or anxiety
Increased appetite
Weight loss
Neurofibromatosis
Fundoscopic changes
Nausea and vomiting
Tuberous sclerosis
Previous catastrophic anesthesia or surgery
Pressor response to beta blockers or to induction of anesthesia
Family history of pheochromocytoma, medullary thyroid carcinoma, or hyperparathyroidism

Laboratory and Diagnostic Tests

Routine laboratory screening for pheochromocytoma in the work-up of every hypertensive patient is not recommended. Testing should be reserved for those who exhibit signs that would suggest pheochromocytoma or those with adrenal masses.

The simplest screening procedure is a metanephrine assay of a spot urine preferrably while the patient is medication free (Kaplan, 1998). Metanephrine is a catecholamine metabolite that is least affected by various interfering agents. The assay of urinary catecholamines (total and fractioned), metanephrines, vanilmandelic acid (VMA), and creatinine detects most pheochromocytomas, especially if specimens are obtained immediately after an attack. A 24-hour urine collection is usually obtained, although a shorter collection can be used (Fitzgerald, 1995). In most patients, excretion of all metabolites is elevated, but normal values of one may be seen. Since these tumors may secrete only epinephrine or only norepinephrine, both should be measured to confirm elevated metanephrine levels. Elevated basal plasma levels of both norepinephrine and epinephrine have been found in most patients with pheochromocytoma. It is, however, reported that as many as 10 to 30% of pheo patients have falsely normal levels. False–positive plasma epinephrine and NE levels make plasma assays worthless for screening purposes.

CT scan and MRI have been helpful in confirming and localizing pheochromacytomas but should not be used to replace urinary catecholamine assays because nonpheochromocytoma lesions (i.e., adrenal adenoma) are seen in approximately one-third of abnormal scans and may lead to misdiagnosis. The most accurate way to localize the tumor is by using ^{131}I-MIBG scan which provides 88% sensitivity and 99% specificity, a 95% positive predictive value, and a negative predictive value (Kaplan, 1998).

The clonidine suppression test is useful to help differentiate pheochromocytoma from essential hypertension in patients with elevated plasma catecholamines. The purpose of this test is to distinguish between the patient with pheochromocytoma, who has hypersecretion of plasma norepinephrine that does not respond to the drug, and the patient without tumor whose high basal concentration of catecholamines is decreased or returns to normal with the drug. Clonidine suppression tests commonly can have false–negative results in the patient with pheochromocytoma because of low baseline plasma catecholamine levels at the time of the testing. Provacative pharmacological tests are rarely necessary (Hall et al., 1994; Sheps, 1993).

Management

The treatment of choice is surgical removal of the tumor or tumors. Administration of alpha–adrenergic blocking agents preoperatively has reduced complications during surgery. Patients should be treated medically for at least one week prior to surgery or, if possible, until hypertension and symptoms are under control. In a hypertensive crisis, the alpha–adrenergic blocker phentolamine (Regitine) is given IV, 2 to 5 mg every 5 minutes, until the blood pressure is controlled. If serious tachycardia or arrhythmias occur, give propranolol 1 to 2 mg over a 5- to 10-minute period. If the patient is not in crisis, give oral alpha–adrenergic blockers. Oral phenoxybenzamine (Dibenzyline) is preferred because of its prolonged duration of action. The dose should be started at 10 mg daily and advanced to every 12 hours; dose should be increased gradually until hypertension is controlled. The usual maintenance dose is 49 to 120 mg daily.

After appropriate response with the alpha–adrenergic blocker is achieved, the beta blocker propranolol may be added. If the beta blocker is used before adequate alpha–adrenergic blockade is reached, the beta blocker may cause a pressor response. This response is because the beta blockade of the beta$_2$-mediated vasodilator actions of epinephrine leaves the alpha-mediated vasoconstrictor actions unopposed, or pulmonary edema may occur, probably from removal of beta–adrenergic drive to the heart (Kaplan, 1998). There are a few patients who do not respond to an alpha blocker, but do respond well to a calcium-entry blocker or a converting enzyme inhibitor (Kaplan, 1998).

Metyrosine is a competitive blocker that inhibits catecholamine synthesis. It is used primarily with malignant or inoperable tumors. The initial dose is 250 mg four times daily, increased daily by increments of 250 to 500 mg to a maximum of 4 grams/day (Fitzgerald, 1995). This also should not be used without concomitant use of an alpha blocker (Kaplan, 1994). Metastatic or unresectable pheochromocytomas have had the best response with combination chemotherapy of cyclophosphamide, vincristine, and dacarbazine. As much of the tumor mass that can be reached should be resected. Shrinkage of the tumor has been reported with Metyrosine.

Since it is possible that there are multiple tumors, it is very important to recheck urinary catecholamine levels postoperatively (1 to 2 weeks following surgery).

Oral Contraceptive Use

Hypertension is reported to be two to three times more common in women taking oral contraceptives than in those who do not use oral contraceptives. The hypertension is usually mild but can be severe, can persist after discontinuation of the agent, and is a contributing factor in cardiovascular mortality that is seen among young women taking oral contraceptives (JNC VI, 1997; Kaplan, 1992). Although the use of these agents is associated with increased mortality and morbidity, the total numbers are quite small and the risks appear to be dwindling with improved awareness, better selection of patients, and lower doses of hormones (Kaplan, 1992a). Most of the deaths reported were in women who were smokers, had other cardiovascular risk factors, and who were taking estrogen formulations of greater than 50 ug. The smaller doses of estrogen that is currently used (20-35 ug) may induce much less hypertension. Although most cases are mild among these women, a few women have accelerated rapidly into a malignant phase, causing severe irreversible renal damage. In approximately half of the women with oral contraceptive-induced hypertension, the blood pressure will fall to normal within three to six months after stopping the pill (Kaplan, 1992a).

The mechanism for oral contraceptive-induced hypertension is not known. Changes in hemodynamics, renin–angiotensin–aldosterone system, and insulin sensitivity have all been cited as potential causes.

The use of estrogen-containing oral contraceptives should be restricted in women over the age of 35, especially if they are obese, smoke, or are already hypertensive. Women age 35 and older who smoke cigarettes should be counseled to quit. If they cannot quit they should be discouraged from using oral contraceptives. If hypertension develops in women taking oral contraceptives, the patient should be advised to stop their use.

Women on oral contraceptives should be closely monitored. The initial supply of oral contraceptives should be only for three months, then six months thereafter. Also, they should be required to return for a blood pressure check before a renewal is given. If blood pressure rises, an additional form of contraception should be given. If the pill is the only acceptable contraceptive, the hypertension should be treated with appropriate therapy. The use of a diuretic–spironalactone agent is ideal because of the role of aldosterone with oral contraceptive use. In those women who discontinue use of the oral contraceptive, investigation into secondary causes of hypertension should be delayed at least three months until the changes with the renin–angiotensin–aldosterone system return to normal. If the hypertension persists, additional work-up and therapy are recommended (Kaplan, 1992a).

Hypertension in Pregnancy

Hypertension occurs in over 5% of all pregnancies. According to Kaplan (1998), hypertensive disorders are among the leading causes of maternal and perinatal mortality in developed countries. The term "pregnancy-induced hypertension" is being used less often. Table 30–17 lists definitions that are used to describe hypertension during pregnancy.

TABLE 30–17. Classifications of Hypertension Associated with Pregnancy

Chronic hypertension	Hypertension that was present prior to pregnancy, or diagnosed before the 20th week of gestation, or that persists after 6 weeks' postpartum
Preeclampsia	An elevated blood pressure appearing after 20 weeks' gestation, usually associated with edema and proteinuria
Eclampsia	Seizures in the preeclamptic patient that cannot be attributed to any other causes
Preeclampsia superimposed on chronic hypertension	Women with chronic hypertension who have SBP elevations of 30 mm Hg or DBP elevations of 15 mm Hg in addition to the appearance of proteinuria or edema
Transient hypertension	Blood pressure that is elevated during pregnancy or during the first 24 hours postpartum with no previous history of hypertension or signs of preeclampsia

From Kaplan (1998).

The goal of therapy for women with chronic hypertension during pregnancy is to reduce the short-term risks of the elevated blood pressure to the mother and avoiding therapy that will be harmful to the fetus. Most medication for hypertension taken prior to the pregnancy can be continued, that is, diuretics, beta blockers, and most others, *except* ACE inhibitors and A-II receptor blockers. If hypertension is newly diagnosed during pregnancy, methyldopa is the drug of choice because it is the agent that has been studied the most during pregnancy. Beta blockers are considered safe in the latter part of pregnancy; however, their use in early pregnancy is associated with growth retardation of the fetus. ACE inhibitors and A-II receptor blockers should always be avoided because they can cause renal failure and death to the fetus. See Table 30–18 for antihypertensive drugs used during pregnancy.

Postmenopausal Estrogen Replacement

Hypertension rarely occurs with postmenopausal estrogen use. There is a significantly lower mortality rate from coronary artery disease among postmenopausal women using estrogen replacement when compared with nonusers (Kaplan, 1992a).

Hormonal Disturbances

Thyroid and parathyroid dysfunction may be the sole cause or a contributing factor in essential hypertension. The types of thyroid disease that are associated with hypertension are hypothyroidism, hyperthyroidism, hyperparathyroidism, and Cushing's syndrome (Kaplan, 1998; Young, 1993).

Hypothyroidism results from a deficiency of thyroid hormones, causing many metabolic functions (including cardiac output) to slow down. There is also decreased myocardial contractility and impaired diastolic relaxation. Together, these effects cause hypertension. Because cardiac output is low, SNS and alpha–adrenergic activity increases, causing increased peripheral resistance in an attempt to maintain tissue perfusion. Diastolic pressures are elevated more than systolic pressures (Kaplan, 1998; Young, 1993). Thyroid replacement therapy is necessary.

Hyperthyroidism occurs from excessive amounts of

TABLE 30–18. Antihypertensive Drugs Used in Pregnancy[a]

The report of the NHBPEP Working Group on High Blood Pressure in Pregnancy permits continuation of drug therapy in women with chronic hypertension (except for ACE inhibitors). In addition, angiotensin II receptor blockers should not be used during pregnancy. In women with chronic hypertension with diastolic levels of 100 mm Hg or greater (lower when end organ damage or underlying renal disease is present) and in women with acute hypertension when levels are 105 mm Hg or greater, the following agents are suggested.

Suggested Drug	Comments
Central alpha-agonists	Methyldopa (C) is the drug of choice recommended by the NHBPEP Working Group
Beta-blockers	Atenolol (C) and metoprolol (C) appear to be safe and effective in late pregnancy. Labetalol (C) also appears to be effective (alpha- and beta-blockers)
Calcium antagonists	Potential synergism with magnesium sulfate may lead to precipitous hypotension (C)
ACE inhibitors, angiotensin II receptor blockers	Fetal abnormalities, including death, can be caused, and these drugs should not be used in pregnancy (D)
Diuretics	Diuretics (C) are recommended for chronic hypertension if prescribed before gestation or if patients appear to be salt-sensitive. They are not recommended in preeclampsia
Direct vasodilators	Hydralazine (C) is the parenteral drug of choice based on its long history of safety and efficacy (C)

[a] Adapted from Lindheimer, M. D. (1996). Pre-eclampsai–eclampsia 1996: Preventable? Have disputes on its treatment been resolved? *Curr Opin Nephrol Hyperten. 5:* 452–8 and Sibai, B. M. (1996). Treatment of Hypertension in Pregnant Women. *New England Journal of Medicine, 335*, 257–265. There are several other antihypertensive drugs for which there are very limited data. The U.S. Food and Drug Administration classifies pregnancy risk as follows: C, adverse effects in animals; no controlled trials in humans; use if risk appears justified; D, positive evidence of fetal risk. ACE indicates angiotensin-converting enzyme.

circulating thyroid hormone that interact with receptors on peripheral tissues. The result is increased metabolic activity and sensitivity to circulating catecholamines. These patients, in contrast to hypothyroidism, have an increased cardiac output, decreased peripheral resistance, and an elevated systolic blood pressure with a lowered diastolic pressure (Kaplan, 1998; Young, 1993). Treatment of the hyperthyroidism is necessary (see Chapter 39 on endocrine problems).

Outside the fact that increased levels of parathyroid hormone have a possible role in the pathogenesis of primary hypertension, the presence of hyperfunction of the parathyroid gland (primary hyperparathyroidism) is associated with a twofold rate of hypertension and LVH (even in the absence of hypertension) (Kaplan, 1998).

The primary function of the parathyroid hormone is to maintain normal levels of serum calcium. An autonomous overproduction of parathyroid hormone (primary hyperparathyroidism) commonly leads to hypercalcemia, which is associated with an increased incidence of hypertension. Hypercalcemia raises the blood pressure most likely from a direct effect on peripheral resistance that may be caused by an increased reactivity of the vasculature to catecholamines (Kaplan, 1998; Young, 1993).

Most patients with hyperparathyroidism exhibit symptoms related to the effects of chronic hypercalcemia such as polyuria and polydipsia, constipation, osteoporosis, renal lithiasis, peptic ulcer disease, and hypertension. Laboratory testing will reveal hypercalcemia and hypophosphatemia, with elevated serum levels of parathyroid hormone. To diagnose there should be two documented levels of hypercalcemia on separate occasions. In addition, elevated parathyroid hormone levels should be documented. If serum concentrations of parathyroid hormone are not elevated, causes of hypercalcemia should be investigated. These include pheochromocytoma, hyperthyroidism, cancer (including multiple myeloma), vitamin D intoxication, and sarcoidosis (Young, 1993).

Cushing's syndrome is a serious disease with a high mortality rate, mostly related to cardiovascular complications, such as LVH. The hypertension in these patients is difficult to treat and requires prompt diagnosis.

This syndrome is caused by increased levels of glucocorticoids, either from endogenous cortisol (idiopathic) or exogenous steroids (iatrogenic). The severity of the hypertension may be related to the elimination of the normal fall in blood pressure at night that is seen in patients with Cushing's syndrome and glucocorticoid administration. Hypertension is rare in patients taking exogenous glucocorticoid steroids because they have more mineralcorticoid activity than cortisol.

Kaplan (1998) points out the major mechanisms responsible for hypertension in Cushing's syndrome: (1) may be related to sodium-retaining qualities of excessive levels of cortisol that bind to mineralocorticoid receptors or non-receptor mechanisms; (2) increased production of mineralocorticoids; and (3) increased renin levels and reduced vasodepressor action.

Because fluid volume excess is most likely involved, a diuretic in combination with the aldosterone antagonist spironolactone is a logical initial choice. In most cases the hypertension resolves with appropriate antihypertensive therapy, except in longstanding cases. Treatment of the syndrome itself is discussed in Chapter 39.

Obstructive Sleep Apnea

Obstructive sleep apnea (OSA) causes a significant increase in blood pressure that is initially transient but may develop into hypertension during waking hours. OSA has been associated with myocardial infarction, ventricular arrhythmias, LVH, cerebral ischemia and stroke, pulmonary hypertension, and cor pulmonale (Levinson & Millman, 1993).

Drugs and Other Substances that Cause Hypertension

Immunosuppressive Agents

Immunosuppressive agents such as cyclosporin, tacrolimus, and steroids increase blood pressure in 50 to 80% of those patients who are recipients of solid organ transplants. When used in nontransplant recipients, hypertension develops in 25 to 30% of patients. The blood pressure elevation occurs secondary to widespread vasoconstriction. Renal vasoconstriction leads to diminished glomerular filtration and increased sodium reabsorption (JNC VI, 1997).

Within weeks to months of initiating cyclosporine therapy, hypertension occurs and is related to activation of the SNS, blunted natriuresis in response to volume expansion, impaired vasodilation, and release of endothelial factors (Kaplan, 1998).

Treatment should be aimed at vasodilation with ACE inhibitors or dihydropyridine calcium channel blockers. Amlodipine does not alter cyclosporin metabolism like verapamil or diltiazem and is therefore preferred (Kaplan, 1998). Diuretics are effective but may increase prerenal azotemia and precipitate gout (JNC VI, 1997).

Erythropoietin

Recombinant human erythropoietin increases blood pressure in 18 to 45% of patients when used in the treatment of end-stage renal disease. This rise in blood pressure is secondary to an increased systemic vascular resistance from direct vascular effects of the recombinant human erythropoietin and is not related to changes in hematocrit or viscosity. In some cases a reduction in the erythropoietin dose is necessary if blood pressure cannot be controlled with antihypertensive agents.

Cocaine

There is no evidence that continued use of cocaine causes chronic hypertension. According to the JNC VI, the majority of people who are dependent on cocaine are normotensive. However, they recommend that cocaine abuse should always be considered in all patients who present to the emergency room with hypertension-related problems. Cocaine may cause severe coronary and cerebral vasoconstriction in addition to acute renal failure from rhabdomyolysis. The patient may present with chest pain, tachycardia, dilated pupils, combativeness, altered mental status, and seizures.

Nitroglycerin is indicated to reverse coronary vasoconstriction related to the cocaine, though other parenteral agents may be needed to lower blood pressure. Nonselective beta blockers (i.e., propranolol) should be avoided because of the risk of paradoxical rise in blood pressure as well as coronary vasoconstriction from increased effect of catecholamines on unblocked alpha-receptors (JNC VI, 1997).

Amphetamines

Acute amphetamine toxicity is similar to that of cocaine; however, the duration can last up to several hours. Cerebral and systemic vasculitis and renal failure may occur. The treatment is similar to that used with cocaine toxicity.

Other Causes of Secondary Hypertension

Glycyrrhetenic acid is the active ingredient in licorice extract and has been known to cause sodium retention, potassium wasting, and hypertension in rare cases. Excessive amounts of the mineralocorticoid deoxycorticosterone (DOC) may also cause hypertension. This syndrome can either arise from hyperplastic adrenals with enzymatic deficiencies or from DOC-secreting tumors. The entire syndrome can be treated with glucocorticoid therapy, usually cortisol in doses of 10 to 30 mg/day (Kaplan, 1998).

▶ HYPERTENSIVE CRISES

Hypertensive Emergencies

Hypertensive emergencies require immediate reduction to prevent or limit target-organ damage. Patients in these situations may need their blood pressure reduced within minutes if there is immediate danger to the heart, brain, or large vessels. Hypertensive emergencies include: encephalopathy, eclampsia, intracranial hemorrhage, unstable angina pectoris, acute myocardial infarction, dissecting aortic aneurysms, and acute left ventricular failure with pulmonary edema (Kaplan, 1995; JNC VI, 1997). Hypertensive encephalopathy is defined as a severe and abrupt elevation in blood pressure with severe headache and alterations in levels of consciousness, reversible by blood pressure reduction (Kaplan, 1992a).

According to the JNC VI (1997), the initial goal of therapy in hypertensive emergencies is to reduce mean arterial blood pressure by no more than 25% between minutes to two hours. Once this is achieved, the goal is to work toward a blood pressure of 160/100 mm Hg between 2 to 6 hours, avoiding extreme decline in blood pressure trends that may cause ishemia to the vital organs. Elevated blood pressure alone without evidence of new or progressive target-organ damage rarely requires emergency therapy (JNC VI, 1997).

Initial treatment for hypertensive emergencies should be with parenteral administration of the appropriate drugs. Parenteral drugs for hypertensive emergencies are listed in Table 30–19. These patients should be monitored closely in an intensive care unit, preferably with an intraarterial line, to avoid overshooting of blood pressure reduction. Carefully titrated intravenous nicardipine or labetolol are effective and may have less side effects than intravenous nitroprusside. For acute LV failure, enalaprilat is the drug of choice. For symptoms of acute myocardial ischemia, intravenous nitroglycerin is the first choice (Kaplan & Opie, 1997). Intravenous methyldopa is the drug of choice for eclampsia (refer to Table 30–18).

Nitroprusside directly dilates the arteriolar and venous system and has no effect on the autonomic or central nervous systems. Venous return to the heart is decreased and cardiac output and stroke volume are decreased with an increase in heart rate. Increased peripheral vascular resistance is prevented because of arteriolar dilation. In addition, there is an increase in intracranial pressure. For these reasons other parenteral agents are being more widely used, such as labetolol and nicardipine.

The onset of action of nitroprusside is within 30 seconds; the peak hypotensive effect occurs within 2 minutes and the effects of the drug disappear within 3 minutes of discontinuing the infusion (Oates, 1996). Nitroprusside is metabolized by smooth muscle to cyanide in the red blood cells and thiocynate in the liver. Toxic accumulations of cyanide can occur, leading to severe lactic acidosis. By concurrently administering sodium theosulfate to those patients receiving higher than usual doses of nitroprusside, accumulation of cyanide can be avoided. The risk of thiocyanate toxicity increases when sodium nitroprusside is given for greater than 24 to 48 hours, especially in patients who have renal impairment. Toxicity may manifest with the following symptoms: nausea, anorexia, fatigue, disorientation, and psychosis. Plasma levels of thiocyanate should be monitored during prolonged infusions of the drug, and should not exceed 0.1 mg/mL (Kaplan, 1992a; Oates, 1997).

The ACE inhibitor enalaprilat has a rapid onset of action and can be given as an infusion for an extended period of time for a prolonged antihypertensive response. This agent is especially useful in situations where ACE inhibition is thought to offer special advantages, such as severe congestive heart failure (Kaplan, 1992a).

TABLE 30–19. Parenteral Drugs for Treatment of Hypertensive Emergencies[a]

Drug	Dose[b]	Onset of Action	Duration of Action	Adverse Effects[c]	Special Indications
Vasodilators					
Sodium nitroprusside	0.25–10 μg/kg per min as IV infusion[d] (maximal dose for 10 min only)	Immediate	1–2 min	Nausea, vomiting, muscle twitching, sweating, thiocyanate and cyanide intoxication	Most hypertensive emergencies; caution with high intracranial pressure or azotemia
Nicardipine hydrochloride	5–15 mg/h IV	5–10 min	1–4 h	Tachycardia, headache, flushing, local phlebitis	Most hypertensive emergencies except acute heart failure; caution with coronary ischemia
Fenoldopam mesylate	0.1–0.3 μg/kg per min IV infusion	<5 min	30 min	Tachycardia, headache, nausea, flushing	Most hypertensive emergencies; caution with glaucoma
Nitroglycerin	5–100 μg/min as IV infusion[d]	2–5 min	3–5 min	Headache, vomiting, methemoglobinemia, tolerance with prolonged use	Coronary ischemia
Enalaprilat	1.25–5 mg every 6 h IV	15–30 min	6 h	Precipitous fall in pressure in high-renin states; response variable	Acute left ventricular failure; avoid in acute myocardial infarction
Hydralazine hydrochloride	10–20 mg IV 10–50 mg IM	10–20 min 20–30 min	3–8 h	Tachycardia, flushing, headache, vomiting, aggravation of angina	Eclampsia
Diazoxide	50–100 mg IV bolus repeated, or 15–30 mg/min infusion	2–4 min	6–12 h	Nausea, flushing, tachycardia, chest pain	Now obsolete; when no intensive monitoring available
Adrenergic inhibitors					
Labetalol hydrochloride	20–80 mg IV bolus every 10 min 0.5–2.0 mg/min IV infusion	5–10 min	3–6 h	Vomiting, scalp tingling, burning in throat, dizziness, nausea, heart block, orthostatic hypotension	Most hypertensive emergencies except acute heart failure
Esmolol hydrochloride	250–500 μg/kg/min for 1 min, then 50–100 μg/kg/min for 4 min; may repeat sequence	1–2 min	10–20 min	Hypotension, nausea	Aortic dissection, perioperative
Phentolamine	5–15 mg IV	1–2 min	3–10 min	Tachycardia, flushing, headache	Catecholamine excess

[a] These doses may vary from those in the *Physicians' Desk Reference* (51st edition).
[b] IV indicates intravenous; IM, intramuscular.
[c] Hypotension may occur with all agents.
[d] Require special delivery system.
(From the Joint National Committee on Detection, Evaluation, and Treatment of High Blood Pressure [1997].)

Nicadipine is a dihydropyridine calcium channel blockers that produces a consistent and progressive fall in the blood pressure with little change in the heart rate and a slight increase in the cardiac output.

In the past, sublingual or "bite and swallow" nifedipine has been widely used in hypertensive emergencies in place of an intravenous agent; however, several serious side effects have been reported with its use. The greater the initial blood pressure elevation, the greater the blood pressure response will be after nifedipine administration in the acute setting. Many sources agree that the reduction in blood pressure is gradual and consistent by approximately 20% within 20 to 30 minutes (Kaplan & Opie, 1997; Zusman, 1996). Abrupt blood pressure reductions have been reported, especially in those patients who are volume depleted or who already have antihypertensive medications in their system before the hypertensive emergency was recognized. Additionally, these abrupt blood pressure reductions may result in myocardial ischemia in patients with underlying coronary artery disease, or cerebral ischemia in patients with underlying carotid artery disease. The sudden drop in blood pressure and resultant adrenergic discharge can lead to reflex tachycardia which may exacerbate symptoms of unstable angina pectoris or myocardial infarction, and would be contraindicated in patients with a dissecting aortic aneurysm (Zusman, 1996). Because the degree of blood pressure decline with this agent is often unpredictable and too difficult to control, the JNC VI (1997) deem its use in hypertensive emergencies unacceptable.

Hypertensive Urgencies

Hypertensive urgencies are those situations that require blood pressure reduction within a few hours. Examples of hypertensive urgencies include: upper levels of stage 3 hypertension, hypertension with papilledema, progressive target-organ complications, and severe perioperative hypertension (JNC VI, 1997). Other examples include: cerebral thrombosis, MAO-tyramine interaction, sympathomimetic drug overdose, and rebound from abrupt cessation of adrenergic inhibiting drugs (Kaplan, 1995).

REFERENCES

Berecek, K. H. & Wyss, M. (1993). Adrenergic receptors and actions. In J. L. Izzo & H. R. Black (Eds.), *Hypertension primer.* (pp. 7–9). Dallas: American Heart Association.

Carleton, P. F. (1992). Anatomy of the cardiovascular system. In S.A. Price & L. M. Wilson (Eds.), *Pathophysiology: Clinical concepts of disease processes.* (pp. 371–381). St. Louis: Mosby.

Cushman, W. C. (1993). Physical activity, fitness, and blood pressure. In J. L. Izzo & H. R. Black (Eds.), *Hypertension primer.* (pp. 161–163). Dallas: American Heart Association.

Fitzgerald, P. A. (1995). Endocrine disorders. In L. M. Tierney, Jr., S. J. McPhee & M. A. Papadakis (Eds.), *Current: Medical diagnosis & treatment* (34th ed.). (pp. 943–1003). Norwalk, CT: Appleton & Lange.

Frishman, W. H. (1993). Beta-adrenergic blockers. In J. L. Izzo & H. R. Black (Eds.), *Hypertension primer.* (pp. 297–300). Dallas: American Heart Association.

Frolich, E. D. (1994). Pathophysiology of systemic arterial hypertension. In R. C. Schlant, et al. (Eds.), *Hurst's The heart* (8th ed.). (pp. 1391–1401). New York: McGraw-Hill.

Gavras, H. (1993). Angiotensin-converting enzyme inhibitors. In J. L. Izzo & H. R. Black (Eds.), *Hypertension primer.* (pp. 309–310). Dallas: American Heart Association.

Goldstein, D. S. (1993). Autonomic nervous dysfunction in essential hypertension. In J. L. Izzo & H. R. Black (Eds.), *Hypertension primer.* (pp. 61–63). Dallas: American Heart Association.

Graettinger, W. F. (1995). Systemic hypertension. In M. H. Crawford (Ed.), *Current: Diagnosis and treatment in cardiology.* (pp. 163–171). Norwalk: Appleton & Lange.

Hall, W. D., Wollam, G. L., & Tuttle, E. P. (1994). Diagnostic evaluation of the patient with systemic arterial hypertension. In R. C. Schlant, et al. (Eds.), *Hurst's, the heart* (8th ed.). (pp. 1403–1425). New York: McGraw-Hill.

Hoffman, B. B. & Lefkowitz, R. J. (1996). Catecholamines, sympathomimetic drugs, and adrenergic receptor antagonists. In J. G. Hardman, et al. (Eds.), *Goodman & Gilman's The pharmacological basis of therapeutics* (9th ed.). (pp. 199–248). New York: McGraw-Hill.

Jackson, E. K. & Garrison, J. C. (1996). Renin and angiotensin. In J.G. Hardman, et al. (Eds.), *Goodman & Gilman's The pharmacological basis of therapeutics* (9th ed.). (pp. 733–758). New York: McGraw-Hill.

Joint National Committee on Detection, Evaluation, and Treatment of High Blood Pressure. The Sixth Report of the Joint National Committee on Detection, Evaluation, and Treatment of High Blood Pressure. National Institute of Health, National Heart, Lung, and Blood Institute. (1997). NIH Publication No. 98–4080.

Kaplan, N. M. (1992a). Systemic hypertension: Mechanisms and diagnosis. In E. Braunwald (Ed.), *Heart disease: A textbook of cardiovascular medicine* (4th ed.). (pp. 817–851). Philadelphia: W. B. Saunders Company.

Kaplan, N. M. (1992b). Systemic hypertension: Therapy. In E. Braunwald (Ed.), *Heart disease: A textbook of cardiovascular medicine* (4th ed.). (pp. 852–874). Philadelphia: W. B. Saunders.

Kaplan, N. M. (1995). *Management of hypertension* (6th ed.). Durant, OK: Essential Medical Information Systems, Inc.

Kaplan, N. M. (1998). *Clinical hypertension* (7th ed.). Baltimore, MD: Williams & Wilkins.

Kaplan, N. M. & Opie, L. H. (1997). Antihypertensive drugs. In L. H. Opie, et al. (Eds.), *Drugs for the Heart* (4th ed.) (pp. 174–206). Philadelphia: W. B. Saunders.

Khan, M. G. (1995). Hypertension. In M. G. Khan (Ed.), *Cardiac drug therapy* (4th ed.). (pp. 97–148). Philadelphia: W. B. Saunders.

Klatsky, A. L. (1993). Alcohol use and blood pressure. In J. L. Izzo & H. R. Black (Eds.), *Hypertension primer.* (pp. 164–166). Dallas: American Heart Association.

Kuller, L. H. (1993). Calcium, magnesium, and blood pressure. In J. L. Izzo & H. R. Black (Eds.), *Hypertension primer.* (pp. 173–175). Dallas: American Heart Association.

Levinson, P. D. & Millman, R. P. (1993). Sleep apnea: Management. In J. L. Izzo & H. R. Black (Eds.), *Hypertension primer.* (pp. 275–277). Dallas: American Heart Association.

Malseed, R. T., Goldstein, F. J., & Balkon, N. (1995). Antihypertensive Drugs. In M. Belcher (Ed.), *Pharmacology: Drug therapy and nursing considerations.* (pp. 327–348). Philadelphia: J. B. Lippincott.

Massie, B. M. (1995). Systemic hypertension. In L. M. Tierney, Jr., S. J. McPhee, & M. A. Papadakis (Eds.), *Current. Medical diagnosis & treatment* (34th ed.). (pp. 373–390). Norwalk: Appleton & Lange.

Materson, B. J., Reda, D. J., Cushman, W. C., Massie, B. M., Freis, E. D., Kocker, M. S., Hamberger, R. J., Fyhe, C., Lakshman, R. E., et al. (1993). Single-drug therapy for hypertension in men. A comparison of six antihypertensive agents with placebo. *New England Journal of Medicine, 328* (1), 914.

Moore, M. A. (1993). Renal parenchymal disease: Evaluation. In J. L. Izzo & H. R. Black (Eds.), *Hypertension primer.* (pp. 265–267). Dallas: American Heart Association.

Moser, M. (1997). *Clinical management of hypertension* (2nd ed.). Caddo, OK: Professional Communications, Inc.

Nally, J. V. (1993). Renovascular disease: Evaluation. In J. L. Izzo & H. R. Black (Eds.), *Hypertension primer.* (pp. 262–264). Dallas: American Heart Association.

Oates, J. A. (1996). Antihypertensive agents and the drug therapy of hypertension. In J. G. Hardman, et al. (Eds.), *Goodman & Gilman's The pharmacological basis of therapeutics* (9th ed.). (pp. 780–808). New York: McGraw-Hill.

Opie, L. H., Frishman, W. H., & Thadani, U. (1997). Calcium channel antagonists (Calcium entry blockers). In L. H. Opie, et al. (Eds.), *Drugs for the heart* (4th ed.). (pp. 50–82). Philadelphia: W. B. Saunders.

Opie, L. H., Kaplan, N. M., & Poole-Wilson, P. A. (1997). Diuretics. In L. H. Opie, et al. (Eds.), *Drugs for the Heart* (4th ed.). (pp. 83–103). Philadelphia: W. B. Saunders.

Opie, L. H., Poole-Wilson, P. A., Sonnenblick, E., & Chatterjee, K. (1997). Angiotensin-converting enzyme inhibitors. Contrasts with conventional vasodilators. In L. H. Opie, et al. (Eds.), *Drugs for the Heart* (4th ed.). (pp. 105–144). Philadelphia: W. B. Saunders.

Opie, L. H., Sonnenblick, E. H., Frishman, W., & Thadani, U. (1997). Beta-blocking agents. In L. H. Opie, et al. (Eds.), *Drugs for the heart* (4th ed.). (pp. 1–30). Philadelphia: W. B. Saunders.

O'Rourke, M.(1993). Mechanisms of arteriosclerosis and decreased arterial compliance. In J. L. Izzo & H. R. Black (Eds.), *Hypertension primer* (pp. 121–123). Dallas: American Heart Association.

Perry, H. M. (1993). Central and peripheral sympatholytics. In J. L. Izzo & H. R. Black (Eds.), *Hypertension primer* (pp. 306–309). Dallas: American Heart Association.

Porsche, R. (1995). Hypertension: Diagnosis, acute antihypertensive therapy, and long-term management. *AACN Clinical Issues, 4,* 515–525.

Ram, C. V. & Featherston, W. E. (1993). Vasodilators. In J. L. Izzo & H. R. Black (Eds.), *Hypertension primer.* (pp. 314–316). Dallas: American Heart Association.

Ramachandran, E. & Frank, R. N. (1993). The eye in hypertension. In J. L. Izzo & H. R. Black (Eds.), *Hypertension primer.* (pp. 131–133). Dallas: American Heart Association.

Rea, R. F. (1993). Cardiopulmonary baroreflexes and central blood volume. In J. L. Izzo & H. R. Black (Eds.), *Hypertension primer.* (pp. 71–72). Dallas: American Heart Association.

Sheps, S. G. (1993). Pheochromocytoma: Evaluation. In J. L. Izzo & H. R. Black (Eds.), *Hypertension primer.* (pp. 268–270). Dallas: American Heart Association.

Shub, C. (1993). Cardiac evaluation in hypertension. In J. L. Izzo & H. R. Black (Eds.), *Hypertension primer.* (pp. 245–247). Dallas: American Heart Association.

Swartz, S. L. & Moore, T. J. (1996). Nonpharmacologic and pharmacologic treatment of hypertension. In T. W. Smith, et al. (Eds.), *Cardiovascular therapeutics: A companion to Braunwald's heart disease.* (pp. 484–494). Philadelphia: W. B. Saunders.

Treadway, K. K. (1995). Management of hypertension. In A. H. Goroll, L. A. May, & A. G. Mulley (Eds.), *Primary care medicine: Office evaluation and management of the adult patient* (3rd ed.). (pp. 125–138). Philadelphia: J. B. Lippincott.

Weir, M. R. (1993). Calcium entry blockers. In J. L. Izzo & H. R. Black (Eds.), *Hypertension primer.* (pp. 311–314). Dallas: American Heart Association.

Williams, G. H. (1994). Hypertensive vascular disease. In K. J. Isselbacher, et al. (Eds.), *Harrison's principles of internal medicine* (13th ed.). (pp. 1116–1131). New York: McGraw-Hill.

Young, W. E. (1993). Thyroid and parathyroid disorders: Evaluation. In J. L. Izzo & H. R. Black (Eds.), *Hypertension primer.* (pp. 274–275). Dallas: American Heart Association.

Zusman, R. M. (1996). Treatment of hypertensive emergencies. In T. W. Smith et al. (Eds.), *Cardiovascular therapeutics: A companion to Braunwald's heart disease* (pp. 495–502). Philadelphia: W. B. Saunders.

31

Vascular Disease

Andrew B. Roberts
Susan Bradford

"Vascular disease" is a very broad topic. To try to give some order to this chapter, it has been divided into sections on the arterial, venous, and lymphatic systems. The arterial tree's principal function is to act as a conduit for blood from the cardiac ventricles to the capillary beds. This chapter is limited to the systemic circulation, the arteries extending from the left ventricle and the aortic valve to the peripheral capillary beds that transport oxygenated blood. All the arteries are composed of three layers: the innermost intima, the media, and the outer adventitia. In the aorta, the media is largely made up of elastic fibers. As the arteries become progressively smaller, the elastic fibers are replaced by smooth muscle cells that, at the precapillary arteriolar level, become extremely important in the regulation of the peripheral resistance of different perfusion beds. This discussion focuses on diseases of large- and medium-sized arteries that can be endovascularly or surgically manipulated.

The venous system acts as the conduit through which blood returns from the capillary beds to the heart. It is a low-pressure, thin-walled system that has essentially no elastic tissue in its media. Like the arteries, it is composed of three layers, but unlike the arteries, veins have valves. The major veins run with the arteries and peripheral nerves in "neurovascular bundles."

Lymphatics comprise the lowest-pressure and thinnest-walled system. This system of valved channels transports fluid and large proteins from the interstitium back to the central veins.

▶ OCCLUSIVE ARTERIAL DISEASE

Overview

Pathophysiology

Currently, in the United States, the vast majority of large-vessel arterial occlusive disease is secondary to atherosclerosis. Interestingly, despite the fact that atherosclerotic disease is the direct cause of the majority of all deaths in this country, and that the pathology has been well described for almost 100 years, the mechanism of atherosclerosis is not well understood. In simplest terms, the wall of the atherosclerotic artery thickens. The external diameter of the vessel remains relatively stable, and, as the wall becomes thicker, the internal lumen decreases in size. In extreme situations, hemodynamically significant stenosis, or even total occlusion of the vessel, may develop.

The atherosclerotic lesions can be subdivided into fatty streaks, fibrous plaques, and complex lesions. Only the latter two are clinically significant. In these lesions, the plaque is composed of a complex mixture of smooth muscle cells, monocytes, macrophages, lipids, and extracellular matrix (primarily collagen, elastin, and glycosaminoglyans). The more mature "complex lesions" also contain lakes of lipid (triglyceride and cholesterol), hematoma within the plaque, and/or areas of dense calcification. In these complex lesions, the wall itself may outgrow its blood supply, causing it to necrose and ulcerate.

The stimulus for this excessive growth remains unclear; however, the most commonly accepted theory hypothesizes that the initiating event is an injury to the arterial endothelium (Ross, 1986), the innermost layer of cells of the artery. Collagen, which is normally beneath the endothelium, is exposed to the blood elements, and platelets aggregate at the site of injury. The endothelium and platelets release growth factors that have two effects. They stimulate the migration of monocytes and smooth muscle cells (SMC) from the media, the middle arterial layer, to the intima (the inner layer). They also stimulate both cell lines to proliferate and grow, and to produce extracellular material. All of these effects lead to thickening of the arterial wall.

Despite the fact that the exact mechanism of atherosclerosis remains obscure, it is perfectly clear that certain "risk factors" are associated with early development of clinically relevant atherosclerotic occlusive disease. In our society, there are seven major factors, four of which we can influence and three that we cannot. The three we cannot change are family history, gender (women tend to be relatively spared until they go through menopause), and age (atherosclerosis is part of the aging process and is usually more evident the older one gets). The four that we can influence are: smoking (perhaps the biggest health problem in the United States), hypertension, diabetes mellitus, and hyperlipidemia, specifically, hypercholesterolemia (the role of triglycerides is less clear). One of the great frustrations of treating patients with atherosclerotic disease is the knowledge that behavior patterns (specifically, smoking) have had a significant role in the development of their troubles. On the other hand, one of the sources of hope is the realization that by paying attention to risk factors (stopping smoking and getting blood pressure, blood sugar, and cholesterol under control), patients can do much to alter their course and to save themselves.

History and Physical Findings

Whenever a patient presents with an arterial problem, there are certain fundamentals of diagnosis that should be followed. The general principles hold true whether the arteries involved are the coronaries or more peripheral vessels. Except for infrequent life-threatening emergencies, history-taking is the first step. The specifics of the chief complaint vary depending upon the vascular bed involved and the mechanism of the pathologic process, but the examiner should always try to record the presence or absence of the common risk factors. This helps to focus the examiner's inquiries. An elderly, hypertensive, diabetic, hypercholesterolemic, smoking male is much more likely to have arterial insufficiency as the etiology of leg pain than a young, normotensive, nonsmoking, nondiabetic female. The examiner should also inquire for evidence of arterial insufficiency in other vascular beds. It is especially important to ask for symptoms of coronary insufficiency in any potential surgical candidate.

Physical examination of the patient with vascular disease is based on the same principles as the examination of any patient: inspection, palpation, and auscultation. The details of the different pathologic examinations are presented with each section, but the basic questions remain the same. Is an extremity swollen? What color is it? Can the patient move it? Does it have normal hair distribution and skin? What temperature is it? Does it have normal sensation? Are normal pulses felt? What is their quality? Are they widened and abnormally prominent? Are they faint? Is there a thrill? Is there a bruit? If so, what are its characteristics? Is the bruit high-pitched? Does it extend into diastole? Is it continuous?

Bruits are the buzzing or blowing sounds heard with the cardiac cycle over arteries. Bruits occur because turbulent flow in the artery causes the vessel wall to vibrate, and the vibrations produce sound. Turbulent flow occurs when the blood travels at an unusually high speed. This most commonly occurs where an artery narrows or is stenotic, but may also be produced by arteriovenous fistulae or abrupt changes in the direction of flow. When the vibration becomes strong enough to be palpable, there is a thrill. Thrills are palpable vibrations, and bruits are the sounds produced by vibrations. Somewhat imprecisely, thrills can be thought of as palpable bruits.

The normally palpable pulses are presented in Figure 31–1. In the head and neck, the examiner can feel the common carotid pulse between the trachea and sternocleidomastoid muscle. The facial artery pulse can be felt where the artery crosses the edge of the mandible in the mandibular groove. The preauricular temporal arterial pulse is found just in front of the tragus of the ear. One should always listen for cervical bruits, after asking the patient to hold his or her breath.

In the upper extremities, the axillary artery can be palpated against the proximal humerus. The brachial artery pulse is just medial to the biceps tendon, proximal to the elbow crease. The radial artery is palpated over the volar surface of the distal radius. The ulnar artery usually cannot be felt.

The abdominal aorta can usually be appreciated (in thin or small people) above the umbilicus in the midline, or slightly to the patient's left.

The femoral pulses are located just below the inguinal ligament, approximately one-third of the way from the pubic tubercle to the anterior, superior iliac spine (the borders of the inguinal ligament). The popliteal pulse is usually quite deep and may be difficult to feel. It is easiest to find this pulse when patients are supine, with their knees slightly flexed, and their legs relaxed. The posterior tibial pulse is felt behind the medial malleolus, and the dorsalis pedis on the dorsum of the foot, just lateral to the extensor hallucis longus tendon.

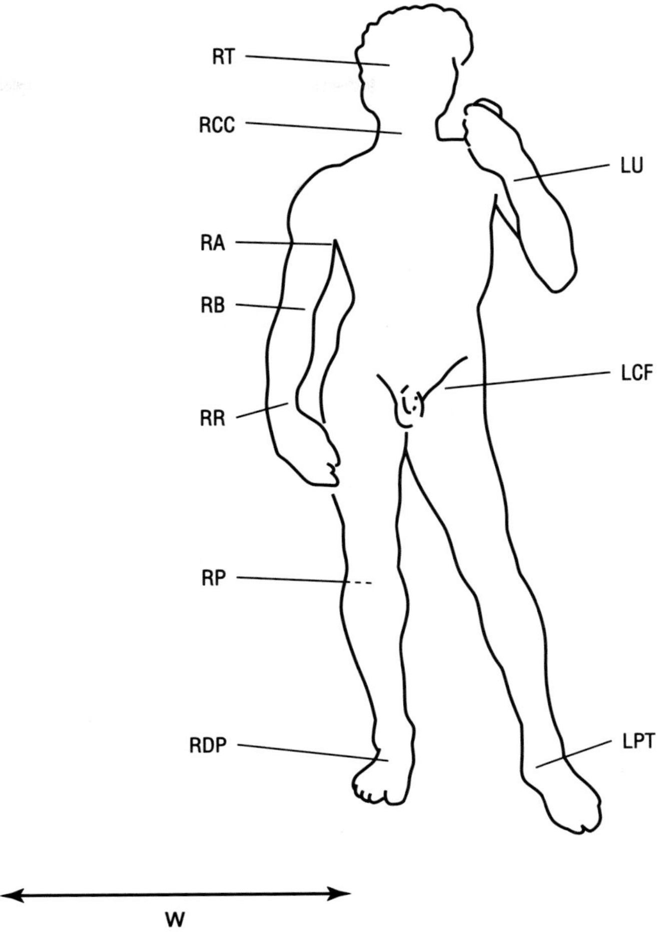

Figure 31–1. Location of superficial arteries and palpable pulses.
RCC - right common carotid artery
RT - right temporal artery
RA - right axillary artery
RB - right brachial artery
RR - right radial artery
LU - left ulnar artery
LCF - left common femoral artery
RP - right popliteal artery
RDP - right dorsalis pedis artery
LTP - left posterior tibial artery
See text for descriptions of pulse locations.

Laboratory and Diagnostic Tests

Vascular Laboratory. Vascular diseases are processes that can very often be diagnosed on history and physical examination alone. However, over the past 20 years, the noninvasive vascular laboratory has developed into a very important adjunct in the diagnosis of arterial and venous disorders. Using ultrasound technology, and waveform and pressure measurements, these laboratories study the anatomy and physiology of vessels and the blood flowing through them noninvasively (no needles or catheters). The indications for vascular laboratory studies are three: (1) to assist in making the diagnosis; (2) to carefully assess a patient over time; and (3) to produce a hard-copy study for the patient's record.

In our laboratory, we rely on five different examinations for the vast majority of our studies. By far the most important is the color-flow Doppler examination. This is the most modern form of the duplex Doppler study. The traditional duplex machine has two components: a B-mode ultrasound and a gaited Doppler. The ultrasound component gives the examiner an image of the anatomic structures being studied. Using the principle of the Doppler shift, in which the frequency of sound waves change when they are deflected off moving structures, these machines use the gaited Doppler to characterize and measure the velocity of blood flow in particular locations. The B-mode ultrasound image defines the exact anatomic location of the velocity measurement. The color Doppler machine uses a linear array of ultrasound elements, Fast Fourier Transformation, and a powerful computer to give the examiner real-time studies of multiple points simultaneously. Color is used in the visual display to indicate flow. This machine has become the mainstay of our laboratory examinations of the carotid bifurcation, venous systems, and specific arterial segments such as the common femoral artery (to rule out a false aneurysm or arteriovenous fistula) or a lower extremity arterial bypass (to look for areas of stenosis).

The pulse volume recorder (PVR) is an instrument that measures the changing extremity volumes with the cardiac cycle (Fig. 31–2). It uses three or four air-filled cuffs placed around the limb at different levels. As a pulse of blood travels down the extremity, the limb's volume transiently increases. The volume changes in the leg or arm produce a pressure change in the air-filled cuffs. These pressure changes are recorded on a strip recorder as an arterial pulse contour. This is a qualitative test that is matched with "sequential pressure measurements." Sequentially measuring peak systolic pressures also uses pneumatic pressure cuffs at different levels in the limb. Using a continuous-wave Doppler probe, the examiner measures the maximal systolic pressure at the different limb levels. These measurements are usually recorded as ratios of the recorded pressure compared with the brachial artery pressure. This quantitative study joins with the qualitative PVR to give a useful resting examination of limb arterial perfusion.

The exercise test is a more provocative study than the resting PVR (Fig. 31–3). Since the normal large-vessel arterial tree is a very low-resistance system, the normal person can exercise vigorously for prolonged periods of time without a change in the ratio between the arm and the leg (the ankle/brachial index or ABI). However, if there is significant large-vessel occlusive disease, the exercising patient is not able to increase distal perfusion in proportion to the increased demand of the exercising muscle. This results in a fall in distal pressure at the ankle. The exercise test is very helpful in sorting out patients who have exercise-induced pain, differentiating those whose pain is secondary to arterial disease from those whose pain is from another etiology.

The final commonly used study in our laboratory is arterial photoplethysmography. A probe that emits infra-red light is taped to the patient's skin. The probe records the intensity of the light reflected back to it. The infra-red light reflects off red cells; the intensity of the reflection is directly related to the cutaneous blood supply. With normal blood flow, this gives a pulsatile wave that varies with the cardiac cycle. This study is qualitative and gives gross observations of flow characteristics to fingers and toes. It can be made quantitative by using digital cuffs to measure the pressure necessary to dampen out the waveforms. This study assesses digital flows to either fingers or toes. This study is very helpful in diagnosing vasospastic disorders and very distal occlusive or embolic disease.

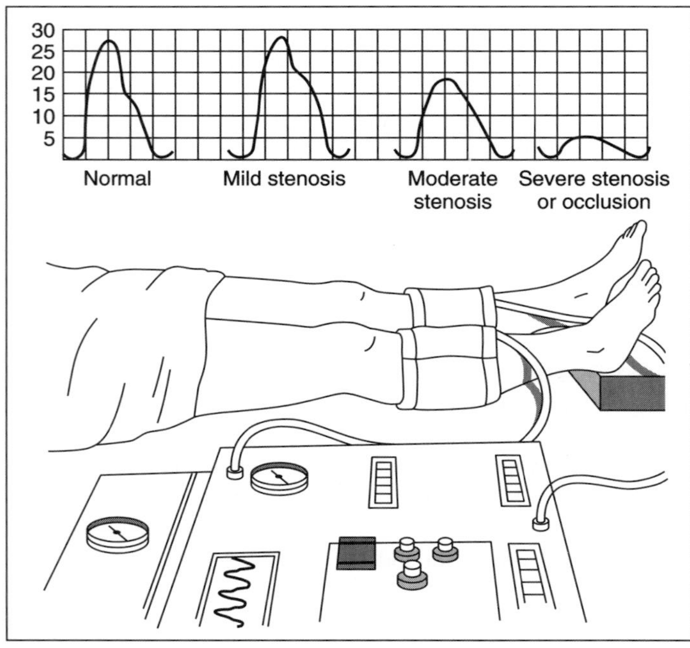

Figure 31–2. Pulse volume recorder machine and representative waveforms.

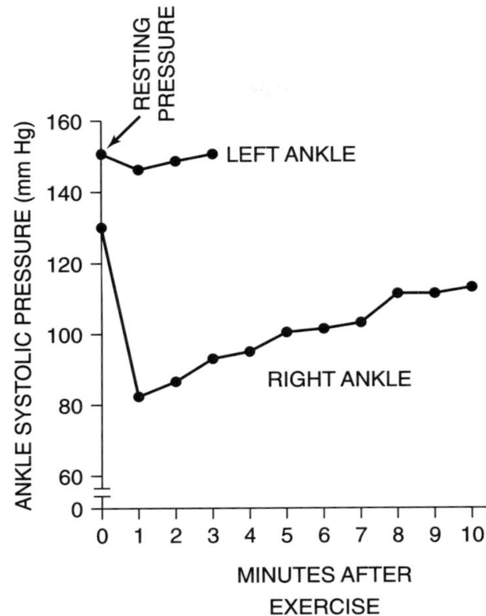

Figure 31–3. Exercise test form showing marked drop in ankle pressures with exercise, consistent with short-distance claudication.

Radiologic Studies. Rapid changes are occurring in vascular radiologic studies. The traditional arteriogram uses an arterial puncture (most commonly the Seldinger technique is used to place an intra-arterial catheter via the femoral artery) and a direct injection of radio-opaque dye into the arterial tree. In contradistinction to the noninvasive vascular laboratory, which studies dynamic flow patterns, the arteriogram defines anatomy. It was, and remains, the gold standard for vascular anatomic diagnosis. Recent advances in digital subtraction technology and nonionic contrast dyes have made these examinations much more comfortable for the patient, and probably safer. Nonetheless, these studies still require intra-arterial manipulation, and because of this, always have the potential of arterial complications, such as bleeding, embolization, thrombosis, and dissection, as well as dye-related toxicity.

The past 25 years have seen remarkable changes and improvements in solid organ imaging. Computerized tomographic imaging (CT scan) was the first major step forward; however, this requires oral and intravenous contrast for optimal delineation. These studies were soon followed by magnetic resonance imaging (MRI). By measuring the electron shifts produced by exposing tissue to powerful electromagnetic fields, accurate anatomic images are generated. These magnetic resonance images have changed the diagnostic method of a number of medical areas (most dramatically in Neurology and Neurosurgery), and over the past 10 years, magnetic resonance imaging technology has advanced rapidly. Magnetic resonance angiography (MRA) was first described in 1989 (Edelman, 1989), and the advantages of this method are obvious: it does not require instrumentation of the arterial tree, and there is no injection of contrast. Despite the fact that there are papers that claim better anatomic definition of the distal lower extremity using MRA rather than angiography (Schiebler, Listerud, Baum, Carpenter, Weigele, Holland et al., 1993), at this time, this is not widely accepted, and angiography remains the anatomic study of choice in most centers. This may change over the next few years.

Management

Risk Reduction. A few general remarks can be made about the treatment of patients with occlusive atherosclerotic arterial disease. There are three levels of treatment: risk reduction and lifestyle changes, medical therapy, and invasive therapy. Although many may ask whether changing behavior patterns and treating chronic diseases helps patients once their atherosclerotic occlusive disease is so advanced that they are symptomatic, the evidence is clear that exercising, smoking cessation, and controlling blood pressure can have a significant effect in stopping progression of the disease process. It does not reverse the basic problem. Plaque does not disappear, but its progression either stops or slows dramatically. This allows collateral circulation to increase and improve distal perfusion, and, in some patients, this may make a remarkable difference. Hopefully it also has a similar effect on the coronary circulation, which may avoid or postpone adverse coronary events. There is very dramatic evidence that in markedly hypercholesterolemic patients, normalization of serum cholesterol leads to reversal of coronary plaques, observations made with repeat angiographic studies (Buchwald, Matts, Fitch et al., 1992). It is reasonable to suspect that similar changes may occur in the peripheral arteries. It should be noted that these dramatic changes have been seen in only very hypercholesterolemic patients. The more routine patients with moderately elevated serum cholesterol probably have their plaque stabilized with cholesterol normalization, rather than have the plaque diminish. The data on control of blood sugar are not so encouraging. Despite a vigorous effort to control blood sugar, the Joslin Clinic's group has not been able to produce a measurable decrease in arterial occlusive disease in its patient population compared with a control group (Ganda, 1984). This may change with increasing use of insulin infusion pumps (The Diabetes Control and Complications Trial Research Group, 1993); however, it is too early to predict this with certainty.

The other "lifestyle" factors that are helpful in patients with symptomatic arterial disease are to be thin and to stay active. Both of these sound easy, but it is very hard to stop smoking and not gain weight, let alone lose it. This is especially true in patients who are limited in their activities because of underlying arterial occlusive disease. Nonetheless, weight control cannot be emphasized enough. When patients are able to lose weight, blood pressure, blood sugar, and serum lipids are all easier to control. Patients who are able to reduce their risks by making these very important changes may profoundly affect their outcomes.

Medical Therapy. Medical therapy for arterial occlusive disease can be broken down into four groups of drugs: antiplatelet drugs, anticoagulant drugs, thrombolytic agents, and rheologic agents. Only the most commonly used are discussed. The most frequently used antiplatelet drug is acetylsalicylic acid, or aspirin. Aspirin irreversibly inactivates cycloxygenase, an enzyme necessary for platelet production of thromboxane A_2. Thromboxane A_2 has many effects, but most important, it is a vasoconstrictor and a stimulator of platelet aggregation and release. Aspirin use has been shown to decrease the rate of stroke and myocardial infarction in men (The Canadian Cooperative Study Group, 1978) and probably increases patency of both coronary and distal bypasses (Chesebro, Foster, & Elvback, 1984). Interestingly, the effects are not so marked in women as in men. The other commonly used antiplatelet drug is ticlopidine (Ticlid). This drug decreases platelet aggregation by inhibiting platelet ADP receptors. It appears to be equally effective in both men and women and decreases the risk of stroke in those with transient ischemic attacks (Hass, Easton, Adams, et al., 1989). Unfortunately, it is quite expensive and may produce dangerous side effects, including pancytopenia and agranulocytosis. When patients begin the drug, their blood counts need to be followed closely for the first three months in case they develop either of these problems, which are reversible with cessation of the drug.

The two most commonly used anticoagulants are heparin and Coumadin. Heparin is a heterogeneous mixture of sulfonated mucopolysaccarides. Heparin inhibits the clotting cascade at a number of places, but most important, it greatly accentuates the effect of anti-thrombin III, which indirectly inhibits conversion of prothrombin to thrombin. Heparin is poorly absorbed from the gastrointestinal tract and must be given parenterally (either intravenously or by subcutaneous or intramuscular injection). The drug is used extensively for both prophylaxis and treatment of venous thrombosis. Its current use in arterial disease is much more limited. Because of its rapid onset, it is used as the anticoagulant when major arteries are clamped during arterial surgery, and as an anticoagulant bridge while awaiting the onset of the effect of warfarin. Warfarin (Coumadin) is an inhibitor of the production of vitamin K-dependent clotting factors: factors II, VII, IX, and X. Like heparin, warfarin is most commonly used for the treatment of venous disease, but it has been used to prevent arterial emboli in patients who are in atrial fibrillation, who have prosthetic heart valves, or who have had previous embolic events. The drug is also used in some patients with severe extracranial occlusive disease or tenuous arterial grafts, but there are no statistically significant studies that support its use in these situations.

In the United States, there are three commonly available thrombolytic drugs: streptokinase, urokinase, and tissue plasminogen activator (tPA). The mechanics of all three are different, but similar, each stimulating the conversion of plasminogen to plasmin. Plasmin is the natural thrombolytic agent that leads to clot dissolution. Streptokinase was the first agent used clinically. It is rarely used now. Compared with urokinase, it has a somewhat diminished effectiveness, an increased rate of complications, and frequent allergic reactions. tPA has a quicker mechanism of action than urokinase, but is much more expensive. Therefore, its use is usually limited to patients with acute cardiac ischemia. Urokinase is the thrombolytic agent of choice for noncardiac uses. It is most commonly used for the treatment of venous disease: upper and lower extremity deep venous thrombosis and pulmonary emboli. Its role in the treatment of acute arterial thrombosis is not clear, and there are ongoing multicenter studies trying to define the indications for its use.

The last medicines used in arterial disease are in the group of rheologic agents. Two are briefly discussed: pentoxifylline and Dextran. Pentoxifylline (Trental), a caffeine derivative, increases the flexibility of the hypoxic erythrocyte, and reduces the tendency of these cells to rouleaux formation. Both of these effects increase the red cell's ease of passage through the microcirculation. Studies have shown that pentoxifylline increases walking distance in approximately 70% of patients who take the drug for at least eight weeks. Unfortunately, the improvement is small in most. Only 25 to 30% of those taking the drug double their walking distance (Taylor & Porter, 1986).

Dextran is a heterogeneous group of long-chain carbohydrates. It comes in two forms: a lower-weight Dextran 40 (mean molecular weight of 40,000 daltons) or a higher molecular-weight Dextran 70 (mean molecular weight of 70,000 daltons). In our hospital, the Vascular Surgery Service uses only Dextran 40. It has three effects: it expands plasma volume, it increases microcirculatory blood flow, and it acts as an antithrombogenic agent. The antithrombogenic effect is multifactorial. Dextran affects vascular surfaces, platelets, and clotting factors. The drug must be given intravenously and is infused intraoperatively and postoperatively in cases in which there is fear of intravascular thrombosis or platelet aggregation, such as distal lower extremity bypasses or carotid endarterectomies. The clinical effectiveness of this agent in both of these circumstances remains a point of contention (Rutherford, Jones, Bergenty, et al., 1984).

Invasive Therapy. Invasive therapy can be subdivided into two categories: endovascular procedures and surgical procedures. Endovascular procedures can, in turn, be separated into three groups: angioplasty, with and without stents; atherectomy; and endovascular graft placement. Endovascular procedures were first introduced by Dr. Charles Dotter in the early 1960s (Dotter & Judkins, 1964). Dr. Andreas Gruntzig developed the balloon angioplasty catheter in the early 1970s. It overcame many of the earlier technical problems of Dotter's techniques (Gruntzig & Hopf, 1974). After 25 years of experience, the indications and limitations of the balloon catheter are well described and generally accepted. Percutaneous placement of endovascular stents has broadened the role of angioplasty. At present, the indications for stent placement are dissections, recurrent stenosis, and difficult dilatations. This endovascular technology in larger arteries has withstood the test of time (Roberts & Ring, 1982). This cannot be said, however, for the same methods at the popliteal or tibial vessels, the atherectomy devices, or laser-assisted angioplasty. Each of these has provoked much early interest, only to have disappointing late results.

The indications for endovascular graft placements remain unclear. This technique has produced a great deal of interest over the last five years (Perochi, Pelman, & Barone, 1991). There is no question that properly selected infrarenal and thoracic aneurysms can be treated with this technique; however, the durability of the procedure remains undetermined. This question will be answered over the next five years as large numbers of patients are followed long enough so the rates of long-term success and late complications are clarified.

Surgical intervention for chronic occlusive disease consists of two basic arterial procedures: endarterectomy and bypass grafting. Endarterectomy is the open surgical removal of the diseased intima and media followed by arterial closure, with or without a patch graft to increase the diameter of the vessel. This procedure is most commonly used at the carotid bifurcation.

Bypass grafts are conduits placed as new arteries around areas of stenosis or occlusion. There are three principles that determine the success of any graft: inflow, outflow, and the graft itself. "Inflow" is arterial pressure and flow at the level of the proximal anastomosis. It must be normal or very close to it. In other words, if a patient has multi-level occlusive disease, one must start at the top, with the proximal anastomosis closer to the heart than the first occlusion or significant stenosis. "Outflow" is the capacity of the arterial tree to drain away the blood that has passed through the graft. It is a reflection of the amount of occlusive disease at and beyond the distal anastomosis. Since blood is a non-Newtonian fluid and clots when the flow becomes too sluggish, outflow can be a very important determinant for long-term patency, especially in distal (infrapopliteal) bypass grafts. The "graft itself" refers to both the graft and the manner in which it is placed. As the graft gets longer and flows slower, the composition of the graft becomes increasingly important. An aortic tube graft for replacement of a short infrarenal aortic aneurysm can be made out of a number of different fabrics and have good long-term patency, since the graft is short and has high rates of blood flow through it. However, a femoral to dorsalis pedis bypass is a very long graft that crosses two joints and has relatively low flows in it. In these situations, the graft material becomes extremely important. Under these difficult conditions, a good-sized, undiseased, autologous saphenous vein gives excellent long-term results. Under similar circumstances, the patency of any other graft that is not autologous tissue is fair to poor at best. The difference is the presence of live endothelium, which has many antithrombogenic properties.

At present, the options for graft material are three: prosthetic material, nonautologous tissue, and autologous tissue. The most commonly used prosthetic grafts are either Dacron or polytetrafluoroethylene (PTFE). The nonautologous tissue grafts are either cadaver vein or umbilical vein. Both veins are treated with glutaraldehyde, essentially tanning them. What is placed is a collagen tube without any living cells.

Autologous vein can come from a number of sites: greater saphenous veins, lesser saphenous veins, or upper extremity veins (cephalic or basilic). The graft can be placed as an *in situ* graft (the greater saphenous is left in its bed and the valves are cut), a nonreversed graft (the free vein graft, usually from the other leg, is placed in its normal direction and the valves cut), or a reversed vein graft (the vein is turned around so the valves are opened by the arterial flow). The advantage of the reversed vein graft is that the inner surface of the graft is not manipulated and potentially injured while cutting the valve cusps. The disadvantage is that in addition to disruption of its external blood supply, there is size mismatch between the graft and the artery: the small end of the vein is sewn to the larger artery. In distal lower extremity bypass grafts, most authors have found that the *in situ* vein graft offers an advantage in long-term patency (Leather, Shah, Chang, et al., 1988); however, there are others who report no significant difference between nonreversed and reversed vein grafts (Taylor, Edward, & Pater, 1990).

CAROTID ARTERY DISEASE

Carotid artery occlusive disease is a major source of strokes, which, in the United States, remain a major cause of mortality (fourth leading cause of death in the United States) and morbidity (more than one million American citizens are disabled to some degree at any one time by strokes).

Three terms need to be clearly defined: stroke, transient ischemic attack (TIA), and amaurosis fugax. Each has two definitions: a clinical definition (the criteria of the clinical diagnosis) and the pathologic definition (what is truly happening at the cellular level). Clinically, a stroke is a localized neurologic deficit, lasting longer than 24 hours. Pathologically, a stroke occurs when there is cerebral infarction. There is loss of brain tissue. In contrast, a TIA is a localized neurologic deficit that lasts less than 24 hours, and there is no brain necrosis. Amaurosis fugax is transient monocular blindness that totally resolves in less than 24 hours. It is the equivalent of a retinal TIA (retinal infarction is the equivalent of a retinal stroke). Until CT scans were developed, these definitions appeared clear and concise. Once CT enabled treating physicians to examine the brains of live patients, it became evident that there was more overlap than had been realized. Some patients with clinical transient ischemic attacks (deficits cleared within 24 hours) were found to have strokes, and others with prolonged deficits were free of detectable infarction.

There are two primary etiologies of stroke: intracranial hemorrhage (hemorrhagic strokes) and intracranial ischemia (ischemic strokes). This discussion focuses on the second group. Acute ischemia of any vascular bed occurs because of either an embolic event or an arterial thrombosis. Embolic events happen when a nonliquid element (usually solid—a piece of plaque or thrombus) enters the arterial bloodstream. It is swept along the vessel until the embolus becomes lodged in the artery, usually at a bifurcation, and occludes it. Spontaneous thrombosis occurs when flow in an artery becomes so sluggish that the blood in the vessel clots or thromboses. This almost always occurs because of an area of stenosis in the artery itself. Either of these mechanisms can produce an abrupt or acute decrease or cessation of blood flow.

In 1951, C. Miller Fisher recognized that most patients with acute ischemic strokes had very severe atherosclerotic disease at the ipsilateral carotid bifurcation. He popularized the idea that carotid occlusive disease was either the source of emboli or the critical stenosis that led to thrombosis of the internal carotid artery or its branches.

He also noted that these lesions could potentially be treated surgically. Subsequent studies have shown that approximately 60% of all patients with ischemic strokes have ipsilateral carotid disease that was the cause of the acute cerebral ischemia. Miller hypothesized that the discovery of these lesions and correction of them before a permanent neurologic event occurred should decrease the rate of stroke. However, such an aggressive prophylactic treatment program involving surgery resulted in complications. Before general acceptance of the merits of this therapeutic approach occurred, the natural history of these lesions had to be defined. It has been recognized for more than forty years that there were groups of patients who were at increased risk for ischemic strokes. They were symptomatic patients who had had previous ischemic infarctions, who had had lateralizing TIAs, or who had had episodes of amaurosis fugax. With improved methods of noninvasive measurement of carotid stenosis, the stroke risk was measured for both symptomatic and asymptomatic patients who had carotid disease. Although the methodology was not perfect, stroke rates were measured in those with severe carotid stenosis. They were found to be approximately 5% per year for asymptomatic patients (Chambers & Norris, 1986); 7-8% per year for patients with amaurosis fugax (Sandok, Trautmann, Ramirez-Lassepas et al., 1974); 9% per year for those with lateralizing TIAs (Whisnant, Matsumoto & Elveback, 1973); and 10% per year for those with previous strokes (Sacco et al., 1982) (Table 31–1). These are the patients who might justify an aggressive prophylactic approach to attempt to reduce their stroke risk.

History and Physical Findings

The common presentation of patients with extracranial carotid occlusive disease is one of three: lateralizing symptoms, nonlateralizing symptoms, or asymptomatic stenosis. Lateralizing symptoms are neurologic deficits that anatomically correspond to the internal carotid artery or to one of its major branches; for example, aphasia, hemiparesis, and monocular blindness. These symptoms can be either transient (TIA) or not (stroke). Non-lateralizing symptoms are those that may be consistent with either global ischemia or brain-stem dysfunction; examples are lightheadedness, vertigo, and diplopia. When the history is taken, specific inquiries should be made about the duration, nature, and associated symptoms of the presenting episode, as well as the number and frequency of similar events.

Physical examination should focus on signs of carotid occlusive disease. These are diminished carotid, facial or preauricular pulses, and a cervical bruit. The patient should also be examined for neurologic deficits and (if the examiner is facile with an ophthalmoscope) for Hollenhorst plaques (pieces of cholesterol-laden plaque in the retinal vessels). Unfortunately, the internal carotid artery cannot be directly assessed on physical examination. The presence

TABLE 31–1. Annual Risk of Stroke

Patient Presentation	Annual Risk	Source
Asymptomatic critical stenosis	5.0%	Chambers & Norris, 1986
Amaurosis fugax	7.0–8.0%	Sandok, Trautmann, & Ramirez-Lassepas, 1974
Lateralizing TIA	9.0 %	Whisnant, Matsumoto, & Elveback, 1973
Previous ischemic stroke	10.0%	Sacco, Wolf, Kannel, & McNamera, 1982

and location of a cervical bruit are helpful, but not diagnostic of internal carotid artery stenosis. This problem has been largely solved by the duplex or color-flow Doppler examination, which can very accurately define the degree of stenosis of the internal carotid artery. As mentioned earlier, patients with lateralizing symptoms and tight carotid stenoses are at increased risk for stroke. The data are much less clear for those with non-lateralizing symptoms, since the possible etiology of these complaints is very diverse. Because of this, our unit treats these patients as if they had asymptomatic carotid stenosis.

Laboratory and Diagnostic Tests

At the present time, all patients who are suspected of having carotid stenosis undergo duplex or color-flow Doppler examinations, whether or not they are symptomatic. If they are found to have a high-grade stenosis (greater than 75%), they are believed to have a hemodynamically significant carotid stenosis and to be at increased stroke risk. If surgical therapy is being considered, most units require substantiation of the degree of stenosis by either magnetic resonance angiography (MRA) or standard angiography.

Management

The therapeutic options for patients with a significant carotid stenosis are varied. The non-surgical options include antiplatelet drugs (commonly, aspirin or Ticlid) or anticoagulation with warfarin. Both families of drugs decrease the rate of TIAs and may reduce the risk of stroke by perhaps as much as 40% (Brousser et al., 1983).

The commonly used surgical option is carotid endarterectomy (CEA). Simplistically, this procedure opens the artery by removing the thickened intima and media. The artery is either directly closed, or else a patch of either vein or fabric is sewn into the arteriotomy to increase the diameter of the vessel (Fig. 31–4). As with any surgical procedure, there are potential complications. The two most feared are a perioperative myocardial event (myocardial infarction, malignant arrhythmia, or episode of congestive heart failure) or stroke. The perioperative stroke rate should be less than 4%. Most of these neurologic events occur because of either embolization from the operative site or internal carotid artery thrombosis. Other complications include infection, bleeding, hoarseness (secondary to vagal dysfunction), and dysphagia (secondary to hypoglossal dysfunction). Luckily, both of these cranial nerve injuries due to retraction during surgery are rarely permanent.

Patient Selection

Until relatively recently, the proper prophylactic therapy for these high-risk patients was disputed; however, in the last 5 years, three studies have done much to clarify the picture. The question asked was whether or not carotid endarterectomy with aspirin reduced the stroke risk more than aspirin alone. The North American Symptomatic Carotid Endarterectomy Trial (NASCET) (North American Symptomatic Carotid Endarterectomy Trial Collaborators, 1991), the VA Trial (Mayberg, Wilson, Yatsu et al., 1991), and the European Stroke Trial (European Carotid Surgery Trialists' Collaborative Group, 1991) all had similar results when comparing symptomatic, high-grade carotid stenoses (Table 31–2). Those who underwent surgical treatment while continuing aspirin did significantly better than those who took aspirin alone. After 2 years the stroke rate of the medically treated group was slightly less than 30%, and of the surgically treated group, approximately 8%. At this time, it is accepted that symptomatic patients (patients who have had an episode of amaurosis fugax, a lateralizing TIA, or a stroke with good recovery) with ipsilateral high-grade carotid stenosis should be offered carotid endarterectomy, as long as they are felt to be reasonable operative risks, and there is an experienced surgical team to do the procedure.

The role of surgery in the asymptomatic patient is less

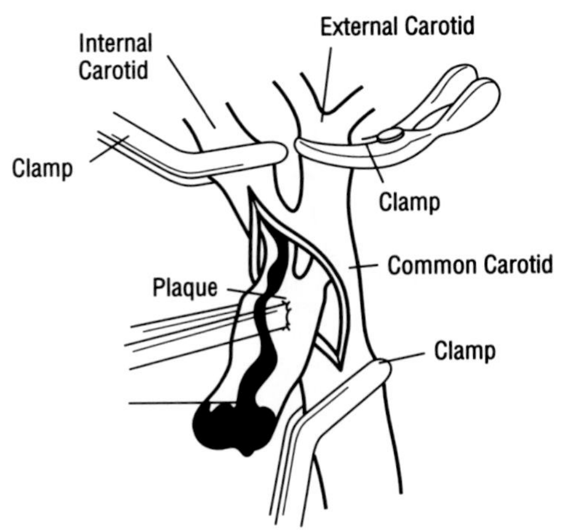

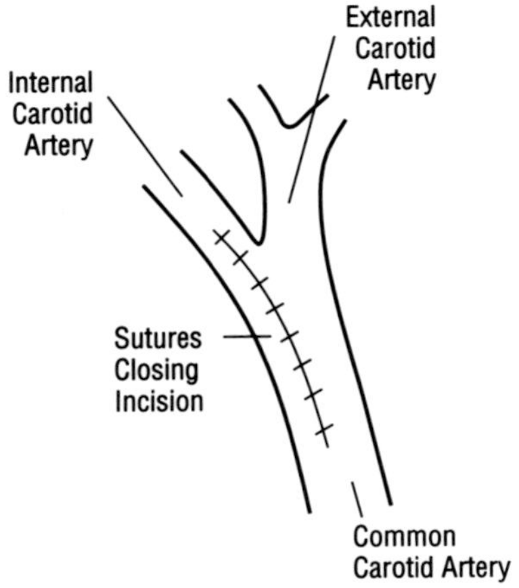

Figure 31–4. Carotid endarterectomy, the surgery.

TABLE 31–2. Prospective, Randomized Carotid Endarterectomy Trials

Symptomatic Patients
North American Symptomatic Carotid Endarterectomy Trial (NASCET) (North American Symptomatic Carotid Endarterectomy Trial Collaborators, 1991)
European Carotid Surgery Trial (ECST) (European Carotid Surgery Trialists' Collaborative Group, 1991)
Veterans Affairs Symptomatic Carotid Stenosis Trial (Mayberg, Wilson, Yatsu et al., 1991)
Asymptomatic Patients
Asymptomatic Carotid Atherosclerosis Study (ACAS) (Executive Committee for Asymptomatic Carotid Atherosclerosis Study, 1995)

clear. An excellent natural history study found that patients with asymptomatic stenoses were at very low risk of stroke until they developed very tight, or "critical," stenoses (greater than 80%) (Roederer, Langlois, Jager, et al., 1984). Therefore, it was generally accepted that asymptomatic patients should not be offered the procedure unless there was a "critical" lesion; however, a recent prospective, multicenter study, the ACAS study (Executive Committee for the Asymptomatic Carotid Atherosclerosis Study, 1995), demonstrated improved stroke rates in patients with a diameter reduction of 60% or more. This study stands alone in demonstrating the surgical advantage to the patients with moderate to severe (60-80%) stenosis, and the role of surgery in this group remains uncertain.

In summary, CEA is a very commonly performed surgical procedure. It is indicated in patients who are reasonable operative risks who have tight carotid stenoses. The operation should be able to be done with a low mortality and morbidity.

▶ MESENTERIC OCCLUSIVE DISEASE

The blood supply of the gastrointestinal tract is rarely so compromised that the viscera are threatened; however, when this does occur, prompt and effective surgical treatment can be truly life-saving.

There are four main sources of blood to the intestines (Fig. 31–5). The fore-gut is primarily perfused by the celiac axis (CA), a short vessel originating from the ventral surface of the aorta, which divides into the splenic, left gastric, and hepatic arteries. The mid-gut (proximal jejunum to mid-transverse colon) depends upon the superior mesenteric artery (SMA) which originates just below the CA. There are large collaterals between these two trunk vessels, involving the pancreaticoduodenal and gastroduodenal arteries. The left colon is supplied by the inferior mesenteric artery (IMA). In turn, it has extensive collaterals with the SMA through the middle colic (a branch of the SMA) and the arch of Riolan. The rectum is perfused through the inferior hemorrhoidal vessels, branches of the internal iliac artery. There are, again, extensive collaterals with branches of the IMA through the middle and superior hemorrhoidal arteries. There are many collateral channels throughout the gut, with the exception of the distal SMA. Once distal to both the pancreaticoduodenal and the middle colic arteries, the SMA usually becomes an end-artery, and its occlusion may result in infarction of the small intestine and right colon.

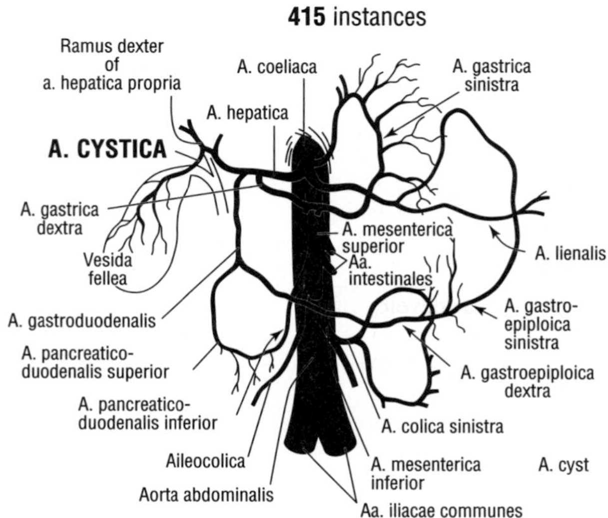

Figure 31–5. Normal intestinal arterial anatomy. Arteria cystica, types of origin, 600 specimens.

Acute Mesenteric Ischemia

As mentioned previously, acute ischemia usually occurs because of either spontaneous thrombosis or embolization. The collateral potential of the central vessels of the gut is so good that acute occlusion of any one of the trunk arteries at its origin on the aorta is rarely symptomatic. However, an acute occlusion of the SMA beyond the middle colic may be catastrophic. The arch of Riolan is rarely well developed in the region of the hepatic flexure, so an acute SMA occlusion results in profound ischemia of the mid-gut, with possible infarction of most of the small bowel, cecum, and right colon. This most commonly occurs because of an embolic event to the SMA. If there is total cessation of midgut perfusion, this part of the intestine begins to infarct within 6 hours of the event.

These patients present dramatically. They have the sudden onset of very severe periumbilical pain. They may vomit or move their bowels, neither of which relieves their symptoms. Early in the course of the disease, their physical examination is very benign. There are no masses. There is no tenderness, and there is no guarding. Bowel sounds are usually hypoactive, but may be normal. Patients with acute mesenteric ischemia are described as having "pain out of proportion" to their physical findings.

Since the gut begins to infarct within 6 hours, speed of diagnosis is of paramount importance. The mandatory first step is that the examiner consider the possibility of acute intestinal ischemia in the differential. Most commonly, these are older patients at increased risk for arterial emboli, patients with atrial fibrillation or who have had a recent myocardial infarction. Once acute mesenteric ischemia is considered in the differential, there is only one reliable examination to make or rule out the diagnosis: an arteriogram. This must be done as a biplanar study with lateral views to adequately examine the celiac axis and SMA (Fig. 31–6). The arteriogram should not be delayed awaiting results of blood studies, which are often normal early in the disease process. Once the diagnosis is seriously considered, an emergent angiogram should be obtained as soon as possible.

Conventional treatment of an SMA embolus is a surgical embolectomy that must be done emergently. If the midgut has not suffered irreparable injury, the results are usually gratifying (Wilson, Gupta, Gilmour et al., 1987). However, if there have been delays, the gut may have developed transmural necrosis. Usually the surgical group has an indication of this preoperatively if the patient has developed abdominal tenderness and a leukocytosis, and a very strong sign of it if the patient has peritoneal signs. Under these discouraging circumstances, proper therapy is largely determined by the amount of viable small bowel. If the length of viable gut is not compatible with life, the patient should be closed (Fig. 31–7). On the other hand, a more limited area of infarction should be resected after embolectomy is performed.

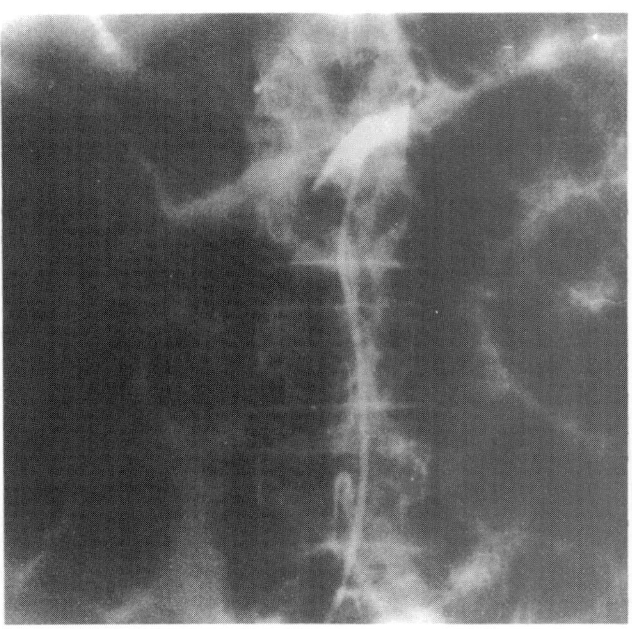

Figure 31–6. Selective injection of superior mesenteric artery showing total occlusion of vessel with convex filling defect, consistent with an embolus. Note the distended loops of small bowel with thickened intestinal walls. *(Used with permission from Rutherford, [1984].)*

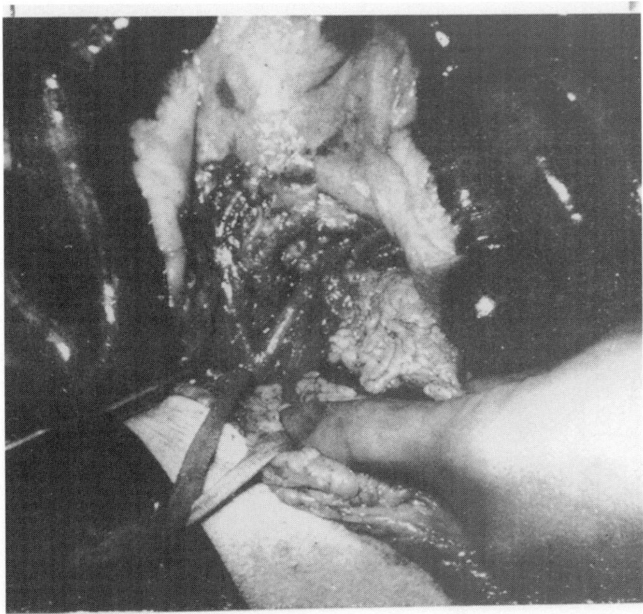

Figure 31–7. Infarcted small bowel found on abdominal exploration of patient with superior mesenteric artery embolus.

The gut may also infarct from venous thrombosis or a nonocclusive ischemic process. Both tend to be more insidious in their presentations. Patients with venous thrombosis tend to be either grossly dehydrated or hypercoagulable. They present with signs and symptoms of ileus, abdominal distention, and pain. The diagnosis is usually made by color-flow Doppler, CT with contrast, or venous phase angiography (Fig. 31–8). Therapy consists of anticoagulation, and observation for signs of bowel infarction, when intestinal surgery is required (Harward, Green, Bergan, et al., 1989).

Nonocclusive intestinal ischemia typically occurs in patients in a low cardiac output state. These very sick patients, who are typically already in an ICU, present with the gradual onset of abdominal pain and, often, mild distention. The diagnosis is made by a characteristic angiographic appearance of the SMA, which is open but with minimal flow and with few distal branches (Fig. 31–9A and Fig. 31–9B). The gut is dying because of intense arterial spasm. The treatment is two-pronged: optimization of cardiac function and direct infusion of vasodilators into the involved artery. Operation is reserved only for resection of infarcted bowel. Even under the best of circumstances, this is a very morbid problem with a mortality rate in excess of 50% (Brandt & Boley, 1991).

Chronic Mesenteric Ischemia

Chronic mesenteric ischemia is, by definition, a more insidious process than acute mesenteric ischemia. It presents as "intestinal angina." Typically, these patients develop postprandial mid-abdominal pain, which may be very severe. These patients present with a good deal of weight loss. They are not anorectic. In fact, most are hungry and would gladly eat if they could do so without discomfort.

Obviously, chronic mesenteric ischemia is not the most common cause of postprandial pain associated with weight loss. However, once one has ruled out benign and malignant diseases of the pancreas, biliary tree and stomach, chronic mesenteric ischemia should be considered, especially if the patient is not anorectic and has other signs of atherosclerotic disease. Once again, the definitive study is a biplanar arteriogram to examine each of the major arteries perfusing the gut (Fig. 31–10). Typically, patients do not develop symptoms unless they have at least two, and usually three, of the proximal vessels severely stenosed or occluded. Treatment is surgical. Basically, two different kinds of procedures can be performed: either bypass grafts from the aorta to the CA, SMA, and IMA (Fig. 31–11) or else a transaortic endarterectomy (Fig. 31–12). Both can lead to excellent short- and long-term results (Yao & Bergan, 1990). It is important to revascularize as many of the diseased vessels as possible.

To summarize, both acute and chronic mesenteric ischemia are unusual clinical problems. It is imperative that the diagnosis be considered early and definitely ascertained with angiography. Once the diagnosis is assured, the surgical goals are urgent and clearly defined.

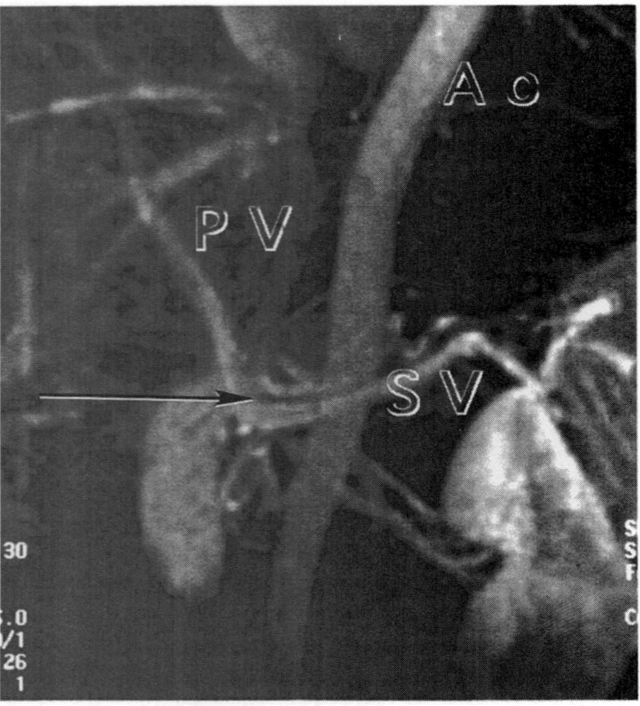

Figure 31–8. CT scan showing thrombus in the portal vein of patient with mesenteric venous infarction.

▶ RENAL ARTERY OCCLUSIVE DISEASE

Obliterative diseases of the renal arteries manifest themselves in two ways: hypertension and loss of renal function. The pathophysiology of renovascular hypertension has been well described (Fig. 31–13; see p. 575). Simplistically presented, the renal juxtaglomerular apparatus (JGA), which is associated with the afferent arterial of the glomerulus, detects intra-arterial pressure. If it senses that the pressure is too low, it excretes renin. Renin catalyzes the conversion of angiotensinogen to angiotensin-I, a mild vasoconstrictor. The angiotensin-I, in turn, is converted to angiotensin-II in the pulmonary circulation by angiotensin-converting enzyme (ACE). In contrast to angiotensin-I, angiotensin-II is a very potent vasoconstrictor. It also stimulates the adrenal production and release of aldosterone, which is a potent stimulator of renal conservation of sodium and water. The mixture of an increased intravascular volume and potent vasoconstriction results in marked hypertension.

The pathophysiology of the loss of renal function is more straightforward. Reduced perfusion of the kidney mass leads to gradual loss of renal tissue, which can result in a small, shrunken, but functional, kidney. The renal artery may also thrombose, which can lead to renal infarction.

The most common etiology of the obliterative disease

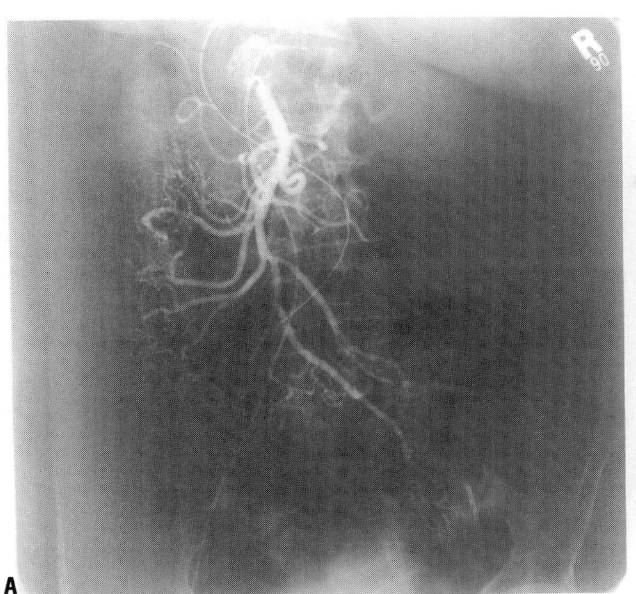

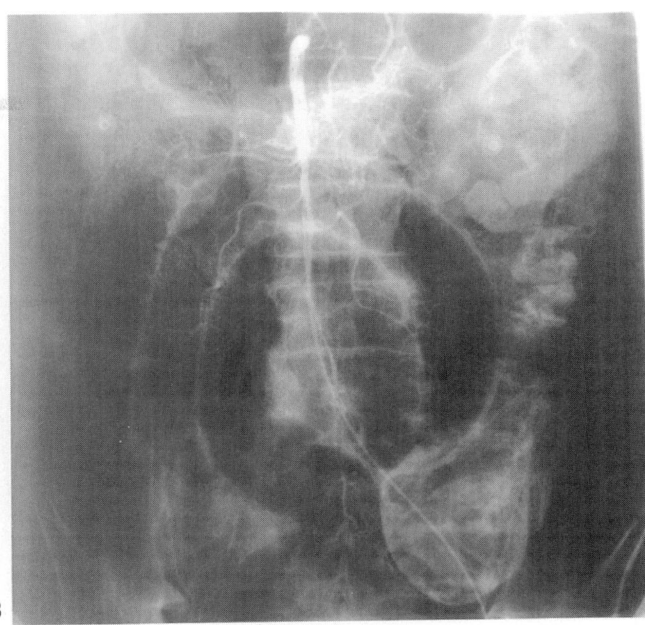

Figure 31–9. Arteriogram of superior mesenteric artery of patient with nonocclusive mesenteric ischemia. Note the lack of branches and small diameter of the artery in **(B)** compared with the normal superior mesenteric artery in **(A)**.

is atherosclerosis. This may be atherosclerotic disease of the aorta involving the ostia of the renal artery (Fig. 31–14) or else of the renal artery itself (Fig. 31–15). The other less common etiology is fibromuscular dysplasia (FMD).

The most common presentation of FMD is multiple stenoses and dilatations—a string of beads (Fig. 31–16). The etiology of this process is unknown. Interestingly, in contrast to atherosclerosis, which is a problem of the elderly, usually of men, FMD is a pathology of the young, most commonly of women.

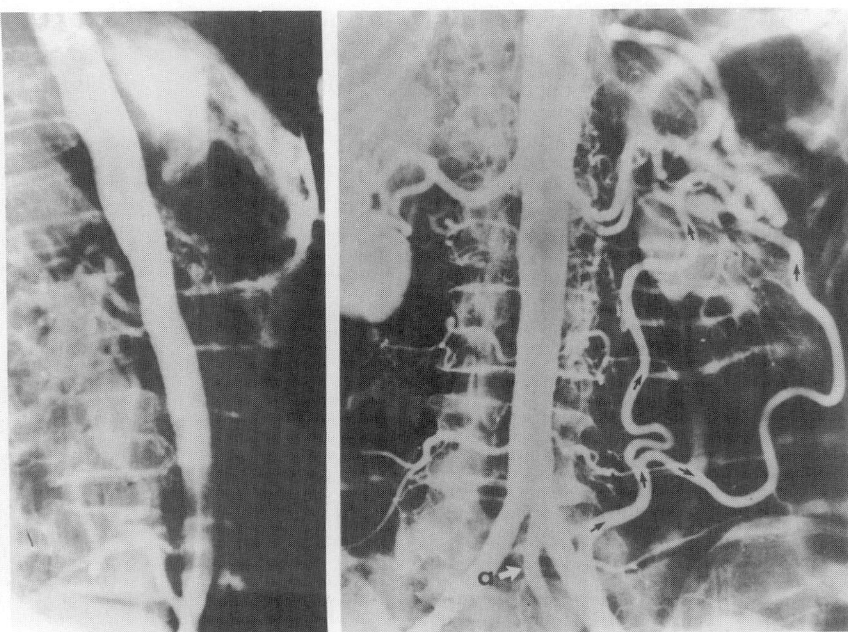

Figure 31–10. Arteriogram of patient with chronic mesenteric ischemia. The film on the *left* is a lateral aortogram which shows no evidence of the celiac axis, superior mesenteric artery, or inferior mesenteric artery. The delayed AP view on the *right* shows a large meandering collateral coming up from the pelvis, which is perfusing the gut.

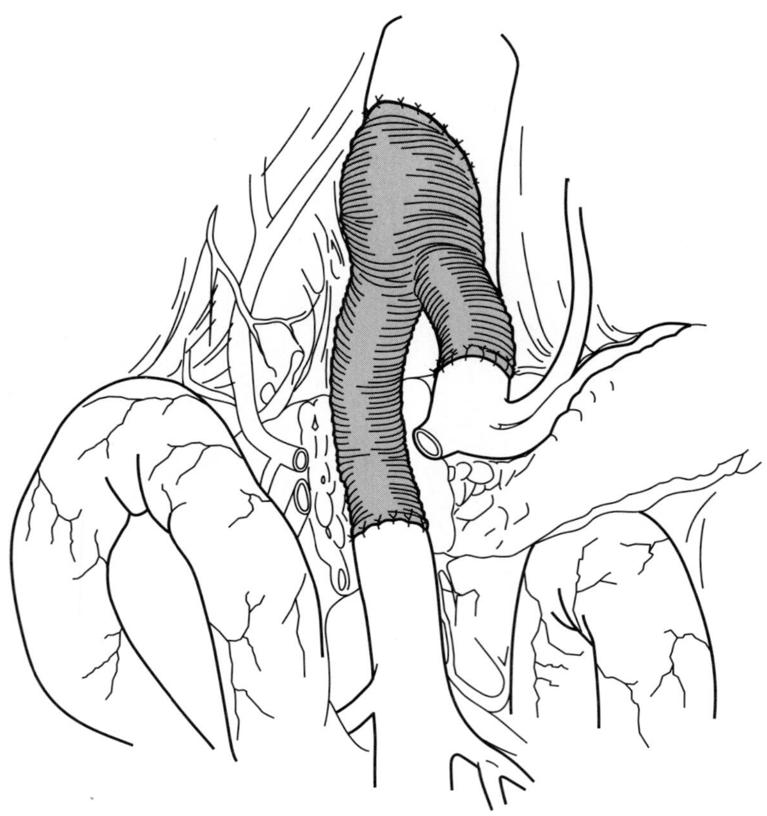

Figure 31–11. Bifurcated prosthetic graft with the proximal anastomosis to the supraceliac aorta and the limbs to the superior mesenteric artery (*left limb*) and CA (*right limb*), used to revascularize the gut in a patient with occlusions of both the proximal celiac axis and superior mesenteric artery.

The presentation of patients with occlusive disease of the renal arteries is mixed. Acute occlusion most commonly occurs after trauma, either blunt or penetrating. The patient may present with hematuria, flank pain, and/or sudden hypertension. The diagnosis is made with an intravenous pyelogram, CT with contrast, MRA, or angiogram. The treatment is emergent renal revascularization. However, if the artery is acutely thrombosed in a patient without previous stimulation for collateral development, the kidney begins to suffer significant injury after only an hour of warm ischemia. Usually these kidneys have been irreparably injured by the time they are revascularized.

Luckily, the outlook is not so grim for chronic renal artery stenosis. These patients present with either renovascular hypertension or progressive loss of renal function. Hypertensive patients with renal artery disease as the driving cause make up about 5% of all hypertensive patients in the United States. Patients who should be examined more closely are those whose hypertension is unusually difficult to control, who have marked diastolic hypertension, or who are unusually young (less than 30 years of age), or who are over 60 years of age when their blood pressure goes out of control. The young are suspected of having FMD; the older, atherosclerotic disease.

Renal artery stenosis should be considered as a cause of loss of renal function in any patient who has evidence of advanced atherosclerotic disease and a rapid and unexplained deterioration of creatinine clearance. This is especially true if there is an asymmetric loss of renal volume.

The evaluation of suspicious patients has been quite clear. Until recently, the only study that could rule out the problem was an arteriogram. If it were normal, the patient did not have renovascular hypertension, nor was large-vessel disease the source of deteriorating renal function. If the patient did have renal artery stenosis of greater than 70%, along with post-stenotic dilatation, increased distal collateralization, and/or a small kidney, then one could be comfortable that there was a hemodynamically significant stenosis. A number of newer diagnostic techniques, including color-flow ultrasound, captopril renal scans, MRA, and spiral CT, have been proposed as either screening or definitive diagnostic studies. The proper role of each of these in the diagnosis of renal artery stenosis remains unclear.

Therapy has three possible modes: medical, endovascular, or surgical. Medical therapy has little role to play in the preservation of renal function, since medical therapy does not improve renal perfusion. However, in patients with renovascular hypertension, blood pressure control can often

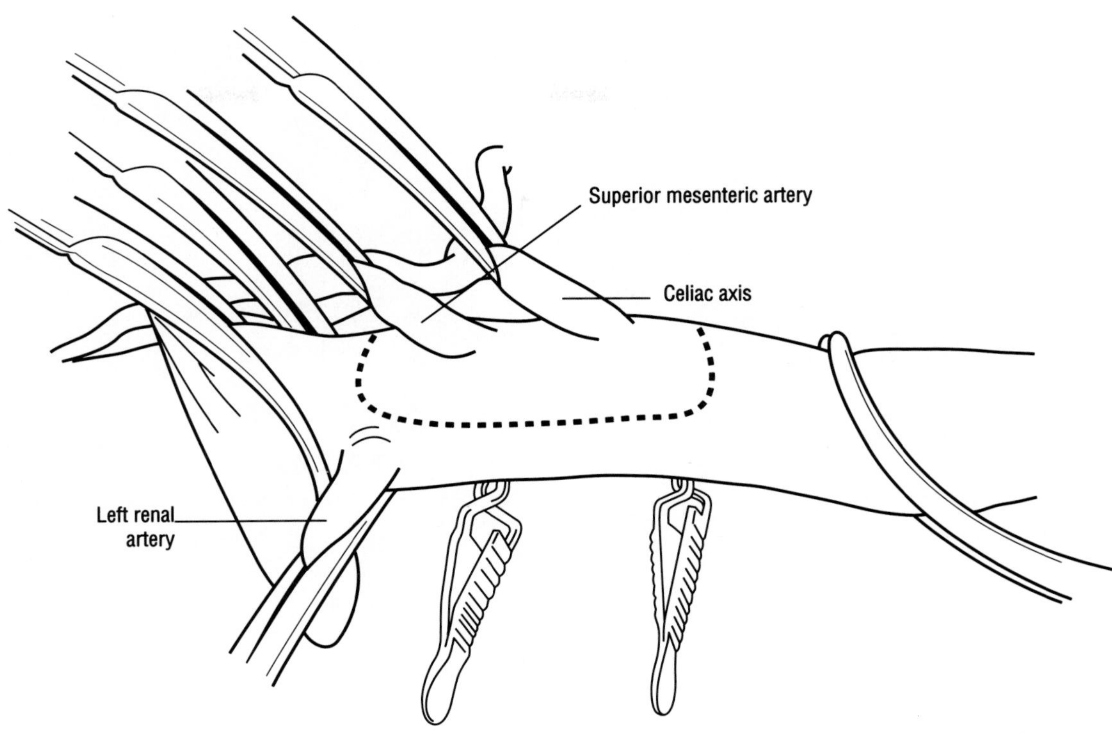

Figure 31–12. Transaortic endarterectomy. The aorta is opened in a "trap door" configuration and an endarterectomy performed, opening stenotic ostia.

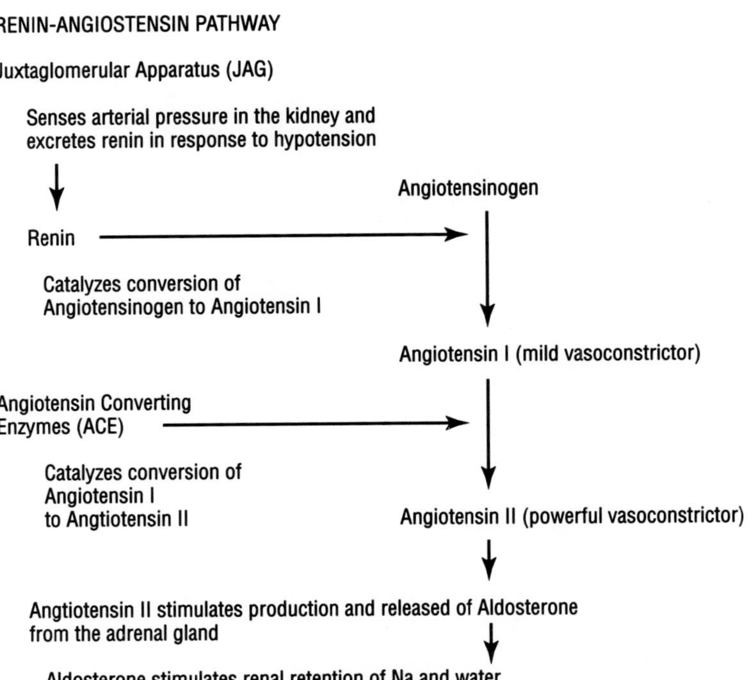

Figure 31–13. Renin–angiotensin system. Stimulation of the production of renin results in both marked vasoconstriction (angiotensin II effect) and salt and water retention (aldosterone effect).

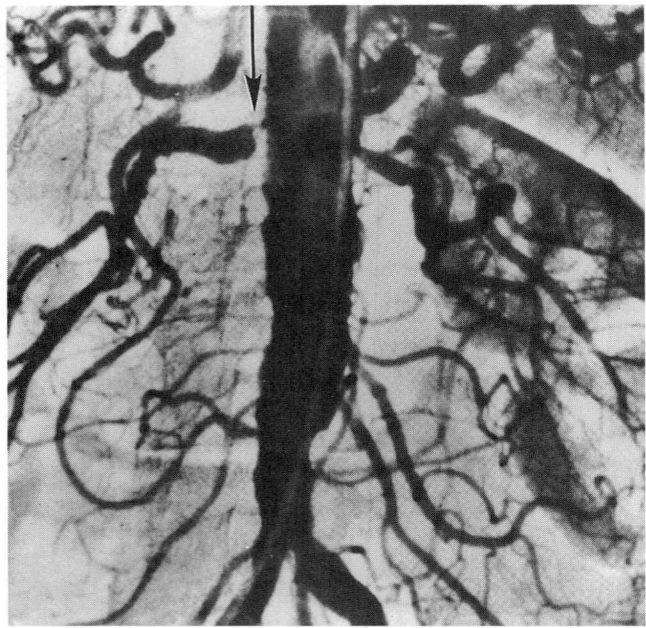

Figure 31–14. Stenosis of the right renal artery (osteal stenosis) (*black arrow*).

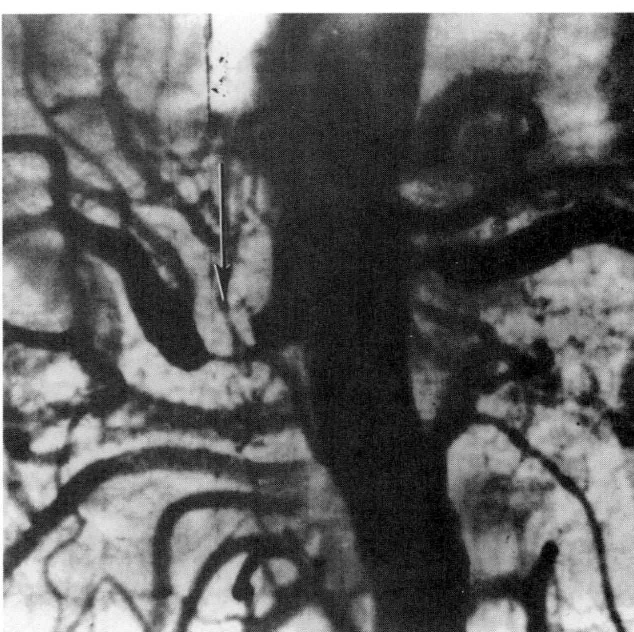

Figure 31–15. Stenosis of the right renal artery within the artery itself (*black arrow*).

be obtained, especially with the use of multi-drug combinations and ACE inhibitors. Medical therapy always remains an option for those not felt to be good candidates for either endovascular or surgical procedures. The endovascular techniques of PTCA with or without stents have had very good results in patients with either FMD or atherosclerotic renal artery disease (Tegtmayer, Kellum, & Ayers, 1984). Ostial lesions have not responded to PTCA as well as renal artery lesions; however, the use of stents may improve long-term results (Blum, Krumme, Flugel et al., 1997).

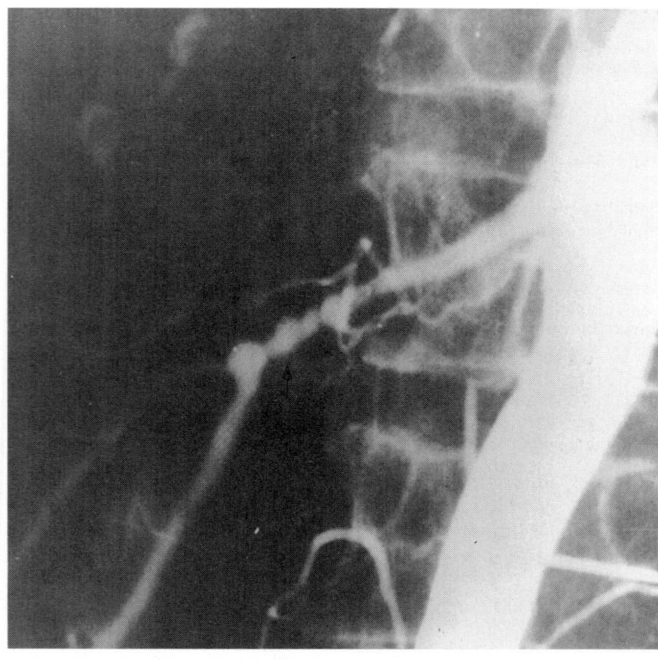

Figure 31–16. Fibromuscular dysplasia of the right renal artery. Note the beaded appearance of the artery (*black arrow*).

Surgical therapy takes a number of forms: aortorenal bypass, direct renal artery reimplantation into the aorta, extraanatomic bypass (hepatorenal on the right and splenorenal on the left), renal artery endarterectomy, or patch angioplasty. The use of these different techniques is dependent upon anatomy, clinical presentation, and surgical preference. Similar results have been reported for all. The most persuasive data on renovascular disease indicate that surgical repair of the renal artery results in either cure of hypertension or ease of treatment in more than 90% of patients, and that these results are durable (Dean, 1993). Recent studies indicate that renal artery PTCA results are similar, but re-stenose at a more rapid rate (Bonelli, McKusick, & Textor, 1995). Both of these techniques preserve renal function compared with medical treatment of renovascular hypertension (Dean, Keiffer, Smith et al., 1981). Logically, this is not a surprise, since medical control of the hypertension does not resolve renal ischemia.

In summary, renal artery disease usually presents itself as either renovascular hypertension or renal ischemia, leading to loss of kidney function. Traditionally, angiography was the critical examining study, but a number of newer techniques may alter this. Mechanical correction of the stenosis, using either endovascular or surgical techniques, remains the treatment of choice.

LOWER EXTREMITY OCCLUSIVE DISEASE

A large percentage of any vascular surgeon's practice deals with ischemia of the lower extremities. Hemodynamically significant occlusive disease rarely involves the aorta above the renal arteries. On the other hand, atherosclerosis may, and frequently does, involve the infrarenal aorta, and all of the more distal arteries. Convention allows these vessels to be divided into two segments: the aorta and iliac arteries, and the infrainguinal vessels (the femoral, popliteal, tibial, and pedal arteries).

Chronic Lower Extremity Ischemia

Patients with chronic lower extremity occlusive disease have characteristic presentations. The least severe is intermittent claudication, which is exercise-induced muscular pain. The pain occurs when the oxygen demands of the muscle outstrip the oxygen delivery, and the muscle bed becomes ischemic. If the occlusive disease involves the superficial femoral or popliteal vessels, the pain is only below the knee. If the blockage is higher, the pain may be in the thigh or buttock as well. It is usually very reproducible, and neither the amount of exercise necessary to produce the pain nor the length of time needed to relieve it vary much on a day-to-day basis.

When the degree of ischemia worsens, the exercise needed to produce symptoms decreases until the patient has pain at rest—ischemic rest pain. In contradistinction to claudication, which is muscular pain, ischemic rest pain involves the most distal part of the extremity—usually the toes and forefoot. Typically, it is relieved or lessened by dependency, and worsened by elevation. It is usually first noted at night when the patient is in bed. Patients with this problem often end up sleeping with their feet hanging over the side of the bed or else sitting in a chair.

The most severe presentation is that of tissue loss: ischemic ulcerations, nonhealing wounds, or gangrene. Ischemic ulcers characteristically are on or between the toes, or in the web spaces. They are usually painful lesions, and the pain again may be somewhat relieved by dependency. Nonhealing wounds refer to the absence of healing of any of the usual blisters, cuts, or scrapes that all of us get on our feet from time to time. If they do not heal in six weeks, the patient should be closely examined to rule out large-vessel occlusive disease as the etiology. Gangrene, secondary to large-vessel arterial disease, typically first involves the toes. It is referred to as "dry gangrene" when there is no infection or putrefaction. Such toes are dark, dry, and horn-like ("mummified"). The infected lesion is called "wet gangrene."

History and Physical Findings

When a patient presents with lower extremity pain at rest, or with exercise, arterial occlusive disease is almost always in the differential. Just as with carotid disease, the presence or absence of the other risk factors increase or diminish the examiner's index of suspicion of ischemia as the symptoms' etiology. The history gives many clues about the severity of the disease and the location of the occlusion. Physical examination clarifies the examiner's perception of both location and severity. The examination usually begins with observation of the distal leg and foot, looking at skin, hair, nails, and color. The chronically ischemic foot has shiny, atrophic skin; the absence of hair; thickened nails; and ruborous color with dependency, which changes to blanching with elevation. These signs are not present in the resting claudicator, who has adequate resting pedal perfusion. Once the ischemia is severe enough for pain at rest or tissue loss, the resting signs are usually found. Decreased temperature and delayed capillary refill also add to the impression of the degree of ischemia. Pulses and bruits do much to localize the proximal extent of the disease. Absence of femoral pulses means that there is at least severe segmental disease in the aorta, iliacs, or common femoral arteries. Femoral bruits indicate common femoral or iliac stenoses. They are usually best heard over their point of origin. Similarly, brisk femoral pulses and absent popliteal and pedal pulses are consistent with superficial femoral artery occlusions.

Laboratory and Diagnostic Tests

The role of the noninvasive studies in this situation is dual-purposed: to help make a confusing diagnosis more secure, and to follow patients over time. As mentioned earlier, the commonly used examinations are pulse volume recordings (PVRs), segmental pressures (including ankle/brachial indices [ABIs]), and the exercise test. These examinations can be very helpful in sorting out patients whose physical examination and history do not fit so well as the examiner would like. Two obvious examples are patients with claudication-like symptoms whose physical examination at rest is normal. Here, an exercise test should clearly define whether or not the pain is secondary to arterial insufficiency; a significant fall in the ABI to less than 0.3 with pain produced by exercise would confirm the diagnosis, while no decrease or a minimal one would rule out the diagnosis. The other example is a diabetic with foot pain at rest and a physical examination compatible with only mild to moderate arterial insufficiency. Is the physical examination misleading and the pain really ischemic, or is the pain neuropathic? PVRs, toe waveforms, and segmental pressures should help answer these questions.

The role of arteriography needs to be clearly defined. Since there is always potential risk, some discomfort, and real expense with angiography, it should be used only when it will be acted upon. Angiography remains the gold standard examination for defining arterial anatomy. This information is critical in making decisions about possible angioplasty or operative procedures. Angiography, or some similar study, remains mandatory prior to consideration of intervention for chronic lower extremity ischemia. The "similar study" in 1997 is a magnetic resonance angiogram, whose role remains controversial under these circumstances.

The natural history of the different presentations of lower extremity ischemia has a critical role in any therapeutic decisions. The amputation rate for claudicators is very low: 5 to 7% at 5 years (Imparato & Kim, 1975) and 10 to 12% at 10 years (Boyd, 1960); however, the mortality rate is high. Approximately one-half of all claudicants die within 10 years of their presentation (Boyd, 1960). Most of these deaths are related to coronary artery disease or stroke. The natural history data are surprisingly scanty for patients with ischemic rest pain or tissue loss; however, traditionally, these have been believed to be "threatened limbs." The amputation rate has been reported to be much higher, especially in those patients who have gangrene as their presenting complaint. Once again, this group has a high mortality rate because of concurrent coronary artery disease.

Management

As with all arterial occlusive disease, there are three levels of treatment: risk reduction, medicinal therapy, and invasive therapy. All patients with symptomatic arterial insufficiency of any arterial bed should be strongly urged to reduce their risk-amplifying behavior: to stop smoking and to get blood sugar, blood pressure, and serum cholesterol within normal limits. Claudicants should also be urged to stay active and to attempt to lose weight, if they are at all overweight. Weight loss accomplishes many things: it reduces the amount of weight carried, enabling the patient to walk further, but it also makes blood sugar, blood pressure, and lipids (especially triglycerides) much easier to control. The desired results are both improved lower extremity perfusion and avoidance of progression of coronary disease.

The next level of treatment is medicinal. At present, the only FDA-approved drug for relief of claudication is pentoxyphylline, which helps about 70% of claudicators, but only 25 to 30% have a doubling of their walking distance (Taylor & Porter, 1986). It is a drug with a slow onset of action, and it must be taken for 6 to 8 weeks to give an adequate therapeutic trial. We usually offer 2 months of treatment before making a determination of efficacy. Approximately 10% of all patients who take it develop gastrointestinal problems, usually nausea, diarrhea, or abdominal pain. A dosage reduction from one tablet, three times a day, to one tablet, twice a day with meals, usually solves the problem. If it does not, we stop the treatment. Because of the slow onset, we rarely offer the drug to patients with limb-threatening disease (rest pain or tissue loss), but instead, move quickly to the third level of treatment: invasive therapy. This next step should be considered in patients with tissue loss and/or ischemic rest pain. The role of invasive therapy in the treatment of claudicants is unclear and largely dependent upon the philosophy of the treating surgeon. Since these patients do not have limb-threatening ischemia, most surgeons recommend surgery for only those with very short-distance ("incapacitating") claudication.

When one contemplates utilizing endovascular, or open surgical techniques, for lower extremity occlusive disease, surgeons divide patients into two groups: those with aortoiliac occlusive disease and those with infrainguinal disease. If there is significant aortoiliac disease, this must be addressed first. This arterial segment is very amenable to endovascular techniques. Many groups have reported excellent long-term results after angioplasty, with or without stent placement (Fig. 31–17), in the distal aorta and iliac systems (Wilson, Wolf, Gross et al., 1989) when dealing with either short stenotic segments or very short occlusions. If the disease is too extensive for endovascular techniques, the surgeon is presented with a choice of an in-line, anatomic graft, an aortobifemoral graft (Fig. 31–18), or else an extra-anatomic graft, usually an axillobifemoral graft (Fig. 31–19), or, under certain circumstances of unilateral iliac occlusion, a femoral–femoral bypass (Fig. 31–20). In general terms, the long-term patency of the aortobifemoral graft is excellent, with a five-year patency of between 85% and 90% (Brewster & Darling, 1978). Obviously, it is a large operation and one that has significant morbidity for patients with very compromised hearts or lungs. These patients, as well as those with a very hostile abdomen, may be better served with an extra-anatomic procedure in which no body cavity is entered. These operations are less stressful

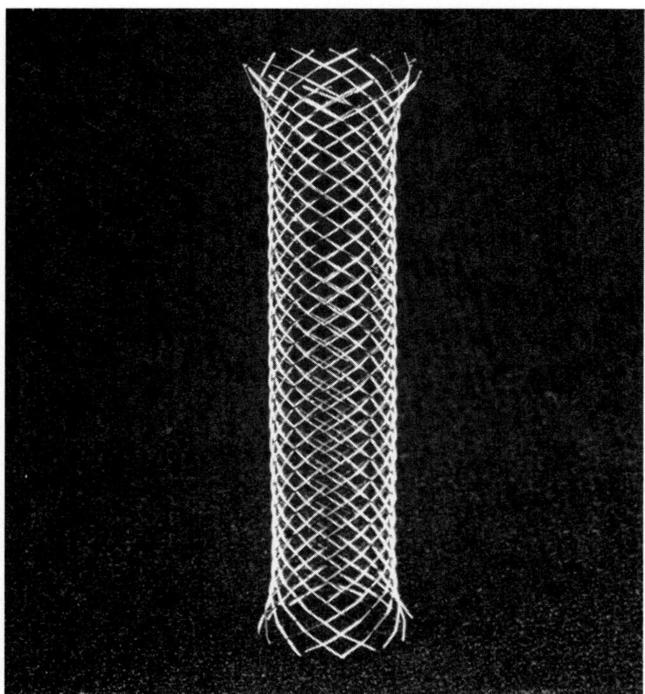

Figure 31–17. Intra-arterial stent.

for the patient, but in most hands, the long-term patency is not as good. However, with the development of a graft exoskeleton that increases the rigidity of the graft, making its compression less likely, much improved patency data have been reported. This has led some to recommend an axillobifemoral graft as the standard procedure for aortoiliac occlusive disease (Harris, Taylor, McConnell et al., 1990).

Endovascular procedures have less of a role for infrainguinal occlusive disease. The extent of the stenosis or length of occlusion, mixed with the small size of the arteries, have resulted in relatively poor long-term results for an-

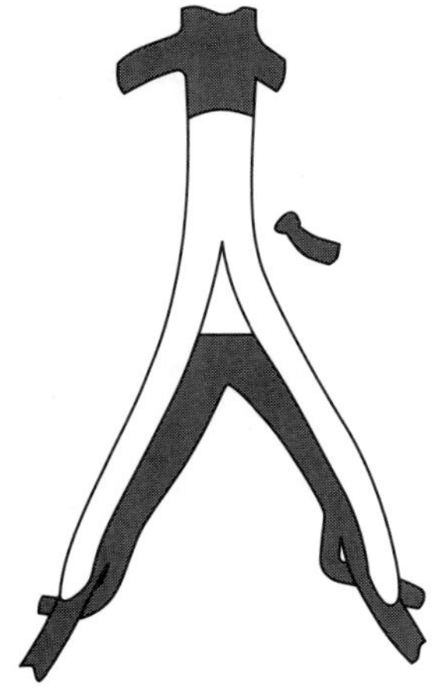

Figure 31–18. Aortobifemoral bypass.

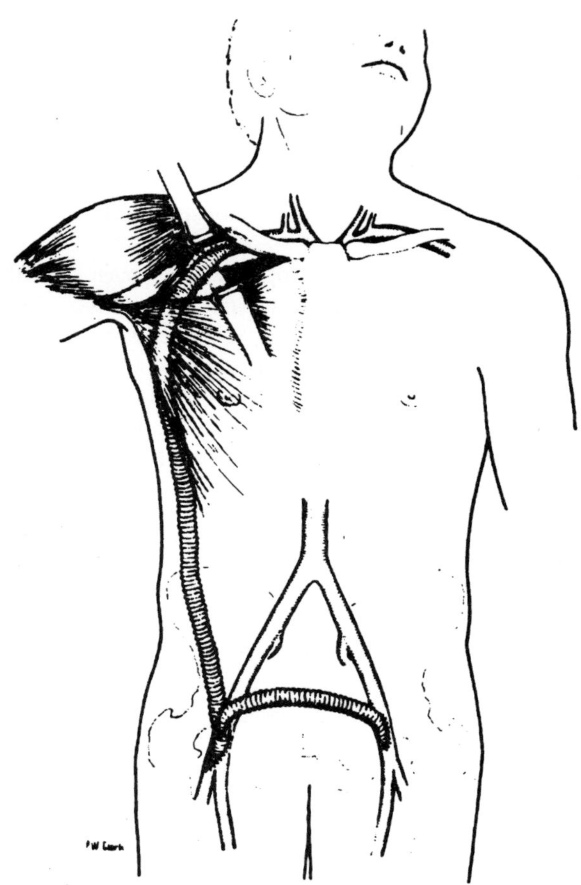

Figure 31–19. Axillobifemoral bypass. *(Used with permission from Rutherford, [1984].)*

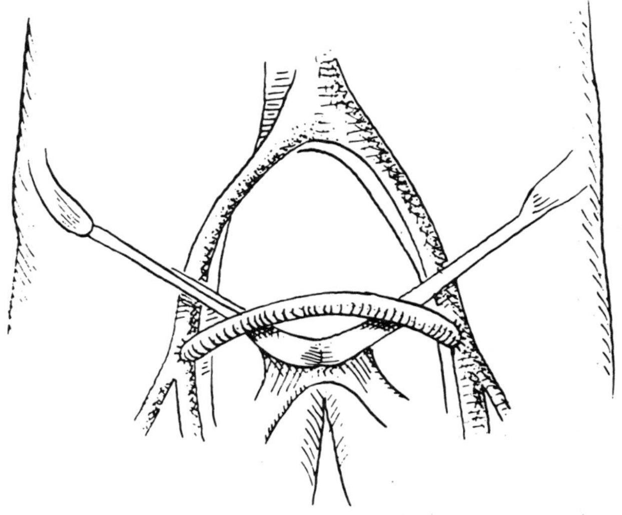

Figure 31–20. Femoral–femoral bypass. *(Used with permission from Moore, [1993].)*

gioplasties. Endarterectomies with patches are often the treatment for common femoral artery occlusions and profunda disease (relatively infrequent beyond the first centimeter of the artery). Most patients coming to operation for chronic infrainguinal occlusive disease require bypass grafting. Ideally, these bypasses should extend to beyond all disease, so that the patient has an unobstructed flow into the foot.

If the distal popliteal is open with at least one tibial vessel clear throughout, the distal anastomosis would be at the below-knee popliteal artery. If there is severe distal popliteal or proximal tibial disease, one would bypass further down to an open tibial artery (Fig. 31–21). As mentioned earlier, the composition of these very distal grafts is of overwhelming importance. Using the *in situ* vein techniques, excellent results have been reported by many groups with patency of greater than 75% at 5 years (Leather, Shah, Chang et al., 1988). These *in situ* tibial bypasses can be very long and tedious cases, and it is generally recommended that they be done by surgeons who do them relatively frequently.

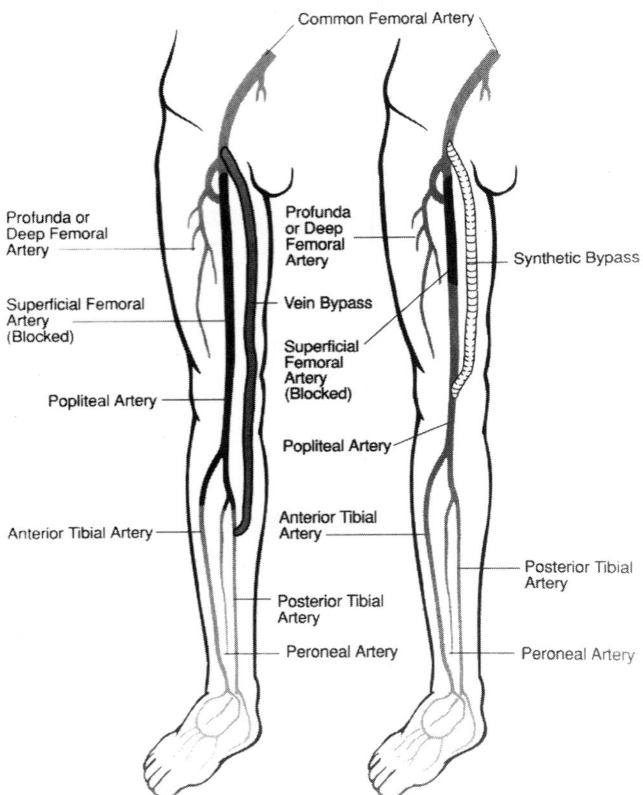

Figure 31–21. Infrainguinal bypasses. The drawing on the *left* shows a femoral-posterior tibial bypass using vein as the conduit. On the *right* is an above-knee femoral-popliteal bypass using prosthetic graft. *(Used with permission from Patient Education Committee, [1990].* Lower Extremity Arterial Disease, *Society of Vascular Nursing.)*

The importance of the *in situ* technique as opposed to reversed vein grafts, or free, nonreversed grafts, remains a point of dispute. Most vascular surgeons believe the *in situ* technique gives the best long-term results, but this is not universally accepted (Taylor, Edward & Pater, 1990). One thing perfectly clear, though, is that the results of vein grafts to the tibial level are significantly better than those of prosthetics (Bergan, Veith, Bernhard et al., 1982). The vast majority of vascular surgeons go to great lengths to obtain reasonable vein rather than use prosthetic grafts to the infrapopliteal level.

In summary, chronic arterial insufficiency of the lower extremity presents with either limb-threatening ischemia (rest pain or tissue loss) or nonthreatening disease (claudication). Most surgeons take a more aggressive posture toward the former group, moving more quickly toward invasive therapy, than they do with the claudication population. Angioplasty can produce excellent results at the aortoiliac level. Severe infrainguinal occlusive disease generally requires surgical bypass.

Acute Lower Extremity Ischemia

The etiology of acute arterial insufficiency to the lower extremity is the same as in the carotid, mesenteric, or renal beds: embolization or spontaneous thrombosis. The most common source of the emboli remains the heart, with the aorta a distant second (Abbott, Maloney, McCabe, Lee, & Wirthlin, 1982).

The presentation is generally quite distinctive (Table 31–3). The most common complaint is the sudden onset of distal pain, which may proceed to paresthesias and even anesthesia. The patient may note weakness that may progress to paralysis of the foot and even the leg. On physical examination, the distal extremity is pale, pulseless, and cool. In the less severe situation, the foot is painful, but the patient has sensation and movement. With more severe ischemia, the foot may be blanched, anesthetic, and paralyzed. This is usually indicative of neuronal dysfunction secondary to local ischemia. Such cases are emergencies that result in permanent neurologic and muscular injury within a few hours unless the blood supply is restored.

When presented with a patient in this predicament, it is very important to initially proceed with anticoagulation to attempt to stop propagation of proximal and distal thrombi. The next step is to attempt to decide if the acute event is embolic or thrombotic. This is an important distinction to

TABLE 31–3. Signs of Acute Arterial Insufficiency

Pain
Pallor
Pulselessness
Paresthesias
Paralysis

make, since the treatment is quite different. Often history and physical examination give the examiner clues. Is there a history of cardiac problems (recent myocardial infarction or atrial fibrillation) that increases the chances of emboli? Is there any history of claudication, indicative of underlying occlusive disease, which may have led to thrombosis? Atherosclerosis is usually symmetrical. Is there evidence of chronic occlusive disease, or the lack of it, in either the ischemic leg or its mate? How severe is the ischemia? Emboli typically produce a more severely compromised extremity, since the embolus typically lodges at major bifurcations, obstructing both the primary channel and its major collaterals. With an embolic event, there is no prolonged stimulus for the development of collaterals, as there is with the more chronic obstructive disease.

If the surgeon is sure that the event is embolic, there is generally no need for an arteriogram, and the proper treatment is a quick trip to the operating room. Since the embolus usually lodges at major bifurcations (aortic, common iliac, common femoral, or distal popliteal), its location is usually clear. Typically there is a very strong pulse (a water hammer pulse) immediately above the embolus. When the embolus is in the extremity, the clot should be approached directly (Fig. 31–22). After removing the embolus itself, Fogarty catheters are used to remove any propagated thrombus, both proximally and distally. Intraoperative thrombolytic therapy is often used to lyse any residual clot. Aortic saddle emboli can usually be removed from below by common femoral artery incisions but this may lead to internal iliac occlusions. Postoperatively, all patients who have had an arterial embolus should be anticoagulated indefinitely to reduce the chances of a second embolic event.

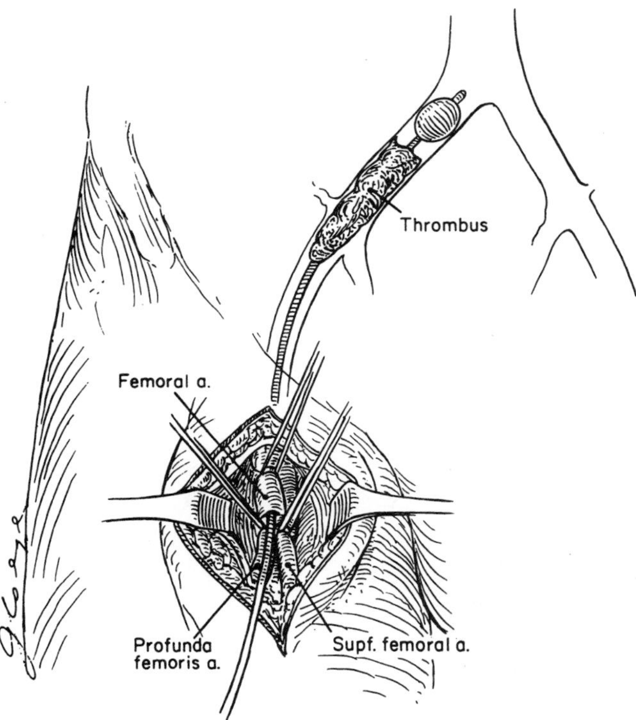

Figure 31–22. Removal of propagated thrombus in the right common iliac artery using a Fogarty catheter after removing embolus to common femoral bifurcation. *(Used with permission from Moore, [1993].)*

These embolectomy procedures are relatively simple and quick, and have predictably good results, as long as the underlying arterial tree is not severely diseased. Unfortunately, there is still a 10 to 15% mortality rate because of either secondary emboli despite anticoagulation or else underlying coronary disease (Kendrick, Thompson, Pearl et al., 1981).

If the ischemic event appears to be a spontaneous thrombosis, then an arteriogram is mandatory to define arterial anatomy. This is important information since a bypass is almost certainly necessary. Luckily, most patients who have had a thrombotic event do not present with such severe ischemia that they need to be taken immediately to the operating room. Instead, they usually continue to have sensation and movement and can, therefore, be evaluated in a slightly less urgent manner.

The role of lytic therapy in the treatment of the acutely ischemic limb remains obscure (McNamara, Bomberger, Merchant et al., 1989). It may well have an important role in the treatment of patients with moderate to severe ischemia, but there is insufficient time to attempt such treatment in patients with a paralyzed, anesthetic foot, which is immediately threatened.

A final note should be made about the role of fasciotomies. When muscle has been severely ischemic for more than 4 to 6 hours, it swells when reperfused. There are four compartments in the leg that are encased by bone and fascia, neither of which are elastic (Fig. 31–23). Muscular swelling in these compartments leads to increased intercompartment pressures, which in turn may stop capillary perfusion of muscle and nerve.

Within a few hours of reperfusion, this can lead to necrosis of both the muscle and nerve within the involved compartment. The common presentation is severe local pain and tenderness over a tense compartment. Passive movement increases the pain. There is usually paralysis of the muscles in the compartment, and there are areas of anesthesia distally in the foot that correspond with sensory nerves that also traversed the enclosed space. Palpable pulses may still be felt distally. The anterior compartment is the most common compartment involved, followed by the lateral compartment and then the two posterior compartments. Clinically the diagnosis of an anterior compartment syndrome is made by local tenderness over the anterior compartment, severe anterior compartment pain with passive extension and flexion of the toes, inability to extend the toes or foot, anesthesia in the first web space, and a tense anterior compartment. If a patient presents like this, the examin-

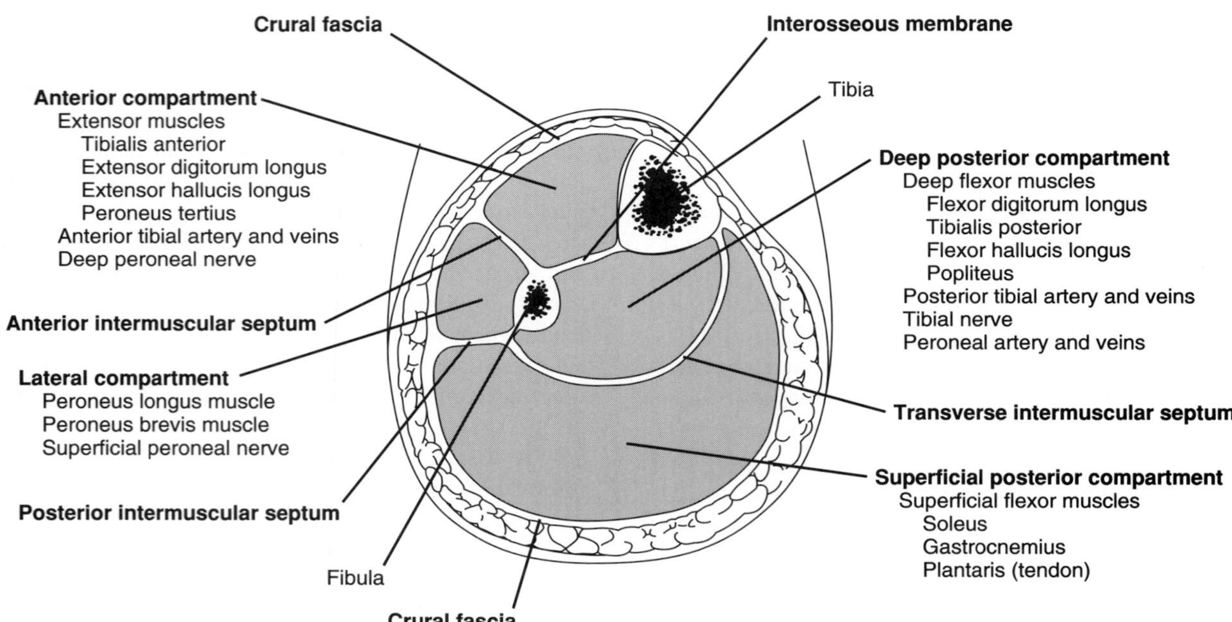

Figure 31–23. The four compartments of the leg (cross-section through the mid-calf).

ers have a choice of measuring compartment pressures to assure themselves of the diagnosis, or else empirically decompressing the compartment, which is the recommendation of our unit. This is done by incising the skin and fascia, which allows expansion of the compartment (Fig. 31–24).

Fasciotomies should either be performed (or seriously considered) with any patient who has had severe ischemia for more than 4 hours. This is especially true if there is underlying arterial insufficiency or some reason to believe that there is an element of venous hypertension. In the prophylactic situation, the compartment can be decompressed and the skin closed with staples, which can easily be removed at the bedside, if necessary.

ANEURYSMAL DISEASE

Pathophysiology

Aneurysms are areas of arterial dilatation that occur because of a weakening in the arterial wall. Aneurysms can be fusiform (Fig. 31–25), where the weakness is circumferential and the artery dilates symmetrically, or saccular (Fig. 31–26), where the weakness is not circumferential. Saccular aneurysms appear like bubbles or sacs on the surface of the artery. "True" aneurysms have all three arterial layers (intima, media, and adventitia) in the dilated segment. "Pseudo" or "false" aneurysms do not. Usually the wall of a

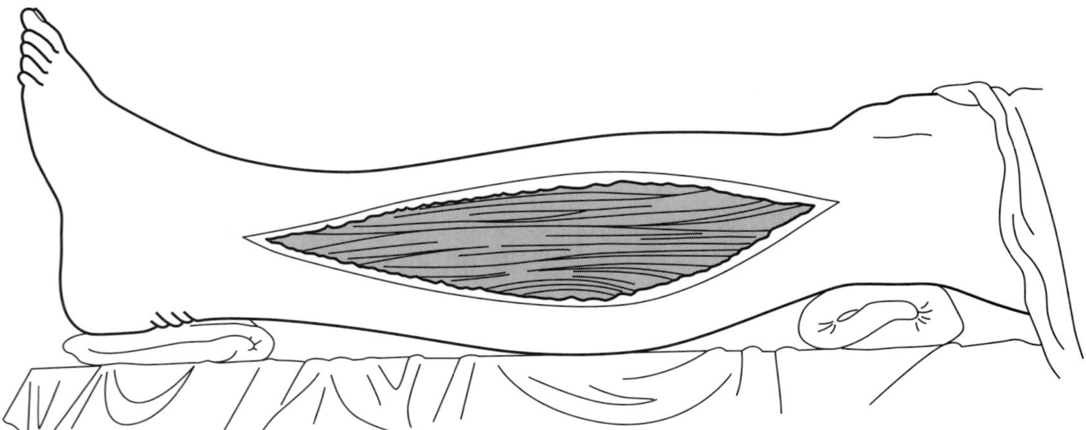

Figure 31–24. Fasciotomy of the anterior compartment.

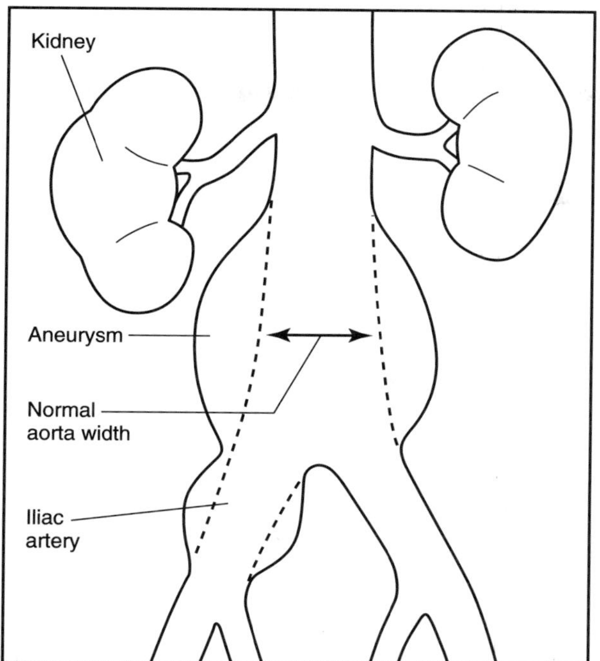

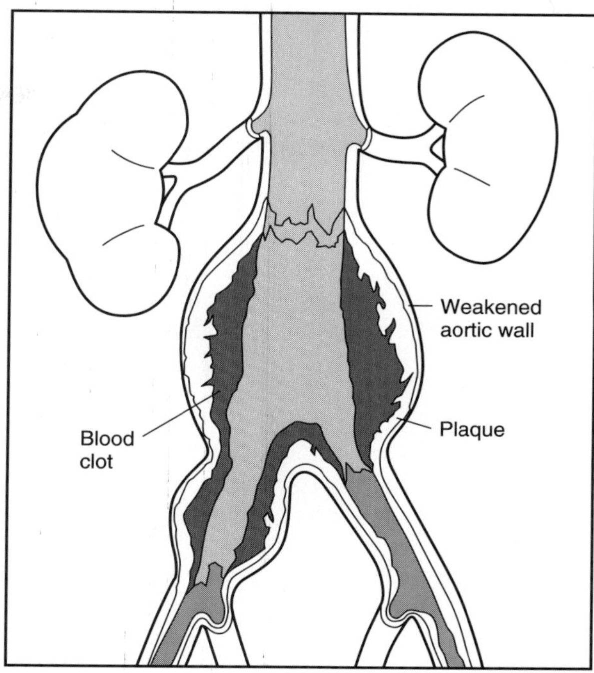

Figure 31–25. Fusiform aneurysm of the aorta secondary to circumferential weakness of the wall.

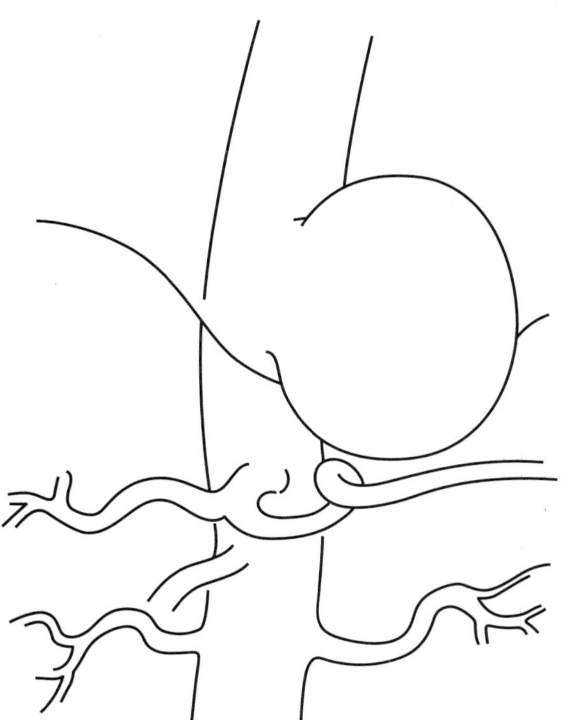

Figure 31–26. Saccular aneurysm of the supradiaphragmatic aorta secondary to a localized, noncircumferential weakness in the aorta. *(Used with permission from Moore, [1986].)*

"false" aneurysm is composed of compressed thrombus or scar. "Septic" aneurysms are those that occur because of arterial wall weakening secondary to an infectious arteritis. A "dissecting" aneurysm is really a misnomer that often causes confusion. An aortic dissection occurs when the aortic intima cracks, and blood, under systemic pressure, enters the aortic wall, separating or "dissecting" the intima and some of the media from the surrounding adventitia. This produces two lumens, a true and a false lumen (Fig. 31–27). Over time, the process may weaken the aorta, which may then become distended and aneurysmal; however, usually the expression "dissecting aneurysm" refers to an aortic dissection, which is unrelated to the standard atherosclerotic aortic aneurysm.

"True" aneurysms have many etiologies; however, these can be grouped into four categories: degenerative, inflammatory, mechanical, and congenital. The congenital causes are largely associated with either segmental weaknesses at bifurcations (almost always found intracranially) or with connective tissue disorders, most commonly Marfan's or Ehlers–Danlos syndromes. Mechanical sources are those situations in which there has been recurrent trauma to the artery that leads to weakness and dilatation, such as the subclavian artery aneurysms associated with thoracic outlet syndrome. Inflammatory aneurysms may be either sterile or infectious (syphilitic, bacterial, or fungal). Sterile inflammatory aneurysms are generally associated with autoimmune diseases, such as polyarteritis nodosa. Degenerative sources are the most common. Most are labeled "atherosclerotic aneurysms." Why some patients manifest athero-

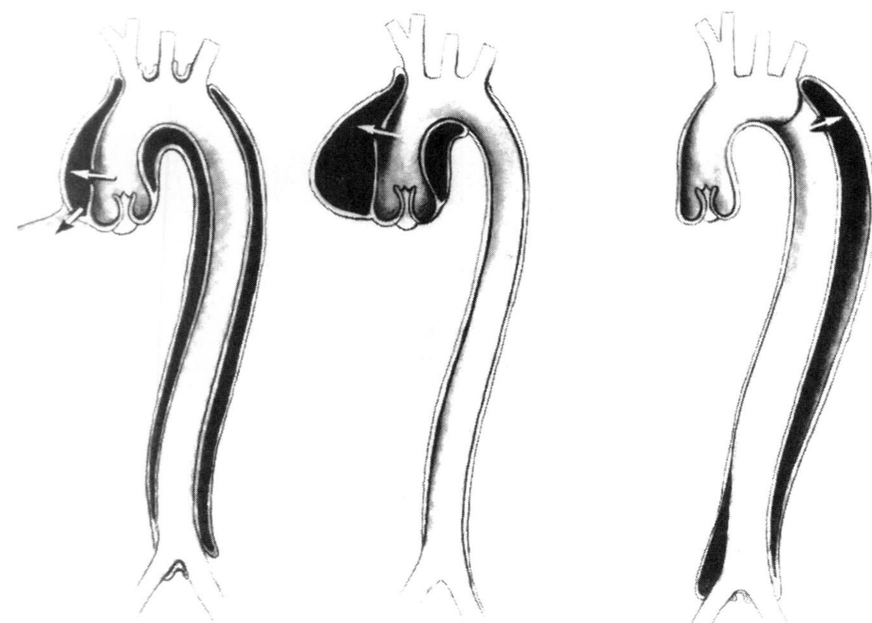

Figure 31–27. Aortic dissections. In the *left* drawing, the entry point is in the ascending aorta and involves the whole aorta. In the *middle* drawing, the dissection is limited to the ascending aorta. On the *right,* the dissection is limited to the descending aorta. In each, there is a true lumen (*white*) and a false lumen (*black*). *(Used with permission from Rob, [1976].)*

sclerotic disease as occlusive and others as aneurysmal disease remains unclear. The most commonly accepted theory is that patients with aneurysmal disease have abnormally high concentrations of elastases and collagenases that gradually weaken the atherosclerotic arterial wall (Dobrin, Baker, & Gley, 1984).

The common complications from aneurysms are rupture, thrombosis, embolization, and compression of contiguous structures.

Abdominal Aortic Aneurysms

Since the discovery of penicillin has made syphilitic aortic aneurysms a rarity, the most common large-vessel aneurysm is the atherosclerotic infrarenal abdominal aortic aneurysm (AAA) (Fig. 31–28). By far, the most common of the complications of AAA is rupture. Unless these patients become symptomatic from either impending or frank rupture, most aneurysms are discovered incidentally.

History and Physical Findings

Abdominal aortic aneurysms may be found on either physical examination or as unexpected findings on imaging studies. The classical physical finding is a pulsatile, epigastric mass. It should be emphasized that the mass is usually epigastric—not midabdominal, as many believe. The aortic bifurcation is usually at L-4, approximately the level of the umbilicus, so AAAs are felt in the upper abdomen. The differential of a pulsatile, epigastric mass is an abdominal aneurysm, an unusually large visceral artery aneurysm, or any mass that overlies the aorta and transmits its pulsations. Examples are pancreatic pseudocysts, gastric carcinoma, and gastrointestinal lymphoma.

Laborabory and Diagnostic Tests

The same imaging modalities used to clarify the origin of epigastric, pulsatile masses are the means of diagnosis when AAA are found incidentally: ultrasound, CT, and MRI (Fig. 31–29). The advantages and disadvantages of these different methods have been discussed previously. The diagnosis is also occasionally made on either AP or lateral abdominal films when a rim of calcium in the aortic wall can be identified (Fig. 31–30). Angiography may be deceptive in the diagnosis of an abdominal aneurysm, since often the aneurysm is often filled with thrombus, and the angiogram shows only the column of blood traversing the lesion. Angiography does define other arterial anatomy, which may be very important. Renal artery stenosis, aberrant inferior pole renal arteries, mesenteric occlusive disease, or iliac occlusive disease can be unexpected and undiagnosed preoperatively without angiography. The role of this invasive procedure in the preoperative evaluation of patients with routine infrarenal abdominal aortic aneurysms without evidence of either marked hypertension or lower extremity occlusive disease is controversial. Some feel that angiography is unnecessary with a high-quality CT or MRI (Gaspar, 1982), while others believe that the information is worth the small risk and expense (Brewster et al., 1975).

The natural history of infrarenal AAA is conceptually

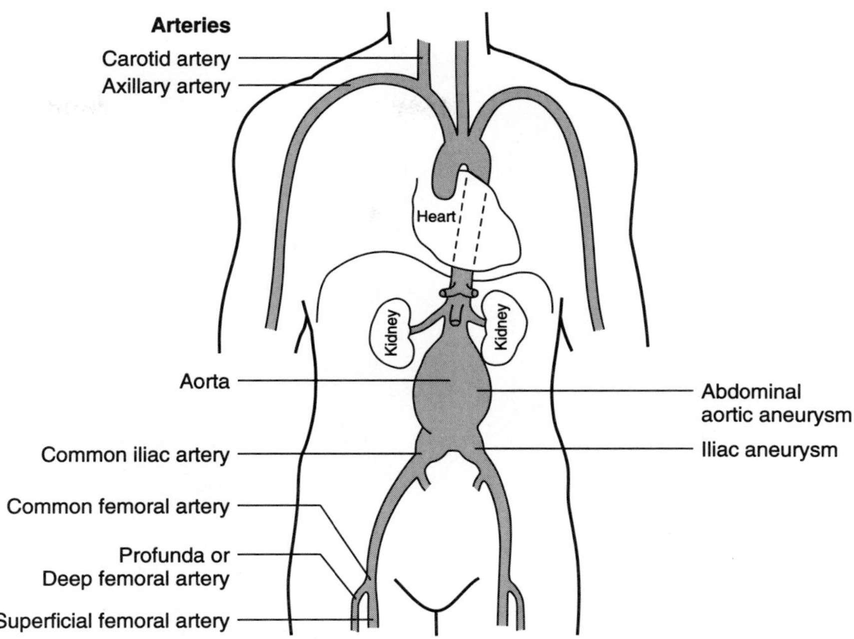

Figure 31–28. Infrarenal abdominal aortic aneurysm involving both common iliac arteries.

well defined, but important details remain contentious. In 1966, Dr. Emmett Szilagyi published an important paper demonstrating a positive association between the risk of rupture and the diameter of the aneurysm (Szilagyi, Smith, DeRusso et al., 1966). He found the risk of rupture very small in aneurysms of less than 4 centimeters in diameter, and significant in those of greater than 6 centimeters. The 4- to 6-centimeter group was of modest risk. As the operative mortality has decreased, the interest in resecting smaller aneurysms has increased, but disagreements persist on what the minimal diameter should be leading to resection. There are very good groups who recommend resection

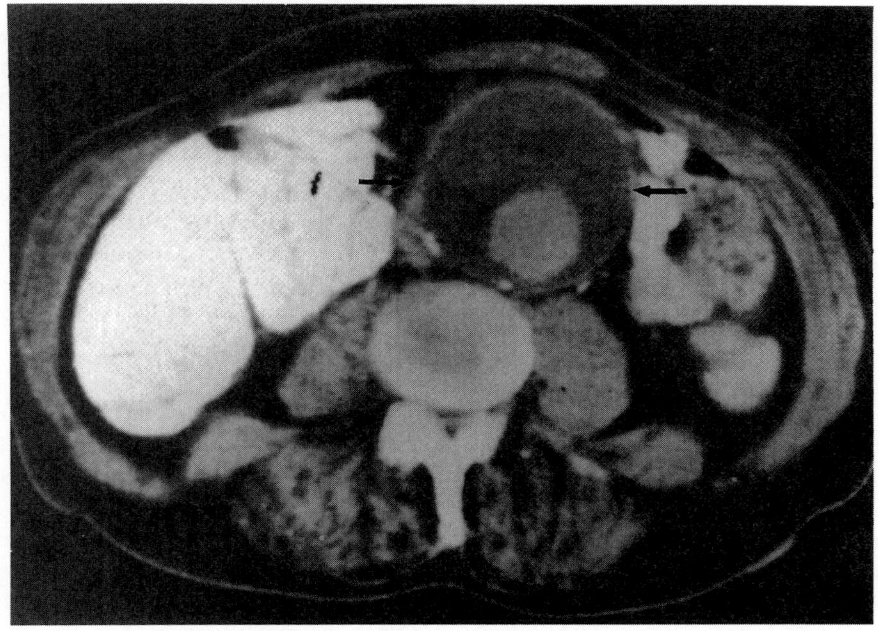

Figure 31–29. CT scan of a large abdominal aortic aneurysm between *arrow heads* with a relatively small lumen *(arrow)* surrounded by laminated clot. *(Used with permission from Rutherford, [1984].)*

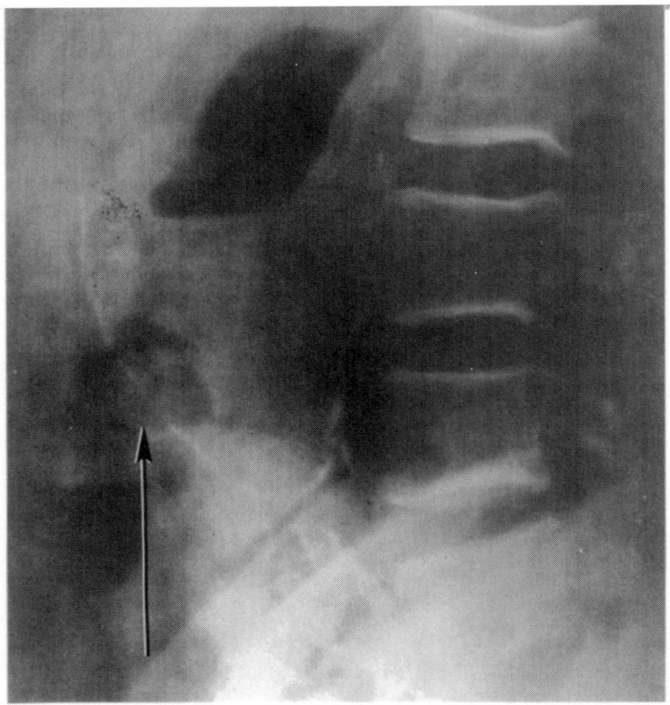

Figure 31–30. Calcified rim of abdominal aortic aneurysm. The calcium in the aortic wall (*arrow*) can be seen on this lateral film. *(Used with permission from Eastcott, [1969].)*

for any AAA of greater than 4 centimeters, while others believe that no aneurysm needs operative intervention until it is at least 5 centimeters (Hollier, Taylor, & Ochsner, 1992).

Management

The nonoperative treatment for small aneurysms, or for aneurysms in those who are at either prohibitively high operative risk or who decline surgery, is the control of atherosclerotic risk factors, with special emphasis on blood pressure control and cessation of smoking. It is of interest that a second significant risk factor for abdominal aortic aneurysm rupture is the presence of emphysema, a disease associated with both tobacco use and high serum elastase levels.

Operative treatment of AAA is conceptually very simple. The weakened aneurysmal segment of aorta is replaced by a cloth graft, placed in an end-to-end fashion (Fig. 31–31). The grafts are either straight or bifurcated, depending upon the aneurysmal involvement of the common iliac arteries. The operative risk depends upon the size of the aneurysm, length of the aneurysm neck (infrarenal segment of normal aorta), and concomitant diseases, most important the presence of significant coronary artery disease. Good surgical units now report a 3 to 5% mortality rate for all resections (Crawford, Saleh, Babb et al., 1981). One-half of the deaths occur because of perioperative myocardial events, and the other one-half from a mixture of bleeding, embolization, infection, and organ failure (heart, renal, hepatic, and/or pulmonary).

Ruptured Abdominal Aortic Aneurysm

A ruptured AAA is a surgical emergency. Although risk of rupture is related to the diameter of the aneurysm and associated with the presence of emphysema, small aneurysms can leak, whether or not the patient has emphysema.

Typically, the patient presents with a relatively short history of severe back, flank, or abdominal pain. This symptom complex can occur with an "impending rupture," in which the artery is acutely distending, as well as with a true rupture itself. However, if the patient gives a history of either a syncopal episode or lightheadedness, then the aneurysm has probably leaked. The critical finding on physical examination is a tender, pulsatile, epigastric mass. If the patient is stable and the examiner unsure of the diagnosis, an emergency ultrasound or CAT scan can clarify the situation.

A patient with a ruptured AAA should be taken to the operating room as soon as possible. The critical factors are that the patient is bleeding, and that the bleeding will continue until the aorta is cross-clamped. The units with the best statistics on survival from this event are those in which the diagnosis is made, the patient transported to the operating room, and the aorta controlled—all quickly. In general, it is reasonable to accept relative preoperative hypotension, since normotension or hypertension leads to increased blood loss (Crawford, 1991).

Although some units have reported mortality rates of

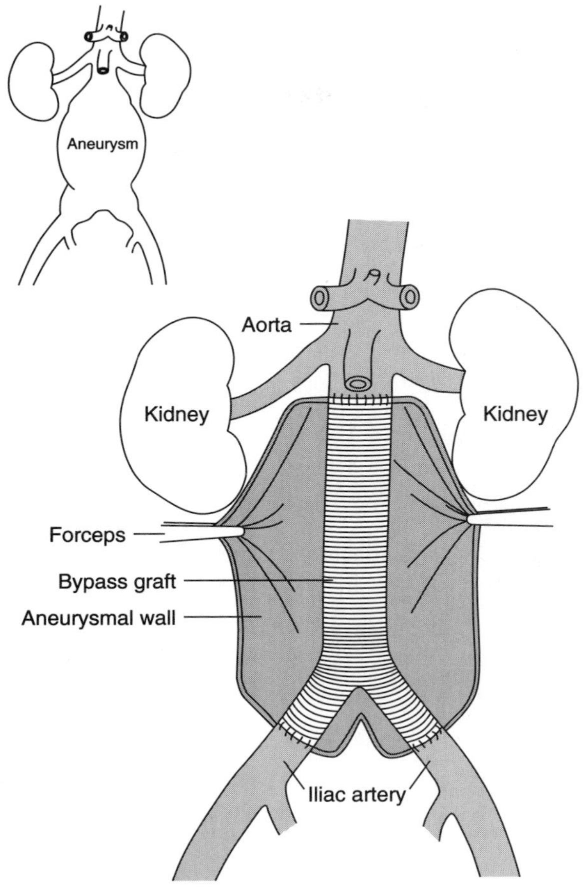

Figure 31–31. Abdominal aortic aneurysm with iliac artery involvement with the aneurysm replaced by a bifurcated prosthetic graft.

less than 30% (Mulherin & Edwards, 1980), in most hands the results are more discouraging: the mortality rate for all patients is approximately 50% and greater than 70% for those who present with shock or anuria (Hiatt, Barker, Machleder et al., 1984).

Peripheral Aneurysms

Peripheral aneurysms are much less common than AAAs. The two most common sites for these lesions are the popliteal artery and the common femoral artery. These are almost always degenerative or atherosclerotic aneurysms. Aneurysms at either site have a high rate of bilaterality and of concomitant aneurysms. In other words, if a popliteal or femoral aneurysm is found, the examiner is obliged to look carefully for other aneurysms in the contralateral leg as well as in other locations, especially the aorta.

The common complications associated with peripheral aneurysms are ischemic (embolization and thrombosis). Rupture can occur, but is rare. The most common presentation is an ischemic symptom: claudication, rest pain, or tissue loss. Any patient with a history and physical examination compatible with pedal embolization should be examined for femoral or popliteal aneurysms. The classic physical finding is an abnormally wide or prominent pulse. Suspicion of a peripheral aneurysm can be confirmed by duplex ultrasound examination of the suspected artery. Other imaging techniques—CT or MRI—can be used to make the diagnosis, but in most hospitals, ultrasound remains the least invasive and least expensive. If the diagnosis is verified and operative intervention is planned, an aortogram is usually performed to define proximal and distal arterial anatomy.

The indications for operative intervention are not completely defined. There is no dispute about large (greater than 2 cm in diameter) or symptomatic aneurysms, but what should be done with small, asymptomatic aneurysms with no evidence of intraluminal thrombus by ultrasound is unclear.

The basic principle of repair is the same as that for AAA. The aneurysmal segment is replaced with a graft. Cloth grafts are usually used in the femoral location (Fig. 31–32) and vein grafts for those at the popliteal level. The popliteal artery can be dissected directly from a posterior approach, with the patient in a prone position, or else a medial approach can be used with the patient supine (Fig. 31–33). The artery is controlled above and below the knee joint, and the aneurysmal segment excluded from the circulation.

When popliteal arteries thrombose, run-off vessels often also occlude. Over the last 10 to 15 years, there has been increasing appreciation that these patients with ischemic legs and no run-off can often be markedly improved by the use of lytic therapy prior to operation. The goal of the thrombolytic therapy is to open the run-off vessels rather than the aneurysm itself, which needs to be resected. The results of peripheral aneurysm resection are dependent upon the presence of open distal vessels. When most, or all, of the tibial vessels are occluded, the long-term patency of popliteal bypasses is poor. Not surprisingly, if the run-off vessels are open, the results are excellent (Lilly, Flinn, McCarthy et al., 1988).

False Aneurysms (Pseudoaneurysms)

False aneurysms (pseudoaneurysms) are aneurysms without the normal three layers of the arterial wall. There are generally three sources of these lesions. The first is trauma, which includes catheter-related injuries. The second is infection; the infected arterial wall weakens and essentially disintegrates. This may occur from direct extension of infection (often from intravenous drug use) or else by hematogenous spread, by either inoculation from a bacteremia or septic embolization. The third source is an anastomotic aneurysm that occurs when an arterial suture line begins to separate. Prosthetic grafts never truly heal to the artery the way a vein graft does. If the suture line breaks

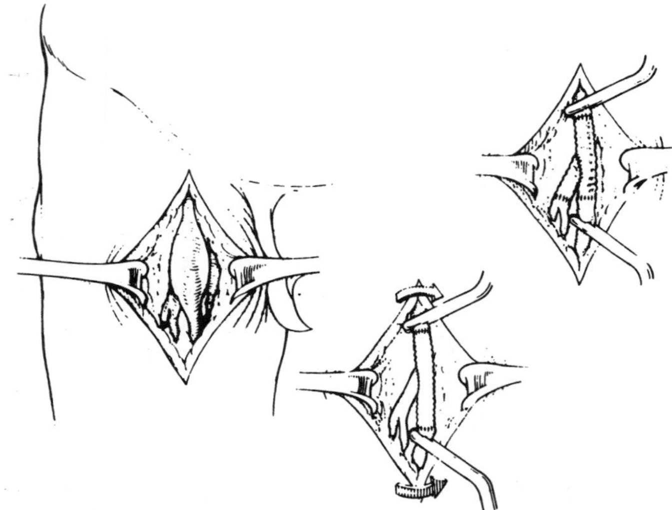

Figure 31–32. Femoral artery aneurysm involving the origin of the profunda femoris artery, which should be reimplanted. *(Used with permission from Moore, [1986].)*

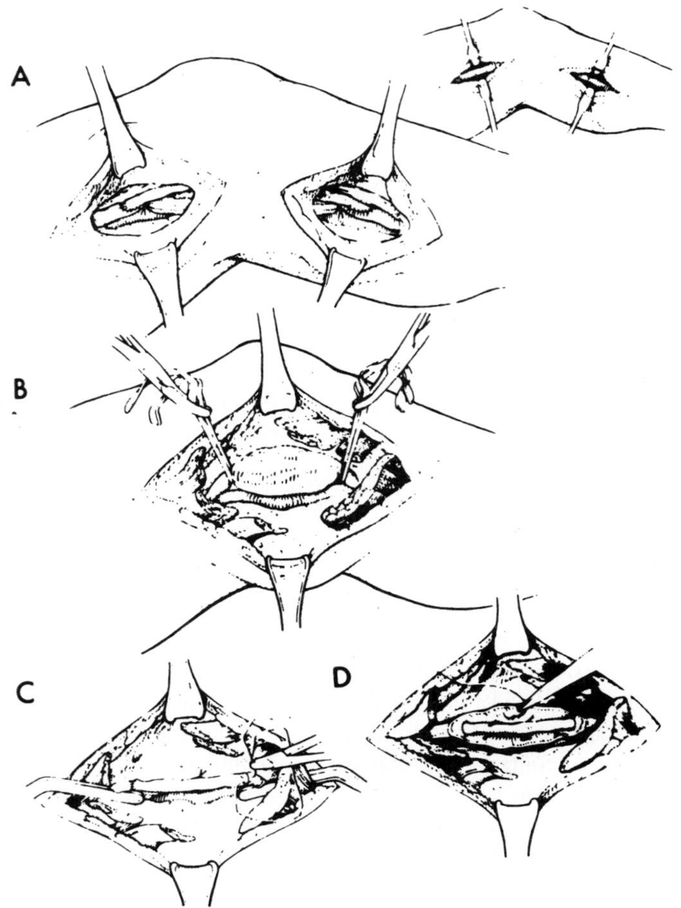

Figure 31–33. Popliteal artery aneurysm repair with a medial approach. *(Used with permission from Moore, [1986].)*

down, the graft begins to separate from the artery, forming a false aneurysm. The wall of the aneurysm is scar, not the normal arterial layers. The reasons for suture line failure are multiple: suture disintegration, arterial weakening secondary to either endarterectomy or infection, inadequate depth of the suture bites, or too much tension on the suture line.

The diagnosis is initially entertained after noting a widened arterial pulse associated with a bruit. If the history and physical examination suggest the diagnosis, it can be substantiated by either ultrasound or other imaging techniques.

In general terms, these lesions increase in size over time and should be repaired. The one exception is small, catheter-produced, false aneurysms. These cases usually have a very small arterial wall defect. If observed, many spontaneously thrombose as long as the patient is not anticoagulated. Another nonsurgical option for catheter-related false aneurysms is ultrasound-guided compression therapy. This technique requires a skilled ultrasound technologist who can use the ultrasound probe to simultaneously compress the neck of the false aneurysm, stopping the turbulent flow into the aneurysm, while at the same time allowing normal distal flow in the artery itself. This compression is sustained for 15 to 20 minutes. If necessary, it may be repeated a number of times prior to declaring the effort unsuccessful. If the aneurysm does not thrombose, surgical repair for puncture wounds is usually quite straightforward. Proximal control is gained prior to exposing the defect, which can usually be closed with a figure-of-eight suture.

Treatment of infected false aneurysms may be very problematic. The diagnosis is generally made in patients who are clinically septic, with localized areas of inflammation. Positive blood cultures, a false aneurysm by CT, MRI or ultrasound, and an obvious inflammatory mass around the false aneurysm, again by imaging, secure the diagnosis. The arterial anatomy needs to be defined (usually by angiography) prior to operation. In general terms, the infected arterial segment needs to be debrided. Often the distal extremity needs to be revascularized. This can be done either extraanatomically through clean fields or *in situ,* using autologous tissue after debridement of all infected material.

Anastomotic false aneurysms are potentially tricky. One must always consider infection as a possible source. If this is the etiology, then correct treatment can be very complex and difficult, depending upon the graft, the extent of infection, location of the false aneurysm, degree of ischemia without the graft, and the patient's overall condition.

A sterile false anastomotic aneurysm is relatively simple to manage. The anatomy of the arterial tree close to the aneurysm needs to be defined. Traditionally, this has been done with angiography, but at the femoral and popliteal levels, either ultrasound or MRA can usually get the same information. The anastomosis needs to be redone, and usually a short interposition graft allows a new anastomosis to be made without tension.

In summary, the most frequent complication of abdominal aortic aneurysm, the most common aneurysm, is rupture. The risk of this complication is associated with aneurysmal diameter. Rupture increases the mortality of resection by at least a factor of ten. The critical elements in the results of AAA rupture are the cardiovascular status of the patient upon presentation, the patient's concomitant diseases, and the speed with which the diagnosis is made and the aorta controlled. On the other hand, peripheral aneurysms rarely rupture, but when symptomatic are most often the source of ischemic complications. False aneurysms and septic aneurysms tend to rupture. In almost all situations, it is preferable to resect these lesions electively, prior to the development of difficulties.

▶ VENOUS DISEASE

Venous disease tends to be overshadowed by arterial pathology, which appears more dramatic and dangerous. Nonetheless, venous disorders are more common than arterial, are potentially life-threatening, and may be the source of significant long-term morbidity.

Anatomy and Physiology

The anatomy and physiology of the venous system of the lower extremities is linked and ingenious. The venous system can be divided into three segments: the deep veins, the superficial veins, and the perforating veins. The "deep veins" are deep to the investing fascia, run with the arteries, and carry the same names as the corresponding arterial segments. The "superficial" system is superficial to the fascia and, in the lower extremity, is composed of the greater and lesser saphenous veins and their branches. The greater saphenous vein empties into the deep system at the level of the common femoral vein, and the lesser saphenous vein does so at the level of the popliteal vein. There are also a variable number of veins that connect the two systems by perforating the fascia, the "perforating veins." All of these veins have valves (Fig. 31–34) that allow blood to go in only one direction. The superficial and deep system valves allow blood to return only towards the heart, and the perforator valves allow blood to go only from the superficial to the deep system.

This system of valves produces an extraordinary method of actively pumping blood back to the heart, using energy from the skeletal muscles. After standing for a period of time, the venous pressure in the foot or lower leg of a normal person is that of a column of blood from the floor to that individual's right atrium. When the person takes a step, the skeletal muscles of the calf contract, compressing the deep venous system and increasing its pressure. Valves

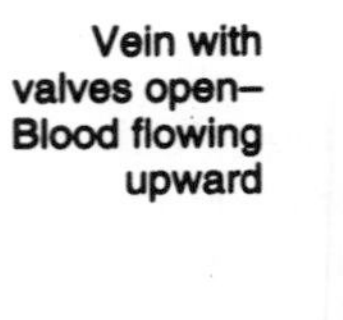

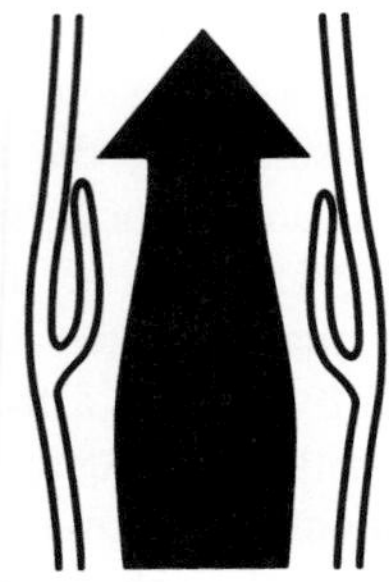

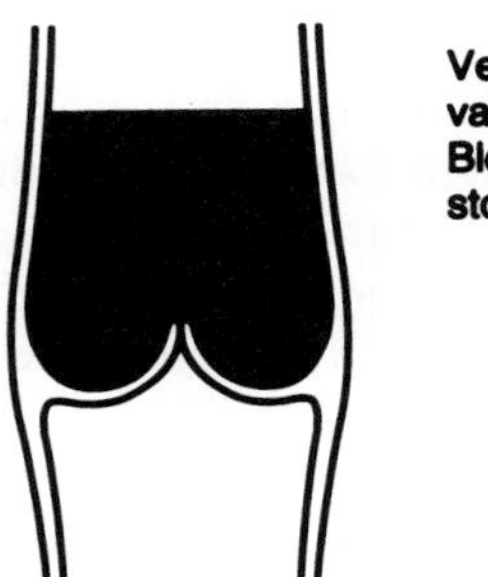

Figure 31–34. Venous valves, which only allow blood to go in one direction. *(Used with permission from Patient Education Committee, [1992].* Venous Disease, *The Society of Vascular Nursing.)*

close in the perforators and in the deep veins beyond the contracting muscles. Valves central to the contracting muscles open, and the full calf veins are emptied centrally. When the muscles relax, the pressure in the calf veins falls, the proximal valves close preventing reflux, and the deep venous system begins to fill with blood from its superficial system and from the capillary beds.

The whole process repeats itself every time a step is taken, as the blood is pumped back to the heart by the skeletal muscles. While exercising, the mean venous pressure at the ankle drops to low levels, with a normally functioning "musculovenous pump." During exercise, approximately 20% of the total energy needed to circulate blood comes from the skeletal muscles in the lower extremities. If the valves do not function properly, the pump is much less effective in returning the blood centrally and in decreasing the mean venous pressure. Without competent valves, blood refluxes during both muscular contracture (retrograde distally into the deep veins and/or into the foot, as well as out to the superficial system through the perforators) and relaxation (from the central veins back down the leg), resulting in high venous pressures and inefficient venous return. If there is a deep venous occlusion, the hemodynamic response to exercise is even more abnormal. Under these circumstances, the venous pressures rapidly rise with exercise, as more blood circulates through the extremity and the muscles attempt to pump that blood centrally against the high resistance of the occluded vein. The different pressure responses to exercise are presented in Figure 31–35.

Acute Venous Disease

Acute venous disease really consists of one problem—acute thrombosis: superficial phlebitis in the superficial system and deep venous thrombosis (DVT) in the deep system. The three main risk factors for the spontaneous development of thrombosis were recognized by Rudolph Virchow well over 100 years ago. "Virchow's triad" is stasis, hypercoagulability, and endothelial injury. These three components still describe the vast majority of those at increased risk.

Superficial Phlebitis

Superficial phlebitis is the acute thrombosis of a superficial vein. There is a sterile inflammatory response to the clot and, typically, these patients complain of a discrete area of pain, redness, and warmth. On physical examination, the clot-filled vein (the cord) can usually be felt.

The cord is tender, warm, and erythematous. There is rarely extremity swelling. This diagnosis is made clinically.

Superficial phlebitis is a surprisingly safe process. These patients almost never embolize from the superficial system and, unless the phlebitis is high in the thigh, the clot rarely extends into the deep system. Associated deep thrombus is rare. Because of these facts, patients with routine su-

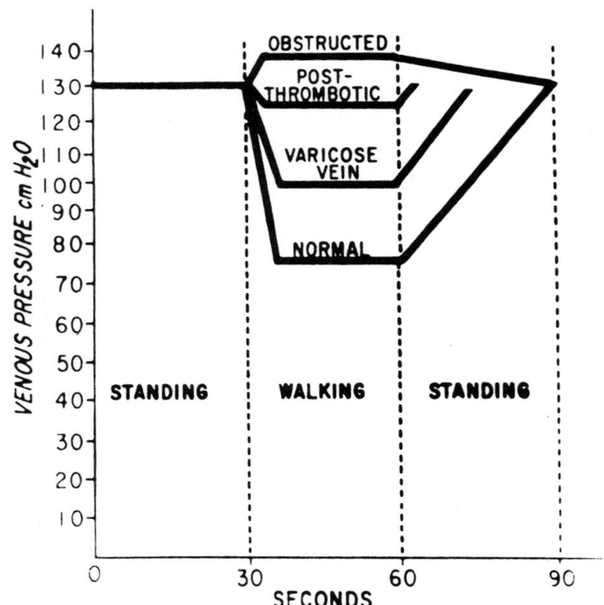

Figure 31–35. Venous pressure responses to exercise. Normally, there is a rapid drop in venous pressure because of the musculovenous pump. Increasingly severe valvular insufficiency progressively decreases this response. If there is venous occlusion, the pressures may even rise with exercise. *(Used with permission from Bergan & Kistner, [1992].)*

perficial phlebitis do not need to be anticoagulated. They are treated symptomatically with nonsteroidal antiinflammatory agents (NSAIDs) and wraps. Untreated, the pain usually disappears in 10-14 days. With high doses of NSAIDs, the symptoms are usually gone in 24 to 36 hours.

Deep Venous Thrombosis

Unfortunately, DVT is not so benign a process as superficial phlebitis. It is a dangerous entity with potentially life-threatening complications and a high probability of chronic morbidity.

Typically, these patients present with complaints of lower extremity pain and swelling. The location of the aching discomfort and the degree of swelling are dependent upon the extent and location of the clot. There are no specific, diagnostic physical findings. Legs with DVTs are variably swollen and inconsistently tender. Homan's sign (calf pain with dorsiflexion of the foot) has low specificity. Because of these and the fact that many swollen, painful legs have causes other than venous disease, the ability to accurately make the diagnosis of DVT on history and physical examination alone is poor. If DVT is being considered, other diagnostic studies are needed to reliably make the diagnosis. In 1997, the most widely used study is ultrasound, either a duplex or a color-flow Doppler study. In the hands of a skilled technologist, these examinations have a high level of sensitivity and specificity for both occlusive and nonocclusive thrombus in the common femoral, superficial femoral, profunda femoris, and popliteal veins. The accuracy decreases in the tibial veins because of the normal anatomic variability of these structures. If the examiner has a very high level of suspicion of clot at the calf level, or does not believe a negative ultrasound study, an ascending venogram (Fig. 31–36) can be performed. Although rarely ordered now, it remains the gold standard for the diagnosis of DVT.

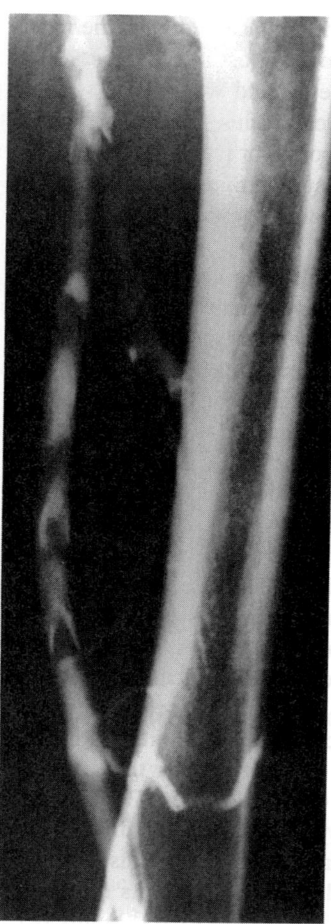

Figure 31–36. Normal ascending venogram. Note the valves seen in the superficial femoral vein.

The natural history of an acute DVT has been studied extensively over the last fifteen years, since ultrasound technology has given us a noninvasive way to do so. When the clot first forms in the deep system, it commonly obstructs the vein, which increases the venous pressures and produces edema.

The risk of pulmonary embolus, the most feared early complication, is greatest in the first 4 to 5 days after the development of the thrombus. During this window of risk, the clot is relatively friable and not very adherent to the vein wall. It is not known what percentage of DVTs embolize, but it is estimated that annually in the United States, more than 50,000 deaths are associated with acute pulmonary emboli. After 5 days, the organization of the thrombus is such that the clot rarely fragments and has become adherent to the vein wall, resulting in a rapid decrease in the rate of embolization. Extension of the clot is common unless the patient is anticoagulated.

Over the same five days, collateral venous channels increase in size and the degree of swelling decreases. Often the leg appears normal when the patient first arises in the morning, but soon swells with dependency and exercise. Over time, most of the clots lyse. Six months after an acute DVT, approximately 80% have recanalized (Johnson, Marryo, Bergelin et al., 1996); however, the veins are not normal. The venous channels are small, noncompliant, and often partially occluded by synechiae or bands of scar. Usually the valves have been destroyed. This leaves a vein that is very different than the vessel before the DVT. After DVT, the vein either remains occluded or else becomes a relatively high-resistant system without valves. Either way, there are frequently high venous pressures that can result in the chronic problems of postphlebitic syndrome. Because of these sobering facts, intense efforts are made to avoid the development of DVT. This is especially true for surgical inpatients where often all three components of "Virchow's triad" (stasis, hypercoagulability, and endothelial injury) exist simultaneously.

DVT prophylaxis focuses on avoidance of stasis and hypercoagulability. There have been a number of approaches

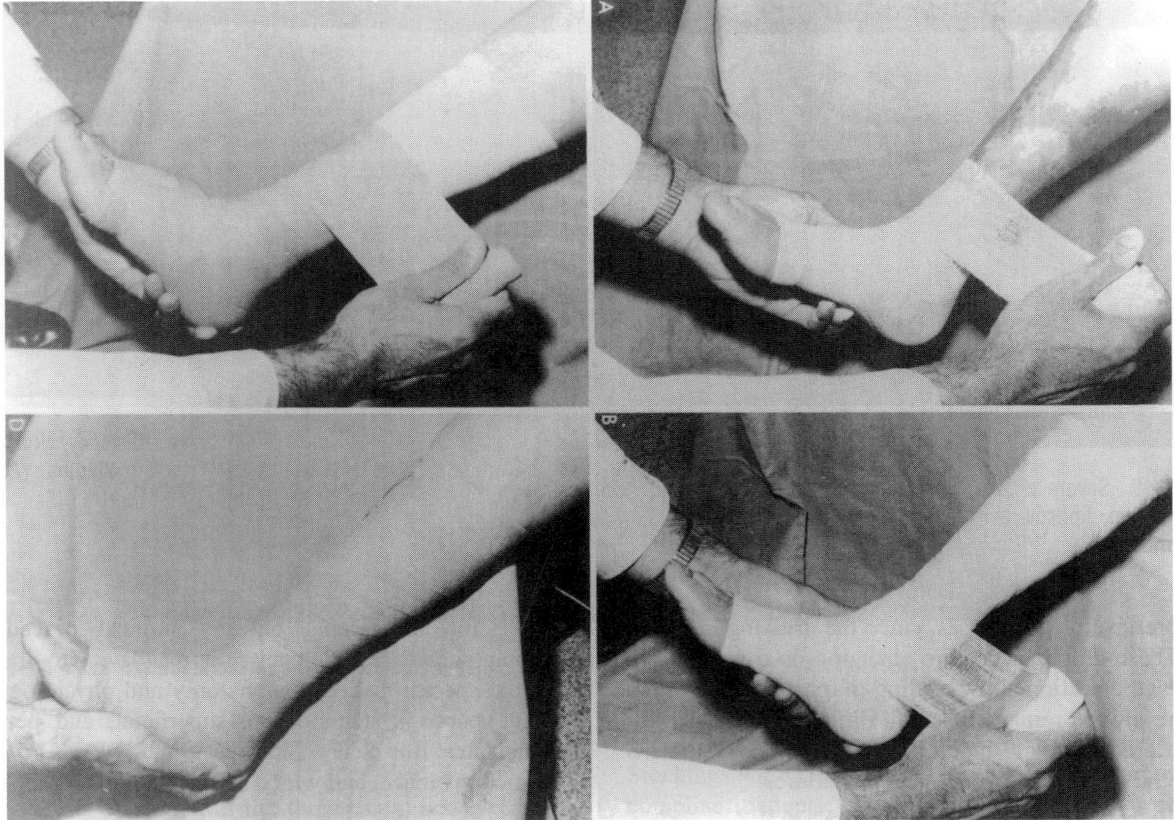

Figure 31–43. Application of Unna boot. The foot and leg are wrapped in three layers: the zinc oxide impregnated wrap, a gauze wrap, and then an elastic wrap. *(Used with permission from Rutherford, [1984].)*

cal procedure can be recommended. If the deep system is normal, the superficial veins and perforators may be ligated and/or removed, with a high expectation of an excellent result. A recent British study indicted that this is a much more common anatomic situation than previously suspected, occurring in approximately 25% of their patients who had venous stasis ulcers (Grabes, Wakely, Nyamekye et al., 1996).

Chronic deep venous occlusive disease can be potentially bypassed if the occlusion is not too extensive (Fig. 31–44). If the deep veins are incompetent, either a valve reconstruction (Fig. 31–45) or a valve translocation from an axillary vein to popliteal vein (Fig. 31–46) may be tried.

There are surgical groups with a special interest in this sort of venous surgery who report excellent long-term results (Raju, 1983), but most surgeons do not have this degree of experience nor so encouraging results.

▶ LYMPHATIC DISEASE

Disorders of the lymphatic system present difficult clinical problems; however, aggressive palliative treatment can be very rewarding, especially if the therapy is instituted early in the natural history of the process.

Anatomically, the lymphatics are divided into three components: terminal, or initial, lymphatics; collecting ducts; and lymph nodes. The terminal lymphatics are very much like capillaries, but with either absent or minimally developed basement membranes. These coalesce into collecting ducts that in turn empty into regional lymph nodes. From there, lymph flows into other lymphatics and ultimately empties into the subclavian veins. In the lower extremities, there are two lymph systems: a superficial and a deep. Unlike the venous system, there are no lymphatic perforators. As in the veins, lower extremity lymphatics have valves.

The physiologic role of the lymphatics is primarily to clear macromolecular proteins and fluid from the interstitial space. Lymph progresses along the lymph channels in the deep system because of a musculolymphatic pump similar to the mechanism of venous return. The lymphatic vessels also have an intrinsic contractile mechanism that is not seen in the venous system.

When the lymphatic system is impaired and unable to clear the extremity of interstitial protein and fluid, lym-

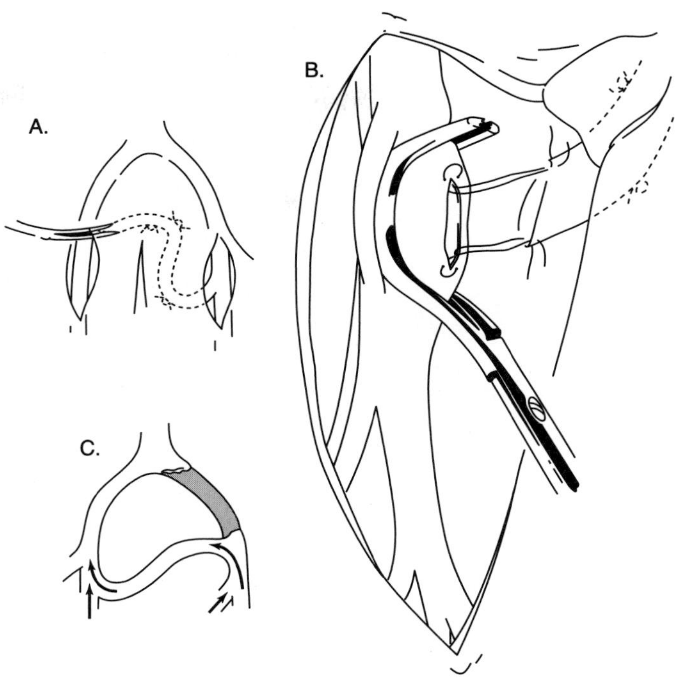

Figure 31–44. A venous femoral-femoral bypass using the ipsilateral greater saphenous vein to improve outflow from a leg with a chronic iliac vein occlusion.

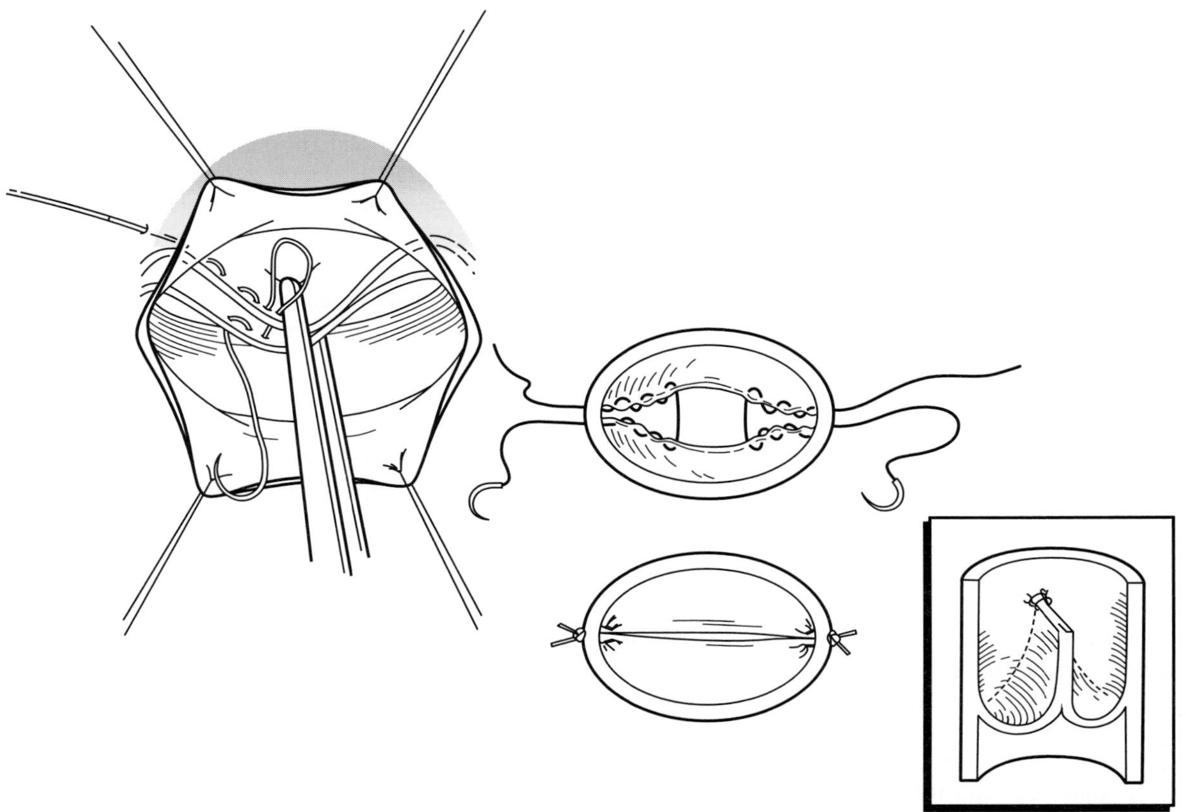

Figure 31–45. Valve reconstruction to render an incompetent valve competent. *(Used with permission from Bergan & Kistner, [1992].)*

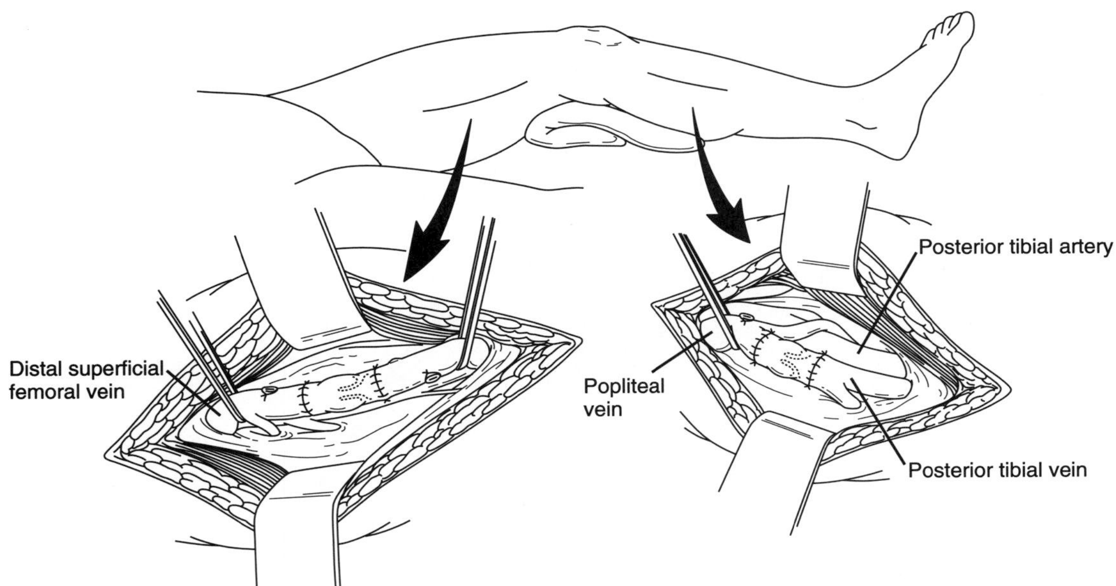

Figure 31–46. Valve translocation from the axillary vein to either the above-knee popliteal vein or the venous tibioperoneal confluence. *(Used with permission from Bergan & Kistner, [1992].)*

phedema develops. Typically the patient gives a history of gradually progressive edema that is initially painless and soft. In the lower extremity, it tends to not resolve with elevation overnight, as edema secondary to venous disease usually does, but instead resolves only after 3 or 4 days of elevation. Because of the high protein content in the interstitial fluid, over time the edema becomes brawny with increasing fibrosis and inflammation. This fluid is a potentially rich culture medium, so these patients often develop cellulitis and lymphangitis.

Lymphedema is subdivided into a primary and a secondary process, depending upon the etiology. Primary lymphedema is further divided into three separate diseases, depending upon the age of onset of the edema. Congenital lymphedema is quite unusual and presents at birth. Lymphedema praecox is by far the most common form of primary lymphedema. It typically appears during adolescence, most often in girls. Lymphedema tarda usually doesn't appear until the fourth decade. Again, it is predominantly seen in women and also usually involves only one lower extremity.

The anatomic abnormality is usually a hypoplastic proximal lymphatic system. It is not known why patients with lymphedema praecox or tarda do not develop edema until relatively late in life. Less than 10% of these patients have what is known as hyperplastic lymphedema. These patients appear to have distal lymphatics that don't empty centrally. The lymphatics are large, tortuous, and varicocele-like, as compared with the small, underdeveloped, or absent lymphatics in the hypoplastic patients, which make up the vast majority.

Secondary lymphedema occurs because of some injury to the lymphatic system. The precipitating event may be an infection (examples are filaria and tuberculosis), a malignant infiltration, a surgical resection, or fibrosis secondary to irradiation. Patients with an acquired lymphedema essentially always have normal distal lymphatics.

The diagnosis of lymphedema can almost always be made by history and physical examination alone. The keys are the gradual onset and persistence in primary lymphedema and the precipitating event in secondary lymphedema. If the diagnosis is questioned after other causes of edema have been ruled out, a definite diagnosis can be made using lymphoscintigraphy, a nuclear medical study in which the rate of lymphatic isotope clearance is measured (Browse, 1986).

Treatment remains largely nonsurgical. Once the diagnosis has been made, the therapeutic goals are to avoid episodes of cellulitis and to control swelling. Patients with lymphedema tend to have recurring episodes of cellulitis that frequently lead to fibrosis of the remaining lymphatics and worsening of the underlying process. Because of this, it is mandatory to minimize the frequency and severity of these infectious episodes.

Cutaneous hygiene cannot be emphasized enough, and many patients are given prescriptions for appropriate antistaphylococcus and antistreptococcal antibiotics, with instructions to begin taking the drug as soon as the first signs of infection appear.

The treatment for the edema is extrinsic compression: elastic compression stockings, mechanical pneumatic pumps (Fig. 31–47) and, most recently, strapped Velcro boots (Fig.

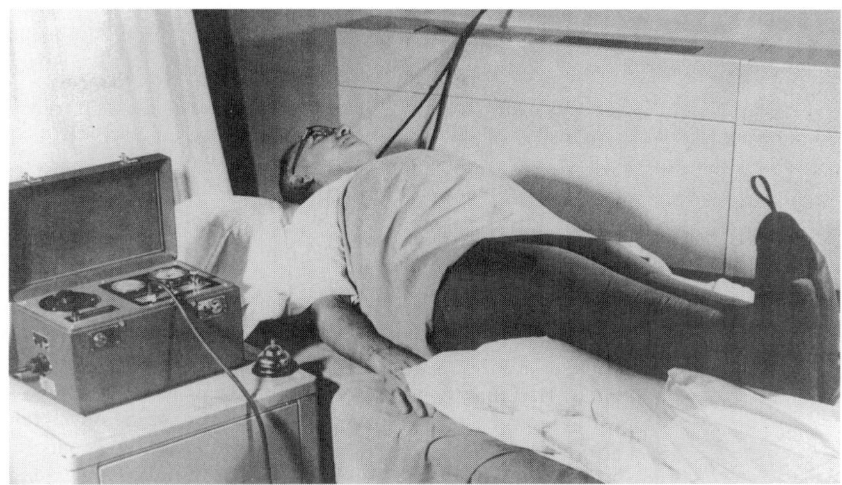

Figure 31–47. Patient using pneumatic compression pump.

31–48). The sooner the therapy is begun, the better. The goal is to minimize interstitial fluid and protein, and, hopefully, fibrosis. This therapy requires perseverance for the patient's lifetime.

Unfortunately, surgical therapy has limited effect. Generally, efforts to reconstruct the lymphatic system by constructing lymphovenous or lympholymphatic anastomoses or shunts have not been successful. When they have worked, the patients have had either hyperplastic lymphedema or normal distal lymphatics. When patients present with grossly enlarged legs that do not respond to nonoperative therapy, staged excisional procedures to remove skin and subcutaneous tissue may palliate the patient (Serville, 1987). Hopefully, with improved pneumatic compression devices and early treatment, these sorts of end-stage extremities will become rare.

In summary, lymphedema is a process that is either congenital or acquired. Therapy is largely palliative and nonsurgical, but with persistence, long-term control may be obtained.

Acknowledgment: Special thanks to Brooke Roberts and Morris Kerstein for their helpful assistance and review, and to Rebecca Shuttleworth for her editorial assistance.

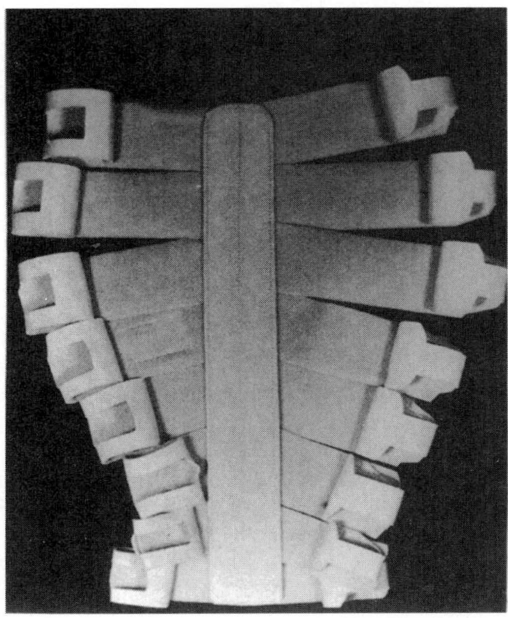

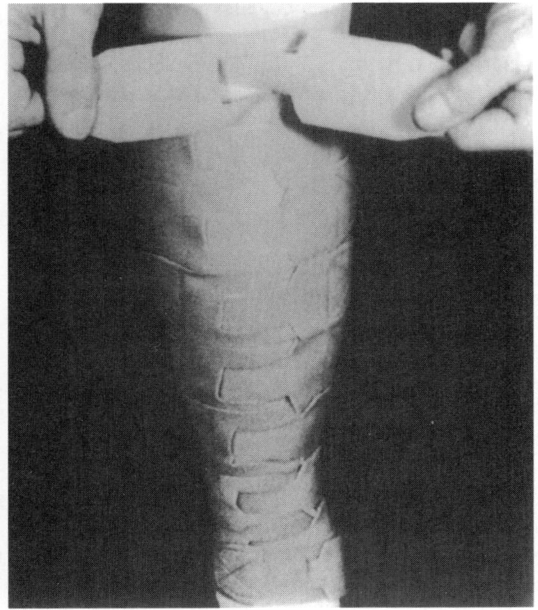

Figure 31–48. Strapped Velcro boot for chronic venous and lymphatic disease.

REFERENCES

Abbott, W. M., Maloney, R. D., McCabe, C. C., Lee, C. F., & Wirthlin, L. S. (1982). Arterial emboli: A 44-year prospective. *American Journal of Surgery, 143,* 460–464.

Bergen, J. J. & Kistner, R. L. (1992). *Atlas of venous surgery.* Philadelphia: W. B. Saunders.

Bergan, J. J., Veith, F. J., Bernhard, V. M., et al. (1982). Randomization of autologous vein and polytetrafluoroethylene grafts in femoral–distal reconstruction. *Surgery, 92,* 921–930.

Blum, V., Krumme, B., Flugel, P., et al. (1997). Treatment of ostial renal artery stenosis with vascular endoprostheses after unsuccessful balloon angioplasty. *New England Journal of Medicine, 336,* 459–465.

Bonelli, F. S., McKusick, M. A., Textor, S. C., et al. (1995). Renal artery angioplasty: Technical results and clinical outcome in 320 patients. *Mayo Clinic Proceedings, 70,* 1041–1052.

Bousser, M. D., et al. (1983). AICLA controlled trial of aspirin and dypyridamole in the secondary prevention of arteriothrombotic cerebral ischemia. *Stroke, 14,* 5–14.

Boyd, A. M. (1960). The natural course of atherosclerosis of the lower extremity. *Angiology, 11,* 10–14.

Brandt, L. J. & Boley, S. J. (1991). Nonocclusive mesenteric ischemia. *Annual Review of Medicine, 42,* 107–117.

Brewster, D. C., et al. (1975). Angiography in the management of aneurysms of the abdominal aorta. Its value and safety. *New England Journal of Medicine, 292,* 822–825.

Brewster, D. C. & Darling, R. C. (1978). Optimal methods of aortoiliac reconstruction. *Surgery, 84,* 739–748.

Browse, N. L. (1986). The diagnosis and treatment of primary lymphedema. *Journal of Vascular Surgery, 3,* 181–184.

Buchwald, H., Matts, J. P., Fitch L. L., et al. (1992). Changes in sequential coronary arteriograms and subsequent coronary events. Surgical control of the hyperlipidemia (POSCH) group. *Journal of the American Medical Association, 286,* 1429.33.

Chambers, B. R. & Norris, J. W. (1986). Outcome in patients with asymptomatic neck bruits. *New England Journal of Medicine, 315,* 860–865.

Chesebro, J. H., Foster, V., Elvback, L. R., et al. (1984). Effect of dipyrididamole and aspirin on late vein graft patency after coronary bypass operation. *New England Journal of Medicine, 310,* 209–214.

Crawford, E. S. (1991). Ruptured abdominal aortic aneurysm: An editorial. *Journal of Vascular Surgery, 13,* 348–350.

Crawford, E. S., Saleh, S. A., Babb III, J. W., et al. (1981). Infrarenal abdomimal aortic aneurysm: Factors influencing survival after operation performed over a 25-Year period. *Annals of Surgery, 193,* 699–709.

Dean, R. H. (1993). Renovascular hypertension. In W. S. Moore (Ed.), *Vascular Surgery.* Philadelphia: W. B. Saunders.

Dean, R. H., Kieffer, R. W., Smith, B. M., et al. (1981). Renovascular hypertension: Anatomic and renal function changes during drug therapy. *Archives of Surgery, 116,* 1408–1415.

Dobrin, P. B., Baker, W. H., & Gley, W. C. (1984). Elastolytic and collagenolytic studies of arteries: Implications for the mechanical properties of aneurysms. *Archives of Surgery, 119,* 405–409.

Dotter, C. T. & Judkins, M. P. (1964). Transluminal treatment of atherosclerotic obstruction. Description of a new technic and a preliminary report of its Application [classical article]. *Radiology,* 904–920.

Eastcott, H. H. (1969). *Arterial surgery.* Philadelphia: Lippincott-Raven.

Edelman, R. R., et. al. (1989). Projection arteriography and venography: Initial clinical results with MR. *Radiology, 172,* 351–357.

European Carotid Surgery Trialists' Collaborative Group. (1991). MRC European carotid surgery trial: Interim results for patients with severe (70-99%) or with mild (0-29%) carotid stenosis. *Lancet, 337,* 1235–1243.

Executive Committee for the Asymptomatic Carotid Atherosclerosis Study. (1995). Endarterectomy for asymptomatic carotid artery stenosis. *Journal of the American Medical Association, 273,* 1421–1428.

Fisher, C. M. (1951). Occlusion of the internal carotid artery. *Archives of Neurology and Psychiatry, 65,* 346–377.

Ganda, O. P. (1984). Pathogenesis of accelerated atherosclerosis in diabetes. In G. P. Kozak, C. S. Hoan, J. L. Rowbotham, et el. (Eds.), *Management of Diabetic Foot Problems. Joslin Clinic and New England Deaconess Hospital.* Philadelphia: W. B. Saunders.

Gaspar, M. R. (1982). Role of arteriography in the evaluation of arotic aneurysms. The case against. In J. J. Bergan and J. S. T. Yao (Eds.), *Aneurysms: Diagnosis and Treatment.* New York: Grune and Stratton.

Grabs, A. J., Wakely, M. C., Nyamekye, I., et al. (1996). Color duplex ultrasonography in the rational management of chronic venous leg ulcers. *British Journal of Surgery, 83,* 1380–1382.

Gruntzig, A. & Hopf, H. (1974). Perkutane rekanalization chronischer arterieller verschlusse mit einen neven dilatationskatheter. *Dtsch. Med. Wochenschrift 99,* 2502–2510.

Harris, E. J., Taylor, L. M., McConnell, B. D., et al. (1990). Clinical results of axillobifemoral bypass using externally supported polytetracluoroethylene. *Journal of Vascular Surgery, 12,* 416–421.

Harward, T. R. S., Green, D., Bergan, J. J., et al. (1989). Mesenteric venous thrombosis. *Journal of Vascular Surgery, 9,* 328–333.

Hass, W. K., Easton, D., Adams, Jr., M. P. et al. (1989). A randomized trial comparing ticlopidine hydrochloride with aspirin for the prevention of stroke in high risk patients. *New England Journal of Medicine, 321,* 501–507.

Hiatt, J. C. G., Barker, W. F., Machleder, H. I., et al. (1984). Determinants of failure in the treatment of ruptured abdominal aortic aneurysms. *Archives of Surgery, 119,* 1264–1268.

Hollier, L. H., Taylor, L. M., & Ochsner, J. (1992). Recommended indications for operative treatment of abdominal aaortic aneurysms. *Journal of Vascular Surgery, 15,* 1046–1056.

Imparato, A. M. & Kim, G. E. (1975). Intermittent claudication: Its natural course. *Surgery, 78,* 795–799.

Johnson, B. F., Marryo, R. A., Bergelin, R. O., et al. (1996). The site of residual abnormalities in the leg veins in long-term follow-up after deep vein thrombosis and their relationship to the development of the post-thrombotic syndrome. *International Angiology, 15,* 14–19.

Kakan, V. V. & Lorenz, D. (1985). Hemodynamic and clinical assessment after therapy for deep venous thrombosis. A prospective study. *American Journal of Surgery, 140,* 54–60.

Kendrick J., Thompson, B. W., Pearl, R. C. et al. (1981). Arterial embolectomy in the leg. Results in a referral hospital. *American Journal of Surgery, 142,* 739–743.

Leather, R. P., Shah, D. M., Chang, B. B., et al. (1988). Resurrection of the in-situ vein bypass. 1000 cases later. *Annals of Surgery, 208,* 435–442.

Lilly, M. P., Flinn, W. R., McCarthy III, W. J., et al. (1988). The effect of distal arterial anatomy on the success of popliteal aneurysm repair. *Journal of Vascular Surgery, 7,* 653–660.

Mayberg, M. R., Wilson, S. E., Yatsu, F., et al. (1991). Carotid endarterectomy and prevention of cerebral ischemia in symptomatic carotid stenosis. Veterans Affairs cooperative studies program 309 trialist group. *Journal of American Medical Association, 266,* 3332–3333.

McNamara, T. O., Bomberger, R. A., Merchant, R. E., et al. (1989). *Intra-Arterial Urokinase Therapy for Acutely Ischemic Limbs.* Paper presented at the Fourth Annual Meeting of the Western Vascular Society, Kanai, Hawaii, June 18–22, 1989.

Moore, W. S. (1986). *Vascular surgery,* (2nd ed.). New York: Grune & Stratton.

Moore, W. S. (1993). *Vascular surgery,* (4th ed.). Philadelphia: W. B. Saunders.

Mulherin, J. L. & Edwards, W. H. (1980). Improved survival after ruptured abdominal aortic aneurysm. *Southern Medical Journal, 73,* 986–989.

North American Symptomatic Carotid Endarterectomy Trial Collaborators. (1991). Beneficial effect of carotid endarterectomy in symptomatic patients with high-grade carotid stenosis. *New England Journal of Medicine, 325,* 445–453.

Patient Education Committee. (1990). *Lower Extremity Arterial Disease.* The Society of Vascular Nursing.

Patient Education Committee. (1992). *Venous Disease.* The Society of Vascular Nursing.

Perochi, J. C., Pelman, J. C. & Barone, H. D. (1991). Transfemoral intraluminal graft implantation for abodminal aortic aneurysms. *Annals of Vascular Surgery, 5,* 491–499.

Porter, J. M., Seaman, A. J., Common, H. H. et al. (1975). Comparison of heparin and stretptokinase in treatment of venous thrombosis. *American Surgeon, 41,* 511–519.

Raju, S. (1983). Venous insufficiency of the lower limb and stasis ulceration: Changing concepts and management. *Annals of Surgery, 97* (6), 688–697.

Rob C. (1976). *Operative surgery.* (3rd ed.). London: Butterworth Heinemann.

Roberts, B. & Ring, E. J. (1982). Current status of percutaneous transluminal angiolasty. *Surgical Clinics of North America, 62,* 357–372.

Roederer, G. O., Langlois, Y. E., Jager, K. A., et al. (1984). The natural history of carotid artery disease in asymptomatic patients with cervical bruits. *Stroke, 15,* 605–613.

Ross, R. (1986). The pathogenesis of atherosclerosis—an update. *New England Journal of Medicine, 314,* 488–500.

Rutherford, R. B. (1984). *Vascular surgery* (2nd ed.). Philadelphia: W. B. Saunders.

Rutherford, R. B., Jones, D. N., Bergenty, S. E., et al. (1984). The efficacy of dextran 40 in preventing early postoperative thrombosis following difficult lower extremity bypass. *Journal of Vascular Surgery, 1,* 765–773.

Sacco, R. L., Wolf, P. A., Kannel, W. B., & McNamara, P. M. (1982). Survival and recurrence following stroke: The Framingham study. *Stroke, 13,* 290–295.

Sandok, B. A., Troutmann, J. C., Ramirez-Lossepas, M., et al. (1974). Clinical-angiographic correlations in amaurosis fugax. *American Journal of Ophthalmology, 78,* 137–142.

Schiebler, M. L., Listerud, J., Baum, R. A., Carpenter, J., Weigele, J., Holland, G., Schnall, M. D., Owen, R. S., Cope, C., Pentecost, M., et. al. (1993). Magnetic resonance imaging arteriography of the pelvis and lower extremities. *Magnetic Resonance Quarterly, 9*(3), 152–187.

Servelle, M. (1987). Surgical treatment of lymphedema: A report on 652 cases. *Surgery, 101,* 484–495.

Szilagyi, D. E., Smith, R. F., DeRusso, F. J., et. al. (1966). Contribution of the abdominal aortic aneurysmectomy to prolongation of life. *Annals of Surgery, 164,* 678–689.

Taylor, L. M., Edward, J. M., & Pater, J. M. (1990). Present status of reversed vein bypass: Five-year results of a modem series. *Journal of Vascular Surgery, 11,* 207–215.

Taylor, Jr., L. M. & Porter, J. M. (1986). Drug treatment of claudication: Vasodilators, hemorrheologic agents, and anti-serotonin drugs. *Journal of Vascular Surgery, 3,* 374–381.

Tegtmayer, C. J., Kellum, D., & Ayers, C. (1984). Percutaneous transluminal angioplasty of the renal artery. Results and long-term follow-up. *Radiology, 153,* 77–84.

The Canadian Cooperative Study Group. (1978). A randomized trial of aspirin and sulfinpyrazone in threatened strokes. *New England Journal of Medicine, 299,* 53–59, 77–84, 153.

The Diabetes Control and Complications Trial Research Group. (1993). The effect of intensive treatment of diabetes on the development and progression of long-term complications in insulin-dependent diabetes mellitus. *New England Journal of Medicine, 329,* 977–986.

Whisnant, J. P., Matsumoto, M., & Elveback, L. R. (1973). The effects of anticoagulant therapy on the prognosis of patients with transient cerebral ischemic attacks in a community: Rochester, Minnesota 1955-1969. *Mayo Clinic Proceedings, 48,* 844–848.

Wilson, C., Gupta, R., Gilmour, D. G., et al. (1987). Acute superior mesenteric ischemia. *British Journal of Surgery, 74,* 279–281.

Wilson, S. E., Wolf, G. L., Cross, A. P., et al. (1989). Percutaneous transluminal angioplasty versus operation for peripheral arteriosclerosis. *Journal of Vascular Surgery, 9,* 1–8.

Yao, J. S. T. & Bergan, J. J. (1990). Operative procedures in visceral ischemia. In J. J. Bergan & J. S. T. Yao (Eds.), *Techniques in Arterial Surgery.* Philadelphia: W. B. Saunders.

32

Coronary Artery Disease

C. Beth Staudenmayer
Margaret A. O'Connell
Mary Malitas
Christine Alberts

Cardiovascular disease is the leading cause of morbidity and mortality in the United States since the early 1900s. The term itself conjures up thoughts of hypertension, myocardial infarction, stroke, even death. Cardiovascular disease prevalence statistics are alarming: 58,200,000 Americans, about one in five, have some form of cardiovascular disease (Heart and Stroke Statistical Update, 1998). Major cardiovascular diseases include coronary artery disease (CAD), high blood pressure, stroke, and rheumatic heart disease. For this portion of the text the area of concentration will be focused on factual content of coronary heart disease and its risk factors.

The majority of coronary heart disease is due to atherosclerotic changes within the coronary vessels. Atherosclerosis or loosely coined "hardening of the arteries" is an age-related degenerative disease, increasing prevalence with advancing age. Statistics published by the American Heart Association in 1997 confirms the increased rate of hospital admissions and death with the aging process (Heart and Stroke Statistical Update, 1997).

Atherosclerosis is due to intimal injury caused by deposits of fatty substances such as cholesterol, calcium, fibrin, and cellular waste products. This infiltration of byproducts causes a buildup on the cell walls and lining leading to an obstruction of flow within the coronary artery. Atheromatous changes, calcifications, and thrombus formation represent the endothelial injury responsible for the pathogenesis of coronary heart disease (Cheitlin, Sokolow, & McIlroy, 1993). The resulting plaque formation causes partial or complete obstruction. Over time, this obstruction inhibits proper myocardial oxygenation resulting in ischemia to the affected vessel and surrounding heart muscle.

Atherosclerotic disease of the coronary arteries is a slow, progressive process causing connective tissue proliferation within the intima of the coronary arteries (Effat, 1995). The major risk factors for atherosclerosis include high-plasma low-density lipoproteins (LDL), low-plasma high-density lipoproteins (HDL), cigarette smoking, diabetes mellitus, and hypertension. Constant exposure to these risk factors are thought to cause vascular endothelial dysfunction and an abnormal interaction with blood monocytes and platelets (Selwyn & Braunwald, 1994).

The normal vascular endothelium lines the luminal surface of the coronary arteries. It is a physiologically active organ that is important in regulating vascular tone as well as preserving the integrity of the lumen surface. Endothelial factors that regulate coronary artery vasomotion include: (1) endothelium derived relaxing factor (EDRF); (2) prostacyclin, also a vasodilator; and (3) thromboxane A2 and endothelin-vasoconstrictors. All of these endothelial-regulating factors work together to maintain vascular tone. EDRF and prostacyclin are also potent and synergistic inhibitors of platelet aggregation and adhesion. In addition, they inhibit neutrophil and monocyte adherence to the vascular wall, and prevent an early step in the formation of atherosclerotic plaque (Abrams, 1997).

Dysfunction of the endothelium has been described as three distinct but parallel processes. The increased adhesion of macrophages, platelets, and leukocytes to endothelial cells activated by cardiac risk factors leads to the release of growth factors and the inflammatory mediators. There is also local accumulation of lipids and failure to inhibit migration and proliferation of smooth muscle cells. This sequence of events leads to plaque formation and stenosis. The paradoxical vasoconstrictive response to normally vasodilating agents is the second distinct process. Multiple research trials have been able to document the failure of normal vasodilators and the development of constrictor responses to acetylcholine and many other substances. Thrombosis is the third process that occurs and results in the increased adhesion of platelets and macrophages to the endothelium, and the failure of normal local anticoagulant functions. With disease progression, there are breaks in the endothelial layer and plaque fracture with exposure of thrombogenic surfaces that initiate the adhesion and aggregation of platelets. This results in a highly thrombogenic surface with insufficient thrombolytic activity to prevent the collection of platelets, thrombin, fibrinogen, and fibrin from clot formation (Selwyn, Yeung, Ryan, et al., 1992).

Burke, Farb, Malcom, Malcom, et al., (1997) describe two mechanisms of acute coronary thrombosis. Plaque rupture, the most frequent cause, has been implicated in the episodic progression of coronary stenosis and is often associated with unstable angina. Atherosclerotic plaques that are vulnerable to rupture have a dense infiltrate of macrophages and lymphocytes within a fibrous cap that overlies a crescentic acellular mass of lipids. Another mechanism, plaque erosion, has recently been identified as an important cause of sudden coronary death. Eroded plaques differ from ruptured plaques in that they have a base rich in smooth muscle cells and proteoglycans.

Coronary artery disease is also affected by a multitude of factors: those that are inherent to our being and those that can be altered by lifestyle modification.

Major risk factors in the development of atherosclerosis are family history, age, gender, increased cholesterol, hypertension, diabetes, and smoking history. Other factors when seen concomitant to those just listed—such as physical inactivity, poor dietary regimen, and obesity—increase the likelihood of a coronary event.

▶ CORONARY RISK FACTORS

Family History

Genetic predisposition is a nonmodifiable risk factor that represents two times the risk of coronary events among first-degree relatives, all other risk factors excluded (Cheitlin et al., 1993). A patient has a positive family history if a primary relative develops CAD before the age of 50 years.

Age/Sex

Based on 1995 data from the American Heart Association, male deaths related to coronary heart disease represent 50.9%; female deaths, 49.1%. Some authorities surmise that the pathogenesis of coronary heart disease is in young adulthood and continues as a progression through the life cycle. Women above the age of 55, particularly those who are postmenopausal, and men above the age of 45 are at risk of CAD.

Diabetes Mellitus

This condition has been identified as an independent cardiac risk and presents increased risk in combination with other factors. More than 80% of persons with diabetes die from some form of heart or blood vessel disease (Heart and Stroke Statistical Update, 1998). Diabetes, therefore, constitutes a substantial risk for CAD.

Hypertension

High blood pressure causes an increased workload on the heart that directly affects coronary vasculature. The intimal linings of the arteries are altered/injured due to these increased forces. It is well documented in the Framingham Heart Study that the development of coronary heart disease rose in the setting of elevated systolic or diastolic pressure in middle-aged and elderly persons (Braunwald, 1992). Hypertension remains a risk factor for CAD even if the blood pressure is well-controlled.

Hypercholesterolemia

High dietary intake of cholesterol and saturated fats results in abnormal HDL-C/LDL-C ratios as well as elevated total cholesterol level. Elevated cholesterol levels in the blood affect atherosclerosis by increasing fatty lipid deposits into the cell lining. Levine, Keaney, & Vita (1995) reviewed epidemiological and observational studies over the past 60 years that demonstrated a direct correlation between baseline serum cholesterol levels and mortality from coronary heart disease. An increased risk was shown with progressively higher cholesterol levels. Cardiac events also correlated with elevated cholesterol levels in patients with established CAD.

Interestingly, while an elevated LDL-C represents a positive risk factor for CAD, a high HDL-C represents a negative risk factor. That is, a high HDL-C "cancels out" an elevated LDL-C as another independent risk factor (e.g., family history, age/sex).

Smoking

Current estimates reveal that almost 26 million American men and over 23 million American women are smokers, thereby increasing their risk of CAD (Heart and Stroke Statistics Update, 1998). Smoking contributes to a narrowing of small myocardial arteries with intimal thickening, endothelial injury, adherence of platelets, smooth muscle cell proliferation, and growth of thrombus. These factors are associated with the pathogenesis of atherosclerosis and are all enhanced by smoking. An exaggeration of thrombus development in the coronary arteries of smokers is consistent with the epidemiologic finding that smokers have an increased risk of unstable angina, myocardial infarction, and sudden death (Jonas, Oakes, Ockene, & Hennekens, 1992).

Smoking also adversely affects other risk factors associated with coronary heart. HDL-C/LDL-C levels in the blood are altered due to the effects of smoking. Hypertension is prevalent among smokers due to the vasoconstrictive effects on coronary vasculature.

Physical Inactivity

Sedentary lifestyle increases the risk of CAD by altering or lowering HDL-C levels in the blood, increasing blood pressure, and increasing the risk of angina by decreasing the pumping efficiency of the heart. There is also increased risk of acute thrombus related to clot formation, and fatal arrhythmias due to increased sensitivity of myocardium to circulating catecholamines (Blair, Powell, Bazzarre, et al., 1993).

It is estimated that 56% of men and 62% of women fail to engage in regular physical activity, and 25% of men and 30% of women perform no leisure-time physical activity (Blair et al., 1993). In a statement prepared by Bijnen, Casperson, and Mosterd (1994), physical inactivity is listed as an important risk factor for developing CAD.

Obesity

Based on data from the National Center for Health Statistic (NCHS) from NHANES III Survey (1988-1994), over 65 million American adults—women greater than men—exceed the ideal weight range defined by United States dietary guidance council, an increase of over 40% from previous data from the early 1960s (Heart and Stroke Statistical Update, 1998). It is alarming that the prevalence of overweight persons in the United States continues to rise, especially among younger generations.

Change in body weight over time is associated with changes in blood pressure. It is estimated that 60% of hypertensive people are more than 20% overweight (Chait, Brunzell, Denke, et al., 1993). Weight reduction is an important lifestyle modification for overweight hypertensive people. Obesity is also associated with other coronary heart disease risk factors including elevated total serum cholesterol levels, decreased HDL levels, and diabetes mellitus.

Management of Coronary Risk Factors

Individually, each risk factor plays an enormous role in the development of atherosclerotic coronary heart disease. The cumulative effect of multiple risk factors is directly related to the incidence of cardiovascular events. It is important to realize that while family history/genetic predisposition, age, and sex cannot be altered, other lifestyle changes, early identification, and modification of the risk factors previously mentioned slow the progression of coronary heart disease. The extent to which people adhere to lifestyle modification recommendation, therefore, is a widespread problem.

Multiple primary and secondary prevention studies have been performed revealing the decline in overall mortality with risk factor/lifestyle modification. Surveillance of community health, with early identification, prevention, and treatment, shows it is possible to decrease the overall rate of coronary heart disease in the United States.

The provider–patient relationship strongly impacts the patient's compliance to lifestyle modifications. Patients who have more counseling about compliance also have better follow through with recommendations suggested by their health-care provider.

Follow-up visits offer opportunities to continue to promote a healthy lifestyle. Health-care providers need to spend more time motivating patients, developing a plan, and offering reinforcement and feedback. Health-care providers need to be able to anticipate questions regarding recommended changes in lifestyle, and convey the importance of the therapy and its relationship to the patient's condition. It is the responsibility of all health-care providers to incorporate health-promotion activities such as smoking cessation and dietary management into practice.

As the twenty-first century nears, it is still quite evident that as much time needs to be spent on primary prevention and identifying ways to increase compliance to lifestyle modifications if reducing the risk of coronary heart disease is to be accomplished.

THE DIAGNOSTIC WORK-UP OF CORONARY ARTERY DISEASE

History and Physical Findings

It has been said that it is the history alone that admits patients to the coronary care unit. One of the reasons for that may be the lack of physical findings that are diagnostic of coronary artery disease. Although such findings as hypertension, S4, systolic ejection murmur, diffuse and sustained PMI (i.e., LVH), and diminished peripheral pulse amplitude may coexist in patients with CAD, none of these findings are seen exclusively in CAD. This undermines the importance of a careful history.

The first encounter with a patient may be in the setting of a routine visit or acute illness. The reason the patient is seeking medical attention is elicited through this initial encounter. Many of the details to determine the onset and progression of symptoms occur during this clinical encounter. The patient's medical history and recollection of symptoms are a key source of information, a crucial element for a complete exam.

The data obtained from a patient assists the clinician in the development of the differential diagnosis. This differential process leads to further diagnostic work-up that may be helpful in ruling out certain disease entities. The complete work-up and evaluation are done to ensure initiation of appropriate treatment.

The key points of the history for CAD involve detailed evaluation of chest pain. Onset, location, duration, characteristics, associated symptoms, aggravating factors, and relieving factors are important points to assess (Table 32–1).

Diagnostic Tests

Exercise Stress Testing

Exercise stress testing (EST) is a widely used test that provides diagnostic and prognostic information about patients with heart disease. Exercise tests are based on the principle of using a progressive physiologic stress to increase myocardial work and oxygen demand while looking for evidence of ischemia. Ischemia as defined by Braunwald and Sobel (1992) is a condition of oxygen deprivation to the myocardium related to decreased perfusion and can be manifested as angina pain, electrocardiogram (ECG) ST segment changes, arrhythmias and ventricular dysfunction, or a combination of all of these.

Most of the published data regarding diagnostic and prognostic ability of the EST are based on a method of exercise treadmill testing called the *Bruce* protocol. During the Bruce protocol a patient is exercised on a treadmill with progressively increasing incline and speed. The ECG and blood pressure are monitored continuously. The exercise protocol can be modified according to the clinical situation by lowering the rate of increase in the grade and speed. This is called the *modified Bruce* protocol. Patients unable to exercise due to physical limitations such as arthritis, amputation, deconditioning, COPD, or PVD, can undergo a pharmacological stress test with a cardiac imaging modality (Braunwald, Mark, Jones, et al., 1994).

Exercise stress testing has several advantages. First, stress testing can be primarily an office-based procedure. Second, as per the American College of Cardiology (ACC) and the American Heart Association (AHA) 1997 guidelines for exercise testing, stress tests can be performed by trained personnel supervised by appropriately trained physicians; the physician may not necessarily be a cardiologist.

Indications for an EST (Gibbons, Balady, Beasley, et al., 1997, ACC/AHA guidelines for exercise testing) include:

- Diagnosis of ischemic heart disease (IHD)
- Risk stratification postmyocardial infarction
- Management of patients with known IHD by monitoring response to medical therapy
- Monitoring response to coronary revascularization
- Determining exercise limitations before and during enrollment in a prescribed cardiac rehab program
- Evaluate functional capacity of patients with valvular disease, arrhythmias, and hypertension

When evaluating the appropriateness of an exercise stress test for a patient, one must always keep in mind the patient's pretest likelihood of having coronary artery disease (CAD) (Table 32–2). Patients with a low to intermediate likelihood for CAD should be scheduled for a stress test; patients with a high likelihood should be referred for cardiac catheterization (Braunwald et al., 1994).

Contraindications for an EST (Gibbons et al., 1997) include:

- Acute myocardial infarction (within 2 days)
- Unstable angina not previously stabilized by medical therapy
- Arrhythmias causing symptoms or hemodynamic compromise
- Severe aortic stenosis
- Symptomatic heart failure
- Pulmonary edema or pulmonary infarction
- Acute myocarditis or pericarditis
- Aortic dissection

TABLE 32–1. Important Components of the History of Present Illness in Stable and Unstable Angina and Acute Myocardial Infarction

	Stable Angina	Unstable Angina	Myocardial Infarction
Onset	Exertional	At rest	At rest or with exertion
Location	Retrosternal, arm, neck, jaw, back	Retrosternal, arm, neck, jaw, back	Retrosternal, arm, neck, jaw, back
Duration	5–20 minutes, may resolve if "worked through"	5–20 minutes	Hours
Characteristics	Heaviness, tightness, pressure, squeezing, feeling of indigestion	Heaviness, tightness, pressure, squeezing, feeling of indigestion	Heaviness, tightness, pressure, squeezing, feeling of indigestion
Associated symptoms	Dyspnea, palpitations, diaphoresis, dizziness, or lightheadedness	Dyspnea, palpitations, diaphoresis, dizziness, or lightheadedness	Dyspnea, palpitations, diaphoresis, dizziness, or lightheadedness
Aggravating factors	Exertion, cold or hot temperatures	Physical activity	Physical activity
Relieving factors	Rest, nitroglycerine	Nitroglycerine	None

TABLE 32–2. Likelihood of Significant Coronary Artery Disease in Patients with Symptoms Suggesting Unstable Angina

High likelihood (e.g., 0.85–0.99)	Intermediate likelihood (e.g., 0.15–0.84)	Low likelihood (e.g., 0.01–0.14)
Any of the following features:	*Absence of high likelihood features and any of the following:*	*Absence of high or intermediate likelihood features but may have:*
History of prior MI or sudden death or other known history of CAD	Definite angina: males < 60 or females < 70 years of age	Chest pain classified as probably not angina
Definite angina: males ≥ 60 or females ≥ 70 years of age	Probable angina: males ≥ 60 or females ≥ 70 years of age	One risk factor other than diabetes
Transient hemodynamic or ECG changes during pain	Chest pain probably not angina in patients with diabetes	T-wave flattening or inversion < 1 mm in leads with dominant R-waves
Variant angina (pain with reversible ST-segment elevation)	Chest pain probably not angina and two or three risk factors other than diabetes[a]	Normal ECG
ST-segment elevation or depression ≥ 1 mm	Extracardiac vascular disease	
Marked symmetrical T-wave inversion in multiple precordial leads	ST depression 0.05 to 1 mm	
	T-wave inversion ≥ 1 mm in leads with dominant R-waves	

[a] Coronary artery disease risk factors include diabetes, smoking, hypertension, and elevated cholesterol.

Note: Estimation of the likelihood of significant coronary artery disease is a complex, multivariable problem that cannot be fully specified in a table such as this. Therefore, the table is meant to illustrate major relationships rather than offer rigid algorithms.

From the Unstable Angina Clinical Practice Guidelines (Braunwald et al., 1994).

Endpoints to Exercise Testing

Commonly used criteria for concluding an EST (Gibbons et al., 1997) include:

- Attainment of a predetermined percentage of predicated maximum heart rate (usually 85% of age-predicted maximum heart rate)
- Patient completes all stages of exercise test protocol
- Presence of abnormal signs and symptoms such as dyspnea, wheezing, pallor, ataxia, or near-syncope
- Complaints of moderate to severe angina
- Exertional hypotension or hypertension (systolic B/P >250 mm Hg and/or diastolic B/P >115 mm Hg, a drop in systolic B/P below baseline value)
- ECG abnormalities such as ventricular arrhythmias, ST elevation or depression (>2 mm), or heart block
- Patients desire to stop

Interpretation of Test Results

Interpretation of EST results involves the evaluation of many factors including the ECG response, hemodynamic response (heart rate and blood pressure), occurrence of symptoms, and the patient's achieved exercise capacity. It is also important to note the specific exercise protocol used and why the test was stopped.

The most commonly used definition for a positive exercise test result or indication of ischemia from an ECG standpoint is horizontal or downsloping ST segment depression or elevation greater than or equal to 1 mm persisting at least 60-80 milli seconds after the end of the QRS complex (Gibbons et al., 1997).

ST segment elevation, although infrequent, can be a serious response. ST segment elevation in leads without Q waves suggests coronary artery spasm or a critical coronary occlusion corresponding to the site of ST change seen on the ECG (Gibbons et al., 1997). An ECG with Q waves from an old infarction along with ST elevation in those leads may be an indication of LV dysfunction or the presence of viable tissue in the infarcted area (Gibbons et al., 1997).

Additional findings during the EST, such as occurrence of angina and a decreased heart rate response, may indicate ischemia. It is important to record all patient symptoms because angina may present as substernal chest pressure radiating across the chest and down the arms, or it may be described as back, jaw, neck, or facial discomfort. Exercise-induced ventricular arrhythmias or inadequate blood pressure response to exercise (peak systolic B/P less than 110 mm Hg or less than 30 mm increase from resting level) may reflect extensive coronary artery disease or left ventricular dysfunction (Chaitman, 1992).

Exercise capacity is an important and complex prognostic variable that is elucidated through exercise stress testing. Exercise capacity is measured by the exercise stage achieved by the patient. Exercise capacity can be influenced by patient's age, general state of health, and presence of anxiety or depression. A decreased exercise capacity may indicate ischemia or LV dysfunction.

The most recent ACC/AHA practice guidelines for EST 1997 report a mean sensitivity of 67% and a mean specificity of 72% for the detection of CAD. Addition of an imaging modality to EST has been reported to increase the mean sensitivity for diagnosing CAD from 67% to approximately 89%, and the specificity from 72% to approximately 76% as well as providing information about LV function (Ritchie, Bateman, Bonow, et al., 1995).

The electrocardiogram obtained by exercise stress testing cannot localize the site of ischemia, or accurately identify the specific coronary artery occluded or the degree of occlusion if present. Myocardial imaging combined with exercise is extremely valuable in providing information regarding location and extent of abnormal perfusion (Gibbons et al., 1997). Initial choice of exercise testing modality is individualized and should be based on evaluation of patient's resting ECG, physical ability to perform exercise, concurrent medical illness, and local expertise and technology.

Factors Interfering with Interpretation

Patients with an abnormal baseline ECG including resting ST depression, left bundle branch block, pacemaker rhythm, left ventricular hypertrophy, Wolf–Parkinson–White syndrome, or who have resting ST abnormalities from taking medications such as digoxin may have an uninterpretable exercise ECG. Hemodynamic, functional, and symptomatic data, however, can still be obtained from the EST. Referral for a combined exercise test with an imaging study should be considered in these patients.

In addition to digoxin, other medications can interfere with interpretation of EST results. The EST results of patients taking beta blockers may have a reduced diagnostic value due to inadequate heart rate response but the study has value when done to test the effectiveness of these medications. Medications affecting blood pressure may alter the hemodynamic response obtained during the test. Another factor that may interfere with results is gender; women have a higher rate of false–positive EST results than men.

Patient Education

Patients should be instructed not to eat or drink caffeinated beverages or smoke for 3 hours prior to the test and to wear comfortable shoes and clothes. Patients should take all medications unless instructed not to do so by their healthcare provider. While it is true that blood pressure medications can interfere with the hemodynamic response to exercise, abnormally high blood pressure can be a contraindication to performing the test.

Pharmacologic Stress Tests

Myocardial perfusion imaging (MPI) studies are usually done in conjunction with an exercise stress test on a treadmill. If a patient cannot exercise due to physical limitations, a pharmacologic stress test with imaging can be ordered. Drugs used for pharmacologic stress testing are dipyridamole (Persantine), adenosine, and dobutamine. These drugs increase blood flow to the heart, mimicking exercise. Blood pressure and ECG monitoring are done continuously along with recording of symptoms.

Dipyridamole, a vasodilator, is most commonly used to dilate the coronary arteries. Significantly stenosed vessels are usually already maximally dilated to maintain normal blood flow. When normal vessels are dilated a heterogeneity of perfusion results, which can be identified by perfusion imaging. Less often, they can actually "steal" blood from stenosed arteries, causing ischemia (Zaret, Wacker, & Soufer, 1992). Adenosine works in the same way but has a shorter half life. Both dipyridamole and adenosine can induce bronchospasm and AV block. Dobutamine is the drug of choice in a patient with a history of asthma. The most common side effects from dipyridamole and adenosine are chest pain, headache, flushing, and nausea, all of which are transient. Due to its short half life, side effects from adenosine quickly resolve. Administering IV aminophylline can reverse dipyridamole. Because aminophylline is an antagonist of dipyridamole and adenosine, patients on theodur or aminophylline should be considered for a dobutamine study.

Dobutamine is a positive inotrope that increases heart rate and contractility. This causes an increase in myocardial oxygen demand, similar to that of exercise. The most common side effects are chest pain and palpitations.

The patient's medication profile should be reviewed at least 24 hours prior to the test. Specific instructions regarding insulin and hypoglycemic agents should be given since patients are NPO 4-6 hours prior to the test. Patients should not be receiving IV nitroglycerin or an IV antiarrhythmic agent. Persantine should be held for 24 hours before a Persantine or adenosine study. For patients undergoing a dobutamine stress test, beta blockers, calcium channel blockers, and nitrates should be held the morning of the test unless instructed to do otherwise. Patients usually return to their room after the stress portion of their study and are allowed a light meal with no caffeinated products before they are called to return to the nuclear lab for rest imaging.

Dobutamine Stress Echo

Dobutamine stress echo (DSE) is another reliable form of nonexertional stress imaging used in the detection and management of coronary artery disease. As with all stress-testing methods, it is important to consider the pretest likelihood of diagnosing coronary artery disease. With stress echo, the diagnostic value is greatest in patients in whom the pretest possibility of coronary artery disease is intermediate (Cheitlin, Alpert, Armstrong, et al., 1997).

In normal patients, the response of the myocardium to stress is an increase in myocardial contractility brought about by catecholamine stimulation. In patients with coronary artery stenoses, dobutamine-induced stress precipitates myocardial ischemia in those segments supplied by stenosed coronary arteries resulting in the development of wall motion abnormalities. Wall motion abnormalities are described in Figure 32–1 and as follows (Beattie, Billiard, Meinhardt, 1989).

- Hypokineses: reduced contractility
- Dyskineses: bulging or paradoxical movement of the myocardium during systole such as occurs with ventricular aneurysm
- Akineses: noncontractile myocardium, an area that fails to contract

Preexisting resting wall motion abnormalities present in patients with coronary artery disease may be caused by nonviable myocardium (scar), which is irreversible. They may also be the result of potentially reversible myocardial processes called stunning and hibernation. Myocardial stunning may occur following an acute ischemic insult, resulting in myocardium which is alive, but not contractile. Stunned myocardium can respond to inotropic stimulation by developing contractility. During a DSE these wall motion abnormalities may improve. Regional dysfunction of stunned myocardium following an ischemic event resolves spontaneously over the course of several days to weeks (Cheitlin et al., 1997).

Myocardial hibernation is thought to be due to chronically reduced myocardial blood flow to levels inadequate to support normal contractile performance but sufficient to preserve viability. In patients with multivessel coronary artery disease and depressed left ventricular function, improvement in left ventricular function during DSE is considered to indicate contractile reserves and is predictive of improved LV function after revascularization (Cheitlin et al., 1997). Hibernating is distinguished from stunned myocardium by demonstrating a "biphasic" response to catechole stimulation. That is, contractility improves with low-dose dobutamine, but becomes hypokinetic with higher doses. Identifying potentially reversible wall motion abnormalities with DSE or nuclear imaging has important clinical value. Left ventricular function is among the most important determinants of long-term prognosis in patients with coronary artery disease (Handel, Bonow, & Chaudhy, 1996). These are the patients who may benefit the most from coronary revasularization.

Procedure. Patients can be prepared for a DSE by reviewing the following. The patient should not eat or drink 3 to 6 hours before the test. They may take all medications. Baseline vital signs, ECG, and ECHO are obtained. Blood pressure and ECG are monitored continuously. The patient lies in the left lateral decubitus position to improve image quality. Patient symptoms are recorded. The dobutamine infusion is titrated every 3 minutes to a maximum of 40 mcg/kg/min or until procedural endpoints are reached. Con-

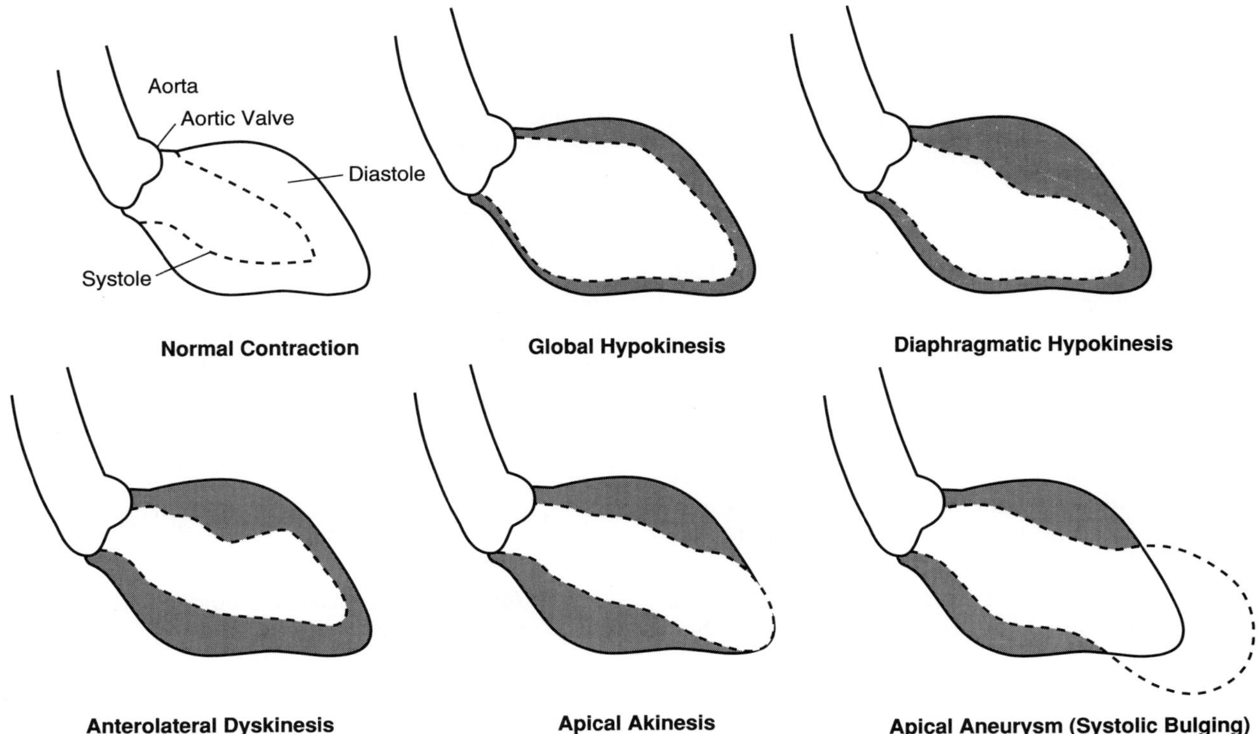

Figure 32–1. Spectrum of abnormal left ventricular (LV) wall motion. *(Reprinted from Beattie, Billiard, Meinhardt, et al. [1990].)*

tinuous acquisition of ECHO images is done throughout the procedure and for up to 20 minutes after the dobutamine infusion has ended. Actual procedure may vary with institution policy.

General DSE endpoints (Thompson, Detwiler, & Nelson, 1996) are as follows:

- New regional wall motion abnormality develops
- Preexisting wall motion abnormality improves then deteriorates during infusion (identifying hibernating myocardium)
- Preexisting wall motion abnormality worsens (indicating induced ischemia)
- Greater than or equal to 2 mm ST segment depression on ECG
- Greater than 25mm Hg decrease in systolic blood pressure from previous stage
- Side effects (nausea, vomiting, severe headache) or arrhythmias develop
- Maximum dose of 40 mcg/kg/min delivered
- Achievement of 85% of age-predicted heart rate

It may be difficult to visualize the myocardium and subsequent interpretation may be difficult if the patient is obese or has chest wall changes related to COPD. These patients should be referred for a myocardial perfusion imaging study.

Conclusion. A DSE is considered positive for myocardial ischemia if new regional or global wall motion abnormalities develop. Segments abnormal at rest that do not improve their contractility during the infusion represent irreversible scar tissue. On the other hand, improvement of a preexisting hypokinetic or akinetic segment suggests the presence of viable myocardium (either stunned or hibernating). On the basis of DSE results, patients may undergo further work-up or treatment. Because the test involves no radiation exposure, is quicker and cheaper, and is generally more accessible than nuclear imaging techniques, it is finding wider application.

Myocardial Perfusion Imaging

General Overview. Myocardial perfusion imaging (MPI) involves the process of intravenous injection of a radioactive isotope or tracer into a patient, recording the process of distribution of the isotope through the coronary arteries and into the heart muscle (perfusion). Viable myocardium is required for the uptake of the isotope. Detecting the radioactivity or "imaging" is done by a computer-generated camera called a "gamma" camera. The camera records the amount of radioactive isotope that has perfused different areas of the heart muscle. Generally a patient is exercised to his or her maximum capacity, a radioisotope is injected, and soonafter images are obtained. Another set of images are taken approximately 3-4 hours later after the patient has rested. Comparisons of isotope uptake are made. Regions of decreased tracer uptake correlate with coronary artery stenosis or infarction (Ritchie et al., 1995).

In patients unable to walk on a treadmill, pharmacologic stress is substituted for exercise. A perfusion study can also be performed at rest with serial imaging done after isotope injection. Variations in imaging protocols are based on patient condition, isotope used, experience of the institution, and information desired by a study.

Thallium-201 and technetium-99m sestamibi (Cardiolite) are the two most commonly used radioactive tracers. Thallium-201, a potassium analog, requires cell integrity and intact sodium–potassium ATPase pump activity for intracellular uptake (Zaret et al., 1992). Thallium distributes in proportion to regional myocardial blood flow and redistribution of ischemic areas generally takes place 3-4 hours after initial injection of the isotope.

Technetium-99m sestamibi is a cationic compound that has a shorter half life (6 hours) compared with thallium-201 (73 hours) (Ritchie et al., 1995). This allows for the administration of a large dose of technetium-99 than thallium-201. A larger dose along with higher energy emission than thallium-201 results in improved imaging characteristics. After initial injection of Cardiolite, there is minimal redistribution of the isotope overtime which means that imaging can be delayed for several hours and still provide accurate information about myocardial perfusion at the time of injection. A second injection of the isotope is required for rest imaging so comparisons of perfusion defects can be made. Cardiolite may be the isotope of choice in obese patients or in women where breast tissue may interfere with imaging quality.

The images are displayed on a computer screen as a series of slices through the heart muscle. Three series are recorded: short-axis slices, horizontal long-axis slices, and vertical long axis slices. Exercise and rest images should be displayed side-by-side for comparison (Fig. 32–2). A slice of the left ventricle and corresponding coronary artery that supplies blood to each area of the image are indicated in Figure 32–3.

Interpretation of images (Zaret et al., 1992) may be described as follows:

- Normal: Equal uptake of isotope throughout the myocardium.

Figures 32–2 and 32–3. Stress and Rest Nuclear SPECT and "Bull's Eye" Images. The SPECT images are arranged with the stress images above the rest images. The vertical long axis is displayed in the *top two rows,* the horizontal long axis is shown in the *second two rows,* and the short axis images are shown in the *last two rows.* The "bull's eye" on the *left* is the stress image, the one on the *right* is the rest image. They are arranged concentrically such that the apex is the center and the base is the outer edge. There are no demonstrable perfusion defects.

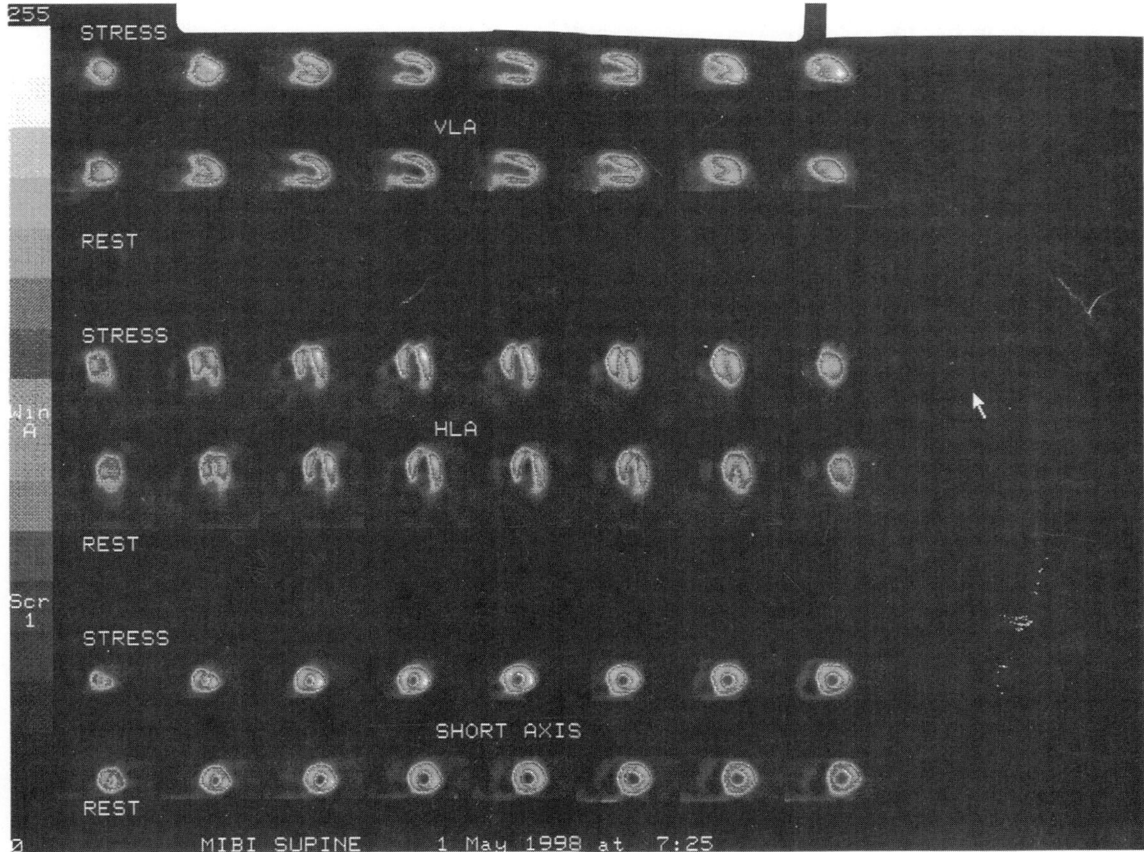

Figure 32–2

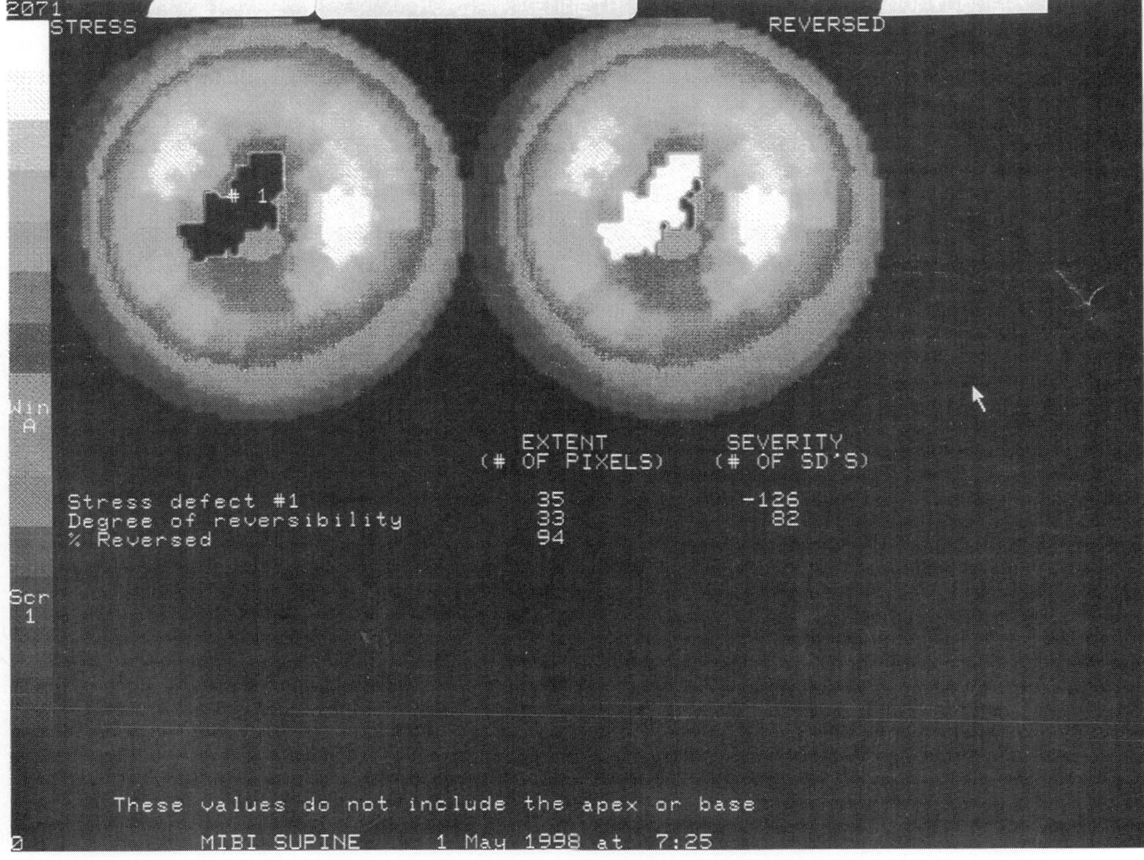

Figure 32–3

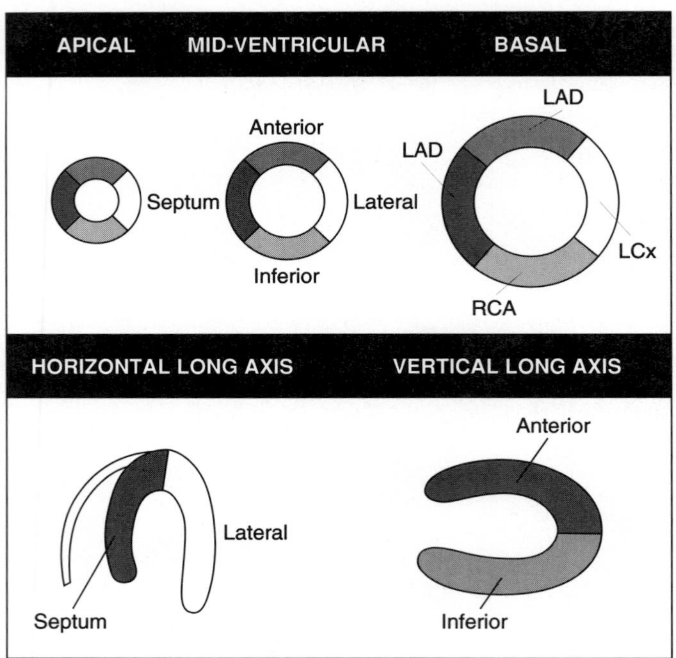

Figure 32–4. Left ventricular anatomy and coronary artery territories on SPECT Slices. *(From Braunwald, E. [1992].* Heart Disease: A Textbook of Medicine. *Philadelphia: W. B. Saunders.)*

- Defect: An area of myocardium with decreased tracer uptake. Defects vary in intensity from slightly reduced activity to total absence of radioactive activity.
- Reversible defect: A defect present on initial stress images and is no longer present (or *fills in*) on the resting (delayed) images. This pattern indicates ischemia. The change over time is called *reversibility of the defect.*
- Fixed defect: A defect that is unchanged and present on both exercise *and* rest images. This pattern usually indicates infarcted or scarred myocardium.

Research into myocardial viability has found that fixed defects seen on the usual stress/rest images may be improved on a 24-hour rest image or with a new rest injection of isotope (Ritchie et al., 1995).

For all cardiac-imaging studies, patients may voice a concern about exposure to radioactive material. They should be reassured that, unless pregnant, exposure is insignificant and no special precautions are necessary.

Indications for Myocardial Perfusion Imaging

There are numerous clinical applications for MPI. First, MPI is useful for the detection of CAD, particularly in patients with resting ECG abnormalities that make interpretation of a standard EST unreliable. Next, in a patient with known CAD such as diagnosed by prior cardiac catheterization, an imaging study can determine whether the myocardium supplied by a given artery becomes ischemic with stress. Physiologic significance of a coronary occlusion is then determined (Cheitlin et al., 1993). This information can assist in determining the treatment plan for the patient. Also, results of a coronary revascularization can be assessed by establishing whether an area of ischemia present before intervention is adequately perfused postprocedure. This is especially informative when a patient has symptoms postrevascularization and restenosis is a possibility. Risk stratification after myocardial infarction is another important use of MPI. It has been shown that event-free survival of a postmyocardial infarction patient is related to the amount of residual myocardial ischemia remaining following an MI. An MPI study that is free of ischemia correlates with a 97 to 99% chance of event-free survival over a coarse of 18 months. As with DSE, the presence of myocardial viability can also be determined with MPI. This may be relevant when considering a patient with LV dysfunction for revascularization. A patient with viable myocardium may benefit from the revascularization procedure with less adverse outcomes due to improvement in LV function after revascularization (Hendel et al., 1996).

Viability Studies

Viability studies, also known as rest–redistribution imaging studies, are designed to answer the question concerning the presence of viable myocardium, not for the detection of ischemia.

Research into myocardial viability has found that fixed

defects seen on the usual stress/rest nuclear images may be improved with a 24-hour rest image or with a new rest injection of isotope (Ritchie et al., 1995). These reversible perfusion defects are caused by stunning or hibernation. Myocardium originally classified as dead or scarred—when found to be viable and revascularized—may show normalization or improved wall motion, thus improving the prognosis of this set of patients with coronary artery disease and left ventricular dysfunction.

Rest–redistribution protocols vary and are still being studied. Generally the patient receives an IV injection of thallium-201 while at rest, with imaging immediately afterwards and then again 3 to 4 hours later and sometimes 24 to 72 hours later. Images are compared for redistribution.

Radionuclide Angiography

First Pass. First-pass radionuclide angiography allows visualization of the atria and ventricles. A bolus of a radioactive isotope is injected IV and sequential images are obtained at a rapid rate during the initial passage of the isotope through the great vessels and chambers of the heart. The change in radioactivity over time is calculated as the bolus passes through the right then left side of the heart. Right and left ventricular ejection fractions and ventricular and pulmonary blood volumes can be measured. The first pass study is most appropriate for intracardiac shunt detection and evaluation of RV function. Cardiolyte is used for first-pass imaging.

Gated-Equilibrium Blood Pool Acquisition

The multiple-uptake gated aquisition (MUGA) approach generates reliable left and right ventricular ejection values and can suggest areas of abnormal wall motion. It can be applied at both rest and during exercise or pharmacologic stress. The term "gated" applies to the acquisition of images that are synchronized to the cardiac cycle, that is, systole and diastole, thus allowing for the most accurate method for ejection fraction determination.

Cardiac Catheterization

Cardiac catheterization has been the gold standard to diagnose heart disease. After being initially developed in the animal laboratory, catheterization was first applied to humans by Werner Forssmann in 1929. At the age of 25, Werner Forssmann performed the first right heart catheterization on himself by placing a catheter into his brachial vein and into his right atrium. He then confirmed the placement of the catheter with a chest x-ray. Forssmann's goal was to develop a therapeutic technique for direct delivery of drugs into the heart. Many of his colleagues realized the importance of this technique as a diagnostic tool and helped him to develop the technique further which won them the Nobel prize (Grossman & Baim, 1991).

Today, a standard cardiac catheterization involves the evaluation of the venous and arterial systems. The right heart catheterization is performed by inserting a ballooned-tipped catheter into the venous system. Pressure measurements and oxygen saturations can be obtained from inside the heart and lungs. Left heart catheterization entails placing a catheter in the aorta, through the aortic valve, into the left ventricle and taking pressure measurements, respectively. Angiography involves selectively injecting contrast dye into each coronary artery. Cardiac catheterization is used as a diagnostic test to determine structural and functional information to allow the clinician to assess prognosis and management of heart disease.

Indications and Contraindications. Cardiac catheterization is used to identify structural cardiac diseases such as atherosclerotic coronary artery disease, myocardial dysfunction (infarction or myopathy), and valvular or congenital heart abnormalities. In adults, the procedure is used to define and diagnose coronary artery disease for the purpose of defining a definitive treatment, such medical therapy, coronary intervention, or coronary artery bypass graph surgery. This procedure is also used to define valvular heart disease such as aortic stenosis or mitral stenosis by measuring the pressure across the diseased valve.

Cardiac catheterization is contraindicated in patients with fever of unknown cause, anemia, and electrolyte imbalance especially hypokalemia predisposing to arrhythmia. It is also contraindicated in patients with coagulopathies either induced by warfarin or other causes (Kern, 1991).

Indications for and contraindications to cardiac catheterization are listed in Table 32–3. Table 32–4 lists the potential complications associated with cardiac catheterization.

Precardiac Catheterization. All medications, cessation of oral intake, and preprocedural medication should be tailored to the timing of cardiac catheterization laboratory. Unfortunately, in a busy lab this is difficult for the practitioner to predict. The patient should be NPO except cardiac medications. If medications such as diuretics are withheld, prior to the procedure the practitioner needs to address fluid status by exam to determine the need for these medications after the procedure.

TABLE 32–3. Indications for and Contraindications to Cardiac Catheterization

Indications	Contraindications
Suspected or known coronary artery disease	Uncontrolled congestive heart failure, high blood pressure, or arrhythmia
Angina, stable or unstable	Recent cerebral vascular accident (< 1 month)
Myocardial infarction	Infection
Sudden cardiovascular death	Electrolyte imbalance
Valvular heart disease	Acute gastrointestinal bleeding or anemia
Congenital heart disease	Pregnancy (relative)
Pericardial constriction	Anticoagulation or uncontrolled bleeding
Cardiomyopathy	Uncooperative patient
	Medication intoxication (digoxin, phenothiazine)

TABLE 32–4. Risks Associated with Cardiac Catheterization

Death < 0.2%
Myocardial infarction < 0.5%
Stroke < 0.5%
Serious arrhythmia <1.0%
Major vascular complications (thrombic, bleeding requiring transfusion or pseudoaneurysm) < 1.0%

Source: Kern. (1991).

Diabetic patients need to be carefully monitored pre- and postprocedure. If the patient is on oral hypoglycemic agent, the oral medication should be held while the patient is NPO. After the patient starts eating, the oral medication should be restarted. If the patient is taking insulin, half the dose of neutral protamine hagedorn (NPH) is routinely given along with a slow $D_5$1/2 NS intravenous drip and the regular insulin is held. If the patient is taking 70/30 insulin, half the NPH dose should be given and the regular insulin held. For example, if the patient is taking 50 units of 70/30, 35 units is NPH and 15 units is regular, the patient should only be given 17.5 units of NPH insulin. Also it is very important to check a glucose level prior to the procedure. The diabetic patient is prone to contrast-induced renal failure. Intravenous fluids should always be ordered on diabetic patients for two reasons: (1) so their glucose does not change drastically and (2) to hydrate their kidneys. Patients taking NPH insulin are also prone to protamine reactions, though not all cardiac catheterization laboratories give protamine postprocedure. Patients taking NPH insulin have an increased sensitivity to protamine. The incidence of protamine reactions of NPH insulin-dependent diabetics is 27% compared with 0.5% in noninsulin diabetics (Kern, 1991).

Patients taking metformin HCL (Glucophage [Bristol-Myers Squibb]) should stop taking the oral agents 2 to 3 days prior to undergoing cardiac catheterization. Metformin affects renal function; therefore, any agent (e.g., contrast dye) that affects renal function should not be given concomitantly. Arterial contrast studies with iodinated materials can lead to acute renal failure and have been associated with lactic acidosis in patients receiving metformin. The manufacture of metformin (Glucotrol) recommends that the medication be withheld for at least 48 hours prior and 48 hours subsequent to the procedure. Metformin should only be restarted after renal function has been reevaluated and found to be normal.

The patient should always be asked preprocedure if he or she is allergic to contrast dye or shellfish and if he or she has ever had prior x-ray procedures with contrast media. Shellfish contains iodine and there is a 15% correlation between shellfish allergy and contrast media. The patient who has an allergy to contrast dye or iodine should be premedicated; usually patients are given 25 to 50 mg of intravenous benedryl and 100 mg of intravenous hydrocortisone (Kern, 1991). Patients may also be treated prior to the day of procedure with prednisone 60 mg q 8 hours for 3 doses 24 to 36 hours prior to the procedure (Kern, 1991). Allergic reactions are classified as either major or minor. Minor reactions include rash, itching, urticaria, nausea, flushing, or hives and the treatment is usually benedryl and steroids. Major reactions includes coughing, dyspnea, sneezing, syncope, and shock. These should be treated with epinephrine, CPR, and ACLS protocol as indicated.

Patients with renal insufficiency and diabetes are at higher risk for contrast-induced renal failure. Advanced preparation includes hydration and maintenance of large volume urine flow (> 200 ml/h). These patients should be hydrated intravenously the night prior to procedures, and after the procedure urine output should be closely monitored. If urine output falls and is not responsive to increased intravenous fluids and lasix, renal insufficiency is probable. The use of different contrast agent (ionic, nonionic, and low osmolarity) does not reduce the incidence of contrast-induced nephropathy; therefore, hydration is extremely important as preventative therapy.

Procedure. Cardiac catheterization is performed while the patient is awake, although sedated. Typical sedatives include diazepam (5-10 mg po prior to procedure) and diphenhydramine (25-50 mg po prior to procedure). Prophylactic antibiotics are not necessary.

There are two approaches to cardiac catheterization. One is to expose the artery and vein (usually the brachial), which is called a Sones procedure. The other is by percutaneous approach, usually via the femoral artery and vein, which is called the Judkins technique. The percutaneous approach can also be used in the brachial approach; and either technique can be used for right and left heart catheterization. The brachial approach has advantages for the patient with peripheral vascular disease involving the abdominal aorta and iliac femoral arteries. Also patients can get out of bed earlier in a brachial approach. The disadvantage of brachial approach is that arterial repair is often necessary because there is direct exposure of the brachial artery. The femoral approach is the approach of choice by most physicians. It is safer and easier to use the femoral artery and vein, and the same site can be used over again usually without a scar. The disadvantage is that infection and thrombophlebitis are greater in the femoral approach.

Right Heart Catheterization. Right heart catheterization is no longer routinely performed on all patients. Therefore, it is important in the precatheterization work-up to assess for heart failure or valvular disease by good physical exam. If murmurs of ventricular septal defect, atrial septal defect, or valvular heart disease are heard, a right heart catheterization may be imperative to the diagnosis. The right heart catheterization is a measurement of each chamber as a ballooned-tipped pressure catheter is passed through the heart. First, the right atrial pressure is measured, where normal is 4 to 8 mmHg. The catheter is then passed to the right ventricle, where normal pressure is 20/2-4 mmHg. The catheter is advanced to the pulmonary artery and then to the "wedge" position in the capillary arteries. The pulmonary capillary wedge pressure is reflective of the left atrium pressure. The measurements are made in each position respectively. Normal pulmonary artery pressure is 20/12 mmHg and the normal pulmonary capillary wedge pressure is 4 to 12 mmHg. Pressures are recorded in each position (Kern, 1991). Cardiac output can also be measured with a thermodilution catheter and pulmonary artery blood gases can be drawn so the cardiac output can be measured by the FICK principle. A more detailed discussion of the right heart catheterization is included in Chapter 33, Valvular and Congenital Heart Disease.

Left Heart Catheterization. During the left heart catheterization, a catheter is placed into the ascending aorta where pressures are measured and the catheter is then advanced in the left ventricle where pressures are measured. The comparison of ascending aorta pressure with left ventricular pressure will determine if there is a systolic gradient. Normally the left ventricle and the ascending aorta should have the same systolic pressure. If right heart catheterization is performed, mitral valve area can be measured and calculated by comparing the left ventricle wave form with the pulmonary capillary wedge pressure (PCWP), since the PCWP reflects the left atrial pressure. There should not be a gradient between the two chambers. The PCWP is compared with the diastolic pressure of the left ventricle.

CORONARY VISUALIZATION. Coronary angiography involves injecting radiopaque contrast into a specific chamber or vessel. Contrast agents are either nonionic or ionic; the nonionic agents have less myocardial depressant effects but are much more expensive than higher osmolar ionic agent. During injection, lower osmolar agents cause less vasodilation and less sensation of warmth.

The most common procedure involves selective injection of the right coronary artery and the left coronary artery. Using different catheters and fluoroscopic guidance, the angiographer is able to specifically inject each artery. Each artery is viewed in several projections because the heart is three-dimensional and, unfortunately, the x-ray camera is two-dimensional. These pictures enable the clinician to view the stenosis and to minimize overlapping of vessels. In addition to detecting coronary artery stenosis, angiography is useful to determine congenital abnormalities, coronary fistulas, and patency of coronary artery bypass grafts.

LEFT VENTRICULOGRAPHY. Injection of radiographic dye into the left ventricle is an important diagnostic test, although with the use of echocardiography it is not always routine. Angiographic assessment of left ventricle at end diastolic and end systolic allow for calculation of left ventricular chamber volume and ejection fraction. The normal left ventricle ejects 50 to 80% of its end diastolic volume with each beat (Kern, 1991). The left ventriculogram provides the ability to assess wall-motion abnormalities, aortic valve function, flow across a ventricular septal defect, and to view the aortic root. Mitral regurgitation is also easily visualized as the appearance of contrast material in the left atrium during systole.

INTRAVASCULAR ULTRASOUND. The development of a small over-the-wire catheter with ultrasound transducers or angioscopic images delivered from the distal ends have introduced the ability to evaluate intravascular procedures from an intraluminal perspective. As these catheters become more affordable and user-friendly, they may help direct interventional therapy more precisely so that better outcomes are achieved. Unlike angiography, which displays the coronary artery as a silhouette of the contrast-filled lumen, intravascular ultrasound generated a cross-sectional, tomographic image of the vessel. The ability of ultrasound to penetrate tissue enables this modality to create an image, not only of the lumen, but also the intramural structure of the vessel wall. With these features of coronary ultrasound, the angiographer is given important insight into diverse phenomena, ranging from the pathophysiology of coronary syndromes to the mechanical effects of each of the interventional devices.

▶ MYOCARDIAL ISCHEMIC SYNDROMES

Myocardial ischemic syndromes are a group of clinical syndromes that result in a spectrum of clinical manifestations, ranging from asymptomatic atherosclerosis and stable angina to the acute coronary syndromes—unstable angina and myocardial infarction. An imbalance between myocardial oxygen supply and demand is the common factor. A reduction in oxygen supply occurs when there is a significant reduction in coronary artery lumen size caused by the presence of plaque, coronary spasm, thrombus, or coronary emboli. A reduction in the oxygen-carrying capacity of the blood, such as severe anemia or carboxyhemoglobin, can precipitate ischemia. Myocardial oxygen demand is increased by physical exertion, stress, and anxiety. Severe ventricular hypertrophy due to hypertension or aortic stenosis can also place abnormally high oxygen requirements on the myocardium (Selwyn & Braunwald, 1994).

In patients with stable coronary artery disease, angina commonly results from increases in myocardial oxygen demand that outstrip the ability of stenosed coronary arteries to increase its delivery. In contrast, in unstable angina, a relatively small fissuring of an atherosclerotic plaque may lead to a sudden change in plaque morphology and a reduction in coronary blood flow, resulting in anginal symptoms. Recurrent episodes of thrombotic vessel occlusion at the site of plaque disruption or residual thrombus may lead to angina at rest. The thrombus is usually labile, causing temporary vessel occlusion that may last only 10 to 20 minutes. In addition, the release of vasoactive substance by the thrombus and vasoconstriction due to endothelial vasodilator dysfunction may further impede coronary flow. In myocardial infarctions, plaque disruption may be associated with deep arterial damage and ulceration. This results in the formation of a fixed and persistent thrombus that is occlusive and leads to an abrupt cessation of myocardial perfusion and eventual necrosis. As in other acute coronary syndromes, the lesion responsible for the infarction is frequently only mildly to moderately stenotic, suggesting that plaque disruption with superimposed thrombus, rather than the severity of the underlying lesion, is the primary determinant of acute occlusion. The pathogenesis is similar in sudden coronary death; however, the absence of collateral blood flow to the myocardium distal to the occlusion may contribute to sudden ischemic death (Fuster, Badiman, Badiman, & Chesebro, 1992).

Chronic Stable Angina

Chronic stable angina is paroxysmal chest pain or discomfort due to transient myocardial ischemia. Symptoms are brought about by a predictable degree of exertion or emotion, characterized by a stable pattern of symptoms. The character of angina is described by the Unstable Angina Guideline Panel (Braunwald et al., 1994) as a deep, poorly localized chest or arm discomfort that is reproducibly associated with physical exertion or emotional stress and relieved promptly by rest or sublingual nitroglycerin. Some patients may have no chest discomfort but present with jaw, neck, ear, arm, or back discomfort. If these symptoms can be correlated to exertion or stress and are relieved with rest or sublingual nitroglycerine, they should be considered an angina equivalent.

Patients with stable angina generally have a relatively good prognosis, with an annual CAD mortality rate < 4% (Alderman et al., 1990). The key to proper diagnosis and successful management of stable angina is a complete, detailed history of the patient's symptoms including precipitating factors and symptom resolution. It is important to identify risk factors for future coronary events. Physical examination is rarely diagnostic and ECG tracings are often normal with stable angina. Exercise stress testing that reproduces the patient's anginal symptoms may reflect ECG changes to suggest coronary artery disease and is helpful in assessing risk level. Patients with chest pain who can exercise into stage III of *Bruce* protocol have an annual CAD related mortality of <1%.

There are several goals in the management of chronic stable angina. The first is the treatment of conditions that worsen angina, such as anemia, thyrotoxicosis, and arrhythmias. The second is risk-factor modification. It is well established that modification of risk factors for CAD is beneficial in reducing cardiovascular morbidity and mortality. Blood pressure reduction, lowering of blood cholesterol levels, and smoking cessation are interventions of proven value and, in addition, appear to improve endothelial function. In postmenopausal women, estrogen replacement therapy has been shown to have a beneficial effect on lipid profile and to reduce CAD-related morbidity and mortality. The third goal is effective relief of angina symptoms. Three classes of antianginal drugs—nitrates, beta–adrenergic blockers, and calcium channel antagonists—along with aspirin are approved for the treatment of stable angina (Thadani, 1997). The pharmacologic management of chronic stable angina will be discussed in detail with unstable angina.

Unstable Angina

Unstable angina has been identified as a syndrome that bridges stable angina and myocardial infarction. It appears to be a good clinical marker for the rapid progression of coronary artery disease (Falk, 1989). Unstable angina is defined by the Unstable Angina Guideline Panel (Braunwald et al., 1994) as a transitory clinical syndrome usually associated with increased intensity and frequency of symptoms thought to be indicative of coronary artery disease. The three principle presentations of unstable angina are listed in Table 32–5.

In unstable angina, the character of the pain is the same as described in stable angina; however, the episodes are either more severe, prolonged, or may occur at rest without a known relationship to exertion or stress. There are some patients who present with isolated, unexplained, new onset, or worsened exertional dyspnea, and ischemia must be considered as a precipitating factor. Rest discomfort with all the features of angina but without an exertional component should be considered definite angina for purposes of estimating CAD likelihood (Braunwald et al., 1994).

Diagnosis of Unstable Angina

Patient History. As previously mentioned, a detailed history is paramount in determining the likelihood of CAD. The following factors provide key information.

TABLE 32–5. Three Principle Presentations of Unstable Angina

Rest angina	Angina occurring at rest and usually prolonged >20 minutes occurring within a week of presentation
New onset angina	Angina of at least CCSC III severity with onset within 2 months of initial presentation
Increasing angina	Previously diagnosed angina that is distinctly more frequent, longer in duration or lower in duration, or lower in threshold (i.e., increased by at least one CCSC class within 2 months of initial presentation to at least CCSC III severity)

Note: CCSC = Canadian Cardiovascular Society classification (See Table 32–6).
Reprinted from the Unstable Angina Clinical Practice Guidelines (Braunwald et al., 1994).

TABLE 32–6. Grading of Angina Pectoris by the Canadian Cardiovascular Society Classification System

Class	Description of Stage
Class I	Ordinary physical activity such as walking, climbing stairs does not cause angina. Angina occurs with strenuous, rapid, or prolonged exertion at work or recreation
Class II	Slight limitation of ordinary activity. Angina occurs on walking or climbing stairs rapidly, walking uphill, walking or stair climbing after meals, or in cold, or in wind, or under emotional stress, or only during the few hours after awakening. Walking more than two blocks on the level and climbing more than one flight of ordinary stairs at a normal pace and in normal conditions
Class III	Marked limitations of ordinary physical activity. Angina occurs on walking one to two blocks on the level and climbing one flight of stairs in normal conditions and at a normal pace
Class IV	Inability to carry on any physical activity without discomfort—anginal symptoms may be present at rest

Used with permission from Campeau, L. (1976). Copyright 1976, American Heart Association, Inc.

Description of Angina. Typical angina pain has been described. Features that support nonanginal pain include pleuritic pain (sharp or knife-like pain brought on by respiratory movements or cough), pain localized with one finger, pain lasting for seconds or for several days, pain reproducible with movement or palpation.

Prior MI. Report by history or presence of significant Q waves on ECG.

Sex and Age. Older patients have a higher likelihood of CAD, and the likelihood of disease and severity increases with age. At any age, men have a higher CAD likelihood than women. Women who have not undergone premature menopause generally lag ten years behind men.

Risk Factors. Risk factors have been found to be only weakly predictive of the likelihood of acute ischemia in men. Diabetes and family history were the strongest followed by smoking history. Ironically, no risk factor was a significant predictor of acute ischemia in women. Therefore, when deciding whether a patient should be treated for unstable angina, it is more important to consider the patient's symptoms and ECG findings and place less consideration on risk factors.

History of Variant Angina. Variant angina is an uncommon clinical syndrome of rest pain and reversible ST-segment elevation which may be difficult to diagnose on initial presentation. The chest discomfort characteristically occurs at rest or awakens the patient from sleep and is caused by focal spasm of proximal epicardial coronary arteries (Selwyn & Braunwald, 1994). Approximately one-fourth of these patients have insignificant CAD and symptoms are due to coronary vasospasm. Calcium channel blockers, nitrates and avoidance of beta blockers are the treatments of choice. The other three fourths of patients have a subtotal stenosis in a coronary artery, and a ruptured plaque is the cause of unstable angina. Management of this group is the same as unstable angina.

History of Cocaine Use. Three possible mechanisms by which cocaine induces myocardial ischemia are: (1) increased myocardial oxygen demand, (2) decreased myocardial oxygen supply secondary to vasospasm or coronary thrombosis, and (3) direct myocardial toxicity. Cocaine use does not rule out underlying significant CAD.

Electrocardiogram. A normal ECG does not exclude the diagnosis of CAD. One-half of the patients with angina have normal rest ECGs. In ischemic tissue, the repolarization process is delayed producing ST-T wave changes; however, these changes are nonspecific and could be caused by other factors (Selwyn & Braunwald, 1994). ST-segment depression typically signifies ischemia or non-Q-wave infarction. Inverted T waves may also indicate ischemia or non-Q-wave infarction, especially with T waves inverted ≥ 1 mm in leads with dominant R waves. Marked symmetrical precordial T-wave inversion strongly suggests acute ischemia, particularly that due to a proximal LAD lesion (Table 32–7) (Braunwald et al., 1994).

Cardiac Enzymes. Since the ECG changes that are present with unstable angina could also be indicative of a non–Q-wave MI, serial cardiac enzymes must be done to diagnose or rule out MI. Cardiac enzymes will be discussed in full in the section on myocardial infarction.

TABLE 32–7. ECG Findings Useful for Establishing the Likelihood of Coronary Artery Disease

Finding	Most Likely Cause	Alternate Causes
ST-segment elevation ≥ 1 mm in two or more contiguous leads	Acute MI	Acute pericarditis; early repolorization; left ventricular aneurysm, coronary spasm
ST-segment depression ≥ 1 mm	Ischemia or acute MI	Normal heart; hyperventilation, LV hypertrophy with strain; digitalis; hypokalemia; hypomagnesemia
Inverted T-waves in two or more contiguous leads (≥ 1 mm in leads with dominant R waves, or marked symmetrical precordial T-wave inversion)	Ischemia or acute MI	Normal heart; central nervous system disease; hypertrophic cardiomyopathy

Reprinted from (Braunwald et al., 1994).

Treatment of Unstable Angina

The severity of the patient's symptoms dictate the treatment course. All treatment should begin in the emergency room and not wait for admission to coronary care or intermediate unit. Patients should be placed on bed rest while the diagnosis of ischemia is being considered. All patients should be placed on continuous ECG monitoring. Supplemental oxygen should be used in patients with cyanosis or respiratory distress and should be monitored with pulse oximetry to confirm adequate oxygenation (Braunwald et al., 1994).

Pharmacologic Management. Drugs to be considered for use at the time of initial evaluation and treatment of patients with symptoms suggestive of unstable angina include aspirin, heparin, nitrates, and beta blockers. The goal of drug therapy is directed at the interruption of the pathophysiologic processes involved in ischemic heart disease. Currently, intravenous (IV) thrombolytic therapy is not indicated in patients who do not have evidence of acute ST-segment elevation or left bundle branch block on 12-lead ECG. See Table 32–8 for a summary of commonly used drugs.

Aspirin. The best-studied, least-toxic, and most widely used antithrombotic agent in acute and chronic coronary artery disease is aspirin (Fuster et al., 1992). Several trials have demonstrated that aspirin administration has reduced the risk of MI and cardiac death in unstable angina by as much as 50% (Matrisciano, 1992). All patients with the diagnosis of unstable angina should receive regular aspirin 160 to 324 mg as soon as possible after presentation unless a definite contraindication is present (Braunwald et al., 1994). Aspirin inhibits platelet aggregation by inhibiting the formation of thrombaxane A2. Plaque rupture leads to platelet aggregation and thrombus formation. Aspirin interrupts one part of this process by the inhibition of platelets, thereby reducing events. No data directly compare the efficacy of different doses of aspirin in patients with unstable angina. However, a broad review and metaanalysis of different doses of aspirin in the treatment of coronary artery disease suggest equal efficacy of daily doses of 75 to 324 mg per day (Antiplatelet Trialists' Collaboration, 1994).

Contraindications to aspirin use include a clear history of hypersensitivity to the drug or evidence of major hemorrhage or significant predisposition to such hemorrhage as bleeding peptic ulcer. Adverse reactions include gastrointestinal upset and bleeding (Braunwald et al., 1994).

Heparin. Various studies have demonstrated a significant reduction in the incidence of myocardial infarction or a recurrent episode of angina when heparin is used in the treatment of unstable angina (Matrisciano, 1992). Heparin exerts its anticoagulant effect by markedly accelerating the action of circulating antithrombin III, a proteolytic enzyme that inhibits thrombin and several other activated factors in the clotting cascade. Heparin acts to prevent thrombus formation but does not lyse existing thrombi (Hirsch, 1991).

The initial weight-based heparin dose is 80 units/kg bolus, followed by an IV infusion of 18 units/kg/hour. An aPTT is drawn six hours after starting the infusion with the goal of keeping the aPTT 1.5 to 2.5 times the control or be-

TABLE 32–8. Summary of Drugs Commonly Used to Treat Patients with Symptoms Suggestive of Unstable Angina

Drug Category	Clinical Condition	When to Avoid[a]	Usual dose
Aspirin	Diagnosis of unstable angina or acute MI	Hypersensitivity, active bleeding, severe bleeding risk	324 mg (160–324)
Heparin	Unstable angina in high-risk and some intermediate-risk patients	Active bleeding, history of heparin-induced thrombocytopenia, severe bleeding risk, recent stroke	80 units/kg IV bolus with constant IV infusion at 18 units/kg/hr titrated to maintain aPTT between 46 and 70 seconds[b]
Nitrates	Ongoing pain or ischemia	Hypotension	Sublingual (1–3 tablets)[c] IV (5–100 mcg/min)
Beta Blockers	Diagnosis of unstable angina	PR segment >0.24 seconds, 2nd- or 3rd-degree AV block, heart rate <60, systolic blood pressure <90 mmHg, shock, left ventricular failure with CHF, severe reactive airway disease	Oral dose appropriate for specific drug IV metoprolol (1–5 mg slow every 5 minutes to 15 mg total) IV propranolol 0.5 to 1.0 mg IV atenolol 5 mg every 5 minutes to 10 mg total
Narcotics	Persistent pain following initial therapy with nitrates and beta blockers	Hypotension, respiratory depression, confusion, obtundation	Morphine sulfate 2 to 5 mg IV

[a] Allergy or prior intolerance contraindication for all.

[b] Dose regimen assumes a mean control aPTT of 30 seconds and a therapeutic goal of 1.5 to 2.5 times control.

[c] Patients with symptoms suggestive of unstable angina and ongoing pain should be given sublingual NTG 0.3 to 0.4 every 5 minutes until discomfort is relieved, three tablets have been given, or limiting symptoms or signs develop. If discomfort is still present after three tablets, IV NTG should be started promptly at a dose of 5 mcg/min and titrated up to 75 to 100 mcg/min or limiting side effects.

Reprinted from the Unstable Angina Guideline Panel (Braunwald et al., 1994).

tween 46 and 70 seconds. Serial hemoglobin and hematocrit and platelet counts should be drawn daily for at least the first three days of heparin therapy. Serial platelet counts are necessary to monitor for heparin-induced thrombocytopenia. Heparin-induced thrombocytopenia with thrombosis is a rare but catastrophic complication that occurs with <0.2% incidence. It is believed to be immunologically mediated and occurs equally with bovine and porcine heparin. A high clinical suspicion mandates immediate cessation of all heparin therapy, including flushes pending further evaluation.

Enoxaparin. Enoxaparin is a low molecular-weight heparin that binds to less plasma and tissue proteins, has higher bioavailability, has a more pronounced effect on factor Xa than on thrombin, and is resistant to platelet factor IV making it more successful in the reduction of thrombin (Armstrong, 1997). Its potential advantages over unfractionated heparin include a more predictable anticoagulant effect than standard heparin, no required laboratory monitoring, a lower incidence of heparin-induced thrombocytopenia, and ease of administration.

The ESSENCE study concluded that when compared with unfractionated heparin, enoxaparin, 1 mg/kg subcutaneously every 12 hours, was more effective in reducing the incidence of ischemic events in patients with unstable angina or non-Q wave MI (Cohen et al., 1997).

Nitrates. Nitrates are given to relieve the symptoms of unstable angina. In vascular injury, thrombin and the platelet products, thrombaxane A2, and serotonin induce direct vasoconstriction of the smooth muscle (Fuster et al., 1992). Nitrates act by causing systemic venodilation and venous pooling, thereby decreasing myocardial pre-load and LV-end diastolic volume. This results in a reduction in myocardial wall tension and oxygen requirements, as well as dilating the epicardial coronary vessels and increasing blood flow in collateral vessels. The action of these agents is most rapid and complete through the mucous membranes and, for this reason, nitroglycerin is administered sublingually. Patients should be instructed to take the drug both to relieve symptoms and to prevent them when an attack is anticipated (Selwyn & Braunwald, 1994). Sublingual nitroglycerin (NTG) should be taken at 5-minute intervals, with patients being aware that they should seek medical attention if the symptoms are not totally relieved after three sublingual nitroglycerin tablets. At that point intravenous (IV) nitroglycerin may be required to relieve symptoms.

Nitroglycerin should be started at a dose of 5–10 mcg/min by continuous infusion and titrated up by 10 mcg/min every 5 to 10 minutes until relief of symptoms or limiting side effects (headache or hypotension with SBP <90 mmHg or more that 30% below starting mean arterial pressure if significant hypertension is present). Patients on IV NTG should be switched to oral or topical therapy once they have been symptom-free for 24 hours. Tolerance to nitrates is dose and duration dependent and typically becomes significant only after 24 hours of continuous therapy. This can be countered by increasing the dose or switching the patient to a nonparenteral form of therapy and using a nitrate-free interval. Topical, oral, or buccal nitrates should be given with a 6- to 8-hour nitrate-free interval (Braunwald et al., 1994). Nitroglycerin deteriorates with exposure to air, moisture, and sunlight and, therefore, should be stored in a cool, dark place. If the drug neither relieves discomfort nor produces a headache or burning sensation at the sublingual site of absorption, the preparation may be inactive and a fresh supply should be obtained (Selwyn & Braunwald, 1992). Reflex tachycardia may result from the use of vasodilators which could increase myocardial oxygen demand. The use of concomitant beta blockers, in the appropriate patient population, would counteract this effect.

Beta Blockers. Beta-blocking agents are competitive antagonists to catecholamines which exert their effects on cell membrane at the beta receptors. Beta-1 receptors are located primarily in the myocardium. Inhibition of catecholamine action on the myocardium reduces cardiac contractility, sinus node rate, and AV node conduction velocity. Beta-2 receptors are located primarily in vascular and bronchial smooth muscle and inhibition of catecholamine action at these sites produces arterial vasoconstriction and bronchoconstriction. In unstable angina the primary benefits of beta-blocker therapy are due to its effect on beta-1 receptors that decrease cardiac work and myocardial oxygen demand. Metaanalyses of the available trials reveal that there is no clear effect on mortality in unstable angina to date. However, randomized trials in acute MI, recent MI, and stable angina with silent ischemia have all shown a mortality benefit for beta blockers. Therefore, the overall rationale for the use of beta blockers is compelling and sufficient to make them a routine part of care for patients with unstable angina.

Choice of beta blocker for a patient is based primarily on pharmacokinetic and side-effect criteria. There is no evidence that any member of this class of agents is more effective in producing beneficial effects in unstable angina than any other. On the basis of side-effect profiles, initial choice of agents favors metoprolol or atenolol, and esmolol can be used if a continuous infusion is required. If there are concerns about patient intolerance due to pulmonary disease or LV dysfunction, a short-acting agent should be considered. Mild wheezing or a history of COPD should prompt a trial of a short-acting beta blocker at a reduced dose rather than complete avoidance.

For patients at high risk for MI, it is recommended that IV beta blockers be started in the abscence of contraindications. Monitoring during IV beta-blocker therapy should include frequent checks of heart rate and blood pressure and continuous ECG monitoring, as well as auscultation for rales or bronchospasm. After the initial IV load, patients may be converted to oral agents. The target heart rate for beta-blocker therapy is 50 to 60 beats per minute. Contraindications to beta-blocker therapy include marked first-degree atrioventricular (AV) block—PR segment > 0.24 seconds, any form of second- or third-degree AV block, a history of asthma, or severe LV dysfunction with congestive heart failure or cardiogenic shock. Significant sinus bradycardia (heart rate < 60) or hypotension should be resolved before initiation of beta-blocker therapy.

Calcium Channel Blockers. Five unique subgroups of calcium channel antagonists are available for the treatment of angina: the dihydropyridines (nifedipine, isradipine, felodipine, amlodipine, and nicardipine), diltiazem, verapamil, tetralol, and bepridil (Clem, 1995). Calcium channel blockers reduce the myocardial cell transmembrane influx of calcium ions which, in turn, affects myocardial and vascular smooth muscle contraction as well as AV conduction. The agents in this class vary in the degree to which they produce clinically important vasodilation, decreased myocardial contractility, and increased AV block. The dihydropyridines generally have the largest peripheral arterial vasodilatory effect, and they lack any effect on the cardiac conduction system. Verapamil has an intermediate vasodilatory effect and diltiazem has the least effect. All four agents appear to have coronary vasodilatory properties that are equivalent. The first-generation dihydropyridines (e.g., nifedipine and nicardipine) may occasionally induce a proischemic effect by a coronary steal mechanism or by inducing hypotension or reflex tachycardia. This does not seem to be a problem with second-generation dihyropyridines such as amlodipine (Thadani, 1997). Each of the dihydropyridines and both verapamil and diltiazem have negative inotropic effects.

Bepridil, a type 4 calcium antagonist, possesses characteristics of the traditional calcium antagonists; however, it also may inhibit fast sodium channels, which may account for some of the serious side effects associated with this drug. It is usually reserved for patients with refractory chronic stable angina who have failed to respond to other agents. The drug prolongs the QT interval making patients more susceptible to torsades de pointes and other ventricular arrhythmias. Electrolytes, especially potassium, and ECGs must be monitored closely when initiating and titrating the drug.

Beneficial effects of the calcium channel blockers in unstable angina are believed due to variable combinations of decreased myocardial oxygen demand relating to decreased afterload, contractility, and heart rate. However, major side effects are also related to exaggeration of these three therapeutic effects: hypotension, worsening CHF, and AV block. These agents may also have a beneficial effect of LV diastolic relaxation and compliance. Other adverse effects include peripheral edema, especially with the dihydropyridine group and constipation with verapamil, especially in the elderly (Thadani, 1997).

The limited randomized trial data available are not consistent with a beneficial effect on mortality or recurrent infarction. In addition, results from randomized trials involving the use of these agents in acute MI patients suggests an overall detrimental effect on mortality, with patients with LV dysfunction being particularly at risk. For these reasons, it is the recommendation of the Unstable Angina Guideline Panel to reserve use of these agents as second- or third-line therapy following nitrates and beta blockers (Braunwald et al., 1994).

Morphine. Morphine sulfate has potent analgesic and anxiolytic effects, as well as hemodynamic effects, that are potentially beneficial in unstable angina. Morphine relieves pain and decreases cardiac work and oxygen consumption. In particular, morphine causes significant venodilation along with modest reduction in heart rate (through increased vagal tone) and systolic blood pressure. Morphine sulfate at a dose of 2 to 5 mg IV is recommended for any patient whose symptoms are refractory to other anti-ischemic therapy. It may be repeated every 5 to 30 minutes as needed and tolerated to relieve symptoms and maintain patient comfort. Adverse reactions to morphine include hypotension (especially in the presence of concomitant vasodilator therapy), nausea, and vomiting. Respiratory depression is the most serious complication of morphine; naloxone may be required to reverse its effect (Braunwald et al., 1994).

Myocardial Infarction

Myocardial infarction is defined as irreversible necrosis of myocardial tissue as a result of inadequate blood flow for a critical period of time (Stewart, 1992). The cessation of blood flow and oxygen supply results first in ischemia, then progression to injury and necrosis. The timetable is variable, ranging from minutes to several hours. During coronary artery occlusion, the myocardial area at risk depends on the culprit coronary artery and its distribution along with the presence and extent of collateral blood supply and myocardial demands. Cellular death in this myocardial region spreads across the ventricular wall over time in a wavefront of necrosis extending from subendocardium to the subepicardium. It is widely accepted that "time is muscle" and that rapid and early treatment to salvage myocardium greatly improves patient outcomes (Coombs & Brinker, 1995).

The initiating event for nearly all cases of acute myocardial infarction is the abrupt instability of an atheromatous plaque in a coronary artery (Davies & Thomas, 1985). One mechanism of plaque disruption is a surge of sympathetic activity that increases blood pressure, heart rate, cardiac contractility, and coronary blood flow (Shah, 1997). The resulting shear stress on the vessel wall causes fissuring of the overlying fibrous capsule which renders the plaque unstable. A sudden increase in coronary narrowing occurs through several mechanisms: platelet adhesion, fibrin clot formation, enlargement of the atheromatous plaque by intraplaque hemorrhage, abnormal vasoconstriction, and an adventitial inflammation (Vincent, 1994). Figure 32–5 shows the pathogenesis of acute MI.

There are certain conditions or activities that are felt to be triggers for up to 50% of MIs. These include vigorous exercise, emotional stress, cold weather, time of the day (early morning), day of the week (Monday), and possibly recent infections (Shah, 1997).

Types of Myocardial Infarction

Q-wave Versus Non-Q-wave MI. The nomenclature for classifying MIs can be confusing. It was previously believed that Q-wave MIs were transmural (involving all layers of heart muscle) while non-Q-wave MIs only affected a layer of myocardium (subendocardial layer). Autopsy results, however, have confirmed that transmural infarctions have occurred in the absence of pathologic Q waves on ECG. In turn, patients with Q waves on ECG have been found to have only subendocardial infarction at autopsy (Lavie & Gersh, 1990a).

The presence of Q waves occurs in 60% of infarcts and typically indicates larger size and an increase in pathologic findings. During cardiac catheterization, total coronary thrombosis was present (Lewis, 1992).

Non-Q-wave MIs occur in about 25 to 40% of all MIs, are smaller in terms of gram weight, and are less pathologic. During cardiac catheterization, partial thrombosis to completely patent vessels were found, possibly secondary to spontaneous reperfusion (Williams & Morton, 1995). Non-Q-wave MIs have lower incidence of CHF, lower cardiac enzyme levels, and an overall lower hospital mortality rate. The 3-year mortality, however, is the same for Q-wave and non-Q-wave MIs at 30%. Non-Q-wave MI patients are at a higher risk for reinfarction with 43% of patients having an extention of the infarct, the theory being that spontaneous reperfusion leaves the viable tissue vulnerable to reinfarction (Lewis, 1992). Patients with non-Q-wave MIs also have more unstable angina, and a higher incidence of angioplasty and coronary artery bypass grafting (Williams & Morton, 1995). Any evidence of recurrent ischemia or extension of infarction warrants emergent cardiac catheterization and prompt revascularization.

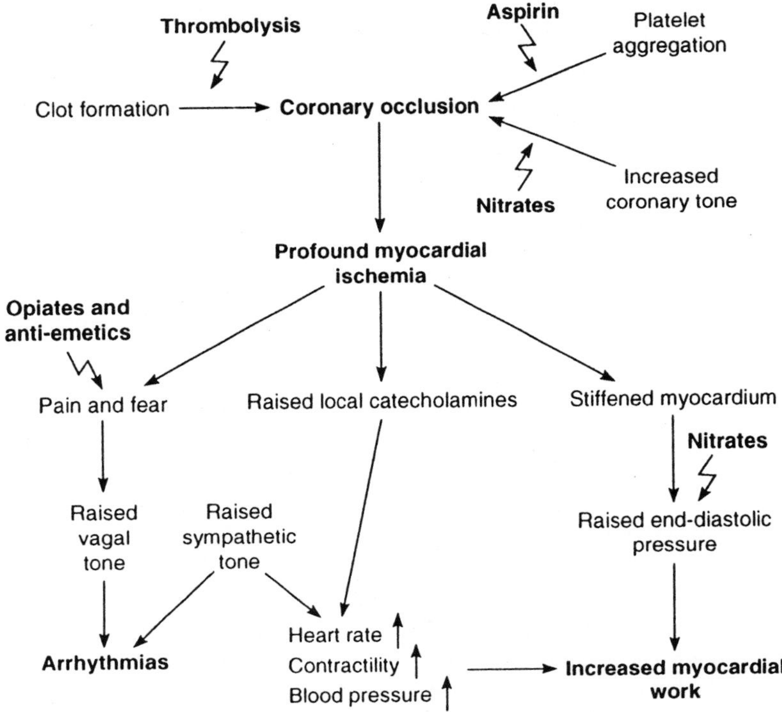

Figure 32–5. The pathogenesis of acute myocardial infarction with potential sites for therapy. *(From Vincent R. [1994]. [pp. 3–28].).*

Right Ventricular Infarction. Right ventricular infarction can occur independently but most commonly is associated with an inferior or posterior wall MI and can result in right ventricular failure and cardiogenic shock. It occurs when there is an occlusion of the right coronary artery proximal to the acute marginal branches, but it may also occur with a left circumflex artery lesion in patients with left dominant coronary circulation (Kinch & Ryan, 1994). Because it almost always occurs in conjunction with a left ventricular infarction and is not easily detected on routine 12-lead ECG, it is often overlooked.

After a right ventricular infarction (RVI), the contractile ability of the right ventricle (RV) is impaired, resulting in an inability of the RV to handle the incoming venous return. This results in an increase in right ventricular end diastolic pressure (RVEDP) and elevated central venous pressure (CVP), causing right-sided filling pressures to exceed the left-sided filling pressures. Concurrently, the impaired RV contractility leads to reduced RV output which decreases LV stroke volume, leading to hypotension and cardiogenic shock (McMillan & Little-Longeway, 1991).

Typical physical signs of RV failure include hypotension, jugular venous distention (JVD), Kussmaul's sign (paradoxical distention of the jugular veins on inspiration), and clear lung fields. Other physical findings that may be present include a right ventricular gallop, the murmur of tricuspid regurgitation, and AV dissociation (Kinch & Ryan, 1994; McMillan & Little-Longeway, 1991).

Since one third of all patients with inferior or posterior infarctions demonstrate at least some degree of RV necrosis, patients who present with these infarct patterns should have a right-sided 12-lead ECG. This is similar to a standard 12-lead; however, the precordial leads are on the right side of the chest. Elevation of the ST segment in V4R greater than 1 mm is usually indicative of RVI. It is important to do a right-sided 12-lead ECG as early as possible since ST-segment elevation in the right precordial leads is often a transient finding that resolves when the patient is pain-free. RVI may also be diagnosed by echocardiography which detects abnormal wall motion of the RV or evidence of a dilated RV (Kinch & Ryan, 1994).

The managment goals of RVI are directed at maintaining RV preload, reducing RV afterload, and improving contractility. Treatment differs from that of LVI in that as opposed to fluid restriction and diuretics, volume expansion is a key goal of therapy. Intravenous fluids enhance RV stroke volume which leads to improved RV output and consequently LV output. Patients should be carefully monitored with a pulmonary artery catheter in place to guide management. If fluid loading alone does not improve hypotension and enhance cardiac output, inotropic support may be needed to enhance contractility. Dobutamine has a positive inotropic effect on both ventricles and produces a decrease in pulmonary vascular resistance which reduces impedance to right ventricular ejection (McMillan & Little-Longeway, 1991).

Atrioventricular block or bradyarrhythmias, common complications of inferior and posterior wall MIs, are usually refractory to atropine and may require pacing. AV sequential pacing is the treatment of choice since it restores AV synchrony which improves stroke volume and cardiac output (Kinch & Ryan, 1994).

If right ventricular infarctions are identified early and treated properly, the outcome is favorable. Patients with RVI generally have a restoration of normal RV function with resolution of hemodynamic abnormalities (Kinch & Ryan, 1994).

Diagnosis of Myocardial Infarction

Patient History. The classic initial manifestations of acute myocardial infarction are prolonged substernal chest discomfort, dyspnea, and diaphoresis; however, not all patients present with these symptoms. Pain can be atypical in quality, for example, sharp or stabbing as opposed to the crushing, constricting, or squeezing pain usually described. Radiation of the pain to the neck, jaw, shoulders, arms, fingers, and back often occur. Associated symptoms of nausea, vomiting, diarrhea, weakness, dizziness, palpitations, and a sense of impending doom need to be elicited during the history as an integral part of the clinical picture (Lavie & Gersh, 1990a). Not all MIs are symptomatic. Undiagnosed MIs occur most often in the elderly and in patients with hypertension and diabetes. In fact, 27.7% of all documented MIs were silent or unrecognized and initially detected during routine physical examination according to the Framingham data (Kannel & Abbott, 1984).

Physical Examination. The physical examination is not diagnostic in determining MI; however, there are findings that may directly reflect myocardial injury and, therefore, give important information to help guide the immediate management plan. Signs of severe left ventricular dysfunction—such as hypotension, tachycardia, pulmonary congestion, S3 or paradoxical splitting of the second heart sound on cardiac auscultation—may be present, along with palpable dyskinesia and pulsus alternans. A systolic murmur not previously noted can result from papillary muscle dysfunction or severe mitral regurgitation secondary to papillary muscle rupture, ventricular dilatation, or ventricular septal rupture (Lavie & Gersh, 1990a; Ryan, Anderson, Antman, et al., 1996). A baseline examination of the patient's peripheral vasculature is important to assess adequacy if invasive procedures are required and also give important baseline information in the event of systemic embolization, a complication of MI.

In right ventricular infarcts, hypotension, elevated jugular venous pressure with clear lung fields may be present (Lavie & Gersh, 1990a). A widely split S2, a right ventricular S3, an S4, or both and the murmur of tricuspid insufficiency may be appreciated on cardiac auscultation (Hanisch, 1991).

Electrocardiogram

Infarct Patterns. Electrocardiographic criteria indicative of an acute myocardial infarction (AMI) include ST-segment elevation and the presence of pathologic Q waves (Table 32–9). Elevation of the ST segment >1 mm along the vertical axis in two contiguous leads is necessary for the diagnosis of AMI. To be pathologic and diagnostic of AMI, Q waves must be greater than 0.04 seconds' duration and greater than 25% of the R-wave amplitude.

Approximately 40 to 60% of AMIs have nonspecific ECG changes and cardiac enzymes are required to make a definitive diagnosis (Williams & Morton, 1995).

INFERIOR MYOCARDIAL INFARCTION. Inferior-wall myocardial infarction (IWMI) generally occurs as a result of occlusion of the right coronary artery (RCA) or the posterior descending coronary artery (PDA), a branch of the RCA in 90% of individuals. Less frequently it is caused by disease in a dominant left circumflex artery. Patients with IWMI with no previous history of an MI have a generally more favorable prognosis than patients with anterior wall MI, most likely because less myocardium is involved. The RCA supplies blood to the atrioventricular (AV) node and the bundle of HIS 90% of the time and the sinus node 55% of the time. It also supplies the inferior (diaphragmatic) myocardium of the left ventricle and the lower third of the interventricular septum. Therefore, conduction abnormalities post-IWMI are reflective of the ischemia to these areas.

ECG changes in inferior MI include ST-wave elevation, T-wave inversion, and Q waves in leads II, III, and AVF (Figs. 32–6 and 32–7). Inferolateral wall MIs have the same changes in II, III, AVF, I, AVL, and possibly V5 and V6. Inferobasal or inferoposterior MIs have ST-segment elevation, T-wave inversion, and Q waves in II, III, AVF, and a positive T wave and R/S ratio in V1 that is less than or equal to one.

Sinus node disturbances, first-degree AV block, AV Wenchebach, complete AV block, and atrial arrhythmias are conduction complications associated with IWMI. Nausea, vomiting, vasovagal syncope caused by enhanced vagal stimulation, bronchospasm, and tracheal burning are also common.

RIGHT VENTRICULAR INFARCTION. Often found in the presence of an IWMI, right ventricular MI occurs from the occlusion of the proximal right coronary artery. A right-sided ECG must be recorded with all inferior wall MIs, especially if RVI is suspected. ST-segment elevation in V1r–V3r is present along with the ECG criteria for IWMI. The ST-segment elevation seen in the right precordial leads typically lasts only 10 to 24 hours.

The complications that arise from a right ventricular infarct are caused by RV pump failure resulting in the inability of the RV to provide the left ventricle with adequate filling pressures. This results in a decreased cardiac output, elevated central venous pressures, and no pulmonary congestion. A pulmonary artery catheter is usually indicated to guide management.

Conduction disturbances common to IWMI, such as heart block and symptomatic brady arrhythmias, are also common and a transvenous pacer may be required. AV sequential pacing has been shown to be more beneficial than ventricular pacing alone; it effectively increases stroke volume and, therefore, cardiac output.

Papillary muscle dysfunction often occurs with IWMI. With RVI, therefore, it is important to be cognizant of the signs and symptoms of papillary muscle dysfunction or rupture.

POSTERIOR WALL INFARCTION. The right coronary artery, or less commonly, the mid and posterior marginal branches of the left circumflex artery supply the posterior wall of the heart. None of the conventional surface ECG leads face the posterior surface of the heart. "Mirror image" changes in leads V1–V3, which are opposite the posterior segment, are used to diagnose posterior wall infarcts (Figs. 32–8 and 32–9). In these leads, ST-segment depression, tall symmetric T waves, reversal of T-wave polarity, and tall broad initial R-wave upswing are diagnostic of posterior infarcts.

Complications include the possibility of symptomatic bradycardia and heart block. These conditions are usually transient and disappear as the infarction heals.

ANTERIOR WALL INFARCTION. The main left coronary artery originates in the left sinus of valsalva and branches

TABLE 32–9. Electrocardiographic Infarction Patterns

Location of MI	Involved Vessel	ECG Changes	Complications
Inferior	RCA	II, III, AVF	Bradycardia, AV conduction disturbances; AV block
Right ventricular	RCA	II, III, AVF, ST ↑ V1r–V3r	↑ CVP; ↓ CO; clear lung fields; possible papillary muscle dysfunction; heart block and bradycardia
Posterior	RCA or less common LCFx branch	ST segment↓, tall, symmetric T waves, reversal of T-wave polarity, tall and broad R-wave upswing	Bradycardia, heart block
Anterior	LM, LAD, LCFx	ST seg ↑ & T wave↓ V1–V4, Q waves V3 & V4; loss of R waves V2–V6	CHF, cardiogenic shock, arrhythmias, R & L BBB, Mobitz II–CHB
Lateral	LCFx, diagonal branches of LAD	ST seg↑ & T wave↓, Q waves I, AVL, V5, V6	Isolated lateral wall MI uncommon—typically smaller, least likely to cause complications

Source: P. J. Hanisch (1991).

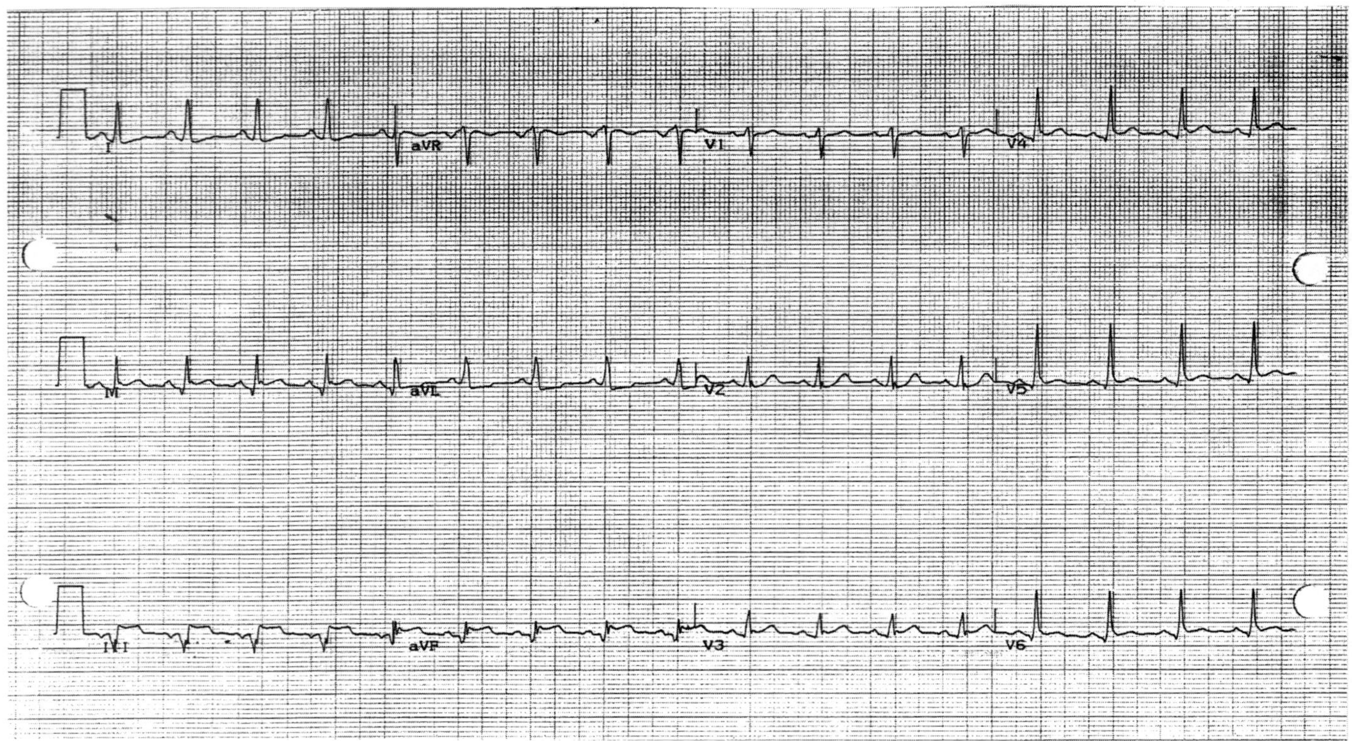

Figure 32–6. Inferior myocardial infarction. Q waves are present in leads II, III, and aVF. There is also mild ST elevation suggesting that the MI is recent or ongoing.

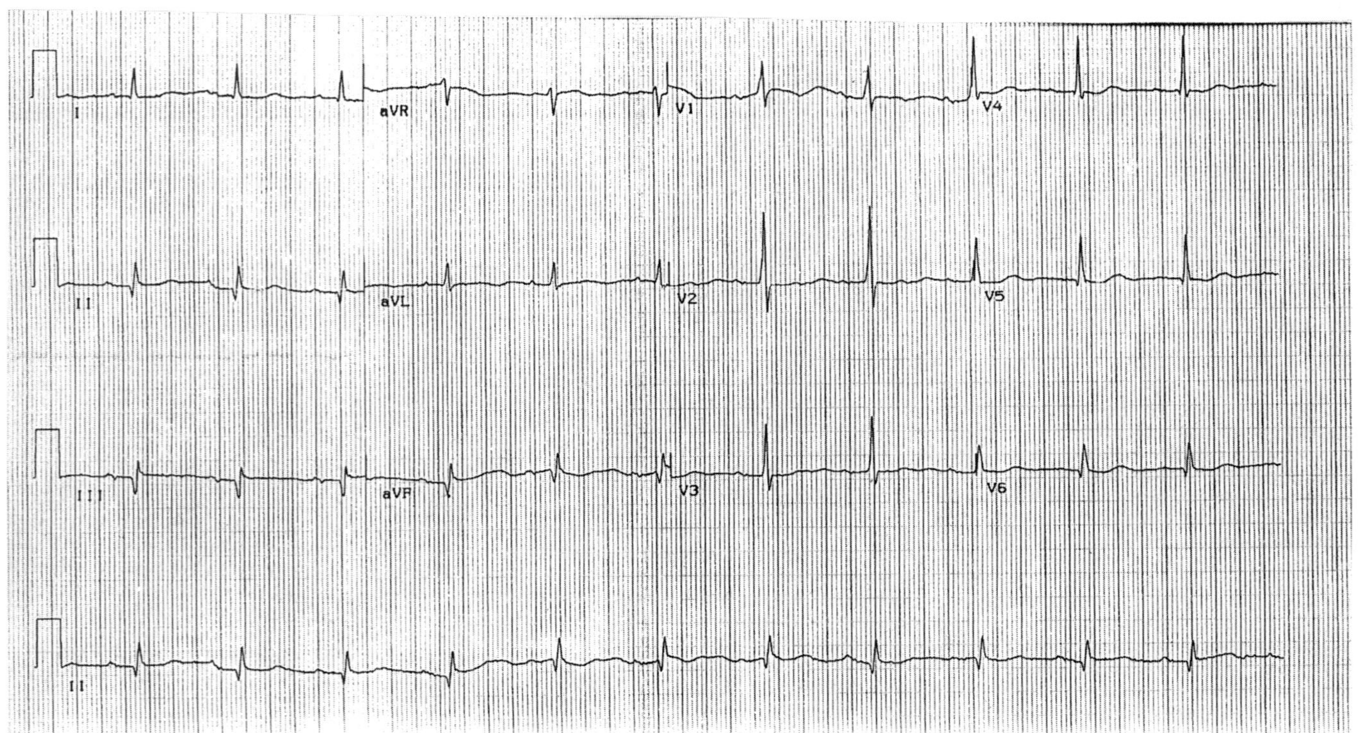

Figure 32–7. Inferior (Q's in II, III, and aVF) and posterior (tall R's in V1 and V2) myocardial infarction of indeterminate age.

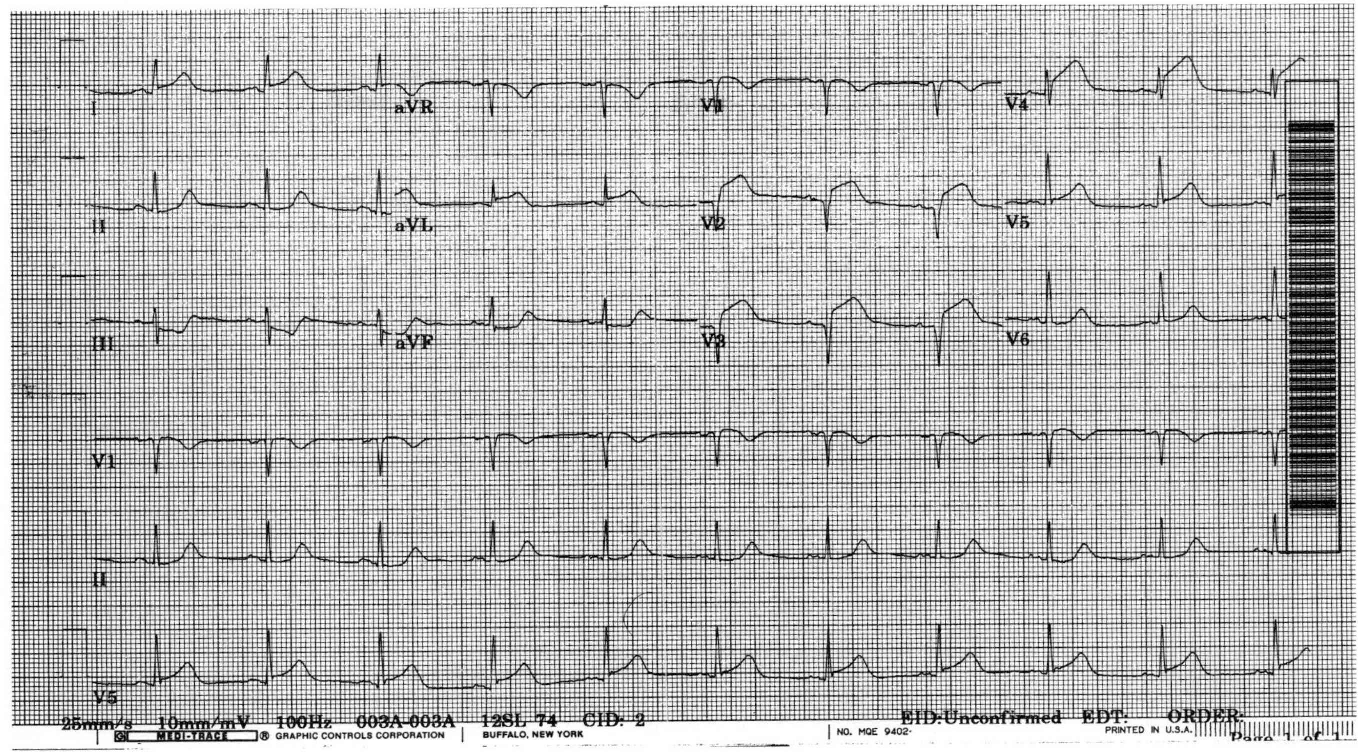

Figure 32–8. Acute anterior myocardial infarction with reciprocal ST depression in inferior leads. There is also lateral ST elevation that likely represents ischemia.

into the left anterior descending and left circumflex. It supplies the right bundle branch, part of the posteroinferior branch, and anterior two thirds of the ventricular septum.

ECG changes suggestive of anterior ischemia include ST-segment elevation and T wave inversion in leads V1–V4. Q-waves in V1–V4 indicate MI. Similarly, anterolateral ischemia is characterized by ST elevation and T inversion in I, AVL, V5–V6, while Q-waves represent infarction. Septal leads are considered V1–V2.

Anterior wall MIs are typically associated with large muscle mass involvement and, therefore, the complications and prognosis are significantly worse than an IWMI. Pump failure may occur and include CHF and cardiogenic shock. Arrhythmias such as sinus tachycardia, premature ventricular contractions, ventricular tachycardia, and atrial fibrillation may occur. Intraventricular conduction defects such as right and left bundle branch blocks, Mobitz II, and complete heart block are also associated with anterior MIs. The development of bundle branch block and hemiblock in the setting of an MI worsens the prognosis.

LATERAL WALL INFARCTION. The circumflex artery and the diagonal branches of the left anterior descending supply the lateral, and sometimes part of the inferior, myocardium.

Due to the standard 12-lead EKG method, the lateral wall has few leads. The lateral wall, then, is quite electrically "silent," making identification of lateral infarcts challenging. Lateral infarcts reveal Q waves and ST-segment elevation in leads V5–V6. Inferolateral infarcts are suggested by Q waves and ST-segment elevation in leads II, III, AVF, V5, V6. Anterolateral infarcts are characterized by Q waves and ST-segment elevation in I, AVL, V5, V6.

MI localized only in the lateral wall is uncommon and generally benign as far as significant complications. It usually accompanies anterior or inferior infarcts (Conover, 1988; Hanisch, 1991).

Cardiac Enzymes. For the early diagnosis of acute MI, the diagnostic value of physical examination and the electrocardiogram is often limited. Myocardial necrosis releases intracellular cytoplasmic and mitochondrial structural elements, such as myosin and enzymes, into the interstitial space and then into the venous blood. After an acute MI, enzymes such as creatine kinase (CK), serum aspartate transaminase (AST), and lactate hehydrogenase (LDH) are released in amounts related to the volume of infarcted myocardial muscle (Figueredo & Cheitlin, 1994). Myoglobin, a small molecular-mass protein abundant in skeletal and cardiac tissue and troponin T and I, polypeptide subunits of the myofibrillar regulatory troponin complex, are also released from damaged myocardial cells (Bakker, Koelemay, Gorgels, et al., 1994).

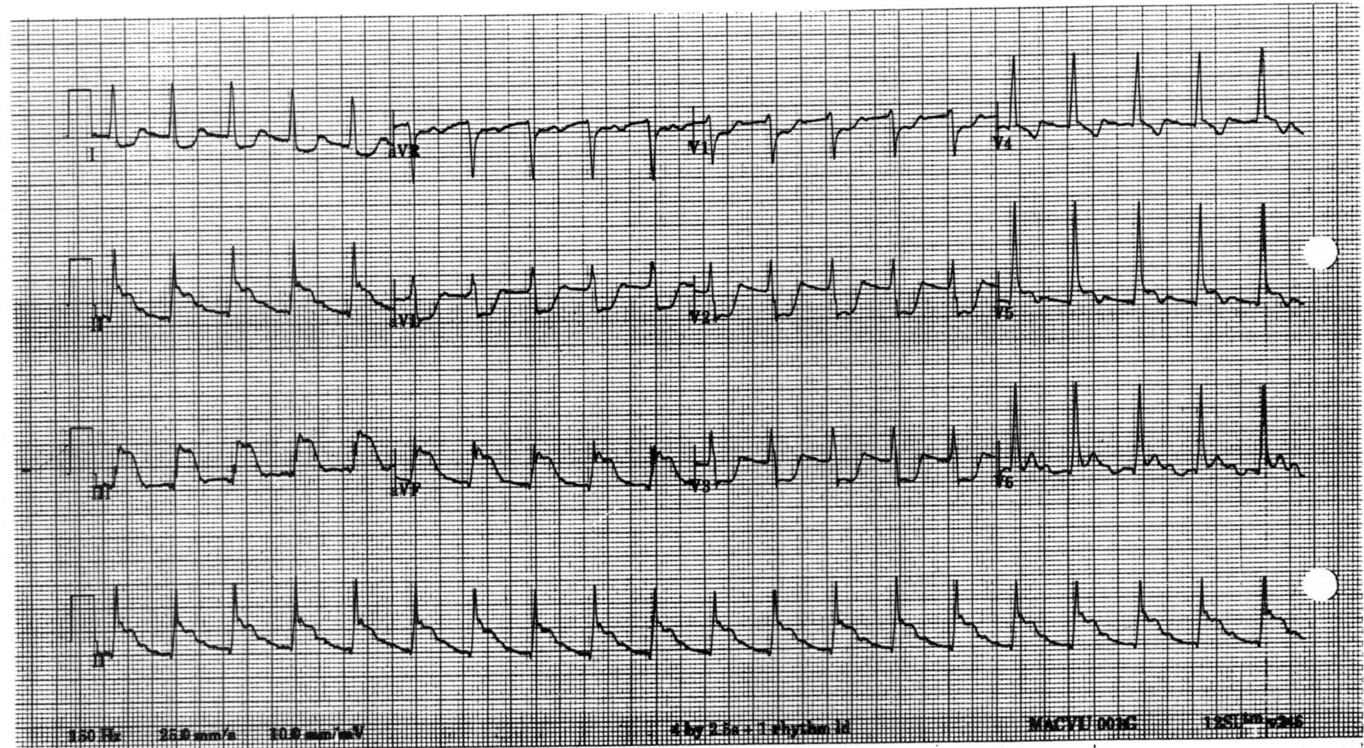

Figure 32–9. Evolving infero posterior myocardial infarction. Note the ST segment elevation in leads II, III, AVL, and ST depression in V1–V3.

Creatine Kinase. Creatine kinase (CK) is the current laboratory test for the confirmation of MI. It is elevated in the serum 3 to 4 hours following a MI, reaches its peak of activity between 18 to 30 hours and is followed by a sharp drop to normal levels by the third or fourth day. Because CK elevation is not specific for myocardial injury, a CK isoenzyme, CK–MB, is concurrently evaluated. CK–MB is very specific for myocardial infarction. It will not rise in patients with transient cardiac chest pain; it will, however, rise post cardioversion, cardiac contusion, cardiac surgical procedures, myocarditis, and acute pericarditis with myocardial involvement. CK–MB is elevated in the serum 2 to 4 hours following acute MI, reaches its peak in 12 to 24 hours, and returns to normal in 24 to 36 hours. CK–MB should be 4% greater than total CK for definitive diagnosis of MI (Bakerman, 1994).

Lactate Dehydrogenase. Normally elevated within 8 to 12 hours, lactate dehydrogenase (LDH) peaks in 2 to 4 days, and lasts for 10 to 14 days. This enzyme is also not specific to myocardial tissue, therefore, isoenzymes are concurrently evaluated. The typical myocardial infarct exhibits a rise in LDH levels (LDL1 > LDL2) beginning at 8 to 12 hours, peaks at 24 to 72 hours, and remains elevated for 7 to 12 days. LDH1 can be increased by conditions other than MI, including hemolytic and megaloblastic anemias, acute renal infarction, hemolysis, and testicular cancer. If serum CK–MB levels are increased, it is not considered cost effective or necessary to measure LDH isoenzymes unless patients present with symptoms 24 to 48 hours after their onset (Bakerman, 1994; Lavie & Gersh, 1990a).

Serum Myoglobin. This is a small molecular-mass protein abundant in skeletal and cardiac tissue. Elevated concentrations of myoglobin are also encountered in skeletal muscle injury. The release is limited to a rather narrow time window after MI (Bakker et al., 1994). It is highly sensitive, however, making it possible to safely exclude MI if the serum myoglobin is normal within 4 hours of the onset of symptoms.

Troponin. Cardiac-specific Troponin I (cTnI) is a recently discovered marker for acute MI. Levels rise early after muscle damage and, in contrast to CK–MB, remain elevated up to 1 to 2 weeks post infarction, making it a useful tool for early and late diagnosis of AMI (Ryan et al., 1996).

The clinical implications of cardiac enzymes are summarized in Table 32–10.

Treatment of Myocardial Infarction

The goals of treatment of myocardial infarction involve the restoration of the oxygen supply and demand equation. This includes reducing infarct expansion, maximizing myocardial salvage, preserving ventricular function, and minimizing reperfusion injury (Williams & Morton, 1995).

TABLE 32–10. The Times to Earliest Rise, Peak, and Normalization of Cardiac Enzymes After Myocardial Infarction

Serum Enzyme	Earliest Rise	Peak	Normalization
Myoglobin	1–2 hr	4 hr	~ 8 hr
Cardiac Troponin I (cTnI)	3–6 hr	12–24 hr	7 days
Creatine kinase (CK)	4–6 hr	8–24 hr	48–72 hr
Lactic dehydrogenase (LDH)	24–48 hr	24–48 hr	7–14 days

General Measures. Patients admitted to the hospital with an MI or suspicion of an MI must have continuous ECG monitoring to diagnose and treat life-threatening arrhythmias (Ryan et al., 1999). IV access and supplemental oxygen are also necessary.

Generally, it is recommended that patients activity level be restricted to bed rest with bedside commode privileges for the first 6 to 12 hours after MI since physical exercise increases the area of myocardial damage when coronary blood flow is limited. However, several randomized trials have revealed that early mobilization (after 12 hours in the uncomplicated MI) has resulted in a reduction of serious complications. Patients should be encouraged to participate in self-care activities progressing to light ambulation with appropriate staff supervision to prevent physiological deconditioning (Antman, 1994).

The valsalva maneuver should be avoided. Forced expiration against a closed glottis causes sudden and intense changes in systolic blood pressure and heart rate and may predispose the patient to ventricular arrhythmias. Stool softeners should be prescribed routinely and a bedside commode used rather than a bedpan (Ryan et al., 1996).

Pharmacologic Management. See the section on pharmacologic management of unstable angina.

Oxygen. Patients presenting with myocardial infarction typically have some degree of hypoxia as a result of ventilation–perfusion abnormalities secondary to left ventricular dysfunction. Supplemental oxygen should be administered in the initial hours of presentation, although it is not known whether this therapy limits myocardial damage or reduces morbidity and mortality. If oxygen saturation is less than 90%, supplemental O_2 is indicated but is probably not beneficial if the saturation on room air is near 100%. Experimental studies have shown that breathing oxygen may limit ischemic myocardial injury and there is evidence that supplemental O_2 reduces ST-segment elevation in acute MI. In cases of severe congestive heart failure or pulmonary edema, mechanical ventilation may be required (Ryan et al., 1996).

Analgesics. The relief of pain and anxiety may lead to a decrease in circulating catecholamines and a possible reduction in associated arrhythmias. Morphine reduces preload and afterload and decreases myocardial oxygen demand, making it the drug of choice in treating the pain and anxiety associated with AMI (Ryan et al., 1996).

Nitrates. Nitrates relieve pain from myocardial ischemia by decreasing myocardial O_2 demand (lowering preload) and increasing O_2 supply by dilating infarct-related coronary or collateral vessels (Pasternak & Braunwald, 1994). Several clinical trials have reported a > 40% reduction in mortality with IV nitroglycerine use post MI by decreasing infarct size and reducing the incidence of ventricular fibrillation (Lavie & Gersh, 1990b). In the absence of hypotension, it is recommended that patients with acute MI and CHF, large anterior infarctions, persistent ischemia, or hypertension receive intravenous nitroglycerin for the first 24 to 48 hours, and continued if postinfarct angina is present (Ryan et al., 1996).

Heparin and Aspirin. Heparin and aspirin are administered together to reduce the incidence of reocclusion after successful reperfusion and to decrease infarct extension. The combined use may increase the likelihood of bleeding complications; however, the actual risk of short-term concomitant use is quite low and the benefits outweigh the risks (Clem, 1995; Ryan et al., 1996).

Heparin prevents reocclusion by inactivating free thrombin formed in the area of a lysing clot. This free thrombin may otherwise interact with fibrinogen to form fibrin and reestablish the thrombus (Williams & Morton, 1995).

Intravenous heparin is recommended in patients undergoing percutaneous or surgical revascularization, and in patients who are treated with thrombolytic therapy. The specific thrombolytic agent dictates the heparin recommendation. The PTT should be between 1.5 and 2 times control values. In the absense of more aggressive anticoagulation, all patients with suspected MI should be given low-dose heparin, 7500 units subcutaneously every 12 hours until they are fully ambulatory to prevent deep venous thrombosis. In patients who are high risk for systemic emboli, IV heparin is recommended (Ryan et al., 1996).

Aspirin inhibits the synthesis of thromboxane A2, a powerful platelet activator and vasoconstrictor implicated in the formation of coronary thrombosis. This results in a decrease in platelet aggregation and clot formation (Williams & Morton, 1995).

The ability of aspirin to reduce the risk of recurrent cardiovascular complications in patients with previous myocardial infarctions has been studied in numerous trials. An overview of these trials reveals that aspirin can reduce the risk of fatal and nonfatal cardiovascular events by one-fourth (Patrono, 1994). The AHA/ACC recommend an initial dose of 160 mg of nonecteric-coated aspirin which should be continued indefinitely (Ryan et al., 1996).

Warfarin. Warfarin (Coumadin) should be used in patients who have had a large anterior wall infarction, and when there is a risk of developing a LV thrombus. When a thrombus has been clearly demonstrated by echocardiography, the use of coumadin markedly lowers the incidence of embolic complications. The likelihood of arterial embolism appears to increase with the extent of infarction and the resultant inflammation and endocardial stasis due to akinesis. Therefore, the indication for coumadin therapy for the prevention of embolic complications increases wtih the extent of the infarct. The approximate duration of therapy is 3 to 6 months (Pasternak & Braunwald, 1994). The previous ACC/AHA guidelines of 1990 supported this and recommended that an international normalized ration (INR) of approximately 2.5 should be maintained. The current ACC/AHA guidelines of 1996, however, allow that although there are a number of small observational studies that support the previous information, randomized controlled trials are not available to support this recommendation.

Beta Blockers. Beta blockers are an integral component of the management of an acute myocardial infarction. By reducing myocardial contractility and heart rate, they reduce myocardial oxygen consumption. In the setting of an acute MI, beta blockers have been shown to reduce infarct size and mortality rate (Clem, 1995). As evidenced by several drug trials, chronic beta blockage begun in the early phase of infarction improves survival and decreases the incidence of reinfarction for at least the first several months after an acute infarction. This includes a reduction in the frequency of sudden cardiac deaths (Ryan et al., 1996).

The favorable effects of beta blockade in patients without contraindications to therapy occur with both cardioselective and nonselective agents. Agents with intrinsic sympathomimetic activity (ISA), however, such as acebutalol and pindolol, should be avoided (Clem, 1995; Ryan et al., 1996).

Calcium Channel Blockers. Calcium channel blockers inhibit the influx of calcium into cells, reducing the amount of calcium available for contraction. The resulting physiologic effects are coronary and peripheral vasoconstriction, decrease in peripheral vascular resistance, decrease in afterload, and a reduction in heart rate (Williams & Morton, 1995).

The known cardiovascular properties of these drugs suggest a rationale for their use in the treatment of acute MI; however, the AHA/ACC guidelines for the management of AMI report that there is no clear evidence to support the use of calcium channel blockers in the treatment of MI, with the exception of the subset of patients with non–Q-wave infarction in whom diltiazem was found effective in preventing early reinfarction and recurrent severe angina (Ryan et al., 1996). Immediate-release nifedipine may be particularly detrimental in patients with hypotension and/or tachycardia, causing a reduction in coronary perfusion pressure, disproportionate dilatation of the coronary arteries adjacent to the ischemic area, reflex activation of the sympathetic nervous system, with an increase in myocardial oxygen demands (Ryan et al., 1996).

ACE Inhibitors. Postmyocardial infarction, thinning of the ventricular muscle in the infarct area and left ventricular dilatation may occur. This is known as ventricular remodeling and ACE inhibitors are thought to prevent this phenomenom from occurring. Although, the exact mechanism of action is unknown, the inhibition of the conversion of angiotensin I to angiotensin II (a very potent vasoconstrictor) leads to a reduction in afterload that reduces left ventricular dilatation.

As reported in The Survival and Ventricular Enlargement Trial group, the use of ACE inhibitors post MI have been proven beneficial in improving mortality, as well as heart failure and recurrent MI prevention, in patients with ejection fractions < 40% (Pfeffer, 1992).

ACE inhibitors are usually well tolerated. They should be started post MI once the patient is hemodynamically stable and titrated to optimal dose (Pasternak & Braunwald, 1994). Common adverse reactions include dry, chronic cough; hypotension; worsening of renal dysfunction; electrolyte imbalances (hyperkalemia and hyponatremia); and hypersensitivity reactions. Patients should have regular evaluation of blood pressure, renal function, signs of developing heart failure, and complete blood count and serum electrolytes (Clem, 1995).

Magnesium. Clinical trials suggest that the early use of intravenous magnesium may have a favorable effect on cardiac arrhythmias, coronary blood flow, platelet aggregation, as well as myocardial metabolism. It is felt to reduce total mortality in patients post MI (Pasternak & Braunwald, 1994). It is inexpensive and has few side effects. In patients with arrhythmias, an infusion of 2 to 4 gms of magnesium sulfate over 30 to 60 minutes should be considered (Lavie & Gersh, 1990b). There are conflicting data about the benefit of magnesium, though.

Thrombolytic Agents. Acute myocardial infarction is the most common cause of death in the United States (Pasternak & Braunwald, 1994). One of the most important developments in the care of patients with acute myocardial infarction is the recognition that early reperfusion of ischemic myocardium can potentially salvage tissue before it becomes irreversibly injured. Most infarctions are caused by a sudden thrombotic occlusion overlying an atherosclerotic plaque in a major coronary artery. Recent attention has been placed on either pharmacologically or mechanically recanalizing the "culprit" vessel. Thrombolytic agents such as streptokinase, urokinase, tissue plasminogen activator (tPA), and anisoylated plasminogen streptokinase activator complex (APSAC) have been approved by the Federal Drug Administration. Efforts have been made to study the benefits and the time in which these agents are administered

(Pasternak & Braunwald, 1994). Thrombolytic therapy has been shown to reduce in-hospital mortality for myocardial infarction by up to 50% when administered within the first hour of the onset of symptoms. Much of this benefit is maintained for one or more years. Appropriately employed thrombolytic therapy appears to improve mortality by reducing infarct size and limiting left ventricular dysfunction. Since salvage of myocardium can only occur before the myocardium is irreversibly injured, timing of thrombolytic therapy is of extreme importance in achieving maximum benefit. Patients treated within 1 to 3 hours of the onset of symptoms stand to benefit most. However, therapy remains of benefit in many patients seen 3 to 6 hours after the onset of infarction.

Criteria for thrombolytic agents vary, but the multicenter thrombosis in myocardial infarction (TIMI) study used the following: at least 30 minutes of ischemic pain, ST-segment elevation of at least 0.1 mV in at least two contiguous ECG leads, less than 7 hours from the onset of symptoms, and 75 years old or less (Ross, 1990). Thrombolytic exclusion criteria include any recent surgery or trauma, pregnancy, bleeding, poorly controlled hypertension, prolonged cardiopulmonary resuscitation, or severe advanced illness (Table 32–11).

Streptokinase (SK) is an exogenous plasminogen activator that lysis thrombin by first complexing with plasminogen k; the resulting complex then converts other plasminogen to plasmin. Plasmin disrupts the thrombus by severing the fibrin strands into fragments known as fibrin degradation products. However, the plasmin produced also destroys fibrinogen as well as coagulation factors V and VIII, resulting in a systemic lytic state. This systemic lytic state last 23 to 36 hours, and it exposes the patient to potential major bleeding complications. Plasmin dissolves the clot. The approximate cost of streptokinase is $200. Streptokinase is often not effective in patients who recently have had a streptococcal infection. It is also not very effective if given after 6 hours of the onset of symptoms. The lytic state last about 24 hours.

TABLE 32–11. Absolute and Relative Contraindications to Thrombolysis

Absolute Contraindications	Relative Contraindications
Active internal bleeding	Recent (< 10 days) major surgery biopsy or trauma
Intracranial or intraspinal surgery or trauma within 2 months	Previous recent cerebrovascular accident with residual symptoms
Intracranial neoplasm, or arteriovenous malformation or cerebral aneurysms	Postpartum period or pregnancy
Uncontrolled hypertension with diastolic blood pressure ≥ 120 mmHg	Cardiopulmonary resuscitation < 10 days or > 10 minutes
Severe blood dyscrasia	Thoracentesis, paracentesis, lumber puncture
	Recent serious trauma
	Uncontrolled coagulation defects, potentially serious bleeding

Urokinase (UK) is synthesized from fetal kidney cell cultures or isolated from urine. Urokinase is a native human plasminogen activator that is different from activators appearing in plasma following the stimulation of the intrinsic or extrinsic mechanism of fibrolysis. There are several advantages of UK: (1) it is nonantigenic and true allergy is rarely seen; (2) there are no antiurokinase antibodies present to interfere with its action; and (3) there is a greater affinity to fibrin-bound plasminogen compared with streptokinase. Generally, it is believed there is no clinical significant difference between the two. The cost of UK is approximately $1300.

Tissue plasminogen activator (tPA) is a naturally occurring serum protease present in endothelium, circulating blood, and human tissue. Unlike SK, which activates plasminogen systemically, tPA is fibrin-specific and activates plasingogen that is incorporated into the thrombus. This produces a local supply of plasmin to clot; therefore, clotting factors are not depleted and the incidence of bleeding complications is reduced. Tissue plasminogen activator must be given within 8 hours of onset of symptoms and is more effective than SK in clot that has been present for more than 6 hours. The cost of tPA is approximately $2200. The lytic state lasts 30 minutes to 7 hours.

Anisoylated plasminogen streptokinase activator complex (APSAC) is a complex of streptokinase and human blood-bound plasminogen to which a P-amisoyl group has been added to mask the catalytic center of the complex. It converts plasminogen to plasmin at the site of the thrombus, and is more site-specific than streptokinase, although systemic production of plasmin does occur. Plasmin dissolves the clot. The lytic state lasts about 48 hours. Occasional allergic reactions do occur, about the same as streptokinase (15-30%). The cost is approximately $1700.

Evidence-Based Use of Thrombolytic Therapy. Many studies have been done to determine the effectiveness of thrombolytic therapy. Table 32–12 summarizes the results of some of the major clinical trials.

From the studies, general guidelines for giving thrombolytics have been determined (Fuster, 1993):

1. Patients with acute myocardial infarctions seen within the first 6 hours and who have no contraindications should immediately receive chewable aspirin and an IV thrombolytic agent. It is more important that *a* thrombolytic agent is given rather than *which* one. If tPA is given, heparin should be added. But, if SK is given there is no data that adding heparin is beneficial.

TABLE 32–12. Comparison of Major Clinical Trials on Thrombolytic Therapy

Trial	Variables	Conclusions
GISSI (1986)[a]	SK Placebo	• 18% overall decrease in mortality
ISIS-2 (1988)[b]	SK, ASA, SK + ASA Placebo	• 42% reduction in mortality was seen in the SK + ASA group
GISSI-2 (1990)[c]	SK + SQ heparin, SK alone tPA + SQ heparin, tPA alone (all patients got ASA and atenolol)	• No significant difference among treatment groups • Criticized for use of SQ heparin
ISSIS-3 (1992)[d]	SK + ASA ± SQ heparin tPA + ASA ± SQ heparin Eminase + ASA ± SQ heparin	• No difference observed among treatment groups
GUSTO (1993)[e]	SK + SQ heparin SK + IV heparin Accelerated tPA + IV heparin Standard tPA + SK	• Accelerated tPA better than SK • Slightly increased stroke rate with tPA

Key: SK = streptokinase; ASA = aspirin; SQ = subcutaneous; tPA = tissue plasminogen activator

Sources: [a] *GISSI (1986);* [b] *ISIS-2 Collaborative Group (1988);* [c] *GISSI (1990);* [d] *ISSIS-3 Collaborative Group (1992); and* [e] *The GUSTO Investigators, 1993.*

2. Streptokinase may be appropriate in patients over 75 and in those with inferior infarcts presenting more than 4 hours after the onset of symptoms.
3. tPA may be preferable for those < 75 who have anterior infarcts and present within 4 hours of onset of symptoms. It may also be the preferable agent in those with previous exposure to streptokinase.
4. Patients with contraindication to thrombolytic therapy or severe hemodynamic compromise should be considered for immediate coronary angioplasty.

Adjunctive Therapies. Platelets have a key role in atherosclerosis, thrombosis, and acute coronary syndromes. Therapeutic manipulation of platelet function has focused principally on the use of aspirin.

Aspirin is the first line of choice for adjunctive therapy, especially after the ISIS-2 study which showed that aspirin alone was equal in efficacy to IV streptokinase in reducing mortality. The acetyl group binds to an inactive platelet cyclooxygenase. This inhibition of cyclooxygenase leads to a decreased thromboxane A_2 production, therefore decreasing platelet aggregation. Aspirin is indicated in patients with unstable angina, myocardial infarction prophylaxis, postcoronary bypass surgery, history of transischemic attacks, and artificial graphs such as with dialysis patients. Aspirin affects platelet aggregation for the life of the platelel (10 days).

Persantine inhibits phosphodiesterase by increasing cyclic AMP and increasing platelet prostacyclin. Studies have shown there is no benefit to giving persantine and aspirin to patients with unstable angina or myocardial infarction.

Finally, ticlopidine (Ticlid) has become increasingly more important in patients with coronary artery stent placement. Ticlid works by inhibiting ADP-induced platelet-fibrinogen binding and subsequent platelet aggregation. Ticlid is indicated in patients with TIA symptoms and with interventional coronary artery procedures. It is not indicated for patients with unstable angina or for myocardial infarction prophylaxis. It is important to check a complete blood count every 2 weeks for the first 3 months because ticlopidine can cause neutropenia. Plavix is a newer agent that is similar to ticlopidine, but is not associated with the risk of neutropenia. Additionally, Plavix carries an indication for use in patients with recent MI.

Intravenous therapy includes the use of heparin, hirudin, hirugen, and Reopro. Heparin is the gold standard following myocardial infarction or interventional procedures. Heparin works by accelerating the formation of complexes by antithrombin III and serum proteases of the coagulation system. Heparin blocks enzymatic activity of several coagulation factors especially thrombin. Hirudin is a polypeptide isolated form of the saliva of the medicinal leech. Hirugen is fragments of parent hirudin that works by directly inhibiting thrombin, unlike heparin. It is superior to heparin for enhancing thrombolysis and delaying or preventing reocclusion.

Recently a new platelet glycoprotein IIb/IIIa receptor (Reopro) has been identified as the pivotal mediator of platelet aggregation (Bennett, 1992). The glycoprotein Ib receptor exists in a complex with glycoprotein IX and glycoprotein V on the platelet surface, which binds with the von Willebrand factor and is the principal glycoprotein involved in the initial contact between platelets and the vessel wall. The glycoprotein IIb/IIIa integrin, in addition to its function in platelet aggregation, has a secondary role in platelet adhesion. Platelet activates causes changes in the shape of platelets and conformation changes in glycoprotein IIb/IIIa receptors, transforming the receptors from a ligand-unreceptive to a ligand-receptive state. Ligand-receptive glycoprotein IIb/IIIa receptors bind fibrinogen molecules, which form bridges between adjacent platelets and facilitate platelet aggregation. Inhibitors of glycoprotein IIb/IIIa receptors also bind to glycoprotein IIb/IIIa receptors, blocking the binding of fibrinogen and thus preventing platelet aggregation. The development of these drugs parallel the revolution of thrombolytic therapy 10 years ago: the initial demonstration of their potency, the lack of understanding of a number of their mechanisms of action and nuances of their administration, and bleeding are the principal drawbacks to their use. Inhibitors of glycoprotein IIb/IIIa (reopro) receptors are likely to be the first " anti-integrins" to be used widely and should lead to the development of other clinically useful agents direct against cellular adhesion molecules. In the future, Reopro will be used out of the catheterization laboratory and for long-term management of coronary syndromes (Lefkovits, Plow, & Topol, 1995).

Interventional Techniques. The beginning of interventional cardiology started in 1964 when two radiologists introduced a technique called "transluminal angioplasty." They placed a diagnostic catheter through a high-grade stenosis of an iliac artery and, after pulling the catheter out, it was discovered that the stenosis was decreased. After several years of research in the United States and Europe, the technique was refined. Initially, angioplasty was researched on peripheral arteries only; the first coronary angioplasty to be performed on a human was in 1977. By 1981, there were 3000 cases performed; in 1993 alone, 350,000 cases were performed. In current practice, interventional cardiology provides a safe and effective alternative to conventional coronary bypass graft surgery (Gruntzig, 1978).

Percutaneous Transluminal Coronary Angioplasty. The indication for percutaneous transluminal coronary angioplasty (PTCA) is the presence of one or more coronary stenosis not involving the left main coronary artery. The procedure involves placing a guide wire into the coronary artery through the stenosis. A balloon catheter is then placed over the guide wire across the lesion and the balloon is inflated. The plaque is then redistributed to improve the lumen of the vessel in the stenosed area.

There are three prevalent mechanisms by which PTCA improves luminal blood flow. The first is plaque compression. This usually occurs when a relatively soft plaque material is compressed against the media. Plaque rupture is the second mechanism in which the plaque is broken by the force exerted by the balloon. Finally, the media of the artery is mechanically stretched by the balloon. The combination of these three mechanisms leads to a larger vessel lumen at the end of balloon angioplasty (Fig. 32–10).

Almost always, a certain degree of dissection occurs in the intima separating from the media, which results in an intimal flap. If the intimal flap is large enough, it can be seen on the angiographic image and may cause immediate or late impairment to flow, leading to abrupt or subacute vessel closure.

Restenosis and acute closure occur in several different ways. Acute elastic recoil, which usually occurs immediately or shortly after arterial dilation, is related to the elastic nature of the arterial wall, (primarily the media containing the smooth muscle cells, the collagen and elastic fibers). Another reason for closure is intimal hyperplasia which is a proliferative response of the intima and media to arterial wall injury and results from growth of smooth muscle wall within the internal elastic lamina, not usually acute. Also, arterial contracture corresponds to shrinkage of the media, again not usually acute. In general, arterial wall injury and mechanical trauma to the endothelium initiates thrombus formation and platelet adhesion to the injured wall which locally releases platelet-derived growth factor and transforms growth factors, provoking the cellular proliferative response. This proliferative response, usually limited to 6 months' duration, is the major contributing factor to restenosis (Beyer, 1996).

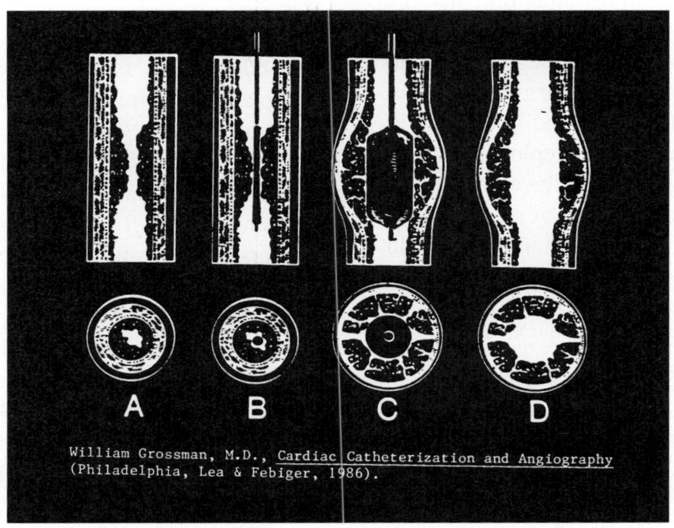

Figure 32–10. The mechanisms by which angioplasty achieves patentcy. *(From Grossman, 1986.)*

Angiographers use the Thrombolysis in Myocardial Infarction (TIMI) flow scale to describe angiographically the flow of blood through a coronary artery (Table 32–13).

The patients who should receive cardiac catheterization or PTCA are those who present with intermediate or high-risk unstable angina and history of a prior PTCA within the past year. These patients have a higher risk of restenosis, which often can be effectively treated by repeat angioplasty. Noninvasive testing is not sufficiently accurate to detect restenosis in these patients. Coronary artery bypass grafts can also have interventional procedures performed in them.

Intracoronary Stents. Today, stents play a key role in interventional cardiology. Stents are used far more than any other type of atherectomy catheter. Just a few years ago, stents initially were approved as a "bridge" to the operating room from the cath lab; however, stents are now used along with PTCA for long-term use. In the early 1980s, when stents where first used, there was a high rate of restenosis because of thrombus. Because of this thrombus formation around the stent, there were many acute closures and bleeding complications. Today stents and anti-platelet medications have improved.

Stents are used to compress dissected vessel flaps against the wall of the vessel and—because of its radial force—prevent elastic recoil of the artery. Initial coverage of the stent with fibrin and platelet within hours of deployment leads to a proliferative response of the intima. Because the stent becomes part of the artery wall, there is less chance of thrombus formation and an inflammatory response. The incidence of thrombus formation usually is higher in the initial days after implantation but is almost nonexistent once the stent is covered with the neointima. During the thrombogenic period, the incidence of stent thrombosis is multifactorial and probably related to the final lumen size, coronary flow rate, anticoagulation, and the presence of residual thrombus.

There are now many stents being used. Intracoronary stents are balloon-expandable metal devices inserted into the coronary lumen. Once the stent is placed within the lesion, the balloon is inflated so the stent is deployed over the plaque. The balloon is then pulled out and the stent remains in place. The Palmaz–Schatz stent is made of stainless steel and is a slotted tube which works well in long straight lesion. The Gianturco–Roubin–Cook stent is also made of stainless steel, but is made of a winding coil design that allows the stent to bend slightly in the artery.

TABLE 32–13. TIMI Classification of Coronary Blood Flow

TIMI Class	Description
0	No flow through artery
1	Blood flow slows at the occlusion and does not completely fill the distal artery
2	Blood goes down the artery, slows at the blockage, and slowly fills the distal artery completely
3	Normal blood flow

Stents are used in almost in any lesion, but in lesions with thrombus there is a higher risk of intrastent thrombus. The presence of calcium could prevent adequate stent expansion and, therefore, increase the risk of restenosis.

Atherectomy. The aim of any atherectomy device is to debulk the lesion. There are three main types of atherectomy catheter used in clinical practice: the directional atherectomy, the high-speed rotational atherectomy, and the transluminal extraction atherectomy.

DIRECTIONAL ATHERECTOMY. In 1990, the FDA approved the use of the Sampson AtheroCath for directional atherectomy. The device is designed to cut and remove atherosclerotic plaque. The AtheroCath consists of stainless-steel housing made up of a rotating cutter and cutting chamber, a balloon on the opposite side of the cutting chamber, and a distal nose cone to store atherosclerotic debris (Smith, Hanley, & Sheridan, 1995). A guide wire is placed into the coronary artery through the lesion. The cutting chamber is directed towards the plaque and the balloon is then inflated at low inflation pressure to secure the cutting chamber over the plaque. With the cutter rotating at 2000 rpm, the catheter is slowly advanced to remove the plaque and push the debris to the nose cone. The device is ideally suited for focal, eccentric lesions in the proximal portion of a large coronary artery. The advantage of direction coronary atherectomy (DCA) is that the plaque is removed. One disadvantage is that the guide catheter is large in diameter, therefore causing more peripheral vascular complications because of the large sheath size. Another disadvantage is the relative inflexibility of the device, which makes it difficult to advance in small distal vessels or around corners.

ROTATIONAL ATHERECTOMY. This device is a high-speed, diamond-studded, football-shaped rotating burr that abrades the plaque into microscopic particles that are flushed downstream into distal microcirculation, eventually being taken up by the endothelial system. The burr is mounted onto a flexible driveshaft that rotates 180,000 rpm and is powered by compressed gas. The rotational atherectomy device works on the principle of differential cutting, much like a bone saw. Normal, relatively elastic endothelium is deflected away from the spinning burr while fibrotic atheroma is abraded. This provides a smooth, polished lumen (Beyer, 1996).

The reason for choosing rotational atherectomy is it benefits calcified lesions. Balloon angioplasty is considered high risk for calcified lesions. Also, occasionally lesions that are fibrotic but not calcified will not dilate with conventional balloon angioplasty.

The major disadvantage is cost. Most rotational atherectomy procedures require the use of two relatively expensive burrs, a pacing lead, and at least one angioplasty balloon. This is an increased equipment cost, especially if long-term benefits prove to be equal.

TRANSLUMINAL EXTRACTION CATHETER. The transluminal extraction catheter (TEC) uses a slowly rotating cutter (750 rpm) in combination with continuous vacuum suction through the inner case of the catheter. The distal cutting tip shaves soft plaque and thrombus while the continuous vacuum suction is applied through the inner lumen to extract the thrombus and atheromatous material. The energy source is a hand-held battery-powered motor-drive unit. Because the TEC eliminates material from the vessel, it is usually used in saphenous vein grafts. In some centers the TEC is used on vessels filled with thrombus such as after an acute myocardial infarction (Beyer, 1996).

Laser. The excimer laser is a short "excited dimmer" (which describes the state of 2 atoms in the lasting medium that is comprised of a gas, usually xenon chloride). The excimer laser emits ultraviolet radiation in short pulses rather than continuously. High-energy pulses theoretically allow vaporization of tissue with minimal tissue penetration and therefore limited thermal diffusion and damage. The pulsed excimer laser is thought to ablate plaque by nonthermal disruption of peptide bonds. Initially, guide-wire placement across a lesion is the same as traditional angioplasty. The laser catheter is advanced over the guide wire to the plaque and lasing is performed in 2- to 3-second pulses. Since the excimer laser is opaque to blood, it only ablates tissue in direct contact (Smith, Hanley, & Sheridan, 1995).

The ideal type of lesions for laser therapy are long, osteal, calcified, and totally occluded. Unfortunately, the initial reports of the results show a higher rate of restenosis and higher cost than conventional angioplasty.

In the Future. A thrombectomy system (AngioJet) is an angioplasty catheter that removes thrombus. The system of self-contained high-velocity saline "waterjets" creates suction at the tip that simultaneously attracts, breaks up, and removes thrombus. The AngioJet uses tiny high-velocity saline jets to create a low pressure region around the catheter tip. The difference between the low pressure at the catheter tip and the high pressure present in the vessel forms a near-perfect vacuum which draws in thrombus material. Once the clot material is broken up into microscopic fragments, it is immediately drawn out of the patient's body for disposal in a collection bag (Smith, Hanley, & Sheridan, 1995).

Other research is currently being directed toward changing the coronary arterial vascular wall locally in an effort to decrease the 30 to 40% restenosis rate which continues to plague all interventional efforts. Experiments are underway to deliver a vast array of drugs, genetic material, or radiation to the luminal surface of the disrupted artery after intervention to inhibit processes thought to be central to restenosis–endothelial dysfunction, smooth muscle proliferation, platelet activation, and thrombus formation. Coated or porous balloons, coated or radioactive stents, and microspheres bonded with monoclonal antibodies are examples of methods that have been proposed to deliver such local therapies.

Complications of Myocardial Infarction

Mechanical

Cardiogenic Shock. Cardiogenic shock is a complication of acute MI caused by severe ventricular dysfunction. The advent of thrombolytics, rescue angioplasty, and other measures that restore coronary blood flow have reduced the frequency of occurrence. However, when it does occur, it is generally associated with a greater than 70% mortality rate and is the primary cause of inhospital death from acute MI (Pasternak & Braunwald, 1994). This clinical syndrome is characterized by hypotension (systolic arterial pressure < 80 mmHg); peripheral vasoconstriction with cool, clammy extremities; urine output less than 20 to 30 ml/hr; and altered mental status. Hemodynamic measurements reveal a low cardiac index (1.8-2.0 L/min), arterial hypotension, elevated left ventricular filling pressures, tachycardia, and elevated systemic vascular resistance (Lavie & Gersh, 1990b).

The Killip classification groups patients into four categories according to the clinical degree of pump failure post MI with the associated hospital mortality rate (Table 32–14). With the improvement in the treatment of myocardial infarctions, there has been a reduction in the severity and rate of complications with a resulting decrease in the mortality rate by as much as one third to one half in each classification since its initial conception (Pasternak & Braunwald, 1994).

The prognosis of cardiogenic shock can be greatly improved by the early diagnosis of the underlying cause and the prompt restoration of coronary and tissue perfusion by the use of thrombolytic therapy, percutaneous transluminal coronary angioplasty, or coronary artery bypass grafting (Califf & Bengtson, 1994).

Key elements in the management of cardiogenic shock include adequate oxygenation and ventilation, correction of fluid, electrolyte, and acid–base disturbances, relief of pain, and restoration of coronary blood flow and adequate tissue perfusion (Califf & Bengtson, 1994). The use of a pulmonary artery (PA) catheter is helpful in the pharmacologic management of cardiogenic shock. The use of PA catheters is not without risk; however, when inserted and used by experienced professionals and removed within 72 hours, the complications are minimized.

Hypovolemia may be caused by over-diuresis, vomiting, or decreased PO intake during acute infarction. IV hydration should be administered cautiously while monitoring oxygenation and cardiac output (Pasternak & Braunwald, 1994).

Vasopressors are often required in patients with adequate intravascular volume but inadequate tissue perfusion.

TABLE 32–14. The Killip Classification

Class	Clinical Symptoms	Mortality Rate
Class I	No signs of pulmonary or venous congestion	0–5%
Class II	Moderate heart failure as evidenced by rales at lung bases, S3, tachypnea, right-sided heart failure	10–20%
Class III	Severe heart failure, pulmonary edema	35–40%
Class IV	Cardiogenic shock	85–95%

From Pasternak & Braunwald. (1994).

Dobutamine, a sympathomimetic, stimulates predominantly B1 adrenergic receptors to increase myocardial contractility, increases cardiac output, and lowers left ventricular filling pressures. It also augments diastolic coronary blood flow and collateral blood flow to the ischemic area. When significant hypotension is present, dopamine is preferable, since vasoconstriction in the peripheral vessels is often needed to maintain vital organ perfusion. Caution must be used in higher doses of dopamine that the myocardial oxygen supply and demand ratio is not adversely affected (Califf & Bengtson, 1994; Lavie & Gersh, 1990b).

Vasodilators should be used cautiously in patients in shock since they can precipitate further hypotension and reduce coronary blood flow. In patients with adequate blood pressure but hypoperfusion, vasodilators such as nitroprussside and nitroglycerine reduce preload and afterload, thereby improving left ventricular systolic function and improving tissue perfusion. Nitroglycerine, in particular, increases coronary flow to areas of ischemia, promotes collaterol flow, and decreases the ST-segment elevation. It also reduces the mortality associated with AMI, making it the vasodilator of choice in cardiogenic shock (Lavie & Gersh, 1990b).

An intraaortic balloon pump (IABP) provides counterpulsation which augments diastolic pressure and cardiac output. Although use of the IABP can provide temporary clinical and hemodynamic stability, survival is improved only in patients who subsequently undergo revascularization (Califf & Bengtson, 1994).

Ventricular assist devices (VADs) are used to reduce myocardial workload, increase perfusion to vital organs, and maintain adequate preload. A VAD is used to partially or totally support circulation until the heart recovers, or as a bridge to cardiac transplantation in patients with intractable pump failure (Ryan et al., 1996; Williams & Morton, 1995).

Ventricular Remodeling. Ventricular remodeling occurs in a large number of patients with myocardial infarctions, particularly those that are anterior or apical in location, large in size, and transmural in thickness. There is a loss of contractile force at the scarred infarct site and the compensatory response of the remaining myocardium results in an enlarged, spherical-shaped heart that has reduced contractility. Hypertrophy also occurs as a response to the altered stress–strain relationship brought about by the geometric distortions of a segmental ventricular scar. The process is mediated by activation of the sympathetic nervous system and the renin–angiotensin–aldosterone (RAA) system which becomes activated during an acute MI. Early use of ACE inhibitors post MI have proven to attenuate the left ventricular remodeling and dilatation that causes congestive heart failure, decreased exercise tolerance, and increased mortality as shown by several large clinical trials (Gorlin, 1994).

Papillary Muscle Rupture. Papillary muscle rupture is an infrequent but catastrophic complication of AMI producing mitral incompetence. It may arise from ischemia or muscle necrosis but an abnormal alignment of the papillary muscle and chordae secondary to LV dysfunction is probably the underlying pathology (Lavie & Gersh, 1990b; Ryan et al., 1996).

Rupture of the papillary muscle usually occurs 2 to 7 days after AMI and usually involves the posteromedial papillary muscle, which gets its blood supply from the posterior descending coronary artery. The IABP is used to stabilize patients; however, coronary artery bypass graft surgery and mitral valve repair or replacement are indicated (Lavie & Gersh, 1990b; Ryan et al., 1996).

Cardiac Rupture. Cardiac rupture is a dramatic and rare event in acute myocardial infarction, occurring in 1 to 3% of all patients with infarcts, and causes about 10% of all infarct-related deaths. It usually occurs during the first week after an MI. It is more common with the elderly, women, first infarctions, no history of angina, and history of systemic hypertension, especially if present post MI.

The clinical features occur acutely with loss of blood pressure, heart rate, and apparent electromechanical dissociation. The myocardium continues to contract but there is no forward flow. The blood escapes into the pericardium. The only definitive treatment is surgical intervention; however, few patients survive to undergo surgery (Lavie & Gersh, 1990b).

Ventricular Septal Rupture. Rupture of the ventricular septum occurs in about 2% of all acute infarctions and accounts for about 10% of all cardiac ruptures. It often occurs in patients with single vessel disease and poor septal collateral flow (Lavie & Gersch, 1990b).

Patients present with severe heart failure in association with the sudden onset of pansystolic murmur, often accompanied by a parasternal thrill. The presence of a left-to-right shunt is a diagnostic factor that differentiates this complication from papillary muscle rupture. Ventricular septal rupture is a life-threatening complication and requires immediate surgical repair (Pasternak & Braunwald, 1994).

Left Ventricular Aneurysm. This is defined by the ACC/AHA guidelines for the management of acute MI as a demarcated diastolic deformity of the left ventricle appearing with systolic dyskinesia (Ryan et al., 1996). The complications of LV aneurysm include congestive heart failure, arterial embolism, and ventricular arrhythmias, which can occur weeks to months after an MI. Apical aneurysms are the most common and most easily detected by a double, diffuse, or displaced apical impulse on physical exam. ST-segment elevation in the precordial leads is found on 12-lead ECG in 25% of patients with apical or anterior aneurysms (Pasternak & Braunwald, 1994).

Surgical intervention may be required if refractory ventricular tachycardia or CHF is present (Ryan et al., 1996).

Electrical

Ventricular Tachycardia. During the onset of myocardial ischemia and up to 48 hours after an MI, patients are at increased risk for development of ventricular dysrhythmias. This derangement is caused by damaged but surviving cells in the infarct zone that exhibit abnormal electrical behavior. Ventricular tachycardia (VT) is defined as at least three consecutive ventricular beats with a ventricular rate between 110 to 250. It occurs in 3 to 15% of patients with AMI; however, patients with LV failure post MI, with an ejection fraction of < 40%, have a 20 to 25% incidence of sustained VT or sudden death (Nicolai, 1995).

The VT is usually short lived, self limiting, and asymptomatic. Sustained VT, however, causes hemodynamic instability and often degenerates into ventricular fibrillation (VF). At one time, lidocaine was used prophylactically to prevent arrhythmias; however, this use has never been shown to reduce overall mortality with AMI and may predispose to bradycardia and asystole. The early and more frequent use of beta blockers post MI appears to have contributed to the decline in the incidence of ventricular arrythmias (Pasternak & Braunwald, 1994).

For sustained VT, the initial treatment is lidocaine, a 1 mg/kg bolus followed by an infusion of 1 to 4 mg/min administered for 24 to 36 hours. In patients with CHF or liver disease, or the elderly, the dose should be reduced by half. If the lidocaine bolus is not successful, cardioversion (following Advanced Cardiac Life Support [ACLS] guidelines) should be employed. If the patient is hemodynamically unstable or the rhythm deteriorates into ventricular fibrillation, immediate defibrillation is warranted (Pasternak & Braunwald, 1994; Nicolai, 1995). Lidocaine levels should be monitored to prevent toxicity. Low levels of potassium and magnesium may predispose patients post MI to ventricular arrythmias, so care must be taken to monitor serum electrolytes and replace them when warranted (Campbell, 1994).

Ventricular Fibrillation. Ventricular fibrillation (VF) is the most critical arrhythmic complication of an AMI; however, if corrected promptly, the prognosis is favorable (Campbell, 1994). VF is the most common arrhythmia recorded in patients who have out-of-hospital cardiac arrest and is responsible for about 200,000 to 250,000 deaths per year. Rapid defibrillation is the treatment of choice and ACLS protocols should be promptly initiated for successful restoration of sinus rhythm (Nicolai, 1995).

In patients who have primary ventricular arrhythmias as a result of acute ischemia, the prognosis is generally good: > 90% survival at one year. However, in patients who develop VT/VF later in their hospitalization, the predisposing factors could be pump failure or ventricular aneurysm. The mortality in these cases can be as high as 85% and a further electrophysiologic evaluation is warranted (Pasternak & Braunwald, 1994).

Accelerated Idioventricular Rhythm. Accelerated idioventricular rhythm (AIVR) is characterized by a wide QRS complex with a rate of 60 to 120 beats per minute and is hemodynamically stable. It occurs in about 30% of patients with AMI, most commonly during the first 48 hours; after IWMI; post reperfusion with thrombolytics; and during sleep. The rhythm is generally benign and does not require treatment other than careful monitoring (Nicolai, 1995). When AIVR is associated with hemodynamic compromise or it precipitates VT or VF, atropine or overdrive pacing is usually effective (Winters & Eisenberg, 1995).

Sinus Bradycardia. The incidence of sinus bradycardia (SB) in patients with AMI ranges from 14 to 36%; about 70% of these patients have an inferoposterior wall infarction. Ischemic damage to the sinus node may contribute to the incidence of SB but it is not the primary causative reason. Stimulation of the lower interatrial septum between the ostium of the coronary sinus and the posterior atrioventricular node results in bradycardia and hypotension. In inferoposterior MI, this area is vulnerable to ischemia and could precipitate an automatically mediated vasodilatation and bradycardia (Lavie & Gersh, 1990b).

Treatment is indicated if there is hemodynamic compromise. Atropine is most useful for increasing heart rate; 0.5 mg initially repeated every 5 minutes for a total of 2 mg may be given if necessary. If symptomatic bradycardia persists, a temporary pacing wire may be warranted (Pasternak & Braunwald, 1994).

Atrioventricular Conduction Disturbances. The mortality rate of patients with AV block when associated with AWMI is 60 to 70% as compared with the 25 to 40% associated with IWMI. This disparity appears to be related to the amount of involved myocardium. Heart block in inferior ischemia is related to AV nodal ischemia. In AWMI, heart block is usually related to ischemia of all three fascicles of the conduction system that results from extensive myocardial necrosis (Pasternak & Braunwald, 1994). Transvenous temporary pacing or noninvasive pacing is the most effective treatment of symptomatic, hemodynamically unstable conduction disturbances (Lavie & Gersh, 1990b).

Supraventricular Tachycardias. Sinus tachycardia is common in patients with AMI and is frequently associated with anxiety, pain, hypoxemia, hypovolemia, or heart failure. Treatment is directed at correction of the underlying cause; however, if the tachycardia is felt to be sympathetic overstimulation, treatment with a beta blocker should be considered (Pasternak & Braunwald, 1994).

Atrial fibrillation (AF) complicates up to 20% of acute MIs usually associated with either atrial infarction or with large ventricular infarcts, particularly when the right ventricle is involved. AF is deleterious to ischemic myocardium because the ventricular response is usually rapid and the atrial component of ventricular filling (atrial kick) is lost. When AF occurs with a controlled ventricular response, it is generally asymptomatic and self terminating, requiring only close monitoring (Winters & Eisenberg, 1995).

In AF with a rapid ventricular response, hemodynamic compromise dictates prompt therapy directed at controlling the ventricular rate and ideally the restoration of sinus rhythm. Rate control can be achieved by using digoxin, beta blockers, and IV cardizem. Cardioversion may be required to restore normal sinus rhythm (Winters & Eisenberg, 1995).

Paroxysmal supraventricular tachycardia (PSVT) occurs infrequently in patients with AMI, but should be treated to prevent exacerbation of myocardial ischemia. If the patient is stable, digoxin, beta blockers, or IV diltiazem can be given or vagal maneuvers may be attempted. In hemodynamically unstable patients, synchronized cardioversion is the treatment of choice (Winters & Eisenberg, 1995).

Risk Stratification

Risk stratification in patients with CAD is necessary to assess the probability of future coronary events and guide appropriate therapy. The ACC/AHA task force on the management of patients with acute MI recommend a submaximal exercise stress test before discharge or a symptom-limited stress test three weeks after discharge in patients with an uncomplicated post MI course (Ryan et al., 1996). Patients who can exercise into stage III of *Bruce* treadmill protocol have an annual CAD-related mortality of less than 1% (Thadani, 1997). Several studies have shown that revascularization offers no benefit over medical management in the low-risk population; therefore, pharmacologic management with risk-factor modification should be the first treatment option (Thadani, 1997). The ACC/AHA recommend medical therapy for patients who can achieve at least five metabolic equivalents (METS); however, if there are signs of severe ischemia at a low level of exercise, the patient should go on to have coronary arteriography (Fig. 32–11).

Patients who are considered high risk for future cardiac events include those with postinfarct angina, previous MI, CHF, left ventricular dysfunction, and the presence of ventricular arrhythmias. Patients with these prognostic factors may benefit from early coronary arteriography and revascularization when necessary, along with aggressive management of LV dysfunction and arrhythmias (Kulick & Rahimtoola, 1991).

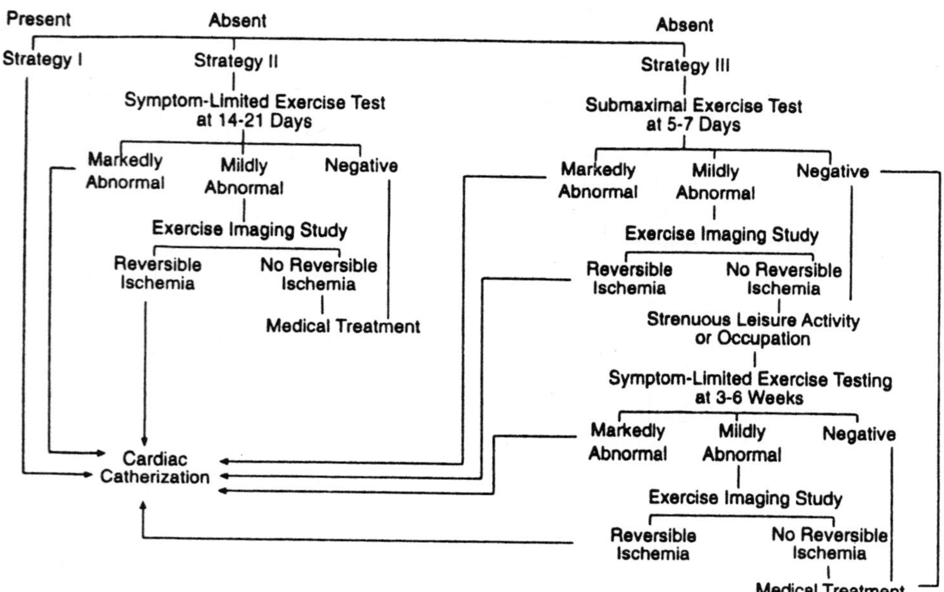

Figure 32–11. Strategies of exercise stress test evaluation soon after myocardial infarction. *(From Ryan, et al. [1996]. [5].)*

Risk-Factor Modification

Regardless of the treatment option—revascularization or medical management—attention must be paid to the alteration of lifestyle or risk-factor modification to reduce cardiovascular morbidity and mortality.

Several studies have shown that lowering blood cholesterol with a statin resulted in reduction in overall mortality, cardiovascular morbidity and mortality, and the need for revascularization (Thadani, 1997). The National Cholesterol Education Panel II has recommended that all patients with coronary artery disease have a complete lipid profile. A low-cholesterol, low-saturated fat diet should be instituted in all patients with elevated lipids; however, if the low density lipoprotein (LDL) remains greater than 130 mg/dL despite diet, drug therapy should be instituted. The goal of therapy in patients with CAD is a LDL less than 100 mg/dL (Ryan et al., 1996). More detail is provided in Chapter 29.

Smoking triggers coronary spasm, reduces the effects of beta blockers, and doubles mortality after acute MI. Cigarette smoke appears to contribute to the degradation of EDRF, resulting in endothelial dysfunction. Smoking cessation reduces rates of reinfarction and death within a year of quitting (Ryan et al., 1996; Thadani, 1997).

Estrogen replacement therapy has been shown to improve the lipid profile and lower fibrinogen and is most likely of benefit in both primary and secondary prevention of coronary artery disease. The apparent increased risk of breast cancer associated with estrogen use must be taken into consideration before initiating therapy (Ryan et al., 1996).

Long-Term Management

Along with modification of the risk factors previously listed, patients with coronary artery disease should be strongly encouraged to make positive lifestyle changes. Participation in an exercise program along with healthy eating habits help in weight management, control of hypertension, and lipid management. Smoking-cessation programs and stress management contribute to the reduction of morbidity and mortality. In patients post acute MI, aspirin, beta blockers, and ACE inhibitors should be continued indefinitely if they are tolerated (Ryan et al., 1996).

Patients should be referred to, and strongly encouraged to participate in, a formal cardiac rehabilitation program. Aside from monitored prescriptive exercise training, patients receive education, support, and reinforcement about coronary risk-factor modification techniques. Cardiac rehab has been shown to effectively improve functional capacity, improve quality of life, reduce cardiovascular mortality, and reduce the risk of future coronary events. Formal programs promote social integration and social support which have proven to positively effect outcomes after an acute MI (Ryan et al., 1996).

In the uncomplicated MI patient, return to previous level of activity can usually occur safely within 2 weeks. This includes return to work, sexual activity with the usual partner, driving, and air travel if accompanied with a companion. Return to physically demanding activities can be determined by evaluating the energy level requirements of the activity with a graded exercise stress test.

For patients with a complicated post MI course, driving should be delayed 2 to 3 weeks after symptoms resolve. Patients should be stabilized at least 2 weeks before traveling by air because of the lowered oxygen tension experienced above 5000 feet (Ryan et al., 1996).

REFERENCES

Abrams, J. (1997). Role of endothelial dysfunction in coronary artery disease. *American Journal of Cardiology, 79,* 2–9.

Alderman, E. L., Bourassa, M. G., Cohen, L. S., Davis, K. B., Kaiser, G. G., Killip, T., Mock, M. B., Pettinger, M., & Robertson, T. L. (1990). Ten-year follow-up of survival and myocardial infarction in the randomized coronary artery surgery study. *Circulation, 82,* 1629–1646.

American Heart Association. Guideline: Cardiac Catheterization and Myocardial Revascularization 93–99.

Antiplatelet Trialists' Collaboration. (1994). Collaborative overview of randomised trials of antiplatelet therapy—I: Prevention of death, myocardial infarction, and stroke by prolonged antiplatelet therapy in various categories of patients. *British Medical Journal, 308,* 81–98.

Antman, E. M. (1994). General hospital management. In D. G. Julian and E. Braunwald (Eds.), *Management of acute myocardial infarction* (pp. 29–70) London: W. B. Saunders Company Ltd.

Armstrong, P. W. (1997). Heparin in acute coronary disease—Requium for a heavyweight? *New England Journal of Medicine, 337,* 492–494.

Bakerman, S. (1994). *Bakerman's ABC's of Interpretive Laboratory Data* (3rd ed.). (pp. 182–185, 322–326). Myrtle Beach, SC: Interpretive Laboratory Data, Inc.

Bakker, A. J., Koelemay, M. J. W., Gorgels, J. P., van Vlies, B., Smits, R., Tijssen, J. G., & Haagen, F. D. (1994). Troponin t and myoglobin at admission: Value of early diagnosis of acute myocardial infarction. *European Society of Cardiology, 15,* 45–53.

Bates B. (1991). *A guide to physical examination and history taking* (5th Ed.). Philadelphia: J. B. Lippincott.

Beattie, S., Billiard, S. J., & Meinhardt, B. S. (1989). The use of cardiac catheterization data to design nursing care plans. *Critical Care Nurse, 10* (6), 43–52.

Bennett, J. S. (1992). Mechanisms of platelet adhesion and aggregation: An update. *Hospital Practice, 27,* 124–138.

Beyer, R. (1996). New devices in interventional cardiology: Present and future. *Israel Journal of Medical Science, 32,* 515–525.

Bijnen, F. C., Casperson, C. J., & Mosterd, W. L. (1994). Physical inactivity as a risk factor for coronary heart disease: A WHO and International Society and Federation of Cardiology position statement. *Bulletin of the World Health Organization, 72* (1), 1–4.

Blair, S. N., Powell, K. E., Bazarre, T. L., Early, J. L., Epstein, L. H., Green, L. W., Harris, S. S., Haskell, W. L., King, A. C., Kaplan, J., Marcus, B., Puffenberger, R. S., & Yeager, K. K. (1993). Physical inactivity. *Circulation, 1988* (3), 1402–1404.

Braunwald, E. (1992). Heart Disease: Textbook of Cardiovascular Medicine (4th Ed.). (Chaps. 28–37). Philadelphia: W. B. Saunders Company.

Braunwald, E. & Sobel, B. (1992). Coronary blood flow and myocardial ischemia. In E. Braunwald (Ed.) *Heart Disease* (pp. 1161–1199). Philadelphia: W. B. Saunders Company.

Braunwald, E., Mark, D. B., Jones, R. H. et al. (1994). Unstable angina: Diagnosis and management. Clinical Practice Guideline Number 10 (amended). AHCPR Publication No. 94-0602. Rockville, MD: Agency for Health Care Policy and Research and the National Heart, Lung, and Blood Institute, Public Health Service, U.S. Department of Health and Human Services.

Burke, A. P., Farb, A., Malcom, G. T., Liang, Y., Smialek, J., & Virmani, R. (1997). Coronary risk factors and plaque morphology in men with coronary disease who died suddenly. *New England Journal of Medicine, 336,* 1276–1281.

Califf, R. M. & Bengtson, J. R. (1994). Cardiogenic shock. *New England Journal of Medicine, 330,* 1724–1730.

Campbell, R. W. (1994). Arrhythmias. In D. G. Julian & E. Braunwald (Eds.), *Management of Acute Myocardial Infarction* (pp. 223–240). London: W. B. Saunders Company Ltd.

Campeau, L. (1976). Grading of angina pectoris [letter]. *Circulation, 54,* 522–523.

Chait, A., Brunzell, J. D., Denke, M. A., Eisenburg, D., Ernst, N. D., Franklin, F. A., Ginsberg, H., Kotchen, T. A., Kuller, L., Mullin, R. M., Nichaman, M. Z., Nicolosi, R. J., Scharfer, E. J., Stone, N. J., & Weidman, W. H. (1993). Rationale of the diet heart statement of the American Heart Association. *Circulation, 88* (6), 3008–3025.

Chaitman, B. (1992). Exercise stress testing. In E. Braunwald (Ed.), *Heart disease* (pp. 161–179). Philadelphia: W. B. Saunders Company.

Cheitlin, M. D., Sokolow, M., & McIlroy, M. B. (1993). *Clinical Cardiology* (6th Edition) Norwalk, CT: Appleton and Lange.

Cheitlin, M. D., Alpert, J. S., Armstrong, W. F., Aurigemma, G. P., Beller, G. A., Bierman, F. Z., Davidson, T. W., Davis, J. L., Douglas, P. S., Gillam, L. D., Lewis, R. P., Pearlman, A. S., Philbrick, J. T., Shah, P. M., & Williams, R. G., (1997). ACC/AHA guidelines for the clinical application of echocardiography: A report of the American College of Cardiology/American Heart Association Task Force on Practice Guidelines (Committee on Clinical Application of Echocardiography). *Circulation, 95,* 1686–1744.

Clem, J. R. (1995). Pharmacotherapy of ischemic heart disease. *AACN Clinical Issues. Advanced Practice in Acute and Critical Care, 6,* 404–417.

Cohen, M., Demers, C., Gurfinkel, E. P., Turpie, A. G., Fromell, G. J., Goodman, S., Langer, A., Califf, R. M., Fox, K. A., & Premmereur, J. (1997). A comparison of low-molecular weight heparin with unfractionated heparin for unstable coronary artery disease. *New England Journal of Medicine, 337,* 447–452.

Conover, M. B. (1988). Myocardial infarction. In *Understanding Electrocardiography. Arrhythmias and the 12-lead ECG* (5th Ed.). (pp. 319–349). St. Louis: Mosby.

Coombs, V. J. & Brinker, J. A. (1995). Primary angioplasty in the acute myocardial setting. *AACN Clinical Issues. Advanced Practice in Acute and Critical Care, 6,* 387–397.

Davies, M. J. & Thomas, A. C. (1985). Plaque fissuring—the cause of acute myocardial infarction, sudden ischemic death, and crescendo angina. *British Heart Journal, 53,* 363–373.

Effat, M. A. (1995). Pathophysiology of ischemic heart disease: An overview. *AACN Clinical Issues. Advanced Practice in Acute and Critical Care, 6,* 369–374.

Falk, E. (1989). Morphologic features of unstable atherothrombotic plaques underlying acute coronary syndromes. *American Journal of Cardiology, 63,* 114E–119E.

Figueredo, V. & Cheitlin, M. D. (1994). Risk stratification. In D. Julian & E. Braunwald (Eds.), *Management of acute myocardial infarction* (pp. 361–391). London: W. B. Saunders Company Ltd.

Fuster, V. (1993). Coronary thrombolysis—a perspective for the practicing physician. *New England Journal of Medicine, 329,* (10), 723–725.

Fuster, V., Badiman, L., Badiman, J., & Chesebro, J. (1992). The pathogenesis of coronary artery disease and the acute coronary syndromes—part 2. *New England Journal of Medicine, 326,* 310–316.

Gibbons, R. J., Balady, G. J., Beasley, J. W., Bricker, J. T., Duvernoy, W. F. C., Froelicher, V. F., Mark, D. B., Marwick, T. H., McCallister, B. D., Thompson, P. D., Winters, W. L., Jr., & Yanowitz, F. G. (1997). ACC/AHA guidelines for exercise testing: A report of the American College of Cardiology/American Heart Association Task Force on Practice Guidelines (Committee on Exercise Testing). *Journal of American College Cardiology, 30,* 260–315.

GISSI. (1986). Effectiveness of intravenous thrombolytic treatment in acute myocardial infarction. *Lancet, 1,* 397–401.

GISSI. (1990). GISSI-2: A factorial randomized trial of alteplase versus streptokinase and heparin versus no heparin among 12,490 with acute myocardial infarction. *Lancet, 336,* 65–71.

Gorlin, R. (1994). Late use of ACE inhibitors. In D. Julian & E. Braunwald (Eds.), *Management of acute myocardial infarction* (pp. 343–359). London: W. B. Saunders Company Ltd.

Grossman, W., & Baim, D. S. (1991). *Cardiac catheterization, angiography and intervention* (4th Ed.). Philadelphia: Lea & Febiger.

Grossman, W., Baim, D. (1994). Diagnostic cardiac catheterization and angiography. In K. J. Isselbacher, E. Braunwald, J. D. Wilson, J. B. Martin, A. S. Fauci & D. L. Kasper (Eds)., *Harrison's principles of internal medicine* (13th Ed.). (pp. 980–983). New York: McGraw-Hill.

Gruntzig, A. R. (1978). Transluminal dilation of coronary artery stenosis. *Lancet, 1,* 263.

Gruntzig, A. R., Turina, M. I., & Schneider, J. A. (1976). Experimental percutaneous dilation of coronary artery stenosis. *Circulation, 54,* 81.

The GUSTO Investigators. (1993). An international randomized trial comparing four thrombolytic strategies for acute myocardial infarction. *New England Journal of Medicine, 329,* 673–682.

Hanisch, P. J. (1991). Identification and treatment of acute myocardial infarction by electrocardiographic site classification. *Focus on Critical Care, 18,* 480–488.

Heart and Stroke Facts. (1996). Dallas, TX: American Heart Association.

Heart and Stroke Statistical Update. (1997). Dallas, TX: American Heart Association.

Heart and Stroke Statistical Update. (1998). Dallas, TX: American Heart Association.

Handel, R. C., Bonow, R. O., and Chaudhy, F. A. (1996) Myocardial Viability. *Current problems Cardiology,* 21(3), 151–185.

Hirsch, J. (1991). Heparin. *New England Journal of Medicine, 324,* 564-574.

ISIS-2 Collaborative Group. (1988). Randomized trial of intravenous streptokinase, oral aspirin, both, or neither among 17,187 cases of suspected acute myocardial infarction. *Lancet, 2,* 349–360.

ISSIS-3 Collaborative Group. (1992). ISSIS-3: A randomized comparison of streptokinase versus tissue plasminogen activator versus anistreplase and of aspirin plus heparin versus aspirin alone among 41,299 cases of suspected acute myocardial infarction. *Lancet,* 339: 753–770.

Jonas, M. A., Oakes, J. A., Ockene, J. K., Hennekens, C. H. (1992). Statement on smoking and cardiovascular disease for health care professionals. *Circulation, 1986* (5), 1664–1660.

Kannel, W. B. & Abbott, R. B. (1984). Incidence and prognosis of unrecognized myocardial infarction: An update of the Framingham study. *New England Journal of Medicine, 311,* 1144–1147.

Kern, M. J. (1991). *The cardiac catheterization handbook.* (pp. 1–20). St. Louis: Mosby.

Kern, M. J., Deligonul, U., & Gudipati, C. (1991). Hemodynamics and ECG data. In M. J. Kern (Ed.), *The cardiac catheterization handbook.* (pp. 98–132). St. Louis: Mosby.

Kern, M., Deligonul, U. & Roth, R. (1991). Introduction to the catheterization laboratory. In M. J. Kern (Ed.), *The cardiac catheterization handbook.* (pp. 1–20). St. Louis: Mosby.

Kinch, J. W. & Ryan, T. J. (1994). Right ventricular infarction. *New England Journal of Medicine, 330,* 1211–1216.

Kulick, D. L. & Rahimtoola, S. H. (1991). Risk stratification in survivors of acute myocardial infarction: Routine cardiac catheterization and angiography is a reasonable approach in most patients. *American Heart Journal, 121,* 641–651.

Lavie, C. J. & Gersh, B. J. (1990a). Acute myocardial infarction: Initial manifestations, management, and prognosis. Symposium on myocardial ischemia—part III. *Mayo Clinic Proceedings, 65,* 531–548.

Lavie, C. J. & Gersh, B. J. (1990b). Mechanical and electrical complications of acute myocardial infarction. Symposium on myocardial ischemia—part IV. *Mayo Clinic Proceedings, 65,* 709–728.

Lefkovits, J., Plow, E. F., & Topol, E. J. (1995). Platelet glycoprotein IIb/IIIa receptors in cardiovascular medicine. *New England Journal of Medicine, 332,* 1553–1559.

Levine, G. N., Keaney, J. F., & Vita, J. A. (1995). Cholesterol reduction in cardiovascular disease. *New England Journal of Medicine, 332* (8), 512–519.

Lewis, P. S. (1992). Clinical implications of non–Q-wave (subendocardial) myocardial infarctions. *Focus of Critical Care, 19,* 29–33.

Matrisciano, L. (1992). Unstable angina: An overview. *Critical Care Nurse, 12,* 30–38.

McMillan, J. Y. & Little-Longeway, C. D. (1991). Right ventricular infarction. *Focus on Critical Care, 18,* 158–163.

Nicolai, C. (1995). Ventricular dysrhythmias in ischemic heart disease. *AACN Clinical Issues. Advanced Practice in Acute and Critical Care, 6,* 452–463.

Nissen, S. E., DeFranco, A. C., Moliterno, D. J., & Tuzcu, E. M. (1995). Coronary intravascular ultrasound: Diagnostic and interventional applications. *Coronary Artery Disease, 6,* 355–367.

Oparil, S. (1994). Cardiovascular Health at the Crossroads: Outlook for the 21st Century. *Scientific Statement.* Dallas, TX: American Heart Association.

Pasternak, R. C. & Braunwald, E. (1994). Acute myocardial infarction. In K. J. Isselbacher, E. Braunwald, J. D. Wilson, J. B. Martin, A. S. Fauci, & D. L. Kasper (Eds.), *Harrison's principles of internal medicine* (13th Ed.). (pp. 1066–1076). New York: McGraw-Hill.

Patrono, C. (1994). Aspirin as an antiplatelet drug. *New England Journal of Medicine, 330,* 1287–1293.

Pfeffer, M. A. (1992). Effect of captopril on mortality and morbidity in patinets with left ventricular dysfunction after myocardial infarction. Results of the survival and ventricular enlargement trial. *New England Journal of Medicine, 327,* 669–674.

Ridker, P., O'Donnel, C., Marder, V. & Hennekins, C. (1993). Large scale trials of thrombolytic therapy for acute myocardial infarction: GISSI II, ISIS III, and GUSTO I. *Annals of Internal Medicine, 119* (6), 530–532.

Ritchie, J. L., Bateman, T. M., Bonow, R. O., Crawford, M. H., Gibbons, R. J., Hall, R. J., O'Rourke, R. A., Parisi, A. F., & Verani, M. S. (1995). ACC/AHA guidelines for clinical use of cardiac radionuclide imaging: A report of the American College of Cardiology/American Heart Association Task Force on Assessment of Cardiovascular Procedures (Committee on Nuclear Imaging). *Journal of American College Cardiology, 24,* 521–547.

Ross, A. (1990). Implications of TIMI trials. *Advanced Experiments of Medicine and Biology, 281,* 361–366.

Ryan, T. J., Anderson, J. L., Antman, E. M., Braniff, B. A., Brooks, B. H., Califf, R. M., Hillis, L. D., Hiratzka, L. F., Rappaport, E., Riegel, B. J., Russell, R. O., Smith III, E. E., & Weaver, W. D. (1996). ACC/AHA guidelines for the management of patients with acute myocardial infarction: A report of the American College of Cardiology/American Heart Association Task Force on Practice Guidelines (Committee on Management of Acute Myocardial Infarction). *Journal of American College of Cardiology, 28,* 1328–1428.

Selwyn, A. P. & Braunwald, E. (1994). Ischemic heart disease. In K. J. Isselbacher, E. Braunwald, J. D. Wilson, J. B. Martin, A. S. Fauci, & D. L. Kasper (Eds.), *Harrison's principles of internal medicine* (13th Ed.). (pp. 1077–1084). New York: McGraw-Hill.

Selwyn, A. P., Yeung, A. C., Ryan, Jr., T. J., Raby, K., Barry, J., & Ganz, P. (1992). Pathophysiology of ischemia in patients with coronary artery disease. *Progress in Cardiovascular Diseases, 35,* 27–39.

Shah, P. K. (1997). New insights into the pathogenesis and prevention of acute coronary syndromes. *American Journal of Cardiology, 79,* 17–23.

Smith, J. F., Hanley, H. G., & Sheridan, F. M. (1995). Percutaneous interventions for ischemic heart disease. *Journal of Louisiana State Medical Society, 147,* 223–229.

Special Investigations: Noninvasive. In M. D. Cheitlin, M. Sokolow, & M. B. McIlroy (Eds.), *Clinical Cardiology* (pp. 88–113). Norwalk, CT: Appleton & Lange.

Stewart, S. L. (1992). Acute MI: A review of pathophysiology, treatment, and complications. *Journal of Cardiovascular Nursing, 6,* 1–25.

Thadani, U. (1997). Management of patients with chronic stable angina at low risk for serious cardiac events. *American Journal of Cardiology, 79,* 24–29.

Thompson, E. J., Detwiler, D. S., & Nelson, C. M. (1996). Dobutamine stress echocardiography: A new, noninvasive method for detecting ischemic heart disease. *Heart and Lung, 10*(2), 87–97.

Vincent, R. (1994). Pre-hospital management. In D. G. Julian & E. Braunwald (Eds.), *Management of Acute Myocardial Infarction* (pp. 3–28). London: W. B. Saunders Company Ltd.

Volpi, A., Divita, C., Franzosi, M., Geraci, E., & Maggioni, G. (1993). Determinants of six month mortality in survivors of myocardial infarction after thrombolysis: Results of the GISSI II database. *Circulation, 88* (2), 416–429.

Williams, K. & Morton, P. G. (1995). Diagnosis and treatment of acute myocardial infarction. *AACN Clinical Issues. Advanced Practice in Acute and Critical Care, 6,* 375–384.

Winters, K. J. & Eisenberg, P. R. (1995). Ischemic heart disease. In G. A. Ewald & C. R. McKenzie (Eds.), *Manual of medical therapeutics. The Washington manual* (28th Ed.), (pp. 85–113). Boston: Little, Brown and Company.

Zaret, B., Wackers, F., & Soufer, R. (1992). Nuclear cardiology. In E. Braunwald (Ed.), *Heart disease* (pp. 276–311). Philadelphia: W. B. Saunders Company.

33

Valvular and Congenital Heart Disease

Paul Logan
Yvonne A. Ruddy-Stein
C. Beth Staudenmayer

This chapter is an overview of valvular heart conditions and two congenital malformations that are encountered in clinical practice. Emphasis is on diagnosis and the medical and surgical management. Aortic, mitral, and tricuspid regurgitation are discussed, as are stenotic lesions of the aortic and mitral valves. Because of their extremely low incidence in the adult population of the United States, pulmonic stenosis and regurgitation and tricuspid stenosis are not covered in this chapter. Finally, two congenital lesions that cause shunting—atrial and ventricular septal defects—are discussed.

▶ ANATOMY AND PHYSIOLOGY

Conceptually, it is convenient to think of the heart as having six chambers. On the right side are the right atrium, right ventricle, and the pulmonary artery. On the left side are the left atrium, left ventricle, and the aorta. Each of these chambers has distinct hemodynamic characteristics and unique pressure waveforms (Fig. 33–1) that are useful when considering valvular heart disease.

The atria and ventricles are separated by atrioventricular valves. The chordae tendinae connect the atrioventricular valves to the papillary muscles that arise from the ventricular myocardium (Fig. 33–2). The papillary muscles prevent prolapse of the valve leaflets into the atria, and resultant regurgitation, during ventricular contraction.

The pulmonary artery and aorta are separated from the ventricles by the semilunar valves (Fig. 33–2). The valves prevent regurgitation into the ventricles during diastole. The semilunar valve leaflets arise from the endocardium and are suspended by fibrous tissue connected to the aortic wall. The leaflets meet to form the cup-shaped sinuses of Valsalva. In the aorta the sinuses of Valsalva fill the right and left coronary arteries during ventricular diastole.

▶ DIAGNOSTIC TESTING

Echocardiography and cardiac catheterization are the diagnostic tests for confirming valvular or congenital heart disease.

Transthoracic Echocardiography

Echocardiography is high frequency ultrasound that can be used to assess structural, functional, and hemodynamic indices. Echocardiography was developed in the late 1960s and early 1970s. Initially, the tools were crude and not user-friendly. Since then, the technology has developed substantially, making echocardiography among the best overall tests of cardiac function.

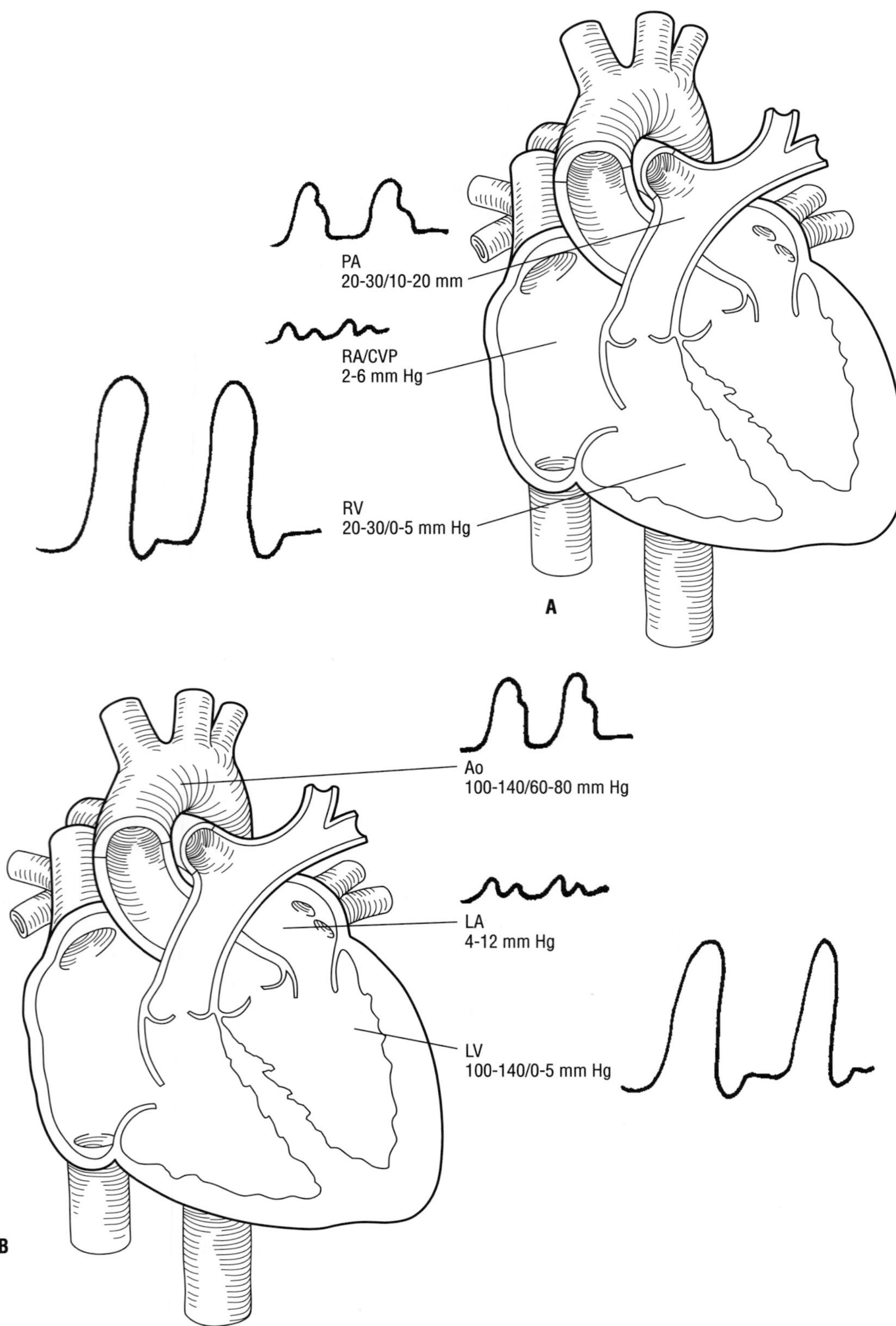

Figure 33–1. Pressures and waveforms of the heart and great vessels. **A,** Filling pressures of the right-heart. RA—right atrium, CVP—central venous pressure, RV—right ventricle, PA—pulmonary artery. **B,** Filling pressures of the left-heart chambers. LA—left atrium, LV—left ventricle, Ao—aorta. *(Adapted from J. G. Alspach. [1991]. [p. 190].)*

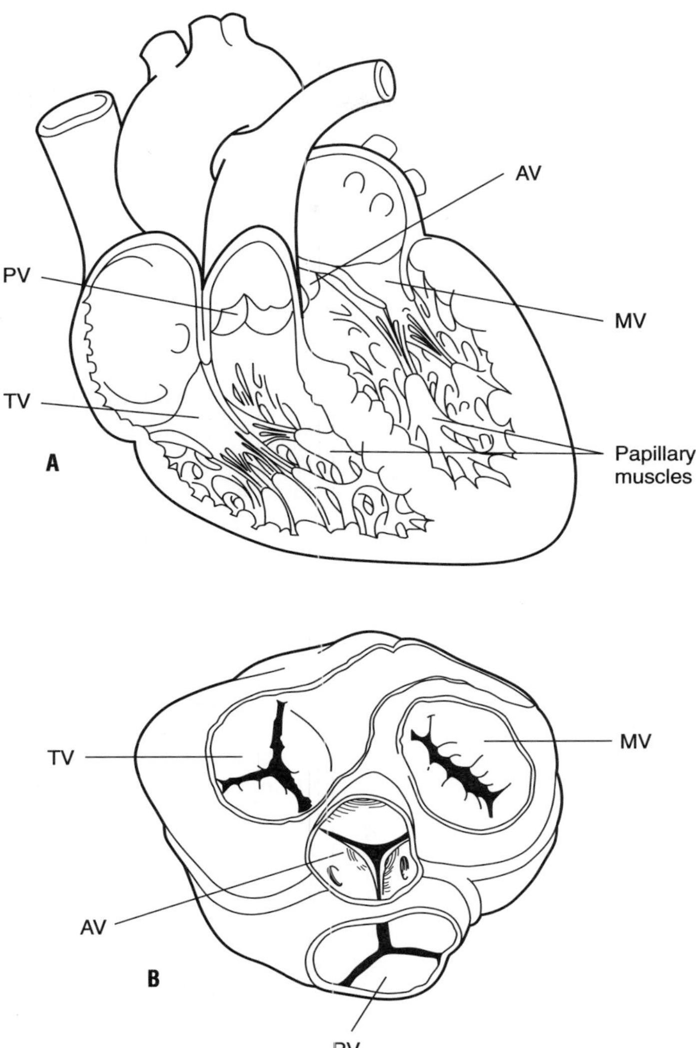

Figure 33–2. Anatomy of the heart and great vessels. **A,** Anterior view of the heart in cross section showing each of the four valves. Note the three cusps of the aortic valve and the anterior and posterior leaflets of the mitral valve. AV—aortic valve, PV—pulmonic valve, MV—mitral valve, TV—tricuspid valve.

The clinical utility of echocardiography is vast. Because it is noninvasive and risk-free, echocardiography can provide rapid assessment of cardiac function in almost all clinical settings. It is equally as beneficial in emergencies as in controlled settings. Table 33–1 lists the clinical uses of echocardiography.

Today, the M-mode, two-dimensional, color Doppler, and continuous- and pulsed-wave Doppler comprise the standard echocardiogram. M-mode (Fig. 33–3) is useful for measuring cardiac dimensions and evaluating the opening and closing of the aortic and mitral valves.

Two-dimensional echocardiography (2D echo) provides high-resolution images of cardiac structures in two-dimensional planes so that detailed anatomic and functional information can be obtained (Fig. 33–4). The ultrasound probe is placed in four transducer positions that allow various views of the heart. The structures of the heart and vasculature are visible in real-time, allowing 2D echo to be valuable in evaluating wall motion.

The Doppler effect is the phenomenon in which wave frequency increases as the source moves towards the observer, and decreases as the source moves away. In echocardiography, the ultrasound beam reflects off of red blood cells. The frequency, then, increases when the red blood cells move toward the ultrasound source and decreases when the red blood cell moves away.

Doppler echocardiography is most useful in assessment of valvular and congenital heart disease. Continuous wave (CW) and pulsed wave (PW) Doppler are used to produce graphic displays of the Doppler effect. In CW

TABLE 33–1. Clinical Uses of Echocardiography

- Quantification of:
  - Cardiac dimensions
  - Myocardial thickness
- Systolic function
  - Global wall motion
  - Regional wall motion (e.g., coronary artery disease)
- Diastolic function
  - Abnormal relaxation
  - Restrictive physiology
  - Venous flow pattern in diastolic filling
- Prosthetic valve evaluation
- Pulmonary hypertension
- Hemodynamic assessment
  - Stroke volume
  - Cardiac output
  - Valve areas
  - Intracardiac pressures
- Coronary artery disease
  - Evaluation of acute MI
- Chest pain syndromes
  - Helps rule out other causes such as aortic dissection
- Pericardial disease
  - Pericardial effusion
  - Tamponade
- Congenital heart disease
  - Atrial–septal defect
  - Ventricular–septal defect
  - Outflow obstruction
  - Patent ductus arterious
  - Overriding aorta

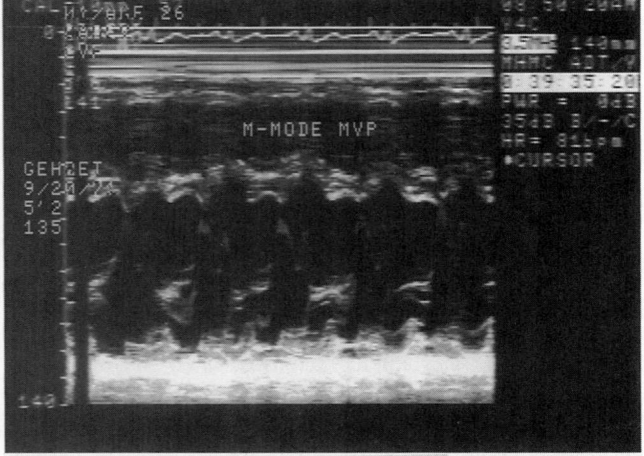

Figure 33–3. M-mode echocardiogram showing mitral valve prolapse. Note the M-shaped pattern created by the motion of the mitral valve leaflets.

(Fig. 33–5), the transducer emits a continuous wave of ultrasound waves. Once the beam strikes any reflective surface, be it red blood cell or myocardium, it is reflected back to the transducer. The result is that flow velocities from each point along the ultrasound wave are sampled. This is ideal for conditions such as aortic stenosis. But, if one wants to sample data from one specific area (e.g., the pulmonary vein) CW does not suffice. Instead, PW (Fig. 33–6) is used to send a pulsed wave of ultrasound energy to the area of interest. The reflected waves that are sampled, then, are known to come from the specified area. PW is used to "map" the Doppler signals in the cardiac chambers. By convention, CW and PW signals that move toward the probe are plotted above the baseline, while signals that move away from the probe are plotted below the baseline.

Color-flow Doppler uses the same principles, but displays the data as color superimposed over the 2D echo image (Fig. 33–7). In color-flow Doppler, signals that move toward the probe are red and signals that move away from the probe are blue.

Transesophageal Echocardiography

Transesophageal echocardiogram (TEE) is a useful modality in valvular and congenital heart disease. Unlike transthoracic echo, TEE provides very clear images of the heart and shows posterior structures such as the pulmonary veins. These characteristics make TEE particularly useful in evaluating mitral valve disease and atrial septal defects (Fig. 33–8), among others. Like transthoracic echocardiography, M-mode and 2D echocardiography and PW, CW, and color-flow Doppler are possible with TEE.

TEE is safe, having relatively few potential complications. The major potential complication is perforation of the esophagus. Patients with swallowing difficulty or a history of esophageal stricture should not undergo TEE. Aspiration and hypoxemia are other potential complications of TEE related to sedation. To minimize risk, a pulse oximeter should be used and a nurse should monitor the sedated patient (Feigenbaum, 1994).

After the procedure is explained to the patient and informed consent is obtained, the patient is prepared for the procedure. An intravenous line is inserted to administer sedatives. A pulse oximeter is applied and baseline vital signs are recorded. Viscous lidocaine and/or lidocaine spray are used to anesthetize the oropharynx. The sedative is administered in small doses until an adequate level of sedation is achieved. The TEE probe (i.e., transducer) is then inserted into the esophagus while the patient swallows. The study is performed, during which the patient is carefully monitored and additional sedatives are administered as necessary. TEEs generally take between 10 and 30 minutes, depending on operator skill, patient cooperation, difficulty passing the probe, and so on.

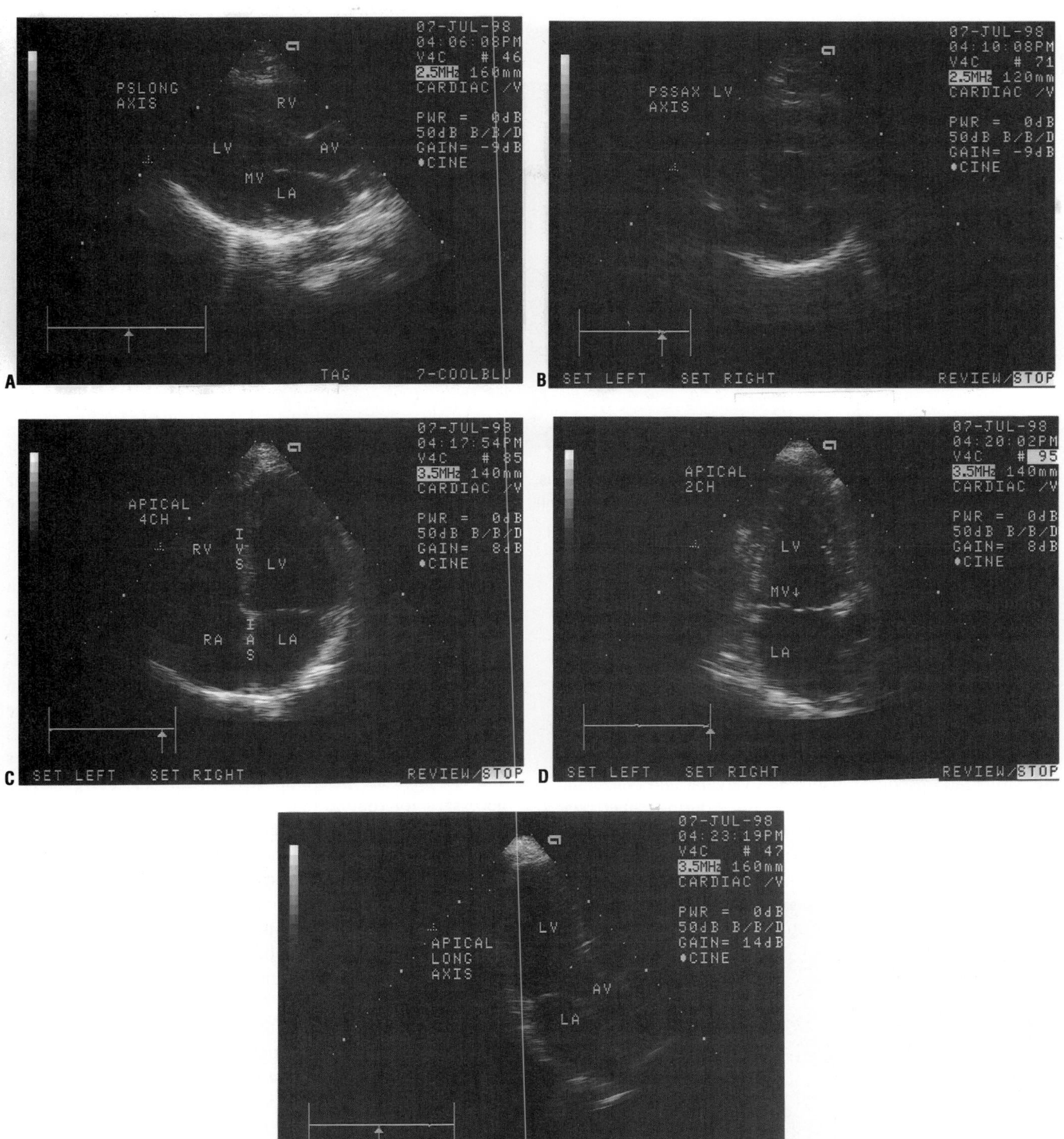

Figure 33–4. Five standard transthoracic two-dimensional echocardiogram views. **A,** Parasternal long axis showing the right ventricle (RV), left ventricle (LV), left atrium (LA), mitral valve (MV), and aortic valve (AV). The anteroseptal and posterior walls are visualized. **B,** Parasternal short axis view showing the right and left ventricles in cross section. At 12 o'clock to 2 o'clock is the midanterior wall, 3 o'clock is the midlateral wall, 6 o'clock is the midinferoposterior wall, and 9 o'clock is the midseptum. Note the papillary muscles in the midinferoposterior wall of the left ventricle. **C,** Apical four-chamber view showing the right and left ventricles, right atrium (RA), interventricular septum (IVS), and interatrial septum (IAS). The lateral wall of the left ventricle is visualized opposite the IVS. **D,** Apical two-chamber view showing the left ventricle, left atrium, and mitral valve. The inferior wall is seen on the left, and the anterior wall is seen on the right of the image. **E,** The apical long axis, or three-chamber view shows the left atrium and ventricle and the aorta. Like the parasternal long-axis view, the left ventricular walls visualized are the anteroseptal and posterior walls.

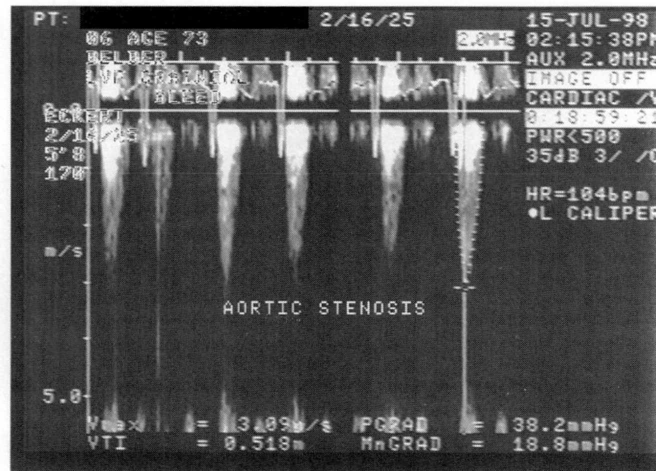

Figure 33–5. Continuous-wave doppler recording of aortic stenosis. Here, a Pedoff (nonimaging) transducer is placed at the apex of the heart. The negative deflections represent the velocities of blood moving away from the transducer. In this case, aortic stenosis is noted with a peak gradient of 38.2 mm Hg and mean gradient of 18.8 mm Hg.

Cardiac Catheterization

Cardiac catheterization combines direct measurement of hemodynamic indices, calculation of shunts, measurement of transvalvular gradients, calculation of valve areas, and visualization of anatomic structures. Together, these observations create a representative indication of heart function and are helpful in confirming diagnoses.

Measurement of hemodynamic indices and oxygenation are particularly useful in diagnosing valvular and congenital heart disease. From the raw data acquired during catheterization cardiac output, transvalvular gradients, shunts, and valve areas can be calculated.

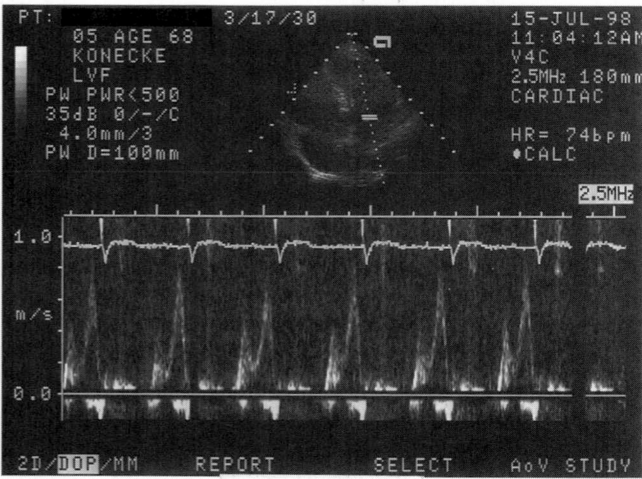

Figure 33–6. Pulsed-wave doppler of mitral inflow area. Normally, the E-wave is taller than the A-wave. When the ventricle hypertrophies, however, diastolic compliance is reduced. E: A reversal, as shown in the illustration, suggests diastolic noncompliance. The sampling area is shown in the two-dimensional image.

Once informed consent has been obtained the patient is moved to the catheterization table. EKG leads are then placed on the chest and limbs. Sedation may, or may not, be administered, depending upon the preference of the operator. The operator then injects lidocaine to numb the skin over the right femoral artery and vein, or other site. Once the skin is numb, the Seldinger technique (Fig. 33–9) is used to insert the sheaths, through which the guide-wires and catheters are inserted. Heparinization is not generally necessary for routine diagnostic catheterization, but if angioplasty will be performed the patient can be safely heparinzed after the introducer sheaths are in place. If the patient requires right heart catheterization, it is done first. Otherwise, the left heart catheterization is performed. The length of the procedure varies among operators, but a right and left heart catheterization, including left ventriculography and coronary angiography, is generally completed in within 30 minutes.

After catheterization, the introducer sheaths must be removed. The patient is usually moved to the bed or litter for sheath removal. The best method of achieving hemostasis is contested. In some institutions manual pressure is used to achieve hemostasis, requiring the nurse, technician, or physician to hold pressure over the arterial and/or venous puncture site until hemostasis is achieved, sometimes more than 30 minutes. Mechanical devices have also been shown to be safe and effective (Simon, Bumgarner, Clark, & Israel, 1998), though time to hemostasis may be prolonged and the overall cost may be greater (Bogart, 1995). Once hemostasis is achieved, the patient is confined to bedrest for a period of time. One study showed that bedrest for as short as 4 hours after sheath removal is sufficient to prevent bleeding (Keeling, Taylor, Nordt, Powers & Fisher, 1996). During the period of bedrest sandbags placed over the

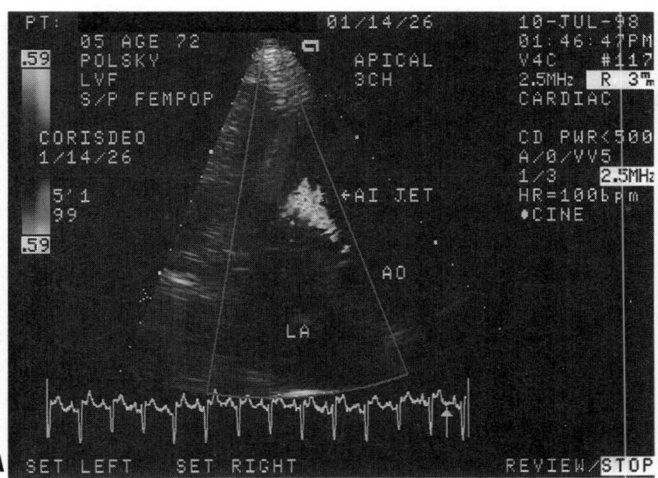

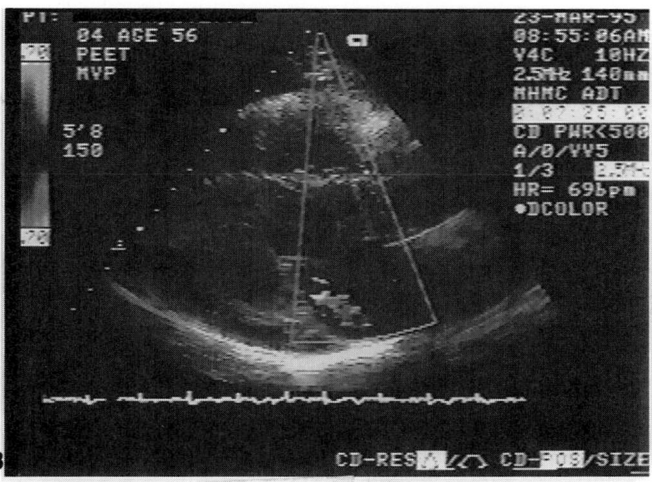

Figure 33–7. Color flow Doppler images of aortic and mitral regurgitation. **A,** Apical long-axis view showing mild aortic regurgitation (AI). **B,** Parasternal long-axis view showing mitral regurgitation (blue "flame"). (See Color Plate 1.)

catheterization site are probably not necessary (Hogan-Miller, Rustad, Sendelbach, & Goldenberg, 1995), and may be dangerous since bleeding can occur and be masked by the opaque sandbag. If there are no complications, the patient can safely be discharged following the bedrest period.

Catheterization is generally safe, with a complication rate of about one per thousand (Wyman, Safian, Portway, et al., 1988). Among the most feared complications of cardiac catheterization are embolization of clot or atheromatous debris to the coronary arteries, brain, gut, or periphery, resulting in myocardial infarction, stroke, or other catastrophic events. Death can also result. Complications at the catheter insertion site, however, are more common and include

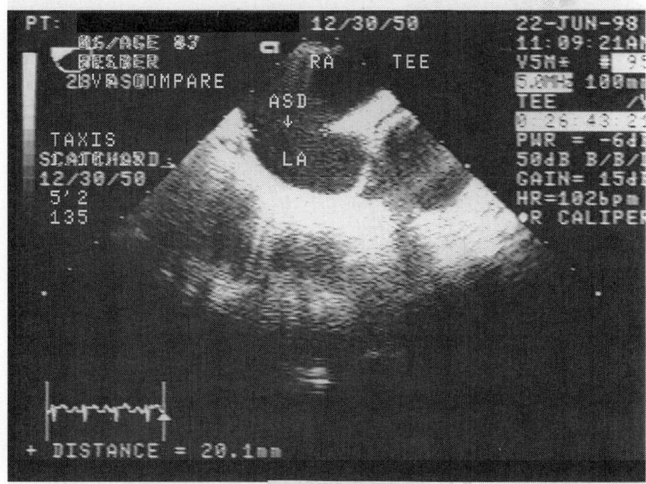

Figure 33–8. Two-dimensional transesophageal echocardiogram atrial septal defect. TEE—transesophageal echocardiogram, RA—right atrium, LA—left atrium, ASD—atrial septal defect.

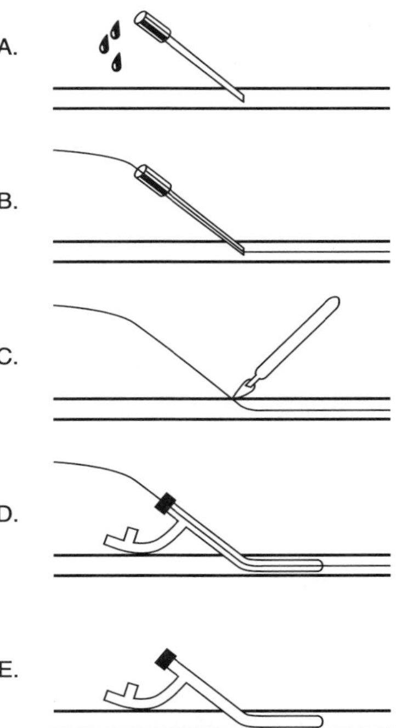

Figure 33–9. Seldinger technique for percutaneous insertion of introducer sheaths. **A,** A needle is inserted, at a 45 degree angle, into the vessel until blood returns through the needle. **B,** A wire is passed through the needle and into the vessel. **C,** A knife is used to make an 1/8 to 1/4 inch incision adjacent to the wire. **D,** An introducer sheath is threaded over the guide wire into the vessel. The wire is held at all times during the insertion of the sheath. **E,** Finally, the wire is removed and the sheath is flushed and secured with sutures. Catheters are inserted through the sheath.

bleeding, arterial dissection, arteriovenous fistula, and pseudoaneurysm.

Cardiac Output

Thermodilution Method. In 1971 Ganz and colleagues described the thermodilution method of determining cardiac output. This method involves injecting saline (at a known temperature) into the proximal port of a pulmonary artery catheter, then measuring the temperature of the blood as it passes the catheter tip. When the injectate mixes with the blood in the right ventricle, the blood is cooled. In high output states the cooled blood reaches the catheter tip quickly. When the cardiac output is low, however, it takes longer for the cooled blood to reach the catheter tip. Taking into account the temperatures of the injectate and the patient and the size of the catheter, a computer calculates the cardiac output.

Fick Method. Fick determined that if the rate of oxygen consumption (Vo_2) and the oxygen content of the blood entering (Cao_2) and returning from (Cvo_2) the system are known, the flow of the system (cardiac output) can be readily calculated. Because direct measurement of oxygen consumption is awkward and must be measured *in vivo,* this value is assumed.

The oxygen content of arterial blood is calculated using the following equation:

$$Cao_2 = \left(\frac{[Hb](1.34)(Sao_2)}{100} \right) + (Pao_2)(0.003)$$

where [Hb] is the concentration of hemoglobin in mg %, Sao_2 is the percent arterial oxygen saturation, and Pao_2 is the partial pressure of oxygen in mm Hg.

The oxygen content of venous blood (Cvo_2) is calculated similarly, but the venous oxygen saturation and partial pressure are substituted for the arterial.

Once the variables are known, cardiac output (Q) is calculated using the Fick equation:

$$Q = \frac{Vo_2}{(Cao_2) - (Cvo_2)}$$

Intracardiac Pressures and Waveforms

Among the most important information obtained from catheterization are the intracardiac pressures and waveforms. The intracardiac pressures indicate the severity of various cardiac anomalies. Waveform tracings can also give valuable information.

Each cardiac chamber has unique pressures and characteristic waveforms (refer to Fig. 33–1). The right atrial pressure is measured directly with a catheter in the atrium. Left atrial diastolic blood flow precludes the passage of a catheter from the left ventricle into the left atrium. If it is necessary to measure the left atrial pressure directly, a catheter may be passed transseptally from the right atrium. Ordinarily, though, because there is no valve between the left atrium and the pulmonary veins, the pulmonary capillary wedge pressure (PCWP) is an accurate estimation of the left atrial pressures. (Therefore, an important point is that when reading the PCWP it is essential that *a* and *v* waves are visible. Merely observing the diminuation of the PA waveform is not sufficient.)

The right ventricular systolic and diastolic pressures are lower than the left ventricular pressures (refer to Fig. 33–1). There are two characteristics that are useful in differentiating a ventricular from a pulmonary artery or aortic waveform. First, the ventricular end diastolic pressure is normally near zero. Although the end-diastolic pressure may be elevated (suggesting heart failure), it is never as high as the diastolic blood pressure (or the diastolic pulmonary pressure, if right sided). The shape of the waveform is the best indicator of catheter placement. The ventricular end diastolic waveform dips below the baseline. No other hemodynamic waveform shares this characteristic.

The pulmonary artery and aortic waveforms are best characterized by the presence of a dicrotic notch, which is caused by the closure of the pulmonic and aortic valves, respectively (refer to Fig. 33–1).

Transvalvular Gradients

The severity of valvular stenoses are gauged by the gradient—the difference between the prevalvular and postvalvular pressures—across the valve. Across a normal aortic valve, for instance, the gradient is zero. That is, the peak aortic pressure is equal to the peak left ventricular systolic pressure.

To calculate the peak aortic valvular gradient, simply subtract the peak systolic ventricular pressure from the peak systolic aortic pressure. It is important to measure the pressures using simultaneously-recorded waveforms (Fig. 33–10).

Calculation of the mean aortic valvular gradient is done by calculating the area between the aortic and ventricular pressure tracings (refer to Fig. 33–10). Today computers in the catheterization laboratory readily perform this cumbersome calculation.

Like the aortic valvular gradient, calculation of the mitral valve gradient requires simultaneous recordings of the pulmonary capillary wedge (i.e., left atrial) and left ventricular pressures (Fig. 33–11). Again, the mean gradient is calculated by measuring the area between the left atrial and left ventricular tracings. Generally, the mean left atrial pressure is inferred from the pulmonary wedge pressure, though direct measurement of the left atrial pressure is possible. To obtain the direct left atrial pressure, the left atrium is entered from the right atrium via the interatrial septum. Because this method is somewhat riskier than the alternative, it is typically performed only when the left atrial pressure is suspected of being substantially different than the pulmonary wedge pressure (e.g., pulmonary hypertension).

The pulmonic and tricuspid valvular gradients are not

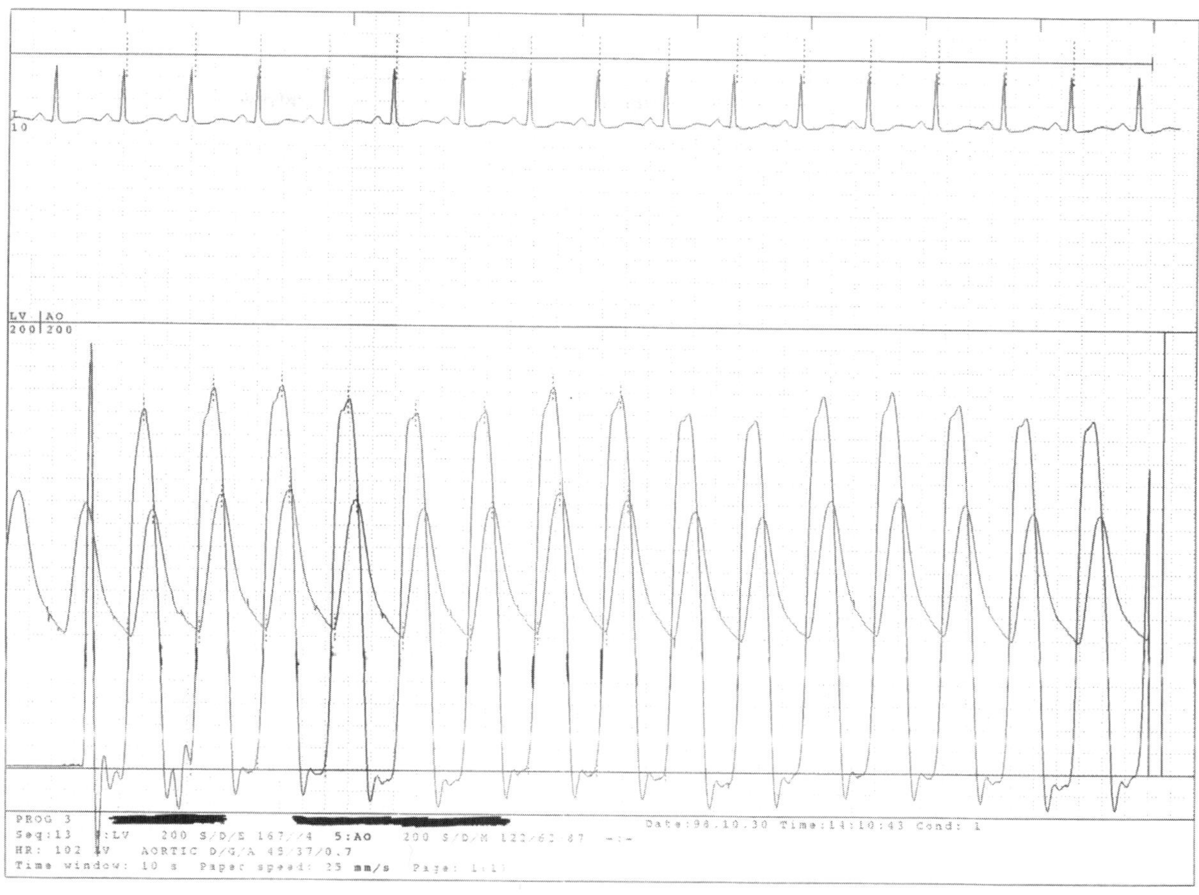

Figure 33–10. Simultaneously recorded aortic and left ventricular waveforms showing the peak-to-peak aortic valve gradient. Catheters are placed in the left ventricle and aorta. Simultaneous recordings are made of the pressure waveforms in each chamber. The peak-to-peak aortic valve gradient is the difference between the peak aortic pressure and the peak left ventricular pressure.

routinely measured during cardiac catheterization. The pulmonic valvular gradient is the difference between the peak systolic pulmonary artery and right ventricular pressures. The tricuspid valvular gradient is the difference between the right atrial and right ventricular pressures.

Valve Areas

In addition to determination of valve gradients, calculation of the valve area is important for such stenotic lesions as aortic and mitral stenoses. The Gorlin equation is used to calculate valve areas:

$$\text{Aortic valve area} = \frac{F}{44.3\sqrt{\Delta P}}$$

$$\text{Mitral valve area} = \frac{F}{37.7\sqrt{\Delta P}}$$

where F is flow (a function of cardiac output, diastolic filling period, and systolic ejection period) and ΔP is the difference between the prevalvular and postvalvular pressures.

A normal aortic valve area is greater than 1 cm^2 and a normal mitral valve area is greater than 2 cm^2. Severe aortic stenosis is defined as an aortic valve area of 0.7 cm^2 or less. Severe mitral stenosis is defined as 1.0 cm^2 or less.

Shunts

By obtaining blood samples from the superior and inferior vena cavas, right atrium, right ventricle, and pulmonary artery, the operator can see "step-up" in the oxygen content of the right heart (Fig. 33–12). For example, assume that the normal oxygen saturation is 70% in right atrium, right ventricle, and pulmonary artery. If the catheterization reveals 70% saturation in the right atrium, 85% in the right ventricle, and 90% in the pulmonary artery, then a step-up, or left-to-right (e.g., ventricular septal defect) shunt, is likely present. Additional studies such as transesophageal echocardiogram can be employed to identify the particular defect.

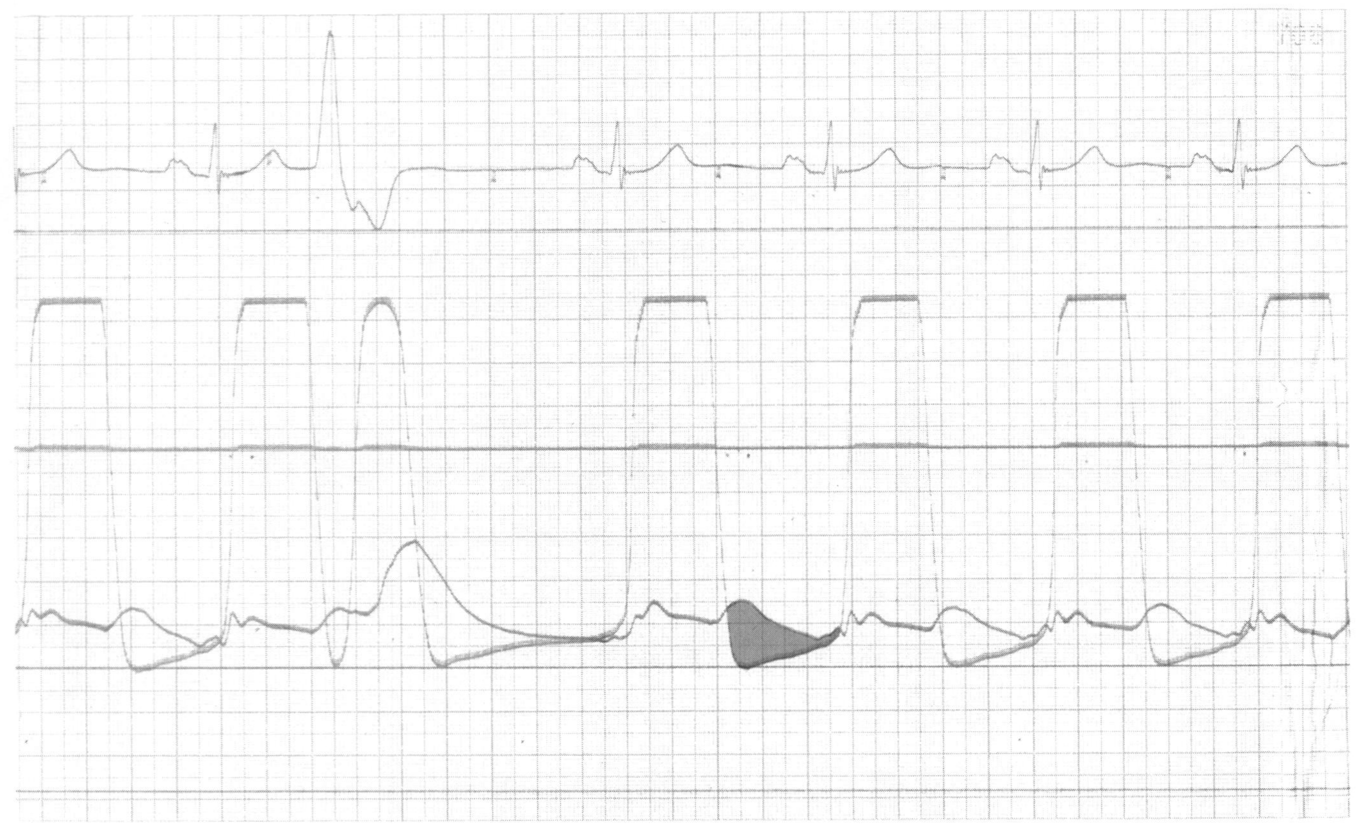

Figure 33–11. Simultaneously recorded pulmonary capillary wedge and left ventricular pressures showing mitral stenosis. The gradient is shown by the shaded area between the wedge and LV tracings.

Visualization of Structures

In addition to hemodynamic measurements and calculations, direct visualization of anatomic structures is useful for select valvular and congenital lesions. Left ventriculography is helpful in determining the extent of mitral regurgitation. In the cath lab a catheter is inserted into the left ventricle. Radiopaque dye is then injected into the ventricle while filmed fluoroscopically. Normally no dye flows across the plane of the mitral valve in sinus rhythm. When mitral regurgitation is present, however, the left atrium is opacified.

Similarly, dye can be injected into the aortic root. If the aortic valve is competent, no dye regurgitates into the left ventricle. The appearance of dye in the ventricle is diagnostic of aortic regurgitation. The degree of opacification is graded on a scale of 1 to 4 where 1 is mild and 4 is severe.

▶ DEGENERATIVE VALVULAR DISEASE—MITRAL VALVE PROLAPSE

Pathophysiology

Mitral valve prolapse (MVP) results from a variety of mechanisms—including myxomatous degeneration of the mitral valve apparatus and papillary muscle dysfunction—and can range in severity from mild to severe. Myxomatous degeneration of the mitral valve leaflet and chordae tendineae is the most common cause of MVP. Myxomatous degeneration causes redundant tissue of the valve apparatus and is associated with an increase in the concentration of acid micropolysaccharides. Generally, the redundant valve leaflets function well and cause no hemodynamic consequences. In some cases, however, severe MVP causes regurgitation. This process is usually progressive, but if one or more chordae rupture, acute regurgitation can occur.

Myxomatous degeneration is frequently found in patients who have connective tissue disorders such as Marfan's syndrome. In most patients, the myxomatous degeneration is confined to the mitral valve, and usually involves only the posterior leaflet. Some patients, however, also have involvement of the tricuspid valve.

In MVP due to papillary muscle dysfunction, ischemia is generally the cause. The papillary muscles are supplied by the obtuse marginal branch of the circumflex coronary artery in most patients. At rest, the papillary muscle may be nonischemic, in which case MVP is absent. If the muscle is made ischemic, however, MVP may occur. This is a poten-

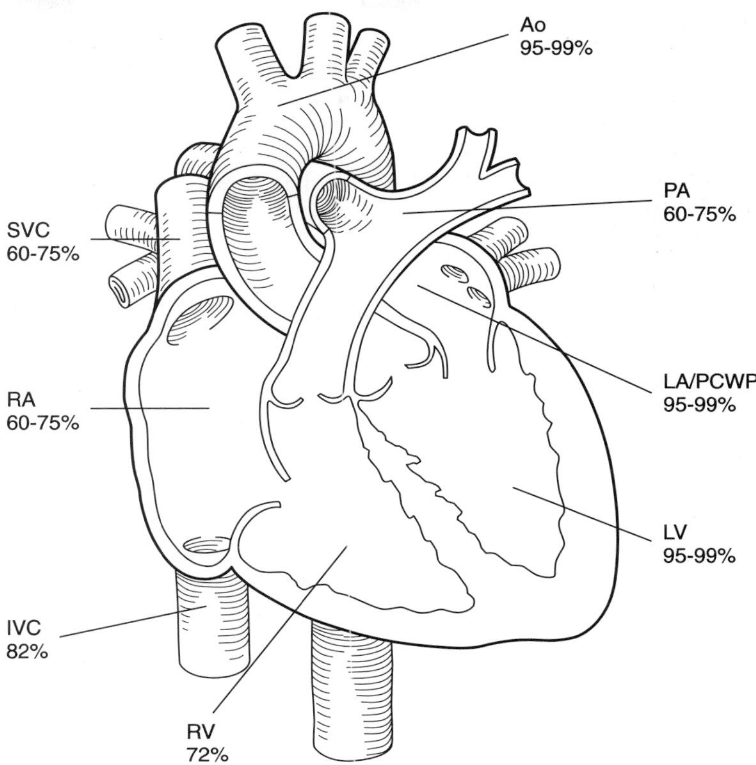

Figure 33–12. Normal oxygen saturations of blood in the heart and great vessels. The oxygen saturations in the left heart are higher than those in the right heart. A left-to-right shunt causes "step-up" of the right-sided saturations at and distal to the level of the shunt.

tially dangerous situation. If the papillary muscle becomes necrotic, acute regurgitation can result.

History and Physical Findings

MVP is more common in females, usually between the ages of 14 and 30 years. The majority of patients with MVP are entirely asymptomatic. In some cases, however, symptoms include palpitations, arrhythmias, light-headedness, syncope, and chest pain. In severe MVP with concomitant mitral regurgitation, symptoms of heart failure may occur.

Harvey & Canfield (1997) say that "we must listen very carefully to our patients since, in some, the telltale auscultatory findings are heard only on inspiration, in others only on expiration. The findings may be transient, intermittent, varying at times, with some heartbeats having: No click or murmur, only a click or clicks, only a murmur, combinations of click and murmur, or a musical murmur termed a 'whoop' or 'honk'."

A mid-late systolic click is produced when the valve leaflets billow into the left atrium during systole. The click is the physical finding diagnostic of MVP. One or more clicks may be heard during systole. Clicks may be followed by a late systolic murmur caused by mitral regurgitation. This is an important diagnostic finding, as the indication for endocarditis prophylaxis in MVP is the presence of mitral regurgitation.

Maneuvers provide important clues. The click and murmur occur earlier in systole, and may be louder, with standing. Valsalva maneuver increases the intensity of the murmur and click, while squatting and isometric exercise decrease the intensity. Commonly, a murmur is not heard while the patient is lying. When the patient stands, however, the murmur becomes evident.

Laboratory and Diagnostic Tests

MVP can be verified with two diagnostic tests: ventriculography and echocardiography. Because it is an invasive procedure, and because the usefulness of the images is limited, ventriculography is not a primary diagnostic tool. Rather, MVP is often found incidentally during cardiac catheterization.

The echocardiogram is the best tool for evaluating MVP. It can both identify prolapse of the leaflets and quantify mitral regurgitation. The parasternal long axis view is the gold standard used to diagnose MVP (Reynolds, 1993). MVP is present when the leaflets prolapse past the mitral annulus into the left atrium. This is a highly subjective test, but is clearly evident in patients with severe MVP.

Management

Undoubtedly, the ubiquity of echocardiography has led to a greater number of MVP diagnoses. MVP is sometimes found incidentally on an echocardiogram done for other reasons. The fact that few patients complain of symptoms prior to being given the diagnosis is testament that MVP is often asymptomatic.

MVP typically has an excellent prognosis, and for many patients treatment is unnecessary. In patients with chest pain or palpitations, beta blockers are often effective in alleviating symptoms and are generally benign. Only in a minority of patients is surgical valve repair necessary.

Follow-Up

Patients with severe myxomatous MVP may, at some time in their life, require surgical valve repair. For this reason, close follow-up for severe MVP is necessary. Annual echocardiograms are common, with 3-month follow-up visits.

As with all structural heart disease, MVP can place patients at risk of endocarditis. According to the American Heart Association guidelines, patients with MVP should have endocarditis prophylaxis only if mitral regurgitation is present (Dajani, Taubert, Wilson, Bolger, Bayer, Ferrieri, et al., 1997).

▶ REGURGITANT VALVULAR LESIONS—VOLUME OVERLOAD

Regurgitant valvular lesions cause volume overload; stenotic valvular lesions cause pressure overload. The distinction between volume and pressure overload is clinically important. In aortic regurgitation, for instance, the incompetent aortic valve allows regurgitation of blood from the aorta into the ventricle during diastole. Similarly, in mitral regurgitation blood flows from the left ventricle backward into the atrium during ventricular systole. Consequently, a larger volume of blood is returned from the atrium to the ventricle during diastole. Over time, the ventricular cavity dilates to accommodate the large volume of blood produced by regurgitant lesions. Late in the natural history of volume overload conditions, the ventricle dilates to such a point that it can no longer adequately contract. Heart failure results.

Aortic Regurgitation

Pathophysiology

Rheumatic heart disease is perhaps the most common etiology of aortic regurgitation (AR) (Garver et al., 1995), but congenital valvular abnormalities, aortic root dilatation (e.g., Marfan's), aortic dissection, and endocarditis also cause regurgitant lesions of the aortic valve (Table 33–2). Rheumatic, congenital, and degenerative etiologies of AR generally cause chronic regurgitation. Acute AR—a more serious condition—is typically seen in acute aortic dissection and aortic valve endocarditis.

TABLE 33–2. Some Causes of Aortic Regurgitation

Rheumatic fever
Congenitally bicuspid (or unicuspid) valve
Endocarditis
Aortic dissection (acute AR)
Marfan's syndrome
Syphilis

Chronic AR is well-tolerated by most patients (Ishii et al., 1996). Early in the course of the disease the body easily compensates for the increased ventricular volume. Because the aorta allows regurgitation of blood backward into the ventricle during diastole, there is a relatively low afterload on the ventricle. The heart has little peripheral resistance to overcome, so systolic function is not compromised.

As the disease progresses the persistent volume overload increases left ventricular wall tension. Left ventricular hypertrophy occurs and, eventually, the ventricular cavity dilates. The remodeling that occurs may also cause the mitral apparatus to stretch, resulting in abnormal closure of the mitral leaflets and resultant mitral regurgitation.

History and Physical Findings

In mild or moderate AR patients are typically asymptomatic. As the disease progresses, however, fatigue, paroxysmal nocturnal dyspnea (PND), orthopnea, and exertional dyspnea develop over several months. In acute AR patients may present with frank pulmonary edema and respiratory failure. Patients in whom dissecting thoracic aneurysm is suspected should be evaluated for AR.

Previous history of endocarditis or rheumatic fever may provide clues to the diagnosis of AR. These diseases damage the structure of the valve and cause regurgitation.

Among the most sensitive findings in AR is a wide pulse pressure, that is, a difference between the systolic and diastolic blood pressure of 70 mm Hg or more. If the patient has a normal pulse pressure (less than 70 mm Hg), it is unlikely that there is severe AR.

Marfan's syndrome is sometimes associated with dilatation of the aortic root and, hence, aortic regurgitation. Findings such as high arched palate, arachnodactyly, and hyperextendability of joints should prompt the clinician to consider Marfan's syndrome and a work-up for AR.

Patients with chronic heart failure from AR may exhibit signs of "wasting." Unexplained weight loss, fatigue, abdominal distension, and loss of muscle bulk are indications that metabolic demand chronically exceeds the heart's ability to supply necessary nutrients. Other general findings suggestive of AR are head bobbing and a pulsatile uvula. These phenomena are related to the increased stroke volume that accompanies AR.

Jugular venous distension, a sign of right heart failure, does not typically occur in chronic AR. Increased pulmonary artery pressures due to left heart failure may cause right ventricular failure. This is a late finding, however, and does not precede symptoms of left heart failure.

Examination of the carotid arteries in patients with AR may reveal one of three important findings: Pulsus bisferens, pulsus alternans (Fig. 33–13), or water hammer pulse. Water hammer pulse is a bounding pulse palpable throughout the systemic arterial system. Over the femoral artery "pistol shot" sounds may be heard. These are the result of increased stroke volume. Although these findings may be present in mild or moderate AR, they typically disappear as ventricular function deteriorates. Pulsus bisferens is the presence of two carotid upstrokes during each cardiac cycle. The first upstroke is caused by ejection of blood in early systole, the second is caused by regurgitation into the ventricle. Lastly, pulsus alternans is the beat-to-beat alternation of pulse amplitude. This is a late finding that always indicates severe ventricular systolic dysfunction and is accompanied by symptoms of heart failure.

In mild AR the point of maximum intensity (PMI) is typically located at the fourth or fifth intercostal space, midclavicular line. As the ventricle hypertrophies, the PMI becomes diffuse and sustained. The characteristic dime-sized PMI that normally strikes the chest wall is replaced with a more diffuse PMI that persists against the chest wall during systole. As the ventricle dilates, the PMI moves inferolaterally to the sixth intercostal space, anterior axillary line. Also, the impulse bocomes hypokinetic.

AR produces a characteristic decrescendo diastolic murmur that is typically heard with the diaphragm of the stethoscope along the left sternal border (refer to Fig. 33–13). The murmur starts simultaneously with S_2 and ends well before S_1. It is helpful to conceptualize the AR murmur as a "prolonged S_2." In mild or moderate AR the murmur may be inaudible. To accentuate the murmur have the patient lean forward, exhale, and hold his or her breath.

Systolic ejection murmurs, such as would be heard in other "high output states," are commonly heard in AR. Although the murmur may be the result of such a mechanism,

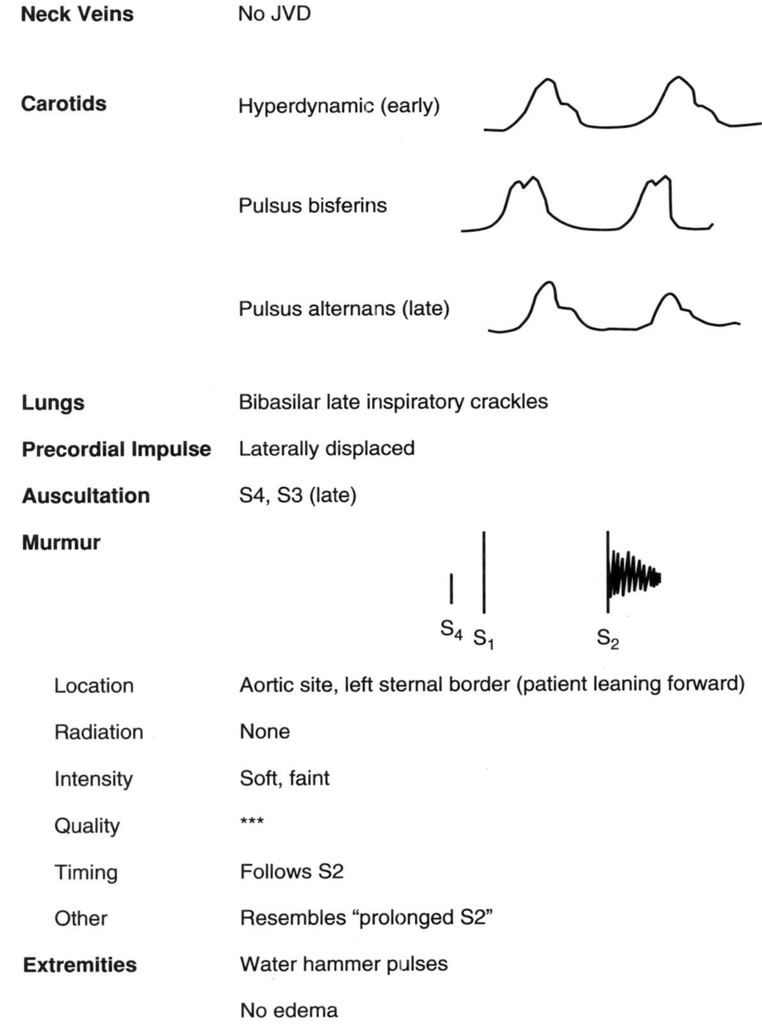

Figure 33–13. Summary of physical findings in aortic regurgitation.

it is important to evaluate the patient for concomitant aortic stenosis which can be present in rheumatic heart disease.

An interesting phenomenon occurs in severe AR. An Austin–Flint murmur occurs when the regurgitant AR jet forces the anterior mitral valve leaflet to close prematurely. The resultant murmur occurs well after S_2 and mimics the murmur of mitral stenosis.

Laboratory and Diagnostic Tests

The chest x-ray in aortic regurgitation may reveal left ventricular dilation and evidence of congestive heart failure. Typically, the left atrium is not enlarged. Depending upon the etiology of the AR, a dilated aortic root may be present.

The electrocardiogram is of limited value in diagnosing AR. Because AR is a problem of volume overload, left ventricular dilatation occurs. The dilated ventricle is closer to the chest wall resulting in higher voltage in the chest leads. There are, however, no criteria that differentiate left ventricular dilation from left ventricular hypertrophy (Wagner, 1994). Electrocardiographic evidence of ventricular dilation include large S waves in V1 and V2 and large R waves in V5 and V6. Late in the disease there may be a loss of R wave progression in the precordial leads.

Echocardiography. M-mode echocardiography is used to measure the cardiac dimensions. An end-systolic dimension of 50-55 mm is an indication for surgery. Color-flow Doppler is one of the best echocardiographic tools for estimating AR (refer to Fig. 33–7). The width of the AR jet at the valve orifice and the length of the jet correlate directly with the severity of the regurgitation. Also, continuous-wave Doppler is used to measure the pressure half-time, "the time required for the peak gradient to be reduced to one-half" (Feigenbaum, 1994). A pressure half-time less than or equal to 300 msec suggests severe AR (Reynolds, 1993).

Cardiac Catheterization. In mild or moderate AR, hemodynamic function is preserved. The left atrial pressure and left ventricular end-diastolic pressures remain normal and the cardiac output may be supranormal. Severe AR is associated with elevated left atrial and left ventricular end-diastolic pressures. As ventricular function deteriorates the cardiac output falls.

The gold standard diagnostic tool in AR is the aortogram. A catheter is placed in the ascending aorta and radiopaque dye is injected while the aorta is filmed. The appearance of dye in the left ventricle during the injection is diagnostic of AR. The degree of regurgitation is graded on a scale of 1 to 4, where 1 is mild and 4 is severe.

Management

Medical Therapy. Because asymptomatic chronic AR carries an annual mortality rate that is less than 0.5% (Bonow, 1994), medical therapy is generally sufficient early in the disease. Vasodilators are the mainstay of medical therapy for AR. Nifedipine, angiotensin converting enzyme (ACE) inhibitors, and hydralazine improve ventricular function and delay the need for aortic valve surgery (Lin et al., 1994; Schon, 1994; Scognamiglio et al., 1994). Although medical therapy should be instituted early (Carabello, 1996), the maximal benefits are seen in patients with the "largest and sickest hearts" (Levine & Gaasch, 1996).

Vasodilators should be instituted early and titrated upwards as the patient tolerates. In patients with evidence of heart failure, diuretic therapy should be instituted until valve replacement surgery is performed. Digoxin should be added in severe AR to improve contractile function. The importance, too, of sodium restriction should not be overlooked.

Acute AR due to aortic dissection is generally treated with intravenous beta blockers such as esmolol and intravenous vasodilators such as sodium nitroprusside to control blood pressure. Once stabilized, the patient can be taken to the operating room, if necessary.

Surgical Treatment. Despite maximal medical therapy, all patients with chronic AR eventually require aortic valve surgery. Although some surgeons favor early operation for AR, the studies, to date, have not supported this practice. A recent study showed no difference in operative mortality or length of stay between patients who underwent early versus late aortic valve surgery (Rao et al., 1996).

Two endpoints indicate the need for aortic valve surgery in chronic AR: worsening ventricular systolic function or clinical heart failure (Bonow, 1994). Symptoms of heart failure should be evaluated thoroughly and the patient referred for surgery, if appropriate. Asymptomatic patients, on the other hand, are followed with serial echocardiograms and referred for aortic valve replacement surgery as soon as ventricular function begins to deteriorate.

Acute AR is often lethal if untreated, but may respond well to urgent surgery. In one study, the in-hospital mortality for patients with class IV (severe) congestive heart failure due to acute AR was 9.4%. The overall survival was 82% at 5 years and 74% at 10 years (Kadri et al., 1994). The highest mortality occurred in patients with aortic valve endocarditis.

Once the decision is made to operate, the patient and provider must select a prosthetic valve—bioprosthesis or mechanical valve. Essentially, the benefit of a bioprosthesis is freedom from long-term anticoagulation, but longevity is sacrificed. The longevity of bioprostheses is generally considered to be 10 years or less. That long-term anticoagulation is unnecessary, and the longevity is about 10 years, makes bioprostheses nearly ideal for octogenarians. It is not so likely that an 85-year-old would outlive his or her valve as it is that a 70-year-old would. It can be complicated, however, when an 88-year-old returns for replacement of a deteriorating bioprosthesis.

The advantage of mechanical valves is greater longevity. Because of the greater longevity, it is estimated that two-thirds of patients receive mechanical valves (Garver et al., 1995). The disadvantage is that life-long anticoagulation is necessary.

Recently, homografts and stentless bioprosthetic valves have been used. These devices may combine the advantages of bioprostheses and mecahanical valves. The benefit of stentless valves is that they have better hemodynamic profiles than mechanical valves. In the first two years of follow-up, recipients of stentless prosthetic valves showed better regression of left ventricular hypertrophy and more improvement of ventricular function (Jin et al., 1996). It is theorized that, in addition to better hemodynamics, stentless prosthetic valves may experience fewer shear forces, thus improving their longevity.

Follow-Up

Close follow-up of patients with AR is essential. Typically, office visits at three-month intervals is adequate (Braunwald, 1994). The patient should be instructed to notify the provider of any symptoms that suggest progression of the disease. Fatigue, although highly subjective, may be the earliest symptom of worsening ventricular function. Paroxysmal nocturnal dyspnea, orthopnea, and exertional dyspnea signal heart failure and, when they occur, require immediate attention.

Echocardiography is a convenient, harmless, noninvasive method of monitoring progression of AR. Asymptomatic patients with an end-systolic dimension less than 45 mm are well-served by annual echocardiograms. Those with end-systolic dimensions 45–55 mm should have semiannual echos and be referred for catheterization and surgery when the end-systolic dimension reaches 50–55 mm (Carabello, 1996).

Mitral Regurgitation

Pathophysiology

Mitral regurgitation (MR) can occur acutely or it can develop and worsen over long periods of time. Acute MR is frequently the result of injury to the papillary muscles or chordae tendineae, though direct damage to the valve leaflets by endocarditis can also occur.

Papillary muscle dysfunction or rupture is usually related to coronary artery disease, particularly the circumflex coronary artery that supplies the inferoposterior and lateral walls. During ventricular contraction the papillary muscle normally contracts to prevent prolapse of the mitral valve leaflets into the atrium. Ischemia of the papillary muscle, however, prevents papillary contraction during systole. Hence, there is regurgitation through the otherwise structurally normal mitral valve. Once the ischemia is relieved, the papillary muscle and, subsequently, the mitral valve function normally. Nevertheless, the effects of transient papillary muscle dysfunction may be sufficient to cause "flash" pulmonary edema.

In addition to cardiorexus (cardiac rupture) and ventricular septal defect, papillary muscle rupture is a serious complication of myocardial infarction that occurs in less than 1 percent of patients experiencing myocardial infarction. When papillary muscle rupture occurs, it is typically 3 days after inferoposterior or lateral transmural (Q-wave) myocardial infarction. The physiological consequences are dramatic, immediate, and often fatal.

Similarly, degenerative disease of the mitral valve can lead to rupture of the chordae. Because of the structure of the mitral valve apparatus, the location of chordal rupture is of particular importance. Like papillary muscle rupture, chordal rupture near the papillary muscle compromises valvular function and can induce heart failure. A chordal rupture near the valve leaflet, however, often causes little hemodynamic effect.

In some cases MR develops slowly over years. Degenerative myxomatous conditions such as mitral valve prolapse (MVP) are particularly likely to cause chronic mitral regurgitation. Rheumatic heart disease can also lead to MR.

MR can also occur when the left ventricle dilates. In this case, the valve remains structurally normal. But, because the valve apparatus is stretched, the leaflets do not coapt correctly and regurgitation results. When the dilatation occurs from aortic regurgitation, for example, aortic valve replacement is often sufficient to relieve the MR.

As the disease progresses, the amount of regurgitant flow increases and the volume of blood in the left heart increases. The result of this volume overload is ventricular dilatation and heart failure. Also, atrial arrhythmias like atrial fibrillation can occur and complicate heart failure.

History and Physical Findings

Mild chronic MR is generally well tolerated. Patients may remain asymptomatic for years. As the disease progresses, however, increased left atrial pressures may cause symptoms of left heart failure—exertional dyspnea, orthopnea, and paroxysmal nocturnal dyspnea. Late in the course of the disease left heart failure may become severe enough that the hemodynamics of the right heart are compromised. Peripheral edema, diarrhea, nausea and vomiting, abdominal cramping, and ascites may result.

Whereas mild or moderate chronic MR may be easily managed and well tolerated, acute MR is poorly tolerated. The dramatic hemodynamic effects of acute MR cause symptoms of heart failure to develop abruptly. Patients with acute MR may present with "flash" pulmonary edema and may die without immediate life-saving interventions.

Important clues regarding the etiology of symptoms may be obtained from a careful patient history. Acute MR is often associated with endocarditis, ischemia or necrosis (and subsequent rupture) of the papillary muscle, or rupture of the chordae tendineae. Chronic MR caused by myxomatous mitral valve disease often remains stable for many years, but can worsen acutely when a chordae ruptures.

The general appearance of patients with chronic MR is

variable. As with many valvular heart disorders, the compensation in the early stages of the disease prevents marked physical findings and symptoms. A late finding associated with heart failure is cachexia, or wasting.

Jugular venous distention suggests elevated pulmonary artery pressures and severe MR. The jugular venous pulsation may be markedly elevated, particularly in acute MR. In mild and moderate MR the carotid pulsation is normal. Pulsus alternans (Fig. 33–14), a finding associated with severe left ventricular failure, suggests severe MR. As ventricular function worsens and the left ventricle dilates, the point of maximum intensity moves inferolaterally. Initially, however, precordial motion may be normal.

The classic auscultatory finding in MR is a holosystolic murmur heard best at the apex. The murmur begins with S_1, lasts throughout systole, and ends with the second heart sound (refer to Fig. 33–14). The murmur of MR generally radiates to the axilla and to the back. A systolic murmur that radiates to the back is almost certainly caused by MR.

MR due to prolapse of the mitral valve produces a characteristic murmur that is preceded by one or more midsystolic clicks.

Unlike aortic stenosis in which the characteristics of the murmur help distinguish a moderate from severe lesion, it is the events of diastole that confirm the severity of MR. In mild MR diastolic flow across the mitral valve is not heard. As the disease progresses, the diastolic flow across the mitral valve increases. In severe MR the anterograde flow of blood across the mitral valve causes either an S_3 or a diastolic rumble. Although not always present, these diastolic sounds indicate severe MR.

Laboratory and Diagnostic Testing

Electrocardiographic clues to MR include left atrial enlargement and atrial arrhythmias such as atrial flutter and fibrillation (Fig. 33–15). Chest x-ray may reveal left ventricular dilation, left atrial enlargement, and evidence of congestive heart failure.

Echocardiogram. The echocardiogram is among the most useful diagnostic tools in MR. M-mode echo is used to measure the end-systolic dimension. An end-systolic dimension greater than 45 is indication for surgery (Carabello, 1996). Two-dimensional echocardiography is used to assess wall motion and evaluate the structure of the mitral valve apparatus. Patients with MR and severely reduced left ventricular systolic function are not generally candidates for mitral valve replacement surgery. For those patients who go on to surgery, the two-dimensional echo can reveal which leaflet is involved and can identify ruptured chordae.

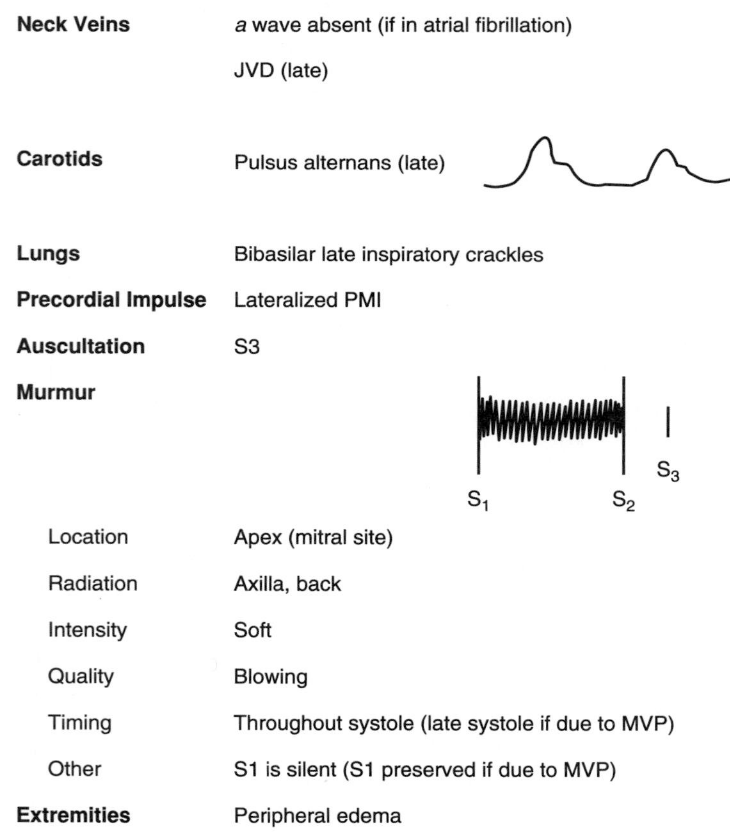

Figure 33–14. Summary of physical findings in mitral regurgitation.

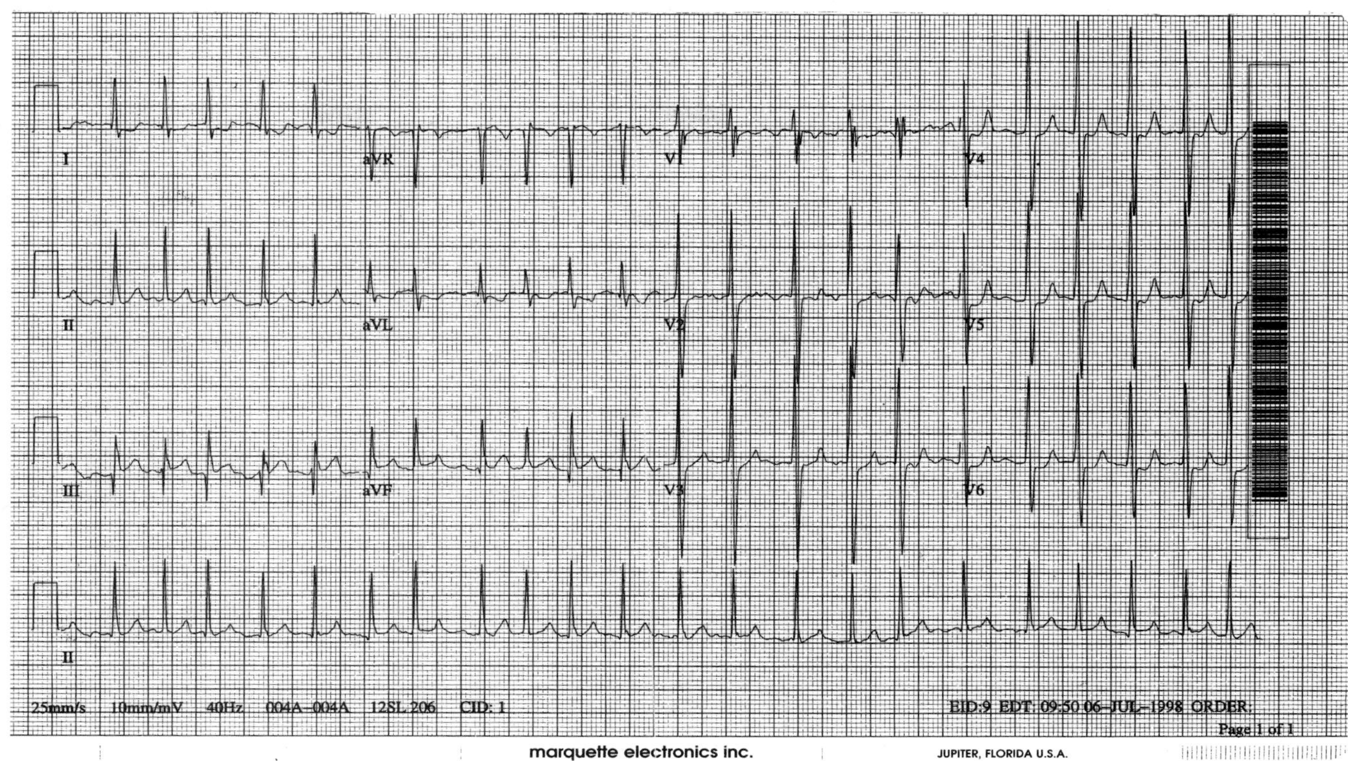

Figure 33–15. Electrocardiogram of patient with severe mitral regurgitation, showing atrial fibrillation and right-sided conduction abnormality.

Color-flow Doppler imaging is used to evaluate the regurgitant jet produced by the incompetent valve. The density of the continuous-wave Doppler signal also helps define the severity of the regurgitant lesion—the denser the spectral display, the more severe the regurgitation.

Transesophageal echocardiography (TEE) is another useful tool. The pictures of the valve that are obtained from TEE have much better resolution than the transthoracic pictures. The valve leaflets, therefore, can be better visualized on TEE (refer to Fig. 33–8). Frequently, mechanical abnormalities such as flail leaflet that are missed on transthoracic echo are visualized on TEE. Also, the severity of MR can be better assessed on TEE. A doppler recording is made with the cursor in the pulmonary vein. If retrograde (from atrium to lung) flow is observed during ventricular systole, severe MR is present.

Cardiac Catheterization. In MR, important cardiac catheterization data include pulmonary arterial, left atrial (pulmonary capillary wedge), and left ventricular pressures and waveforms; cardiac output; and, left ventriculogram. It is often helpful to combine the cath data with the results of transthoracic and transesophageal echocardiograms.

Pulmonary artery pressures and cardiac output are preserved in mild to moderate MR. As the disease progresses, backward flow from the left ventricle causes elevation of the left atrial and pulmonary pressures. Large *v* waves that represent ventricular systole may be visible on the left atrial tracing (Fig. 33–16).

Left ventriculography is useful in quantifying the severity of MR. With the camera in the right anterior oblique position, radiopaque contrast dye is injected into the left ventricle. Blushing of the left atrium indicates MR. Regurgitant flow, then, is graded on a scale of 1 to 4—1+ MR is mild, 4+ is severe. Also, during ventriculography prolapse of the mitral valve leaflets can be observed.

Management

Medical Therapy. Medical therapy of chronic MR is directed at afterload and preload reduction. Afterload reduction allows more blood to flow forward into the aorta than would otherwise occur due to the low-resistance of the left atrium. Vasodilators such as nifedipine and ACE-inhibitors are used at doses as high as the patient tolerates. In hospitalized patients it is advisable to begin therapy with a short-acting agent, then switch to a long-acting agent, particularly if there is concomitant heart failure. It is not an unusual goal for the systolic blood pressure to be less than 100 mm Hg, as long as the patient does not have dizziness, lightheadedness, or syncope.

The Frank–Starling curve shows that fluid volume overload (high preload) worsens cardiac output (Fig. 33–17).

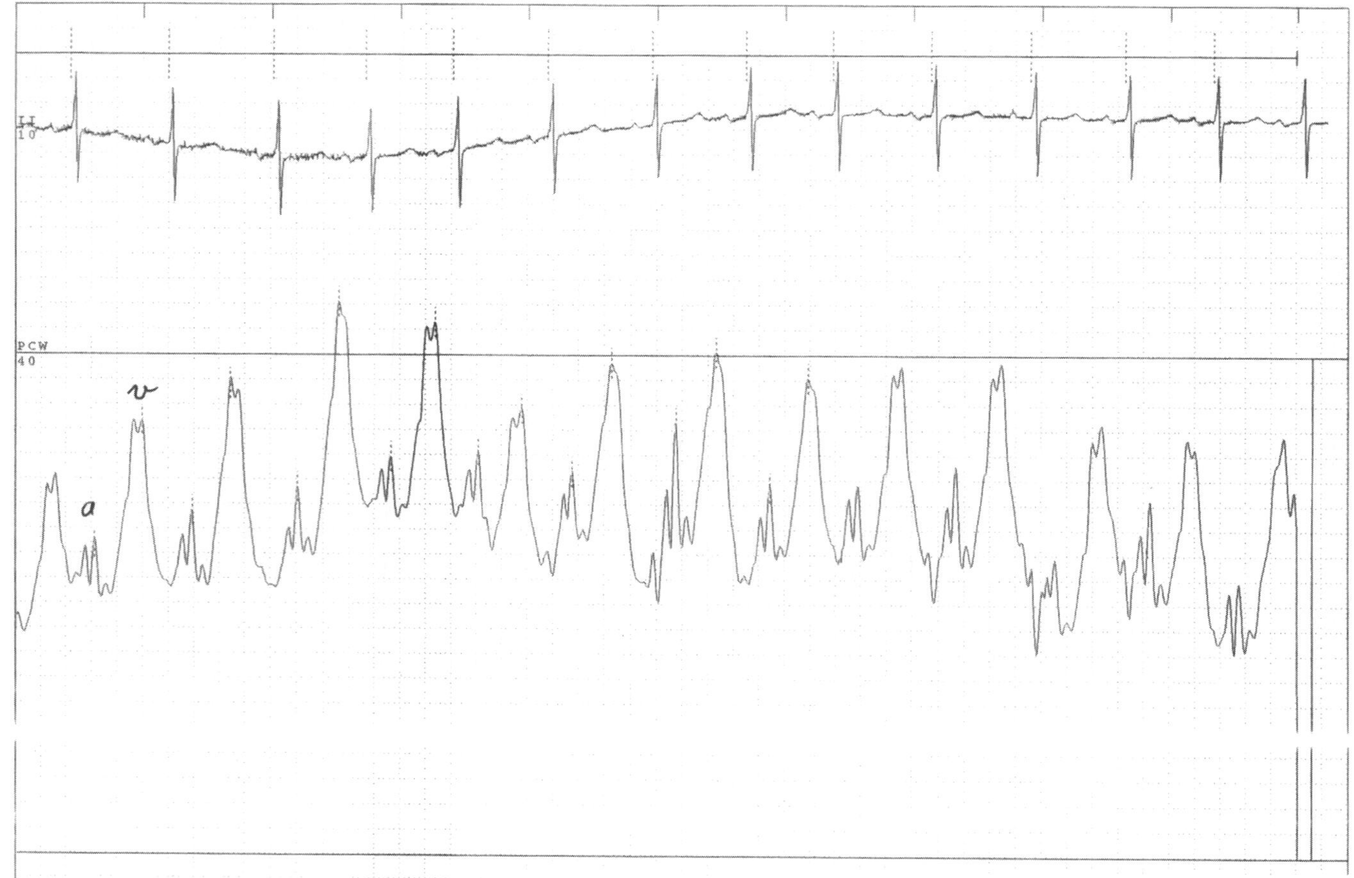

Figure 33–16. Pulmonary capillary wedge tracing in mitral regurgitation, showing large *v* waves.

Diuretics are used to combat the effects of excessive preload and prevent exacerbations of heart failure. Nitrates, too, provide some preload reduction benefit.

Frequently, due to left atrial enlargement, atrial fibrillation complicates MR. In this case, digoxin may be of particular benefit, for both rate control and inotropic support. Other AV nodal drugs, such as beta blockers, diltiazem, and verapamil, also have negative inotropic effects and may exacerbate heart failure. Although they are not absolutely contraindicated, they must be used with caution. Table 33–3 lists drugs that are used to treat MR.

Acute MR may present as flash pulmonary edema. Emergent afterload reduction with sodium nitroprusside and diuresis are necessary to save the patient's life. Intubation may be required to oxygenate the patient. Surgery is necessary to correct the underlying pathology.

Surgical Treatment. Traditionally, mitral valve surgery was delayed until left ventricular systolic function began to fail. This approach is advocated by many experts (Carabello, 1996). Neverthelss, due to improved operative techniques and the favorability of valve repair over replacement, the indications for mitral valve surgery are changing. Some surgeons now favor early valve surgery in hopes of returning the patient to normal sinus rhythm (Obadia et al., 1997).

Following the decision to operate, it must be determined what procedure will be performed. Mitral valve repair? Mitral valve replacement with a bioprosthesis? Or, mitral valve replacement with a mechanical valve? Recently, it has been noted that, for patients with MR due to MVP, outcomes are more favorable if the mitral valve is repaired, not replaced. Patients who undergo mitral valve repair are spared the necessity of lifelong anticoagulation. Additionally, there is no functional gradient such as would be induced by a mechanical valve. Most important, survival and the need for reoperation are improved by mitral repair surgery (Akins, Hilgenberg, Buckley, Vlahakes, Torchiana, Daggett, & Austen, 1994). Early intervention may improve the likelihood of successful mitral valve repair.

The decision whether to repair or replace the valve is often made in the operating room. Frequently, the patient and surgeon plan mitral valve repair with the understanding that valve replacement may be required. The patient should, with recommendation from the provider, choose whether he or she wants a bioprosthesis or mechanical valve, though it is ultimately the surgeon's choice which specific valve will be used.

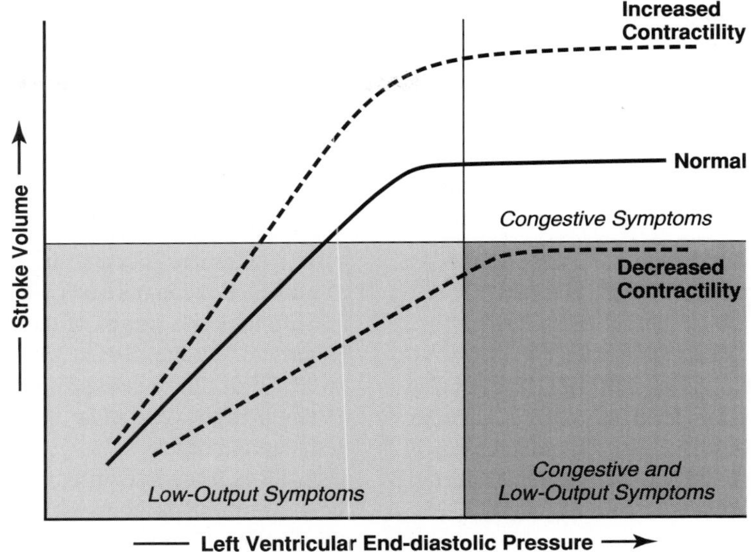

Figure 33–17. The Frank–Starling mechanism. *(From Chulay, Guzetta, & Dossey. [1997]. [p. 259].)*

Because mechanical mitral valves are particularly prone to thromboembolism, adequate anticoagulation is essential. Therefore, patients in whom long-term anticoagulation is risky (e.g., elderly patients or those who are prone to falls) should generally receive bioprosthetic valves. The tradeoff, however, is shorter longevity. And, even with bioprostheses most surgeons anticoagulate the patient for up to 3 months immediately following mitral valve replacement.

Follow-Up

Close follow-up of the medically managed patient with MR is necessary to determine when surgery is indicated. Echocardiograms are recommended every 6 to 12 months for asymptomatic patients. When symptoms or atrial fibrillation occur, or the end-systolic dimension reaches 45 mm, cath and subsequent surgery are recommended (Carabello, 1996). Braunwald (1994) recommends surgery for patients with NYHA class II heart failure.

Because stress-induced wall motion abnormalities may be the earliest signs of diminishing ventricular function, some clinicians advocate serial stress echocardiography. Stress echocardiography is ideal for gauging the degree of LV dysfunction that occurs at peak exercise.

Following surgery, particularly mitral valve repair, a baseline echocardiogram should be obtained. Subsequent studies should be done as the patient's condition warrants.

TABLE 33–3. Drugs Used in the Treatment of Chronic Mitral Regurgitation

	Usual Dosage	Comments
Calcium Channel Blockers		
Nifedipine (Adalat CC, Procardia XL)	30–90 mg daily	No AV node effects
ACE Inhibitors		
Captopril (Capoten)	6.25–100 mg TID	Short-acting
Enalapril (Vasotec)	2.5–10 mg TID	Relatively short-acting; also available in IV form
Fosinopril (Monopril)	10–40 mg daily	Long-acting
Lisinopril (Prinivil, Zestril)	5–20 mg daily	Long-acting
Quinapril (Accupril)	5–40 mg BID	BID dosing most effective
Diuretics		
Furosemide (Lasix)	20–80 mg PO daily or BID	Inexpensive
Torosemide (Demadex)	5–40 mg PO daily	Sustained diuresis over most of day
Bumetanide (Bumex)	0.5–2 mg daily	40 times more potent than furosemide
Cardiac Glycosides		
Digoxin (Lanoxin)	0.125–0.25 mg daily	AV node-blocking effects, inotropic support

Lifelong endocarditis prophylaxis is essential, particularly after mitral valve replacement.

Tricuspid Regurgitation

Nearly everyone has some degree of tricuspid regurgitation (TR) on echocardiogram. This trace amount of TR is "functional." That is, the regurgitation causes no hemodynamic sequelae. Clinically significant TR, however, is rare. When present, TR is almost always associated with either endocarditis or pulmonary hypertension.

Pathophysiology

Tricuspid regurgitation (TR) can occur due to primary valvular problems, such as endocarditis, or extra-valvular problems. Endocarditis is likely the most common cause of primary valvular TR in this country. Interestingly, tricuspid endocarditis is associated almost exclusively with intravenous drug abuse. Additionally, tricuspid valve disease may be due to myxomatous degeneration of the valve apparatus or to previous rheumatic fever.

Among the most common causes of tricuspid regurgitation are extravalvular conditions such as pulmonary hypertension and right ventricular dilatation.

The most harm that can come of severe TR is right-sided fluid overload, a non–life-threatening condition. In fact, one can live without a tricuspid valve. Thankfully, though, TR by itself is rarely severe enough to cause right-sided heart failure. When heart failure does occur, it is usually easily treated with diuretics. These features make medical therapy the best treatment option for TR. Unless there is a compelling reason to do so, tricuspid replacement surgery is generally not performed.

Patients with pulmonary hypertension, by definition, have TR. Other patients likely to have TR are those with histories of endocarditis (particularly intravenous drug abusers).

History and Physical Findings

The symptoms of severe tricuspid regurgitation are those of right-sided heart failure—peripheral edema, nausea and vomiting, diarrhea, abdominal distention and cramping, and ascites.

Patients with moderate or severe TR have discernable physical findings. Normally, veins of the upper extremities are visible only when the limb is dependent, or below the level of the heart. In TR the veins of the upper extremities may be visibly engorged when the limb is positioned above the level of the heart.

Edema, too, suggests TR, particularly late in the course of the disease when right ventricular failure may occur.

Like venous engorgement of the upper extremities, jugular venous distention is present in TR. During each cardiac cycle in sinus rhythm, there are two impulses: the *a* wave, representing atrial contraction, and the *v* wave, representing ventricular contraction. Ordinarily, the larger *a* wave is followed by a smaller *v* wave during each cardiac cycle. The hallmark of TR is the presence of large *v* waves in the jugular venous pulsations. The large *v* waves are the result of ejection of regurgitant blood through an incompetent tricuspid valve. Therefore, if the *a* wave is larger than the *v* wave, there is no significant TR.

The carotid pulsations are generally unaffected by TR. It is only in the very late stages of the disease—when right ventricular failure has caused left ventricular failure—that pulsus alternans occurs. It is unlikely that the clinician would ever encounter such a finding.

In the early stages of the disease the precordial motion is normal. As the disease progresses, however, the volume overload of the right ventricle produces right ventricular dilatation. Right ventricular dilatation is palpable at the lower left sternal border.

TR is frequently difficult to hear. When heard the diagnostic murmur is holosystolic and varies in intensity with respiration. Figure 33–18 provides the diagnostic findings of TR.

Laboratory and Diagnostic Testing

Right atrial enlargement may be the only obvious electrocardiographic and radiologic finding of TR. Right ventricular enlargement due to pulmonary hypertension is also possible.

Echocardiogram. Like the use of echo to quantify MR, continuous-wave (CW) Doppler and color Doppler are used to quantify TR. A dense CW tracing suggests severe TR. Color Doppler is used to identify the length and width of the regurgitant jet, which are directly related to the severity of the regurgitation.

Cardiac Catheterization. Although TR is generally diagnosed by history, physical findings, and echocardiography, cardiac catheterization is helpful in evaluating the severity of TR. The right heart catheterization reveals the atrial, ventricular, and pulmonary arterial pressures and waveforms. In addition to elevated right atrial pressure, large *v* waves are present on the right atrial tracing in TR. The right ventricular and pulmonary artery pressures remain normal. Rarely, right ventriculography is employed to visualize the regurgitant jet.

Management

Medical Therapy. Frequently, TR can be managed without surgery. Medical therapy is aimed at alleviating the signs and symptoms of right heart failure, primarily peripheral edema. Because the main pathology of TR involves right-sided volume overload, the treatment is diuresis.

Surgical Treatment. Surgery is indicated when symptomatic right heart failure persists despite maximal medical therapy. Or, in the case of tricuspid endocarditis, surgery is indicated for persistent fever or persistent pulmonary emboli. Many surgeons are hesitant to operate for tricuspid endocarditis because there is little difference in outcome between medical and surgical management (Hecht & Berger, 1992).

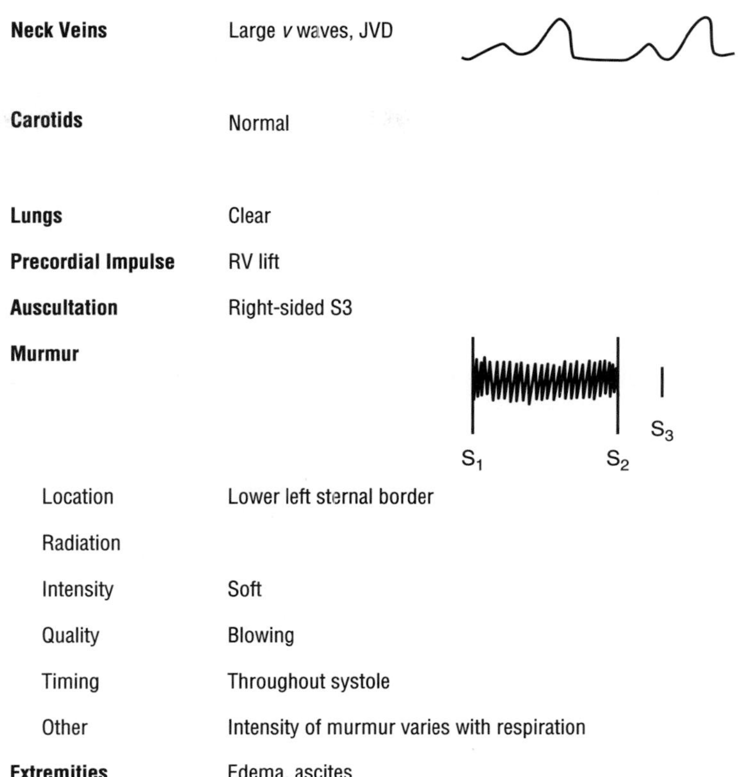

Figure 33–18. Summary of physical findings in tricuspid regurgitation.

STENOTIC VALVULAR LESIONS—PRESSURE OVERLOAD

Stenotic lesions such as aortic stenosis are pressure overload problems. As the ventricular orifice narrows, a greater relative pressure is required to overcome the obstruction and eject blood into the aorta. Just as muscle mass increases when one lifts weights regularly, so too does the myocardium hypertrophy when required to contract against chronically high pressures.

Aortic Stenosis

Pathophysiology

The etiologies of AS are many. Typically, AS that occurs in patients under age 50 is due to a congenital bicuspid valve, whereas AS in the elderly is typically the result of valvular calcification. Other causes of AS are listed in Table 33–4.

Normally, the aortic valve opens freely during left ventricular contraction. Stenosis of the aortic leaflets due to calcification, however, restricts their ability to open. A higher intraventricular pressure is, therefore, required to open the valve. The heart compensates for this pressure overload by increasing the left ventricular mass (hypertrophy). This compensatory mechanism allows the heart to adequately meet the metabolic demands of the body.

Although left ventricular hypertrophy (LVH) is initially compensatory, it has detrimental effects later in the course of the disease. The degree of hypertrophy is directly related to the compliance of the ventricle. That is, the thicker the myocardium, the less elastic it is. This so-called diastolic noncompliance compromises left atrial emptying. Consequently, left atrial pressure is elevated in LVH. Eventually, contractile dysfunction occurs and the ventricle fails.

Congestive heart failure generally occurs late in the course of AS and is frequently multifactorial. When heart failure occurs, it is an ominous sign. Diastolic failure can occur secondary to ventricular hypertrophy. Diastolic failure results from diminished diastolic filling.

History and Physical Findings

The classic triad of symptoms associated with severe aortic stenosis is angina, dyspnea on exertion, and syncope. Angina is generally the result of increased myocardial oxygen demand due to myocardial hypertrophy. Dyspnea and syncope are the result of heart failure and fixed cardiac out-

TABLE 33–4. Causes of Aortic Stenosis
Congenital bicuspid aortic (or unicuspid) valve
Myxomatous degeneration
Rheumatic fever
Valvular calcification

put, respectively. The presence of any of these symptoms ought to prompt the clinician to consider AS.

Because AS is a pressure overload problem, jugular venous distention is not typically present in mild or moderate AS. But, jugular venous distention is a late finding of severe AS and suggests congestive heart failure.

Evaluation of the carotid impulse is critical. As the valve orifice narrows over time, the ejection of blood during systole is further impeded. The aortic pressure peaks later and the amplitude is less (Fig. 33–19). This effect is palpable as a "sluggish" carotid upstroke and is termed pulsus tardus. Pulsus tardus may not be detectable in mild AS, but is diagnostic of moderate or severe aortic stenosis.

There are specific diagnostic precordial pulsations that suggest AS. First, left ventricular hypertrophy (LVH) occurs to help the heart overcome the outflow gradient; the larger myocardial mass contributes a more forceful contraction. Instead of the normal dime-sized impulse that strikes the chest wall sharply, the impulse of a hypertrophied ventricle is diffuse and sustained. Another palpable feature of LVH is a presystolic impulse. This presystolic impulse occurs just before the systolic impulse and is, in fact, a palpable S_4. It is only felt in sinus rhythm and occurs when the atria contract and fill the noncompliant ventricle.

The AS murmur is a diamond-shaped, or crescendo–decrescendo, murmur that occurs during systole (refer to Fig. 33–19). The murmur is harsh and generally heard best over the aortic site. The first heart sound is always heard clearly because the murmur does not begin until the ejection sound, which is well after the first heart sound. In mild and moderate AS the murmur peaks relatively early and the second heart sound is well-preserved. As AS worsens, however, it takes longer for the ventricle to overcome the outflow obstruction. The hallmark of severe AS is a late peaking murmur that "overtakes" the second heart sound and makes the pulmonic component better heard than the aortic component.

Over time the increased afterload precipitates left ventricular hypertrophy. The diminished compliance of the hypertrophied ventricle causes an S_4. Figure 33–19 summarizes the physical findings in AS.

Laboratory and Diagnostic Tests

As previously detailed, the presence of an elevated afterload over long periods stimulates myocardial hypertrophy,

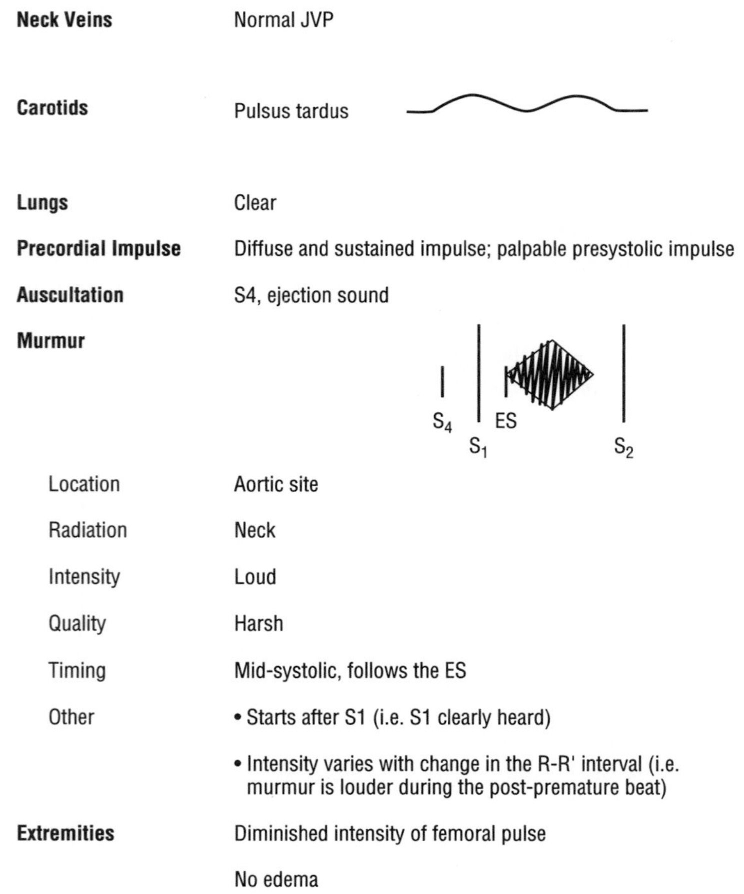

Figure 33–19. Summary of physical findings in aortic stenosis.

the effects of which are often seen on the electrocardiogram. The most specific electrocardiographic manifestation of LVH is an R wave in aVL that measures 1.1 mV. In the absence of this clue, however, a point system may be applied to diagnose LVH. Using the Romhilt–Estes criteria (Table 33–5), a score of 5 points is diagnostic of LVH; a score of 4 points may or may not represent LVH. In addition to LVH, left atrial enlargement may also be noted on the cardiogram. Left atrial enlargement occurs due to diastolic noncompliance.

The chest x-ray is normal in mild to moderate AS. Poststenotic dilatation of the aorta, left atrial enlargement, and evidence of congestive heart failure can be seen in severe AS.

Echocardiography. It is said that echo overestimates the severity of AS. This is due to the difference in measurement techniques between catheterization and echo. Echo measures the maximum instantaneous gradient, while the peak-to-peak gradient is measured in the catheterization laboratory. The instantaneous gradient is higher than the peak-to-peak gradient (Fig. 33–20) (Feigenbaum, 1994). So, comparing the gradient obtained by echo with the gradient obtained at cath amounts to comparing apples with oranges. The valve area, however, is more easily compared.

Blood ejected from a narrowed aortic valve moves faster than that ejected through a nonstenotic valve. The peak aortic velocity, therefore, is an adequate estimate of severity of AS. When applied to the Bernoulli equation,

$$\Delta P = 4v^2$$

the peak aortic velocity allows calculation of the instantaneous gradient. For instance, a peak aortic velocity of 4.0 m/sec yields an instantaneous gradient of 64 mm Hg. Generally, a peak aortic velocity greater than or equal to 4.0 m/sec, or an instantaneous gradient greater than 75 mm Hg, indicates severe AS (Reynolds, 1993).

TABLE 33–5. Romhilt-Estes Scoring System for LVH

1. R or S in any limb lead ≥ 0.20 mV *or* S in lead V1 or V2 *or* R in lead V5 or V6 ≥ 0.30 mV	3 points[a]
2. Left ventricular strain ST segment and T wave in opposite direction to QRS complex	
without digitalis	3 points
with digitalis	1 point
3. Left atrial enlargement Terminal negativity of the P wave in lead V1 is ≥ 0.10 mV in depth and ≥ 0.04 sec in duration	3 points
4. Left axis deviation of ≥ –30°	2 points
5. QRS duration ≥ 0.09 sec	1 point
6. Intrinsicoid deflection in lead V5 or V6 ≥ 0.05 sec	1 point
Total	13 points

[a] LVH, 5 points; probable LVH, 4 points.

Modified from D. W. Romhilt, K. E. Bove, R. J. Norris, E. Conyers, S. Conradi, D. T. Rowlands, & R. C. Scott. (1969). p. 185.

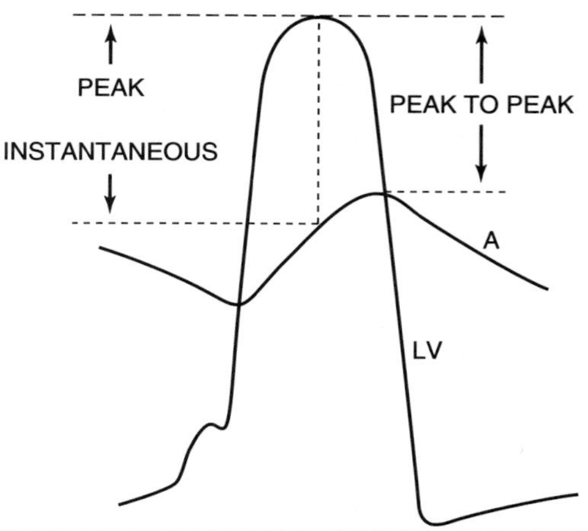

Figure 33–20. Comparison of peak-to-peak and instantaneous gradients in aortic stenosis. *(From H. Feigenbaum. [1994]. [p. 281].)*

Aortic valve area is calculated by applying the continuity equation,

$$\text{Aortic valve area} = \frac{CSA_{(LVOT)} \times V_{max(LVOT)}}{V_{max(AOV)}}$$

where $CSA_{(LVOT)}$ is the cross-sectional area of the left ventricular outflow tract (LVOT) and V_{max} are the peak velocities at the LVOT and aortic valve (these measurements are made in the 2D echo). The aortic valve area is normally 3–5 cm^2. Valve area less than 0.75 is diagnostic of severe AS (Reynolds, 1993).

Cardiac Catheterization. Cardiac catheterization reveals important data about the severity of aortic stenosis. One of the most important measurements is the transaortic (peak-to-peak) gradient. Once the aortic valve is crossed with a wire—which is often very challenging in severe AS—a catheter is inserted into the ventricle and the left ventricular pressure waveform is recorded. Then, using simultaneous left ventricular and aortic recordings, the aortic and ventricular pressure waveforms are compared and the gradient is calculated (refer to Fig. 33–10). A peak-to-peak gradient of 50 mm Hg is considered severe aortic stenosis.

Using the thermodilution cardiac output and the transaortic gradient, the aortic valve area is then calculated using the Gorlin equation. Recall, however, that, in part, the velocity of the jet determines the valve area. In the presence of substantial left ventricular systolic dysfunction, the ventricle cannot generate a high pressure to eject blood from the ventricle. The result is a low cardiac output and low peak-to-peak gradient. This is Gorlin's conundrum; that, in association with severe LV dysfunction, the peak-to-peak gradient does not accurately estimate the valve area. When left ventricular systolic function is reduced, the continuity equation (used in echocardiogram) may yield a more reliable estimate of aortic valve area (Feigenbaum, 1994).

Management

Medical Therapy. Medical management of AS is directed at minimizing the transaortic gradient and maximizing cardiac output. Digoxin, ACE inhibitors, and antihypertensives (such as beta blockers) all adversely affect the gradient and should generally not be used in AS. Rather, maximizing the preload to exploit the Frank–Starling curve is beneficial. In severe AS, however, diuretics and/or digoxin may be necessary to avert heart failure. Extreme caution must be exercised when prescribing diuretics.

The mainstays of medical therapy, then, are cautious use of diuretics and avoidance of antihypertensives. Patients with AS should be diuresed only if they display symptoms of heart failure. Otherwise, medications are generally not indicated.

Because the ventricle is dependent upon the atrial kick (10–20% of total cardiac output) in AS, atrial fibrillation, although rare, is a particularly problematic arrhythmia. Loss of atrial kick causes decreased LV filling—a condition that already exists due to LVH—and may result in acute heart failure. Braunwald (1994) advocates prophylactic antiarrhythmic therapy if there is suspicion that the patient will develop atrial fibrillation.

Surgical Treatment. Because catheter-based procedures such as balloon valvuloplasty have limited benefit in calcified aortic valves, and because stenoses are not amenable to surgical repair, valve replacement surgery is required for definitive treatment of AS. Mechanical valves, bioprostheses, stentless bioprostheses, and aortic homografts are all used in aortic valve replacement surgery. As with any valve replacement surgery, the decision of which valve to use is largely based on the patient's projected lifespan and his or her candidacy for lifelong anticoagulation.

Follow-Up

Serial echocardiograms are helpful in evaluating progression of AS and timing surgery. Carabello (1996) recommends annual office visits for asymptomatic patients with Doppler gradients less than 50 mm Hg and semiannual office visits if the Doppler gradient is greater than 50 mm Hg. The echo should be repeated when symptoms develop.

Following AVR, a baseline echocardiogram should be obtained. Sometimes the anatomy limits the surgeon to a smaller valve orifice than would otherwise be used. In this case, it is important to know the degree of residual AS that exists.

Endocarditis is required for all patients with AS. Because prosthetic valve endocarditis carries a poor prognosis, lifelong prophylaxis is necessary for patients who have undergone AVR.

Mitral Stenosis

Pathophysiology

In the United States mitral stenosis (MS) is exclusively the result of rheumatic fever. In developing nations, however, MS may be caused by other infectious or parasitic agents.

History and Physical Findings

As with most valvular abnormalities, patients with MS may remain asymptomatic for long periods. The symptoms of MS are due to elevated left atrial pressures and include dyspnea, orthopnea, and paroxysmal nocturnal dyspnea. Additionally, fatigue may be a common feature of MS.

In mild to moderate MS the physical findings may be scant. As the disease progresses, more findings appear. Jugular venous distension, for instance, is generally not present until late in the course of the disease. Due to pulmonary hypertension, and the resultant tricuspid regurgitation, large *v* waves may be visible. The carotid upstroke may be blunted due to reduced stroke volume. In severe heart failure, pulsus alternans may be palpable.

The classic auscultatory findings of MS are an early diastolic opening snap (OS) and characteristic diastolic crescendo murmur (Fig. 33–21), both of which are best heard in the left lateral recumbent position.

Laboratory and Diagnostic Testing

Left atrial enlargement is a frequent finding on the EKG and chest x-ray. Atrial arrhythmias such as atrial fibrillation and atrial flutter may be present and are the result of atrial enlargement.

Echocardiogram. Echocardiography is useful for determining the cardiac chamber sizes, the transvalvular gradient, and the valve area. Particularly in severe MS, the left atrium is dramatically enlarged. Of special importance is excluding intraatrial thrombus or its predecessor, spontaneous echo contrast (SEC), also known as "smoke" (Fig. 33–22). The presence of SEC or intraatrial thrombus places the patient at risk of embolic stroke.

Mitral valve area is calculated using either the pressure half-time or the continuity equation. A pressure half-time less than or equal to 220 msec, or a calculated mitral valve area of less than 1.0 cm^2, indicates severe mitral stenosis.

Cardiac Catheterization. The measurement of a transmitral gradient and the calculation of the mitral valve area are essential components of the catheterization findings of MS. To measure the gradient, catheters are placed in the pulmonary artery wedge position and in the left ventricle. Simultaneous recordings are made of the two pressure waveforms. From these tracings the area between the curves is measured and recorded as the transmitral gradient. Calculation of the mitral valve area is then performed. From these two measurements, the clinician plans medical therapy or definitive intervention.

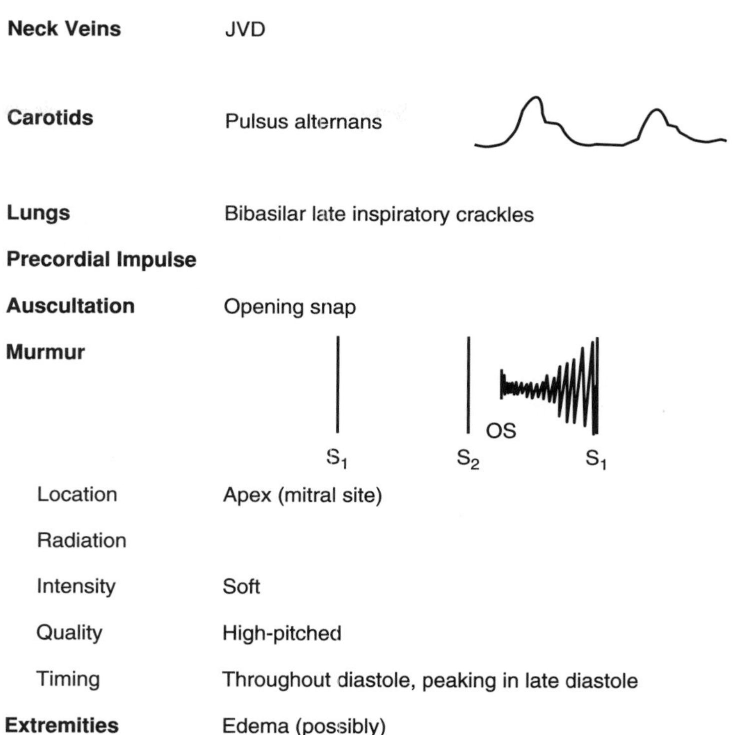

Figure 33–21. Summary of physical findings in mitral stenosis.

Management

Medical Therapy. The goal of medical therapy of MS is management of symptoms until intervention is deemed necessary. Because the mitral valve allows little blood to enter the left ventricle, preload reduction is very important in MS. Diuretics are useful in early stages of the disease, but are less effective in later stages.

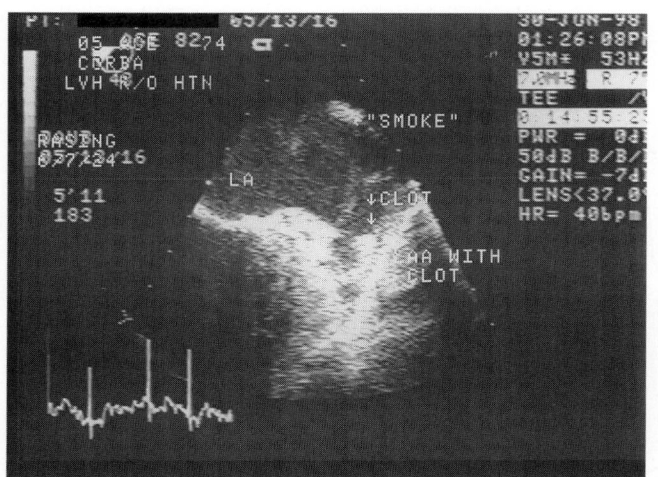

Figure 33–22. Spontaneous echo contrast and left atrial thrombus noted by transesophageal echocardiogram (TEE). TEE shows spontaneous echo contrast (e.g., "Smoke") in the left atrium (LA) and clot in the left atrial appendage (LAA).

Due to left atrial congestion, blood is prone to clot in the left atrium. This puts patients with MS at risk for embolic stroke. Serious consideration should be given to anticoagulation. If the echocardiogram reveals intraatrial clot or SEC, anticoagulation is essential to lessen the risk of neurological events.

Because the ventricle is highly dependent upon the atrial kick, atrial arrhythmias such as atrial fibrillation and flutter are poorly tolerated. These arrhythmias should be aggressively treated if they occur.

Surgical Treatment. In severe MS mechanical intervention is necessary—balloon valvuloplasty, surgical commissurotomy, or mitral valve replacement. Because mitral stenosis in the United States has exclusively a rheumatic etiology, it is common for other valve lesions to be present simultaneously. In this case, surgery may be the wisest decision.

When MS presents alone, however, or when the other valvular lesions do not require intervention, balloon mitral valvuloplasty is equally effective as surgical commissurotomy (Ben Farhat et al., 1998; Glazier & Turi, 1997).

Follow-Up

Patients with asymptomatic MS should have a baseline echocardiogram and be followed annually with detailed history and physicals (Carabello, 1996).

Following mechanical intervention a baseline echocardiogram is warranted. Repeat echos should be performed as symptoms demand.

▶ LESIONS THAT CAUSE SHUNTING

Two lesions that cause shunting are atrial septal defect (ASD) and ventricular septal defect (VSD). ASD and VSD are congenital cardiac defects that result from incomplete embryonic development of the atrial and ventricular septum, respectively.

Congenital cardiac defects can be caused by maternal medication use (amphetamines, thalidomide, progesterone, estrogen, and others) and alcohol use. Maternal illnesses such as rubella and diabetes may cause congenital heart disease. Inherited diseases such as Holt–Oram syndrome or Zellweger syndrome are often associated with congenital cardiac defects, including ASD and VSD.

ASD, VSD, and other congenital heart defects are often associated with chromosomal abnormalities such as Trisomy 13, Trisomy 18, and Trisomy 21. Noninherited syndromes may also have associated ASD or VSD: congenital diaphragmatic hernia, DiGeorge syndrome, and fetal alcohol syndrome (FAS).

Congenital malformations of certain organ systems are associated with an increased incidence of congenital heart defects, hydrocephalus, tracheo–esophageal fistula, esophageal atresia, and imperforate anus.

Atrial Septal Defects

Pathophysiology

Atrial septal defects (ASDs) are classified by their location in the atrial septum (Fig. 33–23). Sinus venosus defects are located high in the atrial septum, at the entry of the superior vena cava into the right atrium. They may be located less commonly at the entry of the inferior vena cava into the right atrium. Partial anomalous pulmonary venous return is often present. Ostium primum defects are located immediately adjacent to the atrioventricular (AV) valves, often with clefts or other deformities in the AV valves. Ostium secundum defects, the most common ASD, are located at the fossa ovalis, in the midportion of the septum.

ASDs allow shunting of blood from the left atrium to the right atrium, causing an increase in pulmonary blood flow. Small ASDs often have little or no hemodynamic effect in childhood or early adulthood. Late in the disease, however, severe hemodynamic effects such as pulmonary hypertension and heart failure may result. Additionally, the shunt reverses to right to left, putting patients at risk of stroke or other catastrophe due to systemic embolization.

History and Physical Findings

ASDs are asymptomatic in infancy and childhood. In adulthood, the most common symptoms suggesting ASD are fatigue and dyspnea—both, symptoms of left-sided failure. Additionally, atrial arrhythmias are common with ASD.

The classic physical finding in ASD is a fixed, widely split second heart sound. Ordinarily, A_2 and P_2 are split only during inspiration. This phenomenon is due to the variation in venous return that occurs during respiration. In ASD, however, the interatrial shunt precludes the normal venous return from being interrupted by the changes in intrathoracic pressure during respiration. The result is a prolonged A_2:P_2 interval that does not change with respiration.

The larger right-sided blood volumes may also cause a diastolic flow murmur across the tricuspid valve or a systolic flow murmur across the pulmonic valve. These murmurs are secondary phenomena, though, and are not, by themselves, diagnostic of ASD.

Laboratory and Diagnostic Tests

EKG often shows right bundle branch block, suggestive of right ventricular dilation, and left anterior hemiblock (Wagner, 1994). The echocardiogram allows direct visualization

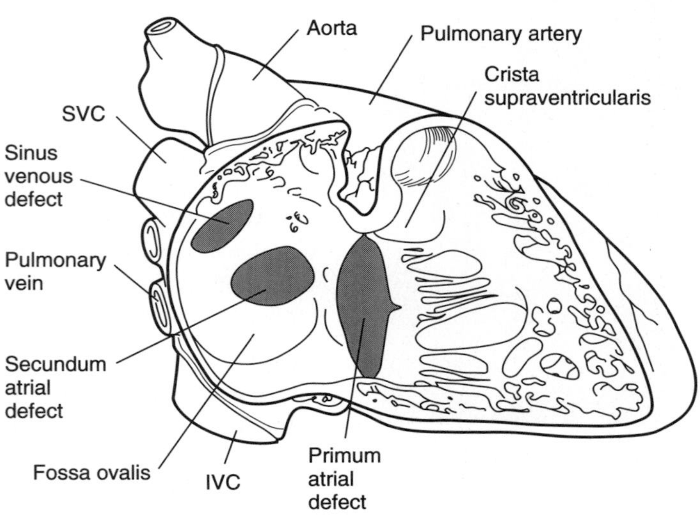

Figure 33–23. Anatomic classification of atrial septal defects.

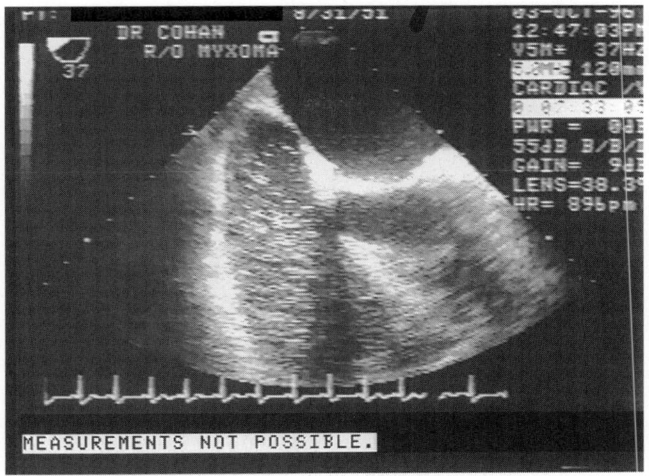

Figure 33–24. Bubble study to exclude atrial septal defect. The right atrium is opacified when agitated saline is injected intravenously. In this case, the absence of bubbles in the left atrium (*top*) excludes hemodynamically significant ASD.

of ASDs. Also, associated right ventricular enlargement, right atrial enlargement, and pulmonary artery dilation may be evident. Cardiac catheterization reveals step-up in RA saturations.

The diagnostic tool that best shows ASD is the echocardiogram. The bubble study is useful for finding ASD. Saline is agitated in a syringe, then injected intravenously. The continuous 2-D echo is recorded as the bubbles reach the right atrium (Fig. 33–24). In the presence of ASD, some bubbles pass into the right atrium. Transesophageal echocardiography is particularly useful for visualizing ASD (refer to Fig. 33–8).

Management

Medical management of ASD includes treatment for heart failure with ACE inhibitors, digoxin, and diuretics. As with most valvular diseases, medical therapy has limited effectiveness in patients with severe defects. In such cases, surgery is the only definitive treatment.

Transcatheter techniques of ASD repair are attractive alternatives to surgery for some patients, particularly those with significant comorbidity. According to Landzberg & Lock (1996), patients with ostium secundum defects less than 22 mm and small left-to-right shunts may benefit from transcatheter repair. Suture or patch closure of ASDs remains standard for nonsecundum lesions.

Ventricular Septal Defects

Pathophysiology

Ventricular septal defects (VSDs) represent the most common form of congenital heart disease. There are many different types of VSDs, classified by their location in the ventricular septum (Fig. 33–25). Outlet or infundibular defects are located in the outlet septum; inlet defects are located in the inlet septum; and central muscular, apical muscular, and marginal defects are located in the trabecular or muscular septum. Perimembranous defects involve the membranous septum, located immediately below the aortic valve, and variable amounts of tissue adjacent to the membranous septum.

In a small minority of patients with myocardial infarction (MI), VSD may occur. This serious complication of MI

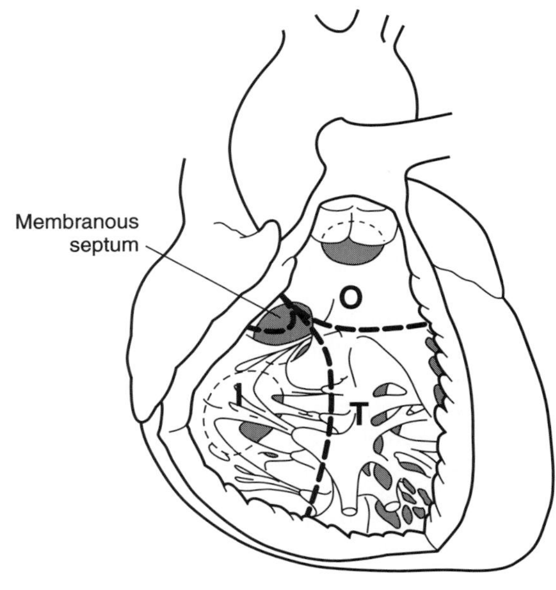

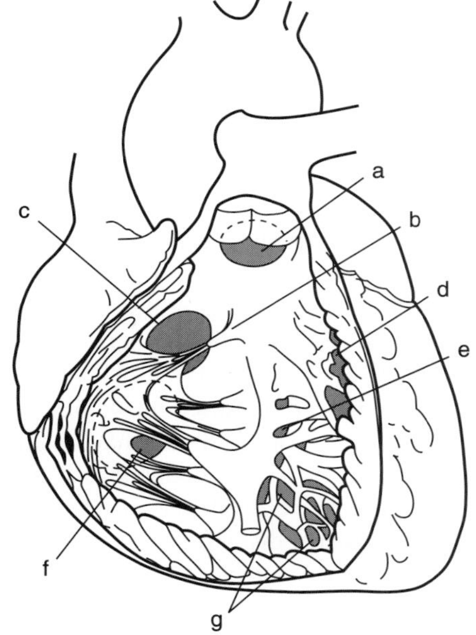

Figure 33–25. Anatomic classification of ventricular septal defect.

typically occurs within 72 hours of an anteroseptal or inferoseptal MI. When it occurs, the presentation is acute pulmonary edema.

History and Physical Findings

Because large VSDs are discovered and repaired in infancy and childhood, small VSDs are more likely to be newly diagnosed in adulthood. Patients with small VSDs are asymptomatic. In the rare cases where large VSDs have not been discovered until adulthood, the patient may have symptoms of right heart failure. If the patient has developed a right-to-left shunt, they may report dyspnea, chest pain, syncope, or hemoptysis.

VSDs cause harsh holosystolic murmurs that are heard along the left sternal border. These murmurs are typically very loud and accompanied by a thrill. Other physical findings in VSDs may include jugular venous distension and evidence of right heart failure such as peripheral edema or ascites.

Laboratory and Diagnostic Tests

In patients with small VSDs, the EKG is normal. In a moderate VSD, the EKG shows LVH. In a large VSD, the EKG reveals biventricular hypertrophy. If the VSD is due to myocardial infarction, left or right bundle branch block or hemiblock may be seen. The chest x-ray shows variable degrees of left atrial enlargement and LVH, depending on the amount of left-to-right shunting. The 2-D echo and color-flow Doppler (Fig. 33–26) identify the location and size of the VSD. Pulse-wave Doppler is used to estimate the flow across the defect. Cardiac catheterization reveals step-up in RV saturations.

Management

Heart failure is treated with digoxin and diuretics, though this is only palliative. Definitive therapy is suture or patch repair. Surgery is usually reserved for patients who have not developed right-to-left shunting.

▶ ENDOCARDITIS PROPHYLAXIS

The incidence of endocarditis in the healthy, nonintravenous drug-abusing adult population is low. Although the presence of structural heart disease increases the risk of endocarditis, the overall risk for patients with structural heart disease is also relatively low (Dajani et al., 1997). All patients with structural heart disease, including congenital anomalies and valvular lesions, should have endocarditis prophylaxis for any high-risk or moderate-risk procedure. Additionally, because the survival rate of prosthetic valve endocarditis is particularly dismal, all patients with prosthetic heart valves—mechanical, tissue, and homograft valves—must be well-informed of the importance of antibiotic prophylaxis.

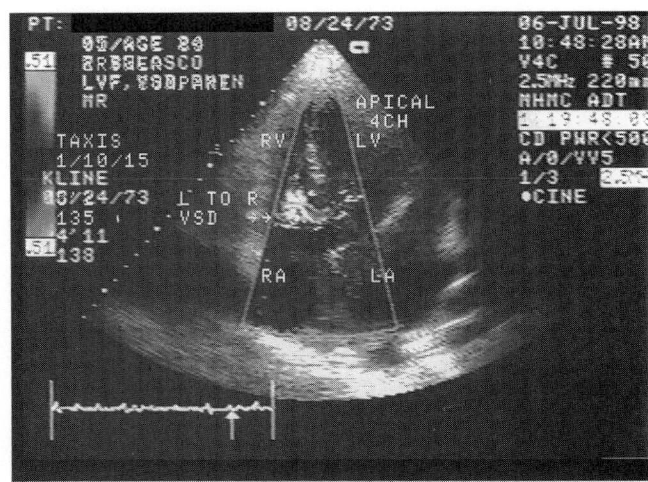

Figure 33–26. Apical four-chamber color Doppler view showing ventricular septal defect. (See Color Plate 2.)

Current recommendations are that patients with mitral valve prolapse do not need antibiotic prophylaxis unless they also have mitral regurgitation or another structural heart problem. Patients with innocent murmurs, pacemakers, or cardioverter–defibrillators do not require routine an-

TABLE 33–6. Cardiac Conditions Associated with Endocarditis

Endocarditis Prophylaxis Recommended
High-Risk Category
Prosthetic cardiac valves, including bioprosthetic and homograft valves
Previous bacterial endocarditis
Complex cyanotic congenital heart disease (e.g., single ventricle states, transposition of the great arteries, tetralogy of Fallot)
Surgically constructed systemic pulmonary shunts or conduits
Moderate-Risk Category
Most other congenital cardiac malformations (other than above and below)
Acquired valvular dysfunction (e.g., rheumatic heart disease)
Hypertrophic cardiomyopathy
Mitral valve prolapse with valvular regurgitation and/or thickened leaflets
Endocarditis Prophylaxis Not Recommended
Negligible-Risk Category (no greater risk than the general population)
Isolated secundum atrial septal defect
Surgical repair of atrial septal defect, ventricular septal defect, or patent ductus arteriosus (without residua beyond 6 mo)
Previous coronary artery bypass graft surgery
Mitral valve prolapse without valvar regurgitation
Physiologic, functional, or innocent heart murmurs
Previous Kawasaki disease without valvar dysfunction
Previous rheumatic fever without valvar dysfunction
Cardiac pacemakers (intravascular and epicardial) and implanted defibrillators

Reprinted from Dajani, Taubert, Wilson, Bolger, Bayer, Ferrieri, et al. (1997).

TABLE 33–7. Dental Procedures and Endocarditis Prophylaxis

Endocarditis Prophylaxis Recommended[a]
- Dental extractions
- Periodontal procedures including surgery, scaling and root planing, probing, and recall maintenance
- Dental implant placement and reimplantation of avulsed teeth
- Endodontic (root canal) instrumentation or surgery only beyond the apex
- Subgingival placement of antibiotic fibers or strips
- Initial placement of orthodontic bands but not brackets
- Intraligamentary local anesthetic injections
- Prophylactic cleaning of teeth or implants where bleeding is anticipated

Endocarditis Prophylaxis Not Recommended
- Restorative dentistry[b] (operative and prosthodontic) with or without retraction cord[c]
- Local anesthetic injections (nonintraligamentary)
- Intracanal endodontic treatment; postplacement and buildup
- Placement of rubber dams
- Postoperative suture removal
- Placement of removable prosthodontic or orthodontic appliances
- Taking of oral impressions
- Fluoride treatments
- Taking of oral radiographs
- Orthodontic appliance adjustment
- Shedding of primary teeth

[a] Prophylaxis is recommended for patients with high- and moderate-risk cardiac conditions.
[b] This includes restoration of decayed teeth (filling cavities) and replacement of missing teeth.
[c] Clinical judgment may indicate antibiotic use in selected circumstances that may create significant bleeding.
Reprinted from Dajani, Taubert, Wilson, Bolger, Bayer, Ferrieri, et al. (1997).

TABLE 33–8. Other Procedures and Endocarditis Prophylaxis

Endocarditis Prophylaxis Recommended
- Respiratory tract
  - Tonsillectomy and/or adenoidectomy
  - Surgical operations that involve respiratory mucosa
  - Bronchoscopy with a rigid bronchoscope
- Gastrointestinal tract[a]
  - Sclerotherapy for esophageal varices
  - Esophageal stricture dilation
  - Endoscopic retrograde cholangiography with biliary obstruction
  - Biliary tract surgery
  - Surgical operations that involve intestinal mucosa
- Genitourinary tract
  - Prostatic surgery
  - Cystoscopy
  - Urethral dilation

Endocarditis Prophylaxis Not Recommended
- Respiratory tract
  - Endotracheal intubation
  - Bronchoscopy with a flexible bronchoscope, with or without biopsy[b]
  - Tympanostomy tube insertion
- Gastrointestinal tract
  - Transesophageal echocardiography[b]
  - Endoscopy with or without gastrointestinal biopsy[b]
- Genitourinary tract
  - Vaginal hysterectomy[b]
  - Vaginal delivery[b]
  - Cesarean section
  - In uninfected tissue:
    - Urethral catheterization
    - Uterine dilatation and curettage
    - Therapeutic abortion
    - Sterilization procedures
    - Insertion or removal of intrauterine devices
- Other
  - Cardiac catheterization, including balloon angioplasty
  - Implanted cardiac pacemakers, implanted defibrillators, and coronary stents
  - Incision or biopsy of surgically scrubbed skin
  - Circumcision

[a] Prophylaxis is recommended for high-risk patients; it is optional for medium-risk patients.
[b] Prophylaxis is optional for high-risk patients.
Reprinted from Dajani, Taubert, Wilson, Bolger, Bayer, Ferrieri, et al. (1997).

tibiotic prophylaxis against endocarditis. Nor, do patients who have had coronary artery bypass grafting or intracoronary stents need prophylaxis (Table 33–6).

The American Heart Association periodically issues guidelines on the prevention of endocarditis. These recommendations are produced by a committee of experts who review the endocarditis literature and draw conclusions about the minimally effective preventive prophylaxis regimens. Tables 33–6 through 33–10 are reproduced from the American Heart Association guidelines.

Patients at high or moderate risk of endocarditis require antibiotic prophylaxis for certain dental, upper respiratory, gastrointestinal, and genitourinary procedures (Tables 33–7 and 33–8). These procedures are commonly associated with transient bacteremia that can cause endocarditis in patients with structural heart disease.

The antibiotic regimens for endocarditis prophylaxis are shown in Tables 33–9 and 33–10.

TABLE 33–9. Prophylactic Regimens for Dental, Oral, Respiratory Tract, or Esophageal Procedures

Situation	Agent	Regimen
Standard general prophylaxis	Amoxicillin	*Adults:* 2.0 g; *children:* 50 mg/kg orally 1 h before procedure
Unable to take oral medications	Ampicillin	*Adults:* 2.0 g IM or IV; *children:* 50 mg/kg IM or IV within 30 min before procedure
Allergic to penicillin	Clindamycin or	*Adults:* 600 mg; *children:* 20 mg/kg orally 1 h before procedure
	Cephalexin[a] or cefadroxil[a] or	*Adults:* 2.0 g; *children;* 50 mg/kg orally 1 h before procedure
	Azithromycin or clarithromycin	*Adults:* 500 mg; *children:* 15 mg/kg orally 1 h before procedure
Allergic to penicillin and unable to take oral medications	Clindamycin or	*Adults:* 600 mg; *children:* 20 mg/kg IV within 30 min before procedure
	Cefazolin[a]	*Adults:* 1.0 g; *children:* 25 mg/kg IM or IV within 30 min before procedure

IM = intramuscularly, IV = intravenously.
[a] Cephalosporins should not be used in individuals with immediate-type hypersensitivity reaction (urticaria, angioedema, or anaphylaxis) to penicillins.
Reprinted from Dajani, Taubert, Wilson, Bolger, Bayer, Ferrieri, et al. (1997).

TABLE 33–10. Prophylactic Regimens for Genitourinary/Gastrointestinal (Excluding Esophageal) Procedures

Situation	Agents[a]	Regimen[b]
High-risk patients	Ampicillin plus gentamicin	*Adults:* ampicillin 2.0 g IM or IV plus gentamicin 1.5 mg/kg (not to exceed 120 mg) within 30 min of starting procedure; 6 h later, ampicillin 1 g IM/IV or amoxicillin 1 g orally *Children:* ampicillin 50 mg/kg IM or IV (not to exceed 2.0 g) plus gentamicin 1.5 mg/kg within 30 min of starting the procedure; 6 h later, ampicillin 25 mg/kg IM/IV or amoxicillin 25 mg/kg orally
High-risk patients allergic to ampicillin/amoxicillin	Vancomycin plus gentamicin	*Adults:* vancomycin 1.0 g IV over 1–2 h plus gentamicin 1.5 mg/kg IV/IM (not to exceed 120 mg); complete injection/infusion within 30 min of starting procedure *Children:* vancomycin 20 mg/kg IV over 1–2 h plus gentamicin 1.5 mg/kg IV/IM; complete injection/infusion within 30 min of starting procedure
Moderate-risk patients	Amoxicillin or ampicillin	*Adults:* amoxicillin 2.0 g orally 1 h before procedure, or ampicillin 2.0 g IM/IV within 30 min of starting procedure *Children:* amoxicillin 50 mg/kg orally 1 h before procedure, or ampicillin 50 mg/kg IM/IV within 30 min of starting procedure
Moderate-risk patients allergic to ampicillin/amoxicillin	Vancomycin	*Adults:* vancomycin 1.0 g IV over 1–2 h complete infusion within 30 min of starting procedure *Children:* vancomycin 20 mg/kg IV over 1–2 h; complete infusion within 30 min of starting procedure

IM = indicates intramuscularly, IV = intravenously.
[a] Total children's dose should not exceed adult dose.
[b] No second dose of vancomycin or gentamicin is recommended.
Reprinted from Dajani, Taubert, Wilson, Bolger, Bayer, Ferrieri, et al. (1997).

Acknowledgment: Thanks to Cecelia Cary for assistance with the figures.

REFERENCES

Akins, C. W., Hilgenberg, A. D., Buckley, M. J., Vlahakes, G. J., Torchiana, D. F., Dagget, W. M., & Austen, W. G. (1994). Mitral valve reconstruction versus replacement for degenerative or ischemic mitral regurgitation. *Annals of Thoracic Surgery, 58* (3), 668–675.

Ben Farhat, M., Ayari, M., Maatouk, F., Betbout, F., Gamra, H., Jarra, M., et al. (1998). Percutaneous balloon versus surgical closed and open mitral commissurotomy: seven-year follow-up results of a randomized trial. *Circulation, 97* (3), 245–250.

Bogart, M. A. (1995). Time to hemostasis: A comparison of manual versus mechanical compression of the femoral artery. *American Journal of Critical Care, 4* (2), 149–156.

Bonow, R. O. (1994). Asymptomatic aortic regurgitation: Indications for operation. *Journal of Cardiac Surgery, 9* (2 suppl), 170–173.

Braunwald, E. (1994). Valvular heart disease. In Braunwald, E. (Ed.), *Heart disease: A textbook of cardiovascular medicine* (4th ed.). Philadelphia: W. B. Saunders.

Carabello, B. A. (1996). The timing of valve surgery. In Smith, T. W. (Ed.), *Cardiovascular therapeutics: A companion to braunwald's heart disease.* Philadelphia: W. B. Saunders.

Dajani, A. S., Taubert, K. A., Wilson, W., Bolger, A. F., Bayer, A., Ferrieri, P., et al. (1997). Prevention of bacterial endocarditis: Recommendations by the American Heart Association. *Circulation, 96* (1), 358–366.

Feigenbaum, H. (1994). *Echocardiography.* (5th ed.). Philadelphia: Lea & Febiger.

Ganz, W., Donoso, R., Marcus, H. S. et al. (1971). A new technique for measurements of cardiac output by thermodilution in man. *American Journal of Cardiology, 27* (392), 392–396.

Garver, D., Kaczmarek, R. G., Silverman, B. G., Gross, T. P., & Hamilton, P. M. (1995). The epidemiology of prosthetic heart valves in the United States. *Texas Heart Institute Journal, 22* (1), 86–91.

Glazier, J. J. & Turi Z. G. (1997). Percutaneous balloon mitral valvuloplasty. *Progress in Cardiovascular Diseases, 40* (1), 5–26.

Harvey, W. P. & Canfield, D. C. (1997). Mitral valve prolapse (Number 1). In *Clinical Auscultation of the Cardiovascular System.* pp 9–10. Fairfield, NJ: Laennec Publishing.

Hecht, S. R. & Berger, M. (1992). Right-sided endocarditis in intravenous drug users. Prognostic features in 102 episodes. *Annals of Internal Medicine, 117* (7), 560–566.

Hogan-Miller, E., Rustad, D., Sendelbach, S. & Goldenberg, I. (1995). Effects of three methods of femoral site immobilization on bleeding and comfort after coronary angiogram. *American Journal of Critical Care, 4* (2), 143–148.

Ishii, K., Hirota, Y., Suwa, M., Kita, Y., Onaka, H., & Kawamura, K. (1996). Natural history and left ventricular response in chronic aortic regurgitation. *American Journal of Cardiology,* 78 (3), 357–361.

Jin, X. Y., Zhang, Z. M., Gibson, D. G., Yacoub, M. H., & Pepper, J. R. (1996). Effects of valve substitutes on changes in left ventricular function and hypertrophy after aortic valve replacement. *Annals of Thoracic Surgery, 62* (3), 683–690.

Kadri, M. A., Levy, R. D., Nashef, S. A., & Jones, M. T. (1994). Aortic valve replacement for end-stage aortic valve disease. *Thoracic and Cardiovascular Surgeon, 42* (6), 321–324.

Keeling, A., Taylor, V., Nordt, L. A., Powers, E., & Fisher, C. (1996). Reducing time in bed after cardiac catheterization (TIBS II). *American Journal of Critical Care, 5* (4), 277–281.

Landzberg, M. J. & Lock, J. E. (1996). Interventional approaches to congenital heart disease and intracardiac shunts. In Smith, T. W. *Cardiovascular Therapeutics,* Saunders: Philadelphia.

Levine, H. J. & Gaasch, W. H. (1996). Vasoactive drugs in chronic regurgitant lesions of the mitral and aortic valves. *Journal of the American College of Cardiology, 28* (5), 1083–1091.

Lin, M., Chiang, H. T., Lin, S. L., Chang, M. S., Chiang, B. N., Kuo, H. W., & Cheitlin, M. D. (1994). Vasodilator therapy in chronic asymptomatic aortic regurgitation: Enalapril versus hydralazine therapy. *Journal of the American College of Cardiology, 24* (4), 1046–1053.

Obadia, J. F., El Farra, M., Bastien, O. H., Lievre, M., Martelloni, Y., & Chassignolle, J. F. (1997). Outcome of atrial fibrillation after mitral valve repair. *Journal of Thoracic and Cardiovascular Surgery, 114* (2), 179–185.

Rao, V., Christakis, G. T., Weisel, R. D., Buth, K. J., Ikonomidis, J. S., Shirai, T. et al. (1996). Changing pattern of valve surgery. *Circulation, 94* (9 suppl), II 113–120.

Reynolds, T. (1993). *The Echocardiographer's Pocket Reference.* Phoenix: Arizona Heart Institute Foundation.

Schon, H. R. (1994). Hemodynamic and morphologic changes after long-term angiotensin converting enzyme inhibition in patients with chronic valvular regurgitation. *Journal of Hypertension, 12* (4 suppl), 95–104.

Scognamiglio, R., Rahimtoola, S. H., Fasoli, G., Nistri, S. & Dalla Volta, S. (1994). Nifedipine in asymptomatic patients with severe aortic regurgitation and normal left ventricular function. *New England Journal of Medicine, 331* (11), 689–694.

Simon, A., Bumgarner, B., Clark, K., & Israel, S. (1998). Manual versus mechanical compression for femoral artery hemostasis after cardiac catheterization. *American Journal of Critical Care, 7* (4), 308–313.

Wagner, G. S. (1994). *Marriott's Practical Electrocardiography.* (9th ed.). Baltimore: Williams & Wilkins.

Wyman, R. M., Safian, R. D., Portway, V., Skillman, J. J., McKay, R. G., & Baim, D. S. (1988). Current complications of diagnostic and therapeutic cardiac catheterization. *Journal of the American College of Cardiology, 12* (6), 1400–1406.

34

Cardiac Surgery

Barbara Asorian

Over the last 50 years, the field of cardiothoracic surgery has made huge technological strides. Currently, there are no known cardiothoracic surgical diseases for which there is not some type of surgical palliation. With the explosion of capabilities has come an enormous proliferation of knowledge, technology, and management protocols (Bojar, 1992).

The purpose of this chapter is to introduce the acute care nurse practitioner (ACNP) to the intricacies of perioperative management of the patient with acquired cardiac surgical diseases including: coronary artery disease, valvular heart disease, and diseases of the thoracic aorta. This chapter has electively excluded the more "niche" areas of cardiothoracic surgery such as adult congenital disease, trauma, and cardiac tumors.

▶ HISTORY OF CARDIAC SURGERY

The first successful use of cardiopulmonary bypass by Gibbon in 1953 opened the door for the explosive growth in cardiac surgery that has occurred during the past four decades. Isolation of the heart from the circulation by means of a heart–lung machine permitted correction of congenital and acquired valvular abnormalities that were previously not accessible (Dillard & Miller, 1983).

In the early years of open heart surgery, most procedures were done for congenital heart disease. Prosthetic heart valves became commercially available in the early 1960s, permitting a more aggressive surgical approach for patients with acquired valvular heart disease. Initial clinical reports of coronary artery bypass surgery first appeared in the literature in 1969 and by the early 1970s it was being performed nationwide (Dillard & Miller, 1983).

During the past decade, the art and science of cardiac surgery continued to evolve. Nearly 300,000 procedures were performed worldwide in 1990, predominantly for the treatment of coronary artery disease and valvular heart disease (Bojar, 1992). The typical profile of a patient under-going cardiac surgery is also changing. With advances in the nonsurgical treatment of cardiac diseases, we are now encountering a patient population with far advanced medical and surgical problems. Most cardiac surgery programs are now faced with a patient population that is older, has increased morbidities, and poorer ventricular function along with performing more redo and emergency operations. Therefore, the ACNP working in cardiac surgery may often be managing patients at the end of the clinical spectrum (Bojar, 1992; Jones, Weintraub, Craver, Guyton, & Cohen, 1991).

▶ PREOPERATIVE EVALUATION OF THE CARDIAC SURGICAL PATIENT

Most often patients are admitted to the hospital on the day of planned cardiac operation. Same-day admission is appropriate for patients with low perioperative risk; however, it requires efficiency, organization, and a focused evaluation to ensure that the patient is adequately prepared for the intended surgery. The following section represents a focused yet systematic approach to preoperative evaluation of the cardiac surgical patient.

The goal is to identify any potential "red flags" that

may signal the need for further evaluation and/or treatment prior to proceeding with surgery. Attention to noncardiac problems as well as any new cardiac abnormalities that may have arisen since the time of initial consultation and/or cardiac catheterization not only allows for preventive measures to minimize postoperative morbidity and mortality, but also affords the cardiothoracic surgical team and patient an insight into the operative risk (Bojar, 1994; Moreno-Cabral, Mitchell, & Miller, 1988). To summarize, a thorough preoperative evaluation should include: (1) interview and assessment of patient, (2) review of all diagnostic test results, (3) identification of patient's baseline knowledge, his or her support systems, and living arrangements so that appropriate discharge planning can be initiated, and (4) preparation and education of the patient for the planned operation.

History of Present Illness

Get a detailed history of the patient's signs and symptoms of heart disease as well as the patient's functional status. It is important to differentiate the primary presentation as angina versus heart failure. Note the presence or absence of dyspnea on exertion, paroxysmal nocturnal dyspnea, orthopnea, peripheral edema, palpitations, and (pre) syncope as well as the patient's exercise tolerance and the characteristics of the angina if present. Tables 34–1 and 34–2 show two commonly used classification systems.

Medications

Preoperative medications should be evaluated and modified as necessary. Be sure to ask the patient about over-the-counter medications as well as prescription medications and any known drug allergies.

Cardiac Medications

Most cardiac medications are continued until the day of surgery. In particular, those drugs used to control hypertension, angina, or arrhythmias should be continued because abrupt cessation can precipitate rebound hypertension and myocardial ischemia as well as intraoperative lability.

TABLE 34–1. New York Heart Association's Functional Classification System

I: Patients with cardiac disease but without resulting limitation of physical activity. Ordinary physical activity does not cause undue fatigue, palpitation, dyspnea, or angina pain

II: Patients with cardiac disease resulting in slight limitation of physical activity. They are comfortable at rest. Ordinary physical activity results in fatigue, palpitation, dyspnea, or anginal pain

III: Patients with cardiac disease resulting in marked limitation of physical activity. Less than ordinary physical activity results in fatigue, palpitation, dyspnea, or anginal pain

IV: Patients with cardiac disease resulting in inability to carry on any physical activity without discomfort. Symptoms of cardiac insufficiency or of anginal syndrome may be present even at rest

TABLE 34–2. Canadian Cardiovascular Society's Functional Classification System

I: Ordinary physical activity, such as walking or climbing the stairs, does not cause angina. Angina may occur with strenuous, rapid, or prolonged exertion at work or recreation

II: There is slight limitation of ordinary activity. Angina may occur with walking or climbing stairs rapidly, walking uphill, walking or stair climbing after meals or in the cold, in the wind, or under emotional stress, or walking more than two blocks on the level, and climbing more than one flight of stairs at normal pace under normal conditions

III: There is marked limitation of ordinary activity. Angina may occur after walking one or two blocks on the level or climbing one flight of stairs under normal conditions at normal pace

IV: There is inability to carry on any physical activity without discomfort. Angina may be present at rest

Digitalis and Diuretics

In general, digoxin and diuretics should be discontinued the day before surgery. Digoxin is withheld the day of surgery because of its low therapeutic index and, thus, the propensity towards digoxin toxicity with intraoperative potassium shifts. Diuretics are discontinued to avoid potentiating intraoperative fluid and electrolyte imbalances.

Anticoagulants

Medications affecting hemostasis should be identified and stopped at an appropriate time interval preceding surgery. Warfarin depresses the synthesis of prothrombin by the liver and, because of its long half life, it is generally held for three to five days before the date of surgery (Moreno-Cabral et al., 1988). Depending on the indication for warfarin, it may be necessary to administer intravenous heparin during this time period to prevent thromboembolic complications. Heparin can be stopped safely "on call" to the operating room, especially in the setting of unstable angina.

Drugs affecting platelet function should be stopped to allow for physiologic recovery of platelet activity (Moreno-Cabral et al., 1988). Aspirin irreversibly acetylates platelet cyclooxygenase, impairing thromboxane A^2 formation, and inhibiting platelet aggregation and platelet plug formation. The effects of aspirin persist for the life of the platelet and therefore, aspirin should be stopped 5 to 7 days before a planned surgery. If cessation is impossible because of an emergent or urgent operation, platelet transfusion should be anticipated and available (Moreno-Cabral et al., 1988). Those patients who report a more recent aspirin use should also undergo a preoperative bleeding time to evaluate platelet function (Bojar, 1994; Finkelmeier, 1995).

Conversely, nonsteroidal antiinflammatories (NSAIDs) have a reversible effect on platelet function. They only impact platelet function while in the circulation and, therefore, only need to be stopped a few days before surgery.

Oral Hypoglycemic Agents and Insulin

Oral hypoglycemic agents are generally withheld the day of surgery only. Patients who are insulin dependent should receive half their usual dose on the morning of surgery and intravenous fluids of dextrose should be given to avoid hypoglycemia. It is also important to note that patients who take protamine-based insulins such as NPH are at increased risk for protamine reactions upon termination of cardiopulmonary bypass and reversal of heparin (Bojar, 1994; Finkelmeier, 1995).

Steroids

Chronic steroid use for such conditions as rheumatoid arthritis and chronic obstructive pulmonary disease also needs to be identified preoperatively. Although a predictor for postoperative problems with wound healing, abrupt cessation of steroids preoperatively can lead to acute adrenal insufficiency. Parenteral steroids should be administered perioperatively until the patient can resume preoperative dosing.

Personal Habits

Smoking

Patients with a known history of smoking need to be appropriately counseled to stop at least two weeks and preferably two months before surgery. It is well documented that smoking within two months of surgery is associated with a fourfold increase in the risk of developing postoperative pulmonary complications when compared with patients who have stopped (Warner et al., 1989). Pulmonary function tests should be obtained to assess the patient's pulmonary risk when the history elicits decreased exercise tolerance due to poor pulmonary function coupled with a significant tobacco history. Baseline room air arterial blood gases should also be considered in this patient subset.

Alcohol use

Eliciting a significant history for alcohol use identifies potential problems with intraoperative bleeding as well as postoperative hepatic dysfunction and delirium. In patients who need valve replacement, it should also be considered a relative contraindication to anticoagulation with warfarin; therefore, if valve replacement surgery is anticipated, selection of a mechanical valve in this subset of patients as a replacement option is probably not a good choice.

Presence of Comorbid Diseases

Diabetes

Diabetes mellitus is a relative contraindication to bilateral internal mammary artery use due to the increased risk of nonunion of the sternum and mediastinitis (Cosegrove et al., 1988; Bojar, 1994). Healing of the saphenous vein harvest site may also be delayed in the diabetic patient and minor superficial wound infections including cellulitis are more common in this patient population (Shaffer, Schulkers, & Wexler, 1991).

Cerebrovascular Disease

Five percent of patients undergoing cardiac surgery for coronary artery bypass have associated cerebrovascular abnormalities. Conversely, 26% of all patients undergoing complete work-up for cerebrovascular disease are found to have coronary artery disease that warrants surgical intervention. While each of these two disease entities is important in and of itself, their coexistence is commonly encountered and merits special attention (Baue, Geha, Hammond, Laks, & Naunheim, 1991).

Neurologic symptoms and/or a documented history of transient ischemic attack (TIA), cerebrovascular accident, or previous carotid endartarectomy should alert the nurse practitioner to a potential increased risk for an intraoperative neurologic event. These patients should be evaluated with a preoperative carotid duplex.

Peripheral Vascular Disease

A history of peripheral vascular disease, claudication pain, prior coronary artery bypass surgery with vein harvest, saphenous vein stripping, or ligation should alert the nurse practitioner to a potential problem obtaining a sufficient amount of conduit for coronary artery bypass surgery. If there is a history of severe lower extremity claudication or advanced manifestations of ischemic peripheral vascular disease, harvesting saphenous vein from the lower leg should be avoided since delayed healing and other wound complications are likely, especially in the diabetic patient (Moreno-Cabral et al., 1988). Preoperative venous mapping of the greater and lessor saphenous systems as well as ankle brachial indices should be considered in this patient subset.

Renal Dysfunction

It is frequently said that the best cure is prevention. Nowhere is this more appropriate than with kidney function in response to an insult like open heart surgery. It has been estimated that the frequency of renal failure in the setting of open heart surgery ranges from 5 to 40%. Patients at high risk include those with preexisting renal dysfunction, diabetes (types I and II), significant peripheral vascular disease, congestive heart failure receiving diuretics, elderly (i.e., >75 years of age), and those with a prior history of acute renal failure (Paganini & Bosworth, 1991). Baseline blood urea nitrogen and creatinine should be obtained preoperatively. It is important to differentiate acute renal dysfunction due to the nephrotoxicity of angiogram contrast versus chronic renal insufficiency. High-risk patients need to be adequately hydrated, which may seem obvious; however, the cardiac surgery patient is often "kept dry" due to deminished left ventricular function, and in fact is frequently receiving diuretic therapy.

Male patients with a documented history and/or symptoms suggestive of benign prostatic hypertrophy or urethral stricture need to be identified. This may signal the need for special perioperative urinary drainage catheters as well as the need for prolonged postoperative urinary drainage.

Peptic Ulcer Disease or History of Gastrointestinal Bleed

A history of peptic ulcer disease predisposes the patient to upper gastrointestinal bleeding with cardiac operations. This is especially significant if the patient requires postoperative anticoagulation.

Chronic Obstructive Pulmonary Disease

Chronic obstructive pulmonary disease (COPD) is an important risk factor for pulmonary dysfunction postoperatively. It has been speculated to be a risk factor that may prolong intensive care unit stay as well as require mechanical ventilation. COPD increases the overall risk of the operation because it predisposes to an increased work of breathing and air trapping after surgery. This patient subset may also have difficulty in weaning from mechanical ventilation (Kirklin & Barratt-Boyes, 1993).

Previous Surgery or Radiation to Chest Wall

Previous surgery or radiation to the chest wall make surgical exposure of the heart more difficult and increase the risk of catastrophic hemorrhage upon opening the sternum (Loop, 1994). The presence of adhesions can cause the heart to adhere to the surrounding tissues. Previous bypass grafts, if present on the anterior surface of the heart, as well as the right ventricle itself can become adherent to the posterior table of the sternum making re-entry more difficult because of the risk of inadvertently lacerating them (Finkelmeier, 1996).

Physical Examination

Active Skin Infection or Rash

Perform a head-to-toe visual inspection of the preoperative cardiac surgery patient to identify any active skin lesions that could be secondarily infected, thus increasing the risk of surgical wound infection.

Carotid Bruit

Carotid bruits are detected in approximately 10% of patients undergoing cardiac surgery. Although a bruit is a good marker for potential cardiac and cerebral ischemia, it is not a sensitive or specific-enough indicator of extracerebral carotid disease. More than half of the patients with bruits do not have significant carotid disease and approximately 30% of patients with significant stenosis have no bruits. Evaluation of carotid bruits with noninvasive Doppler should be done preoperatively. In general, most surgeons forgo further evaluation if noninvasive studies demonstrate unilateral stenosis less than 90% or bilateral stenosis less than 75%, especially in the absence of symptoms or complex/ulcerated plaque (Bojar, 1992).

Dental Carries

For any cardiac surgical procedures in which there will be placement of prosthetic material such as valves or aortic grafts, the nurse practitioner should elicit a complete dental history as well as perform a visual inspection of the patient's oral mucosa and teeth. Significant dental caries, abscess, or severe gingival gum disease should be treated prior to proceeding with surgery to reduce the risk of endocarditis.

Differential Arm Pressures

Differential arm blood pressures may signify subclavian artery stenosis. This assessment finding may preclude use of a pedicled internal mammary artery graft for coronary operations (Bojar, 1994).

Severe Peripheral Vascular Disease

Evidence of severe peripheral vascular disease on physical examination identifies the lower extremity from which the saphenous vein should not be harvested because of potential impairment in wound healing. Assessment of peripheral pulses is also helpful in planning for potential site placement of an intraaortic balloon pump should it be necessary (Bojar, 1994).

Laboratory Assessment

General preoperative laboratory assessment should include the following:

1. *Complete blood count.* Patients with unstable angina and a hematocrit less than 30 should receive preoperative blood transfusion.
2. *Prothrombin time and partial thromboplastin time.* Prolonged coagulation may predict increased risk for excessive bleeding. It may warrant postponing surgery or guide preparation for blood products.
3. *Chemistries.* These aid in evaluation of preoperative renal function as well as critical electrolytes.
4. *Liver function tests.* Abnormal liver function may suggest chronic passive congestion due to low cardiac output versus hepatitis or cirrhosis.
5. *Urinalysis.* Broad spectrum antibiotic coverage should be instituted for suspected urinary tract infection, especially if the planned surgical procedure involves placement of prosthetic materials.
6. *Electrocardiogram.* This provides a baseline for postoperative comparison.
7. *Chest x-ray.* Two-view chest x-ray helps identify the proximity of cardiac structures to the posterior sternal table.

Preoperative Blood Preparation

Advances in intraoperative blood salvaging techniques as well as postoperative autotransfusion systems have minimized the need for perioperative homologous transfusion requirements. Aside from the intrinsic risks that are associated with blood bank products such as febrile and allergic transfusion reactions, most patients are more concerned about the risk of contracting hepatitis or HIV.

In some select patient groups undergoing cardiac surgery, preoperative autologous blood donation may be possible; however, in the higher risk surgical patient, it is generally discouraged since lowering the hemoglobin and hematocrit impairs oxygen-carrying capacity and, therefore, can precipitate ischemia or symptoms of heart failure.

Conversely, directed donations from family or friends with compatible blood types is a desirable alternative for some patients undergoing cardiac surgery despite the existence of no clear-cut evidence of a statistical difference in the potential for disease transmission.

A thorough review and explanation of both the potential need for transfusion as well as blood donation options should be presented to the patient before surgery unless an urgent/emergent situation makes it impossible to do so.

Preoperative Orders and Progress Note

Before surgery, a brief preoperative progress note should be written summarizing the essential information that should be reviewed prior to proceeding with the operation (Table 34–3). Writing a note helps prevent important details from being inadvertently overlooked. Preoperative orders should also be written at this time and should include antibiotic prophylaxis as well as surgical skin preparation.

The original intent of antibiotic prophylaxis in cardiothoracic operations was to reduce the prevalence of prosthetic valve endocarditis. Since the widespread adoption of antibiotic prophylaxis for cardiothoracic surgery, however, and the development of coronary artery bypass procedure, wound infection has become the primary marker of prophylaxis efficacy.

The choice of prophylactic agent has shifted through the years as new drugs have become available and the microbiology of wound infection has shifted. In general, choosing an anti-staphylococcal penicillin or first-generation Cephalosporin is appropriate. Second-generation Cephalosporins such as Cefamandole and Cefuroxime may be associated with a decreased prevalence of wound infection when compared with Cefazolin. Published trials comparing first- and second-generation Cephalosporins as prophylactic antibiotics for infection after cardiothoracic operations have shown a trend towards this (Kreter & Woods, 1992).

The question of whether different methods of preoperative shaving have an effect on wound infection rates have also been addressed extensively. Manual skin shaving with a razor has been shown to cause microscopic breakage in the epithelial barrier, leading to bacterial contamination of the surgical wound. Data suggests that the closer the preparation to the time of surgery as well as the use of either clippers or depilatory are associated with a lower wound infection rate (Ko, Lazenby, Zelano, Isom, & Krieger, 1992).

TABLE 34–3. Components of the Preoperative Progress Note

Diagnosis:
Planned Operative Procedure:
Surgeon:
Labs:
Urinalysis:
EKG:
CXR:
Other:
Blood Type: Donor Directed Blood: Autologous Blood:
____ Type & Cross ____ PRC ____FFP ____Platelets
____ OR Consent ____ Anesthesia Consent

Surgical risks, benefits, and alternatives—including the risks of bleeding, infection, myocardial infarction, stroke, irreversible brain damage, multi-system organ failure, and death—have been discussed with the patient. The potential need for a transfusion and blood donation options have also been reviewed. The patient states that he/she understands and is in agreement to proceed with surgery using blood bank blood if necessary.

____
Signature and date

▶ INTRAOPERATIVE TECHNIQUES

Cardiopulmonary Bypass

Purpose

The development of cardiopulmonary bypass (CPB) is largely attributed to the pioneering research of Dr. John Gibbon. He performed the first successful intracardiac operation using CPB bypass in May of 1953. CPB, also known as extracorporeal circulation or the heart–lung machine, describes an apparatus used to assume the pumping action of the heart and gas exchange function of the lungs during surgery of the heart and great vessels.

Components

The basic components of the CPB circuit include: venous and arterial cannulae, a reservoir, an oxygenator, a heat exchanger, an arterial pump, a cardiac vent, the cardiotomy suction system, and a cell saver device.

Venous cannulae drain blood by gravity from the patient to the extracorporeal circuit. One or more venous cannulae are used depending on the type of operative procedure and the surgeon's preference. Cannulation of the right atrium and inferior vena cava via the right atrial appendage using a two-stage cavoatrial cannula is usually employed for coronary and aortic valve surgery. Alternatively, for surgeries during which the right heart must be entered (e.g., mitral valve, tricuspid valve), bicaval (inferior and superior vena cava) cannulation is performed. This technique is employed to prevent entry of air into the venous lines (Bojar, 1992).

Blood drained from the patient's body enters the venous reservoir or the oxygenating column of a bubble oxygenator. The reservoir functions to hold a volume of blood in the extracorporeal circuit. It also allows for escape of air and manipulation of blood return to the patient as well as containing a port for intraoperative volume replacement and medication administration.

The oxygenator is the apparatus where gas exchange occurs. There are two types: bubble and membrane. The bubble oxygenator employs direct contact between the blood and thousands of small oxygen bubbles that are dispersed directly into the venous blood. The venous blood must then be defoamed to prevent gas emboli. In this system, gas exchange occurs across a thin film at the blood–gas interface around each bubble. The membrane oxygenator employs a semipermeable membrane across which oxygen and carbon dioxide diffuse due to the concentration gradient. In this system, the venous blood does not come in direct contact with gas. Both membrane and bubble oxygenators cause blood trauma and produce microemboli; however, membrane oxygenators are preferred for CPB cases lasting longer than two hours because this system has been shown to have superior oxygenation capabilities with less trauma to blood components during prolonged use (Baue et al., 1991) (Fig. 34–1).

The heat exchanger is usually incorporated into the oxygenator. It is used to cool and rewarm the blood during CPB. Water circulates within the heat exchanger to achieve the desired temperature control.

There are two types of pumps that can be employed in the CPB circuit: the roller pump and the centrifugal pump. They are both considered non-physiologic in that they both produce non-pulsatile blood flow. The purpose of these pumps is to propel oxygenated blood into the arterial circulation. The roller pump is the more common and achieves blood return by external compression of the arterial tubing with two rotating rollers positioned 180 degrees apart. Conversely, the centrifugal pump consists of a rapidly rotating impeller. The impeller causes blood to rotate at high speed within the compartment and the centrifugal force propels blood forward through an outlet port (Baue et al., 1991).

The arterial filter is designed to trap particulate matter and gas emboli in the blood before it re-enters the patient. An arterial filter is required for a bubble oxygenator and optional for a membrane oxygenator perfusion system.

Oxygenated blood is most commonly returned from the extracorporeal circuit to the patient via an arterial cannula placed in the distal ascending aorta, just proximal to the origin of the innominate artery. Femoral arterial cannulation is an alternative site and most commonly employed for aortic operations or when severe aortic calcifications preclude safe ascending aortic cannulation due to the risk of calcium embolization into the cerebral circulation. Cannulation of the femoral artery also allows for rapid initiation of CPB in emergent situations.

The purpose of venting the left ventricle during CPB is to prevent distention of the ventricle during the period of aortic cross clamp. The vent catheter is placed either in the superior pulmonary vein or directly into the left atrium across the mitral valve and into the left ventricle. It may also be placed through the aortic root in a retrograde fashion across the aortic valve into the left ventricle. Although left ventricular venting is not universally employed for all cardiac operations, distention of the left ventricle for even limited periods of time can result in damage to the lungs due to increased pulmonary venous pressures, as well as severe,

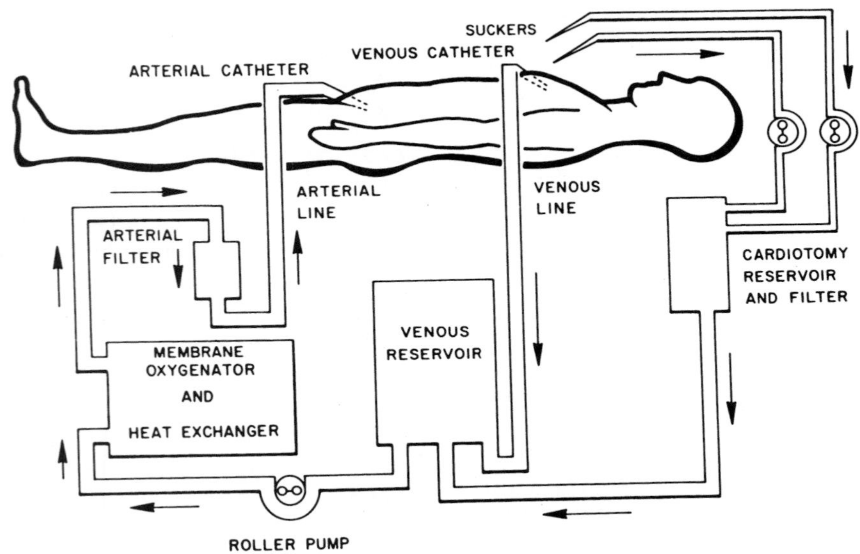

Figure 34–1. Diagram of a typical cardiopulmonary bypass set-up with a membrane oxygenator. *(Used with permission from Baue et al., [1991].)*

sometimes irreversible damage to the left ventricle due to overstreching of myocardial fibers (Finkelmeier, 1995).

The cardiotomy suction system allows heparinized blood to be scavenged from the operative field and be returned back to the extracorporeal circuit. Conversely, cell saving devices scavenge shed non-heparinized blood from the surgical field. They are used to salvage operative blood losses that occur both before initiation of systemic anticoagulation and after reversal of heparin with protamine. As blood enters the cell saver sucker tip, heparin is immediately added to prevent clotting. The blood then passes through a filter where the cells are washed and concentrated using a centrifuge. The washed, concentrated red blood cells can be reinfused as needed and provide blood with a hematocrit of 70% (Baue et al., 1991; Finkelmeier, 1995).

Initiation of Cardiopulmonary Bypass

CPB is initiated by giving the patient a 300 unit/kg bolus of heparin. Heparin is mandatory for all extracorporeal circuits to prevent clotting when the blood is exposed to non-biologic surfaces. Although some synthetic materials may be relatively thromboresistent, the endothelial cell is the only known nonthrombogenic surface. Since heparin sensitivity and metabolism vary from patient to patient, activated clotting time (ACT) is measured at 30-minute intervals and supplemented throughout surgery to maintain the ACT greater than 400 (Baue et al., 1991).

Once systemic anticoagulation is achieved, the CPB circuit is "primed" with 2 liters of a crystalloid solution that is similar in composition to plasma electrolytes. This fluid is then circulated for several minutes to ensure proper functioning of the system as well as to filter out all air and particulate matter.

Once the surgeon has inserted the venous and arterial cannulae, they are connected to the CPB circuit. To begin CPB, the perfusionist initiates venous drainage and activates the arterial pump. Core cooling (systemic hypothermia) is initiated to achieve moderate hypothermia (i.e., 28-30°C). Core cooling helps to minimize ischemic damage to vital organ systems by decreasing metabolic demands. Metabolic rate decreases 7% for each 1°C reduction in body temperature. More complex cardiac operations, such as surgery of the aortic arch, require circulatory arrest and employ profound hypothermia (i.e., 18°C) to safely extend the duration of cerebral protection.

As the patient's blood circulates through the extracorporeal circuit, it mixes with the crystalloid priming solution causing hemodilution, lowering the hematocrit to 25 to 30%. This is well tolerated during hypothermia because of the decreased oxygen demands. In fact, hemodilution is desirable because it decreases blood viscosity, thus counteracting the effects of hypothermia.

Maintenance of Cardiopulmonary Bypass

During CPB, the perfusionist controls systemic blood flow. The "ideal" flow rate during CPB is still debated. In general, at normothermia, flows exceeding 1.8 L/min/m^2 are acceptable with regard to total body oxygen consumption; however, flows of 2.2 to 2.5 L/min/m^2 are more securely adequate. Flow rates can safely be decreased to 1.8 L/min/m^2 during periods of moderate hypothermia because of the decreased metabolic demands (Baue et al., 1991; Finkelmeier, 1995; Sabiston & Spencer, 1995). Conversely, excessive flow rates during CPB should be avoided because they can contribute to blood element trauma, increase the potential for gas emboli formation, and increase noncoronary collateral/systemic venous flow in the heart which may impair myocardial protection (Bojar, 1992).

Weaning and Termination of Cardiopulmonary Bypass

When the surgeon is nearing completion of the operation, he or she instructs the perfusionist to begin rewarming. Several maneuvers are employed to de-air the heart and—with the patient in trendelenburg—the aortic cross clamp is removed. This position is used so that any residual air is directed into the descending thoracic aorta, rather than the cerebral circulation. Pump reservoir volume is adjusted to ensure adequate circulating volume and mechanical ventilation is initiated allowing air in the pulmonary veins to escape.

Once the operative procedure is completed and the heart is rewarmed sufficiently to resume a spontaneous cardiac rhythm, weaning from CPB is begun by slowly reducing flow rates through the circuit. When the heart is functioning effectively enough to sustain adequate arterial pressure, CPB is discontinued. If ventricular function is impaired and low cardiac output ensues, several attempts at weaning from CPB may be necessary. Various combinations of inotropes, vasodilators, and antiarrhythmic medications, an intraaortic balloon pump, as well as temporary pacing via epicardial wires to increase heart rate and ensure atrioventricular synchrony, should be readily available as they are used frequently to maximize cardiac output. When the patient is clearly able to sustain adequate arterial pressure and cardiac output without support from CPB, protamine is given at a usual dose of 1 milligram per 100 units of heparin to return the ACT to baseline. The venous and arterial cannulae are removed, the purse strings are tied, the chest is closed, and the patient is transferred to the intensive care unit (Finkelmeier, 1995).

Catastrophic Sequelae of Cardiopulmonary Bypass

The ten most commonly occurring perfusion incidents by frequency include: protamine reactions, hypoperfusion, inadequate oxygenation, electrical failure, drug errors, gas emboli, blood clotting, transfusion reaction, line separation, and blood leaks (Bojar, 1992). Most perfusion incidents are a result of human error and are completely preventable; however, protamine reactions are unpredictable, fairly common, and potentially life threatening.

Bojar (1992) describes three types of protamine reactions. The first is hypotension related to histamine release. The second type of reaction is anaphylaxis caused by immunoglobulin-mediated histamine release. This type of reaction may be seen in patients receiving NPH insulin or having fish allergies. The most life-threatening protamine reaction, however, is that of catastrophic pulmonary vasoconstriction. It is characterized by an acute increase in pulmonary pressure, a decrease in left atrial pressures, systemic hypotension, and right ventricular dysfunction. Although the cause is unclear, it has been hypothesized to be the result of complement activation by the heparin–protamine complex causing release of thromboxaine A^2 leading to pulmonary vasoconstriction. Prevention of protamine reactions has thus far not been possible. Catastrophic pulmonary vasoconstriction is treated with pharmacologic agents to counteract its hemodynamic effects and occasionally reinstitution of CPB is necessary.

Physiologic Derangements Associated with CPB

Diversion of systemic blood flow through the extracorporeal circuit ultimately effects every organ system, some more subtly than others. This happens as a result of the circulating blood volume being exposed to nonbiologic (i.e., nonendothelial) surfaces which in turn activates the humoral and cellular components of the inflammatory response. As a result of this whole body inflammatory response, biologically active substances are released into the circulation leading to a multitude of physiologic derangements including: both a qualitative and quantitative platelet dysfunction, increased capillary permeability, increased circulating catecholamines, and impaired immune function. These physiologic derangements all contribute to the common clinical scenarios typically seen in the early hours following cardiac surgery. They are collectively referred to as Post Perfusion Syndrome (Kirklin & Barratt-Boyes, 1993). Post Perfusion Syndrome is heralded by fluid, electrolyte, and metabolic imbalances, along with hypertension, bleeding, and low cardiac output. Although most patients demonstrate minimal clinical evidence of this syndrome, some patients have severe physiologic derangements such as pulmonary and renal dysfunction, bleeding diathesis, increased interstitial fluid (i.e., persistent capillary leak), leukocytosis, fever, vasoconstriction, and hemolysis. In general, it is the patient subset exposed to a prolonged duration of cardiopulmonary bypass that is most susceptible to experience Post Perfusion Syndrome.

Myocardial Protection

Perioperative myocardial damage remains the leading cause of morbidity and mortality in patients undergoing cardiac surgery. Myocardial protection refers to the specific intraoperative techniques employed to protect the heart from ischemic injury and infarct (Bojar, 1992). Optimal myocardial protection remains controversial, as excellent results can be achieved by many different techniques.

Principles

There has been a tremendous amount of research focused on how to best protect the heart during cardiac operations. Current perioperative techniques of myocardial protection are based on several principles. First, blood flow to the heart is regulated by aortic pressure, myocardial wall tension, and coronary vascular resistance. All of these protective regulatory factors are altered during cardiopulmonary bypass. Second, both ischemia and hypoxia are damaging to the myocardium because both conditions result in anaerobic metabolism, which in turn produces hydrogen ions and lactate. However, hypoxia is tolerated better than ischemia because the lack of adequate blood flow associated with ischemia allows for harmful metabolites to accumulate instead of being washed out. Third, the left ventricular endocardium is most vulnerable to ischemic damage because it receives oxygenated blood flow only during diastole. Diastolic blood flow can be compromised in the face of left ventricular hypertrophy or coronary artery disease and ischemic tissue injury increases exponentially with time. Lastly, hypothermia is known to decrease the deleterious consequences of ischemia by decreasing metabolic demands and thereby allowing existing energy stores to maintain cell viability (Bojar, 1992; Finkelmeier, 1995).

Techniques

Almost all cardiac operations are performed using hypothermia, cardioplegia, and a period of aortic cross-clamp. These techniques allow the surgeon a still, bloodless operative field. Without the use of an aortic clamp, blood flow to the coronary arteries would not be interrupted and, therefore, the heart would continue to be perfused and beat; the disadvantage being that the myocardium would be more vulnerable to ischemic damage. It is the induction of electromechanical arrest in combination with topical and systemic hypothermia that help to greatly reduce myocardial oxygen demands during cardiac operations.

Although the aortic cross-clamp isolates the coronary circulation from the circulating blood volume within the CPB circuit, not all blood flow to the myocardium is eliminated. Noncoronary collaterals in the pericardial attachments and pulmonary vein walls continue to provide some blood flow during the period of aorta cross-clamping. Blood flow through these collateral vessels produces an ischemic rather than an anoxic state in the myocardium. Therefore, myocardial preservation techniques are aimed at preventing the heart from global myocardial ischemia. The most commonly employed methods used to protect the heart include: moderate systemic hypothermia, profound myocardial hypothermia, and infusion of cardioplegia solution.

Hypothermia. Three techniques are used in combination to achieve moderate systemic and profound myocardial hypothermia: (1) systemic cooling of blood as it is pumped through the CPB circuit, (2) intermittent topical bathing of the heart with a cold saline solution placed in the pericardium, and (3) infusion of cold cardioplegia solution into the coronary arteries.

Systemic Hypothermia. Systemic hypothermia is also referred to as core cooling. Core cooling is initiated at the onset of CPB to reduce cellular metabolic demands of all vital organs including the heart. When moderate systemic hypothermia (i.e., 28-30°C) is achieved, an occlusive clamp is applied to the proximal ascending aorta, just above the coronary ostia. Once the aortic clamp is applied, further temperature reduction is accomplished with topical bathing of the heart and infusion of cardioplegia solution. With the addition of these measures, myocardial temperature is lowered to approximately 15°C (Finkelmeier, 1995).

Topical/Surface Cooling. Topical cooling contributes to myocardial protection by minimizing rewarming between doses of cardioplegia. It is accomplished by bathing the heart with ice-cold saline or ringers lactate that is dripped over the anterior surface of the heart. An alternative to bathing the heart with cool solution is to use a cooling pad that can be wrapped around the heart. Some surgeons prefer this method because they believe it minimizes the risk of hypothermic phrenic nerve injury.

Cardioplegia. Cold cardioplegic arrest has become the preferred method of myocardial protection for nearly all cardiac operations performed today. It involves cross-clamping of the aorta and administration of a chilled solution infused directly into the coronary circulation. The exact composition of the cardioplegia solution varies among surgeons; however, all cardioplegia solutions are designed with specific goals in mind. They include: arrest of the heart, continued energy production by the myocardium, and avoidance of ischemia. The merits of specific components of cardioplegia solutions also remains controversial. In general, the significant components of cardioplegia include: an ingredient (usually potassium) to induce rapid diastolic arrest of the heart, a solution temperature of 4 to 8°C to induce profound hypothermia of the myocardium, a substrate that provides a source for energy production, a buffering agent to maintain pH, a membrane-stabilizing agent, and appropriate osmolarity and colloid oncotic pressure to prevent myocardial edema (Finkelmeier, 1995).

There are two basic types of cardioplegia solution: blood and crystalloid. The superiority of one over the other remains controversial; however, evidence suggests that blood cardioplegia provides better cellular protection with greater preservation of ATP, less creatinine phosphokinase release, and improved post ischemic ventricular performance. This is thought to be related to the fact that blood cardioplegia provides oxygen for aerobic metabolism during the period of cardiac arrest (Bojar, 1992).

Several techniques are employed for the administration of cardioplegia. The most common method is antegrade infusion, in which the solution is infused via a catheter placed into the aortic root proximal to the aortic cross-clamp. As long as the aortic valve is competent, the cardioplegia solution passes via the coronary ostia into the coronary arteries. The rate of administration is determined by aortic root pressure. Ideal aortic root pressure is maintained between 80 to 100 mm Hg. Global cardiac arrest usually occurs within 30 seconds of cardioplegia infusion; however, it can take up to 2 minutes in the presence of stenotic or totally occluded coronary arteries. Since blood flow from noncoronary collaterals washes away infused cardioplegia solution and gradually rewarms the heart, intermittent infusion of 300 to 500 milliliters every 15 to 20 minutes is necessary during the period of aortic cross-clamp.

There are several clinical situations in which antegrade delivery of cardioplegia solution into the aortic root or coronary ostia may provide suboptimal myocardial protection (e.g., severe triple vessel disease, left main disease, aortic regurgitation). In these situations, retrograde cardioplegia via the coronary sinus is employed.

Standard Versus Minimally Invasive Techniques

The morbidity and mortality of open heart procedures are largely attributed to the use of CPB, global cardiac arrest, and hypothermia. In the early 1990s, two developments inspired the exploration of alternative treatment strategies for patients requiring coronary surgery. First, data were being collected from two centers in South America that had been performing coronary artery bypass (CAB) without CPB for ten years in selected patient groups. Second, thoracoscopic surgery was now being performed on other structures in the chest. It was the advent of thoracoscopic chest surgery that inspired the initiative at Stanford in 1991 to develop closed chest, port access, video-assisted CAB and mitral valve surgery on the arrested heart using peripheral cannulation for CPB. This strategy, however, remained unattractive to many surgeons because the major cause of procedure-related morbidity had not been removed (i.e., CPB) (Borst, Jansen, & Grundeman, 1997) (Figs. 34–2 through 34–5).

Renewed interest in the potential value of CAB surgery on the beating heart off CPB led to a fresh look at the coronary motion problem in 1993. It was then that research involving use of mechanical immobilization devices began. The beating heart creates two obstacles to CAB. First, motion of the distal target site hampers accurate anastomosis suturing, and second, to reach posterior anastomosis sites, the beating heart needs to be dislocated, which causes a precipitous drop in blood pressure. The purpose of mechanical immobilization devices is to stabilize the operative portion of the heart during minimally invasive surgery.

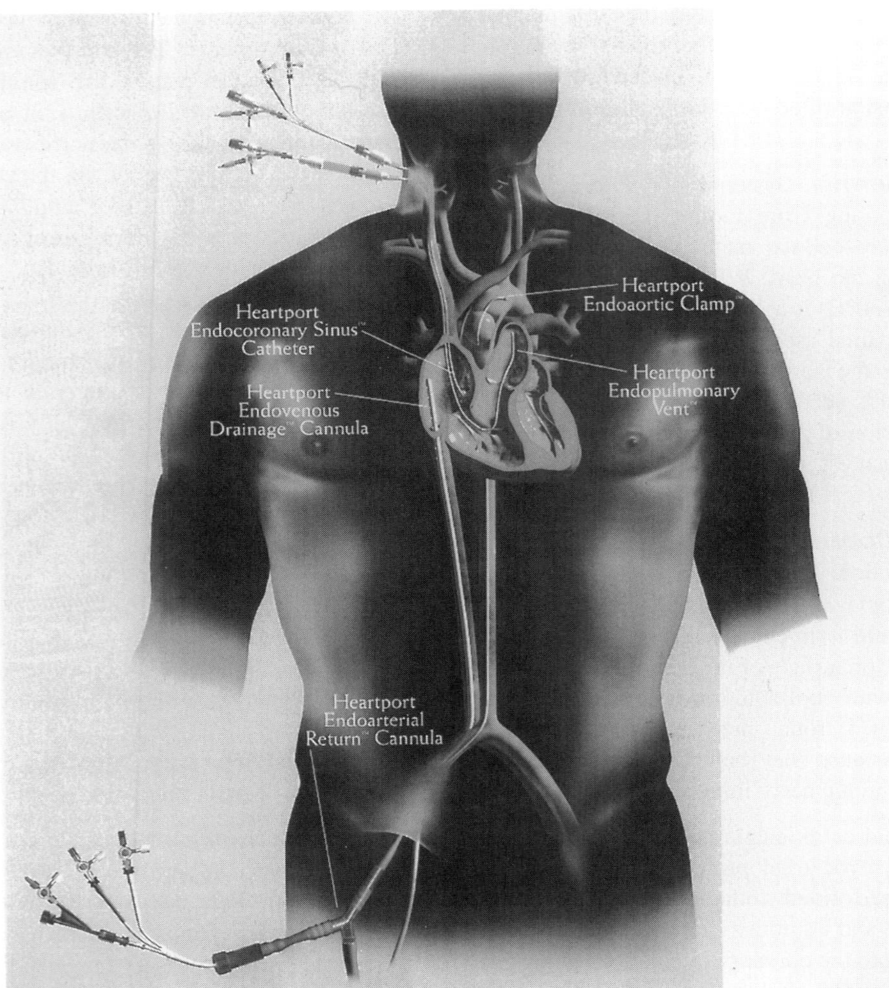

Figure 34–2. Diagram of the Heartport endovascular cardiopulmonary bypass system (endoCPB™). *(Used with permission from the Heartport Training Manual, 1996.)*

The Medtronic Octopus is one example of a mechanical immobilizer. It consists of two suction arms placed on either side of the anastomosis site resulting in a still field for suturing while the remainder of the heart continues to beat (Figs. 34–6 and 34–7).

Currently, minimally invasive cardiac surgery is performed using one of two approaches. Port access CAB and mitral valve replacement are performed using a series of small holes or "ports" in the chest. The femoral vessels are cannulated for cardiopulmonary bypass. As with other minimally invasive surgeries, the cardiothoracic surgeon views the operation on video monitors rather than directly. The acronym MIDCAB is used to describe minimally invasive direct vision CAB where surgical anastomosis are done under direct vision. Unlike port access cardiac surgery, MIDCAB is performed with the intention of avoiding cardiopulmonary bypass. The procedure was designed for bypassing one or two coronary arteries and the arteries must be directly beneath the incision (Hartz, 1996). A variety of smaller incisions such as partial sternotomy, transverse sternotomy, parasternal thoracotomy, and limited anterolateral thoracotomy are also being employed now for a variety of valvular heart surgeries. Since Antonio Calafiore and colleagues (1996) described their techniques and results on MIDCAB in a series of 155 patients (left internal mammary artery to left anterior descending coronary artery in a beating heart via left anterior small thoracotomy), interest for this approach has dramatically increased worldwide.

In summary, both the technology and terminology for minimally invasive cardiac surgery are evolving. Despite tremendous enthusiasm, widespread adoption of minimally invasive cardiac surgery is pending accumulation of suitable data and will ultimately be defined by comparative studies. Some of the potential benefits include: (1) shorter length of stay, (2) faster recovery, (3) less bleeding—hemostasis management is improved without CPB, (4) improved

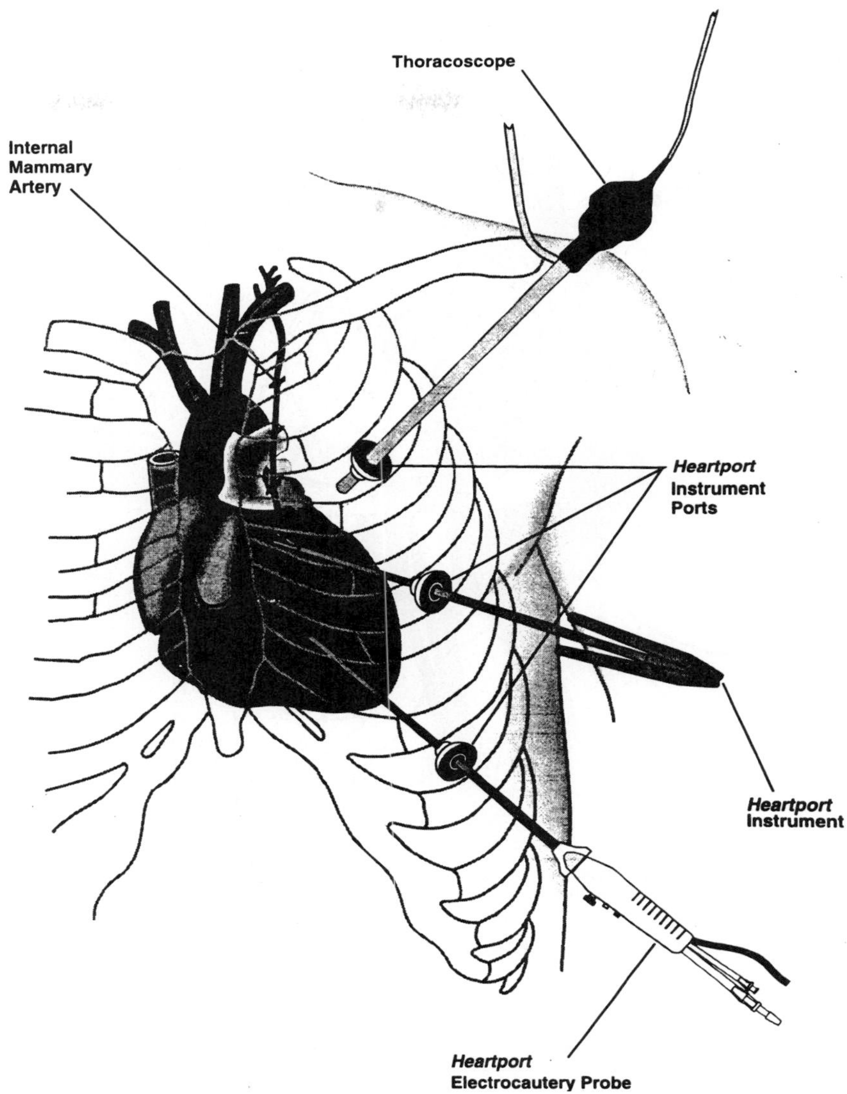

Figure 34–3. Schematic view of port-access coronary artery bypass procedure: internal mammary artery takedown. *(Used with permission from Heartport Training Manual, 1996.)*

patient satisfaction—smaller incisions are more cosmetically appealing, and (5) less cost—minimally invasive cardiac surgery is one-third to one-half the cost of conventional cardiac surgery.

IMMEDIATE POSTOPERATIVE CARE OF THE CARDIAC SURGERY PATIENT

It is essential that the nurse practitioner caring for the postoperative cardiac surgery patient has a thorough understanding of each individual patient's cardiac anatomy and pathophysiology as well as the known causes of morbidity and mortality associated with the specific surgical procedure performed. Communication with the cardiothoracic surgeon regarding significant intraoperative findings or events and any specific postoperative treatment strategies to be employed is imperative for optimal patient outcomes.

The goals of immediate postoperative care can be summarized as: (1) safe and efficient transport of the patient from the operating room to the intensive care unit, (2) smooth, uneventful emergence from anesthesia, (3) maintenance of and/or achievement of hemodynamic stability, (4) short-term respiratory support (i.e., early extubation), and (5) monitoring for and immediate treatment of bleeding or tamponade (Hendren & Higgins, 1991).

In most intensive care units standardized protocols provide nurses with flexibility to respond to common postoperative scenarios such as bleeding, arrhythmias, and fluid and electrolyte imbalances.

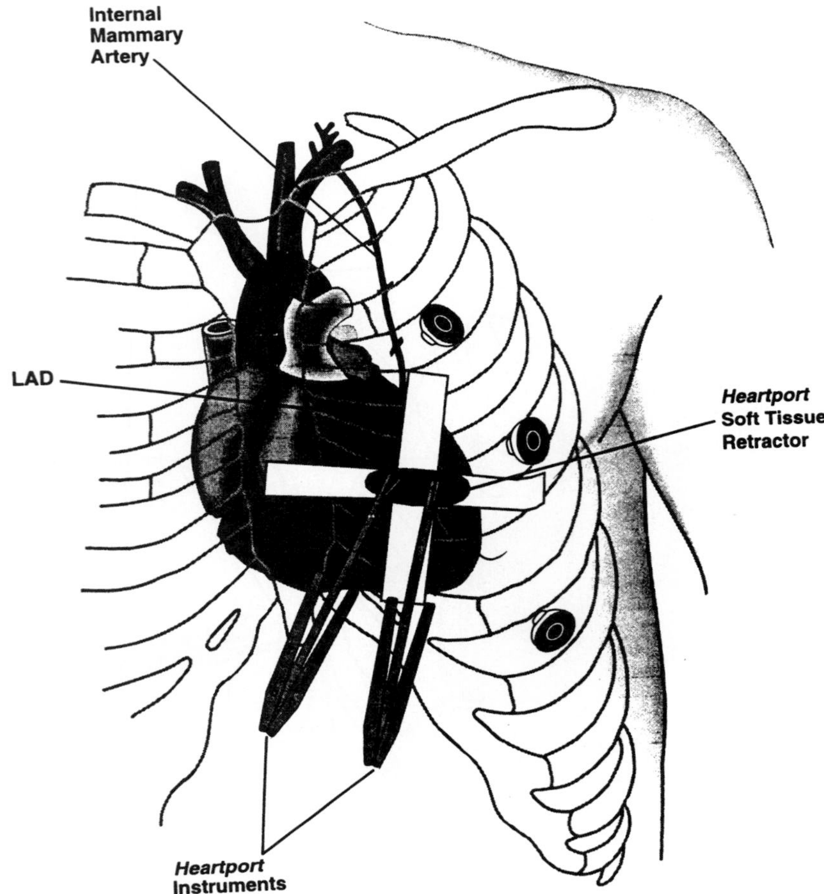

Figure 34–4. Schematic view of port-access coronary artery bypass procedure: anastomosis. *(Used with permission from Heartport Training Manual, 1996.)*

COMPLICATIONS ASSOCIATED WITH CARDIAC SURGERY

The patient recovering from a routine cardiac surgical procedure and having an uneventful postoperative course is usually extubated within several hours and off inotropic support by postoperative day one, at which point he or she is transferred to an intermediate care or postoperative cardiac surgery floor. Invasive monitoring is no longer available; however, telemetry is commonly used for arrhythmia surveillance.

Never be lulled into complacency! Despite being out of the intensive care unit, these patients still require scrupulous attention to prevent, identify, and treat postoperative complications that may have developed either during surgery, in the intensive care unit, or during convalescence on the floor. Daily examination of the patient using a systems approach is a must.

The development of postoperative complications is more likely to occur in patients with multiple comorbidities as well as in those patients who experienced a stormy postoperative course with an associated low cardiac output state; however, complications can also occur unpredictably in low risk, otherwise healthy patients despite an uneventful surgery and early postoperative course. In general, elderly patients are more susceptible to complications and do not tolerate them as well. Baseline left ventricular dysfunction, redo procedures, and emergent procedures are also powerful predictors of postoperative complications (Bojar, 1994).

Some problems such as atrial arrhythmias are quite common, usually benign, and have little influence on length of stay or long-term outcomes. Conversely, more serious complications such as stroke, renal insufficiency, or deep wound infection may result in multisystem organ failure, prolonged length of stay, and early death. The following section summarizes the major postoperative complications associated with cardiac surgery and is presented in a systems format.

Cardiac Complications

Arrhythmias

Supraventricular. Most arrhythmias that occur in the early postoperative period are supraventricular, in origin

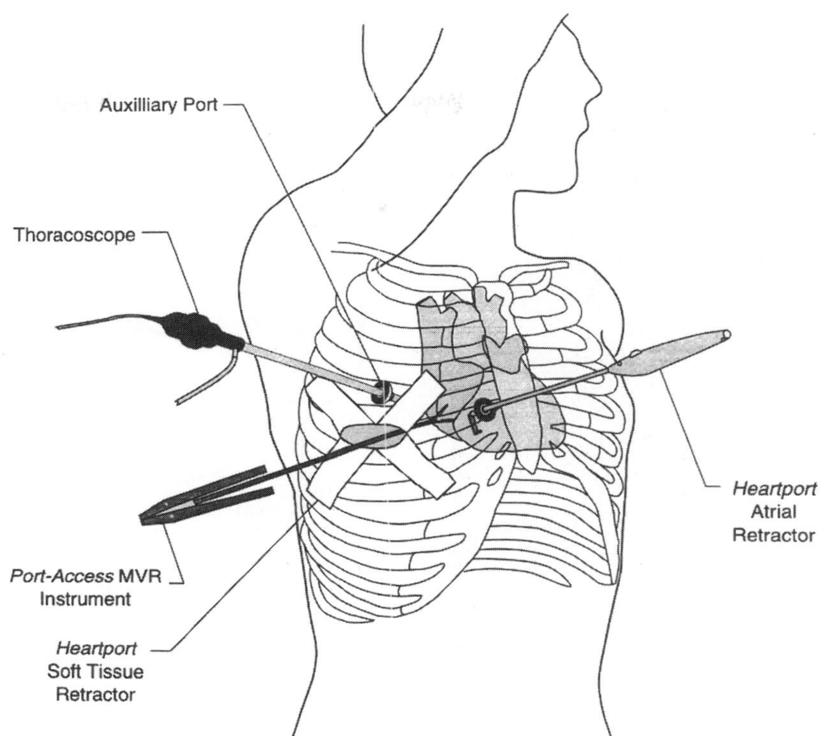

Figure 34–5. Schematic view of port-access mitral valve replacement procedure. *(Used with permission from Heartport Training Manual, 1996.)*

with atrial fibrillation being the most common. Atrial arrhythmias occur in 30% of all patients undergoing open heart surgery. They most commonly occur on postoperative day two or three. Keep in mind that although they are usually benign and self-limiting, loss of atrial contraction is poorly tolerated in patients with marginal left ventricular function. Common etiologies of postoperative atrial arrhythmias include: cannulation trauma of the atria, adrenergic rebound in patients taking preoperative beta blockers, pericarditis, atrial distention, hypoxia, and hypokalemia. Atrial arrhythmias are usually converted pharmacologically; however, electrical cardioversion is indicated for refractory or hemodynamically unstable rhythms. In patients with intermittent atrial fibrillation or in those patients whose arrhythmias persists greater than 72 hours, anticoagulation should be considered due to the risk of a thromboembolic event.

Ventricular. Ventricular arrhythmias can develop any time after cardiac surgery. They are usually related to myocardial ischemia and/or infarction. Ventricular arrhythmias may also occur transiently related to acute reperfusion of ischemic myocardium, hypoxia, electrolyte imbalances, or acid–base disturbances. In the absence of an obvious, treatable source, the patient should be reevaluated by an electrophysiologist regarding appropriate treatment therapy.

Heart Block. Heart block is common following open heart surgery with use of cardioplegic arrest and usually resolves within several hours postoperatively. Most centers use temporary epicardial pacemaker wires for this purpose. Heart block most commonly occurs after aortic valve surgery due to the proximity of the conduction system to the aortic valve annulus. In general, any heart block that persists beyond one week postoperatively warrants evaluation for a permanent dual-chamber pacemaker.

Myocardial Dysfunction

Transient myocardial dysfunction in the early postoperative period may be related to hypoxemia, acidosis, and decreased left ventricular compliance postcardiopulmonary bypass. In the face of persistent myocardial dysfunction, be suspicious for ongoing ischemia or infarct (Shinn, 1992).

Myocardial Ischemia

Postoperative myocardial ischemia usually manifests itself by significant electrocardiogram changes, return of angina, ventricular arrhythmias, or low cardiac output. In the worst-case scenario, sudden death! Contributing factors include: incomplete revascularization due to lack of sufficient amount of conduit or—more commonly—poor distal targets and acute graft thrombosis or spasm. Maximizing the medical regime is frequently the most appropriate treatment option and includes the use of nitrates, calcium channel

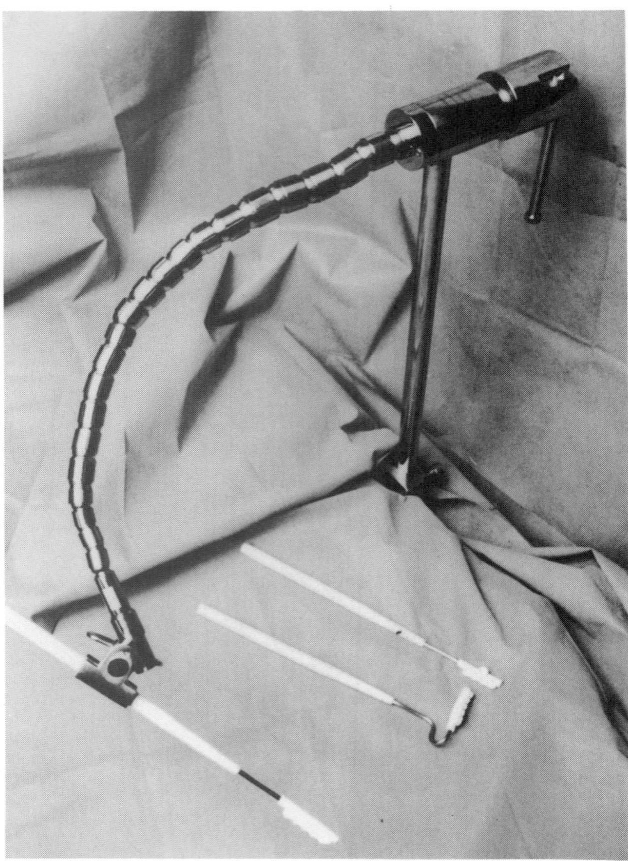

Figure 34–6. Medtronic Octopus™ system for minimally invasive cardiac surgery. This photograph shows the table-mounted arm holder and three variations of suction heads. Two suction heads, each held in place by the arm holder, are placed on either side of the anastomosis site. *(Used with permission from Medtronic News Release Packet, 1997.)*

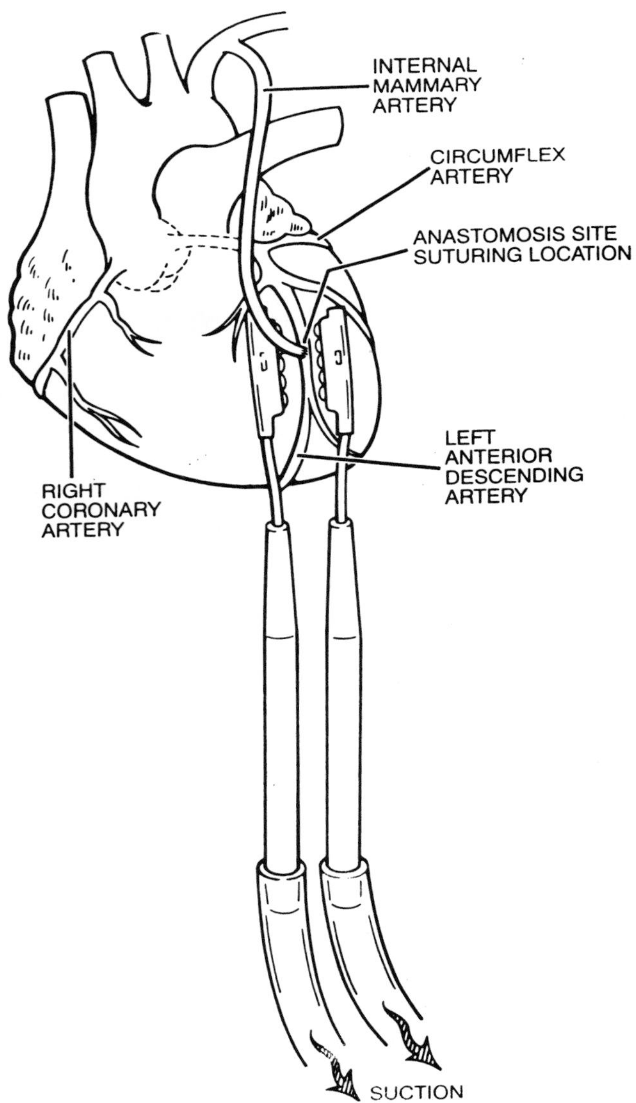

Figure 34–7. Schematic of Medtronic Octopus™ system with suction heads positioned on the heart. *(Used with permission from Medtronic News Release Packet, 1997.)*

blockers, and beta blockers. Occasionally, urgent coronary angiogram may be done to confirm the diagnosis (Bojar, 1994).

Postpericardiotomy Syndrome

Postpericardiotomy Syndrome (PPS) is one of the most common postoperative complications related to open heart surgery. It occurs in anywhere from 10 to 50% of all patients. It may occur as early as postoperative day 3, or as late as 6 months after surgery, as well as occurring repetitively. The etiology is thought to be an autoimmune inflammatory response to a foreign protein (i.e., blood) remaining in the pericardium after surgery. PPS has a variable presentation and the diagnosis is based on clinical findings that include: fever with a negative work-up, leukocytosis, anterior chest wall pain that increases with inspiration or lying supine, and an audible pericardial friction rub. PPS can cause considerable postoperative discomfort, prolong length of stay, and—in the worst-case scenario—cause cardiac tamponade. It has also been suggested as a cause of premature coronary artery bypass graft closure (Bojar, 1994; Miller, Horneffer, Gardner, Rykiel, & Pearson, 1988). Treatment of PPS is symptom oriented and most commonly involves use of nonsteroidal antiinflammatories or steroids.

Pericardial Effusion and Cardiac Tamponade

Pericardial effusions occur in approximately 50% of patients following open heart surgery. Fortunately, the vast majority are asymptomatic and resolve completely. A small percentage of effusions do, however, increase in size becoming hemodynamically significant. Etiologies include: intrapericardial bleed related to anticoagulation or antiplatelet therapy, removal of epicardial pacemaker wires, postpericardiotomy syndrome, postoperative coagulopathy, and true surgical bleeding.

Cardiac tamponade occurs in less than 1% of patients after cardiac surgery. Patients who have excessive bleeding from their mediastinal chest tubes are at greatest risk for acute cardiac tamponade due to the increased incidence of clot formation or blood accumulation not drained by the tubes. Be especially suspicious when there is an abrupt decrease or cessation of drainage that occurs (Shinn, 1992). Conversely, delayed or late tamponade usually occurs as a result of postpericardiotomy syndrome. It can occur weeks to months following surgery and is often more difficult to diagnose because often the symptoms are vague and insidious, making it difficult to differentiate them from a "slow" postoperative recovery.

Signs and symptoms associated with pericardial effusion and tamponade include jugulovenous distention, pericardial rub, muffled heart sounds, pulsus paradoxus, and hypotension. Be suspicious if chest x-ray demonstrates an increased cardiac sillouhette. Diagnosis is usually made by echocardiogram. Pericardiocentesis under fluoroscopy is the least invasive intervention and is a reasonable approach for a patient with a nonloculated, pericardial effusion. Initiation of nonsteroidal antiinflammatories or steroids is often effective for effusions caused by postpericardiotomy syndrome. Mediastinal exploration is indicated for acute tamponade associated with active bleeding.

Pulmonary

Atelectasis

Atelectasis is the most common, minor respiratory abnormality following cardiac surgery. In fact, is also one of the most common culprits of early postoperative fever. Some degree of atelectasis is almost an expected postoperative finding. The cause is multifactorial including fluid overload, splinting on inspiration due to chest wall discomfort, and decreased surfactant production while the lungs are deflated on cardiopulmonary bypass. Atelectasis is easily treated with aggressive pulmonary hygiene.

Pneumonia

Pneumonia occasionally occurs due to colonization of the upper respiratory tract in patients requiring prolonged intubation. Its typical presentation includes fever, leukocytosis, increased oxygen requirements, and new infiltrate on chest x-ray. Pneumonia is usually treated with aggressive pulmonary hygiene coupled with an organism-specific antimicrobial drug (Finkelmeier, 1995).

Pleural Effusion

Pleural effusion is a common postoperative finding, especially on the left side if the left internal thoracic artery was harvested (i.e., requires entry into pleural space). Most postoperative pleural effusions are small, stable, and resolve over time; however, occasionally, they are either persistent, increase in size, or the patient develops respiratory compromise. In that scenario, the effusion may be treated with either thoracentesis or chest tube drainage (Finkelmeier, 1995).

Diaphragm Dysfunction

Injury to the phrenic nerve resulting in paresis or paralysis can occur after cardiac surgery because of the anatomic proximity of the nerve to the operative field. The phrenic nerve runs along the parietal pericardium. Hypothermic injury can result from intraoperative topical cooling of the heart using ice slush solution. The nerve can also be directly damaged during takedown of the internal thoracic artery. Most patients usually have unilateral phrenic nerve paresis with resultant minor respiratory symptoms, unless the patient had marginal baseline pulmonary function. The diagnosis of phrenic nerve injury is suggestive by persistent elevation of the diaphragm on chest x-ray. However, this can sometimes be obscured by concomitant left lower lobe atelectasis or pleural effusion. The diagnosis can be confirmed by the "sniff test" (i.e., diaphragmatic fluoroscopy) which would demonstrate paradoxical motion of the diaphragm on inspiration. Treatment is usually supportive until phrenic nerve function recovers. Ventilatory support may be necessary if there is bilateral nerve involvement. Diaphragmatic plication may also provide significant relief of symptoms in these cases (Bojar, 1994).

Neurologic

Central Neurologic Deficit

Central neurologic deficit following cardiac surgery is usually related to cerebral hypoperfusion or particulate embolization. Preoperative risk factors include age greater than 75, diabetes mellitus, preexisting cerebrovascular disease (known atheromatous/calcified plaques), left heart mural thrombus, and atrial fibrillation. Clinical presentation depends on the site and extent of the cerebral insult. Common presentations include: transient ischemic attack (TIA) or focal deficits (e.g., hemiparesis/plegia, aphasia, visual deficits). In the worst-case scenario, a postoperative central neurological deficit manifests itself as coma. Methods of evaluation include neurological examination, transesophageal echocardiogram, and CAT scan. Once an intracranial bleed is ruled out, anticoagulation is indicated for embolic strokes. Other treatment modalities include standard measures to decrease intracranial pressure, carotid endartarectomy for significant cerebrovascular disease, and physical therapy.

Peripheral Neurological Damage

Compression of the lower trunk of the brachial plexus during retraction of the sternum may produce brachial plexus injury. Patients usually present with numbness and parasthesia in the ulnar nerve distribution (i.e., fourth and fifth digits). Electromyelogram may be useful in assessing the extent of deficit but is not performed routinely. Treatment usually consists of physical therapy. Tegretol is also often helpful for pain associated with nerve injury (Bojar, 1994; Finkelmeier, 1995).

Recurrent laryngeal nerve injury is a rare complication associated with internal thoracic artery mobilization; however, it is seen more commonly in surgeries involving the transverse aortic arch because of the anatomic proximity of the two structures. Patients usually present with hoarseness or difficulty swallowing with associated aspiration. The diagnosis of recurrent laryngeal nerve damage is confirmed by laryngoscopic examination of the vocal cords. Treatment with fat injection of the cords as a temporizing measure is often employed until nerve function returns (Bojar, 1994).

Delirium

Acute changes in a patient's mental status after cardiac surgery are fairly common with an incidence approaching 30%. Risk factors include increased age, recent alcohol use, preoperative organic brain syndrome, complex prolonged surgery on cardiopulmonary bypass, and prolonged intensive care unit stay. Although the cause is often multifactorial, it is important to rule out common treatable things such as medication, alcohol withdrawal, low cardiac output, hypoxia, sepsis, and cerebral vascular accident.

Other neuropsychological problems are common after cardiac surgery. They are frequently subtle and transient, occurring in the form of cognitive dysfunction. In fact, cognitive dysfunction occurs in up to 70% of all heart surgery patients and persists for up to three weeks postoperatively. These types of neurological deficits have been shown to decrease over time and most patients return to their preoperative level of functioning within six months (Bojar, 1994; Shinn, 1992).

Renal

Fluid and Electrolyte Imbalances. A multitude of physiologic derangements associated with the use of cardiopulmonary bypass are responsible for the fluid and electrolyte imbalances so commonly seen in the early postoperative period. Some of the more common alterations include: (1) increased release of renin and aldosterone resulting in sodium retention and potassium excretion, (2) elevation in angiotensin II levels producing vasoconstriction, (3) increased vasopressin secretion which increases systemic vascular resistance and produces a sodium diuresis by directly impairing tubular absorption, (4) elevation of plasma-free cortisol contributing to sodium retention and enhancing potassium excretion, and (5) other vasoactive substances released during cardiopulmonary bypass altering vascular tone and producing the generalized inflammatory response that increases capillary permeability (Bojar, 1994).

Renal Failure. Extracorporeal circulation during open heart surgery produces dramatic changes in both fluid distribution and renal function. Hypothermia, nonpulsatile perfusion, and hemodilution all contribute to a decreased renal blood flow, decreased glomerular filtration rate, and some degree of tubular injury. Transient renal dysfunction affects approximately 5 to 7% of patients undergoing cardiac surgery. It is most likely to occur in those patients with preoperative renal insufficiency, left ventricular dysfunction, age greater than 75, and concomitant comorbidities such as hypertension, diabetes, or peripheral vascular disease. Oliguric renal failure requiring some form of dialysis develops in approximately 2% of patients and carries an operative mortality of 30 to 50% (Bojar, 1994).

Management of postoperative renal dysfunction is tricky at best. The overall goal is to maintain adequate intravascular volume in order to prevent prerenal azotemia without producing pulmonary edema, while simultaneously using diuretics to create a negative fluid balance with a rising BUN and creatinine. Treatment is especially difficult in patients who have borderline myocardial function. Despite the complex array of contributing factors, low cardiac output remains the number one culprit in the development of postoperative renal failure. General management strategies of oliguria include: ensuring Foley catheter patency, optimizing cardiac output, initiation of renal dose Dopamine, diuretics, and consideration of dialysis if there is evidence of hyperkalemia, hypervolemia, metabolic acidosis, or progressive uremia (Bojar, 1994).

Gastrointestinal

Gastrointestinal (GI) complications affect approximately 1 to 2% of all patients undergoing cardiac surgery. Although they are relatively uncommon, abdominal complications can be quite serious. Patients with GI complications require on the average a fourfold increase in length of stay when compared with those patients with uncomplicated courses. Also, a large percentage of patients who develop GI complications require surgical intervention, with an associated operative mortality as high as 40% (Halm, 1996).

Paralytic Ileus. Paralytic ileus occasionally persists for several days after surgery. It is usually a benign, self-limiting process, but occasionally it may reflect sepsis or severe intraabdominal pathology. The most common contributing factors in the postoperative period are immobility and narcotics. Postoperative ileus is characterized by abdominal distention, absent bowel sounds, failure to pass flatus or stool, and radiographic evidence of dilated loops of bowel. Keeping the patient NPO with nasogastric decompression until peristaltic activity returns are the most common treatment modalities (Bojar, 1994; Finkelmeier, 1995).

Gastrointestinal Bleeding. Of all the GI complications, GI bleeding is most amenable to prevention. Prophylaxis consists of antacid therapy, histamine receptor antagonists, and sulcralfate. Most episodes of GI bleeding occur around postoperative day four. The majority of upper GI bleeding occurs from gastroduodenal sources such as esophagitis, preexisting peptic ulcer disease, and stress ulceration. Conversely, lower GI bleeding is usually the result of mesenteric ischemia, diverticulosis, colonic lesion (e.g., polyp or tumor), and colonic angiodysplasia (Heyde's syndrome) which is associated with aortic stenosis. Clinical manifestations of GI bleeding may include: hematemesis and melana (upper GI), hematochezia and bright red blood per rectum (lower GI), epigastric distress, decreased hemoglobin and hematocrit, and elevation of blood urea nitrogen. Endoscopy is the definitive diagnostic tool for upper GI bleeding and colonoscopy is the diagnostic tool used most commonly for lower GI bleed. Treatment consists of correction of any coagulopathy, lavage, fluid resuscitation, supplemental oxygen, endoscopic sclerotherapy, and surgery (Halm, 1996).

Intestinal Ischemia. For unknown reasons, the superior mesenteric artery, which supplies the small intestine and right half of the colon, is most frequently associated with perioperative ischemia and infarction. Postoperative intestinal ischemia is most commonly associated with prolonged low cardiac output states in combination with use of alpha adrenergic agents; however, it may also be caused by embolism or mesenteric thrombosis. The clinical spectrum of intestinal wall damage goes from mucosal edema to transmural necrosis, which may lead to perforation, peritonitis, and sepsis. Intestinal ischemia produces severe abdominal pain. In critically ill, sedated, or moribund patients be suspicious of metabolic acidosis, watery/bloody diarrhea, peritoneal signs, fever, leukocytosis, and shock-like symptoms. Diagnosis can be made by angiogram of the abdominal aorta but more commonly, the patient in whom there is a high index of suspicion is taken to the operating room for exploratory laparotomy and possible bowel resection.

Acute Symptomatic Cholecystitis. Normal gallbladder function is disrupted following cardiac surgery most likely as a result of hypoperfusion. In addition, fasting, parenteral nutrition, and narcotics all decrease gallbladder contraction producing biliary stasis. Acalculous (as opposed to calculous) cholecystitis occurs more frequently with an overall incidence of 3 to 5% (Halm, 1996). Diagnosis can be difficult because of non-specific findings. Right upper quadrant ultrasound and HIDA scan can identify a dilated gallbladder and biliary obstruction. Cholecystectomy is usually the treatment of choice unless the patient is considered too critically ill to tolerate the procedure.

Hepatic Dysfunction. Clinical jaundice may occur in the absence of other GI findings. There are several etiologies associated with the development of postoperative jaundice. An increased pigment load due to administration of large amounts of bank blood and increased red blood cell hemolysis is a common prehepatic etiology. However, hypotension and hypoxia are the two predominant and often coexistent causes of hepatic dysfunction leading to jaundice. Hepatotoxic drugs, positive pressure ventilation, congestive heart failure, and sepsis are other significant causes of clinical jaundice. Preoperative right heart failure predisposes the patient to jaundice because of hepatic congestion and decreased ability of the liver to conjugate bilirubin. Most postoperative cases of hepatic dysfunction are mild and self-limiting. It is imperative that adequate urine output be maintained in these patients to prevent renal failure from hemoglobinuria.

Pancreatitis. Hyperamylasemia is noted in approximately 35% of patients following cardiopulmonary bypass; however, it is associated with clinical pancreatitis in only 1 to 3% of all patients (Halm, 1996). Subclinical pancreatitis is suggested by the presence of anorexia, nausea, and ileus coupled with elevation in serum amylase and lipase. In fact, many times this subclinical form of pancreatitis may go undiagnosed. It usually resolves spontaneously and is not associated with significant morbidity or mortality. Although a brief period of bowel rest may be beneficial in these patients, no specific treatment is necessary unless there is evidence of overt pancreatitis or GI tract dysfunction (Bojar, 1994). Overt pancreatitis usually occurs as a result of ischemic necrotic injury from hypoperfusion. Acute symptomatic postoperative pancreatitis may take two forms: interstitial or hemorrhage. Interstitial pancreatitis is characterized by pancreatic edema and usually responds well to conservative treatment (i.e., nasogastric drainage and antibiotics). Hemorrhagic pancreatitis carries a much higher morbidity and mortality. It is associated with other organ systems injury due to low cardiac output. Exploratory laparotomy with debridement and drainage is usually a last resort; however, it may be the only hope for survival in patients with necrotizing pancreatitis.

Hematological

Hemorrhage postcardiac surgery is characterized by sustained chest tube output greater than 100 ml/h or greater than 300 mL in any one hour. The patient subset most prone to postoperative bleeding includes those who: (1) have undergone previous cardiac operations, (2) have liver dysfunction, (3) have an underlying bleeding disorder, (4) have received recent antiplatelet or anticoagulant therapy, (5) required a long operation with associated prolonged period of CPB, and (6) have friable tissue or an underlying pathologic process likely to be associated with hemorrhage (e.g., aortic dissection or aneurysm) (Finkelmeier, 1995). Postoperative bleeding can be broadly categorized into surgical or non-surgical (i.e., coagulopathy). Surgical bleeding is the culprit in approximately half the patients who require reexploration. Conversely, the qualitative and quantitative platelet dysfunction associated with CPB is the most common cause for postoperative coagulopathy. Nonsurgical bleeding may also be caused by inadequate heparin reversal at the end of CPB as well as fibrinolysis, complement activation, and depletion of factors V, VIII, and XIII. Coagulopathy is more common in patients who have received antiplatelet agents, thrombolytic therapy, or heparin in the preoperative period (Finkelmeier, 1995).

Infectious Complications

Leg Wounds. Superficial infection of the leg incision (saphenous vein harvest site) is a problem most commonly encountered in those patients who are obese, diabetic, have severe peripheral edema, or peripheral vascular disease. Leg wound infections may also occur as a result of poor surgical technique resulting in creation of flaps, failure to eliminate dead space, or hematoma formation (Bojar, 1994). Clinical presentation includes cellulitis, wound breakdown with purulent drainage, or skin necrosis from flaps or subcutaneous hematoma. Leg wound infections are treated with local drainage, debridement, and frequent dressing changes. Infections are treated with organism-specific antibiotics.

Sternal Wounds. Sternal dehiscence is defined as the separation of the wired sternal halves. Although dehiscence is usually associated with deep infection of the sternal wound, it may also occur in the absence of wound infection. A sterile sternal dehiscence can be caused by initial surgical division of the sternum that is off center, erosion of the sternal wires through the bone, wires that are not tight enough, excessive and forceful postoperative coughing, and patient noncompliance with limitations on activities involving the upper extremities (Finkelmeier, 1995). Mechanical dehiscence usually occurs earlier in the postoperative course than does dehiscence associated with infection and is corrected with reoperation and sternal rewiring.

Sternal wound infections complicate approximately 2% of all cardiac operations. Staphylococcus aureus and Staphylococcus epidermis are the most common offending organisms despite perioperative antibiotic prophylaxis with agents having excellent gram positive coverage. Loop et al. (1990) describe the most common risk factors associated with the development of postoperative sternal wound infections to include: (1) duration of the operative procedure, (2) diabetes is an independent risk factor and the risk is significantly greater among patients who receive bilateral thoracic artery grafts, (3) obesity, (4) mediastinal reexploration for bleeding, (5) redo surgeries, (6) prolonged episodes of low cardiac output, and (7) prolonged ventilatory support.

Sternal wounds can be either superficial (i.e., confined to the subcutaneous tissue) or deep in which the infection extends down to and involves the sternum and mediastinum. An unstable sternum with serous or purulent wound drainage is often the first warning sign of infection. Other indicators include: fever, leukocytosis, and gram positive bacteremia. Keep in mind that elderly, diabetic, and malnourished patients are notorious for mounting a very poor inflammatory response and may present several weeks following surgery with extensive purulent mediastinitis and few systemic signs (Bojar, 1994).

Most superficial sternal wound infections respond to local wound care and long-term (i.e., six weeks) intravenous antibiotics; however, deep sternal wound infections usually require mediastinal reexploration. The goal of treatment is to debride all infected and avascular tissue as well as obliterate all dead space. The closed method of treatment entails placement of substernal drainage catheters for mediastinal irrigation. Irrigation is usually continued for three to five days or until the effluent becomes sterile. Irrigants include antibiotic solutions or dilute povidone–iodine. Povidone–iodine is probably used more frequently because of its effectiveness and because reports that continuous mediastinal lavage with antibiotics may predispose the patient to fungal infection and antibiotic toxicity. Caution should be used, however, when using povidone–iodine because its use has been associated with the development of constrictive pericarditis (Loop et al., 1990). The open method of treatment for deep sternal wound infection and sternal osteomyelitis involves radical debridement, sternectomy, and placement of muscle flaps (e.g., pectoralis major or rectus abdominus). Applying muscle flaps brings a rich network of blood supply to the poorly vascularized bone. This is thought to increase oxygen tension as well as intravascular delivery of antibiotics to the infected area. In addition to enhancing regional blood supply, the muscle flap also serves to eradicate empty space within the mediastinum.

Deep sternal wound infection necessitates meticulous attention to wound management and antibiotic administration. Bacteremia with the potential to develop septic shock is a possible complication associated with surgical debridement. Other complications associated with mediastinitis include spread of infection to the aortic or cardiac suture lines, especially if felt pledgets were used at the time of surgery. Hospital mortality rates approach 14% (Loop et al., 1990) and multisystem failure involving renal failure is reported to be the most common mode of death.

Discharge Planning and Ambulatory Postoperative Care

With the advent of "patient care pathways" and "fast tracking," patients are being discharged from the hospital progressively earlier after open heart surgery, sometimes as early as postoperative day three or four. The ACNP plays a key role in discharge planning as well as attentive outpatient care.

Discharge Planning

Getting discharged from the hospital is usually a great relief to the patient, but can often also be quite stressful. Patients need reassurance that it is safe for them to leave the hospital environment. They also need education regarding what are common signs and symptoms that are a normal part of recovery versus problems that should be reported right away to the surgeon or nurse practitioner. Written and verbal instructions should also be given regarding medications, activity, restrictions, diet, wound care, risk factor modification, follow-up appointments, as well as instructions as to what to do and who to call if they are experiencing a problem.

Discharge medications vary from patient to patient depending on the type of surgery and the patient's underlying pathology. In general, all CAB patients are discharged on antiplatelet therapy (e.g., aspirin) for graft patency and all patients with mechanical valves are discharged on warfarin. It is essential that any patient receiving an anticoagulant gets explicit instructions regarding follow-up anticoagulation blood studies. Also, any patient at risk for endocarditis (e.g., valve repair or replacement, aortic grafts) must be educated according to the American Heart Association guidelines regarding antibiotic prophylaxis.

Although activity also varies among patients, most patients should be able to perform self care prior to discharge. They should be instructed on a home walking program, increasing up to 1 mile/day by the fourth postoperative week.

There are very few activity restrictions in the early postoperative recovery period. Heavy lifting (i.e., anything greater than 5 pounds) is absolutely contraindicated for 6 to 8 weeks, which is the usual length of time needed for the sternum to heal. Likewise, any exercise or sport that involves vigorous arm movements (e.g., golf, tennis, bowling, swimming, weight lifting, rowing machines, push-ups, chin-ups, and sit-ups) should be avoided for 6 to 8 weeks. Female patients with large breasts should be instructed to wear a bra at all times to reduce tension on the sternal incision (Finkelmeier, 1995). Most surgeons also instruct patients not to drive for at least 4 weeks. This prevents the patient from attempting to drive when reaction times may still be slowed as well as avoiding potential injury to the sternum should an accident occur and result in blunt trauma to the chest (Finkelmeier, 1995).

Outpatient Follow-Up

Patients are usually seen in the outpatient setting 2 to 4 weeks following discharge from the hospital. Postoperative patients commonly present at this point in their recovery with a complex array of complaints. Most complaints, however, are expected, self-limiting alterations in both their physical and psychological state that are associated with open heart surgery.

Fatigue is probably the number one patient complaint following cardiac surgery and because it causes patients to be less active during the day, insomnia is also a universal problem. To combat fatigue and insomnia, patients should be instructed to space their activities, allow for rest periods, and avoid late afternoon naps.

All of the surgical incisions should be healing without evidence of erythema, edema, or wound drainage and the sternum should be assessed for any evidence of nonunion. It is normal to have mild distal saphenous vein graft harvest site edema for several weeks to months following surgery because of disruption of the lymphatic channels. To combat this problem, remind patients to wear support stockings during the day and to always elevate the affected leg higher than the hips when sitting or lying supine. To assess for sternal stability, apply firm pressure with your hands on either side of the sternotomy incision and ask the patient to cough. Nonunion manifests itself as a palpable movement or "clicking." It occurs most frequently in patients who are obese, diabetic, receiving steroids, or in those who have had previous sternotomy, postoperative reexploration of incision, or closed chest massage.

Mild to moderate incisional discomfort is expected. It is important, however, to get a thorough pain history and differentiate musculoskeletal or pleuritic pain from return of angina. Be suspicious of infection and/or sternal wire irritation if the patient has persistent moderate to severe wound pain reproducible with palpation and start looking for other clinical evidence to substantiate or refute this.

In summary, convalescence continues for several months after the patient has been discharged from the hospital. Most postoperative problems are self-limiting and can be easily managed by a competent nurse practitioner. Postoperative assessment should take into consideration the patient's underlying pathology as well as the type of surgical procedure performed. This enables the nurse practitioner to differentiate between expected consequences and significant complications that may warrant further evaluation, rehospitalization, and/or consultation with attending surgeon.

ACQUIRED CARDIAC SURGICAL DISEASES

Coronary Artery Disease

Coronary artery bypass (CAB) surgery is the consequence of continuous evolution starting in 1910 with the work of Alexis Carrel, evolving up to 1968 when Favaloro and Effler at the Cleveland Clinic reported on 171 coronary operations with a 4.6% patient mortality (Favaloro, 1994). Over the next several years, surgical techniques were refined and expanded to include all branches of the coronary arteries. By the mid 1970s, CAB was widely performed and the relative advantage of surgical revascularization versus the natural history of coronary artery disease was beginning to be defined.

Today, CAB is the most common procedure performed in adult cardiac surgery. Most cardiac surgical programs are now faced with a patient population that is older, has increased comorbidities, poorer left ventricular function, and more redo procedures. Along with this shift has come an evolution in surgical techniques, myocardial protection, and conduit choice. The benefit of using the left internal mammary artery to bypass the left anterior descending coronary artery appears irrefutable at this time. Data from multiarterial grafts are still evolving and conduit choice for other than mammary to LAD is still debated (Reardon, Conklin, Reardon, & Baldwin, 1997).

Goals of Surgery

The objectives of CAB are to relieve ischemia by providing increased blood flow to the myocardium beyond the area of coronary artery stenosis and to improve long-term survival by preventing myocardial infarction and preserving left ventricular function.

Indications for Surgery

Three large randomized, prospective, clinical studies were initiated in the 1970s to evaluate the outcome of CAB on survival and to clarify the indications for surgery. They included the Veterans Administrative Cooperative Study (1972–1974), the European Coronary Surgery Study (1973–1976), and the Coronary Artery Surgery Study (1975–1979). In the 20 some years since these study results have been reported, however, several important changes in both the conduct of coronary surgery as well as perioperative patient monitoring and management strategies have occurred. Therefore, previously reported results are of limited value in the current era of surgical revascularization. Unfortunately, no comparable studies have been carried out since then. Robert Bojar (1992) summarizes some of the most notable changes that have occurred since these studies as: (1) widespread use of cardioplegia which was not available then, (2) many patients managed with one or two vessel CAB at the time of these studies are now undergoing coronary angioplasty, (3) the internal mammary artery was not used in any study—the decreasing benefit of surgery with time in all three studies reflects attrition of saphenous vein grafts, (4) anesthetic regimes and intraoperative monitoring techniques were less sophisticated in the 1970s—now we routinely use Fentanyl-based anesthesia, Swan-Ganz catheters, and intraoperative transesophageal echocardiogram, (5) the surgical techniques themselves have improved, (6) there is increased sophistication and availability of postoperative monitoring as well as pharmacologic agents, and (7) intraaortic balloon pumps as well as other circulatory-assist devices are now widely available. Currently accepted indications for CAB surgery are outlined in Table 34–4 (ACC/AHA Task Force Report, 1991; Baue et al., 1995; Bojar, 1992; Finkelmeier, 1995; Sabiston & Spencer, 1995).

Criteria for Suitable Target Vessel

There are several anatomic findings during cardiac catheterization that determine suitability of a vessel for bypass grafting, including: (1) percent stenosis of the arterial lumen, (2) diameter of the coronary artery distal to the stenosis (target vessel), and (3) myocardial viability in the areas supplied by the artery in question.

The current surgical strategy for coronary artery disease is to obtain complete revascularization by bypassing all severe stenosis (i.e., greater than 50%) in all coronary artery trunks and branches except those of trivial (i.e., less than 1 millimeter in diameter) size (Kirklin & Barratt-Boyes, 1993). If preoperative assessment of ventricular function demonstrates an area of akinesia, noninvasive viability studies should be obtained to differentiate hibernating myocardium from dead myocardium.

Cab Conduits

Traditional Conduits for CAB. CAB is performed in the vast majority of patients using a combination of saphenous vein and internal thoracic artery (ITA), also called the internal mammary artery (IMA).

Saphenous Vein. Saphenous vein has been the gold standard for CAB since its inception in the 1960s. It is easily harvested, has a diameter similar to that of the coronary artery, is generally available in substantial quantities, and has a better flow rate than ITAs (Reardon et al., 1997). The rapidity with which the saphenous vein can be harvested makes it the conduit of choice in emergent situations such as failed coronary angioplasty or acute myocardial infarction.

Over the years, however, it has become increasingly evident that the greater saphenous vein has several distinct disadvantages. Early patency studies have demonstrated a 1-month occlusion rate of approximately 10%, a 2 to 4% per year occlusion rate in the first 5 years, and a 4 to 8% per

TABLE 34–4. Indications for Coronary Artery Bypass Surgery

Clinical Indications	Anatomic Indications
1. Class III–IV angina refractory to medical management	1. Left main stenosis > 50% either alone or in combination with other lesions
2. Post-infarction angina	2. Three-vessel disease with impaired left ventricular function
3. Acute ischemia or hemodynamic instability following unsuccessful coronary angioplasty (PTCA)	3. Three-vessel disease with normal left ventricular function but inducible ischemia
4. Acute evolving infarction within 6 hours of onset of pain with/without failed PTCA or thrombolytic therapy	4. Two-vessel disease with significant proximal LAD stenosis before the first septal perforator
5. Cardiogenic shock and/or mechanical complications from acute myocardial infarction	5. Coronary anomalies associated with risk of sudden death
6. Ischemic pulmonary edema	6. Complex lesions not suitable for interventional procedures

year occlusion rate after the fifth year. Occlusion within the first month of surgery appears to be most closely related to technical factors such as poor anastomosis, poor vein quality, and/or poor distal target. From 1 month to 3 years intimal hyperplasia plays the predominant role in graft closure, and after 3 years accelerated atherosclerosis is the main mode of saphenous vein graft failure (Reardon et al., 1997).

For removal of the greater saphenous vein, the patient's leg is abducted anterolaterally and the knee is flexed at 45 degrees (Fig. 34–8).

Approximately 15 centimeters in length is needed to bypass the diagonal branches of the left anterior descending coronary artery, 20 centimeters for the marginal branches of the circumflex artery, and 18 centimeters for the right coronary artery and its branches (Kirklin & Barratt-Boyes, 1993). The importance of atraumatic technique in dissection, removal, and preparation of the saphenous vein cannot be overemphasized. Excessive traction and/or high pressure distention are associated with endothelial injury with resultant premature intimal hyperplasia.

Internal Thoracic Artery. The internal thoracic artery (ITA) has now become the preferred conduit because its long-term patency rates are superior to that of the saphenous vein. Data clearly demonstrates that use of ITA lowers the risk of late deaths, myocardial infarction, and reoperation. Histologically, the ITA has qualities that make it relatively immune to the three biologic modes of graft failure affecting veins: early thrombosis, subintimal fibrosis, and late atherosclerosis. Consequently, the benefit of using the ITA to bypass the left anterior descending coronary artery, or alternatively, the vessel judged to be the most critical to myocardial function, is irrefutable at this time. The greatest limitation to using ITA is that it is more tedious to takedown, has limited length, and there are only two of them.

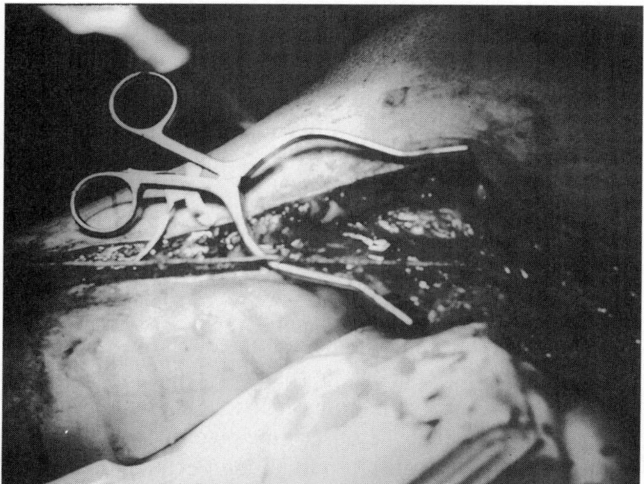

Figure 34–8. Correct positioning of leg for harvest of greater saphenous vein. Notice that the leg is abducted anterolaterally and that the knee is flexed at 45°.

ITA can be harvested as either a pedicle or free graft. When used as a pedicle graft, the vessel is dissected from the underside of the chest wall in its fat pedicle (Fig. 34–9).

The origin is left intact at its anatomic connection to the subclavian artery and the distal end is attached to the target vessel using an end-to-side anastomosis. Free flow is checked prior to anastomosis. Flow rates less than 120 mL/min indicate either vessel spasm, subclavian disease, intimal disease, or vessel injury. If free flow is diminished, a pedicle graft should not be used. Conversely, an ITA free graft is anastomosed proximally to the aorta in the same fashion as the saphenous vein and the distal end is attached to the target coronary artery vessel (Fig. 34–10). ITA free and pedicle grafts appear to have similar long-term patency rates, greater than 90% at 10 years.

Since unilateral grafting has proven so effective, many surgeons have begun performing bilateral ITA grafting; however, while it has been well documented that one ITA decreases cardiac morbidity and mortality, it has been more difficult to document improved long-term outcome when both ITAs are used. Most current data suggest that use of both ITAs reduces occurrence of ischemic events, but not mortality rates, when compared with left ITA placement to the left anterior descending coronary artery. This benefit applies to patients under 60 years of age.

Alternative Arterial Conduits. As the incidence of redo coronary operations continues to increase, the problem of conduit availability has become an important issue. The primary argument for use of the "newer" alternative arterial conduits, even when the ITAs or saphenous vein are available, is based on the assumed long-term patency that is extrapolated from the excellent long-term patency of the ITA (Barner, 1994). There is no data to suggest that use of three or more arterial conduits reduces ischemic events or improves survival rates, mostly because numbers are small and follow-up is limited. All arterial grafts have in common that inadequate flow can occur postoperatively due to vessel spasm, caliber mismatch (i.e., arteries are smaller in diameter than veins which can limit blood flow relative to demand, especially in the postischemic state when demand is increased), and steal phenomenon, which results in the so-called malperfusion syndrome (Schmid & Scheld, 1996).

Radial Artery. The radial artery was the second arterial conduit introduced into clinical practice by Carpentier and associates in 1973. Early patency for this conduit was dismal in comparison with the saphenous vein and ITA and, consequently, 2 years later, Carpentier abandoned use of the radial artery because of severe diffuse narrowing in 35% of the grafts. At the time, this was attributed to spasm of the denervated artery. Recently, however, the radial artery is being revived with encouraging early results after gaining more knowledge on how to overcome vessel spasm.

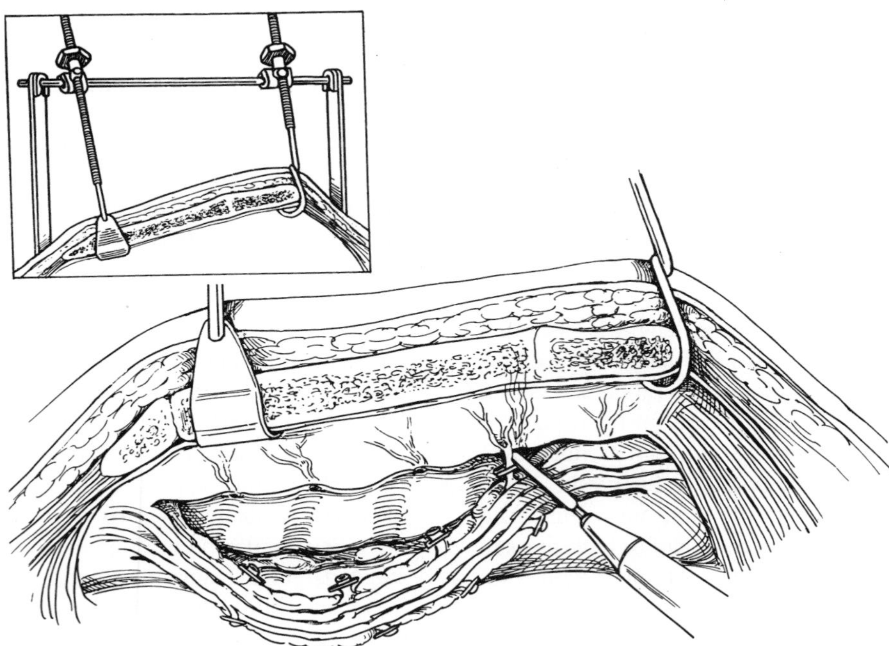

Figure 34–9. Takedown of the right internal thoracic artery using a modified Favaloro retractor (Navco Pilling Co., Fort Washington, PA.). *(Used with permission from* Operative Techniques in Cardiac and Thoracic Surgery, *Philadelphia: W. B. Saunders Company, 1996.)*

Preoperative Allen test is routinely performed on all patients considered candidates for radial artery harvest. The ulnar and radial arteries are occluded at the wrist, the hand is vigorously opened and closed several times, and the ulnar artery is then released. Intense capillary refilling of the palmar surface of the hand and digits should occur within 3 to 5 seconds. Calcium blocking agents, beginning with intraoperative intravenous infusion, followed by intravenous infusion postoperatively with a transition to oral therapy for 3 to 6 months, is a common therapy to avoid vessel spasm. To minimize the risk of infection or hematoma, no intravenous or arterial lines should be placed in the donor arm.

Because the radial artery is a so-called "obligatory free graft," it is necessary to perform a proximal anastomosis either to the aorta or to an *in situ* arterial conduit (Barner, 1996).

The incision to harvest the radial artery is made from the wrist to the mid antecubital fossa (over the radial pulse extending to over the brachial pulse). The antebrachialis fascia is incised, the brachioradialis muscle is retracted laterally in its entire length, and then the radial artery is dissected (Fig. 34–11). Emphasis on proper harvesting technique to avoid spasm and intimal hyperplasia is a must (Dietl & Benoit, 1995). Possible complications related to harvest of the radial artery include hand claudication.

In summary, reasons for early poor patency in contrast to the recent good results probably relate to better understanding of the need for atraumatic harvest, use of Papaverine to overcome graft spasm, and avoidance of intragraft saline that destroys endothelium. Additionally, intraoperative and postoperative use of calcium channel blocking agents have proven valuable in treating or preventing graft spasm (Barner, 1994).

Gastroepiploic Artery. The right gastroepiploic artery (GEA) was first used in the 1960s as a substitute for the left ITA in the Vineberg operation. Many surgeons began using it in the early 1980s for CAB, but it was Suma who popularized its clinical use in 1984 (Califiore & DiGiammarco, 1996). The GEA continued to gain popularity with demonstrated patency rates of 95% at 5 years in two series (Barner, 1994). Although the GEA is easier to harvest than the ITA and has short-term patency rates similar to the ITA, it is still considered a relatively new conduit for revascularization and there is lack of long-term follow-up studies (Fig. 34–12).

The GEA can be used as either a pedicled or a free graft. It is exposed by extending the sternotomy incision by 5 to 8 centimeters into the epigastrum and entering the peritoneal cavity (Figs. 34–13 and 34–14). A pedicled right GEA can be anastomosed to all three coronary arteries. There is increased patient morbidity related to harvest of the GEA due to the laparotomy incision which is necessary to retrieve the graft. There is also the potential risk of bleeding or incisional hernia. Reported complications, however, are virtually nonexistent. Early fears of gastric ischemia, pancreatitis, and ileus have not materialized (Barner, 1994).

There are several disadvantages to using the GEA including: (1) it should not be used in patients who have had

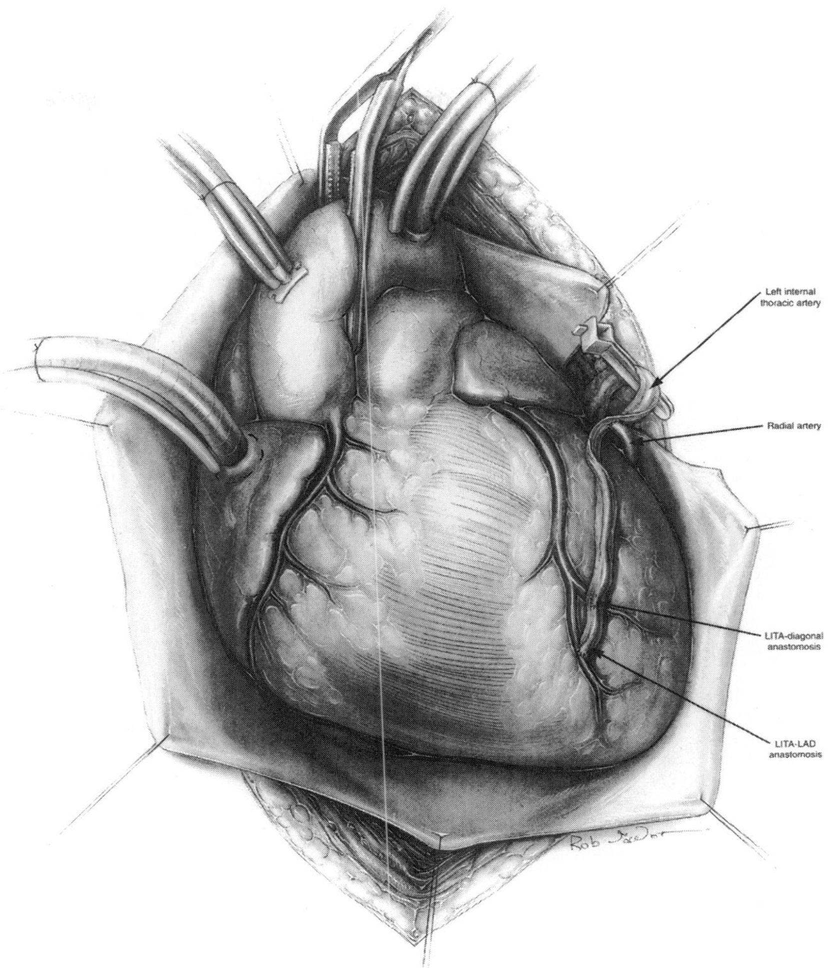

Figure 34–10. The left ITA is used as a sequential bypass graft to the left anterior descending and diagonal coronary arteries. The radial artery is used to bypass the circumflex coronary artery. The proximal end of the radial artery is anastomosed end-to-side to the *in situ* ITA graft. *(Used with permission from* Operative Techniques in Cardiac and Thoracic Surgery, *Philadelphia: W. B. Saunders Company, 1996.)*

previous gastric surgeries, (2) it is technically difficult to harvest in obese patients, and (3) there is the potential for graft damage during future abdominal operations. Nevertheless, many cardiothoracic surgeons support this vessel as the third alternative after the saphenous vein and ITA (Reardon et al., 1997).

Inferior Epigastric Artery. The inferior epigastric artery (IEA) is one of the most recent arterial conduits under trial as an alternative graft for CAB and published results are scarce. Preliminary patency rates of the IEA are lower than those of pedicled ITA grafts (Buche & Dion, 1996). Patency is somewhat less than the GEA and reported to be 88% at 10 days and 85% at 6 months. Recent data demonstrate at 1 year, 25% of these grafts were either occluded or significantly diseased (Schmid & Scheld, 1996).

Harvesting the IEA does not require laparotomy and bilateral use of the vessel is feasible. Midline or paramedian incision from the umbilicus to the symphysis pubis is used to harvest the IEA (Figs. 34–15 and 34–16). The midline approach with lateral retraction of the rectus muscle allows for one or both IEAs to be mobilized, but the paramedian incision with medial rectus retraction or splitting of the muscle provides better exposure (Barner, 1994).

A significant percentage of IEAs bifurcate before reaching the umbilicus, thereby limiting conduit length. As with the radial artery, the IEA is used as a free graft. The only difference is in length (i.e., 6 to 8 centimeters for the IEA versus approximately 18 centimeters for the radial artery). The shorter length limits placement of the IEA to the diagonal branches, ramus intermedius, or obtuse marginals, although distal sites can be reached by using the IEA as a composite graft with another arterial conduit.

Complications related to harvesting the IEA include bleeding and wound hematomas. They are best prevented

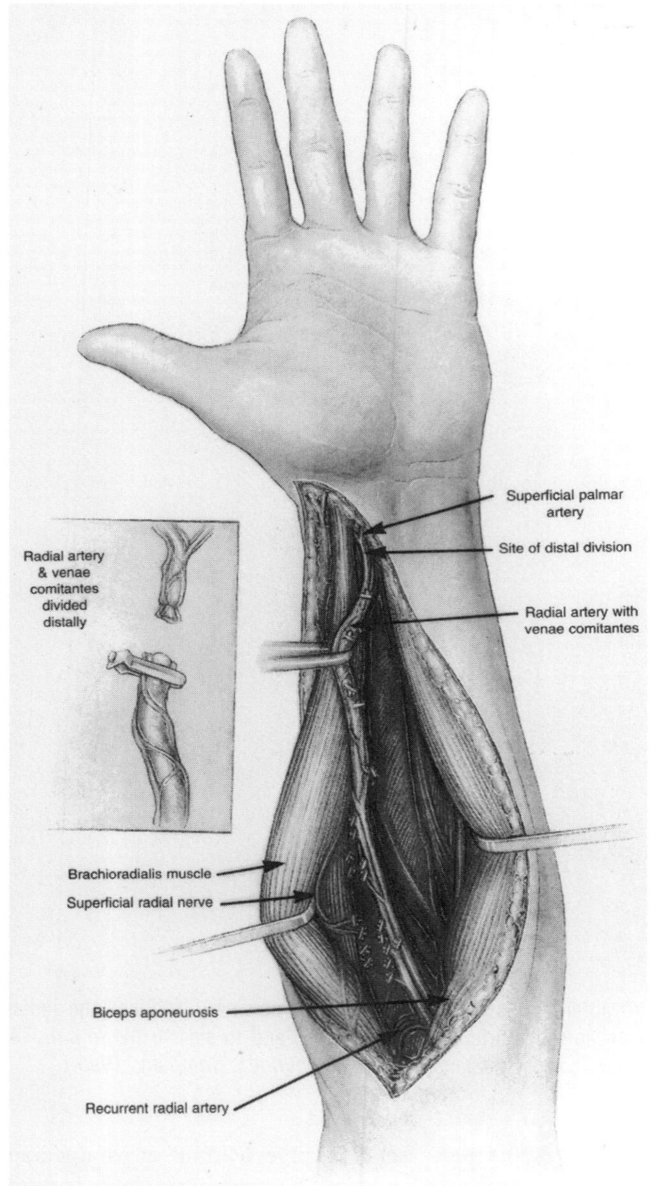

Figure 34–11. Dissection of the radial artery for use as an alternative arterial conduit for coronary artery bypass surgery. *(Used with permission from* Operative Techniques in Cardiac and Thoracic Surgery, *Philadelphia: W. B. Saunders Company, 1996.)*

by closing the incision after reversal of heparin with protamine. Injury to the ductus deferens, genitocrural nerve, and external iliac artery or vein is also possible (Barner, 1994).

Additional Venous Conduits

Arm Vein. Cephalic vein was first used for CAB in 1969. Although early follow-up studies were promising, it was soon discovered that after 6 months, patency rates declined dramatically until only 10% of these vessel remain patent at 6 years (Reardon et al., 1997). Consequently, this data would suggest that use of cephalic vein should be reserved for situations in which there are no other superior alternative conduits available to harvest.

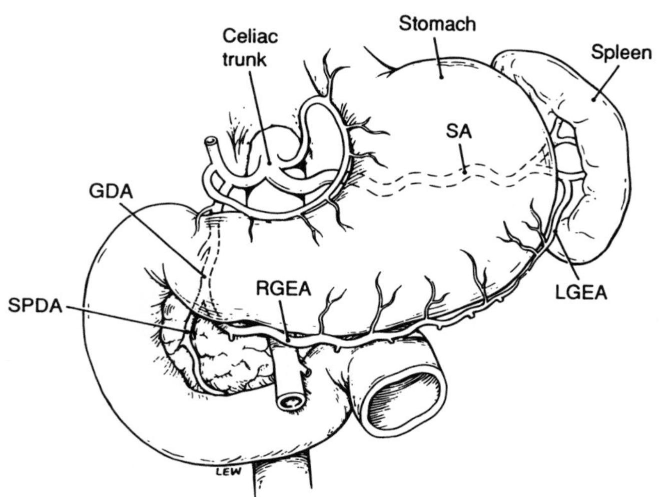

Figure 34–12. Depiction of the anatomic location of the gastroepiploic artery (GEA). The GEA is a branch of the gastroduodenal artery that arises from the common hepatic artery. The GEA runs posterior to the duodenum and then along the greater curvature of the stomach. *(Used with permission from* Operative Techniques in Cardiac and Thoracic Surgery, *Philadelphia: W. B. Saunders Company, 1996.)*

Cryopreserved Vein. Current data indicate that cryopreserved veins have poor patency rates when used as conduits for CAB. These data concur with earlier studies that demonstrated a 41% patency rate at 7 to 9 months postoperatively. The etiology of poor patency rates likely involves problems of tissue viability and immunologic rejection. It has been proposed that immunosuppressive agents could possibly improve graft survival; however, the clinical risks may outweigh the potential benefits. In conclusion, cryopreserved veins have poor short- and long-term patency rates and, therefore, the use of this graft should be restricted, especially in light of the good results with alternative arterial conduits (Iaffaldano, Lewis, Johnson, Piffare, & McKiernan, 1995).

Conclusions Regarding Conduit Selection. When determining which conduit to use for CAB, the cardiothoracic surgeon must take into account patient age and clinical status at the time of surgery. The primary conduits are still considered to be the ITAs and the greater and lesser saphenous veins. The left ITA to the left anterior descending coronary artery can be supported in all age groups of patients without brachiocephalic or subclavian artery stenosis. For patients less than 45 years of age, and particularly those with hyperlipidemia, all arterial bypass grafts should be attempted due to a documented poor long-term patency of vein grafts. In patients less than 60 years of age, it becomes more difficult to demonstrate improvement; how-

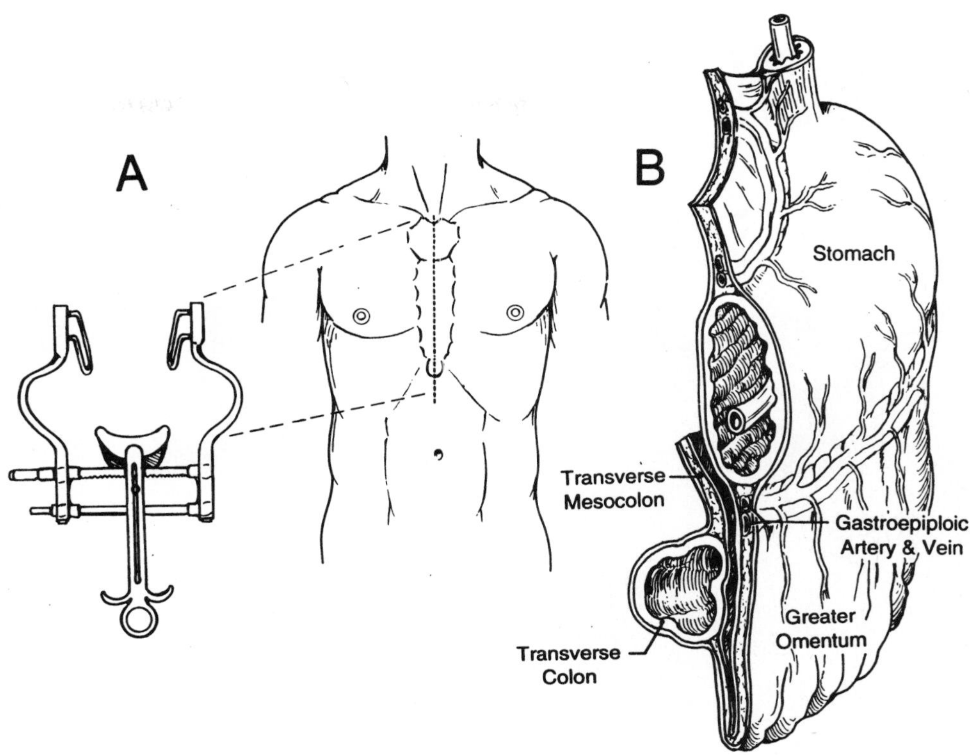

Figure 34–13. A, Extension of the sternotomy for harvest of the GEA. **B,** Shows the anatomic location of the right GEA found between the most anterior and second serosal layer of the stomach. *(Used with permission from* Operative Techniques in Cardiac and Thoracic Surgery, *Philadelphia: W. B. Saunders Company, 1996.)*

ever, no negative long-term results have been reported from the use of all arterial grafts. It is generally accepted that the GEA is the second arterial conduit of choice. The IEA and radial artery have adequate short-term results, but their long-term effectiveness has not yet been established (Reardon et al., 1997).

Special Postoperative Consideration Following Coronary Artery Bypass

Coronary vasospasm has become increasingly recognized as a cause of postoperative morbidity and mortality following CAB. It can affect normal coronary arteries, bypassed vessels, saphenous vein grafts, and arterial grafts. The etiology is speculative, and most likely multifactorial to include: calcium infusions, increased alpha-adrenergic tone, release of platelet thromboxane A^2, and rebound withdrawal from calcium channel blockers used preoperatively (Bojar, 1994). The diagnosis of spasm can be difficult to make. It is generally manifested by ischemic EKG changes, hemodynamic collapse, and ventricular arrhythmias. These symptoms can also indicate myocardial ischemia due to incomplete revascularization, poor myocardial protection, or acute graft thrombosis. Treatment modalities include intravenous nitroglycerin, calcium channel blockers, and, if necessary, an intraaortic balloon pump. If severe ischemia is felt to be caused by a problem with a bypass graft, emergency coronary angiography or reexploration may be indicated.

Valvular Heart Disease

The decision to recommend surgery in a patient with valvular heart disease (VHD) remains a challenge. It requires a thorough understanding of the pathophysiology of the particular valve lesion as well as the natural history of such a lesion in a given patient. The overall goals of surgery for VHD are prolongation of event-free survival, improved functional status, and avoidance of subclinical deterioration in left ventricular function (Assey & Spann, 1990). Since preoperative ventricular dysfunction can persist even after a "successful" operation, surgical intervention should be carried out before ventricular function deteriorates irreversibly.

Valve Repair Versus Valve Replacement

The repair of cardiac valves dates back to the beginning of surgical treatment for heart disease. However, once prosthetic valves became available, interest in valve reconstruction decreased sharply in the United States for over 20 years. Fortunately, a few groups continued reconstructive techniques in selective patients. During the 1970s major contributions to valve reconstruction surgery were made by

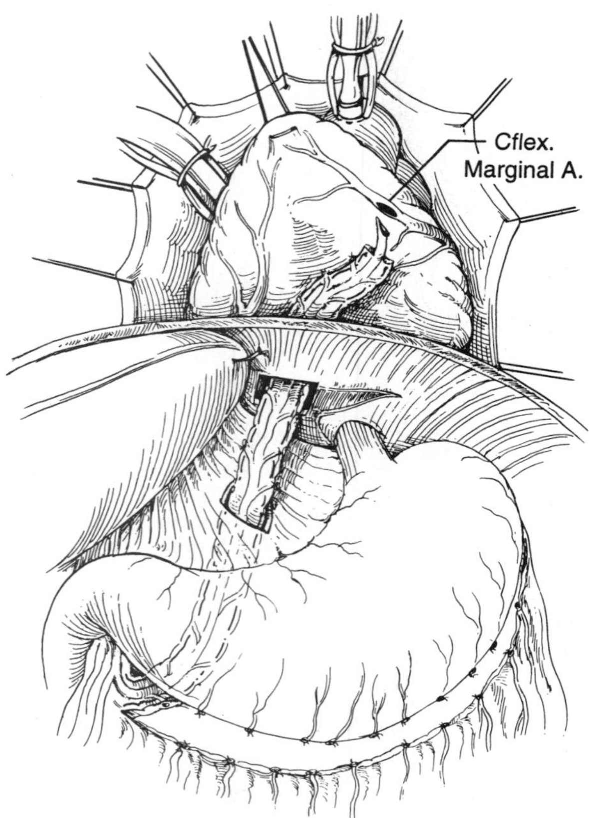

Figure 34–14. The right GEA is routed posterior and lateral to bypass the circumflex coronary artery branches. *(Used with permission from* Operative Techniques in Cardiac and Thoracic Surgery, *Philadelphia: W. B. Saunders Company, 1996.)*

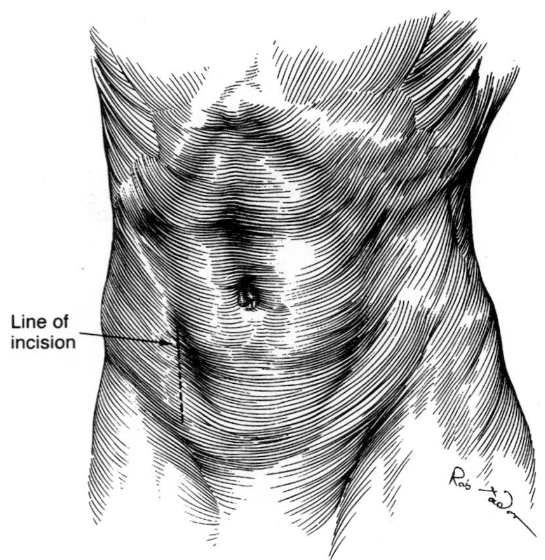

Figure 34–15. The line of incision for harvest of the inferior epigastric artery (IEA) is right sided, 2–3 cm below the umbilicus and three fingers lateral to midline extending to the groin. *(Used with permission from* Operative Techniques in Cardiac and Thoracic Surgery, *Philadelphia: W. B. Saunders Company, 1996.)*

Carpentier in France and Duran in Spain. Reconstructive techniques were combined with annuloplasty rings to correct annular dilatation. The Carpentier and Duran techniques were used to a limited extent in the United States until 1979 when Colvin at New York University began applying the Carpentier technique with reported excellent results. Since then, valve reconstruction has been performed with increasing frequency (Sabiston & Spencer, 1995).

Today, it is more apparent than ever that salvaging a native cardiac valve is always the more desirable option

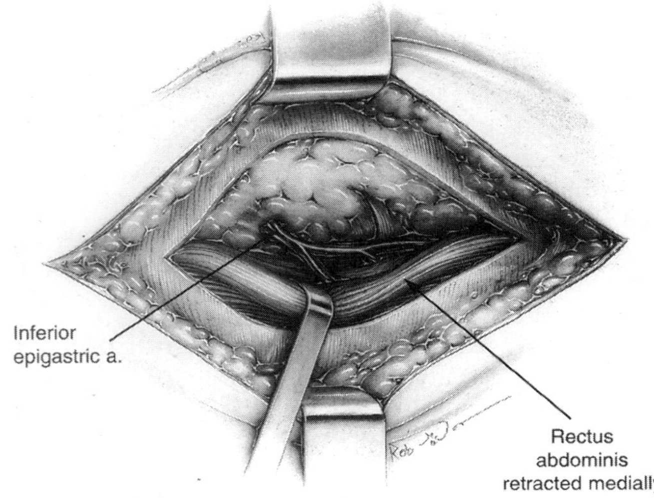

Figure 34–16. The IEA is found in the lateral fat and courses upward and medially into the posterior surface of the rectus abdominus muscle. *(Used with permission from* Operative Techniques in Cardiac and Thoracic Surgery, *W. B. Saunders Company, 1996.)*

when feasible because of the inherent complications associated with virtually every prosthetic valve design. As Bojar (1992) states, replacing a diseased native valve with a prosthetic valve is like trading one problem for another because patients then become susceptible to prosthetic valve endocarditis, thromboembolism, hemolysis, valve deterioration, and anticoagulant-related hemorrhage. Awareness of these limitations has refocused attention on developing techniques to preserve the patient's native valve. In summary, when practical, valve repair should be considered preferable to valve replacement in the mitral, tricuspid, and aortic positions. Unfortunately, aortic valve repair has not yet stood the test of time (Grunkemeier, Starr, & Rahimtoola, 1992).

Review of Prosthetic Valves

The variety of available prostheses attests to the imperfections of all existing designs. Each type of valve has inherent advantages and disadvantages that make it particularly suited for an individual patient. Although currently available valves on the market are the only ones relevant with regard to valve selection, some discontinued models are still implanted in large numbers of patients and, therefore, they are important with regard to patient management.

Mechanical Valves. Mechanical valves are the oldest type of prosthetic valves available. They account for approximately 60% of all prostheses implanted. Mechanical valves are constructed of varying combinations of metal, plastic, and dacron. These materials make mechanical valves very durable over long periods of time; however, these same design features are associated with a high incidence of thromboembolism, especially in the mitral position. Therefore, chronic anticoagulation, a high-risk therapy in and of itself, is a must with all mechanical valves. Today, only four mechanical valves are approved by the FDA for use in the United States: Starr–Edwards, St. Jude, Medtronic–Hall, and Omniscience.

Caged-Ball Valves. The Starr–Edwards mechanical valve (Fig. 34–17) is an example of a caged-ball valve in which a cage attached to a sewing ring houses a ball inside. Various models have been in use since its original design in 1961. Experience with the current model spans over 20 years, so information about this valve is most secure. Although these valves have excellent durability, the valve design produces turbulent flow due to central obstruction by the ball. Because of their bulky, high-profile design, they are also difficult to use in patients with small ventricles or small aortic roots. Thromboembolic events are reported to be the highest with this valve design. Approximately 4.5% of patients per year experience their first thromboembolic event (Sabiston & Spencer, 1995).

Tilting Disc Valves. The tilting disc valves were the second generation of mechanical valves. They have better flow characteristics than the caged-ball design. The Medtronic–Hall is one example of a tilting disc valve. It was first introduced in 1977, has excellent hemodynamics, and a thromboembolic rate of approximately 2% per patient year.

The Bjork–Shiley tilting disc valve was first introduced in 1982; however, it is no longer available because of structural design flaws that resulted in strut fracture and disc embolization. The Bjork–Shiley valve was withdrawn from the market in 1986. Although valve replacement is indicated for strut fracture, prophylactic valve replacement is not warranted because the overall incidence of strut fracture remains very low, thus the risk of reoperation outweighs the potential benefits of changing the valve.

The Omniscience mechanical valve was introduced in 1978 and is reported to have hemodynamics similar to other tilting disc valves. The thromboembolic complication rate associated with this valve remains controversial, but appears to be increased when compared with other tilting disc devices.

Bileaflet Valves. Bileaflet mechanical valves are the least obstructive to central flow and thus have the best reported hemodynamics of all mechanical valves; however, they also have the highest regurgitation fraction. The St. Jude bileaflet valve (Fig. 34–18) is currently the most commonly implanted prosthetic valve. It has been available in the United States since 1977.

Ninety percent of patients with St. Jude valves are reported to be free from thromboembolic complications at 5 years from implantation. The overall rate of a first-time

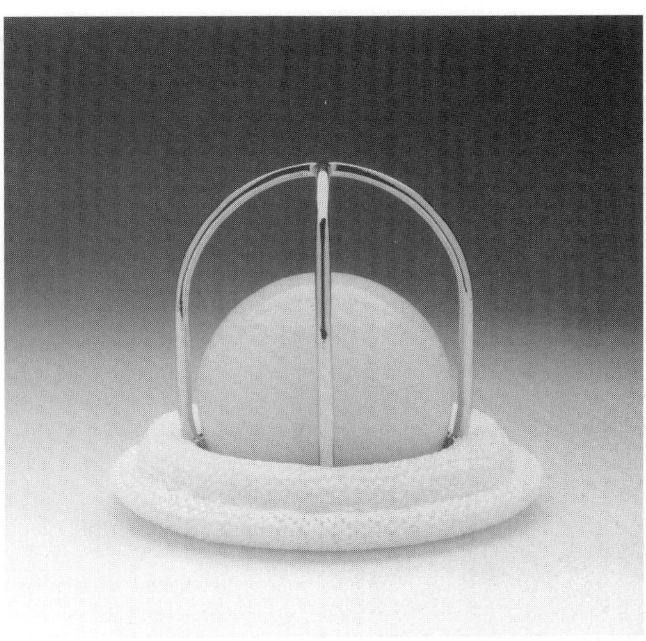

Figure 34–17. Starr–Edwards™ Silastic Ball valve, mitral model 6120. *(Photograph: courtesy of Baxter Healthcare Corporation, Edwards CVS Division.)*

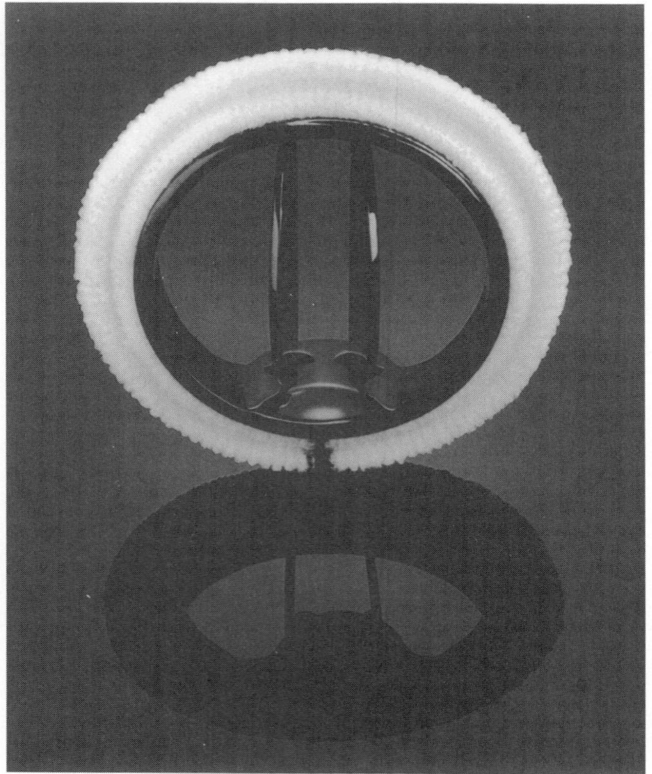

Figure 34–18. St. Jude Medical® mechanical heart valve. St. Jude Medical® is a registered trademark of St. Jude Medical, Inc. *(Photograph: courtesy of St. Jude Medical, Inc. All rights reserved.)*

thromboembolic event is reported to be 2 to 8 per 100 patient years (Sabiston & Spencer, 1995). The Carbomedics mechanical valve is another example of a low-profile bileaflet valve that became available in the United States in 1986.

Tissue Valves

Xenografts. Biologic tissue valves were introduced in the early 1970s. They are derived from animal cardiac tissue (xenograft/heterograft) or harvested from human cadaver hearts (homograft/allograft). Xenograft tissue valves are derived from two sources: porcine aortic valves or bovine pericardium.

Porcine valves have been used extensively since the early 1970s. Porcine valves are preserved in a buffered glutaraldehyde and mounted on a flexible, lightweight frame. Glutaraldehyde fixation reduces antigenicity and increases tissue stability. Except in small sizes, porcine valves have hemodynamics comparable with mechanical valves. The major drawback to porcine valves is the well-documented incidence of valve failure. Primary valve degeneration can be expected at 10 years in 73% of patients younger than 30 years of age at the time of implant; in 23% of patients aged 30 to 59, and 17% of patients age 60 or older. Primary valve failure occurs more frequently in the mitral position (i.e., 28% at 10 years) as opposed to the aortic position (i.e., 21%). Aside from the durability problem, the valve itself is rarely a cause of mortality, thromboembolism, or permanent morbidity (Sabiston & Spencer, 1995).

Currently there are two porcine valves available for use: the Carpentier–Edwards and the Hancock. The Hancock porcine bioprosthesis became available in 1970. Current data on freedom from prosthetic valve dysfunction are reported to be 82% (plus or minus 3%) at 10 years. The Carpentier–Edwards porcine bioprosthesis (Fig. 34–19) became available in 1975 and is reported to have a 79% (plus or minus 5%) durability at 10 years.

Several pericardial valves have been used in the United States, including the Ionescu–Shiley and Hancock bioprostheses. However, both of these valves have been withdrawn from the market because of structural dysfunction (i.e., early valve failure due to tears in valve cusps). The Carpentier–Edwards aortic bioprosthesis (Fig. 34–20) is the only remaining pericardial valve being implanted today. It has been available in the United States since 1991 and has demonstrated good intermediate (7-year follow-up) durability as well as low rates of valve-related morbidity. Preliminary data suggest durability to be superior to existing porcine bioprostheses with freedom from prosthetic valve dysfunction reported to be 97% at 7 years (Sabiston & Spencer, 1995).

The newest generation of tissue valves are the stentless porcine valves. They have been available in the United States since 1995 are designed to offer superior hemodynamic performance and increased durability over conventional stented bioprosthetic valves. Stentless valves do not have frames or sewing rings and, therefore, provide for a larger central ori-

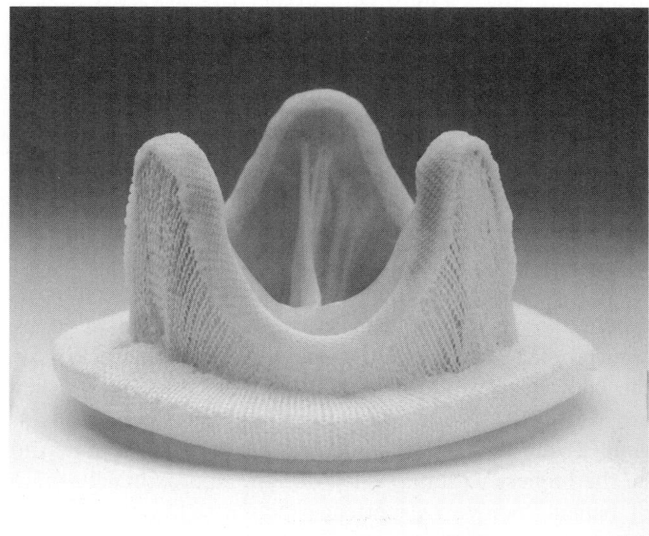

Figure 34–19. Carpentier–Edwards® porcine bioprosthesis, aortic model 2625. *(Photograph: courtesy of Baxter Healthcare Corporation, Edwards CVS Division.)*

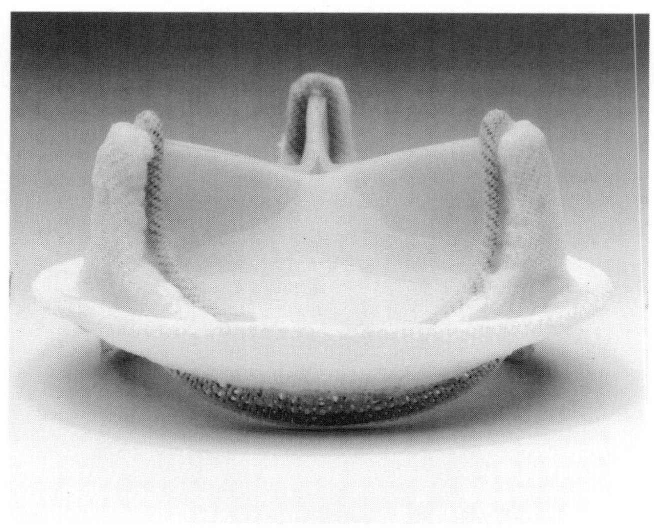

Figure 34–20. Carpentier–Edwards® Perimount® RSR Pericardial Bioprosthesis, Aortic Model 2800. *(Photograph: courtesy of Baxter Healthcare Corporation, Edwards CVS Division.)*

fice area and improved transvalvular blood flow. Both Medtronic and St. Jude are currently manufacturing stentless porcine valves.

Homografts. In the early 1960s several investigators began work preserving and implanting homograft valves. Initial results of attempting to preserve and store homograft valves for later use were disappointing. Issues revolved around preservation techniques that could preserve cell viability. Experimentation was done with gamma irradiation, lyophilization, and chemical preservatives. Within the last 10 years, major innovations in the prefreezing process, the cryopreservation technique, and the thawing process have enabled homograft valves to be preserved for extensive periods without losing cell viability. Both aortic and pulmonary valves are harvested as a valve-conduit with a portion of the corresponding great vessel (aorta or pulmonary artery) then cryopreserved. The current cryopreservation technique consists of: (1) treatment of homograft valves with broad spectrum antibiotics immediately following dissection, (2) after 24 hours of antibiotic storage, they are placed in culture media with fetal calf serum and dimethyslfoxide at 4°C, and (3) the valve is then packaged in a sterile envelope where it undergoes cryogenic freezing in a liquid nitrogen freezer for long-term storage at −196°C.

Current data suggests that the cryopreserved aortic homografts have the greatest durability with freedom from valvular degeneration at ten years being 100%. The incidence of endocarditis with homografts is extremely low because of the absence of foreign material. Like other bioprosthetic valves, they have a very low incidence of thromboembolism. The primary disadvantages of homograft valves include: limited availability, cost of procurement and handling, and the greater technical demands of insertion as opposed to stented prosthesis. Current indications for homografts include: (1) life expectancy greater than 10 years with a contraindication to warfarin, (2) aortic root replacement, (3) small aortic annulus, (4) endocarditis, and (5) reoperation for other failed bioprosthesis. Current contraindications for use of aortic homografts include: (1) severe annular calcification and (2) connective tissue disorders (e.g., Marfan's syndrome).

The Ross Procedure. The first Ross operation was performed over 30 years ago in 1967 and was inspired by the desire to provide young patients with a better aortic valve replacement as disenchantment with available prostheses grew. The operation was regarded with suspicion and not well accepted by the surgical community until impressive long-term results were published in 1988 (Joyce, Tingleff, & Pattersson, 1996). Donald Ross showed an overall surgical mortality of 6.6%, which was truly a remarkable statistic considering the time frame in which these operations were performed. The majority of operative deaths in this series of 241 patients occurred early in the procedure's evolution, implicating factors related to inadequate myocardial protection and unfamiliarity with regional coronary anatomy. The series contained no reported operative deaths since 1976 (Oury, 1996). The long-term durability of the pulmonary autograft was also answered in these published results. The reported 20-year freedom from autograft replacement was 75% and the reported freedom from pulmonary homograft replacement was 80% (Ross, 1996).

The surgical technique can best be looked upon as two standard procedures: translocation of the patient's own pulmonary valve to the aortic position with reimplantation of the coronary ostia and reconstruction of the right ventricular outflow using a pulmonary homograft valve (Fig. 34–21). Problems with early cases were related to the vulnerability of the first septal coronary artery and its close relationship to the root of the pulmonary artery. Damage to this vessel gave rise to septal infarcts and sometimes fatal arrhythmias (Ross, 1996).

Present mainstream indications for the Ross procedure continue to broaden as familiarity with the procedure grows. The mean age for patients undergoing the Ross procedure is currently 28 with a majority (81%) between ages 11 and 50. Although there are cases reported of patients undergoing the Ross procedure in their 70s, it seems unnecessary to subject patients in this age group to a higher risk procedure with no proven long-term benefit. Current indications for aortic valve replacement with a pulmonary autograft include: (1) patients under age 50, (2) single valve pathology, (3) mechanical or bioprosthetic valve failure, (4) endocarditis limited to aortic root, and (5) athlete or young adult in whom anticoagulation is contraindicated and optimal hemodynamics are desired (Oury, 1996). Present-day

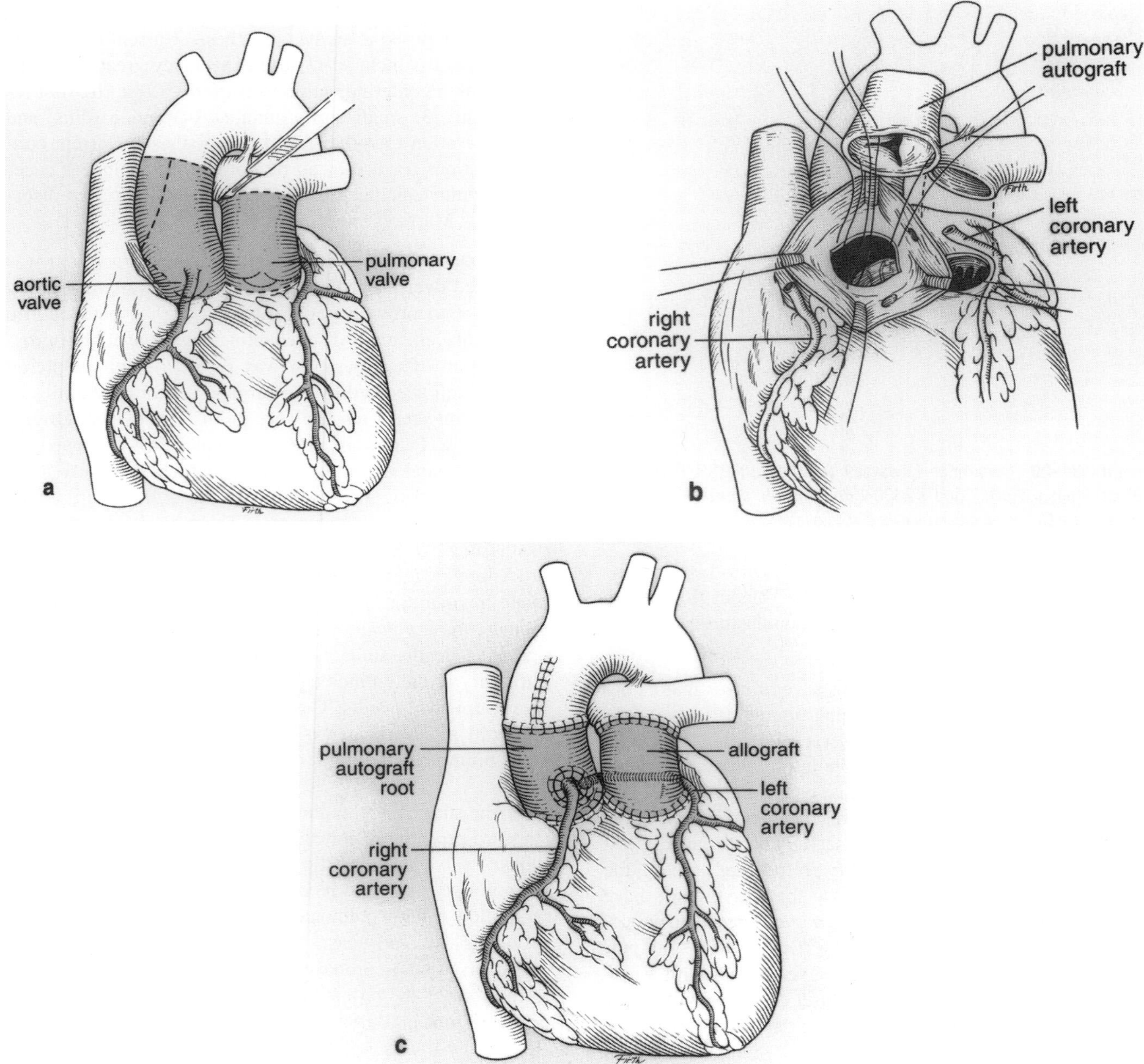

Figure 34–21. In the Ross procedure, the patient's own pulmonary valve is removed and placed in the aortic position (autograft) with reimplantation of the coronary ostia. Then a pulmonary homograft is placed in the pulmonary position. **A,** Depicts the pulmonary valve and a segment of pulmonary artery being excised. **B,** The diseased native aortic valve along with the proximal portion of the aortic root is removed leaving the coronary arteries with a small button of tissue. **C,** The pulmonary autograft is placed in the aortic position and the coronary arteries are reimplanted. The pulmonary homograft is positioned to replace the excised segment. *(Photograph: courtesy of the USC University Hospital.)*

contraindications to the Ross procedure include: (1) advanced three-vessel coronary artery disease, (2) extensive other valve pathology, (3) extremes of age, (4) multisystem organ failure, (5) pulmonary valve pathology, and (6) Marfan's syndrome (Oury, 1996)

Considerations for Prosthetic Valve Selection

Hemodynamics. Hemodynamic performance is determined by transvalvular gradients. In general, all of the currently available mechanical valves demonstrate comparable hemodynamic function in equivalent sizes. The hemodynamic performance of porcine valves is not quite so good because of their basic design. The Carpentier–Edwards pericardial valve that became available in 1991 demonstrates superior opening characteristic. In general, the hemodynamic performance of all prosthetic valves becomes important only when using a small size (i.e., less than 21 millimeters in the aortic position and less than 25 millimeters in the mitral position) because the valve sewing ring reduces the effective orifice area. All prosthetic valves manifest some resting gradient because of the sewing ring which reduces the effective orifice. An excellent alternative for the use of a very small prosthetic valve is placement of a homograft valve or the newer generation, low-profile, stentless porcine valves. These valves produce no gradient because they have no sewing ring.

Thromboembolism. All prosthetic valves are susceptible to the formation of thrombus that can subsequently embolize. A prosthetic-related thromboembolic event is defined as any new permanent or transient focal or global neurologic deficit, or a peripheral embolus in the absence of another clear-cut source (Bojar, 1992). Currently, the Starr–Edwards prosthetic valve has the highest thromboembolism rate of any valve available. All of the other mechanical valves have a relatively similar incidence of thromboembolism and all require chronic anticoagulation with warfarin, which is a risk in and of itself. Tissue valves are more resistant to thromboembolism but the sewing ring can be a nidus for thrombus formation in the early postoperative period; therefore, some surgeons choose to use short term (i.e., 2 to 3 months) of anticoagulation in patients with tissue valves until the sewing ring endothelializes. Conversely, thromboembolism is extremely unusual on homograft valves and, therefore, they do not require anticoagulation.

Valve Thrombosis. Although the risk of mechanical valve thrombosis is very low during satisfactory anticoagulation, it has been reported in patients with therapeutic prothrombin times. In the left heart, the risk is higher in the mitral as opposed to the aortic position and greatest with the caged-ball valve. The incidence of mechanical valve thrombosis is greatest overall in the tricuspid position due to the lower pressure/flows. Therefore, use of mechanical valves should be avoided in the tricuspid position. Thrombosis of a mechanical valve may occur as a catastrophic event with acute onset of heart failure, pulmonary edema, and cardiogenic shock; however, it is more often heralded by nonspecific cardiac complaints and/or progressive symptoms of congestive heart failure. Valve thrombosis almost always requires reoperation which is associated with a mortality rate of up to 50% depending on the acuteness of the patient presentation.

Anticoagulation Related Hemorrhage. The use of anticoagulants to reduce thromboembolic events occasionally results in bleeding that can cause the need for blood product transfusions, hospitalization, reoperation, stroke, and even death. The annual risk of a major bleeding episode related to anticoagulation therapy averages 0.5% per year and is cumulative with time. The risk of bleeding is also increased in the elderly (i.e., greater than 70 years of age). Careful pre-operative history of potential contraindications to warfarin should be obtained to guide in prosthetic valve selection.

Prosthetic Valve Endocarditis. Prosthetic valve endocarditis can occur both early and late after surgery. It has a similar incidence of 1 to 2% per year following valve replacement with either a mechanical or tissue valve. The development of prosthetic valve endocarditis within the first two months after surgery (i.e., early) is usually associated with a Staphylococcal infection and carries a very poor prognosis. The mortality rate approaches 50% even when treated with intravenous antibiotics and reoperation. Conversely, prosthetic valve endocarditis that develops after the first 2 months following surgery (i.e., late) usually involves organisms similar to native valve endocarditis such as Streptococcus viridan, Staphylcoccus aureus, and Enterococcus. It can often be treated with antibiotics alone. Nonetheless, the overall mortality in patients with late prosthetic valve endocarditis is approximately 25%. Infections with tissue valves may be limited to the valve leaflets and can occasionally be sterilized with antibiotics. Infections involving mechanical valves tend to produce periannular abscesses and nearly always require surgical intervention. The incidence of endocarditis on a homograft valve is extremely low because of the absence of foreign material.

Hemolysis. Cellular destruction from transvalvular forward flow is very unusual with all the current prosthetic valve designs. Hemolysis is almost always associated with periprosthetic leak or a stenotic/regurgitant valve which creates turbulent flow. Hemolysis can be detected by new onset and/or progressive cardiac murmur, persistent anemia requiring blood transfusions, elevated LDH, and hemoglobinuria. Definitive diagnosis can be made by echocardiogram. Significant perivalvular leak almost always requires reoperation.

Durability. Although there are isolated causes of structural failure of mechanical valves, their lifespan is usually limited by the development of thromboembolism, endocarditis, or bleeding requiring reoperation. Conversely, tissue valves' durability is predominantly compromised by the development of structural deterioration. Structural deterioration results from collagen degeneration and calcification of the leaflets. Degeneration of tissue valves has been reported to occur more rapidly with mitral valves due to higher transmitted pressure during leaflet closure. There is also a higher incidence of bioprosthetic valve deterioration in patients with renal failure or abnormalities in calcium metabolism, in younger patients, in women, and in patients in whom endocarditis has been successfully treated with antibiotics.

Availability, Cost, and Ease of Insertion. The majority of prosthetic valves cost between $3000 to $4000. The overall cost of homografts is about one and a half times that of a prosthetic valve. Homograft valves are also more technically challenging to implant and their supply is limited.

Conclusions Regarding Prosthetic Valve Selection. In summary, when matching a prosthetic valve to a patient situation, consider the following: patient's age (i.e., less than 65 years of age because durability is a factor) and comorbidities, potential interference of warfarin with patient's current lifestyle, patient compliance and/or ability to take warfarin reliably, any absolute or relative contraindications to warfarin, and the patient's cardiac anatomy.

When valve replacement is necessary, an argument can be made for a particular type of valve depending on the patient's physical and psychological circumstances. A bioprosthetic valve should be used when the patient cannot tolerate or will not take warfarin, desires pregnancy, or has a short (i.e., 8- to 10-year) life expectancy. Conversely, a mechanical valve should be used if the patient requires chronic anticoagulation for a concomitant disease (e.g., chronic atrial fibrillation or a mechanical valve in another position), is in renal failure or on dialysis, or has a long (greater than 15-year) life expectancy. For patients who do not fit these criteria, valve selection remains somewhat subjective (Grunkemeier et al., 1992).

Aortic Stenosis

Natural History and Indications for Surgery. Natural history studies of asymptomatic patients with aortic stenosis have shown that 70% of patients with moderate aortic stenosis (i.e., an aortic valve area of 0.7-1.2 cm^2) remain free of complications at four years. Conversely, 40% of patients with severe, hemodynamically significant aortic stenosis will develop symptoms within 6 months to 1 year of diagnosis. Patients with hemodynamically significant aortic stenosis may have symptoms of congestive heart failure (60%), angina (50%), or syncope (40%). Natural history studies show that symptomatic aortic stenosis carries a prohibitive mortality. Average survival is only 2 years for heart failure, 3 years for syncope, and 5 years for angina (Assey and Spann, 1990; Bojar, 1992). This data clearly indicate that aggressive surgical intervention should be offered to patients with symptomatic aortic stenosis to improve long-term survival. Indications for surgery in patients with aortic stenosis include any patient who is symptomatic. Symptoms are usually noted in patients who have an aortic valve area less than 1 cm^2, a mean aortic valve gradient greater than 40 mm Hg, or a peak systolic gradient greater than 50 mm Hg. In general, no patient with hemodynamically significant aortic stenosis should be deemed inoperable because of congestive heart failure or low ejection fraction.

Surgical Options for Aortic Stenosis. Aortic valves' repair for aortic stenosis has yielded relatively poor-long-term results in comparison with aortic valve replacement. With the exception of stenotic lesions in children and regurgitation due to septal defects, most cardiothoracic surgeons treat all aortic valve lesions with replacement (Duran, Kumar, & Halees, 1991).

In children with aortic stenosis, aortic valve repair (primarily commissurotomy) continues to have a clear role as a palliative procedure until the patient grows larger. In the adult, aortic valve repair for aortic stenosis involves both aortic valve commissurotomy and debridement of aortic valve calcium deposits. Duran reports acceptable results with valve repair. Unfortunately, few centers have been able to duplicate these results. In general, aortic valve repair for aortic stenosis in adults has a high incidence of early recurrent stenosis or progression of aortic valve regurgitation and, therefore, the current role for aortic valve repair in the adult with aortic stenosis is very limited (Sabiston & Spencer, 1995).

Since it was first performed in 1960, aortic valve replacement has been the treatment of choice for patients with symptomatic aortic stenosis. The operative mortality averages 5%, but several factors have been found to increase the operative risk including: urgent or emergent operations, class III or IV symptoms preoperatively, impaired left ventricular systolic function, and co-morbidities such as renal insufficiency (Bojar, 1992). Through a median sternotomy incision, using cardiopulmonary bypass, the aorta is opened and the native aortic valve is excised. A sizing instrument is then used to measure the native valve annulus and select an appropriate-size prosthetic valve. A series of sutures are placed around the circumference of the native valve annulus and brought through the corresponding location on the sewing ring of the prosthesis. The prosthetic valve is then positioned in the annulus and the sutures are tied (Finkelmeier, 1995).

Postoperative Considerations for Patients with Aortic Stenosis. Early postoperative care of the patient undergoing aortic valve replacement must address the residual pathophysiologic changes of left ventricular hypertrophy. Maintenance of a supraventricular rhythm is crucial to ensure adequate filling of the left ventricle, which tends to be stiff and noncompliant in these patients. Control of postoperative hypertension is also paramount in order to prevent bleeding from the aortotomy (Bojar, 1994).

In addition to the usual complications associated with open heart surgery, there are procedure-specific complications associated with aortic valve surgery. Complete heart block may result from extension of calcific disease into the septum near the conduction system or from aggressive debridement and suture placement in that region. Heart block related to edema should resolve several days postoperatively; however, heart block persisting greater than 1 week is usually an indication for a dual-chamber pacemaker.

Aortic Regurgitation

Natural History and Indications for Surgery. Most patients with chronic aortic regurgitation have a natural history that encompasses a lengthy asymptomatic period during which there may be undetected deterioration of left ventricular systolic function due to progressive dilatation. Generally accepted indications for aortic regurgitation include: any patient with moderate to severe symptoms or asymptomatic patients in whom there is sufficient documentation of progressive left ventricular chamber enlargement (i.e., left ventricular end-diastolic dimension greater than 70 millimeters or left ventricular end-systolic dimension greater than 55 millimeters). Conversely, acute aortic regurgitation is generally not well tolerated because the heart is unable to dilate acutely to accommodate the regurgitant volume. Therefore, acute aortic valve insufficiency almost always required urgent surgical intervention.

Surgical Options for Aortic Regurgitation. Patients with chronic aortic regurgitation may have several underlying valvular pathologies that are potentially amenable to aortic valve repair. In particular, patients with bicuspid aortic valves have undergone successful aortic valve repair with resection or plication of a redundant leaflet as well as aortic valve annuloplasty. Resuspension of the aortic valve for aortic regurgitation due to acute type A aortic dissection has also proven to be successful with both short- and long-term results (Sabiston & Spencer, 1995).

Aortic valve replacement is performed for the patient with indications for surgical intervention. When significant aortic root enlargement (i.e., greater than 5 cm) is present, aortic valve replacement is done either in conjunction with a supracoronary ascending aortic interposition graft or as a composite aortic graft using a valve conduit with reimplantation of the coronary arteries. The operative mortality of aortic valve replacement performed for aortic regurgitation is slightly higher than in patients with aortic stenosis.

Postoperative Considerations for Patients with Aortic Regurgitation. Aortic regurgitation produces both a volume and pressure overload of the left ventricle, resulting in a dilated and frequently hypertrophied chamber. Maintenance of a supraventricular rhythm is important for a stable hemodynamic status. Filling pressures often rise minimally, despite large fluid challenges because of the large compliant left ventricle (Bojar, 1994)

Heart block may complicate aortic valve replacement because of edema, hemorrhage, suturing, or debridement near the conduction system which lies adjacent to the base of the right coronary cusp (Bojar, 1994).

Mitral Stenosis

Natural History and Indications for Surgery. Mitral stenosis is caused almost exclusively by rheumatic fever after which there is generally a long latent period of approximately 20 years before the development of symptoms occurs. Many patients who present with longstanding mitral valve stenosis also have pulmonary hypertension with resultant functional tricuspid valve regurgitation. Natural history studies have shown that the 10-year survival rates for class I to II patients is 85% and class III patients is 40%. In general, indications for surgery include: NYHA class III to IV symptoms, NYHA class II symptoms if the calculated mitral valve area is less than 1 cm^2, and a history of a thromboembolic event.

Surgical Options for Mitral Stenosis. Surgical therapy for mitral stenosis is directed at increasing the valve orifice area without producing or significantly worsening mitral regurgitation (Carabello, 1993). Open mitral commissurotomy has traditionally been considered the procedure of choice for patients with mitral stenosis. It allows for direct visualization and repair of both the valvular and subvalvular apparatus which is involved in approximately 30% of all patients with mitral stenosis. Typical valves that respond well to repair are ones with limited calcification, good leaflet mobility, little subvalvular stenosis, and moderate mitral regurgitation (Carabello, 1993).

Mitral valve replacement is indicated when the degree of valvular or subvalvular disease precludes open commissurotomy. This is usually determined at the time of surgery by examining the amount of valve thickening, calcification, and deformity as well as the amount of chordae shortening and thickening. The most common approach is to perform a transverse right atriotomy. Once the valve is examined and deemed unsuitable for repair, it is excised. The conventional wisdom has been to preserve the posterior and/or anterior leaflet of the native mitral valve with its chordal attachment because of the growing evidence that this contributes to preserved left ventricular function in the postoperative period. Data suggest that there are better surgical outcomes with mitral valve replacement for mitral stenosis as opposed to mitral regurgitation. This is probably attributed to the fact that there is usually less antecedent left ventricular dysfunction with stenotic lesions.

Postoperative Considerations for Patients with Mitral Stenosis. Most patients with pure mitral stenosis have a small left ventricular cavity with preserved function. Hemodynamic function following mitral valve surgery for mitral stenosis is influenced by the degree of pulmonary hypertension and the quality of right ventricular protection during surgery. Pulmonary artery pressures usually decrease substantially following surgery; however, elements of irreversible pulmonary hypertension, interstitial edema, decreased lung compliance from CPB, and mechanical ventilation all contribute to right ventricular dysfunction in the early postoperative period by increasing afterload. Use of inotropes with vasodilator properties or use of afterload reducing agents are helpful in improving cardiac performance.

Postoperative ventilatory failure with prolonged mechanical ventilation is not uncommon in patients with chronic mitral stenosis as a result of pulmonary hypertension, fluid overload, and chronic cachexia with poor ventilatory reserve. Most patients with mitral stenosis are also diuretic dependent and despite surgical correction of their valvular abnormality, they usually require diuretics for several months postoperatively.

Left ventricular rupture is the dreaded complication of mitral valve replacement. It occurs in approximately 1% of all cases. Small, elderly women with small left ventricular cavities seem to be at highest risk for this complication. Rupture usually occurs upon termination of CPB or within hours of arrival to the intensive care unit. Technical factors are usually responsible for the occurrence of left ventricular rupture post mitral valve replacement and include: excessive resection of tissue around the valve annulus, suturing deep into the left ventricular myocardium, using an oversized valve, and elevating the left ventricular apex after valve replacement (Bojar, 1994).

Mitral Regurgitation

Natural History and Indications for Surgery. Despite all available diagnostic tools, determining the proper timing for mitral valve surgery in the patient with mitral regurgitation remains difficult. Because compliance of the left ventricle cannot change acutely, severe acute mitral valve insufficiency causes an abrupt rise in left atrial pressures, resulting in acute pulmonary edema. This net reduction in forward flow usually results in rapid hemodynamic deterioration and cardiogenic shock. Although medical management to reduce afterload may help, urgent surgical intervention is indicated for acute, severe mitral valve regurgitation.

Conversely, the volume load that accompanies chronic mitral regurgitation is well tolerated and patients usually remain asymptomatic for years despite the insidious development of left ventricular decompensation. Natural history studies of patients with rheumatic mitral valve regurgitation have demonstrated 5-year survival rates of 80% and 10-year survival rates of 60%. Survival is really dependent, however, on the phase of mitral valve regurgitation during which the patient seeks medical attention. Traditionally, operation was not recommended for mitral regurgitation until significant disability was present. However, clinical results have shown that once significant congestive heart failure is present, there is often a certain degree of irreversible ventricular injury. This is demonstrated by 5-year survival rates of 90% with preoperative NYHA class II symptoms versus 50-60% with NYHA class IV symptoms. The presence of poor left ventricular function with chronic mitral regurgitation is evidence of decompensation. Patients may have normal ejection fractions despite the presence of left ventricular dysfunction. The reduced systolic function is unmasked once valve competence is restored. Surgical indications for mitral regurgitation include: acute mitral valve regurgitation with congestive heart failure of cardiogenic shock, acute endocarditis, class III to IV symptoms, class I to II symptoms with evidence of deteriorating left ventricular function, and left atrial size greater than 4.5 to 5 cm with new onset atrial fibrillation.

Surgical Options for Mitral Regurgitation. Until the mid 1980s, most cardiothoracic surgeons considered mitral valve replacement to be the procedure of choice for patients with mitral regurgitation. Today, accumulation of evidence suggests that mitral valve repair is superior to mitral valve replacement. There are four basic annuloplasty techniques used to repair a regurgitant mitral valve including: (1) use of an annuloplasty ring (Fig. 34–22), (2) quadrangular segmental resection of the diseased posterior leaflet, (3) shortening of the chordae, and (4) transposition of the posterior leaflet chordae to the anterior leaflet.

Success of mitral valve reconstruction is highly operator dependent; however, the operative mortality for mitral valve repair is lower than that of replacement regardless of the cause of insufficiency, and independent of the prosthesis used; thus, mitral valve repair should be performed whenever possible over mitral valve replacement (Fenster & Feldman, 1995). Unfortunately, repair cannot be guaranteed until it is attempted so any patient scheduled for a repair procedure should also be ready to accept valve replacement if repair cannot be performed.

Mitral valve repair is theoretically possible as long as a

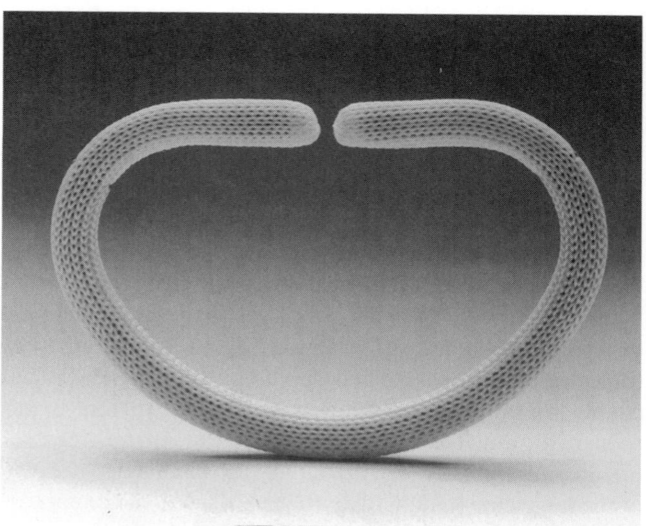

Figure 34–22. Carpentier–Edwards Classic™ Annuloplasty Ring, model 4400 mitral. *(Photograph: courtesy of Baxter Healthcare Corporation, Edwards CVS Division.)*

functioning anterior leaflet is present because the cross section of the anterior leaflet alone is greater than the orifice area of most prosthetic valves. When annular or posterior leaflet calcification is present, valve reconstruction is possible if sufficient calcium can be removed safely to permit subsequent annular repair and ring annuloplasty. Mitral valve repair is clearly feasible in most patients with mitral regurgitation from degenerative/myxomatous disease. With rheumatic valves, the feasibility of repair varies with the relative degree of stenosis or insufficiency. If insufficiency is the predominant lesion and the leaflets are mobile, repair is possible in greater than 50% of rheumatic cases. Statistics show that 10-year freedom from reoperation rates are approximately 90% in nonrheumatic versus 67% in rheumatic mitral valves (Sabiston & Spencer, 1995). Mitral regurgitation due to endocarditis can be repaired if the disease is discrete. Ischemic mitral regurgitation is also usually amenable to a ring annuloplasty.

Survival advantage of repair versus replacement is difficult to demonstrate. Left ventricular function is probably better with repair due to preservation of the subvalvular apparatus. However, this difference is small with the advent of newer surgical techniques allowing chordal preservation with valve replacement. The primary advantage of valve reconstruction seems to be the lower incidence of prosthetic valve-related complications

Postoperative Considerations for Patients With Mitral Regurgitation. Early postoperative care addresses similar issues as previously discussed for mitral valve replacement in the patient with mitral stenosis. The big difference in mitral valve surgery for mitral regurgitation when compared with other cardiac operations is the deterioration of left ventricular function postoperatively. The standard explanation for why left ventricular ejection fraction falls after mitral valve surgery for regurgitant lesion is that restoring mitral valve competence removes one of the pathways for ejection; thereby increasing afterload. Mitral regurgitation reduces left ventricular wall stress by systolic unloading through the incompetent valve into the left atrium. With restoration of a competent mitral valve, systolic unloading of the left ventricle is eliminated and there is an "unmasking" of left ventricular dysfunction because it now must generate a higher wall stress to produce forward flow. Inotropic agents coupled with afterload reducing agents are the hallmark of postoperative management. Again it has been shown that preservation of the integrity of the subvalvular apparatus is critical to the preservation of left ventricular function. The subvalvular apparatus helps maintain the normal left ventricular geometry and muscle function. Therefore, it is recommended the mitral valve replacement should be performed with preservation of at least the posterior leaflet and its associated subvalvular apparatus. This can be done by plicating the posterior leaflet into the suture line. Preservation of the posterior leaflet and subvalvular apparatus may also minimize the potential for postoperative left ventricular rupture. The most important determinant of long-term survival is the status of preoperative left ventricular systolic function (Bojar, 1994; Carabello, 1995).

Tricuspid Valve Disease

Natural History and Indications for Surgery. Tricuspid valve disease rarely occurs as an isolated lesion; it most commonly is a mixed valvular pathology (i.e., stenosis and regurgitation). Tricuspid valve disease can be classified as either functional or organic in origin. Surgery is indicated for severely symptomatic tricuspid valve disease or during correction of left-sided valvular pathologies. In general, organic tricuspid valve disease does not improve during left-sided valve surgery and therefore must be corrected with annuloplasty or replacement, whereas functional tricuspid valve disease often improves when the left-sided problem is corrected. Surgical indications for tricuspid valve disease include: development of class III to IV symptoms with hepatic congestion, ascites, or peripheral edema that cannot be managed medically.

Surgical Options for Tricuspid Valve Disease. Annuloplasty procedures on the tricuspid valve produce clinical improvement in approximately 90% of all patients. Residual but mild degrees of either stenosis or regurgitation are noted in 30 to 50% of patients postoperatively, but are usually of no hemodynamic significance. There are three basic annuloplasty techniques: (1) the Kay or Wooler technique uses mattress or figure-of-eight sutures to obliterate the commissure and annulus between the anterior and posterior tricuspid valve leaflet, (2) the De Vega annuloplasty uses a double purse-string suture to narrow the annulus from the anterior commissure to the posterior–septal commissure, and (3) the Carpentier–Edward C-shaped annuloplasty configuration which is open at the area of the bundle of HIS.

Since the introduction of these techniques, many cardiothoracic surgeons have attempted correction of moderate to severe tricuspid valve regurgitation especially in the absence of organic lesions. Results from the Kay and Wooler types of annuloplasty have been unpredictable. Both the De Vega and Carpentier methods are successful. However, whereas the shape of the C ring conforms to the tricuspid valve, De Vega's method narrows the annulus by placement of circumferential sutures, produces semicircular deformation of the orifice, and, for purely geometric reasons, causes infolding of the leaflets with the potential for impairment of long-term function (Rivera, Duran & Ajuria, 1985).

Tricuspid valve replacement is indicated for tricuspid valve disease when repair procedures cannot be performed successfully. Most cases of mixed stenosis and regurgitation can be treated with commissurotomy and annuloplasty, but when the valve is severely distorted, replacement may become necessary. Prosthetic valve selection in the tricuspid position is usually limited to a tissue valve since mechanical valves are particularly prone to thrombosis in the low pressure system of the right heart.

Postoperative Consideration for Patients with Tricuspid Valve Disease. The bundle of HIS is adjacent to the tricuspid valve annulus and its septal leaflet. Therefore, postoperative heart block may occur more commonly with this operative procedure. Placement of epicardial ventricular pacing leads should be strongly considered in this patient subset because use of a transvenous pacemaker in the event of complete heart block will impair the tricuspid valve function (Bojar, 1994).

Surgical Diseases of the Thoracic Aorta

Thoracic Aortic Dissection

Dissection of the aorta has been known since the sixteenth century; however, despite various forms of surgical intervention, it was not until 1954 when DeBakey performed the first successful repair of an aortic dissection of the descending thoracic aorta. Today, aortic dissections still present one of the most challenging problems in cardiac surgery. Successful surgery for aortic dissection has lagged behind that for most other acquired cardiovascular abnormalities. This is in part due to the fact that acute aortic dissections often go undiagnosed. Patients also frequently present to a facility unequipped to handle the complexity of the problem. As a result, many patients die before adequate treatment is initiated or may reach the operating room, but in moribund condition.

Aortic dissection results from a sudden tear in the aortic intima. Blood then escapes from the true lumen and passes into the outer half of the media creating a longitudinal separation called a false lumen. Pulsatile flow generated by ventricular contraction causes the dissection channel to propagate retrograde and/or antegrade throughout the aorta. The clinical and pathologic consequences of aortic dissection are determined by the path that the dissection takes as it progresses between layers of the aorta. Dissections usually involve approximately half the circumference of the aorta and tend to spread along the greater curvature.

Expansion of the false lumen may compress the true lumen and, because the outer medial and adventitial layers of the aorta are thin, pressure necrosis from an expanding hematoma may result in external rupture. The majority of dissections do have reentry sites in the distal aorta or iliacs, most commonly on the left side.

Etiologies of Aortic Dissection. Etiologies of aortic dissections include: (1) congenital anomalies (e.g., Marfan's syndrome and coarctation of the aorta), (2) arterial hypertension, (3) third trimester pregnancy, (4) atherosclerosis, (5) inflammatory disease (e.g., aortitis, syphilis), and (6) trauma, both blunt and iatrogenic catheter induced.

Classification of Aortic Dissection. Aortic dissections have been classified by several different systems in an attempt to identify the location and extent of dissection as well as the acuity of the presentation (Bojar, 1992). Dissections are described as acute versus chronic based upon weather the patient presents less than or greater than 2 weeks from the onset of dissection (Bojar, 1992). The first 14 days after onset is designated the acute phase and approximately 74% of deaths from complications of the dissection occur within these 2 weeks. After 2 weeks, the chronic stage begins and surviving patients are more stable with a better prognosis (Crawford, 1990). The first classification was described by DeBakey in 1965 (Fig. 34–23). The Stanford group modified this classification and proposed a simplified version based on whether or not the ascending aorta was involved (Fig. 34–24). Stanford type A dissections are twice as common as type B. Approximately 90% of type A dissections originate in the ascending aorta with distal propagation, and 10% extend retrograde from the arch or descending thoracic aorta. Eighty-five percent of type B dissections originate in the descending thoracic aorta and 15% originate in the arch.

Incidence of Aortic Dissection. The true incidence of aortic dissection is hard to determine because many clinical cases are not diagnosed correctly. Dissections occur

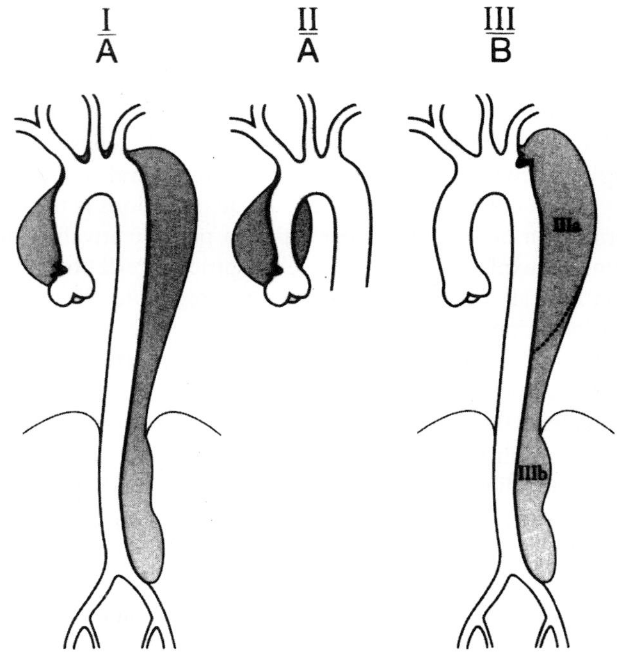

Figure 34–23. Commonly used classifications of aortic dissections. DeBakey types I = involvement of the ascending, arch, and descending aorta; II = involvement of the ascending aorta only; IIIa = limited to the thoracic aorta; and IIIb = involvement of the thoracic and abdominal aorta. Stanford type A = involvement of the ascending aorta regardless of the site of tear and Stanford type B = no involvement of the ascending aorta. *(Used with permission from Borst et al., [1996].)*

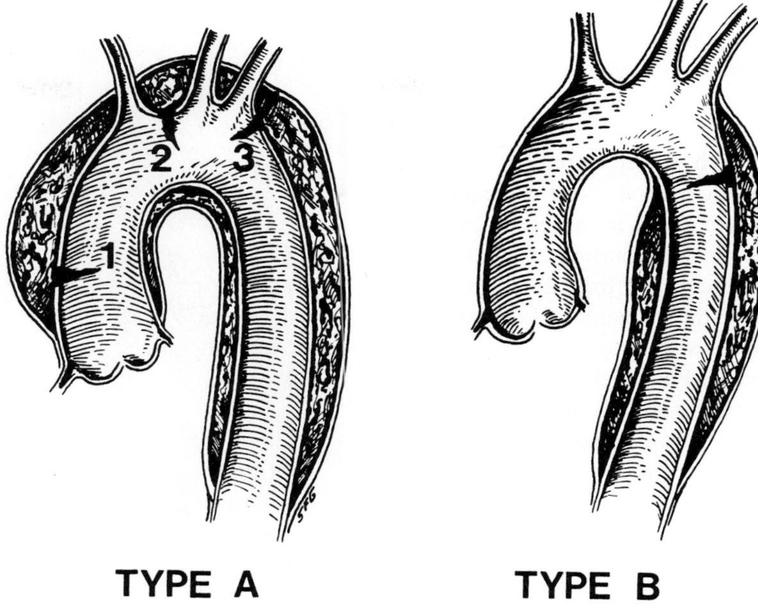

Figure 34–24. Stanford classification of aortic dissection is based upon the presence or absence of involvement of the ascending aorta. Type A involves the ascending aorta regardless of where the dissection originates. Type A dissections include DeBakey types I and II. Stanford type B dissection does not involve the ascending aorta and includes DeBakey types IIIa and IIIb. *(Used with permission from McCauley et al., [1985].)*

more frequently in males than females (3:1) and most commonly occur in the fifth decade of life. Patients with dissection of the descending thoracic aorta are about ten years older than those with ascending aortic lesions and are more likely to have concomitant atherosclerosis or cardiopulmonary disease (Cohn, 1994). An estimated 24,000 acute aortic dissections occur annually, surpassing even the incidence of abdominal aortic aneurysms. Unfortunately only 2,000 cases are correctly diagnosed before the patient dies! Despite remarkable recent advances in the diagnostic accuracy and the availability of advanced imaging modalities, the most important factor leading to a successful antemortem diagnosis is a high clinical index of suspicion by the examining clinician (Borst, Heinemann, & Stone, 1996).

Natural History of Aortic Dissection. Patients with acute aortic dissections have a very poor prognosis due to the propensity of the aorta to rupture at the site of tear. In fact, rupture accounts for over 90% of deaths resulting from acute aortic dissection. Type A dissections tend to rupture in the intrapericardial aorta resulting in cardiac tamponade. Conversely, in type B dissections, the tear usually originates just beyond the left subclavian artery with rupture most commonly occurring into the left pleural space. In patients with healed or chronic dissections, approximately 56% of deaths result from rupture of an expanding aneurysmal aortic wall. The natural history of untreated dissections is: 25% mortality within the first 24 hours, 50% at 1 week, and 90% within the first 3 months (Bojar, 1992).

Clinical Presentation of Aortic Dissection. Aortic dissections can almost always be traced to an acute event of severe chest and back pain coinciding with the onset of the process (Borst et al., 1996). The pain is cataclysmic and maximal at its inception (Cohn, 1994). In fact, severe "tearing" type chest pain is the cardinal feature of aortic dissection occurring in over 90% of all patients. The pain tends to be anterior for type A dissections and intrascapular for type B dissections; however, patients with Marfan's commonly develop silent dissections (Bojar, 1992). Most patients present either normotensive or hypertensive. When hypotension is present, suspect leakage or rupture into the pericardium, thoracic cavity, or retroperitoneum. Hypotension can also occur from severe sudden onset of congestive heart failure due to acute aortic regurgitation or compromise of the coronary arteries. Either a pulse deficit or absent pulses from an expanding false lumen are also common. Specific signs and symptoms of aortic dissection depend on the size of dissection channel and the degree of compromise of the true lumen and its branches (Bojar, 1992).

Type A Dissections. Although the dissection can spread proximally towards the aortic valve or distally toward the arch, it is convenient to think of the complications associated with type A dissections as starting at the level of the aortic valve and proceeding distally. All of the complications discussed with type B dissection can also occur with type A dissection if it extends distally to involve the descending thoracic aorta (Bojar, 1992).

Aortic regurgitation occurs in 50 to 60% of patients caused by loss of commisural support of the aortic cusps. Myocardial infarctions may result from compression of the coronary ostia by the dissection channel and the right coronary artery is most commonly effected. The overall incidence of myocardial infarction, however, is only 1 to 2%. Cardiac tamponade is the most common cause of death in patients with acute type A dissection. It is caused by external rupture through the intrapericardial portion of the aorta. Superior vena cava syndrome can result from compression of the superior vena cava by the expanding hematoma. Look for neck distention along with progressive cyanosis and edema of the head and neck. Pulse deficit results from compression of the brachiocephalic vessels and is noted in 50% of patients with type A dissections. Involvement of the innominate or left subclavian artery may produce arm ischemia or a discrepancy in upper extremity blood pressures. There may also be diminished or absent carotid pulses with associate neurologic deficits such as syncope or mental status changes or stroke.

Type B Dissections. Type B complications are localized to the intrathoracic or intraabdominal aorta and its distal branches. Aortic rupture into the chest is the most common cause of death for acute type B dissections. Intrathoracic rupture may occur into the mediastinum or pleural space (left more common than right). Infradiaphragmatic rupture occurs into the retroperitoneum or peritoneal space. Branch artery compromise can produce ischemia or infarction of the bowel by involvement of the celiac or mesenteric vessels (severe abdominal pain), renal artery compromise producing oliguria (left renal artery more commonly perfused off the false lumen while the right kidney is perfused by the true lumen), paraplegia if the intercostal or lumbar arteries are involved (2% of patients present with paraplegia), or lower extremity ischemia if the false channel extends beyond the aortic bifurcations (Bojar, 1992).

Evaluation of Aortic Dissection. Imaging objectives are to view the intimal tear and entry site, view the aortic valve, view the true and false lumens as well as any sites of communication, and to view the major branch vessels including the coronary arteries, great arteries, abdominal viscera, and renal arteries. The most important diagnostic tools for the detection and evaluation of the extent of aortic disease encompass CT scanning with contrast enhancement, MRI, transesopahgeal echocardiogram, and aortography (Figs. 34–25 through 34–27). These tests have a diagnostic accuracy rate approaching 99%.

Management of Aortic Dissection. The keys to successful outcome are being aware of symptoms of dissection, early diagnosis, and prompt treatment. During the diagnostic evaluation process, medical therapy must be instituted for all patients with suspicion of dissection because of

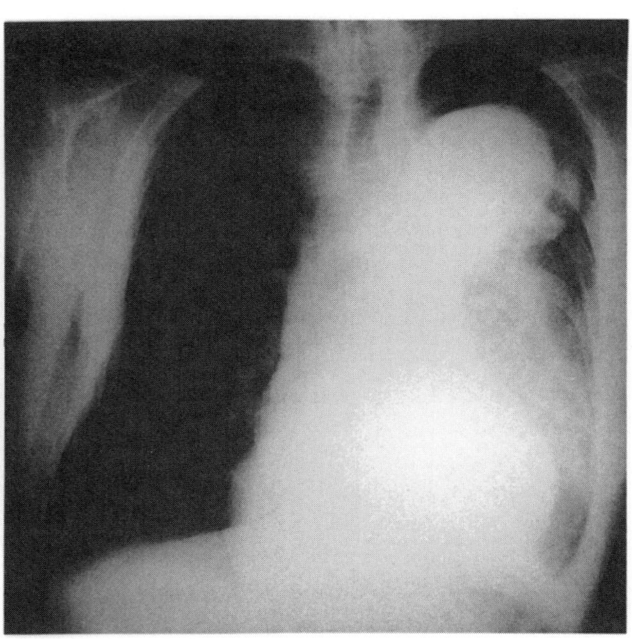

Figure 34–25. Typical chest radiograph from a patient with an aortic dissection. Several findings typical for dissection are shown including enlargement of the aortic shadow, a double shadow at the aortic knob, cardiomegaly, displacement of the left mainstem bronchus, and loss of distinct aortic shadows. *(Used with permission from Borst et al., [1996].)*

the high risk of rupture. This usually consists of intravenous morphine to control the pain in combination with beta blockers and vasodilators to control blood pressure. The goals for medical therapy were established by M.W. Wheat and associates at the University of Florida College of Medicine in the 1960s. They emphasize the importance of lowering not only blood pressure but also the velocity of left ventricular ejection, which was found to be a major factor contributing to the pathogenesis and propagation of aortic dissection (Cohn, 1994).

There is general consensus among the experts that acute type A dissections are best treated with immediate operation. Surgery should also be considered electively for all chronic type A dissections if they are either symptomatic or greater than 6 cm in diameter. The principles of surgery for type A dissections include: elimination of aortic valve insufficiency by either resuspension or replacement, obliteration of the false lumen at the proximal extent of the dissection which is the most likely site of rupture, and reestablishment of intimal continuity of the aorta by resecting or excluding the entry site and interposing a vascular graft. It is not possible to eliminate all distal fenestrations between the true and false lumens. In approximately 70% of patients, the false lumen remains patent distally because of multiple reentry sites. This is actually beneficial because organ perfusion through major blood vessels may depend on

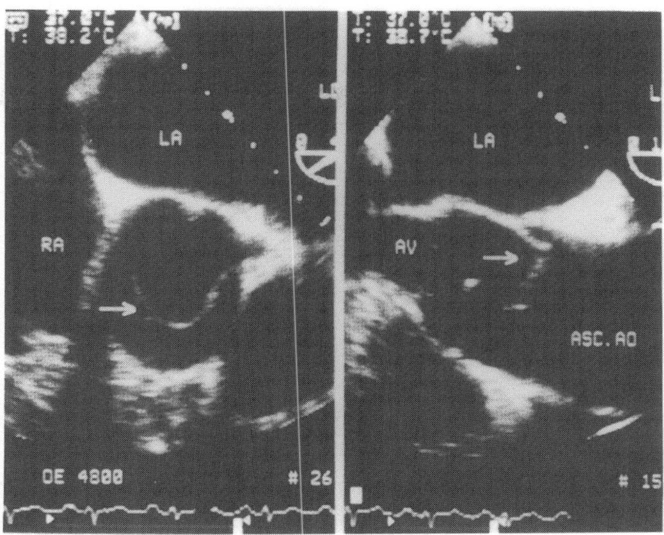

Figure 34–26. Transesophageal echocardiogram images from a patient with an acute type A aortic dissection. The arrow points to the dissecting membrane in the proximal ascending aorta. RA, right atrium; LA, left atrium; AV, aortic valve; ASCAO, ascending aorta. *(Used with permission from Borst et al., [1996].)*

false lumen flow (Bojar, 1992). Conversely, treatment of uncomplicated type B dissections is medical.

Surgical intervention is warranted however, for those patients with persistent pain, uncontrolled hypertension, visceral or peripheral arterial compromise, neurologic deficits, expansion, or rupture (Bojar, 1992).

Operative Techniques. Surgical repair of a type A dissection is performed through a median sternotomy incision with use of cardiopulmonary bypass and cold cardioplegic solution. If aortic regurgitation is present due to loss of commissural support, resuspension of the commissures or replacement of the aortic valve is performed (Fig. 34–28).

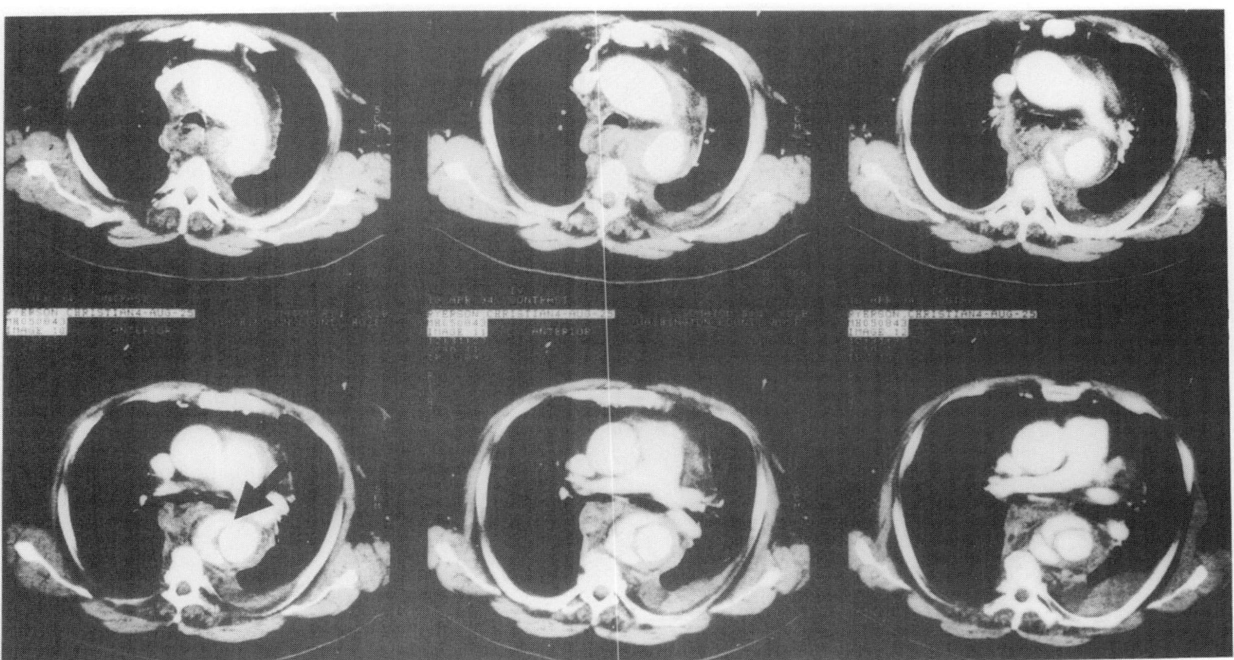

Figure 34–27. CAT scan images from a patient with an acute type B aortic dissection, involving a chronically aneurysmal ascending and descending thoracic aorta. The ascending aorta is dilated but not dissected. The descending portion contains a complex dissection with three distinct lumens and is leaking retroperitoneally. *(Used with permission from Borst et al., [1996].)*

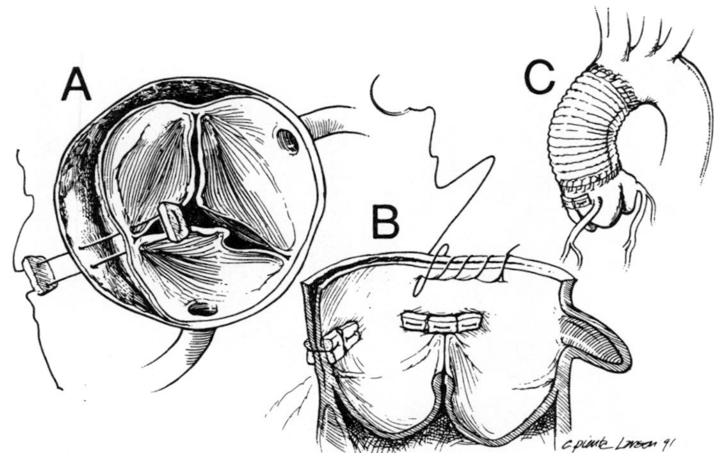

Figure 34–28. **A** and **B,** In patients with aortic regurgitation due to aortic dissection because the commissures have dissected away from the aortic wall, the commissures are resuspended with interrupted sutures pledgeted with either Teflon or pericardial pledgets. **C,** The proximal aorta is reapproximated and the repair is complete. *(Used with permission from Svensson & Crawford, [1997].)*

When the intimal tear extends proximally to the coronary ostia or the dissection produces marked dilatation of the aortic annulus with aortic regurgitation, placement of a composite aortic graft with reimplantation of the coronary ostia (valved conduit) is indicated. The three most common surgical techniques for composite aortic grafting include the Bentall procedure, the Cabrol procedure, and the modified Bentall button technique (Figs. 34–29 through 34–32).

Surgery for type B aortic dissection is approached through a left thoracotomy incision. The aorta is clamped proximally and distally to exclude the section containing the intimal tear. Once this area is resected, aortic continuity is restored with a tubular dacron graft, obliterating the false lumen at the proximal and distal ends. If blood flow to arterial branches has been compromised, adequate blood supply to organs supplied by the branches must be restored (Finkelmeier, 1995).

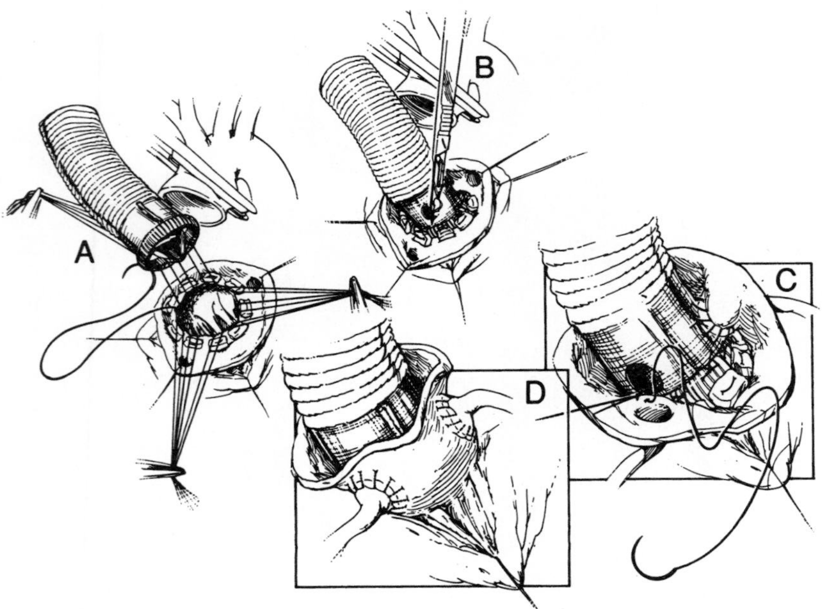

Figure 34–29. Steps in the classic technique of composite valve graft insertions by the Bentall method. **A,** Seating of the composite valve graft. **B,** Excision of holes in the graft opposite the coronary ostia. **C,** Anatomosis of the ostia to the graft. **D,** Completion of the operation. Wrapping of the graft with the residual native aorta has been shown to be associated with a higher incidence of false aneurysm formation. *(Used with permission from Svensson & Crawford, [1997].)*

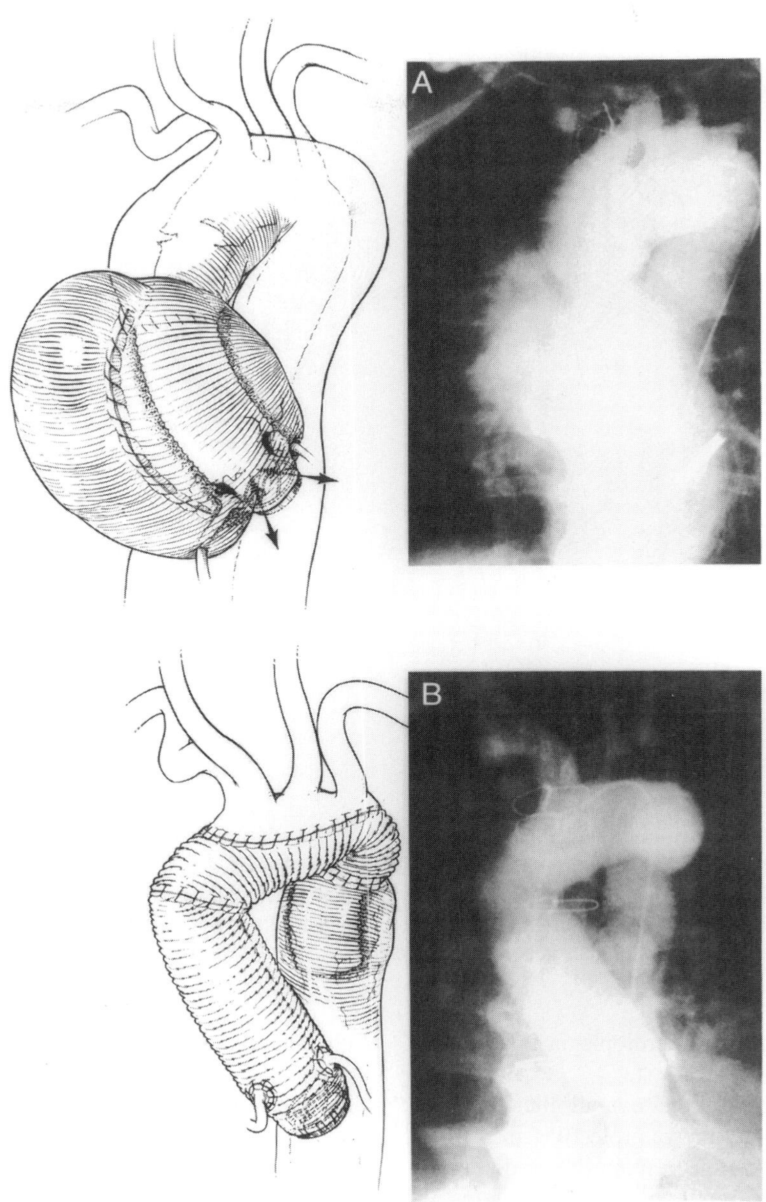

Figure 34–30. A, Diagram and angiogram showing the not uncommon complications of a false aneurysm developing after the classic Bentall procedure with direct reimplantation of the coronary ostia into the tube graft. **B,** Postoperative illustrations after reimplantation of the coronary ostia as aortic buttons and replacement of the aortic arch by the elephant trunk technique. *(Used with permission from Svensson & Crawford, [1997].)*

Maintenance of Adequate Circulation During Aortic Operations. Surgery of the aorta requires temporary interruption of blood flow through the involved segment making maintenance of adequate perfusion to vital organs a challenge. Operations of the ascending aorta are done using standard cardiopulmonary bypass with cold cardioplegia solution via the coronary arteries for myocardial protection. Depending on the specific location of aortic pathology, the arterial cannulation site can be either the distal ascending aorta or the femoral artery.

Operations involving the transverse arch require special attention to protection of the cerebral circulation because blood flow through the carotid arteries is interrupted during the period of surgical repair. As opposed to the moderate hypothermia and standard cardiopulmonary bypass techniques used during most other cardiac operations, profound hypothermia and circulatory arrest are used in aortic arch operations (Finkelmeier, 1995). With the patient on cardiopulmonary bypass, core body temperature is lowered to 18 to 20°C, clamps are placed on the proximal aorta and

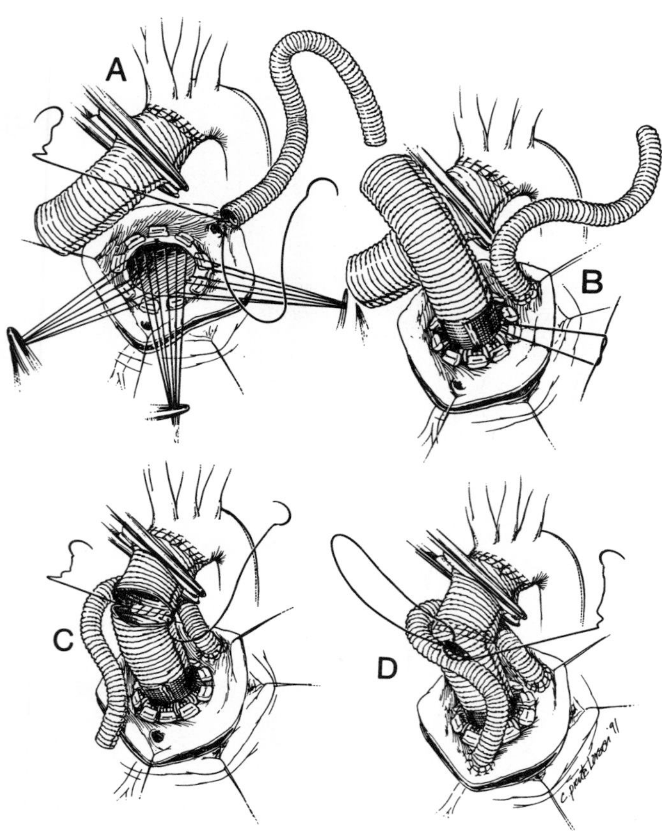

Figure 34–31. Insertion of a composite valve graft by the Cabrol technique. **A,** The valve annular sutures are placed and the tube graft is sutured to the left main ostium. **B,** The tube graft is seated and tied into position. **C,** The tube graft to the left main ostium is brought behind the composite graft and then the composite graft is sutured the aortic arch. **D,** Finally, the coronary interposition graft is sutured to the right coronary artery ostium and the side-to-side anastomosis is performed. *(Used with permission from Svensson & Crawford, [1997].)*

brachiocephalic arteries, and cold cardioplegia is administered to establish total circulatory arrest.

These techniques decrease the overall incidence of neurologic sequelae. Despite these protective measures, however, neurologic complications remain the predominant cause of morbidity associated with operative procedures on the aortic arch (Finkelmeier, 1995). Over the past 5 years, there has been increasing support for the use of retrograde cerebral perfusion (RCP) as an adjunct to hypothermic circulatory arrest. Use of RCP is thought to extend the safety of hypothermic circulatory arrest during operations involving an open aortic arch by preventing cerebral rewarming. RCP provides between 10 to 30% of cerebral blood flow when administered through a superior vena cava cannula (Bavaria & Pochettino, 1997) (Fig. 34–33).

Operations on the descending thoracic aorta are associated with the potential for impaired perfusion to organs and tissue distal to the clamp. The spinal cord, however, is the most vulnerable to ischemic damage with resultant paraplegia. Spinal cord injury following aortic surgeries is largely due to the duration and degree of ischemia, failure to reestablish blood flow after the aortic repair, and a biochemically mediated reperfusion injury as a result of the ischemia to the spinal cord (Svensson, 1997). Several factors have been found to correlate with the incidence of postoperative paraplegia including: duration of aortic cross-clamping (when no provisions are made to increase distal perfusion, risk of paraplegia increases with aortic cross clamping greater than 30 minutes), the level of proximal aortic cross clamp, the extent of the excluded aortic segment (the incidence of paraplegia increases with extensive aneurysms or dissections and reimplantation of the intercostal vessels has been shown to decrease the incidence of paraplegia), and the adequacy of the distal perfusion (a distal perfusion pressure of 60 to 70 mm Hg should be maintained and monitored by a femoral arterial line) (Bojar, 1992). The most common intraoperative techniques used in descending aortic operations for spinal cord protections include left heart (partial) bypass and cerebral spinal fluid drainage. In left heart bypass blood is drained via a cannulae in the left atrium and returned to the systemic circulation via a femoral arterial cannula. Because circulation is maintained through the right heart, it is not necessary to use an oxygenator in this circuit and only low doses of heparin are re-

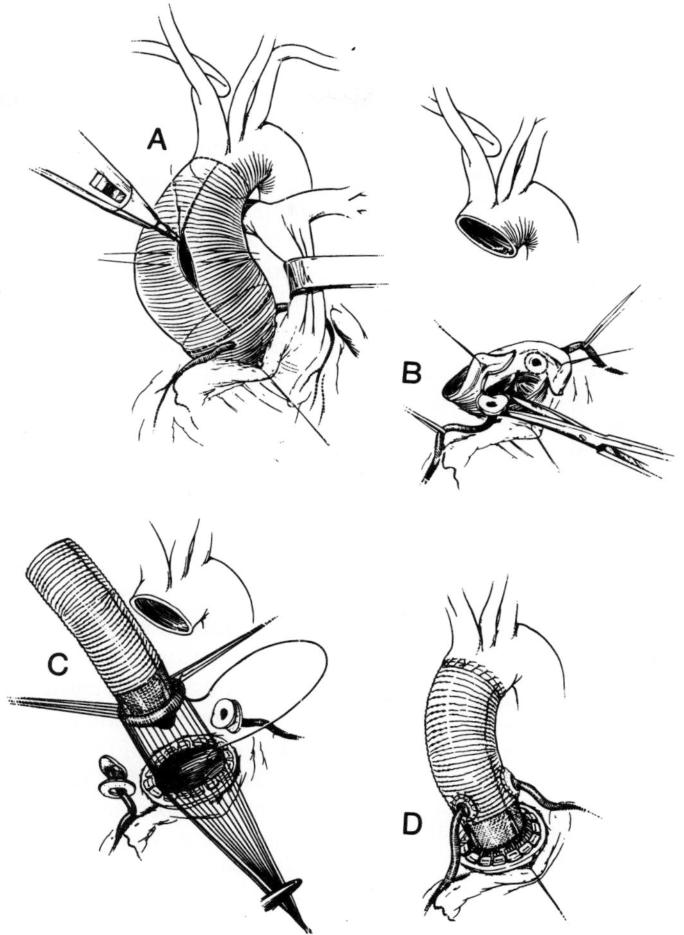

Figure 34–32. Insertion of a composite graft by the button technique. **A,** The aorta is incised and the coronary ostia are mobilized. **B,** The composite graft is seated. **C,** The coronary buttons with Teflon doughnut-shaped collars are sutured to the graft. **D,** The repair is complete. *(Used with permission from Svensson & Crawford, [1997].)*

quired. Cerebral spinal fluid (CSF) drainage decreases the risk of paraplegia postoperatively by decreasing CSF pressure which in turn enhances cord perfusion pressure.

Special Postoperative Considerations. The most common complications of aortic surgery are bleeding and ischemic organ injury. Control of hypertension remains as important after surgery as it was pre-operatively. The re-establishment of vascular continuity involves extensive suturing of dacron graft material to the very fragile native aortic tissues with the potential for extensive bleeding from the suture lines. In addition, surgical repair of dissections is predicated on stabilization of the entry site of the dissection, but does not completely eliminate the distal false channel. Thus, surgery is palliative and leaves the patient predisposed to aneurysmal formation within the false channel. Continued antihypertensive treatment is critical to improving long-term survival (Bojar, 1994). The most common antihypertensive regimes in the early postoperative period are esmolol and nitroprusside with transition to oral agents.

Long-Term Follow-Up of Aortic Dissection. Diligent follow-up of patients with aortic dissection includes controlling blood pressure, decreasing the velocity of left ventricular contraction with beta blockers, monitoring the size of the residual aorta with serial CT/MRI, and taking appropriate action if redissection, aneurysm, or rupture occurs (Crawford, 1990). The development of aneurysms in the dissected segment is the most common problem encountered in the chronic stage. Rupture of these aneurysms are size dependent and rarely occur in patients with an aortic diameter less than 5 cm. Patients with Marfan's should have aortic root and entire aortic monitoring regularly to assess for aneurysms and dissections. Elective graft replacement is indicated when the aortic diameter exceeds 5 cm or twice the diameter of the normal aorta (Crawford, 1990).

Aortic Aneurysms

An aneurysm is a localized area of thinning and dilatation of the aortic wall that exceeds the normal diameter for the

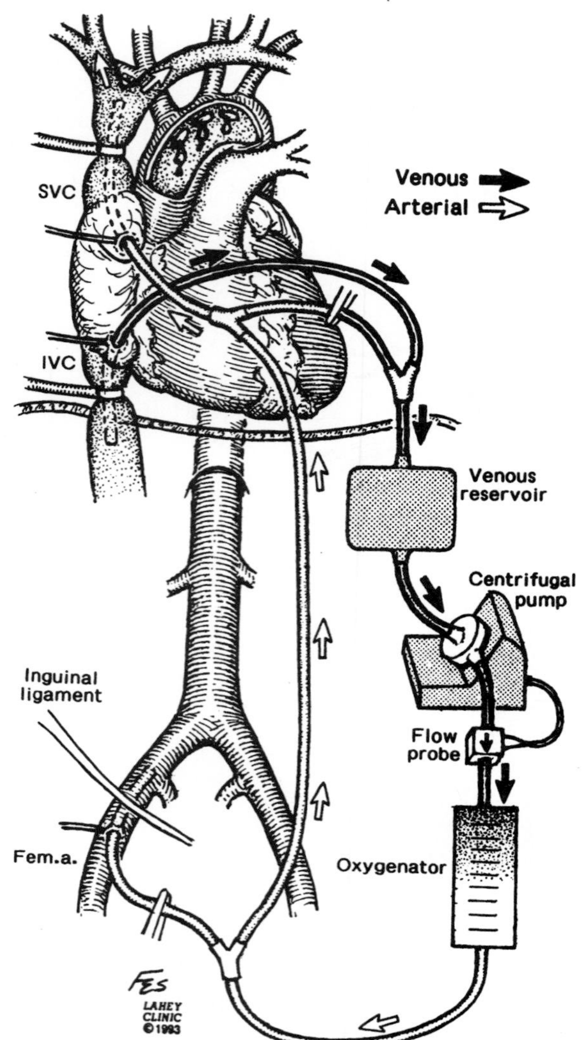

Figure 34–33. Cannulation arrangement for cardiopulmonary bypass with deep hypothermic arrest and retrograde cerebral perfusion. Note the Y connection of the arterial line to the superior vena cava cannula. *(Used with permission from Svensson & Crawford, [1997].)*

patient's age and height (Svensson & Crawford, 1997). Over 75% of all aortic aneurysms occur in patients who are asymptomatic and are detected incidentally either during routine physical examination, chest x-ray, or ultrasound. True aortic aneurysms are associated with a degenerative aortic media, aortic dissection, disorders of connective tissue, blunt trauma, aortitis, mycotic infections, previous graft insertion, and congenital abnormalities. Aneurysms not lined with the intima of the aortic wall are known as false or pseudoaneurysms. They tend to occur at sites of previous aortic anastomosis, infection, or post-trauma (Svensson & Crawford, 1997). Aneurysms are generally described according to their shape (i.e., fusiform or saccular) and their location (i.e., ascending aorta, transverse arch, descending aorta, thoracoabdominal aorta). The natural history for all types of aortic aneurysms regardless of site or cause is rupture. In fact, 75% of patients with thoracic aneurysms die within 5 years of diagnosis, with 50% of the deaths due to rupture (Finkelmeier, 1995). Although rupture is somewhat unpredictable, the risk is known to increase proportionately to the diameter of the aorta. The decision to operate prophylactically to prevent rupture is dependent upon the risk of rupture causing death versus the risk of other comorbid conditions.

Ascending Aortic Aneurysms. Aneurysms of the ascending aorta are usually the result of degenerative changes in the aortic media that is often associated with connective tissue disorders such as Marfan's syndrome. Atherosclerotic aneurysms are relatively infrequent in the ascending aorta. Aneurysms may be localized to the supracoronary aorta and may extend to the level of the innominate artery or may extend more distally to include the transverse arch or descending thoracic aorta. Chronic type A aortic dissections with gradual expansion of the false lumen are the second most common cause of ascending aortic aneurysms. Other causes include trauma, infections, and poststenotic dilatation associated with aortic stenosis. Overall, about 25% of thoracic aortic aneurysms occur in the ascending aorta. The vast majority of patients are asymptomatic. Nonspecific chest discomfort may be present and severe chest pain may occur with an acute dissection (Bojar, 1992). Often, the diagnosis of an ascending aortic aneurysm is suggested by routine chest x-ray. Diagnosis should, however, be confirmed by either CT or MRI of the chest.

Indications for surgery of an ascending aortic aneurysm include: (1) aneurysm of any etiology in which there is documented rapid growth rate from serial diagnostic imaging studies, (2) aneurysms of any etiology larger than 6 cm or greater than twice the diameter of the "normal" aorta, (3) aneurysms greater than 5 cm in patients with progressive, symptomatic aortic regurgitation (annuloaortic ectasia), (4) all acute type A dissections, (5) asymptomatic aneurysms exceeding 5 cm in patients with Marfan's syndrome, and (6) mycotic aneurysms. (See Fig. 34–34.)

Transverse Aortic Arch Aneurysms. The transverse aortic arch is involved in about 25% of all thoracic aortic aneurysms and nearly 70% of arch aneurysms have either proximal or distal aortic involvement that requires either simultaneous or staged surgical repair. The most common etiology associated with arch aneurysms is medial degeneration; however, they are occasionally caused by type A dissections that extend or originate within the arch. Aneurysms involving the distal arch are most frequently associated with atherosclerosis. Like ascending aortic aneurysms, the vast majority of arch aneurysms are asymptomatic and identified incidentally by a widened medistinum on routine chest x-ray (Bojar, 1992).

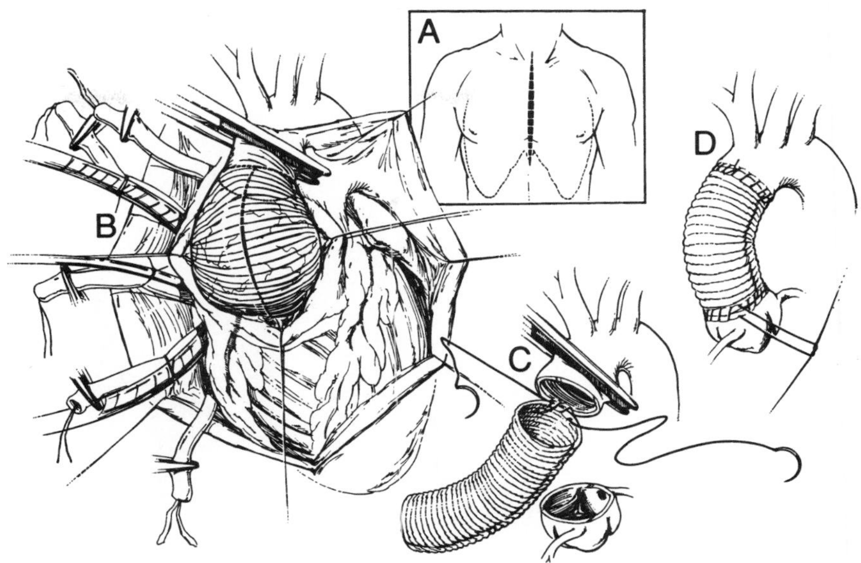

Figure 34–34. Steps in the repair of an ascending aortic aneurysm. **A,** A midline sternotomy incision is made. **B,** The aneurysm is incised and the aorta is transected both proximally and distally. **C,** The tube graft is sutured into position distally. **D,** The proximal anastomosis is completed. *(Used with permission from Svensson & Crawford, [1997].)*

Surgical intervention is indicated to prevent rupture due to expansion or dissection in the following situations: (1) transverse arch aneurysm that is symptomatic or greater than 6 cm, (2) acute arch dissection, or (3) ascending aortic aneurysms that involve the arch. (See Fig. 34–35.)

Descending Aortic Aneurysms. Nearly 50% of all aortic aneurysms are located in the descending thoracic aorta. The vast majority are a result of atherosclerotic degenerative changes. The diagnosis is most commonly made from an abnormal chest x-ray that demonstrates a widened mediastinum with a prominent descending aorta. Patients are usually asymptomatic; however, symptoms can occur as the aorta continues to expand and compress adjacent structures. Common symptoms include: chest pain due to compression of spine and ribs, hoarseness due to compression of the recurrent laryngeal nerve, dysphagia due to compression of the esophagus, cough or hemoptysis due to compression of the airway, or Horner's syndrome due to compression of the cervical ganglia (Bojar, 1992).

As with other aneurysms of the thoracic aorta, the natural history of descending aortic aneurysms is one of progressive expansion. Eventually rupture into the airway, esophagus, mediastinum, or pleural space occurs. Rupture accounts for approximately 50% of all deaths in patients with atherosclerotic aneurysms, with a 5-year survival rate ranging between 20 to 50%. (See Fig. 34–36.)

Thoracoabdominal Aneurysms. Around 10% of descending thoracic aortic aneurysms extend across the diaphragm to involve portions of the abdominal aorta. One of

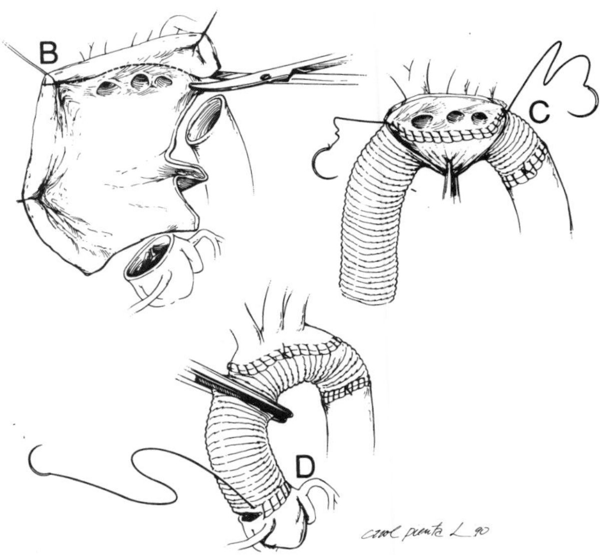

Figure 34–35. Replacement of the aortic arch with a distal end-to-end anastomosis. **A,** Note the thrombus in the ascending aorta and aortic arch on the CT scan, a more unusual finding in the ascending aorta than in the descending aorta. **B,** Opening of the aortic arch and transection of the distal aorta in the descending aorta as well as proximal aorta above the level of the aortic valve. **C,** Insertion of the posterior suture line for reattachment of the arch vessels after the distal anastomosis has been performed. **D,** Completion of the repair by doing the proximal anastomosis above the aortic valve. *(Used with permission from Svensson & Crawford, [1997].)*

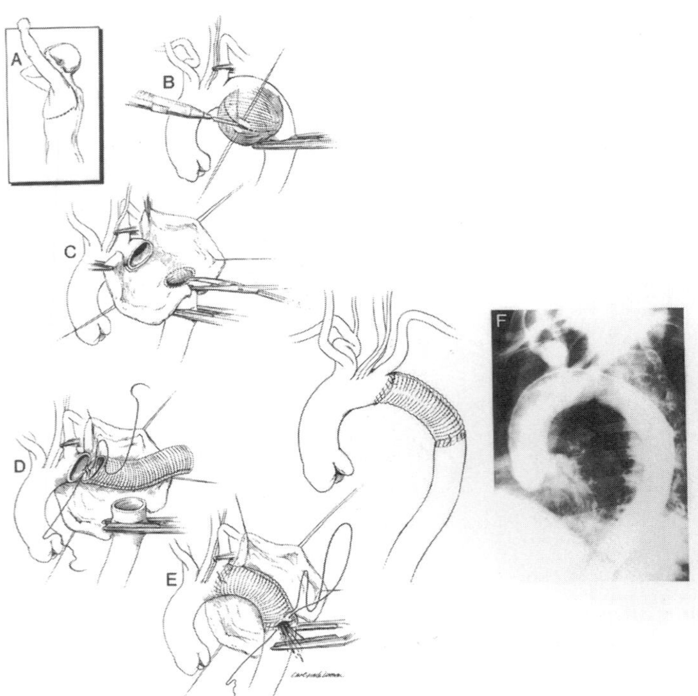

Figure 34–36. **A,** Positioning of the patient for a left thoracotomy. **B,** A proximal descending thoracic aortic aneurysm is opened. **C,** The aneurysm is transected. **D** and **E,** A tube graft is sutured into position beyond the left subclavian artery and distally the descending thoracic aorta. **F,** Postoperative aortogram after the repair. *(Used with permission from Svensson & Crawford, [1997].)*

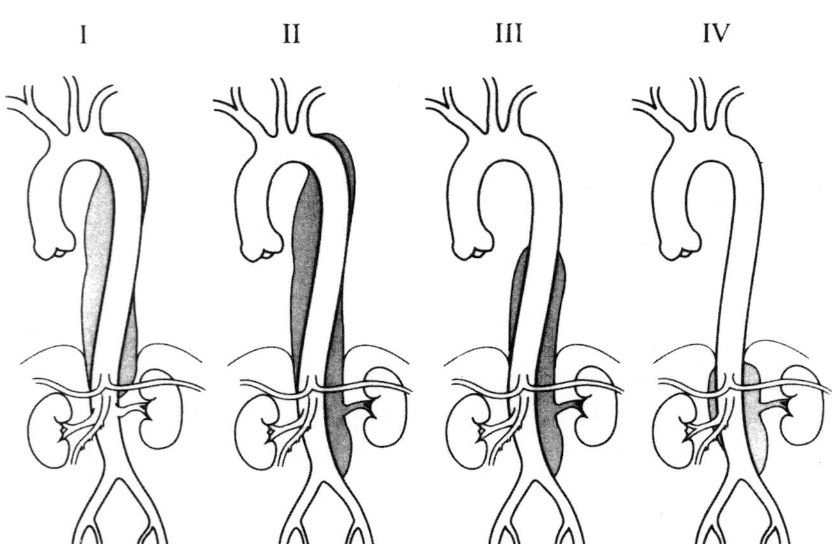

Figure 34–37. Crawford classification of thoracoabdominal aneurysms. Type I = originates in the proximal descending thoracic aorta and ends above the renal arteries; Type II = originates in the proximal descending thoracic aorta and terminates below the renal arteries; Type III = originates in the distal descending thoracic aorta, below T6; and Type IV = involves most of the abdominal aorta. *(Used with permission from Borst et al., [1996].)*

the more common ways to describe the location and extent of these aneurysms is the Crawford classification system (Fig. 34–37).

Again, the most common cause of these types of aneurysms is atherosclerotic degeneration. Unlike other aortic aneurysms, patients frequently complain of chest or abdominal pain. The natural history in unoperated patients is death resulting from rupture. Therefore, surgery is indicated for any symptomatic thoracoabdominal aneurysm as well as those with a diameter twice that of the uninvolved proximal aorta (Bojar, 1992) (Fig. 34–38).

Special Postoperative Considerations. Thoracic aneurysms tend to develop in patients with hypertension, chronic lung disease, and diffuse atherosclerosis including cerebrovascular, cardiovascular, and renovascular disease. Prevention and/or recognition of problems involving these organ systems in the early postoperative period is paramount to decrease the overall incidence of morbidity and mortality associated with these operations.

Knowledge and early recognition of procedure-specific complications are also crucial to an uneventful surgical recovery. Repair of ascending and arch aneurysms using hypothermic circulatory arrest carries a significant incidence of coagulopathy and potential neurologic insult. Aggressive management of mediastinal bleeding and careful neurologic examination is imperative. Conversely, repair of descending and thoracoabdominal aneurysms involves a thoracotomy incision that can make postoperative pain control a chal-

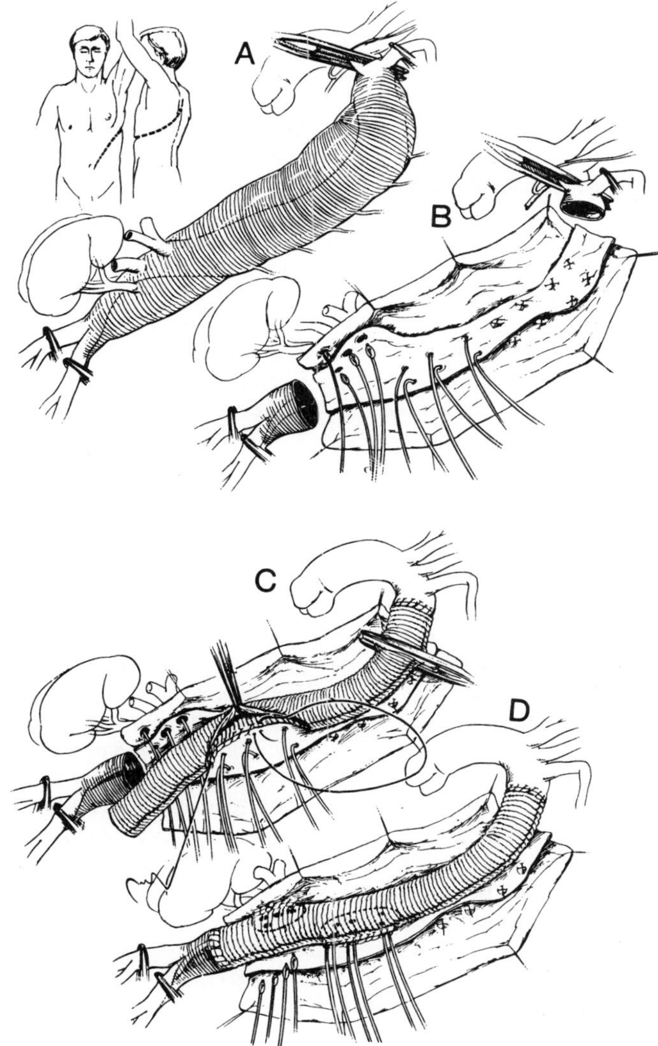

Figure 34–38. Steps in repair of the thoracoabdominal aorta. **A,** The line of incision is indicated and the aorta is then cross clamped. **B,** The upper intercostal arteries are oversewn and the intercostal arteries below T7 are preserved. **C,** The intercostal arteries are reimplanted followed by the visceral arteries. **D,** The distal aortic anastomosis is performed. Whenever possible atrial to femoral artery bypass is used and a segmental repair is performed in descending thoracic aortic resections. *(Used with permission from Svensson & Crawford, [1997].)*

lenge that ultimately impacts on postoperative pulmonary function. Also, cross-clamping of the descending aorta can result in paraplegia or renal failure. Particular assessment and support of these systems is a must in the early postoperative period (Bojar, 1994).

Long-Term Follow-Up of Aortic Aneurysms. Follow-up of patients who have undergone surgical resection of a thoracic aortic aneurysm includes careful monitoring and treatment of their commonly associated comorbidities. It is generally recommended that serial evaluations of the residual aorta and the dacron graft be done with either CT or MRI. A suggested schedule for follow-up scans is six months postoperatively and annually thereafter.

REFERENCES

American College of Cardiology & American Heart Association Task Force Report (1991). Guidelines and indications for coronary artery bypass graft surgery. *The Journal of the American College of Cardiology, 17* (3), 543–589.

Assey, M. E. & Spann, J. F. (1990). Indications for heart valve replacement. *Clinical Cardiology, 13,* 81–88.

Barner, H. B. (1994). New arterial conduits for coronary bypass surgery. *Seminars in Thoracic and Cardiovascular Surgery, 6* (2), 76–80.

Baue, A. E., Geha, A. S., Hammond, G. L., Laks, H., & Naunheim, K. S. (Eds.). (1991). *Glenn's thoracic and cardiovascular surgery* (5th ed.). East Norwalk, CT: Appelton & Lange.

Bavaria, J. E. & Pochettino, A. (1997). Retrograde cerebral perfusion (RCP) in aortic arch surgery: Efficacy and possible mechanisms of brain protection. *Seminars in Thoracic and Cardiovascular Surgery, 9* (3), 222–232.

Bojar, R. M. (1992). *Adult cardiac surgery.* Cambridge, MA: Blackwell Scientific Publications.

Bojar, R. M. (1994). *Manual of perioperative care in cardiac and thoracic surgery* (2nd ed.). Cambridge, MA: Blackwell Scientific Publications.

Borst, H. G., Heinemann, M. K., & Stone, C. D. (1996). *Surgical treatment of aortic dissection.* New York: Churchill Livingstone Inc.

Borst, C., Jansen, E. W., & Grundeman, P. F. (1997). Less invasive coronary artery bypass grafting: Without cardiopulmonary bypass and via reduced surgical access. *Heart, 77* (4), 302–303.

Buche, M. & Dion, R. (1996). Current status of the inferior epigastric artery. *Seminars in Thoracic and Cardiovascular Surgery, 8* (1), 10–14.

Calafiore, A. M. & DiGiammarco, G. (1996). Complete revascularization with three or more arterial conduits. *Seminars in Thoracic and Cardiovascular Surgery, 8* (1), 15–23.

Calafiore, A. M., DiGiammarco, G., Teodori, G., Bosco, G., D'Annunzio, E., Barsotti, A., Maddestra, N., Paloscia, L., Vitolla, G., Sciaria, A., Fino, C., & Conti, M. (1996). Left anterior descending grafting via left anterior small thoracotomy without cardiopulmonary bypass. *Annals of Thoracic Surgery, 61,* 1658–1665.

Carabello, B. A. (1993). Mitral valve disease. *Current Problems in Cardiology, 17* (7), 421–480.

Cohn, L. H. (1994). Aortic dissection: New aspects of diagnosis and treatment. *Hospital Practice, 15,* 47–56.

Cosgrove, D. M., Lytle, B. W., Loop, F. D., Taylor, P. C., Stewart, R. W., Gill, C. C., Golding, A. R., & Goormastic, M. (1988). Does bilateral internal mammary artery grafting increase surgical risk? *The Journal of Thoracic and Cardiovascular Surgery, 95* (5), 850–856.

Crawford, E. S. (1990). The diagnosis and management of aortic dissection. *The Journal of the American Medical Association, 264,* (19), 2537–2541.

Dietl, C. A. & Benoit, C. H. (1995). Radial artery graft for coronary revascularization: Technical considerations. *Annals of Thoracic Surgery, 60,* 102–110.

Dillard, D. H. & Miller, D. W. (1983). *Atlas of cardiac surgery.* New York: Macmillan Publishing Company.

Duran, C., Kumar, N., Gometza, B., & Al Halees, Z. (1991). Indications and limitations of aortic valve reconstruction. *Annals of Thoracic Surgery, 52,* 447–454.

Favaloro, R. G. (1994). Current status of coronary artery bypass graft (CABG) surgery. *Seminars in Thoracic and Cardiovascular Surgery, 6* (2), 67–71.

Fenster, M. S. & Feldman, M. D. (1995). Mitral regurgitation: An overview. *Current Problems in Cardiology, 20* (4), 193–280.

Finkelmeier, B. A. (1995). *Cardiothoracic surgical nursing.* Philadelphia: J. B. Lippincott.

Grunkemeier, G. L., Starr, A., & Rahimtoola, S. H. (1992). Prosthetic heart valve performance: Long term follow-up. *Current Problems in Cardiology, 17* (6), 331–406.

Halm, M. A. (1996). Acute gastrointestinal complications after cardiac surgery. *American Journal of Critical Care, 5* (2), 109–118.

Hartz, R. S. (1996). Minimally invasive heart surgery. *Circulation, 94* (10), 2669–2670.

Hendren, W. G. & Higgins, T. L. (1991). Immediate postoperative care of the cardiac surgery patient. *Seminars in Thoracic and Cardiovascular Surgery, 3* (1), 3–11.

Iaffaldano, R. A., Lewis, B. E., Johnson, S. A., Piffare, R., & McKiernan, T. L. (1995). Patency of cryopreserved saphenous vein grafts as conduit for coronary artery bypass surgery. *Chest, 108* (3), 725–729.

Jones, E. L., Weintraub, W. S., Craver, J. M., Guyton, R. A., & Cohen, C. (1991). Coronary bypass surgery: Is the operation different today. *The Journal of Thoracic and Cardiovascular Surgery, 101* (1), 108–115.

Joyce, F., Tingeloff, J., & Pettersson, G. (1996). Changing indications for the Ross procedure. *Seminars in Thoracic and Cardiovascular Surgery, 8* (4), 336–344.

Kirklin, J. W. & Barratt-Boyes, B. G. (1993). *Cardiac surgery* (2nd ed.). New York: Churchill Livingstone Inc.

Ko, W., Lazenby, D., Zelano, J. A., Isom, W., & Krieger, K. H. (1992). Effects of shaving methods and intraoperative irrigation on suppurative mediastinitis after bypass opeartions. *Annals of Thoracic Surgery, 53,* 301–305.

Kreter, B. & Woods, M. (1992). Antibiotic prophylaxis for cardiothoracic surgery operations: Metaanalysis of thirty years of clinical trials. *The Journal of Thoracic and Cardiovascular Surgery, 104* (3), 590–599.

Loop, F. D., Lytle, B. W., Cosgrove, D. M., Mahfood, S., McHenry, M. C., Goormastic, M., Stewart, R. W., Golding, L. A., & Taylor, P. C. (1990). Sternal wound complications after isolated coronary bypass grafting: Early and late mortality, morbidity, and cost of care. *Annals of Thoracic Surgery, 49,* 179–187.

Loop, F. D. (1994). The value and conduct of reoperations for cornary atherosclerosis. *Seminars in Thoracic and Cardiovascular Surgery, 6* (2), 116–119.

McCauley, K. M., Brest, A. N., & McGoon, D. C. (1985). *McGoon's cardiac surgery: An interprofessional approach to patient care.* Philadelphia: F. A. Davis Company.

Miller, R. A., Horneffer, P. J., Gardner, T. J., Rykiel, M. F., & Pearson, T. A. (1988). The epidemiology of postpericardiotomy syndrome: A common complication of cardiac surgery. *American Heart Journal, 116* (5), 1323–1329.

Moreno-Cabrol, C. E., Mitchell, R. S., & Miller, D. C. (1988). *Manual of postoperative management in adult cardiac surgery.* Baltimore: Williams & Wilkins.

Oury, J. H. (1996). Clinical aspects of the Ross procedure: Indications and contraindications. *Seminars in Thoracic and Cardiovascular Surgery. 8* (4), 328–335.

Paganini, E. P. & Bosworth, C. P. (1991). Acute renal failure after open heart surgery: Newer concepts and current therapy. *Seminars in Thoracic and Cardiovascular Surgery, 3* (1), 63–69.

Reardon, M. J., Conklin, D., Reardon, P. R., & Baldwin, J. C. (1997). Coronary artery bypass conduits: Review of current status. *The Journal of Cardiovascular Surgery, 38* (3), 201–209.

Rivera, R., Duran, E., & Ajuria, M. (1985). Carpentier's flexible ring versus De Vega's annuloplasty. *The Journal of Thoracic and Cardiovascular Surgery, 89* (2), 196–203.

Ross, D. (1996). The pulmonary autograft: History and basic techniques. *Seminars in Thoracic and Cardiovascular Surgery, 8* (4), 350–357.

Sabiston, D. C. & Spencer, F. C. (1995). *Surgery of the chest* (5th edition). Philadelphia: W. B. Saunders.

Schmid, C. & Scheld, H. H. (1996). Trends and strategies for myocardial revascularization. *Thoracic and Cardiovasular Surgeon, 44,* 113–117.

Shaffer, J. A., Schulkers, N. M., & Wexler, L. (1991). Ambulatory postoperative care of patients following coronary artery bypass and valve replacement surgery: Discussion and algorithms. *Progress in Cardiovascular Nursing, 6* (1), 3–12.

Shinn, J. A. (1992). Management of a patient undergoing myocardial revascularization: Coronary artery bypass surgery. *Nursing Clinics of North America, 27* (1), 243–255.

Svensson, L. G. (1997). New and future approaches for spinal cord protection. *Seminars in Thoracic and Cardiovascular Surgery, 9* (3), 206–221.

Svensson, L. G. & Crawford, E. S. (1997). *Cardiovascular and vascular disease of the aorta.* Philadelphia: W. B. Saunders.

Warner, M. A., Offord, K. P., Warner, M. E., Lennon, R. L., Conover, M. A., & Jansson-Schumacher, U. (1989). Role of preoperative cessation of smoking and other factors in postoperative pulmonary complications: A blinded prospective study of coronary artery bypass patients. *Mayo Clinic Proceedings, 64,* 609–616.

Yun, K. L. & Miller, D. C. (1997). Ascending aortic aneurysm and aortic valve disease: What is the most optimal surgical technique. *Seminars in Thoracic and Cardiovascular Surgery, 9* (3), 233–245.

35

Heart Failure and Cardiomyopathy

Carol Twomey
Paul Logan

The incidence of heart failure (HF) has increased over the past 10 years. According to the Agency for Health Care Policy and Research, about 2 million patients are currently treated for HF and 400,000 new cases are documented every year. More than $10 billion is spent on the treatment of HR annually, including $2.4 billion paid by the Medicare program in 1992 (Konstam, Dracup, Baker, et al., 1994).

The cause for the rise in HF cases is multifactorial. One reason is better recognition of the disease, especially in young patients and those without history of ischemic heart disease. Better treatment of HF is another reason for the high prevalence of HF cases.

It is estimated that 20,000 patients with HF could benefit from heart transplantation; experience has shown, however, that there are only 2000 heart transplants done each year (Schroeder, 1994). This leads to a great discrepancy in the number of transplants needed versus the number of patients who receive them.

▶ OVERVIEW OF HEART FAILURE

Heart failure is defined as a pathologic state in which an abnormality of cardiac function is responsible for the failure of the heart to pump blood at a rate necessary for the metabolizing tissues. Many conditions can lead to decreased cardiac function. Acute MI, hypertension, or valvular heart disease are among the many etiologies that result in HF. Commonly, idiopathic cardiomyopathy is the cause of HF, in which case no etiology is identified. Regardless, the reason for HF is not so important as the fact that the cardiac output and, consequently, the perfusion to the rest of the body are diminished.

Determinants of Cardiac Function

Preload

Preload is defined as the amount of blood that is available to the ventricles for each contraction. It is the amount of stretch on the myocardial fibers prior to systole. The Frank–Starling Law states that an intact ventricle has the capacity to vary the force of contraction as preload or ventricular filling increases (Fig. 35–1). For example, a rubber band illustrates the Frank–Starling relationship very well. Initially, the more a rubber band is stretched, the better the "snap." The same principle applies to myocardial fibers. In the early stages of HF, the ventricular myocardial fibers hypertrophy, or stretch, so that they are able to increase the force of contraction and therefore increase cardiac output. But, just as a rubber band becomes overstretched when overused, so too does the left ventricle. As it overstretches, the fibers are unable to produce a good contraction, and cardiac output is adversely affected.

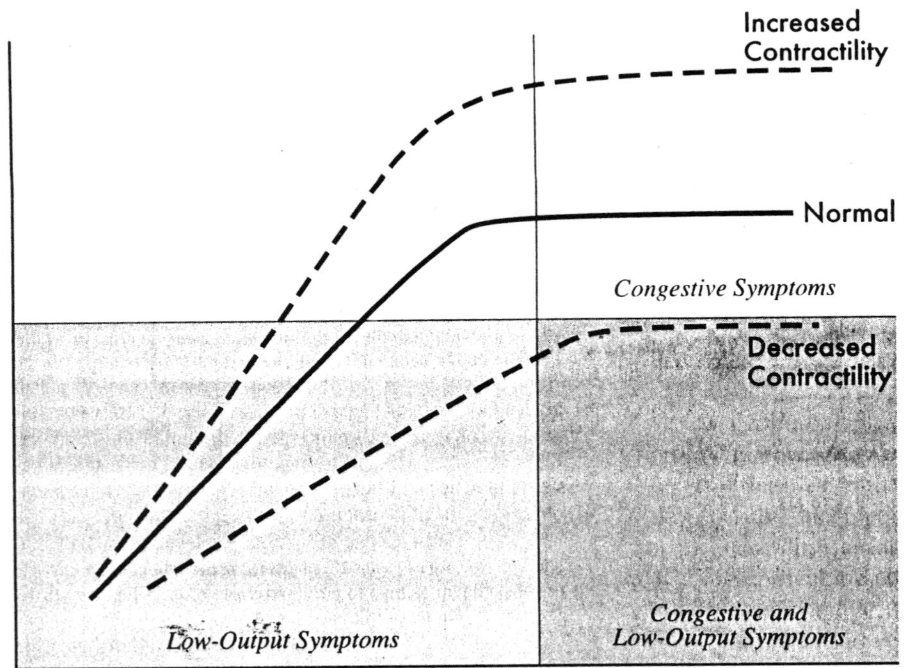

Figure 35–1. The Frank–Starling mechanism. *(From Chulay, Guzetta, & Dossey. [1997]. [p. 259].)*

The determinants of preload are many. First is the atrial contribution to filling, or atrial kick. Atrial kick contributes 10 to 20% of the cardiac output in sinus rhythm. Total blood volume, muscular contraction, and venous tone are important components of preload. Exercises such an walking increase muscular activity and subsequently increase venous return to the heart. Intrathoracic and intrapericardial pressure also influence preload. Intrathoracic pressure changes with inspiration and expiration, and has an affect on preload. Upon inspiration, preload is decreased and upon expiration preload is increased. In patients with large pericardial effusions, right ventricular filling and right atrial filling are compromised. Right ventricular output, therefore, is also affected.

Finally, body positions can affect preload. Normally, patients placed in Trendelenberg position (head down, feet up) experience increased ventricular preload due to augmented venous return. Patients in end-stage HF, however, do not benefit from being placed in this position. Trendelenberg should be avoided, therefore, as management for hypotension in the patient with HF unless it has been documented that low circulating volume or vasodilation has caused decreased preload to the heart.

Afterload

Afterload is the amount of resistance that the ventricle must overcome to eject blood during systole. An analogy can be made to opening a door in a windstorm. It is difficult to open a door against a very strong wind that is trying to push it shut. Similarly, if the pressure in the aorta is high (i.e., elevated systemic vascular resistance), it is more difficult for the left ventricle to generate force sufficient to eject blood into the aorta.

Contractility

Contractility is the force of contraction, or the ability of the ventricular muscle fibers to shorten. Contractility is influenced by many factors including end-diastolic volume, ischemia. Circulating catecholamines due to sympathetic nervous system (SNS) activation, and exogenous inotropic agents such as dobutamine and milirone augment the cardiac output. Pharmacologic agents such as beta blockers and many calcium channel blockers can decrease contractility.

Heart Rate

The last determinant of heart function is heart rate. The cardiac output is a function of the heart rate and stroke volume ($CO = HR \times SV$). Therefore, for any given heart rate the cardiac output is maintained as long as ventricular filling remains constant.

In patients who can no longer maintain stroke volume, such as those with compromised ventricles from HF or large MI's, the heart rate increases to maintain the cardiac output. In patients with very poor ventricular function, a heart rate greater than 120 may be needed to maintain the cardiac output.

Preload, afterload, contractility, and heart rate are not independent forces. Rather, they are interrelated mechanisms that, together, contribute to the overall cardiac output (Fig. 35–2).

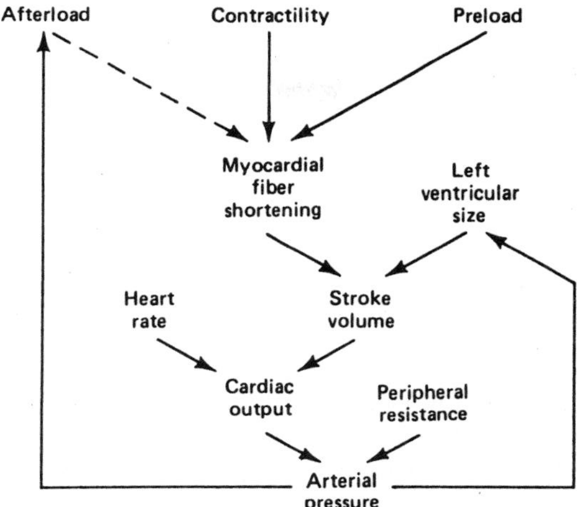

Figure 35–2. Interactions between the components that regulate cardiac output and arterial pressure. *(From Ganong. [1993]. [p. 517].)*

Compensatory Mechanisms in Heart Failure

The consequences of left ventricular failure are cyclical and are often referred to as "the cycle of heart failure." The renin–angiotensin system (RAS) and the sympathetic nervous system (SNS) are affected by decreased cardiac output. If the kidneys do not receive enough blood due to low cardiac output, the RAS is activated. The results of RAS activation are conservation of volume (i.e., water) and sodium.

When the heart fails, decreased glomerular filtration is sensed by the kidney. The RAS is then activated. Activation of the RAS stimulates conversion of aldosterone into angiotensin-I (A-I) and subsequently angiotensin-II (A-II) (Fig. 35–3). A-II stimulates secretion of vasopressin, which increases blood volume through sodium and water reabsorption in the renal tubules. The effect of volume expansion, however, is increased myocardial workload. The use of angiotensin converting enzyme (ACE) inhibitors was shown in the late 1980s to prolong survival of patients with end-stage HF.

The second compensatory mechanism activated by end-stage HF is the sympathetic nervous system (SNS). As mentioned previously, RAS activation causes an increased systemic vascular resistance or afterload. The sympathetic nervous system is also activated, further increasing vasoconstriction and resultant afterload. The adrenergic nervous system, when stimulated, increases heart rate and strengthens myocardial contractility by increasing cardiac output. The further increase in afterload decreases left ventricular emptying and causes the HF to worsen.

In the long term, however, when HF is prolonged, adrenergic nervous system increases afterload, decreases stroke volume, and precipitates arrthymias with the constant bombardment by the sympathetic nervous system. Because of this effect of the SNS, there is intense research in the suppression of the SNS with beta blockade for the treatment of HF.

In summary, the cyclical nature of HF can cause worsening of the condition. It is the recognition and treatment of these two responses to end-stage HF that currently are at the "heart" of treatment of HF.

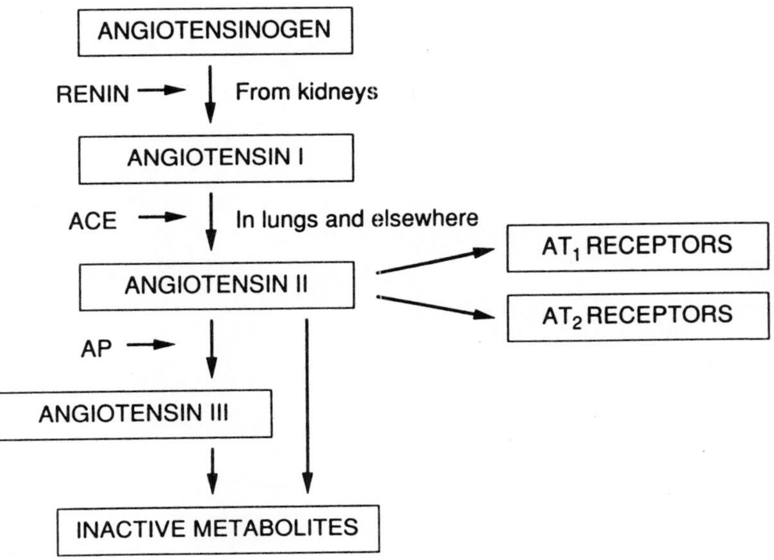

Figure 35–3. The Renin-Angiotensin system. *(From Ganong. [1993]. [p. 415].)*

LEFT SIDED VS. RIGHT SIDED FAILURE

Left sided HF can certainly occur without right sided HF, especially in acute MI. Right ventricular failure can also occur without left ventricular failure, as in the case of an acute proximal right coronary artery occlusion. In most patients with HF there is a degree of both right and left sided HF, thus making it biventricular failure.

Left sided failure is failure of the left ventricle. Symptoms of left sided HF include dyspnea, orthopnea, proximal nocturnal dyspnea (PND), fatigue, weakness, mental confusion, and cool clammy skin. In severe cases, pulmonary edema may develop. Late inspiratory crackles in the bases of the lungs are diagnostic of left heart failure. Symptoms of right sided HF include dependent edema, right upper quadrant pain from liver engorgement, anorexia, nausea, bloating, early satiety, constipation, abdominal pain, diarrhea, fatigue, dyspnea, orthopnea, and syncope. Biventricular failure may manifest with a combination of right and left sided symptoms.

SYSTOLIC VS. DIASTOLIC FAILURE

Left ventricular ejection fraction (LVEF)—as determined by echocardiogram, MUGA scan, or ventriculogram—is normally 60 to 80%. Subnormal LVEF is diagnostic of systolic failure.

It is not only systolic dysfunction, however, that causes HF. Diastolic dysfunction can also produce an inability of the heart to meet the metabolic demands of the body and is another important factor in evaluating overall ventricular function. It is during diastole that the heart relaxes and fills. If diastolic relaxation is affected, the ventricle cannot properly relax or fill. Cardiac output is adversely affected. This can be easily illustrated in a patient who has a tachycardia of greater than 130. Since systole is usually two thirds of the ventricular contraction, it is easy to see that when a patient has an extremely high heart rate, there really is not enough "time" for diastole, and therefore diastolic abnormalities can exist.

Diastolic dysfunction is diagnosed by E:A reversal on the Doppler echocardiogram (Fig. 35–4). Normally, the E-wave, representing passive ventricular filling in early diastole, is greater than the A-wave, representing active ventricular filling (atrial kick). In conditions such as persistent tachycardia or ventricular hypertrophy due to chronic hypertension or aortic stenosis, ventricular relaxation is adversely affected. This is evident on Doppler echocardiography as E:A reversal.

CLASSIFICATIONS OF HEART FAILURE

Cardiomyopathies, whether due to systolic or diastolic disease, are primary disorders of the myocardium. Dilated cardiomyopathy causes systolic failure, and is by far the most common cause of heart failure in the United States. Hypertrophic and restrictive cardiomyopathies are characterized by diastolic heart failure. Table 35–1 summarizes the pathophysiologic and clinical features of cardiomyopathies. Figure 35–5 shows the pathophysiologic features of dilated, hypertrophic, and restrictive cardiomyopathy.

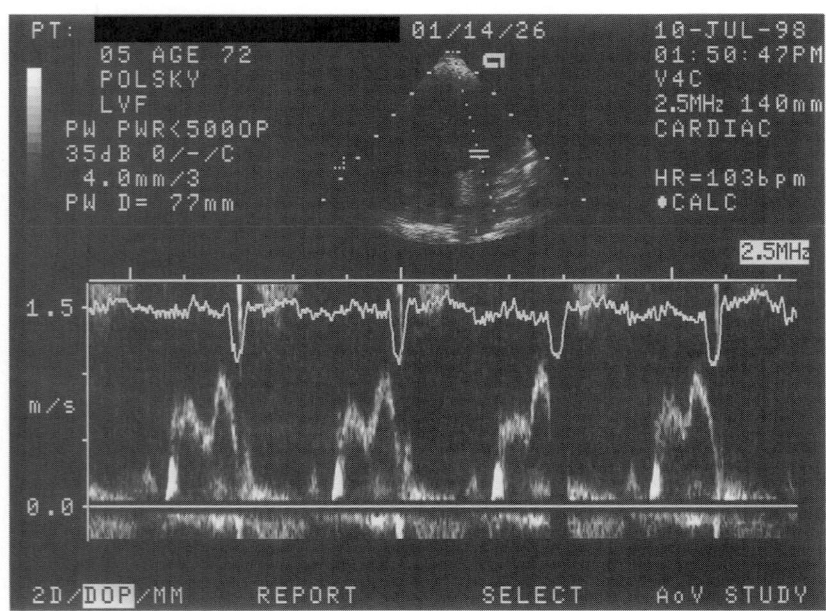

Figure 35–4. E:A Reversal. Pulsed-wave Doppler at the mitral inflow area showing E:A reversal. E:A reversal suggests diastolic dysfunction.

TABLE 35–1. International Classification of Cardiomyopathies

	Pathophysiologic Features	Clinical Features	Causes
Dilated cardiomyopathy (DCM)	Myocytes replaced with fibrous tissue causing decreased systolic function	Systolic heart failure, arrhythmia	Idiopathic, genetic, toxic, viral, immunologic, valvular, hypertensive, ischemic
Hypertrophic cardiomyopathy (HCM)	Myocytes in disarray causing diastolic noncompliance	Diastolic heart failure, arrhythmia	Genetic (familial)
Restrictive cardiomyopathy (RCM)	Infiltrative process causing diastolic noncompliance	Diastolic heart failure, arrhythmia	Idiopathic, infiltrative processes such as amyloidosis
Arrhythmogenic right ventricular cardiomyopathy (i.e., right ventricular dysplasia)	Fatty infiltrates in the right ventricular myocardium	Arrhythmia, sudden death	Genetic (familial)
Unclassified cardiomyopathies		One or more features of the other cardiomyopathies	

Dilated Cardiomyopathy

Pathophysiology

Genetic, toxic, viral, and immunologic causes of dilated cardiomyopathy (DCM) have been identified, though many cases are classified as idiopathic. The pathologic features of DCM are loss of myocardiocytes and the proliferation of fibrotic tissue. Together, these processes lead to a diminished ability of the myocardium to contract during systole.

History and Physical Findings

A careful history is necessary to identify the etiology of the HF, though, in reality, no definite etiology may be determined. For many subtypes of DCM there is no diagnostic test that always identifies the cause. In this case a careful history is essential. Clues regarding recent viral illness, immune disorders, alcohol dependence, pregnancy, and metabolic abnormalities are particularly important. Occasionally, a family history of HF guides the clinician toward the appropriate diagnosis.

Specific cardiomyopathies are generally identified through diagnostic tests that are carried out later in the diagnostic evaluation. It is particularly important that valvular, ischemic, and hypertensive cardiomyopathies be identified early so that curative therapies can be instituted.

Patients with DCM may present with pulmonary symptoms, volume overload symptoms, or both, depending on the etiology. Pulmonary symptoms are caused by left-sided failure and include dyspnea, orthopnea, and paroxysmal nocturnal dyspnea (PND). The dyspnea of DCM occurs initially only with exertion, and later is also present at rest. Patients with orthopnea often describe the need to use several pillows that progresses over several days. Sometimes sleeping in bed is impossible and they are able only to sleep in a chair, perhaps using a table to prop themselves up. These descriptions are very diagnostic.

The presence of PND leaves little for the clinician to guess at. A typical description of PND is awakening from sleep with dyspnea that forces the patient to sit up. The dyspnea then persists for roughly 20 minutes. True PND is among the best diagnostic clues of elevated left atrial pressure due to left ventricular failure.

Patients with right-sided failure due to DCM often present with several days of worsening edema. In more severe cases the fluid volume overload produces abdominal symptoms such as abdominal pain and distension, diarrhea, nausea, and vomiting.

In severe cases of DCM, right-sided failure and left-sided failure may occur together. In fact, right-sided failure may worsen left-sided failure.

Proctor Harvey advocates the "five fingered approach" to cardiac exam. Using this approach, the clinician notes the patient's general appearance, examines the neck veins and the carotid pulsations, palpates the precordial impulses, and auscultates the heart. This method provides a systematic approach to physical examination and reduces the chance that important physical findings are missed.

The general appearance of the patient with DCM is remarkable. By the time the patient presents for treatment, he or she may have severe dyspnea and air hunger. In chronic HF there may be evidence of wasting due to long-term inability of the heart to meet the metabolic demands of the body and absorb nutrients.

The neck veins are distended in patients with right- or left-sided failure. There is some disagreement about the accuracy of estimating central venous pressure (CVP) by examining the neck veins, though most clinicians agree that examination of the neck veins is a valuable screening tool. To assess jugular venous distension, it is usually not necessary to use tangential lighting and sit the patient at 45 degrees, as many are taught in physical examination courses. Instead, it is generally sufficient to sit the patient up 90 degrees and look for venous pulsations (i.e., two pulsations per cardiac cycle). If no jugular venous pulsations are seen with the patient at 90 degrees, the CVP is not elevated. If

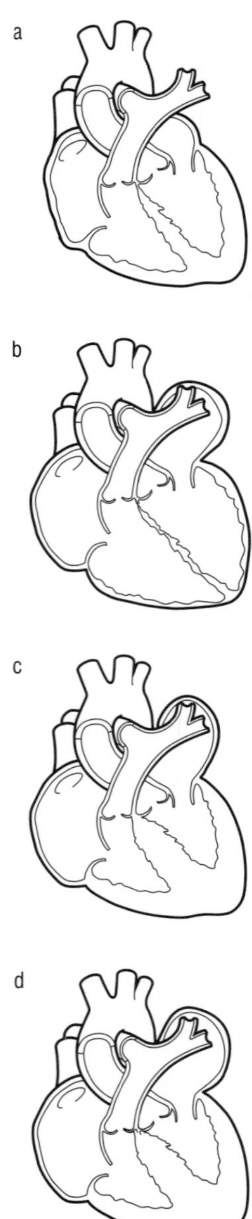

Figure 35–5. Pathophysiologic features of dilated, hypertrophic, and restrictive cardiomyopathy. **A,** Normal heart. **B,** DCM—four-chamber dilatation. **C,** HCM—dilated atria, reduced ventricular cavity size, and thickened muscle. **D,** RCM—dilated atria and normal sized ventricular cavity and muscle.

pulsations are visible above the clavicle, the clinician can safely assume that the CVP is elevated. The distance from the sternal notch to the level of the pulsations (measured in cm) can then be measured and added to 10 to estimate the CVP (in cm of water, not mm Hg) (Fig. 35–6).

Much additional information can be determined from careful evaluation of the jugular pulsations. In normal sinus rhythm there are two jugular pulsations per cardiac cycle. The *a* wave corresponds to atrial contraction and normally is the larger of the two pulsations. The *x* descent represents atrial diastole. The *v* wave, which corresponds to ventricular contraction, is normally smaller than the *a* wave and is followed by the *y* descent. Figure 35–7 illustrates the components of the jugular venous pulsations.

A skilled clinician can determine other abnormalities by assessing the jugular pulsations. In atrial fibrillation, for example, the *a* wave is absent and the *v* wave occurs irregularly. Cannon *a* waves occur when the atrium contracts against a closed tricuspid valve, as in complete heart block and junctional rhythm. Finally, the *v* wave is larger than the *a* wave in tricuspid regurgitation. This may occur in pulmonary hypertension due to severe left sided failure. Palpation of the carotid impulse also yields valuable diagnostic information. Pulsus alternans, the beat-to-beat alternation of the carotid intensity, is diagnostic of severe left heart failure.

The precordial impulse is useful in determining ventricular cavity size. A Point of Maximum Intensity (PMI) that is laterally displaced suggests a dilated left ventricle. When the right ventricle is dilated, a right ventricular impulse is felt at the lower left sternal border.

Ausultation of the heart can also reveal important diagnostic clues. A third heart sound is a normal finding in children, but when heard in adults it suggests volume overload and left ventricular failure. The S3 (Fig. 35–8) is caused by passive ventricular filling at the end of systole. It is heard with the bell of the stethoscope placed lightly over the PMI, occurs following the second heart sound, and sounds like "LUB da-boom." In some patients the S3 is heard easily, but frequently it is very faint. In addition to listening for the cadence, one trick for differentiating an S3 from other similarly-timed sounds is to listen first for the "LUB da-boom" with the bell, then pressing firmly on the chest. The firm pressure of the stethoscope on the chest wall filters out the low-pitched S3 and produces "LUB dub."

Ventricular dilatation changes the shape of the ventricular cavity and, in moderate and severe cases, causes the mitral and/or tricuspid valves to coapt poorly during ventricular systole. Mitral regurgitation, a holosytolic murmur heard at the apex that radiates to the axilla and back, can often be heard in DCM. Tricuspid regurgitation (TR), too, can sometimes be heard at the lower left sternal border. The intensity of the TR murmur varies with respiration.

Diastolic rumbles may also be heard in DCM (refer to Fig. 35–8). Diastolic rumbles are produced by increased volumes of blood flowing through the mitral or tricuspid valves.

Laboratory and Diagnostic Tests

The purposes of laboratory and diagnostic tests in DCM are to determine the cause of the HF and define the severity of the pathophysiologic process. Baseline laboratory data are obtained to guide therapy. Table 35–2 lists the routine laboratory tests for newly diagnosed DCM.

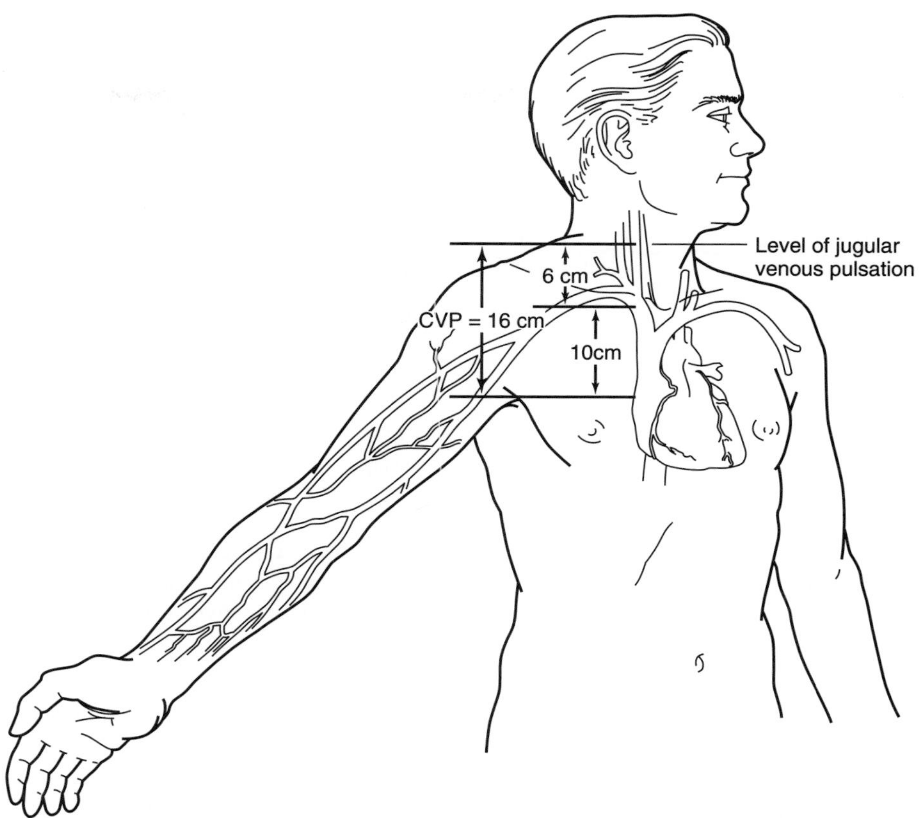

Figure 35–6. Estimating central venous pressure. Assume that the distance from the right atrium to the sternal notch is 10 cm. With the patient upright, measure the distance from the sternal notch to the level of the jugular venous pulsations. Add the two numbers for the estimated right atrial pressure.

In newly diagnosed DCM, the role of viral titers and myocardial biopsy are controversial. In a National Institutes of Health (NIH) study done in the early 1980s, it was shown that, to be of benefit, myocardial biopsy must be done within the first 2 weeks of the onset of HF symptoms. Even with early biopsy, the yield for diagnosing viral myocarditis is low (Becker, Heijmans, Essed, 1991). Rarely is the causative virus identified in cases of viral cardiomyopathy. When a virus is identified, the management is not affected. For these reasons, routine testing for viral etiologies is not standard at all centers. Myocardial biopsy, if performed, typically reveals loss of myocytes and presence of myocardial fibrosis.

Electrocardiogram (EKG), chest x-ray (CXR), and echocardiogram are mandatory for all patients presenting with HF. The EKG may reveal atrial fibrillation or other arrhythmias, chamber enlargement, or conduction abnormalities. A normal EKG generally excludes DCM, particularly chronic DCM.

Exercise testing may also be used to determine the degree of HF and to quantify the functional capacity. V02 exercise oxygen consumption measurement may be done simultaneously. While the normal is greater than 20mL/kg/min, patients with end-stage HF can have V02 of less than 10 mL/kg/min.

The CXR is used to assess the degree of pulmonary congestion and chamber enlargement and to look for extracardiac etiologies of HF. Normally, the pulmonary vessels in the apices (cephalic) are not well visualized on an upright CXR. In HF, however, the pulmonary vessels are easily seen. This pattern is called cephalization. In severe HF, Kerley B lines and peribronchial cuffing may be seen (Fig. 35–9). Fluid may also be visualized in the fissures or at the lung bases (pleural effusion).

The echocardiogram (echo) is among the most valuable tools for assessing cardiac function. Information about chamber size, wall motion, overall contractile function, valvular function, and diastolic function can be obtained by a skilled sonographer. Pericardial and pleural effusions can also be visualized. Serial echos are useful in following the patient's response to therapy.

Cardiac catheterization is typically performed on all patients with newly diagnosed HF. Like echo, catheterization allows assessment of wall motion and valvular function. Catheterization is also used to measure intracardiac pressures and the cardiac output. Additionally, catheteriza-

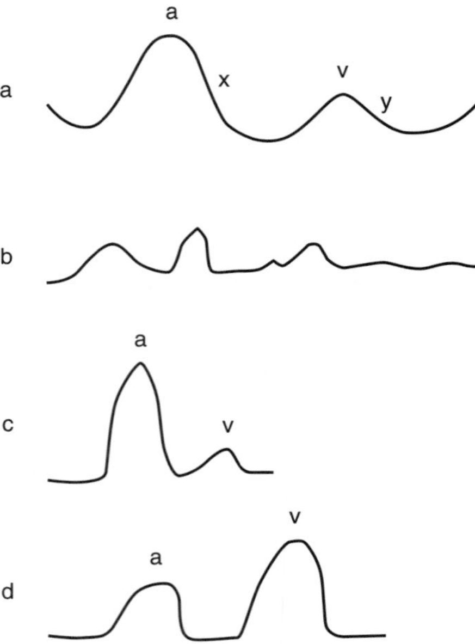

Figure 35–7. Jugular venous pulsations. The jugular venous pulsations are akin to right atrial pressure tracings. **A,** Normal components of the right atrial tracing. The *a* wave corresponds with atrial contraction and is followed by the *x* descent. The *v* wave occurs during ventricular contraction and is followed by the *y* descent. **B,** Absence of *v* waves in atrial fibrillation. **C,** Cannon *a* wave, as seen in junctional rhythm. **D,** Large v waves as seen in tricuspid regurgitation due to pulmonary hypertension.

tion can be used to visualize the coronary arteries. This is particularly useful in older patients in whom coronary artery disease must be excluded.

In patients with coronary artery disease, exercise or pharmacologic stress testing should be performed to determine whether ischemia is present. Viability testing (i.e., rest–rest nuclear imaging) is also useful to identify patients with hibernating myocardium (see also Chapter 32, Coronary Artery Disease).

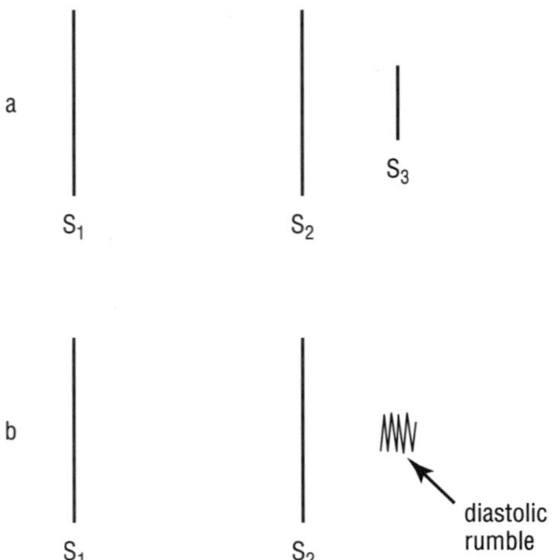

Figure 35–8. Heart sounds in heart failure. **A,** The S3 occurs after S2 and indicates fluid volume overload. **B,** The diastolic rumble is a low-pitched sound heard after S2.

TABLE 35–2. Routine Laboratory Tests for Newly Diagnosed DCM

Laboratory Test	Rationale
Complete blood count	Exclude anemia
Liver function tests	Evaluate liver dysfunction due to hepatic congestion
Thyroid function tests	Exclude thyrotoxicosis
Cardiac enzymes	Exclude myocardial infarction
Electrolytes	Evaluate electrolyte abnormalities
BUN and creatinine	Evaluate renal function
Prothrombin time (PT) and partial thromboplastin time (PTT)	Evaluate liver dysfunction due to hepatic congestion; obtain baseline coagulation studies before instituting anticoagulation
Urinalysis	Proteinuria

Cardiac Output. The thermodilution and Fick methods of determining cardiac output are discussed in Chapter 33, Valvular and Congenital Heart Disease. In patients acutely ill with HF, a pulmonary artery (e.g., Swan–Ganz) catheter is useful to monitor the cardiac output and hemodynamic indices.

Which cardiac output method to use is an important consideration. Interestingly, in low-output states the thermodilution method is less accurate than the Fick method. The reason is this: When the output is low, the cooled injectate takes longer to reach the tip of the catheter. Consequently, the injectate is warmed by the blood into which it is injected.

It seems reasonable, then, to use the Fick method in critically ill patients. But, this is not usually practical. To accurately know the oxygen consumption, it must be measured directly. Because of the complexity of measuring oxygen consumption nomograms based on normal patients in the resting state have been developed. Such nomograms do not apply, however, to postoperative patients and those who are critically ill. In this case, it is acceptable to infer the Fick output from the mixed venous oxygen saturation (Mvo_2). A normal Mvo_2 is 60 to 80%. Low Mvo_2 suggests that it is taking longer for blood to return to the heart, causing more oxygen to be removed from the hemoglobin molecule at the tissue level. High Mvo_2, on the other hand, is indicative of a left to right shunt, such that oxygenated blood is injected from the left heart chambers into the pulmonary circulation (e.g. ventricular septal defect, atrial septal defect).

Management

Medical Therapy. The AHCPR Clinical Practice Guidelines include an algorhythm for medical management of HF

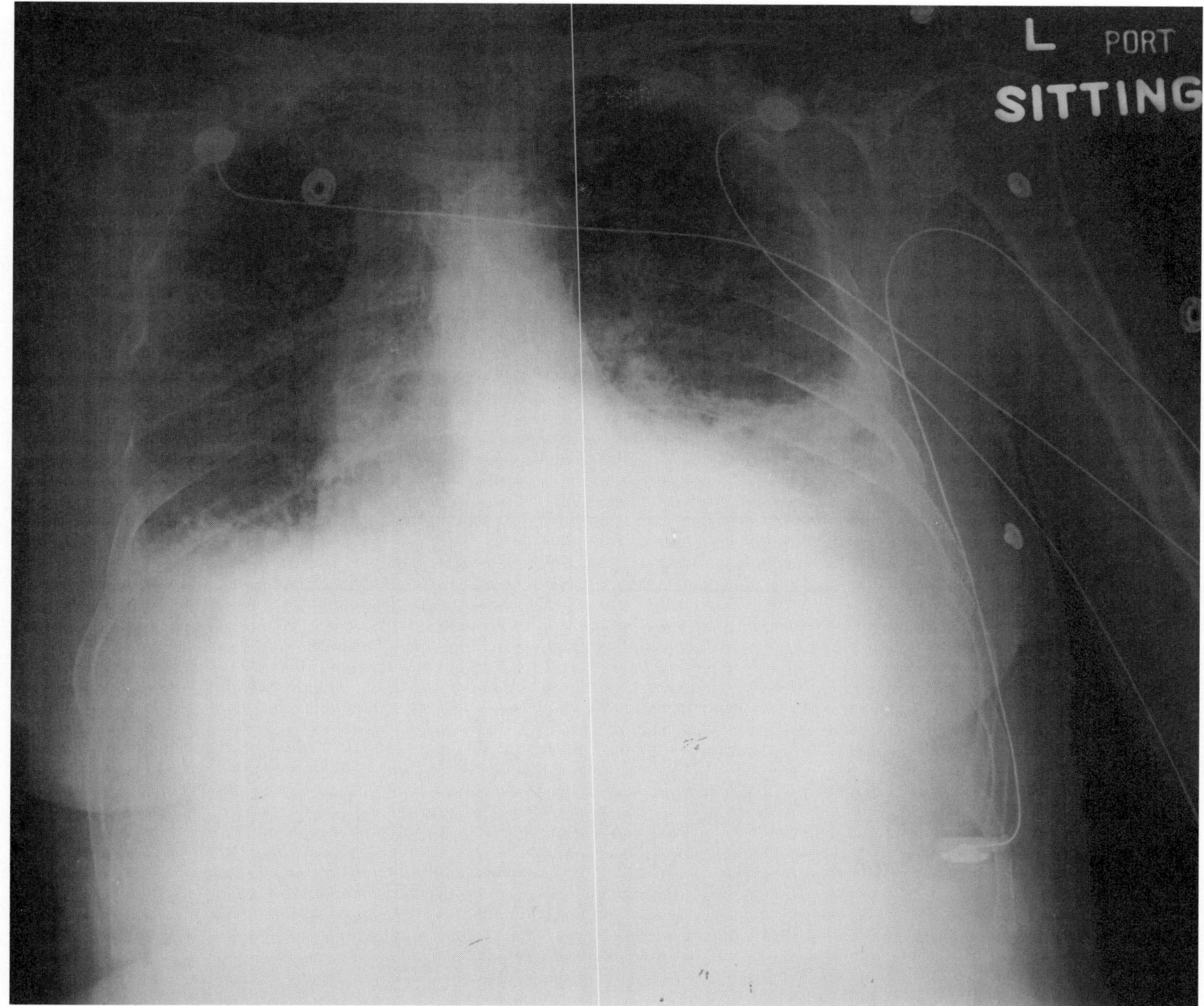

Figure 35–9. PA and lateral chest x-ray showing congestive heart failure.

(Fig. 35–10). Angiotensin converting enzyme (ACE) inhibitors are first-line therapy for HF, particularly HF associated with DCM. Diuretics can be added if moderate dyspnea on exertion (DOE) exists. If the patient has severe DOE, then digoxin should be added. Consideration should also be given to adding nitrates to reduce preload and afterload and improve symptoms.

In addition to ACE inhibitors, diuretics, and digoxin, other agents are available for patients with HF (Table 35–3). Since the publication of the guidelines in 1994, angiotensin II (A2) receptor blockers (e.g., losartin, irbisartin, valsartin) and the alpha/beta blocker carvedilol have become available. Currently, A2 blockers are not indicated for the treatment of HF, but clinical trials have been implemented to investigate the use of these agents. It is unclear, therefore, whether A2 blockers are beneficial in HF. Because they do not affect the bradykinin pathway, the incidence of cough is less than that associated with the ACE inhibitors. Many clinicians substitute A2 blockers for ACE inhibitors in patients who are intolerant of the cough sometimes associated with ACE inhibitors.

The availability of carvedilol (COREG) is an exciting development in the treatment of HF. In the past it was theorized that the compensatory sympathetic stimulation that occurs in chronic HF may have deleterious effects in the long run. Early studies of beta blockers in HF had mixed results and did not show improved survival. Carvedilol, however, has been shown to improve survival in randomized

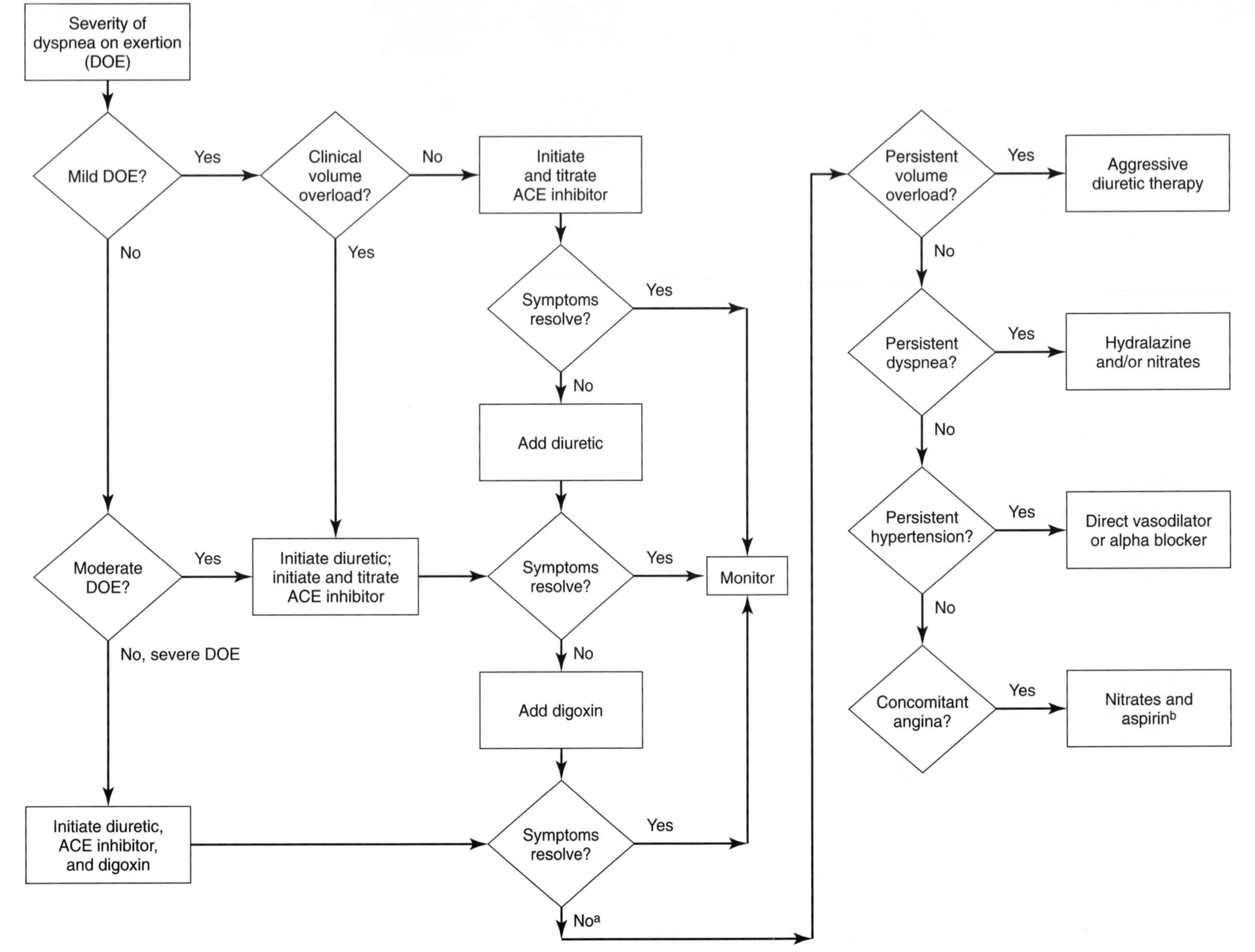

[a] Obtain cardiology consult if not already done.
[b] Beta blockers and calcium-channel blockers may also be effective but should be considered investigational.

Figure 35–10. Pharmacological management of patients with heart failure. *(From Konstam, Dracup, Baker, et al. [1994]. [pp. 50–51].)*

TABLE 35–3. Medications Commonly Used for Heart Failure

Drug	Initial Dose (mg)	Target Dose (mg)	Recommended Maximal Dose (mg)	Major Adverse Reactions
Thiazide Diuretics				
Hydrochlorothiazide	25 QD	As needed	50 QD	Postural hypotension, hypokalemia, hyperglycemia, hyperuricemia, rash. Rare severe reaction includes pancreatitis, bone marrow suppression, and anaphylaxis.
Chlorthalidone	25 QD	As needed	50 QD	
Loop Diuretics				
Furosemide	10–40 QD	As needed	240 BID	Same as thiazide diuretics.
Bumetanide	0.5–1.0 QD	As needed	10 QD	
Torosemide	20 QD	As needed	40 BID	
Thiazide-Related Diuretic				
Metolazone	2.5[a]	As needed	10 QD	Same as thiazide diuretics.
Potassium-Sparing Diuretics				
Spironolactone	25 QD	As needed	100 BID	Hyperkalemia, especially if administered with ACE inhibitor; rash; gynecomastia (spironolactone only).
Triamterene	50 QD	As needed	100 QD	
Amiloride	5 QD	As needed	40 QD	
ACE Inhibitors				
Enalapril	2.5 BID	10 BID	20 BID	Hypotension, hyperkalemia, renal insufficiency, cough, skin rash, angioedema, neutropenia.
Captopril	6.25–12.5 TID	50 TID	100 TID	
Lisinopril	5 QD	20 QD	40 QD	
Quinapril	5 BID	20 BID	20 BID	
Digoxin	0.125–0.25 QD	0.125–0.25 QD	0.375 QD	Cardiotoxicity, confusion, nausea, anorexia, visual disturbances.
Hydralazine	10–25 TID	75 TID	100 TID	Headache, nausea, dizziness, tachycardia, lupus-like syndrome.
Isosorbide Dinitrate	10 TID	40 TID	80 TID	Headache, hypotension, flushing.

[a] Given as a single test dose initially.
ACE = angiotensin-converting enzyme, BID = twice a day, QD = once a day, TID = three times a day.
Adapted from Konstam, Dracup, Baker, et al. (1994). (pp. 52–53).

clinical trials of patients with HF. Carvedilol has both alpha blocking (vasodilatory) effects and nonselective beta blocking effects. The United States Carvedilol Heart Failure Trials Program was stopped prematurely when it was noted that patients who were randomized to carvedilol showed a 65% risk reduction. Patients in this study had heart failure for at least 3 months and had ejection fractions of less than 35% (Packer et al., 1996).

Carvedilol seems best suited for use in patients with mild or moderate HF. When starting carvedilol, patients should have no overt symptoms of heart failure. The starting dose is 3.125 mg twice daily and is titrated every 2 to 4 weeks to a maximum of 50 mg twice daily. Initially, patients feel worse due to the beta blockade. Table 35–4 shows patient selection criteria, dosage, and side effects of carvedilol therapy.

For patients with severely decreased LV function (ejection fraction < 20%), intraventricular thrombus can form. For these patients anticoagulation should be considered. Anticoagulation is essential when there is concomitant atrial fibrillation or a history of thromboembolism.

Surgical Therapy. Even with maximal medical therapy, patients with HF eventually succumb to the disease process. This has spurred interest in finding surgical approaches to the treatment of HF.

Revascularization. Revascularization, whether angioplasty or coronary artery bypass, is indicated for patients who have evidence of ischemia by nuclear stress testing or hibernating myocardium by viability study.

Transmyocardial Revascularization. In those patients who are not candidates for angioplasty or coronary artery bypass, transmyocardial revascularization (TMR) may someday be an option. Studies are ongoing to determine the efficacy of TMR in patients who have poor target vessels. TMR involves the use of a laser to perforate the myocardium, producing small channels from the ventricle

TABLE 35–4. How to Use Carvedilol in Heart Failure

Patient selection
- Mild to moderate heart faliure
- Already receiving angiotensin-converting enzyme inhibitors, a diuretic and digoxin
- Not recommended in patients hospitalized for decompensated heart failure, or who have significant hypotension or pulmonary congestion

Dosage
- Start with 3.125 mg twice a day for 2 weeks
- Observe the patient for side effects 1 to 2 hours after initial dose and each dose increase or have the patient take these doses at bedtime
- If first dose is tolerated well, increase to 6.25 mg twice a day after 2 weeks
- Double the dose every 1–2 weeks until target reached
  - 25 mg twice a day in patients weighing 85 kg or less
  - or 50 mg twice a day in patients weighing more than 85 kg
- Tell the patient to take carvedilol with meals

Side effects during upward titration
- Vasolidator effects (dizziness or light-headedness)
  - Give the drug with food
  - Give drug 2 hours before other agents
  - Consider reducing diuretic or vasodilator doses temporarily
  - Reduce carvedilol dose
  - May require no attention, as symptoms are often self-limiting
- Worsening heart failure (edema, weight gain, dyspnea)
  - Intensify salt restriction
  - Increase diuretic dose
  - Reduce carvedilol dose
- Significant bradycardia (consistently < 60–65/minute with symptoms)
  - Reduce carvedilol dose
  - Monitor digoxin levels
  - Reduce digoxin dose

From Young, J. B. (1997). (p. 421).

to the epicardium. It is theorized that TMR may stimulate growth of collateral vessels within the myocardium.

Intraaortic Balloon Counterpulsation. There are multiple surgical treatments for HF that can be considered. The first mechanical intervention often employed in HF is intraaortic balloon counterpulsation. Intraaortic balloon pumps (IABP) work by hyperperfusing the coronary arteries during balloon inflation, and decreasing afterload during balloon deflation. IABPs contribute approximately 0.8 liters per minute to cardiac output. In patients with severe end-stage HF, less than one liter of cardiac output will be of little help in the long term. However, if the HF is due to an acute ischemic event, IABP may be helpful because of its ability to hyperperfuse the coronary arteries.

Ventricular Assist Device. Another surgical option that it is becoming increasingly important to patients with HF is the ventricular assist device (VAD). There are many types of ventricular assist devices within use in the United States. There are both univentricular and biventricular support systems. There are permanent, semipermanent (meant for use for months to years), and temporary (meant for use for less than 1 month) VADs. In general, VADs shunt blood from the heart into a pump and then pump back into the systemic circulation by an extracorporeal device (Fig. 35–11), thereby assisting the ventricle.

In general, semipermanent VADs are becoming more mainstream. Studies in which the patients leave the hospital with the VAD in place to await transplantation are ongoing. Most of these devices are now electrically powered. The equipment to run them is quite compact, and the power pack can be worn around the waist. The ventricle or pumping unit itself is usually implanted under the skin and only the battery and controls are outside the body. Presently, these semipermanent devices are being used as a bridge to transplant. In the near future, however, they may be an alternative to cardiac transplant.

Biventricular devices may also be used, though most are temporary devices. They are usually cannulated from the right atrium into the pump and from the pump into the pulmonary artery and then from the left atrium into the pump and from the pump into the ascending aorta. Biventricular devices are external devices and sit on the abdomen outside the body or on a pole next to the bed. They can be driven electrically or pneumatically, or they can be gravity drained.

The risk of infection with most of these devices is great as there are multiple exit sites that need meticulous care to prevent infection from going into the body.

Cardiac Reduction Surgery. There are many new surgical options being considered for patients with HF. Cardiac reduction surgery, or the Batiste procedure, is a surgical option that has received much recent media attention. Originally designed by Brazilian surgeon R. J. Batista, the surgery consists of removal of excess, dilated myocardium of the left ventricle to decrease surface area and surface tension and allow the heart to pump more efficiently. The myocardial mass is usually removed from the posterior portion of the muscle between the two heads of the papillary muscle of the left ventricle. Studies are underway to assess the long-term effects on survival and functional capacity. Partial left ventriculectomy may be a corrective and permanent solution for some patients with HF (McCarthy, McCarthy, Starling, Smedira, Scalia, Wong, et al., 1998).

Complications of ventricular reduction surgery can include malignant arrrythymias, to which some patients succumb. Suppression of potential malignant ventricular arrthymias should be undertaken before the patient has the surgery, with drugs such as amiodarone.

Cardiomyoplasty. Cardiomyoplasty has also had limited exposure in treatment of HF. Cardiomyoplasty is the removal of latissimus dorsi muscle, which is wrapped around the heart and innervated to aid in ventricular contraction. It has limited success in patients with higher ejec-

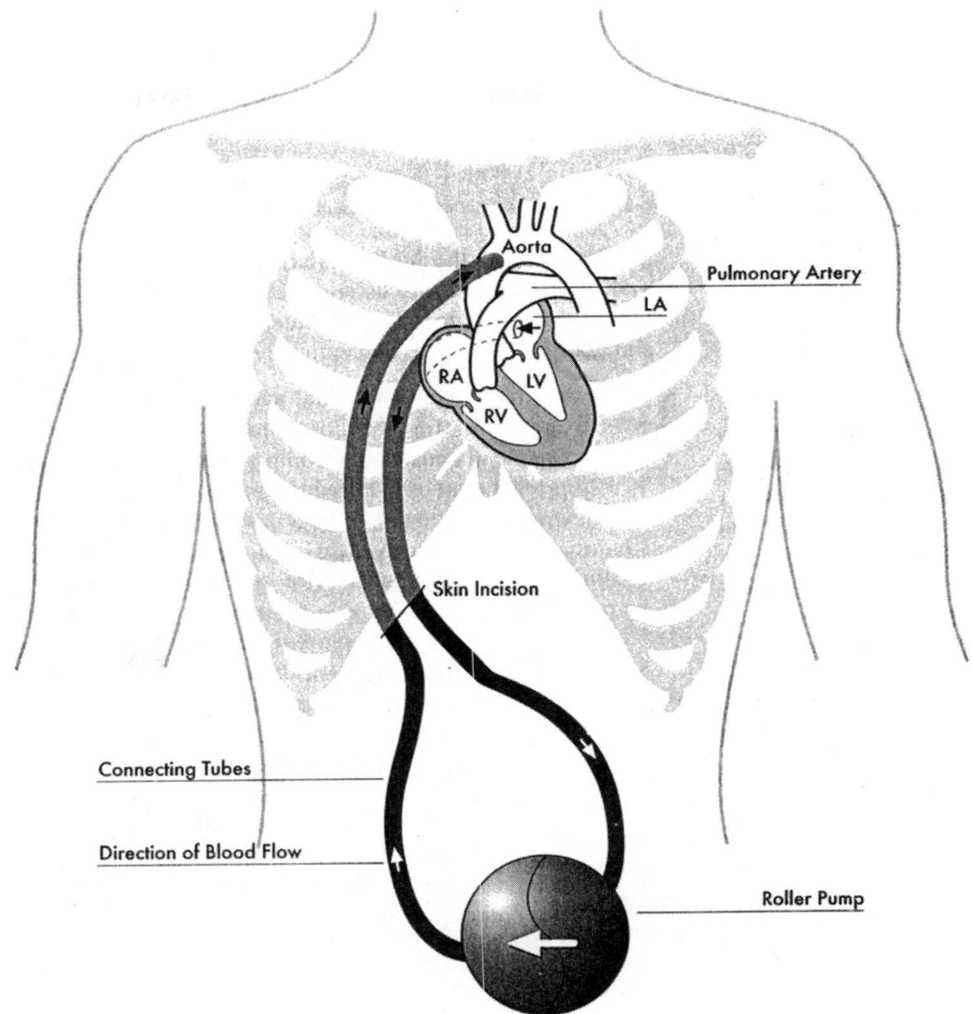

Figure 35–11. Left ventricular assist device. The venous anastamosis is made at the left atrium, the arterial anastamosis is made at the aorta. *(From Chulay, Guzetta, & Dossey. [1997]. [p. 483].).*

tion fractions, usually over 20%. It is now being done as an randomized study for those patients who are refractory to HF treatment and who are not cardiac transplant candidates.

Cardiac Transplantation. Cardiac transplantation is available for patients with end-stage HF who have exhausted medical treatment. Cardiac transplantation carries with it high risk of complications in the time posttransplant but will also return heart functions to normal and allow the patient to live a fairly normal life.

There are multiple contraindications to heart transplant, including irreversible pulmonary hypertension, ongoing infections, pulmonary infarction, malignancy, and social factors, such as alcohol and drug use, which would make the patient not a transplant candidate. After transplant, patients are relegated to taking immunosuppressive rejection drugs for the rest of their lives as well as having surveillance biopsies and cardiac catheterization to assist how the heart is working.

Peripartum Cardiomyopathy

Peripartum cardiomyopathy is another form of DCM that occurs generally in the last month of pregnancy or up to 6 months postpartum. The cause is unknown, and the incidence varies internationally. It is estimated that one case occurs in the United States in every 1300 to 4000 deliveries; one third of patients with peripartum cardiomyopathy die from progressive heart failure, one third remain the same, and one third improve (Homans, 1985). In those cases where the HF improves, functional capacity improves and the heart can return to normal size within 6 months.

The treatment of peripartum cardiomyopathy is the same as the treatment for DCM, including heart transplantation if necessary. Women with peripartum cardiomyopathy are usually advised to not become pregnant again, as the exact mechanism of the disease is not well understood and it is unknown whether HF would recur in subsequent pregnancies.

Hypertrophic Cardiomyopathy

Pathophysiology

Hypertrophic cardiomyopathy (HCM), also known as idiopathic hypertrophic subaortic stenosis (IHSS), is an autosomal dominant genetic disease that has variable phenotypic expression. That is, there are multiple presentations and clinical manifestations of the disease. Some patients present in infancy or early childhood, though many present in the teenage years or in early adulthood.

The pathology of the disease involves disarray of the myocardial fibers, which is the diagnostic pathologic finding at myocardial biopsy. Severe left ventricular hypertrophy (LVH) is often present and is generally asymmetric, involving the septum more than the ventricular free wall. Asymmetric septal hypertrophy can cause obstruction of the left ventricular outflow tract and can be worsened by decreased afterload, decreased preload, or increased contractility. Not all patients with HCM have outflow obstructions.

LVH causes poor diastolic compliance. Diastolic failure is a clinical feature of the disease. Left atrial enlargement occurs due to the resistance of the ventricle to diastolic filling. Atrial fibrillation is common. But, because patients with HCM are preload dependant, the loss of the atrial kick causes worsening of the HF. Also, conduction abnormalities (e.g., bundle branch block, fascicular block, heart block) and ventricular arrhythmias are common in HCM due to the primary myocardial pathology. Sudden death is common and may be the first presenting symptom. It may be due to either left ventricular outflow tract obstruction or ventricular arrhythmia.

The natural history of obstructive HCM is progressive HF, persistent arrhythmias, and eventual ventricular dilatation. In many cases, however, non-obstructive HCM can be managed adequately for many years.

History and Physical Findings

Patients with HCM may recall previous episodes of dizziness, light-headedness, palpitations, syncope, or near-syncope. These symptoms may be more pronounced immediately following maximal exertion when the vasculature is vasodilated and the venous return to the ventricle is low. In this instance, the symptoms are likely due to left ventricular outflow tract obstruction. If symptoms occur at rest, however, the etiology is likely arrhythmogenic.

Chest pain is a common complaint of patients with obstructive HCM. It is usually nonexertional and may last hours. Nitrates do not relieve the pain, and indeed are contraindicated due to their preload-reducing effects.

Because HCM is a genetic disorder, there is often a family history of sudden death in adolesence or early adulthood. If no family history of sudden death exists, the family history should be further explored for other evidence of familial transmission of the disease.

Physical findings in HCM are similar to those seen in other conditions associated with LVH. An irregular pulse suggests atrial fibrillation. The jugular veins are typically nondistended in patients with HCM. The carotid pulsations may be hyperdynamic due to the LVH or hypodynamic due to outflow obstruction. Pulsus alternans can occur due to severe left ventricular systolic failure. It is a late finding, however, and does not occur until the ventricle has dilated. At this point the patient has DCM.

Initially, the point of maximal intensity (PMI) is felt in the normal location (4th intercostal space, mid-clavicular line), but is diffuse and sustained. Additionally, a presystolic component that represents an S4 is also palpable immediately prior to the diffuse and sustained PMI. Late in the course of the disease the ventricle dilates. In this case the PMI becomes laterally displaced.

The "murmur of HCM" is a systolic murmur that may be multifactorial. Part of the murmur is caused by the ejection of blood through the ventricular outflow tract. The murmur peaks in mid to late systole, depending upon the degree of the obstruction. The intensity increases during Valsalva. The second component of the murmur is due to mitral regurgitation. During systole, the anterior leaflet of the mitral valve enters the outflow tract causing it to remain open during all or part of systole. The "murmur of HCM" is harsh and is typically heard throughout the precordium.

Laboratory and Diagnostic Tests

The EKG in patients with HCM is always abnormal, often dramatically so. Left bundle branch block is frequently present, as are other conduction abnormalities. The cardiogram often mimics myocardial infarction.

The echocardiogram demonstrates LVH. Diagnostic features of HCM include asymmetric LVH (septal thickness greater than ventricular free wall), asymmetric septal hypertrophy (ASH), and systolic anterior motion (SAM) of the mitral valve. A subvalvular gradient is also present in hypertrophic obstructive cardiomyopathy (HOCM). The gradient is dynamic in that it increases with Valsalva and premature beats, when the ventricular preload is low.

Myocardial biopsy is diagnostic in HCM. "Disarray" of myocardial fibers is seen.

Management

The distinction between HOCM and HCM (nonobstructive) is important when considering treatment. Although patients with either HCM or HOCM can have HF, the management is substantially different. Those with HOCM are preload-dependant and are at risk for potentially fatal outflow tract obstruction if preload is compromised. Patients with nonobstructive HCM, on the other hand, can be safely managed with standard diastolic failure regimens such as beta blockers and diuretics.

Beta blockers and verapamil are useful for minimizing diastolic dysfunction and are safe for both obstructive and nonobstructive forms of HCM. Often, high doses of these agents are necessary to control symptoms. Once the decision to implant a dual-chamber pacemaker is made, the medications can be maximized, without concern of bradycardia.

Because they have structural heart disease, patients with HOCM and nonobstructive HCM are at risk for arrhythmias. While atrial fibrillation is generally well-tolerated in healthy patients without structural heart disease, those with diastolic dysfunction can become ill due to the loss of atrial kick. Every effort is made to preserve sinus rhythm in patients with HCM. Amiodarone, disopyrimide, and sotalol are among the favored antiarrhythmic agents due to their negative inotropic features. Disopyrimide, however, is not often well-tolerated due to the anticholinergic effects.

Obstructive HCM

Medical Therapy. Diuretics must be used cautiously. Because patients with HOCM are preload-dependant, overaggressive diuresis can precipitate acute outflow tract obstruction. Nevertheless, patients with HOCM can become volume overloaded. ACE inhibitors and digoxin, while the mainstays of therapy for systolic failure, are absolutely contraindicated in HOCM, as are nitrates and beta agonists.

Patients with HOCM must never become dehydrated, even mildly. Water should be consumed regularly throughout the day, particularly in conditions where the liklihood of dehydration is greater (e.g., hot/humid weather). Stool softeners may be added to prevent straining due to constipation, though sufficient water intake also helps. Heavy exertion should always be avoided and patients should generally refrain from competitive sports.

Acute obstruction is a life-threatening medical emergency. The signs and symptoms include pale and dusky skin, extreme hypotension, chest pain, dyspnea, diaphoresis. Patients who are obstructing should first be placed in Trendelenberg position or have their feet elevated. Supplemental oxygen should be given and fluids should be infused rapidly. Simultaneously, a phenylephrine infusion should be started. Phenylephrine is a pure alpha–agonist and has no beta–agonist properties. Dobutamine, epinephrine, levophed, isuprel, and other beta agonists are absolutely contraindicated due to their positive inotropic properties.

Dual-Chamber Pacing. Electrophysiologists and echocardiographers long ago discovered paradoxical septal motion during pacing from the right ventricular apex. It was later learned that chronic dual-chamber pacing improves symptoms in patients with HOCM (Fananapazir et al., 1992).

The mechanism by which dual-chamber pacing relieves outflow tract obstruction is simple. The pacemaker is programmed to DDDR mode and is set to allow the patient's intrinsic atrial rhythm to establish the heart rate. The P wave then triggers the pacemaker to stimulate the ventricle before the intrinsic conduction can. The rhythm, then, is almost entirely V-paced with atrial tracking, also known as "P-synchronous" pacing. The effect of P-synchronous pacing is paradoxical septal motion, resulting in reduction of the outflow tract obstruction (Fig. 35–12).

P-synchronous pacing for patients with HOCM has been shown to improve symptoms and functional class (Fananapazir et al., 1992). No studies to date, however, have shown improved survival in patients who are paced. It appears that the disease progresses to ventricular dilatation, regardless.

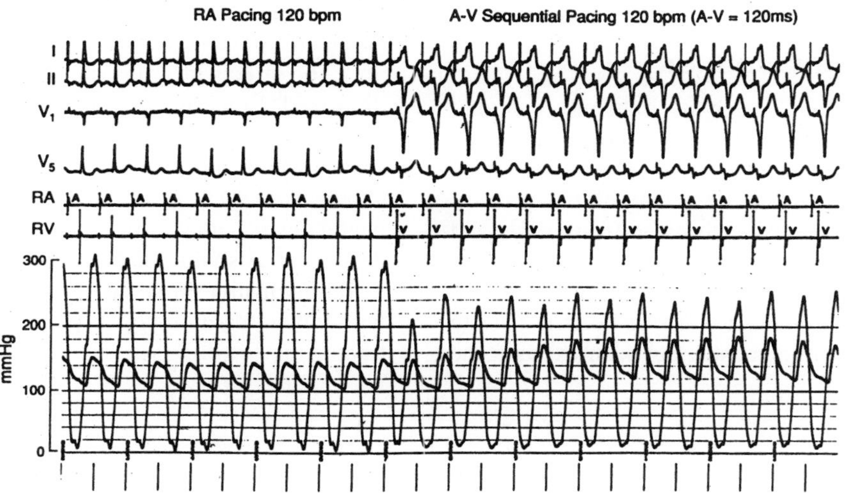

Figure 35–12. Effect of P-synchronous pacing on outflow tract gradient in hypertrophic cardiomyopathy. *(From Fananapazir, Cannon, Tripodi, & Panza. [1992]. [p. 2155].)*

Surgical Therapy. Other treatments for HOCM have also been shown effective. Septal myectomy is the surgical removal of part of the interventricular septum. It is a blind procedure that requires the surgeon to gauge by touch the amount of septum to remove. Even in the hands of the most experienced surgeons, the perioperative mortality rate is as high as 11% (Morrow et al., 1975). The possibility exists that the surgeon will remove an insufficient amount of tissue and the patient will be left with a residual outflow tract gradient. Alternatively, too much tissue may be removed and a ventricular septal defect or conduction abnormality will result.

Because the mitral valve apparatus contributes to the outflow tract obstruction, mitral valve replacement (MVR) is another option in some patients. In recent years we have learned, however, that MVR is not ideal. Patients who undergo MVR are subject to either reoperation (tissue prosthesis) or lifelong anticoagulation (mechanical prosthesis). Additionally, those who receive mechanical prostheses "trade one disease for another," as there is always a gradient across the valve.

With the success of pacing and the availability of medications and surgical palliation, heart transplantation is not generally necessary until ventricular dilatation occurs.

Nonobstructive HCM. ACE inhibitors, digoxin, and nitrates are safely used in patients who have HCM without an outflow tract gradient. These agents are useful in improving diastolic noncompliance.

Restrictive Cardiomyopathy

Restrictive cardiomyopathy (RCM) is rare in the United Sates. It is due to an infiltrative process that, in the end, causes diastolic dysfunction and leads to diastolic failure. Causes of RCM include sarcoidosis, amyloidosis, hemochromotosis, and infiltrative eosinophilia. Definitive diagnosis is by myocardial biopsy.

Specific Cardiomyopathies

"Specific cardiomyopathies," such as ischemic, valvular, and hypertensive cardiomyopathies, have known cardiovascular causes (Richardson et al., 1996). These cardiomyopathies frequently respond to treatment of the primary cause. Valvular heart diseases, such as aortic stenosis and mitral regurgitation, can cause HF in their most severe forms. The fixed cardiac output of aortic stenosis, for example, can cause HF symptoms. At rest, the heart is able to meet the body's metabolic demands, but with exertion the heart fails. Aortic valve replacement cures cardiomyopathy due to aortic stenosis. Similarly, mitral regurgitation causes volume overload. Surgical repair or replacement of the valve is curative.

Table 35–5 lists the specific cardiomyopathies and their known causes.

TABLE 35–5. Definitions of Specific Dilated Cardiomyopathies

Ischemic cardiomyopathy	DCM with impaired contractile performance out of proportion to the extent of ischemia or myocardial damage
Valvular cardiomyopathy	DCM in the presence of valvular heart disease, but out of proportion to the loading conditions
Hypertensive cardiomyopathy	Left ventricular hypertrophy with features of either restrictive or dilated cardiomyopathy
Inflammatory cardiomyopathy	Ventricular dysfunction associated with myocarditis
Metabolic cardiomyopathy	Myocardial dysfunction caused by metabolic/endocrine abnormalities (e.g., thyrotoxicosis, pheochromocytoma, etc.)
Sensitivity and toxic reactions	Myocardial dysfunction caused by alcohol, irradiation, and others
Peripartum cardiomyopathy	Myocardial dysfunction in the last month of pregnancy or within 6 months postpartum[a]

[a] Homans, D. C. (1985). (1432–1437).
From Richardson, McKenna, Bristow, Maisch, Mautner, O'Connel, et al. (1996).

Other Causes of Heart Failure

Other causes of HF do not involve the myocardial muscle fibers. Rather, the heart is unable to meet the body's metabolic demands due to other problems. Included in this group are pericardial disease and cardiac tumors.

The effects of drugs on the myocardium must also be discussed. Some drugs such as cocaine actually increase or interfere with myocardial oxygen supply by causing spasm which may cause an acute myocardial infarction. Other drugs such as adriamycin, a common chemotherapeutic agent, may cause cardiotoxicity, which is dose-dependent. Also the use of alcohol has been known to cause cardiomyopathy. In some of these cases when the drug is withdrawn, cardiomyopathy may somewhat respond to treatment.

REFERENCES

Becker, A. E., Heijmans, C. D., & Essed, C. E. (1991). Chronic non-ischaemic congestive heart disease and endomyocardial biopsies worth the extra? *European Heart Journal, 12* (2), 218–223.

Chulay, M., Guzetta, C., & Dossey, B. (1997). *AACN Handbook of critical care nursing* (pp. 259, 483). Norwalk, CT: Appleton & Lange.

Fananapazir, L., Cannon, R. O., Tripodi, D., & Panza, J. A. (1992). Impact of dual-chamber permanent pacing in patients with obstructive hypertrophic cardiomyopathy with symptoms refractory to verapamil and beta–adrenergic blocker therapy. *Circulation, 85* (6), 2149–2161.

Ganong, W. F. (1993). *Review of medical physiology,* 16th ed. (pp. 415–517). Norwalk, CT: Appleton & Lange.

Homans, D. C. (1985). Current concepts: Peripartum cardiomyopathy. *New England Journal of Medicine, 312* (22), 1432–1437.

Konstam, M., Dracup, K., Baker, D., et al. (1994). *Heart Failure: Evaluation and Care of Patients with Left-Ventricular Systolic Dysfunction.* Clinical Practice Guideline No. 11. AHCPR Publication No. 94-0612. Rockville, MD: Agency for Health Care Policy and Research, Public Health Service, U.S. Department of Health and Human Services. (pp. 50–53).

McCarthy, J. F., McCarthy, P. M., Starling, R. C., Smedira, N. G., Scalia, G. M., Wong, J., Kasirajan, V., Goormastic, M., & Young, J. B. (1998). Partial left ventriculectomy and mitral valve repair for end-stage congestive heart failure. *European Journal of Cardio-Thoracic Surgery, 13* (4), 337–343.

Morrow, A. G., Reitz, B. A., Epstein, S. E., Henry, W. L., Conkle, D. M., Itscoitz, S. B., et al. (1975). Operative treatment in hypertrophic subaortic stenosis: Techniques, and the results of pre- and postoperative assessments in 83 patients. *Circulation, 52* (1).

Opie, L. H. (1991). *The heart: Physiology and metabolism,* (2nd ed.). (p. 411). New York: Raven Press.

Packer, M., Bristow, M. R., Cohn, J. N., et al. (1996). The effect of carvedilol therapy on morbidity and mortality in patients with chronic heart failure. *New England Journal of Medicine, 334* (21), 1349–1355.

Richardson, P., McKenna, W., Bristow, W., Maisch, B., Mautner, B, O'Connel, J., et al. (1996). Report of the 1995 World Health Organization/International Society and Federation of Cardiology Task Force on the definition and classification of cardiomyopathies. *Circulation, 93* (5), 841–842.

Schroeder, J. S. (1994). Cardiac transplantation. In K. J. Isselbacher, E. Braunwald, J. D. Wilson, J. B. Martin, A. S. Fauci, & D. L. Kasper (Eds.), *Harrison's principles of internal medicine* (13th ed.). New York: McGraw-Hill.

Young, J. B. (1997). Carvedilol for heart failure: Renewed interest in beta blockers. *Cleveland Clinic Journal of Medicine, 64* (8), p. 421.

36

Arrhythmias

David J. Callans

▶ BASIC ELECTROPHYSIOLOGY

An understanding of the physiology of impulse formation and conduction in the heart is essential to the study of cardiac arrhythmias and their treatment. This section focuses on the following topics: (1) the structure and function of the specialized conduction system; (2) the cellular electrophysiology of impulse generation and propagation; and (3) mechanisms of arrhythmogenesis, and how antiarrhythmic agents can effect these processes. Interested readers can find a more comprehensive discussion of this elsewhere (Callans, 1993; Hoffman & Cranefield, 1960; Zipes, 1997).

The Specialized Conduction System

Although all myocytes are electrically active, a distinction is made between working (contracting) cells and those functioning primarily for conduction of cardiac impulses. This latter group of cells is organized into the specialized conduction system, which provides uniform, rapid activation of the working myocardium and ensures atrial–ventricular synchrony (Fig. 36–1). In addition, the autonomic nervous system influences cardiac function largely through its interface with the specialized conduction system.

Sinus Node

Under most circumstances, each heart beat is initiated in the cells of the sinus node. The sinus node is a 10 to 20 mm long by 2 to 3 mm wide thick collection of cells located beneath the epicardial surface of the lateral, superior aspect of the right atrium near the junction of the base of the atrial appendage and the root of the superior vena cava. Because sinus node cells are richly interconnected by intercellular gap junctions, no single cell but rather an entire region of cells act as the "pacemaker." Blood is supplied to the sinus node by the sinus node artery, a proximal branch of the right coronary artery in 55 to 60% and of the left circumflex in 40 to 45% of cases. Resting heart rate and response to physiologic stress is determined by autonomic input to the sinus node cells. An extensive network of postganglionic adrenergic and cholinergic nerve terminals enter the nodal region. Parasympathetic stimulation via the vagus nerve slows the sinus discharge rate and prolongs conduction within the node, potentially even to the point of block. Sympathetic stimulation increases heart rate and improves intranodal conduction.

Internodal Tracts

The presence of specialized pathways from region of the sinus node to the atrioventricular (AV) node has been suggested, mostly on the basis of anatomic studies. The cells of these "tracts," however, have never been demonstrated to possess unique histologic or physiologic properties. In contrast, Bachmann's bundle, a band of muscle that traverses the atrial septum, probably does provide a specialized pathway for intra-atrial conduction.

Atrioventricular Node

The AV node is located beneath the right atrial endocardium of the atrial septum between the tricuspid annulus and the coronary sinus os. The AV node is responsible for the majority of the delay associated with conduction between the atrium and the ventricles. This delay may be helpful in providing the proper synchrony for electrical–mechanical cou-

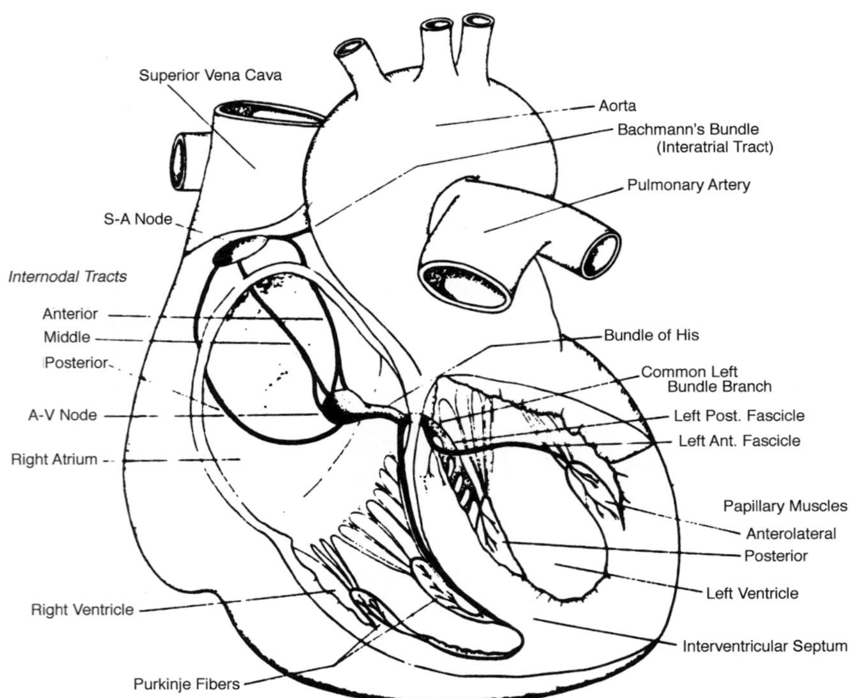

Figure 36–1. A schematic representation of the specialized conduction system. Although specialized internodal tracts (electrically connecting the sinus and atrioventricular nodes) are shown here, most investigators doubt that they exist. See text for discussion. *(Used with permission from Dunn & Lipman. [1989].)*

pling. In addition, slow conduction and a relatively long refractory period in the AV node prevent excessively rapid ventricular rates during supraventricular arrhythmias, particularly in atrial fibrillation. Slow conduction in the AV node is due to several factors. First, the action potentials in this region are calcium dependent, which are not so favorable for conduction as sodium-dependent action potentials. Second, AV nodal cells are relatively isolated electrically because of the scarcity of intracellular gap junctions and the presence of connective tissue between adjacent cells. Finally, the conduction in the AV node is carefully controlled by autonomic nervous system inputs. In the resting state, vagal influences predominate, favoring slow conduction and a long refractory period in AV nodal tissue. In 80 to 90% of cases, the AV node artery arises from the right coronary artery after a peculiar "U-turn" at the posterior intersection of the AV and intraventricular grooves; it originates from the left circumflex in the remaining cases.

Bundle of His

The bundle of His is formed by the continuation of the AV node fibers as they pass through the central fibrous body and the membranous portion of the interventricular septum. Cells in the proximal portion of the bundle of His closely resemble cells of the compact portion of the AV node. The distal bundle of His is composed of cells identical to those of Purkinje fibers, which continue distally as the right and left bundle branch. Arterial blood is supplied by an arcade of septal perforators from the left anterior descending and the posterior descending branch of the right coronary artery. This dual blood supply protects this critical junction of the conduction system from all but extensive (or multiple) myocardial infarction. Bundle of His impulse conduction is essentially unaffected by autonomic nervous system input, and its conduction time is fairly constant (normally 35-55 msec) irrespective of heart rate.

Bundle Branches and Distal Purkinje System

The distal bundle of His divides at the superior margin of the muscular interventricular septum to give rise to a discrete right bundle branch and a fan-like network, collectively called the left bundle branch. The right bundle runs within the septal myocardium to the right ventricular apex. The left bundle branch functions as though it were separated into distinct anterior and posterior fascicles, even though distinct fascicles are not apparent anatomically. The construct is used to explain fascicular rhythms and the electrocardiographic pattern of fascicular block. The left anterior descending coronary artery supplies blood to the bundle branches along with the septal myocardium. Bundle branch block is a recognized complication of extensive anterior infarction. Both bundle branches further subdivide to form the Purkinje network which penetrates the inner third of the endocardium throughout both ventricles. Due to the extensive ramifications of the Purkinje system, the entire surface of the endocardium is activated within 30 to 50 msec in the normal heart.

Cellular Electrophysiology

The Cellular Basis for the Action Potential

There are several cellular characteristics that are essential for the genesis of the cardiac action potential. A necessary property of all electrically active tissue is the presence of a selectively permeable outer membrane. The cell membrane, or sarcolemma, is a phospholipid bilayer that provides a high resistance to the flow of ions across the membrane. This allows for the establishment of an electrochemical gradient between intracellular and extracellular spaces (inside -90 mV in normal myocytes). Because ions are charged, the flow of ions across the membrane generates electric current. Ions can pass through the membrane only at certain sites, called channels, which are formed by relatively specific transmembrane proteins. Channels are regulated, or gated, in such a way that the probability of being "open" (for the passage of a specific ion) is not constant. Changes in the channel gating status can occur with changes in the transmembrane voltage (voltage-dependence), or with passage of time from an event, such as the initiation of an action potential (time-dependence).

The cellular action potential is an "all or none" response that provides the essential "language" for the intracellular propagation of electrical impulses. The characteristics of the action potential are determined by the types of channels that are present in a particular type of myocyte, and can be described as one of two types: sodium-dependent and calcium-dependent action potentials.

The Sodium-Dependent Action Potential

Sodium-dependent action potentials are observed in all working atrial and ventricular myocardium, and in the entire conduction system with the exception of sinus and AV nodal tissue. Sodium-dependent action potentials are also observed in accessory bypass tracts. The sodium-dependent action potential is described in five phases, each of which is determined by a dominant ionic current (Fig. 36–2).

Rapid Depolarization (Phase 0). Phase 0 is the most distinctive feature of the sodium-dependent action potential, in which the intracellular voltage changes from resting membrane potential (–90 mV) to a positive potential (10-20 mV) in a matter of several milliseconds. At resting membrane potential, the cell membrane is essentially impermeable to sodium ions. When a stimulus is applied to the cell that is sufficient to bring the membrane voltage to threshold (such as an action potential in a neighboring cell),

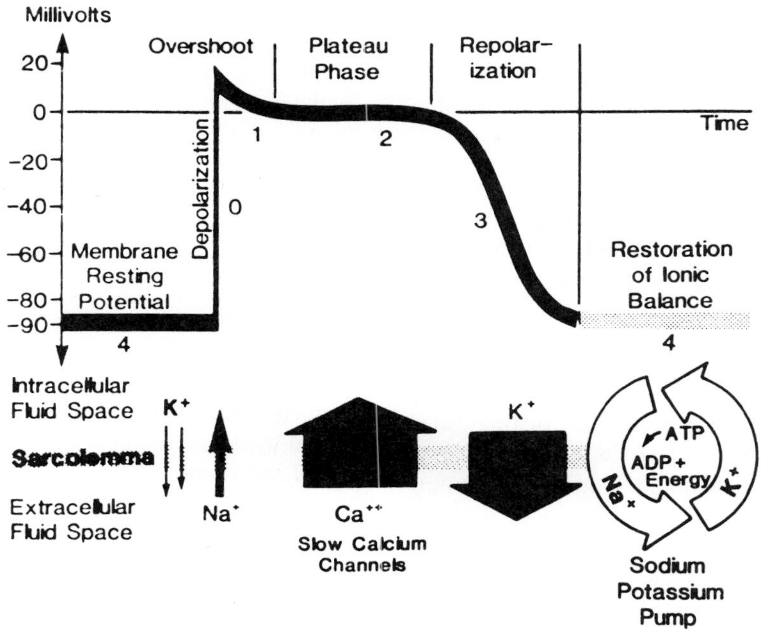

Figure 36–2. The sodium dependent action potential. An electrical impulse of sufficient intensity (such as current from the action potentials of upstream cells) starts the flow of sodium current (phase 0), rapidly changing the intracellular potential to positive. The sodium channels close, and the membrane potential returns to near zero potential (phase 1). The plateau phase (phase 2), mediated mainly by inward calcium current, maintains the potential near zero for sufficient time to facilitate excitation-contraction coupling. Repolarization (phase 3) restores the cell to resting potential, and is mediated primarily by outward potassium current. In contrast to calcium dependent cells, which exhibit phase 4 depolarization (see text and Fig. 36–3), phase 4 in sodium-dependent tissue is devoted to restoration of ionic balance is most sodium dependent cells. *(Used with permission from Dunn & Lipman. [1989].)*

the sodium channel opens suddenly, and sodium ions enter the cell driven by the force of both a concentration gradient and the electrical field. When the sodium channels close, the membrane is no longer permeable to sodium, and phase 0 is complete. Closing of individual channels occurs because of the change in transmembrane voltage to positive (voltage dependence) and the time elapsed since channel opening (time dependence).

It is important to realize the voltage change of phase 0 occurs with the passage of very few sodium ions (4×10^{-12} moles/cm^2). Because of this, even after hundreds of action potentials, the sodium concentration gradient remains intact, and does not need to be regenerated for the cell to return to resting membrane potential. Sodium and potassium homeostasis is maintained by ion pumps. The sodium–potassium ATPase pump exchanges 3 sodium ions (out) for 2 potassium ions (in), in both cases against the transmembrane concentration gradient. This process requires energy, provided by high energy phosphate groups in ATP. One of the first manifestations of cellular damage is the inability for this pump to function effectively, resulting in less negative resting membrane potential. Digitalis inhibits the sodium–potassium exchange pump, an effect that is indirectly responsible for its hemodynamic effects and directly responsible for many of its proarrhythmic effects.

The rapid change in transmembrane potential provided by phase 0 of the action potential is a key determinant of the conduction velocity with which the impulse is propagated. If the amplitude of phase 0 is blunted or its slope is decreased, as may occur in damaged myocardium or with the use of antiarrhythmic agents that block the sodium channel, conduction velocity within the heart decreases.

Early Rapid Repolarization (Phase 1). Following the "overshoot" when the intracellular space becomes transiently positive, the membrane quickly repolarizes to near 0 mV. This change in voltage is due to the inactivation of the inward sodium current and the activation of a repolarization current carried either by outward movement of potassium ions and/or inward movement of chloride ions.

Plateau (Phase 2). The plateau phase distinguishes myocytes from electrically active cells in the nervous system; it is marked by a low membrane conductance to all ions. The transmembrane potential may remain near 0 mV for more than 100 milliseconds. Small inward fluxes of chloride are balanced by a background slow inward current carried by calcium ions. It is thought that this "waiting period" is important to facilitate the proper synchrony for excitation–contraction coupling.

Rapid Repolarization (Phase 3). Rapid repolarization returns the transmembrane potential to values close to the resting potential and is largely due to two currents: the slow inward current carried by calcium is inactivated, and an outward movement of positive charges (carried by potassium) is activated. Sodium channels are still closed during this period, and thus an action potential cannot occur, no matter the intensity of the stimulus. The amount of time before the sodium channels have the capacity to open again is called the absolute refractory period—the minimal time period between action potentials.

Diastolic Depolarization (Phase 4). The membrane potential returns to near resting potential at the conclusion of phase 3. In atrial and ventricular muscle, the transmembrane voltage remains constant throughout diastole under normal conditions. Certain cells have the normal capacity to spontaneously depolarize and may reach threshold in the absence of an external stimulus, leading to another action potential. This phenomenon is called automaticity, and is responsible for the ability of cells in several locations (most notably cells within the sinus and AV nodes and the His–Purkinje network) to act as "pacemakers." Under pathologic conditions, this ability can also develop in working myocytes (abnormal automaticity). The ionic basis of the current(s) responsible for diastolic depolarization is complex and probably requires the interaction of a number of currents carried by sodium, potassium, and chloride ions.

The Calcium-Dependent Action Potential

Calcium-dependent or "slow response" action potentials are observed in cells of the sinus and AV nodes (Fig. 36–3). Calcium-dependent action potentials are also seen in damaged myocardium (particularly in the setting of ischemia) which have less negative resting membrane potentials, causing inactivation of the sodium channel (because of its voltage dependent gating behavior). In nodal tissue, the concepts of resting membrane and threshold potential still apply; however, the upstroke of the action potential (phase 0) is not mediated by sodium current, but by the slow inward current carried by calcium. The channel responsible for this ionic current opens and closes slowly, thus recovery of excitability (i.e., ability for the Ca^{2+} channel to open in response to another stimulus) is prolonged and the absolute refractory period is longer. In addition, the slow upstroke of the action potential in nodal tissue results in low conduction velocity, and explains the "physiologic delay" that is provided by the AV node and is necessary for the synchrony of atrial and ventricular pump function.

Once an action potential is generated, it provides a stimulus to depolarize adjacent patches of cell membrane to threshold so that a wave of activation spreads sequentially to all nonrefractory tissue. The velocity of this transmission, and whether it occurs, depends on several factors. To establish current flow under any circumstances, a circuit must be formed. Positive charges crossing the membrane into the cell during the action potential upstroke must eventually return to the current source. Intracellular passage of current is facilitated by the presence of intracellular connections called gap junctions. In addition, ions cross the cell membrane to return to the source and complete the circuit.

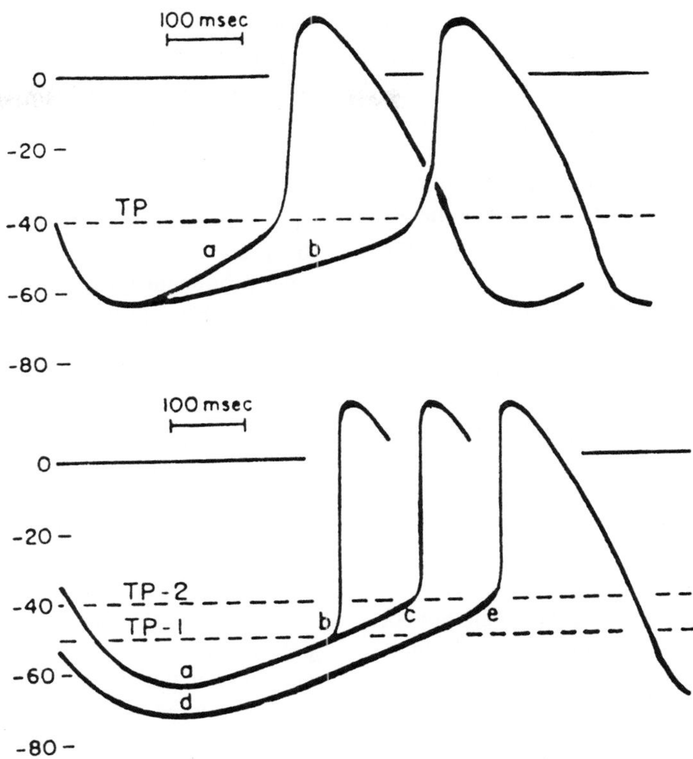

Figure 36–3. The calcium dependent action potential and phase 4 depolarization. Resting membrane potential in calcium dependent cells is less negative (approximately - 60 mV). After reaching threshold, phase 0, mediated by inward calcium current, is slower and smaller in amplitude than in sodium dependent cells. There is no distinct overshoot or plateau phase, and repolarization (phase 3) is mediated by outward potassium current. Phase 4 depolarization, which is determined by a complex combination of ionic currents, is much more prominent, and may result in bringing a cell to threshold potential (TP) spontaneously. Factors that effect the time required to pass from resting membrane potential to threshold potential influence the spontaneous discharge rate (pacemaker rate) of a given cell. These factors include: (1) the slope of phase 4 depolarization (*top panel*), (2) the transmembrane voltage at threshold potential (*bottom panel*), and the transmembrane voltage at resting potential (*bottom panel*). *(Used with permission from Hoffman & Cranefield. [1960].)*

This extracellular movement of ions is recorded at the body surface as the electrocardiogram. The conduction velocity of an impulse is a reflection of ability of a local action potential to depolarize adjacent patches of membrane to threshold, resulting in perpetuation of the spread of action potentials downstream. It is directly related to the magnitude of the current generated in phase 0, and indirectly related to the degree of resistance offered by the intracellular space; the greater the resistance, the more current "leaks" to the extracellular space and is unavailable to depolarize other portions of the membrane. Electrolyte and acid/base disturbances, tissue ischemia, and cellular death, as well as antiarrhythmic drugs can effect these parameters and alter characteristics of the action potential and its intracellular conduction. These changes may effect the likelihood of arrhythmogenesis.

Mechanisms of Arrhythmogenesis

Cardiac arrhythmias are caused by disorders of impulse formation, impulse conduction, or combinations of both. Often the precise mechanism of a clinically observed arrhythmia cannot be proven. Based on the clinical behavior of the arrhythmia and its response to interventions, however, it can usually be classified within one of the broad categories discussed below.

Disorders of Impulse Formation

The usual focus of impulse formation is phase 4 depolarization within the cells of the sinus node. Normal sinus rhythm has a rate of 60 to 100 impulses per minute and is under strict control by the autonomic nervous system. Other cardiac cells are capable of automaticity as well. Lower pacemakers are usually kept from spontaneously reaching threshold because of overdrive suppression by the more rapidly depolarizing sinus nodal cells. In the event of failure of sinus node automaticity, cells of the AV node (40-60 beats/min), bundle of His (30-50 beats/min), or Purkinje system (15-40 beats/min) may provide an escape rhythm, each with its own characteristic rate.

Tachycardias can occur when cells develop a spontaneous rate of discharge faster than the autonomically controlled, appropriate rate of the sinus node. This can occur under normal cellular conditions in the atrium and the ventricle, or under pathologic conditions (normal and abnormal automaticity, respectively). Many conditions (ischemia, electrolyte imbalance, and certain antiarrhythmic drugs) facilitate abnormal automaticity by elevating the resting membrane potential to less negative values; this has the effect of bringing these cells closer to threshold potential. Clinical examples of tachycardias caused by normal or abnormal automaticity include certain atrial tachycardias, accelerated junctional tachycardia (which occurs in the setting of valve surgery, ischemia, or digitalis overdosage), and many fascicular or idioventricular rhythms.

Another mechanism of abnormal impulse formation that probably has clinical significance is triggered activity due to early and delayed afterdepolarizations. Afterdepolarizations represent "spikes" of positive current after the onset of the action potential, but prior to full repolarization (Fig. 36–4). Depending upon their timing, the current responsible for afterdepolarizations is either calcium or sodium. If afterdepolarizations reach sufficient amplitude, the membrane voltage may reach threshold "triggering" another action potential. Triggered activity has been demonstrated in experimental preparations of tissue made abnormal by ischemia, hyperkalemia, digitalis intoxication, and catecholamine superfusion. Clinical rhythm disorders that may be due to triggered activity include many of the tachycardias of digitalis intoxication and torsades de pointes.

Disorders of Impulse Conduction

Most clinically important tachyarrhythmias are caused by disorders of impulse conduction, of which reentry is the most prominent type.. Under normal circumstances, a cardiac impulse is propagated along the specialized conduction system until every cell within the heart is activated. At this point, all cells are refractory, and the impulse extinguishes. If conduction block prevents an area of tissue from being depolarized, this protected region may be available for impulse propagation when the remainder of the heart is refractory. A delayed wave of activation may pass through this region and serve to reactivate the rest of the myocardium just after it recovers from refractoriness and long before the next expected impulse is due.

In order for reentry to occur, three conditions must be present (Fig. 36–5). First, there must be two distinct anatomic or functional pathways of conduction, arranged in such a way that a closed loop could join their proximal and

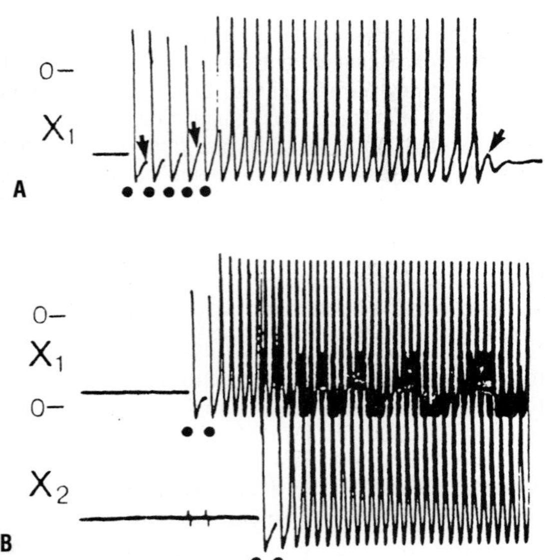

Figure 36–4. Triggered activity caused by delayed afterdepolariztions. Intracellular recordings from isolated myocytes in diseased human ventricle are shown. The first several action potentials in each tracing are paced (*indicated by the dots*). The arrows refer to afterdepolarizations, increases in membrane potential that occur during phase 4 that are not caused by stimulation. In panel **A,** the afterdepolarizations increase in amplitude and reach threshold resulting in sustained, unstimulated rhythm. In panel **B,** triggered activity develops independently in two separate cells (X1 and X2). Even though these cells were separated by only 4 mm, they remained dissociated from one another. *(Used with permission from Gilmour et al. [1983].)*

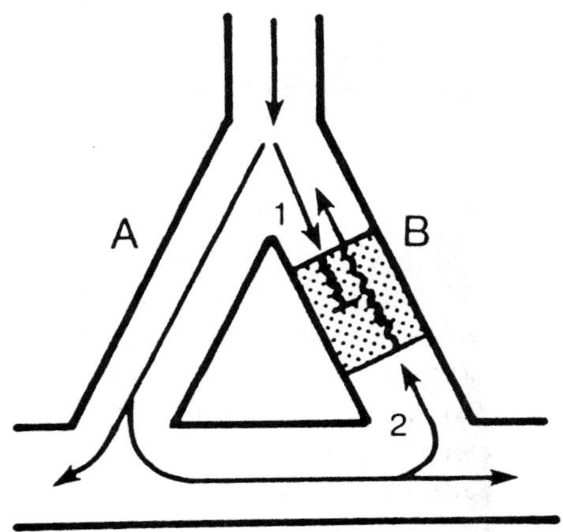

Figure 36–5. The conditions required for reentry, shown in schematic form at a branch point in the distal Purkinje system. First, two pathways for impulse propagation must be present. Second, the pathways must differ in their recovery from refractoriness. This causes initial block of the impulse in limb B (1) because the refractory period in limb B is longer than that of limb A. Third, sufficient slow conduction (indicated by the stippled zone in limb B) must be present in order to allow the tissue within limb B at site 1 to recover from refractoriness by time the impulse returns in the retrograde direction (i.e., from site 2 to site 1). If conditions are appropriate, the "circle" that is established may lead to sustained arrhythmias. *(Used with permission from Hoffman et al. [1981].)*

distal ends. Second, the propagating impulse must block in one pathway (unidirectional block) because of differences in refractoriness between the two pathways. Third, conduction must be sufficiently slow in the pathway that is capable of conduction to allow enough time for recovery in the pathway where the initial impulse blocked, allowing for the formation of a reentrant circuit. If continuous reentry occurs, the resulting impulse generated by the circuit may be conducted to the rest of the heart. Common examples include AV nodal reentry, AV reciprocating tachycardia in the Wolff–Parkinson–White syndrome, and ventricular tachycardia arising from the border zone of surviving tissue near an area of a prior infarction.

▶ ANTIARRHYTHMIC DRUGS

As discussed, disorders of impulse formation and impulse conduction are more likely to occur in areas of myocardium with abnormal cellular electrophysiology. Antiarrhythmic agents further effect conduction and/or the propensity for automaticity in cardiac tissue. Because of these effects, antiarrhythmic drugs can have either antiarrhythmic or proarrhythmic consequences. However, because they tend to change the electrophysiologic properties of abnormal tissue to a greater extent than normal tissue, they more often than not have a beneficial effect.

The major classes of antiarrhythmic drug and representative examples are listed in Table 36–1. They are classified by their predominant actions, either ion channel blockade (sodium, potassium, or calcium) or beta-adrenergic receptor blockade. Class I agents slow conduction by blocking sodium channels and decreasing the magnitude of the action potential upstroke. The agents within class I are subdivided based on their effects on action potential duration and refractoriness, effects that are mediated by blocking potassium channels to a greater or lesser extent. The class II agents interfere with beta-adrenergic receptors. Their effects are directed at the sites of sympathetic nervous system innervation, primarily the sinus and AV nodes, where they cause a reduction in the rate of impulse formation and slow the rate of conduction. Class III drugs block potassium channels and thus prolong the time required for repolarization and recovery from refractoriness. Finally, members of class IV are calcium antagonists. Several agents do not fit neatly into this schema. Digitalis blocks the sodium–potassium pump, leading to less negative cellular resting potentials and conduction slowing or block in sinus and AV nodal tissue. Atropine blocks the action of parasympathetic innervation at the sinus and AV nodes and can lead to improved nodal conduction. Adenosine has several electrophysiologic effects, particularly in atrial myocardium. Its most useful clinical property is its effect on slowing conduction within the AV node.

▶ ELECTROCARDIOGRAPHY

Like many other clinical skills, interpretation of the surface electrocardiogram depends on pattern recognition. Proficiency depends on being exposed to these patterns over the course of years. Displaying all of the patterns—normal and abnormal—is beyond the scope of this chapter; interested readers are referred to several excellent textbooks on the subject (Chou, 1996; Dunn & Lipman, 1989; Marriott, 1983). Instead, a systematic approach to the ECG is presented, so that patterns can begin to be established with every ECG that is encountered.

The electrocardiogram represents the extracellular vector summation of all the individual intracellular action potentials within the chambers of the heart. The 12 lead ECG "surrounds" the heart in space (although the posterior portion of the heart is quite underrepresented), so that each lead group interrogates a separate region (Figs. 36–6 and 36–7). The limb leads view the heart in the frontal plane; leads II, III, and aVF are especially sensitive to changes in the inferior wall, and leads I and aVL to the lateral wall of the left ventricle. The precordial leads view the heart in the transverse plane; leads V1 and V2 focus on right ventricle and the intraventricular septum; leads V3 and V4, the anterior wall; and leads V5 and V6, the lateral wall of the left ventricle.

Systematic evaluation of the ECG includes consideration of the following variables (Table 36–2): rate, rhythm,

TABLE 36–1. Antiarrhythmic Drug Classification

Class	Channel Effected	Prototype Agent	ECG Effects	Clinical Uses
IA	sodium channel	quinidine	incr QT	SVT, VT, AF
IB	sodium channel	lidocaine	none	VT (ischemia)
IC	sodium channel	flecainide	incr QRS	SVT, VT, AF
II	β receptor	propranolol	decr heart rate	SVT (AF)
III	potassium channel	sotalol	incr QT	SVT, VT, AF
IV	calcium channel	verapamil	decr heart rate	SVT (AF)
"others"				
	NA-K ATPase	digoxin	digoxin effect	SVT (AF)
	A2 receptor	adenosine	none	SVT

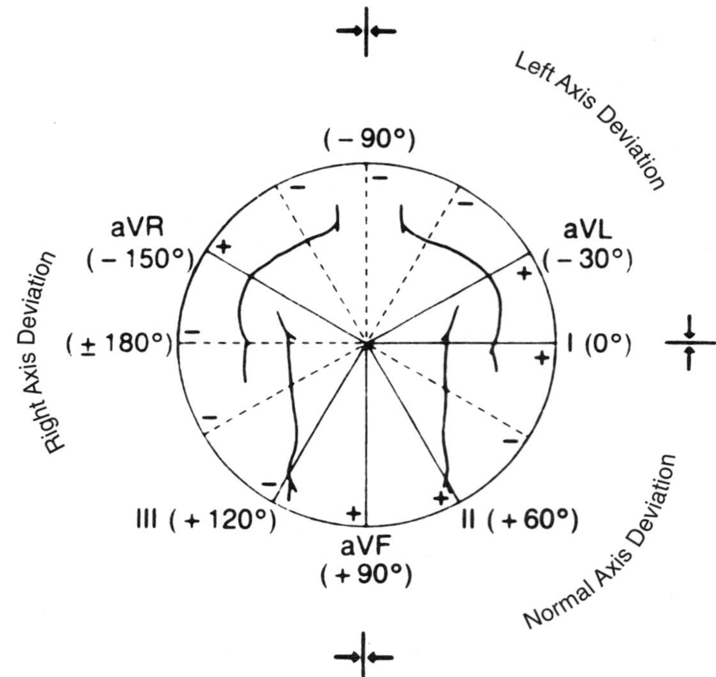

Figure 36–6. The position of the limb leads and the frontal plane axis. The vectors of the limb leads are depicted in space as they relate to the position of the heart. This has two implications. First, different lead groupings (i.e., inferior, anterior, lateral) cooperate to investigate different aspects of the heart more closely. Second, this arrangement allows determination of the electrical axis of the heart. See text for discussion. *(Used with permission from Atlee [1985].)*

relationship of p waves and QRS complexes, intervals, axis, and morphology of the QRS, ST segment, and T waves. The rate can be quickly estimated, as ECG recording paper is calibrated such that the interval between heavy vertical lines is 200 msec; the number of boxes between QRS complexes is related to the heart rate and can be rapidly assessed (Fig. 36–8). By convention, rates between 60 and 100 are "normal"; faster rates are considered tachycardias; slower rates, bradycardias.

The cardiac rhythm refers to what structure is generat-

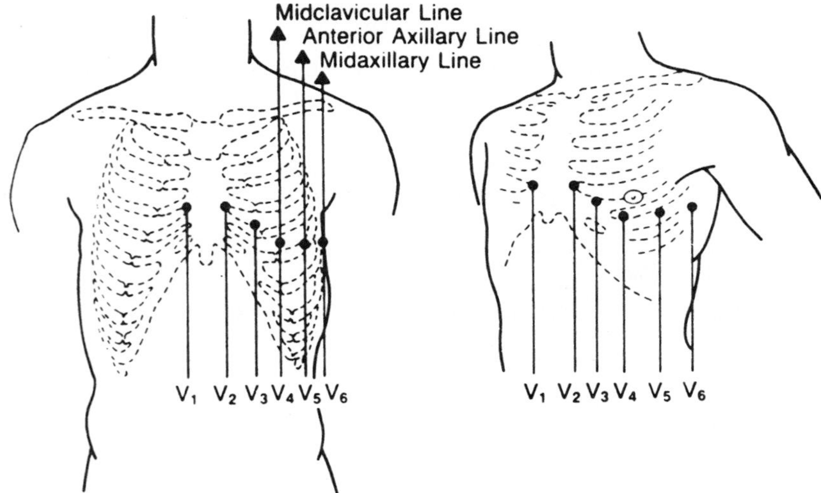

Figure 36–7. The chest leads are positioned as shown diagrammatically, from the midsternum to the left midaxillary line. The chest leads view the heart in the transverse plane and the anterior wall of the left ventricle is the area most closely examined. See text for discussion. *(Used with permission from Atlee [1985].)*

TABLE 36–2. Systematic ECG Reading Checklist

1. Rate
2. Rhythm
3. Relationship of *p* waves and QRS complexes
4. Intervals (PR, QRS duration, QT interval)
5. Axis
6. Morphology of the QRS
7. Morphology of the ST segment and T waves

ing the pacemaker impulse. Sinus rhythm (recognized by upright p waves in leads I, II, and III) implies normal conduction to the ventricles; however, in the event of heart block, the atrial rhythm and the ventricular rhythm may be altogether different (e.g., sinus rhythm in the atria, with a junctional escape rhythm driving the ventricular rate). Central to the determination of the rhythm is deciding the relationship of the p waves to the QRS complexes. It can be very difficult to determine which event is the "driving force" particularly in tachycardias (i.e., if the p wave is responsible for the subsequent QRS or if it occurs because of retrograde conduction from the previous QRS). Often, electrophysiologic study with intracardiac recordings is necessary to determine the mechanism of a tachycardia. The important intervals to consider include the PR interval, the QRS duration, and the QT interval. These intervals are the ECG manifestations of conduction through the atrium–AV node–bundle of His, the His–Purkinje system, and completion of ventricular repolarization respectively (Fig. 36–9).

The axis usually refers to the frontal plane axis (refer to Fig. 36–6). In general, the axis of the p waves, the QRS, and the T waves should all be approximately the same; variations from this rule are seen in abnormalities in the conduction system (bundle branch block, fascicular blocks), chamber hypertrophy, and coronary artery disease. Finally, the morphology of the QRS, ST segment, and the T waves needs to be evaluated. Morphologic abnormalities are particularly important in diagnoses of acute ischemia and infarction (Fig. 36–10) and in the differential diagnosis of wide complex tachycardias.

BRADYARRHYTHMIAS

Bradyarrhythmias may result from dysfunction of the sinus node or disturbances of atrioventricular (AV) conduction (Josephson, Marchlinski, & Buxton, 1991; Sutton, 1995; Wharton & Ellenbogen, 1995). Although 60 beats per minute is often defined as the lower boundary of normal resting heart rate, many normal patients observed on telemetry have occasional sinus rates in the 40 to 50 beats-per-minute range, particularly during sleep. Clinically significant bradyarrhythmias, therefore, cannot be defined by rate alone. Instead, the diagnosis depends on linking the observed bradycardia to symptoms of decreased cardiac output. These disorders are typically episodic, and may be difficult to diagnose on this account, but may also be permanent. Bradyarrhythmias most commonly occur in patients with structural heart disease, and cardiovascular medications often facilitate their development. In addition, bradycardias develop in relatively normal hearts, particularly in older adults, due to replacement fibrosis of working conduction system tissue. Bradyarrhythmias may be characterized into two causes: sinus node dysfunction and disorders of atrioventricular conduction.

Sinus Node Dysfunction

Pathophysiology

The sinus node usually determines the heart rate because the cells of the sinus node complex have the fastest intrinsic rate of impulse formation. The sinus node region is also

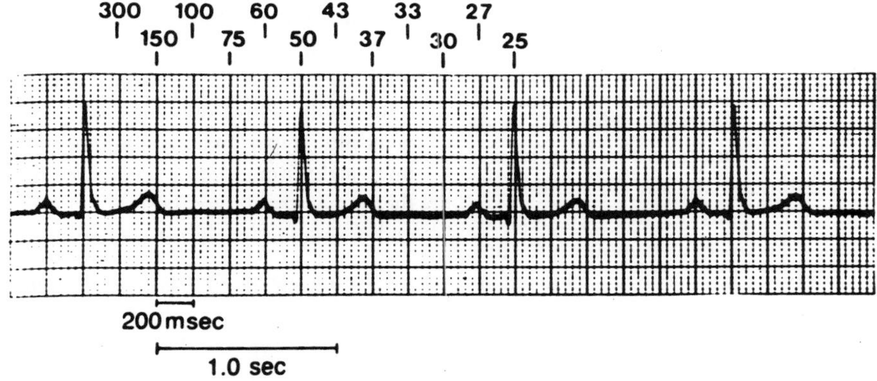

Figure 36–8. Estimation of rate from the electrocardiogram. Because ECG paper is calibrated (25 mm/sec), each small box is equivalent to 0.04 seconds and each large box 0.2 seconds. The heart rate can be estimated rapidly by counting the boxes between QRS complexes and converting interval to rate. If one large box separated successive QRS complexes, the rate would be 300/min (60 seconds divided by 0.2 seconds = 300/min); if two large boxes separated QRS complexes, the rate would be 150/min, and so on. *(Used with permission from Atlee [1985].)*

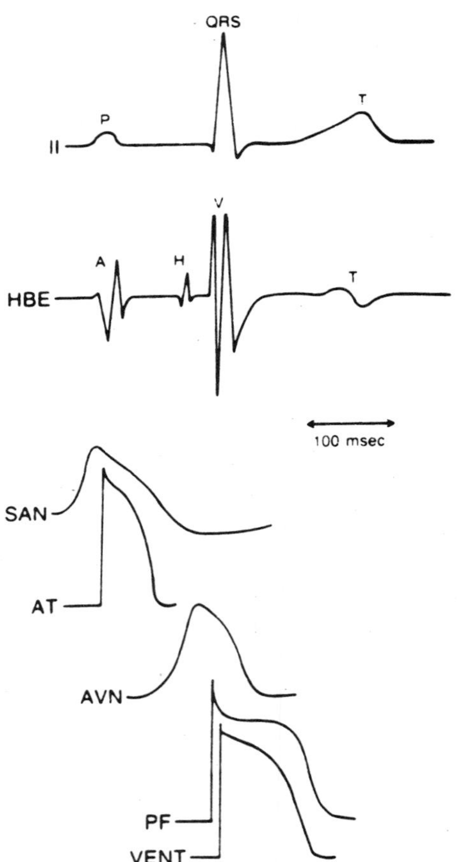

Figure 36–9. The intervals important in ECG interpretation. The surface ECG lead II is shown with a simultaneous His bundle electrogram (HBE, recorded with intracardiac electrodes) and action potentials from different regions within the heart. The PR interval (from the start of the P wave to the start of the QRS), corresponds to activation of the atrium and conduction through the AV node and the His bundle. The QRS duration represents the amount of time required for the Purkinje network to activate each ventricular myocyte. The QT interval (from the start of the QRS to the end of the T wave) represents the total time required for repolarization to occur in both ventricles. *(Used with permission from Atlee [1985].)*

richly innervated with autonomic system efferents, and physiologic demands for higher heart rates are usually directed to this region. In the event the sinus node should fail to initiate the heart beat, other cells capable of normal phase 4 automaticity should take over this function. A "hierarchy of pacemakers" exists within the heart, and each cell type has a characteristic rate of impulse formation (Fig. 36–11). In significant sinus node dysfunction, often not only the sinus node pacemaker, but often many of the subsidiary pacemakers fail to function. This can lead either to sustained low heart rates or significant pauses (Fig. 36–12).

The condition generally referred to as sinus node dysfunction or "sick sinus syndrome" encompasses sinus pauses, sinus arrest, sinus bradycardia, sino–atrial exit block, in which sinus node impulse formation is normal, but the impulse is not conducted to the remainder of the heart because of block at the boundary of the sinus node complex (Fig. 36–13). Although all of these syndromes can potentially be differentiated on the ECG, the distinction is not always clinically relevant as all of these conditions cause similar symptoms and have similar pathophysiologic mechanisms. The pathophysiology of sinus node dysfunction involves the replacement of sinus node cells or the cells at the junction between the sinus node and the atrium with fibrotic scar. Rarely, sinus node dysfunction occurs as a direct result of occlusion of the sinus node artery or due to manipulation of the heart during open heart surgery (particularly valve replacement surgery). Antiarrhythmic drugs of all classes, including digoxin, beta-adrenergic blockers and calcium antagonists, can cause or exacerbate sinus node dysfunction.

It is important to recognize that sinus bradycardia is commonly seen in young patients, particularly athletes, during sleep or other conditions associated with high vagal tone (pain, nausea, vomiting, bowel movements). These episodes are almost uniformly transient and asymptomatic. Sinus node dysfunction (and AV block) can also be observed in the sleep apnea syndrome, presumably secondary to increased vagal tone during pharyngeal obstruction.

Frequently sinus node dysfunction coexists with atrial fibrillation (or other clinically significant SVTs) producing the tachycardia–bradycardia syndrome. In the "tachy–brady" syndrome, paroxysmal atrial fibrillation terminates suddenly, resulting in profound sinus bradycardia, sinus pauses, or sinus arrest associated with a junctional escape rhythm (Fig. 36–14). In this setting, the mechanism of sinus node dysfunction is called overdrive suppression. The resting membrane potential of sinus node cells becomes more negative (and thus farther away from the phase 4 threshold for activation) with each of the rapid impulses from the tachyarrhythmia. Symptoms may be produced by either the tachycardia or the offset pause, which may be associated with syncope. This syndrome is typically seen in older patients with some evidence of atrial disease and/or longstanding hypertension. Obviously, since therapy of the tachyarrhythmia only exacerbates bradycardia, combination therapy with antiarrhythmic or AV nodal blocking agents and permanent pacing is often required.

History and Physical Findings

Patients with sinus node dysfunction may have a variety of complaints, ranging from vague symptoms of personality changes and apparent dementia to recurrent syncope. Exercise intolerance, usually expressed as exertional dyspnea, can also represent a subtle manifestation of sinus node dysfunction. Physical findings are typically limited, although signs of trauma should be excluded in patients with sudden syncope.

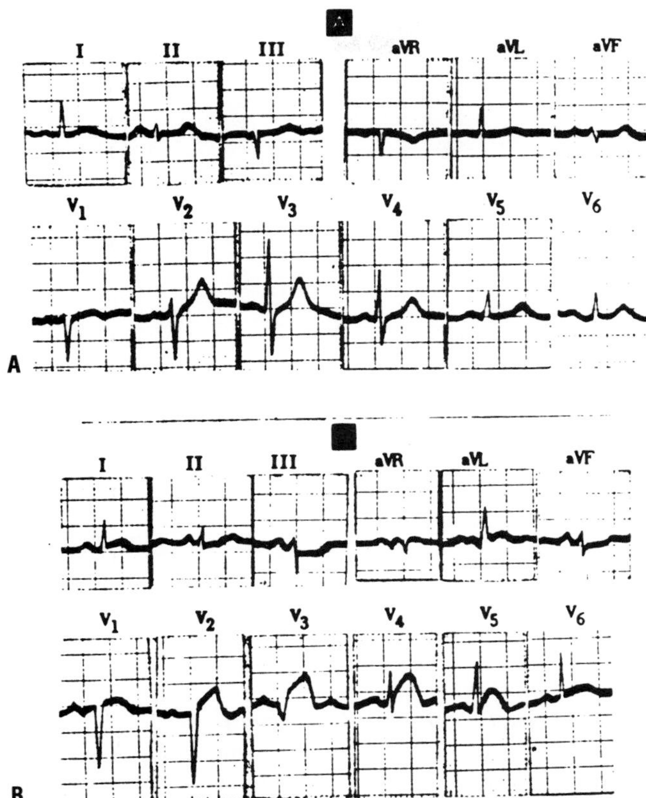

Figure 36–10. Acute anteroseptal myocardial infarction. The tracing in panel **A** is normal. In **B**, recorded during chest pain, demonstrates ST segment elevation in leads I, aVL and V1 through V6, with the development of q waves in V1 through V3. *(Used with permission from Dunn & Lipman. [1989].)*

Laboratory and Diagnostic Tests

Electrolyte disturbances seldom contribute to sinus node dysfunction. Antiarrhythmic drugs certainly do, but serum levels are typically not helpful in determining causality. The ECG may be helpful, but may fail to be diagnostic unless sinus bradycardia is constant. Telemetry monitoring is more likely to discover transient abnormalities, but even several days of normal telemetry does not definitively exclude clinically relevant sinus node dysfunction, particularly in the setting of syncope. Long-term ambulatory loop monitors are useful, but only if the patient is aware of symptomatic episodes. Electrophysiologic studies for formal sinus node testing may be required in some cases when ECG monitoring does not deliver a diagnosis.

Management

Symptomatic sinus bradycardia can be resolved temporarily with pharmacologic agents such as atropine or isoproterenol. Nonessential medications that might effect sinus node function should be discontinued. When causative medications cannot be discontinued, or in patients who have persistent sinus node dysfunction after all such medications have been stopped, permanent pacing therapy is required.

Follow-Up

Patients with sinus node dysfunction treated with permanent pacing generally have relief of symptoms related to end-organ hypoperfusion. Often patients realize substantial gains in exercise tolerance or mental performance only retrospectively after regaining the capacity to do things they no longer noticed they could not do prior to implantation.

Disturbances of Atrioventricular Conduction

Pathophysiology

As discussed, the specialized conduction system usually ensures conduction of the sinus impulse from the atria to the ventricles in a synchronized fashion. Damage to the conduction system may be caused by degenerative diseases (Lev's and Lenegre's diseases), infiltration (sarcoid, amyloid, Lyme carditis, infectious material in endocarditis with abscess formation), or myocardial infarction. The upper conduction system (AV node) is richly supplied with autonomic system input. AV block at the level of the AV node may be observed in normal subjects during sleep. Transient complete AV block can complicate the early course of acute inferior myocardial infarction. This AV conduction disturbance responds to atropine and is due to excess vagal tone.

Although it is an imperfect system, AV block is often classified as first-, second-, and third-degree. This classification is based on the electrocardiographic pattern of the conduction disturbance, not the underlying anatomic substrate. This is unfortunate, as the most important characteristic of AV block is the level within the conduction system at which it occurs. Block occurring in the AV node generally signifies a more benign prognosis than block due to disease of the His–Purkinje system, which more frequently accompanies advanced structural heart disease and is more prone to progress to complete heart block.

First-degree AV block, defined as a PR interval greater than 20 seconds, rarely results in symptoms or significant hemodynamic compromise. It is most often due to delay of the electrical impulse as it conducts through the AV node. Delayed AV nodal conduction can be the result of high vagal tone or cardiovascular medications as well as intrinsic AV nodal disease. Since every sinus impulse is conducted to the ventricle, first-degree AV *delay* is a more accurate description.

Second-degree AV block, defined as intermittent failure of AV conduction, is divided into Mobitz I and Mobitz II block. Mobitz I block, or Wenckebach block, is characterized by progressive PR prolongation prior to AV block (Fig. 36–15). This pattern is characteristic of block at the level of the AV node and may be observed in normal subjects. The majority of patients with Wenckebach block are

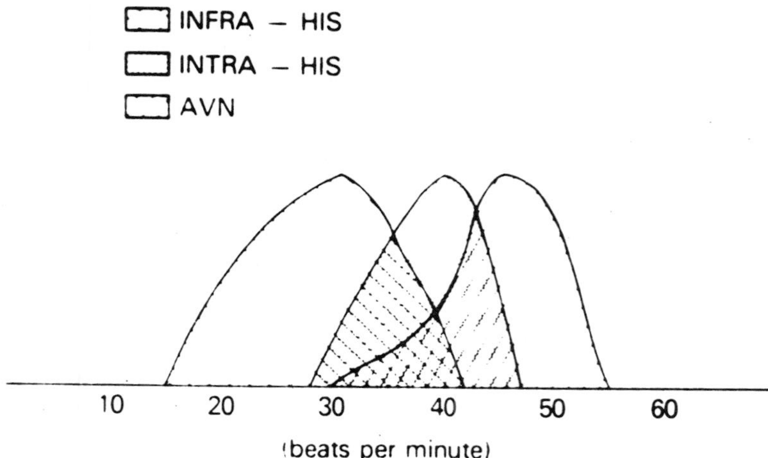

Figure 36–11. "Hierarchy of pacemakers." Depending on the site that fails to generate the cardiac impulse (or the site of block), lower pacemakers are expected to function at characteristic rates. There is considerable overlap between the rates generated by lower pacemakers at various sites. *(Used with permission from Josephson [1993].)*

asymptomatic, and treatment is rarely required. Mobitz II block is characterized by intermittent failure of conduction without preceding prolongation of the PR interval. Mobitz II block (Fig. 36–16) indicates significant His–Purkinje system disease and implies a risk of progression to complete heart block. Other signs of conduction system disease, such as fixed bundle branch block, are typically present.

Third-degree heart block, or complete heart block (CHB), defined as the complete absence of conduction between the atria and ventricles, may be intermittent or persistent (Fig. 36–17). The ventricular rate in complete heart block depends on the level of block and the intrinsic rate of the remaining pacemaker foci (refer to Fig. 36–11). Third-degree heart block usually is a complication of advanced structural heart disease. On the other hand, complete heart block can also be congenital, and several decades may pass before symptoms or incidental detection bring patients to medical attention.

History and Physical Findings

Transient AV block can be asymptomatic, and is typically detected as an incidental finding. High-degree AV block can be episodic, and patients may present with sudden syncope, particularly with exertion. Exercise intolerance is also an occasional complaint, particularly in third-degree AV block. This is due to the fact that the escape rhythm, even if it is sufficient to provide cardiac output during rest, is not responsive to the demands for increased output during exertion. Physical exam may provide diagnostic clues for the etiology of conduction disorders, such as sarcoidosis, Lyme carditis, and/or His–Purkinje damage that accompanies advanced structural heart disease.

Laboratory and Diagnostic Tests

Hyperkalemia can cause high-grade AV block, although typically other signs of hyperkalemia are apparent prior to its development. Digitalis toxicity can also cause AV block, and in elderly or other susceptible patients, even "therapeu-

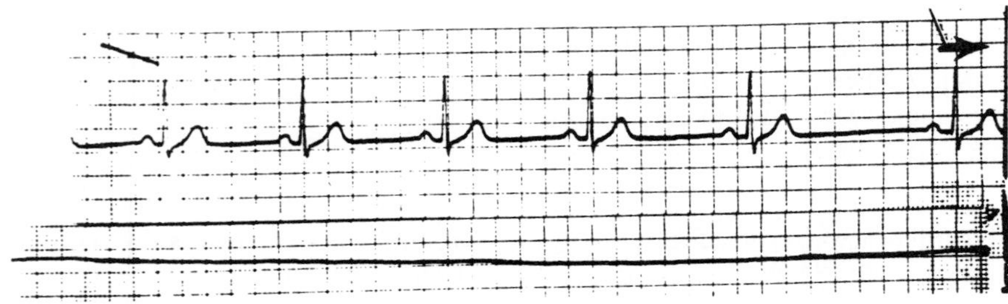

Figure 36–12. Sinus arrest. Continuous rhythm strips are shown. The sequence starts with sinus bradycardia at a rate of 53 bpm. After slight sinus slowing, sinus arrest occurs, resulting in asystole without escape rhythm (*bottom panel*) for 8 seconds. *(Used with permission from Sutton [1995].)*

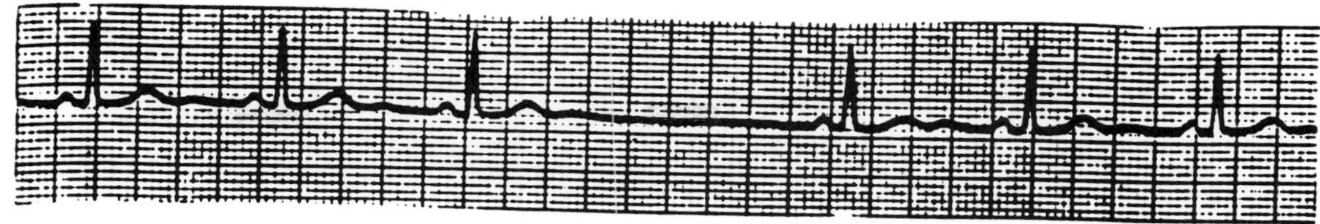

Figure 36–13. Sino-atrial exit block. After three sinus complexes, there is a sudden absence of a P wave, producing a pause. The interval of the pause is exactly twice the baseline sinus interval. This suggests that the sinus node did generate an impulse on time, but the pause was caused by failure of the impulse to conduct to the atrium. The distinction between sinus arrest and sino-atrial exit block is interesting from an electrocardiographic standpoint, but is usually not clinically important. *(Used with permission from Josephson et al. [1987].)*

tic" serum levels of digoxin or other antiarrhythmic agents can exacerbate preexisting conduction system disease. As described earlier for sinus node dysfunction, episodic disorders of AV conduction may not be apparent on a single ECG. Prolonged telemetry monitoring or ambulatory loop recording may be necessary. In patients with a history of syncope and paroxysmal high-degree AV block that is not diagnosed with noninvasive testing, electrophysiologic studies may be helpful.

Management

Atropine (1-3 mg, IV) is helpful in the acute treatment of symptomatic AV block that occurs at the level of the AV node due to excessive vagal tone. In patients with AV block below the level of the AV node, atropine may paradoxically worsen the level of block because of its chronotropic effect on the sinus node (e.g., 2:1 block may become 3:1 or 4:1). Isoproterenol can relieve block at the level of the AV node and can have a mild chronotropic effect on lower escape foci. Typically isoproterenol is not useful for prolonged periods of time, as tachyphylaxis to its effects is common. The transcutaneous pacemaker works by delivering high current through two large surface electrode pads placed on the anterior chest wall and over the right scapula. Long-term use is limited by patient tolerance, often because of capture of the chest wall musculature as well as the heart. Significant bradycardia caused by high-grade AV block that is unresponsive to atropine is usually treated with a transvenous pacing catheter, placed at the right ventricular apex under fluoroscopy or using a balloon flotation mechanism.

Follow-Up

Patients with symptomatic AV block not due to reversible causes are treated with permanent pacing. Although disorders of AV conduction are "cured" with pacing, patients with AV block may have high mortality rates when AV conduction disturbances occur on the basis of accompanying structural heart disease.

Permanent Pacemakers

Indications

As discussed earlier, medical therapies for bradyarrhythmias are extremely limited, and unless medications' negative chronotropic effects can be discontinued, pacemaker implantation represents the sole treatment option for chronic symptomatic bradycardia. Many of the indications for permanent pacing are somewhat controversial, mostly due to the difficulty in providing a secure definition of *symptomatic* bradycardia. Particularly in elderly patients, clinically relevant manifestations of the low cardiac output state may be fairly subtle. Occasionally, mild personality changes or signs of apparent dementia are the only clues of the need for intervention. Often, the benefit can be recognized only retrospectively. One pitfall that is important to avoid is assuming that bradycardia is not hemodynamically significant if the systolic blood pressure is preserved. End-organ perfusion is related more directly to cardiac output, which is the product of stroke volume and heart rate. In addition, many patients with symptomatic bradyarrhythmias are asymptomatic at rest. In these patients, symptoms may occur only with physical exertion that produces the demand

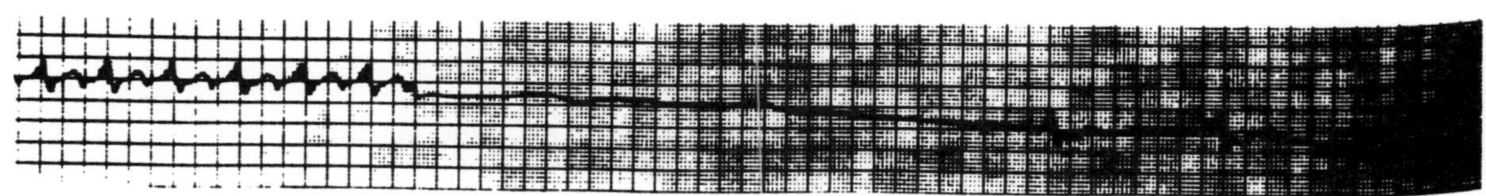

Figure 36–14. Tachycardia-bradycardia syndrome. A lead II rhythm strip is shown. After the spontaneous termination of a regular supraventricular tachycardia (atrial tachycardia with 2-to-1 AV block), a 5.6 second pause occurs before the resumption of sinus activity. *(Used with permission from Josephson et al. [1987].)*

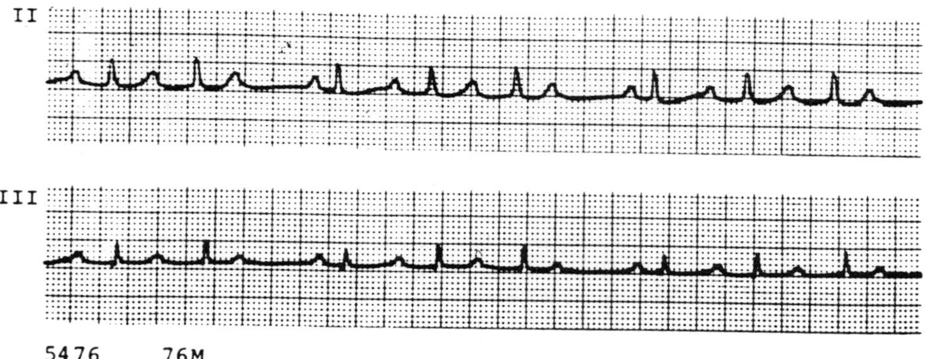

Figure 36–15. Mobitz I second degree AV block. Two simultaneous rhythm strips (leads II and III) are shown. The sinus rate is regular at 110 bpm and every fourth sinus complex is not conducted to the ventricles. There is progressive PR prolongation prior to the development of block. After the dropped beat, the PR shortens once again ("the pause that refreshes," e.g., the PR intervals corresponding to the 3rd and 6th QRS complexes). This physiology is characteristic for block at the level of the AV node. *(Used with permission from Chou [1996].)*

for additional cardiac output, which would be supplied in the normal situation by increases in heart rate.

On the other hand, disorders that are transient in nature, even if they result in symptomatic bradycardia, are not appropriately treated with pacemaker implantation. Examples of these situations are the transient heart block that may occur early after inferior myocardial infarction that is responsive to atropine, heart block complicating Lyme carditis, and bradyarrhythmia caused by side effects of nonessential medications. Pacing is considered for asymptomatic patients at high risk of developing complete heart block (such as patients with bifascicular block complicating acute myocardial infarction) or patients with symptomatic bradycardia caused by medications that are required for treatment of other conditions (e.g., patients with tachy–brady syndrome who require negative chronotropic medications for the treatment of tachycardias). A comprehensive set of guidelines, classified as well accepted (class I), controversial (class II), and unnecessary (class III) indications for permanent pacing was published by an ACC/AHA joint task force (Dreifus, Fisch, Griffin, et al., 1991).

Pacemaker Functionality—ICHD Code

To be useful, pacemakers generally need to function in two ways. First, they must be able to pace (capture) the appropriate chamber. Second, they need to sense intrinsic events in the appropriate chamber to withhold pacing when it is not required. This functionality is expressed in the ICHD code (Table 36–3) which is a 5-position code, although in common parlance, only the first three positions are used. These three positions describe the chamber(s) that are paced, the chamber(s) that are sensed, and how the pacemaker responds to sensed information. Consideration of the most common examples make the code easier to understand. A VOO pacemaker paces the ventricle and does not attempt to sense intrinsic cardiac events. VOO pacing provides ventricular stimulation at a constant rate independent of the spontaneous rhythm. A VVI pacemaker paces the ventricle at a programmed lower rate as well, but because it senses the ventricle (second position in the code), it can inhibit the delivery of pacing stimuli if spontaneous QRS complexes are sensed (third position in the code, Fig. 36–18).

DDD function is more complicated (Fig. 36–19), particularly in the response to sensed information (third position in the code); depending on the type of information sensed, the response is dual—that is, either inhibited or triggered (e.g., a sensed event in the atrium "triggers" the pacemaker to pace in the ventricle if spontaneous conduction does not occur in a predetermined period of time). Put another way, a DDD pacemaker has four modes of function, all aimed at preserving AV synchrony and ensuring that the heart rate is always above a programmed lower rate: (1) atrial sensing, ventricular sensing; (2) atrial pacing, ventricular sensing; (3) atrial sensing, ventricular pacing; and (4)

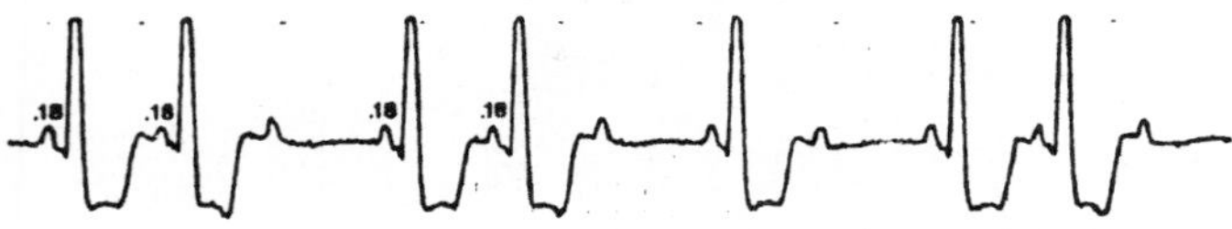

Figure 36–16. Mobitz II second degree AV block. AV block occurs in this instance without a reproducible pattern and without progressive PR prolongation. This type of AV block usually occurs in the setting of other His Purkinje system disease, here manifest by the bundle branch block present on conducted beats. *(Used with permission from Wharton & Ellenbogen [1995].)*

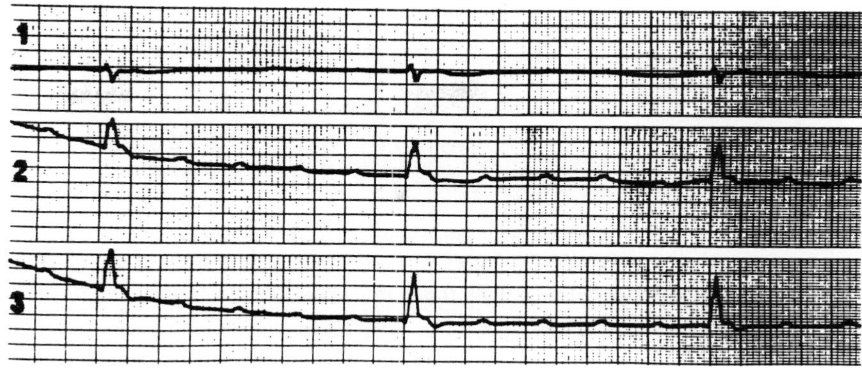

Figure 36–17. Third degree AV block. The sinus rate is 150 bpm, but there is no relationship between the P waves and the QRS complexes. The ventricular rhythm is slow (approximately 30 bpm), regular and wide complex in morphology, most likely signifying an idioventricular escape mechanism. *(Used with permission from Josephson et al. [1987].)*

atrial pacing, ventricular pacing. The typical pacing mode depends on the indication for pacing (sinus node dysfunction versus complete heart block) and whether the condition is episodic or permanent. Because dual chamber pacing more closely duplicates the natural physiology of cardiac conduction, it is preferred in almost all situations, except chronic atrial fibrillation.

Pacemaker Troubleshooting

Modern pacemaker generators are extremely reliable and much of the component failure observed in the early days of pacing, such as sudden failure of output or "run-away pacing" (ultra-rapid delivery of pacing stimuli), was eliminated with advancement in technology. Pacemaker system malfunction, relating to both failure to pace (capture) or failure to sense, does occur, but is usually related to problems in the pacing lead or at the lead–myocardial interface. Causes of transient or sustained pacemaker malfunction include: (1) fracture of the lead conductor or erosion of the insulator (particularly at the area of venous entry, so called "subclavian crush"); (2) lead dislodgment, which is extremely unusual except within the first 4 to 6 weeks post implantation; (3) battery depletion; and (4) inappropriate programming. Pacing dysfunction may be induced in systems with marginal function baseline by the addition of medications, particularly antiarrhythmic drugs, which increase the pacing threshold and decrease the sense amplitude of spontaneous cardiac potentials. Apparent pacing malfunction can often be explained by appropriate programmable behaviors (e.g., hysteresis, safety pacing) that may be different in devices produced by different vendors. Because of the complexity involved, cardiology consultation should be obtained for evaluation of suspected pacemaker malfunction. Part of the complexity is due to the fact that communication with the pacemaker is possible only with the use of manufacturer-specific (and sometimes model-specific) pacemaker analyzer systems.

TABLE 36–3. ICHD Code for Pacemakers

Position	Category	Letters Used
I	chamber(s) paced	V: ventricle, A: atrium, D: dual
II	chamber(s) sensed	V: ventricle, A: atrium, D: dual, O: none
III	response to sensed events	O: none, T: triggered, I: inhibited D: dual (triggered plus inhibited)
IV	programmability	R: rate responsive
V	antitachycardia functions	

One important bedside intervention that can be rapidly employed without the need for a specific analyzer is magnet application. Applying a magnet over the top of the pacemaker generator results in suspension of sensing function resulting in single- or dual-chamber asynchronous pacing (VOO or DOO). This is helpful in situations when the pacing rate is inappropriately slow because of oversensing. Magnet application can also be used to terminate pacemaker mediated tachycardia. This tachycardia is caused when ventricular activation not preceded by atrial activation occurs (such as with a spontaneous PVC) and retrograde conduction to the atrium is present. The pacemaker senses the atrial activity, triggering ventricular pacing, followed by retrograde conduction, and so on. This produces a tachycardia mediated by ventricular pacing near the programmed upper rate limit. Temporary suspension of sensing function with magnet application interrupts the cycle and terminates the arrhythmia.

Pacemaker function can be adversely effected by accidental exposure to high-intensity electromagnetic sources. External cardioversion, surgical electrocautery, and lithotripsy often inhibit or reset the programming of pacemaker generators. MRI scanning can have more profound and unpredictable effects on permanent pacemaker function and is generally considered to be contraindicated.

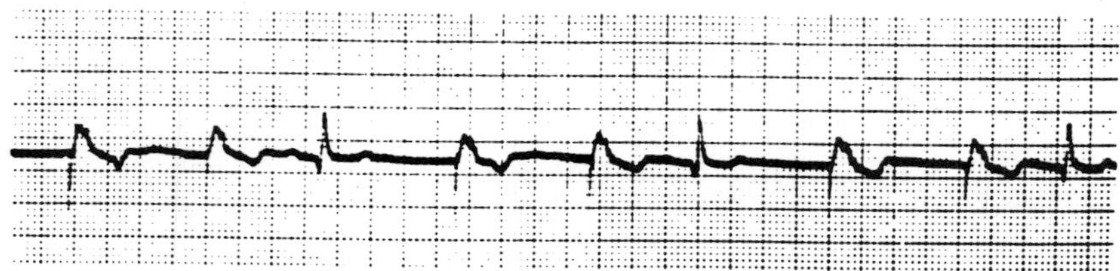

Figure 36–18. VVI pacing function. Stimulation from the pacemaker (note pacemaker spikes) generate the 1st, 2nd, 4th, 5th, 7th and 8th QRS complexes). The pacemaker senses spontaneous QRS complexes (the 3rd, 6th and 9th complexes) and inhibits the delivery of pacing stimuli. The underlying atrial rhythm (sinus bradycardia) is ignored. *(Used with permission from Chou [1996].)*

▶ TACHYARRHYTHMIAS

Atrial Fibrillation and Atrial Flutter

Atrial fibrillation is the most common supraventricular arrhythmia, occurring in 0.4% of all adult patients in the United States and as many as 20% of people over the age of 80 (Kerr & Chung, 1985). Atrial flutter is considerably less common, although actual statistics for its incidence are not available, as atrial fibrillation and atrial flutter are often lumped together as the same arrhythmia. Although atrial fibrillation and flutter share many pathophysiologic features and may even coexist in individual patients, their arrhythmia mechanisms and response to therapy may be quite different.

Atrial fibrillation is recognized by the absence of organized atrial activity on the 12-lead ECG and by its irregular ventricular response (Fig. 36–20). Atrial activation in atrial fibrillation is chaotic and extremely rapid, ranging in frequency from 350 to 600 per minute. Atrial flutter is characterized by an atrial rate of 250 to 350 beats per minute with a "sawtooth" pattern in the inferior leads (Fig. 36–21). The ventricular rate in atrial flutter is usually regular and typically one half the atrial rate. A regular supraventricular tachycardia with a ventricular rate of 150 beats per minute should be considered atrial flutter until proven otherwise.

Pathophysiology. The incidence of atrial fibrillation increases markedly with advancing age. This characteristic seems to be the only unifying theme in the variety of underlying conditions that can lead to atrial fibrillation, including hypertensive heart disease, chronic coronary artery disease, valvular heart disease (particularly rheumatic mitral stenosis), atrial septal defect, and chronic lung disease. Atrial fibrillation is observed in approximately 40% of patients following cardiac surgical procedures, presumably caused by inflammation of the atrial and overlying pericardial tissues. Lone atrial fibrillation, which occurs in young patients without identifiable structural heart disease, accounts for approximately 2.7% of patients with atrial fibrillation (Kopecky, Gersh, McGoon, et al., 1987). Other conditions, such as thyrotoxicosis, acute alcohol intoxication, emotional stress or lack of sleep, can also contribute.

Although the "causes" of atrial fibrillation seem disparate at first glance, they all represent conditions that either increase atrial dimensions or slow conduction in the atrium. Both effects are important in accommodating the mutual existence of multiple reentrant wavelets that are thought to be the root cause of atrial fibrillation. The "size" of these wavelets are determined by conduction velocity and properties of refractoriness in the atrium (to prevent the wavelet "head" from encroaching upon its "tail," resulting is extinction). According to this multiple wavelet hypothesis (Moe, 1962), "true" atrial fibrillation is maintained by the presence of several independent wavelets that wander randomly though around islets of tissue made refractory in the wake of previous wavelets. These wavelets can extinguish, divide, or combine with neighboring wavelets, such that they constantly change direction and size. In this sense,

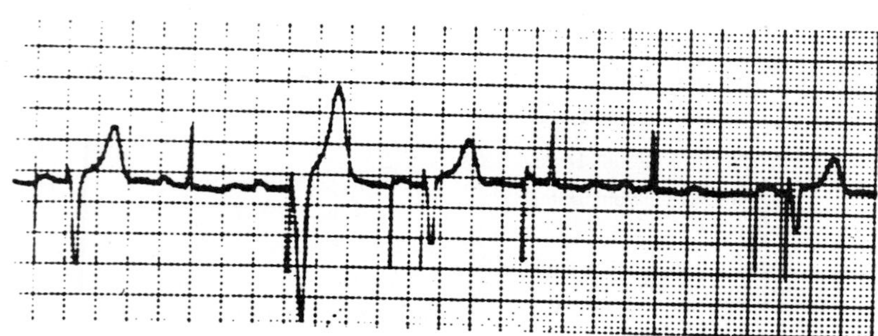

Figure 36–19. DDD pacing function. The underlying rhythm is sinus at 100 bpm. Each of the four modes of DDD function is demonstrated in this panel. See text for discussion. *(Used with permission from Harthorne et al. [1989].)*

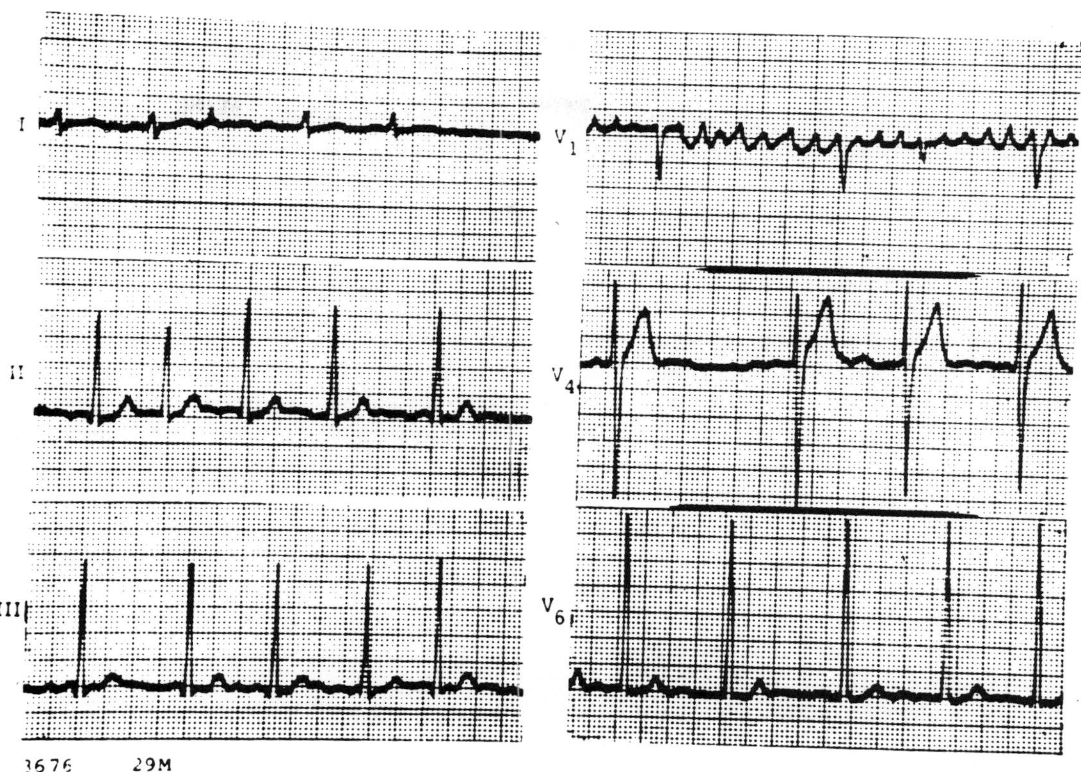

Figure 36–20. Atrial fibrillation. Salient features include the irregular ventricular response and the undulating baseline without evidence of organized atrial activation. Note the coarse "fibrillatory waves" in V1. These should be distinguised from the atrial activity seen in atrial flutter by the following characteristics: (1) they are typically present only in lead V1, (2) the atrial rate is > 300 bpm, and (3) the atrial rate is irregular and the morphology of fibrillatory waves is constantly changing. *(Used with permission from Chou [1996].)*

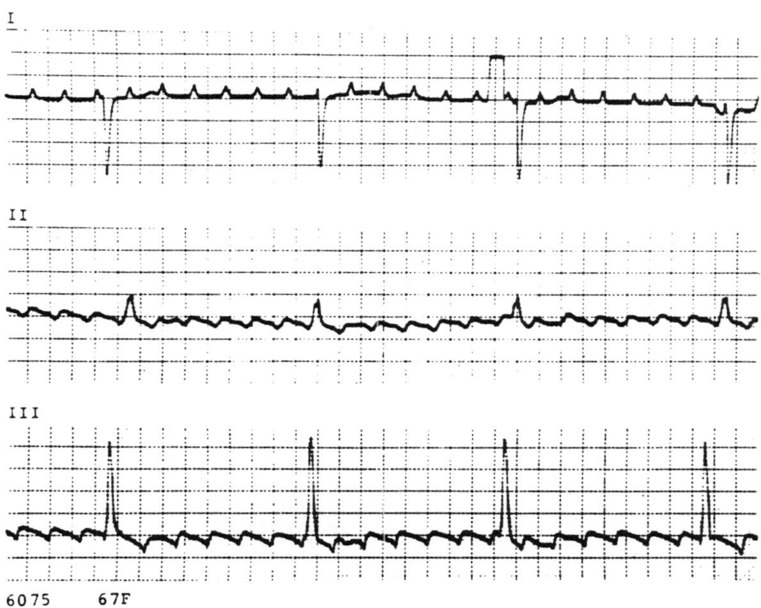

Figure 36–21. Atrial flutter. Note the characteristic "saw tooth" pattern of atrial activation at a rate of 214 bpm. Although the ventricular rate is usually an even fraction of the atrial rate (i.e., 2:1, 4:1, etc.), in this circumstance complete heart block with an idioventricular escape is present. *(Used with permission from Chou [1996].)*

atrial fibrillation is not a focal arrhythmia, but arises from the entire mass of atrial tissue.

Atrial flutter is caused by macroreentry within the right atrium (Fig. 36–22). Similar pathophysiologic conditions appear to contribute to atrial flutter; again, presumably because this single reentrant wave must be facilitated by conduction slowing in the atrium or right atrial dilatation until it can "fit" within the confines of its predetermined anatomic circuit. Until recently, atrial flutter was generally considered an "unstable" rhythm, lasting only briefly before termination to sinus rhythm or degeneration to atrial fibrillation. These observations were based on the behavior of atrial flutter in the postoperative period following cardiac surgery. In other situations atrial flutter can be paroxysmal or persistent and can last several weeks to months (or even longer) if efforts are not made to restore sinus rhythm.

The symptoms caused by atrial fibrillation are related to the following pathophysiologic mechanisms. First, patients with atrial fibrillation usually have a rapid ventricular rate at rest and an exaggerated increase in ventricular rate in response to physiologic stress. This results in symptoms of palpitations, exercise intolerance, fatigue and angina and heart failure in susceptible individuals. Patients with severe conduction system disease may have an inappropriately slow ventricular response to atrial fibrillation, with exercise intolerance or syncope on this account. The rapid ventricular rate is also the key determinant of symptoms in atrial flutter, although the ventricular response is regular and usually does not increase with exertion.

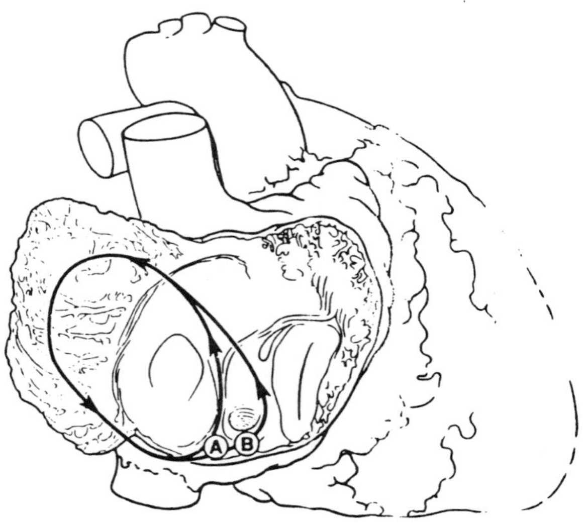

Figure 36–22. Schematic cut-away view of the right atrium from a right anterior oblique projection. The typical direction of activation during atrial flutter is noted (→). The usual locations where radiofrequency ablation terminated atrial flutter are indicated by the open circles posterior (A) or inferior (B) to the ostium of the coronary sinus. Ablation at site (A) was successful in seven patients and at site (B) in three patients. *(Used with permission from Feld et al. [1992].)*

Rarely, sympathetic stimulation (or antiarrhythmic drugs that slow the atrial cycle length) converts 2:1 AV block to 1:1 conduction during atrial flutter; this produces ventricular rates that approach 300 beats per minute and usually causes hemodynamic collapse. Second, the loss of effective atrial contraction during atrial fibrillation can result in a considerable decrease in cardiac output in patients with diastolic dysfunction (hypertensive heart disease, coronary artery disease, mitral stenosis, hypertrophic cardiomyopathy). The resultant pooling of blood in the atrium and particularly the left atrial appendage also contributes to thrombus formation, which can result in systemic embolism. Patients with atrial fibrillation have a five fold increase in risk of embolic stroke compared with age-matched controls (Wolf, Abbott, & Kannel, 1987). The major portion of this increased risk is abolished with long-term anticoagulant therapy (Stroke Prevention in Atrial Fibrillation Investigators, 1991). Until recently, the risk of thromboembolic complications of atrial flutter was not appreciated. Although the risk is not so great, patients with atrial flutter are also at increased risk of stroke, particularly surrounding spontaneous or therapeutic cardioversion to sinus rhythm (Lanzarotti & Olshansky, 1997). Finally, as discussed earlier, atrial fibrillation can cause symptoms related to the "offset pause" in patients with the tachy–brady syndrome (refer to Fig. 36–14).

History and Physical Findings. The history in patients with atrial fibrillation and flutter should focus on establishing the presence and severity of the symptoms and the underlying conditions (acute or chronic) that precipitated the episode. The duration of the arrhythmia should also be estimated, as this has important implications for management of cardioversion and anticoagulation. Symptoms related to manifest or silent systemic emboli should be elicited. Acute myocardial infarction is commonly "ruled out" in patients presenting with their first episode of atrial fibrillation. Although atrial fibrillation can accompany acute MI, it occurs for the first time only in patients with extensive infarction.

The physical exam in atrial fibrillation is most notable for rapid heart rate and the irregularly, irregular (that is irregular in both timing and amplitude) nature of the peripheral pulses. The *a* wave of the jugular venous pulse is absent, and the intensity of the first heart sound is variable. A fourth heart sound (S4), which corresponds ventricular filling during atrial contraction, cannot be present during atrial fibrillation.

Laboratory and Diagnostic Tests. Electrolyte abnormalities do not contribute to atrial fibrillation and flutter, but should be corrected particularly in patients with structural heart disease. Hyperthyroidism should be excluded, particularly because untreated hyperthyroidism can thwart all attempts at treatment of atrial fibrillation. Careful study of the ECG is sometimes necessary to distinguish atrial flutter from "coarse" atrial fibrillation, especially when catheter ablation therapy is being considered (refer to Fig. 36–20). Telemetry monitoring is used in all patients with atrial arrhythmias, to assess the effects of antiarrhythmic therapy (rate control and restoration of sinus rhythm) and to investigate the potential for associated bradyarrhythmias. Evaluation for the presence of coexisting structural heart disease is typically performed in patients with atrial fibrillation, particularly when chronic antiarrhythmic drug therapy is planned. Measurement of left ventricular function (echo, MUGA) is indicated, and exercise testing to diagnose incipient coronary artery disease may be useful in selected patients.

Management. The acute treatment of persistent episodes of atrial fibrillation and atrial flutter focuses on the following considerations: (1) control of the ventricular rate; (2) assessment of the risk of thromboembolic complications and establishment of anticoagulant therapy; and (3) cardioversion to sinus rhythm.

Control of Ventricular Rate. Since the majority of the symptoms arise directly from the inappropriately rapid ventricular rate during atrial fibrillation and flutter, the first step in treatment is usually aimed at controlling the rate. Immediate synchronous cardioversion is used in patients with poorly tolerated atrial fibrillation or flutter and loss of consciousness or hemodynamic embarrassment. Poorly tolerated atrial fibrillation can occur in patients with severe structural heart disease, other serious illnesses (particularly chronic obstructive lung disease), or in those with Wolff–Parkinson–White syndrome. Digoxin is often used in this setting, although, in general, this strategy has little to recommend it. Digoxin, even if given intravenously, has slow onset of action (> 30 minutes). More important, digitalis at doses that produce "therapeutic" serum levels works primarily due to vagomimetic effects; these effects are quickly overwhelmed by any sympathetic stimulation. Even when effective at controlling the ventricular response at rest, digoxin has been demonstrated to be no more effective than placebo at rate control during normal physical exertion (Sarter & Marchlinski, 1992). More potent agents to slow conduction in the AV node, such as beta blockers or calcium antagonists, are much more effective. For patients in whom hypotension is a concern, intravenous diltiazem—which has a short half life and can be discontinued abruptly—can be very useful.

Atrial flutter is almost invariably conducted to the ventricles with an even integral proportion to the atrial rate (i.e., 2:1, 4:1 6:1 AV block), depending on the status of the AV conduction system. It is often difficult to change the ventricular rate during atrial flutter, and ventricular rates may remain 150/min even after maximum tolerated doses of AV nodal blockers are administered.

Anticoagulant Therapy. As discussed earlier, atrial fibrillation and flutter increase the risk of thromboembolic complications, including embolic stroke. Cardioversion, independent of mechanism (spontaneous, chemical, electrical), increases the short-term risk of stroke; again the majority of this risk is mitigated by anticoagulation therapy. Formal recommendations by the American College of Chest Physicians recommend elective cardioversion only after at least 4 weeks of therapeutic anticoagulation in all patients with atrial fibrillation > 48 hours in duration (Laupacis, Albers, Dalen, et al., 1995). Although the situation is in evolution, recommendations for cardioversion of atrial flutter are presently similar. If the duration of atrial fibrillation or flutter is not clear, as in patients without symptoms of palpitations who have these arrhythmias detected incidentally, a duration of > 48 hours should be assumed. Recent observational data and a single, small randomized trial suggests the safety of an alternative approach using transesophageal echocardiography to document the absence of intracardiac thrombus before pursuing early cardioversion (Manning, Silverman, Keighley, et al., 1995). With either approach, long-term anticoagulation with warfarin is used in all patients who can take it safely. One exception to this general rule is in patients with lone atrial fibrillation, defined by the absence of structural heart disease, hypertension, and diabetes who are less than 65 years of age. The event rate in this group of people is sufficiently low that the risk/benefit ratio for anticoagulation may no longer be favorable (Laupacis, et al., 1995).

Restoration of Sinus Rhythm. Many episodes of atrial fibrillation terminate spontaneously, particularly in the early stages of the disease. As atrial fibrillation progresses, the episodes become more frequent and of longer duration, requiring cardioversion for termination. Later still in the process, atrial fibrillation may become permanent (i.e., resistant to cardioversion). Most experts believe that prompt termination of atrial fibrillation early in the disease process may prevent the gradual evolution to permanent atrial fibrillation, although no real data is available to address this question directly.

Sinus rhythm can be restored pharmacologically or electrically. In previous years, type IA agents (particularly quinidine or intravenous procainamide) were given for a "trial" with electrical cardioversion if these agents were not effective. Because these agents were more likely to maintain sinus rhythm once restored but had rather low cardioversion rates, this practice is not so frequent presently. New agents, particularly the class III drug ibutilide (1 mg, IV over 10 minutes; a second 1-mg dose may be given if the first does not result in termination) may revive the practice of pharmacologic cardioversion. Ibutilide restores sinus rhythm within 90 minutes in approximately 40 to 60% of cases (and an even higher proportion of atrial flutter), depending on the duration of the arrhythmia. The most important side effect of ibutilide is QT prolongation, which can result in torsades de pointes, even hours after administration. Obviously, telemetry monitoring is required for its use. Electrical cardioversion is highly effective in terminating atrial fibrillation and flutter. Usually 200 joules of energy delivered in the synchronous mode promptly restores sinus rhythm. Because atrial flutter is more organized, it may be terminated with even smaller amounts of energy (10-50 joules).

For atrial flutter, but not atrial fibrillation, overdrive pacing is also effective in restoring sinus rhythm. Burst pacing at 115 to 130% of the atrial flutter rate typically restores sinus rhythm, but may also change the rhythm disturbance to atrial fibrillation. This method is particularly useful following cardiac surgery (when epicardial pacing wires are present) or in patients with permanent pacemakers that offer rapid pacing functions.

Follow-Up. After termination of the acute episode of atrial fibrillation, consideration should be given to the strategy for preventing recurrence (Prystowsky, Benson, & Fuster, 1996). The overwhelming majority of patients with an episode of atrial fibrillation have recurrent episodes, particularly if they are older or have coexisting structural heart disease. Exceptions to this rule include "situational" atrial fibrillation (precipitated by lack of sleep, caffeine, or alcohol) or atrial fibrillation due to thyrotoxicosis. With the possible exception of amiodarone, all antiarrhythmic agents appear to have similar effects in preventing atrial fibrillation. Approximately 50% of patients are free from any recurrent episodes at 12 months, compared with 25% of untreated patients. Viewed in this way, antiarrhythmic therapy is not very appealing; however, chronic antiarrhythmic drug therapy seems to confer the following benefits. First, even in the event of recurrence, in all studies of antiarrhythmic therapy the frequency of episodes decreases in treated patients. Second, the 50% total freedom from atrial fibrillation refers to single agents. Often "step therapy" with a substitution of agents after drug failure identifies a regimen that provides long-term control. Finally, total freedom from recurrence is not absolutely necessary for successful treatment. Infrequent recurrences can be managed with outpatient cardioversion.

The possibility of drug failure raises two other important implications for therapy. First, anticoagulants and agents for ventricular rate control (unless this effect is "built into" the antiarrhythmic drug, such as in propafenone, sotalol, and amiodarone) are started and continued indefinitely. Second, and even more important, antiarrhythmic regimens are chosen with convenience, safety, and avoidance of side effects first in mind. In patients without structural heart disease, class IC agents are often better tolerated than the traditional class IA agents quinidine and procainamide. Sotalol is also well tolerated, although monitoring is required during initiation of therapy to prevent drug-induced torsades de pointes. Amiodarone is useful in patients with structural heart disease because the incidence of proarrhythmia is very low, even in the sickest subjects.

Surprisingly, data about the success of antiarrhythmic drug therapy is essentially unavailable for atrial flutter. Many authorities feel that recurrent atrial flutter is unlikely to respond to pharmacologic therapy, and curative treatment with catheter ablation is increasingly becoming first-line therapy.

In patients with permanent atrial fibrillation, or in those who cannot tolerate chronic antiarrhythmic drug therapy, an alternative strategy is to provide adequate rate control and anticoagulation without concern over continued atrial fibrillation. The relative benefits of maintaining sinus rhythm and providing rate control only are being investigated in the NIH-sponsored AFFIRM trial, which is still enrolling patients at time of writing. Some patients, particularly those with LV dysfunction, cannot tolerate sufficient doses of AV nodal blocking agents to provide adequate rate control. In these patients, intentional ablation of the AV conduction system, with implantation of a permanent pacemaker, can be effective.

Paroxysmal Supraventricular Tachycardias

Supraventricular tachycardia (SVT) refers to any tachyarrhythmia that originates above the ventricles and includes sinus tachycardia, atrioventricular nodal reentry, bypass tract-mediated reentry, atrial tachycardia, atrial fibrillation, and atrial flutter. Atrial fibrillation and atrial flutter are considered separately; the remaining tachycardias are considered together because, for the most part, all occur in similar types of patients. They can all be recognized on the ECG as *regular* narrow QRS complex tachycardias, usually with 1 to 1 A:V relationships. At sufficiently fast rates, SVT with superimposed left or right bundle branch block causes a regular wide complex tachycardia that can be confused with ventricular tachycardia. Careful analysis of the 12-lead ECG can usually distinguish SVT and VT (Kindwall, Brown, & Josephson, 1988; Wellens, Bar, & Lie, 1978), although occasionally electrophysiologic testing with intracardiac recordings is required to provide a definitive diagnosis. The presence of these SVTs does not necessarily imply coexisting heart disease, and in fact most often occur as isolated electrical abnormalities in an otherwise normal heart. On the other hand, SVT is often tolerated very poorly in patients with structural heart disease, particularly in diseases such as chronic hypertension with diastolic dysfunction in which ventricular filling is compromised by the short diastolic interval during tachycardia. A wide range of symptoms may be encountered in patients with SVT—from incidental detection to syncope. Catheter ablation is the treatment of choice in many patients with paroxysmal SVTs. This therapy has been used with good success rates and allows for the avoidance of the side effects of long-term antiarrhythmic drug therapy, particularly important in otherwise healthy young patients.

Pathophysiology. As briefly considered earlier, structural heart disease is not required for the creation and maintenance of SVT. Instead, electrophysiologic abnormalities, functioning independently of structural heart disease, are the primary cause of most SVTs. One exception to this generality is reentrant atrial tachycardia, which often depends on the presence of abnormally slow conduction in the atrium produced by fibrotic replacement that accompanies exposure to high atrial pressures (as in chronic hypertension and valvular heart diseases). These electrophysiologic abnormalities responsible for SVTs can take various forms. Abnormalities in impulse formation (normal or abnormal automaticity) are responsible for sinus tachycardia and automatic forms of atrial tachycardias. Reentry, caused directly by the presence of extra conduction pathways is responsible for the genesis of AV nodal reentry and bypass tract-mediated reentry.

SVTs are responsible for some interesting secondary pathophysiologic phenomena. Some patients have severe chest pain syndromes, present only during SVT, which occurs in the absence of myocardial ischemia. It is often difficult to distinguish this syndrome from angina, particularly because most such patients focus on their chest pain and ignore the presence of lightheadedness and palpitations. SVTs that occur very frequently (typically automatic atrial tachycardias and some bypass tract mediated SVTs) can cause cardiomyopathy simply on the basis of chronic heart rate elevations. Patients with this tachycardia-related myopathy are very important to identify, as control of the SVT syndrome leads to eventual recovery of normal LV systolic function (Case, Gillette, Oslizlok, et al., 1992).

History and Physical Findings. Patients interviewed during episodes of SVT may complain of a wide spectrum of symptoms, depending primarily on the rate of the tachycardia, the relative A/V interval timing, and the presence or absence of structural heart disease. Some patients are not aware of tachycardia; in others, symptoms range from palpitations, lightheadedness, chest pain (either due to angina or the syndrome described earlier), or syncope. Syncope due to SVT is rather unusual, but has two possible etiologies. First, at the onset of paroxysmal SVTs, there is a sudden, abrupt drop in systolic pressure, caused by a paradoxical response of the autonomic nervous system, which resolves within minutes. Second, patients with diastolic dysfunction (e.g., healed myocardial infarction, chronic hypertension, valvular heart disease) require relatively long diastolic times (low heart rates) to facilitate LV filling. The abrupt shortening of diastolic interval with the onset of SVT can lead to syncope on the basis of low cardiac output based on this mechanism.

Depending on the arrhythmia mechanism, individual SVT episodes are often provoked by exercise or emotional upset. In some patients, caffeine or nicotine exposure can prompt episodes. Many patients complain of similar symptoms, sometimes of shorter duration, occurring frequently over the course of many years. All too often, particularly in women with SVT, symptoms due to arrhythmias are attributed to anxiety for many years in lieu of appropriate evaluation.

The physical examination during SVT may be unrevealing, except of course for the rapid heart rate. In AV nodal reentry, cannon A waves are frequently observed; unlike during VT, where they are seen intermittently, cannon waves occur on every beat in AV nodal reentry. This is because the atrium and ventricles are activated essentially simultaneously in this arrhythmia, so that atrial systole consistently occurs when the AV valves are closed.

Laboratory and Diagnostic Tests. Electrolyte abnormalities usually do not contribute to the pathophysiology of SVT. One minor exception is that hypokalemia may predispose patients to the tachycardias that can be produced with digitalis intoxication (most notably atrial tachycardia with AV block). Serum levels of digitalis should be assessed in patients receiving this agent. The most important part of the evaluation of a patient in SVT is recording the 12-lead electrocardiogram. This is far superior to single monitor leads because the presence of multiple leads often allows the detection of *p* waves that might not be observed in a random lead. As is discussed under the specific types of SVT, determination of the relationship between the *p* waves and the QRS complexes, as well as the morphology of the *p* wave, is the basis for differential diagnosis of SVT. In patients with temporary epicardial atrial leads (or in patients with permanent pacemakers that allow for telemetry from the sensing lead system), direct atrial recordings can be performed and often complement surface ECG tracings. Monitor recordings that demonstrate SVT initiation or termination should be studied, as these events also provide clues to the diagnosis. The laboratory evaluation is otherwise noncontributory.

Bedside techniques may be applied to "interact" with the tachycardia; these may have additional diagnostic or even therapeutic effects. Vagal maneuvers, such as instructing the patient to perform Valsalva maneuver or carotid sinus massage, may produce transient AV block, allowing for either better elucidation of the *p* wave morphology and relationships or termination of the SVT if the AV node is an integral part of the arrhythmia circuit.

Management. All attempts at therapy for SVT should be performed in a monitored setting, with ready access to resuscitative drugs (atropine, pressor agents) and external defibrillation. Reliable intravenous access should be secured. The majority of patients with SVT are hemodynamically stable during tachycardia episodes. In the event that SVT causes unconsciousness or severe hypotension, immediate synchronous cardioversion should be performed. For stable SVTs, after obtaining the 12-lead electrocardiogram, vagal maneuvers during continuous monitoring can be a useful first step, as described earlier.

Adenosine (6-18 mg IV bolus) is also very useful in termination of acute SVTs that require the AV node as part of the arrhythmia circuit (AV nodal reentry and AV reentry). Adenosine has a rather specific effect in slowing conduction in the AV node and causes transient AV block leading to SVT termination. When adenosine is delivered during atrial tachycardia, the expected response is transient AV block with continuation of the tachycardia in the atrium. This response, which demonstrates that the tachycardia circuit is confined to the atrium, is diagnostic of atrial tachycardia. In many cases, however, adenosine terminates atrial tachycardia as well, due to specific effects on atrial cellular electrophysiology. Although this is a limitation in the use of adenosine as a diagnostic probe, it adds to its usefulness in terminating SVT. The side effects of adenosine are limited, mostly due to the extremely short half life of the agent. Transient AV block and precipitation of atrial fibrillation (which is short lived and terminates spontaneously) are seen frequently, but rarely are clinically important.

Other agents that effect conduction in the AV node, such as beta blockers and calcium antagonists, produce similar results. These agents have both the advantage and disadvantage of longer duration of action. This is advantageous in that recurrent episodes may be prevented, but may be a limitation because of the potential for longer duration of drug-related side effects, particularly hypotension. If SVT persists despite the administration of adequate amounts of AV nodal blocking drugs, or if a diagnosis of atrial tachycardia is made with certainty, intravenous procainamide (15 mg/kg IV, given at 25 mg/min) may terminate the arrhythmia. Procainamide is also useful in the treatment of AV reentry as it slows conduction over the bypass tract, although AV nodal conduction is not directly effected. Incidentally, procainamide can also be useful in the event of tolerated wide complex tachycardias when the diagnosis (i.e., SVT with aberrancy versus VT) is not established. The most important side effect of intravenous procainamide is hypotension, which can be ameliorated with a slower rate of administration.

Follow-Up. After termination of the acute episode, management of patients with SVTs focuses on the prevention of recurrent episodes. Most patients with an episode of SVT eventually have recurrent SVT, although some estimation of the frequency of recurrence can be determined by the likelihood of reproducing the events that appeared to trigger the index episode. Prevention of recurrent episodes is best approached if the specific tachycardia mechanism is known. The management of individual SVT syndromes is considered later. In general, particularly in younger patients, catheter ablation therapy is increasingly becoming the first line of therapy for many SVT syndromes; this choice avoids the side effects and the often incomplete efficacy of chronic antiarrhythmic drug therapy (Callans, Schwartzman, Gottlieb & Marchlinski, 1995, 1996; Kay, Epstein, Dailey, et al., 1993).

Although the pathophysiology of most SVTs does not depend on the presence of structural heart disease, patients with SVT are evaluated with echocardiography at some point. This is particularly true in patients with syncope or presyncope during SVT episodes. Evaluation for coronary artery disease is not necessary in general, but is difficult to avoid in patients with chest pain syndromes during SVT.

AV Nodal Reentrant Tachycardia

AV nodal reentrant tachycardia (AVNRT) is the most common paroxysmal SVT. It typically presents as a narrow complex regular tachycardia with rates ranging from 120 to 250 beats per minute. AVNRT can occur in patients of either sex at any age, and episodes are commonly precipitated by exertion or emotional stress. Nearly simultaneous activation of the atrium and ventricles occurs in AVNRT because the circuit acts as a "rotor" within the AV node, spinning off impulses in both directions. Because of this, *p* waves can be difficult to discern on the surface ECG, which in itself is a clue to its diagnosis. Retrograde *p* waves can be recognized in some cases as late negative deflections in the inferior leads, or positive deflections in V1 that can mimic incomplete right bundle branch block (Fig. 36–23).

The mechanism of AVNRT, as for all forms of reentry, depends on the following features: (1) the presence of more than one physical route for conduction (dual AV node pathways); (2) a difference in the refractory properties of the two pathways; and (3) the presence of slow conduction. These features are diagrammed schematically in Figure 36–24. Most atrial impulses are conducted in the AV node through the fast pathway. Since the fast pathway has a relatively long refractory period, early atrial premature beats block in the fast pathway and conduct through the AVN using the slow pathway. This event is implied on the surface ECG by a large increment in the PR interval. If conduction in the antegrade direction is sufficiently slow, the fast pathway may recover to conduct in a retrograde direction, which produces an atrial echo. If additional conduction slowing is introduced in the circuit (such as provided by an earlier atrial premature beat, which produces greater prolongation in the PR interval), the slow pathway can recover sufficiently to maintain sustained reentry.

Many patients with infrequent, mild episodes of AVNRT can be managed by learning Valsalva maneuvers to terminated episodes. Patients with frequent episodes or more substantial symptoms usually require some form of preventative therapy. Pharmacologic therapy is aimed at slowing conduction within the AV node and agents such as beta blockers

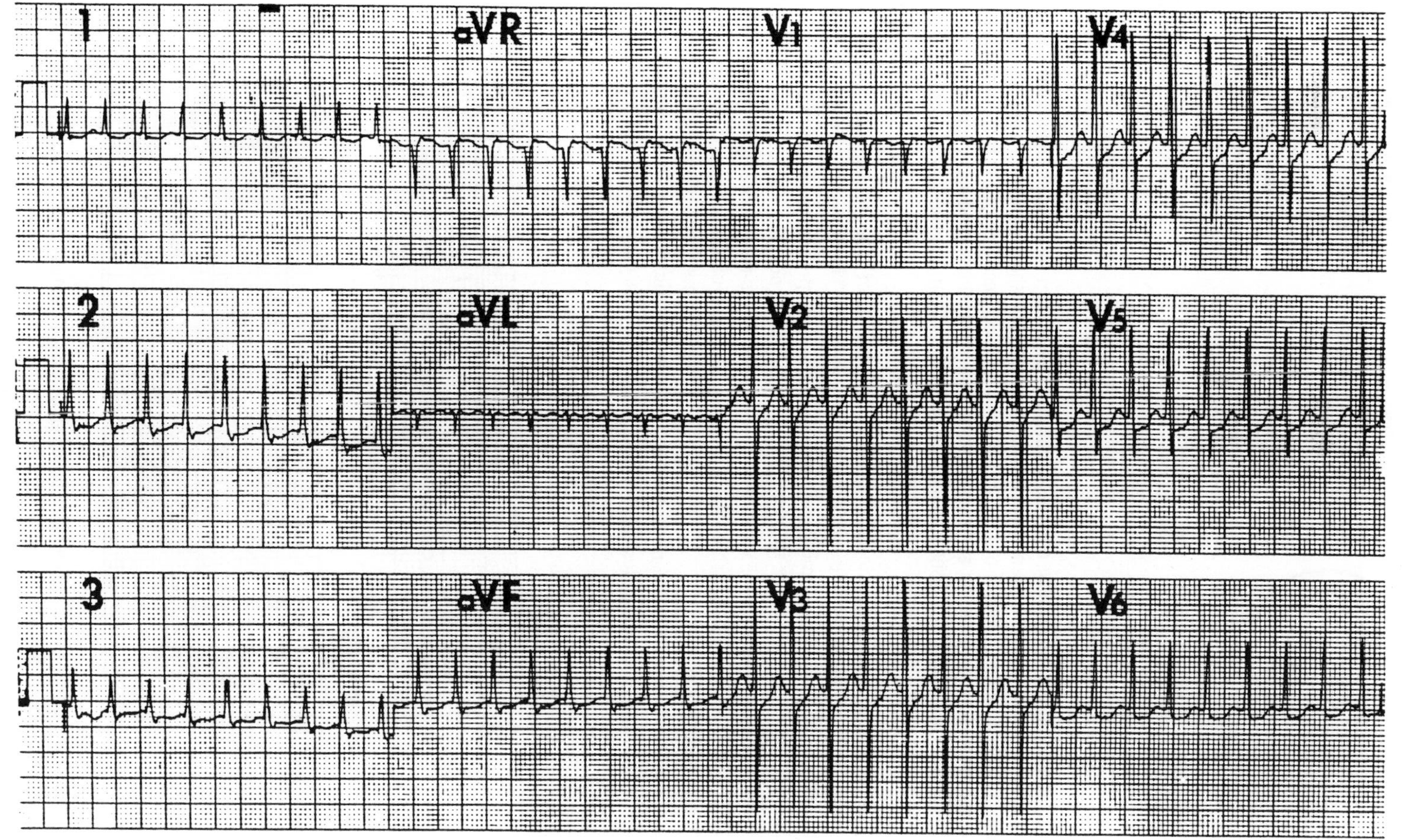

Figure 36–23. Typical AV nodal reentry. The 12-lead electrocardiogram shows a regular, narrow complex tachycardia at a rate of 188 bpm. At first glance, *p* waves cannot be discerned. On closer examination, retrograde *p* waves produce characteristic "pseudo S waves" in the inferior leads, and "pseudo r prime" complexes, mimicking incomplete right bundle branch block, in lead V1. *(Reproduced with permission from Josephson & Wellens. [1990].)*

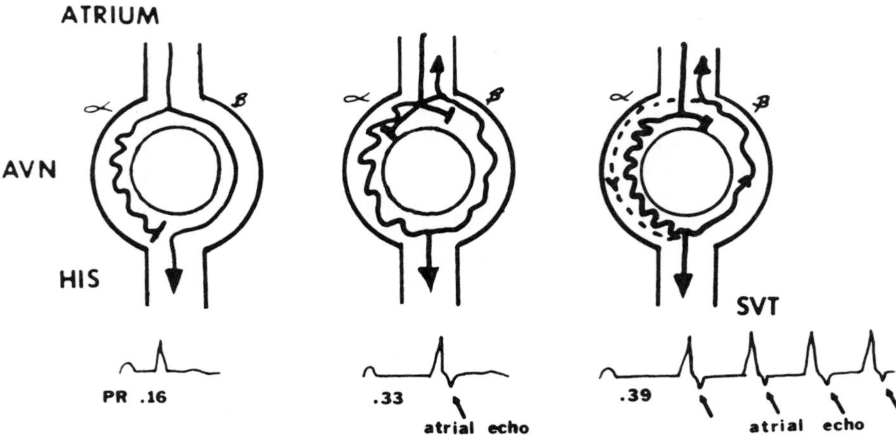

Figure 36–24. A schematic view of the mechanism of AVNRT. During sinus rhythm (*left panel*), the impulse conducts using the fast (beta) pathway, producing a short PR interval. An atrial premature beat produces block in the fast pathway (*middle panel*), conducting to the ventricle using the slow pathway. If a sufficient amount of time has elasped to allow recovery of the fast pathway, retrograde activation of the atrium, producing an atrial echo beat can result. An earlier premature beat (*right panel*), produces more conduction slowing and allows sustained reentry within the AV node to become established. *(Used with permission from Josephson et al. [1987].)*

and calcium antagonists are useful. In some patients, digitalis is sufficient to control recurrence, although the weak vagomimetic effects of this agent are easily overcome by sympathetic stimulation. Catheter ablation is effective in over 95% of patients with AVNRT and is first-line therapy in patients with significant symptoms (Kay et al., 1993).

AV Reentrant Tachycardia

AV reentrant tachycardia (AVRT) uses the AV node for antegrade conduction (i.e., atrium to the ventricles) and a bypass tract for retrograde conduction (ventricles to the atrium). The bypass tract can be manifest in sinus rhythm, causing preexcitation of the ventricles (Wolff–Parkinson–White syndrome), or concealed, in which bypass tract conduction is only possible in the retrograde direction. Because the tachycardia circuit is larger than that of AVNRT, the *p* wave is inscribed after the QRS (Fig. 36–25). As atrium and the ventricles are part of the tachycardia circuit, both PACs and PVCs can initiate and terminate SVT episodes.

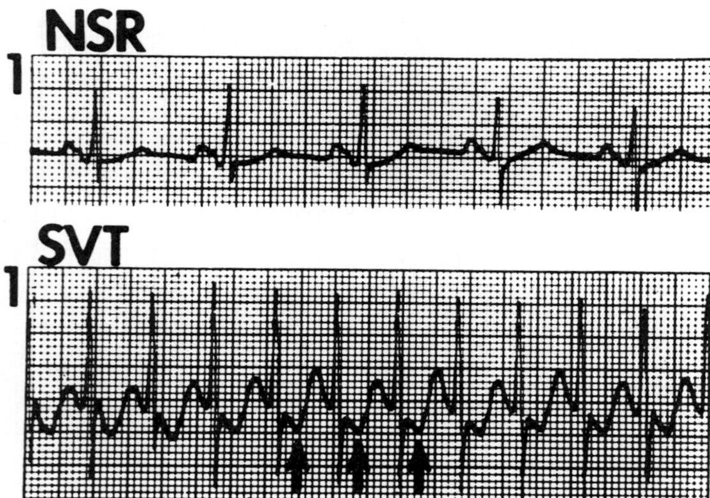

Figure 36–25. AV reentrant tachycardia using a left lateral bypass tract. Lead I is shown both in normal sinus rhythm (*top*) and SVT (*bottom panel*). Note that there is no indication of antegrade bypass tract conduction in sinus rhythm (normal conduction to the ventricles without the presence of a delta wave). This indicates the presence of a “concealed” accessory pathway. During SVT, the *p* wave occurs farther away from the preceding QRS than is the case with AVNRT. This is due to the fact that the impulse has to travel for a longer distance (His–Purkinje system and ventricular myocardium) before engaging the bypass tract, which is responsible for retrograde activation of the atria. *(Reproduced with permission from Josephson & Wellens. [1990].)*

The larger circuit in AVRT offers two strategies for pharmacologic management. Therapy may be targeted at slowing conduction in the AV node (digoxin, beta blockers, calcium antagonists) or in the bypass tract (antiarrhythmic agents, particularly flecainide). Catheter ablation of the bypass tract is effective in management of AVRT, and success rates of > 95% are observed (Callans et al., 1996; Kay et al., 1993).

Wolff–Parkinson–White Syndrome

When a bypass tract capable of antegrade conduction is present, ventricular preexcitation occurs in sinus rhythm (Fig. 36–26). Wolff–Parkinson–White (WPW) syndrome is defined by the presence of ventricular preexcitation and recurrent SVTs, typically AV reentry. Patients with WPW are prone to more severe and even life-threatening arrhythmias, however. Atrial fibrillation and flutter conducted to the ventricles over the bypass tract without the decremental conduction characteristic of the AV node can produce extremely rapid ventricular rates and even precipitate ventricular fibrillation.

AV reentry in patients with manifest preexcitation during sinus rhythm is managed both acutely and chronically in the same way as for patients with concealed bypass tracts. One caveat regards the use of adenosine for termination of acute episodes, as this agent may precipitate atrial fibrillation which could potentially lead to disastrous consequences. Management of patients with preexcited atrial fibrillation and a rapid ventricular response can be difficult. Immediate cardioversion is required for unstable tachycardias. Digoxin should be avoided, not because it slows AV nodal conduction (which would be advantageous, but have negligible effect because bypass tract conduction is much more efficient), but because it can directly enhance bypass tract conduction and increase the ventricular rate. Verapamil is also contraindicated, because the hypotension it may cause results in sympathetic activation that may improve bypass conduction indirectly. Procainamide (15 mg/kg, IV) can be helpful, as it slows conduction in the bypass tract and may cause termination of the atrial fibrillation. Intravenous procainamide should be used with caution because it can cause hypotension.

Chronic management of WPW is similar to that described earlier for AVRT except that ablative therapy is even more desirable in patients with symptomatic SVT and particularly those with documented atrial fibrillation. The risk of atrial fibrillation and subsequent syncope and sudden death in patients with asymptomatic ventricular preexcitation is very low, and intervention is probably not indicated, unless the patient works in a high-risk profession (such as commercial drivers or pilots).

Atrial Tachycardia

Atrial tachycardia may be caused by automatic or reentrant mechanisms and occur paroxysmally or be essentially incessant. Digitalis intoxication can cause atrial tachycardia, typically with 2:1 or variable AV block. Incessant atrial tachycardia is one of the more common causes of tachycardia-induced cardiomyopathy. As discussed earlier, the diag-

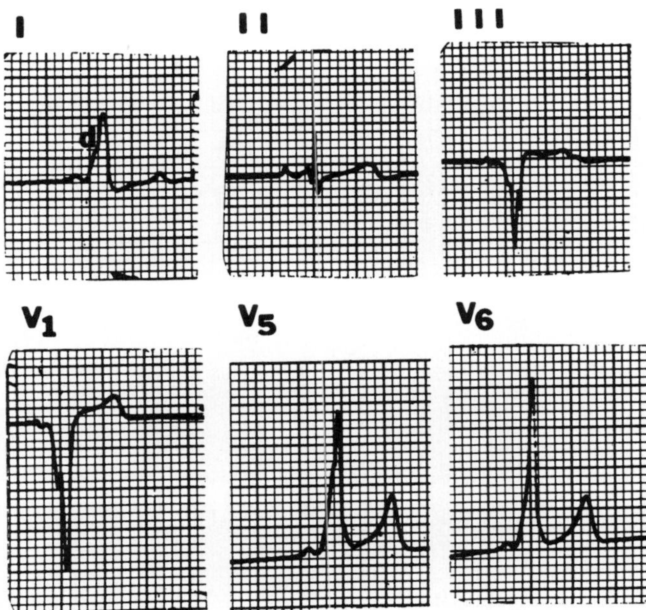

Figure 36–26. Ventricular pre-excitation in the Wolff-Parkinson-White syndrome. Characteristic features include: (1) a short (< 0.11 sec) PR interval, (2) slurring of the upstroke of the QRS caused by the presence of a delta wave (d), (3) prolonged QRS duration, and (4) ST-T wave changes. The delta wave is caused by eccentric activation of a portion of the ventricular myocardium by the bypass tract. *(Used with permission from Josephson et al. [1987].)*

nosis of atrial tachycardia depends on demonstrating that the tachycardia persists despite the development of AV block (Fig. 36–27). Pharmacologic control of atrial tachycardia may be possible with antiarrhythmic drugs such as flecainide, sotalol, or amiodarone. Catheter ablation is also used for cure of atrial tachycardias; although often successful, the efficacy is somewhat less than that observed for other SVT mechanism, owing at least in part to the fact that atrial tachycardias can arise from anywhere in either atrium (Callans et al., 1995).

Sinus Tachycardia

In adult patients, sinus tachycardia is said to be present when the heart rate exceeds 100 beats per minute and the *p* waves on the 12-lead ECG match the sinus morphology; rates greater than 200 beats per minute are unusual, and should prompt consideration of another diagnosis. In sinus rhythm, *p* waves are typically upright in leads I, II, and III, and VI has an initial positive deflection followed by a terminal negative component (corresponding to right and left atrial vectors of activation, respectively). In addition to this "signature" on the ECG, sinus tachycardia can be distinguished from many of the paroxysmal SVTs by its automatic mechanism. Automatic tachycardias typically "warm up" and "warm down" in terms of rate, rather than starting and stopping abruptly. Sinus tachycardia is seldom a primary arrhythmia, but instead almost always represents a physiologic response to stimuli such as pain, fever, hypovolemia, hypoxia, or emotional stress. As such, treatment of sinus tachycardia should be directed to the root cause of the physiologic stress, rather than with the use of antiarrhythmic drugs.

Two SVTs that arise from the sinus node can break this pattern; both are very unusual. Sinus node reentry is a paroxysmal tachycardia that is typically initiated with an APC and stops abruptly with vagal maneuvers or drugs that are active against nodal tissue (adenosine, beta blockers, calcium antagonists). The *p* wave recorded in tachycardia matches the morphology in slow sinus rhythm. Inappropriate sinus tachycardia (IST) is a fairly recently recognized condition in which the sinus node seems to be exquisitely sensitive to sympathetic stimulation (Morillo, Klein, Thakur, et al., 1994). This can produce abnormally fast sinus rates at rest and/or exaggerated increments in rate in response to exertion or emotional stress. IST can cause symptoms of palpitations, chest pain, fatigue, and exercise intolerance or even abrupt syncope. The physiologic mechanisms for IST and the symptoms it produces are far from fully characterized.

Ventricular Tachyarrhythmias

Ventricular tachyarrhythmias, including ventricular tachycardia and ventricular fibrillation, are the most frequent cause of sudden cardiac death, which claims 350,000 to 400,000 lives per year in the United States (Gillum, 1989). Viewed in another way, approximately 50% of total mortality in patients with symptomatic congestive heart failure is caused by ventricular arrhythmias. Only a fraction of patients who suffer out-of-hospital cardiac arrest survive to hospital discharge. Even those who survive often have significant neurologic deficits caused by anoxic encephalopathy during the arrhythmia. Uniform VT may also present less dramatically, with a wide spectrum of symptoms ranging from incidental detection, palpitations, chest pain, and syncope. With few exceptions, ventricular arrhythmias are a

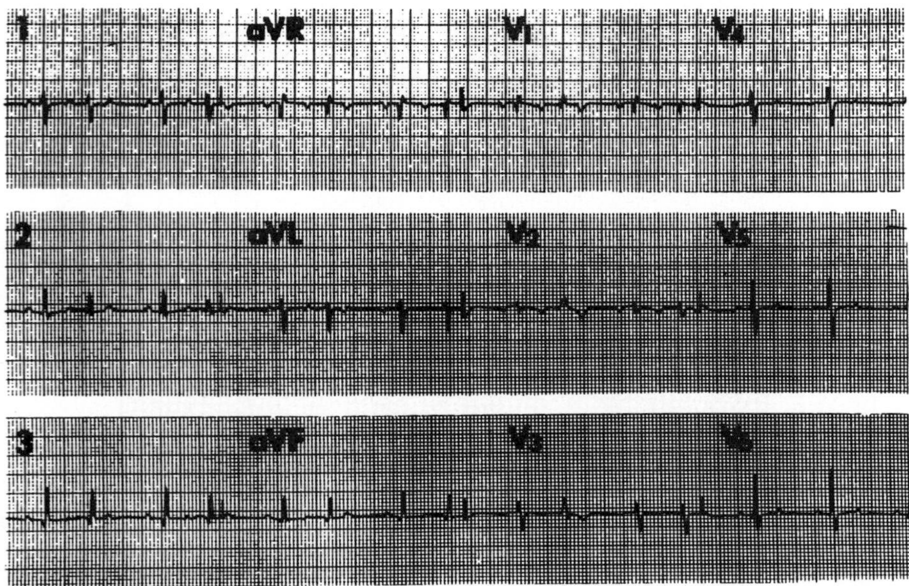

Figure 36–27. Atrial tachycardia with variable AV block. Supraventricular tachycardia that continues in the setting of AV block is by definition confined to the atrium. *(Reproduced with permission from Josephson & Wellens. [1990].)*

consequence of advanced structural heart disease or acute coronary occlusion, with resultant myocardial infarction or ischemia. Treatment of patients with ventricular arrhythmias must focus on acute termination of the arrhythmia, prevention of recurrence, and evaluation of the structural heart disease that serves as the arrhythmia substrate.

Premature Ventricular Contractions

Occasionally, isolated ventricular premature beats are considered ventricular arrhythmias. Although single PVCs may cause symptoms of palpitations, and deserve treatment on this basis, therapy should consist of agents with negligible proarrhythmic risk, such as beta blockers. PVCs are widely considered as "harbingers" of sustained ventricular arrhythmias, a view that was only partially dispelled by the CAST study (Echt, Liebson, Mitchell, et al., 1991). Although the presence of frequent PVCs should prompt evaluation to ensure that electrolytes are normal and that ischemia is well controlled, PVCs usually signal more about the severity of the underlying heart disease than a risk of sustained ventricular arrhythmias per se.

Ventricular Fibrillation and Polymorphic Ventricular Tachycardia

Ventricular fibrillation (VF) refers to extremely rapid (> 300 beats per minute) and disorganized ventricular activation which always causes loss of consciousness and death if not promptly terminated (Fig. 36–28). Polymorphic ventricular tachycardia (PMVT) is essentially indistinguishable from VF electrocardiographically and is observed in the same patient subsets. The distinction is difficult to define, except that PMVT implies a rhythm that is slightly more organized (or has larger amplitude QRS complexes) and is more likely to terminate spontaneously under certain conditions. Torsades de pointes represents a relatively small proportion of episodes of PMVT which, by definition, occurs in the setting of a prolonged QT interval, typically as a complication of antiarrhythmic drug therapy, although other drugs have also been implicated (Fig. 36–29).

Pathophysiology. PMVT (aside from torsades de pointes) and VF occur primarily in the setting of acute ischemia and infarction or as a result of ventricular tachycardia that degenerates into PMVT/VF after producing ischemia. Most episodes of sudden death resulting from PMVT/VF that have been recorded on telemetry or holter monitor actually start as uniform VT (Kempf & Josephson, 1984). As discussed later, this observation has significant implications for the treatment of PMVT/VF with implantable cardioverter–defibrillator therapy. The mechanism of PMVT/VF is reentry, and the rhythm is usually conceptualized as consisting of several small, migrating reentrant wavelets (similar to the multiple wavelet hypothesis for atrial fibrillation). Under most circumstances, PMVT/VF only occurs in the setting of either acute, severe ischemia/infarction or advanced structural heart disease, either in the form of healed myocardial infarction or nonischemic dilated cardiomyopathy. Rarely, idiopathic VF occurs in patients who have no recognizable structural heart disease and normal coronary arteries. This syndrome is referred to as primary electrical disease, and despite the absence of structural heart disease, recurrent PMVT/VF is common. The pathophysiologic mechanism that supports the development and continuation of PMVT/VF is not well understood. Sustained PMVT/VF does not occur in patients without heart disease or ischemia. It is possible that, again like atrial fibrillation, ventricular enlargement and/or slow conduction (which is worsened in the setting of acute ischemia) may be required for the development of enough simultaneous wavelets to maintain VF and allow it to sustain. Once established, VF is the ultimate downward spiral: the extremely rapid rate that it fosters drives continued myocardial energy expenditure in the face of essentially absent coronary perfusion. Even if ischemia was not the root cause of VF induction, ischemia or infarction may be a secondary result of a prolonged VF episode. It is often difficult to sort out which came first—ischemia/infarction or VF. This consideration may have important prognostic and management implica-

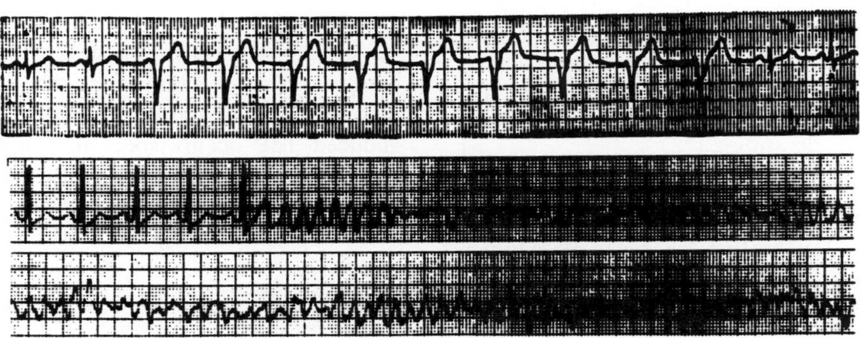

Figure 36–28. Ventricular fibrillation. A lead II rhythm strip starts as sinus rhythm with competing accelerated idioventricular rhythm. In the *middle panel,* a premature ventricular complex occurring on the T wave of a sinus complex induces polymorphic ventricular tachycardia, which degenerates to ventricular fibrillation. *(Used with permission from Josephson et al. [1987].)*

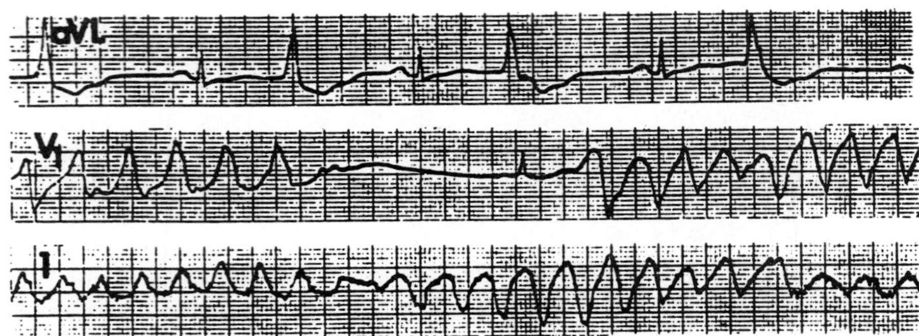

Figure 36–29. Torsades de pointes. In the *top* tracing, sinus rhythm with a markedly prolonged QT (0.74 seconds) alternates with PVCs in a bigeminal pattern. After a short run of nonsustained VT, PMVT arising from the crest of a sinus T wave is observed (*middle panel*). Despite widespread belief to the contrary, after initiation of the arrhythmia (*bottom panel*), torsades has no characteristic features that distinguish it from other PMVTs. *(Used with permission from Josephson et al. [1987].)*

tions, as is discussed later. Obviously, ischemia also occurs in other organ systems as well, and anoxic encephalopathy, acute renal failure, and shock liver may result even after successful resuscitation.

Torsades de pointes (TdP) refers to PMVT that occurs in the setting of a prolonged QT interval, either in the setting of a congenital abnormality or as a result of reversible causes such as drugs or electrolyte disturbances (refer to Fig. 36–29) (Jackman, Friday, Anderson, et al., 1988). The syndrome was named for a sewing technique ("twisting of the points") and refers to the tendency for the arrhythmia to pivot through the isoelectric line on the electrocardiogram. However, all PMVT looks rather similar in this regard and this variability in axis is not specific for TdP, although this is very often a point of confusion. By definition, TdP occurs in the setting of a prolonged QT interval and this is the key distinguishing factor. Although there is no "threshold" value for a QT duration that is likely to result in TdP, the risk of ventricular arrhythmias increases directly with increases in the QT, particularly as it exceeds 500 msec (or corrected QT 550 msec). In addition, the first "beat" of TdP seems to arise from the peak of the T wave, a subtle but specific observation. Often TdP starts as single premature beats, again arising from the peak of the T wave of the preceding beats. The pause that follows premature beats accentuates the QT prolongation on the following sinus beat, aggravating the situation. In fact, short runs of NSVT engender longer pauses, facilitating longer nonsustained runs and finally sustained episodes of TdP PMVT. TdP is thought to be caused by triggered activity due to early afterdepolarizations, at least for the first few beats after initiation. After initiation, it is thought that other mechanisms, such as reentry, may be responsible for continuing the arrhythmia. Finally, although TdP can occur in patients with otherwise normal hearts, preexisting structural heart disease, particularly healed myocardial infarction, is a significant risk factor for drug-induced TdP.

History and Physical Findings. Patients with PMVT/VF can be characterized in two patient subsets: (1) those with preceding structural heart disease, who typically have PMVT/VF as a consequence of uniform VT that degenerates to PMVT/VF; and (2) those without a history of preceding structural heart disease who develop PMVT/VF due to acute ischemia. Often the latter group has objective findings of ischemia immediately prior to the event, such as symptoms of severe chest pain or ST changes in monitored patients. Patients with sustained PMVT/VF uniformly suffer cardiac arrest. Depending on the time elapsed prior to restoration of sinus rhythm, and particularly if cardiac arrest occurred in a nonmonitored or out-of-hospital setting, findings of anoxic encephalopathy may be present. Occasionally, PMVT/VF can be nonsustained, and cause symptoms of palpitations or syncope without cardiac arrest. Patients with witnessed PMVT/VF become unconscious after approximately 15 seconds of this rhythm disturbance, and may have seizure-like movements caused by acute cerebral ischemia. Peripheral pulses and spontaneous respiratory efforts are uniformly absent, although slow (and ineffective) agonal breathing may persist.

In patients with torsades de pointes, the most important part of the history focuses on the medications that the patient has been taking, both prescription and nonprescription. A listing of medications that can cause QT prolongation and TdP is shown in Table 36–4. Usually the drug-induced TdP occurs soon after initiating the responsible medication; this observation has led to the typical practice of initiating antiarrhythmic agents in the hospital during telemetry monitoring. However, electrolyte disturbance (particularly hypokalemia), changes in drug excretion as may occur with decreased renal function, or drug combinations may upset a situation that had been previously stable.

Laboratory and Diagnostic Tests. Electrolyte abnormalities may be an important "trigger" for the occurrence of both PMVT/VF and TdP; hypokalemia is the most

TABLE 36–4. Medications that Can Precipitate Torsades de Pointes

Antihistamines	Seldane, Hismanol
Antibiotics	Erythromycin, Pentamidine, Bactrim, Septra
Antiarrhythmics	Quinidine, Procainamide, Disopyramide, Sotalol
Antifungal Agents	Ketoconazole, Fluconazole, Itraconazole
Cardiac Agents	Probucol, Bepridil
Gastrointestinal	Propulsid
Psychotropics	Tricyclics, Phenothiazines, Haloperidol, Resperdal

important contributing factor. On the other hand, the catecholamine surge that accompanies these life-threatening events causes spurious hypokalemia by forcing potassium from the serum to the intercellular space. Nonetheless, careful correction of electrolyte abnormalities is prudent if not curative. The electrocardiogram is diagnostic in TdP, in demonstrating the presence of QT prolongation as discussed earlier. Serial electrocardiograms and cardiac enzymes are important to determine if myocardial infarction either produced or resulted from a sustained episode of PMVT/VF. Additional evaluation of the coronary anatomy with cardiac catheterization as well as an assessment of LV function is an important part of planning treatment strategy in all patients with sustained ventricular arrhythmias, unless TdP is diagnosed with certainty.

Management. Treatment of acute episodes of sustained PMVT/VF is focused on immediate defibrillation. Other portions of the ACLS protocol cannot be ignored, but the ultimate outcome of the episode of cardiac arrest is determined by the amount of time required for restoration of sinus rhythm; with each additional minute of VF, the mortality of the event increases by 10%. High energy (360 joules) should be used as soon as possible and repeatedly if necessary in the asynchronous mode. If sinus rhythm does not result after the initial shock(s), a distinction must be made between defibrillation with subsequent recurrence of VF versus failure to restore sinus rhythm even transiently. Antiarrhythmic drugs (lidocaine, bretylium, amiodarone) may prevent acute recurrence of VF whereas epinephrine, oxygenation, and especially repeated defibrillation may allow eventual success in the latter situation.

After successful defibrillation, in addition to supportive measures such as mechanical ventilation and blood pressure support as needed, attention is directed to prevention of recurrent episodes. If PMVT/VF was caused by acute ischemia, antianginal therapy and immediate coronary catheterization and revascularization are appropriate in selected patients. Antiarrhythmic drugs are administered, and the first-line agent is typically lidocaine (100 mg IV bolus), particularly in the setting of acute ischemia and infarction. In patients with recurrent PMVT/VF despite lidocaine or in those whose arrest occurred because of degeneration of uniform VT (which is not caused by acute ischemia) intravenous amiodarone has been demonstrated to be extremely effective (Scheinman, Levine, Cannon, et al., 1995).

The acute treatment of TdP differs from other forms of PMVT particularly as it is usually caused by an "excess" rather than a deficiency of antiarrhythmic drugs (Jackman et al., 1988). Nonsustained runs of PMVT presage the development of sustained events unless the offending agent is withdrawn. Potassium repletion is also critical, and intravenous magnesium is beneficial independent of whether the serum magnesium concentration is low. Because the QT interval increases at slow rates and particularly following pauses caused by PVCs, isoproterenol or pacing to increase the heart rate to 80-100 beats per minute often prevents recurrent episodes. By definition, the QT returns to normal with the removal of the offending agent.

Follow-Up. The long-term therapy for patients with sustained PMVT/VF depends on whether the etiology was acute ischemia. In patients with previously normal LV function who have objective evidence of severe ischemia or infarction as the cause of the episode, treatment is directed to coronary revascularization without specific antiarrhythmic therapy. When PMVT/VF occurs as a consequence of prolonged episodes of uniform VT, or if it occurs in the setting of preexisting heart disease, directed antiarrhythmic therapy is required in addition to appropriate treatment of coronary artery disease. Implantable cardioverter–defibrillators are presently the therapy of choice in this setting, as recent trials have demonstrated superior efficacy of the ICD compared with empiric amiodarone or guided therapy with other agents (Epstein for AVID, 1997; Moss, Hall, Cannon, et al., 1996). Often "adjuvant" antiarrhythmic drug therapy is also prescribed, with the objective to reduce the frequency of VT/VF episodes to prevent unnecessary ICD shocks.

The long-term prognosis for patients with PMVT/VF also depends on the etiology of the event, whether it was determined by ischemia/infarction or if it occurred as a consequence of poorly tolerated VT. The incidence of recurrent cardiac arrest in the latter group may be as high as 40-50% in two years; treatment with ICD therapy decreases the annual risk of sudden death in follow-up to 1 to 2% (Zipes & Roberts, 1995). Once protected from the risk of sudden death, the prognosis for total mortality is largely determined by the degree of structural heart disease and the chance of recurrent myocardial infarction.

Ventricular Tachycardia

Pathophysiology. Ventricular tachycardia (VT) is a wide complex, regular tachycardia, ranging in rate from 120 to <300 beats per minute (Fig. 36–30) (Callans & Josephson, 1995). VT typically occurs in the setting of healed myocardial infarction, although it can occur in dilated cardiomyopathy and even in patients without structural heart disease. The mechanism of VT is reentry occurring in the border

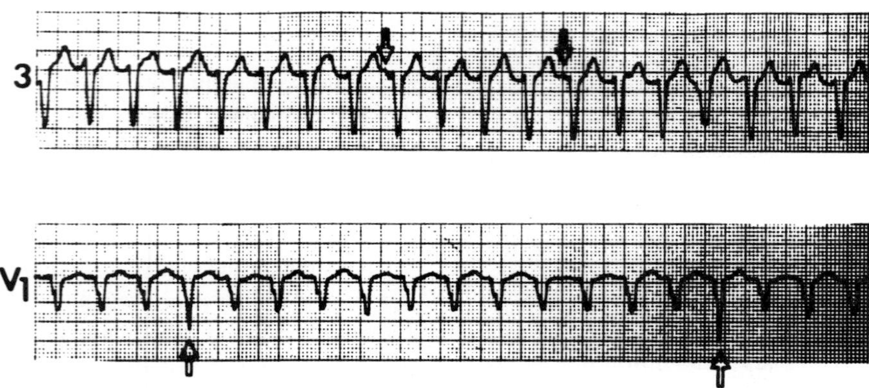

Figure 36–30. Ventricular tachycardia. Characteristic features include a wide complex regular tachycardia with evidence of AV dissociation, indicated by *p* waves that do not effect ventricular depolarization (*top panel, arrows*), and narrow complex capture beats (*bottom panel, arrows*). *(Used with permission from Josephson et al. [1987].)*

zone of surviving tissue around a healed infarction. The slow conduction produced by poor cell-to-cell connections because of ingrowth of fibrous tissue secondary to infarct healing is the major determinant. Depending on the heart rate during VT, the clinical syndrome can range from tachycardias that are discovered incidentally to cardiac arrest. The major determinant of hemodynamic compromise during VT is not deterioration of systolic function, but insufficient time for diastolic filling and the intervening effects of secondary ischemia. Unlike PMVT, VF, uniform VT is never exclusively caused by acute ischemia, although ischemia may serve as a "trigger" and influence the time when a certain VT episode occurs.

History and Physical Findings. Patients with VT almost invariably have a history of healed myocardial infarction. Sometimes the first episode of VT can occur 10 to 20 years after the index infarction, in the absence of recurrent angina or symptoms of heart failure. The incidence of VT is highest, however, in the first 6 months following infarction. Evidence of previous episodes of VT, causing symptoms such as palpitations, syncope, or sudden onset of heart failure, should be sought. A wide range of systolic pressures can be recorded during VT, and in patients with relatively slow rates (< 150/min), VT can be tolerated for hours or even days. The occurrence of tolerated tachycardia in a patient with known structural heart disease should not lead one to suspect a diagnosis of supraventricular tachycardia. The most salient feature of the physical examination during VT is cannon A waves, caused by atrial systole against closed AV valves when AV dissociation is present.

Laboratory and Diagnostic Tests. The diagnosis of VT traditionally centers on interpretation of the electrocardiogram. The differential diagnosis of a regular, wide complex tachycardia includes VT and SVT with aberrancy. Interested readers are referred to classic descriptions of the fine points of making this distinction (Kindwall et al., 1988; Wellens et al., 1978). Briefly, VT can be recognized by the presence of AV dissociation (refer to Fig. 36–30) or by a bizarre QRS morphology that does not match the pattern produced by either left or right bundle branch block (Fig. 36–31). A wide complex tachycardia in a patient with prior myocardial infarction should be assumed to be VT unless certain evidence is provided to the contrary; often a mistaken diagnosis of SVT with aberrancy leads to treatment with verapamil, turning a stable situation into an emergency.

Management. Even in the most stable situations, all attempts at therapy for VT should be performed in a monitored setting, with ready access to resuscitative drugs (atropine, pressor agents) and external defibrillation. Reliable intravenous access should be secured. The choice of therapy for sustained VT depends on the degree of hemodynamic compromise. Patients who are unconscious require immediate synchronous cardioversion. With synchronous cardioversion, the defibrillator coordinates the delivery of energy to the QRS complex. If the energy delivery is not timed (asynchronous) and is delivered on the T wave, ventricular fibrillation may result. On the other hand, synchronous cardioversion is not used in termination of VF because the surface QRS complexes are small and erratic and might remain undetected by the defibrillator, delaying energy delivery. In patients with hemodynamically tolerated VT, antiarrhythmic drug infusion (lidocaine, procainamide, amiodarone) may be used. Although lidocaine is traditionally the drug of choice in this situation, procainamide is superior in efficacy. Problems with intravenous procainamide or amiodarone include hypotension during loading; this may be reduced if the administration rate is decreased. Alternatively, overdrive pacing (via a permanent pacemaker or a temporary catheter) or cardioversion after appropriate sedation can be used to restore sinus rhythm. Most episodes of VT

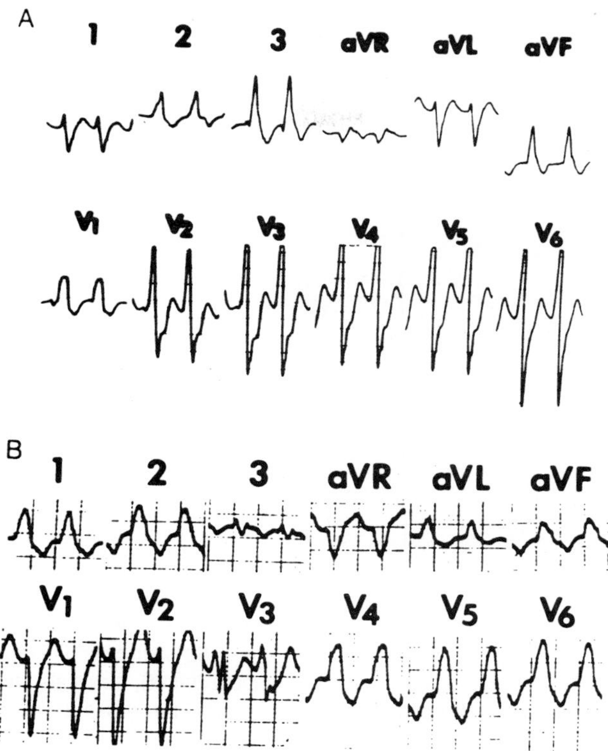

Figure 36–31. QRS morphologies during ventricular tachycardia. In the *top panel,* the QRS morphology resembles the pattern of right bundle branch block. In the *bottom* panel, the QRS morphology resembles the pattern of left bundle branch block. Variations from the expected patterns of bundle branch block allow a diagnosis of ventricular tachycardia in the majority of cases. *(Used with permission from Josephson & Wellens. [1990].)*

are sporadic, and infrequent. In some patients, however, events may be "clustered" over the course of 24 to 48 hours or even become incessant, with immediate VT recurrence following cardioversion. Aggressive loading with amiodarone can be helpful in this situation (Scheinman et al., 1995), although urgent catheter or surgical ablation is sometimes required.

Follow-Up. After restoration of sinus rhythm, the long-term management focuses on (1) long-term prevention of symptomatic VT recurrence and protection from the risk of sudden death and (2) evaluation of the underlying structural heart disease that served as the substrate for the initial VT episode (Callans, 1997). Until recently, the standard of care dictated that chronic antiarrhythmic drug therapy be prescribed based on the results of programmed stimulation in the electrophysiology laboratory. Using this paradigm, patients with inducible VT in the drug-free state were given a series of antiarrhythmic drugs until VT was no longer inducible. This response appeared to correlate with long-term freedom from VT recurrence on the same drug. The ESVEM study (Mason, 1993) demonstrated that drug therapy selected on this basis was not significantly better than regimens selected on the basis of noninvasive testing (Holter and exercise testing). More important, both strategies were demonstrated to have a high rate of arrhythmia recurrence and an unacceptable risk of sudden death. This uncertainty has led to increased use of implantable defibrillators in this setting, particularly since the development of overdrive pacing to allow for VT termination without requiring the delivery of high-energy shocks (Fig. 36–32). As discussed earlier, "adjuvant" antiarrhythmic drug therapy is often prescribed for patients with VT who are primarily treated with implantable defibrillator therapy. Patients with frequently recurrent VT of a single QRS morphology may also benefit from catheter ablation (Callans, Schwartzman, Gottlieb, & Marchlinski, 1994; Marchlinski, Gottlieb, Callans, et al., 1997).

The cardiac evaluation in patients with VT should also include determination of LV function and an assessment of the presence of active ischemic heart disease. Similar to patients with PMVT/VF, once protected from risk of recurrent arrhythmias, the prognosis of patients with VT is largely determined by the extent of their structural heart disease. Patients with VT typically have more advanced LV dysfunction than those with PMVT/VF and symptomatic heart failure is more common. Optimal therapy for CHF and prevention of recurrent ischemia is also critical for the long-term management of these patients.

Ventricular Tachycardia in Patients Without Structural Heart Disease

Several specific morphologies of VT can occur in the absence of structural heart disease (Callans et al., 1994). Although these syndromes are somewhat unusual, they are important to recognize for several reasons: (1) idiopathic VT does not confer a negative prognosis; (2) extensive cardiac evaluation, particularly coronary angiography, is not indicated; and (3) idiopathic VT often responds to medication that would be unhelpful or even contraindicated in VT associated with structural heart disease. Approximately 10% of patients referred for evaluation of VT do not have structural heart disease (Brooks & Burgess, 1988). In these patients, the VT is termed idiopathic and, for the most part, represents one of the following patterns: repetitive monomorphic VT (RMVT) or idiopathic LV midseptal VT (ILVT). RMVT typically originates from the right ventricular outflow tract, and has a very distinctive inferiorly directed electrocardiographic appearance (Fig. 36–33). Episodes are usually provoked by exercise or emotion and may be very frequent "bursts" of nonsustained VT, or paroxysmal episodes of sustained VT. This syndrome typically responds to therapy with beta blockers, although catheter ablation is frequently used successfully (Callans et al., 1994). ILVT also has a distinctive morphology on ECG (Fig. 36–34), with a "normal" appearing right bundle

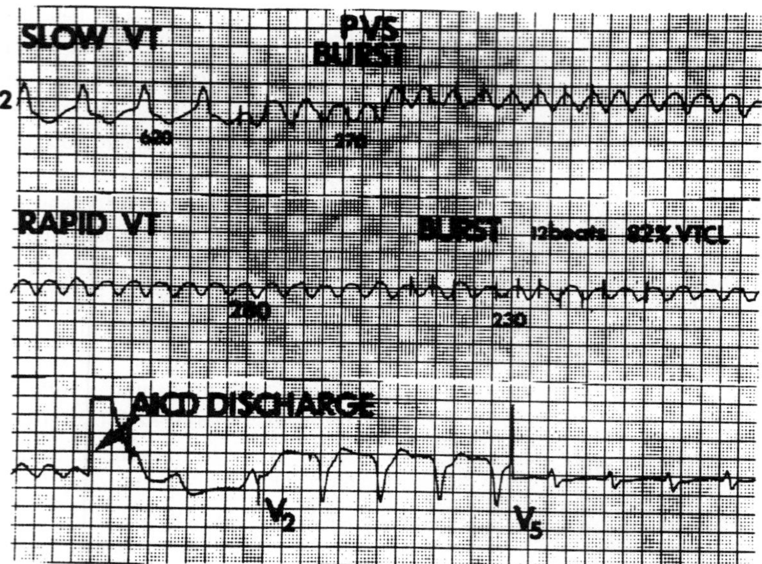

Figure 36–32. Tiered therapy delivery from an implantable cardioverter-defibrillator (ICD). The sequence starts with slow ventricular tachycardia, which the ICD attempts to treat with antitachycardia pacing (PVS burst). Although this mode of therapy is over 90% successful, in this instance it results in acceleration of the arrhythmia to rapid VT. Antitachycardia pacing at a different rate is attempted (burst), but is also unsuccessful. After failure of less aggressive treatment modes, back up defibrillation (AICD discharge) restores sinus rhythm. *(Used with permission from Marchlinski. [1990].)*

branch block morphology. This VT is unique in that acute episodes consistently terminate with intravenous verapamil (note that the diagnosis must be secure before administration of verapamil for VT!). Verapamil is also effective in preventing VT recurrence, and catheter ablation is used in patients with refractory episodes.

Implantable Cardioverter–Defibrillators

As mentioned earlier, implantable defibrillators have revolutionized the treatment of patients with life-threatening ventricular arrhythmias. Sudden death mortality is markedly reduced; many studies have documented a 1 to 2% annual risk of sudden death, even in the highest risk populations,

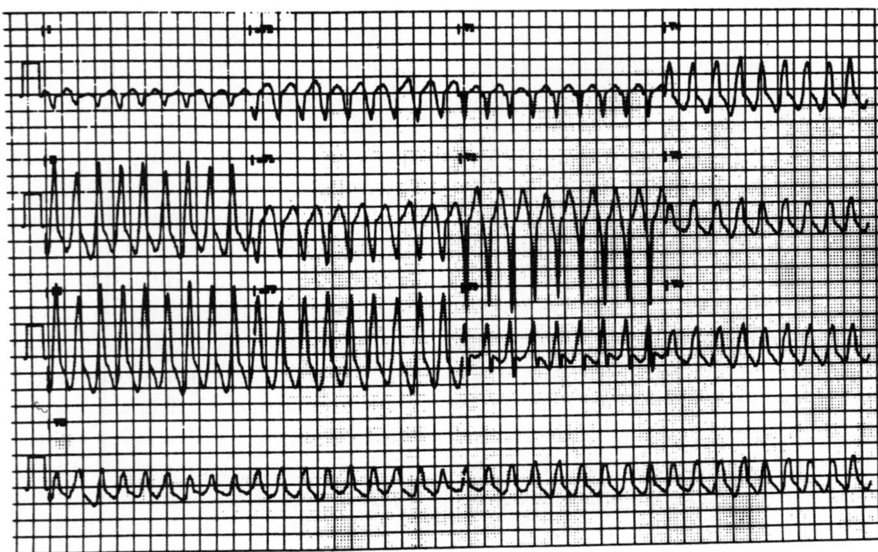

Figure 36–33. Idiopathic ventricular tachycardia from the right ventricular outflow tract (RVOT). The characteristic morphology of this VT is a relatively narrow left bundle branch block pattern with high amplitude positive QRS complexes in the inferior leads. *(Used with permission from Callans et al. [1994].)*

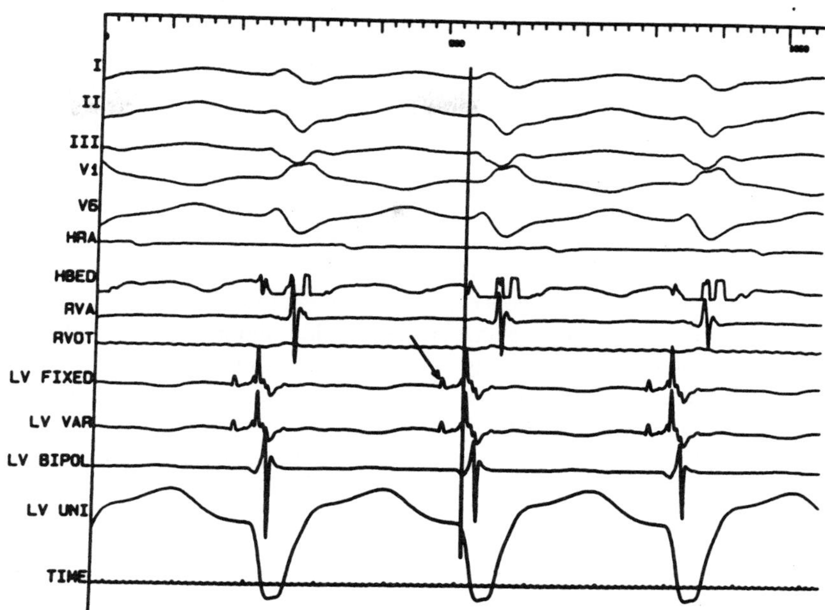

Figure 36–34. Idiopathic ventricular tachcyardia from the left ventricular septum. Surface ECG tracings and intracardiac recordings from various sites are shown. This form of VT has a right bundle branch block morphology on the surface ECG. A catheter placed at the VT site of origin typically records a sharp potential (*arrow*) that precedes ventricular activation. This spike implies that the Purkinje system activation may be essential for the genesis of this type of VT. *(Used with permission from Callans et al. [1994].)*

compared with 30 to 40% 2-year sudden death mortality using conventional antiarrhythmic therapy (Zipes & Roberts, 1995). With recent improvements in device technology, such as the development of nonthoracotomy lead systems and generators small enough to be implanted in the pectoral position, ICD implantation is no more complicated than pacemaker implantation. Tiered therapy—the combination of antitachycardia pacing, low-energy cardioversion, and high-energy defibrillation—allows for the termination of many episodes of VT without the need for painful shock delivery (refer to Fig. 36–32).

Despite enthusiasm for ICD therapy, there is still need for device troubleshooting. Although complex diagnostic algorithms are now available, for the most part, the ICD "diagnoses" life-threatening ventricular arrhythmias on the basis of ventricular rate. Sinus tachycardia and atrial fibril-

TABLE 36–5. Antiarrhythmic Drug Doses

	Intravenous (mg)		Oral (mg)	
Drug	***Loading***	***Maintenance***	***Loading***	***Maintenance***
Quinidine	6–10 mg/kg	600–1000/day	300–600 q6h	300–600 q6–8h
Procainamide	6–13 mg/kg	2–6 mg/min	500–1000	1000–2000 bid
Disopyramide				100–400 q6–8h
Lidocaine	1–3 mg/kg	1–4 mg/min		
Mexiletine			400–600	150–300 q6–8h
Tocainide			400–600	400–600 q6–8h
Flecainide				50–200 q12
Propafenone			600–900	150–300 q8h
Moricizine			300	100–400 q8h
Propranolol	0.25–0.5 q5 min			10–200 q6–8h
Sotalol				80–160 q12h
Amiodarone	150	0.5 mg/min	800–1600 qd	200–400 qd
Ibutilide	1–2			
Bretylium	5–10 mg/kg	0.5–2 mg/min		
Verapamil	10			80–120 q6–8h
Adenosine	6–12			

lation with rapid ventricular rates may prompt inappropriate therapy delivery (Hook, Callans, Kleiman, et al., 1993). This is a significant problem for patients, particularly because shocks are almost uniformly perceived as uncomfortable. In addition, if the rhythm disturbance is not terminated by the first shock, the increase in sympathetic tone caused by the pain of the shock only increases the rate of the ventricular response. This futile cycle is even worse in the setting of lead fracture. In this circumstance, rapid ventricular rates are "mimicked" by the electrical noise generated by the "make–break" connections in the rate sensing leads. In all situations where inappropriate therapy is being delivered, additional shocks can be prevented by magnet application. Analogous to the effect on pacing systems, a magnet placed over an ICD suspends sensing function as long as contact is maintained.

It is important to recognize that ICD therapy is delivered very rapidly if an appropriate diagnosis is made by the device. If therapy is delayed, inappropriate programming or device dysfunction is probably to blame. In this event, therapy should be initiated as if the patient did not have an ICD. External cardioversion delivered to the device can rarely damage ICD circuitry; however, this consideration is not important compared with patient outcome. Unlike the case with external cardioversion, caregivers in contact with a patient who receives an ICD shock are not harmed.

Even more sophisticated ICD systems are presently available, combining tachyarrhythmia therapies and dual-chamber pacing, or even dual-chamber antitachycardia therapy (i.e., for atrial and ventricular tachyarrhythmias). Although this increase in functionality provides great benefits for selected patients, it also increases the complexity of troubleshooting.

REFERENCES

Brooks, R., & Burgess, J. H. (1988). Idiopathic ventricular tachycardia: A review. *Medicine, 67,* 271.

Callans, D. J. (1993). Cellular electrophysiology of cardiac function. In E. B. Savage, S. J. Fishman, & L. D. Miller (eds.). (pp. 81–90). *Essentials of basic science in surgery.* Philadelphia: J. B. Lippincott.

Callans, D. J. (1997). Sustained monomorphic ventricular tachycardia: Immediate evaluation and management, long-term management. *Cardiac Electrophysiology Review, 1,* 105–109.

Callans, D. J., & Josephson, M. E. (1995). Ventricular tachycardias in the setting of coronary artery disease. In D. P. Zipes & J. Jalife (eds.). *Cardiac electrophysiology: From cell to bedside.* 2nd ed. (pp. 732–743). Philadelphia: W. B. Saunders Company.

Callans, D. J., Schwartzman, D., Gottlieb, C. D., & Marchlinski, F. E. (1994). Insights into the electrophysiology of ventricular tachycardia gained by the catheter ablation experience: "Learning while burning." *Journal of Cardiovascular Electrophysics, 5,* 877–894.

Callans, D. J., Schwartzman, D., Gottlieb, C. D., & Marchlinski, F. E. (1995). Insights into the electrophysiology of atrial arrhythmias gained by the catheter ablation experience: "Learning while burning, part II." *Journal of Cardiovascular Electrophysics, 6,* 229–243.

Callans, D. J., Schwartzman, D., Gottlieb, C. D., & Marchlinski, F. E. (1996). Insights into the electrophysiology of accessory pathway-mediated arrhythmias gained by the catheter ablation experience: "Learning while burning, part III." *Journal of Cardiovascular Electrophysics, 7,* 877–904.

Case, C. L., Gillette, P. C., Oslizlok, P. C., et al. (1992). Radiofrequency catheter ablation of incessant, medically resistant supraventricular tachycardias in infants and children. *Journal of the American College of Cardiology, 20,* 1405.

Chou, T-C. (1996). Electrocardiography in clinical practice (4th ed.). Philadelphia: W. B. Saunders.

Dreifus, L. S., Fisch, C., Griffin, J. C., et al. (1991). Guidelines for implantation of cardiac pacemakers and anti-arrhythmic devices. *Journal of the American College of Cardiology, 18,* (1).

Dunn, M. I., & Lipman, B. S. (1989). Lipman-Masse clinical electrocardiography (8th ed.). Chicago: Yearbook Medical Publishers.

Echt, D. S., Liebson, P. R., Mitchell, B., et al. (1991). Mortality and morbidity in patients receiving encainide, flecainide, or placebo: The Cardiac Arrhythmia Suppression Trial (CAST). *New England Journal of Medicine, 324,* 781.

Epstein, A. E. for the AVID Investigators. Results presented at the 18th Annual Scientific Sessions, North American Society of Pacing and Electrophysiology, May 1997.

Feld, G. K., Fleck, R. P., Chen, P. S., et al., (1992). Radio frequency catheter ablation for the treatment of human type I atrial flutter. Identification of a critical zone in the reentrant circuit by endocardial mapping techniques. *Circulation, 86,* 1233.

Gillum, R. F. (1989). Sudden coronary death in the United States. *Circulation, 79,* 756.

Hoffman, B. F. & Cranefield, P. F. (1960). Electrophysiology of the heart. New York: McGraw-Hill.

Hook, B. G., Callans, D. J., Kleiman, R. B., et al. (1993). Implantable cardioverter defibrillator therapy in the absence of significant symptoms: Rhythm diagnosis and management aided by stored electrogram analysis. *Circulation, 87,* 1897.

Jackman, W. M., Friday, K. J., Anderson, J. L., et al. (1988). The long QT syndromes: A critical review and a unifying hypothesis. *Progress in Cardiovascular Diseases, 31,* 115.

Josephson, M. E., Marchlinski, F. E., & Buxton, A. E. (1991). Bradyarrhythmias: Disorders of sinus node function and AV conduction disturbances. In Harrison's principles of internal medicine (12th ed.). New York: McGraw-Hill.

Kay, G. N., Epstein, A. E., Dailey, S. M., et al. (1993). Role of radiofrequency catheter ablation in the management of supraventricular arrhythmias: Experience in 760 patients. *Journal of Cardiovascular Electrophysics, 4,* 371.

Kempf, F. C., & Josephson, M. E. (1984). Cardiac arrest recorded on ambulatory electrocardiograms. *American Journal of Cardiology, 53,* 1577.

Kerr, C. R., & Chung, D. C. (1985). Atrial fibrillation: Fact, controversy and future. *Clinical Prog Electrophysiol Pacing, 3,* (319).

Kindwall, K. E., Brown, J., & Josephson, M. E. (1988). Electrocardiographic criteria for ventricular tachycardia in wide complex left bundle branch block morphology tachycardias. *American Journal of Cardiology, 61,* 1279.

Kopecky, S. L., Gersh, B. J., McGoon, M. D., et al. (1987). The natural history of lone atrial fibrillation: A population-based study over three decades. *New England Journal of Medicine, 317,* 669.

Lanzarotti, C. J., & Olshansky, B. (1997). Thromoembolism in chronic atrial flutter: Is the risk underestimated? *Journal of the American College Cardiology, 30,* 1506.

Laupacis, A., Albers, G., Dalen, J., et al. (1995). Antithrombotic therapy in atrial fibrillation. *Chest, 108,* 352S.

Manning, W. J., Silverman, D. I., Keighley, C. S., et al. (1995). Transesophageal echocardiography facilitated early cardioversion from atrial fibrillation using short-term anticoagulation: Final results of a prospective 4.5 year study. *Journal of the American College of Cardiology, 25,* 1354.

Marchlinski, F. E., Gottlieb, C. D., Callans, D. J., et al. (1997). Ablative therapy for ventricular tachycardia in the setting of chronic coronary artery disease. In K. Ellenbogan & A. Epstein (eds.). (pp. 199–224). *Sudden cardiac death: Past, present and future.* Armonk NY: Futura Publishing Company.

Marriott, H. J. L. (1983). Practical electrocardiography (7th ed.) Baltimore: Williams & Wilkins.

Mason, J. W. (1993). A comparison of electrophysiologic testing with Holter monitoring to predict antiarrhythmic drug efficacy for ventricular tachyarrhythmias. *New England Journal of Medicine, 329,* 445.

Moe, G. K. (1962). On the multiple wavelet hypothesis of atrial fibrillation. *Archives Internationales de Pharmacodynamie et de Therapie, 140,* 183–188.

Morillo, C. A., Klein, G. J., Thakur, R. K., et al. (1994). Mechanism of inappropriate sinus tachycardia. *Circulation, 90,* 873.

Moss, A. J., Hall, W. J., Cannon, D. S., et al. (1996). Improved survival with an implanted defibrillator in patients with coronary disease at high risk for ventricular arrhythmia. *New England Journal of Medicine, 335,* 1933.

Prystowsky, E. N., Benson, W., & Fuster, V. (1996). Management of patients with atrial fibrillation. *Circulation, 93,* 1262.

Sarter, B. H., & Marchlinski, F. E. (1992). Redefining the role of digoxin in the treatment of atrial fibrillation. *American Journal of Cardiology, 69,* 71G.

Scheinman, M. M., Levine, J. H., Cannon, D. S., et al. (1995). Dose-ranging study of intravenous amiodarone in patients with life-threatening ventricular tachyarrhythmias. *Circulation, 92,* 3264.

Stroke Prevention in Atrial Fibrillation Investigators. (1991). Stroke prevention in atrial fibrillation study: Final results. *Circulation, 84,* 527.

Sutton, R. (1995). Sinus node disease. In K. A. Ellenbogan, G. N. Kay, B. L. Wilkoff (eds.). Clinical cardiac pacing. Philadelphia: W. B. Saunders.

Wellens, H. J. J., Bar, F. W. H. M., & Lie, K. I. (1978). The value of the electrocardiogram in the differential diagnosis of a tachycardia with a widened QRS complex. *American Journal of Medicine, 64,* 27.

Wharton, J. M. & Ellenbogen, K. A. (1995). Atrioventricular conduction system disease. In K. A. Ellenbogan, G. N. Kay, B. L. Wilkoff (eds.). Clinical cardiac pacing. Philadelphia: W. B. Saunders.

Wolf, P. A., Abbott, R. D., & Kannel, W. B. (1987). Atrial fibrillation: A major contributor to stroke in the elderly: The Framingham study. *Archives of Internal Medicine, 147,* 1561.

Zipes, D. P. (1997). Genesis of cardiac arrythmias: Electrophysiological considerations. In E. Braunwald (ed.). *Heart disease: A textbook of cardiovascular medicine.* 5th ed. (pp. 548–592). Philadelphia: W. B. Saunders.

Zipes, D. P. & Roberts, D. (1995). Results of the international study of the implantable pacemaker cardioverter-defibrillator. A comparison of epicardial and endocardial lead systems. The Pacemaker Cardioverter-Defibrillator Investigators. *Circulation, 92,* 59.

37

Pulmonary Problems

Nancy P. Blumenthal

Pulmonary problems may arise from structural or functional defects in any aspect of ventilation or respiration. Care of the patient with pulmonary problems requires an organized approach to collecting pertinent history, acquiring supportive diagnostic studies, formulating a diagnosis and treatment plan, and evaluating the patient's response to therapy. This chapter is designed to serve as a reference for the acute care nurse practitioner with questions regarding pulmonary care of the adult patient. Supporting references have been carefully selected to guide further study where more detailed information is sought.

▶ ANATOMY AND PHYSIOLOGY

Ventilation and respiration are achieved through the complex interaction between the respiratory, neuromuscular, and circulatory systems. Control of breathing is orchestrated by the respiratory center of the brainstem. Communication occurs via central and peripheral sensory and chemoreceptors, and afferent and efferent nerves. The medulla responds to metabolic needs by regulating the rate and timing of breaths. The pons controls inspiration via the apneustic center and limits inspiration via the pneumotaxic center.

In response to the efferent sensory message, the respiratory muscles contract to alter the intrapleural and intraabdominal pressures which, in turn, change the intrapulmonary volumes. The ventilatory pump is driven by the chest wall, pleura, and respiratory muscles. During inspiration, the diaphragm contracts, expanding the superior–inferior diameter of the lung and raising the lower ribs. The intercostal muscles increase the anterior–posterior (AP) diameter of the chest. In distress, the accessory muscles (scalenes, sternocleidomastoids, and abdominals) may also contribute to expanding the AP diameter by pulling upward on the sternum and ribs. With thoracic expansion, intrapulmonary pressure is dropped below atmospheric pressure. This results in air being entrained through the upper respiratory tract, through the conducting airways, the bronchioles and the alveolar ducts to the alveoli where gas exchange occurs. When enough air has been inspired, the intrapulmonary pressure equals atmospheric pressure and inspiration ceases. Expiration is normally a passive process with lung recoil being the primary driving mechanism.

Perfusion through the lung is driven by the right side of the heart, through the arborizing pulmonary arteries to the capillaries. Gas exchange occurs at the terminal respiratory unit across the alveolar–capillary membrane. The oxygenated blood then returns to the left side of the heart to be pumped to the rest of the body. Gas exchange occurs between peripheral capillaries and the cells of tissues throughout the body. The deoxygenated blood (carrying CO_2) is then returned to the right side of the heart to begin the process again.

To perform its function in the setting of constant exposure to noxious respirable agents such as dust, smoke, bacteria, toxins, and viruses, the lung has highly developed defense and clearance mechanisms. The defense mechanism varies depending on where the respiratory tract particles are deposited. Particle deposition is influenced by whether the individual is mouth- or nose-breathing, the size of the particle, rate of air flow, and depth of breathing. Large particles are usually deposited, by impaction, in the upper airways. Smaller particles are carried by the airstream to the lower respiratory tract where they impact in the bronchial tree. The mucociliary escalator and the cough reflex are responsible for clearance of the airways. The smallest particles may reach the alveolar level where macrophages provide the primary defense. Macrophages phagocytize the particulate matter which is then transported from the distal areas of the lung by the expansive pulmonary lymphatic system.

The Aging Patient

Several changes occur with aging. Musculoskeletal changes include the loss of muscle tone and strength, decalcification of the ribs and vertebrae, calcification of the costal cartiledges, and arthritic changes in the joints between the vertebrae and the ribs. These changes result in the stiffening of the thoracic cage, kyphosis, and an increased AP diameter. Although the basic architecture of the lung is preserved, there is a progressive loss of elasticity and collagen content of the structures of the lung. This results in the dilatation of the alveolar ducts, flattening and reduction of the alveolar surface area, and the progressive loss of lung compliance. Reduction in total lung capacity and vital capacity result in an increase in dead space and are normal findings in the aging patient (Bates, 1995).

Neural changes with aging include diminished ventilatory responses to hypoxia and hypercapnea and increased ventilatory responses to exercise. There is also a heightened sensitivity to the respiratory depressant effects of narcotics and sedatives (Conrad, Jayr & Peper, 1995). An increase in the frequency of nocturnal awakenings and episodes of apnea are also attributed to the aging process (Pack & Millman, 1988).

▶ THE PULMONARY DATABASE

Obtaining Pertinent Clinical History

Beyond gathering the details of a patient's chief complaint, it is necessary to obtain a comprehensive pulmonary history. Done thoroughly, the history guides the formulation of the differential diagnosis and streamlines the diagnostic evaluation. Furthermore, it may reveal risk factors and self-care deficiencies that warrant patient education, preventive care or ongoing monitoring, and follow-up.

When the chief complaint suggests a pulmonary process, it is important to obtain a detailed chronology of respiratory symptoms. Other valuable aspects of the pulmonary history are the past medical, social, family, and environmental histories. Salient features of the past medical history detail all known diagnoses, how they were made, and how they have been treated. This aspect of history taking can be quite revealing about the patient's approach to health maintenance. The astute nurse practitioner takes note of how the individual obtains and institutes medical advice. As care is later planned, understanding the patient's style is very useful in designing a plan that can be readily integrated into the individual's lifestyle. Patients who prefer to "follow orders," viewing the clinician in a parental role, may decline the opportunity to hear about the mechanism of action of newly prescribed drugs. On the other end of the spectrum, those who are accustomed to managing their own health, viewing their clinician as a partner in their care, may require detailed information about every aspect of their therapy.

Past medical history may reveal patterns of recurrence or may link one disease process with another. Many chronic illnesses are characterized by cycles of exacerbation and remission. Several pulmonary complaints are indicative of extrapulmonary disorders and, conversely, there are many extrapulmonary complaints that may be suggestive of pulmonary pathology. Information about current and past medications is useful in determining likelihood of respiratory side effects or drug-induced lung disease. Drugs associated with adverse pulmonary reactions are detailed in Table 37–1.

Information regarding prior hospitalizations and emergency room visits may be revealing. This encompasses details about admission to intensive care as well as frequency and duration of intubations for mechanical ventilation.

TABLE 37–1. Drugs Associated with Adverse Pulmonary Reactions

Cancer Chemotherapeutic Agents	**Antiinflammatory Agents**
Radiation	Nonsteroidal antiinflammatory agents
Bleomycin	Salicylates
Busulfan	Penicillamine
Mitomycin-C	Gold
Nitrosourea (BCNU)	Corticosteroids
Methotrexate	**Illicit Drugs**
Cyclophosphamide	Heroin
Cytosine arabinoside (Ara-C)	Methadone
Chlorambucil	Propoxyphene
Melphalan	Cocaine
Vinblastine	**Toxic Gases**
Cardiac Medications	O_2
Amiodarone	SO_2
Procainamide	NO_2
Tocainide	**Miscellaneous Agents**
Propanolol	Tocolytics
Hydralazine	Diphenylhydantoin
Antimicrobial Drugs	Methylsergide
Nitrofurantoin	Blood transfusions
Sulfonamides	Talc
Penicillins	Lymphangiography dye
Cephalosporins	Hydrochlorothiazide

From Marti, II. (1997).

Last, it is worthwhile to inquire about the patient's functional status; that is, to determine the extent to which the individual is limited by the presenting symptom. Though subjective, it is a useful measure and monitoring tool of the impact of a disorder on the patient's lifestyle. Objective support of this data can be acquired with exercise testing.

Social history establishes the quantification and route of recreational substances including tobacco, alcohol, and illicit drugs. Date and method of cessation should be noted as should the circumstances surrounding any relapse. Given the deleterious effects of cigarette smoking, the opportunity to encourage a smoker to quit should be taken at each encounter (Agency for Health Care Policy and Research [AHCPR], 1996). Sexual history and practices may also contribute medically relevant information about the patient's lifestyle and risk factors when developing or ordering a list of differential diagnoses.

Family history of genetic pulmonary diseases (e.g., cystic fibrosis, alpha–1 antitrypsin deficiency) and familial thromboembolic disorders (e.g., Protein C or S deficiencies, factor V Leiden) are rare yet noteworthy. Frequently, patients do not know specific details of the health of their ancestors. Unexplained ancestral death at an early age should raise suspicion for the possibility of genetic disorders. More commonly, useful information may be gleaned regarding immediate family history of illness from or exposure to infectious organisms. Children and pets may be vectors for viral and bacterial infections.

Environmental toxins may be encountered through the workplace, hobbies, residence, or travel. These toxins include asbestos, coal, silica, beryllium, solvents, dust, and particulate matter. Time and duration of exposure as well as protective measures employed are important factors to note when documenting exposures. Environmental lung disease is discussed in greater detail later in this chapter.

A thorough history should raise clinical suspicions that guide pertinent physical examination. This information is essential to the discriminating selection of diagnostic studies and the precise interpretation of their results.

Understanding the Symptom

As in any clinical setting, patients typically seek attention for a respiratory complaint when self-care measures have been exhausted, when they fear serious underlying pathology, or when routine health screening has identified an abnormality. The most common respiratory complaints for which patients seek medical attention are cough, sputum production, hemoptysis, chest pain, and dyspnea. Other complaints frequently associated with pulmonary pathology are anxiety, sleep disturbance, anorexia, weight loss, hoarseness, post-nasal drip, fever, and night sweats. Understanding the mechanism or pathology of the presenting symptom is essential to both the diagnosis and the treatment.

Cough

Coughing is a protective response that clears the large bronchi of accumulated secretions and foreign material. A cough may be caused by disorders of the upper respiratory tract, lower respiratory tract, or the upper gastrointestinal tract. The cough mechanism may be reflexive or voluntary. Sensory branches of the trigeminal, glossopharyngeal, superior laryngeal, and vagus nerves are stimulated by a defect that may be inflammatory, mechanical, chemical, or thermal in nature. The efferent limb of the cough reflex uses the recurrent laryngeal and spinal nerves. Changes in the surface epithelium cause the hypersensitivity of the airways to mild irritants such as cold air, dust, deep breathing, or pulmonary secretions (Pratter, Bartter, Akers, & DuBois, 1993).

It is important to gather information about the temporal features (duration, pattern over a 24-hour period, seasonal variations) as well as influencing factors (position, self-care measures). The most common cause of the acute cough is viral tracheobronchitis. Current medications may also provide insight to the source of cough. New exposure to drugs such as beta–adrenergic antagonists or angiotensin converting enzyme (ACE) inhibitors may cause a cough. This side effect is usually relieved by the discontinuation of the drug. Many smokers have a chronic cough, due to chronic irritation from cigarette smoke, to which they are oblivious until its qualities change.

Though rare, a forceful cough can cause serious complications. Patients with decreased bone density are at risk for rib fractures. Known or occult bullous disease provides the setting for spontaneous pneumothorax. Cough syncope occurs when a patient coughs so hard that increased intrathoracic pressures cause decreased cardiac output and, consequently, diminish cerebral perfusion. This finding may be a clue to underlying occult pulmonary hypertension.

By definition, a chronic cough is an unexplained cough lasting more than three weeks. Some common causes of chronic cough are post-nasal drip, asthma, gastroesophageal reflux, and chronic bronchitis.

Postnasal Drip (Rhinitis and Sinusitis). The diagnosis of postnasal drip should be suspected when the patient reports sinus congestion, morning cough, or frequent voluntary clearing of the throat throughout the day. Physical examination reveals sinus tenderness, boggy nasal mucosa, or drainage spilling into the posterior pharynx. When supine, sinus drainage increases and this material may be aspirated into the lower respiratory tract and become a source of chronic bronchial irritation. Treatment is geared toward reducing or relieving the sinus drainage. Patients with postnasal drip associated with sinusitis are treated with a combination of antibiotics (against *H influenzae, S pneumoniae,* and upper respiratory tract anaerobes), a decongestant nasal spray, and an antihistamine. If the source of sinus drainage is felt to be allergic or seasonal rhinitis, antihistamine therapy and avoidance of the allergen is recommended. The addition of intranasal steroids is indicated when antihistamine therapy alone is ineffective in the treatment of rhinitis or sinusitis.

Asthma. Asthma, defined by airway hyperreactivy, may be acute or chronic in presentation. While wheezing and chest tightness are classic symptoms, cough is frequently the only manifestation. Pulmonary function testing using methacholine challenge to provoke bronchospasm is the standard assessment for airway reactivity. This diagnosis and its treatment modalities is discussed in greater detail later in this chapter.

Gastroesophageal Reflux Disorder. When the patient history is notable for heartburn that worsens with bending over or lying supine or for complaints of "sour taste" upon waking, gastroesophageal reflux (GERD) should be suspected. GERD is confirmed by gastroesophogography or acid reflux testing. Choking during or after meals, waking up coughing, and recurrent, dependent lobar pneumonias are all indicators that aspiration is occurring. Though prokinetic motility agents and H_2 blockers are commonly used to treat reflux, the problem is frequently relieved by modifying lifestyle factors. Recommended is a high-protein, low-fat diet. Patients are instructed to avoid oral intake within two hours of sleep, to avoid foods that relax the lower esophageal sphincter (such as alcohol, caffeine, and chocolate) and to elevate the head of the bed to a 30-degree angle.

Chronic Bronchitis. Cigarette use and advanced age are the major risk factors associated with chronic bronchitis. By definition, the symptom of cough with increased sputum production must be present for at least three consecutive months each year for at least 2 years for bronchitis to be considered chronic. The recommended therapy for chronic bronchitis is modifying any contributing factors. In many cases, this means cessation of cigarette smoking. Because of the overlap between chronic bronchitis and chronic obstructive pulmonary disease, this subject is discussed in greater detail later in this chapter.

Sputum Production

Sputum production is a common presenting symptom that has a broad differential diagnosis. Sputum is the collection of secretions formed by the mucous glands and goblet cells of the tracheobronchial tree. The mucociliary escalator is responsible for rhythmically propelling the secretions and the impurities of inspired air upward. The timing of onset and duration of sputum production and its characteristics are important to note. Furthermore, the presence of other complaints (e.g., fever, malaise, wheeze, hemoptysis, chest pain) and risk factors (e.g., smoking, known pulmonary disease, malignancy) must be assessed. Microscopic evaluation of sputum is a useful diagnostic tool and is discussed in greater detail later in this chapter.

Hemoptysis

The report of hemoptysis may indicate the expectoration of gross blood or blood-tinged sputum. It is important to try to quantify the amount of blood expectorated and whether it was bright red, dark, or contained blood clots. Patients frequently mistake hematemasis or bleeding from the upper respiratory tract (e.g., epistaxis) for hemoptysis. The three most common causes of frank hemoptysis are infection, neoplasm, and cardiovascular disorders. Blood-streaked sputum is associated with both acute and chronic bronchitis. Bleeding may emanate from the bronchial circulation, the pulmonary arterial circulation, or the pulmonary alveolocapillary circulation. Etiologies of each are described in Table 37–2.

Massive hemoptysis is arbitrarily defined as expectoration of 400 mL to 600 mL of blood in a 16- to 24-hour period (Cahill & Ingbar, 1994; Goldman, 1989). It is important to be aware that a patient may bleed into the lung without actually expectorating blood, so monitoring the hemoglobin and hematocrit levels is important. This is more common in the setting of a bleed at the alveolar level than with a bleed involving the airways. Chest x-ray, oxygen saturation monitoring, and bronchoscopy are necessary diagnostic tools used in the initial and ongoing evaluation of the patient with hemoptysis. The mortality associated with massive hemoptysis is high and is caused not by exsanguination, but by asphyxiation (Hapopnik, 1997).

Chest Pain

Distinct from dyspnea or chest tightness, chest pain arises from two major sources: the chest wall and the viscera

TABLE 37–2. Sites of Bleeding in Hemoptysis and Common Etiologies

Bronchial Circulation
Chronic bronchitis
Bronchiectasis
Neoplasm
Tracheoesophageal fistula
Foreign body aspiration
Pulmonary Arterial Circulation
Pulmonary arteriovenous malformation
Aspergilloma
Tuberculosis
Tumor
Vasculitis
Lung abscess
Pulmonary hypertension
Pulmonary Alveolocapillary Circulation
Mitral stenosis
Left ventricular failure
Pulmonary infarct
Goodpasture's Syndrome
Idiopathic pulmonary hemosiderosis

(Branch & McNeil, 1983). Chest wall pain arises from the musculoskeletal structures of the thorax (e.g., rib fractures, costochondritis) and is typically sharp, well localized, and exacerbated by coughing or deep breathing. The lung parenchyma has few pain receptor fibers and, so, is insensitive to painful stimuli. On the contrary, the parietal pleura is very sensitive to painful stimuli. Pleuritic pain is associated with diseases that inflame the parietal pleura, such as infections, trauma, or tumor. Visceral chest pain occurs with malignancy or inflammation of any of the thoracic structures as well as with subdiaphragmatic processes such as pancreatitis or choleycystitis (George, 1995).

Dyspnea

Dyspnea, or breathlessness, is the uncomfortable awareness of breathing or difficulty taking a deep breath. The patient may describe the sensation of choking, chest tightness, shortness of breath, or inability to get enough air. Because this is a subjective finding, it is difficult to quantitate. The Borg Scale of Breathlessness (Table 37–3) was devised for the purpose of assessing and monitoring patient reports of dyspnea. This symptom may be the cause or effect of anxiety. It is associated with increased work of breathing due to obstructive or restrictive lung diseases or dysfunction of the ventilatory pump due to disorders of the respiratory, neural, or musculoskeletal structures (George, 1995). Clinical history must include temporal features as well as positional factors. Chest x-ray, physical exam, and cardiopulmonary testing are important to the evaluation of this symptom.

Diagnostic Studies

Diagnostic tests are indicated to provide support for a suspected diagnosis, to exclude a diagnosis from further consideration, to stage a disease process, or to monitor the effectiveness of an intervention. Before a study is ordered, clinicians should know what they are looking for and what they will do with the results.

TABLE 37–3. The Borg Scale of Perceived Exertion

0	Nothing at all	
0.5	Very, very weak	(just noticeable)
1	Very weak	
2	Weak	(light)
3	Moderate	
4	Somewhat strong	
5	Strong	(heavy)
6		
7	Very strong	
8		
9		
10	Very, very strong	(almost max)
	Maximal	

From Borg. (1982).

Sputum Examination

Sputum assessment is germane to the work-up of pulmonary symptoms or abnormal chest x-ray findings. Cytologic examination is used to confirm the presence of malignancy. Microbiologic examination is used to identify infectious organisms and their sensitivities. A Gram stain is performed in the instance when bacterial infection is suspected. Special stains identify fungal, viral, and atypical bacterial infections. Sputum assessment also serves as a tool to monitor chronic bronchial diseases. The physical descriptors of sputum include the color, or mucopurulence, the amount, and the tenacity. As a rule, sputum collected with the first expectoration in the morning tends to give the best diagnostic yield due to the high constituence of sputum versus saliva.

Although there are a variety of collection methods, each allows for some degree of contamination by organisms that colonize the upper airway. The most common means of acquiring sputum is expectoration into a sterile cup. This is noninvasive and repetitively available for serial specimens, though frequently results in collection of saliva rather than true sputum. Tracheobronchial aspiration, or suctioning, allows access to sputum in the intubated or sedated patient. For alert patients who are unable to expectorate adequate specimens for collection, hypertonic 3% saline can be administered via nebulizer to incite sputum production. Transtracheal needle aspiration through the cricothyroid membrane into the trachea is used to obtain lower respiratory tract samples while avoiding upper respiratory tract contamination. This method has limited utility in patients who suffer from chronic bacterial colonization of the lower respiratory tract due to chronic bronchitis, bronchiectasis, or bronchogenic carcinoma. This technique is rarely employed because of its serious complications of hemmorhage, worsening hypoxemia, and death.

Chest Imaging

Imaging of the structures of the thorax is an integral part of the work-up of most pulmonary complaints. Imaging techniques range from the "plain film," meaning the standard PA and lateral chest radiograph, to more elaborate computed tomography (CT) scan and magnetic resonance imaging (MRI). The selection of study is done in a step-wise fashion, starting with the least invasive and relatively inexpensive plain film.

There are four distinct densities found on a radiograph: bone, fluid, fat, and air (Fig. 37–1). The denser tissue absorbs more of the x-ray beam resulting in a more opaque or white appearance on film. Conversely, less dense tissue is radiolucent and gives a black appearance on film. Calcium-containing bones are most dense and therefore appear opaque or white. Similarly, metal—such as jewelry, electrodes, or bullet fragments—also give a dense white image. Fluid (blood)-filled structures such as the heart, the great vessels and the liver, are less dense, but still opaque. Fat is

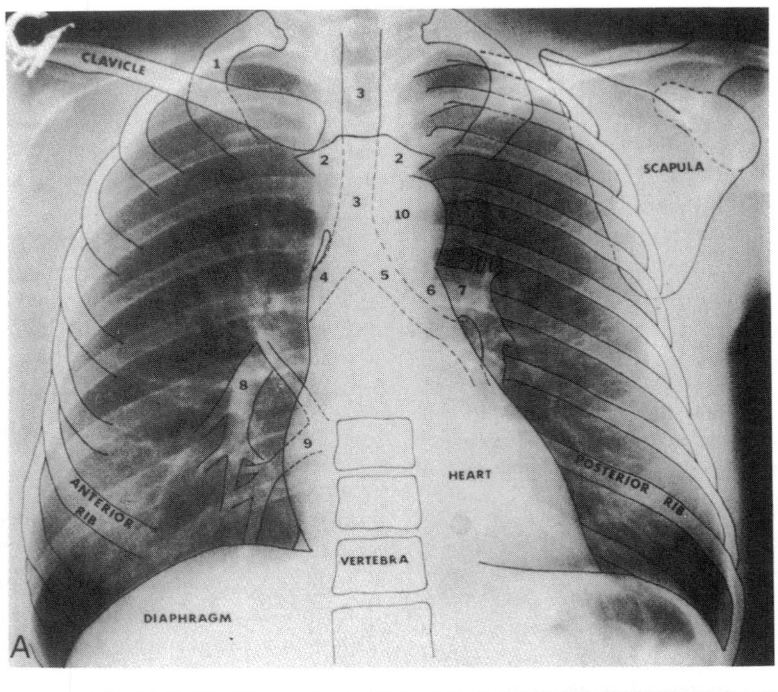

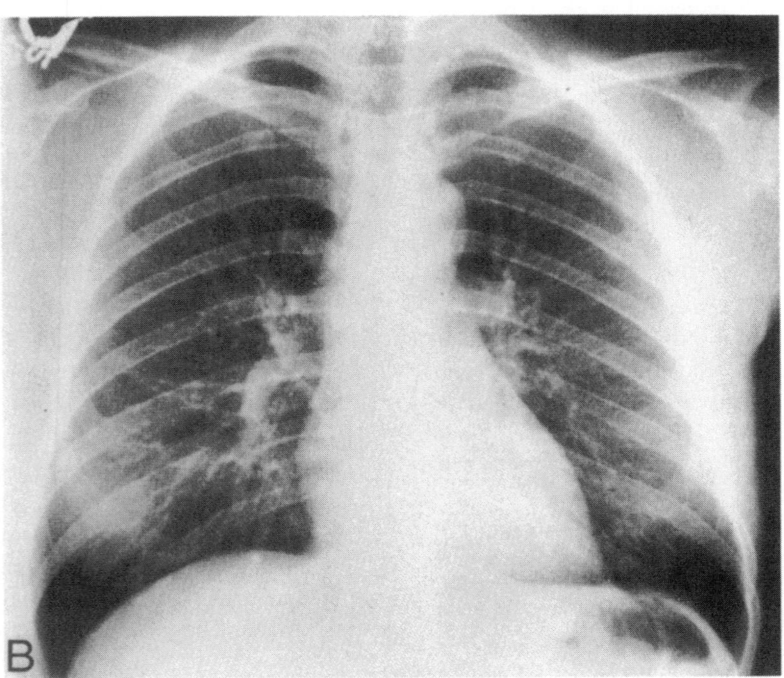

Figure 37–1. A, Posteroanterior (PA) chest radiograph with diagrammatic overlay. Various structures are identified by label or numbers: (1) first rib; (2) upper portion of manubrium; (3) trachea; (4) right main bronchus; (5) left main bronchus; (6) main pulmonary artery; (7) left pulmonary artery; (8) right interlobar pulmonary artery; (9) right pulmonary vein; (10) aortic arch. **B,** Chest radiograph of the same subject without the diagrammatic overlay. *(Reprinted with permission from Sostman & Matthay. [1995]. [p. 111].)*

less dense and, so, more lucent than bone or fluid. It is typically noted as breast tissue or extrathoracic fat surrounding the rib cage or abdomen. The normally air-filled parenchyma of the lungs is radiolucent, or dark, because it absorbs very little of the x-ray beams. When evaluating any radiographic study, it is important to understand that structures are identifiable because they are surrounded by air. This is true for normal anatomic structures as well as most abnormalities. Table 37–4 defines terms frequently used in chest radiology.

TABLE 37–4. Frequently Used Terms in Chest Radiology

Air bronchogram: air-filled bronchi made visible by consolidation of adjacent alveoli; a hallmark of alveolar disease
Alveolar pattern: fluffy, cloud-like density suggestive of alveolar disease; typically conforms to anatomic subdivisions of the lung
Atelectasis: volume loss of alveoli secondary to resorption of air by the pulmonary circulation
Batwing pattern: perihilar or central distribution of pulmonary edema suggestive of cardiogenic pulmonary edema; butterfly pattern
Cephalization: vascular redistribution toward the apices
Diffuse pattern: widespread abnormality that uniformly or near uniformly involves both lungs
Empyema: infected or pus-filled pleural effusion
Focal pattern: an abnormality that involves only a portion of a lung
Honeycombing: pattern of coarse polygonal cystic lesions; a hallmark of end-stage fibrotic disease
Infiltrate: nonspecific opacification of the parenchyma representing a spectrum of pathologic entities; may be acute or chronic, focal or diffuse, alveolar or interstitial in nature
Interstitial pattern: linear or nodular parenchymal shadows that do not correspond to anatomic structures
Kerley B lines: parenchymal septae that are thickened and made visible by the presence of interstial pulmonary edema; suggestive of congestive heart failure
Nodule: well-circumscribed rounded density; may be suggestive of neoplasm or infection
Pleural effusion: abnormal collection of fluid in the pleural space caused by a variety of pathologic entities (e.g., infection, malnutrition, congestive heart failure, trauma)
Pneumonia: infection of the pulmonary parenchyma
Pneumothorax: air in the pleural space secondary to disruption of the integrity of the parietal or visceral pleurae
Silhouette sign: the absence or obscuration of a normally seen thoracic structure caused by fluid in the adjacent alveoli
Tracheal deviation: the displacement of the trachea to the right or left of the normally midline position; may be caused by retraction of the ipsilateral structures (e.g., atelectasis, resected parenchyma), displacement by a mass (e.g., lymphadenopathy, cardiomegaly, tumor), or positive pressure (e.g., pneumothorax)

Chest Radiographs

Posterior–Anterior and Lateral Views. The most common chest radiographic study, the posterior–anterior (PA) and lateral views are typically used for screening and diagnostic purposes. Malignancies, tuberculosis, and asymptomatic pulmonary disease may be detected on screening films. The diagnostic utility of the PA and lateral chest x-ray is vast. The clinician can visualize the presence, locality, and extent of an abnormality. It is noninvasive, comparably inexpensive, and readily repeated for the sake of serial monitoring.

As its name suggests, this study includes two views of the chest: the posterior to anterior view and the lateral view. When the x-ray beam is shot from posterior to anterior, the shadows of the heart and mediastinum (housed in the anterior aspect of the chest) cast a lesser shadow or silhouette. This results in a view of a greater portion of the lung fields. Ideally, the patient is able to sit upright and hold a deep inspiration while the picture is being taken. This, too, promotes maximal visualization of the lung fields. Figure 37–1B demonstrates a PA film with no abnormalities.

The lateral view augments the information obtained in the PA film by providing an image of the retrosternal structures obscured by bony and vascular structures (Fig. 37–2). On the PA view, the most dependent aspect of the lung bases and pleura are obscured by the diaphragm and liver. The lateral view offers a vantage point to evaluate the presence of fluid or thickening of the dependent sulcus. Commonly, the lateral film is used to determine the exact location (i.e., depth) of a lesion seen on the two-dimensional PA film.

Anterior–Posterior View. The anterior–posterior (AP) view is usually only taken when a patient is unable to travel to the radiology department to have the higher quality PA and lateral film shot. The patient's condition may make consistent, correct positioning and holding full inspiration difficult or impossible. This decreases the utility of serial films for comparison. The portable x-ray generator is smaller (for the purposes of mobility) and less powerful and is positioned much closer to the patient's thorax. Because the x-ray beams are sent a shorter distance and from anterior to posterior, the shadows of the heart and mediastinum obscure a greater portion of the lung fields than those in the PA view (Fig. 37–3).

Oblique Views. On the standard plain film it is frequently difficult to discern a pulmonary or mediastinal lesion from an anomaly of the pleura or chest wall. Similarly, it may be difficult to discern whether the location of an abnormality is anterior or posterior. In this instance, the clinician may chose to order an oblique view radiograph. X-ray beams for the right anterior oblique view are shot at a 45-degree angle to the right hemithorax. To avoid the heart, the left anterior oblique is shot at a 60-degree angle to the left hemithorax.

Lateral Decubitus View. The lateral decubitus film is used to detect the presence, amount, and mobility of air or fluid in the pleural space. Using the principles of gravity (fluid falling and air rising), this view requires that the patient hold a side-lying position while the picture is being taken. The side on which the patient is positioned depends upon the information that is sought. If the intent is to move air in the pleural space, the patient is positioned on the contralateral side. Conversely, the patient is placed on the ipsilateral side if the goal is to move fluid within the lateral aspect of the pleural space. If the fluid or air is loculated, or trapped, the lateral decubitus film is of little utility.

Lordotic View. This view of the lung fields allows for visualization of the apices, lingula, and right middle lobe

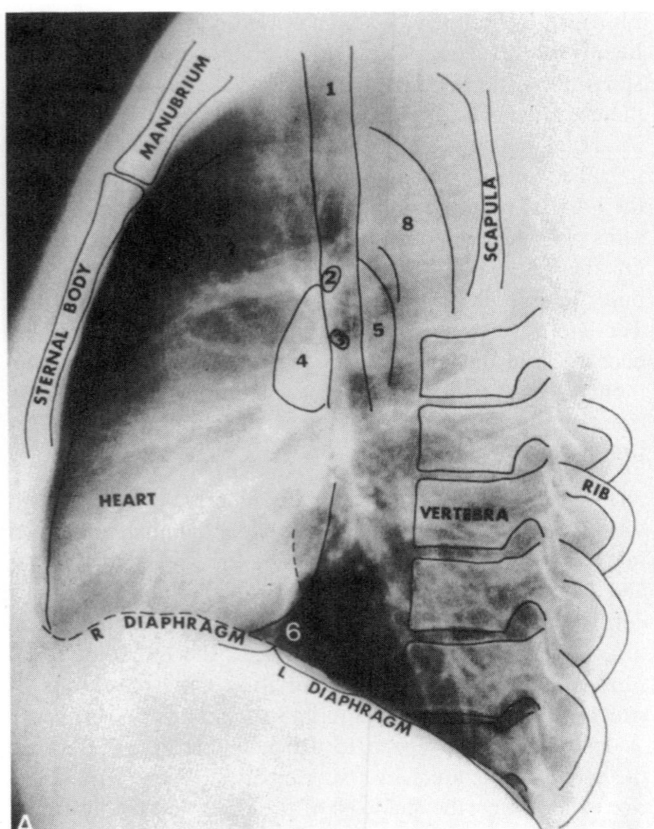

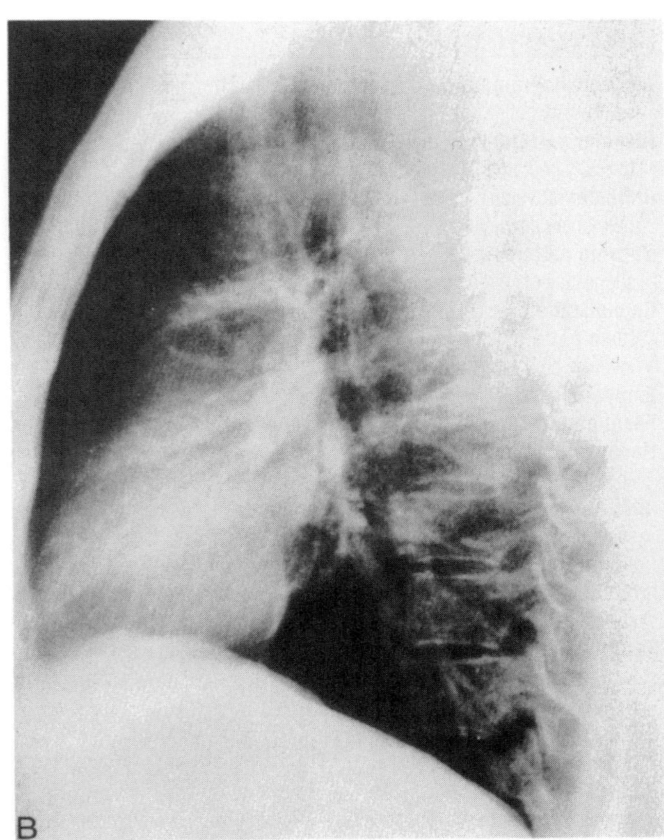

Figure 37–2. A, Lateral chest radiograph of the same patient as in Figure 37–1, with diagrammatic overlay. Structures are identified by labels or numbers: (1) trachea; (2) right upper lobe bronchus; (3) left upper lobe bronchus; (4) right pulmonary artery; (5) left pulmonary artery; (6) inferior vena cava; (7) ascending aorta; (8) descending aorta. **B,** Lateral chest radiograph without the diagrammatic overlay. *(Reprinted with permission from Sostman & Matthay. [1995]. [p. 112].)*

which are normally difficult to appreciate on the plain film. When taking the lordotic film, the x-ray beams are sent upward at a 45-degree angle. The result is an upward projection of anterior structures and a downward projection of posterior structures. This position raises the clavicle and first ribs out of the field of view of the apices and gives a broader field of visualization for the lingula and right middle lobe.

Expiratory View. Occasionally, the patient's condition warrants assessment of the thorax during expiration to evaluate the presence of retained, or trapped, air. Such situations include evaluation of pneumothorax or the assessment of lung distal to an airway obstructed by tumor or foreign body.

Computed Tomography Scan. When the precise morphology and density of a lesion is sought, the computed tomography (CT) scan can provide valuable information where plain films are indistinct. The standard CT provides images of 10 mm transverse cross sections, or slices, of the thorax. While standard films are two dimensional (height and width), this view eliminates the shadows of overlying structures and adds the third dimension, depth to the picture (Fig. 37–4).

Better definition of parenchymal lesions is achieved using 1 mm cross-sections. This technique is referred to as a high resolution CT scan (HRCT). IV contrast is used in the evaluation of mediastinal contents when it is necessary to differentiate vascular structures from lymph nodes or tumors.

Magnetic Resonance Imaging. Similar to the CT scan, magnetic resonance imaging (MRI) provides information about the density and extent of a lesion by supplying a cross-sectional image. However, this technique does not use x-ray beams or contrast material, but rather magnetizes the protons in the body tissues which are then met by a radiofrequency pulse and then constructed into cross-sectional (transverse, sagital, or coronal) images. Variations in density are determined by the tissue's concentration of protons. While MRI scanning is ideal for scanning the brain, spinal cord, and musculoskeletal structures, its use in pulmonary scanning is limited to visualization of the vasculature of the mediastinum and hila in the assessment of soft tissue anomalies or lymphadenopathy.

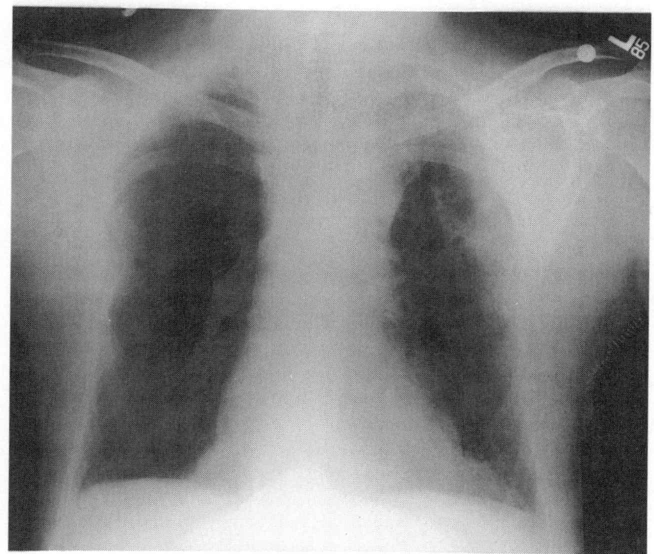

Figure 37–3. Portable anterior-posterior (AP) chest radiograph. Generally a lesser quality view than the PA, the AP view allows for imaging of patients who are unable to be moved to the radiology department. Note that the cardiac and aortic silhouettes obscure a greater portion of the lung fields than do those on the PA view. Also, note the skin staples at the left axilla and apical pleural effusion related to recent thoracotomy.

Fluoroscopy. Fluoroscopy demonstrates the structures of the thorax in motion. It is most frequently used at the bedside to confirm line placement, to localize an anomaly for needle aspiration, and to place forceps for transbronchial biopsy. Fluoroscopy is extremely useful in the assessment of diaphragmatic function. With a short, deep inspiration (or "sniff"), the paralyzed hemidiaphragm moves paradoxically rather than downward. Fluoroscopy exposes both the patient and the clinician to a great deal of radiation, so protective measures should be taken by all individuals within proximity.

Ventilation–Perfusion Scanning. The ventilation–perfusion (V/Q) scan is a nuclear medicine study that examines the distribution and uniformity of air movement and blood flow throughout the lung so that comparisons may be made (Fig. 37–5, see p. 787). During the ventilation phase of scanning, radioactive particles are inhaled. Similarly, the evaluation of perfusion is achieved by the intravenous injection of a radionucleotide contrast. V/Q scanning is most commonly used to assess the probability of acute pulmonary embolism (Fig. 37–6, see p. 788). The utility of this technique has been enhanced by the ability to quantify perfusion in thirds. The quantitated V/Q scan reports percentages of air and blood flow to the upper, middle, and lower regions (not lobes) of the lung. This is useful in the preoperative evaluation for lung transplantation and lung resectional surgery (e.g., pneumonectomy, lung resection, lung volume reduction surgery).

Invasive Procedures

Once the information gathered from noninvasive studies has been exhausted, the clinical situation may warrant proceeding to data-collection methods that require the violation of airways or pleural space. Though the associated risk with invasive studies is notably higher, the diagnostic yield can be far superior to that of noninvasive tests.

Pulmonary Angiography. Pulmonary angiography images the pulmonary vasculature using contrast injected directly into the pulmonary artery (Fig. 37–7). This procedure is most commonly used for the detection and evaluation of an obstructive lesion, such as a pulmonary embolism. Other uses include the evaluation of a pulmonary arteriovenous fistula or malformation. The risks associated with this procedure are cardiac dysrhythmia, allergic reaction, and nephrotoxicity caused by the contrast material. Embolization is indicated when shunting due to pulmonary arteriovenous malformation is severe. Should the embolus migrate systemically, this intervention places the patient in danger of devastating spinal artery infarction or cerebral vascular accident.

Bronchial Arteriography. Bronchial arteriography is indicated to assess hemoptysis emanating from the bronchial circulation. It is important to understand that this procedure is only useful when the patient is actively bleeding. Bronchial arteriography is typically used in the evaluation of a patient with major hemoptysis associated with bronchiectasis or mycatoma. Because this requires arterial puncture for injection of the dye, there is a significant risk for bleeding. The risks associated with use of contrast dye and embolization are the same as those in pulmonary arteriography.

Nasopharyngeal Laryngoscopy. The nasopharyngeal laryngoscope is used to inspect the upper respiratory tract. This has a role in the evaluation of sinus disease, upper airway obstruction or inflammation, or vocal cord pathology. This low-risk procedure is done in the office or at the bedside and requires little or no sedation.

Fiberoptic Bronchoscopy. When the clinical situation requires direct visualization of the airways, fiberoptic bronchoscopy is used. This procedure has extensive diagnostic value (Table 37–5). It allows inspection of the airways to the subsegmental level and provides access for lung fluid analysis and tissue samples.

The fiberoptic scope is approximately 5 mm in diameter and is passed through the nose, mouth, tracheostomy, or endotracheal tube to the area of interest. This procedure can be done at the bedside in the intensive care unit or in an outpatient procedure area and requires local anesthesia of the gag reflex and conscious sedation. The associated risks are hypoxemia and, when biopsies are taken, pneumothorax and hemmorhage. The bronchoscopist has complete control over the direction and movement of the flexible scope. Saline and tissue-sampling instruments can be passed

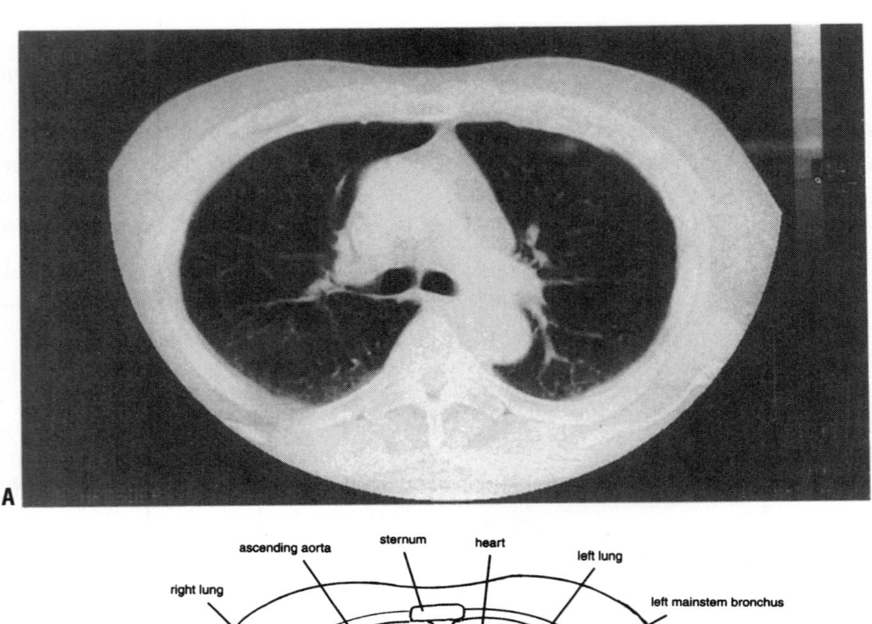

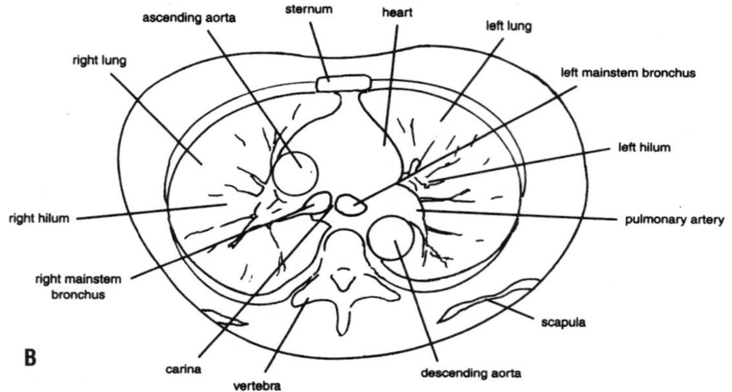

Figure 37–4. CT scan of the normal chest at the level of the carina. **A,** Radiographic view. **B,** Diagrammatic view. *(Reprinted with permission from Farzan & Farzan. [1997]. [p. 31].) Stamford, CT: Appleton & Lange.)*

through the scope to acquire material for microbiologic, cytologic, and pathologic examination.

A bronchial wash requires the instillation of 10 mL to 30 mL of saline through the bronchoscope and subsequent aspiration back through the scope into a sterile collection cup. By the same route, a transbronchial brush can be inserted, and brushed back and forth over a lesion to obtain cells for evaluation. Similarly, biopsy forceps can be used, with fluoroscopic guidance, to sample the parenchyma or a visualized lesion. To obtain a bronchial alveolar lavage (BAL), the scope must be wedged into a subsegmental bronchus while large amounts of saline are systematically instilled and aspirated. The aspirate represents the cell population of the alveoli and is analyzed for cell counts, morphology, and typing.

The therapeutic potential of fiberoptic bronchoscopy is vast (refer to Table 37–5). Guided access to areas of obstruction, malacia, or neoplasm has supplanted modes of treatment that were more invasive or less effective.

Rigid Bronchoscopy. There are instances when the bronchoscopist may require more control over the patient's airway. A larger channel for biopsy, suctioning, or foreign body retrieval is available using the rigid bronchoscope. This straight scope has a large diameter through which a patient can be ventilated. Though the upper lobe bronchi and smaller peripheral airways cannot be assessed with the rigid bronchoscope, this instrument is ideal for the assessment and treatment for massive hemoptysis, bronchial strictures, and neoplasms requiring laser therapy. Both the higher risks and costs of this procedure are attributable to it being done in the operating room under general anesthesia.

Transthoracic Needle Aspiration and Biopsy. As its name suggests, this technique involves a percutaneous needle approach to lesions or fluid of the parenchyma, pleura, and mediastinum. Under fluoroscopy, a flexible spinal needle is passed to the site where specimens are then aspirated into a sterile needle. The collected fluid is then sent to microbiology, cytology, and pathology labs for evaluation. Because of the risk for pneumothorax, this procedure should not be attempted in the patient who is uncooperative or coagulopathic or who has significant emphysema.

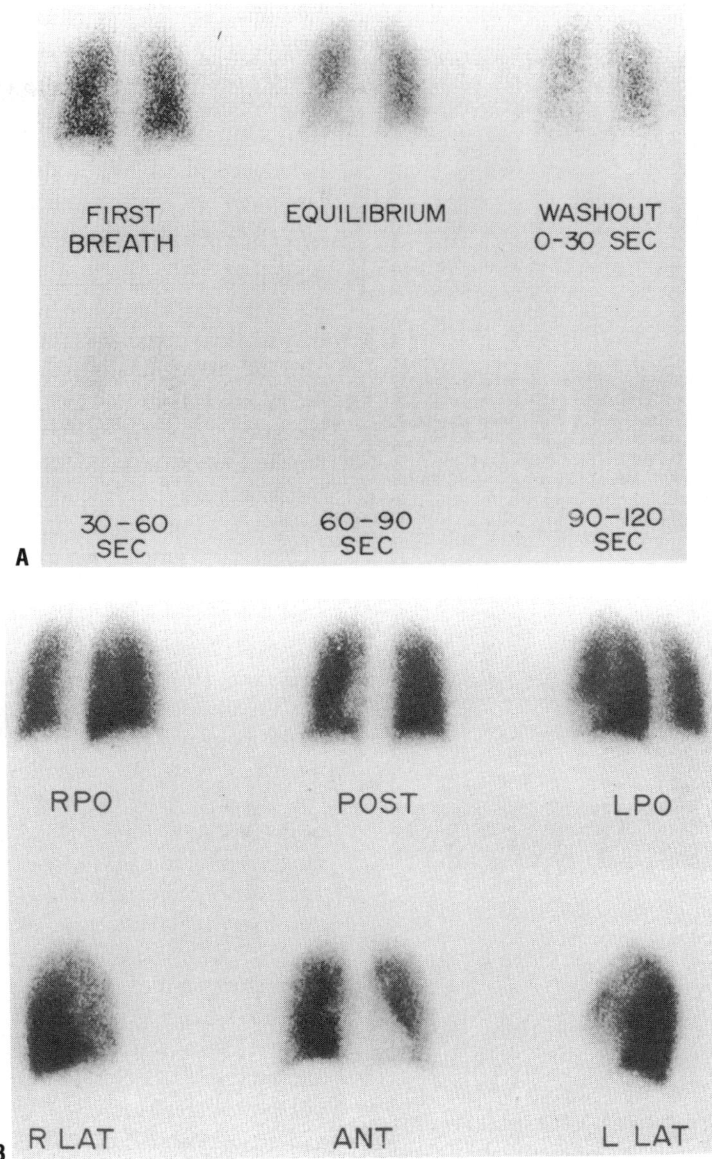

Figure 37–5. A, Ventilation phase of a ventilation–perfusion scan. Note that in the "first breath" and "equilibrium" images there is homogenous distribution of the radioactivity in both lungs. Note that in the "wash-out" phase (which is performed by serial imaging when the patient is no longer breathing in radioactive gas, so that the gas already in the lungs is imaged as it exits from the lungs), there is no evidence of abnormal retention of radioactive gas. **B,** Perfusion images of the same patient. It is important to obtain at least six views of the lungs. In this patient the perfusion is normal, with no focal defects seen in the images. The radioactive particles are injected with the patient lying supine. Note on the right and left lateral views that there is more perfusion in the posterior (dependent) portions of the lungs. This is a graphic demonstration of the effect of gravity on the pulmonary perfusion gradient. *(From Sostman & Matthay. [1995]. [p. 127].)*

Video-Assisted Thorocoscopy. This procedure, performed by a surgeon under general anesthesia, allows for the direct visualization of the pleural space, pleural structures, pleural surfaces, and anomalies. Larger tissue samples can be obtained through this method than by the lower cost, lower risk procedures. Video-assisted thorocoscopy has replaced open lung biopsy for diagnostic purposes. This subject is covered in more detail in Chapter 38, Thoracic Surgery.

Functional Testing

Pulmonary Function Testing. One of the mainstays of pulmonary assessment, pulmonary function testing (PFT) can determine whether lung function is normal,

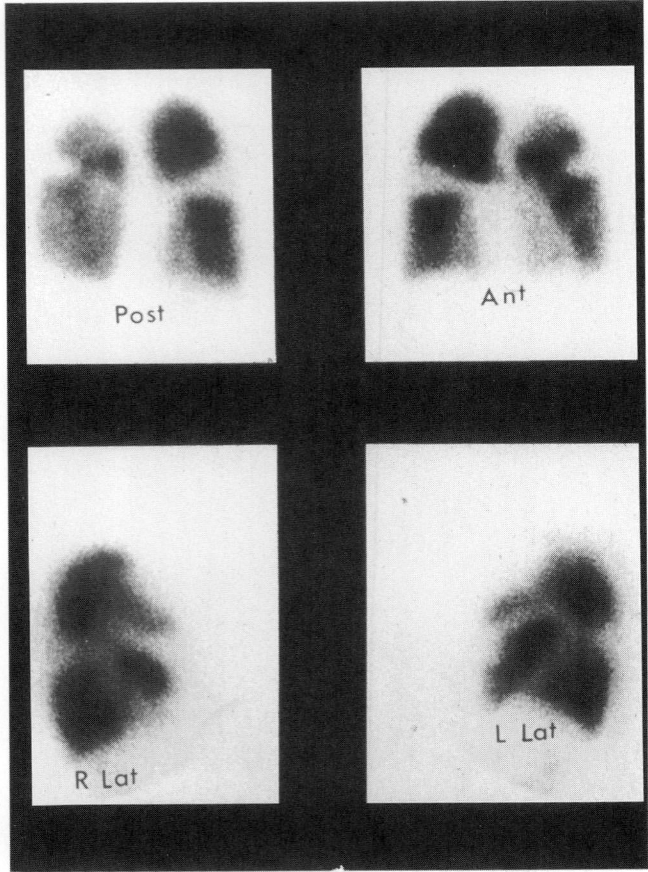

Figure 37–6. This perfusion scan demonstrates areas of loss of perfusion secondary to acute pulmonary embolism.

obstructed, or restricted. PFTs measure the many aspects of ventilation and respiration in objective, quantitative terms (Table 37–6). Information is gathered about lung volumes, air flow rates, diffusion capacity, respiratory muscle strength, and response to bronchodilator therapy. Values are then compared with the patient's cohort matched for gender, age, and height. Serial testing is essential to monitor the progression of disease and the response to treatment.

Inspiratory and expiratory flow volumes are recorded using a graphic format called a flow volume loop (Fig. 37–8A). Volume is plotted on the horizontal axis and flow is plotted on the vertical axis. Examples of abnormal flow–volume loops are found in Figure 37–8B.

In an obstructive pattern, the expiratory flow rate (FEV_1) is reduced in comparison with the vital capacity. That is, the FEV_1/FVC ratio is less than 70%. Criteria for quantifying degree of obstruction are described in Table 37–7A. Because air is trapped distal to the airways in chronic obstruction, the patient hyperinflates the lungs. This is evidenced by an elevated total lung capacity (TLC) and residual volume (RV). Small airways disease, the earliest sign of smoking-induced lung disease (e.g., emphysema), is indicated by a decrement in the FEF_{25-75}.

A restrictive pattern is characterized by diminished lung volumes. Marked reduction is seen in vital capacity and total lung capacity. Because the forced vital capacity (FVC) is reduced, the FEV_1 is also low. The ratio (FEV_1/FVC) is preserved or higher than normal. Criteria for quantifying degree of restriction are described in Table 37–7B.

Arterial Blood Gas. While the main function of the respiratory system is to maintain a physiologic exchange between oxygen and carbon dioxide, it also plays an integral role in maintaining the body's acid–base balance. The arterial blood gas (ABG) describes the blood pH as well as the arterial content of oxygen, carbon dioxide, and bicarbonate. Frequently done in conjunction with pulmonary function testing, this study is also one of the most common lab studies ordered in critical care and emergency settings. Because the lungs have tremendous compensatory reserve, a normal ABG does not rule out pulmonary disease. However, an abnormal ABG in the absence of extrapulmonary disease is highly indicative of pulmonary pathology (Farzan & Farzan, 1997).

Interpretation of ABG results begins with assessment of the patient's acid–base balance. This balance reflects to the ratio between carbonic acid (CO_2) and bicarbonate (HCO_3). Normally between 7.35 and 7.45, a low pH defines acidosis and a high pH defines alkalosis. Acid–base derangements are caused by either a primary respiratory abnormality (characterized by a high or a low PCO_2) or by a primary metabolic process (characterized by a high or a low HCO_3). When an acid–base balance is abnormal, the body compensates by using the system opposite that causing the imbalance (i.e., altering the level of CO_2 to normalize the pH that is deranged by a metabolic disorder or altering the secretion of HCO_3 to normalize the pH that is deranged by a respiratory process). Common causes of respiratory and metabolic acidosis and alkalosis are described in Tables 37–8A and 37–8B.

The measure of PaO_2 reflects the association between oxygen and hemoglobin. When the PaO_2 is greater than 80, the oxygen readily transfers (or dissociates) from the hemoglobin to the cells of the tissues. However, as the PaO_2 drops below this norm, this process of cellular gas exchange is impaired. Factors influencing oxyhemoglobin dissociation include pH, PCO_2, extreme temperature, and abnormal levels of 2,3,DPG. To compensate for hypoxemia, patients are given supplemental oxygen until the underlying cause can be corrected.

Pulse Oximetry Monitoring. Pulse oximetry, or oxygen saturation (SaO_2) monitoring, is a noninvasive and dynamic measure of what percentage of hemoglobin is transporting oxygen. This tool is integral to the cardiopulmonary monitoring from the critical care to the outpatient settings. Normal values range from 93% to 98%, though

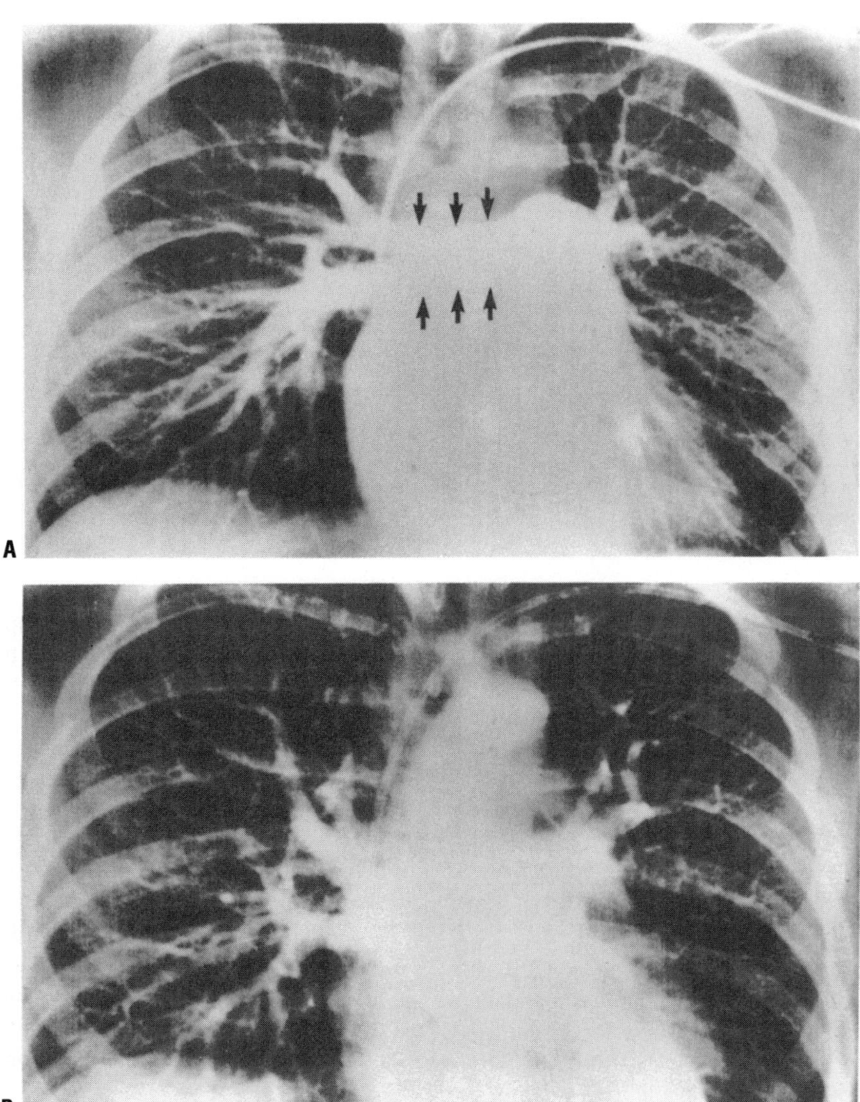

Figure 37–7. A, Pulmonary angiogram during arterial phase. Normal pulmonary artery anatomy is shown on the arterial phase of a normal pulmonary arteriogram. Note the long course of the main right pulmonary artery (arrows). Branches of the left pulmonary artery, in contrast, are given off almost immediately. **B,** Pulmonary angiogram during venous phase. Levophase (venous and left-heart phase of the same pulmonary arteriogram). Note the differing course of the pulmonary veins as compared with the pulmonary arteries. *(From Matthay & Sostman. [1990]. [p. 89].)*

patients with chronic disease may have individualized norms. When the PaO_2 falls below 80, the SaO_2 falls rapidly (Fig. 37–9). Because of the relationship between SaO_2 and PaO_2, information about the patient's tissue oxygenation is readily available. This data has less reliability in pathologic states that alter hemoglobin function (i.e., anemia, polycythemia, carbon monoxide poisoning). The clinician must also be mindful that this data bears no reflection on the patient's acid–base balance or CO_2 level.

Exercise Testing. While the subjective description of pulmonary limitation is captured in the patient's history, objective and quantitative functional data are gathered in formal exercise testing. During exercise, there is an increase in the workload of the respiratory, metabolic, and cardiovascular systems. Physiologic and biochemical changes in these systems are coordinated to facilitate increased oxygen uptake and CO_2 production and clearance. A physiologic defect in any of these systems may manifest itself with respiratory symptoms. Exercise testing is used to determine and quantify the nature of exercise limitations. Measurements are made of O_2 and CO_2 concentrations in expired gas, minute ventilation, and heart rate. Progressive, staged exercise protocols, wherein workload is incrementally in-

Table 37–5. Indications of Bronchoscopy

Diagnostic
Unexplained abnormality on chest radiograph
Unexplained or persistent cough
Hemoptysis
Localized wheeze
Positive sputum cytology
Phrenic or recurrent laryngeal nerve paralysis
Superior vena cava syndrome
Chylothorax
Unexplained pleural effusion
Lung abscess unresponsive to therapy
Evaluation of endotracheal tube placement or complications
Staging of lung cancer
Obtaining culture material
Obtaining tissue for biopsy
Assessment of extent of airway trauma
Tracheoesophalgeal fistula
Assessment of injury secondary to inhalation injury or aspiration
Assessment of response to therapy
Assessment of diffuse lung disease
Therapeutic
Extraction of secretions not mobilized by lesser means
Removal of foreign bodies
Removal of abnormal endobronchial tissue
Endobronchial stent placement
Laser or brachytherapy
Difficult endotracheal tube placement
Lung lavage

Reprinted with permission from Anderson & Light. (1995).

creased, are most often used in clinical practice. Clinical implications of the findings can determine the patient's need for supplemental oxygen, qualification for disability, or suitability for lung transplantation. Several protocols by which to conduct this assessment are available. Most use a treadmill, stationary bicycle, or upper body ergometer to grade exertion. Each measures the patient's perceived exertion and cardiopulmonary response to varying external workloads (Wasserman, Hansen, Sue, Whipp, & Casaburi, 1994).

In the setting of significant debility, certain patients are unable to tolerate comprehensive exercise testing. Serial monitoring of function may not require the expense (financial or physical) associated with full exercise protocols. Adaptations to formal exercise testing are described.

Exercise Desaturation Testing. This study incorporates a subset of the measures from the formal exercise test and is generally better tolerated by more debilitated patients. Monitored by single-lead electrocardiography and pulse oximetry, the patient is exercised on a graded protocol to the point of fatigue, desaturation, or development of limiting symptoms. After recovery, the test is sequentially repeated on a higher level of oxygen (FiO_2), until symptoms, fatigue, or desaturation recur. This study is very useful in determining the appropriate dose of supplemental oxygen at rest and with exertion.

6-Minute Walk Test. This test is a standard baseline assessment and monitoring tool used in outpatient practices and pulmonary rehabilitation programs. While connected to electrocardiography and pulse oximetry, the patient is instructed to walk for 6 minutes (or as much of that time as possible) on level ground at the swiftest, comfortable pace possible. The essential measures include the total time walked, total distance covered, lowest SaO_2, amount of supplemental oxygen, and patient's perceived level of dyspnea (Wasserman, Hanse, Sue, et al., 1994).

▶ PULMONARY DISEASES

Obstructive Lung Diseases

There are five basic mechanisms of airflow obstruction: expiratory airway collapse, bronchospasm, mucosal inflammation with edema, mucous gland hypertrophy, and external compression of the airway (Prakash, 1996). Expiratory airway collapse is the result of progressive loss of elastic recoil. Bronchospasm can be the reaction to vagal stimulation, allergens, hypothermia, or external physical or chemical injury. Mucous gland hypertrophy results from the chronic stimulation of the mucous glands. Tumor compression or structural derangement of the airway are the mechanisms for extrinsic compression of the airway.

Patients with obstructive lung disease may suffer from a single mechanism or a combination of mechanisms. The common disease entities in this category are chronic obstructive pulmonary disease (emphysema and chronic bronchitis), asthma, cystic fibrosis, and bronchiectasis.

Emphysema and Chronic Bronchitis

As previously described, chronic bronchitis is defined by persistent productive cough for a duration of at least three consecutive months for two successive years. Emphysema is characterized by the pathologic dilatation of the air sacs distal to the bronchioles in conjunction with progressive destruction of alveolar walls. Because of the similarities in symptomatology, etiology, and treatment, emphysema and chronic bronchitis must be discussed as a complex known as chronic obstructive pulmonary disease (COPD). It is difficult, and clinically insignificant, to determine whether a patient suffers from one of these processes or both (Burrows, 1990).

COPD is one of the leading causes of death and disability in the United States (ATS, 1995). Although environmental factors are believed to play a small role in the predisposition for COPD, cigarette smoking is felt to be responsible for nearly 90% of all cases (Burrows, 1991). There is a direct relationship between the quantity and duration of cigarette use and the severity of disease. Because

Table 37–6. Frequently Used Measurements in Pulmonary Function Testing

Measurement	Description
Lung Volumes	
Tidal Volume (V_T)	Amount of air inspired and expired during normal breathing. Usually about 5 cc/kg of body weight or 10% of VC. Decreased V_T is suggestive of restrictive disease.
Minute Volume (Ve)	Total amount of air inspired per minute. Ve equals V_T multiplied by respiratory rate.
Inspiratory Reserve Volume (IRV)	The amount of air that can be inspired following normal inspiration. IRV is the V_T subtracted from the inspiratory capacity (IC). IRV is normally reduced during exercise.
Expiratory Reserve Volume (ERV)	The amount of air that can be expired following normal expiration.
Residual Volume (RV)	The amount of air remaining in the lungs following forced expiration. RV equals the ERV subtracted from functional residual capacity (FRC). Markedly elevated RV is indicative of obstructive disease.
Lung Capacities	
Vital Capacity (VC)	Total volume of air that can be expired after maximal inspiration. Typically 70 cc/kg body weight, this is directly measured or can be calculated by adding V_T, IRV, and ERV.
Inspiratory Capacity (IC)	The amount of air that can be inspired after a normal expiration. This is directly measured or can be calculated by adding IRV and V_T. Reduced IC indicates restrictive disease.
Functional Residual Capacity (FRC)	The amount of air in the lungs after a normal expiration. Measured using helium dilution or calculated by adding ERV and RV. Increased FRC indicates hyperinflation of the lungs, which is suggestive of obstructive disease.
Total Lung Capacity (TLC)	The amount of air in the lungs following maximal inspiration. TLC is calculated by adding VC and RV; or FRC and IC; or V_T, IRV, ERV, and RV. Reduced TLC is suggestive of restrictive disease. Elevated TLC is suggestive of obstructive disease.
Forced Vital Capacity (FVC)	This is a direct spirographic measurement. Decreased FVC is suggestive of flow resistance due to obstructive disease.
Forced Expiratory Volume (FEV_1, FEV_2, FEV_3)	Volume of air expired in the first 1, 2, and 3 seconds of the FVC maneuver. This is a direct spirographic measure. Diminished FEV_1 is suggestive of obstructive disease. This value may be reduced or normal in restrictive disease.
FEV_1/FVC Ratio	Expressed as a percentage, this value is normally between 75% and 85%. The FEV_1/FVC tends to decrease to 65% to 75% with normal aging. A reduction in this value is the most important marker for obstructive disease. The FEV_1/FVC may be normal or elevated in restrictive disease.
Flow Rates	
Forced Expiratory Flow (FEF_{25}, FEF_{50}, FEF_{75})	The amount of air forcibly expired at 25%, 50%, and 75% points of the FVC.
Forced Expiratory Flow $_{25\text{–}75}$ ($FEF_{25\text{–}75}$)	The average flow during the middle half (25% and 75% points) of an FVC maneuver. Recorded in liters per second, this value is reduced in the setting of obstructive small airways disease.
Maximal Voluntary Ventilation (MVV)	The greatest amount of air breathed into and out of the lungs in a 10- to 15-second interval with voluntary effort. This is a direct spirographic measurement. The MVV is diminished in the setting of severe obstructive disease or respiratory muscle dysfunction.
Peak Expiratory Flow Rate (PEFR)	The maximal flow rate achieved during the FVC maneuver. This effort-dependent measure primarily measures large airway function.
Diffusion Capacity	
Diffusion Capacity of Carbon Monoxide (DL_{CO})	The milliliters per minute of carbon monoxide (CO) diffused across the alveolar–capillary membrane in one minute. This is measured by subtracting the amount of CO exhaled from the amount inhaled in one minute. A diminished value reflects a thickened alveolar capillary membrane, which is highly suggestive of interstitial disease.
Pulmonary Pressures	
Maximal Inspiratory Pressure (MIP)	This assesses inspiratory muscle strength. Normally greater than −60 cm H_2O, the MIP measures the greatest negative pressure that can be generated against an occluded airway. Decreased MIP is suggestive of disorders of the diaphragm, intercostal, or accessory muscles. This may also be seen in obstructive disease with hyperinflation of the lungs imposing upon the movement of the diaphragm.
Maximal Expiratory Pressure (MEP)	This assesses expiratory muscle strength by measuring the highest pressure generated during the forced expiration against an occluded airway. Normally greater than 80 to 100 cm H_2O, this value is influenced by the strength of the accessory muscles, the abdominal muscles, and the elastic recoil of the lungs and thorax.

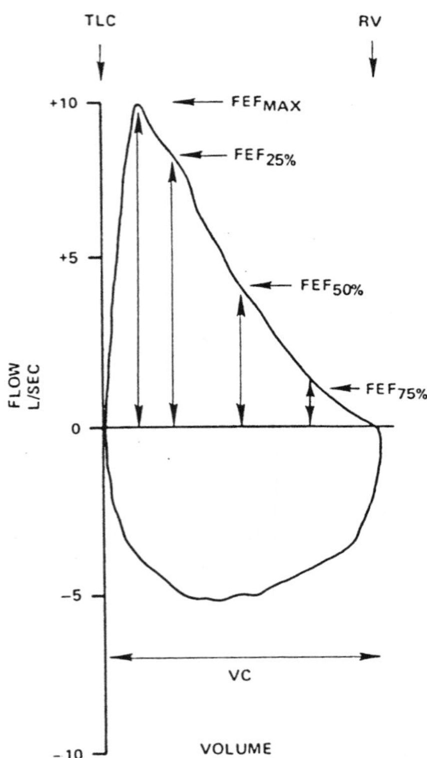

Figure 37–8A. A typical flow-volume loop from a normal subject showing both expiratory (upper) and inspiratory (lower) portions. Instantaneous flows may be measured after 25% ($FEF_{25\%}$), 50% ($FEF_{50\%}$), and 75% ($FEF_{75\%}$) of the vital capacity has been exhaled. The peak flow is easily measured as the value of the peak of the graph.

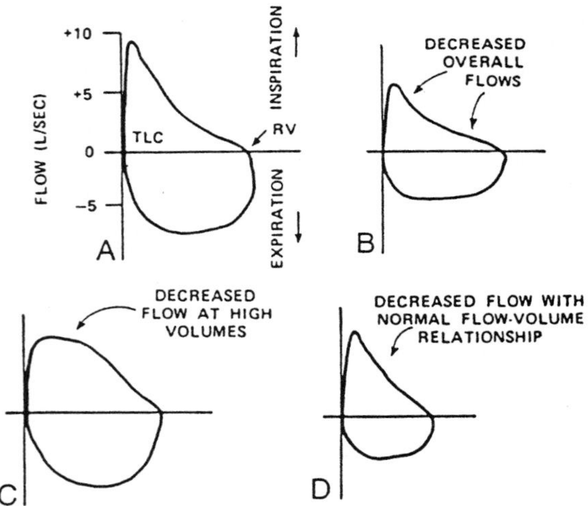

Figure 37–8B. Common examples of abnormal flow volume loops. **A,** Mild obstructive airway disease characterized by decreased flow at low lung volume when elastic support is reduced. **B,** Significant obstructive airway disease characterized by decreased overall flows with a further decrease at low lung volumes. **C,** Variable intrathoracic large airway obstruction in which peak flow is decreased at higher lung volumes with preservation of normal flow–volume relationship at lower lung volumes. **D,** Restrictive pulmonary disease with decreased vital capacity and flows but preservation of normal flow–volume relationships. *(Reprinted with permission from Light. [1995]. [p. 134].)*

of the large reserve of the lung, symptoms generally do not appear until the sixth and seventh decades of life. Evidence of COPD may be present, even if cessation of smoking took place years earlier. Following chronic irritation of the bronchial mucosa, mucous-producing glands become hypertrophied and hyperplastic. Loss of cilia and altered pulmonary secretions impair airway clearance which contributes to hypersensitivity of irritant receptors, bronchial hyperreactivity, and chronic cough.

Symptomatology, morbidity, and mortality are progressive, though the course of COPD is unpredictable. It is marked by recurrent episodes of intercurrent bacterial infections, exacerbations of airways obstruction, loss of functional capacity and, in advanced stages, hypercarbia and hypoxemia (Ries, 1997).

The natural history of this disease process is highly variable, so an individual's prognosis is difficult to predict. The measurement of the FEV_1 is considered the best prognostic indicator, with more severe decrements suggesting shorter survival. The development of cor pulmonale and right heart failure portends an extremely poor prognosis. Smoking cessation and supplemental oxygen use are the only interventions shown to favorably alter survival in COPD. Strategies to assist patients in smoking cessation are discussed later in this chapter. Respiratory failure is the most common cause of death in this patient population (Panettieri & Murray, 1994).

The most common presenting symptom is dyspnea on

TABLE 37–7A. Criteria for Quantitating Degree of Obstruction

Grade	FEV_1/FVC	FEV_1 (ml)
Very severe	<0.30	<600
Severe	0.3–0.4	600–1000
Moderate	0.4–0.6	1000–2000
Mild	0.6–0.7	2000–3000
Very mild	0.7–predicted value	>3000

Reprinted with permission from Light. (1995). (p. 152).

TABLE 37–7B. Criteria for Quantitating Degree of Restriction

Grade	VC % Predicted	TLC % Predicted
Very mild	>80	>90
Mild	60–80	70–90
Moderate	30–60	50–70
Severe	<30	<50

Reprinted with permission from Light. (1995). (p. 153).

TABLE 37–8A. Common Causes of Respiratory Acidosis and Alkalosis

Respiratory Acidosis	Respiratory Alkalosis
Causes	Causes
Hypoventilation	Hyperventilation
COPD	Pulmonary embolism
Sedation	Severe pain
Clinical manifestations	Anxiety
Dyspnea	Brain-stem disease
Headache	Chronic overventilation on controlled ventilator
Mental confusion	Clinical manifestations
Pallor	Dizziness
Sweating	Tingling, numbness
Apprehension, restlessness	Restlessness, agitation
ABG measurements (example)	Tetany
pH 7.24	ABG measurements (example)
$PaCO_2$ 60	pH 7.48
HCO_3^- 24	$PaCO_2$ 30
Treatment	HCO_3^- 22
Determine and treat cause	Treatment
Maintain adequate respiratory minute volume	Identify and treat cause
Increase tidal volume or increase respiratory rate	Sedate patient
Suctioning	Reduce respiratory minute volume
	Decrease tidal volume or decrease respiratory rate
	Reassure and support patient

ABG: arterial blood gas; COPD: chronic obstructive pulmonary disease.

TABLE 37–8B. Common Causes of Metabolic Acidosis and Alkalosis

Metabolic Acidosis	Metabolic Alkalosis
Causes	Causes
Cardiac arrest	Vomiting
Diabetic ketoacidosis	Gastric suctioning
Poisoning (acetylsalicylic acid, methyl alcohol, ethylene glycol, paraldehyde)	Sodium bicarbonate overload
Renal failure	Diuretics
Diarrhea (loss of HCO_3^-)	Adrenal disease
Clinical manifestations	Corticosteroids
Lethargy	Clinical manifestations
Nausea, vomiting	Dullness
Dysrhythmias	Weakness
Coma	Dysrhythmias
ABG measurements (example)	Tetany
pH 7.30	Hypokalemia
$PaCO_2$ 40	ABG measurements (example)
HCO_3^- 15	pH 7.50
Treatment	$PaCO_2$ 40
Identify and treat cause	HCO_3^- 40
Give sodium bicarbonate	Treatment
	Identify and treat cause
	Correct dehydration
	Correct hypokalemia
	Acetazolamide (Diamox)
	Ammonium chloride
	Arginine monohydrochloride

ABG: arterial blood gas.
Reprinted with permission from Guzetta. (1992). (p. 299).

exertion. Other important historical features are cough, sputum production and frequent lung infections and, of course, cigarette use. Anxiety, restlessness, sleep pattern disturbance, and early satiety are all secondary symptoms of this disorder that warrant attention. Frequently, the patient's history reveals chronic progressive exertional dyspnea that may be attributed, by the patient, to advancing age or decline in fitness. Patients may also describe a critical event, like a cold, from which they never fully recovered. Individuals who ignore their symptoms often come to medical attention during crisis associated with an exacerbation of their disease (Farzan & Farzan, 1997). During an exacerbation, airways are further narrowed, causing further obstruction, in response to noxious exposures (e.g., virus, allergenic substance).

The physical findings of COPD are dependent upon the stage and severity of the disease. Early in the disease process, clinical examination may be unremarkable. Diminished breath sounds, a widened anterior–posterior thoracic diameter (barrel chest), and reduced thoracic excursion are clinical features of this process. Breath sounds may be absent over areas with airflow obstruction or severe bullous disease. Wheezing is heard in the setting of bronchospasm. Coarse rhochi indicate secretions in the large airways. Pa-

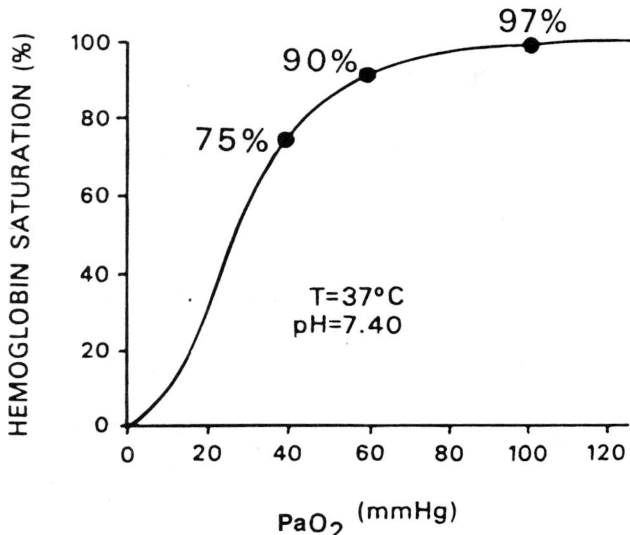

Figure 37–9. The normal oxyhemoglobin dissociation curve at pH 7.4 and temperature 37°C. Saturations at three key points are marked. Hyperthermia shifts the curve to the right and hypothermia shifts it to the left. Acidemia shifts it to the right and alkalemia to the left (Bohr effect). *(Reprinted with permission from George. [1995]. [p. 67].)*

tients with COPD frequently report a daily cough productive of clear to yellow sputum. The use of accessory muscles, pursed-lip breathing, tachypnea, and tripod positioning (leaning forward with elbows out and neck extended) may be demonstrated by patients with severe COPD. Signs of right heart failure (e.g., pedal edema, hepatomegaly, or cyanosis) are suggestive of longstanding hypoxemia.

The diagnosis of COPD is made on the basis of clinical history, chest radiograph, and pulmonary function tests. Pulmonary function tests demonstrate a reduction in expiratory flow rates (due to narrowing of the airways) and the FEV_1/FVC ratio is less than 70% (indicating an obstructive pattern). The FEV_1 is the most sensitive measure of disease severity as it correlates with exercise tolerance and survival (Ries, 1997). A bronchodilator, typically albuterol, is administered during the study to assess reversibility of airways obstruction.

In early stages, the PA and lateral chest x-ray may have a normal appearance. However, in advanced stages, chest x-ray can confirm the presence of obstructive lung disease. Hyperinflated lung fields with flattened diaphragms and widening of the anterior–posterior diameter and hyperlucency (Fig. 37–10) are highly suggestive of chronic air trapping. Changes seen on baseline chest radiograph do not regress. On the contrary, hyperinflation, noted during an exacerbation, may improve with resolution of the crisis.

Treatment for COPD begins with cessation of cigarette use. Benefit from other therapy is very limited in the setting of persistent smoking. The goals of treatment are to slow the loss of function and prevent intercurrent infections while minimizing the severity of symptoms. A step-by-step guide to pharmacologic therapy for COPD is detailed in Table 37–9A. Precautions regarding these agents are detailed in Table 37–9B. Because of their predisposition to lung infections, COPD patients are advised to be immunized against influenza and pneumococcal pneumonia. For those patients who demonstrate a diminished functional capacity, pulmonary rehabilitation (discussed later in this chapter) is strongly indicated. Pharmacotherapy typically involves a combination of bronchodilators, corticosteroids and, when indicated, antibiotics (Ferguson & Cherniak, 1993).

When airway responsiveness has been established by PFTs, bronchodilators can be prescribed. The drugs that may be used alone or in combination are sympathomimetic beta-agonists, anticholinergics, and methylxanthines (Theophylline). Drugs administered by nebulizer or metered-dose inhaler must be introduced to the patient and family with thorough teaching (Fig. 37–11). The effectiveness of these agents is frequently compromised by improper administration technique (Lindell & Mazzocco, 1990). For this reason, it is strongly advised that patients demonstrate their inhaler technique at each clinical encounter (NAEPP, 1997).

The role of systemic corticosteroids in the treatment of COPD is somewhat controversial. Long-term use of these drugs is associated with many serious side effects. How-

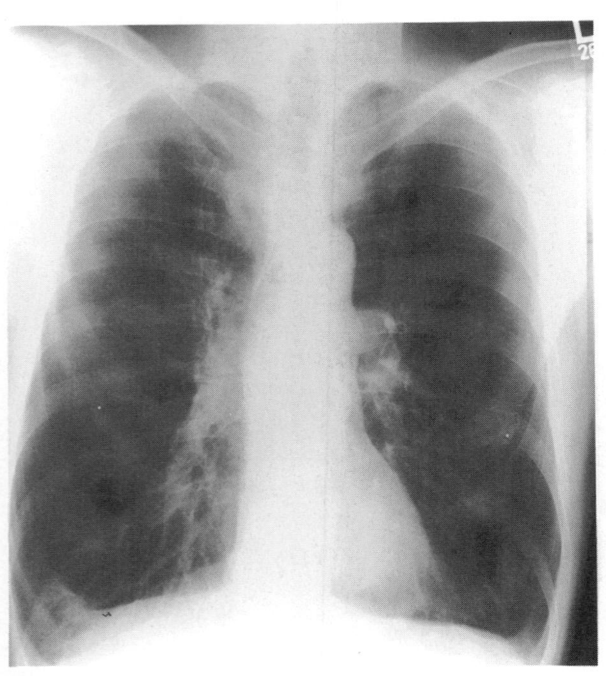

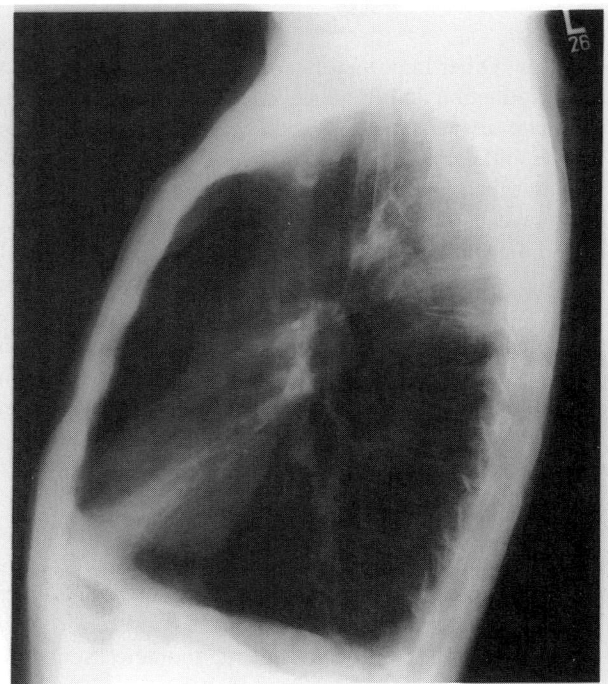

Figure 37–10. Chest radiograph of a 58-year-old white male ex-smoker with severe emphysema. **A,** Flattening of the diaphragm with hyperinflation of the lung fields, hyperlucency of the upper lung fields, and vascular attenuation are classic radiographic features of COPD. **B,** A wide anterior–posterior (AP) diameter is noted on the lateral view.

TABLE 37–9A. Step-by-Step Pharmacologic Therapy for COPD

1. For mild, variable symptoms:
   - Selective β_2-agonist metered dose inhaler (MDI) aerosol, 1–2 puffs every 2–6 h as needed not to exceed 8–12 puffs per 24 h
2. For mild to moderate continuing symptoms:
   - Ipratropium MDI aerosol, 2–6 puffs every 6–8 h; not to be used more frequently

   plus
   - Selective β_2-agonist MDI aerosol, 1–4 puffs as required four times daily for rapid relief, when needed, or as regular supplement
3. If response to step 2 is unsatisfactory, or there is a mild to moderate increase in symptoms:
   - Add sustained release theophylline, 200–400 mg twice daily or 400–800 mg at bedtime for nocturnal bronchospasm

   and/or
   - Consider use of sustained release albuterol, 4–8 mg twice daily, or at night only

   and/or
   - Consider use of mucokinetic agent
4. If control of symptoms is suboptimal:
   - Consider course of oral steroids (e.g., prednisone), up to 40 mg/d for 10–14 d
     —If improvement occurs, wean to low daily or alternate-day dose, e.g., 7.5 mg
     —If no improvement occurs, stop abruptly
     —If steroid appears to help, consider possible use of aerosol MDI, particularly if patient has evidence of bronchial hyperreactivity
5. For severe exacerbation:
   - Increase β_2-agonist dosage, e.g., MDI with spacer 6–8 puffs every 1/2–2 h or inhalant solution, unit dose every 1/2–2 h or subcutaneous administration of epinephrine or terbutaline, 0.1–0.5 mL

   and/or
   - Increase ipratropium dosage, e.g., MDI with spacer 6–8 puffs every 3–4 h or inhalant solution of ipratropium 0.5 mg every 4–8 h

   and
   - Provide theophylline dosage intravenously with calculated amount to bring serum level to 10–12 μg/mL

   and
   - Provide methylprednisolone dosage intravenously giving 50–100 mg immediately, then every 6–8 h; taper as soon as possible

   and add:
   - An antibiotic, if indicated
   - A mucokinetic agent if sputum is very viscous

From American Thoracic Society Statement. (1995). (p. 586).

ever, many patients report subjective improvement of their symptoms. A short tapering course of corticosteroids may help a patient who is suffering with an exacerbation of his or her symptoms. The role of inhaled steroids has not been well-defined (Ries, 1997).

Secretion management is largely nonpharmacologic. Coughing techniques and postural drainage are useful to some patients. Because of the protective mechanism of the cough, cough suppressants are not recommended. When the mucopurulence of the sputum changes, indicating infection,

TABLE 37–9B. Precautions for Use of Medications for COPD

Precautions when using beta-agonists
- Watch for nonimprovement or paradoxical deterioration with aerosol use
- Use spacers to improve compliance and reduce systemic side effects
- Avoid overuse; check number of metered dose inhalers (MDIs) used per month against number of puffs per MDI (200 to 300+ depending on brand).
- Instruct patient on maximum number of puffs per day (usually 8–12) and on number allowed during an exacerbation (e.g., 12–24 over 3–4 h) before additional intervention is required
- If a long-acting agent is used, caution patient that frequent use must be avoided
- Home updraft nebulizers with inhalant solutions that provide large dosages are rarely needed

Precautions when using theophylline
- Initiate treatment with a low dose (e.g., 400 mg/d) and adjust after a few days
- Reduce dosage if drug clearance is likely to be impaired because of illness, liver malfunction, or concomitant drugs.
- Do not allow any additional theophylline preparation to be taken
- Drug must be taken at the same time each day with respect to meals
- When symptoms change, acute illness develops, new drugs are added, or symptoms suggestive of toxicity develop, check serum level of theophylline
- Aim for a serum level of 8–12 μg/mL; adjust dosage and follow serum level when indicated

Precautions when using ipratropium
- Patients should generally use a spacer and should avoid spraying into eyes
- Be prepared to increase dose if necessary from 2–3 puffs 3–4 times a day to 6–8 puffs 3–4 times a day, if tolerated
- Caution patient that onset of effect is relatively slow; additional doses should not be taken for acute symptom relief
- Monitor for side effects, e.g., tachycardia, dry mouth, glaucoma, prostatism, or bladder neck obstruction

Precautions when using oral steroids
- Reduce dosage to lowest effective daily dose or to alternate-day dosing as quickly as symptoms allow
- Monitor for hypertension, diabetes, weight gain, mental changes, infections, central polar cataracts, skin thinning, purpura, osteoporosis, and osteonecrosis
- Distinguish psychological benefit from true pulmonary benefit by following FEV_1 for 2 wk after initiating therapy
- Administer prophylactic calcium therapy to women; treat osteoporosis appropriately
- Steroid-dependent patients require steroid coverage during any crisis for many months after stopping steroids
- Repeatedly evaluate patient to determine if steroid therapy can be discontinued

Precautions when using aerosol steroids
- Seek objective evidence of the value of this therapy because its use may decrease compliance with other aerosol usage
- Standard dosing (2–4 puffs 2–4 times a day) should not be exceeded
- Use a spacer; monitor for oral thrush and laryngeal dysfunction
- Be aware that aerosol steroid side effects may occur in skin, bone, etc.
- When introducing aerosol steroids in a patient on an oral steroid, wean slowly off the oral drug

From American Thoracic Society Statement. (1995). (p. 588).

Please demonstrate your inhaler technique at every visit.

1. Remove the cap and hold inhaler upright.
2. Shake the inhaler.
3. Tilt your head back slightly and breathe out slowly.
4. Position the inhaler in one of the following ways (A or B is optimal, but C is acceptable for those who have difficulty with A or B. C is required for breath-activated inhalers):

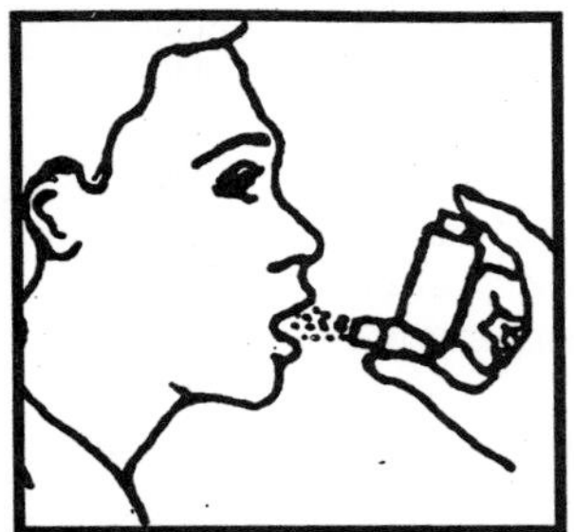

A. Open mouth with inhaler 1 to 2 inches away.

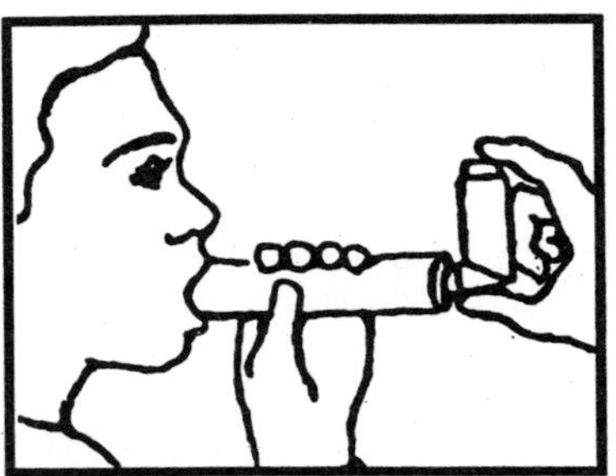

B. Use spacer/holding chamber (that is recommended especially for young children and for people using corticosteroids).

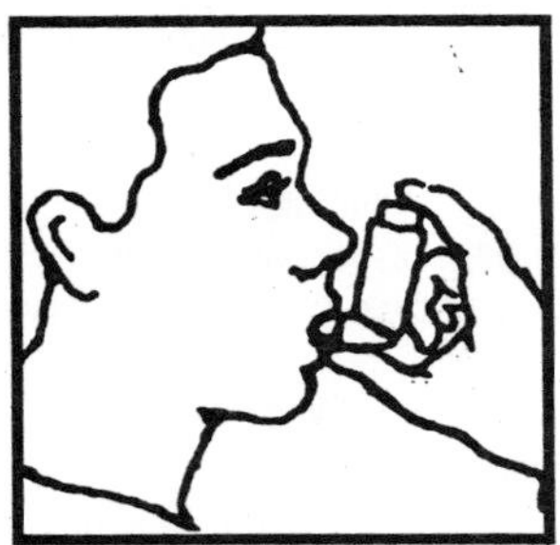

C. In the mouth. Do not use for corticosteroids.

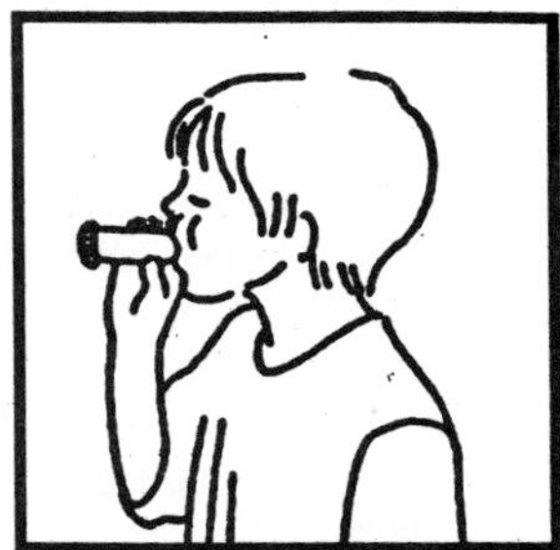

D. NOTE: Inhaled dry powder capsules require a different inhalation technique. To use a dry powder inhaler, it is important to close the mouth tightly around the mouthpiece of the inhaler and to inhale rapidly.

5. Press down on the inhaler to release medication as you start to breathe in slowly.
6. Breathe in slowly (3 to 5 seconds).
7. Hold your breath for 10 seconds to allow the medicine to reach deeply into your lungs.
8. Repeat puff as directed. Waiting 1 minute between puffs may permit second puff to penetrate your lungs better.
9. Spacers/holding chambers are useful for all patients. They are particularly recommended for young children and older adults and for use with inhaled corticosteroids.

Avoid common inhaler mistakes. Follow these inhaler tips:

- Breathe out *before* pressing your inhaler.
- Inhale *slowly*.
- Breathe in through your mouth, not your nose.
- Press down on your inhaler at the *start* of inhalation (or within the first second of inhalation).
- Keep inhaling as you press down on inhaler.
- Press your inhaler only *once* while you are inhaling (one breath for each puff).
- Make sure you breathe in evenly and deeply.

NOTE: Other inhalers are becoming available in addition to those illustrated above. Different types of inhalers may require different techniques.

Figure 37–11. Steps for proper use of the multi-dose inhaler (MDI). *(From the National Asthma Education and Prevention Program [NAEPP]. [1997]. [p. 73].)*

a 7- to 10-day course of antibiotics is recommended. The common pathogens that colonize the airways are *H influenzae, S pneumoniae,* and *M catarrhalis* (Murphy & Sethi, 1992).

Other therapy is aimed at the extrapulmonary sequelae of this disease. Because of hyperinflation of the lungs, the diaphragm may impose upon the stomach causing early satiety. If weight loss or muscle loss is noted, the patient should be seen by a dietician for recommendations regarding protein supplementation. A regular exercise regimen is important in maintaining functional capacity. Anxiolytic therapy may be necessary to reduce the anxiety associated with dyspnea.

Serial measures of spirometry are used to monitor the disease's progression and the patient's response to treatment. In certain severe situations, patients should be referred for consideration for lung volume reduction surgery or lung transplantation. Surgical intervention for emphysema is discussed in greater detail in Chapter 38.

Alpha-1 Antitrypsin Deficiency. Alpha-1 antitrypsin (A1AT) deficiency is a rare, autosomal recessive, genetic abnormality that leads to the development of precocious emphysema. Synthesized by hepatocytes, A1AT is a glycoprotein that protects the elastin content of the lung by inhibiting proteolytic enzymes. Cigarette use is a catalyst for lung destruction. The chronic inflammation caused by cigarette use attracts neutrophils. Neutrophils release proteolytic enzymes that are normally inhibited by A1AT. In the absence of sufficient A1AT, the proteolytic enzymes overwhelm the antineutrophil elastase defense mechanisms of the lung resulting in progressive destruction of elastin and premature development of emphysema. Patients who present with COPD in the fourth and fifth decades of life, particularly if there is a strong family history of COPD, should be suspected of having A1AT deficiency. Chest x-ray typically demonstrates hyperinflated lung fields with hyperlucency most notable at the bases. Confirmation of clinical suspicions are made by sending serum for alpha-1 antitrypsin level. Treatment is essentially the same as common emphysema. Though long-term results are not as yet available, there is hope that administration of synthetic A1AT (Prolastin), through weekly intravenous infusion, may slow the rate of decline in pulmonary function (ATS, 1989).

Asthma

Asthma is characterized by recurrent episodes of reversible airway obstruction secondary to smooth muscle contraction and bronchial hyperactivity, airway inflammation, and increased airway responsiveness to certain stimuli. It may be accompanied by mucosal inflammation or mucous plugging of the lumen of the bronchi. This disease entity is estimated to effect between 5% and 7% of the population, with half of the reported cases beginning earlier than age 10 (ATS, 1995). The incidence and associated morbidity and mortality of asthma have risen 31% over recent decades (Osbone & Deffebach, 1997). Among African-Americans, the death rate is nearly three times higher than among white Americans. Prevalence and mortality are increased in urban areas, particularly in school-aged children. Factors contributing to the increased mortality and morbidity of asthma are described in Table 37–10.

The precise mechanism of asthma is not well understood. Increased airway resistance reduces the forced expiratory flow rates (peak expiratory flow rate and FEV_1) which causes hyperinflation. This leads to an increase in the respiratory workload, requiring use of accessory muscles. In severe cases, mucous plugging and bronchoconstriction can result in ventilation–perfusion mismatch. Untreated, this can cause hypoxemia and progressive hypercapnea. In the absence of effective therapy, hypercapnea is followed by rapid deterioration and death (Farzan & Farzan, 1997).

The National Asthma Education and Prevention Program (NAEPP) was established to develop strategies and make recommendations to better serve this population. This expert panel set forth clinical practice guidelines for the diagnosis and management of asthma. These guidelines delineate the four components necessary to the care of patients with asthma (National Asthma Education and Prevention Program [NAEPP], 1997). Recommendations are detailed in Table 37–11, though any clinician working with asthmatic patients should be familiar with the original document.

Asthma is described as extrinsic or intrinsic in nature. Extrinsic asthma is characterized by the association between exposure to certain "triggers" (antigens or external factors) and episodes of bronchospasm. The most common provocative factors to extrinsic asthma are outlined in Table 37–12. If not withdrawn, triggers may also exacerbate an asthma attack. Though the pathophysiology is identical, intrinsic asthma is not associated with specific triggers. It presents in older individuals and tends to run a persistent course of unrelenting decline.

The clinical presentation may be acute or chronic. Commonly, patients complain of a triad of symptoms including cough, wheeze, and dyspnea. The presence of any singular symptom warrants the inclusion of asthma in the differential diagnosis. The classic physical exam finding is diffuse wheezing heard throughout the lung fields. Characteristically, paroxysmal episodes of airway obstruction are reversible and are interspersed with asymptomatic periods. In assessing the patient's history, it is crucial to differentiate extrinsic asthma from occupational lung disease. Variation in severity and duration of episodes may be reported. Patients frequently report that symptoms are worse late at night and early in the morning. Most asthma attacks start with mild symptoms, a cough or wheeze, that escalate to the point of dyspnea, accessory muscle use, and respiratory compromise (Osborne & Deffebach, 1997).

The suspected diagnosis of asthma is confirmed by relief of symptoms with bronchodilator therapy. Pulmonary function testing is used to quantify responsiveness to therapy (typically albuterol). Provocation of airway hyperreactivity, though rarely done, examines the degree of airway response to histamine or methacholine and the subsequent reversibility of airway obstruction with time or bronchodilator therapy. This study is known as a methacholine challenge.

TABLE 37–11. Guidelines for the Diagnosis and Management of Asthma

Component 1:	Initial Assessment and Diagnosis of Asthma Periodic Assessment and Monitoring
Component 2:	Control of Factors Contributing to Asthma Severity
Component 3:	Pharmacologic Therapy
Component 4:	Education for a Partnership in Asthma Care

From National Asthma Education and Prevention Program (NAEPP). (1997).

TABLE 37–10. Factors Contributing to the Increased Morbidity and Mortality of Asthma

Increased allergen exposure
Increased incidence of viral infections
Inadequate access to health care
Improper assessment of severity of episodes by patient and/or clinician
Inappropriate therapy
Improper medication delivery (i.e., improper use of inhalers)

TABLE 37–12. Common Triggers of Asthma

Viral infection of respiratory tract
Respirable irritants or allergens
Tobacco smoke
Exercise
Cold air
Certain food additives (sulfites, preservatives, or dyes)
Certain medications (especially aspirin, NSAIDs, or beta blockers)
Extreme emotions
Gastroesophageal reflux

The treatment of asthma is based on the severity of the individual case. The NAEPP (1997) categorizes asthma severity as: severe persistent, moderate persistent, mild persistent, or mild intermittent. Essential aspects of care include long-term control, quick relief, and patient education. The stepwise approach for managing asthma, from the clinical practice guidelines of the NAEPP, is found in Table 37–13. The usual medication dosages for both quick relief and long-term control of asthma are outlined in Tables 37–14A and 37–14B.

Acute asthma exacerbations, or attacks, are categorized as mild, moderate, or severe. Table 37–15 provides guidelines for making the clinical distinction among these categories. Initial treatment requires the use of a short-

TABLE 37–13. Stepwise Approach for Managing Asthma in Adults and Children Older Than 5 Years of Age

<table>
<tr><th></th><th colspan="2">Treatment</th><th>Preferred Treatments Are in Bold Print</th></tr>
<tr><th></th><th>Long-Term Control</th><th>Quick Relief</th><th>Education</th></tr>
<tr><td>STEP 4
Severe Persistent</td><td>Daily medications:
■ Anti-inflammatory: inhaled corticosteroid (high dose)
AND
■ Long-acting broncholdilator: either long-acting inhaled beta$_2$-agonist, sustained-release theophylline, or long-acting beta$_2$-agonist tablets
AND
■ Corticosteroid tablets or syrup long term (2 mg/kg/day, generally do not exceed 60 mg per day).</td><td>■ Short-acting bronchodilator: inhaled beta$_2$-agonists as needed for symptoms.
■ Intensity of treatment will depend on severity of exacerbation; see component 3—Managing Exacerbations.
■ Use of short-acting inhaled beta$_2$-agonists on a daily basis, or increasing use, indicates the need for additional long-term-control therapy.</td><td>Steps 2 and 3 actions plus:
■ Refer to individual education/counseling</td></tr>
<tr><td>STEP 3
Moderate Persistent</td><td>Daily medication:
■ Either
Anti-inflammatory: inhaled corticosteroid (medium dose)
OR
Inhaled corticosteroid (low-medium dose) and add a long-acting bronchodilator, especially for nighttime symptoms: either long-acting inhaled beta$_2$-agonist, sustained-release theophylline, or long-acting beta$_2$-agonist tablets.
■ If needed
Anti-inflammatory: inhaled corticosteroids (medium-high dose)
AND
Long-acting bronchodilator, especially for nighttime symptoms; either long-acting inhaled beta$_2$-agonist, sustained-release theophylline, or long-acting beta$_2$-agonist tablets.</td><td>■ Short-acting bronchodilator: inhaled beta$_2$-agonists as needed for symptoms.
■ Intensity of treatment will depend on severity of exacerbation; see component 3—Managing Exacerbations.
■ Use of short-acting inhaled beta$_2$-agonists on a daily basis, or increasing use, indicates the need for additional long-term-control therapy.</td><td rowspan="2">Step 1 actions plus:
■ Teach self-monitoring
■ Refer to group education if available
■ Review and update self-management plan</td></tr>
<tr><td>STEP 2
Mild Persistent</td><td>One daily medication:
■ Anti-inflammatory: either inhaled corticosteroid (low doses) or cromolyn or nedocromil (children usually begin with a trial of cromolyn or nedocromil).
■ Sustained-release theophylline to serum concentration of 5–15 mcg/mL is an alternative, but not preferred, therapy. Zafirlukast or zileuton may also be considered for patients ≥ 12 years of age, although their position in therapy is not fully established.</td><td>■ Short-acting bronchodilator: inhaled beta$_2$-agonists as needed for symptoms.
■ Intensity of treatment will depend on severity of exacerbation; see component 3—Managing Exacerbations.
■ Use of short-acting inhaled beta$_2$-agonists on a daily basis, or increasing use, indicates the need for additional long-term-control therapy.</td></tr>
</table>

TABLE 37–13. Stepwise Approach for Managing Asthma in Adults and Children Older than 5 Years of Age *(Continued)*

	Treatment	Preferred Treatments Are in Bold Print	
	Long-Term Control	**Quick Relief**	**Education**
STEP 1 Mild Intermittent	■ No daily medication needed.	■ Short-acting bronchodilator: **inhaled beta$_2$-agonists** as needed for symptoms. ■ Intensity of treatment will depend on severity of exacerbation; see component 3—Managing Exacerbations. ■ Use of short-acting inhaled beta$_2$-agonists more than 2 times a week may indicate the need to initiate long-term-control therapy.	■ Teach basic facts about asthma ■ Teach inhaler/spacer/ holding chamber technique ■ Discuss roles of medications ■ Develop self-management plan ■ Develop action plan for when and how to take rescue actions, especially for patients with a history of severe exacerbations ■ Discuss appropriate environmental control measures to avoid exposure to known allergens and irritants (See component 4.)

Step down
Review treatment every 1 to 6 months; a gradual stepwise reduction in treatment may be possible.

Step up
If control is not maintained, consider step up. First, review patient medication technique, adherence, and environmental control (avoidance of allergens or other factors that contribute to asthma severity).

NOTE:

- **The stepwise approach presents general guidelines to assist clinical decisionmaking; it is not intended to be a specific prescription. Asthma is highly variable; clinicians should tailor specific medication plans to the needs and circumstances of individual patients.**
- Gain control as quickly as possible: then decrease treatment to the least medication necessary to maintain control. Gaining control may be accomplished by either starting treatment at the step most appropriate to the initial severity of the condition or starting at a higher level of therapy (e.g., a course of systemic corticosteroids or higher dose of inhaled corticosteroids).
- A rescue course of systemic corticosteroids may be needed at any time and at any step.
- Some patients with intermittent asthma experience severe and life-threatening exacerbations separated by long periods of normal lung function and no symptoms. This may be especially common with exacerbations provoked by respiratory infections. A short course of systemic corticosteroids is recommended.
- At each step, patients should control their environment to avoid or control factors that make their asthma worse (e.g., allergens, irritants); this requires specific diagnosis and education.
- Referral to an asthma specialist for consultation or comanagement is *recommended* if there are difficulties achieving or maintaining control of asthma or if the patient requires step 4 care. Referral may be *considered* if the patient requires step 3 care (see also component 1—Initial Assessment and Diagnosis).

From National Asthma Education and Prevention Program (NAEPP). (1997).

acting beta$_2$-agonist (a single nebulizer treatment or up to three doses of 2 to 4 puffs by MDI at 20-minute intervals). Patients who achieve a good response are encouraged to contact their clinician for follow-up instructions. Those who achieve an incomplete response are instructed to contact their clinician urgently (i.e., same day) for care. Those who achieve a poor response to this therapy are instructed to proceed immediately to the local emergency department (NAEPP, 1997). Emergency department and hospital-based care of the patient with an asthma exacerbation is described in the flow chart in Figure 37–12.

Optimal care of the asthmatic requires ongoing patient education. Salient features of the teaching plan are outlined in Table 37–16. It is imperative that asthmatic patients be educated as partners in their care. Patient education should begin at the time of initial diagnosis and be reinforced with each subsequent encounter by all members of the health-care team. Concepts to be covered are: basic facts about asthma, the roles of medication and self monitoring, proper use of inhalers, environmental control tactics, and emergency protocols as well as the importance of follow-up care (NAEPP, 1997).

Bronchiectasis

Bronchiectasis is a chronic disease defined by the irreversible dilatation of the bronchi and bronchioles with inflammation and destruction of the segmental or subsegmetal conducting airways. This process more commonly involves a localized portion of the lung, but may be diffuse throughout all lung fields. Repeated secondary infection is a result of impaired clearance of bronchial secretions. Ongoing infection contributes to progressive destruction of the bronchi

TABLE 37–14A. Usual Dosages for Long-Term Control Medications

Medication	Dosage Form	Adult Dose	Child Dose	Comments
Inhaled Corticosteroids				
Systemic Corticosteroids		(Applies to all three systemic corticosteroids)		
Methylprednisolone Prednisolone Prednisone	2, 4, 8, 16, 32 mg tablets 5 mg tablets, 5 mg/cc, 15 mg/cc 1, 2.5, 5, 10, 20, 25 mg tablets; 5 mg/cc solution	■ 7.5–60 mg daily in a single dose or qid as needed for control ■ Short-course "burst": 40–60 mg per day as single or 2 divided doses for 3–10 days	■ 0.25–2 mg/kg daily in single dose or qid as needed for control ■ Short course "burst": 1–2 mg/kg/day, maximum 60 mg/day, for 3–10 days	■ For long-term treatment of severe persistent asthma, administer single dose in a.m. either daily or on alternate days (alternate-day therapy may produce less adrenal suppression). If daily doses are required, one study suggests improved efficacy and no increase in adrenal suppression when administered at 3:00 p.m. (Beam et al. 1992). ■ Short courses or "bursts" are effective for establishing control when initiating therapy or during a period of gradual deterioration. ■ The burst should be continued until patient achieves 80% PEF personal best or symptoms resolve. This usually requires 3–10 days but may require longer. There is no evidence that tapering the dose following improvement prevents relapse.
Cromolyn and Nedocromil				
Cromolyn	MDI 1 mg/puff Nebulizer solution 20 mg/ampule	2–4 puffs tid-qid 1 ampule tid-qid	1–2 puffs tid-qid 1 ampule tid-qid	■ One dose prior to exercise or allergen exposure provides effective prophylaxis for 1–2 hours.
Nedocromil	MDI 1.75 mg/puff	2–4 puffs bid-qid	1–2 puffs bid-qid	■ See cromolyn above.
Long-Acting $Beta_2$-Agonists	***Inhaled***			
Salmeterol	MDI 21 mcg/puff, 60 or 120 puffs DPI 50 mcg/blister	2 puffs q 12 hours 1 blister q 12 hours	1–2 puffs q 12 hours 1 blister q 12 hours	■ May use one dose nightly for symptoms. ■ **Should not be used for symptom relief or for exacerbations.**
Sustained-Release Albuterol	***Tablet*** 4 mg tablet	4 mg q 12 hours	0.3–0.6 mg/kg/day, not to exceed 8 mg/day	
Methylxanthines				
Theophylline	Liquids, sustained-release tablets, and capsules	Starting dose 10 mg/kg/day up to 300 mg max; usual max: 800 mg/day	Starting dose 10 mg/kg/day; usual max: ■ <1 year of age: 0.2 (age in weeks) + 5 = mg/kg/day ■ ≥1 year of age: 16 mg/kg/day	■ Adjust dosage to achieve serum concentration of 5–15 mcg/mL at steady-state (at least 48 hours on same dosage). ■ Due to wide interpatient variability in theophylline metabolic clearance, routine serum theophylline level monitoring is important. ■ See factors below that can affect levels.

TABLE 37–14A. Usual Dosages for Long-Term-Control Medications *(Continued)*

Factors Affecting Serum Theophylline Concentrations[a]

Factor	Decreases Theophylline Concentrations	Increases Theophylline Concentrations	Recommended Action
Food	↓ or delays absorption of some sustained-release theophylline (SRT) products	↑ rate of absorption (fatty foods) products	Select theophylline preparation that is not affected by food.
Diet	↑ metabolism (high protein)	↓ metabolism (high carbohydrate)	Inform patients that major changes in diet are not recommended while taking theophylline.
Systemic, febrile viral illness (e.g., influenza)		↓ metabolism	Decrease theophylline dose according to serum concentration level. Decrease dose by 50 percent if serum concentration measurement is not available.
Hypoxia, cor pulmonale, and decompensated congestive heart failure, cirrhosis		↓ metabolism	Decrease dose according to serum concentration level.
Age	↑ metabolism (1 to 9 years)	↓ metabolism (<6 months, elderly)	Adjust dose according to serum concentration level.
Phenobarbital, phenytoin, carbamazepine	↑ metabolism		Increase dose according to serum concentration level.
Cimetidine		↓ metabolism	Use alternative H_2 blocker (e.g., famotidine or ranitidine).
Macrolides: TAO, erythromycin, clarithromycin		↓ metabolism	Use alternative antibiotic or adjust theophylline dose.
Quinolones: ciprofloxacin, enoxacin, pefloxacin		↓ metabolism	Use alternative antibiotic or adjust theophylline dose. Circumvent with ofloxacin if quinolone therapy is required.
Rifampin	↑ metabolism		Increase dose according to serum concentration level.
Ticlopidine		↓ metabolism	Decrease dose according to serum concentration level.
Smoking	↑ metabolism		Advise patient to stop smoking; increase dose according to serum concentration level.
Leukotriene Modifiers			
Zafirlukast	20 mg tablet	40 mg daily (1 tablet bid)	■ For zafirlukast, administration with meals decreases bioavailability; take at least 1 hour before or 2 hours after meals.
Zileuton	300 mg tablet 600 mg tablet	2400 mg daily (two 300 mg tablets or one 600 mg tablet, qid)	■ For zileuton, monitor hepatic enzymes (ALT).

[a] This list is not all inclusive; for discussion of other factors, see package inserts.

From National Asthma Education and Prevention Program (NAEPP). (1997).

TABLE 37–14B. Usual Dosages for Quick-Relief Medications

Medication	Dosage Form	Adult Dose	Child Dose	Comments
Short-Acting Inhaled Beta$_2$-Agonists				
	MDIs			
Albuterol	90 mcg/puff, 200 puffs	■ 2 puffs q 5 minutes prior to exercise	■ 1–2 puffs 5 minutes prior to exercise	■ An increasing use or lack of expected effect indicates diminished control of asthma. ■ Not generally recommended for long-term treatment. Regular use on a daily basis indicates the need for additional long-term-control therapy. ■ Differences in potency exist so that all products are essentially equipotent on a per puff basis. ■ May double usual dose for mild exacerbations. ■ Nonselective agents (i.e., epinephrine, isoproterenol, metaproterenol) are not recommended due to their potential for excessive cardiac stimulation, especially in high doses.
Albuterol HFA	90 mcg/puff, 200 puffs	■ 2 puffs tid-qid prn	■ 2 puffs tid-qid prn	
Bitolterol	370 mcg/puff, 300 puffs			
Pirbuterol	200 mcg/puff, 400 puffs			
Terbutaline	200 mcg/puff, 300 puffs			
	DPI			
Albuterol Rotahaler	200 mcg capsule	1–2 capsules q 4–6 hours as needed and prior to exercise	1 capsule q 4–6 hours as needed and prior to exercise	
	Nebulizer solution			
Albuterol	5 mg mL (0.5%)	1.25–5 mg (.25–1 cc) in 2–3 cc of saline q 4–8 hours	0.05 mg/kg (min 1.25 mg, max 2.5 mg) in 2–3 cc of saline q 4–6 hours	May mix with cromolyn or ipratropium nebulizer solutions. May double dose for mild exacerbations.
Bitolterol	2 mg mL (0.2%)	0.5–3.5 mg (.25–1 cc) in 2–3 cc of saline q 4–8 hours	Not established	May not mix with other nebulizer solutions.
Anticholinergics	***MDI***			
Ipratropium	18 mcg puff, 200 puffs	2–3 puffs q 6 hours	1–2 puffs q 6 hours	Evidence is lacking for anticholinergics producing added benefit to beta$_2$-agonists in long-term asthma therapy.
	Nebulizer solution			
	0.25 mg mL (0.025%)	0.25–0.5 mg q 6 hours	0.25 mg q 6 hours	
Systemic Corticosteroids		(Applies to all three systemic corticosteroids)		
Methylprednisolone	2, 4, 8, 16, 32 mg tablets	■ Short course "burst": 40–60 mg/day as single or 2 divided doses for 3–10 days	■ Short course "burst": 1–2 mg/kg/day, maximum 60 mg/day, for 3–10 days	■ Short courses or "bursts" are effective for establishing control when initiating therapy or during a period of gradual deterioration. ■ The burst should be continued until patient achieves 80% PEF personal best or symptoms resolve. This usually requires 3–10 days but may require longer. There is no evidence that tapering the dose following improvement prevents relapse.
Prednisolone	5 mg tabs, 5 mg/5 cc, 15 mg/5 cc			
Prednisone	1, 2.5, 5, 10, 20, 25 mg tabs; 5 mg/cc, 5 mg/5 cc			

From National Asthma Education and Prevention Program (NAEPP). (1997).

and is thereby a self-perpetuating pathologic process (Stanford & Galvin, 1988).

As both the cause and result of chronic infection, bronchiectasis classically presents with a cough that is productive of large amounts of mucopurulent (yellow to green) sputum. Past medical history may be notable for recurrent diffuse or localized pulmonary infections (bacterial, fungal, or TB) or mucociliary clearance abnormalities. Patients frequently report dyspnea with exertion, recurrent fever, or hemoptysis. In diffuse bronchiectasis, physical examination

TABLE 37–15. Classifying Severity of Asthma Exacerbation

	Mild	Moderate	Severe	Respiratory Arrest Imminent
Symptoms				
Breathlessness	While walking	While talking (infant–softer, shorter cry; difficulty feeding)	While at rest (infant–stops feeding)	
	Can lie down	Prefers sitting	Sits upright	
Talks in	Sentences	Phrases	Words	
Alertness	May be agitated	Usually agitated	Usually agitated	Drowsy or confused
Signs				
Respiratory rate	Increased	Increased	Often >30/min	
		Guide to rates of breathing in awake children: *Age* — *Normal rate* <2 months — <60/minute 2–12 months — <50/minute 1–5 years — <40/minute 6–8 years — <30/minute		
Use of accessory muscles; suprasternal retractions	Usually not	Commonly	Usually	Paradoxical thoracoabdominal movement
Wheeze	Moderate, often only end expiratory	Loud; throughout exhalation	Usually loud; throughout inhalation and exhalation	Absence of wheeze
Pulse/minute	<100	100–120	>120	Bradycardia
		Guide to normal pulse rates in children: *Age* — *Normal rate* 2–12 months — <160/minute 1–2 years — <120/minute 2–8 years — <110/minute		
Pulsus paradoxus	Absent <10 mm Hg	May be present 10–25 mm Hg	Often present >25 mm Hg (adult) 20–40 mm Hg (child)	Absence suggests respiratory muscle fatigue
Functional Assessment				
PEF % predicted or % personal best	80%	Approx. 50–80%	<50% predicted or personal best or response lasts <2 hr	
PaO_2 (on air)	Normal (test not usually necessary)	>60 mm Hg (test not usually necessary)	<60 mm Hg: possible cyanosis	
and/or PCO_2	<42 mm Hg (test not usually necessary)	<42 mm Hg (test not usually necessary)	≥42 mm Hg: possible respiratory failure (see text)	
SaO_2 % (on air) at sea level	>95% (test not usually necessary)	91–95%	<91%	

Hypercapnia (hypoventilation) develops more readily in young children than in adults and adolescents.

NOTE:
- The presence of several parameters, but not necessarily all, indicates the general classification of the exacerbation.
- Many of these parameters have not been systematically studied, so they serve only as general guides.

From National Asthma Education and Prevention Program (NAEPP). (1997).

reveals clubbing of the digits, diffuse rhonchorous breath sounds and, in advanced stages, evidence of cor pulmonale. Mechanism of debility and death from bronchiectasis is by cor pulmonale, respiratory failure, and overwhelming infection (Nicotra, 1994).

The diagnostic evaluation of bronchiectasis begins with the standard chest x-ray. Air bronchograms, air fluid levels, and hyperinflated lung fields are classic radiographic findings. Where the extent of bronchiectasis is pertinent, a high-resolution CT scan (HRCT) is indicated. The hallmark "signet ring" sign describes the radiographic appearance of dilated airways and their associated pulmonary artery

(Text continued on p. 806)

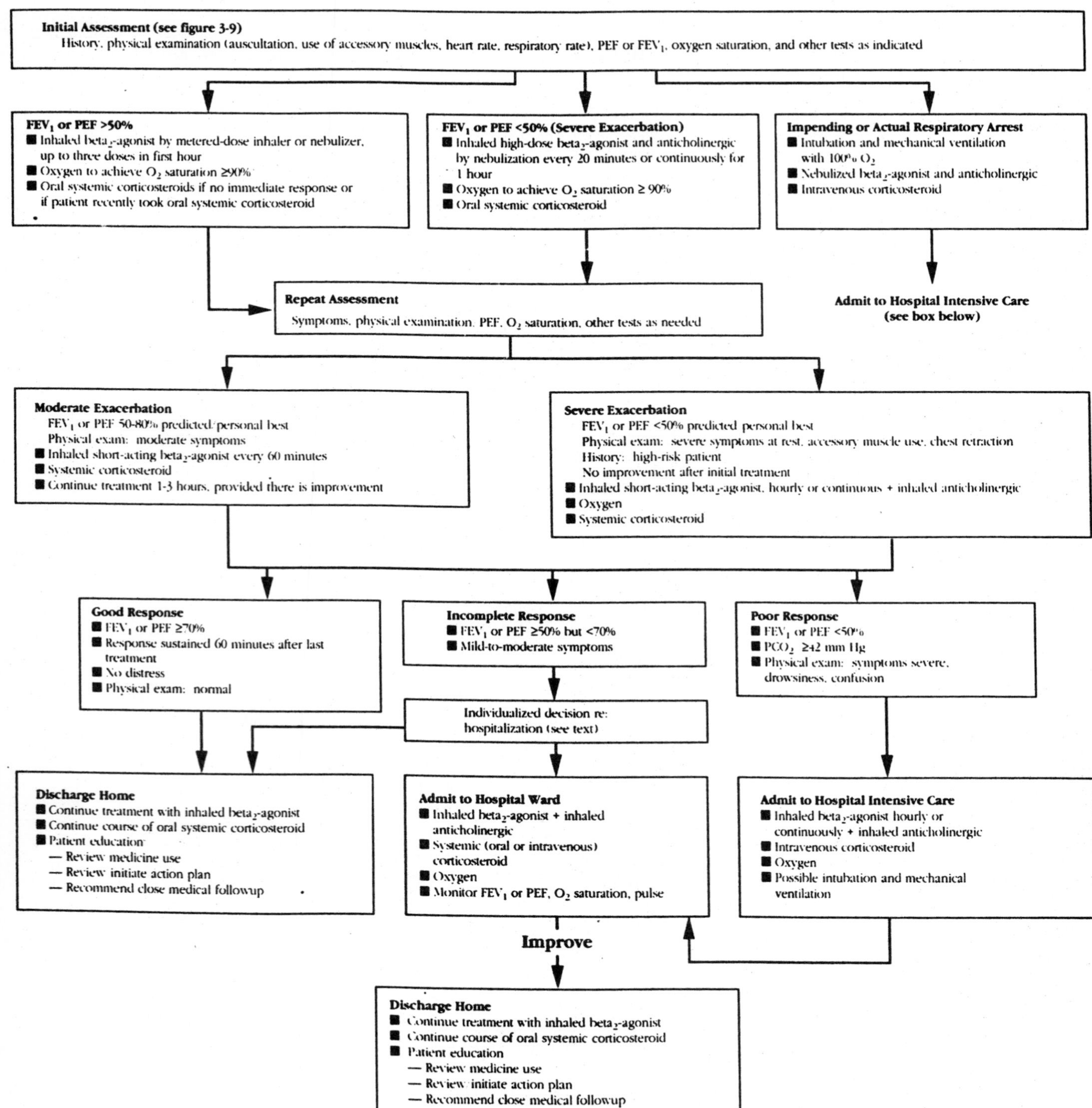

Figure 37–12. Management of asthma exacerbations: emergency department and hospital-based care. *(From the National Asthma Education and Prevention Program (NAEPP). [1997]. [p. 64].)*

TABLE 37–16. Delivery of Asthma Education by Clinicians During Patient Care Visits

Assessment Questions	Information	Skills
Recommendations for Initial Visit		
Focus on: ■ Concerns ■ Quality of life ■ Expectations ■ Goals of treatment	Teach in simple language:	Teach and demonstrate:
"What worries you most about your asthma?" "What do you want to accomplish at this visit?" "What do you want to be able to do that you can't do now because of your asthma?" "What do you expect from treatment?" "What medicines have you tried?" "What other questions do you have for me today?"	What is asthma? A chronic lung disease. The airways are very sensitive. They become inflamed and narrow; breathing becomes difficult. Asthma treatments: two types of medicines are needed: ■ Long-term control: medications that prevent symptoms, often by reducing inflammation ■ Quick relief: short-acting bronchodilator relaxes muscles around airways Bring all medications to every appointment. When to seek medical advice. Provide appropriate telephone number.	Inhaler and spacer/holding chamber use. Check performance. Self-monitoring skills that are tied to an action plan: ■ Recognize intensity and frequency of asthma symptoms ■ Review the signs of deterioration and the need to reevaluate therapy: Waking at night with asthma Increased medication use Decreased activity tolerance Use of a simple, written self-management plan and action plan
Recommendations for First Follow-up Visit (2 to 4 weeks or sooner as needed)		
Focus on: ■ Concerns ■ Quality of life ■ Expectations ■ Goals of treatment	Teach or review in simple language:	Teach or review and demonstrate:
Ask relevant questions from previous visit and also ask: "What medications are you taking?" "How and when are you taking them?" "What problems have you had using your medications?" "Please show me how you use your inhaled medications."	Use of two types of medications. Remind patient to bring all medications and the peak flow meter to every appointment for review. Self-evaluation of progress in asthma control using symptoms and peak flow as a guide.	Use of a daily self-management plan. Review and adjust as needed. Use of an action plan. Review and adjust as needed. Peak flow monitoring and daily diary recording Correct inhaler and spacer/holding chamber technique.
Recommendations for Second Follow-up Visit		
Focus on: ■ Expectations of visit ■ Goals of treatment ■ Medications ■ Quality of life	Teach or review in simple language:	Teach or review and demonstrate:
Ask relevant questions from previous visits and also ask: "Have you noticed anything in your home, work, or school that makes your asthma worse?" "Describe for me how you know when to call your doctor or go to the hospital for asthma care." "What questions do you have about the action plan?" "Can we make it easier?" "Are your medications causing you any problems?"	Relevant environmental control/avoidance strategies ■ How to identify home, work, or school exposures that can cause or worsen asthma ■ How to control house-dust mites, animal exposures if applicable ■ How to avoid cigarette smoke (active and passive) Review all medications. Review and interpret from daily diary: ■ Peak flow measures ■ Symptom scores	Inhaler/spacer/holding chamber technique. Peak flow monitoring technique. Use of daily self-management plan. Review and adjust as needed. Review use of action plan. Confirm that patient knows what to do if asthma gets worse.

(Continued)

TABLE 37–16. Delivery of Asthma Education by Clinicians During Patient Care Visits *(Continued)*

Recommendations for All Subsequent Visits		
Focus on: ■ Expectations of visit ■ Goals of treatment ■ Medications ■ Quality of life	Teach or review in simple language:	Teach or review and demonstrate:
Ask relevant questions from previous visits and also ask: "How have you tried to control things that make your asthma worse?" "Please show me how you use your inhaled medication."	Review and reinforce all: ■ Educational messages ■ Environmental control strategies at home, work, or school ■ Medications Review and interpret from daily diary: ■ Peak flow measures ■ Symptom scores	Inhaler/spacer/holding chamber technique. Peak flow monitoring technique. Use of daily self-management plan. Review and adjust as needed. Review use of action plan. Confirm that patient knows what to do if asthma gets worse. Periodically review and adjust written action plan.

From National Asthma Education and Prevention Program (NAEPP). (1997).

(Fig. 37–13). Degree of airflow obstruction is measured by pulmonary function testing. Response to bronchodilator therapy should be assessed and, if hypoxemia and hypercarbia are suspected, an arterial blood gas should be drawn. Two-dimensional echocardiogram is used to confirm the presence of cor pulmonale if suspicion has been raised by electrocardiogram. Periodic sputum culture and sensitivity is essential to guide therapy.

Antibiotics are the mainstay of treatment for bronchiectasis. The route of delivery may be oral, intravenous, or local with nebulized inhalation. The role of chronic antibiotic therapy is controversial, though intermittent therapy for exacerbations is quite effective. Intermittent antiobiotic treatment is begun when a patient reports worsening dyspnea, hemoptysis, or increased mucopurulence of sputum. Duration of treatment may be 2 to 6 weeks depending on patient response and provider preference. *S pneumoniae, H influenzae,* and *S aureus* are the most common infectious organisms. In advanced bronchiectasis, strains of Pseudomonas may predominate and develop resistance to antibiotics. Other therapeutic measures include use of mucolytics, bronchodilators, and airway clearance techniques.

Bronchodilators are indicated to provide symptomatic relief only if reversibility of airflow obstruction is seen on

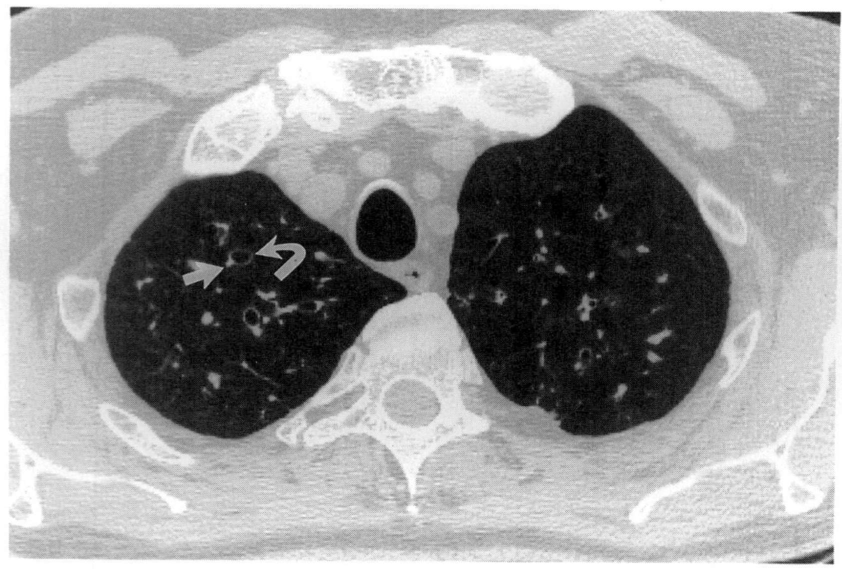

Figure 37–13. High-resolution CT scan (HRCT) of the chest in this patient with bronchiectasis. The normally smaller bronchiole is very dilated *(curved arrow)* appearing larger than its associated pulmonary artery *(straight arrow),* giving rise to the finding described as the signet ring sign. Multiple other signet ring signs are appreciated in this image.

PFTs. Serial PFTs are valuable for monitoring the disease process and response to therapy. Chest percussion, postural drainage, and airway clearance maneuvers are used to promote secretion clearance. Chest percussion using cupped hands or a mechanical percussion device is used to dislodge thick, tenacious secretions. During acute respiratory infections, the need for more vigorous and frequent chest percussion and postural drainage is increased. Proper positioning for postural drainage of the various segments of the lungs are demonstrated in Figs. 37–14 through 37–20. Surgical resection is considered for patients with severe focal disease or for patients who develop recurrent life threatening hemoptysis (Stockley, 1987).

Evaluation of therapy and monitoring of pathophysiology is achieved by following serial PFTs, chest x-ray, and sputum cultures. In advanced stages of bronchiectasis (FEV_1 less than 30% predicted) referral for lung transplantation should be considered for younger patients with diffuse bronchiectasis.

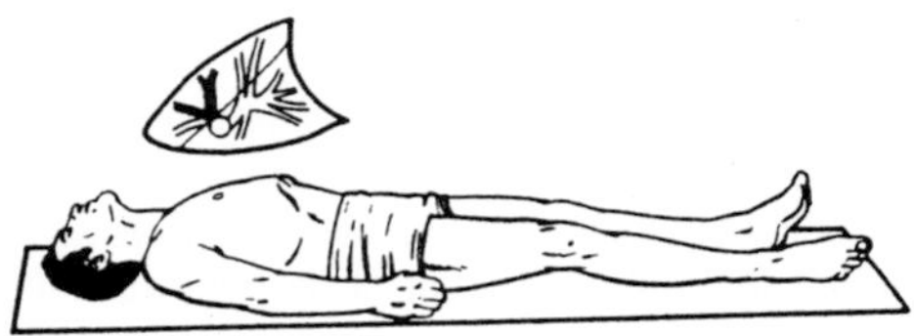

Figure 37–14. Postural drainage. Optimal position for drainage of anterior and superior segments of the upper lobes. *(Reprinted with permission from Farzan & Farzan. [1997]. [p. 182].)*

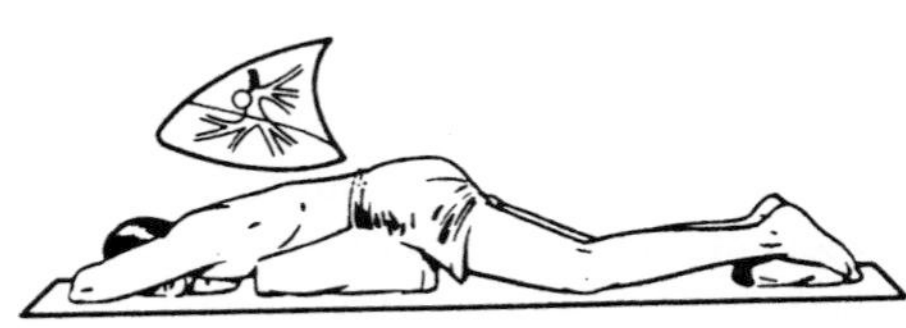

Figure 37–15. Postural drainage. Optimal position for drainage of superior segments of lower lobes. *(Reprinted with permission from Farzan & Farzan. [1997]. [p. 182].)*

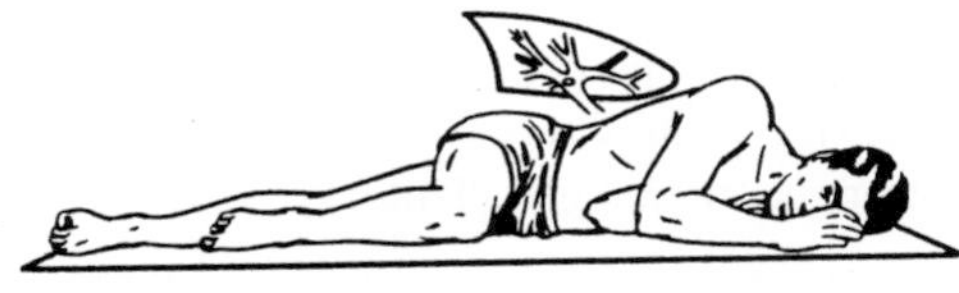

Figure 37–16. Postural drainage. Optimal position for drainage of posterior segment of the right upper lobe. *(Reprinted with permission from Farzan & Farzan. [1997]. [p. 182].)*

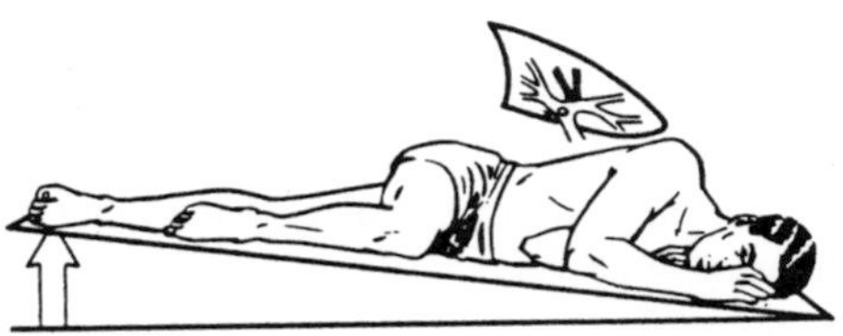

Figure 37–17. Postural drainage. Optimal position of the right middle lobe. *(Reprinted with permission from Farzan & Farzan, [1997]. [p. 182].)*

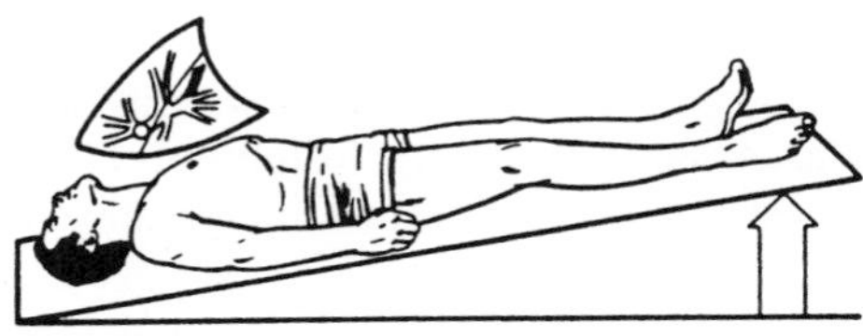

Figure 37–18. Postural drainage. Optimal position for drainage of the anterior basilar segments. *(Reprinted with permission from Farzan & Farzan. [1997]. [p. 183].)*

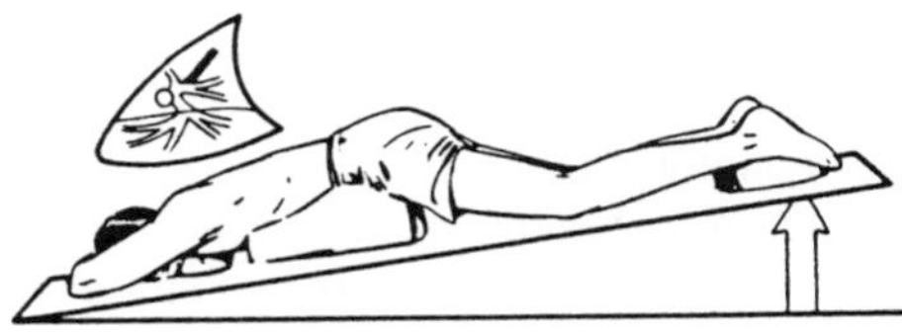

Figure 37–19. Postural drainage. Optimal position for drainage of the posterior basilar segments. *(Reprinted with permission from Farzan & Farzan. [1997]. [p. 183].)*

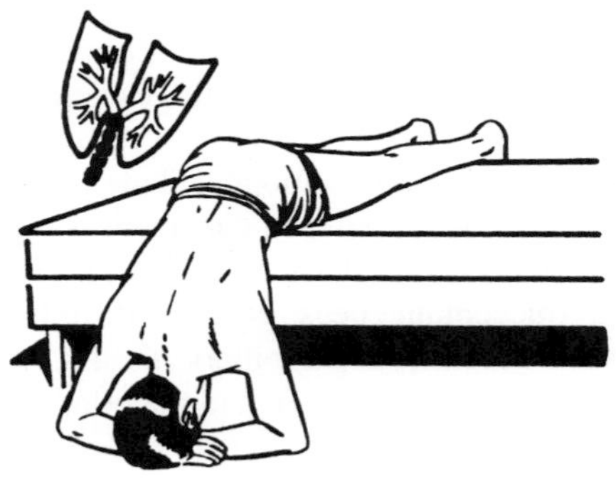

Figure 37–20. Postural drainage. Optimal position for drainage of the trachea. *(Reprinted with permission from Farzan & Farzan. [1997]. [p. 183].*

Cystic Fibrosis

Cystic fibrosis (CF) is a hereditary disorder characterized by dysfunction of the exocrine glands. Associated manifestations affect the lungs, sinuses, pancreas, gastrointestinal tract, hepatobiliary system, sweat glands, and reproductive systems. An autosomal recessive disorder, CF is the most common lethal genetic disease in Caucasians. In the United

States, it is estimated to affect 1 in 2500 caucasians, 1 in 17,000 African-Americans, and 1 in 90,000 Asian-Americans. Though CF has traditionally been considered a pediatric disorder, therapeutic advances have extended median life expectancy to 28 years (Aitken, 1997).

The diagnosis of CF is made on the basis of positive sweat test or genetic testing. The diagnosis is suspected in children with neonatal meconium ileus, GI malabsorption, and failure to thrive or recurrent pulmonary infections within the first years of life. Occasionally, older patients come to medical attention due to sinusitis, chronic pulmonary infections, hepatobiliary disorders (biliary cirrhosis, gallstones, pancreatitis), or male infertility secondary to azospermia. A positive family history of CF (or unexplained ancestral childhood deaths) is suggestive of this disorder.

The mechanism of pathogenesis is the defective transport of sodium and chloride across the epithelial membrane. The result is an increase in sweat electrolyte concentration and dysfunctional mucous secretion and clearance. The pulmonary consequence is related to abnormal mucosal fluid composition. Tenacious secretions and impaired mucociliary function provide the setting for airway obstruction and chronic infection. Acute exacerbations are characterized by worsening symptoms of cough, dyspnea, and sputum production. Recurrent treatment of chronic infections contributes to the development of resistant strains of bacterial pathogens. Chronic air trapping and infection place patients at risk for pneumothorax and hemoptysis, either of which may be life threatening. The radiographic feature of cystic fibrosis is bronchiectasis (Fig. 37–21). Progressive airflow obstruction and hypoxemia mark the course of deterioration. The finding of PCO_2 greater than 50 torr portends a 2-year survival of approximately 50%. Respiratory failure with or without cor pulmonale are the causes of eventual death (Aitken, 1997).

Extrapulmonary complications include chronic sinusitis (with or without nasal polyps), pancreatic disease (insufficiency, pancreatitis, and diabetes mellitus), gastrointestinal disease (meconium ileus equivalent, reflux, peptic ulcers, bowel strictures), hepatobiliary disease, arthropathy (particularly of the lower limbs), and male infertility (Fiel, 1991).

Pulmonary treatment strategies are aimed at chronic suppression of infection and maximization of airway clearance. Ongoing therapy includes chest percussion with postural drainage and combination drug therapy. Bronchodilators are appropriate for patients with hyperreactive airways demonstrated by bronchodilator response on PFTs. DNase is a nebulized mucolytic agent that promotes airway clearance by reducing the tenacity of sputum. Antibiotic use is guided by sputum culture and sensitivity. Intravenous antibiotics are given for exacerbations of pulmonary symptoms.

Malabsorption, electrolyte loss, and dehydration put CF patients at high risk for nutrition deficiency. Anorexia and increased metabolic requirements occur during exacerbations because of increased work of breathing. Enteral supplementation (orally or by jejunostomy tube) is frequently required to meet the high nutritional and caloric requirements of these patients. Improved nutrition is felt to sustain respiratory muscle strength and pulmonary function (Scanlin, 1988).

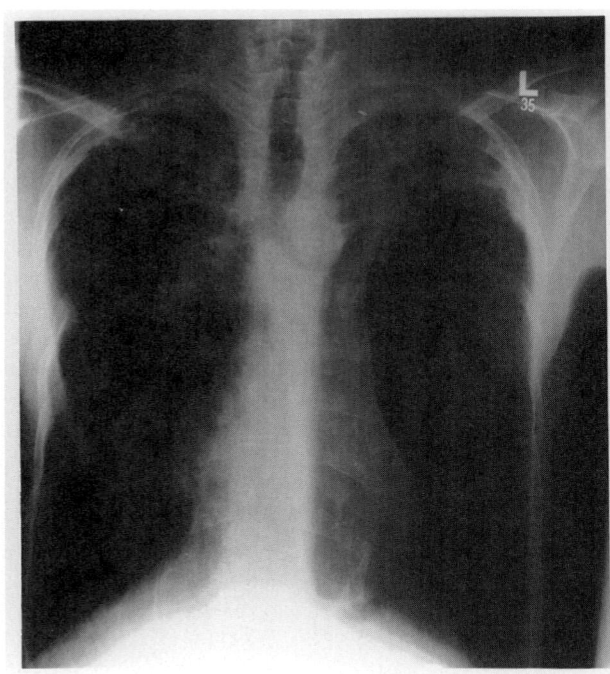

Figure 37–21. PA chest radiograph of a 31-year-old male with cystic fibrosis. Multiple ring shadows are seen at the upper lobes. This is characterisitic of bronchiectasis. The hila are retracted superiorly due to upper lobe fibrosis. Lung fields are hyperinflated due to chronic airways obstruction.

Ongoing treatment and follow-up of patients is ideally achieved in a multidisciplinary setting because the disease process affects multiple aspects of patient wellness (i.e., nutrition, fitness, psychosocial). Physiologic parameters that are monitored include pulmonary function tests (particularly FEV_1), sputum culture and sensitivity, and body weight. Frequency of testing is based on the individual patient's course.

Referral for Lung Transplantation. Patients with advancing disease should be referred for lung transplantation. Increased frequency of infection, rapid weight loss, and hemoptysis along with a fixed decrement in FEV_1 (less than or equal to 30% predicted) all portend failure. Because of the increasing waiting times for suitable donors, early referral is strongly encouraged (Trulock, 1997).

Gene Therapy. Correction of the genetic defect responsible for cystic fibrosis will be necessary to achieve a cure. Gene therapy, though still in the early stages of *in vivo* testing, holds a great deal of promise to this end. The goal is to correct the dysfunction of the chloride secretory mechanism of the lung. Recombinant forms of adenovirus serve as the vehicle by which a normal version of the gene responsible for CF is transferred into the patient's airway epithelial cells. Despite problems related to immune responses against both the vehicle and the genetically corrected gene, early results are very encouraging (Wilson, 1997).

Sleep-Disordered Breathing

In recent decades, scientific understanding of sleep and sleep-related disorders has blossomed. As a consequence, sleep has become a rapidly growing subspecialty within pulmonary medicine. Sleep disorders that are studied by such specialists include (but are not limited to) narcolepsy, idiopathic hypersomnia, periodic leg movement disorder, and sleep apnea syndromes (Phillipson, 1988). Because the subject of sleep is far too broad to be sufficiently covered in this context, discussion is limited to sleep-disordered breathing, specifically, sleep apnea syndromes.

Apnea is defined as episodic airflow cessation lasting at least ten seconds. Recurrent episodes of apnea, or hypopnea, that occur during sleep can cause clinically significant hypoxemia, sleep pattern disturbance, and daytime hypersomnolence. This condition, called sleep apnea, is the manifestation of occlusion of the airway, absence of ventilatory effort, or both. When coincidental with systemic hypertension or COPD, sleep apnea places patients at increased risk for cardiac dysrhythmias, cerebral vascular events, and sudden death during sleep (Strollo & Rogers, 1996).

Obstructive Sleep Apnea

Obstructive sleep apnea (OSA) is caused by increased upper airway resistance. It is characterized by anatomic and functional occlusion of the airway that causes cessation of airflow despite persistent respiratory muscle effort. The most common type of sleep apnea, OSA is caused by a structural deformity causing pharyngeal occlusion of the airway (Berry, 1995). Contributing factors include obesity with large neck circumference, hypertrophic tonsils and adenoids, large tongue, or edema of the pharyngeal mucosa.

Presenting symptoms of sleep apnea include sonorous snoring, abnormal motor behavior during sleep, nocturnal arousals, and daytime hypersomnolence. Cognitive deterioration, morning headaches, and loss of libido may also be reported. Male gender, advanced age, obesity, use of alcohol or sedating drugs, and history of COPD are all contributing or exacerbating factors of this disorder (Berry, 1995). Pertinent features of the clinical scenario may be obtained from the patient's bed partner.

The diagnosis and precise nature of sleep apnea is confirmed by polysomnography. This provides the simultaneous recording of central nervous system, respiratory, and cardiac functions during sleep. Results describe the nature, severity, and physiologic impact of the disorder.

Treatment priorities begin with modification of risk factors. Patients should eliminate excess body weight and use of alcohol and CNS depressants. Constant positive airway pressure (CPAP) by nasal mask is used to provide a pneumotactic splinting of the upper airway designed to maintain its patency. Though quite effective, this measure has significant lifestyle implications and therefore often fails due to nonadherence (Strollo & Rogers, 1996). In extreme cases of structural deformity, reconstructive surgery of the pharynx and palate and use of prosthetic devices or tracheostomy are effective in restoring airway patency (Hudgel, 1996).

Central Sleep Apnea

Central sleep apnea is differentiated from OSA by the absence of respiratory muscle contractions. It is rare that patients have pure central sleep apnea. Central sleep apnea accounts for only 10% to 15% of sleep apneas that come to medical attention (Sullivan & Issa, 1985). Frequently, patients suffer from a combination, or mixed, sleep apnea in which the initial disruption in ventilatory effort is followed by resumption of effort with absence of airflow due to interceding obstruction of the upper airway. Presenting features and treatment modalities are identical to those of OSA. However, respiratory stimulants are administered to patients felt to have a predominantly central component to their sleep apnea.

Obesity Hypoventilation Syndrome

A subset of patients with obstructive sleep apnea who are very obese manifest daytime hypoventilation (increased PCO_2). Formerly described as "Pickwickian"—named for the pathologically somnolent, obese, and plethoric character "Joe the fat boy" in Charles Dickens's novel, *The Postumous Papers of the Pickwick Club*—these patients have reduced ventilatory responses to hypercapnia and hypoxemia and demonstrate decreased respiratory compliance. The episodes of apnea demonstrated by these patients during sleep may be obstructive or mixed obstructive and central. Unlike other sleep-disordered breathing, the blood gas abnormalities noted during sleep persist with wakefulness. These patients are at significant risk for cor pulmonale and its associated morbidity and mortality. Treatment is similar to that of OSA; however, supplemental oxygen may be added to treat hypoxemia and diminish its sequelae (Berry, 1995).

Restrictive Lung Diseases

Commonly referred to as interstitial lung diseases (ILD), restrictive disorders of the lung share common pathologic processes despite an array of etiologies. While physiologic restriction can be the result of thoracic cage abnormalities (e.g., kyphoscoliosis, pectus excavatum) or neuromuscular disorders (e.g., phrenic nerve impairment, Guillian–Barre Syndrome), interstitial lung disease refers only to pathophysiology of the parenchyma. Injury to the structures of the interstitial space, the alveolar space, or both precipitate the influx of inflammatory and immune cells. The number and activity of alveolar macrophages is enhanced. This process is ultimately replaced by the deposition of fibrous tissue in the interstitium. The fibrosis, or scarring, may affect the alveolar wall, the airways, or the capillary bed. Increased thickness of the alveolar–capillary membrane alters permeability and results in gas transport abnormalities. Eventually, the normal architecture of the lung is remodeled into thick bands of scar tissue separating cystic spaces. For this reason, the patient develops progressive hypoxemia. An early indicator of this process is the reduction in diffusion capacity (DLCO) on pulmonary function tests. Longstanding hypoxemia and fibrosing of the pulmonary vascular bed cause increased pulmonary vascular resistance and cor pulmonale. As the disease process advances, lung compliance is reduced and elastic recoil is enhanced. Patients demonstrate rapid shallow breathing and frequently have low PCO_2 due to hyperventilation. In late stages, respiratory muscle fatigue results in an increased PCO_2. The ventilatory capacity of "stiff" lungs is limited, hence, the categorical designation of restrictive lung disease.

There are several processes that can incite the cascade of pulmonary fibrosis. The degree of impairment reflects the degree of physiologic distortion. Comorbid conditions as well as exposure to agents found in the home or workplace can be responsible. For this reason, a thorough history becomes essential in making the diagnosis and attempting to halt disease progression. Common systemic diseases, environmental toxins, and primary disorders related to interstitial lung disease are described.

Idiopathic Pulmonary Fibrosis

As its name implies, the etiology of idiopathic pulmonary fibrosis (IPF) is not well understood. Genetic, viral, and immune factors have all been implicated. Because the etiologic process has not been clearly defined, cure has been elusive. Also known as cryptogenic fibrosing alveolitis, IPF is a clinical term used to describe several histologic entities including usual interstitial pneumonitis (UIP), desquamative interstitial pneumonitis (DIP), lymphocytic interstitial pneumonitis (LIP), bronchiolitis obliterans with interstitial pneumonia (BIP), and giant cell interstitial pneumonia (GIP).

IPF primarily affects adults between the fifth and seventh decades of life. There is no apparent racial, geographic, or seasonal prevalence of the disease. The incidence is 5 in 100,000 individuals, men being slightly more affected than women. Clinical features include insidious onset of dyspnea and, in some patients, a nonproductive cough. Though frequently hard to ascertain, specific details about initial onset of symptoms may provide important clues to inciting factors (Kotloff, 1994). Physical examination may initially be normal, but eventually reveals coarse bibasalar crackles (called "Velcro rales" because of the likeness to the sound of Velcro strips being separated) and digital clubbing. As previously described, pulmonary function tests demonstrate restrictive physiology notable for a reduced DLCO. The degree of hypoxemia worsens with exercise and can be used to monitor disease progression. Chest radiograph shows a basilar predominant interstitial process that gradually extends upward over the course of serial films (Fig. 37–22). For this reason, every effort should be made to obtain previous chest radiographs of a patient suspected of having IPF. High-resolution CT scan demonstrates honeycombing at the level of the interstitial disease (Fig. 37–23).

Because many disease processes can produce nonspecific pulmonary fibrosis, IPF is a diagnosis of exclusion (King, 1997). Before labeling a patient with IPF, the clinician must first rule out primary lung diseases, connective tissue disorders, and exposure-related lung diseases. Table 37–17 outlines the differential diagnosis of idiopathic pulmonary fibrosis. Surgical biopsy reveals nonspecific interstitial fibrosis without granuloma formation (Raghu, 1995).

Treatment of IPF is aimed at disruption of the inflammatory process that results in fibrosis. No measure is capable of restoring normal lung architecture once scarring has occurred, so the goal is to halt disease progression. First-line therapy is high-dose corticosteroids (40-60 mg/d) for two to three months followed by gradual taper. Other immunosuppressive agents, such as azathiaprine or cytoxan,

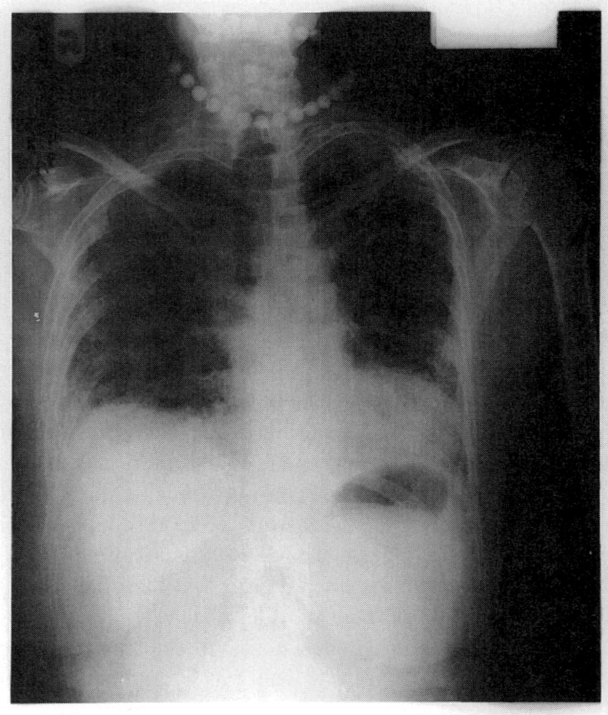

Figure 37–22. Posterior–anterior (PA) chest radiograph of a 61-year-old woman with end-stage idiopathic pulmonary fibrosis. The diffuse, bilateral interstitial changes with a basilar predominence and diminished lung volumes are classic findings for IPF.

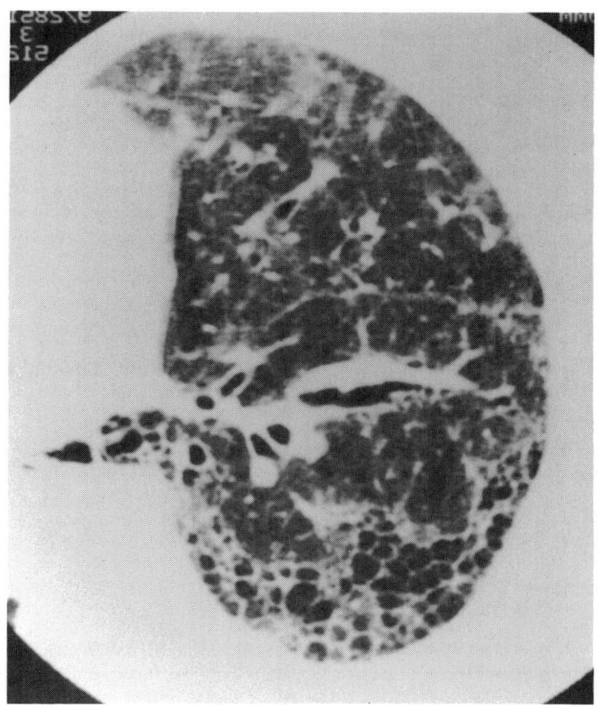

Figure 37–23. High-resolution CT (HRCT) scan of the chest of a patient with idiopathic pulmonary fibrosis. The coarse, reticular network of lines reflects thickening of the interstitium consistent with advance interstitial disease. This finding, known as honeycombing, is the radiographic correlate of end-stage fibrotic disease.

may be added to the regimen if no response has been appreciated (Kotloff, 1994). It is essential that the patient be closely monitored for side effects of the therapy. Diabetes mellitus, hyperlipidemia, cataracts, bone loss, and compression fractures can result from steroid use and opportunistic infections can be seen with all immunosuppression therapy. Other management strategies are geared toward alleviating the manifestations of IPF. As for any immunocompromised patient, vaccinations should be given for pneumococcal pneumonia and influenza. Smoking cessation is essential. Supplemental oxygen is instituted and dosed to maintain SaO_2 above 90% at rest and with exertion. Codeine or other antitussive agents may provide symptomatic relief of cough. In advanced stages, diuretic therapy may be necessary to relieve the symptoms of cor pulmonale. Change in symptoms or development of focal abnormalities on chest radiograph should be evaluated for malignant and infectious causes. For unclear reasons, IPF patients have an increased risk of developing lung cancer. While assessing the response to therapy, appropriate patients should be referred for consideration for lung transplantation (Trulock, 1997).

TABLE 37–17. Differential Diagnosis of Idiopathic Pulmonary Fibrosis (IPF)

Primary Lung Diseases
Sarcoidosis
Eosinophilic Granuloma
Connective Tissue Disorders
Scleroderma
Rheumatoid Arthritis
Environmental Disorders
Hypersensitivity Pneumonitis
Pneumoconiosis
Drug-Induced Lung Disease

Hypersensitivity Pneumonitis

Diffuse inflammatory lung disease caused by an immune reaction to an inhaled antigen is known as hypersensitivity pneumonitis. Also known as extrinsic allergic alveolitis, this entity was first described in workers who stripped bark from maple logs. It subsequently presented in other individuals whose hobbies or occupations required work in proximity to particulate matter of molds, fungi, animal proteins, or chemicals (Table 37–18). Most of the causative antigens are spores that are small enough to reach the alveoli where they initiate the immunologic cascade. Clinical presentation of this disorder may be acute, subacute or chronic (Farzan, 1997).

Acute hypersensitivity pneumonitis is characterized by the onset of symptoms 3 to 6 hours after exposure. Symptoms may include fever, chills, malaise, headache, chest tightness, and cough. Physical exam findings and severity of symptoms are highly individual and may range from those of a flu-like syndrome to fulminate acute respiratory distress syndrome (ARDS). Although the insult occurs at the level of the alveoli and small airways, patients with a history of asthma may demonstrate wheezing. This finding indicates large airway involvement.

Subacute hypersensitivity pneumonitis features a more vague constellation of complaints beginning at the point of exposure to the antigen. With recurrent exposure, patients may report worsening cough and chest tightness as well as anorexia, weight loss, night sweats, and hemoptysis. In most cases, removal of the patient from source of exposure for several days results in resolution of the symptoms. This diagnosis is strongly favored in individuals who report improvement in symptoms while on leave from their home or worksite and in whom symptoms recur upon return.

Without relief from exposure to the causative antigen, the chronic inflammatory process eventually causes scarring of the parenchyma. With disease progression, symptoms are persistent and unrelenting. Chronic fibrosis occurs and the clinical scenario is indistinguishable from idiopathic pulmonary fibrosis.

Making the diagnosis of hypersensitivity pneumonitis relies upon a supportive clinical history. Information should be elicited regarding the patient's work, hobbies, home, pets, and travel. Curiously, this disease has a predilection for nonsmokers. The mechanism is not understood.

TABLE 37–18. Hypersensitivity Pneumonitis: Disorders, Antigens, and Sources

Disease	Antigen	Source of Particles
Farmer's lung	Thermophilic actinomycetes	Moldy hay, grain, silage
Bird fancier's, breeder's, or handler's lung	Parakeet, budgerigar, pigeon, chicken, turkey proteins	Avian droppings or feathers
Humidifier or air-conditioner lung	Thermophilic actinomycetes, *Aureobasidium pullulans,* or other	Contaminated water in humidification and air-conditioning systems
Bagassosis	Thermophilic actinomycetes	Moldy bagasse (sugar cane)
Malt worker's lung	*Aspergillus fumigatus* or *A clavatus*	Moldy barley
Mushroom worker's lung	Thermophilic actinomycetes	Mushroom compost
Sequoiosis	*Pullularia, Graphium* species	Redwood sawdust
Maple bark disease	Cryptostroma corticale	Maple bark
Woodworker's lung	Wood dust; *Alternaria*	Oak, cedar, and mahogany dusts; pine and spruce pulp
Cheese washer's lung	*Penicillium casei*	Moldy cheese
Suberosis	Cork dust mold	Cork dust
Sauna taker's lung	Unknown	Contaminated sauna water
Pituitary snuff taker's lung	Animal proteins	Heterologous pituitary snuff
Coffee worker's lung	Coffee bean dust	Coffee beans
Miller's lung	Infested wheat flour	*Sitophilus granarius* (wheat weevil)
Fish meal worker's lung	Fish meal dust	Fish meal
Furrier's lung	Animal fur dust	Animal pelts
Lycoperdonosis	Puffball spores	*Lycoperdon* puffballs
Chemical worker's lung	Isocyanates	Polyurethane foam, varnishes, lacquer, foundry casting

Adapted with permission from Richerson. (1988). (p. 668).

The diagnostic work-up should include bloodwork, allergy testing, chest x-ray, and, if necessary, bronchial alveolar lavage (BAL) and lung biopsy. Bloodwork may feature a slightly elevated white blood cell count and elevated ESR, an increase in eosinophils and polyclonal hypergammaglobulinemia. Chest radiograph may be normal or demonstrate patchy alveolar infiltrates or miliary (seed-like) nodules. Prior to the development of chronic fibrosis, circulating antibodies may be detected using antigen screening panels. BAL reveals lymphocytosis and increased polymorphonuclear leukocytes (PMNs) in subacute and acute diseases respectively. BAL is useful in ruling out sarcoidosis and infectious disorders of the lung. Transbronchial biopsies reveal granulomas in most patients (Merrill, 1997).

The primary treatment strategy is to avoid or limit exposure to the offending antigen. In many cases this requires the patient to change jobs or residence. For those patients whose disease advances to the point of declining lung function, a short course (2 months at 30-60 mg/d) of corticosteroid therapy followed by taper may be useful in disrupting the immune reaction central to this disorder (Merrill, 1997).

Sarcoidosis

Sarcoidosis is a multisystem idiopathic granulomatous disorder that most commonly affects the lungs, skin, eyes, reticuloendothelial system, liver, and myocardium. While no causative infectious or inflammatory agent has been associated with this disorder, it is believed to be related to a hypersensitivity response in patients with an inherited or acquired predisposition. It tends to affect young adults and, in the United States, is 12-fold more common in African-Americans than in caucasians. In the black population, the incidence in women is twice that of men; in the white population, gender has no significance (James & Hosoda, 1994). Because this disease is multisystemic, patients may present to a variety of specialists with complaints related to sarcoidosis.

Pulmonary involvement is found in over 90% of patients. Dyspnea, dry cough, and chest pain are common complaints. Many patients report nonspecific constitutional complaints such as fever, anorexia, fatigue, weight loss, chills, and night sweats. Others have asymptomatic disease identified because of an abnormal chest radiograph. Palpable peripheral lymph nodes or splenic enlargement are found in about one third of all patients with sarcoidosis. Myocardial involvement may present with findings as benign as premature atrial contractions or as serious as intractable heart failure and sudden death. Granulomas of the liver are present in a majority of patients. Though many patients demonstrate elevated serum bilirubin and alkaline phosphatase, the development of portal hypertension or liver failure is rare. Granulomatous uveitis is a common occular lesion attributed to sarcoidosis. Erythema nodosum, plaques, maculopapular eruptions, and alopecia are all cutaneous manifestations of this disorder. Granulomatous basilar meningitis is responsible for the majority of neurologic sequlae, though defects can be seen throughout the nervous system (Kotloff & Rossman, 1992). The multisystemic clinical manifestations of sarcoidosis are described in Table 37–19.

The pulmonary radiographic manifestations of sarcoidosis are described by stages. In stage I, the chest radiograph

TABLE 37–19. Clinical Manifestations of Sarcoidosis

Organ or System	Manifestations
Lungs	Interstitial lung disease, bronchial stenosis, bronchiectasis, pleural effusion (rare), pneumothorax, aspergilloma
Lymph nodes	Hilar/mediastinal adenopathy, peripheral adenopathy
Skin	Erythema nodosum, lupus pernio, papules, nodules, plaques, enlargement and tenderness of previous traumatic or surgical scars
Eyes	Uveitis, scleral and conjunctival lesions, lacrimal gland enlargement, optic neuritis, papilledema, keratoconjunctivitis sicca syndrome
Liver	Asymptomatic abnormalities in liver function studies, hepatomegaly, cirrhosis and portal hypertension, intrahepatic cholestasis
Endocrine	Hypercalcemia, hypercalciuria, panhypopituitarism
Musculoskeletal	Arthralgias, acute and chronic arthritis, osseous lesions, granulomatous myopathy
Heart	Cor pulmonale, arrhythmias, heart block, congestive cardiomyopathy, mitral regurgitation
CNS	Chronic basilar meningitis, space-occupying lesions, hydrocephaly, increased intracranial pressure, peripheral and cranial neuropathies, diabetes insipidus secondary to hypothalamic involvement, pituitary involvement
Kidney	Nephrolithiasis, interstitial nephritis, glomerulonephritis

Reprinted with permission from Kotloff. (1994). (p. 37).

reveals bilateral hilar lymphadenopathy. In stage II, parenchymal infiltrates are added to the previous picture (Fig. 37–24). In stage III, pulmonary infiltrates persist though the hilar lymphadenopathy resolves. In the final stage of pulmonary sarcoidosis, cystic lesions and bullae may be present with evidence of advanced fibrosis (Siltzbach, 1967).

Confirming a suspected diagnosis of sarcoidosis requires not only compatible clinical and radiographic features, but also tissue biopsy demonstrating noncaseating granulomas and negative bacterial and fungal cultures (Kotloff & Rossman, 1992). Transbronchial biopsy is the tissue-sampling method most frequently used in the work-up of pulmonary sarcoid. When that fails to acquire the necessary information, mediastinoscopy for lymph node biopsy is performed. Because the abnormalities of the chest radiograph may represent a spectrum of pathologic entities, and inflammatory or infectious disorders can induce the development of noncaseating granuloma, stepwise measures to obtain adequate tissue is necessary to make the diagnosis.

Prognosis is generally good. In one third of all patients evidence of sarcoid resolves, and in one third of patients the disease stabilizes. On the contrary, patients who have unremitting pulmonary infiltration and sarcoid involvement of three or more organ systems have poorer outcomes (James & Hosoda, 1994). Mortality in this patient population is most frequently due to respiratory failure, cor pulmonale,

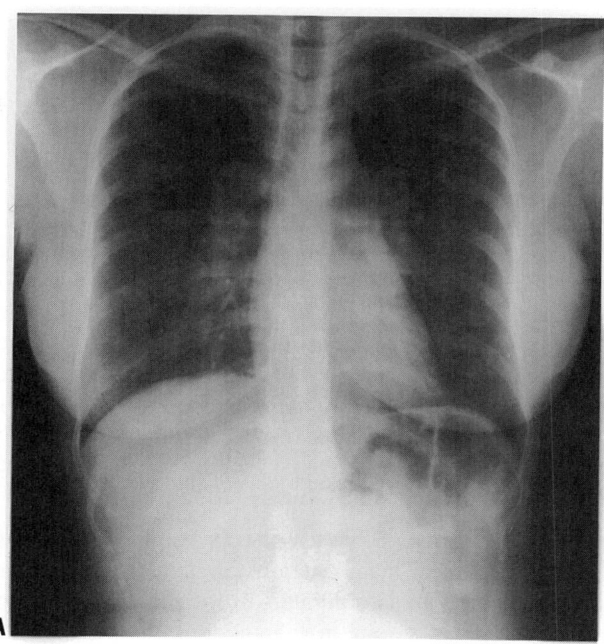

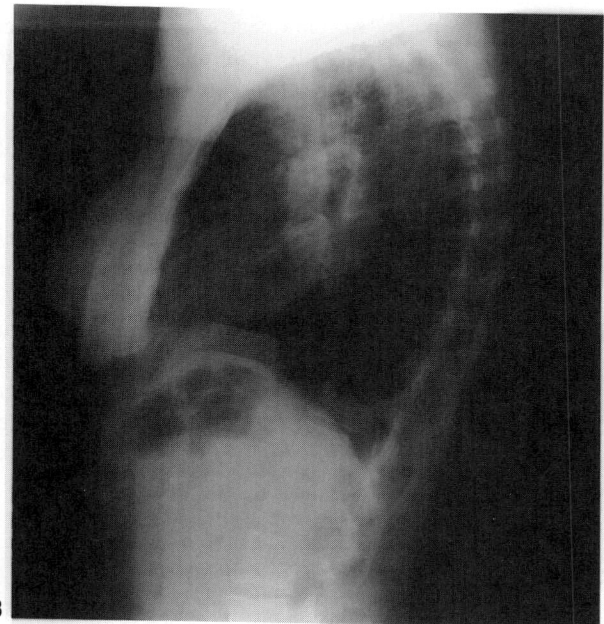

Figure 37–24. Posterior–anterior (PA) and lateral chest radiograph of a 41-year-old patient with stage II pulmonary sarcoidosis. **A,** Bilateral hilar lymphadenopathy is the typical finding at this stage. **B,** The lateral view also demonstrates a lobular density in the midlung. This is the characteristic appearance of adenopathy on the lateral view.

and aspergillus-associated massive hemoptysis (Kotloff, 1994). Treatment is not necessary in those patients who are asymptomatic. Patients with pulmonary compromise or significant extrapulmonary findings should be treated with corticosteroid therapy. A 3- to 6-month course of 30 to 40 mg per day of prednisone followed by a taper to a standing dose of 5 to 10 mg per day is usual treatment (Sharma, 1997). Interestingly, pregnancy has a favorable effect on this disease process. Without teratogenic effect, the sarcoidosis usually remits during pregnancy allowing patients to curtail or discontinue corticosteroids.

Collagen Vascular Diseases

There are several systemic immunologic disorders that can involve the lungs. While the precise etiologies of these disorders are not well understood, it is apparent that the immune system is the mechanism of pathogenesis. These autoimmune diseases are recognized by the presence of antibodies against certain proteins or cell types found in connective tissue and blood vessels throughout the body. The pulmonary manifestations of common collagen vascular diseases are detailed in Table 37–20.

Systemic Lupus Erythematosus. Presenting with a variety of clinical manifestations, systemic lupus erythematosus (SLE) is an autoimmune disorder that primarily affects the skin and serous membranes resulting in vascular and connective tissue changes. This disorder is seen most commonly in women of childbearing age. The clinical course tends to be chronic with symptoms waxing and waning over periods of exacerbation and remission.

Pulmonary consequences of SLE may be acute or chronic in presentation. The disease involves the vascular and serous structures of the parenchyma and pleura. Lupus pneumonitis and alveolar hemmorhage are both forms of acute pulmonary manifestations. Lupus pneumonitis closely mimics the clinicoradiographic features of bacterial pneumonia. It may have a rapid course resulting in acute respiratory failure. Alveolar hemmorhage results from inflammation of the pulmonary capillaries. Because patients with autoimmune disorders are particularly vulnerable to infection, respiratory tract infections should always be included in the differential diagnosis cough, sputum production, or fever (Mills, 1994).

The clinical course and pathogenesis of chronic pulmonary SLE is similar to that of pulmonary fibrosis. With an insidious onset, slowly progressive fibrosis causes worsening dyspnea. Pulmonary functions tests are often the first indicator of pulmonary involvement, demonstrating restrictive impairment with reduction in vital capacity and DLCO. As in other fibrotic diseases of the lung, hypoxemia may be present with hypocapnia due to hyperventilation. With persistent pulmonary involvement, chest radiograph shows increased interstitial markings and small lung fields. Patients may develop pleural effusions or chest pain associated with pleural manifestations of the disease. Because of the assault on vascular structures, patients with SLE are at increased risk for pulmonary thromboembolism (Von Feldt & Callegari, 1994).

Immunosuppression is the foundation of treatment of this immune disorder and its consequences. High-dose corticosteroids are used, sometimes in combination with other immunosuppressive agents, to quiet the immune activity. Pulmonary management is driven by the severity of compromise. Patients may require supplemental oxygen, or in severe acute exacerbations, mechanical ventilatory support (Farzan & Farzan, 1997).

Rheumatoid Disease. Similar to SLE, rheumatoid disease is an autoimmune disorder with poorly understood etiology. Confirmation of the diagnosis is made by the presence of rheumatoid factor antibodies. These hallmark antibodies are found in serum and joint fluid. Though predominantly manifested in the joints, this systemic disorder can cause vasculitic lesions in the eye, subcutaneous structures, and in the parenchyma and pleura of the lung (Von Feldt & Callegari, 1994).

Exudative pleural effusion featuring a low glucose content is characteristic of rheumatoid disease. Parenchymal sequellae may be nodular or diffuse infiltrates. Nodular lesions, described radiographically as necrobiotic lesions, are clinically insignificant causing no symptoms or defect

TABLE 37–20. Pulmonary Manifestations of the Major Collagen Vascular Diseases

Pulmonary Manifestations	Rheumatoid Arthritis	Systemic Sclerosis	Polymyositis and Dermatomyositis	Systemic Lupus Erythematosus
Pleural				
Thickening	++	+	0	++
Effusion	++	0	0	+++
Parenchymal				
Acute pneumonia	0	0	0	+
Diffuse intersititial fibrosis	++[a]	+++	++[a]	+
Nodules	++	0	0	0
Primary pulmonary vasculopathy	0	++	0	+
Aspiration	0	++	+++	0
Ventilatory insufficiency	0	+	++	+

[a] A rapidly progressing variant may occur.

NOTE: 0 = Absent or rare; + = uncommon; ++ = recognized manifestation; +++ = important feature of disease.

Reprinted with permission from Dickey & Myers (1988). (p. 646).

in lung function. The presentation of diffuse disease closely mimics that of pulmonary fibrosis with a progressive restrictive physiology as fibrosis of the parenchyma occurs. Pulmonary toxicity may also be seen related to the drugs used to treat rheumatoid arthritis. Treatment regimens include combination therapy with corticosteroids, gold therapy, methotrexate, or penicillamine (Lynch & Hunninghake, 1992). To monitor for the presence of pulmonary manifestations of this disease or adverse reactions to its treatment, serial chest radiographs should be followed.

Scleroderma. Also known as progressive systemic sclerosis, this devastating disorder affects connective tissues and vasculature resulting in the vascular insufficiency and progressive fibrosis of multiple systems. Believed to be an autoimmune defect, the pathogenesis of scleroderma involves the unregulated deposition of collagen fiber throughout the body. Commonly affected systems include the skin, the GI tract, the kidneys, the heart, and the lungs. Characteristic skin changes are diagnostic in most patients. The skin manifestations are thickening, fibrosis, hypo- and hyperpigmentation telangectasis, and cutaneous calcinosis. This renders the appearance of the face taught and expressionless as the natural wrinkles and folds are replaced by skin with excess collagen. This is a progressive disease with a poor prognosis. Death usually occurs secondary to cardiac, renal, or respiratory failure (Von Feldt & Callegari, 1994).

CREST syndrome is a limited variant of scleroderma. Its features are *c*alcinosis, *R*eynauds' phenomenon, *e*sophageal dismotility, *s*clerodactily, and *t*alangectasias. In comparison with widespread scleroderma, CREST syndrome has a more favorable prognosis.

Anatomic derangements related to scleroderma include interstitial fibrosis and vascular changes. Clinical manifestations of pulmonary distortion include progressive dyspnea, cough, and basalar rales. Primary involvement of the pulmonary vasculature causes narrowing and occlusion of the vessels that, in turn, cause pulmonary hypertension and cor pulmonale (Farzan & Farzan, 1997). This process may be present with or without fibrosing of the lung parenchyma. Radiographic appearance reflects the pathology. Diffuse fibrosis appears radiographically similar to IPF with an early fine interstitial pattern advancing to marked destruction and honeycombing in later stages. Prominent central pulmonary vasculature is evident on the chest radiograph of patients with pulmonary hypertension.

Pulmonary function test and arterial blood gas results are similar to those in other chronic interstitial lung diseases. Restrictive physiology with reduced DLCO is noted on pulmonary function testing. ABGs reveal hypocarbia and exercise-induced hypoxemia. Patients may develop hypercarbia with respiratory muscle fatigue. While, to date, there is no curative treatment for this disease, immunosuppression therapy is frequently used in the hope of disrupting the immune activity (Legerton, Smith, & Silver, 1995).

Pulmonary Vascular Diseases

The anatomical structures of pulmonary circulation are, in order of flow, the right heart chambers, the pulmonary arteries and arterioles, the capillary bed, and the venules and pulmonary veins. An understanding of the factors that determine blood flow, vascular pressures, and vascular resistance is essential to recognition of pulmonary vascular disorders and their consequences.

The pulmonary vasculature is a low-resistance system, therefore, low pressure is sufficient to circulate blood through it. The average pulmonary artery pressure is 25 mm Hg systolic and 10 mm Hg diastolic, with a mean of 15 mm Hg. The surface area of the pulmonary vasculature is approximately four times that of the rest of the body. The walls of the pulmonary vessels are thin and highly distensible, so they distend and recoil according to cardiac output without causing pressure changes. Factors that affect cardiac output also influence pulmonary circulation. Vasoactive substances, altered alveolar oxygen tension, and acidosis alter the hemodynamics of the lung. Changes in ventilation of the lung result in regional changes in circulation. For example, areas of atelectatic lung demonstrate reduced perfusion. Likewise, areas of reduced perfusion are matched by diminished ventilation. Blood supply to the bronchi and bronchioles is delivered through the bronchial arteries, which arise from the thoracic aorta.

Pathology of the pulmonary circulation can be the consequence of abnormalities of the heart, the blood vessels, vascular flow, permeability, or the pulmonary parenchyma. The physiologic symbiosis of the heart and lungs often results in disorders of one influencing function of the other.

Pulmonary Hypertension

Under normal circumstances, the pulmonary vascular system is able to adapt to increased cardiac output without changes in pulmonary artery pressures . There are, however, several mechanisms that can disrupt or exhaust this adaptability resulting in pulmonary hypertension. Causes of pulmonary hypertension are described as either postcapillary or precapillary (Rubin, 1997). Table 37–21 details etiologies of pulmonary hypertension according to the site of primary defect.

Impaired function of structures distal to the pulmonary capillary bed cause postcapillary pulmonary hypertension. Left ventricular failure, mitral valve disease, and pulmonary venous occlusion are all postcapillary sources of capillary congestion and hypertension.

Precapillary hypertension is more common and is caused by decreased surface area of the pulmonary arterioles. Mechanisms include vascular destruction, constriction, or obstruction. Because of the high reserve and distensibility of the pulmonary vessels, the total area of the normal vascular bed must be compromised by at least 50% before any pressure changes occur. Pulmonary embolism, discussed later in this chapter, is a classic example of pre-

TABLE 37–21. Classification of Pulmonary Hypertension Based on Site of Primary Defect

Postcapillary
- Left ventricular failure
- Mitral valve disease
- Aortic valve disease
- Left atrial myxoma or thrombus
- Pulmonary venoocclusive disease

Precapillary
- Respiratory disorders
  - Parenchymal lung disease (obstructive, restrictive, or mixed)
  - Restrictive chest wall diseases
  - Sleep apnea and hypoventilation syndromes
  - High altitude disease
- Occlusive pulmonary vascular disease (tumor, air, amniotic fluid, intravenously injected foreign material, schistosomiasis)
- Congenital heart disease
  - Intracardiac septal defects
  - Peripheral pulmonic stenosis
- Pulmonary vasculitis
- Primary pulmonary hypertension

Reprinted with permission from Rubin. (1997). (p. 468).

capillary hypertension due to obstruction. Pulmonary vasculitis, an inflammatory disorder of the vasculature, causes pulmonary hypertension by destruction of significant surface area. The most common cause of pulmonary hypertension is chronic pulmonary parenchymal disease. Hypoxic vasoconstriction occurs at the capillary level with acute alveolar hypoxia. Chronic hypoxemia causes increased pulmonary artery resistance by causing constriction and eventual remodeling of pulmonary vessels. This increases the burden and pressure of remaining vessels. When no causative factor can be identified, the patient is labeled as having primary pulmonary hypertension (American College of Chest Physicians [ACCP], 1993).

Pulmonary hypertension typically is unrecognized until the development of right heart failure, or cor pulmonale (Palevsky & Fishman, 1993). Exertional dyspnea, chest pain, weakness, and syncope are common presenting symptoms. Hypoxemia is a common feature of pulmonary hypertension, particularly in the setting of underlying lung disease.

Prominent central pulmonary arteries are the radiographic indicators of pulmonary hypertension (Fig. 37–25). Two-dimensional echocardiogram can be used to estimate the pulmonary artery pressure. Once a patient's baseline is established, echocardiography is used to monitor pulmonary artery pressures in a low-risk, noninvasive way. Right-heart catheterization allows precise measurement of pulmonary arterial pressure at rest and during exercise. Pulmonary angiogram is used to confirm suspected thromboembolism as the etiology of pulmonary hypertension.

Treatment of pulmonary hypertension lies in resolution or modification of the underlying cause. In the setting of chronic hypoxemia secondary to chronic lung disease, supplemental oxygen should be dosed to maintain SaO_2 above 90% at rest and with exertion. Diuretic therapy should be judiciously used to reduce preload in the setting of right-heart failure. The advent of new pulmonary vasodilator strategies and medications hold great promise for alleviation of symptoms and improved survival. Lung transplantation or heart–lung transplantation may be an option

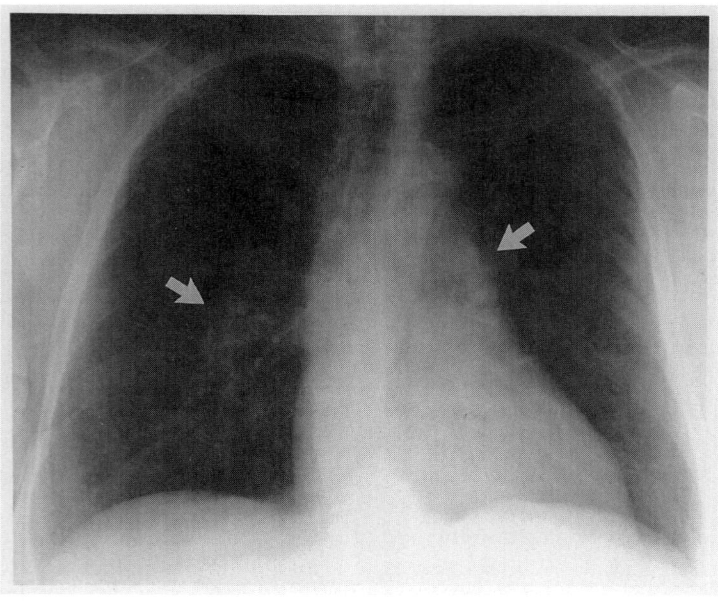

Figure 37–25. Posterior–anterior (PA) chest radiograph of a 32-year-old woman with severe pulmonary hypertension and cor pulmonale. Large central pulmonary arteries and a wide cardiac silhouette are features of this disorder.

for patients with primary pulmonary hypertension and some forms of congenital heart disease (Palevsky, 1997).

Cor Pulmonale

Right-heart failure secondary to chronic pulmonary hypertension is called cor pulmonale. As previously described, any pulmonary disease that causes the destruction, constriction, or obstruction of the pulmonary vasculature can cause an increase in pulmonary vascular resistance, or right-heart afterload. After chronically pumping against increased pulmonary vascular resistance, the right heart remodels. It becomes hypertrophic and dilated as both wall thickness and chamber size are enlarged. In many cases, the intraventricular septum may be recruited to work for the right ventricle rather than the left. The heart becomes predisposed to dysrhythmias. Eventual failure of the right ventricle ensues (Palevsky & Fishman, 1993).

Physical findings of cor pulmonale include jugular venous distention, an increased second heart sound over the pulmonic valve (loud P_2), peripheral edema, and hepatomegaly. Radiographic evidence is not apparent until advanced stages (refer to Fig. 37–25). Enlarged central pulmonary arteries with attenuation of distal branches and a large cardiac silhouette are characteristic radiographic findings of cor pulmonale. P-pulmonale is a classic electrocardiographic finding indicative of right-heart hypertrophy (Fig. 37–26). Both echocardiography and radionucleotide imaging are useful in the assessment of ventricular size and contractility. In addition, echocardiogram is used to ascertain myocardial wall thickness. Once the diagnosis of cor pulmonale is established, the latter three diagnostic studies are used to monitor disease progress and response to treatment.

In devising a treatment strategy, it must be recognized that cor pulmonale is a consequence of primary pulmonary pathology. For this reason, treatment of this disorder is directed at correction of the underlying cause. Supplemental oxygen is indicated when the cause of increased pulmonary vascular resistance is chronic hypoxemia. Diuretics, antiarrhythmics, and anticoagulation may each have a role in modifying the complications of cor pulmonale (Palevsky, 1997; Rubin, 1997). A prescribed exercise regimen may improve symptoms associated with this disorder.

Acute Pulmonary Thromboembolism

Pulmonary embolism (PE) is a common and potentially fatal consequence of blood clot migration to the pulmonary vascular bed. In the vast majority of cases, thromboemboli originate in the large proximal capacitance vessels of the lower extremities. As such, PE is considered a complication of deep vein thrombosis (DVT). Less common vascular sources of clot are the upper extremities, pelvic veins, and the right ventricle. Amniotic fluid (pregnancy), septic thrombi (sepsis), fat (long bone fracture), air (central line mismanagement), and talc (intravenous drug use) are the constituents of rare types of emboli. Venous thrombi from systemic veins are, by far, the most common sources of PE (Tino & Kelley, 1997).

Patients at risk for venous clot formation have any combination of venous stasis, hypercoaguability, and endothelial injury. The most common risk factors for PE are detailed in Table 37–22. Iatrogenic sources of thromboembolism include indwelling venous catheters and certain medications, such as oral contraceptives.

Consequences of pulmonary emboli depend largely on the extent and site of the PE and whether blood flow distal to the clot is partially or completely obstructed. The patient may demonstrate profound hemodynamic compromise, mild chest pain, and dyspnea, or may remain asymptomatic. Hypoxemia may be a feature of PE and is due to ventilation–perfusion (V/Q) mismatch. Massive PE is associated with shunting and severe hypoxemia for which the patient may not be able to compensate. Obliteration of more than 50% of the pulmonary vascular bed results in significant increase in pulmonary vascular resistance by exceeding the capacitance of the remaining patent vasculature. This results in precapillary pulmonary hypertension and cor pulmonale. Because the right heart does not have the capacity to acutely alter its stroke volume, it fails, which causes systemic venous congestion. In the presence of a patent foramen ovale, increased right-heart pressures can result in an intracardiac shunt across the intraatrial septum to the left heart and systemic circulation. This is one mechanism by which massive PE results in intractable hypoxemia and death (Tino & Kelley, 1997).

The clinical presentation of pulmonary embolism can be enigmatic. As in any situation, the clinical setting has enormous bearing on suspicion of this disorder (Palevsky, 1994). Complaints of dyspnea, pleuritic chest pain, or hemoptysis are typical of the patient with PE. Other common, equally nonspecific symptoms are cough, fever, syncope, and orthopnea. The most common feature of the physical exam is tachypnea. Tachycardia and hypotension are seen with massive PE. Elevation of the neck veins (jugular venous distention) suggests right-heart failure and is extremely worrisome in the presence of risk factors for PE.

The initial diagnostic evaluation for PE includes chest radiograph, ABG, ECG, and V/Q scan (Kelley, Carson, Palevsky, & Schwartz, 1991). The value of chest radiography is in ruling out other entities that can mimic the clinical presentation of PE. Atelectasis, pleural effusion, or parenchymal infiltrate may be present, but are nondiagnostic. ABG may reveal hypoxemia with respiratory alkalosis. However, the absence of hypoxemia does not rule this diagnosis out. Any patient suspected of having a PE should have an ECG to rule out myocardial infarction. The most common ECG finding in acute PE is sinus tachycardia. Signs of right-heart abnormalities and nonspecific ST segment changes on ECG are common in this setting. V/Q scanning is most frequently used in the evaluation of PE (refer to Fig. 37–7B). A normal V/Q scan does rule out PE. Probability of PE is described as

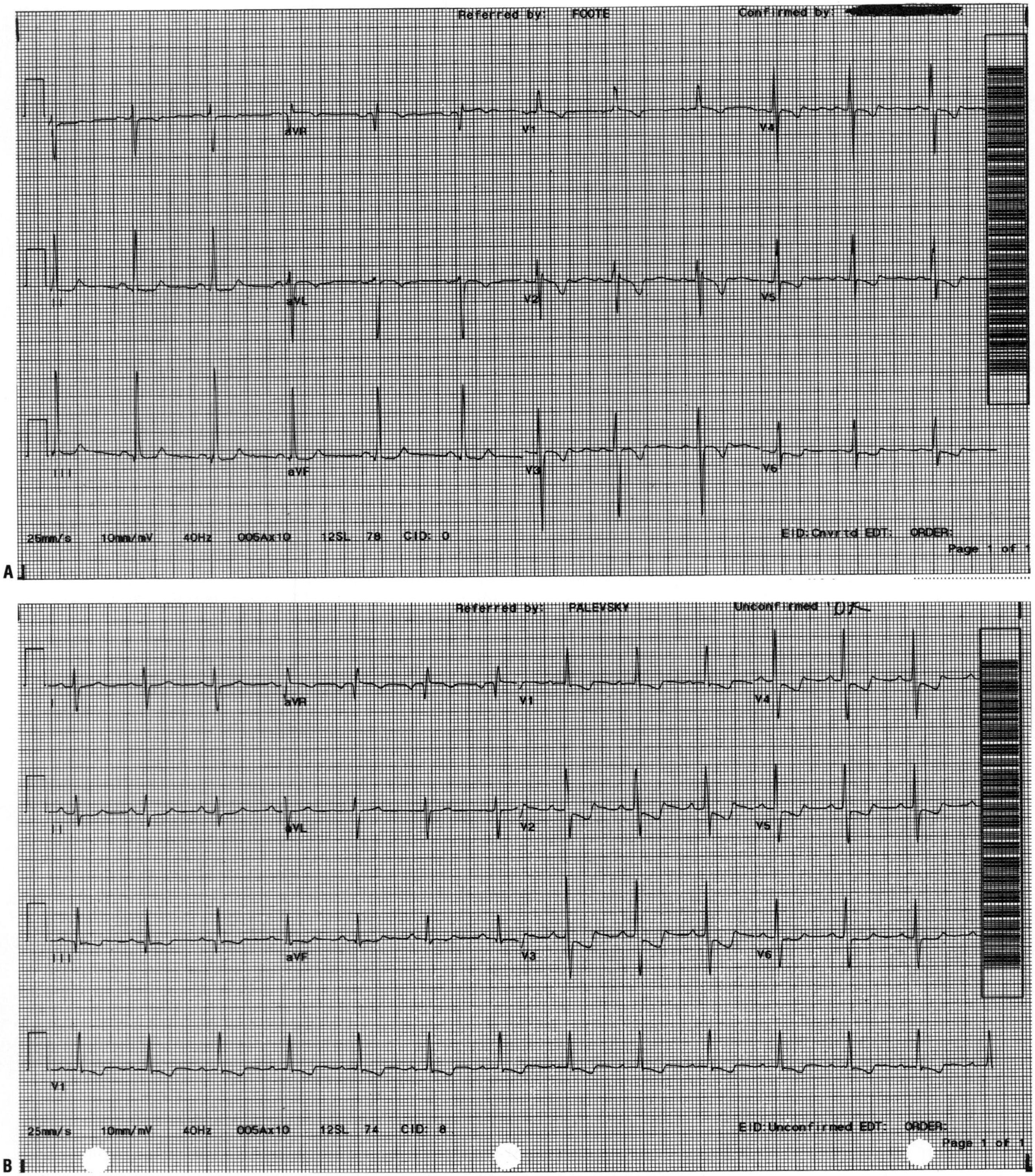

Figure 37–26. Electrocardiograph evidence of right ventricular hypertrophy. **A,** ST depressions seen in anterolateral and inferior leads suggest severe right ventricular hypertrophy. **B,** Severe right ventricular hypertrophy with associated incomplete right bundle branch block (wide QRS) is seen best in leads V_1-V_5. Inverted T-waves represent the right ventricle, not the left ventricle; therefore, the computer interpretation of anterolateral ischemia is in error.

TABLE 37–22. Risk Factors for Pulmonary Embolism

Venous Stasis
- Bed rest longer than 7 days
- Immobility
- Paralysis of lower extremities
- Congestive heart failure
- Cor pulmonale
- Prior venous thrombosis
- Recent major surgery requiring general anaesthesia

Endothelial Injury
- Trauma
- Surgery

Hypercoagulopathy
- Malignancy
- Estrogen therapy
- Inflammatory bowel disease
- Disemminated intervascular coagulopathy (DIC)
- Nephrotic syndrome
- Thrombocytopenia/thrombocytosis

low, intermediate, or high. When combined with sound clinical judgment, this is a highly effective diagnostic tool that is relatively low-risk (Kelley, Carson, Palevsky, & Schwartz, 1991; PIOPED, 1990). The gold standard to evaluate the presence of PE is pulmonary angiography.

By selectively injecting contrast dye into the branches of the pulmonary arterial system, pulmonary angiography is used to image the patency of the vascular lumen (Fig. 37–27). This invasive procedure has an increased risk in the setting of pulmonary hypertension due to right heart failure associated with infusion of the contrast. Renal toxicity of the dye, vascular injury, and dysrhythmias are other adverse reactions. Pulmonary angiography is expensive and not available at all institutions. Because of the risks, cost, and lack of availability, noninvasive testing is generally preferred despite the high sensitivity and specificity of this tool (Tino & Kelley, 1997).

Because most PEs originate in the deep veins of the lower extremities, noninvasive studies of these vessels are quite useful in the evaluation of thromboembolism. Documentation of deep venous thrombosis (DVT) is very supportive of the diagnosis of PE as it defines a source. The two most common diagnostic procedures used to evaluate for DVT are impedance plethsmography (IPG) and Doppler ultrasound (also known as "duplex"). Both of these diagnostic procedures are described in Chapter 31, Vascular Disease. MRI is used to evaluate the presence of venous thrombosis in the pelvic vasculature. Though a superior imaging technique, the cost and limited availability of MRI prohibit its use in the evaluation of lower extremity vessels. The presence of clot in the proximal venous system justifies intervention with antithrombotic therapy (Palevsky, 1994).

Interrupting further clot formation and migration from the proximal veins is the first therapeutic goal. Failure to intervene places the patient at high risk for recurrent PE. Despite common misperception, anticoagulation therapy does not dissolve clot; rather, it inhibits the expansion of the thrombosis while the endogenous lytic system dissolves the original obstruction. Standard treatment requires the intravenous administration of heparin (bolus of 5K to 10K units followed by continuous drip titrated to PTT of 1.5 to 2

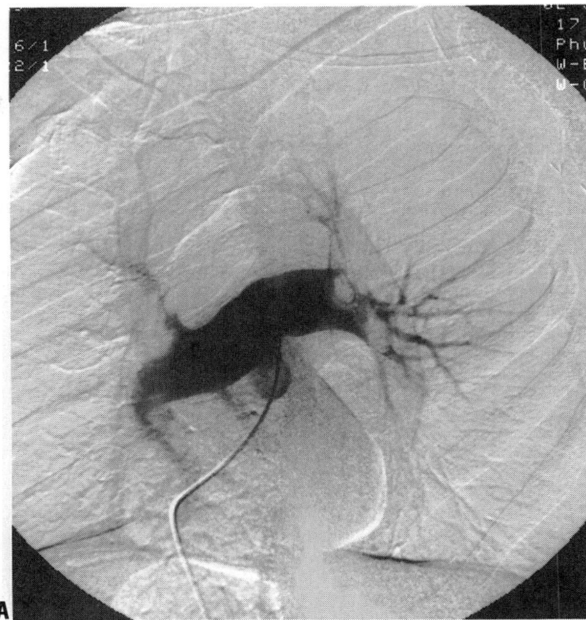

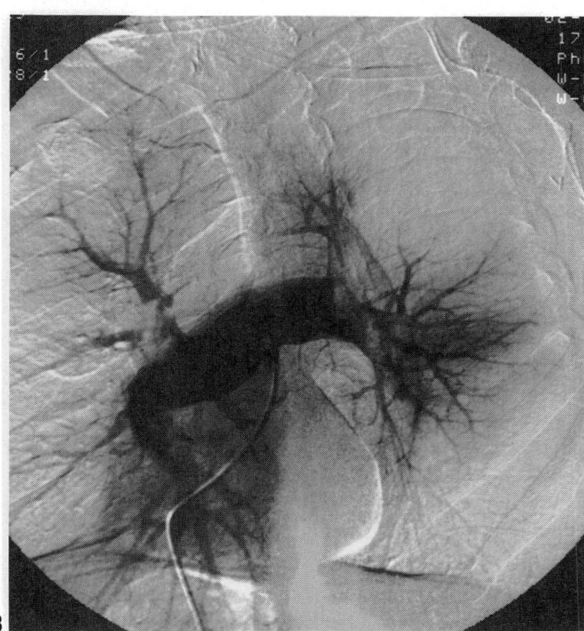

Figure 37–27. A, A picture of the arterial phase of an angiogram done on a 66-year-old man who presented with acute shortness of breath and chest pain. **B,** Obstruction of flow confirms the diagnosis of acute pulmonary embolism.

times the control) followed by oral anticoagulation using warfarin (dose titrated to PT of 1.25 to 1.5 baseline or INR of 2 to 3). Duration of therapy is a minimum of 3 months; longer as dictated by the perpetuation of predisposing factors (Tino & Kelley, 1997).

The role of thrombolytic therapy remains highly controversial. The three agents available for this approach are streptokinase, urokinase, and recombitant tissue-type plasminogen activator (tPA). These drugs are reserved for treating PE that causes cardiopulmonary crisis including profound, refractory hypoxemia, or right-heart failure. Major contraindications are cerebral vascular disease, invasive procedures, surgery, or trauma within the week that precipitates PE. After a course of thrombolytic therapy, chronic anticoagulation therapy is still necessary to prevent recurrent thromboemboli.

The major adverse effect of anticoagulation is bleeding. In patients for whom anticoagulation is contraindicated or insufficient, placement of a filter in the inferior vena cava (IVC) is the best option (Becker, Philbrick, & Selby, 1992). IVC filter placement is also recommended for patients who have suffered a life-threatening PE in whom recurrent embolism might be fatal. Placed percutaneously the IVC filter is designed to trap thromboemboli en route to the right heart and pulmonary vascular bed. Associated risks are filter dislodgement or migration, caval perforation, or clot propagation in the IVC. This option is frequently used in conjunction with anticoagulants for patients at high risk for recurrent thromboembolism.

In patients with life-threatening PE, surgical embolectomy may be indicated (Palevsky & Edmunds, 1997). This high-risk technique is reserved for severely compromised patients as it requires cardiopulmonary bypass. Pulmonary thromboendartarectomy is typically available only at tertiary hospitals.

Chronic Pulmonary Embolism

Uncommonly, pulmonary embolism fails to resolve despite appropriate therapy. In this setting, a scar forms within the pulmonary vasculature. This may, in time, result in the development of chronic thromboembolic pulmonary hypertension. There are no signs or symptoms specific to this disorder. As in other scenarios manifesting pulmonary hypertension, the most common presenting symptom is exertional dyspnea (Rubin, 1984). Patients with advanced disease or higher pulmonary arterial pressures may also report syncope or pre-syncope with exertion, angina-like chest pain, hemoptysis, or symptoms associated with cor pulmonale (Palevsky & Edmunds, 1997).

Physical exam findings of pulmonary hypertension are the same regardless of underlying pathophysiology. Diagnostic evaluation includes chest radiograph, electrocardiogram, pulmonary function testing, ventilation–perfusion (V/Q) scanning, and pulmonary angiogram. Chest radiograph is consistent with right ventricular hypertrophy with prominent central arteries. The electrocardiogram corroborates right ventricular hypertrophy with right axis deviation and a dominant R-wave in V_1. Pulmonary function tests may demonstrate normal (or slightly restricted) lung volumes and flows. This is useful in ruling out intrinsic parenchymal obstructive or restrictive disease as a potential cause of pulmonary hypertension. A reduction in diffusion capacity (DLCO) may be the only abnormality identified on PFTs. The V/Q scan is crucial in the determination of unresolved PE (Palevsky & Edmunds, 1997). A normal V/Q scan rules out both acute and chronic PE. However, the finding of subsegmental or larger perfusion defects obligate the clinician to pursue pulmonary angiogram to confirm or exclude thromboembolic disease. Pulmonary angiogram demonstrates organized thrombi appearing as atypical filling defects, webs or bands, or completely thrombosed vessels (Auger, Feullo, Moser, et al., 1992).

Medical management with anticoagulation and thrombolytic therapy is of little value in the setting of chronic PE. Because clots are organized and fibrotic, they are no longer amenable to pharmacologic intervention (Moser, Auger, Fedullo, & Jamieson, 1992). Inferior vena caval filter placement is indicated to prevent recurrent thromboembolization.

Once this diagnosis is established, referral should be made for consideration of surgical thromboendartarectomy (Palevsky & Edmunds, 1997). This operation has been developed to relieve vascular obstruction, improve pulmonary circulation, and reduce pulmonary arterial pressures and right heart afterload. In the absence of surgical intervention, the natural history of this disease leads to progressive right-heart failure and death. Following surgery, patients require lifelong anticoagulation, but improvement in their clinical situation can be dramatic (Palevsky & Edmunds, 1997).

Environmental Lung Diseases

This category of lung disorders result from the inhalation of particulate matter or noxious gases. Frequently used synonymously with environmental lung disease, occupational lung diseases are actually a category within this group of disorders. With each breath, the lungs are exposed to the hostile elements of the environment. Environmental pulmonary exposures are divided into four categories: infectious agents, organic dusts, inorganic dusts, and gases. Inorganic dusts and gases are primarily responsible for the disorders recognized as occupational lung diseases. The physiologic reaction to such an exposure include asthma or bronchitis, parenchymal disease, and neoplastic disorders. This disease category may include hypersensitivity pneumonitis, wherein there is granulomatous response to antigen exposure (Redlich & Balmes, 1995). Table 37–23 describes a variety of environmental lung diseases and their causative agents. The most common environmental lung diseases are discussed.

Precise history-taking is crucial in the evaluation of suspected environmental lung disorders. It is important to remember that exposure may have taken place outside of the work setting. Many hobbies employ substances that can

TABLE 37–23. Classification of Occupational Lung Disorders

Disease/Problem	Example of Causative Agent
Major acute or subacute diseases	
Upper respiratory tract irritation	Irritant gases, solvents
Airway disorders	
Occupational asthma	
Sensitization	Diisocyanates, animal dander
Irritant-induced, RADS	Irritant gases
Byssinosis	Cotton dust
Grain dust effects	Grain
Inhalation injury	
Toxic pneumonitis	Irritant gases, metals
Metal fume fever	Metal oxides—zinc, copper
Polymer fume fever	Plastics
Smoke inhalation	
Hypersensitivity pneumonitis	Microbial agents
Infectious disorders	Tuberculosis
Acute pleural disease	Asbestos
Major chronic diseases	
Interstitial fibrotic diseases (pneumoconioses)	Asbestos, silica, coal
Beryllium/hard metal-related disease	Beryllium, cobalt
Chronic bronchitis/COPD	Mineral dusts, coal
Malignancies of the respiratory tract and pleura	
Sinonasal cancer	Wood dust
Laryngeal cancer	Asbestos?
Lung cancer	Asbestos, radon
Mesothelioma	Asbestos
Air pollution	
Ambient air pollution	Sulfur oxides, particulates
Indoor air pollution	Environmental tobacco smoke

Reprinted with permission from Redlich & Balmes. (1995). (p. 360).

become airborne pathogens, so recreational details must be included in a thorough history. Exposures to pathogens may have been remote or, even, indirect. The patient may have been exposed to dust particles carried in the clothing of the spouse or children. In most cases, duration and intensity of exposure have direct bearing on severity of illness (Weill & Jones, 1988).

Asbestos-Related Lung Disease

Asbestos is an industrial material that, until recently, was widely used in construction materials, insulation, automotive parts, and fire-resistant clothing. It is a silicate fiber that is heat resistant and flexible, yet durable. Although there is now legislation limiting its use, asbestos is still present in old buildings and ships. Asbestos fibers are released into the environment with demolition or renovation of such structures. When inhaled, these fibers may be deposited in the pulmonary parenchyma. The most common findings in asbestos exposure are pleural placques that are of minimal clinical significance. Asbestosis is the parenchymal reaction to asbestos fibers that results in interstitial fibrosis. Other complications of asbestos exposure are pleural effusion, pleural fibrosis and/or pleural thickening, mesothelioma, and bronchogenic carcinoma.

As in IPF, the mechanism of injury is persistent inflammatory response. Following an initial insult to the terminal airways, the smaller particles are phagocytized and cleared from the lung. The longer fibers, however, remain in the alveolar bed perpetuating the inflammatory process and fibrous tissue deposition. This process, in the presence of cigarette smoking, is estimated to increase the patient's risk for pulmonary cancers by 50 to 100 times (Weill & Jones, 1988).

The clinical presentation of the patient with asbestosis is similar to that of the patient with other restrictive defects. Progressive dyspnea, persistent dry cough, and pleuritic chest pain are common symptoms. Physical exam may reveal clubbing, bibasalar rales, and cyanosis. Pulmonary function testing may range from normal to restricted, though typically, the greatest decrement is seen in the DLCO. Diagnosis is made on the basis of CXR, CT scan, BAL, and, if necessary, lung biopsy (Redlich & Balmes, 1995).

The chest radiograph of a patient with asbestosis has a "ground glass" appearance with changes predominantly in the lower lung fields (Fig. 37–28). Bilateral pleural fibrosis, pleural plaques, pleural thickening, or pleural effusions may also be radiographically apparent. Asbestos bodies (also

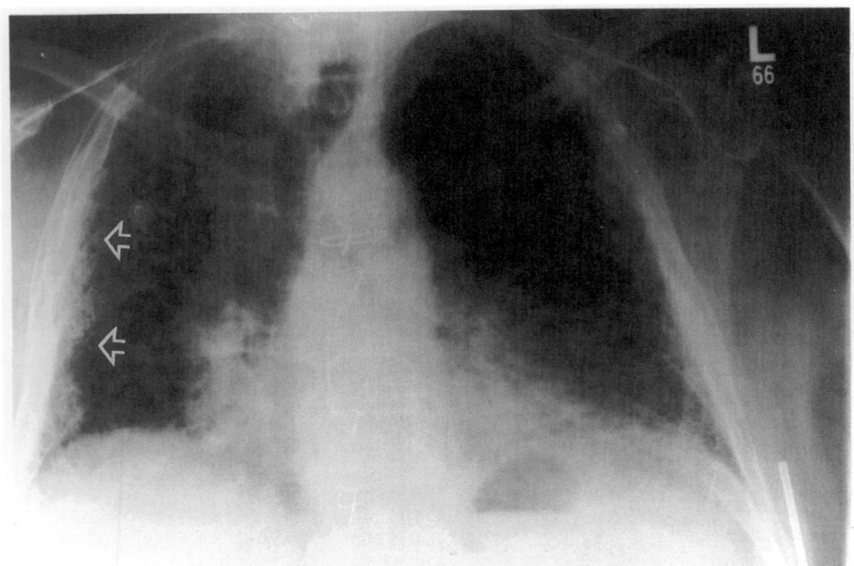

Figure 37–28. Posterior–anterior (PA) chest radiograph of a 59-year-old shipyard worker. Bilateral interstitial markings with reticular densities in the peripheral and basalar lung (marked with arrows on the right side only) are typical of asbestosis. The indistinct borders of the heart and diaphragm are described as "shaggy" and are indicative of interstitial lung disease in the lung adjacent to the heart. (Note: Sternal wires from prior medianstemotomy for cardiac surgery.)

known as ferrugenous bodies) found on either bronchial alveolar lavage or tissue biopsy confirm this diagnosis.

By virtue of its pathogenesis, asbestosis is a progressive and unrelenting disease. Treatment principles are identical to those of pulmonary fibrosis. It is important to protect the patient from further exposure to asbestos. Because of the dramatic increase in incidence of bronchogenic carcinomas and pulmonary fibrosis, it is imperative that cigarette smokers be strongly urged to quit.

Silicosis

Silica is the main constituent of most of the Earth's rocks. There are a variety of industrial settings wherein crystalline silica becomes a respirable dust. Depending on the particle size, the concentration in the air, and the intensity of exposure, people who entrain this dust into the airways can develop silicosis, a chronic fibrosing disorder of the lung. Miners, tunnel diggers, sandblasters, masons, foundry workers, potters, and road construction workers are all at risk for silicosis. Though there is an acute form of silicosis, it typically progresses slowly after decades of low to moderate exposure (Lapp & Castranova, 1993). The disease has been seen to progress even if the exposure is terminated.

Silica particles deposited in the alveoli provoke macrophage activity. A series of inflammatory events ensues during which the silica is ingested by the macrophage but never destroyed. When the macrophage is lysed, inflammatory mediators are released and the silica is reintroduced to the cell membrane. The inflammatory process continually cycles resulting in fibrosis. With recurrent inflammation, collagen fibers are deposited in concentric layers, rendering a whorled nodule encased in collagen. The appearance of the chest radiograph varies with the different manifestations of silicosis. The functional impairment depends on the extent of the disease and the individual susceptibility. PFTs may reveal restrictive, obstructive, or mixed patterns.

There are four clinical manifestations of this disease process: chronic uncomplicated silicosis, accelerated silicosis, acute silicosis, and silicotuberculosis (Weber & Banks, 1994). The distinction is important in predicting clinical outcomes. Chronic uncomplicated silicosis has the most indolent clinical presentation. It occurs after decades of low to moderate exposure. In the initial stages, it tends to be accompanied by no respiratory symptoms other than a mild cough. As it advances, the patient may complain of dyspnea and productive cough. Frequently, it is detected on routine chest radiograph which shows a varying degree of the size and number of rounded symmetric nodules (Fig. 37–29). Calcified hilar lymph nodes are described as "eggshell calcification" and are a classic feature of silicosis. The degree of radiographic abnormality depends on the intensity of exposure.

When the nodules enlarge and coalesce, they destroy vasculature and bronchi, resulting in progressive massive fibrosis. This is the hallmark of complicated silicosis. The bilateral and symmetrical upper lobe masses tend to cavitate and are associated with tuberculosis, atypical mycobacterial disease, and other anaerobic infections. Chest radiographic shows upper lobe fibrosis and retraction with splaying of the hila. Lower lung fields may demonstrate emphysematous changes (Redlich & Balmes, 1995).

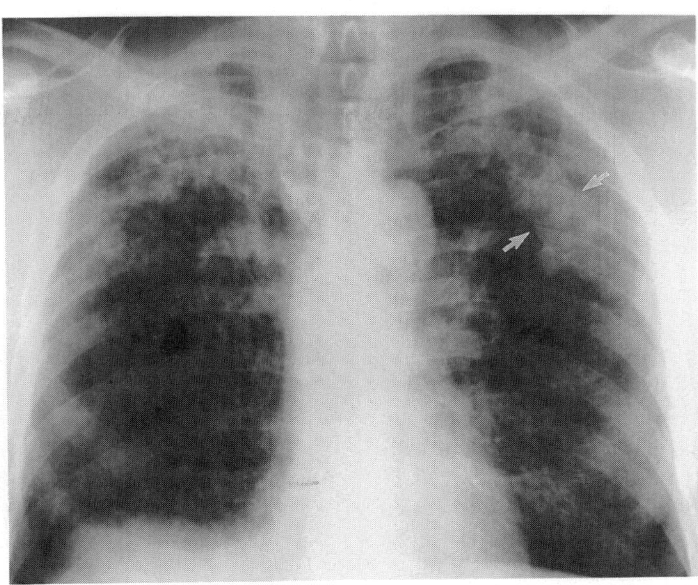

Figure 37–29. Posterior–anterior (PA) chest radiograph of a 72-year-old man with silicosis. There are diffuse, bilateral nodular densities and a conglomerate mass *(arrows)* in the left upper lobe. These are characteristic radiographic features of this disorder.

Accelerated silicosis occurs in the setting of exposure to moderately high-dust concentrations over a shorter period of time (4-8 years). The radiographic presentation shows small stellate opacities mixed with linear and irregular forms. The progression to massive pulmonary fibrosis is more rapid and more frequent than in chronic silicosis.

Acute silicosis is a rare entity that rapidly progresses to death by respiratory failure. It is seen in individuals (e.g., sandblasters) who have had a heavy and concentrated exposure to silica dust. Within months of the exposure, patients present with severe dyspnea, weight loss, and fatigue. Chest radiograph demonstrates an ill-defined consolidation in the mid and lower lung zones without nodulations. BAL reveals lung fluid that is high in surfactant, lipids, and proteinaceous material.

Because silica is toxic to pulmonary alveolar macrophages, the lung becomes vulnerable to mycobacteria. Species of mycobacteria include *M kansasi, M avium,* and *M tuberculosis* (Balmes, Cullen, & Gee, 1981). Symptoms of chest pain, hemoptysis, or fever may be attributed to superimposed infection rather than the original process of silcosis. The risk of tuberculosis is 4 to 6 times normal in the patient with silicosis (Snider, 1978). The development of tuberculosis in this setting is termed "silicotuberculosis." Patients should be monitored with bacteriologic evaluation of the sputum and annual PPD skin tests. Positive results may require a prolonged course of anti-tuberculin therapy because relapse rates are higher in this population.

Coal Workers' Pneumoconiosis

Prolonged exposure to coal dust results in the development of coal workers' pneumoconiosis (CWP). This entity is better recognized by the lay public as "black lung." The incidence of CWP has been significantly reduced by the mechanization of coal mining over the past several years. Chronic bronchitis is a lesser, though more common, manifestation of exposure to the mineral dust (Lapp & Parker, 1992).

With heavy exposure to coal dust, the clearance mechanisms of the lung are overwhelmed. The pathogen accumulates and settles in the terminal air spaces. The aggregation of coal dust, macrophages, fibroblasts, and reticulin fibers are described histologically as coal macules. Coal macules collect around small airways causing bronchiolar dilatation and focal centrilobular emphysema. Radiographically, the coal macules appear as tiny nodular infiltrates with an upper lobe predominance. In the absence of cigarette smoking, there are generally no PFT abnormalities. FEV_1 may be slightly reduced in relation to centrilobular emphysema (Redlich & Balmes, 1995). Patients who have simple, uncomplicated CWP should terminate their exposure to the inciting dust, but require no further treatment. Unlike silicosis, this disease is halted by the cessation of dust exposure. The report of melanoptysis, the production of black sputum, should raise clinical awareness of the patient's risk for CWP, but does not confirm its presence.

This disease rarely advances (Lapp & Parker, 1992). The development of progressive massive fibrosis distinguishes the pathologic process as "complicated CWP." The complaint of exercise-induced dyspnea is common in this setting. Patients with complicated CWP have a reduced DLCO and evidence of restriction on PFTs. The PFTs rarely demonstrate a mixed picture of restriction and obstruction. As in silicosis, patients with progressive massive fibrosis are at risk for mycobacterial infections, especially tuberculosis. Treatment is guided by the patient's symptoms. The most important interventions are the patient's removal from site of the exposure and avoidance of irritants, such as cigarette smoke. Interestingly, there is no evidence to suggest that CWP predisposes the patient to pulmonary malignancies.

Infectious Lung Diseases

Most infectious disorders of the lung arise from inhalation or aspiration of an infectious organism. The pathogens involved in acute infections are bacteria, viruses, and mycoplasmas. Chronic pulmonary infections are related to mycobacteria or fungi. Immunocompromised individuals are further susceptible to opportunistic infections. When the intrinsic pulmonary defense mechanisms are overwhelmed by the number and aggressiveness of the organisms, infection ensues. Depending on the site of inflammation, infections are categorized as upper or lower respiratory tract infections. They are further identified by their location within the respiratory tract. Common pathogens indigenous to sites within the upper and lower respiratory tract are detailed in Table 37–24A and 37–24B, respectively. Lower respiratory tract infections are discussed here.

Acute Bronchitis

Acute inflammation of the mucous membrane that lines the lumen of the bronchi is called acute bronchitis. The term "tracheobronchitis" is used to describe inflammation that extends to incorporate the trachea. Physical or chemical irritation of the bronchi cause noninfectious bronchitis. Infectious sources of acute bronchitis in the otherwise healthy individual are usually viruses (Neiderman & Sarosi, 1995). The same viruses frequently cause upper respiratory tract infections that precipitate lower respiratory tract infections. The only mycoplasma frequently identified in this process is *M pneumoniae.* Primary infection by bacteria is rare in the healthy individual. However, in patients with underlying COPD, impaired airway clearance renders increased vulnerability to superimposed bacterial infections.

Acute bronchitis is typically associated with low-grade fever and productive cough. Cough is the universal feature of bronchitis. Alteration of the surface epithelium makes the nerve endings very sensitive to mild irritants. The stimulation of the sensory receptors in the airways results in cough. Cold air, dust, deep breathing, talking, or laughing may incite a coughing spell. Initially, the cough is dry and may be accompanied by mild, retrosternal chest pain. As the virus runs its course, the bronchial mucosa secretes excessive mucous. This causes a productive cough with varying degrees of mucopurulence. The irritation of the bronchial mucosa can cause bronchial hyperreactivity; hence, acute bronchitis may precipitate bronchospasm in asthmatic patients (Farzan, 1997).

In most cases, this infection is self-limited and has no sequelae. Diagnosis is made on the basis of clinical features. In the absence of underlying lung disease, breath sounds and chest radiograph are unremarkable. Treatment is guided by the patient's symptoms. Patients are advised to avoid bronchial irritants. The role of cough suppressants and expectorants are merely comfort measures and are not believed to speed recovery. Antibiotic therapy is indicated only when a bacterial infection is suspected (Neiderman & Sarosi, 1995). Sputum culture and sensitivity is used to identify a bacterial pathogen and guide antibiotic selection. This process rarely progresses to pneumonia. Abnormal findings on physical exam, including significant fever, should prompt the clinician to obtain a chest x-ray to rule out pneumonia.

TABLE 37–24A. Common Pathogens for Upper Respiratory Tract Infections

Pharyngitis
Group A streptococci
Viruses
Adenovirus
Enteroviruses
Influenza
Epstein-Barr virus
Herpesvirus hominis
Laryngitis
Viruses
Common cold
Viruses
Rhinovirus
Adenovirus
Coronavirus
Influenza
Sinusitis
Haemophilus influenzae
Pneumococcus
Anaerobes
Rhinovirus
Epiglottitis
H. influenzae
Haemophilus parainfluenzae
Staphylococcus aureus
Group A streptococcus
Croup
Viruses
Parainfluenza virus
Respiratory syncytial virus
Adenovirus
Mycoplasma pneumoniae

Reprinted with permission from Niederman & Sarosi. (1995). (p. 426).

Pneumonia

By definition, pneumonia is the acute inflammation of the gas-exchanging units (bronchioles, alveolar ducts, alveolar sacs, and alveoli) of the lung. The mechanism of the inflammation is usually infectious, though chemical sources (e.g., aspiration of gastric contents) can cause pneumonia as well.

TABLE 37–24B. Common Pathogens for Lower Respiratory Tract Infections

- Bronchitis
  - *Haemophilus influenzae*
  - Pneumococcus
  - *Branhamella catarrhalis*
  - *Mycoplasma pneumoniae*
  - Viruses
    - Adenovirus
    - Influenza
    - Rhinovirus
    - Respiratory syncytial virus
- Bronchiolitis
  - Viruses
    - Respiratory syncytial virus
    - Parainfluenza virus
    - Adenovirus
    - Rhinovirus
- Pneumonia
  - Pneumococcus
  - *Legionella pneumophilia*
  - *M pneumoniae*
  - *H influenzae*
  - Anaerobes
  - *Staphylococcus aureus*
  - Enteric Gram-negatives
  - Viruses
    - Influenza
    - Respiratory syncytial virus
    - Adenovirus
  - *Chlamydia psittaci (TWAR)*
  - *Pneumocystis carinii*
- Bronchiectasis
  - *Pseudomonas aeruginosa*
  - *S. aureus*
  - Mucoid *Escherichia coli*
  - *H influenzae*

Reprinted with permission from Niederman & Sarosi. (1995). (p. 427).

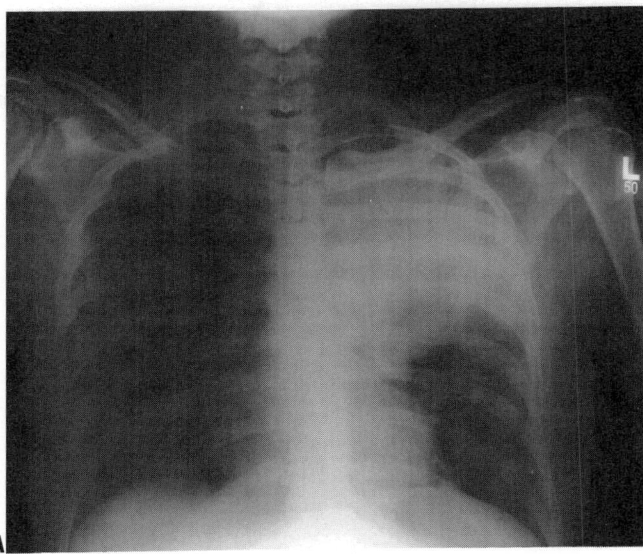

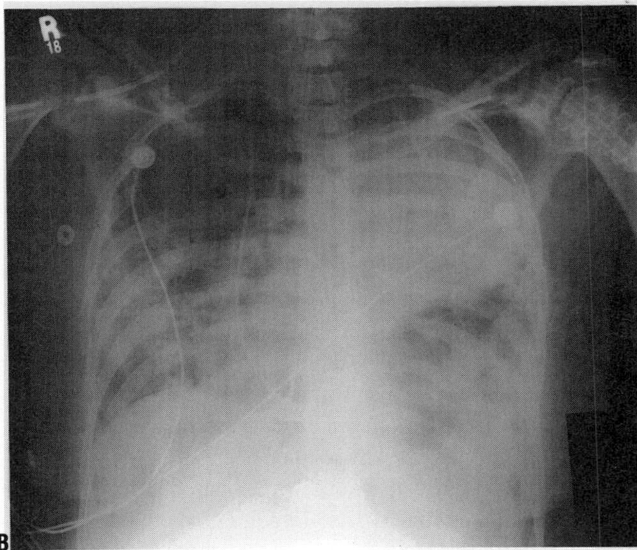

Figure 37–30. A, Anterior–posterior (AP) chest radiograph of a 50-year-old woman with fever, dyspnea, and productive cough. The fluffy alveolar infiltrate represents pneumonia. **B,** A repeat AP radiograph of the same patient 24 hours later demonstrates the presence of new diffuse and bilateral infiltrates. This is one of the criteria necessary to confirm acute respiratory distress syndrome (ARDS). Note endotracheal tube in place.

Patients at risk for pneumonia are those with impaired pulmonary defenses. Individuals who are elderly, chronically ill, immunocompromised, or have altered mental status are prone to this potentially life-threatening disorder.

The chest radiograph of a patient with pneumonia typically reveals an alveolar infiltrate (Fig. 37–30). Depending on the organism and the condition of its host, the infiltrate may be focal or diffuse. Sputum and blood cultures are important in the identification of the offending organism and its sensitivities. Unfortunately, clinical decision making cannot wait for culture growth and sensitivity testing, which can take as long as 72 hours to complete. For this reason, diagnostic assumptions are based on the patient's clinical scenario (Neiderman & Sarosi, 1995).

Presenting symptoms of bacterial pneumonia may include cough, purulent sputum production, hemoptysis, pleuritic chest pain, dyspnea. Physical examination typically reveals fever, tachycardia, and tachypnea. Crackles may be appreciated over the affected area. An elevated white blood cell count (15,000 to 30,000/mL) is found in most patients with pneumonia. Atypical pneumonias present with a gradual onset of constitutional symptoms (fever, malaise, headache, sore throat) that precede pulmonary symptoms by as much as three to four days. Cough is dry or scantly productive, but may be severe. Physical examination is frequently unremarkable, though rales may be present. In early stages, radiographic presentation of atypical pneumonia usually shows an ill-defined interstitial infiltrate. Later, the chest radiograph reveals alveolar consolidation similar to that seen in bacterial pneumonia. Infections are categorized as community-acquired, nosocomial, or pneumonia in the immunocompromised host. This is the basis for therapeutic intervention, including antibiotic selection. The principles behind recognizing and treating pneumonia are discussed at length in Chapter 16, Fever and the Hospitalized Patient.

Lung Abscess

A lung abscess is a localized, suppurative, necrotizing lesion within the pulmonary parenchyma. Most abscesses result from necrosis associated with an existing pulmonary lesion, such as pneumonia or neoplasms. Secondary abscesses stem from septic emboli, aspirated foreign bodies, or rupture of an extrapulmonary abscess into the lung (Wiedemann & Rice, 1995).

Though most abscesses contain mixed bacterial flora, anaerobes are the most common infectious organisms involved. Precipitating factors of the development of a lung abscess are aspiration, bronchial obstruction, or septic embolism from a remote infected site (Cassiere & Niederman, 1997). Individuals with altered mental status or oropharyngeal–esophageal dysmotility are at greatest risk for aspiration. Risk of abscess formation is enhanced in patients with poor dentition or gingival disease due to the high bacterial load of the aspirate. Postobstructive abscesses develop distal to bronchial obstruction. The normal clearance mechanism of the lung becomes defunct when a foreign body or neoplasm blocks airway clearance. Trapped infectious secretions fester, cause local necrosis, and become pyogenic. Rarely, penetrating chest wounds or suppurative lesions below the diaphragm can extend to the parenchyma to cause an abscess. Direction of the bronchi and gravitational effects at the time of aspiration cause most abscesses to occur in the superior segments of the lower lobes or in the posterior segments of the upper lobes (Niederman & Sarosi, 1995).

Most patients present with insidious onset of symptoms. History of aspiration may be remote (greater than 2 weeks), if present or recalled. Common complaints include cough, sputum production, fever, chills, anorexia, weight loss, pleuritic chest pain, or hemoptysis. Information about risk factors for aspiration or bronchial obstruction should be elicited. The most common finding on physical exam is foul-smelling sputum which is indicative of an anaerobic infection. Another noteworthy finding (requiring follow-up care) is poor oral hygiene.

The classic finding of a lung abscess on chest radiograph is a cavitary lesion with an air-fluid level (Fig. 37–31). Elevated white blood cell count and mild anemia may be present. Sputum culture may be of limited value because of obfuscation by oral contaminants. In most cases,

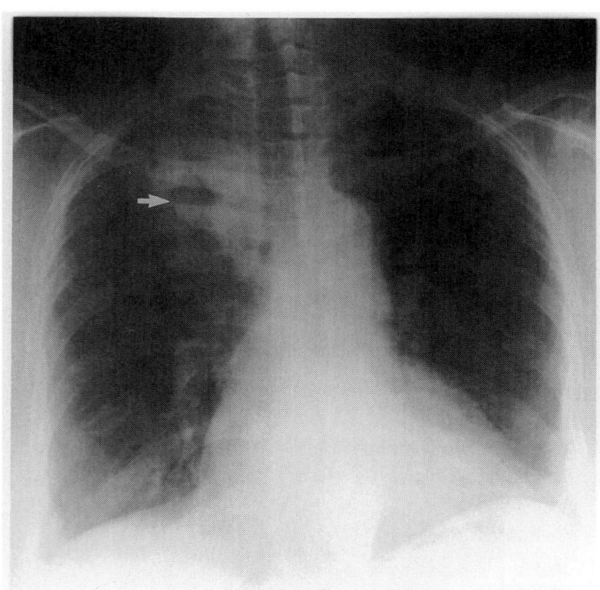

Figure 37–31. Posterior–anterior (PA) chest radiograph of a 29-year-old intravenous drug user with a history of low-grade fevers and 20-pound weight loss over the previous 3 months. The cavitary lesion containing an air-fluid level (*arrow*) is the classic finding supportive of the diagnosis of lung abscess.

the diagnosis is made on the basis of chest radiograph and supportive clinical history. Treatment includes antibiotic therapy and abscess drainage. Antibiotics are selected for their specificity against anaerobic organisms. Typically patients are started on intravenous penicillin or clindamycin and subsequently converted to oral amoxicillin, clindamycin, or penicillin for a prolonged course until the abscess resolves. Pulmonary toilet is achieved with postural drainage and, unless the patient has hemoptysis, chest percussion. This process is gradual but essential in resolution of the abscess (Cassiere & Niederman, 1997).

When empiric antibiotic therapy fails, definitive diagnosis is established by percutaneous needle aspiration, transtracheal needle aspiration, or bronchoscopy. Fiberoptic bronchoscopy is also indicated by the suspicion of endobronchial obstruction, the absence of risk factors for aspiration, or microbiologic evaluation in the immunocompromised host (Sosenko & Glassroth, 1985). In patients with large air–fluid levels, percutaneous drainage with a pigtail catheter may speed resolution of fever and other symptoms. This procedure eliminates the risk of decanting the contents of the abscee into other regions of the lung. Bronchoscopy is not utilized for the drainage of an abscess due to the risk of hemoptysis or abscess rupture and subsequent aspiration and spread of infection.

The development of an empyema is a serious complication of lung abscess. Rupture of the abscess into the pleural space causes a pyopneumothorax. Either of these perilous circumstances indicates referral to a thoracic surgeon for surgical drainage. This procedure is covered in detail in Chapter 38, Thoracic Surgery.

Fungal Infections

Fungi are found throughout the environment. Different species of fungi are endemic to certain climates or geographic regions. Fungal organisms grow as molds in soil and release spores into the atmosphere. These spores are respirable particles that require heat and moisture to reproduce. Once established in the infected host, fungi change to yeast where they multiply by budding. Budding yeast provide pathogenic evidence of fungal infection. Individuals with impaired pulmonary defenses or those exposed to a large innoculum are at risk for fungal infection, invasion, and dissemination. The degree to which the host is affected depends largely upon the status of the immune system. In all fungal infections, those individuals who suffer disseminated disease are at much higher risk for critical illness and death than those who only develop acute uncomplicated infections. Common fungi associated with pulmonary infection include aspergillus, *H capsalatum, B dermatitidis,* and *C immitis.*

Aspergillosis. There are many species of this ubiquitous fungus. Grown as mold on organic materials, aspergillus becomes airborne when its medium is disturbed. Construction sites with building renovations are notorious for inciting aspergillosis epidemics, particularly near hospitals where there is a higher population of medically vulnerable individuals. This fungus may also be found as a saprophyte, or colonizer, in the airways of people with chronic lung disease. Complications of exposure to aspergillus include hypersensitivity pneumonitis (discussed earlier in this chapter) as well as the following disorders.

Allergic Bronchopulmonary Aspergillosis. In the presence of longstanding asthma, patients can develop an allergy-mediated asthmatic response to the aspergillus organism. The clinical features of allergic bronchopulmonary aspergillosis (ABPA) are episodic asthma attacks, mucous plugging of the airways, atelectasis, and transient infiltrates on chest radiograph. Recurrent episodes can cause fibrosis of the upper lobes or bronchiectasis of the central bronchi.

Diagnosis is made on the basis of clinical history and supportive laboratory evidence. Sputum culture that is positive for aspergillus may merely indicate airway colonization. Blood tests that reveal high IgE, eosinophilia, and high specific antibodies to the fungal antigen are indicative of ABPA. A positive skin test indicates exposure to the fungal antigen and may support the diagnosis of ABPA (Levitz, 1989).

Patients with ABPA are treated with systemic corticosteroids, bronchodilators, and aggressive pulmonary hygiene. The goal of treatment is to prevent distortion of the bronchial architecture and to control bronchospasm (Richman, 1994). There is no proven role for oral antifungal agents (e.g., itraconazole) in the treatment of this disorder.

Aspergilloma. Cavitary or cystic lesions in the lung provide a dark, warm, moist environment in which fungus can thrive. The aggregation of fungal mycelia, fibrin, mucous, and cellular debris in such a setting constitutes an aspergilloma. More aptly described as a "fungus ball," aspergillomas are most commonly found in the cavitating lesions created by underlying tuberculosis or sarcoidosis.

Standard chest radiograph is usually diagnostic of this entity (Fig. 37–32). Typically located in the upper lobes, the fungus ball is identified by the crescent of air that surrounds it. It appears as a freely movable density within a preexisting cavity. Prior chest radiographs are extremely useful in determining the presence of a preexisting cavity. CT scanning is used to image the abnormality in more subtle disease.

Though rarely invasive, aspergillomas occasionally erode through a vessel wall and cause hemoptysis. Drug therapy is not indicated unless local invasion is suspected. In this circumstance, the patient is treated with systemic anti-fungal therapy (Niederman & Sarosi, 1995) or local delivery of mucomyst and amphotericin. Surgical resection of the mass and its cavity may be indicated by massive or recurrent hemoptysis.

Chronic Necrotizing Pulmonary Aspergillosis. Because of their impaired immunity and clearance mechanisms, patients with underlying diabetes, malnutrition, or COPD are at risk for chronic indolent aspergillus infection (Levitz,

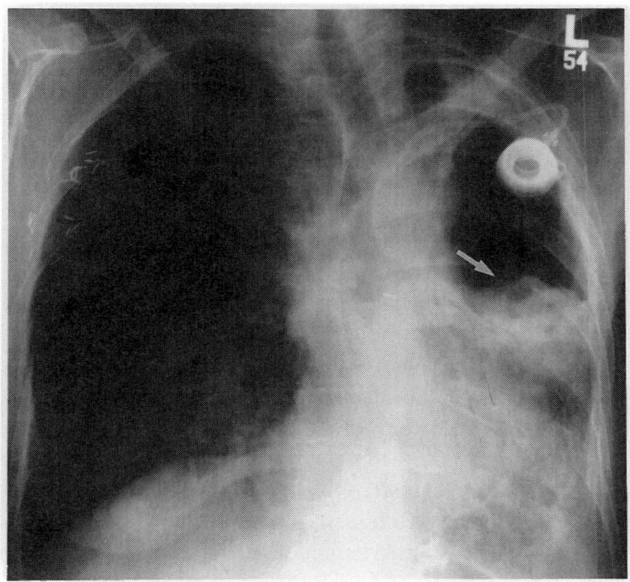

Figure 37–32. Posterior–anterior (PA) chest radiograph of a 39-year-old woman status-post breast cancer, status-post radiation to the left lung who is being treated with chemotherapy and corticosteroids and presents with a fever. Chest radiograph demonstrates a large cavity with a dependent intracavitary mass (*arrow*). This is the radiographic appearance of an aspergilloma.

1989). Persistent localized invasion of the parenchyma can lead to necrosis of the involved tissue.

The chest radiograph of the individual with this disorder demonstrates an upper lobe infiltrate with cavitation and fibrosis. An aspergilloma may or may not be present. Fiberoptic bronchoscopy is used to obtain sputum and tissue biopsies from the area of concern. Histologic evidence of tissue invasion confirms the diagnosis (Niederman & Sarosi, 1995).

This serious complication is treated with intravenous antifungal therapy (amphotericin B). The role of chronic suppressive therapy with oral agents is unclear.

Invasive Aspergillosis. Also known as "disseminated aspergillosis," this process is the most serious complication of aspergillosis. Granulocytopenia, compromised immunity, and critical illness are typical risk factors for this entity. Uncontrolled pulmonary infection leads to seeding of the bloodstream, or fungemia, which spreads the disease to extrapulmonary structures and causes severe systemic and neurologic sequelae. Locally, the injured vasculature becomes occluded causing infarction and necrosis of the associated parenchyma.

Profound compromise of the patient necessitates aggressive diagnostic evaluation. Tissue biopsy, obtained by transbronchial biopsy or surgical resection, provides pathologic evidence to confirm the diagnosis.

Like many other fungal infections, invasive aspergillosis is treated with intravenous antifungal therapy. It is important that granulocytopenia be corrected so as to bolster the patient's defense against this highly fatal process (Levitz, 1989).

Histoplasmosis. *Histoplasma capsalatum (H capsalatum)* is the organism responsible for histoplasmosis. It is prevalent in the Ohio River and Mississippi River valleys and is found in soil, bird, and bat droppings. Once the spores are inhaled, they germinate in 2 to 3 days. An infiltrate develops and causes regional lymph node involvement. Fungus is then spread to the bloodstream where, in the immunocompetent host, cellular immunity is established. Necrosis of infected tissue and granuloma formation then calcifies the lesions, thereby arresting its activity and spread at primary and metastatic sites. Subsequent exposures are met with the previously established immunity that are not harmful to the host. Patients who suffer from impaired cellular immunity, particularly those with AIDS, are at high risk for disseminated histoplasmosis. Young children are also susceptible to disseminated disease. In this setting, there is multisystemic invasion by the fungus and significant risk for death. Complications of primary histoplasmosis include erosion or distortion of central bronchial and vascular structures by calcified lymph nodes or massive mediastinal fibrosis (Fishman, 1994).

In acute primary infection, the patient is generally asymptomatic, but thereafter renders a positive skin test reaction to histoplasmin. Heavy innoculum can cause flulike symptoms (malaise, headache, fever) for a few days. Chest x-ray shows patchy diffuse parenchymal infiltrates and bilateral hilar lymphadenopathy. Positive serology studies for complement fixation and immunodiffusion are consistent with active disease (Wheat, 1994). Evidence of the organism in body fluids, bone marrow, or in tissues provides definitive diagnosis.

The majority of cases of histoplasmosis are self-limited and require no medical intervention (Davies, 1994). Disseminated disease, however, requires aggressive therapy with an intravenous anti-fungal agent (e.g., amphotericin B) followed by chronic oral anti-fungals (e.g., itraconazole) (Dismukes, Bradsher, Cloud, et al., 1992; Niederman & Sarosi, 1995).

Blastomycosis. Blastomyces dermatitidis, the organism responsible for blastomycosis, is found in the soil in the south central and Great Lakes states. This fungal infection affects ten times as many men as women and is seen most commonly in the middle-aged. Following inhalation, the fungus converts to yeast. It is then disseminated to the skin, the skeletal structures, central nervous system, and, in men, the genitourinary system distal to the kidneys (Fishman, 1994).

Acute infection is characterized by influenza-like symptoms (fever, chills, arthralgias, myalgias) and a nonproductive cough that eventually becomes mucopurulent. Chest radiograph in this setting shows lobar or segmental consolidation. From this point, the patient either recovers without intervention or progresses to chronic or disseminated infection (Niederman & Sarosi, 1995).

Chronic disease has an indolent onset but results in chronic pneumonia, productive cough, hemoptysis, weight loss, and pleuritic chest pain. Cavitary lesions may be present on chest radiograph, though the typical feature is upper lobe predominant fibronodular disease.

The diagnosis is made by the presence of characteristic budding yeast organisms on smear or culture from sites of infection. Skin lesions are the most common extrapulmonary site of blastomycosis infection. Found on exposed skin, lesions are chronic and progressive and have a wart-like crusting appearance with microabscess formation (Fishman, 1994).

Like the other pulmonary fungal infections, the treatment of choice is amphotericin B intravenously (Dismukes, Bradsher, Cloud, et al., 1992). Immunocompromised patients require chronic suppressive therapy with an oral agent such as itraconazole. Disseminated disease that remains untreated places the patient at high risk for developing acute respiratory distress syndrome (ARDS).

Coccidiomycosis. Coccidioides immitis, the fungus that causes coccidiomycosis, is endemic from northern California as far south as Argentina. Most infections are seen during the dry hot months that follow the rainy season in these areas. Following initial infection by this organism, a nonspecific immune response incites a granulomatous reaction that walls off the infection, prohibiting its spread. Failure of this response results in dissemination of the infection and is most often seen in black and hispanic males as well as immunocompromised individuals (Fishman, 1994). Dissemination involves spread through the reticuloendothelial system (lymph nodes, spleen, liver, skin), bone, and central nervous system.

The majority of infected patients remain asymptomatic. Of those who become symptomatic, most complain of general malaise, headache, fever, and cough. This syndrome, referred to as "desert fever" or "valley fever," is self limited and resolves within several days. These patients generally do not suffer prolonged illness and are at low risk for developing disseminated disease (Patterson, 1997).

The most common chest radiographic finding during acute infection is localized parenchymal consolidation with or without hilar lymphadenopathy. Single or multiple nodules may be present and can develop into thin-walled cavities. Disseminated disease is radiographically represented by a diffuse bilateral micronodular pattern.

The diagnosis of coccidiomycosis is based on clinicoradiographic findings in the appropriate epidemiologic setting. Positive complement fixation serologic findings support the diagnosis (Stevens, 1995).

Acute infection is generally self-limited and therefore requires no medical intervention. Patients who develop cavitary lesions should be followed closely for secondary infections. Patients with disseminated disease are given intravenous anti-fungal therapy (amphotericin B) (Niederman & Sarosi, 1995). Unfortunately, extrapulmonary dissemination, particularly to the central nervous system, is associated with a very poor prognosis.

Mycobacterial Infections

Tuberculosis. Tuberculosis (TB) is one of the most common infections in the world. It is estimated that each year there are 8 million new cases and 3 million deaths associated with TB worldwide. Infection rates in the United States have been on the rise over the past decade due to an increase in the most vulnerable populations and the emergence of drug-resistant strains of the infectious organism (American College of Chest Physicians [ACCP] & American Thoracic Society [ATS], 1995). In this country, the people at greatest risk are the homeless, the elderly, foreign-born individuals from high incidence countries, the nutritionally compromised, the HIV infected, and intravenous drug users.

The organism responsible for this infection is Mycobacterium tuberculosis. This rod-shaped (bacilli) bacteria enters the pulmonary tree be inhalation of droplet nuclei expelled from the airways of infected individuals. Interestingly, the infection cannot be picked up through contact with contaminated surfaces or fomites. The host's response may range from subclinical findings to death depending on the status of the immune system and the virulence of the infectious organism. Active infection may occur shortly after innoculation or can be suppressed for years only to be reactivated when comorbidity causes immunity to wane (Silibovsky, 1994). While the lung is both the port of entry and the primary site of infection, extrapulmonary sites may also be involved. Clinical stages of tuberculosis are described as primary TB or reactivation TB.

Because TB may be quiescent in its early phases, infection is often identified on routine health screening. Chest radiography and PPD testing are mainstays in detection of this public health hazard. A PPD test involves the intradermal injection of the purified protein derivative of tuberculin to which the sensitized, or previously exposed, individual reacts. A positive result is manifested by a palpable induration within 48 to 72 hours. Guidelines for interpreting a positive tuberculin skin test reaction are described in Table 37–25.

Where health screening or clinical scenarios are suspicious for active TB, confirmation via culture of appropriate specimens is always necessary. Acid-fast bacilli (AFB) are found in the sputum, bronchoscopic specimens, or fluid samples from sites of extrapulmonary involvement. Thoracentesis and pleural biopsy may be required to evaluate fluid from a pleural effusion suspected to be secondary to TB. Massive hemoptysis, bronchopleural fistula, bronchial stenosis, trapped lung, and destroyed lung with persistently positive sputum are all manifestations that may necessitate

TABLE 37–25. Guidelines for Interpreting a Positive Tuberculin Skin Test Reaction

5-mm Induration	10-mm Induration	15-mm Induration
HIV-positive Immunosuppressed Recent contacts of TB case Abnormal CXR c/w TB	Foreign born from high-prevalence countries Low-income populations IV drug users Residents of institutions Persons > 70 y HCWs who directly care for patients at high risk or with active TB Mycobacteriology lab personnel Persons with medical conditions that make them high risk	No risk factors for TB

Reprinted with permission from Dunlap & Kimerling. (1997). (p. 1998).

surgical intervention (which provides a tissue specimen for culture) (Dunlop & Kimerling, 1997). If positive for *M tuberculosis,* the specimen is then tested for drug sensitivities.

In the immunocompetent patient, alveolar macrophages eliminate the bacillus organisms, thereby limiting initial infection. As the organism multiplies, cell-mediated immunity is established. This process occurs over 2 to 10 weeks and is evidenced by positive skin test to purified protein derivative (PPD). By virtue of ongoing immune activity, the infected lung tissue develops a granuloma that may contain a necrotic center. This process is referred to as "primary TB" and typically takes place at the mid lung fields. Regional lymph nodes may also be involved. The small granuloma and enlarged lymph node is a radiographically feature of this disease process recognized as a "Ghon complex." Frequently, the infection is stifled at this stage and confined by fibrosis, leaving the patient cured. Over time a radiographically apparent scar develops as this lesion calcifies (ATS, 1990).

When the immune system fails to contain it, the bacillus organism is spread via the bloodstream to areas with high oxygen tension. Here, the infection lays dormant until the host's immunity is weakened. Given the opportunity, these viable organisms incite secondary infection known as "reactivation TB." By far, the most common site of reactivation of TB infection is the apex of the lung. Other sites include lymph nodes, the kidneys, the meninges of the brain, the vertebral columns, and the long bones.

The clinical manifestations of primary TB are variable. While some patients are asymptomatic, others present with fever, nonproductive cough, or pleuritic chest pain. Crackles may be appreciated on physical examination. Chest radiograph typically demonstrates a mid or lower lung field infiltrate with unilateral hilar lymphadenopathy. Pleural effusion denotes pleural involvement of the infection.

Clinical presentation of reactivation TB largely depends on the site of infection and the point at which the patient comes to medical attention (Niederman & Sarosi, 1995). Early on, common complaints are fever, cough (which may be productive of sputum), or hemoptysis. There are no specific physical exam findings associated with this entity in the early stages of reactivation TB. Chest radiograph demonstrates scattered, ill-defined infiltrates at the apices or posterior bronchopulmonary segments. These infiltrates represent granulomas or tubercles surrounding necrotic tissue. Extrapulmonary disease requires more complex imaging or biopsy.

Patients with reactivation TB report night sweats, weight loss, and chronic wasting in addition to the earlier symptoms. Chest radiographic findings classically show upper lobe cavities with infiltrates in other lung zones (Fig. 37–33). The finding of diffuse small nodular densities is described as miliary TB. In the absence of therapy, the process of chronic wasting leads inexorably to death.

Care of patients with TB is threefold: pharmacotherapy, education, and follow-up (ATS, 1994). Understanding

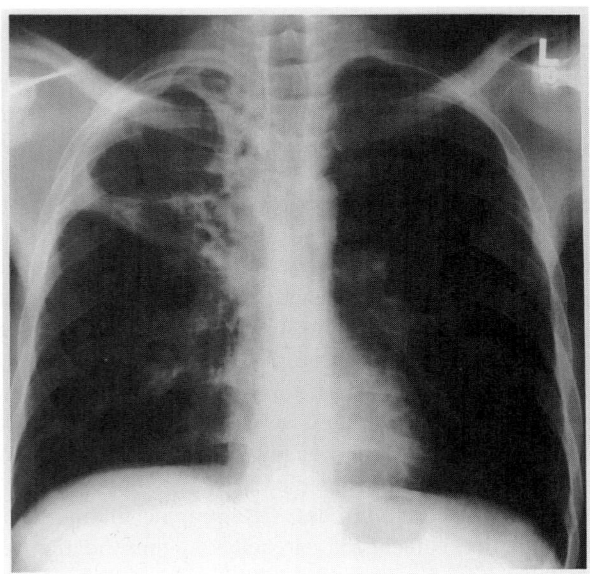

Figure 37–33. Posterior–anterior (PA) chest radiograph of a 46-year-old patient with upper lobe cavitation, a feature strongly supportive of the diagnosis of reactivation TB.

the indications and implications of drug therapy for TB is essential for any clinician who works with populations at risk, including health-care colleagues. Preventive therapy is indicated for any patient who demonstrated a positive PPD without signs of active infection. Every patient being considered for prophylaxis should be evaluated for active disease. Standard therapy is isoniazid (INH) 300 mg daily for 6 to 12 months; immunocompromised individuals may require a longer course. Patients exposed to INH-resistant TB must be prophylaxed with other agents. These individuals must be closely supervised for the development of organism resistance.

Patients with active infection, either primary or reactivation, must be treated with at least two agents to which the organism is susceptible. Often, treatment is initiated before culture and sensitivity results are known. In this setting, the patient must be treated with three or four drugs to assure sensitivity to at least two drugs. The dosage recommendations for adults and children being treated for TB infection are detailed in Table 37–26. Drug resistance is an enormous problem in the epidemiology of this disease. Contributing to the emergence of resistant strains of TB is the sequential or intermittent use of individual drugs. The goal of therapy is to prevent communication or relapse of infection. All patients receiving drug therapy should be monitored for drug sensitivity of the organism as well as drug tolerance by the host. Drug interactions with any previously prescribed medications must be identified. Table 37–27 describes the adverse reactions to the most commonly used anti-TB drugs as well as the typical clinical features and recommendations for monitoring.

TABLE 37–26. Dosage Recommendations for the Treatment of TB in Children and Adults

Drug	Daily Dosage		Twice-Weekly Dosage	
	Children	*Adults*	*Children*	*Adults*
Isoniazid	10–20 mg/kg Max 300 mg	5 mg/kg Max 300 mg	20–40 mg/kg Max 900 mg	15 mg/kg Max 900 mg
Rifampin	10–20 mg/kg Max 600 mg	10 mg/kg Max 600 mg	10–20 mg/kg Max 600 mg	10 mg/kg Max 600 mg
Pyrazinamide	15–30 mg/kg Max 2 g	15–30 mg/kg Max 2 g	50–70 mg/kg Max 4 g	50–70 mg/kg Max 4 g
Ethambutol	15–25 mg/kg	15–25 mg/kg	50 mg/kg	50 mg/kg
Streptomycin	20–40 mg/kg Max 1 g	15 mg/kg Max 1 g	25–30 mg/kg Max 1.5 g	25–30 mg/kg Max 1.5 g
Ofloxacin		800 mg qd		
Ciprofloxacin		750 mg BID		

Children are defined as being 12 y old or less.
Ethambutol is not recommended for children who are too young to be monitored for changes in their vision (<8 y old).
Streptomycin should not be used in children too young to evaluate hearing acuity.
Quinolones (ofloxacin and ciprofloxacin) are not recommended for children. Also, twice-weekly dosages have not been defined.
Reprinted with permission from Dunlap & Kimberling. (1997). (p. 1998).

Before initiating therapy, baseline measures of liver enzymes, bilirubin, blood urea nitrogen, serum creatinine, complete blood count, and uric acid level should be obtained. Monthly sputum cultures are sufficient to document ongoing sensitivity of the organism to the prescribed regimen. Should sensitivity patterns change, so, too, should the drug regimen. If sputum cultures remain positive after three months of treatment, the regimen must be reassessed (ATS, 1995). Patients who are immunocompromised must be followed life-long for recurrence of the disease.

It is imperative that the clinician not only prescribe an adequate anti-TB regimen, but also ensure that the patient has tools to follow it. The resources necessary to follow this complex regimen begin with access to medications and follow-up. Equally vital is the patient's understanding of the consequences of untreated or undertreated disease and the responsibility for preventing the spread of infection. All patients started on anti-TB medications must be reported to the local department of public health. This is so that the contacts of the patient may be informed of their risk and urged to seek medical evaluation. Collaboration between sensitive, savvy clinicians and the public health department offers the best hope for containing this epidemic.

Nontuberculous Mycobacteria. The variety of atypical mycobacteria, known as nontuberculous mycobacteria (NTM), or alternatively, as mycobacteria other than tuberculosis (MOTT), have only recently earned recognition as important infectious pathogens in humans. Most of the NTM occur naturally in soil, water supplies, and dust.

TABLE 37–27. Adverse Reactions to Anti-TB Medications

Drug	Common Adverse Reactions	Signs and Symptoms	Recommended Regular Monitoring
Isoniazid	Abnormal results for liver function tests; hepatitis; peripheral neuropathy; other effects on nervous system; drug interactions	Nausea, vomiting, abdominal pain, weakness, fatigue, dark urine, tingling sensations in hands and feet	Liver function tests if baseline results are abnormal or if symptoms of adverse reactions occur
Rifampin	Orange discoloration of urine and other body fluids; drug interactions; hepatitis; bleeding problems due to thrombocytopenia	Nausea, vomiting, abdominal pain, weakness, fatigue, dark urine, flu-like symptoms	Liver function tests if baseline results are abnormal or if symptoms of adverse reactions occur
Pyrazinamide	Abnormal results for liver function tests; rash; gout	Stomach upset, joint aches	Liver function tests if baseline results are abnormal or if symptoms of adverse reactions occur; uric acid if joint sx occur
Ethambutol	Damage to the nerve of the eye; elevation of uric acid	Changes in vision and color vision; joint aches	Monthly vision tests
Streptomycin	Damage to the nerves of the ear; abnormal kidney function	Hearing loss, balance problems	Hearing tests and kidney function tests
Quinolones	GI upset is most common; hypersensitivity and mild CNS reactions have been reported		

Reprinted with permission from Dunlap & Kimerling. (1997). (p. 1999).

Though poorly understood, it is believed that most respiratory infections with NTM result from inhalation of infectious droplets that have been aerosolized from environmental sources. This is in direct contrast to the human-to-human transmission by respiratory droplet recognized in TB.

To date, 16 different organisms have been identified as NTM that cause infection in humans (Table 37–28). These organism have been found to be frequent colonizers of the airways and, as such, may confound the evaluation of a patient with underlying lung disease. The epidemic of HIV, increased prevalence of nosocomial infections, and increased use of immunosuppression therapy have all contributed to the increase of infection caused by these organisms (Areno & San Pedro, 1996). The prevalence of NTM infection has been estimated to be 1.8 in 100,000 individuals in the United States, a rate one-fifth that of TB (Kotloff, 1993). However, because of the frequency of colonization, NTM are now more frequently isolated in hospital mycobacterium laboratories than is TB. Of note, *M avium complex* infection has been reported in 15% to 24% of AIDS patients (Horsburgh, 1991).

Chronic pulmonary disease resembling TB is the most common manifestation of NTM infection in immunocompetent patients (Kotloff, 1993). Cough and sputum production are the typical presenting complaints though fever, night sweats, weight loss, and hemoptysis may also be present. The course of NTM infection is slowly progressive or may wax and wane over the course of months to years. In patients with underlying lung disease, it may be impossible to distinguish symptoms of NTM pulmonary infection from that of the undelying pulmonary process. Extrapulmonary manifestations of NTM infection are lymphadenitis involving the cervical, submaxillary, and submandibular lymph nodes (more common in children); cutaneous infection; and infection of the joints, bursae, tendon sheaths, and bone.

TABLE 37–28. Nontuberculous Mycobacteria That Cause Infection in Humans

M avium complex
M kansasii
M fortuitum complex
M chelonae
M scrofulaceum
M xenopi
M leprae
M simiae
M szulgai
M malmoense
M gordonae
M marinum
M ulcerans
M haemiphilum
M terrae
M smegmatis

Recovery of NTM organisms from a sterile space (i.e., joint fluid, pleural fluid) confirms infection.

Establishing a diagnosis of pulmonary infection due to NTM is difficult. Because these organism have a tendency to colonize the airways of individuals with underlying lung disease, their isolation from sputum cultures is not definitive evidence of infection. Similarly, clinicoradiographic features may also be ascribed to either underlying lung disease or superimposed NTM infection.

Definitive diagnosis of NTM pulmonary infection requires biopsy specimen with granulomatous inflammation and the recovery of an organism from tissue or sputum culture. Given the indolent nature of this type of infection, noninvasive diagnostic strategies are generally preferred. If the chest radiograph demonstrates a cavitary infiltrate and other etiologies have been ruled out, two or more sputum cultures with moderate to heavy growth of acid-fast bacilli are supportive of this diagnosis. The same criteria must be met if the chest radiograph has a noncavitary infiltrate. However, sputum cultures should be followed. If the culture clears of AFB within 2 weeks of starting antibiotics and pulmonary toilet, it is likely that the NTM is colonizing, rather than infecting, the airway. The latter group of patients do not require treatment but warrant close monitoring and reassessment for infection if clinicoradiographic deterioration is noted (American Thoracic Society, 1990). PPD skin testing has not been useful in the diagnostic evaluation for NTM infection. Given the similar clinicoradiographic resentation, however, it can help to distinguish TB (positive result) from NTM infection.

The treatment of NTM infections is evolving rapidly as this disorder becomes more prevalent. For those patients at risk for rapid progression of infection, a multidrug regimen should be considered. Empirically, patients should be started on a four-drug regimen and subsequently narrowed to two-drug therapy once sensitivities are available. A minimum of two drugs are necessary to prevent the emergence of resistance. Drug selection is made on the basis of culture and sensitivity findings. Patients with a more indolent course can be observed while the presence and extent of infection is confirmed. Bronchodilators, smoking cessation, and routine antibiotics may also have therapeutic benefit. Depending on the organism, treatment should continue for at least 12 months after the sputum culture converts to negative (Kotloff, 1993).

Lung Cancer

Lung cancer is, by far, the most common cause of cancer death in our country. A steady rise in the incidence of lung cancer has been seen since the 1940s. In that time, there has been an alarming rise in the percentage of women being diagnosed, equilibrating their rates to those of their male cohorts (Wingo, Tong, & Bolden, 1995). While the exact cause and pathogenesis of cancer is, as yet, unknown, certain risk factors have been identified.

Cigarette smoking has been implicated in 85% of cases. Cigarette smokers with underlying COPD are at particularly high risk for developing lung cancer. This addiction should be discouraged by each clinician at every encounter with a smoker (Department of Health and Human Services [DHHS], 1996). Smoking-cessation programs include counseling, nicotine replacement therapy and, as indicated by the patient's needs, anxiolytic therapy. It has been clearly established that the risk for cancer drops significantly in nonsmokers the longer they remain smoke-free (Beckett, 1993). In 1964, the U.S. Surgeon General's Advisory Committee on Smoking and Health first publicly described the causal relationship between cigarette smoking and lung cancer as well as several other cardiopulmonary maladies. Since that time, extensive research has defined the negative effects of cigarettes on smokers and the people around them (DHHS, 1996). Legal sanctions have recently mandated that tobacco companies restrict their marketing to reduce the number of new and adolescent smokers.

Family history and exposure histories are important to ascertain. There is believed to be a genetic predisposition to lung cancer. This has been noted in nonsmoking relatives of patients with early development of disease. Occupational history may reveal exposure to other carcinogens. Asbestos is the most common environmental risk factor. Other agents include radon gas, aluminum, arsenic, chromium, nickel, and mustard gas (Beckett, 1993). Routine screening should be performed for any individual who describes exposure to these elements (Wolpaw, 1996). The incidence of lung cancer becomes exponentially higher with each additional risk factor (Davila & Williams, 1993; Matthay & Carter, 1995).

Most pulmonary malignancies are detected as incidental findings on chest x-rays or when studies are ordered to evaluate symptoms such as cough, hemoptysis, chest pain, or unexplained weight loss. Chest x-ray and sputum cytology are the mainstays of screening for lung cancers. Although obtaining these studies on a routine basis promotes the detection of malignancy, there is no evidence to suggest that screening has a positive impact on survival.

Neoplasms of the lung arise from the bronchial epithelium, and so the term "bronchogenic carcinoma" is frequently used. There are four major cell-types encountered in this setting. They are small-cell carcinoma, adenocarcinoma, squamous-cell carcinoma, and large-cell carcinoma. The latter three are categorized as "non–small-cell" lung cancers and, because of the similarities in their prognosis and treatment, are discussed as one entity (D'Amico & Sabiston, 1995).

Clinical manifestations of lung tumors are determined by anatomic location and spread. Tumor growth or lymphadenopathy may impinge upon the adjacent structures compressing the airway, vasculature, or nerves. The primary tumor or its metastases may secrete hormonal intermediates that cause a constellation of signs and symptoms referred to as paraneoplastic syndromes. Persistent cough, which is caused by endobronchial irritation, is the most common presenting symptom of bronchogenic carcinoma. The location of tumors within the lung is described as central or peripheral. The symptoms associated with each site are described in Table 37–29. The symptoms caused by peripherally located malignancies are, in large part, manifestations of pleural and chest wall involvement. Hemoptysis is caused by erosion into a blood vessel or rupture of the highly vascular tumor wall. Compression or obstruction of the airway predisposes the patient to atelectasis or localized infection. Secretions trapped distal to an obstruction may cause postobstruction pneumonia or lung abscess. An abscess may also be caused by the cavitation of a large peripheral tumor (Matthay & Carter, 1995).

Persistent cough, wheeze, hemoptysis, or pain are frequently the presenting symptoms when patients with undiagnosed lung cancer pursue medical attention. By the time the diagnosis of lung cancer is made, most patients already have regional lymph node involvement or metastatic spread (Kern & Clamon, 1997). Metastases may extend into local or distant regions (Fig. 37–34). Spread occurs via direct extension or by the bloodstream or the lymphatics. Prognosis and plan of care are driven by the extent of local disease, the presence of metastases, and the category of cell type (i.e., small cell versus non–small-cell carcinoma).

The diagnosis and staging of lung cancer is discussed at length in Chapter 38, Thoracic Surgery. Table 37–30 describes the 5-year survival and recommended therapy for each category and stage of lung cancer. An overview of the chemotherapy and radiation therapy is detailed in Chapter 26, Cancer Treatment.

Small-Cell Carcinoma

Accounting for approximately 25% of lung cancers, small-cell carcinoma features aggressive growth and rapid spread. There is a high frequency of metastatic disease already established at the time of diagnosis. The preponderance of patients with small-cell carcinoma present with extensive disease (Kern & Clamon, 1997). Common sites of metastasis are the liver, bone marrow, brain, and peritoneum.

Surgical resection is not an option in this setting. This cell type demonstrates a greater responsiveness to chemotherapy and radiation therapy. Combination chemotherapy with three or more agents for a minimum of 6 months is standard (Lazaar & Pilewski, 1994). Agents with specificity against

TABLE 37–29. Symptoms Associated with Location of Bronchogenic Problems

Central	Peripheral
Cough	Chest pain
Stridor	Cough
Wheeze	Dyspnea
Hemoptysis	
Dyspnea	
Chest pain	

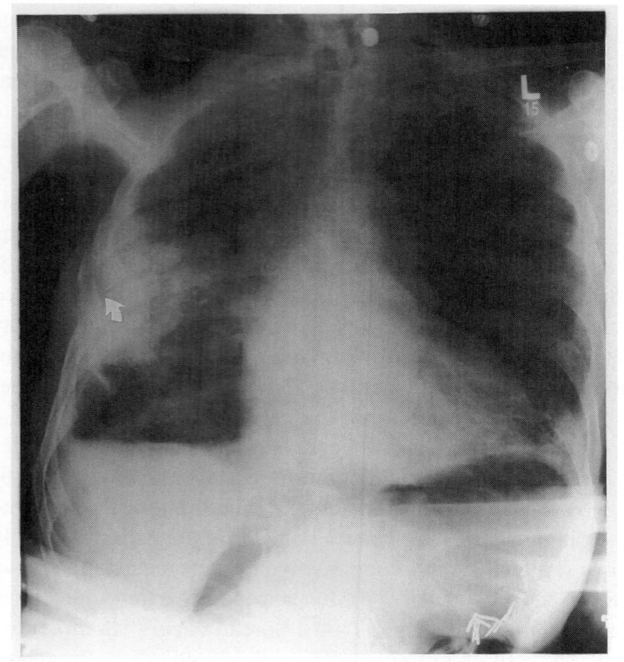

Figure 37–34. Posterior–anterior (PA) chest radiograph of a 79-year-old former-smoker with lung cancer. Chest radiograph demonstrates a large rounded mass in the right lung. Note the destruction of the right 6th rib (*arrow*) indicating chest wall invasion.

this cell type are described in Table 37–31. The addition of radiation therapy to the regimen improves locoregional control of the primary site. At the risk of added toxicity, this may help relieve symptoms associated with the tumor.

The goal of therapy is typically palliation. Median survival for treated patients with limited disease is 14 to 16 months. Those without treatment have a median survival of 3 months. In the setting of metastatic spread of small cell, treatment improves the median survival from less than 2 months to less than 1 year (Goodman & Livingston, 1989).

In rare instances, prophylactic brain irradiation is used to reduce the incidence of metastasis. This is a controversial issue in disease and symptom management. It does not contribute to overall survival, but is believed to reduce the incidence of brain metastasis. It is indicated only for those rare individuals who achieve complete response to chemotherapy (Lazaar & Pilewski, 1994). Poor responders are likely to succumb to the cancer before brain lesions become symptomatic.

Non-Small-Cell Carcinoma

Surgical resection is the cornerstone of therapy for the vast majority of non-small-cell carcinomas. Criteria for surgical resection are discussed at length in Chapter 38, Thoracic Surgery. For those patients who are deemed inoperable by virtue of far-advanced disease or contraindications to surgery, radiotherapy offers potential for symptom relief, palliation, and, rarely, cure (Ihde & Minna, 1991).

TABLE 37–30. Management of Lung Cancer

Stage	% of Population	Goal	Recommended Therapy	5-Year Survival
NSLC				
I				
Operable	20–30	Cure	Resection Adjuvant therapy not indicated	60–75%
Inoperable		Cure	Curative radiation therapy Adjuvant therapy not indicated	20%
II				
Operable	<10	Cure	Resection Adjuvant therapy not indicated	40–50%
Inoperable		Palliation	Radiation therapy	—
III	30			
Operable IIIA		Cure	1) Resection 2) Neoadjuvant chemotherapy followed by resection and radiation therapy	10–35% Under study (25–45%)
Inoperable IIIA and IIIB		Palliation	1) Combined chemotherapy and radiation therapy for prolonged survival 2) Radiation therapy for symptom palliation or 3) None	19%
IV	50	Palliation	Radiation therapy for symptom palliation	
SCLC				
LIMITED	30	Cure	Combination chemotherapy with radiation therapy	30%
EXTENSIVE	70	Palliation (rare cures)	Combination chemotherapy/radiation therapy for symptom palliation	Median survival <1 y

Reprinted with permission from Kern & Clamon. (1997). (p. 2056).

TABLE 37–31. Chemotherapeutic Agents Used in the Management of Small-Cell Carcinoma

Cyclophosphamide
Vincristine
Cisplatin
Etoposide
Doxorubicin
Methotrexate
Lomustine

The major side effect of radiation therapy is esophagitis. The associated dysphagia is treated symptomatically. This treatment modality is associated with cure when given in high doses to inoperable individuals with early stage disease. More often, it is indicated for palliation of symptoms caused by tumor compression. Hemoptysis, cough, and postobstructive disorders may be relieved by radiotherapy. Likewise, symptoms due to metastatic disease, such as brain or bone lesions, may be temporarily ameliorated.

Radiation therapy delivered endobronchially is called "brachytherapy." This intervention allows for the direct delivery of radiation to the site of an endobronchial lesion. Airway obstruction may also be relieved by laser resection of endobronchial tissue or stent placement to offset malacia, stenosis, or compression of the bronchus (Kern & Clamon, 1997).

Acute Respiratory Failure

Ventilation of the lungs and transfer of oxygen and carbon dioxide across the alveolar capillary membrane are the two major physiologic processes that complete the work of respiration. If the mechanisms that support either of these processes fail, acute respiratory failure (ARF) ensues. ARF describes the clinical scenario wherein a rapid deterioration in gas exchange results in failure to meet the metabolic demands of the body. The defining feature of this condition is profound hypoxemia ($PaO_2 < 55$ mm Hg at rest) which may or may not be associated with hypercapnea ($PaCO_2 > 50$ mm Hg) and acidosis. If precipitating factors and blood gas derangements are not corrected, ARF can lead to tissue hypoxia and the patient's rapid demise.

In the setting of an isolated gas transfer abnormality, PaO_2 levels drop precipitously while baseline $PaCO_2$ values are preserved (until the condition is severe). This is described as "hypokemic respiratory failure." Singularly, or in combination, hypoventilation and impaired gas exchange can cause hypoxemia with hypercapnea. Acidosis occurs when the acute rise in $PaCO_2$ remains uncompensated. ARF featuring hypercapnia is termed "hypercapneic respiratory failure." It is important to distinguish the nature of ARF as the pathophysiology determines the patient's treatment and prognosis.

Hypoxemic (Normocapnic) Respiratory Failure

Frequently affecting individuals with no preexisting lung disease, hypoxemic respiratory failure is characterized by arterial hypoxemia and a markedly widened alveolar–arterial (A–a) gradient. The pathologic process occurs at the level of the parenchyma; hence, the disorder is also described as "lung failure." The mechanisms for this distortion include V/Q mismatch, right-to-left shunt, and diffusion abnormalities.

V/Q mismatch arises from an increase in the pulmonary dead space. Dead space refers to alveoli that are underventilated in relation to their blood flow. Clinical scenarios where V/Q mismatch occurs acutely are pneumothorax or pulmonary embolus. Both disorders give rise to areas of partial atelectasis. Hypoxemia in this setting is usually effectively managed with low doses of supplemental oxygen.

Perfusion of nonventilated alveoli is described as right-to-left shunt. This physiology is distinguished from V/C mismatch by its failure to correct arterial hypoxemia with an increase in FiO_2. Shunting occurs in the setting of pneumonia, cardiogenic pulmonary edema (CHF), and noncardiogenic pulmonary edema (ARDS). Treatment of the precipitating disease process is crucial to the reversal of this abnormality.

Diffusion anomalies, as seen in end-stage fibrotic disease, frequently contribute to ARF. They are rarely the primary cause of this disorder (Beers, 1994).

Hypercapnic Respiratory Failure

Any disorder that hinders airflow into and out of the alveolar space (i.e., global alveolar ventilation) can impair the ventilatory pump. This causes subnormal minute ventilation or V/Q mismatch that without intervention provokes hypercapnic respiratory failure. This scenario is seen in the patient with an exacerbation of chronic obstructive disease. During the exacerbation, airflow obstruction reduces alveolar ventilation while perfusion remains essentially stable. Increased dead space in the setting of V/Q mismatch impedes excretion of CO_2. As previously discussed, this is evidenced by a widened A–a gradient.

On the contrary, if the pathologic process is global alveolar hypoventilation, the A–a gradient is preserved. Disorders of the neuromuscular system, central nervous system, or chest bellows precipitate subnormal minute ventilation that can cause global alveolar hypoventilation and, in turn, escalate to hypercapnic respiratory failure.

Clinical Presentation

The clinical manifestations of ARF are multisystemic and nonspecific. For this reason care must be taken to avoid misinterpretation of the findings. Fatigue is a common and early warning sign of hypoxemia. As the tissues of the body are deprived of oxygen, mental status changes and cardiovascular repercussions (tachycardia, hypotension, dysrhythmias) may be seen. CNS sequelae of hypercapnia range from a mild headache to lethargy, seizures, psychosis, or even coma. Neuromuscular effects can include muscle weakness, hyporeflexia, asterixis, or tremor. Obvious respiratory distress is a more specific and less subtle manifestation of ARF. New onset of accessory muscle use, paradoxical motion of the diaphragm, poor air movement, or unexplained adventitious breath sounds should prompt further investigation.

The goals of diagnostic testing in ARF are to define the precipitating factors and to monitor the efficacy of the intervention. As previously described, the hallmark features of ARF are hypoxemia, hypercapnea, or both as documented by arterial blood gas. Chest x-ray is used to identify the nature and the course of the underlying disease process. Sputum culture is useful in determining the presence of infection and guiding antibiotic therapy. Because myocardial ischemia, dysrhythmias, and pericardial disease may contribute to the development of ARF, electrocardiograms should be monitored. If the patient is able to perform the maneuvers, valuable information regarding airflow may be gleaned from bedside spirometry. Toxin screen may reveal the presence of drugs or poisons in a patient with otherwise unexplained CNS depression causing hypercapnic respiratory failure.

Management

As in any urgent care scenario, the first priority in management of the patient in ARF is to ensure an adequate and stable airway. Once that is ascertained, respiratory acidosis is corrected by relieving hypercapnea. This is accomplished by reducing CO_2 production (e.g., reducing fever, treating infection, reducing carbohydrate intake) or by increasing CO_2 excretion (i.e., increasing alveolar ventilation by improving respiratory muscle function or providing mechanical ventilation). Supplemental oxygen is given to improve oxygenation. The goal for PaO_2 is greater than 50 to 60 mm Hg, yet care must be taken to avoid oxygen toxicity. When less aggressive forms of treatment are inadequate and the patient develops signs of respiratory muscle fatigue, mechanical ventilation is indicated (Table 37–32). Finally, the underlying cause of ARF must be differentiated and treated. The patient's prognosis is largely dependent upon the reversibility of underlying disease process, the ability to avoid complications during management, and the patient's baseline pulmonary status.

Acute Respiratory Distress Syndrome

Often described as "noncardiogenic pulmonary edema," acute respiratory distress syndrome (ARDS) is an acute lung injury that causes abrupt onset of respiratory failure. Once described as adult respiratory distress syndrome, this pathologic scenario is now understood to occur in children as well as adults. Hence, the preferred nomenclature is acute respiratory distress syndrome.

There are several processes that may culminate in respiratory failure by different pathways. In developing a treatment strategy, it is important to differentiate these processes from ARDS (Hansen-Flaschen, 1994). Cardiogenic pulmonary edema, indicated by pulmonary capillary wedge pressures above 18 mm Hg, must be ruled out as a cause of diffuse alveolar infiltrates. The clinical criteria used to define ARDS are detailed in Table 37–33.

ARDS occurs as a result of an array of etiologies. Table 37–34 lists many of the precipitants to ARDS and the relative incidence. The major risk factors are sepsis, aspiration extensive trauma, and multiple blood transfusions. The reported incidence in this country ranges from 1.5 to 5.3 cases per 10,000 people per year (Garber, Herbert, & Yelle, 1996). The American–European Consensus Conference on ARDS estimated mortality to be 50% (Bernard, Artigas, Brigham, et al., 1994).

TABLE 37–32. Common Modes of Ventilation in Acute Respiratory Failure

Modes of Ventilation	Abbreviation	Description	Indications
Controlled Mandatory Ventilation or Assist Control	CMV or AC	• Fixed ventilatory rate • Patient can initiate additional breaths • Fixed tidal volume for spontaneous and controlled breaths	Patients who need support of the work of breathing (e.g., ARF, coma, sedation, ARDS)
Synchronized Intermittent Mandatory Ventilation	SIMV or IMV	• Fixed minimum ventilatory rate • Patient can initiate additional breaths • Mandatory breaths have fixed tidal volume; Tidal volume for spontaneous breaths is dependant on patient's respiratory effort	Awake and alert patients; those ready for weaning from mechanical ventilation
Continuous Positive Airway Pressure	CPAP	• No mandatory breaths • Patient initiates each breath • Tidal volume is dependant upon patient's inspiratory effort	Awake and alert patients; those ready for extubation
Pressure Support Ventilation	PSV	• Overcomes the resistance of the tubing • Allows patient to obtain large tidal volumes with low inspiratory effort • Can be instituted in either SIMV or CPAP mode	Awake and alert patients; those ready for weaning from mechanical ventilation

ARF = acute respiratory failure; ARDS = acute respiratory distress syndrome.

TABLE 37–33. Criteria for ARDS

1. Onset of respiratory failure occurs secondary to acute injury of the lungs.
2. There is rapid progression to respiratory failure within 6 to 48 hours of injury to the lungs.
3. Chest radiograph demonstrates extensive, bilateral "fluffy" alveolar infiltrates.
4. Severe disturbances in gas exchange necessitate mechanical ventilation and FiO_2 concentration in excess of 50% (PaO_2:FiO_2 ratio < 200).

ARDS usually evolves within 6 to 72 hours of the predisposing event to the point of requiring intubation for mechanical ventilation. The pathogenesis from systemic insult to arterial hypoxemia is shown in Figure 37–35. Hypoxemia is caused by the shunting of blood through atelectatic or fluid-filled alveoli. Because there is an increase in physiologic dead space (i.e., the area of lung not contributing to the work of gas exchange), a high minute ventilation must be achieved to rid the body of CO_2. As demonstrated on chest radiograph (refer to Fig. 37–30), the alveolar airspaces become filled with alveolar fluid or obliterated by inflammatory material. This congestion causes the lungs to become stiff, or less compliant, and so higher pressures are needed to inflate the lungs during ventilation. A 5 to 10 mm

TABLE 37–34. Causes of Acute Respiratory Distress Syndrome (ARDS)

Cause	Frequency[a]	Cause	Frequency[a]
Infections		**Drugs and Ingested Toxins**	
Bacterial sepsis	F	Phenytoin	R
Gonococcemia	R	Protamine	R
Legionnaires' disease	I	Salicylates	I
Mycoplasma pneumonia	I	Toxic oil	I
Pneumococcal pneumonia	I	**Diagnostic and Therapeutic Agents**	
Adenovirus pneumonia	I	Granulocyte transfusion	I
Babesiosis	R	Leukoagglutinin transfusion reaction	I
Blastomycosis	R	Lymphangiography contrast medium	R
Coccidioidomycosis	I	Radiologic contrast media	R
Cytomegalovirus pneumonia	I	Thoracic radiotherapy	R
Falciparum malaria	I	**Embolic Disorders**	
Influenza pneumonia	I	Amniotic fluid embolism	I
Pneumocystis pneumonia	F	Fat embolism	F
Rocky Mountain spotted fever	R	Venous air embolism	I
Tuberculosis	I	**Inflammatory and Neoplastic Disorders**	
Inhalation Injuries		Diffuse pulmonary hemorrhage	I
Ammonia	I	Granulocytic leukemia	I
Aspiration of gastric contents	F	Pancreatitis	I
Chlorine gas	I	Thrombotic thrombocytopenic purpura	I
Near-drowning	F	**Physical Injuries**	
Nitrogen dioxide	I	Bilateral lung contusion	F
Oxygen toxicity	I	Burns (extensive)	F
Phosgene	I	Heart lung transplantation	F
Smoke inhalation	I	Heat stroke	R
Sulfur dioxide	I	High altitude pulmonary edema	I
Drugs and Ingested Toxins		Neurogenic pulmonary edema	I
Cytosine arabinoside	I	Radiation	R
Denatured rapeseed oil	I	Reperfusion pulmonary	F
Ethchlorvynol	I	Suicidal hanging	F
Ethylene glycol	I	Trauma	F
Hydrochlorothiazide	R		
Lidocaine	R		
Narcotics	I		
Nitrofurantoin	I		
Paraldehyde	R		
Paraquat	F		

[a] Estimated frequency among individuals at risk: F = frequent; I = infrequent; R = rare.
Adapted with permission from Hansen-Flaschen & Fishman. (1998). (p. 2206).

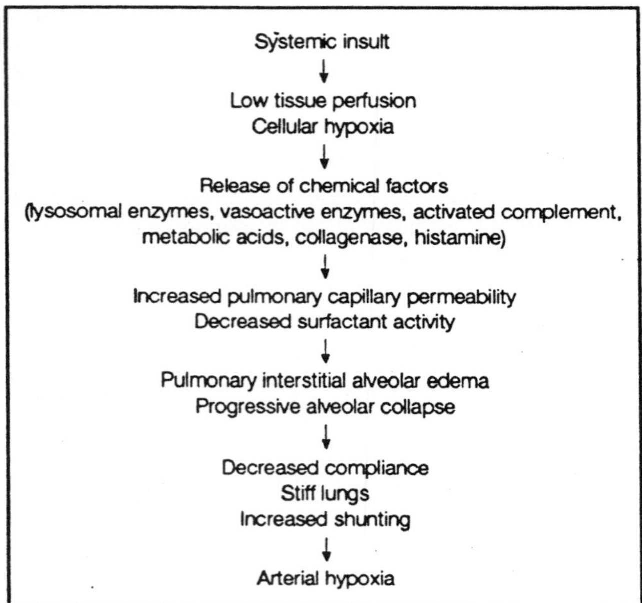

Figure 37–35. Pathogenesis and pathophysiology of ARDS. *(Re-printed with permission from Rieman & Wagner. [1992]. [p. 315].)*

Hg rise in the pulmonary artery pressures is frequently revealed by right-heart catheterization (i.e., Swan–Ganz catheterization).

The clinical course of ARDS has three phases: the exudative phase, the proliferation and fibrosis phase, and the repair and recovery phase (Hansen-Flaschen, 1994). The initial injury to the alveolar–capillary membrane causes acute inflammatory changes and increased permeability pulmonary edema. This damage leads to leakage of protein-rich edema fluid into the interstitial spaces. Some alveoli fill with fluid while others become atelectatic and collapse under the pressure. Alveolar macrophages respond to this influx by secreting cytokines, which, in turn, magnify the inflammatory response to acute lung injury.

The proliferative and fibrosis phase begins as early as 3 to 4 days after the initial injury. During this phase, epithelial cells and fibroblasts multiply to begin the restructuring of the alveolar walls and the adjacent interstitium. Granulation tissue may be deposited within the alveolar spaces. In the best-case scenario, this phase begins to repair the damage to the architecture of the lung. However, when this process persists without regulation, the alveolar units are at risk for becoming obliterated by granulation tissue. Seen in varying degrees, this progressive fibrosis prevents restoration of effective gas exchange and can lead to widespread pulmonary fibrosis. This process may be radiographically apparent within two weeks of the onset of ARDS. The return of lung function is dependent upon the tissue's ability to heal. Some patients remain too sick with the underlying pathology or sustain such extensive injury to the lung that recovery is impossible. These patients require ventilatory support for the rest of their lives (Hansen-Flaschen, 1994).

Patients fortunate enough to advance from the second phase of ARDS enter the repair and recovery phase. This phase occurs weeks to months after the initial development of ARDS. Serial chest x-rays demonstrate gradual clearing of the dense cystic infiltrates that characterize the second phase. It is believed that these changes reflect the resorption or rearrangement of the fibrous tissue (Hansen-Flaschen, 1994). Though most patients are left with some permanent decrement in lung function, the chest x-ray may return to normal.

Treatment of ARDS requires meticulous intensive care and patience (Matthay, 1995). The precipitating factor must be identified and treated. The extremely vulnerable patient must be protected from superimposed infections. Judicious use of antibiotics is necessary to prevent drug resistance. Minimizing indwelling foreign bodies limits the available ports of entry, preventing line-related sepsis. Provision of adequate nutrition promotes healing and prevents tissue breakdown.

It is estimated that 50% of patients with ARDS die before leaving the hospital (Bernard, Artigas, Brigham et al., 1994). Mortality is associated with age, etiologic factors, and development of complications. Those who survive generally have a protracted course that includes weaning from mechanical ventilation, physical rehabilitation, and the psychological markers of critical illness.

▶ SPECIAL INTERVENTIONS

Throughout this chapter, nonpharmacologic interventions have been described as key aspects of comprehensive care of the patient with pulmonary disease. Home oxygen therapy is prescribed when a patient's disease renders atmospheric FiO_2 inadequate to maintain physiologic requirements. Pulmonary rehabilitation has been deemed effective in helping patients to achieve a maximal fitness level and independence in the setting of progressive pulmonary disease. The benefits of smoking cessation are, of course, universal. Acute care nurse practitioners may be responsible for prescribing or administering these special interventions.

Home Oxygen Therapy

Several studies have demonstrated that supplemental oxygen therapy results in an improved quality of life marked by increased exercise tolerance and neuropsychiatric function (Neff & Petty, 1970; Petty & Finigan, 1968; Woodcock, Gross, & Geddes, 1981). Furthermore, this intervention has been shown to increase survival in COPD patients with hypoxemia when used continuously or near continuously (Nocturnal Oxygen Therapy Trail Group [NOTT], 1980; Anthonisen, Wright, Hodgkin, & IPPB Trial Group, 1986).

The Health Care Financing Administration (HCFA), which funds Medicare, has established guidelines by which this therapy may be prescribed. These guidelines are based on those used in the NOTT (1980) study; they are outlined in Table 37–35. Both the oxygen and the equipment necessary for its administration are reimbursed by HCFA as durable medical equipment (not as a medication). In prescribing this therapy, the clinician must prove, for the sake of financial coverage, that it is indicated.

There are a variety of delivery systems available to patients who require supplemental oxygen. The categories of home oxygen delivery systems are stationary, portable, and ambulatory. Unless a portable, or ambulatory system is prescribed with appropriate justification, DME suppliers are reimbursed only for a stationary system.

Stationary systems are appropriate for patients who remain within 50 feet (the length of standard oxygen tubing) of their system. Individuals who only require supplemental oxygen during sleep may be best served by stationary systems. The three types of delivery systems in this category are oxygen concentrators, compressed gas cylinders, and liquid oxygen reservoirs. Oxygen concentrators are electrically powered and use a molecular sieve to separate nitrogen from oxygen. They are the most widely used delivery system, and require a backup system to be available in the event of a power failure. Compressed gas cylinders (H or K tanks) are rarely used anymore because they are less efficient than the other available systems. These large cylinders must be replaced every 2 to 3 days when used continuously at usual flow rates (2 to 4 liters per minute). Today, they are used primarily in rural areas or as backup units. Liquid oxygen tanks are also quite large. They require refilling approximately once a week at usual flow rates. They serve the dual purpose of stationary oxygen system and reservoir from which ambulatory liquid systems may be filled by the patient.

TABLE 37–35. Guidelines for Prescribing Supplemental Oxygen Therapy

Use Continuously

PaO_2 equal to or less than 55 mm Hg or SaO_2 less than 88%, or
PaO_2 56 mm Hg to 59 mm Hg or SaO_2 equal to 89% with:
- ECG evidence of cor pulmonale, or
- edema secondary to congestive heart failure, or
- erythrocytosis with hematocrit greater than 56%

Use During Exercise

PaO_2 equal to or less than 55 mm Hg or SaO_2 less than 88% with exertion

Use During Sleep

PaO_2 equal to or less than 55 mm Hg or SaO_2 less than 88% during sleep, or

Decrease in PaO_2 of greater than 10 mm Hg or in SaO_2 more than 5% with signs or symptoms of hypoxemia (e.g., restlessness, insomnia, cognitive impairment)

Portable systems are those that weigh 10 pounds or more and are designed to be moved, but not easily carried by the patient. An example of a portable oxygen system is the steel cylinder (E tank) which can be placed in a metal carrier with wheels (known as a "stroller"). They are indicated for patients who go beyond the reach of the stationary system for at least 2 hours per week but not more than 2 hours per day. These systems allow for some degree of mobility for patients, but are awkward and cumbersome compared with ambulatory systems.

Ambulatory systems are indicated for those patients who are away from their stationary system for more than 2 hours per day for at least 6 hours per week. These systems weigh less than 10 pounds (filled) and are designed to be carried by the patient. They may be used with or without oxygen-conserving devices and last for at least 4 hours at usual flow rates.

Oxygen-conservation devices have been developed to maximize the length of time between system refills. This has helped to reduce the cost of such therapy. Furthermore, conserving devices extend the duration of the portable and ambulatory systems, thereby allowing patients to be away from their homes (i.e., stationary systems) for greater lengths of time. All conservation devices are believed to extend the oxygen savings by 50% at rest. The degree of conservation may vary significantly with exercise and may require individual titration to maintain adequate oxyhemoglobin saturation (O'Donohue, 1997).

There are two different types of oxygen-conservation devices: reservoirs and bolus pulsation. Reservoir devices (e.g., nasal reservoir cannula and pendant reservoir cannula) fill with oxygen from the system during exhalation. During subsequent inspiration, the oxygen in the reservoir is inhaled. This type of device prevents oxygen flow from being wasted during the time that a patient is exhaling. Transtracheal oxygen (TTO) is a variation of this mode of oxygen conservation. Rather than using an external reservoir, this mode delivers oxygen through a transtracheal catheter and uses the upper airway as a reservoir for oxygen.

The more commonly used method of oxygen conservation is the delivery of a pulsation of a bolus of oxygen during the first part of inspiration. Most devices that manipulate oxygen flow in this manner are battery operated and may be built into or attached onto portable and ambulatory systems. The device may be set to deliver a bolus with each breath or at variable frequency based on the flow setting.

Following the initiation of supplemental oxygen therapy, it is important to monitor the patient for response to treatment and adequacy of dose and delivery system. Patients should be retested every 1 to 3 months to determine ongoing need for this therapy. The dose of oxygen (i.e., liter per minute flow rate) is titrated according to findings at rest, with activity, and, when appropriate, during sleep (O'Donohue, 1997). Because of the lifestyle and body image implications of this therapy, it is important to ascertain the patient's level of adherence to the prescribed regimen. Poor adherence warrants reassessment of the delivery system as well as the reinforcement of patient education. Cigarette smoking is dangerously incompatible with this intervention. Patients who continue to smoke are threatened by two scenarios. If they remove their oxygen cannula while smoking, they risk sequelae from repeated episodes of hypoxemia. If they continue to use the oxygen while smoking, they risk ignition of the flammable oxygen and are a fire hazard to themselves and others in close proximity. In situations of misuse or disuse, the cost and risk of oxygen therapy must be weighed against potential benefit (O'Donohue, 1997).

Smoking Cessation

In 1996, the Agency for Health Care Policy and Research (AHCPR) published a clinical practice guideline for smoking cessation. The introduction of this document notes that, "indeed, it is difficult to identify a condition in the United States that presents such a mix of lethality, prevalence, and neglect, and for which effective interventions are so readily available." The goal of the AHCPR guidelines is to provide recommendations regarding the treatment of tobacco addiction. Though the guidelines are summarized here, any clinician working with smokers is strongly encouraged to obtain this essential resource.

The first major recommendation of the AHCPR guideline is that every clinician should assess the cigarette use of every patient at every encounter. It has been suggested that outpatient practices employ a system whereby tobacco use be measured in the same context as the vital signs (Kottke & Solberg, 1995). Those patients who are actively smoking should be strongly urged to quit and should be offered smoking-cessation treatment. This encouragement should be clear and personalized. Every smoker should be asked about his or her willingness to make a quit attempt.

Those patients who are unwilling to quit should be given information about the risks of cigarette use and the rewards of smoking cessation as they pertain to the individual's situation (e.g., concerns about health, beauty, finance, family or social well-being). This message should be repeated with every clinical encounter. If the patient is willing to make a quit attempt, assistance should be provided. For those individuals who may need more intensive assistance, a referral to individual counseling or a smoking-cessation specialist is appropriate. Hospitalized patients must be encouraged to remain abstinent from cigarette use during and after the hospitalization.

Establishing a plan for quitting smoking is recommended. The first step in devising this plan is to have the patient set a "quit date" that occurs within 2 weeks of the decision to quit. To prepare to quit, the patient is encouraged to tell the people in close daily contact about the intention to quit and request understanding and support. The patient should prepare the environment by getting rid of cigarettes and ashtrays. Prior to quitting, patients are advised to avoid smoking in places where they spend a lot of time (e.g., car, office, living room). It is valuable to review previous quit attempts to learn what factors led to relapse and what influences were supportive. Having done this, it is important to anticipate obstacles to cessation, particularly in the first few weeks.

Smoking-cessation counseling is delivered in a variety of forums. Brief encounters with health-care providers may be sufficient for some patients. Others may prefer to enroll in a smoking cessation program run by a counselor well-versed in the behavioral and pharmacologic strategies associated with overcoming this addiction. Certain patients require intensive, individual treatment. The choice of support should be made collaboratively between the patient and the care provider.

Essential components of smoking-cessation treatment are nicotine-replacement therapy (nicotine gum or nicotine patches), skill training, and clinician-delivered social support. Nicotine-replacement therapy is advised unless the patient is pregnant, has cardiovascular disease, or develops a local skin reaction. Dosing of nicotine replacement is based on previous experience with the drug, number of cigarettes smoked, and degree of addiction.

Nicotine replacement must be prescribed with very clear instructions for use. The first patch should be applied as soon as the patient wakes up on the scheduled quit date. It should be placed on a relatively hairless location on the body between the neck and the waist and should be replaced at the beginning of each day. While using the patch, the patient must absolutely refrain from smoking.

It is supportive to give a patient advice on successful quitting. Total abstinence after the quit date is imperative. Even "a single puff" is a violation of smoking cessation. Because alcohol use is highly associated with relapse, patients should be encouraged to minimize or forego alcohol during the quit process. The potential for weight gain is a serious concern to many individuals. Nutrition counseling and nicotine gum should be available to address this risk. The presence of other smokers in the household is associated with lower success rates. Patients should be advised to anticipate a plan to maintain abstinence in the setting of temptation. Better still, other members of the household should consider quitting at the same time.

Written material regarding the dangers of smoking and the benefits of cessation are considered useful supplements. Such information should be readily available in every clinical setting. The material must be written at a level that is understandable and meaningful to the patient.

Follow-up contact with the patient, either in person or via telephone, should occur within the first week following quit date. A second follow-up contact is ideally made within the ensuing month. Further follow-up contacts are made as needed. During such encounters, success is reinforced with congratulations. If smoking has occurred, it is useful to review the circumstances and elicit recommitment to cessation. Episodes of relapse ought to be examined for learning value rather than being considered failure.

Problems identified during the review of relapse episodes can be used to create strategies to deal with future challenges. Nicotine-replacement therapy must be examined for appropriateness of dose, use, and problems. Referral to a more intensive program should be considered for each patient who encounters difficulty maintaining abstinence.

Pulmonary Rehabilitation

Pulmonary rehabilitation has become an integral part of care of patients with severe symptomatic lung disease. It is intuitive that individuals who are dyspneic with activity, engage in less activity, thereby losing physical fitness. The result is a vicious cycle of worsening dyspnea with exertion, inactivity, loss of function, and psychosocial isolation. By interrupting that cycle with monitored, individualized physical conditioning and teaching, pulmonary rehabilitation is designed to help restore the individual to the maximal level of physical and psychosocial health.

Ideally provided by a multidisciplinary team, pulmonary rehabilitation addresses the influence of lung disease on the many aspects of a patient's health. The goals of a pulmonary rehabilitation program are to help patients achieve maximal fitness level, an understanding of their lung disease, and improvement in their symptomology. Physical rehabilitation incorporates muscle training for strength and flexibility, and supervised aerobic exercise for conditioning. The educational content of such programs include energy-conservation techniques, anxiety-alleviation strategies, respiratory-therapy techniques (e.g., use of oxygen, nebulizers, and multidose inhalers), proper nutrition, smoking cessation, as well as anatomy and (patho)physiology.

There is a great deal of data to support that a comprehensive pulmonary rehabilitation program improves quality of life and the capacity to complete activities of daily living (Make, 1986; Celli, 1995). Though most studies include only patients with advanced COPD, findings are broadly applied to all patients with symptomatic lung disease. Factors that may negatively impact upon an individual's success in pulmonary rehabilitation are disabling extrapulmonary disease, lack of adequate support system, and lack of motivation (Celli, 1997).

▶ NURSING CONSIDERATIONS

To varying degrees, the presence of pulmonary disease influences every other aspect of a patient's health. Concepts of wellness such as self-esteem, family and community role, and sexuality are fundamental to quality of life and, yet, are frequently overlooked in the clinical setting. It is the traditional role of the physician to assess the patient from the context of pathophysiology. Nursing has the unique responsibility to address the meaning of that process to the patient and the system from which he or she comes. Accepting a new diagnosis, learning the meaning of specific symptoms, and adhering to complicated medical regimens are all clinical challenges that can determine a patient's success. Helping patients to integrate necessary medical regimens into their particular lifestyles is the foundation of our practice. Perhaps the most important contribution the ACNP can make to the clinical setting is fulfilling this responsibility.

REFERENCES

The Agency for Health Care Policy and Research Smoking Cessation Clinical Practice Guideline. (1996). *Journal of the American Medical Association, 275,* 1270–1280.

Aitken, M. L. (1997). Cystic Fibrosis. In W. N. Kelley (Ed.), *Textbook of internal medicine.* (3rd ed.). (pp. 2002–2007). Philadelphia: Lippincott-Raven.

American College of Chest Physicians. (1993). Consensus statement: Primary pulmonary hypertension. *Chest, 104,* 236–250.

American College of Chest Physicians & American Thoracic Society Consensus Conference. (1995). Institutional control measures for tuberculosis in the era of multiple drug resistance. *Chest, 108,* 1690–1710.

American Thoracic Society. (1989). Guidelines for the approach to the patient with severe hereditary alpha-1 antitrypsin deficiency. *American Review of Respiratory Diseases, 140,* (pp.1494–1497).

American Thoracic Society (1990). Diagnosis and treatment of disease caused by nontuberculous mycobacteria. *American Review of Respiratory Diseases, 142,* 940–953.

American Thoracic Society. (1990). Diagnostic standards and classification of tuberculosis. *American Review of Respiratory Diseases, 142,* 725–735.

American Thoracic Society. (1994). Treatment of tuberculosis and tuberculosis infection in adults and children. *American Journal of Respiratory and Critical Care Medicine, 149,* 1359–1374.

American Thoracic Society. (1995). Standards for the diagnosis and care of patients with chronic obstructive pulmonary disease. *American Journal of Respiratory and Critical Care Medicine, 152 (supplement),* S77-S121.

Anderson, W. M. & Light, R. W. (1995). Invasive diagnostic procedures. In R. B. George, R. W. Light, M. A. Matthay, & R. A. Matthay (Eds.). *Chest medicine: Essentials of pulmonary and critical care medicine* (3rd ed.). (p. 62). Baltimore: Williams & Wilkins.

Anthonisen, N. R., Wright, E. C., Hodgkin, J. E., & IPPB Trial Group. (1986). Prognosis in chronic obstructive pulmonary disease. *American Review of Respiratory Diseases, 133,* 14–20.

Areno, J. P. & San Pedro, G. S. (1996). Atypical mycobacterial pulmonary infections in the non-immunocompromised patient. *Mediguide to Pulmonary Medicine, 3(5),* 1–7.

Auger, W. R., Fedullo, P. F., Moser, K. F., et al. (1992). Chronic major vessel thromboembolic pulmonary artery obstruction: Appearance at angiography. *Radiology, 182,* 393–398.

Balmes, J., Cullen, M. R., & Gee, J. B. L. (1981). What infections occur with occupational lung disease? *Clinics in Chest Medicine, 2,* 111–120.

Bates, B. (1995). *A guide to physical examination and history taking* (6th ed.). Philadelphia: J. B. Lippincott.

Becker, D. M., Philbrick, J. T., & Selby, J. B. (1992). Inferior vena cava filters: Indications, safety, effectiveness. *Archives of Internal Medicine, 152,* 1985–1994.

Beckett, W. S. (1993). Epidemiology and etiology of lung cancer. *Clinics in Chest Medicine, 14,* 1–15.

Beers, M. (1994). Acute respiratory failure. In A.P. Fishman (Ed.), *Pulmonary diseases and disorders companion handbook* (2nd ed.). (pp. 411–418). New York: McGraw Hill.

Bernard, G. R., Artigas, A., Brigham, K. L., Carlet, J., Falke, K., Hudson, L., Lamy, M., Legall, J. R., Morris, A., & Spragg, R. (1994). The American–European consensus conference on ARDS: Definitions, mechanisms, relevant outcomes and clinical trial coordination. *American Journal of Respiratory and Critical Care Medicine, 149,* 818–824.

Berry, R. B. (1995). Sleep related breathing disorders. In R. B. George, R. W. Light, M. A. Matthay, & R. A. Matthay (Eds.), *Chest medicine: Essentials of pulmonary and critical care medicine* (3rd ed.). (pp. 247–270). Baltimore: Williams & Wilkins.

Bone, R. C. (1996). Goals of asthma management: A step-care approach. *Chest, 109,* 1056–1065.

Borg, G. A. V. (1982). Psychophysical bases of perceived exertion. *Medicine and Science in Sports and Exercise, 14,* 377–381.

Branch, W. T. & McNeil, B. J. (1983). Analysis of the differential diagnosis and assessment of pleuritic chest pain in young adults. *American Journal of Medicine, 75,* 671–679.

Burrows, B. (1990). Airways obstructive diseases: Pathogenetic mechanisms and natural histories of the disorders. *Medical Clinics of North America, 74,* 547–559.

Burrows, B. (1991). Epidemiologic evidence for different types of chronic airflow obstruction. *American Review of Respiratory Diseases, 143,* 1452–1454.

Cahill, B. C. & Ingbar, D. H. (1994). Massive hemoptysis: Assessment and management. *Clinics in Chest Medicine, 15,* 147–168.

Cassiere, H. A. & Niederman, M. S. (1997). Lung abscess. In W. N. Kelley (Ed.), *Textbook of internal medicine.* (3rd ed.). (pp. 1992–1995). Philadelphia: Lippincott-Raven.

Celli, B. R. (1995). Pulmonary rehabilitation. *American Journal of Respiratory and Critical Care, 152* (3), 861–864.

Celli, B. R. (1997). Pulmonary rehabilitation for patients with advanced lung disease. *Clinics in Chest Medicine, 18,* 521–534.

Conrad, S. A., Jayr, C., & Peper, E. A. (1995). Thoracic trauma, surgery and perioperative management. In R.B. George, R. W. Light, M. A. Matthay, & R. A. Matthay (Eds.), *Chest medicine: Essentials of pulmonary and critical care medicine* (3rd ed.). (pp. 629–657). Baltimore: Williams & Wilkins.

D'Amico, T. A. & Sabiston, Jr., D. C. (1995). Neoplasms of the lung: Carcinoma of the lung. In D. C. Sabiston, Jr. & F. C. Spencer (Eds.), *Surgery of the chest.* (6th ed.). (pp. 634–648). Philadelphia: W. B. Saunders.

Davies, S. F. (1994). Fungal pneumonia. *Medical Clinics of North America, 78,* 1049–1065.

Davila, D. G. & Williams, D. E. (1993). The etiology of lung cancer. *Mayo Clinics Proceedings, 68,* 170–182.

Dickey, B. F. & Myers, A. R. (1988). Pulmonary manifestations of collagen-vascular diseases. In A. P. Fishman (Ed.), *Pulmonary diseases and disorders,* (2nd ed.). (p. 646). New York: McGraw-Hill.

Dismukes, W. E., Bradsher, Jr., R. W., Cloud, G. C., Kauffman, C. A., Chapman, S. W., George, R. B., Stevens, D. A., Girard, W. M., Saag, M. S., & Bowles-Patton, C. (1992). Itraconazole therapy for blastomycosis and histoplasmosis. *American Journal of Medicine, 93,* 489–497.

Dunlap, N. E. & Kimerling, M. E. (1997). Pulmonary tuberculosis. In W. N. Kelley (Ed.), *Textbook of internal medicine.* (3rd ed.). (pp. 1995–2000). Philadelphia: Lippincott-Raven.

Farzan, S. & Farzan, D. (1997). *A Concise handbook of respiratory diseases* (4th ed.). Stamford, CT: Appleton and Lange.

Ferguson, G. T. & Cherniak, R. M. (1993). Management of chronic obstructive pulmonary disease. *New England Journal of Medicine, 328,* 1017–1022.

Fiel, S. B. (1993). Clinical management of pulmonary disease in cystic fibrosis. *Lancet, 341,* 1070–1074.

Fishman, N. O. (1994). Endemic fungal pneumonias. In A. P. Fishman (Ed.), *Pulmonary diseases and disorders: Companion handbook.* (2nd ed.) (pp. 375–382). New York: McGraw-Hill.

Garber, B. G., Herbert, P. C., Yelle, J. D., Hodder, R. V., & McGowan, J. (1996) Adult respiratory distress syndrome: A systemic overview of incidence and risk factors. *Critical Care Medicine, 24,* 687–695.

George, R. B. (1995). History and physical examination. In R. B. George, R. W. Light, M. A. Matthay, & R. A. Matthay (Eds.), *Chest medicine: Essentials of pulmonary and critical care medicine* (3rd ed.). (pp. 81–91). Baltimore: Williams & Wilkins.

George, R. B. (1997). Approach to the patient with acute respiratory failure. In W. N. Kelley (Ed.), *Textbook of internal medicine* (3rd ed.). (pp. 1932–1937). Philadelphia: Lippincott-Raven.

Goldman, J. M. (1989). Hemoptysis. *Emergency Medicine Clinics of North America, 7,* 325–338.

Goodman, G. E. & Livingston, R. B. (1989). Small cell lung cancer. *Current Problems in Cancer, 13,* 1–55.

Guzzetta, C. E. (1992). Cardiopulmonary arrest and resuscitation. In B. M. Dossey, C. E. Guzzetta, & C. V. Kenner (Eds.). *Critical care nursing: Body-mind-spirit,* (3rd ed.). (p. 299). Philadelphia: J. B. Lippincott.

Hansen-Flaschen, J. (1994). Acute respiratory distress syndrome (ARDS). In A. P. Fishman (Ed.), *Pulmonary diseases and disorders: Companion handbook.* (2nd ed.) (pp. 419–430). New York: McGraw-Hill.

Hansen-Flaschen, J. & Fishman, A. P. (1988). Adult respiratory distress syndrome: Clinical features and pathogensis. In A. P. Fishman (Ed.), *Pulmonary diseases and disorders* (2nd ed.). (p. 2206). New York: McGraw-Hill.

Hapopnik, E. F. (1997). Approach to the patient with hemoptysis. In W. N. Kelley (Ed.), *Textbook of internal medicine.* (3rd ed.). (pp. 1918–1922). Philadelphia: Lippincott-Raven.

Horsburgh, Jr., C. R. (1991). Mycobacterium avium complex infection in acquired immunodeficiency syndrome. *New England Journal of Medicine, 324,* 1332–1338.

Ihde, N. H. & Minna, J. D. (1991). Non-small cell lung cancer. *Current Problems in Cancer, 15,* 63–104, 107–154.

James, D. G. & Hosoda, Y. (1994). Epidemiology. In D. G. James (Ed.), *Sarcoidosis and other granulomatous disorders: Lung biology in health and disease, Vol 73.* New York: Marcel Dekker.

Kelley, M. A., Carson, J. L., Palevsky, H. I., & Schwartz, J. S. (1991). Diagnosing pulmonary embolism: New facts and strategies. *Annals of Internal Medicine, 114,* 300–306.

Kern, J. A. & Clamon, G. (1997). Lung cancer. In W. N. Kelley (Ed.), *Textbook of internal medicine.* (3rd ed.). (pp. 2047–2058). Philadelphia: Lippincott-Raven.

Kotloff, R. M. (1993). Infection caused by nontuberculous mycobacteria: Clinical aspects. *Seminars in Roentgenology, 28,* 131–138.

Kotloff, R. M. (1994). Sarcoidosis. In A. P. Fishman (Ed.), *Pulmonary diseases and disorders: Companion handbook.* (2nd ed.). (pp. 35–41). New York: McGraw-Hill.

Kotloff, R. M. & Rossman, M. D. (1992). Sarcoidosis. *Immunology and Allergy Clinics of North America, 12,* 421–449.

Kottke, T. E. & Solberg, L. I. (1995). Is it not time to make smoking a vital sign? *Mayo Clinic Proceedings, 70,* 303–304.

Lapp, N. L. & Castranova, V. (1993). How silicosis and coal worker's pneumoconiosis develop: A cellular assessment. *Occupational Medicine: State of the Art Review, 8,* 35–55.

Lapp, N. L. & Parker, J. E. (1992). Coal workers' pneumoconiosis. *Clinics in Chest Medicine, 13,* 243–252.

Lazaar, A. & Pilewski, J. (1994). Lung cancer. In A. P. Fishman (Ed.), *Pulmonary diseases and disorders: Companion handbook.* (2nd ed.). (pp. 227–239). New York: McGraw-Hill.

Legerton III, C. W., Smith, E. A., & Silver, R. M. (1995). Systemic sclerosis (scleroderma): Clinical management of its major complications. *Rheumatic Disease Clinics of North America, 21,* 203–216.

Levitz, S. M. (1989). Aspergillosis. *Infectious Disease Clinics of North America, 3,* 1–18.

Light, R. W. (1995). Clinical pulmonary function testing, exercise testing, and disability evaluation. In R. B. George, R. W. Light, M. A. Matthay, & R. A. Matthay (Eds.), *Chest medicine: Essentials of pulmonary and critical care medicine,* (3rd ed.). (p. 152–153). Baltimore: Williams & Wilkins.

Lindell, K. O. & Mazzocco, M. C. (1990). Breaking bronchospasm's grip with MDI's. *American Journal of Nursing, 90(3),* 35–39.

Lynch III, J. P. & Hunninghake, G. W. (1992). Pulmonary complications of collagen vascular disease. *Annual Review in Medicine, 43,* 17–35.

Make, B. J. (1986). Pulmonary rehabilitation: Myth or reality? *Clinics in Chest Medicine, 7,* 519–540.

Marti II, W. J. (1997). Drug-induced lung disease. In W. N. Kelley (Ed). *Textbook of internal medicine* (3rd ed.). (p. 2059). Philadelphia: Lippincott-Raven.

Matthay, M. A. (1995). Acute hypoxemicrespiratory failure: Pulmonary edema and ARDS. In R. B. George, R. W. Light, M. A. Matthay, & R. A. Matthay (Eds.), *Chest Medicine: Essentials of Pulmonary and Critical Care Medicine* (3rd ed.). (pp. 593–608). Baltimore: Williams & Wilkins.

Matthay, R. A. & Carter, D. C. (1995). Lung neoplasms. In R. B. George, R. W. Light, M. A. Matthay, & R. A. Matthay (Eds.), *Chest Medicine: Essentials of Pulmonary and Critical Care Medicine* (3rd ed.). (pp. 393–422). Baltimore: Williams & Wilkins.

Merrill, W. W. (1997). Hypersensitivity pneumonitis. In W. N. Kelley (Ed.), *Textbook of internal medicine.* (3rd ed.). (pp. 2014–2017). Philadelphia: Lippincott-Raven.

Mills, J. A. (1994). Systemic lupus erythematous. *New England Journal of Medicine, 330,* 1871–1879.

Moser, K. M., Auger W. R., Fedullo, P. R., & Jamieson, S. W. (1992). Chronic thromboembolic pulmonary hypertension: Clinical picture and surgical treatment. *European Respiratory Journal, 5,* 334.

Murphy, T. F. & Sethi, S. (1992). Bacterial infection in chronic obstructive pulmonary disease. *American Review of Respiratory Diseases, 146,* 1067–1083.

National Asthma Education and Prevention Program (NAEPP). (1997). Expert panel report 2: *Guidelines for the diagnosis and management of asthma.* National Heart, Lung and Blood Institute. National Institutes for Health Publication No. 97-4051.

Neff, T. A. & Petty, T. L. (1970). Long-term continuous oxygen therapy in chronic airway obstruction. *Annals of Internal Medicine, 72,* 621–626.

Niederman, M. S. & Sarosi, G. A. (1995). Respiratory tract infections. In R. B. George, R. W. Light, M. A. Matthay, & R. A. Matthay (Eds.), *Chest medicine: Essentials of pulmonary and critical care medicine* (3rd ed.). (pp. 423–478). Baltimore: Williams & Wilkins.

Nicotra, M. B. (1994). Bronchiectasis. *Seminars in Respratory Infections, 9,* 31–40.

Nocturnal Oxygen Therapy Trial Group. (1980). Continuous or nocturnal oxygen therapy in hypoxemic chronic obstructive lung disease: A clinical trial. *Annals of Internal Medicine, 93,* 391–398.

O'Donohue, W. J. (1997). Home oxygen therapy. *Clinics in Chest Medicine, 18,* 535–545.

Osborne, M. L. & Deffebach, M. E. (1997). Asthma. In W. N. Kelley (Ed.), *Textbook of internal medicine.* (3rd ed.). (pp. 1974–1979). Philadelphia: Lippincott-Raven.

Pack, A. I. & Millman, R. P. (1988). The lungs in later life. In A. P. Fishman (Ed.), *Pulmonary diseases and disorders.* (2nd ed.). (pp. 79–90). New York: McGraw-Hill.

Palevsky, H. I. (1994). Thromboembolic disease. In A. P. Fishman (Ed.), *Pulmonary diseases and disorders: Companion handbook.* (2nd ed.). (pp. 139–149). New York: McGraw-Hill.

Palevsky, H. I. (1997). Therapeutic options for severe pulmonary hypertension. *Clinics in Chest Medicine, 18,* 595–609.

Palevsky, H. I. & Edmunds, Jr., L. H. (1997). Pulmonary thromboembolism. In L. H. Edmunds (Ed.), *Cardiac surgery in the adult.* (pp. 1319–1344). New York: McGraw-Hill.

Palevsky, H. I. & Fishman, A. P. (1994). Pulmonary hypertension and cor pulmonale. *Heart Disease and Stroke, 2,* 335–341.

Panettieri, R. A. & Murray, R. K. (1994). Chronic obstructive pulmonary disease (COPD). In A. P. Fishman (Ed.), *Pulmonary diseases and disorders: Companion handbook.* (2nd ed.) (pp. 170–180). New York: McGraw-Hill.

Patterson, T. F. (1997). Infections caused by dimorphic fungi. In W. N. Kelley (Ed.), *Textbook of internal medicine.* (3rd ed.). (pp. 1719–1723). Philadelphia: Lippincott-Raven.

Petty, T. L. & Finigan, M. M. (1968). Clinical evaluation of prolonged ambulatory oxygen therapy in chronic airway obstruction. *American Journal of Medicine, 45,* 242–252.

Phillipson, E. A. (1988). Sleep disorders. In J. F. Murray & J. A. Nadel (Eds.), *Textbook of respiratory medicine,* (pp. 1841–1860). Philadelphia: W. B. Saunders.

The PIOPED Investigators. (1990). Value of the ventilation/perfusion scan in acute pulmonary embolism: Results of the Prospective Investigation of Pulmonary Embolism Diagnosis (PIOPED). *Journal of the American Medical Association, 263,* 2753–2759.

Prakash, U. B. S. (1996). Pulmonary diseases. In U. B. S. Prakash (Ed.), *Mayo international medicine board review: 1996–1997.* Rochester, MN: Mayo Foundation for Medical Education and Research.

Rachelefsky, G., Fitzgerald, S., Page, D., & Santamaria, B. (1993). An update on the diagnosis and management of pediatric asthma. *Nurse Practitioner, 18,* 51–52, 55, 59–62.

Redlich, C. A. & Balmes, J. (1995). Occupational and environmental lung disease. In R.B. George, R. W. Light, M. A. Matthay, & R. A. Matthay (Eds.), *Chest medicine: Essentials of pulmonary and critical care medicine* (3rd ed.). (pp. 357–392). Baltimore: Williams & Wilkins.

Reinman, M. D. & Wagner, Y. L. (1992). Acute respiratory failure: The patient with adult respiratory distress syndrome. In R. M. Dossey, C. E. Guzzetta, & C. V. Kenner (Eds.), *Critical care nursing: Body-mind-spirit* (3rd ed.). (p. 315). Philadelphia: J. B. Lippincott.

Richardson, H. B. (1988). Hypersensitivity pneumonitis (extrinsic allergic alveolitis). In A. P. Fishman (Ed.), *Pulmonary diseases and disorders,* (2nd ed.). (p. 668). New York: McGraw-Hill.

Richman, P. (1994). Eosinophilic pneumonias. In A. P. Fishman (Ed.), *Pulmonary diseases and disorders: Companion handbook. (2nd ed.). (pp. 64–70). New York: McGraw-Hill.*

Ries, A. L. (1997). Chronic obstructive pulmonary disease. In W. N. Kelley (Ed.), *Textbook of internal medicine.* (3rd ed.). (pp. 1979–1984). Philadelphia: Lippincott-Raven.

Rubin, L. J. (1984). Clinical evaluation. In L. J. Rubin (Ed.), *Pulmonary heart disease.* Boston: Marinus Nijhoff.

Rubin, L. J. (1997). Pulmonary hypertension and cor pulmonale. In W. N. Kelley (Ed.), *Textbook of internal medicine.* (3rd ed.). (pp. 467–473). Philadelphia: Lippincott-Raven.

Scanlin, T. F. (1988). Cystic fibrosis. In A. P. Fishman (Ed.), *Pulmonary diseases and disorders.* (2nd ed.). (pp. 1273–1294). New York: McGraw-Hill.

Sharma, O. P. (1997). Sarcoidosis. In W. N. Kelley (Ed.), *Textbook of internal medicine.* (3rd ed.). (pp. 2018–2021). Philadelphia: Lippincott-Raven.

Silibovsky, R. (1994). Infection due to mycobacterium tuberculosis. In A. P. Fishman (Ed.), *Pulmonary diseases and disorders: Companion handbook.* (2nd ed.). (pp. 353–365). New York: McGraw-Hill.

Siltzbach, L. E. (1967). Sarcoidosis: clinical features and management. *Medical Clinics of North America, 51,* 483–502.

Snider, D. E. (1978). The relationship between tuberculosis and silicosis. *American Review of Respiratory Diseases, 118,* 455–460.

Sosenko, A. & Glassroth, J. (1985). Fiberoptic bronchoscopy in the evaluation of lung abscesses. *Chest, 87,* 489–494.

Sostman, H. D. & Matthay, R. A. (1995). Chest imaging. In R. B. George, R. W. Light, M. A. Matthay, & R. A. Matthay (Eds.), *Chest medicine: Essentials of pulmonary and critical care medicine* (3rd ed.). (p. 111). Baltimore: Williams & Wilkins.

Stanford, W. & Galvin, J. R. (1988). The diagnosis of bronchiectasis. *Clinics in Chest Medicine, 9,* 691–699.

Steinberg, K. P. & Hudson, L. D. (1997). Approach to the management of the patient with acute respiratory distress syndrome. In W. N. Kelley (Ed.), *Textbook of internal medicine.* (3rd ed.). (pp. 1937–1942). Philadelphia: Lippincott-Raven.

Stevens, D. A. (1995). Coccidiomycosis. *New England Journal of Medicine, 332,* 1077–1082.

Stockley, R. A. (1987). Bronchiectasis: New therapeutic approaches based on pathogenesis. *Clinics in Chest Medicine, 8,* 481–494.

Sullivan, C. E. & Issa, F. G. (1985). Obstructive sleep apnea. *Clinics in Chest Medicine, 6* (4), 633–650.

Tino, G. & Kelley, M. A. (1997). Pulmonary thromboembolism. In W. N. Kelley (Ed.), *Textbook of internal medicine.* (3rd ed.). (pp. 2062–2068). Philadelphia: Lippincott-Raven.

Trulock, E. P. (1997). Lung transplantation. *American Journal of Respiratory and Critical Care Medicine, 155,* 789–818.

von Feldt, J. M. & Callegari, P. E. (1994). Pulmonary manifestations of collagen vascular disease. In A. P. Fishman (Ed.), *Pulmonary diseases and disorders: Companion handbook.* (2nd ed.). (pp. 42–51). New York: McGraw-Hill.

Wasserman, K., Hansen, J. E., Sue, D. Y., Whipp, B. J., & Casaburi, R. (Eds.). (1994). *Principles of exercise testing and interpretation (2nd ed).* Philadelphia: Lea & Febiger.

Weber, S. L. & Banks, D. E. (1994). Silicosis. In L. Rosenstock & M. R. Cullen (Eds.), *Clinical occupational and environmental medicine.* (pp. 264–274). Philadelphia: W. B. Saunders.

Weill, H. & Jones, R. N. (1988). In A. P. Fishman (Ed.), *Pulmonary diseases and disorders.* (2nd ed.). (pp. 819–860). New York: McGraw-Hill.

Wheat, L. J. (1994). Histoplasmosis: Recognition and treatment. *Clinical Infectious Disease, 19 (supplement),* S19-S27.

Wiedemann, H. P. & Rice, T. W. (1995). Lung abscess and empyema. *Seminars in Thoracic and Cardiovascular Surgery, 7,* 119–128.

Wilson, J. M. (1997). Human gene therapy. In W. N. Kelley (Ed.), *Textbook of internal medicine.* (3rd ed.). (pp. 2314–2315). Philadelphia: Lippincott-Raven.

Wingo, P. A., Tong, T., & Bolden, S. (1995). Cancer statistics 1995. *Ca: A Cancer Journal for Clinicians, 45,* 8–30.

Wolpaw, D. R. (1996). Early detection in lung cancer. *Medical Clinics of North America,* 80(1), 63–82.

Woodcock, A. A., Gross, E. R., & Geddes, D. M. (1981). Oxygen relieves breathlessness in "pink puffers." *Lancet, 1,* 907–909.

38

Thoracic Surgery

Angela B. Wurster

Thoracic surgery has been a recognized specialty since 1948, having grown from the recognition that surgical diseases of the chest required special expertise. Though having begun as a field dealing with diseases primarily of the lungs, esophagus, and mediastinum, the monumental developments in cardiac surgery all but usurped the entire specialty. Over the past 15 years, general thoracic surgery, sometimes referred to as "noncardiac surgery," has carved out a distinct niche as a number of board-certified practitioners have chosen to pursue this area exclusively. This has greatly advanced the entire specialty and resulted in better patient care.

Additionally, nurse practitioners have developed expertise in general thoracic surgery by training with thoracic surgeons. Few nursing schools offer general thoracic surgery as a distinct part of the curriculum at the undergraduate level and even fewer, if any, offer it as a specialized tract for graduate students. The hope is, however, that this subspecialty will grow.

This chapter provides acute care nurse practitioners with an introduction to the dynamic field of general thoracic surgery. Full understanding of thoracic surgery requires a solid understanding of pulmonary medicine and oncology, which are covered separately within this book. Naturally, a detailed explanation of every aspect of thoracic surgery is not possible within the limitations of this text.

▶ ANATOMY

It has been said that anatomy is "the gateway to medicine" (Crocco, 1977). It is most often the first course taught in nursing schools and serves as the foundation of our practice. While a complete review of anatomy and physiology of the chest is impractical, a brief review is warranted.

The Thorax

The thorax by definition is an airtight cage that enables the alternating changes in pressure required for ventilation. Comprised of the sternum, 12 pairs of ribs, and 12 vertebrae, this bony structure protects the underlying viscera and provides support for the upper extremities.

The sternum, located in the anterior midline of the chest, is usually about 15 to 20 centimeters long and has three components: the manubrium, the body, and the xiphoid process. The manubrium has a central indentation known as the suprasternal notch. Just lateral and slightly distal to the suprasternal notch is the second intercostal space. The notch of the manubrium enables quick location of the second intercostal space in emergent situations such as chest tube placement for a tension pneumothorax. The body of the sternum is slanted at a steeper angle than the manubrium, thus the term the sternal angle. It is almost completely subcutaneous and is therefore easily accessible for surgery. The cartilaginous xiphoid process is the flexible end of the sternum.

The size and shape of the thorax are determined by the ribs and their intercostal spaces. The first seven pairs of ribs articulate directly with the sternum by costal cartilage. The remaining five pairs of ribs are known as "false ribs." They do not articulate with the sternum, but rather, communicate with the cartilage above them. The spaces between the ribs, known as intercostal spaces, provide a means of entry into the chest. Each intercostal space is numbered by the rib above it and is comprised of distinct layers: external intercostal muscles, internal intercostal muscles, intercostal veins– arteries–nerves, and innermost intercostal muscles. In addition to the intercostal nerves, the thoracic wall is innervated by 12 pairs of thoracic spinal nerves substantiating the tremendous pain that is experienced postoperatively in this patient population.

The Airway

The trachea begins at the lower border of the cricoid cartilage and extends to the carina. In the adult, the trachea is approximately 10 cm long with a diameter equivalent to the index finger. There are two cartilaginous rings per cm (Allen, 1996). Anteriorly, the trachea is covered by the isthmus of the thyroid and laterally by the thyroid gland. Posteriorly, in the cervical region, the trachea sits against the cervical esophagus and is surrounded by the innominate artery. Therefore, should a tracheostomy tube be placed too low, there is an increased likelihood of a tracheoinnomanate fistula. Continuing distally, the trachea is surrounded by structures of equal importance: the left carotid, subclavian artery, vagus nerve, and phrenic nerve, as well as the aorta and pulmonary artery.

The bronchus divides at the level of the carina into the right and left mainstem bronchi. The left mainstem is longer than the right as it passes under the aortic arch before attaching to the lung. Each mainstem divides before entering the lung at each lobe. Within each lobe is further branching within each bronchopulmonary segment and continued branching to the alveoli. It is at this alveolar level that gas exchange occurs (Fig. 38–1).

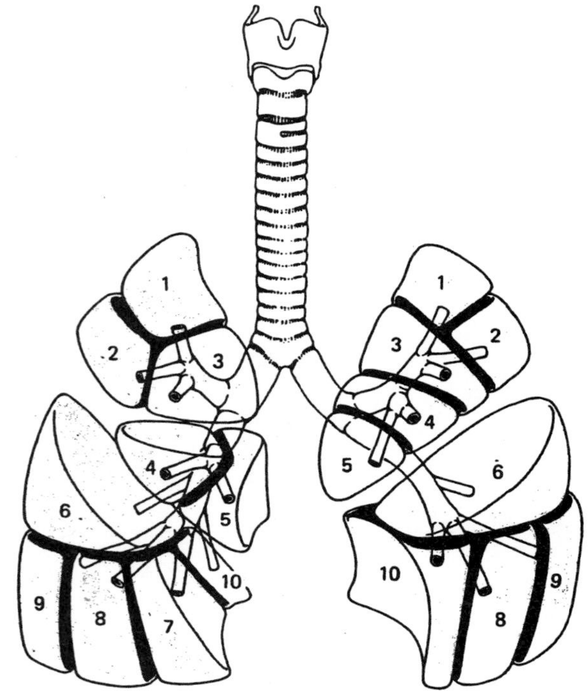

Figure 38–1. The airway and bronchopulmonary segments of the lungs. Bronchopulmonary segments of human lungs. Left and right upper lobes: (1) apical, (2) posterior, (3) anterior, (4) superior lingular, (5) inferior lingular segments. Right middle lobe: (4) lateral and (5) medial segments. Lower lobes: (6) superior (apical), (7) medial-basal, (8) anterior-basal, (9) lateral-basal, and (10) posterior-basal segments. The medial-basal segment (7) is absent in the left lung. NOTE: The lungs are represented as slightly turned inward in order to display part of the lateral face. *(Reprinted with permission from Weibel & Taylor. [1988]. [p.12].)*

The Mediastinum

The mediastinum is best defined as the area that encompasses the paratracheal region, aortopulmonary window, spinal cord, and retrosternal air space. It includes the heart, great vessels, tracheobronchial tree, esophagus, and spinal structures. Many have deemed it one of the most complex areas of the body. Benign and malignant abnormalities may occur in this region.

The Lungs

Upon complete exhalation, the lungs are comprised of 80% air, 10% blood, and 10% tissue (Weibel & Taylor, 1988). As the lungs form, they assume the shape of the pleural cavity and maintain that position if inflated and excised. They maintain their position within the chest due to attachment at the hilum and via the pulmonary ligament. The hilum is defined as the area where the blood vessels and airways attach to the mediastinum. The pulmonary ligament attaches the visceral pleura to the mediastinum. The right lung is the larger, with three lobes and two fissures. On the right, the oblique, or so-called major fissure, separates the lower lobe from the upper and middle lobes. The horizontal, or minor fissure, separates the upper and middle lobes. The left lung has two lobes and one fissure, the oblique or major fissure. Knowledge of the relation of lobes and fissures is critical for assessment and treatment. Within the lungs are ten bronchopulmonary segments (refer to Fig. 38–1).

The Diaphragm

The diaphragm is divided into two sections, the peripheral muscular section and the central tendinous section, which is attached to the pericardium (van Trigt, 1995). There are three major openings in the diaphragm, which allow for certain structures within the chest to continue into the abdominal cavity. The aorta opening allows for passage of the aorta, azygous vein, and thoracic duct. The esophageal opening contains the esophagus and vagus nerve. The vena caval opening facilitates passage of the inferior vena cava. The blood supply to the diaphragm comes from the right and left phrenic arteries off the abdominal aorta, the superior phrenic artery off the thoracic aorta, and the pericardiophrenic and musculophrenic arteries off the internal mammary artery. Venous drainage is by way of the right and left inferior phrenic veins. Motor and sensory input to and from the diaphragm occurs by way of the right and left phrenic nerves. The right phrenic nerve enters the diaphragm just lateral to the inferior vena cava. The left phrenic nerve is located at the border of the left heart. Once the phrenic nerves enter the diaphragm, they divide into four branches and line the inferior surface of the diaphragm (Fig. 38–2). It is relatively easy to injure the phrenic nerves during chest procedures, resulting in a paralysis of the diaphragm.

▶ PREOPERATIVE EVALUATION: THE BLUEPRINT

The preoperative evaluation of a thoracic surgery patient varies according to procedure and surgeon preference. According to Ginsberg (1995a), "there is no formula, no absolute criterion and in the case of curable lung cancer, no absolute contraindication" to thoracic surgery. The goals of the pre-operative evaluation are to determine operability, resectability, and to anticipate and prevent perioperative complications. The preoperative evaluation is the blueprint that enables the surgeon to ascertain if an operation is feasible and, if so, if it is reasonable.

Operability and Resectability

No chapter on thoracic surgery would be complete without clarification of the terms "operability" and "resectability." Frequently misused, these two words have distinct meanings and by no means does one guarantee the other. The determination of both operability and resectability are critical to the preoperative assessment. A condition that is "operable" is one in which there are clinical and physiologic criteria that indicate the patient will tolerate the stress of surgery, loss of tissue, as well as have no evidence of distant disease. To determine operability requires assessment of the patient's comorbid disease status, age, pulmonary function, and absence of distant disease.

"Resectable" refers to a lesion that a surgeon can remove in total. There are many factors that affect resectability including tumor size, location and proximity to the adjacent structures, and lymph node involvement. The determination of resectabilty should rest with the surgeon, as the surgeon is the only one with the knowledge and expertise to make this determination. It must be stated, however, that "resectable" to one surgeon may be "unresectable" to another, but this determination depends only on characteristics of the lesion and the surgeon's experience and technical expertise (Table 38–1).

Patient History

The majority of the first patient visit should be devoted to obtaining an accurate and complete history. An accurate

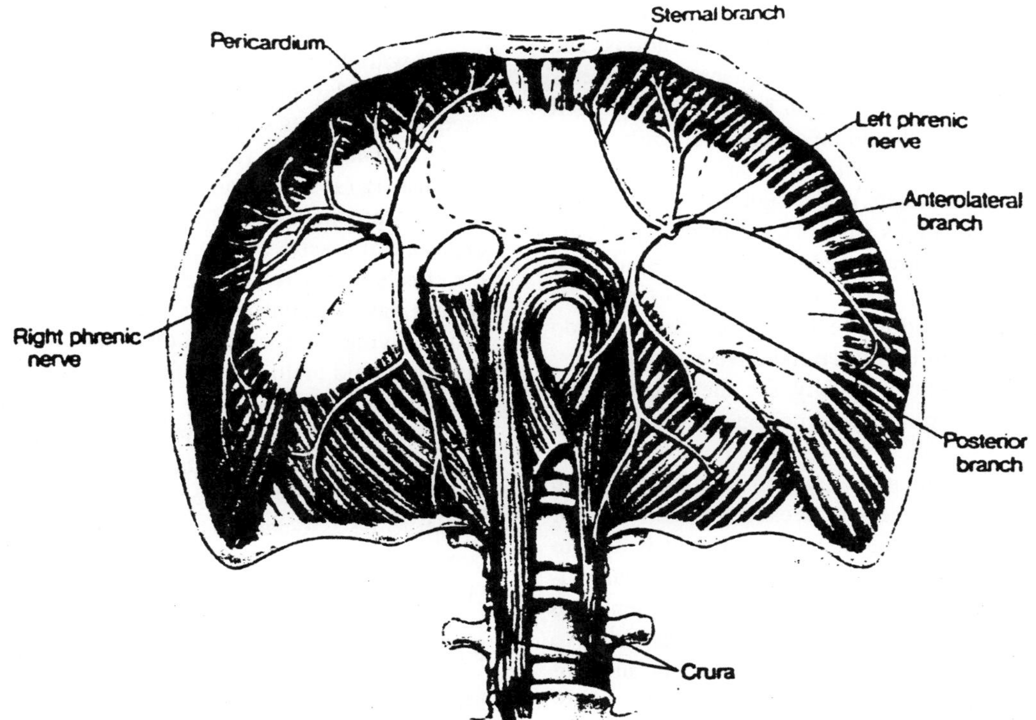

Figure 38–2. The diaphragm. Innervation of the diaphragm. *(From van Trigt III. [1995]. [p.1082].)*

TABLE 38–1. Factors Affecting Resectability

Factor	Considerations
Tumor size (diameter)	A larger lesion has greater likelihood of regional or distant spread.
Proximity to the tracheal carina	Lesions too close to the carina may not be technically amenable to pneumonectomy.
Involvement of the pleural space	Lesions reaching the pleural space with effusion containing malignant cells are unresectable.
Involvement of the mediastinum	Spread of lesion to mediastinum of opposite hemithorax renders it unresectable.
Involvement of distant sites	Metastasis to brain, bone, liver, or adrenal gland precludes resection in all but exceptional circumstances.

Reprinted with permission from Grippi et al. (1988). (p. 2423).

history assists in confirming a diagnosis, determining operability and resectability, as well as indicating the need for additional testing, if necessary. The patient referred to a thoracic surgeon usually has been seen by one, if not several, health-care providers, and thus often presents with written documentation of his or her history. While useful, this in no way obviates the need to obtain a history from the patient.

The history and physical examination of a new patient being referred for thoracic surgery should be problem-focused, bearing in mind the need to determine operability, resectability, and potential perioperative complications. The history should include a detailed assessment of the events that led the patient to see a physician in the first place. All thoracic surgery patients should be asked specifically about shortness of breath at rest or with exertion, cough, hemoptysis, pain, fever, night sweats, and weight loss. A complete review of systems as well as past medical history, past surgical history, allergies, current medications, and family history should be taken. Any premorbid conditions should be optimized prior to operation. Technical complications do not account for the majority of perioperative complications; rather, comorbid conditions usually are the culprit. (See Table 38–2 for the determinants of postoperative morbidity and mortality.)

Assessment of pulmonary function may be made, in part, by determining shortness of breath with activities of daily living in addition to the distance a patient is able to walk at a comfortable pace on level ground. Formal pulmonary function studies should be done for any patient who is a candidate for pulmonary resection. Patients unable to walk at least a block without becoming acutely short of breath may require further evaluation with formal exercise testing. In a few cases a preoperative pulmonary rehabilitation program that incorporates monitored treadmill walking, stationary bicycling, and upper body exercises may be warranted.

TABLE 38–2. Determinants of Postoperative Morbidity and Mortality[a]

Cardiac disease
Pulmonary disease
Tumor characteristics
  Stage
  Type
General medical conditions
  Diabetes
  Creatinine level
  Hemoglobin level
  Serum albumin level
  Immunosuppressed status
    Steroids
    Chemotherapy
    Other chronic illnesses
  Weight loss > 10%
  Age > 70
Anticipated surgery
Extent of resection
Additional procedures
Side of pulmonary resecton (R > L)
Previous surgery

[a] Significant cardiopulmonary disease and tumor stage and extent of resection appear to be the most significant determinants.
Reprinted with permission from Ginsberg. (1995a). (p. 30).

It is estimated that 90% of lung cancers occur in individuals who have a history of cigarette smoking (Shopland, Eyre, & Peckalek, 1991). A thorough social history is required with attention to smoking history including number of packs per day, number of years, and date of last cigarette. Frequently patients who "quit" years ago had "just one cigarette" the day of the visit "to calm their nerves." According to Ginsberg (1995a), smoking cessation for a period of 1 to 2 weeks preoperatively should be mandatory. In addition, exposure to passive smoke should be assessed. While all of the effects of passive smoke have not been fully elucidated, studies have demonstrated a higher incidence of cancer in people living with smokers (Yessner, 1993). Occupational history should include specific questions about exposure to asbestos and radon.

A complete assessment also needs to include the patient's attitude toward surgery. Patient attitude toward disease and the desire to have a favorable outcome have been shown to be associated with a successful operation (Ginsberg, 1995a). No patient should be talked into an elective operation.

Physical Examination

The physical examination of a preoperative thoracic surgery patient should routinely include palpation of cervical, supraclavicular, and axillary lymph nodes. A thorough chest examination including auscultation, percussion, and palpation should be completed. Physical findings characteristic of atelectasis or lobar collapse should be sought as should manifestations of pleural fluid. Wheezing, especially on inspiration, should be carefully assessed. Finally, an abdominal assessment should be included to rule out an enlarged liver or spleen as well as any palpable masses.

Chest Radiograph

According to Shields (1992) the posterior–anterior (PA) and lateral chest radiographs (x-ray) are the foundation of the evaluation of the chest. Proper interpretation of the chest radiograph both preoperatively and postoperatively is critical in the management of the thoracic surgery patient. Chest radiographic findings may be used to diagnose and to guide decision making, often decreasing the need for more costly studies.

The radiologist's interpretation is useful, but the actual film should always be reviewed by the clinician. If the patient brings films to the office, the originals should always be requested as copies are often of poor quality and important findings may be either absent on the copy or distorted. A patient who is unable to bring the original film should have a new film taken at the time of the visit. Every patient who goes to the operating room should have a film within 30 days of surgery to make sure the perceived pathology is still present and to detect any additional problems that may have arisen that might influence the planning of the surgical procedure.

Review of the chest radiograph should be done systematically. Every structure should be reviewed, not just the area(s) in question. Ideally the film should be read by at least two people as the observer rate of error has been documented to be as high as 30% (Garland, 1949). Commonly now, films are read by the radiologist, the nurse practitioner, and then the surgeon. It is important to remember that the radiologist knows about the patient only by what is visualized on the film. Pertinent clinical information should be made available to the radiologist when the film is requested to maximize the value of the interpretation.

While a complete review of chest radiographic interpretation is not possible here, some important features are relevant. First, there are many ways to view the chest radiographically. The standard views are the posterior–anterior (PA) and lateral projections. Three other views used in evaluation of the thoracic surgery patient are the lordotic, inspiratory and expiratory, and lateral decubitus projections. The lordotic view enables a more precise view of the apices, as the bony structures are displaced upward. The inspiratory and expiratory views are helpful in patients with air trapping and diapragmatic fixation. The lateral decubitus film, taken with the patient lying on the side, is valuable in the diagnosis and evaluation of a suspected pleural effusion as the fluid visibly layers out.

Histologic examination of a resected specimen remains the last word, but there are common radiographic findings in lung cancer as well as certain benign processes. Consolidation presents as an opacification *without* loss of lung volume. Atelectasis is an opacification *with* a loss of volume. The exact characteristics that distinguish a nodule from a mass are not agreed upon. Nodules have been described as varying between 3 and 6 centimeters (Swenson, Jett, Payne et al., 1990; Cummings, Littington & Richard, 1986). They are usually spherical or ovoid and well demarcated. While histologic examination remains the only definitive method of distinguishing benign from malignant, calcification occurs more commonly but not exclusively in benign nodules. Malignant nodules tend to be larger with less distinct margins and usually double rapidly, in less than 35 days (Shields, 1992b). The differential diagnosis of the solitary pulmonary nodule is broad and varied (Table 38–3).

Finally, assessment of the chest radiograph provides information regarding the staging of lung cancer. Any suspicious finding on chest radiograph may be an indication for a computed tomography of the chest. A pleural effusion in a patient with known or suspected lung cancer may indicate the possibility of T4 disease, rendering the patient inoperable and mandating the sampling of fluid.

Computed Tomography

The computed tomography (CT scan) offers a more detailed method of detection and characterization of abnormalities within the chest. Cross-sectional computer-reconstructed imaging enables identification of densities that might not be able to be visualized on a chest radiograph. The two main advantages of CT scan are the ability to eliminate superimposition of densities and the greater than tenfold increase in resolution over routine chest radiograph (Naidich, 1992).

Preoperatively the CT scan is valuable in assessing both resectability and operative approach. The CT scan provides detailed information on the size and location of lymph nodes, mainly mediastinal, and gives an excellent and detailed view of the lung parenchyma. The American Thoracic Society has established a lymph node staging map for reporting CT results (Tisi, Friedman, & Peters, 1983). "Normal" lymph nodes are defined as those that are 10 millimeters in size or less with the exception being subcarinal nodes where the upper limit of normal is 12 millimeters. Lymph nodes greater than 1.5 centimeters in diameter have a greater than 80% chance of being malignant, but an invasive procedure remains the only definitive way to assess whether a lymph node contains tumor. Magnetic resonance imaging (MRI) is no better at distinguishing benign from malignant. Positron emission tomography (PET) may offer an increased ability to make this distinction.

The chest CT scan also images the liver and adrenal glands, two common sites for metastatic disease. The CT scan of the chest with thick cuts of the upper abdomen, liver, and adrenals should be part of a routine examination

TABLE 38–3. Causes of Solitary Peripheral Nodules

Neoplasms	**Inflammatory lesions**	**Malformations**
Primary carcinoma	Tuberculoma and tuberculous lesions	Arteriovenous malformation
Solitary metastasis	Histoplasmosis	Vascular endothelioma
Hamartoma	Coccidioidomycosis	Sequestrated segment
Primary sarcoma	Cryptococcosis	**Traumatic lesions**
Bronchial carcinoid	Nonspecific granuloma	Hematoma
Reticuloses	Chronic lung abscess	**Hernias**
Fibroma	Lipoid pneumonia	**Cysts**
Myxoma	Massive fibrosis	Bronchogenic
Neurogenic tumor	Rheumatoid granuloma	Pericardial
Lipoma	Gumma	Dermoid
Myoblastoma	**Parasitic lesions**	Teratoma
Hibernoma	Echinococcosis	**Pulmonary infarct**
Solitary fibrous tumor of the pleura	Ascariasis	**Rounded atelectasis**
Leiomyoma	Dirofilariasis	
Plasmacytoma		
Sclerosing hemangioma		
Thymoma		
Endometriosis		
Sugar tumor		

Reprinted with permission from Shields. (1992). (p. 457).

of a patient with suspected bronchogenic carcinoma. The delineation of metastatic disease is especially important in patients with locally advanced lung cancer where the role of operation is in question and in the patient where the physiologic status is such that an operation may carry a higher risk (Naidich, 1992).

The preoperative CT scan plays an important role in the assessment of the solitary pulmonary nodule. The presence of calicification with the absence of growth over a 2-year period signifies the likelihood of a benign process. The most important information to be gained from the CT scan, however, is the confirmation that the nodule is truly solitary and not one of many that just were not detected by the plain chest radiograph.

Magnetic Resonance Imaging of the Chest

There are two primary indications for obtaining magnetic resonance imaging (MRI) in the patient with suspected lung cancer. The MRI provides information in the assessment of apical lung tumors where the brachial plexus, subclavian vessels, or vertebral bodies may be involved. The extent of chest wall invasion is shown better with MRI than CT due to better contrast on T1 and T2 weighted images between tumor, chest wall, and muscle (Musset, Grenier, Carette, et al., 1986). MRI also enables assessment of the involvement of the subclavian artery or brachial plexus in patients with Pancoast tumors (Heelan, Demas, Caravelli, et al., 1989). The MRI provides valuable information about the extent of the involvement of the vertebral bodies, thus enabling accurate assessment of resectability and need for neurosurgical participation in the operating room.

MRI's second application is in the assessment of the mediastinum. It has been shown that MRI may be more accurate than CT in documenting presence of mediastinal invasion, in part because of the ability to perform sagittal and coronal reconstruction, but only at operation can invasion be truly defined. Where invasion is obvious, the MRI may be better but there is a large group of patients where the invasion is indeterminate on MRI as well as CT scan. It is particularly valuable for patients who cannot tolerate iodinated agents or contrast and in those who have undergone previous radiation to the mediastinum.

Evaluation for Metastatic Disease

Patients with known or suspected lung cancer and signs or symptoms of metastatic disease should undergo a complete "extent of disease evaluation" that includes a total body bone scan and brain imaging, preferably MRI of the brain. The chest CT scan as mentioned earlier includes the liver and adrenal glands, the other common sites of metastatic disease. The findings of metastatic disease obviate the need for operation to remove the primary tumor. Routine testing for metastatic disease is not cost effective and the decision to perform these tests should be based on the presence of either organ-specific or nonspecific findings such as weight loss, anemia, or fatigue.

Ventilation Perfusion Scan

The ventilation perfusion (V/Q) scan has an important role in the preoperative evaluation of patients with poor lung function defined by an $FEV_1 < 2.0$ liters as well as those being evaluated for lung transplantation, pneumonectomy, and lung volume reduction surgery.

In lung transplantation the preoperative V/Q scan has an invaluable role. In the case of single-lung transplant, the V/Q scan determines which lung to transplant. In bilateral lung transplantation, the V/Q scan determines which lung to transplant first. The lung with the poorer function is transplanted first as the procedure is done with single-lung ventilation and the patient breathes off of the nonoperative lung during the procedure.

Traditionally the V/Q scan was quantitated in terms of total ventilation and perfusion to right and left lungs. Now, the V/Q scan is more commonly quantitated for upper, middle, and lower lung on each side. Separating the lung into thirds allows for better assessment of operability and resectability. This is particularly true for patients with emphysema. Patients with a dominant bulla have significantly decreased ventilation/perfusion to the area of the bulla. In emphsyema patients with diffuse lung disease being considered for lung volume reduction surgery, the V/Q scan assists in determing heterogeneity. Typically the scan shows areas of decreased ventilation perfusion to the apices with preserved ventilation perfusion to the middle and lower thirds.

For patients undergoing pneumonectomy, the V/Q scan may be required to assist in the evaluation of potential postoperative pulmonary function. Relative pulmonary perfusion correlates well with actual postoperative pulmonary function tests (Boysen, Block, Olsen, et al., 1977; Olsen, Block, & Tobias, 1977).

Pulmonary Function

In 1977 Dripps, Eckenhoff, and Vandam presented a risk classification system based on the general health and physical status of the patient obtained during a history (Table 38–4). It has been well documented that in the immediate postoperative period, surgery decreases the forced vital capacity 25% to 50%, increases the respiratory rate, decreases tidal volume and PaO_2, as well as impairs pulmonary defense mechanisms (Gamsu, Singer, Vincent, et al., 1976; Tisi, 1979). Thus, while the Dripps classification is helpful and still utilized, more specific information is required to fully assess the preoperative thoracic surgery patient.

TABLE 38–4. Dripps–American Society of Anesthesiologists Classification of Physical Status

Class	Type of Patient
I	Patients in normal health with no restrictions on activity
II	Patients with mild systemic diseases with no restrictions on activity
III	Patients with severe systemic diseases that limit activity but are not incapacitating
IV	Patients with incapacitating life-threatening systemic diseases
V	Moribund patients not expected to survive 24 hours

Reprinted with permission from Bechard. (1992). (p. 567).

Pulmonary Function Tests

The most common method of assessing pulmonary function is the pulmonary function test, a measure of volumes and capacities. Pulmonary function tests are reliable, informative, and generally well tolerated; thus, an ideal screening test (Tisi, 1979). This test enables assessment of the patient's current pulmonary function and a reasonable prediction of pulmonary function after surgery (Table 38–5).

Among the most important pulmonary function indices in thoracic surgery patients are forced vital capacity (FVC), forced exhaled volume over one second (FEV_1), FEV_1/FVC ratio, residual volume (RV), total lung capacity (TLC), maximum voluntary ventilation (MVV), and diffusing capacity (DLCO). The FVC is obtained by having the patient take a full inspiration to total lung capacity and then exhale maximally, rapidly and forcefully. A reduced FVC indicates a restrictive process. The FEV_1 is the volume of

TABLE 38–5. Characteristic Alterations in Pulmonary Function Tests According to the Major Patterns of Abnormality

Pattern	Airflow (FEV_1/FVC,%)	Airflow Response to Bronchodilators	Lung Volumes	DL_{CO}
Obstructive				
Irreversible	↓	↔	↑	↔ or ↓
Reversible	↓	↑	↑	↔
Small airway disease	↓	↔	↔	↔
Upper airway obstruction	↓	↔	↔ or ↑	↔
Restrictive				
Parenchymal disease	↔ or ↑	↔	↓	↓
Surgical resection	↔	↔	↓	↓
Pleural, chest wall disease	↔	↔	↓	↔
Reduced expiratory force generation	↔	↔	↓	↔
Mixed obstructive-restrictive	↓	↔ or ↑	↓	↓
Isolated reduction in efficiency of gas transfer	↔	↔	↔	↓

NOTE: ↓ = decreased; ↑ = increased; ↔ = no change or normal.
Reprinted with permission from Grippi et al. (1988). (p. 2511).

air expelled in the first second during the FVC maneuver and in normal patients is the largest amount of air exhaled. A reduced FEV_1 suggests obstruction. Evaluating the FEV_1/FVC ratio further enables classification of obstruction (Table 38–6). The RV, obtained by measuring the amount of air remaining in the lung after the FVC maneuver is completed, and the TLC, obtained by measuring the amount of air in the lung at the peak of inspiration during the FVC maneuver, enable the practitioner to estimate the degree of hyperinflation (Table 38–7). Further comparison of the TLC to VC enables quantification of restriction (Table 38–8).

Spirometry before and after bronchodilators should be requested for anyone in whom obstruction is suspected. Improved flow rates after bronchodilator administration indicate a reversible process as seen in asthma as opposed to fixed obstruction, more commonly found in emphysema.

The DLCO estimates the rate at which O_2 and CO_2 move by diffusion from alveolar gas to combine with hemoglobin in red blood cells. It indicates the surface area of the lung that is participating in alveolar capillary diffusion (Table 38–9). There are many disorders that may affect the DCLO: anemia, decreased lung volumes, or ventilation perfusion mismatch. Conversely, the DCLO may be increased due to polycythemia or intrapulmonary hemorrhage.

Finally, the MVV measures the movement of air into and out of the lungs during continued maximum effort. It provides an overall assessment of effort, coordination, and elasticity. A normal value indicates an intact respiratory system (Grippi, Metzger, Krupinski, & Fishman, 1988).

Pulmonary Exercise Test

Another method of assessing pulmonary function is the pulmonary exercise test using a formal exercise evaluation or 6-minute walk test. This not only provides a global measure of cardiopulmonary function but also indicates the patient's determination and willingness to persevere in the face of discomfort (Bechard, 1992). Most common indications for exercise testing include evaluation of dyspnea, covert pulmonary disease, response to treatment, guide to oxygen therapy or disability, and determination of operability. Dyspnea that is more severe with exercise may be due to arterial hypoxemia or inadequate cardiac performance. This is best differentiated by an exercise evaluation.

Exercise evaluations may be performed one of three ways: treadmill walking, bicycle ergometry, or 6-minute walk test. When using the treadmill or bicycle ergometry, measurements of VO_2 max, VCO_2, VE, and heart rate are obtained. The VO_2 max is a quantifiable measure of the limit of performance during exercise. Normal values are predicted based on age. Normal individuals can achieve 85% of predicted. Measuring VO_2 and VCO_2 during exercise enables determination of anaerobic threshold or the point at which the metabolic demands of muscle exceed oxygen delivery. In normal individuals anaerobic threshold occurs at 60% of VO_2 max (Kelley & Fishman, 1988).

The 6-minute walk test is a simplified exercise evaluation that is particularly useful for severely deconditioned patients or for a quick assessment of response to treatment. The patient is asked to walk for 6 minutes at his or her own pace over a flat premeasured course. The patient may stop and rest as often as necessary for as long as necessary. Oxygen saturation, dyspnea, and distance are all measured. Patients should be able to walk a minimum of 600 feet in 6 minutes prior to undergoing surgery. If unable to do so, a formal pulmonary rehabilitation program is warranted prior to surgery.

TABLE 38–7. Categorization of Hyperinflation

Category	% Predicted TLC or RV
Normal	< 120
Mild	121–134
Moderate	135–149
Severe	> 150

Adapted with permission from Grippi et al. (1988). (p. 2507).

Cardiac Evaluation

Recognizing that the majority of complications following thoracic surgery are cardiopulmonary in nature, the cardiac evaluation is critical to determining operability. Patients who report recent myocardial infarction (within 3 months), hemodynamic changes such as hypertension or tachycardia, angina, or arrhythmias are at greatest risk for cardiac complications perioperatively (Fintel & Mir Taqui Ali, 1992).

The electrocardiogram (ECG) is a simple, noninvasive, easily performed and well-tolerated test that enables detection of myocardial infarction, resting ischemia, arrythmias, and conduction abnormalities. It is estimated that 28% of

TABLE 38–6. Categorization of Obstruction by FEV_1/FVC

Category	% Predicted FEV_1/FVC
Normal	> 69
Mild	61–69
Moderate	45–60
Severe	< 45

Adapted with permission from Grippi et al. (1988). (p. 2507).

TABLE 38–8. Quantitation of Restriction

Category	% Predicted TLC and VC
Normal	> 81
Mild	66–80
Moderate	51–65
Severe	< 50

Adapted with permission from Grippi et al. (1988). (p. 2507).

TABLE 38–9. Categorization of Reduction in Efficacy of Gas Transfer: Measurement of DL_{CO}

Category	% Predicted DL_{CO}
Normal	81–140
Mild	61–80
Moderate	41–60
Severe	< 41

Adapted with permission from Grippi et al. (1988). (p. 2510).

infarcts are discovered by new ECG changes in the form of new Q waves or R waves (Kannell & Abbott, 1984). For these reasons, patients with a significant cardiac history and any patient over the age of 40 should have a preoperative ECG. Patients with a significant cardiac history and those with ECG changes should be referred to cardiology for further evaluation and treatment prior to surgery.

Laboratory Evaluation

Routine preoperative labs including chemistry battery, CBC, PT, PTT, and type and screen should be obtained within one week of surgery. Therapeutic drug levels should be obtained if the patient is on any medications. Coumadin should be discontinued 3 days prior to operation and aspirin should be discontinued 7 days prior to operation.

▶ THE AIRWAY—TRACHEA AND BRONCHUS

Diagnostic Procedures

Bronchoscopy

Since the late 1800s the use of the bronchoscope as a diagnostic tool has increased dramatically. The development of the flexible bronchoscope has enabled this procedure to be done not only in the operating room but in the outpatient setting as well as at the bedside. Bronchoscopy is routinely used by many specialties including Thoracic Surgery, Pulmonary Medicine, Otolaryngology, and Emergency Medicine. A complete review of bronchoscopy is not possible within the limits of this chapter.

Flexible Bronchoscopy. The indications for flexible bronchoscopy include direct visual examination of the airway, tissue diagnosis, or for transbronchial needle aspiration of extraluminal areas suspicious for nodal metastases (Borchers & Beamis, 1996). For central lesions, the diagnostic yield is as high as 80%; for peripheral lesions, 33% (Steiner, Liu, Goldberg, & Cohn, 1995).

The standard equipment for flexible bronchoscopy includes not only the bronchoscope itself but also a light source, suction apparatus, camera, and often a computer. The scope itself is usually 58 cm long and up to 6 mm in diameter. The diameter of the scope varies for adults from 3 mm to 6 mm. The distal tip of the scope may be flexed up to 180 degrees and downward to 130 degrees. Most units now have photographic and video capability enabling the operator to clearly document the findings at the time of the procedure.

Anesthesia for the procedure varies according to the purpose for the bronchoscopy, the setting in which it is being performed, and practitioner preference. The goals are always the same: to provide patient comfort, safety, and suppression of cough and gag reflex. The patient is usually premedicated with an anxiolytic such as Midazolam. Atropine is often given prior to the procedure to reduce secretions, prevent bradycardia, and inhibit vagal responses. A topical anesthetic is then given to inhibit cough and gag. Most commonly lidocaine is used and is administered via a spray, swab, or jelly depending on practitioner preference. The bronchoscopy may be performed either transorally or transnasally, enabling examination of the nasopharynx and upper airway (Borchers & Beamis, 1996).

The contraindications to flexible bronchoscopy are outlined in Table 38–10. There are few absolute contraindications to this procedure. The relative contraindications must be weighed against the potential complications (Table 38–11). Flexible bronchoscopy has a complication rate of 0 to 5% and a 0% mortality rate (Borchers & Beamis, 1996). Complications may arise from the anesthesia or from the procedure itself. Some complications are expected and generally resolve quickly once the procedure is completed. A decrease in arterial oxygenation of 10 to 20 mm Hg during the procedure is expected due to airway obstruction from the scope, bronchospasm, and suctioning. Bronchospasm occurs more commonly in patients with asthma or COPD. Laryngospasm may occur when the bronchoscope is passed

TABLE 38–10. Contraindications to Flexible Bronchoscopy

Absolute
- Absence of consent from patient
- Bronchoscopy by an inexperienced person
- Inadequate facilities for handling complications
- Inability to oxygenate patient

Increased risk
- Uncontrolled asthma
- Hypoxemia
- Unstable angina
- Recent myocardial infarction
- Partial tracheal obstruction
- Cardiac arrhythmia
- Uncooperative patient
- Coagulopathy
- Uremia
- Pulmonary hypertension
- Positive pressure ventilation

Reprinted with permission from Borchers & Beamis. (1996). (p. 186).

TABLE 38–11. Complications of Flexible Bronchoscopy

Anesthesia	Bronchoscopy
Respiratory failure	Hypoxemia
Hypoxia	Laryngospasm
Hypotension	Bronchospasm
Syncope	Fever
Seizure	Pneumonia
Methemoglobinemia	Pulmonary hemorrhage
Arrhythmia	Pneumothorax
	Cardiac arrhythmia

Reprinted with permission from Borchers & Beamis. (1996). (p. 187).

through the cords but with good sedation this is usually avoided. Ten to twenty percent of patients experience fever post bronchoscopy, which usually resolves within 24 hours. Antibiotics are not routinely given except in the high-risk patient with a prosthetic valve, the immunocompromised patient, or in a patient who has an invasive procedure at the time of bronchoscopy. Hemorrhage occurs most commonly with biopsy. The risk of hemorrhage is increased in a patient with thrombocytopenia or vascular tumor. Hemorrhage that does not resolve spontaneously may require endobronchial tamponade, instillation of 2 ml 1:10,000 epinephrine, or bronchial artery embolization. Pneumothorax occurs most frequently with biopsy and most are successfully aspirated (Borchers & Beamis, 1996).

Rigid Bronchoscopy. The primary indications for rigid bronchoscopy in thoracic surgery include hemoptysis or hemorrhage, removal of foreign body, dilation of stricture, stent placement, and tumor biopsy or excision. There are no absolute contraindications to this procedure.

Hemoptysis greater than 25 mL warrants investigation with a rigid scope. A rigid bronchoscope allows for control of the airway and enables the practitioner to pinpoint the site of bleeding. If necessary a fiberoptic scope may be passed through the rigid scope to reach a distal site. A rigid scope is the ideal way to retrieve foreign bodies from the trachea, mainstem bronchus, and lobar bronchi. Tracheal strictures may be treated by tracheal dilatation through a rigid scope. This may be accomplished either with the tip of the scope itself or by using Bougies, which range in diameter from 6F to 20F (Helmers & Sanderson, 1995).

Ideally, rigid bronchoscopy is performed in the operating room or endoscopy suite. It is only performed at the bedside in emergency situations. The standard adult scope ranges from 4 to 9 mm in diameter and averages 40 cm in length.

Prior to the procedure, if done electively, the patient should be made NPO for 12 hours. The same premedication is given that is used for flexible bronchoscopy. Rigid bronchoscopy may be performed under local anesthesia, but general anesthesia is preferred. Ventilation during the procedure is provided either intermittently or continuously (Miller, 1996). Potential complications include injury to gums or teeth, respiratory depression, laryngospasm, bronchospasm, arrhythmia, hypoxia, pneumothorax, or hemorrhage.

Sputum Cytology

Sputum cytology is the least invasive method of diagnosing lung cancer. It is associated with low cost and no discomfort or risk. Location and size of the lesion affect the ability to obtain a diagnosis. If the lesion is more central, the likelihood of diagnosis is greater than if the lesion is peripheral. Larger lesions also tend to be more likely to yield a diagnosis. It is important to note that a negative cytological result does not necessarily exclude malignancy as the false negative rate is as high as 40% (Mehta, Marty, & Lee, 1993). According to Mehta, Marty, & Lee (1993), squamous-cell carcinoma may be diagnosed with sputum cytology in up to 84% of cases. Sputum cytology to date has not been associated with increased survival when used as a screening test in "high risk" populations. With newer, more sensitive molecular diagnostic techniques, this may change and is currently being evaluated.

Therapeutic Procedures

Tracheostomy

The tracheostomy dates back to 2000 B.C. and is now commonly used for patients who require prolonged mechanical ventilation as well as for those with upper airway obstruction, head and neck tumors, trauma, sleep apnea, and management of secretions (Wood, 1996). This procedure is often considered trivial as it can be performed by surgeons from various specialties and even residents in training. However, if one recalls the anatomy involved and acknowledges the potential complications, it is evident that while simple to perform, it should not be trivialized.

Indications. Perhaps the most common indication for tracheostomy is prolonged ventilation. Today, with advances in hemodynamic monitoring, antibiotics, hemodialysis, nutritional care, and respiratory support, more patients are able to survive respiratory failure (Wood, 1996). The tracheostomy provides a more secure airway with less incidence of self-extubation. It allows for increased mobility, increased comfort, improved oral hygiene, and increased ability to communicate. Additionally there is evidence that it allows for more effective suctioning (Astrachan, Kerchner, & Goodwin, 1988). Many believe it increases the ability to wean a patient by decreasing dead space and airway resistance. The only controversy that remains is the timing of performing a tracheostomy. In situations where it is evident that the patient will require ventilation longer than 14 days, it is generally agreed that tracheostomy is indicated.

Upper airway obstruction was the original indication

for the tracheostomy. Types of airway obstruction include trauma, tumor, foreign body, bilateral vocal cord paralysis, inflammation, edema, and sleep apnea. Additionally tracheobronchial toilet is an indication for the tracheostomy including secretion management, pneumonia or chronic aspiration.

Technique. The tracheostomy is performed in the operating room under general anesthesia. The patient is placed in a supine position and a roll is placed underneath the neck and shoulders to increase neck extension. A 3- to 5-cm incision is made 1.5 cm below the cricoid cartilage (Fig. 38–3). The thyroid isthmus is either divided or retracted. The tracheostomy tube is then placed through either the second or third tracheal ring. Placement into the first tracheal ring leads to subglottic stenosis and placement too low increases the likelihood of a tracheoinnominate fistula (Fig. 38–4). The tracheostomy flanges are sutured to the skin (Wood, 1996).

Postoperative Care. Postoperatively the sutures should be left in place for 5 to 7 days. The site should be cleansed and dressed twice a day. Gentle catheter irrigation and suctioning should be done at least four times a day. It is important to use lightweight ventilator tubing and to minimally inflate the balloon. Humidified ventilation is preferred. If the tracheostomy is in place for a prolonged period of time, a fenestrated trach may be utilized to allow for speech and oral intake.

Complications may be broken down into intraoperative, early, or late (Table 38–12). Bleeding is the most common intraoperative complication and is usually easily corrected. Tracheal laceration or tracheoesophageal fistula may occur if placement is difficult. This is suspected when pneumothorax or pneumomediastinum occurs with ventilation; it requires immediate surgical repair. Malpositioning of the tube is suspected with difficulty ventilating, pneumothorax, and difficulty suctioning. When suspected, the tube should be removed and oral intubation reestablished.

Early complications of tracheostomy include bleeding with coughing or from coagulation disorders. Abscess formation may occur as the result of closing the skin too tightly preventing drainage; in this case, antibiotics are instituted and the wound is opened. Pneumothorax or subcutaneous emphysema is often due to an improperly inflated

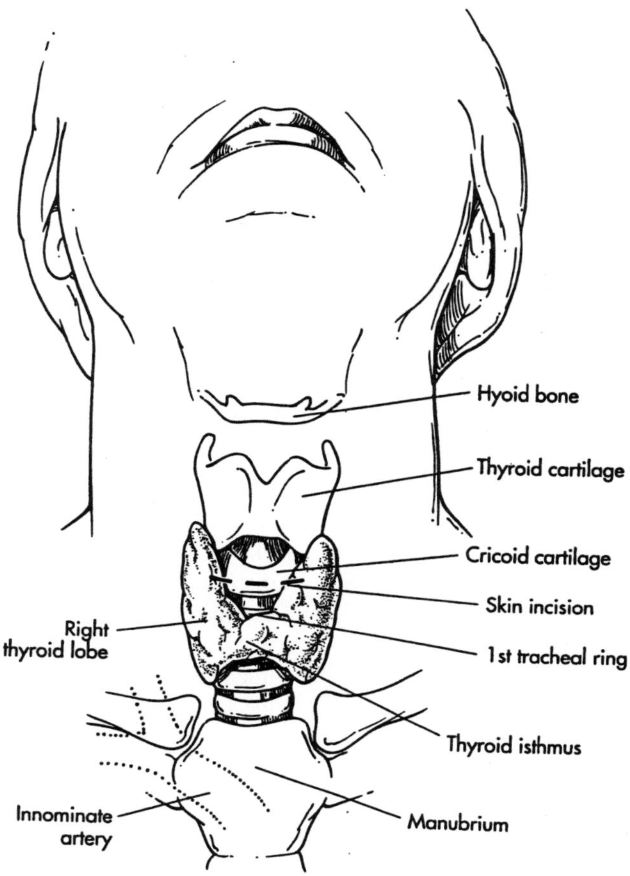

Figure 38–3. Tracheostomy incision. A 3–5 cm incision located 1.5 cm below the cricoid cartilage enables insertion of a tracheostomy tube. *(Reprinted with permission from Kaiser. [1997]. [p. 31].)*

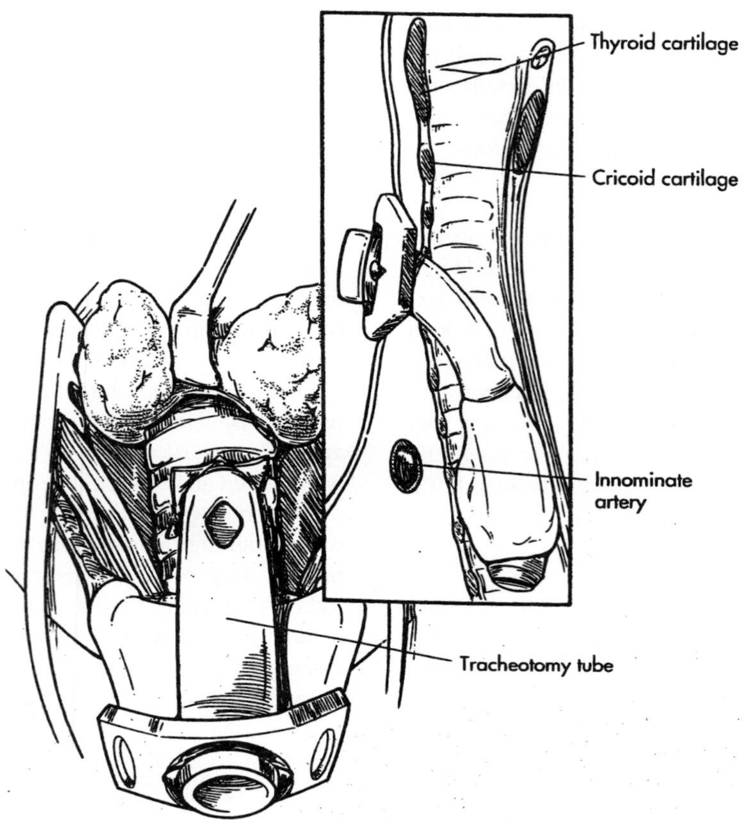

Figure 38–4. Tracheostomy tube. Tracheostomy tube in position and location of cuff to Innominate artery. *(From Kaiser. [1997]. [p. 33].)*

cuff and requires reconfirmation of tube placement. Tube obstruction from blood clot, mucous plug, or secretions may be managed with suctioning or bronchoscopy if necessary. Late complications, while relatively rare, certainly have more serious consequences.

TABLE 38–12. Complications of Tracheostomy

Intraoperative	Late (> 7 days)
Bleeding	Tracheoinnominate artery fistula
Tracheal laceration	Tracheoesophageal fistula
Tracheoesophageal fistula	Tracheal stenosis
Tube malposition	Tracheal malacia
Recurrent laryngeal nerve injury	Persistent tracheocutaneous fistula
Pneumothorax	
Pneumomediastinum	
Cardiorespiratory arrest	
Early (< 7 days)	
Bleeding	
Peristomal abscess or cellulitis	
Subcutaneous emphysema	
Pneumomediastinum	
Tube malposition	
Tube obstruction	

Reprinted with permission from Wood. (1996). (p. 757).

Percutaneous Tracheostomy

The indications for a percutaneous tracheostomy are similar to that of a tracheostomy. Contraindications are the inability to palpate normal laryngeal cartilage and cricoid rings, enlarged thyroid, calcified tracheal rings, bleeding abnormalities, and the need for an emergent airway (Anderson & Bartlett, 1991). The advantage is that this procedure may be performed at the bedside; however, visualization of the landmark for cannulation is limited compared with tracheostomy. The procedure is done with the neck extended and the skin anesthetized with local anesthesia. A 1- to 2-cm incision is placed 1.5 cm below the cricoid cartilage. A catheter introducer needle is placed in the anterior tracheal wall between the second and third tracheal rings. A J-tipped guide wire is inserted followed by sequential dilators. The percutaneous tracheostomy is advanced over the guide wire and secured in the same manner as a tracheostomy (Wood, 1996).

Crichothyroidotomy

The cricothyroidotomy is an ideal alternative to a tracheostomy in an emergency situation. A 1- to 2-cm incision is made over the cricothyroid membrane. Dilation is performed with a hemostat and the tube is inserted. It enables quick establishment of an airway but the complication rate is a high as 25%, which is why it is not used as an elective procedure. Conversion of the cricothyroid tube to a formal tracheostomy within 24 to 72 hours significantly reduces the incidence of complications (Burkey, Esclamado, & Morganroth, 1991).

Minitracheotomy

The minitracheotomy was first described in 1984 for the management of secretions (Matthews & Hopkinson, 1984). This procedure is easily performed at the bedside and many kits are now available. These should be readily available on the general thoracic surgery unit. It is performed by a 1-cm stab incision into the cricothyroid membrane after the injection of local anesthesia. While not recommended for prolonged ventilation, minitracheotomy has been shown to be an ideal method of managing secretions often obviating the need for a formal tracheostomy and significantly decreasing the incidence of pneumonia (Wood, 1996).

Tracheal Resection

Disorders of the trachea make up a very small percentage of the cases in general thoracic surgery and thus are only discussed briefly. Successful management of the trachea may result in elimination of the need for a chronic tracheostomy, preservation of voice, and in some cases may be lifesaving. The most common indications for tracheal surgery are tracheal tumors, postintubation tracheal stenosis, tracheoinnominate fistula, and tracheoesophageal fistula.

Tracheal Tumors. Tracheal tumors are relatively uncommon (Mathisen, 1996). They are generally very slow-growing tumors and often go undiagnosed for a long period of time. There are three categories of tracheal tumors: malignant or squamous-cell carcinoma, intermediate malignant or adenoid cystic, and benign. Wheezing is often the first symptom before there is radiographic evidence, so patients are often initially treated for asthma. Other symptoms include one if not all of the following: dyspnea, hemoptysis, cough, dysphagia, change in voice or hoarseness, stridor, and/or pneumonia.

Evaluation of a tracheal tumor requires a chest radiograph with an AP view to evaluate the extent of tumor. Fluoroscopy of the larynx and trachea assist in evaluating the involvement of recurrent laryngeal nerves, airway, and esophagus. If there is any question of involvement of the superior vena cava, innominate artery, and/or pulmonary artery, an angiogram is warranted. There is no consensus as to the added value of obtaining a CT scan. Endoscopy is helpful for both evaluation of the tumor itself and in obtaining a tissue diagnosis, but is usually done at the time of operation due to the potential of edema and/or hemorrhage resulting in sudden airway compromise (Mathisen, 1996).

No matter what the type of tracheal tumor, surgical excision is the treatment of choice (Briselli, Mark, & Grillo, 1978). Surgical excision is performed through an anterior collar incision. The patient should be prepped from chin to xiphoid in the event that a median sternotomy incision is ultimately required. The trachea is resected with the patient intubated distal to the site of resection. Once the excision is complete, the patient is reintubated. Suction drains are placed substernal and paratracheal. A chin stitch is placed from the chin to the presternal area as a reminder to the patient not to hyperextend the neck. Patients are usually able to be extubated in the operating room (Mathisen, 1996).

Postintubation Tracheal Stenosis. Postintubation tracheal stenosis, a preventable complication, is the primary indication for tracheal resection and reconstruction. It is most often caused by pressure necrosis from the endotracheal tube, tracheostomy tube, or the cuff of either. Simply not inflating the cuff beyond its maximal resting volume prevents this condition, yet it is still common (Cooper & Grillo, 1969).

The patient with postintubation tracheal stenosis presents with dyspnea, wheezing, stridor, and/or obstruction even with minimal mucous. Often the patient is misdiagnosed with asthma. At the time of onset the chest radiograph may be clear. Pneumonia often ensues. Bronchoscopic examination and CT scan make diagnosis. Pulmonary function tests rarely provide necessary confirmatory diagnostic information.

Definitive treatment is surgical resection and reconstruction. A successful operation is dependent upon the timing of the operation and the level of the anastamosis. Reasons to delay operation include medical condition, inflammation, high steroid dose, and mechanical ventilation. Acute obstruction may be managed with dilation through a rigid scope (Grillo & Donahue, 1996).

Tracheal resection for postintubation stenosis is done through a collar incision. During the procedure the patient is ventilated through the distal trachea. Ideally patients are extubated in the operating room. If unable to extubate, the cuff must be placed above or below the suture line. Complications from this operation include the formation of granulation tissue, dehiscence, restenosis, permanent tracheostomy, infection, and death (Grillo & Donahue, 1996).

Tracheoinnominate Fistula. Tracheoinnominate fistula may be caused by necrosis or separation of a suture line after tracheal resection or stent placement or pressure necrosis from the cuff or tip of the tube following tracheostomy (refer to Fig. 38–4) (Wright, 1996). Early diagnosis and management are the key to survival. Tracheoinnominate fistulas should be suspected with any post-tracheostomy hemorrhage, but particularly in the case of new onset hemorrhage within the first 48 hours. Definitive diagnosis is made by rigid bronchoscopy.

Control of bleeding must occur before the patient is moved to the operating room. Overinflation of the cuff to produce a tamponade effect has been reported to work in 85% of cases (Jones, Reynolds, Hewitt, et al., 1976).

Should bleeding persist despite overinflation of the cuff, the trach should be withdrawn and the patient should be intubated either orally or nasally. The innominate artery should be digitally compressed by placing a finger in the trach site and manually compressing the artery against the sternum. The surgical repair is performed by either a full or partial sternotomy. Twenty-five percent of the patients who make it to the operating room ultimately die due to mismanagement, underlying illness, or comorbid conditions (Wright, 1996).

Tracheoesophageal Fistula. Tracheoesophageal fistulas (TE fistula) may be caused by mediastinal infections, immunodeficiency syndrome, complications from anterior cervical spine procedures, complications from total laryngectomy or cervical esophageal procedures, trauma including blunt or penetrating, or it may have an iatrogenic etiology. By far the most common cause of a TE fistula is pressure necrosis from an endotracheal or nasogastric tube in a mechanically ventilated patient (Dartevelle & Macchiarini, 1996). The risk is substantially increased with excessive motion of the tube, infection, hypotension, steroid use, and diabetes.

TE fistula should be suspected in any ventilated patient who has a sudden abdominal distention, abnormal secretions, unexplained pneumonia (especially the right lower lobe), or who is suddenly difficult to ventilate. Bronchoscopy is the most definitive method of diagnosis. Instillation of methylene blue into the esophagus while performing the bronchoscopy assists in the diagnosis of small fistulas that would be difficult to visualize otherwise (Dartevelle & Macchiarini, 1996).

Operative closure should be attempted in all patients as spontaneous closure rarely, if ever, occurs. Surgical options include direct closure with or without a muscle flap, tracheal closure with esophageal patch, segmental tracheal resection, or esophageal diversion. Experience with repair of TE fistulas is limited, however relatively successful, with recurrence reported to be less than 6% and mortality less than 10% (Dartevelle & Macchiarini, 1996).

Complications of Tracheal Surgery. Complications of tracheal surgery occur due to improper patient selection, improper timing of operation, lack of technical skill, or improper postoperative management. Several specific factors have been shown to increase the likelihood of postoperative complications. Mechanical ventilation in all cases except tracheostomy place the patient at risk for anastomotic complications. Steroids interfere with tracheal healing and lead to the potential for dehiscence. Preoperative radiation has been implicated in poor tracheal healing as well. The most common complications following tracheal surgery include the formation of granulation tissue, dehiscence, restenosis, laryngeal dysfunction, tracheomalacia, hemorrhage, anastamotic edema, and infection (Mathisen, 1996).

Airway Stents for Stenosis. Tracheobronchial stenosis may result from a benign or malignant process and leads to respiratory compromise or distress. Common causes include malignancy, poor anastamotic healing, tracheobronchial malacia, infection, or granulomatosis formation. Patients may be asymptomatic even after radiographic evidence of stenosis is present. The most common presenting symptom is dyspnea. In addition, patients may present with cough, hemoptysis, wheezing, or chest pain. Therapeutic options include dilation, radiation therapy, surgery, stent placement, or a combination of these (Nesbitt & Carrasco, 1996). The goal is always to achieve airway patency.

Evaluation for stent placement consists of a chest radiograph, CT scan, and flexible bronchoscopy. Pulmonary function tests are interesting for comparison but not necessary for evaluation (Colt & Dumon, 1995). There are three categories of stents: silicone, metal, or dynamic (combination of silicone and metal) (Fig. 38–5). The advantages and disadvantages of the most commonly used stents are shown in Table 38–13.

Stents are placed in the operating room under general anesthesia. A rigid bronchoscope is used to predilate the trachea and then the stent is placed through the scope. Some patients are discharged the day of the procedure while others stay overnight for observation. Complications include obstruction and migration, both of which are rare, tumor or granulation, and perforation by metal stents (Colt & Dumon, 1995).

▶ THE MEDIASTINUM

Diagnostic Procedures—Mediastinoscopy

Mediastinoscopy allows for endoscopic examination and sampling of the lymph nodes in the pretracheal, paratracheal, subcarinal, and tracheobronchial nodes. It is generally well tolerated and consequently may be performed as a same-day procedure. The pulmonary lymphatic system, like other organs, has lymphatic drainage along the vascular system as well as through lymph nodes. The decision to biopsy these nodes is usually made after review of a CT scan, though some surgeons routinely biopsy. Most omit the mediastinal lymph node biopsy in the presence of a peripheral tumor where the CT does not demonstrate any mediastinal nodes greater than 1 cm.

The patient is placed supine with the neck extended by an interscapular roll. The head of the operating table is elevated 20 to 30 degrees. General anesthesia is required. A 3-cm horizontal incision is centered just above the sternoclavicular heads and a scope is placed (Fig. 38–6). At the time of biopsy or resection, the lymph nodes are identified by color and consistency and then referenced on a map enabling staging (Fig. 38–7). Usually nodes are sampled at

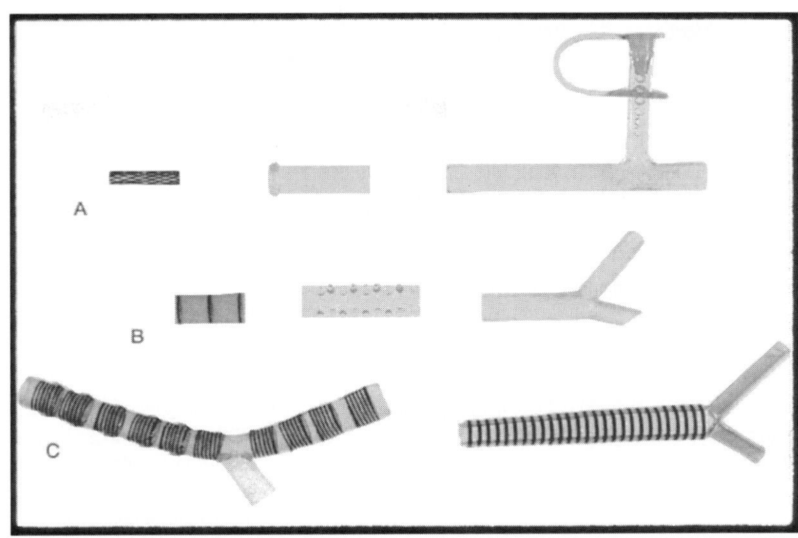

Figure 38–5. Airway stents. Examples of currently available stents: **A,** Palmaz Stent, Hood Stent with proximal Flange, Montgomery T Tube. **B,** Novastent, Dumon studded silicone stent, and bifurcated Y stent. **C,** Orlowski stent and Dynamic Y Stent. *(From Colt & Dumon. [1995]. [p. 465].)*

levels 2, 4, 7, and sent for frozen section. Frozen section enables prompt diagnosis and allows the surgeon to proceed with surgical resection of the tumor in the same sitting.

Rarely is there need for chest tube placement as the pleural space is not entered. The possibility of puncture of this space, however, necessitates the need to check for an air leak prior to closure; if present, chest tube placement is indicated. At the time of closure of the mediastinoscopy incision, sutures are placed subcutaneously and steri strips are placed on the closed wound. If a simple mediastinoscopy is performed without additional resection, the patient is recovered for 2 to 3 hours and then discharged. A postoperative chest radiograph is indicated if there was any entry into the pleural cavity, or in the presence of bleeding or hypoxemia in the immediate postoperative period.

Complications are rare and reported to occur less than 2.5% of the time. Potential complications include hemorrhage, recurrent laryngeal nerve injury, pneumothorax, esophageal perforation, chylous leak, wound infection, mediastinitis, air embolus, phrenic nerve injury, or seroma (Kirschner, 1996).

Therapeutic Procedures

Thymoma

Thymoma is perhaps one of the most common tumors of the mediastinum. It is a tumor of the thymus gland that is composed of epithelial, lymphocytic, or spindle cells (Warren & Gould, 1992). It may be either benign or malignant depending on microscopic or gross invasion. Thymomas are more commonly referred to as encapsulated (benign) or invasive (malignant). A staging system has been developed. Stage I thymomas are well-encapsulated tumors without any microscopic invasion. Stage II thymomas have evidence of growth into adjacent pleura or pericardium. Invasion into the adjacent organs or evidence of intrathoracic metastasis occurs in stage III. Stage IV thymomas have extrathoracic metastases.

Thymomas occur most commonly in the fifth or sixth decades of life, but may occur at any age. Approximately 50% of patients are asymptomatic (Warren & Gould, 1992). The rest of the patients present with a variety of symptoms including weight loss, fatigue, fever, night sweats, chest pain, cough, and/or shortness of breath. Evaluation requires a chest radiograph that demonstrates a smooth, lobulated mass in the anterior mediastinum with or without calcification. A CT scan is necessary to evaluate the relationship of the mass to surrounding structures. Some surgeons further evaluate the patient with an MRI as a means of evaluating the great vessels and the hilum (Warren & Gould, 1992).

Once the diagnosis of thymoma is made, complete resection is the goal. The diagnosis cannot be confirmed without histology. While some advocate the use of biopsy with transthoracic needle biopsy or mediastinotomy to obtain a tissue diagnosis, in general this is discouraged due to the potential implantation of tumor. Video thoracoscopy enables the surgeon to obtain a tissue diagnosis by minimally invasive means and then proceed to complete resection via either a thoracotomy or median sternotomy if frozen section confirms a thymoma.

Recurrence is rare after complete resection. For those patients with extensive involvement of mediastinal structures, sometimes only debulking of the tumor is possible. Postoperative radiation therapy is offered for either invasive thymomas with complete resection or in situations where tu-

TABLE 38–13. Advantages and Disadvantages of Currently Available Airway Stents

Stent	Advantages	Disadvantages
Silicone		
Montgomery T tube	Allows maintenance of a tracheotomy. Suctioning and cleaning are possible through external limb. Provides simultaneous palliation of immediate subglottic stenosis and of more distal tracheal strictures.	Requires a tracheotomy. Easily obstructed by dried secretions, if external limb is uncapped. Frequent formation of granulation tissue in subglottis.
Dumon	Studs on external surface prevent migration and reduce chance for mucosal edema by limiting contact to small surfaces only. Easily removed during rigid or flexible bronchoscopy.	Insertion requires rigid bronchoscopy and dilatation. Proper selection of length and width is essential to assure a snug fit and to avoid obstructing peripheral bronchi. Migration may occur. Relatively thick stent wall reduces airway lumen.
Hood	Smooth-walled, can be custom designed in Y, L, or straight shapes of various lengths and diameters. Easily removed during rigid or flexible bronchoscopy.	Insertion requires rigid bronchoscopy and dilatation. Smooth external surface may lead to greater incidence of stent migration. Stents with distal or proximal flanges, however, are available. Y stents may be difficult to insert.
Metal		
Gianturco Z stent	Simple insertion during bronchoscopy and fluoroscopy. Highly visible on chest radiograph. Excellent fixation to airway walls by small hooks placed at each extremity of the stent. Stents can be attached to each other to obtain adequate length. Maximum diameter usually predefined.	Deployment may be asymmetric. Potential risks of wall perforation with erosion into mediastinum or vessels. Inflammatory granulation tissue formation is frequent. Removal is nearly impossible.
Schneider (Wallstent)	Fine wire mesh stent comes in different lengths and diameters. Self-expanding cylindrical stent easily placed through loading catheter. Self-expandability makes prior dilatation of strictures unnecessary. Highly visible on chest radiograph. Allows re-epithelialization and subsequent incorporation into airway wall. Probably better tolerated than Gianturco Z stents	Potential for inflammatory granulation tissue formation until re-epithelialization is complete. Tumor may grow through the spaces between the wire mesh, thereby causing further stenosis. Removal is impossible. Insufficient long-term clinical follow-up.
Palmaz	Wire mesh cylinder requiring balloon dilatation for maximal expansion, thereby limiting self-expandability and risks for perforation because the ultimate diameter of the stent is controlled. Simple insertion technique through loading catheters. Highly visible on chest radiograph.	Potential inflammatory granulation tissue formation. Airway obstruction caused by tumor overgrowth or granulation through the spaces between the wire mesh. Risk of perforation because of sharp metal edges at distal and proximal extremities of the stent. Insufficient long-term clinical follow-up.
Others		
Freitag (Dynamic stent)	Silicone stent for trachea, usually Y shaped, with anterior wall that is reinforced by metal hoops preventing extrinsic compression. May improve secretion clearance because of malleable posterior wall adjacent to pars membranosa. Well tolerated, easily removable during rigid bronchoscopy.	Y-shaped stent difficult to insert. Especially long tracheal component, but small diameter of left and right main bronchial branches. Insufficient clinical studies available.
Orlowski	Solid, provides simultaneous tracheal and bronchial airway patency. Made of silicone with circular metal armor inside.	Insertion may be tricky without adequate preliminary dilatation. Insufficient clinical or experimental studies available.
Novastent	Rolled silicone sheet with metal armor. Stent wall has minimal thickness. May be self-expanding. Simple insertion through loading catheter.	Insufficient clinical or experimental studies available.

Reprinted with permission from Colt & Dumon. (1995). (p. 472).

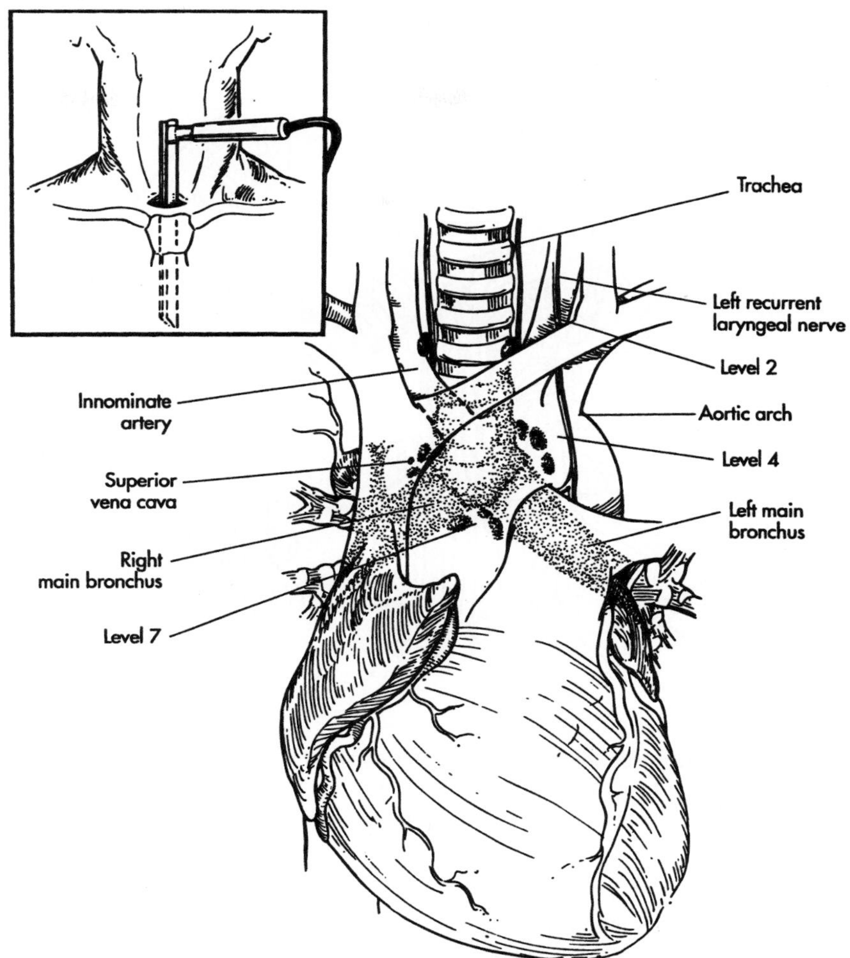

Figure 38–6. Mediastinoscopy. A 3 cm incision is centered above the sternoclavicular heads enabling insertion of a scope. Lymph nodes are then able to be sampled in the areas depicted; commonly Levels 2, 4, and 7. *(Reprinted with permission from Kaiser. [1997]. [p. 6].)*

mor is left behind. The role of chemotherapy remains controversial (Warren & Gould, 1992).

Thymectomy

Myasthenia gravis is an autoimmune disorder that occurs as the result of the destruction of postsynaptic acetylcholine receptors (Blossom, Ernstoff, Howells, Bendick, & Glover, 1993). This results in generalized weakness and fatigue of the affected muscle groups. Ocular symptoms occur in almost every patient, frequently as the presenting symptom. Periods of stress (emotional, physical, or both) exacerbate symptoms. Approximately 18% of patients develop thymomas likely to be invasive (Kirschner, 1992).

Medical management includes the use of steroids, immunosuppression, and plasmapheresis. Medical management may lead to complete control of symptoms, though this is rare. Additionally, the potential for invasive thymoma to develop often necessitates surgical resection. In the case of nonthymomatous myasthenia, if symptoms are well controlled, surgery may be deferred if the patient prefers. If symptoms persist despite maximal medical therapy, thymectomy is recommended. For patients with thymomatous myasthenia, surgery is indicated as soon as symptoms are controlled (Kirschner, 1992). There is no age limit in either case. The only true contraindication to surgery is myasthenic crisis.

The goal of surgical resection is complete removal of the thymus. Surgical approaches vary according to surgeon preference. Transcervical and median sternotomy are the two most common incisions used. However, some advocate a transsternal approach or partial upper sternotomy and some use a thoracotomy. The transcervical approach is the least invasive, has the least potential for postoperative complications, is associated with a decreased length of stay, and is preferable to most patients. There has been some hesitancy in accepting this approach due to the concern that not all of the thymus may be removed. However, this has not been well documented.

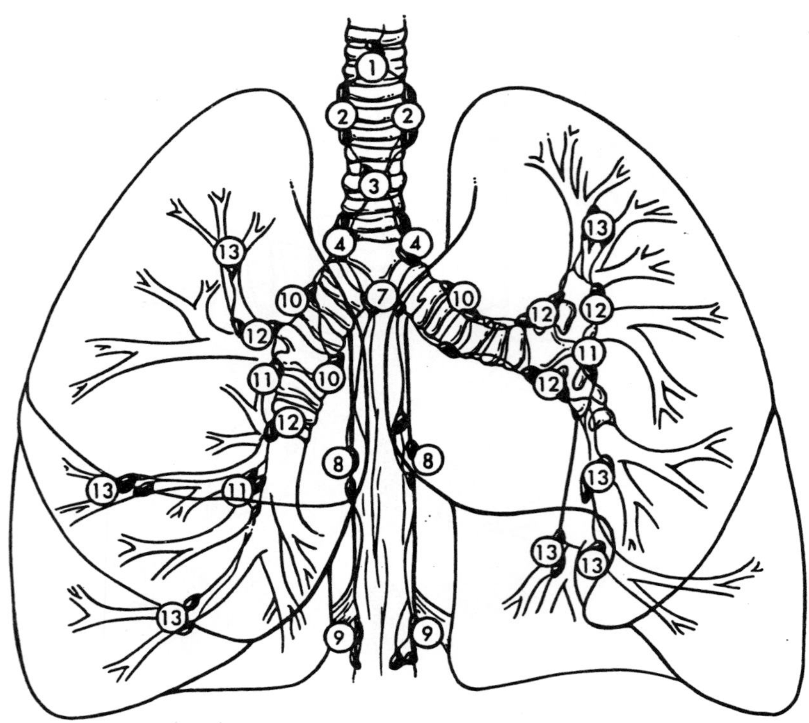

Figure 38–7. Lymph node map. (1) Highest mediastinal node; (2) upper paratracheal; (3) pretracheal; (4) lower paratracheal; (5) aortopulmonary window (*left*); (6) paraaortic (*left*); (7) subcarinal; (8) paraesophageal; (9) inferior pulmonary ligament; (10) tracheobronchial angle; (11) interlobar (N1); (12) lobar (N1); (13) segmental (N1); (14) subsegmental (N1) (not shown). *(Reprinted with permission from Kaiser. [1997]. [p. 115].)*

The perioperative management of the patient undergoing thymectomy for myasthenia gravis is critical. Plasmapheresis may be implemented within 72 hours prior to surgery as it has been demonstrated to control generalized weakness (Kirschner, 1992). Anticholinergic medications are discontinued the day of the surgery and resumed postoperatively at the discretion of the neurologist based on the patient's symptoms. Stress-dose steroids are required for anyone who has been on steroids preoperatively. Standard weaning and extubation parameters are used. Patients should be monitored for respiratory muscle strength by bedside spirometry for the first few days.

Patient response to surgical resection is variable and often not fully appreciated for several months. Approximately 10 to 20% have a complete drug-free remission. Between 15 and 30% achieve a drug-maintained remission. An additional 35 to 50% experience some improvement (Kirschner, 1992).

Lymphoproliferative Disorders

Lymphoproliferative disorders often present as either bulky mediastinal nodes, a mediastinal mass, or the combination of both (Yellin, 1992). The most common lymphoproliferative disorders are Hodgkin's disease, non-Hodgkin's disease and leukemia. Hodgkin's is staged according to the Ann Arbor System. There are four stages based on the lymph node regions involved and their location above or below the diaphragm. Further classification is based on the patient's symptoms and metastatic involvement. Non-Hodgkin's is classified based on cell origin: B cell, T cell, or null cells (Yellin, 1992).

The clinical presentation of a patient depends on the size of the mass. Most commonly patients complain of chest heaviness or pain, cough, and shortness of breath. Evaluation requires a chest x-ray and CT scan that demonstrate a mediastinal tumor, most commonly in the anterior mediastinum, lymphadenopathy, or both. The mass, if present, is usually small and well circumscribed. The primary question at the time of evaluation is whether to obtain a diagnosis or proceed with resection for those masses that prove to be something other than lymphoma. Mediastinoscopy allows a diagnosis and the ability to proceed with resection under one anesthetic depending on the frozen section diagnosis. While some prefer to attempt diagnosis via bronchoscopy with biopsy or transthoracic needle biopsy, adequate tissue samples are difficult to obtain by these approaches and most patients ultimately are referred to a thoracic surgeon for a definitive tissue diagnosis.

Cystic Fore-Gut Malformations

Cystic fore-gut malformations include duplication cysts, bronchoesophageal cysts, bronchogenic cysts, and esophageal cysts. Together they comprise about 20% of all mediastinal masses (Wychulis, Payne, Clagett, et al., 1971). The two most common are bronchogenic cysts and esophageal cysts.

Bronchogenic Cysts. A bronchogenic cyst occurs secondary to abnormal lung growth producing a cystic lesion in the mediastinum. This lesion is most commonly found in a subcarinal location. Most patients are completely asymptomatic; however, if the lesion becomes large enough to compress surrounding structures, pneumonia may ensue due to obstruction. Additionally, a bronchial communication may develop leading to infection.

The evaluation of a bronchogenic cyst includes a chest radiograph that demonstrates a smooth round mass near the carina. Calcification is rare. CT scan is often necessary to specify the location of the lesion with respect to surrounding structures. Treatment is complete surgical resection via a posterolateral thoracotomy or median sternotomy. Preoperatively, patients with pneumonia or infection should be treated with aggressive antibiotic therapy to minimize complications perioperatively. The procedure is generally well tolerated; postoperative complications, if they do occur, include atelectasis, pneumonia, and wound complications. Complete excision provides a cure (Allen & Payne, 1992).

Esophageal Cysts. Esophageal cysts are very similar to bronchogenic cysts. Without pathologic examination they are difficult to distinguish from bronchogenic cysts. They are further defined by an attachment to the esophagus and the presence of gastrointestinal epithelium (Allen & Payne, 1992).

Not unlike bronchogenic cysts, patients are usually asymptomatic but may present with infection or dysphagia depending on the size and location of the cyst. Evaluation includes a chest radiograph that demonstrates a smooth round mass usually located near the carina. Again, CT scan is helpful in determining the exact location of the cyst with respect to surrounding structures.

Treatment is complete surgical resection and is very necessary due to the potential for complications of infection or spontaneous hemorrhage. The surgical approach is thoracotomy or median sternotomy.

▶ THE LUNGS

Diagnostic Procedures

Transthoracic Needle Biopsy

The role of transthoracic needle biopsy (TTNB) for the evaluation of a pulmonary nodule remains controversial. Transthoracic needle biopsy done under high-resolution fluoroscopy enables lesions of the lung, hilum, or mediastinum to be sampled with a diagnostic rate as high as 68% (Weisbord, 1992). The most common indication is for the diagnosis of a pulmonary nodule, mass, or infiltrate when there is a contraindication to operation for medical reasons or there is clinical evidence of metastatic disease. The question remains, why perform TTNB if the patient is going to require an operation regardless of the findings of the needle biopsy? There are a few situations in which the diagnosis might obviate the need for an operation. With the advent of video thoracoscopy enabling a high diagnostic yield and the ability to remove the lesion with a minimally invasive procedure, the needle biopsy may be redundant.

Contraindications to transthoracic needle biopsy include emphysema (with the increased risk of pneumothorax), pulmonary hypertension, and coagulation disorders. Complications from TTNB include a 30% incidence of pneumothorax, hemoptysis, hemorrhage, air embolism, and rare seeding of the needle tract (Weisbord, 1992).

Video-Assisted Thoracoscopic Surgery

Video-assisted thoracoscopic surgery (VATS) has emerged with tremendous popularity as it has been shown to be cost effective with decreased length of stay and hospital costs, is less painful than standard thoracotomy incisions, and is cosmetically appealing (Trastek, Deschamps, Allen, & Pairolero, 1993). There are many indications for the VATS incision including diagnosis and therapy for malignant pleural effusions, treatment of pneumothorax, evacuation of empyema, resection of pulmonary nodules, biopsy of mass or parenchymal disease, and staging of lung cancer. VATS enables conversion from a diagnostic procedure to a therapeutic procedure if necessary. It is important to recognize that the incisions are easily connected to form a thoracotomy incision.

The patient is placed in the standard posterolateral thoracotomy position. The posterolateral thoracotomy incision is drawn on the chest to provide landmarks. Many have described the location of the incisions using the analogy of a baseball diamond. The tip of the scapula is the pitcher's mound. Anterior to the scapula is first base and posterior to the scapula is third base (Trastek, Deschamps, Allen, & Pairlero, 1993). Each incision is approximately 1 to 3 centimeters. One incision is used for the telescopic camera and the others for instruments. Often the surgery may be performed with two incisions, though up to four may be needed depending on the location and complexity of the operation (Fig. 38–8).

Open Lung Biopsy

Anterior Mediastinotomy/Chamberlain Procedure. The anterior mediastinotomy or Chamberlain procedure, not to be confused with the mediastinoscopy, provides access for biopsy in superior mediastinum, hilar region, and upper lobes (Olak, 1996).

The patient is placed supine with arms secured at the sides. A small 4- to 5-cm incision is made just over the second rib in a horizontal fashion. At the time of closure a small chest tube is inserted only if the pleural space has been opened and there is evidence of a leak.

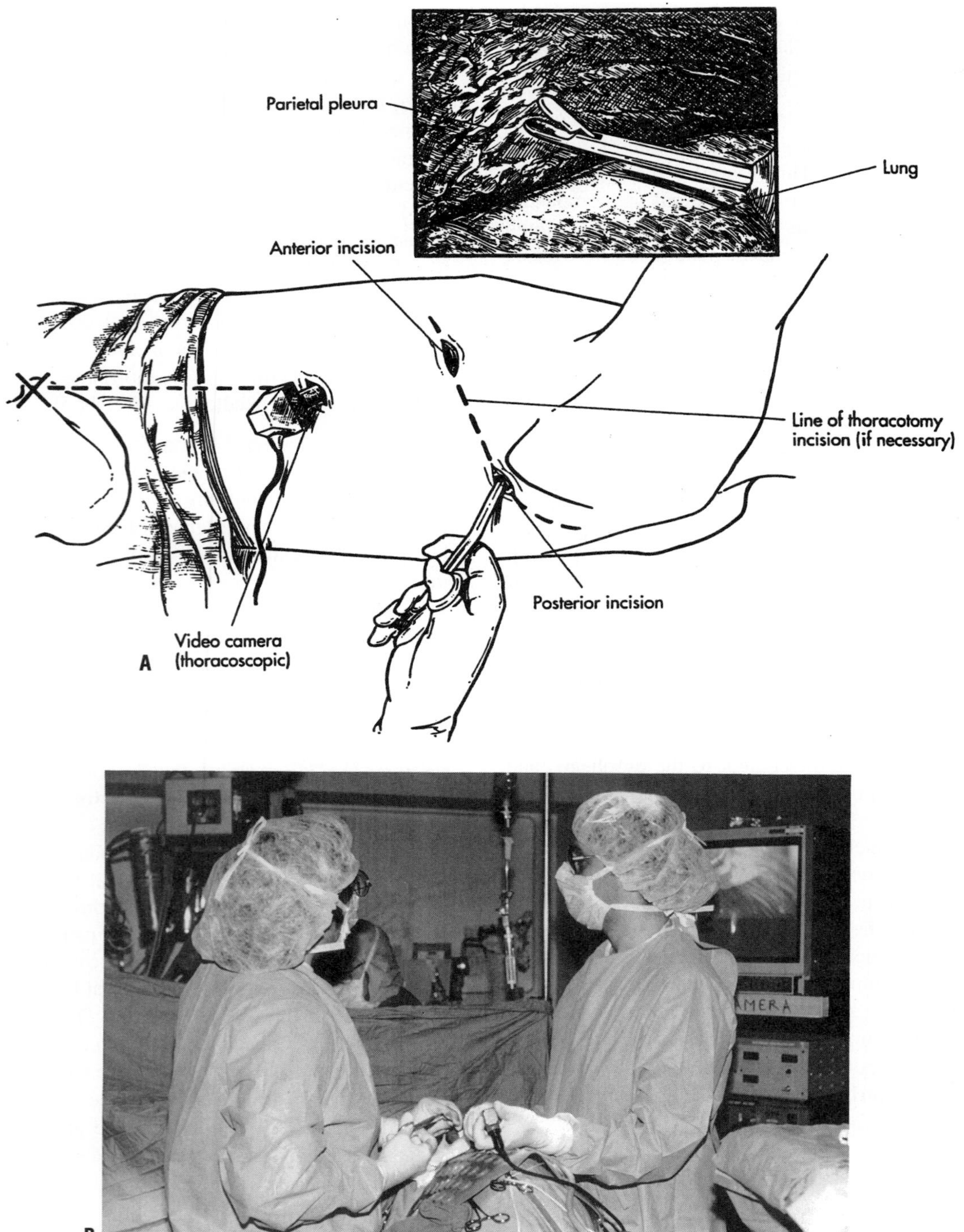

Figure 38–8. Video thoracoscopic surgery. **A,** A posterolateral thoracotomy incision is drawn and three smaller incisions made. **B,** The operation is performed by visualizing the chest on television screens as depicted in photograph. *(Reprinted with permission from Kaiser. [1997].)*

Pathology

Numerous benign and malignant processes may inflict the lung parenchyma necessitating surgical resection. A brief review of the most common entities is presented here.

Neoplasms

Pulmonary Nodules. Pulmonary nodules may be solitary or multiple and may represent a spectrum of pathologic entities. The solitary pulmonary nodule is a single spherical lesion located with the lung parenchyma. It is estimated that 50% of these are malignant, most commonly bronchogenic carcinomas and carcinoid tumors (Lillington & Caskey, 1993). The benign solitary pulmonary nodule is almost always a granuloma, but many other possibilities exist (refer to Table 38–3).

Multiple pulmonary nodules may be the result of a variety of benign or malignant processes, or both. If two or more nodules are present, one should not exclude the possibility of independent pathologic processes. Metastatic spread is the most common cause of multiple pulmonary nodules. Benign processes—both infectious and noninfectious—may precipitate multiple pulmonary nodules as well.

The criteria for resection of pulmonary metastatic disease are listed in Table 38–14. The histology of the tumor has an impact on the benefit derived from pulmonary resection. Metastatic disease that occurs from tumors characterized by long periods of disease-free intervals, like renal cell carcinoma, are more amenable to resection than those with rapid dissemination, such as melanoma. Preoperatively a complete "extent of disease work up" is mandatory in all patients to ensure that the metastatic disease in the lung is the only site of metastasis.

Lung Cancer. Lung cancer, by far, remains the most prevalent diagnosis in the practice of General Thoracic Surgery. Histologically, lung cancer is divided into two types: small cell and non-small cell. Small-cell lung cancers are treated medically and thus are not a surgical problem except for diagnosis. Histologic types further subdivide non–small-cell carcinomas: squamous cell, adenocarcinoma, and large cell. Neuroendocrine tumors (tumors with endocrine expression) have been divided into both small-cell and non–small-cell groupings. A complete discussion of these types of cancer may be found in Chapter 37, Pulmonary Problems.

TABLE 38–14. Criteria for Resection of Pulmonary Metastatic Disease

Control of primary tumor
Metastatic disease confined to the lung
Patient is deemed operable and resectable
No superior treatment is available
Complete resection must be possible

From D'Amico & Sabiston. (1995). (pp. 669–674).

Staging of Lung Cancer

The International Staging System for lung cancer has been in place since the 1970s and is used universally. This staging system was revised in 1997 to provide greater specificity for patients with similar prognoses and treatment options (Mountain, 1997). The international system of staging lung cancer enables identification of the stage of cancer based on the tumor (T), lymph node (N) involvement, and distant metastases (M); thus, the acronym TNM staging. A complete description of the TNM classification is presented in Table 38–15 (Mountain, 1993).

Primary Tumor

The primary tumor is classified according to size, location, and extent of invasion. Tumor that is found by cytology but is not present radiographically is classified as Tx. T0 is the absence of primary tumor. TIS stands for carcinoma *in situ.* T1 is also known as the "coin lesion." It is a tumor less than 3 cm in size that does not invade the bronchus or pleura. A T2 tumor is greater than 3 cm in size, may invade visceral pleura or bronchus, and may cause atelectasis or obstructive pneumonia extending to the hilar region. Tumor that invades parietal pleura or chest wall, mediastinum, or pericardium is classified as T3. T4 represents tumor that invades mediastinal structures or causes pericardial or pleural effusions.

Lymph Nodes. Tumor in the lymph nodes (N) is classified according to location. A complete definition of lymph node stations is provided in Table 38–16. N0 refers to the absence of tumor in the lymph nodes. N1 represents tumor in the intrapulmonary or hilar nodes. Tumor in the ipsilateral mediastinal nodes including paratracheal, tracheobronchial, aortic, paraesophageal, or subcarinal region is classified as N2. N3 defines tumor in contralateral mediastinal or hilar nodes and any scalene or supraclavicular nodes.

Distant Metastases. Distant metastases (M) refers to metastases to organ sites including lung, brain, bone, liver, and adrenal glands. Additionally, cancer may metastasize to nodes of the contralateral lung, axilla, abdominal region, or inguinal chain.

The TNM classifications have been combined to create the five stages of lung cancer. This staging classification remains invaluable in determining treatment and overall prognosis.

Clinical Staging. Stage I lung cancers are contained within the lung and/or visceral pleura without evidence of metastatic disease. For non–small-cell stage I cancers the treatment with the greatest impact on survival is surgical resection. In the original staging sytem, stage I was all-inclusive; however, in the revised system it has been separated into stage IA and stage IB. Stage IA is comprised of the T1N0M0 tumors. Sixty-seven percent of these patients survive 5 years following complete resection (Mountain, 1997). Stage IB, those with T2N0M0, have a 5-year sur-

TABLE 38–15. TNM Descriptors

Primary Tumor (T)

TX	Tumor proved by the presence of malignant cells in bronchopulmonary secretions but not visualized roentgenographically or bronchoscopically, or any tumor that cannot be assessed as in a retreatment staging.
TO	No evidence of primary tumor.
TIS	Carcinoma in situ.
T1	A tumor that is 3 cm or less in greatest dimension, surrounded by lung or visceral pleura, and without evidence of invasion proximal to a lobar bronchus at bronchoscopy.
T2	A tumor more than 3 cm in greatest dimension, or a tumor of any size that either invades the visceral pleura or has associated atelectasis or obstructive pneumonitis extending to the hilar region. At bronchoscopy, the proximal extent of demonstrable tumor must be within a lobar bronchus or at least 2 cm distal to the carina. Any associated atelectasis or obstructive pneumonitis must involve less than an entire lung.
T3	A tumor of any size with direct extension into the chest wall (including superior sulcus tumors), diaphragm, or the mediastinal pleura or pericardium without involving the heart, great vessels, trachea, esophagus, or vertebral body; or a tumor in the main bronchus within 2 cm of the carina without involving the carina; or associated atelectasis or obstructive pneumonitis of entire lung.
T4	A tumor of any size with invasion of the mediastinum or involving heart, great vessels, trachea, esophagus, vertebral body or carina or presence of malignant pleural effusion.

Nodal Involvement (N)

N0	No demonstrable metastasis to regional lymph nodes.
N1	Metastasis to tymph nodes in the peribronchial or the ipsilateral hilar region, or both, including direct extension.
N2	Metastasis to ipsilateral mediastinal lymph nodes and subcarinal lymph nodes.
N3	Metastasis to contralateral mediastinal lymph nodes, contralateral hilar lymph nodes, ipsilateral or contralateral scalene, or supraclavicular lymph nodes.

Distant Metastasis (M)

M0	No (known) distant metastasis
M1	Distant metastasis present. Specify site(s).
	Footnote to the TNM definitions
T1	The uncommon superficial tumor of any size with its invasive component limited to the bronchial wall that may extend proximal to the main bronchus is classified as T1.
T4	Most pleural effusions associated with lung cancer are due to tumor. There are, however, some few patients in whom cytopathological examination of pleural fluid (on more than one specimen) is negative for tumor, the fluid is nonbloody and is not an exudate. In such cases in which these elements and clinical judgment dictate that the effusion is not related to the tumor, the patients should be staged T1, T2, or T3, excluding effusion as a staging element.

Reprinted with permission from Mountain. (1993). (p. 52).

vival rate of 57%. The recurrence rate for both stages is relatively low; 5% with lobectomy and 15% with wedge resection or segmentectomy. No adjuvant chemotherapy or radiation therapy is recommended for stage I tumors (D'Amico & Sabiston, 1995).

Stage II lung cancers are contained within the ipsilateral lung and/or pleura but may have metastases to the intrapulmonary or hilar nodes. There are no distant metastases. In the case of non–small-cell carcinoma, surgical resection offers the best chance of long-term survival. Not unlike stage I, stage II has been updated to have two distinct groupings: IIA and IIB. Stage IIA, or T1N1M0, are now

TABLE 38–16. Defintions of Lymph Node Stations

2R	**Right upper peritracheal (suprainnominate) nodes:** nodes to the right of the midline of the trachea between the intersection of the caudal margin of the innominate artery with the trachea and the apex of the lung (includes highest R mediastinal node).
2L	**Left upper peritracheal (supraaortic) nodes:** nodes to the left of the midline of the trachea between the top of the aortic arch and the apex of the lung (incudes highest L mediastinal node).
4R	**Right lower peritracheal nodes:** nodes to the right of the midline of the trachea between the cephalic border of the azygos vein and the intersection of the caudal margin of the brachiocephalic artery with the right side of the trachea (includes some pretracheal and paracaval nodes).
4L	**Left lower peritracheal nodes:** nodes to the left of the midline of the trachea between the top of the aortic arch and the level of the carina, medial to the ligamentum arteriosum (includes some pretracheal nodes).
5	**Aortopulmonary nodes:** subaortic and paraortic nodes, lateral to the ligamentum arteriosum or the aorta or left pulmonary artery (LPA), proximal to the first branch of the LPA.
6	**Anterior mediastinal nodes:** nodes anterior to the ascending aorta or the innominate artery (includes some pretracheal and preaortic nodes).
7	**Subcarinal nodes:** nodes arising caudal to the carina of the trachea but not associated with the lower lobe bronchi or arteries within the lung.
9	**Right or left pulmonary ligament nodes:** nodes within the right or left pulmonary ligament.
10R	**Right tracheobronchial nodes:** nodes to the right of the midline of the trachea from the level of the cephalic border of the azygos vein to the origin of the right upper lobe bronchus.
10L	**Left peribronchial nodes:** nodes to the left of the midline of the trachea between the carina and the left upper lobe bronchus, medial to the ligamentum arteriosum.
11	**Intrapulmonary nodes:** nodes removed in the right or left lung specimen plus those distal to the main stem bronchi or secondary carina (includes interlobar, lobar, and segmental nodes). Post-thoracotomy staging may designate 11 interlobar, 12 lobar, 13 segmental, 14 subsegmental.

Reprinted with permission from Mountain. (1993). (p. 53).

separated from stage IIB due to the higher survival rates. After complete resection, 5-year survival is 55%. Stage IIB has two groups, T2N1M0 and T3N0M0, as there was little difference in 5-year survival. After complete resection, the 5-year survival is 39% and 38%, respectively (Mountain, 1997). Adjuvant therapy with chemotherapy or radiation remains controversial.

Stage III originally separated into two categories: IIIA and IIIB. Stage IIIA includes tumors that have limited extrapulmonary extension to pericardium, pleura, chest wall, and mediastinal lymph nodes. Stage IIIA has four groupings: T3N1M0, T1N2M0, T2N2M0, and T3N2M0 (Mountain, 1997). Stage IIIA disease is associated with a poor prognosis even with complete resection. In fact, while most surgeons advocate surgical resection, there are some who believe it is not worthwhile. With complete resection and lymph node dissection, 5-year survival is 20 to 30% (D'Amico & Sabiston, 1995).

Stage IIIB disease is considered to be unresectable. In previous attempts at resection, there were no identifiable 5-year survivors; consequently, it remains a disease of medical management with chemotherapy and radiation (D'Amico & Sabiston, 1995). Stage IIIB disease is defined by tumors that have more extensive extension into carina, trachea, esophagus, great vessels, or heart. It is most simply defined as a T4 lesion with any N. Survival is limited even if complete resection is accomplished.

Stage IV is simply defined as any M regardless of T or N and is always fatal. Treatment is palliative and implemented only to limit discomfort.

Therapeutic Procedures

Surgical resection of lung tissue may be done a variety of ways including wedge resection, segmentectomy, lobectomy, and pneumonectomy. Typically the thoracic surgeon aims to leave as much viable tissue as possible without predisposing the patient to advancement of disease. Conservation of tissue often results in a more technically challenging operation.

The goal of surgical resection is to provide a complete resection while preserving as much lung as possible. Wedge resection is usually the procedure of choice, though larger resections are sometimes indicated.

Incisions

Until recently the two most common ways to enter the chest were either posterolateral thoracotomy or median sternotomy. Today, with the refinement of single-lung anesthesia and improved instrumentation, there has been a renewed interest in using smaller incisions or so-called minimally invasive surgery. There are a number of ways to gain entry into the chest and choice of incision is based on underlying pathologic process, location of the abnormality, and patient considerations such as postoperative pain and cosmetics.

Posterolateral Thoracotomy. The posterolateral thoracotomy has been the incision of choice for many years. This incision affords excellent exposure and is able to be placed anatomically in several locations supporting its use in a variety of procedures. The placement of this incision depends on the resection being performed.

It is agreed that the posterolateral thoracotomy incision is the thoracic incision associated with the most postoperative pain. Prior to positioning, an epidural catheter is placed. The patient is placed in the lateral decubitus position and a roll is placed in the axilla to prevent pressure on the brachial plexus. A pillow is placed between the straight upper leg and bent lower leg and all bony prominences are padded. Entry into the pleural space is obtained either through the bed of the resected rib or through an intercostal incision. Once the procedure is completed, two chest tubes are placed: one apically and one at the base. The ribs are reapproximated and closed with pericostal absorbable sutures. The soft tissues and muscles are closed in layers. The incision is then either closed with subcutaneous sutures or staples (Fig. 38–9).

Muscle Sparing Thoracotomy/Lateral Thoracotomy/Axillary Thoracotomy. The muscle-sparing thoracotomy incision, also known as the lateral thoracotomy or axillary thoracotomy incision, provides exposure for many of the same procedures while having many advantages over the posterolateral thoracotomy. The opening and closing times are shorter, there is decreased postoperative pain, and decreased postoperative arm and shoulder immobility. Additionally no division of latissimus dorsi or serratus anterior muscles is necessary and it is more comestically pleasing (Fry, 1995).

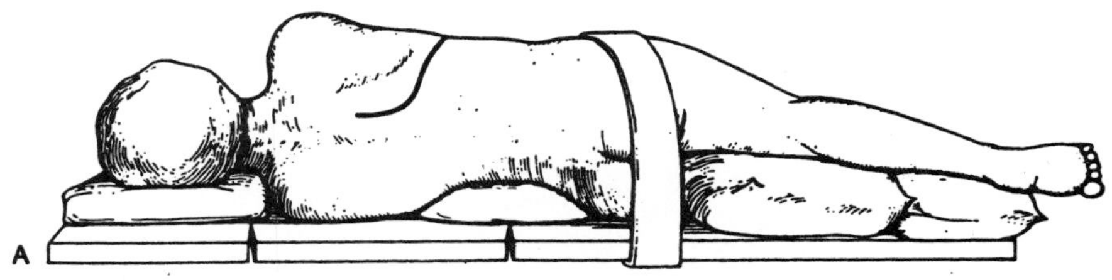

Figure 38–9. Posterolateral thoracotomy incision. Posterolateral thoracotomy. The patient is placed in the lateral decubitus position and the incision placed as shown. *(From Moores, Foster, & McKneally. [1995]. [p. 118].)*

The patient receives an epidural prior to positioning. The arm on the operative side is placed on a sling and abducted 90 degrees to facilitate exposure. The incision may be made vertically or horizontally and placed over the desired interspace (Fig. 38–10). Chest tube placement and closure are done in the same fashion as the posterolateral thoracotomy.

Anterolateral Thoracotomy. The anterolateral thoracotomy is a curved submammary incision that is rarely used today. It was most often used for middle lobe resections or lung biopsy but does not provide adequate exposure for the lower lobe. It is very cosmetically appealing especially to women. Additionally, it is often the choice in emergency situations as it may be made quickly and easily and may be extended across the midline of the chest to provide significant exposure (Moore, Foster, & McKneally, 1995).

The patient is placed in the supine position with the operative side elevated 20 to 45 degrees and is supported by a roll or inflatable sandbag. The arm on the operative side is flexed at the elbow, internally rotated at the shoulder and placed behind the small of the back or placed across the chest in a sling. A curved submammary incision is placed in the fourth or fifth intercostal space (Fig. 38–11). Closure is similar to that of the posterolateral thoracotomy.

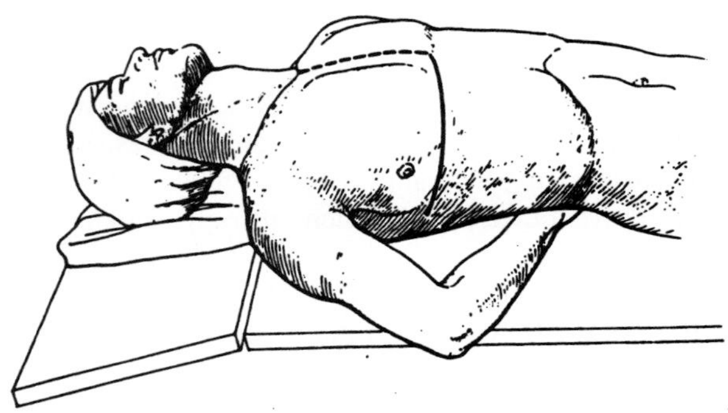

Figure 38–11. Anterolateral thoracotomy incision. Anteriolateral thoracotomy. Patient supine; a curved submammary incision in the 4th or 5th intercostal space. *(Reprinted with permission from Moores, Foster, & McKneally. [1995].)*

Median Sternotomy. The median sternotomy incision has a significant role, not only in cardiac surgery, but thoracic surgery as well. Indications for this incision include resection of mediastinal tumors, thymectomy, bilateral lung resections, lung volume reduction procedures, and repair of traumatic injuries. While often intimidating to the patient, the median sternotomy is good for patients with decreased pulmonary function, as it is less painful than the thoracotomy incision.

The patient is placed in a supine position with arms both abducted and secured on arm boards or secured at the patient's sides. The incision is made in the midline of the chest and extends from the suprasternal notch to a midpoint between the xiphoid process and the umbilicus. The sternum is divided using an oscillating saw (Fig. 38–12). The preoperative lateral chest x-ray is invaluable in determining the proximity of the heart to the sternum. Closure with sternal wires is one of the most critical steps as wound dehis-

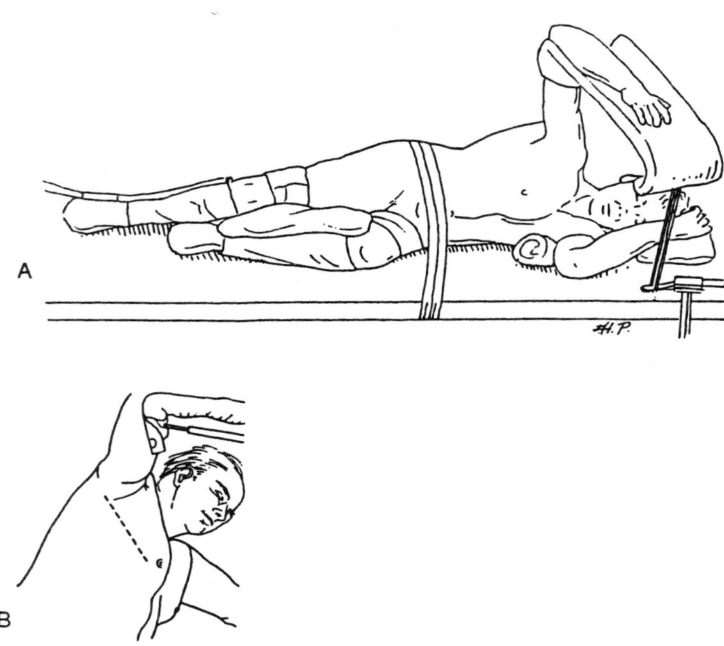

Figure 38–10. Muscle sparing or axillary thoracotomy. Axillary thoracotomy. **A,** The arm is abducted 90 degrees. **B,** The incision is made directly over the interspace selected for entry into the chest. *(Reprinted with permission from Fry. [1995].)*

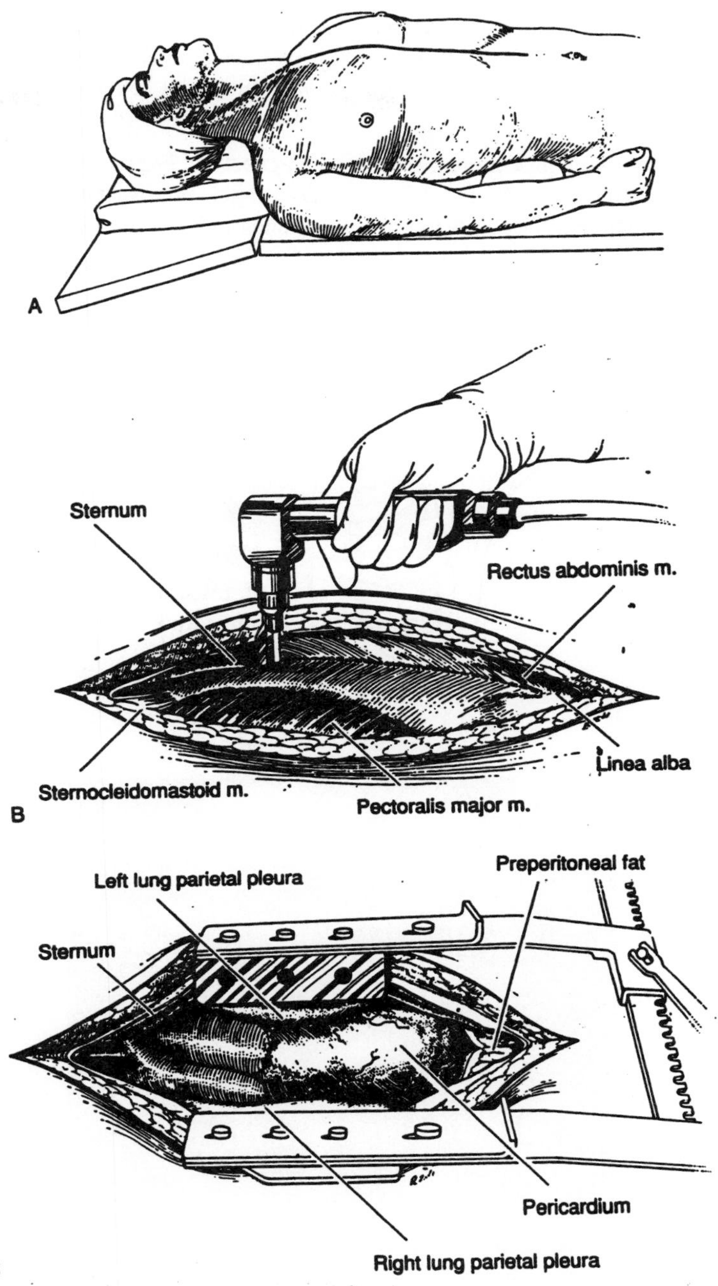

Figure 38–12. Median sternotomy incision. **A,** Median sternotomy; **B,** Division of sternum; **C,** Sternal retractors in place. *(Reprinted with permission from Moores, Foster, & McKneally. [1995].)*

cence and sternal wound infections are among the most serious of complications in the postoperative period.

Bilateral Thoracosternotomy/Clamshell/Costotransverse Sternotomy. The bilateral thoracosternotomy incision, also known as the clamshell or costotransverse sternotomy incision, regained popularity with the advent of bilateral lung transplantation. Because the incision provides such excellent exposure, it is now used for large anterior mediastinal tumors and for excision of multiple bilateral pulmonary nodules.

The patient has an epidural catheter placed and then is positioned supine. The arms are either placed laterally or flexed to 90 degrees and attached to the ether screen at the head by the anesthesiologist. Bilateral inframammary incisions are extended from one axillary line to the other. A sternal or Gigli saw is used to divide the sternum. The rib cage is then lifted as one would the hood of a car. At the time of closure, chest tubes are placed. Pericostal sutures are used to close the chest. Sternal wires are placed in an "X" fashion to secure the sternum. Closure is completed (Fig. 38–13).

Transcervical. The transcervical incision is used by some thoracic surgeons for thymectomy procedures. The patient is placed supine on the operating table. An inflatable bag or pillow is placed behind the patient's shoulders to position the neck in an extended manner. A 4- to 6-cm transverse incision is made. By retracting the sternum anteriorly with a special retractor, the thymus can be removed completely (Fig. 38–14).

Types of Resections

Wedge Resection. The wedge resection is what it sounds like: the removal of a nonanatomical wedge of lung

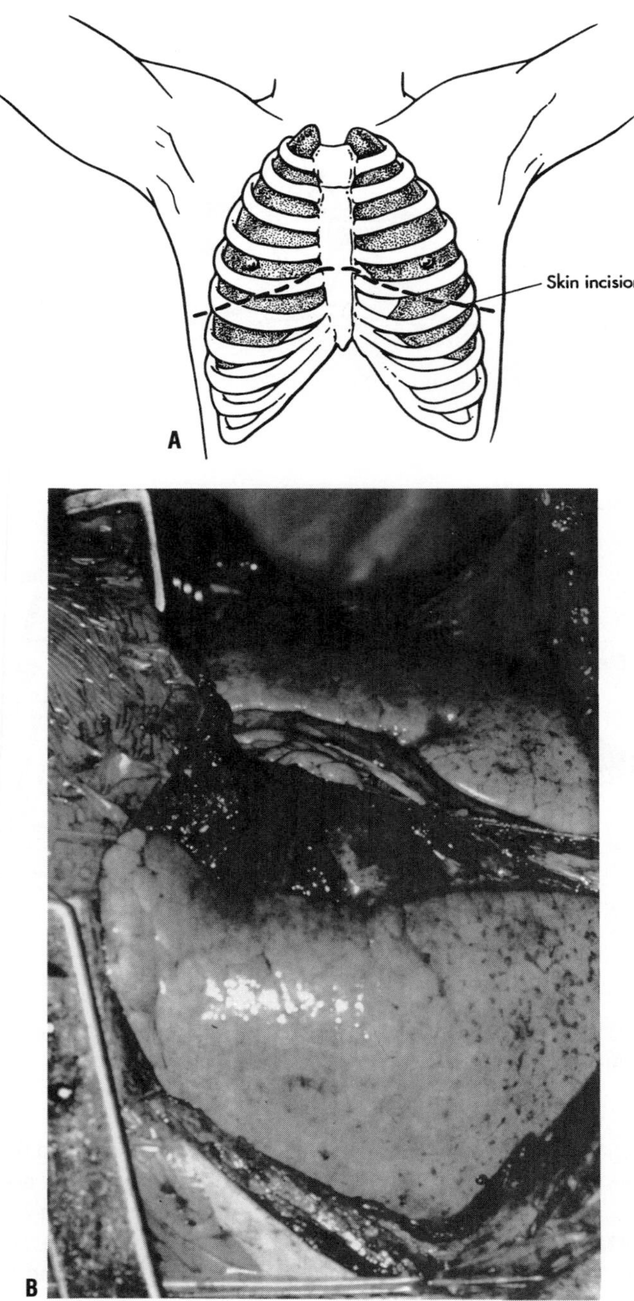

Figure 38–13. The bilateral thoracosternotomy incision. **A,** The bilateral thoracotomy sternotomy incision. **B,** The bilateral thoracotomy sternotomy incision allows for excellent exposure of the lung parenchyma. (Actual photograph of lungs.) *(Reprinted with permission from Kaiser. [1997].)*

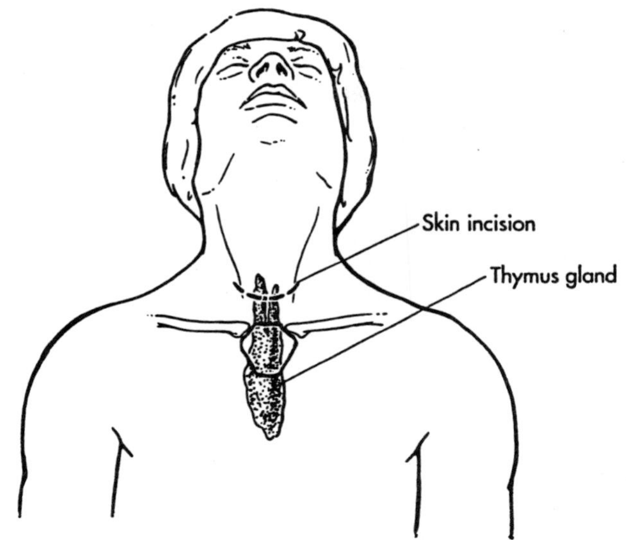

Figure 38–14. The transcervical incision. Transcervical incision and its relationship to the thymus gland. *(Reprinted with permission from Kaiser. [1997].)*

tissue (Fig. 38–15). It is commonly used for the surgical management of a pneumothorax, lung biopsy, removal of nodules both benign and malignant, removal of metastatic lesions, and lung volume reduction surgery. It is important to note that while wedge resection offers the advantage of leaving viable lung tissue, if a significant clean margin of resection is not identified, further resection should be completed. Wedge resections are most often performed via video thoracoscopy but may require a thoracotomy. In the event that bilateral wedge resections are required, a sternotomy may be indicated. Closure of the parenchymal defect is done with staples or sutures depending on size and location.

The physiologic consequences of a wedge resection are more related to the incision than the amount of lung tissue removed (Shields, 1989). The morbidity from a wedge resection is minimal. Most often, complications, if they do occur, are the result of retention of secretions. Restrictive lung physiology is seen in the early postoperative period. Oxygen desaturation and mild carbon dioxide retention are fairly normal. The mortality rate is 0.5% in patients other than those undergoing lung volume reduction (Shields, 1989).

Segmental Resection. Segmental resection is the anatomical resection of one or more bronchopulmonary segments of a lobe of the lung (Fell, 1995). It is used for the resection of lung cancer—both metastatic and primary—as well as benign disease such as bronchiectasis. Considerable controversy has taken place regarding the use of segmental resections in the treatment of primary lung cancer. Jensik (1986) reported local recurrence rates as high as 12%. Current recommendations are that it should be done in a patient with primary lung cancer who can tolerate a lobectomy. Segmental resection should be reserved for T1N0 tumors in patients with compromised pulmonary function, or patients with benign or metastatic disease.

The segmental resection is more technically difficult than a more extensive resection. The thoracic surgeon must be well versed in broncho–arterial relationships. An intraoperative bronchoscopy is performed at the initiation of the procedure to ensure that the bronchus is free of disease. Entry into the chest is accomplished either with a video thoracoscopic approach or thoracotomy. The bronchus and pulmonary vessels serve as initial landmarks. The borders of the bronchopulmonary segment are defined by the intersegmental veins (Fig. 38–16). Once identified, the lung is deflated and the segmental bronchus is occluded. The lung is

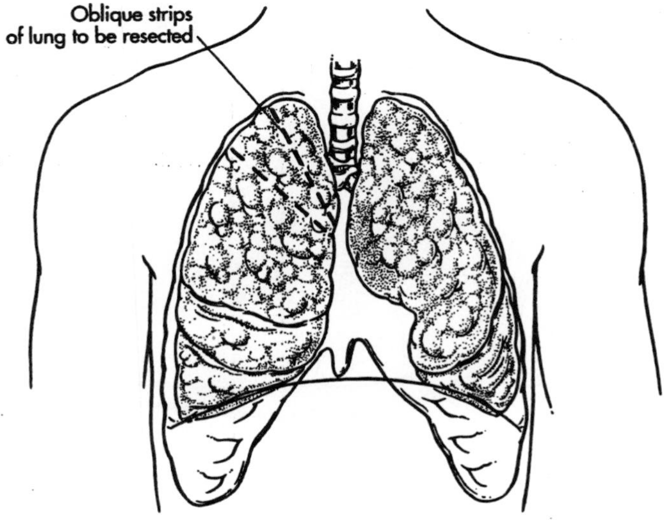

Figure 38–15. Wedge resection. A nonanatomical "wedge" resection. *(From Kaiser. [1997].)*

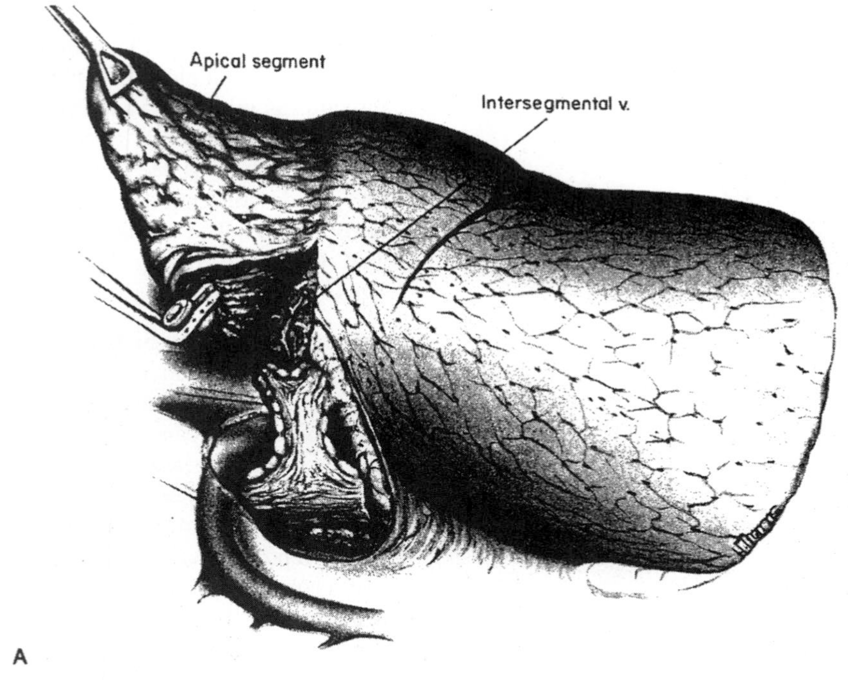

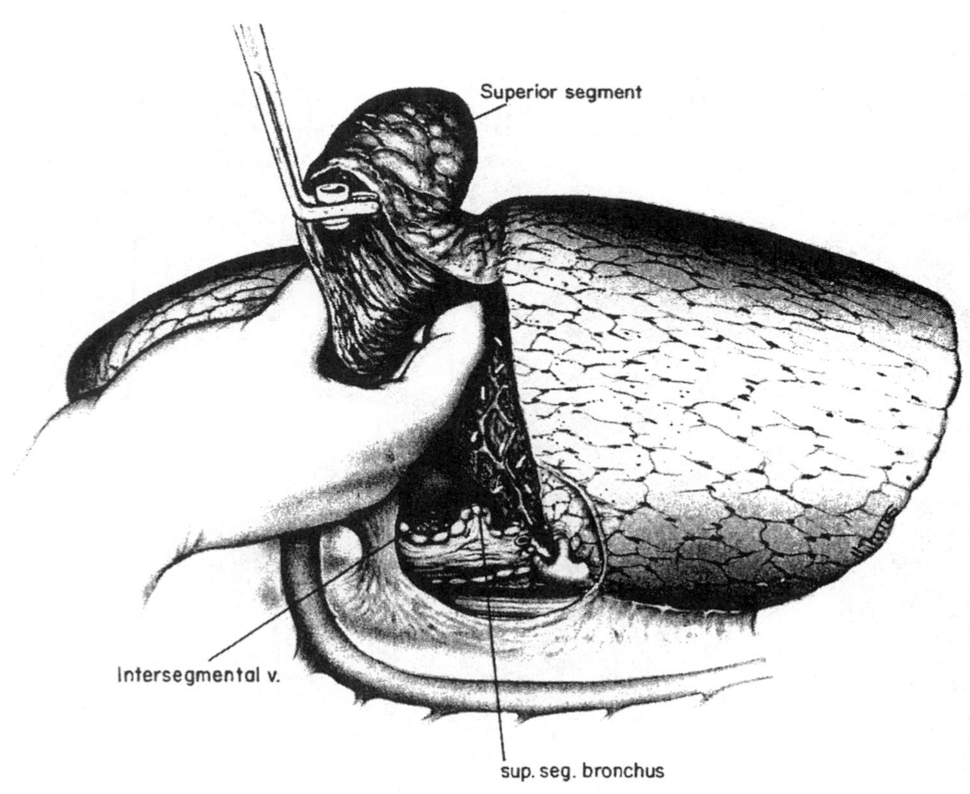

Figure 38–16. Segmentectomy. **A,** Dissection of the intersegmental plane between apical and posterior segments is commenced. **B,** Finger dissection of intersegmental plane, preserving the intersegmental vein.

(Continued)

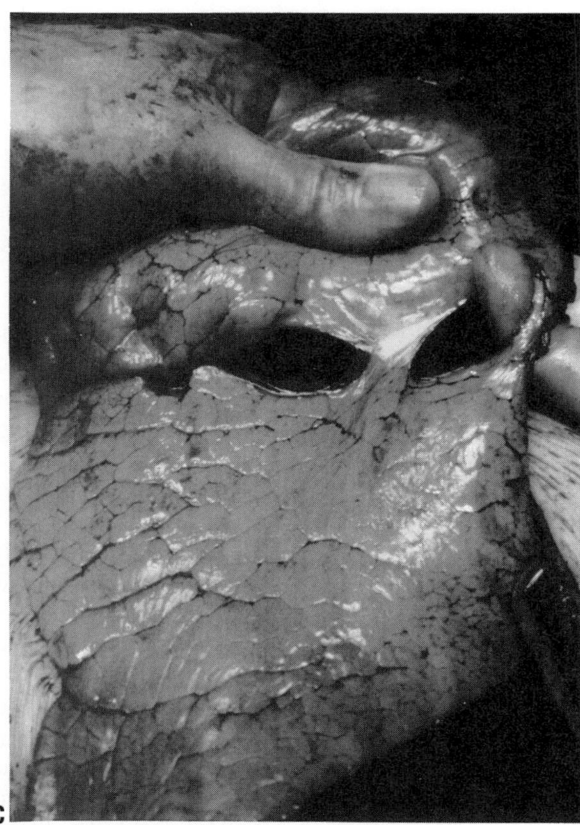

Figure 38–16. *(Continued).* **C,** Intraoperative photograph of segmentectomy. *(Reprinted with permission from Fell & Kirby. [1995].)*

reinflated and the segment that remains airless is ready for excision. Closure of the parenchyma is done by suture or staples (Fell, 1995).

The physiological consequences of segmental resection are similar to that of lobectomy. The functional loss correlates with the number of segments removed (Shields, 1989). Postoperative morbidity results from prolonged air leak, incomplete expansion of the lung, BPF, empyema, or pleural space problems. Prolonged air leak is by far the most common complication. Bronchoscopy may be necessary in the initial postoperative period to assist with reexpansion of the lung. Mortality from segmental resection is estimated to be 1% in patients with satisfactory pulmonary function and early stage disease (Shields, 1989). In patients with poor pulmonary function, mortality may be as high as 4 to 6% (Jensik, 1986).

Lobectomy. A lobectomy is the removal of an entire lobe of the lung. Occasionally a bilobectomy is performed, whereby usually the right middle lobe and right lower lobe, but in some situations the right upper lobe and right middle lobe, are both removed. The indications for lobectomy include malignancy (both primary and metastatic), TB, bronchiectasis, and infection. Recently lobectomy has been accomplished using a video thoracoscopic approach. As an alternative to pneumonectomy, the so-called sleeve lobectomy is often utilized.

Standard Lobectomy. The standard operative approach for lobectomy is the thoracotomy incision, although sternotomy and video thoracoscopic approaches may be warranted in certain patients. After the initial dissection the arterial branches and veins are ligated. The lobar bronchus is divided and closed with interrupted nonabsorbable sutures or staples. The removal of the lobe is completed by dividing any remaining connections to the lobe or lobes (Shields, 1989). Lymph node dissection may or may not be performed.

Lobectomy via Video Thoracoscopy. The video thoracoscopic lobectomy is the same procedure as a standard lobectomy, but it is performed through smaller incisions with endoscopic visualization. It is technically more challenging than a standard lobectomy. The indications and contraindications for this procedure are listed in Table 38–17.

The procedure requires four small incisions. One is a utility thoracotomy incision placed in the anterior midaxil-

TABLE 38–17. Indications and Contraindications for Video Thoracoscopic Lobectomy

Indications	Contraindications
Stage I Tumors < 5 cm	Tumor < 5 cm
Peripheral Tumors	Preoperative Chemotherapy or Radiation Therapy
No Lymph Nodes on CT Scan	Central Tumors
No Endobronchial Tumor	Sleeve Resections
	Tumor Invading Chest Wall

From McKenna. (1995). (pp. 223–232).

lary line. It is a small incision that enables resection with standard instruments without any division of muscles. Visualization is accomplished through the scope to a television screen. If the procedure takes too long, intraoperative complications occur, or a complete resection is unable to be performed due to inadequate exposure, and the incisions are converted to a thoracotomy incision (McKenna, 1995). Video thoracoscopic lobectomy is still in the initial stages of development. It remains to be seen how the advantages of this minimally invasive technique compare with other approaches, such as the muscle sparing thoracotomy.

Sleeve Lobectomy. The sleeve lobectomy provides an alternative to pneumonectomy. It consists of a resection of a portion of the mainstem bronchus with a subsequent re-anastamosis of the remaining lobe. Sleeve lobectomy is indicated in patients who have disease of the lobar orifice (Fig. 38–17). The need for sleeve lobectomy is always determined intraoperatively either upon initial bronchoscopy or at the time of frozen section. If the intraoperative bronchoscopy (done immediately prior to the initiation of the procedure) reveals erythema or dilated submucosal vessels, microscopic invasion should be considered (Faber, 1995). If frozen section reveals a positive margin, additional tissue must be resected using either pneumonectomy or sleeve lobectomy. In patients over the age of 65 or those with underlying lung disease, sleeve lobectomy is preferred as it preserves functional lung tissue.

The approach is through a thoracotomy incision and single lung ventilation is used. After the dissection has been carried out, the vessels are ligated. The appropriate lobar bronchi and mainstem bronchus are cut with a knife to leave a clean, smooth edge.

The remaining lobar bronchus is intussuscepted into the mainstem and sutured with nonabsorbable monofilament sutures. Depending on surgeon preference, the anastomosis may be wrapped with pleura or pericardial fat to provide additional support and vasculature (Faber, 1995). Postoperative complications are most often related to the anastomotic site. Bronchoscopy is indicated postoperatively for patients who are wheezing, have loss of volume on chest x-ray, or who demonstrate a persistent leak.

The physiological consequences of lobectomy regardless of approach correlate with volume loss and depend on the number of segments actually removed with the lobe (Shields, 1989). In the initial postoperative period the functional loss is greater than the proportion of lung removed. Initially there is overinflation of the ipsilateral and contralateral lung. The remaining lung receives increased ventilation that, over time, results in improved ventilatory efficiency as the tidal volume is better used by the remaining lung. There is also an increase in perfusion to the remaining lung, but there is a reduction in the diffusion surface area due to the loss of tissue. Thus, the overall diffusing capacity is reduced (Shields, 1989).

Morbidity following lobectomy is more common with

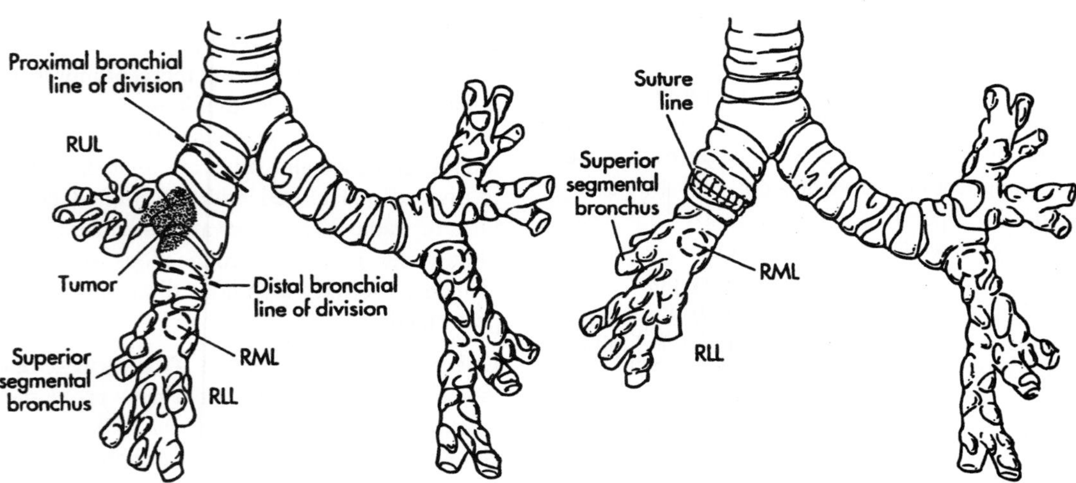

Figure 38–17. Sleeve lobectomy. Tumor at bronchus and right upper lobe take off. Bronchus is divided proximal to tumor and distal to tumor. Bronchus with remaining right middle lobe and right lower lobes is then anastamosed to remaining segment of right mainstem. *(From Kaiser. [1997]. [p. 95].)*

cancer resections, resections in elderly patients, and extended resections such as sleeve lobectomies. The most common complications are cardiopulmonary. Arrythmias, primarily atrial fibrillation, account for 20% of the complications and are quite prevalent in patients over the age of 60; so much so, in fact, that many advocate the use of preoperative Digoxin in this population (Shields, 1989). Prolonged air leak, effusion, pneumonia, empyema, atelectasis, and retention of secretions account for the majority of the remaining complications. Mortality from lobectomy is usually due to sepsis or cardiopulmonary complications. It is reported to average 2% but may be as high as 10% (Shields, 1989).

Pneumonectomy. In the 1940s pneumonectomy was believed to be the only acceptable surgical procedure for lung cancer (Harvey, Erdman, & Beattie, 1995). Today, it is a procedure reserved for situations where complete excision of disease is not possible with a more limited approach. The profound physiological consequences of this procedure are better understood today and the value of leaving viable lung behind has been proven. There are several types of pneumonectomy: standard, completion, extrapleural, and sleeve.

The approach for a standard pneumonectomy is most often a thoracotomy incision but may be done through a median sternotomy. It is accomplished using single lung ventilation. After the dissection has been completed, the pulmonary ligament is divided. The pulmonary arteries and veins are subsequently ligated either by suture or stapling and the bronchus is cut. The key to success is to keep the bronchus short, flush with the mainstem. The bronchus is poorly vascularized and this prevents an unnecessarily long stump, which is subject to poor healing. Some thoracic surgeons advocate the use of omentum or pericardial fat to provide extra support and vasculature.

Completion pneumonectomy is a pneumonectomy that takes place after a previous resection. It occurs most often in the setting of a postoperative complication or spread of disease. In cancer patients, it is associated with the same morbidity and mortality as a standard pneumonectomy. In patients with inflammatory disease or infection, however, the risk triples as these processes lead to potential sepsis and breakdown of the stump (McGovern, Trastek, Pairolero, et al., 1988).

In extrapleural pneumonectomy the pleura is excised along with the lung in an envelope fashion (Harvey, Erdman, & Beattie, 1995). The indications for extrapleural pneumonectomy include chronic empyema with unsalvageable underlying lung, pleural mesothelioma, and TB.

A sleeve pneumonectomy is indicated for patients with tumor in the hilum, orifice of the mainstem, or lateral aspect of the lower trachea (Deslauriers & Jacques, 1995). Prior to the advent of sleeve pneumonectomy, these patients were deemed unresectable. Sleeve pneumonectomies are relatively uncommon, as most tumors that invade the carina and lower trachea are too extensive to complete a resection. As with sleeve lobectomy, the need for a sleeve pneumonectomy is determined intraoperatively at the time of bronchoscopy or at the time of frozen section. This underscores the importance of the preoperative evaluation and the necessity of being prepared for the largest possible procedure. Local invasion into the subclavian vein or pulmonary artery does not preclude resection as they too may undergo a sleeve procedure (Deslauriers & Jacques, 1995).

The key to a successful sleeve pneumonectomy is a clean, disease-free margin of resection and reconstruction without tension. Intraoperatively, skilled anesthesia is mandatory. The surgery is performed with a double lumen endotracheal tube in place. This is changed to a single lumen tube at the time of reconstruction. The reconstruction is performed using periods of apnea and intermittent ventilation until the reconstruction is complete.

The physiological consequences of pneumonectomy may be divided into the changes that take place in the remaining pleural space and the remaining lung. Management of the pleural space varies among thoracic surgeons. If infection is likely, some advocate the instillation of antibiotics directly into the space prior to closure. Some close the space without a chest tube and perform thoracentesis to adjust the pressure within the space to $^{-}2$ to $^{-}4$ cm. Others use a pneumonectomy tube for 24 hours to allow the pressures to equilibrate and the mediastinum to set.

In all patients the diaphragm on the operative side rises, the mediastinum shifts to the operative side, and the intercostal spaces narrow over time. Serosanguinous fluid fills the space over a period of weeks to months and eventually solidifies. As filling occurs, the air within the cavity is pushed into the subcutaneous tissues causing subcutaneous air.

Pulmonary artery pressures may rise temporarily but return to normal once the healing is complete. The remaining lung receives the increased ventilation and as a result becomes overinflated. However, improved pulmonary function in the remaining lung does occur.

The morbidity associated with pneumonectomy is 0 to 30%. Bronchopleural fistula accounts for 3 to 5% of the morbidity (Shields, 1989). Cardiopulmonary complications are usually the culprit in the remaining cases. Mortality from pneumonectomy is 3 to 30% with an average of 10% (Shields, 1989). The major causes of mortality are pulmonary insufficiency, sepsis, anastomotic complications, and myocardial infarction.

Superior Sulcus Tumor Resection. Superior sulcus (Pancoast) tumor invades apical structures including lung, chest wall, ribs, and the lower trunk of the brachial plexus. Patients present with an apical lung mass and complain of pain around the shoulder that radiates down the inner aspect of the arm. Horner's syndrome may also be evident due to tumor invasion.

Treatment consists of preoperative radiation therapy of 3000 to 4500 cGy over three to four weeks followed by resection. The resection is most commonly performed through a posterolateral thoracotomy incision although the transclavicular approach and hemi-clamshell may be used depending on the location of the tumor and the extent of involvement (Ginsberg, 1995b). The resection involves the en bloc removal of the involved ribs, T1 nerve root, and upper lobe. Often the lateral aspect of the vertebrae may need to be resected as well. Occasionally the C8 nerve root must be taken; this is avoided if at all possible as it results in impaired motor function of the hand. Chest wall reconstruction is not required if the scapula covers the defect.

Postoperatively, rehabilitation is imperative to prevent arm and shoulder immobility. Unfortunately, the cure rate with combined radiation and complete surgical resection remains dismal at 30% at 5 years (Ginsberg, 1995b).

Bronchopleural Fistula

A bronchopleural fistula (BPF) is a tract or opening between the bronchus and pleural space. Precipitating causes include infection, trauma, or, most commonly, a breakdown of the bronchus after partial or complete resection. Risk factors include malnutrition, diabetes mellitus, radiation, devascularization, or residual tumor. It may occur at any time but is most common within the first 2 weeks of surgery. BPF should be suspected in any postoperative patient who presents with sudden fever and a productive cough.

Evaluation of a BPF includes a chest x-ray. In the postoperative patient who underwent partial resection, the chest x-ray demonstrates an air fluid level. In a patient post pneumonectomy, the chest x-ray demonstrates a drop in the normally present air fluid level on the operative side. Bronchoscopy may enable direct visualization of the BPF.

A patient who presents with a BPF in the immediate postoperative period should be positioned on the operative side to prevent infecting the good lung. Within 24 to 48 hours of the initial operation, it may be possible to resuture. This requires an original resection line free of tumor and infection. The new suture line is then reinforced with pleura, pericardium, intercostal muscle, or omentum. Completion lobectomy or pneumonectomy may be required. A chronic BPF, or one occurring late in the postoperative course, requires an open window thoracostomy (see Chest Wall).

▶ THE PLEURA

Therapeutic Procedures

At the time of this writing there is no consensus among state boards of nursing as to procedures that may be performed by ACNPs. Thoracentesis, pleurodesis, and/or chest tube placement may be performed by nurse practitioners in certain states. Chest tube removal in certain states may be done by nurses without advanced degrees. Interestingly, not only are state boards not consistent on whether or not nurses may remove chest tubes, they are also not consistent on the type of tube that may be removed (pleural versus mediastinal).

Thoracentesis

The only major contraindication to thoracentesis is coagulopathy. Prior to positioning the patient, an upright chest x-ray should be obtained to assess the amount of fluid or air present and to identify the exact location for placement. For a pleural effusion, ideally the procedure is performed with the patient sitting upright and leaning over with arms and head supported by a table. If the patient is unable to assume an upright position, the procedure may be done with the patient in a lateral decubitus position. In addition to the chest x-ray, the border of the effusion may be identified by loss of tactile fremitus, vocal fremitus, and a flat percussion note. Thoracentesis should be performed in the interspace beneath this.

In a sterile fashion, the skin is cleansed with an antiseptic solution such as iodine. Xylocaine (1%) is then administered to the underlying tissues and periosteum of the rib. A 20-gauge needle attached to a 60-cc syringe with a three-way stopcock is inserted 5 to 10 cm lateral to the spine in the space previously identified as the border of the effusion. The three-way stopcock enables aspiration and functions as a one-way valve preventing air from entering the chest. The needle should be advanced while applying gentle suction until the parietal pleura is punctured and fluid is obtained. For diagnostic purposes, approximately 50 cc of fluid is necessary. If the thoracentesis is also being done for therapeutic purposes, a catheter may be attached and the effusion drained into a collection bottle. To prevent reexpansion pulmonary edema, no more than 1 liter of fluid should be drained at once. Once the effusion is drained, the tube should be clamped for 2 hours and then another liter allowed to drain. Figure 38–18 demonstrates this process. Once the procedure is complete, the needle is withdrawn and a Band-Aid placed over the needle site. A stat chest x-ray should be obtained to rule out a pneumothorax.

For a pneumothorax, the patient is placed in a supine position. The same cleansing and anesthetic techniques are used as for pleural effusion. However, only a 16-gauge needle is needed and is inserted into the second intercostal space at the midclavicular line. A three-way stopcock is attached to a 60-cc syringe. The needle is inserted and air withdrawn until no more air may be aspirated.

If the thoracentesis is performed for a pleural effusion, the aspiration of air signifies that the lung has been punctured. The needle should be withdrawn immediately and the patient observed for pneumothorax. The thoracentesis may be repeated in the space below the initial site if the patient is asymptomatic and without evidence of a pneumothorax. If a pneumothorax is present, chest tube placement may be necessary.

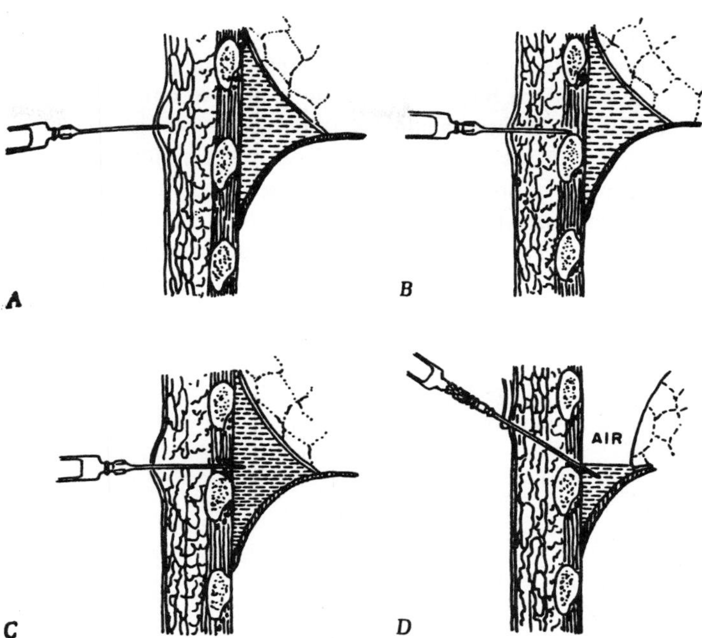

Figure 38–18. Thoracentesis. **A,** The skin is anesthetized with a local anesthetic. **B,** The deeper structures including the periosteum of the rib are infiltrated with anesthetic. **C,** The needle enters the pleural space and fluid is aspirated for diagnostic purposes. **D,** A polyethylene catheter is introduced through the needle and directed inferiorly to perform a therapeutic thoracentesis. *(Reprinted with Permission from Fishman. [1988].)*

Caution should be used when inserting the needle in the tenth intercostal space or below due to the potential to penetrate the diaphragm, spleen, or liver. If bright red blood is aspirated with the needle in this position, the needle should be withdrawn immediately and the patient observed for bleeding and hemothorax.

Pleurodesis

There are many agents available for pleurodesis; the two most commonly used are doxycycline and talc. Doxycycline is preferred in patients who are young or who have benign disease. Iodized talc is the most effective sclerosing agent and thus ideal for malignant effusions (Cohen, DeMeester, & Lafontaine, 1995). However, future entry into the pleural space is difficult due to adhesions and bleeding.

In either case the patient should be premedicated prior to instillation as both agents cause an inflammatory reaction that is excruciatingly painful. When using Doxycycline, 15 mL of Lidocaine is first instilled into the chest tube to provide local anesthesia. A mixture of 500 mg of Doxycycline is dissolved in 30 to 50 mL of 9% saline and instilled in the tube, followed by a 25-mL saline flush. The tube is then clamped. Most clinicians advocate turning the patient every hour to ensure complete coverage of the pleural space with the agent. After 4 hours, the tube is unclamped and ⁻20 cm H_2O of suction applied. When the drainage has decreased to less than 100 cc over a 24-hour period, the tube may be placed on water seal. The procedure is identical for talc slurry, except that the slurry comes already prepared by the pharmacist.

Chest Tube Insertion and Removal

Insertion. Chest tubes range in size from 22 French to 40 French. The choice of size is based on the underlying etiology for placement. For a pneumothorax, a 22 to 26 French is used. Pleural effusions require a slightly larger diameter tube, usually a 28 French. Empyemas or hemothorax require a 36 to 40 French (Kaiser, 1997). No consensus exists as to whether it is necessary to premedicate the patient with intravenous sedation. Many believe that local sedation is sufficient. Nonetheless, it is my opinion that a small dose of a narcotic or anxiolytic rarely, if ever, harms the patient and always proves beneficial.

Patient positioning for the procedure varies among practitioners. Some prefer the lateral decubitus position; however, most place the patient supine. If in the supine position, the ipsilateral hand should be placed behind the head. The skin should be cleansed in a sterile fashion with iodine solution. The incision is made in the seventh intercostal space in line with the anterosuperior iliac spine. Xylocaine (1%) is used to provide local anesthesia to the subcutaneous tissues and intercostal region. The needle should be inserted directly onto the bone and "step down" to the pleura (Kaiser, 1997). An additional anesthetic block is given one interspace above and one below the incision. The skin incision, approximately 1 cm, is made with a scalpel to the intercostal muscle. A hemostat is then used to spread the intercostal muscle until the pleura is visualized. A finger is used to open the pleura. This permits safe entry into the pleural space without puncturing the lung. The tube is inserted and directed apically. Some advocate using a hemostat to direct the tube. Once in place, the tube is sutured to the skin and a dressing is applied according to hospital protocol. A stat chest x-ray is mandatory to assess tube placement (Fig. 38–19).

Removal. Standard criteria for chest tube removal include the absence of an air leak and drainage less than 150 cc over 24 hours. A chest x-ray should be taken to verify complete lung expansion prior to removal. Clamping the tube prior to removal has traditionally been contraindicated due to the risk of tension pneumothorax. In patients who have had a prolonged leak that resolves, however, a trial of clamping the tube simulates the absence of the tube. An x-ray should be taken 30 minutes after clamping to determine if the lung remains hyperinflated. During the trial clamping, the patient should be instructed to notify the nurse if symptoms of shortness of breath develop. In this situation, the tube should be immediately unclamped.

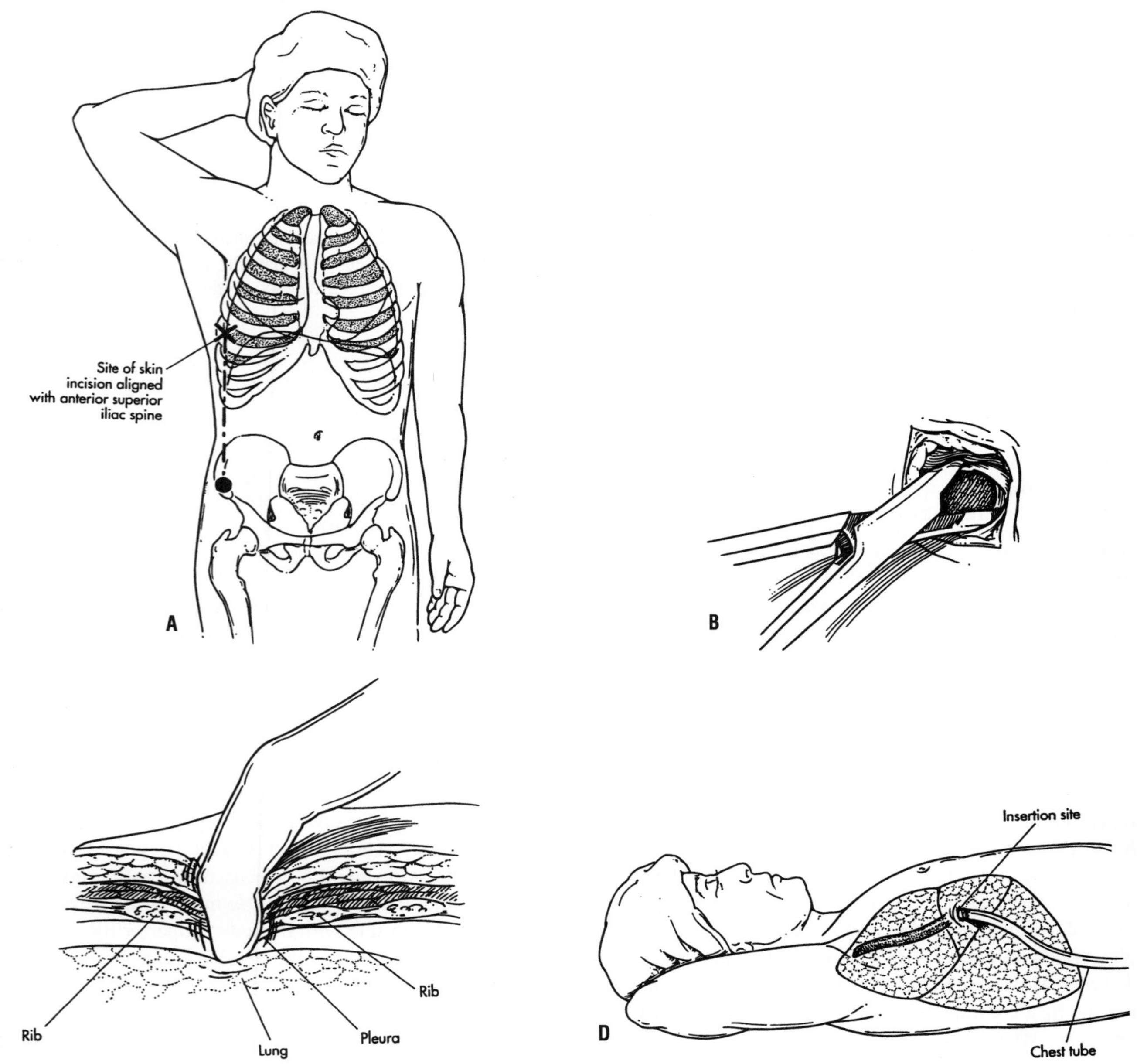

Figure 38–19. Chest tube insertion. **A,** Site of skin incision aligned with anterior superior iliac spine. **B,** Spreading of intercostal muscle with hemostat. **C,** Entry into pleural space with finger. **D,** Chest tube in place. *(Reprinted with permission from Kaiser. [1997].)*

The procedure should be explained to the patient prior to removal and a practice session is often helpful. Premedication is a controversial issue and no consensus exists. It is my recommendation that the patient be given pain medication if due or if the patient has high anxiety and/or a low threshold for pain. The post pull dressing should be prepared by placing sterile Vaseline gauze onto a sterile 4×4 gauge. Strips of tape, enough to provide a secure occlusive dressing, should be readied and placed at the bedside. The old dressing is removed. The sutures are cut and pulled while simultaneously holding the tube in position. The new dressing is placed over the tube and held firmly with one hand. The patient then takes a deep breath in and exhales while performing a Valsalva maneuver. The tube is simultaneously rapidly pulled. The combination of the Valsalva maneuver and rapid pulling of the tube prevent air entry through the holes in the side of the tube, thus preventing a pneumothorax. The dressing is already in place and secured in an occlusive fashion with the remaining tape. Breath sounds should be verified in all lung fields and a stat portable chest x-ray should be taken.

The dressing is left intact for 48 hours to allow a seal to form. Thereafter, it may be removed and the site left uncovered unless it is draining. Controversy still exists as to whether chest tube sites should be sutured closed. Most thoracic surgeons advocate leaving them open to allow for complete drainage. Although the site initially looks unappealing and often raw, it heals with very minimal scar. Continued drainage of straw-colored fluid for a few days post pull is common. A residual pneumothorax is often seen on the first film. If the patient is asymptomatic and if the pneumothorax is small and remains stable, no intervention is needed. Otherwise, reinsertion of the tube is required. Commonly skin-edge bleeding occurs as evidenced by a jelly-like blood clot on the dressing. This resolves spontaneously.

Pathologic Processes

Pneumothorax

By definition a pneumothorax is the accumulation of air within the pleural space. Air enters the pleural space when the integrity of one of the pleural spaces is disrupted. This results in a loss in the negative intrapleural pressure and collapse of the lung. A pneumothorax is described as primary, or spontaneous, when the etiology is unknown. A secondary pneumothorax may be the result of a variety of causes including airway disease, interstitial disease, infection, iatrogenic causes, and neoplasms (Table 38–18).

Primary or Spontaneous Pneumothorax. The primary, or spontaneous, pneumothorax is believed to be the result of the ruptured bleb in otherwise normal lung. A bleb is an air-filled space between the lung parenchyma and the visceral pleura. It develops as a result of the rupture of an alveolar wall (Fig. 38–20). Most often the primary pneumothorax occurs apically, but it may occur in any location.

TABLE 38–18. Causes of Secondary Pneumothorax

Category	
Airway Disease	• COPD—Bullous Disease • Asthma • Cystic Disease—Cystic Fibrosis
Interstitial Disease	• Idiopathic Pulmonary Fibrosis • Eosinophilic Granuloma • Sarcoidosis • Tuberous Sclerosis • Collagen Vascular Disease
Infections	• Pneumonia—Anaerobic, Staphylococcal, Gram Negative, Pneumocystis carinii • Lung Abcesses • Actinomycosis • Nocardiosis • Tuberculosis • Atypical Mycobacterium
Neoplasms	• Primary • Metastatic
Iatrogenic	• Line Placement • Thoracentesis with or without biopsy • Mechanical Ventilation • CPR • Tracheostomy • Bronchoscopy, Esophagoscopy • Malpostioned NGT • Surgery
Others	• Endometriosis • Pulmonary Embolism • Marfan's Syndrome

Adapted with permission from Cohen, DeMeester, & Lafontaine. (1995). (p. 525).

There is some question as to whether or not broad swings in atmospheric pressures may act as a catalyst to the onset of a primary pneumothorax.

Primary pneumothoraces occur primarily in people under the age of 40. They are more common in tall, thin individuals. They occur in men four times more often than women. The incidence is increased in smokers as well as drug abusers. A familial tendency has been found in 10% of cases (Cohen, DeMeester, & Lafontaine, 1995). Recurrence of a primary pneumothorax ranges from 20 to 50% with the highest incidence occurring within the first 6 months. For those that do recur, 90% recur on the same side. After one recurrence, the incidence of recurrence rises to 60 to 80% (Cohen, DeMeester, & Lafontaine, 1995). It is for this reason that surgical intervention is warranted with a second occurrence. With the development of video thoracoscopy, few hesitate to operate for a second recurrence.

Secondary Pneumothorax

The Consequence of Lung Disease. There are many lung diseases that may precipitate the development of a pneumothorax. The primary concern is the potential for respiratory failure due to the already compromised lung

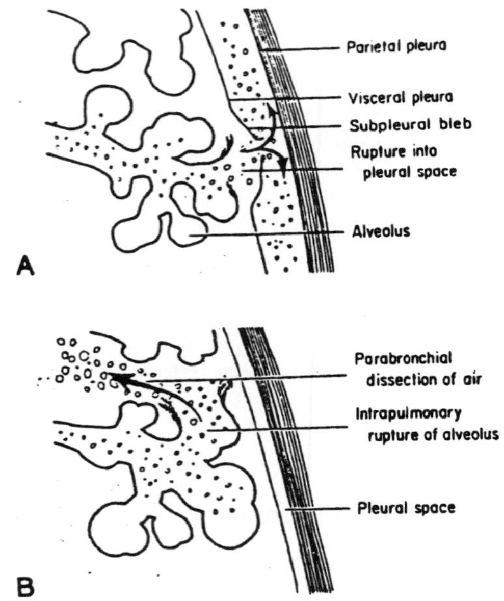

Figure 38–20. Pneumothorax from rupture of alveoli. Schematic drawing of the distended apical alveoli caused by mechanical stress from the weight of the upright lung. Alveolar rupture allows alveolar gas to dissect peripherally and form blebs that eventually rupture into the pleural space and cause a pneumothorax (**A**) or dissect centrally along lobular septa and produce a pneumomediastinum (**B**). *(Reprinted with permission from Cohen, DeMeester, & Lafontaine. [1995].)*

function. Often these pneumothoraces go undetected as the symptoms mimic the underlying disease.

Without question chronic obstructive pulmonary disease is the most frequent culprit. It occurs most often in patients with bullous emphysema. Because emphysema causes a loss of elastic recoil of the lung, the pneumothorax may develop more slowly in these patients. Even a small pneumothorax may result in severe respiratory compromise due to poor lung function. The mortality for a pneumothorax in a patient with COPD is reported to be as high as 16% (Cohen, DeMeester, & Lafontaine, 1995).

Neoplasms may cause a secondary pneumothorax for two reasons. First, rapid growth of a neoplastic lesion causes necrosis that may cause a perforation of the pleura. This has been found to be the case in patients who experience tumor necrosis as the result of chemotherapy. Second, a neoplastic lesion may cause bronchial obstruction that in turn causes alveolar distention and rupture of a bleb (Cohen, DeMeester, & Lafontaine, 1995).

Infectious diseases such as tuberculosis may also precipitate secondary pneumothorax. The concern in these cases is the potential for the development of empyema.

Catamenial Pneumothorax. A catamenial pneumothorax is, by definition, a pneumothorax that occurs during menstruation. Most occur within 48 to 72 hours after the onset of menses. Catamenial pneumothoraces never occur during periods of nonovulation. It is most common in women between the ages of 30 to 40. For reasons unknown, 90% occur on the right side (Cohen, DeMeester, & Lafontaine, 1995).

There remains a great deal of speculation as to the etiology of this condition. Four possible causes have been proposed. First, it is speculated that the rupture of a bleb may be due to the increased levels of prostaglandin during menstruation. Others have proposed that air enters the pleural cavity through the uterus or fallopian tubes during menstruation. A third possibility is diaphragmatic fenestration with the loss of the cervical mucous plug with the onset of menses. Last, it is believed that pleural or pulmonary endometriosis may be the culprit.

Since catamenial pneumothoraces do not occur during periods of nonovulation, treatment may be hormonal, surgical, or both.

Iatrogenic Pneumothorax. Numerous diagnostic and therapeutic procedures such as percutaneous needle biopsy, thoracentesis, bronchoscopy, mechanical ventilation, and central line placement may cause an iatrogenic pneumothorax. Chest radiographs should be ordered routinely after these procedures to definitively rule out a pneumothorax. Additionally, when considering the diagnostic or therapeutic intervention, the possibility of inducing a pneumothorax should be part of the decision-making process.

Percutaneous needle biopsy has a reported incidence of pneumothorax varying from 24% to as high as 57%, therefore making it the procedure associated with the highest risk of iatrogenic pneumothorax (Anthonisen & Filuk, 1988). The risk of pneumothorax from percutaneous needle biopsy increases with age, underlying lung disease, needle size, and depth of penetration required.

Thoracentesis (with or without biopsy) bronchoscopy (with or without biopsy), and mechanical ventilation are all associated with a 2% to 5% risk of pneumothorax (Anthonisen & Filuk, 1988). The risk of pneumothorax with mechanical ventilation is significantly increased with the use of positive pressure ventilation and with right mainstem intubation. Any pneumothorax that occurs in a ventilated patient poses a critical risk for tension physiology. In addition, placement of central lines often leads to pneumothorax, especially when performed by inexperienced personnel.

Clinical Findings of Pneumothorax

Physical Findings. A pneumothorax, regardless of etiology, causes a decrease in lung volumes, compliance, and diffusing capacity. The consequences depend on the size of the pneumothorax, the presence and severity of any underlying lung disease, and the cause of the pneumothorax. Symptoms range from completely asymptomatic to tension pneumothorax physiology. Pain is the most frequent and usually the first complaint. The onset of pain is usually sharp and pleuritic in nature but may progress to a dull ache. Dyspnea is the second most common complaint and varies due to the amount of collapse and underlying lung function. Additionally patients may complain of cough, hemoptysis, orthopnea, and/or syncope.

Findings at the time of physical examination depend on the size of the pneumothorax and thus range from no abnormal findings to tension pneumothorax physiology. Most patients present with decreased or absent breath sounds, tympany to percussion, and decreased or absent tactile fremitus. Cyanosis may or may not be present depending on underlying lung function or tension pneumothorax physiology.

Radiographic Findings. The chest x-ray is the simplest and most efficient method of evaluating a pneumothorax. Ideally a PA and lateral chest film is obtained, but a portable supine film is sufficient. The radiographic signs include the presence of air in the pleural space as evidenced by a hyperlucent area without pulmonary markings. When a pneumothorax is present the visceral parietal pleura is well visualized as a thin white line (Fig. 38–21). Certain conditions such as bullous emphysema or subcutaneous emphysema may obscure the film, making determination of a pneumothorax more difficult.

Estimation of the size of the pneumothorax on the chest x-ray remains a controversial and complicated issue due to the three-dimensional nature of the thorax. Additionally, pneumothoraces may present in any location: apical, basilar, lateral, anterior, posterior, or any combination. While many formulas have been created, it is often easiest and more consistent to describe the location by definition to other structures and approximate size in centimeters. After intervention by either thoracentesis or chest tube placement, a stat portable chest x-ray should be obtained to assess lung reexpansion. The original film is necessary for comparison, particularly in the case of incomplete reexpansion.

Management. The goals of management of a pneumothorax, primary or secondary, are to completely reexpand the lung and thereby alleviate symptoms, and prevent further complications and recurrence. There are many ways to manage a pneumothorax. Selection of an intervention should be made considering the severity of the pneumothorax, duration, underlying disease, past medical history, and occupation. Management techniques include observation, oxygen, thoracentesis, chest tube placement, and surgery.

Observation. Without any intervention, intrapleural air reabsorbs at a rate of 1.25% in a 24-hour period. Patients with small (less than 25%) stable, asymptomatic pneumothoraces are candidates for observation. They may be managed on an outpatient basis with return for a chest x-ray every 24 to 48 hours to assess reexpansion. They should be instructed to limit their activity, stay near a medical facility, and seek medical attention for increasing shortness of breath or pain. An increase in size of the pneumothorax, delayed reexpansion of the lung, and development of symptoms are all indications for chest tube placement.

Oxygen. The use of supplemental oxygen to treat a pneumothorax is controversial. Some believe that supplemental oxygen increases the absorption of air from the pleural space by a rate four times that of the normal 1.25% per day. Oxygen increases the gradient for nitrogen absorption by decreasing the partial pressure of nitrogen in the capillaries (Light, 1993).

Thoracentesis. Thoracentesis is the aspiration of air within the pleural space either by needle or small catheter.

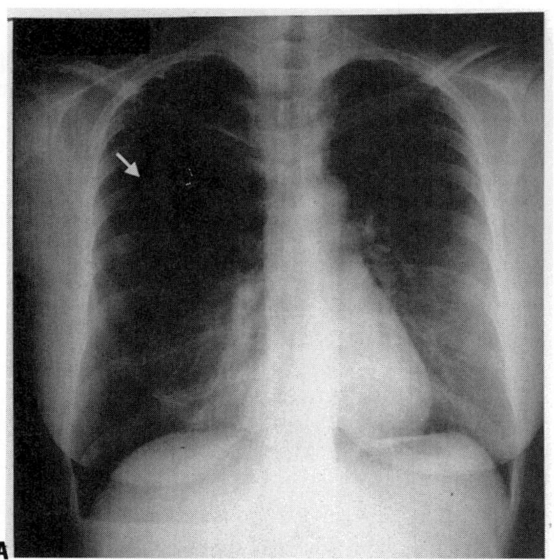

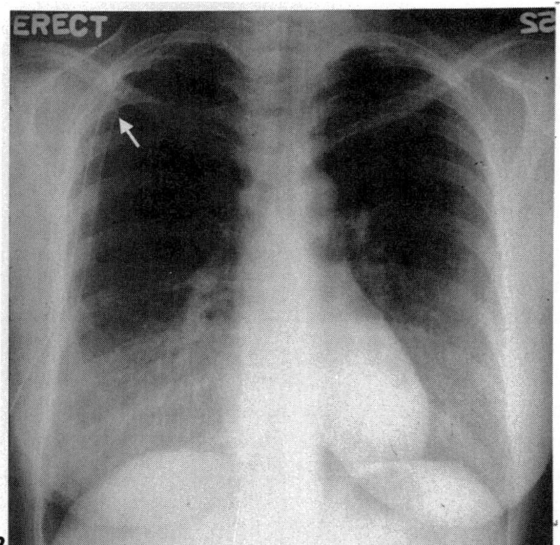

Figure 38–21. Chest x-ray of pneumothorax. **A,** Pneumothorax as evidenced by white line demarcating collapse of lung and absence of lung markings in apex above line. **B,** Resolution of pneumothorax after chest tube placement.

A success rate of 30% to 70% has been reported (Cohen, DeMeester, & Lafontaine, 1995). The only true disadvantage is that, due to the size of the needle or catheter, it is often difficult to evacuate all of the air and completely reexpand the lung. It is an ideal intervention for those patients with a pneumothorax secondary to central line placement or needle biopsy. If need be, the catheter may be attached to a Heimlich valve to allow for continued reexpansion and discharge of the patient. Thoracentesis is contraindicated in patients with an active air leak.

Thoracostomy—Chest Tube Placement. Thoracostomy, or chest tube placement, is by far the most successful way to manage a pneumothorax. For a pneumothorax, the tube is placed in either the fourth or fifth intercostal space posterolaterally or the second intercostal space midclavicular line and directed apically. Suction is applied for an active leak. Once the two pleural surfaces are opposed, the air leak seals. Criteria for removal of the tube include the absence of a leak and complete reexpansion of the lung. A Heimlich valve (a one-way valve) may be attached to a chest tube if the tube is still needed for reexpansion once the leak no longer requires suction and the lung is fully expanded.

Chemical Pleurodesis. Chemical pleurodesis causes an inflammatory reaction between the two pleural surfaces causing apposition, thereby preventing recurrence of a pneumothorax. It is used most frequently in patients with pleural effusions. Chemical pleurodesis is not recommended for patients who may require future surgical intervention; for instance, the patient with cystic fibrosis who may be a candidate for lung transplantation. Entering the pleural space after chemical pleurodesis is technically feasible, but the take down of extensive adhesions often leads to significant blood loss.

Many agents are available for chemical pleurodesis. Doxycycline is the agent that has replaced tetracycline. The most effective agent on the market today is the talc slurry. The procedure is further described in the section on pleural effusions. The potential side effects of both include severe pain and fever of short duration.

Surgery. Surgical intervention for a pneumothorax most often consists of bleb resection and mechanical pleurodesis. This may be accomplished through a thoracotomy, muscle-sparing incision, sternotomy (in the case of bilateral pneumothoraces), or through video thoracoscopy. Video thoracoscopy has become the preferred method due to the ability to use the chest tube site as one of the two or three incisions, decreased hospital stay, decreased pain, and earlier return to work. Parietal pleurectomy or pleural stripping is reserved for patients who experience treatment failure, are of advanced age, or who have undergone a pneumonectomy and experience a pneumothorax in the remaining lung (Cohen, DeMeester, & Lafontaine, 1995). The indications for surgical intervention in patients with pneumothoraces are listed in Table 38–19.

Potential Complications

Tension Pneumothorax. Tension pneumothorax occurs in less than 5% of patients (Cohen, DeMeester, & Lafontaine, 1995). It occurs when air continues to accumulate in the pleural space creating intrapleural pressures that are greater than atmospheric (Paape & Fry, 1994). Patients who progress to tension physiology demonstrate profound hypotension, tachycardia, tachypnea, neck vein distention, a displacement of the trachea, and cardiac impulse to the uninvolved side (Fig. 38–22). This is an emergency situation and failure to act promptly may result in the patient's demise. A tension pneumothorax requires only evaluation by physical findings. Failure to recognize the symptoms and treat them results in impedance of cardiac output and venous return. When suspected, a needle should be inserted anteriorly into the second intercostal space followed by chest tube placement.

Reexpansion Pulmonary Edema. Reexpansion pulmonary edema occurs after rapid reexpansion of the lung. It may occur in the setting of pneumothorax, pleural effusions, or atelectasis. The etiology of this clinical entity remains unclear. Most believe it is caused by an increase in capillary permeability. Rapid reexpansion of the lung, the chronicity of the collapse, loss of surfactant, and pulmonary artery pressure changes are all believed to contribute to this condition (Paape & Fry, 1994).

Empyema. An empyema by definition is an infection within the pleural space. (A complete description of empyema may be found in this chapter under Pleural Effusions.) Empyema may occur in the setting of a pneumothorax of any etiology but is seen most often in the case of secondary pneumothorax due to an abscess, tuberculosis, or bronchopleural fistula. Antibiotic therapy and complete drainage are necessary to prevent further complications of fibrothorax and trapped lung.

TABLE 38–19. Indications for Surgical Intervention in Spontaneous Pneumothorax

1. Second episode
2. Persistent air leak for greater than 7–10 days
3. First episode with unexpanded, "trapped" lung
4. History of contralateral pneumothorax
5. Bilateral pneumothorax
6. Occupation risk (diver, airplane pilot, living in a remote area)
7. Large bulla
8. Large undrained hemothorax
9. First episode in a patient with one lung
10. First episode in a patient with severely compromised pulmonary function

Reprinted with permission from Paape & Fry. (1994). (p. 534).

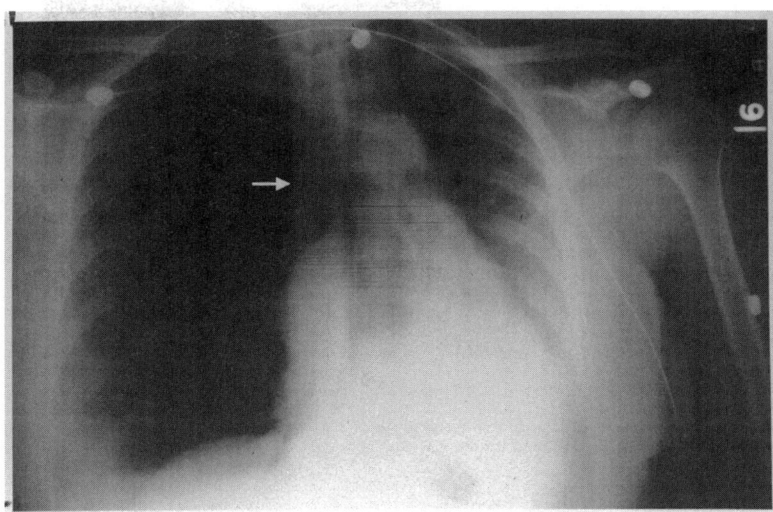

Figure 38–22. Chest radiograph. Tension pneumothorax with arrow indicating mediastinal shift.

Persistent Air Leak. Persistent air leaks (defined as a leak that lasts greater than 7 days) occur most often in patients with primary pneumothorax or those with obstructive airway diseases. After 7 days, surgical intervention is warranted. Prior to the advent of video thoracoscopic procedures, chemical pleurodesis was the treatment of choice. In most cases, stapling of the bleb followed by pleurodesis provides resolution of this condition.

Pleural Effusion

The accumulation of fluid in the pleural space is known as a pleural effusion. Normally, approximately 2 to 3 mL of fluid is present in the pleural space and acts as a lubricant between the visceral and parietal pleura. Table 38–20 lists the many mechanisms by which an excessive amount of fluid may accumulate in the pleural space (Cohen, DeMeester, & Lafontaine, 1995; Kennedy & Sahn, 1994).

Types of Pleural Effusions. There are two types of pleural effusions: transudate and exudate. A transudate occurs as the result of systemic factors that alter the formation or reabsorption of fluid from the pleural space. Transudates are usually clear or straw in color and odorless. They may be caused by a number of clinical conditions (Table 38–21). Exudates occur as the result of disease that affects either the pleural surface or lymphatic system. Exudates are usually cloudy in color and, like transudates, may be caused by a number of clinical conditions (Table 38–22).

Determination of serum and pleural fluid levels of LDH and protein allows differentiation of a transudate from exudate if there is any question. An exudate has a pleural fluid/serum protein ratio of greater than 0.5. The LDH level of an exudate has a pleural fluid/serum protein ratio greater than 0.6 (Cohen, DeMeester, & Lafontaine, 1995).

Chylothorax. A chylothorax is defined by the presence of lymph in the pleural space due to a leak from the thoracic duct (Fig. 38–23). It is estimated that 60 to 70% of fat that is ingested is absorbed by the lymphatic system in the intestines and then transported to the bloodstream via the thoracic duct. The lymph flow through the duct averages 1.5mL per kg body weight per hour (Cohen, DeMeester, & Lafontaine, 1995). The volume of lymph varies with meals and the fat content of the food. In addition to fat, the lymph also contains T cells and fat-soluble vitamins (Cohen, DeMeester, & Lafontaine, 1995). Therefore, impaired immune

TABLE 38–20. Mechanisms of Pleural Effusion

Mechanism	Clinical Entity
Increased hydrostatic pressure	Congestive heart failure
Increased capillary permeability	Pneumonia, inflammtory pleuritis
Decreased plasma colloid oncotic pressure	Hypoalbuminemia
Increased intrapleural negative pressure	Atelectasis, pneumothorax
Impaired lymphatic drainage of pleural space	Tumor, radiation, fungal disease
Movement of ascitic fluid from periotneal space to pleural space	Diapragmatic defects, lymphatics

Adapted from Cohen, DeMeester, & Lafontaine. (1995); and Kennedy & Sahn. (1994).

TABLE 38–21. Causes of Transudates

Congestive heart failure	Peritoneal dialysis
Cirrhosis	Hypoproteinemia
Nephrotic syndrome	Meigs' syndrome
Myxedema	Sarcoidosis

Reprinted with permission from Cohen, DeMeester, & Lafontaine. (1995). (p. 540).

TABLE 38–22. Causes of Exudates

Neoplastic Diseases	Gastrointestinal Diseases
Metastatic disease	Pancreatitis
Mesotheliomas	Pancreatic pseudocyst
Lymphomas	Esophageal rupture
Chest wall tumors	Subphrenic abscess
Meigs' syndrome	Hepatic abscess
Infectious Diseases	**Trauma**
Tuberculosis	Hemothorax
Viral (adenovirus, coxsackie group B mycoplasma)	Chylothorax
Fungal (coccidioidomycosis)	**Miscellaneous**
Parasitic (amebiasis)	Postradiation therapy
Bacterial pneumonia	Postmyocardial infarction syndrome
Pulmonary Infarction	
Collagen-Vascular Diseases	
Rheumatoid arthritis	
Systemic lupus erythematosus	

Reprinted with permission from Cohen, DeMeester, & Lafontaine. (1995). (p. 545).

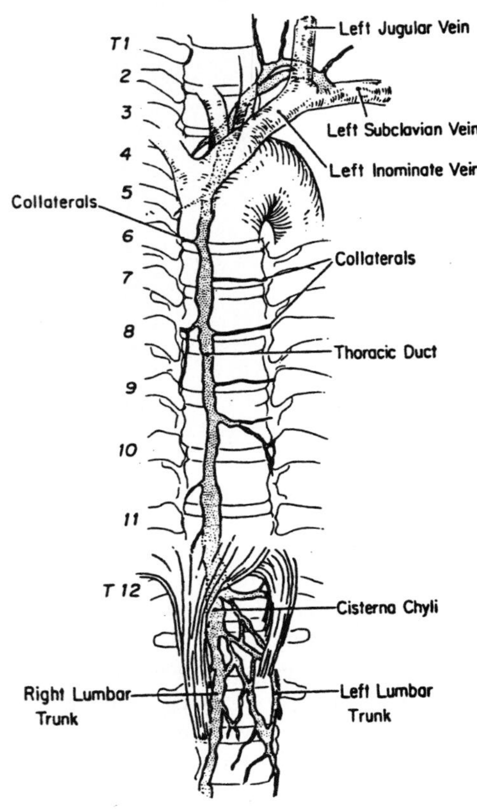

Figure 38–23. Thoracic duct. Schematic drawing of the most usual pattern and course of the thoracic duct. The single duct that enters the chest through the aortic hiatus between T12 and T10 is a relatively consistent finding and the usual site for surgical ligation. *(Reprinted with permission from Cohen, DeMeester, & Lafontaine. [1995]. [p. 536].)*

responses, vitamin K deficiency, and coagulopathy may result with prolonged chylous effusions.

There are many causes of chylous effusions (Table 38–23). Most commonly they are attributable to trauma, neoplasms, and iatrogenic causes due to surgical or diagnostic procedures. Any milky or creamy effusion is suspect. The patient should be given a fatty meal or made to ingest cream or olive oil. Those not tolerating oral intake may be given intravenous lipids. Following ingestion of the lipids, the effusion should be evaluated for lipoprotein analysis to look for chylomicrons.

Treatment consists of conservative management, surgical management, or a combination. Conservative management consists of chest tube placement and complete drainage to prevent fibrothorax along with parenteral nutrition. Oral intake increases the output of the effusion. Should the chylothorax resolve, a high-fat meal should be given to confirm the leak is sealed prior to pulling the chest tube. There is little consensus as to the number of days to attempt conservative management; however, 14 days is generally regarded as sufficient.

There are really two indications for operation: failure of conservative therapy and/or drainage greater that 1500 cc over a 24-hour period (Cohen, DeMeester, & Lafontaine, 1995). Patients should be given a fatty substance such as 100 cc of olive oil or cream 2 to 3 hours prior to the operation. This enables precise visualization of the leak in the operating room. Any fluid remaining in the stomach at the time of operation may be removed with a nasogastric tube.

Video thoracoscopy provides the surgeon with a minimally invasive method of accessing the leak and optimal visualization as the leak is magnified and visualized on a television screen during the procedure. The duct is ligated above and below the tear. There are no major side effects from ligation due to the numerous naturally occurring small lymphatic venous anastomoses (Cohen, DeMeester, & Lafontaine, 1995). Postoperatively serum lipids may fall temporarily. The chest tube is left in place until the drainage is less than 150 cc over 24 hours.

Empyema. By definition, an empyema is pus or infected pleural fluid within the pleural space. The treatment of empyema is where thoracic surgery had its beginnings. Today with the advent of antibiotics, the incidence is decreased but prevalent nonetheless. According to the American Thoracic Society (1962), there are three phases of empyema development. The first phase is an exudative development. Subsequently, a fibrinopurulent phase begins where fibrin is deposited on the pleural surfaces. This forms a peel that encases and traps the lung. Finally, an organizing

TABLE 38–23. Etiology of Chylothorax

Cause	Specific
Congential	• Atresia of the thoracic duct • Birth trauma
Trauma	• Blunt • Penetrating
Iatrogenic	**Surgery** • Cervical • Thoracic • Cardiac • Thoracic **Diagnostic Procedures** • Translumbar arteriography • Subclavian vein catheterization • Heart catherterization
Neoplasms	All
Infections	• Tuberculosis lymphadenitis • Nonspecific mediastinitis

Adapted with permission from Cohen, DeMeester, & Lafontaine. (1995). (p. 537).

or chronic phase ensues where the fibrin begins to organize and the peel becomes complete.

There are many causes of empyema (Table 38–24). It is estimated that over one half of empyemas occur as the result of pneumonia. The second most common cause is after intrathoracic manipulation. The presenting signs and symptoms are often nonspecific and vary with cause and the magnitude of the empyema. More often than not it is difficult to distinguish the symptoms from the underlying etiology. Most commonly the patient complains of pleuritic pain, a heavy sensation on the affected side of the chest, fever, tachypnea, tachycardia, and purulent cough (Cohen, DeMeester, & Lafontaine, 1995).

Evaluation consists of a PA and lateral chest x-ray that often shows pulmonary consolidation with an effusion. A CT scan is usually necessary to identify areas of loculation

TABLE 38–24. Etiology of Empyema

Pneumonia (viral, bacterial, tuberculosis, mycotic)
Lung abscess
Trauma
Postoperative
Extension of subphrenic abscess
Spontaneous pneumothorax
Generalized sepsis

Reprinted with permission from Cohen, DeMeester, & Lafontaine. (1995). (p. 548).

and distinguish the empyema from a lung abscess (Fig. 38–24). Thoracentesis should be performed and the fluid sent for culture and gram stain. If antibiotics have already been initiated, the pleural fluid culture may be negative. In this case, sputum cultures should be obtained, as the organism is usually the same.

The goal of management is to completely evacuate the fluid, resolve the infection, and reexpand the lung. In the very early acute stage, thoracentesis with aggressive antibiotics may be all that is necessary. Rarely is an empyema diagnosed this early. More often than not, a chest tube concomitant with antibiotics are required. The key is a large tube, 28 to 36 French, placed in a dependent position. Often the chest tube is placed in the operating room as video thoracoscopy enables complete drainage, debridement, and tube placement. The chest tube is usually converted to an empyema tube that is gradually withdrawn over several weeks (Fig. 38–25).

Once a pleural peel has completely formed, decortication is necessary. Decortication may be performed either through video thoracoscopy or thoracotomy. Intraoperatively, the surgeon removes the peel taking extra care not to tear the lung (Fig. 38–26). Once freed, the lung should reexpand to fill the space. If complete reexpansion does not occur, muscle transposition or thoracoplasty may be necessary.

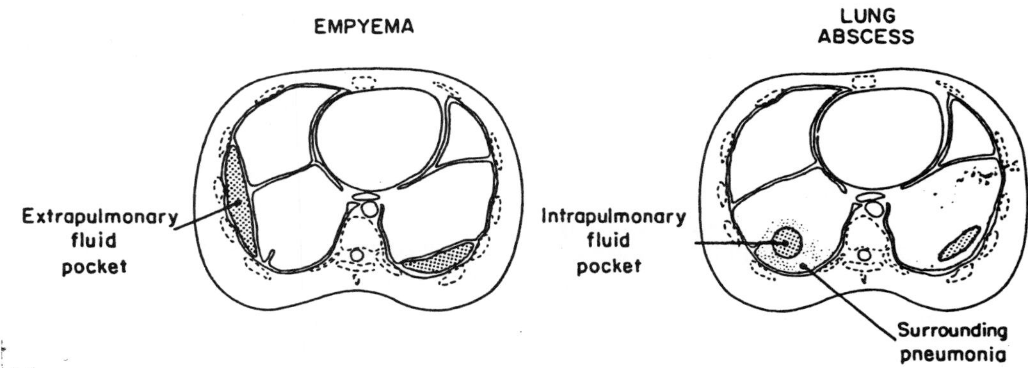

Figure 38–24. CT scan of chest empyema versus lung abscess. Schematic drawing of a chest CT scan showing the difference between an empyema and an abscess in the lung. An empyema conforms to the shape of the adjacent chest wall. An abscess in the lung is usually more spherical, does not extend to or conform with the chest wall, and is surrounded by the pneumonia in which it developed. *(Reprinted with permission from Cohen, DeMeester, & Lafontaine. [1995]. [p. 550].)*

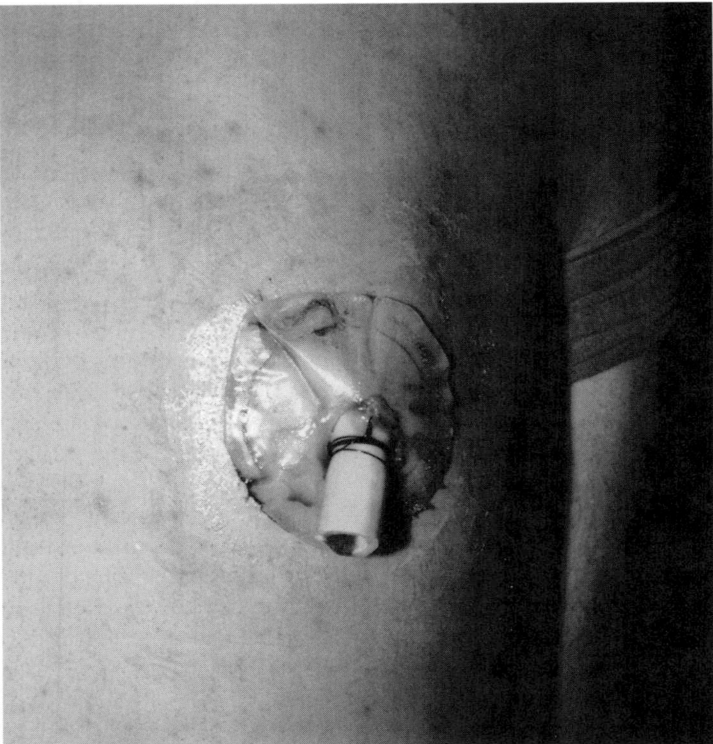

Figure 38–25. Empyema tube.

The management of post pneumonectomy empyema is critical to patient survival. It should be suspected in any pneumonectomy patient who presents with fever and/or malaise. Some surgeons advocate the use of closed tube antibiotic drainage in early cases. In this situation, an antibiotic solution is instilled directly into the space and drained. An open window thoracostomy may also be indicated (see Chest Wall).

Clinical Findings of Pleural Effusions

Physical Findings. Excess fluid in the pleural space inhibits expansion of the lung resulting in dyspnea. The degree of dyspnea depends on the amount of fluid and the patient's underlying lung condition. Often patients also experience pleuritic pain that may subside if the effusion becomes large. Pleural effusions that occur due to malignancy often precipitate a constant dull pain rather than pleuritic pain. Symptoms may range from completely asymptomatic to excruciating and, in addition to dyspnea and pain, may include fever, malaise, a heavy sensation on the affected side, and cough.

Radiographic Findings. The chest radiograph is a simple and effective way of confirming a pleural effusion. A pleural effusion is most often visualized along the diaphragm and obscures the costophrenic angle. It is important to note that 250 mL of fluid must accumulate to obscure the costophrenic angle on an upright film. Pleural thickening may also obscure the costophrenic angle on chest ray. To distinguish a pleural effusion from pleural thickening or to quantify the amount of fluid present, a lateral decubitus film may be necessary. Free fluid may accumulate anywhere in the chest with another fairly common site being the fissure. Ideally an upright film is taken; however, in certain circumstances a supine film may be the only option the patient may tolerate. In this case the fluid is seen on the chest x-ray as a generalized haziness in one hemithorax. A large pleural effusion may be mistaken for atelectasis. Atelectasis results in a loss of volume; pleural effusion does not.

CT scan has replaced ultrasound in the diagnosis of pleural effusion. It has a primary role in determining loculation and enables a distinction to be made between an empyema and lung abscess.

Laboratory Diagnosis. Pleura fluid is easily obtained by thoracentesis and often provides a mechanism of diagnosis. Pleural fluid should routinely be sent for total protein, LDH, white blood cells, glucose, and pH. Serum total protein, LDH, and glucose should be sent simultaneously (Cohen, DeMeester, & Lafontaine, 1995). Additional studies should be requested based on suspicion of the etiology of the effusion (Table 38–25). If infection is suspected, culture, gram stain, and an acid-fast bacilli smear should be or-

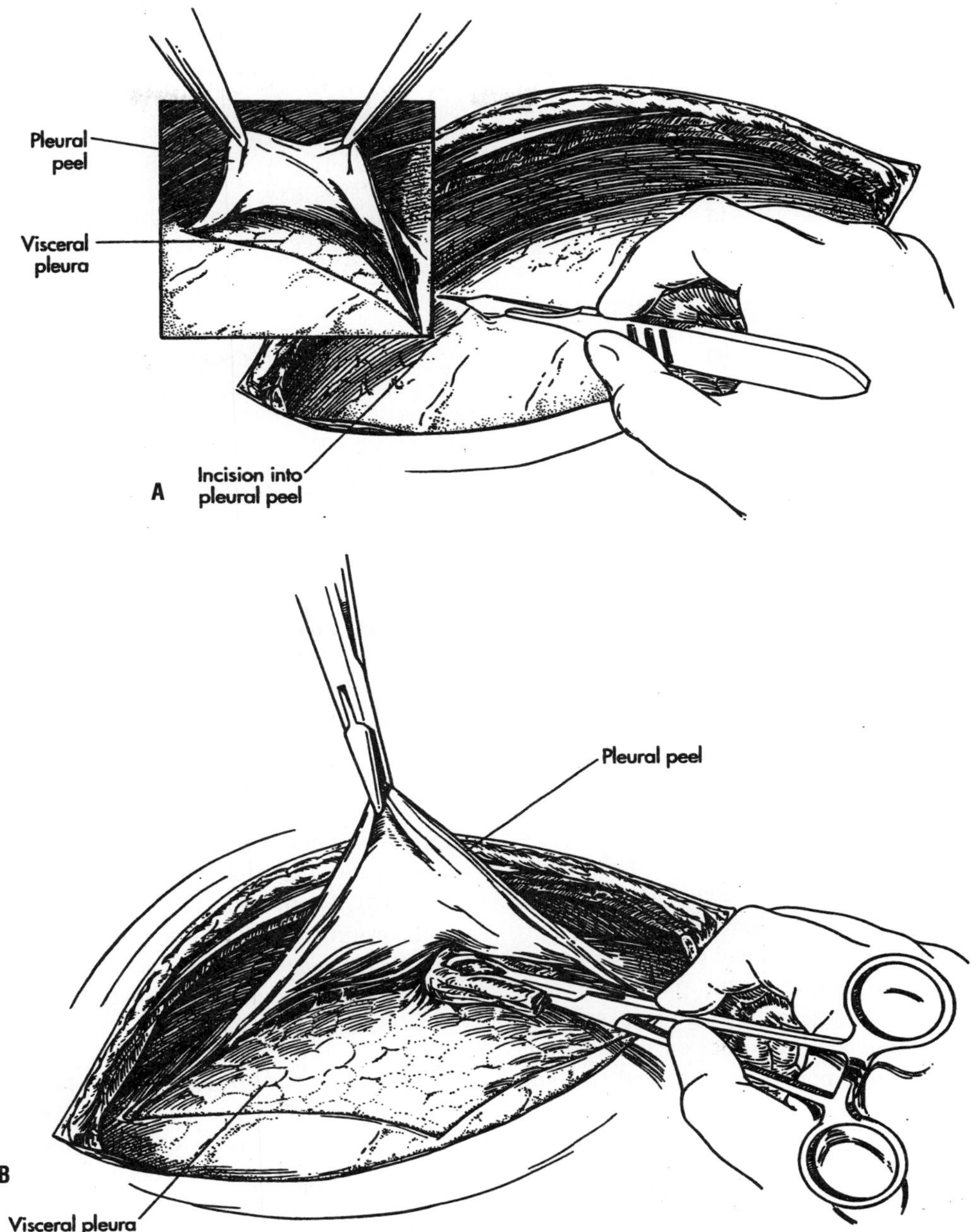

Figure 38–26. Decortication. **A,** Initial incision into pleural peel, separating visceral and parietal pleura. **B,** Removing pleural peel taking great care not to tear lung. *(From Kaiser. [1997]. [pp. 147, 148].)*

dered. Cytology is required to diagnose a malignant effusion. Chylothorax is confirmed by lipids present in the fluid. Immunologic studies are necessary to confirm effusions caused by collagen vascular disease. Obtaining an amylase enables confirmation of an effusion due to pancreatitis or esophageal rupture (Cohen, DeMeester, & Lafontaine, 1995).

Management of Pleural Effusion. Similar to pneumothoraces, small, asymptomatic pleural effusions may be managed with observation, especially when the etiology is known. This is more the exception than the norm. Several management options are available including thoracentesis, thoracostomy with chemical pleurodesis, surgical pleurodesis or pleurectomy, and pleuroperitoneal shunts.

Thoracentesis. There are several advantages to thoracentesis in that it is a relatively simple procedure, may be performed at the bedside or in the outpatient setting, and provides a mechanism for diagnosis and treatment. Additionally

TABLE 38–25. Useful Tests in the Evaluation of Pleural Effusions

Test	Abnormal Values	Frequently Associated Condition
Red blood cells, per mm^3	>100,000	Malignancy, trauma, pulmonary embolism
White blood cells, per mm^3	>10,000	Pyogenic infection
neutrophils, %	>50	Acute pleuritis
lymphocytes, %	>90	Tuberculosis, malignancy
eosinophilia, %	>10	Asbestos effusion, pneumothorax, resolving infection
mesothelial cells	Absent	Tuberculosis
Protein, PF/S[a]	>0.5	Exudate
LDH, PF/S	>0.6	Exudate
LDH, IU[b]	>200	
Glucose, mg/dL	<60	Empyema, TB, malignancy, rheumatoid arthritis
pH	<7.20	Esophageal rupture, empyema, TB, malignancy, rheumatoid arthritis
Amylase, PF/S	>1	Pancreatitis
Bacteriologic	Positive	Etiology of infection
Cytology	Positive	Diagnostic of malignancy

[a] PF/S ratio = pleural fluid to serum ratio.
[b] IU = concentration in international units.
From Fishman, ed. (1988). (p. 2129).

it provides immediate relief of acute symptoms. It does not, however, provide a cure and the underlying etiology must be treated. Furthermore, thoracentesis is not advantageous for those with recurrent effusions or coagulopathy.

Thoracostomy—Chest Tube Pleurodesis. Pleural effusions are most often managed with chest tube placement and chemical pleurodesis. A chest tube is placed in the sixth or seventh intercostal space in the midaxillary line. The pleural fluid should be drained as completely as possible, ideally to less than 200 mL of fluid per day. This prevents dilution of the sclerosing agent and promotes an environment conducive to apposition of the pleura. A chest x-ray should be obtained to assess for lung reexpansion. If complete lung reexpansion does not occur once the fluid is drained, the pleurodesis will not be effective and the fluid will recur.

Surgery—Pleurodesis or Pleurectomy. Traditionally, surgery has been reserved for those patients with significant effusions when all other methods have failed or those with long-term survivability. As more and more thoracic surgeons have become proficient in video thoracoscopic techniques, surgery is generally opted for sooner than it used to be. In most cases, unless a pleural biopsy is needed, chest tube placement followed by sclerosis is attempted first. If this fails, the patient is taken to the operating room and video thoracoscopy is performed.

Video thoracoscopy enables a definitive diagnosis in almost all cases. It has virtually replaced the needle biopsy, with the exception of nonoperative cases. In addition to a definitive diagnosis, video thoracoscopy allows for direct visualization of the pleural space and provides access for biopsy of any suspicious lesions of the pleura, lung, or pericardium. Furthermore, video thoracoscopy provides access for treatment with talc insufflation, debridement of empyemas, ligation of the thoracic duct for chylothorax, and control of bleeding in the hemothorax (Kaiser, 1993). The chest tube site serves as one of the two or three small incisions needed for the procedure. After complete drainage of the effusion, inspection of the pleura by direct visualization is performed. If the pleura is thickened, pleurectomy or pleural stripping may be necessary. If the lung is trapped, decortication, or an unpeeling of the fibrous debris may by indicated. Pleurodesis is accomplished either chemically with insufflation of talc or mechanically by brushing the pleura with a sterile Bovie pad. A chest tube is placed at the end of the procedure and removed when the drainage is less than 150 cc over 24 hours.

Pleural–Peritoneal Shunt. The pleural–peritoneal shunt is a small device that consists of a valve and pumping chamber attached to a pleural catheter on one end and a peritoneal catheter on the other end (Cohen, DeMeester, & Lafontaine, 1995). It is reserved for patients with recurrent effusions after chemical pleurodesis, symptomatic patients with limited life expectancy, and patients who have failed chest tube pleurodesis and who are not operative candidates.

The device is placed in the operating room, although general anesthesia is not necessarily required. The compression valve sits just beneath the surface of the skin. Manual compression of the chamber transfers fluid from the pleural space to the peritoneum. Patients must pump the chamber approximately ten times every hour. The device is usually successful in alleviating the symptom of dyspnea (Fig. 38–27).

Mesothelioma

Mesothelioma is a tumor that originates from the mesothelial cells that line the pleura, peritoneal, and pericardial cav-

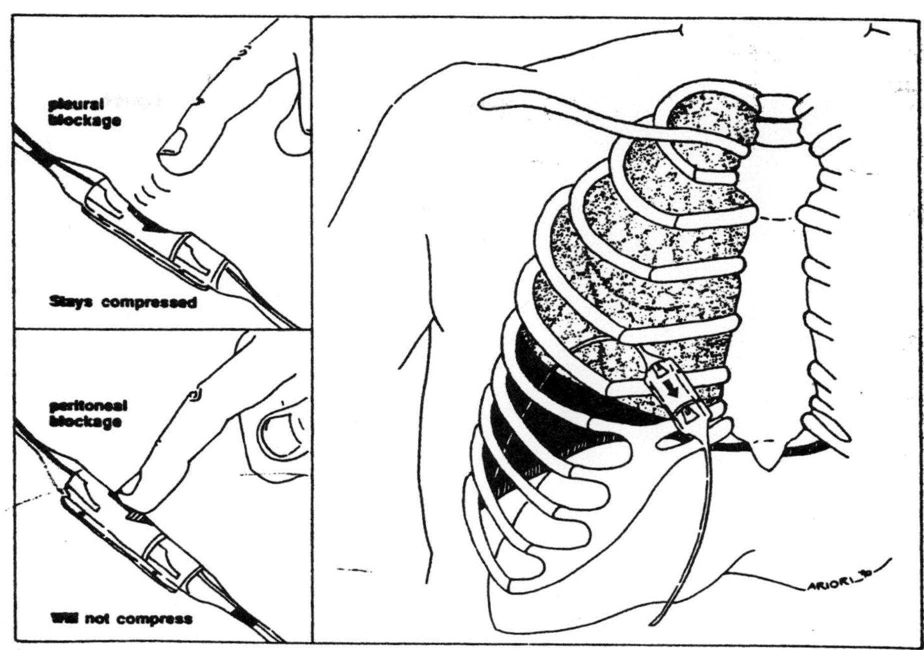

Figure 38–27. Pleural peritoneal shunt. Shunt position and signs of proximal or distal obstruction. *(Reprinted with permission from Ferguson, Sloan, & Steele [eds]. [1991].)*

ities (Cohen, DeMeester, & Lafontaine, 1995). It is relatively uncommon and more prevalent among those who have had extended exposure to asbestos, particularly asbestos mine workers and naval shipmen. Asbestos is not the only precipitating factor as over one half of those with mesothelioma have no prior asbestos exposure. There is usually a latent period from exposure to presentation of 20 to 40 years (Cohen, DeMeester, & Lafontaine, 1995). In the past it was often misdiagnosed as metastatic adenocarcinoma, as the special stains and electron microscopy needed to make the diagnosis were not used. It is estimated that there will be 80,000 new cases of mesothelioma within the next 20 years (Pass, 1994).

There are two types of mesothelioma: localized and diffuse. Localized mesothelioma may be benign or malignant. Localized benign mesothelioma presents as a smooth-walled mass that varies in size. It may be partially calcified or may contain a fluid-filled cyst. Typically patients are asymptomatic unless the tumor is large enough to compress the lung or airway. Associated symptoms include hypertrophic pulmonary osteoarthropy manifested by joint and bone pain, arthralgias, and ankle edema. Additionally patients may have associated hypoglycemia. Evaluation consists of a chest x-ray, which invariably reveals a solitary peripheral mass. A CT scan is helpful in identifying the relationship of the mass to other structures. The diagnosis is made intraoperatively at the time of resection. Complete resection is curative.

Localized mesothelioma may also be malignant. As opposed to localized benign mesothelioma, patients are often symptomatic with pain, cough, dyspnea, and fever. The tumor is firm and encapsulated. Long-term survival is directly correlated with the completeness of the resection (Cohen, DeMeester, & Lafontaine, 1995).

Diffuse malignant mesothelioma originates in the visceral or parietal pleura and often encases the lung and pericardium with extension into the chest wall and even the contralateral chest. It most often presents in the sixth and seventh decades of life. Typically patients present with complaints of dyspnea and an aching pain in the chest.

The diagnosis may be made by pleural biopsy. The management of this disease remains less than optimal. Thus far, it has included radiation, chemotherapy, surgery, or any combination of these. Surgery, if offered, usually consists of pleurectomy or extrapleural pneumonectomy. Thus far, extrapleural pneumonectomy with radiation, chemotherapy, or both offer the best chance of survival over one year (Pass, 1994). There is preliminary evidence that gene therapy may offer new potential for long-term survival.

▶THE CHEST WALL

Pathology

Congenital Abnormalities—Pectus Excavatum

Pectus excavatum or "funnel chest" is the most common congenital deformity of the sternum (Fig. 38–28). The etiology of this deformity is still not well understood. It has

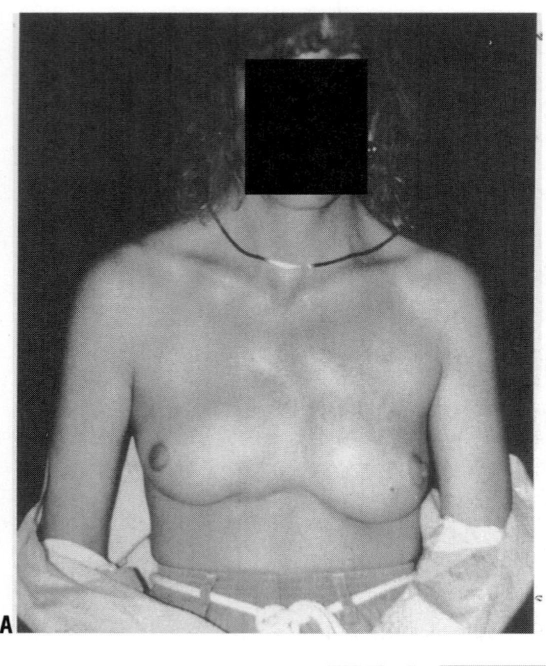

A

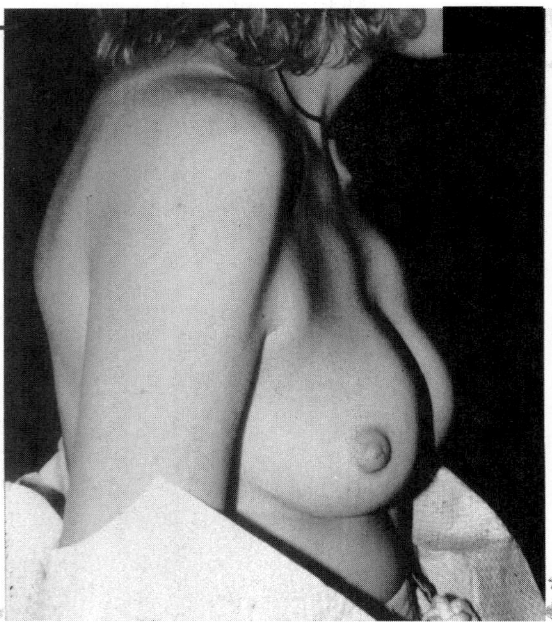

B

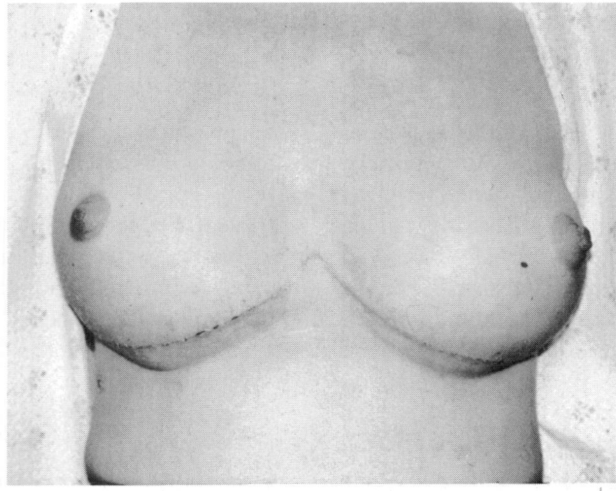

C

Figure 38–28. Pectus excavatum. **A,** Anterior view of pectus excavatum. **B,** Lateral view of pectus excavatum. **C,** Status post surgical repair of pectus excavatum.

been speculated to be the result of a functional abnormality of the anterior diaphragm, the failure of osteogenesis and chondrogenesis, or the abnormal growth of the central tendons. Most believe this deformity is the result of abnormal, rapid growth of the lower costal cartilages that form in an abnormal concave manner, resulting in depression of the sternum (Landolfo & Sabiston, 1995). The resulting deformity may range from very mild to quite severe. While a familial tendency has been questioned, often these defects occur sporadically. In most cases the defect increases in severity with growth; however, the cosmetic effect may diminish with the development of pectoralis muscles and breast development (von Hippel, 1986a).

Clinical Manifestations. The clinical manifestations of pectus excavatum vary among individuals. The most severe depression usually occurs above the xiphoid process resulting in a reduction in the size of the prevertebral space, which displaces the heart to the left and significantly limits pulmonary function. As young children, most patients are completely asymptomatic. As they enter adolescence, if the defect remains unrepaired, many begin to notice a decreased exercise tolerance. Some patients may experience frequent, recurrent lower respiratory tract infections. Many develop asthma. Decreased pulmonary function often occurs due to the restriction and is evidenced by a decreased FVC, VC, TLC, and MVV. Mitral valve prolapse and/or decreased cardiac function occurs in over half of these patients. Scoliosis has also been associated with this deformity (Landolfo & Sabiston, 1995).

Evaluation. Evaluation consists of a chest x-ray that demonstrates the deformity as described. CT scan is required by some surgeons to assess the affect of the deformity on underlying structures. Pulmonary function tests and/or echocardiogram may be necessary to justify medical necessity to the insurance company.

Surgical Repair. Surgical repair is indicated for cosmetic purposes as well as to correct the decrease in respiratory and cardiac function and prevent recurrent infections. Often insurers require clinical justification as cosmetic reasons alone does not always justify reimbursement. The timing of the repair is controversial. Many believe the best results occur between the ages of 2 and 5 as at that stage of development most have not yet developed rib involvement or scoliosis. Often the repair is done in the adolescent once complete growth has occurred.

The repair is done through a midline incision or transverse inframammary incision. The costal cartilages are removed and the sternum is freed from all attachments, enabling repositioning. A wedge of bone or cartilage is placed and secured with transternal sutures.

Complications are rare and a satisfactory repair with resolution of clinical consequences is the norm. Serous drainage often occurs over the first few days and often the patient is sent home with bulb suction in place. A mild fever is not uncommon within the first 24 to 48 hours. It is critical to emphasize the need to avoid contact sports for at least six months and to emphasize correct posture with the spine straight and shoulders rotated back.

Chest-Wall Tumors

Chest-wall tumors include tumors that invade bone, soft tissue, or both. They may be of a primary nature in the bone or soft tissue or may invade from adjacent structure such as breast, lung, pleura, or mediastinum. Primary chest-wall tumors may be either benign or malignant (Table 38–26).

Primary chest-wall tumors are usually very slow growing. Patients often remain asymptomatic until the tumor has reached a significant size at which point pain ensues. The pain is most often described as generalized and vague. Frequently, patients are treated as if they have a neuritis or musculoskeletal condition prior to the discovery of the tumor. Almost all malignant tumors become progressively more painful.

Evaluation. Evaluation consists of a chest x-ray that reveals the tumor. A CT scan is often done to assess the extent of the tumor. MRI is usually the preferred diagnostic test as it enables distinction of tumor from nerves and blood vessels and additionally provides visualization of the tumor from different planes (Pairolero, 1995). Pulmonary function tests are required if the tumor is the result of extension from the parenchyma or if the patient has poor pulmonary function baseline. Needle biopsy should not be done to obtain a tissue diagnosis as the tissue is often inadequate and misdiagnosed as benign.

TABLE 38–26. Primary Chest-Wall Neoplasms

Malignant	Benign
Myeloma	Osteochondroma
Malignant fibrous histiocytoma	Chondroma
Chondrosarcoma	Desmoid
Rhabdomyosarcoma	Lipoma
Ewing's sarcoma	Fibroma
Liposarcoma	Neurilemoma
Neurofibrosarcoma	
Osteogenic sarcoma	
Sarcoma	
Hemangiosarcoma	
Leiomyosarcoma	
Lymphoma	

Reprinted with permission from Pairolero. (1995). (p. 516).

Surgical Treatment. Surgery with or without radiation therapy depending on cell type is the treatment that offers the best chance for long-term survival. Wide surgical resection, defined as a margin free of tumor of at least 4 cm, greatly increases the likelihood of survival (Pairolero, 1995). Any involved bone including ribs, sternum, manubrium, or costal cartilages should be a part of the resection (Fig. 38–29). Likewise, attached structures, lung, thymus, pericardium, and chest-wall muscles should be excised as well. This is all feasible due to the ability to reconstruct the chest wall.

Therapeutic Procedures

Chest-Wall Reconstruction

A critical step in chest-wall resection is to ascertain whether reconstruction will support respiration and protect the underlying organs. Without question successful chest-wall resection depends on adequate reconstruction. When possible a primary closure is preferred. If necessary, chest-wall reconstruction may be accomplished as a joint initiative with a thoracic surgeon and a plastic surgeon.

Chest-wall reconstruction, including both skeletal and soft tissue reconstruction, remains a very controversial issue both in terms of indications and actual procedure. There are many factors to consider when contemplating chest-wall reconstruction (Table 38–27). The size and location of the defect are critical determinants. Defects less than 5 cm in diameter, regardless of location, are generally not reconstructed. If the defect occurs high enough for scapular coverage, there is no need to reconstruct it regardless of size. If the defect is located near the tip of the scapula, it should be reconstructed to avoid catching the tip with arm movement.

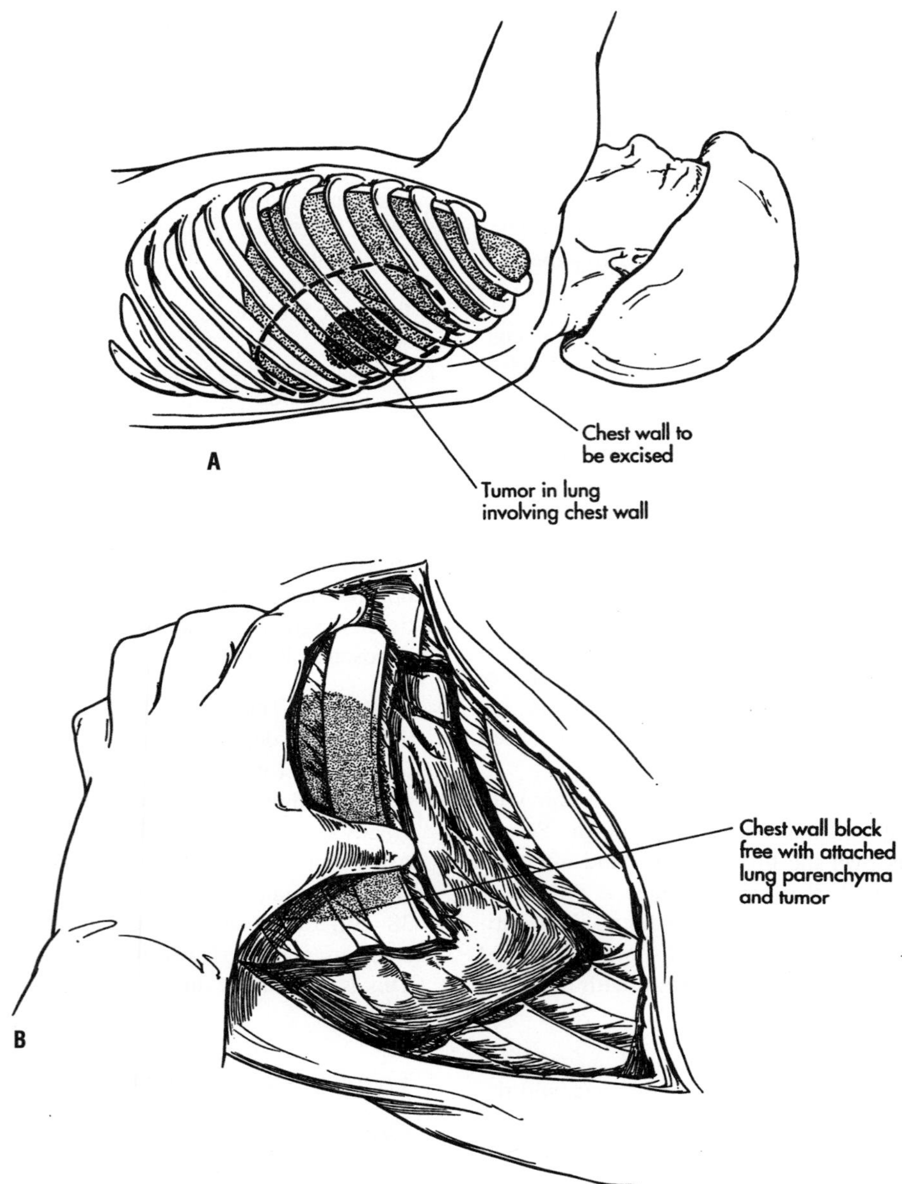

Figure 38–29. Chest wall excision. **A,** Depiction of chest wall tumor. **B,** En bloc resection of chest wall tumor. *(Reprinted with permission from Kaiser. [1997].)*

There are several prosthetic materials available for skeletal reconstruction. The most commonly used materials are prolene mesh, Gore-Tex soft tissue patch, marlex mesh, methyl methacrylate, or a combination of these. Surgeon preference determines selection of material. At our institution marlex mesh and methyl methacrylate are used in combination. The marlex is cut to fit the opening and sutured in place. Methyl methracrylate is painted onto the mesh and then molded to mimic the contours of the chest wall. Another layer of marlex is then placed on top to form a sandwich and sutured in place (Fig. 38–30). Soft tissue reconstruction is done by using either muscle or omentum.

Routine postoperative care is implemented. No special antibiotics are necessary. Complications including poor wound healing and infection are rare.

Thoracoplasty

Thoracoplasty is the removal of the skeletal portion of the chest wall with the intent of obliterating the pleural space. It was originally used in the treatment of empyema and tuberculosis. Currently the primary indication for thoracoplasty is the treatment of chronic empyema when there is no viable tissue to fill the space. Today, it is a procedure of last resort. The original procedure involved the removal of at least seven ribs via a posterior approach. Now limited

TABLE 38–27. Factors to Consider for Reconstruction of Chest-Wall Defects

Location
Size
Depth
Partial thickness
Full thickness
Duration
Condition of local tissue
Irradiation
Infection
Residual tumor
Scarring
General condition of patient
Chemotherapy
Corticosteroid
Chronic infection
Lifestyle and type of work
Prognosis

Reprinted with permission from Pairolero. (1995). (p. 517).

thoracoplasty procedures are performed with the number of ribs resected dependent on the magnitude of collapse needed.

Postoperatively it is critical that patients undergo aggressive physical and pulmonary rehabilitation to prevent scoliosis, shoulder immobility, and pneumonia. Thoracoplasty of any degree may result in retained secretions due to the decreased ability to cough and generate high positive intrapleural pressures. It is estimated that the postoperative mortality from this procedure, due in part to the underlying lung disease, is as high as 13% (Barker, 1994).

Eloesser Flap/Open Window Thoracostomy

The Eloesser flap was designed by Leo Eloesser for the treatment of tuberculosis empyema (Eloesser, 1969). This flap—or open window thoracostomy, as it is more often called now—provides a large, open, dependent space through which purulent material may drain. Indications for this procedure include empyemas, malignant pleural effusions, and chronic bronchopleural fistulas.

The procedure is done by removing a section of chest wall with at least two or three ribs. The remaining flap of skin and subcutaneous tissues are tucked into the pleural space and sutured to the pleura. The result is a U-shaped

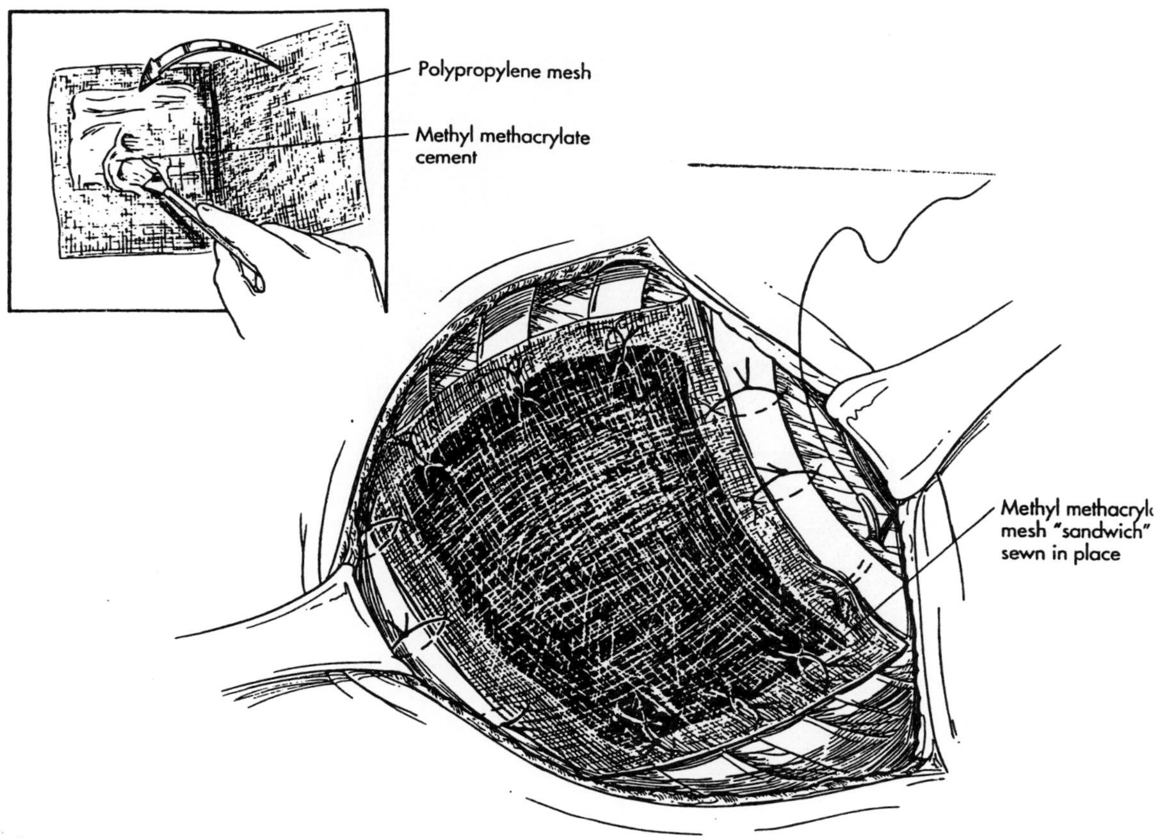

Figure 38–30. Chest wall reconstruction with methyl methacrylate "sandwich." *(Reprinted with permission from Kaiser. [1997].)*

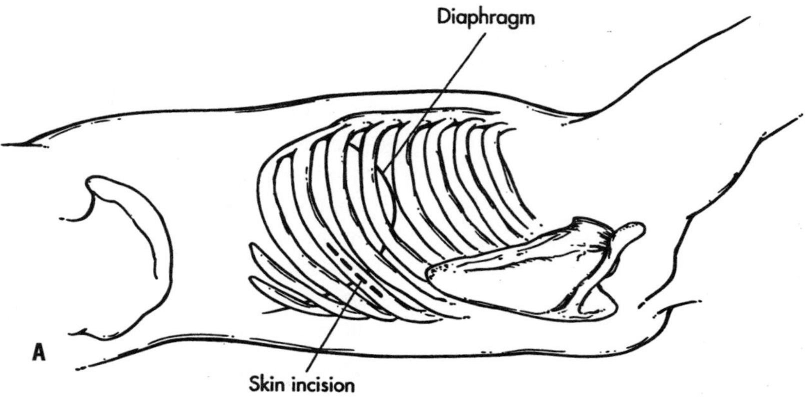

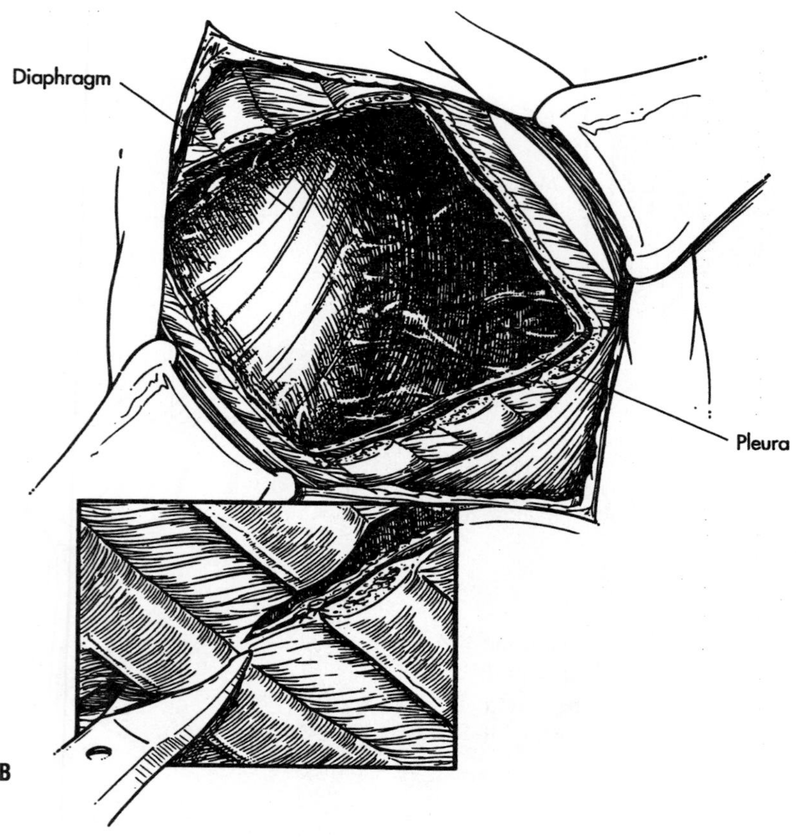

Figure 38–31. Open window thoracostomy. **A, B,** and **C,** Open window thoracostomy in a dependent position. *(Reprinted with permission from Kaiser. [1997].)*

(Continued)

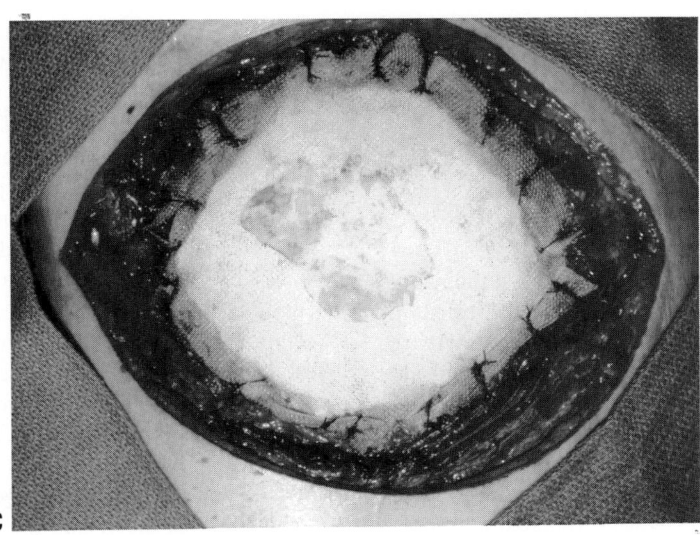

Figure 38–31. Continued.

opening at least 5 cm in diameter. The key to success is to place this open window in a dependent position and make it large (Fig. 38–31).

Postoperatively, the window may be packed loosely in a wet to dry fashion. Ultimately, it may simply be covered. Gradually, over a period of several months to a year, it granulates in and closes. If the precipitating cause for the window has resolved, it may be surgically closed by rotating in muscle to fill the space.

The Eloesser flap, or open window thoracostomy, was designed to provide chronic dependent drainage of the pleural space. It is indicated for empyema, pleural effusions, and most commonly bronchopleural fistula.

The patient is taken to the operating room and placed in the posterolateral thoracotomy position. A transverse incision is placed over the most dependent portion of the area to be drained, identified radiographically. The U-shaped incision is usually 4 to 5 cm and at least two ribs with soft tissues are resected. The skin is sewn down to the pleura, leaving an open draining space.

▶ THE DIAPHRAGM

Diaphragmatic disorders are relatively uncommon. The most common pathologic conditions associated with the diaphragm are eventration and diaphragmatic perforation or tear. Due to the infrequency with which these conditions present, they are only briefly described here.

Morgagni's Hernia or Subcostal Diaphragmatic Hernia

Giovanni Battista Morgagni (1769) was the first to describe the substernal herniation of abdominal contents into the thoracic cavity; thus, the defect bears his name. This defect is also known as a retrosternal hernia, subcostal diaphragmatic hernia, or Larrey's hernia. Dominique Jean Larrey was the surgeon for General Napoleon and the first to describe the surgical approach used to repair this defect (van Trigt, 1995).

This type of herniation is uncommon and represents only 3% of all surgically treated hernias (van Trigt, 1995). It is most often found on routine chest films as patients are generally asymptomatic. The defect occurs just lateral to the xiphoid and predominates on the right. In most cases a well-formed herniated sac is found. On chest x-ray it is often mistaken for a pericardial cyst (von Hippel, 1986b). Surgical repair is indicated as the herniation may precipitate colonic obstruction. Preoperatively patients need upper and lower GI contrast studies. A midline incision or anterior thoracotomy is used for the repair by direct suture.

Eventration

Eventration is defined by an abnormally high position of all or part of the diaphragm. It may be paralytic or nonparalytic depending on the cause. The most common causes include denervation, ascites, pregnancy, obesity, or intraabdominal tumors (van Trigt, 1995).

Denervation of the diaphragm is usually the result of a phrenic nerve injury. Historically phrenic nerve injuries or the so-called phrenic nerve crush was done intentionally in certain patients. It was used in TB patients to "rest" the lung by decreasing the size of the hemithorax. In patients with hiatal hernia, it was believed to decrease esophageal reflux. In pneumonectomy patients, phenic nerve crush was used to decease the size of the empty pleural space (von Hippel, 1986b). Today phrenic nerve injuries are always accidental. Denervation of the diaphragm causes the diaphragm to move paradoxically. It may be confirmed by a sniff test, having the patient sniff under fluoroscopy. Alternatively an inspiratory and expiratory film may be taken and the level of the diaphragm compared. Surgical repair consists of plication.

Traumatic Perforation/Tear

Traumatic perforation of the diaphragm occurs as the result of either blunt or penetrating trauma. In the case of blunt trauma it is believed to be the result of the sudden increase in pleuroperitoneal pressure that results in herniation and subsequent rupture. Automobile accidents are frequently implicated. Ninety percent of traumatic perforations occur on the left. Rarely do they occur on the right due to the cushion of the liver. Perforations of the diaphragm are usually large, posterior, and central. Due to the size and location of the perforation, the abdominal contents easily assume a position within the thoracic cavity.

Perforations of the diaphragm are not easy to diagnose. It should be suspected in any trauma patient who complains of respiratory insufficiency, persistent shoulder pain without obvious cause, epigastric distress, and/or bowel sounds in the chest (von Hippel, 1986b). Inability to completely visualize the diaphragm on a chest film is suspicious for perforation. In most cases the diaphragm is elevated. An air-fluid level may represent a herniated stomach. Haziness may represent blood, the intestines, or the spleen (von Hippel, 1986b).

The mortality from diaphragmatic perforation ranges from 8 to 40% (van Trigt, 1995). Repair is done through a transthoracic incision. The perforation should be directly sutured with a double layer of nonabsorbable suture.

▶ GENERAL THORACIC SURGERY FOR THE NEXT CENTURY

It has been said, "as for the future, the task is not to foresee it, but to enable it." General thoracic surgery continues to evolve at a rapid pace. From scientific research at a cellular level to clinical research and applications at the bedside, great strides are being made to advance the care provided to thoracic surgery patients. It is likely that thoracic surgery procedures will become even more complex. Advances in neoadjuvant therapies will likely increase the number of procedures performed for cancer. Thoracic surgical procedures for benign disease will likely increase as well due to the increased use of immunosuppressive medications, resurgence of mycobacterial disease, and new techniques such as lung volume-reduction surgery (Todd & Ralph-Edwards, 1995). Further, the widespread application of gene therapy and photodynamic therapy are just on the horizon.

Until now, the numbers of nurses specialized in the field of general thoracic surgery has been limited at best. Likely this has been due to the limited integration of this topic in the nursing curriculum and, thus, limited exposure to this specialty. There are both tremendous need and opportunity for acute care nurse practitioners in this field.

▶ ACKNOWLEDGMENT

It is with profound gratitude that this author acknowledges:

- Larry Kaiser, MD, who provided me with an introduction and education in general thoracic surgery—he instilled in me a passion for this specialty.
- John R. Roberts, MD, and Patricia Abbott, PA-C, MHS, for their insightful reviews of this chapter.
- And above all Bill Wurster, who provided the support that made this endeavor possible—one could not ask for a better soul mate.

REFERENCES

Allen, M. S. (1996). Surgical anatomy of the trachea. *Chest Surgery Clinics of North America, 6* (4), 627–635.

Allen, M. S. & Payne, W. S. (1992). Cystic foregut malformations in the mediastinum. *Chest Surgery Clinics of North America: Mediastinal Tumors, 2* (1), 89–106.

American Thoracic Society Subcommitee on Surgery (1962). Management of nontuberculosis emphysema. *American Review of Respiratory Disease, 85,* 935.

Anderson, H. L. & Bartlett, R. H. (1991). Elective tracheostomy for mechanical ventilation by the percutaneous technique. *Clinics in Chest Medicine, 12* (3), 555–560.

Anthonisen, N. R. & Filuk, R. B. (1988). Pneumothorax. In A. P. Fishman (Ed.), *Pulmonary diseases and disorders* (2nd ed.). (pp. 2171–2182). New York: McGraw-Hill.

Astrachan, D. I., Kerchner, J. C., & Goodwin, W. J. (1988). Prolonged intubation versus tracheotomy: Complications, practical and psychological considerations. *Laryngoscope, 98* (11), 1165–1169.

Barker, W. L. (1994). Thoracoplasty. *Chest Surgery Clinics of North America, 4* (3), 593–615.

Bechard, D. E. (1992). Pulmonary function testing. *Chest Surgery Clinics of North America, 2* (3), 565–586.

Blossom, G. B., Ernstoff, R. M., Howells, G. A., Bendick, P. J., & Glover, J. L. (1993). Thymectomy for myasthenia gravis. *Archives of Surgery, 128* (8), 855–862.

Borchers, S. D. & Beamis, J. F. (1996). Flexible bronchoscopy. *Chest Surgery Clinics of North America, 6* (2), 169–192.

Boysen, P. G., Block, A. J., Olsen, G. N., Moulder, P. V., Harris, J. O., & Rawltscher, R. E. (1977). Prospective evaluation for pneumonectomy using the technetium-99m quantitative perfusion lung scan. *Chest, 72* (4), 422–425.

Briselli, M., Mark, G. J., & Grillo, H. C. (1978). Tracheal carcinoids. *Cancer, 42* (6), 2870–2879.

Burkey, B., Esclamado, R., & Morganroth, M. (1991). The role of cricothyroidotomy in airway management. *Clinics in Chest Medicine, 12* (3), 561–571.

Colt, H. G. & Dumon, J. (1995). Airway stents, present and future. *Clinics in Chest Medicine, 16* (3), 465–478.

Cohen, R. C., DeMeester, T. R., & Lafontaine, E. (1995). The pleura. In D. C. Sabiston & F. C. Spencer (Eds.). *Surgery of the chest* (6th ed.). (523–575). Philadelphia: W. B. Saunders.

Cooper, J. D. & Grillo, H. C. (1969). The evolution of tracheal injury due to ventilatory assistance through cuffed tubes: A pathologic study. *Annals of Surgery, 169* (3), 334–348.

Crocco, J. A. (1977). Introduction. In T. P. Pick & R. Howden (Eds.), *Gray's Anatomy.* New York: Crown Publishers.

Cummings, S. R., Littington, G. A., & Richard, R. J. (1986). Managing solitary pulmonary nodules. The choice of strategy is a "close call." *American Review of Respiratory Diseases, 134* (3), 453–460.

D'Amico, T. A. & Sabiston, D. C. (1995). Neoplasms of the lung. In D. C. Sabiston & F. C. Spencer (Eds.), *Surgery of the chest* (6th ed.). (pp. 634–668). Philadelphia: W. B. Saunders.

Dartevelle, P. & Macchiarini, P. (1996). Management of acquired tracheoesophageal fistula. *Chest Surgery Clinics of North America, 6* (4), 819–836.

Deslauriers, J. & Jacques, L. F. (1995). Sleeve pneumonectomy *Chest Surgery Clinics of North America, 5* (2), 297–313.

Dripps, R. D., Eckenhoff, J. E., & Vandam, L. D. (1977). Preanesthethetic consultation and choice of anesthesia. In R. D. Dripps, J. E. Eckenhoff, & L. D. Vandam (Eds.), *Introduction to anesthesia: The principles of safe pracitice* (pp. 11–21). Philadelphia: W. B. Saunders.

Eloesser, L. (1969). [Of an operation for tuberculosis empyema.] *Annals of Thoracic Surgery, 8* (4), 355–357.

Faber, L. P. (1995). Sleeve lobectomy. *Chest Surgery Clinics of North America, 5* (2), 233–251.

Fell, S. C. (1995). Segmental resection. *Chest Surgery Clinics of North America, 5* (2), 205–221.

Fell, S. C. & Kirby, T. J. (1995). Segmental resection. In F.G. Pearson, J. Deslauriers, R. J. Ginsberg, C. A. Hiebert, M. F. McKneally, & H. C. Urschel (Eds.), *Thoracic surgery* (pp. 854–866). New York: Churchill Livingstone.

Fintel, D. & Mir Taqui Ali (1992). Cardiac evaluation of the thoracic surgical patient. *Chest Surgery Clinics of North America, 2* (3), 587–598.

Fry, W. A. (1995). Thoracic incisions. *Chest Surgery Clinics of North America, 5* (2), 177–188.

Gamsu, G., Singer, M. M., Vincent H. H., Berry, S., & Nadel, J. A. (1976). Postoperative impairment of mucous transport in the lung. *American Review of Respiratory Disease, 114* (4), 673–678.

Garland, L. H. (1949). On the scientific evaluation of dignostic procedures. *Radiology, 52,* 309.

Ginsberg, R. J. (1995a) Preoperative assessment of the thoracic surgical patient: A surgeon's viewpoint. In F. G. Pearson, J. Deslauriers, R. J. Ginsberg, C. A. Hiebert, M. F. Mc Kneally, & H. C. Urschel (Eds.), *Thoracic surgery* (pp. 29–36). New York: Churchill Livingstone.

Ginsberg, R. J. (1995b). Resection of a superior sulcus tumor. *Chest Surgery Clinics of North America, 5* (2), 315–331.

Grillo, H. C. & Donahue, D. M. (1996). Postintubation tracheal stenosis. *Chest Surgery Clinics of North America, 6* (4), 725–731.

Grippi, M. A., Metzger, L. F., Krupinski, A. V., & Fishman, A. P. (1988). Pulmonary function testing. In A. P. Fishman (Ed.), *Pulmonary diseases and disorders* (2nd ed.). (pp. 2469–2521). New York: McGraw-Hill.

Harvey, J. C., Erdman, C., & Beattie, E. J. (1995). Pneumonectomy. *Chest Surgery Clinics of North America 5* (2), 253–287.

Heelan, R. T., Demas, B. E., Caravelli, J. F., Martini, N., Bains, M. S., McCormack, P. M., Burt, M., Panicek, D. M., & Mitzner, A. (1989). Superior sulcus tumors: CT and MR imaging. *Radiology, 170* (3), 637–641.

Helmers, R. A. & Sanderson, D. R. (1995). Rigid bronchoscopy the forgotten art. *Clinics in Chest Medicine, 16* (3), 393–399.

Jensik, R. J. (1986). The extent of resection for localized lung cancer: Segmental resection. In C. F. Kittle (Ed.), *Current controversies in thoracic surgery* (pp. 175–182). Philadelphia: W. B. Saunders.

Jones, J. W., Reynolds, M., Hewitt, R. L., & Drapanas, T. (1976). Tracheo–innominate artery erosion: Successful surgical management of a devastating complication. *Annals of Surgery, 184* (2), 194–204.

Kaiser, L.R. (1993). Pleural masses and effusions. In L. R. Kaiser & T. M. Daniel (Eds.), *Thoracoscopic surgery* (pp. 59–74). Boston: Little Brown.

Kaiser, L. R. (1997). Tube thoracostomy. In L. R. Kaiser (Ed.), *Atlas of general thoracic surgery* (pp. 16–19). St. Louis: Mosby.

Kannell, W. B. & Abbott, R. D. (1984). Incidence and prognosis of unrecognized myocardial infarction: An update on the framingham study. *New England Journal of Medicine, 311* (18), 1144–1147.

Kelley, M. A. & Fishman, A. P. (1988). Exercise testing. In A. P. Fishman (Ed.), *Pulmonary diseases and disorders* (2nd ed.). (pp. 2523–2532). New York: McGraw-Hill.

Kennedy, L. & Sahn, S. A. (1994). Noninvasive evaluation of the patient with a pleural effusion. *Clinics in Chest Surgery, 4* (3), 451–479.

Kirschner, P. A. (1992). Myasthenia gravis and other parathymic syndromes. *Chest Surgery Clinics of North America, 2* (1), 183–201.

Landolfo, K. P. & Sabiston, D. C. (1995). Disorders of the sternum and the thoracic wall: Congenital deformities of the chest wall. In D. C. Sabiston & F. C. Spencer (Eds.), *Surgery of the chest* (6th ed.). (pp. 494–515). Philadelphia: W. B. Saunders.

Light, R. W. (1993). Management of spontaneous pneumothorax. *American Review of Respiratory Disease, 148,* 245–248.

Lillington, G. A. & Caskey, C. I. (1993). Evaluation and management of solitary and multiple pulmonary nodules. *Clinics in Chest Medicine, 14* (1), 111–119.

Mathisen, D. J. (1996). Tracheal tumors. *Chest Surgery Clinics of North America, 6* (4), 875–898.

Matthews, H. R. & Hopkinson, R. B. (1984). Treatment of sputum retention by minitracheotomy. *British Journal of Surgery, 71* (2), 147–150.

McGovern, E. M., Trastek, V. F., Pairolero, P. C., & Payne, W. S. (1988). Completion pneumonectomy: Indications, complications, and results. *Annals of Thoracic Surgery, 46* (2), 141–146.

McKenna, R. (1995). VATS lobectomy with mediastinal lymph node sampling or dissection. *Chest Surgery Clinics of North America, 5* (2), 223–232.

Mehta, A. C., Marty, J. J., & Lee, F. Y. (1993). Sputum cytology. *Clinics in Chest Medicine, 14* (1), 69–85.

Miller, J. I. (1996). Rigid bronchoscopy. *Chest Surgery Clinics of North America, 6* (2), 161–167.

Moore, D. W. O., Foster, E. D., & McKneally, M. F. (1995). Incisions. In F. G. Pearson, J. Deslauriers, R. J. Ginsberg, C. A. Hiebert, M. F. McKeally, & H. C. Urschel (Eds.). *Thoracic surgery* (pp. 113–129). New York: Churchill Livingstone.

Mountain, C. F. (1993). Lung cancer staging classification. *Clinics in Chest Medicine: Lung Cancer, 14* (1), 43–53.

Mountain, C. F. (1997). Revisions in the international system of staging lung cancer. *Chest, 111,* 1710–1717.

Musset, D., Grenier, P., Carrette, M. F., Frija, G., Hauuy, M. P., Desbleds, M. T., Girard, P., Bigot, J. M., & Lallemand, D. (1986). Primary lung cancer staging: Prospective comparative study of MR imaging with CT. *Radiology, 160* (3), 607–611.

Naidich, D. P. (1992). Computed tomography of the chest; Surgical correlations. In J. LoCicero (Ed.), *Chest Surgery Clinics of North America, 2* (3), 465–495.

Nesbitt, J. C. & Carrasco, H. (1996). Expandable stents. *Chest Surgery Clinics of North America, 6* (2), 305–328.

Olak, J. (1996). Parasternal mediastinotomy (chamberlain procedure). *Chest Surgery Clinics of North America, 6* (1), 31–40.

Olsen, G. N., Block, A., & Tobias, J. (1974). Prediction of post-pneumonectomy pulmonary function using quantitative macroaggregate lung scanning. *Chest, 66* (1), 13–16.

Paape, K. & Fry, W. A. (1994). Spontaneous pneumothorax. *Chest Surgery Clinics of North America, 4* (3), 517–538.

Pairolero, P. C. (1995). Surgical management of neoplasms of the chest wall. In D. C. Sabiston & F. C. Spencer (Eds.), *Surgery of the chest* (6th ed.). (pp. 516–521) Philadelphia: W. B. Saunders.

Pass, H. I. (1994). Contemporary approaches to malignant pleural mesothelioma. *Chest Surgery Clinics of North America, 4* (3), 497–515.

Shields, T. W. (1989). Pulmonary resections. In T. W. Shield, (Ed.), *General thoracic surgery* (3rd ed.). (pp. 363–377). Philadelphia: Lea & Febiger.

Shields, T. (1992). Radiologic examination of the chest. *Chest Surgery Clinics of North America, 2* (3), 443–464.

Shopland, D. R., Eyre, H. J., & Pechacek, T. F. (1991). Smoking attributable cancer mortality in 1991: Is lung cancer now the leading cause of death among smokers in the United States? *Journal of National Cancer Institute, 83* (16), 1142–1148.

Steiner, R. M., Liu J. B., Goldberg, B. B., & Cohn, J. R. (1995). The value of ultrasound-guided fiberoptic bronchoscopy. *Clinics in Chest Medicine, 16* (3), 519–534.

Swensen, S. J., Jett, J. R., Payne W. S., Viggiano, R. W., Pairolero, P. C., & Trastek, V. F. (1990). An integrated approach to evaluation of the solitary pulmonary nodule. *Mayo Clinic Proceedings, 65* (2), 173–186.

Tisi, G. M. (1979). Preoperative evaluation of pulmonary function: Validity, indications, and benefits. *American Review of Respiratory Diseases, 119* (2), 293–310.

Tisi, G. M., Friedman, P. J., Peters, R. M., et al. (1983). Clinical staging of primary lung cancer. *American Review of Respiratory Diseases, 127,* 659.

Todd, T. R. J. & Ralph Edwards, A. C. (1995). Perioperative management. In F. G. Pearson, J. Deslauriers, R. J. Ginsberg, C. A. Hiebert, M. F. McKneally, & H. C. Urschel (Eds.), *Thoracic surgery* (pp. 69–83). New York: Churchill Livingstone.

Trastek, V. F., Deschamps, C., Allen, M. S., & Pairolero, P. C. (1993). Operative principles. In L. R. Kaiser & T. M. Daniel (Eds.), *Thoracoscopic surgery* (pp. 37–45). Boston: Little Brown.

van Trigt III, P. (1995). Diaphragm and diaphragmatic pacing. In D. C. Sabiston & F. C. Spencer (Eds.), *Surgery of the chest* (6th ed.), (pp. 1081–1099) Philadelphia: W. B. Saunders.

von Hippel, A. (1986a). The chest wall. In A. von Hippel (Ed.), *A manual of thoracic surgery* (2nd ed.). (pp. 25–60). Anchorage: Stone Age Press.

von Hippel, A. (1986b). The diaphragm. In A. von Hippel (Ed.), *A manual of thoracic surgery* (2nd ed.). (pp. 1–24). Anchorage: Stone Age Press.

Warren, W. H. & Gould, V. E. (1992). Epithelial neoplasms of the thymus. *Chest Surgery Clinics of North America, 2* (1), 137–161.

Weibel, E. R. & Taylor, C. R. (1988). Design and structure of the human lung. In A. P. Fishman (Ed.), *Pulmonary diseases and disorders* (2nd ed.). (pp. 11–60). New York: McGraw-Hill.

Weisbord, G. L. (1992). Transthoraic needle biopsy. *Chest Surgery Clinics of North America, 2* (3), 631–647.

Wood, D. E. (1996). Trachesotomy. *Chest Surgery Clinics of North America, 6* (4), 749–764.

Wright, C. D. (1996). Management of tracheoinnominate artery fistula. *Chest Surgery Clinics of North America, 6* (4), 865–873.

Wychulis, A. R., Payne, W. S., Clagett, O. T., & Woolner, L. B. (1971). Surgical treatment of mediastinal tumors: A 40-year experience. *Journal of Thoracic and Cardiovascular Surgery, 62* (3), 379–392.

Yellin, A. (1992). Lymphoproliferative diseases. *Chest Surgery Clinics of North America, 2* (1), 107–120.

Yessner, R. (1993). Pathogenesis and pathology. *Clinics in Chest Medicine, 14* (1), 17–30.

39

Endocrine Problems

Carol A. Offutt

Endocrinology is the study of hormone action and the organs or glands that produce the hormones. The acute care nurse practitioner (ACNP) will encounter several common endocrine problems that will be discussed in this chapter. Because the endocrine system is so vast and complex, this chapter is designed to pinpoint only the most common disorders seen in the hospital setting, namely diabetes mellitus and disorders of the thyroid, pituitary, and adrenal glands.

▶ GENERAL PRINCIPLES OF THE ENDOCRINE SYSTEM

A hormone is a substance usually secreted into the blood in very small amounts by specialized cells or glands and carried by the bloodstream to other parts of the body, where it interacts with specific receptors in target tissue cells to produce a particular biological response (Rhoades & Pflanzer, 1992). Hormones regulate (1) energy production, use and storage, (2) salt and water metabolism, (3) growth and development, and (4) reproductive function. They bind to receptors that have a structure complementary to the specific hormone.

There are hormones produced throughout the body in various tissues. Table 39–1 lists the primary hormones and Figure 39–1 shows the anatomical location of the primary endocrine glands in the body.

The endocrine system has the ability to regulate hormone production via feedback regulation, either positive (stimulating a target cell to produce more product) or negative (inhibiting a target cell to produce product). In simple negative feedback, a cell produces a hormone that has an effect on target tissue. The target tissue in turn generates a biological response. The endocrine cell monitors the response and, if the response is too small, it secretes more hormone. If the response is too great, it secretes less hormone. An example of this is the secretion of insulin from the beta cells of the pancreas in response to glucose.

A more complex negative feedback occurs in some situations. This allows a back-up control system if one element of the loop fails. An example of this complex negative feedback loop is the hypothalamic–pituitary–thyroid axis in regulation of thyroid hormone (Fig. 39–2).

Hormones may be amino acid derivatives, peptides, or steroids. Amino acid derivatives include epinephrine, melatonin, and thyroxine. Peptide hormones vary in structure from single-chain proteins (such as adrenocorticotropic hormone and parathyroid hormone) to large glycoprotein structures (such as thyroid stimulating hormone and human chorionic gonadotropin). Steroid hormones are derived from cholesterol, and include glucocorticoids, mineralocorticoids, androgens, estrogens, and progestins. Steroid hormones and thyroxine are transported on plasma globulins, albumin, and prealbumin.

▶ PITUITARY DISORDERS

The pituitary gland is small, weighing about 600 mg. It consists of two connected parts: the anterior and the posterior. The anterior pituitary makes up about 75% of the pituitary gland, and secretes six hormones of major clinical sig-

TABLE 39–1. Summary of the Primary Hormones in the Body

Hormone	Gland or Source	Target Cells	Primary Biological Effect
Release or release-inhibiting hormones	Hypothalamus	Anterior pituitary	Regulate hormone secretion
Oxytocin	Synthesized in hypothalamus, secreted from posterior pituitary	Breast Uterus	Triggers milk "let down" Stimulates uterine contraction
Vasopressin (antidiuretic hormone) (ADH)	Synthesized in hypothalamus, secreted from posterior pituitary	Kidney Blood vessels	Increases water reabsorption Causes constriction
Growth hormone (GH)	Anterior pituitary	Many; especially bone, fat, and liver	Stimulates growth of skeleton and muscle
Prolactin (PRL)	Anterior pituitary	Breast	Stimulates milk production
Adrenocorticotropic hormone (ACTH)	Anterior pituitary	Adrenal cortex	Promotes adrenal steroid production
Thyroid-stimulating hormone (thyrotropin) (TSH)	Anterior pituitary	Thyroid gland	Promotes thyroid hormone production
Follicle-stimulating hormone (FSH)	Anterior pituitary	Gonads (in females, ovarian follicle cells; in males, Sertoli cells of testes)	Stimulates growth and development
Luteinizing hormone (LH)	Anterior pituitary	Gonads; ovarian follicle cells Leydig cells of testes	Triggers ovulation Stimulates testosterone production
Insulin	Pancreas—islets of Langerhans	Primarily liver, muscle, and fat	Regulates metabolism and blood glucose
Glucagon	Pancreas—islets of Langerhans	Primarily liver	Regulates metabolism and blood glucose
Somatostatin	Hypothalamus Pancreas—islets of Langerhans	Anterior pituitary Other cells of islets	Inhibits growth hormone secretion Regulates insulin and glucagon secretion
Glucocorticoids	Adrenal cortex	Primarily liver, muscle, and fat	Regulate metabolism
Aldosterone	Adrenal cortex	Kidney	Regulates sodium excretion
Epinephrine	Adrenal medulla	Cardiovascular system Muscle, liver, and fat	Stimulates cardiovascular function Regulates energy metabolism
Angiotensin II	Formed by conversion steps involving kidney, blood, and lung	Adrenal cortex	Stimulates aldosterone production
Atrial natriuretic factor (ANF)	Atrial wall of heart	Primarily kidney	Regulates sodium excretion
Thyroid hormones (T_3, T_4)	Thyroid gland	Many cell types	Regulate energy metabolism
Somatomedins			
Insulin-like growth factor I (IGF-I)	Primarily liver	Primarily bone	Promotes bone growth
Insulin-like growth factor II (IGF-II)	Primarily liver	Many tissues	Promotes tissue growth and repair
Parathyroid hormone (PTH)	Parathyroid glands	Bone, kidney	Regulates plasma calcium and phosphate
1,25 Dihydroxyvitamin D_3	Conversion in kidney from precursor formed in liver	Gastrointestinal tract; bone	Regulates plasma calcium and phosphate
Calcitonin (CT)	Parafollicular cells of thyroid gland	Bone	Regulates plasma calcium and phosphate
Gastrointestinal (GI) hormones	Various cells of the GI tract	GI tract; gallbladder and pancreas	Regulates digestive processes, including secretion and motility
Gastrin, secretin, cholecystokinin, gastric inhibitory peptide, and somatostatin			
Androgens	Primarily testes; also adrenal cortex	Reproductive tract	Stimulates growth and development
Estrogens	Ovaries and placenta	Reproductive tract; breasts	Stimulates growth and development
Progesterone	Ovaries and placenta	Uterus; breasts CNS	Promotes proper develpment and function Inhibits ovulation
Placental hormones	Placenta	Various reproductive tissues	Maintains pregnancy
Chorionic gonadotropin, chorionic somatomammotropin, estrogen, and progesterone			
Mullerian inhibitory factor (MIF)	Testes	Mullerian ducts	Causes regression of ducts in fetus
Inhibin	Testes	Hypothalamus and pituitary	Inhibits FSH secretion
Melatonin	Peneal gland	Reproductive system	Influences onset of sexual maturity
Erythropoietin	Kidney	Bone marrow	Stimulates red cell formation
Bradykinin	Kidney and other tissues	Blood vessels	Causes vasodilation

Reprinted by permission from Rhoades & Pflanzer. (1992).

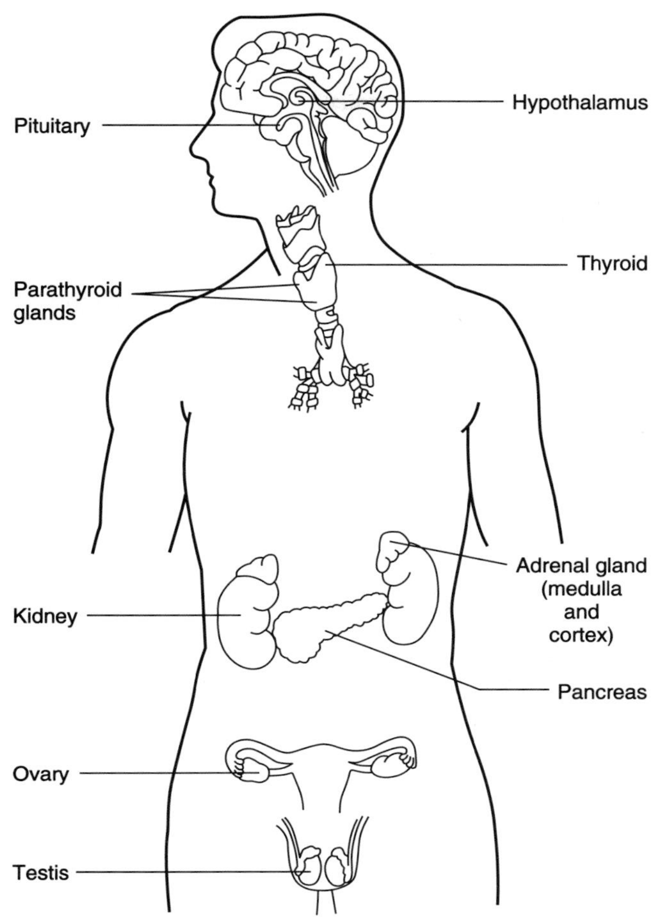

Figure 39–1. The anatomical location of the primary endocrine glands of the human body. *(Reproduced by permission from Rhoades & Pflanzer. [1992].)*

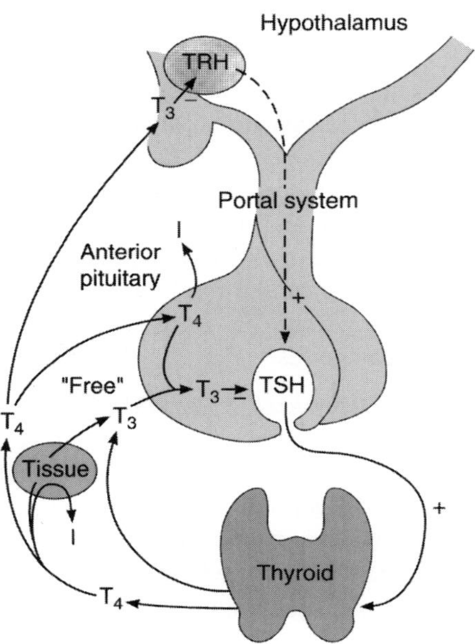

Figure 39–2. The hypothalamic-hypophysial-thyroid axis. (*From Greenspan.* [1997].)

nificance: growth hormone (GH), prolactin (PRL), adrenocorticotropic hormone (ACTH), thyroid-stimulating hormone (thyrotropin, TSH), follicle-stimulating hormone (FSH), and luteinizing hormone (LH). The posterior pituitary makes up the remaining 25% of pituitary size. It secretes arginine vasopressin (also called antidiuretic hormone, ADH, or AVP) and oxytocin (OT), which are synthesized in the hypothalamus and then are transported to the posterior pituitary and stalk.

Disorders of the anterior pituitary are fairly rare, and the ACNP should refer these to an endocrinologist for management. Two clinical syndromes of the posterior pituitary—diabetes insipidus (DI) and syndrome of inappropriate antidiuretic hormone (SIADH)—may be seen in hospitalized patients and, therefore are discussed here.

Diabetes Insipidus

Diabetes insipidus (DI) is a clinical syndrome characterized by excessive amounts of dilute urine, where 24-hour urine volume exceeds 50 ml/kg body weight, specific gravity is less than 1.010, and urine osmolality is less than 300 mOsm/kg (Robertson, 1995). The polyuria of DI is different from a solute diuresis, such as occurs in uncontrolled diabetes mellitus, by absence of glucose in the urine or normal solute excretion rate (Robertson, 1995).

Pathophysiology

Diabetes insipidus is characterized by impairment of renal conservation of water. It may be partial or complete, temporary or permanent.

There are four possible etiologies of DI. The most common cause is a deficiency of the antidiuretic hormone arginine vasopressin (AVP), and may be classified by different names that imply the same disorder—neurogenic, central, neurohypophyseal, pituitary, or cranial DI. This deficiency is usually due to destruction of the AVP-producing cells of the hypophysis (posterior pituitary). There needs to be a loss of approximately 75% of the AVP-producing cells before clinically significant polyuria develops. The most common cause is trauma, either postsurgical or postaccidental injury. Signs and symptoms of DI usually begin 12 to 24 hours posttrauma, but may occur later. Frequently this is a transient condition.

Nephrogenic DI is caused by renal resistence to AVP. This effects the renal collecting tubules where the kidney concentrates urine, with resultant decreased urinary concentration. Plasma AVP levels are usually normal or elevated. Nephrogenic DI can be caused by hypercalcemia, hypokalemia, drugs, and renal parenchymal disease.

Primary polydipsia refers to a decreased production of

AVP secondary to an increased intake of fluid. In this situation, there is no deficiency of AVP or resistance to AVP, such as occurs in the previously mentioned causes. Primary polydipsia may be caused by an abnormality of the thirst mechanism, called dipsogenic DI. Or this may occur due to a cognitive defect, as seen in severe psychosis. This is called psychogenic DI, and results from an irrational belief in the therapeutic value of excessive amounts of water.

Gestational DI is caused by the increased metabolism of AVP in pregnancy. Table 39–2 gives a list of causes of DI in each of these categories.

History and Physical Examination

Careful review of medical history is necessary to determine if DI is a potential problem. Clinically, many patients will not present with dehydration symptoms because they are able to keep up with oral fliud intake. In the comatose or otherwise restricted hospitalized patient, however, signs of intravascular volume depletion may occur (Bianco, 1996).

Laboratory and Diagnostic Tests

The first diagnostic step is to determine if a true polyuria exists, as evidenced by measurement of >50 mL/kg urine output in 24 hours. The next step is to determine if there is a solute diuresis, which would exclude the diagnosis of DI. Solute excretion rate is normal in DI. Normal solute excretion rate is up to 20 mOsm/kg. With solute diuresis, specific gravity is usually >1.010, urine osmolality is >400 mOsm/kg, and daily solute excretion may be >1400 mOsm/kg of solute per day. This can be determined by calculating the product of liters of urine output per 24 hours and urine osmolality in mOsm/kg. If the diuresis is due to solute diuresis from uncontrolled diabetes mellitus, the urine may contain glucose and ketones.

Once polyuria is determined and solute diuresis ruled out, then the cause of DI must be determined—neurogenic, nephrogenic, primary polyuria, or gestational. The acute care nurse practitioner should look at the patient history to determine if this is a setting in which DI can occur. An endocrine consult should be obtained for diagnosis and management of DI.

Sometimes the diagnosis is straightforward. For example, if the urine is not concentrated despite a high plasma osmolality (>295 mOsm/kg) or hypernatremia, primary polydipsia can be ruled out. The determination between neurogenic and nephrogenic can be made by administering a dose of AVP, either as aqueous AVP (Pitressin) or DDAVP (a synthetic analog of AVP). An improvement with AVP administration, exhibited as concentration of urine within 1 or 2 hours, is diagnostic of neurogenic DI. Lack of improvement is indicative of nephrogenic DI.

If there is inconclusive evidence of DI, such as occurs when fluid deprivation results in concentration of urine (>300 mOsm/kg), there may be a partial neurogenic, partial nephrogenic, or dipsogenic DI. The most accurate way to diagnose this is by measuring the plasma AVP level before and during a water deprivation test. Some endocrinologists will try a different approach, giving a clinical trial of DDAVP to differentiate between neurogenic and nephrogenic. A third approach is to obtain an MRI to determine whther the posterior pituitary "bright spot" can be seen. This is a normal finding, but may be absent in patients

TABLE 39–2. Pathogenesis of Diabetes Insipidus

- Neurophypophyseal
  - Acquired
    - Pituitary hypothalamic surgery
    - Head trauma
    - Neoplasms
      - Hypothalamic (craniopharyngioma, germinoma, meningioma)
      - Anterior pituitary (suprasellar, extension)
      - Metastatic (lung, breast, leukemia, lymphoma)
    - Granulomas (neurosarcoid, histiocytosis, xanthoma, disseminatum)
    - Infections (chronic meningitis, encephalitis)
    - Congenital malformations
    - Ischemia (shock)
    - Aneurysms (cavernous part of internal carotid)
    - Hematoma
    - Inflammation (lymphocytic infundibuloneurohypophysitis)
    - Chemical toxins (tetrodotoxin, snake venom)
    - ?Autoimmune
  - Genetic
    - Autosomal dominant (AVP-NPII gene)
  - Idiopathic
- Nephrogenic
  - Acquired
    - Drugs (methoxyflurane, demeclocycline, lithium, amphotericin B, aminoglycosides, cisplatin, rifampin, foscarnet)
    - Electrolyte (hypercalcemia, hypercalciuria, hypokalemia)
    - Obstruction
    - Vascular (sickle cell disease and trait)
    - Granuloma (sarcoid)
    - Neoplasm (sarcoma)
    - Infiltrative (amyloid)
  - Genetic
    - X-linked recessive (AVP_2-receptor gene)
    - Autosomal recessive (aquaporin II gene)
  - Idiopathic
- Psychogenic
  - Acquired
    - Schizophrenia
    - Mania
    - Neurosis (compulsive water drinking)
- Dipsogenic
  - Acquired
    - Granuloma (neurosarcoid)
    - Infection (tuberculous meningitis)
    - Autoimmune (multiple sclerosis)
    - Drugs (lithium, carbamazepine)
    - Head trauma
  - Genetic (?)
  - Idiopathic

AVP-NPII, arginine vasopressin–neurophysin II; AVP_2, arginine vasopressin 2.
Reprinted with permission from Robertson. (1995).

with neurogenic DI. This is prone to false–positives and false–negatives, however, and is not usually the approach of choice.

Once the type of DI is determined, the final step of diagnosis is to determine what caused the specific type of DI. For example, an MRI is helpful in determining cause of neurogenic or dipsogenic DI, attempting to locate a lesion of the pituitary or hypothalamus. Further disease causes should be diagnosed as deemed necessary for each individual case.

Management

The treatment of choice for neurogenic DI is the AVP analogue DDAVP (demopressin acetate). It is usually given via nasal spray at dosages of 0.1 mL (10 mcg) to 0.4 mL (40 mcg) daily in two or three divided doses. There is now an oral tablet form of DDAVP, which may be given instead of nasal spray at dosages of 0.1-0.8 mg/day in two divided doses. For hospitalized patients who are unable to take oral medication or use the nasal spray, there is a parenteral form of DDAVP. The usual dosage for DDAVP injection is 0.5 mL (2.0 mcg) to 1.0 mL (4.0 mcg) SC or IV in two divided doses. Side effects are few, but may include hyponatremia or water intoxication. DDAVP therapy is very expensive, which may prohibit the patient from taking the drug long-term.

Neurogenic DI, and particularly partial DI, can also be managed by administration of oral medications such as chlorpropamide, clofibrate, or carbamazepine. These drugs have the effect of either augmenting secretion of AVP or increasing renal sensitivity to AVP. Robertson (1995) considers the use of chlorpropamide, either alone or with hydrochlorothiazide, to be the safest and most effective choice.

Nephrogenic DI is treated with a low-sodium diet and administration of hydrochlorothiazide, amiloride, or indomethacin at standard doses. Thiazide diuretics paradoxically promote water reabsorption in the proximal tubules and reduce extracellular sodium. Amiloride is potassium sparing, and may enhance the effects of the thiazide diuretic. Indomethacin works by potentiating the action of AVP.

Primary polydipsia may be treated with small doses of DDAVP at bedtime to reduce nocturia, but since AVP production is normal in the patients, DDAVP cannot be used the same as in neurogenic DI due to the danger of water intoxication.

Gestational polydipsia may be treated only with DDAVP, given in the same dosage range as used in neurogenic DI.

In all cases of DI, the acute care nurse practitioner should carefully monitor electrolyte status and fluid balance, attempting to avoid dehydration or water intoxication.

Follow-Up

If DI has not resolved by the time of discharge, the patient should be referred to an endocrinologist for management of DI on an outpatient basis. Discharge instructions for ongoing treatment depend on the individual's DI etiology.

Syndrome of Inappropriate Antidiuretic Hormone

The syndrome of inappropriate secretion of antidiuretic hormone (SIADH) is a disorder characterized by hyponatremia and impaired water excretion in the absence of hypovolemia, hypotension, or a deficiency of cardiac, renal, thyroid, or adrenal function (Kovacs & Robertson, 1992). It is the most commonly recognized form of hyponatremia among hospitalized patients.

Pathophysiology

Most cases of SIADH are due to endogenous secretion of AVP. The following situations may cause this syndrome: (1) malignant tumors that cause ectopic production of ADH, particularly in oat-cell carcinoma of the lung, (2) disorders of the central nervous system that cause inappropriate AVP secretion, (3) pulmonary diseases, particularly acute respiratory failure with marked hypercapnia or hypoxia, (4) physiologic response to surgery may be an increase in AVP secretion, and (5) certain drugs. There is also an idiopathic form of SIADH that may be associated with an AVP leak regulatory defect (Kovacs & Robertson, 1992). Refer to Table 39–3 for a more complete list of disorders and conditions associated with SIADH.

History and Physical Examination

The history and physical examination should focus on manifestations of hyponatremia and hypoosmolemia. Symptoms of lethargy, muscle cramps, anorexia, nausea, and vomiting may be present initially, followed later by coma, convulsions, and the risk of death in the more advanced syndrome. Typically these patients do not have edema or signs of volume depletion.

Laboratory and Diagnostic Tests

To establish diagnosis, the practitioner should first document hyponatremia (plasma sodium <135 mmol/L) and hypoosmolality (plasma osmolality <280 mOsm/kg). If these are present, it should be determined that there is impaired urinary dilution (urine osmolality >100 mOsm/kg).

Next it should be determined that impaired urinary dilution is appropriate or inappropriate. Hypotension; hypovolemia; congestive heart failure; renal, adrenal, or thyroid insufficiency; nephrosis; cirrhosis; or other disorders that cause generalized edema should be ruled out because these conditions are managed differently.

Urinary sodium is typically >20 mmol/L/day in SIADH, although there are exceptions to this. To further clarify diagnosis, other laboratory tests may be helpful, such as plasma renin level, plasma urea, uric acid, and creatinine, which are normal or suppressed in SIADH. Plasma cortisol and TSH levels may help rule out adrenal or thyroid disease, respectively.

TABLE 39–3. Disorders and Conditions Associated with the Syndrome of Inappropriate Antidiuretic Hormone Secretion

1. Malignant tumors (AVP-producing)
   - Carcinoma (bronchogenic, duodenum, pancreas, prostatic)
   - Thymoma
   - Mesothelioma
   - Lymphoma
   - Ewing's sarcoma
2. Pulmonary diseases
   - Asthma
   - Pneumonia (viral, bacterial, or fungal)
   - Pneumothorax
   - Positive pressure breathing
   - Acute respiratory failure
   - Tuberculosis
3. Disorders of the central nervous system
   - Meningitis, encephalitis
   - Guillain-Barré syndrome
   - Head trauma
   - Cerebrovascular accidents
   - Brain abscess
   - Brain tumors (non-AVP producing)
   - Hydrocephalus
   - Neonatal hypoxia
   - Respiratory distress syndrome
   - Delirium tremens
   - Aplasia of corpus callosum
   - Acute intermittent porphyria
4. General Surgery
5. Drugs
   - Vasopressin
   - Desmopressin
   - Oxytocin
   - Vinca alkaloids
   - Cyclophosphamide
   - Carbamazepine
   - Clofibrate
   - Tricyclic antidepressants
   - Monoamine oxidase inhibitors

Reprinted with permission from Kovaes & Robertson. (1992).

Management

Management of the acutely ill hospitalized patient should be based on careful evaluation of fluid balance, such as hydration status, clinical picture, intake and output measurements, and plasma electrolytes. Hyponatremia is often caused by rapid administration of fluid in hospitalized patients.

The management of SIADH is based mostly on the degree and duration of hyponatremia. The goal is to reverse excessive fluid intake, replace sodium, and decrease AVP effects. If the hyponatremia is moderate, asymptomatic, and of some duration (>48 hours), conservative treatment is necessary, including significant fluid restriction (as little as 250 mL/day in many patients), and possibly increasing sodium intake. More severe cases of hyponatremia require emergency measures due to risk of cerebral edema, seizures, coma, and death. A 3% saline solution at a rate of 0.1 mL/kg per minute for 2 hours will raise plasma sodium almost 10 mmol/L safely (Kovacs & Robertson, 1992). Plasma sodium should be monitored frequently, and should not be allowed to rise above 25 mmol/L/day.

Once the emergency period is over, therapy may be slowed. If SIADH does not completely resolve, other drugs may be given that interfere with the renal AVP effect, such as demeclocycline or lithium carbonate. Drugs such as Florinef and salt tablets may also be given to raise sodium level, though these therapies may not work well.

Follow-Up

If the SIADH is not completely resolved, the patient should be followed by an endocrinologist after discharge. Fluid and medication instructions should be individualized to patient situation.

▶ THYROID DISORDERS

The thyroid gland controls the metabolism of the body. Thyroid hormone increases oxygen consumption in all tissues except the brain, testes, and spleen (Streff & Pachucki-Hyde, 1996).

Anatomically, the thyroid gland weighs 15 to 20 gms in the average adult. It consists of two lobes situated on either side of the trachea. An isthmus lies across the trachea below the cricoid, connecting the lobes (Fig. 39–3). Each lobe is approximately 2 to 3 cm in vertical diameter, and 1 cm in width (Safrit, 1992).

The thyroid gland consists of follicular cells that are filled with colloid. The follicles produce thyroglobulin, a glycoprotein-iodide compound. Thyroglobulin is then stored in the colloid material as precursor molecules for thyroid hormone. Follicle cells convert the thyroglobulin to thyroid hormone as needed. The thyroid gland stores enough thyroid hormone for 2 to 3 months of normal secretion.

Thyroglobulin is broken down into two active thyroid hormones: thyroxine (T4) and triiodothyronine (T3). T4 is the major hormone produced by the thyroid gland. T3 is more potent and shorter-acting. Only 20% of T3 is produced by the thyroid gland. The rest (80%) is produced by the conversion of T4 to T3 in the peripheral tissues. T3 then enters the nuclei of the target cells (Lasswell & Burman, 1995). Reverse T3 (rT3) is also formed as a homeostatic mechanism and has no biologic function.

Almost all of the thyroid hormone released from the thyroid gland (about 99.7%) is bound to plasma proteins in the serum. This acts as a reserve of thyroid hormone. More than 80% of the thyroid hormone is bound to thyroxine-binding globulin (TBG) and the rest is bound to prealbumin

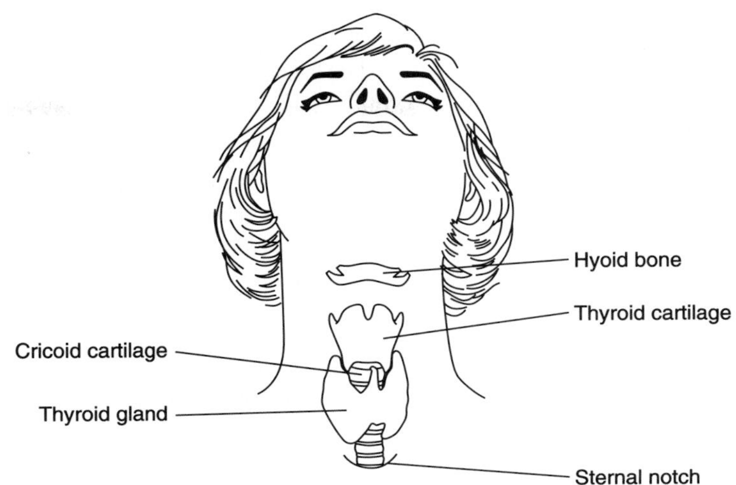

Figure 39–3. Landmarks for the anatomic location of the thyroid gland. *(Used with permission from Becker. [1985].)*

and albumin. The remaining small percentage of thyroid hormone circulates unbound in the plasma, as free T4 (FT4) or free T3 (FT3), the metabolically active hormones.

TBG levels are affected by different disease states. Low TBG may occur in chronic liver disease (inability to synthesize TBG), kidney disease (plasma protein loss), or due to use of certain medications (Table 39–4). High TBG may be caused by pregnancy, estrogen therapy, acute hepatitis, and AIDS in the later stages.

Under normal conditions, the hypothalamic–pituitary–thyroid system regulates thyroid hormone release. The hypothalamus secretes thyrotropin-releasing hormone (TRH), which is transported to the anterior pituitary, and stimulates release of thyroid-stimulating hormone (TSH). TSH is transported through the blood to the thyroid gland, where follicular cells cause breakdown of thyroglobulin to T4 and T3, and secretion into the blood.

A negative feedback mechanism occurs when T4 and T3 levels are high. TRH and TSH levels are then suppressed. Refer to Figure 39–2 for a diagram of this regulatory system.

Thyroid Function Tests and Other Diagnostic Tests

Thyroid function tests are laboratory tests that include measurement of T4 and T3, TSH, and T3 Resin Uptake (T3RU). The most sensitive and accurate measurements of thyroid function are third-generation TSH assays and assays for free T4 and free T3 (Lasswell & Burman, 1995). Major components of thyroid function tests are listed below.

Thyroid-Stimulating Hormone

Thyroid-stimulating hormone is thought to be the most sensitive indicator of thyroid function (Lasswell & Burman, 1995) and is, therefore, usually the single best screening test for thyroid disease. Elevated TSH is the first abnormal lab seen in primary hypothyroidism. Suppressed or undetectable TSH is the most sensitive test for primary hyperthyroidism. Newer third-generation TSH tests are highly sensitive, detecting TSH levels below 0.05 uU/mL.

Free T4 and Free T3

Measurement of Free T4 (FT4) and Free T3 (FT3) is done by equilibrium dialysis or direct assay. It is the most precise determination of the patient's true metabolic status, as it measures the metabolically active hormone, and thus metabolic activity. Changes in plasma protein concentrations do not affect the FT4 and FT3 circulating in the plasma. Figure 39–4 shows a scheme for evaluating thyroid status using TSH and FT4 levels.

Total T4 and Total T3

Total T4 and T3 levels are measured by radioimmunoassay. They are measurements of free thyroid hormone *and* protein-bound hormone, and thus may be affected by levels of plasma proteins that bind T4 and T3. For this reason, they are not so helpful as FT4 or FT3 levels for accurately accessing the amount of metabolically active hormone. If total T4 and T3 levels are used, the free thyroid hormone levels can be calculated by checking the T3RU and calculating the free thyroxine index (see below).

T3 Resin Uptake

T3 Resin Uptake (T3RU) evaluates binding proteins. A resin is added to the patient's serum sample, along with precisely quantitative amounts of radioactive T3. The patient's serum proteins (e.g., TBG, albumin, and prealbumin) and the resin compete for T3 at binding sites. If the patient's TBG is high, there are more binding sites on the plasma proteins and the radioactive T3 binds less to the resin (decreased T3RU). When the TBG is low, there are less plasma

TABLE 39–4. Effects of Some Drugs on Thyroid Hormone Tests[a]

Increase in Binding Protein Concentrations (↑ T_4 and T_3; N, ↑ FT_4; normal TSH) Estrogens Clofibrate Opiates (heroin, methadone) 5-Fluorouracil	**Inhibition of T_4 to T_3 Conversion** (↓ T_3; ↓, N, ↓ T_4 and FT_4; ↑ rT_3; N, ↑ TSH) Glucocorticoids Ipodate, iopanoic acid Propranolol Amiodarone Propylthiouracil
Decrease in Binding Protein Concentrations (↓ T_4 and T_3; normal FT_4, FT_3, TSH) Androgens Glucocorticoids Danazol L-Asparaginase Colestipol-niacin combination	**Increase in TSH Concentration** (↓, N T_4; ↓, N T_3) Iodine Lithium Dopamine antagonists Cimetidine
Inhibition of Binding to Transport Proteins (↓ T_4 and T_3; ↑, ↓ FT_4 and FT_3; N, ↓ TSH) Salicylates, salsalate Phenylbutazone Diphenylhydantoin Furosemide Sulfonylureas Diazepam Heparin Chloral hydrate Fenclofenac	**Decrease in TSH Concentration** (N, ↓ T_4; ↓ T_3; ↓ TSH) Glucocorticoids Dopamine agonists Somatostatin **Inhibition of GI Absorption of Exogenous Hormone** (↓ T_4 and FT_4; ↑ TSH) Cholestyramine Colestipol Soybean flour Iron sucralfate
Inhibition of Thyroid Function (↓ T_4 and T_3; ↓ FT_4; ↑ TSH) Iodine Lithium Sulfonylureas Interleukin-2	

↓, reduced serum level; N, no change; ↑, increased serum hormone level; T_3, triiodothyronine; T_4, thyroxine; FT_3, free T_3; FT_4, free T_4; TSH, thyrotropin (thyroid-stimulating hormone); rT_3, reverse T_3.
[a] Thyroid test results in parentheses indicate the types of changes reported. Not every test result is produced by every drug in a specific category.
Reprinted with permission from Sarkar & Becker. (1995).

protein-binding sites, and more radioactive T3 binds to the resin (increased T3RU).

When there is a protein-binding problem, such as occurs in nonthyroidal illness, T3RU and T4 move in opposite directions. In thyroid hormone disease states, the T3RU moves in the same direction as the thyroid hormone (e.g., decreased T4 and T3RU in hypothyroidism and increased T4 and T3RU in hyperthyroidism).

Free Thyroxine Index

Free thyroxine index is calculated by multiplying the total T4 by the T3RU. This gives as estimation of the FT4. It is not considered so reliable as FT4 measurement by equilibrium dialysis and should be relied on less, as newer techniques for measuring FT4 become more generally available.

Thyroid Antibodies

Elevated thyroid antibodies may be found in patients with autoimmune thyroid disease. Thyroid antibodies include (1) thyroglobulin antibody (Tg Ab), (2) thyroid peroxidase antibody (TPO Ab), formerly called microsomal antibody, and (3) TSH receptor antibody, either stimulating (TSH-R AB [stim]) or blocking (TSH-R Ab [block]) (Greenspan, 1997).

Tg Ab and TPO Ab are measured by hemagglutination, enzyme-linked immunoassay (ELISA), or radioimmunoassay (RIA). High Tg Ab and TPO Ab titers by RIA are found in 97% of patients with Graves' disease or Hashimoto's thyroiditis (Greenspan, 1997). Tg Ab is usually elevated early in the course of Hashimoto's thyroiditis, and decreases over time. TPO Ab is usually measureable over the patient's lifetime, although both antibody levels will decrease after T4 therapy is begun in hypothyroidism, and after antithyroid therapy is begun in Graves' disease.

A positive antibody test indicates only the presence of autoimmune thyroid disease. It does not differentiate the specific type of disease. Low antibody titers, for example, may be seen in subacute thyroiditis, nontoxic multinodular goiter, and thyroid carcinoma (Safrit, 1992).

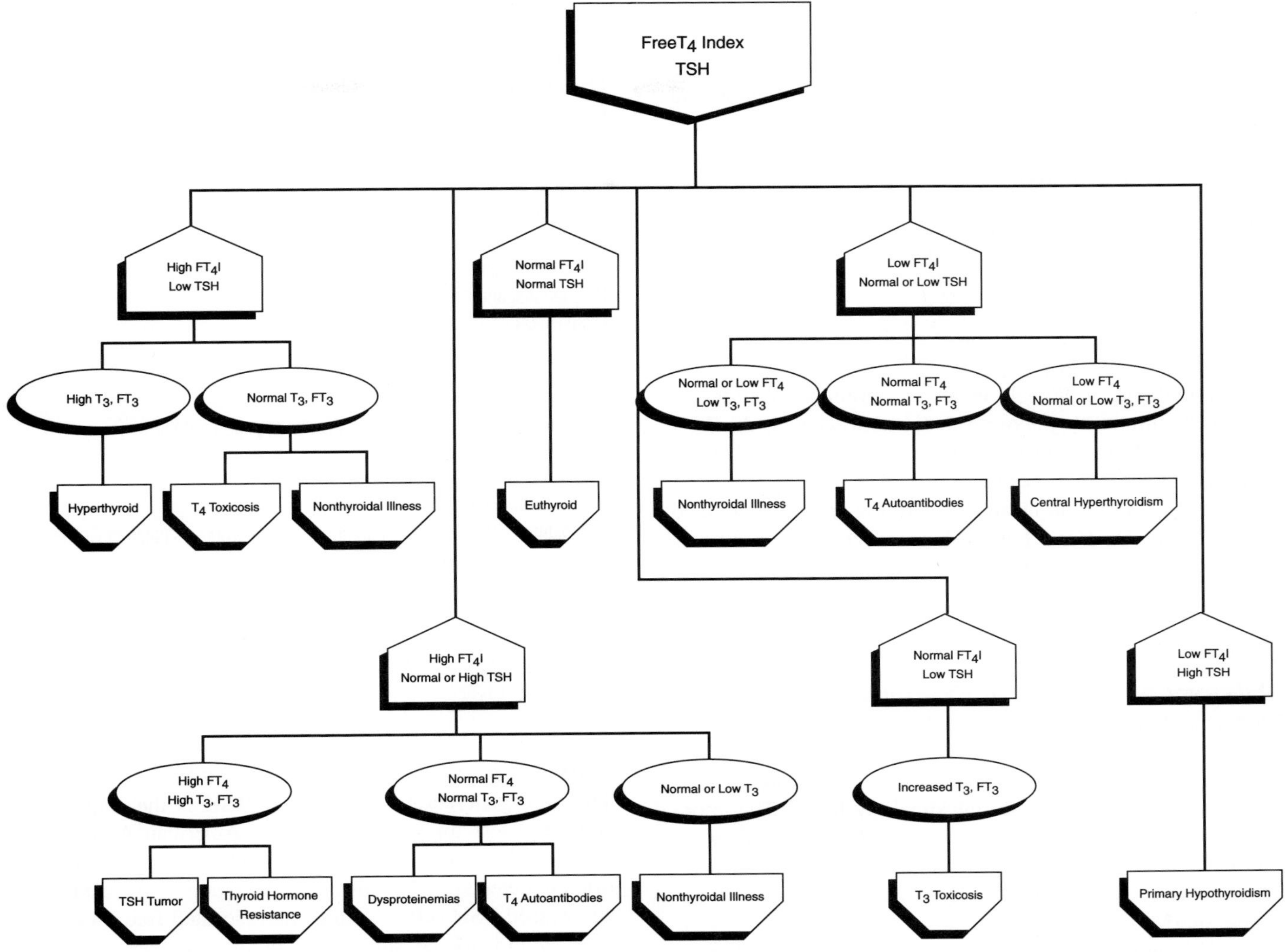

Figure 39–4. Scheme for evaluating thyroid status, using the free T4 index and a thyroid-stimulating hormone (TSH) level as screening tests. *(Used with permission from Becker. [1995].)*

TSH-R Ab (stim) is elevated in 90% of patients with Graves' disease and undetectable in healthy people or patients with Hashimoto's thyroiditis, nontoxic goiter, or toxic nodular goiter (Greenspan, 1997). It is most useful in diagnosing Graves' disease in patients who have ophthalmopathy with normal thyroid function tests.

TSH-R Ab (block) is less sensitive, but a newer test may be helpful in predicting congenital hypothyroidism in newborns of mothers with autoimmune thyroid disease. Only rarely is measurement of both of these TSH-R antibodies useful in clinical situations.

Radioactive Iodine Uptake

Radioactive iodine uptake (RAIU) is a test that measures percentage of a tracer dose of RAI taken up by the thyroid gland at a given time after oral ingestion of the RAI, usually 4 to 6 hours and again 24 hours after ingestion. Normal uptake is 5 to 15% at 5 hours and 10 to 30% at 24 hours (Safrit, 1992).

The major clinical use of RAIU testing occurs in hyperthyroid states. Uptake can be low, normal, or high in hypothyroid patients, and is therefore not helpful in diagnosis. There is increased uptake in Graves' disease, toxic adenoma, toxic multinodular goiter, or in early Hashimoto's thyroiditis. It is low in subacute thyroiditis, silent thyroiditis, with ectopic functioning thyroid tissue, and after exposure to large amounts of iodine (e.g., intravenous contrast).

Thyroid Scans

Thyroid scans use a radioisotope, either technetium Tc99m or radioactive iodine (^{123}I). Imaging is performed 4 and 24 hours after the isotope is given. This type of imaging is most useful in determining function of palpable nodules, pursuing occult thyroid lesions, determining location and size of functional thyroid tissue, and detecting metastases from differentiated thyroid cancer using ^{131}I (Sarkar & Becker, 1995). Previous administration of iodinated contrast radiographic dyes may depress thyroid uptake of isotope for 2 to 10 weeks, and must be considered before ordering this test. RAIU and thyroid scans are contraindicated in pregnancy due to the risk of harm to the developing fetal thyroid.

Hyperthyroidism

Hyperthyroidism is a state of hypersecretion of T4 and/or T3 thyroid hormones. Thyrotoxicosis is a clinical syndrome that results from the metabolic effects of this excess thyroid hormone (Wartofsky, 1996).

Graves' disease is the most common cause of hyperthyroidism, accounting for 60 to 90% of all cases (Schilling, 1997; Dillman, 1996). It is an autoimmune disorder in which the immune system produces antibodies to the TSH receptor. TSH receptor-stimulating antibodies (TSH-R Ab [stim]) are autoantibodies that bind to TSH receptors, stimulating excess thyroid hormone secretion and thyroid gland enlargement (goiter). Graves' disease occurs 5 to 6 times more often in females than males, and usually appears at ages 30 to 50 (Safrit, 1992).

Differential diagnoses of hyperthyroidism are listed in Table 39–5.

History and Physical Examinatioin

Signs and symptoms of hyperthyroidism are associated with increased metabolic effort, and may affect the central and autonomic nervous systems, as well as the cardiovascular, respiratory, and gastrointestinal systems. The more common presenting manifestations (Table 39–6) may be absent in the elderly patient, who may instead present with heart failure, isolated atrial tachyarrhythmias, apathy, or depression (Molitch, 1995).

The signs and symptoms specific to Graves' disease—exophthalmos, proptosis, clubbing, and pretibial myxedema—are felt to be due to autoimmune processes (Laswell & Burman, 1995).

A good history and physical examination should include measurement of weight, pulse rate and rhythm, blood pressure; thyroid palpation and auscultation; assessment for lymphedema, with particular attention to the eye; and neuromuscular, cardiovascular, and dermatologic exams.

TABLE 39–5. Differential Diagnoses of Hyperthyroidism

- Primary thyroid hyperfunction, such as Graves' disease, toxic multinodular goiter, or toxic adenoma
- Secondary thyroid hyperfunction, such as excessive TSH-secreting pituitary tumor, or trophoblastic hCG-secreting tumor
- Subacute thyroiditis, or chronic thyroiditis with transient thyrotoxicosis
- Exogenous iodine excess (such as administration of radiocontrast agents or drugs such as amiodarone) in patients with autonomously functioning thyroid tissue, such as seen in Graves' disease and nodular goiter
- Ectopic thyroid tissue such as struma ovarii or metastatic thyroid cancer
- Excess ingestion of thyroid hormone

TABLE 39–6. Manifestations of Hyperthyroidism

Diffuse thyroid enlargement with thyroid bruit (seen in Graves' disease)
Nervousness, anxiety, and/or irritability
Fine hand tremor, usually bilateral
Brisk deep tendon reflexes with decreased relaxation phase
Heat intolerance
Increased sweating
Fatigue (profound on exertion), muscle weakness
Weight loss despite increased appetite
Sleep disturbances, including insomnia and nightmares
Palpitations, angina pectoris
Dyspnea on exertion
Warm, moist skin
Fine and thin hair and nails, onycholysis
Emotional instability
Oligomenorrhea or menstrual irregularity, impaired fertility
Restlessness and mental disturbance
Increased bowel movements
Photophobia, blurred or double vision, tearing
Ophthalmopathy, including exophthalmos and proptosis (seen in Graves' disease), lid lag and stare
Acropachy (finger clubbing) and pretibial myxedema (seen in Graves' disease)
EKG changes—sinus tachycardia or atrial fibrillation (in 10-15% of all hyperthyroid patients, 25% in hyperthyroid patients >60 years old) (Coffland, 1993)

Laboratory and Diagnostic Tests

The third-generation, ultrasensitive TSH is the single best screening test for hyperthyroidism (American Association of Clinical Endocrinologists, 1995). TSH is suppressed, and often undetectable. Diagnosis can be made on the basis of a suppressed TSH (<0.1 uU/mL) and elevated free T4 (FT4). TSH would not be suppressed in the rare case of TSH-secreting pituitary tumor. Again, measurement of FT4 is preferable to total T4, T3RU, and FTI due to potential for interference from binding proteins with the latter method.

Graves' Disease. Diagnosis of Graves' disease is usually made on the basis of obvious clinical symptoms: diffuse goiter, ophthalmopathy, pretibial myxedema, and acropachy (rare), and confirmed with the findings of thyroid function tests and scans. Elderly patients, however, may appear with only minimal signs and symptoms, such as cardiac manifestations and weight loss. Thyroid function tests show suppressed TSH and elevated FT4. In some rare circumstances, where TSH is suppressed while FT4 is normal, FT3 or T3 radioimmunoassay should be performed. Such a situation occurs in the entity known as T3 toxicosis, and presentation is usually more of mild hyperthyroidism.

As previously mentioned, thyroid antibodies can be checked to confirm diagnosis of Graves' disease. These antibody tests are rarely needed, but can be done when there is uncertainty about the cause of hyperthyroidism. Measurement of TSH receptor stimulating as in pregnant women can also be useful in predicting neonatal thyrotoxicosis.

A thyroid scan is often necessary to differentiate between Graves' disease and thyroiditis or toxic nodular goiter. Uptake is diffuse, homogenous, and markedly elevated at 24 hours in Graves' disease. RAIU is used to determine radioactive iodine dosing for treatment.

Toxic Adenoma. Laboratory findings with a toxic adenoma, or "hot" nodule, are suppressed TSH and elevated FT4 or FT3. A thyroid scan shows a functioning nodule with the remaining tissue relatively or completely suppressed. RAIU may be normal or elevated.

Thyroiditis. Several types of thyroiditis cause a transient hyperthyroidism by causing follicular disruption that releases stored hormones. Subacute thyroiditis initially causes hyperthyroidism for 2 to 8 weeks, followed by a variable period of hypothyroidism. This type of thyroiditis is thought to be caused by a viral infection, and may present with a painful thyroid gland. Postpartum thyroiditis (also called painless, silent, or lymphocytic thyroiditis) may present with a transient thyrotoxicosis as well.

In thyroiditis, the serum T3:T4 ratio is often <20, in contrast to Graves' disease and toxic nodular goiter, where the serum T3:T4 ratio is generally >20 (Molitch, 1995). The hyperthyroid state results in negative feedback to the thyroid gland, where iodine uptake is blocked. This results in low uptake of radioactive tracers, a characteristic finding on thyroid scan which may help further in determining the cause of hyperthyroidism.

Rare Causes of Hyperthyroidism. TSH-secreting pituitary adenomas may be diagnosed by determining elevated FT4 and FT3 levels, with inappropriately elevated or normal TSH levels. A rare hereditary condition, isolated pituitary resistance to thyroid hormone may also produce the same thyroid function test abnormalities. Ectopic production of thyroid hormone may be caused by ovarian teratomas. Thyrotoxicosis can also occur in women with placental tumors (e.g., hydatiform mole or choriocarcinoma). The large amount of HCG secreted by these tumors activates the TSH receptor.

Management

Treatment options include antithyroid medications, radioactive iodine ablation, and surgical ablation. The cause of hyperthyroidism plays a critical role in electing treatment choice.

Antithyroid Medication. The thioamide antithyroid drugs propylthiouracil (PTU) and methimazole (Tapazole) inhibit production of thyroid hormone. They also have an immunosuppressive effect, reducing TSH receptor antibody concentrations. These drugs are most successful at inducing sustained remission of hyperthyroidism when given for (1) small goiter (<50 gm), (2) short disease duration (<6 months), and (3) no previous treatment failure on antithyroid drugs (Wartofsky, 1996).

Each drug has advantages. Methimazole is ten times more potent than PTU, and may be taken with less frequency than PTU, thereby possibly increasing compliance. PTU does not cross the placenta as readily as methimazole, and therefore is used in pregnant women. PTU is used in thyroid storm because of its ability to inhibit conversion of T4 to T3.

Dosage of methimazole begins at 30-60 mg/day in 1 to 2 doses; PTU begins at 300-600 mg/day in 3 to 4 doses. As the hyperthyroidism improves, the dosage is gradually tapered to 100-200 mg PTU/day or 10-20 mg of methimazole/day. Drugs are continued for 6 months to 2 years. They are stopped once the patient no longer needs treatment. Induced remission rates are more than 50% (Wartofsky, 1996), although without definitive treatment, the recurrence rate can be 60 to 70% within 1 year (Molitch, 1995).

Both drugs may cause mild allergic reactions such as skin rash and pruritis, for which an antihistamine may be given concomitantly (Wartofsky, 1996). Agranulocytosis occurs in a small percentage of patients (<0.5%). Although bone marrow suppression resulting in agranulocytosis is extremely rare, all patients taking antithyroid medications should have a complete blood count (CBC with differential) performed whenever they develop fevers or sore throat. The medication should be abruptly discontinued, and hospitalization arranged any time neutropenia is demonstrated.

Other Medications. Beta-blocking agents are used to reduce the adrenergic symptoms of hyperthyroidism, such as tremor, palpitations, tachycardia, benign arrhythmias, sweating, and nervousness. Propranolol in particular is preferred because it also blocks peripheral conversion of T4 to T3. Dosage is usually 10-40 mg every 6 hours. Atenolol is sometimes used because of its cardioselectivity and duration of activity.

Ipodate and iodine are also used in treating hyperthyroidism, usually only when symptoms are severe, such as occurs in thyroid storm. These drugs inhibit synthesis of thyroid hormone. They act rapidly, with dramatic reduction in thyroid hormone levels within 2 to 3 days. They must only be used with antithyroid medications (the thioamides) because the thyroid gland may escape the inhibitory effect of iodine, otherwise causing further hyperthyroidism. This type of iodine-induced thyrotoxicosis is difficult to treat (Burman, 1995).

Glucocorticoids are also used because they block the peripheral conversion of T4 to T3. They suppress inflammation in subacute thyroiditis, and have been used to treat amiodarone-induced thyrotoxicosis with thyroiditis (Bartalena et al., 1996).

Lithium carbonate is a third-line drug of choice. It blocks thyroid hormone release from the thyroid gland. Lithium lowers T4 levels by 30 to 50% in about 10 days, usually at doses of 600-900 mg/day (Burman, 1995).

Radioactive Iodine. Radioactive iodine is the most common initial treatment of Graves' disease once the acute hyperthyroid state has been successfully managed, and it is the treatment of choice for patients who relapse. It may also be used for treatment of an autonomously hyperfunctioning "hot" nodule or toxic multinodular goiter. It is contraindicated in pregnancy. The radioiodine causes destruction of the gland's ability to synthesize thyroid hormone. Dosage is calculated based on RAIU and size of gland.

Complications are due to the release of stored hormone for the initial 1 to 2 weeks after the radioiodine is given. In previously healthy individuals, this surge of hormone may be well tolerated with beta blockers and antithyroid medications. In patients with cardiovascular disease, patients should receive thioamides prior to radioiodine administration to deplete the gland of stored thyroid hormone, thus avoiding the risk of excess hyperthyroidism after treatment. Thioamine drugs should be discontinued for at least 5 days prior to RAI therapy to allow maximum uptake of RAI. Following treatment with radioactive iodine, most patients become hypothyroid and require lifelong hormone replacement therapy.

Surgery. Surgery is the first-choice therapy when the patient has a very large goiter (>100 gm) (Wartofsky, 1996). It also is used when the patient refuses RAI therapy or after failure of antithyroid medication. Surgery should also be the treatment of choice in patients with Graves' disease who have a "cold" nodule (possibly malignant). It should also be considered in some patients with an autonomously hyperfunctioning "hot" nodule or toxic multinodular goiter.

Whenever possible, patients are made euthyroid preoperatively with antithyroid medications. A near-total thyroidectomy is usually performed, leaving 5 to 10 gms of thyroid tissue. Such a surgery preserves the parathyroid glands and recurrent laryngeal nerve. It is crucial that a skilled and experienced surgeon perform this surgery to avoid inadvertent removal of the parathyroid glands and to prevent laryngeal nerve damage. When performed by a competent surgeon, the risk of permanent nerve damage is <1% (Burman, 1995).

Postoperatively, calcium is monitored while the patient is hospitalized to determine if calcium replacement is needed. When it occurs, hypocalcemia is usually transient, and it may not necessarily be the result of parathyroid damage or removal. Often it is due to depletion of serum calcium with increased deposition in bone ("hungry bone syndrome"), and may require temporary calcium supplementation (Burman, 1995).

Most patients become hypothyroid after the surgery, and require lifelong replacement therapy. Therapy usually begins 1 or 2 weeks postoperatively, with the specific timing of postoperative replacement dependent on frequent monitoring of thyroid function. Because TSH values can remain suppressed following prolonged hyperthyroidism even after surgery, serial measurements of FT4 should be used to guide decisions regarding the initiation of thyroid replacement.

Follow-Up

Patients who have undergone surgery and radioactive iodine ablation therapy will require follow-up appointments with an endocrinologist for monitoring of TSH levels and hormone replacement adjustments.

Thyroid Storm

Thyroid storm is a clinical state in which thyrotoxic effects surpass the patient's ability to maintain adequate metabolic, thermoregulatory, and cardiovascular compensatory mechanisms (Burch & Wartofsky, 1993). This condition is a true endocrine emergency that requires prompt aggressive treatment. When not managed appropriately, mortality is 50 to 60% (Wartofsky, 1996). Immediate referral to an endocrinologist should be made.

There are no clear criteria for determining when thyrotoxicosis becomes thyroid storm. Clinical presentation has been extremely variable, although the literature reports that many patients present with hyperthermia, marked tachycardia, and central nervous system dysfunction (Burch & Wartofsky, 1993). Perhaps more important, there is usually a precipitating event or concurrent illness. Thyroid surgery, withdrawal of antithyroid medication, RAI therapy, nonthyroidal surgery, infection, cerebrovascular accidents, and diabetic ketoacidosis are all examples of thyroid storm triggers.

Free T4 levels are significantly increased in thyroid storm, out of proportion to the elevation in total T4. This may be caused by interference in binding of thyroid hormone with binding proteins, and/or TBG deficiency (Wartofsky, 1996). Activation of the adrenergic system may also play a role.

Treatment includes the immediate administration of PTU or methimazole to block hormone synthesis, followed by inorganic iodine (potassium iodide solution or Lugol's solution) or ipodate to inhibit the release of T4 and T3 from the thyroid gland. PTU is usually the thioamide of choice because it inhibits peripheral conversion of T4 to T3. PTU and methimazole may be given per nasogastric tube or rectally in the comatose patient. Beta blockers, such as propranolol, are started immediately to decrease thyrotoxic effects on the cardiovascular system. They are usually given even in congestive heart failure. Propranolol is given either intravenously (0.5-1.0 mg, increased to 2-3 mg, repeated over several hours) or orally (60-80 mg every 4 hours) (Wartofsky, 1996). Glucocorticoids are frequently given to inhibit peripheral conversion of T4 to T3. Also important to treatment is control of hyperthermia, dehydration, and congestive heart failure.

Hypothyroidism

Hypothyroidism is caused by undersecretion of T4. It is fairly common, occurring in 2 to 3% of the population, with a female to male ratio of 10:1 (Haugen & Ridgway, 1995). It occurs more often with increasing age, affecting 5% of the population >60 years old (Smallridge, 1992).

The most common cause of hypothyroidism is Hashimoto's thyroiditis (chronic lymphocytic thyroiditis). In this autoimmune disease, autoantibodies are formed that react with thyroidal antigens. It is unclear whether these antibodies themselves are involved in the pathogenesis of the disease or whether they are merely disease markers. Lymphocytes infiltrate and destroy the thyroid gland. Hashimoto's thyroiditis has a genetic component, and it may be commonly associated with other autoimmune diseases such as diabetes mellitus.

Other causes of hypothyroidism include (1) postablative treatment, either with RAI or surgery, (2) external radiation to the neck, (3) infiltrative disease such as carcinoma, sarcoidosis, lymphoma, and amyloidosis, (4) subacute thyroiditis, (5) postpartum or "silent" thyroiditis, (6) drug-induced from antithyroid medication, amiodarone, or lithium administration, (7) central disorder such as pituitary or hypothalamic disease (called secondary hypothyroidism), and (8) iodine deficiency.

History and Physical Examination

The history and physical examination should focus on the possible manifestations of hypothyroidism listed in Table 39–7.

An EKG may show sinus bradycardia, low voltage, flattened T wave, prolonged QT interval, first-degree AV block, intraventricular conduction defects (Coffland, 1993). The patient should be carefully questioned about other autoimmune diseases in his or her medical history, as well as family history of thyroid disease.

TABLE 39–7. Manifestations of Hypothyroidism

Fatigue
Weight gain
Constipation
Dry skin
Yellow skin (due to increased levels of beta-carotene)
Cold intolerance
Memory or concentration impairment
Depression
Myalgias and joint aches
Coarse or thinning hair
Irregular or heavy menses and infertility
Hyperlipidemia
Goiter
Hoarseness
Delayed relaxation phase of deep tendon reflexes
Bradycardia
Hypothermia
Ataxia
Myxedema fluid infiltration of tissues—face, hands, legs

Laboratory and Diagnostic Tests

Laboratory diagnosis is based upon elevated TSH (>5 mLU/mL) and low FT4 in the otherwise healthy adult. As already mentioned, total T4 and T3 levels may be affected by binding proteins, and are therefore not the preferred method of testing.

Subclinical hypothyroidism is defined as an elevated TSH with normal FT4 (Molitch, 1995). It is suggested that thyroid antibodies (Tg Ab and TPO Ab) be checked to determine the presence of autoimmune thyroid disease. Thyroxine replacement therapy in this population has been shown to improve sense of well being, and to improve associated cardiac abnormalities and hyperlipidemia (Haugen & Ridgway, 1995).

During acute illness, however, diagnosis may require more effort. Acute nonthyroidal illness can cause suppressed T4 and T3 levels, as well as increased TSH during the recovery phase (Haugen & Ridgway, 1995). Severe illness may cause a low FT4. (See the section on euthyroid sick syndrome for further discussion.) The nurse practitioner should rely on assessment of clinical parameters in the setting of hypothyroid lab values. A reverse T3 (rT3) level is seldom necessary but may be helpful if lab tests are not definitive; rT3 is normal or increased in nonthyroidal illness and low in hypothyroidism. A referral for endocrine consult should be made for further evaluation any time a diagnosis remains in doubt.

Other laboratory abnormalities associated with hypothyroidism include hyperlipidemia (particularly increased LDL), hyponatremia, elevated skeletal muscle enzymes (CPK-MM and LDH), and microcytic, normocytic or macrocytic anemia.

Management

Synthetic levothyroxine (LT4) is the recommended treatment for primary hypothyroidism. It is preferred over desiccated thyroid and thyroglobulin, which give unpredictable serum thyroid hormone concentrations. Triiodothyronine (T3) is given only in special circumstances when potency is desired. Brand-name LT4 (Synthroid, Levothroid, Levoxyl) is preferred over generic LT4 because of bioavailability variance (Haugen & Ridgway, 1995), although more recent data casts doubt on this finding—the issue of generic levothyroxine remains controversial (Dong et al., 1997).

In an otherwise healthy adult, LT4 dosage should begin at 1.6 ug/kg/ideal body weight (usually 75-100 mcg/day in women and 100-150 mcg/day in men) (Mandel, Brent, & Larsen, 1993). Serum TSH level is usually sufficient for monitoring the effectiveness of LT4 therapy. FT4 may be checked if compliance issues are involved. TSH levels should be monitored periodically—every 2 to 3 months—until TSH is normal. Once normalization has occurred, patients should have a TSH level done annually (Shapiro & Surks, 1995). If TSH is not normal after 4 months, dosage can be increased in 25-mcg increments. Synthetic T4 has a half-life of approximately 1 week, and may take as long as 1 month to achieve a steady level (Streff & Pachucki-Hyde, 1996). TSH levels, therefore, should not be checked until at least 4 to 6 weeks after an adjustment is made. The goal is to maintain the TSH at 0.5-3.0 mU/L. If the TSH is lower than 0.5 mU/L, dosage should be decreased and rechecked in 2 to 3 months.

LT4 should be given at least 4 hours before or after medications that interfere with absorption of LT4. These include sucralfate, ferrous sulfate, cholestyramine, aluminum hydroxide, rifampin, and carbamazepine.

Patients over age 65 and patients with cardiac disease should be treated more cautiously with LT4, because of its potential effects on increasing myocardial oxygen demand. Initial dosage should begin as low as 25 mcg/day, and TSH levels checked every 8 weeks (Mandel, Brent, & Larsen, 1993). Dosage should be increased by 25 mcg every 8 weeks until TSH is normal. Literature reviews by Becker (1985) and Drucker & Burrow (1985) showed evidence that coronary artery bypass surgery may be safely performed in mild to moderately hypothyroid patients with atherosclerotic heart disease, but LT4 replacement therapy should be postponed until after surgery. The risks and benefits of cardiac surgery in severe hypothyroidism must be weighed on an individual basis.

Myxedema Coma

Myxedema coma is a severe form of hypothyroidism. Like thyroid storm, it is usually precipitated by an event such as infection, surgery, acute illness, drugs (particularly hypnotics or sedatives), trauma, neurologic disorders, or hypothermia. These underlying events must be properly diagnosed and treated. Patients with myxedema coma present with hypothermia, heart failure, fluid and electrolyte problems, hypoventilation, and coma. Distinction between myxedema coma and euthyroid sick patients in coma may be difficult.

This condition is an endocrine emergency, and should be referred to an endocrinologist. Mortality in myxedema coma is high. Treatment begins with intravenous LT4 at a dose of 300-500 ug, followed by 50-100 ug/day (Haugen & Ridgway, 1995). In some cases, LT3 may be administered to achieve prompt thyroid hormone effect.

Thyroid Nodules and Malignancy

Palpable thyroid nodules are common, affecting 4 to 7% of all adults (Molitch, 1995). They occur more often in women and the elderly. The challenge is to determine whether nodules are benign or malignant. Fewer than 10% of solitary thyroid nodules are malignant; however, those occurring in children or in males >60 years of age have a higher risk of malignancy (Singer et al., 1996). Thyroid nodules can by found in (1) thyroid carcinoma, (2) iodine deficiency (nodular goiters), (3) Hashimoto's thyroiditis, and (4) following radiation therapy to the neck (benign or malignant nodules) years to decades after exposure.

History and Physical Examination

History taking is useful but not conclusive in distinguishing between benign and malignant disorders. Table 39–8 lists factors that help distinguish benign from malignant thyroid disease (American Association of Clinical Endocrinologists, 1996).

The clinician should also ask about hoarseness, pain, dysphagia, and obstructive airway symptoms.

Physical examination should include palpation of the thyroid gland and surrounding lymph nodes, as well as assessment for tracheal deviation. Soft, smooth, mobile nodules or multinodular goiter without a dominant nodule favors benign disease. Firm, hard, irregular, and fixed nodules, and/or presence of cervical lymphadenopathy favors a diagnosis of malignancy. Malignancies are more commonly found in patients with a solitary (cold) nodule than in those patients with a multinodular goiter (Wartofsky & Ahmann, 1995).

Laboratory and Diagnostic Tests

Thyroid function tests are of little value in evaluating nodules. TSH and/or FT4 should be measured to determine presence of hypothyroidism or hyperthyroidism. The presence of hypo- or hyperfunction of the gland usually indicates benign disease (Molitch, 1995). Determination of thyroid antibodies may be helpful in diagnosing Hashimoto's thyroiditis, especially if the TSH is elevated. If there is a family history of thyroid medullary carcinoma, the patient should be referred for chromosome analysis since there is a specific oncogene associated with medullary carcinoma.

Fine-needle aspiration and biopsy (FNAB) of the nodule(s) is the main diagnostic tool to distinguish between benign and malignant disease. This is a safe, simple, and accurate test when performed by a skilled endocrinologist and interpreted by a skilled cytologist. FNAB can diagnose the following conditions: Hashimoto's thyroiditis, nodular goiter, subacute thyroiditis, papillary carcinoma, follicular carcinoma, medullary carcinoma, anaplastic carcinoma, malignant lymphoma, and carcinoma metastatic to the thyroid (American Association of Clinical Endocrinologists, 1996). FNAB has reduced the number of surgeries for thyroid exploration by 50% (Wartofsky & Ahmann, 1995).

TABLE 39–8. Distinguishing Features of Benign and Malignant Thyroid Disease

Favors Benign Disease	Favors Malignant Disease
Family history of Hashimoto's thyroiditis or autoimmune thyroid disease	History of external neck irradiation
Family history of benign thyroid nodule or goiter	Family history of multiple endocrine neoplasia (MEN) type IIA or IIB
Symptoms or signs of hyperthyroidism or hypothyroidism	Previous personal or family history of thyroid cancer

Although most endocrinologists advocate use of the FNAB for initial evaluation, the thyroid scan may also be helpful in (1) determining if a nodule in a hyperthyroid patient (Graves' disease or multinodular goiter) is functioning, or "hot," (2) determining whether a nodule found to be follicular neoplasm on FNAB is functioning, (3) determining functional status of nodules in a multinodular goiter, and (4) determining multinodularity, thyroid gland irregularity, or substernal extension of a nodule (Singer et al., 1996). "Hot" nodules are autonomously functioning thyroid nodules that take up more radioisotope. "Warm" nodules function like normal thyroid tissue. "Cold" nodules are either hypofunctioning or nonfunctioning, and are seen as defects on thyroid scan. Although most cold nodules are benign, malignant nodules usually do not take up radioisotope.

Thyroid ultrasonography is useful in differentiating solid and cystic lesions; or in determining multinodularity or monitoring the size of a malignancy. It is especially useful during FNAB to guide biopsy in situations where a nodule is not readily palpated. It may also be used to monitor nodule size serially when the patient is receiving suppression therapy with LT4.

Computerized tomography (CT) and magnetic resonance imaging (MRI) are not typically used for evaluation of thyroid nodules because of the increased cost without yielding significantly different results from the less expensive tests. They are helpful, however, when trying to determine extent of tracheal compression by a substernal goiter.

Management

Figure 39–5 outlines the treatment approach to the solitary thyroid nodule. If the FNAB results indicate a follicular neoplasm, a thyroid scan is helpful in determining whether the nodule is hyperfunctioning, or "hot." A "hot" nodule is almost never malignant. Treatment then focuses on whether the nodule is toxic (the patient is hyperthyroid) or nontoxic (euthyroid). Nontoxic nodules may be followed. Toxic nodules are usually treated with RAI or surgical removal.

If the nodule is benign, a 6-month trial of LT4 suppression therapy may be started. The theory is that by increasing the amount of thyroxine, growth of abnormal thyroid tissue is suppressed. There is controversy about the benefit of suppressive therapy, given its potential risk of cardiostimulatory effects and osteoporosis, although clinical experience has shown that thyroid nodules may shrink in as many as 50% of all patients on suppressive therapy (Molitch, 1995). Dosage of LT4 usually begins at 0.7 mcg/kg/day, and is adjusted upward by 0.025 mcg every 5 to 6 weeks until TSH suppression (0.5-1.0 mU/L) is achieved. Many clinicians choose to observe the nodule without treatment.

Management of nontoxic multinodular goiter may be followed the same as the solitary nodule, with several exceptions. LT4 suppression is not recommended in the elderly because of the risk of thyrotoxicosis from a subsequently appearing autonomous nodule. The goiter size and tracheal compression may necessitate surgical removal. RAI therapy may be used to reduce goiter size when surgery is not appropriate (Singer et al., 1996).

The malignant nodule is always treated by surgical removal. This may be done by lobectomy, near-total, or total thyroidectomy, depending on the situation and clinical preference. LT4 suppression therapy is given after surgery, if appropriate. RAI may be given to ablate any remaining tissue remnants after surgery. RAI may also be used as a pri-

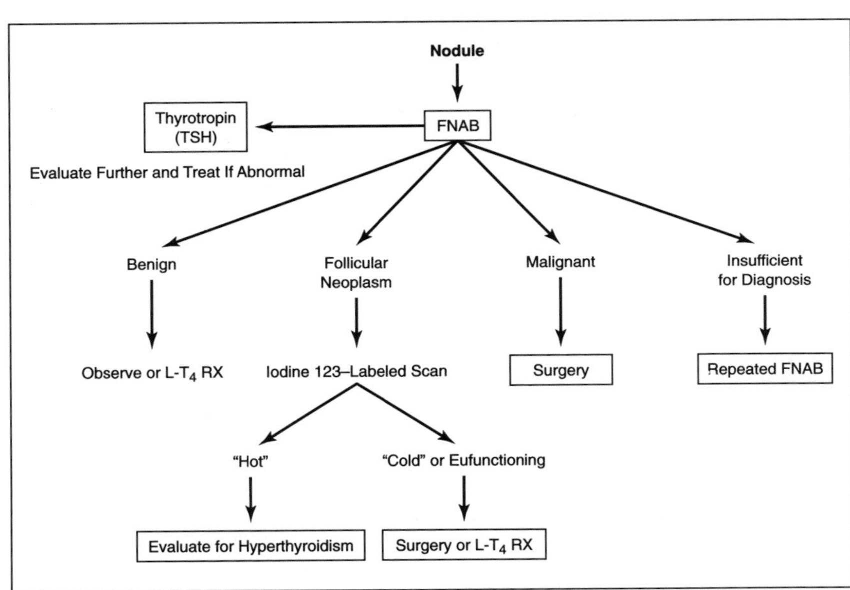

Figure 39–5. Suggested strategy for the management of the patient with a solitary thyroid nodule. *(Used with permission from Singer. et al. [1996].)*

mary choice of ablation if surgery is not appropriate. Chemotherapy has not been shown to be effective.

The four types of thyroid malignancy are papillary, follicular, medullary, and anaplastic. Papillary cancer is the most common, occurring in 75% of all malignancies (Singer et al., 1996). Prognosis is variable, depending on factors such as (1) age >50 at diagnosis, (2) tumor size, (3) extent of local invasion, (4) distant metastases, and (5) poor histologic differentiation (Molitch, 1995). Follicular cancer is found in 10% of all thyroid malignancies. Medullary cancer is found in 5 to 10% of all cases, anaplastic cancer in <1% of all cases, and thyroid lymphoma in 1 to 2% of all cases (Molitch, 1995).

Follow-Up

Follow-up after treatment for thyroid malignancy is individualized, depending on extent of the disease. Some clinicians perform a thyroid scan annually for 1 to 3 years after initial therapy, and RAI is given again if residual tissue or recurrent disease is found. Some clinicians withdraw LT4 and check a thyroglobulin level before determining need for a thyroid scan. Following surgery and radioactive iodine ablation, thyroglobulin levels should be undetectable, making this a useful marker for the presence of recurrent disease.

Nonthyroidal Illness Syndrome

Nonthyroidal illness syndrome (NTIS), or euthyroid sick syndrome, is the phenomenon of abnormal thyroid function tests in patients with nonthyroidal illness. It is a subject of much discussion, as distinguishing between true thyroid disease and NTIS is often difficult. It is important to obtain an endocrine consult for patients when diagnosis is unclear.

NTIS is seen fairly commonly in the acute care setting because it occurs in extremely ill patients, often those seen in the intensive care unit. It is caused by disturbances in the hypothalamic–pituitary–thyroid axis, thyroid hormone binding to serum proteins, tissue uptake of thyroid hormone, and/or thyroid hormone metabolism (Chopra, 1997). There may be decreased peripheral conversion of T4 to T3 in NTIS. Some factors contributing to altered thyroid function tests are listed in Figure 39–6.

The abnormalities seen in thyroid function tests most commonly are (1) low total T3 syndrome (seen in approximately 70% of hospitalized patients), (2) low total T3 and T4 syndrome, and (3) high T4 syndrome, as well as others (Chopra, 1997). The best measurements are ultrasensitive TSH, and FT3 and FT4 by equilibrium dialysis.

Low total T3 is frequently associated with low FT3. Low total T4 is likewise associated with low FT4. Low T4 in patients with NTIS is associated with poorer prognoses (Chopra, 1997; Slag et al., 1981).

These points may be helpful in differential diagnosis:

- For diagnosis of hyperthyroidism TSH is typically undetectable. In NTIS it is rarely undetectable.
- Primary hypothyroidism is the likely diagnosis when TSH >25 uU/mL. TSH is elevated in approximately 12% of patients with NTIS, but rarely >20 uU/mL (Chopra, 1997). Low FT4 in patients not receiving TSH-lowering drugs (dopamine, steroids, and anticonvulsants) suggests primary hypothyroidism. Look for signs of goiter and detection of thyroid autoantibodies, favoring a diagnosis of Hashimoto's thyroiditis.
- Reverse T3 (rT3) may be elevated in NTIS when TSH >10 uU/mL (Burmeister, 1995), and normal in primary hypothyroidism when the TSH >20 uU/mL.
- Low FT4 and low TSH may indicate NTIS, drug-induced lowered TSH, or true hypothalamic–pituitary disease, the later indicating need for a more comprehensive evaluation of pituitary function.

Treatment of NTIS is controversial, mainly because it is unclear as to whether patients with NTIS are clinically hypothyroid during concurrent illness or whether this is simply a physiologic adaptation to the acute illness. In one study, treatment with LT4 was not helpful (Brent & Hershman, 1986). Many studies have shown benefit from T3 replacement therapy (listed in Chopra, 1997).

▶ DIABETES MELLITUS

Diabetes mellitus is a clinical syndrome related to hyperglycemia and altered glucose metabolism. Its manifestations affect essentially all organs and tissues, resulting in neuropathy, retinopathy, nephropathy, and vascular disease. In the United States, 8 million adults have been diagnosed with diabetes mellitus, 90 to 95% of whom have noninsulin-dependent diabetes; an estimated 8 million persons meet diagnostic criteria for diabetes mellitus but remain undiagnosed (Roman & Harris, 1997). Diabetes is the seventh leading cause of disease-related death in the United States, with approximately 150,000 deaths per year (Fain, 1993). The American Diabetes Association (1996) estimates the total cost of diabetes in the U.S. exceeds $90 billion per year. In 1992, 40% of this amount ($37 billion) was spent on hospital care, with 26 million hospital days. With the prevalence of diabetes most likely to increase, there will be even greater numbers of diabetes-related hospitalizations in the future.

In 1979, the National Diabetes Data Group of the National Institutes of Health developed a classification system for diabetes mellitus that is endorsed by the World Health Organization. The Expert Committee on the Diagnosis and Classification of Diabetes Mellitus has recently revised these classifications (1997). Two common classifications are recognized: type 1 (formerly known as insulin-dependent diabetes mellitus or IDDM), and type 2 (formerly known as noninsulin-dependent diabetes mellitus or NIDDM). Type 1 diabetes is characterized by absolute in-

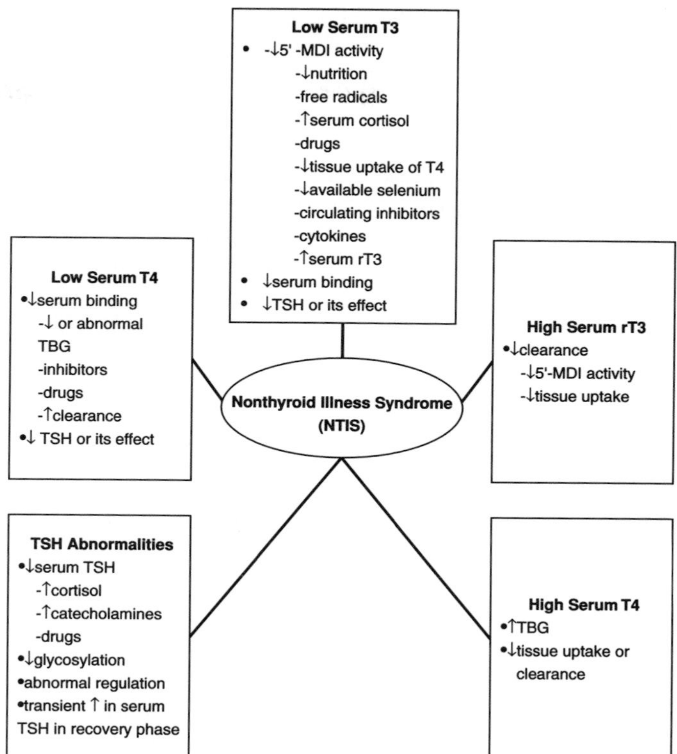

Figure 39–6. Some factors that may contribute to major abnormalities of NTIS. *(Used with permission from Chopra. [1997].)*

sulin deficiency due to autoimmune destruction of the pancreatic insulin-producing beta cells. Type 2 diabetes is characterized by reduced sensitivity to insulin (insulin resistance) and, in its later stages, by insulin deficiency. Table 39–9 lists the classifications of diabetes mellitus.

Pathophysiology of Hyperglycemia

Glucose is the principle carbohydrate used for energy production. Glucose breakdown (glycolysis) is promoted by insulin. Glucose can be used by the cells for energy or may by stored as glycogen in the liver and muscle.

Insulin is an anabolic hormone secreted by the beta cells of the pancreas. It promotes the synthesis of glycogen from glucose (glycogenesis), inhibits the opposite pathways that result in the breakdown of glycogen to glucose (glycogenolysis), and promotes synthesis of proteins and lipids. When insulin is absent, a *catabolic* state exists. This results in glycogenolysis, lipid breakdown (lipolysis), and protein breakdown (proteolysis). A byproduct of lipolysis is ketone formation; generally ketones are excreted through the kidneys, although they may accumulate in the blood.

In low-insulin states, glucose can be formed from noncarbohydrate sources (gluconeogenesis) such as amino acids and glycerol. Gluconeogenesis is stimulated by the following hormones: (1) glucagon, produced by the alpha cells of the pancreas, (2) epinephrine, produced by the adrenal medulla, (3) glucocorticoids, produced by the adrenal cortex, and (4) growth hormone (somatotropin), produced by the anterior pituitary. These four hormones are known as the counterregulatory hormones.

Hyperglycemia, therefore, can occur due to several reasons. Lack of insulin causes increased glycogenolysis and increased gluconeogenesis. There is decreased glycogenesis, as well as decreased glucose utilization by peripheral tissues after food ingestion (Peragallo-Dittko, Godley, & Meyer, 1993).

Pathophysiology of Type 1 Diabetes Mellitus

Type 1 diabetes mellitus is thought to be an autoimmune process that causes destruction of the beta cells of the pancreas. The typical sequence of destruction begins with a genetic susceptibility to the disease, particularly associated with the HLA-DR3 and HLA-DR4 alloantigens. Next, an environmental trigger event is thought to occur, possibly a viral infection. This is followed by an inflammatory response called insulitis, with infiltration of T-lymphocytes into the beta cells. The surface of the beta cell is altered, and is no longer recognized as self. Cytotoxic antibodies act with the immune response to cause beta-cell destruction, insulinopenia, and resultant diabetes (Foster, 1991). While the onset of type 1 diabetes may occur at any age, most cases occur in childhood or adolescence, with peak incidence around puberty. Onset is

TABLE 39–9. Etiologic Classification of Diabetes Mellitus

I. Type 1 diabetes[a] (β-cell destruction, usually leading to absolute insulin deficiency)
   A. Immune mediated
   B. Idiopathic
II. Type 2 diabetes[a] (may range from predominantly insulin resistance with relative insulin deficiency to a predominantly secretory defect with insulin resistance)
III. Other specific types
   A. Genetic defects of β-cell function
      1. Chromosome 12, HNF-1α (formerly MODY3)
      2. Chromosome 7, glucokinase (formerly MODY2)
      3. Chromosome 20, HNF-4α (formerly MODY1)
      4. Mitochondrial DNA
      5. Others
   B. Genetic defects in insulin action
      1. Type A insulin resistance
      2. Leprechaunism
      3. Rabson-Mendenhall syndrome
      4. Lipoatrophic diabetes
      5. Others
   C. Diseases of the exocrine pancreas
      1. Pancreatitis
      2. Trauma/pancreatectomy
      3. Neoplasia
      4. Cystic fibrosis
      5. Hemochromatosis
      6. Fibrocalculous pancreatopathy
      7. Others
   D. Endocrinopathies
      1. Acromegaly
      2. Cushing's syndrome
      3. Glucagonoma
      4. Pheochromocytoma
      5. Hyperthyroidism
      6. Somatostatinoma
      7. Aldosteronoma
      8. Others
   E. Drug- or chemical-induced
      1. Vacor
      2. Pentamidine
      3. Nicotinic acid
      4. Glucocorticoids
      5. Thyroid hormone
      6. Diazoxide
      7. β-adrenergic agonists
      8. Thiazides
      9. Dilantin
      10. α-Interferon
      11. Others
   F. Infections
      1. Congenital rubella
      2. Cytomegalovirus
      3. Others
   G. Uncommon forms of immune-mediated diabetes
      1. "Stiff-man" syndrome
      2. Anti-insulin receptor antibodies
      3. Others
   H. Other genetic syndromes sometimes associated with diabetes
      1. Down's syndrome
      2. Klinefelter's syndrome
      3. Turner's syndrome
      4. Wolfram's syndrome
      5. Friedreich's ataxia
      6. Huntington's chorea
      7. Lawrence Moon Beidel syndrome
      8. Myotonic dystrophy
      9. Porphyria
      10. Prader Willi syndrome
      11. Others
IV. Gestational diabetes mellitus (GDM)

[a] Patients with any form of diabetes may require insulin treatment at some stage of their disease. Such use of insulin does not, of itself, classify the patient.
Reprinted with permission from the American Diabetes Association. The Expert Committee on the Diagnosis and Classification of Diabetes Mellitus. (1997).

frequently abrupt, with signs and symptoms of insulin deficiency and ketosis (Fitzgerald, 1992). Common manifestations are acute weight loss, polyuria, polydipsia, polyphagia, weakness, and fatigue. Approximately 10% of all diabetics in the United States have type 1 diabetes.

Pathophysiology of Type 2 Diabetes Mellitus

The two pathophysiological events that hallmark type 2 diabetes are insulin resistance and impaired insulin secretion. There is debate about which event is the initial one that leads to glucose intolerance (Molitch, 1995), although insulin resistance appears to play the greater role. The beta cells are able to compensate for the insulin resistance to a point, but over years they lose this ability. There is evidence that glucose above normal range may be toxic to the beta cells, causing eventual beta-cell failure (Clement, 1995). When significant beta-cell function is lost, the disease progresses to a syndrome similar to type 1 diabetes. Type 2 diabetics are not prone to ketosis, except in cases of extreme physical stress.

Type 2 diabetes has a strong genetic component. There is a high prevalence of obesity, particularly truncal obesity, which is associated with insulin resistance. First symptoms may appear in mid to late life, and onset is typically gradual. Many people are diagnosed during routine exam and laboratory testing. Approximately 90% of all diabetics in the United States have type 2 diabetes.

Laboratory and Diagnostic Tests

The diagnosis of diabetes mellitus is made based on measurement of the fasting blood sugar. Normal fasting blood glucose is less than 115 mg/dL. The diagnosis of diabetes mellitus is established one of three ways. Each must be confirmed, on a subsequent day, by any one of the methods described in Table 39–10. These criteria have recently been revised (The Expert Committee on the Diagnosis and Classification of Diabetes Mellitus, 1997).

When a diabetic patient is admitted to the hospital, complete laboratory and diagnostic evaluation should be performed. Table 39–11 lists the components of a comprehensive evaluation.

An explanation of certain specific diabetes tests follows.

Glycosylated Hemoglobin (Hemoglobin A1C). This is the measurement of glucose attached to the hemoglobin A1 molecule during its lifespan of 120 days. It is felt to be directly proportionate to the level of blood glucose over the previous two to three months. Therefore, this is a test of long-term control. It provides information about adequacy of treatment or patient compliance to treatment, and accuracy of self-blood glucose monitoring (SBGM). It is not used as a diagnostic tool for diabetes. There are different assay methods used for measuring glycohemoglobin, so it is important to check the hospital laboratory's specific ranges. In general, values under 7% reflect good glycemic control, and values over 9% reflect poor control. Factors interfering with the hemoglobin molecule or lifespan, such as sickle cell anemia or iron deficiency anemia, give erroneous values. Likewise, HgbA1C is invalid after a transfusion. With good continuing diabetes care, HgbA1C is usually checked every 3 to 6 months.

Fructosamine. This assay measures glycosylated serum proteins. Since serum proteins have an average lifespan of 17 days, this test measures blood glucose control over the previous 1 to 3 weeks. Good control is reflected by a value of 2.5 mmol/L or less. Fructosamine is less commonly measured than HgbA1C. It is useful in determining very short-term changes in blood glucose control, such as might be necessary during pregnancy, where the test is most clinically useful. Conditions affecting fructosamine levels include pregnancy, nephrotic syndrome, thyroid dysfunction, hypoalbuminemia, and hyperglobinemia.

TABLE 39–10. Criteria for the Diagnosis of Diabetes Mellitus

1. Symptoms of diabetes plus casual plasma glucose concentration ≥ 200 mg/dL (11.1 mmol/l). Casual is defined as any time of day without regard to time since last meal. The classic symptoms of diabetes include polyuria, polydipsia, and unexplained weight loss.

or

2. FPG ≥ 126 mg/dL (7.0 mmol/l). Fasting is defined as no caloric intake for at least 8 h.

or

3. 2hPG ≥ 200 mg/dL during an OGTT. The test should be performed as described by WHO (2), using a glucose load containing the equivalent of 75-g anhydrous glucose dissolved in water.

In the absence of unequivocal hyperglycemia with acute metabolic decompensation, these criteria should be confirmed by repeat testing on a different day. The third measure oral glucose tolerence testing (OGTT) is not recommended for routine clinical use.

Reprinted with permission from American Diabetes Association. 1997. Diabetes Care, *20, 1190.*

TABLE 39–11. Components of a Comprehensive Diabetes Evaluation

Fasting plasma glucose
Glycosylated hemoglobin (HgbA1C); a fructosamine level is usually not necessary
Fasting lipid profile: total cholesterol, high-density lipoproteins (HDL), low-density lipoproteins (LDL), and triglycerides
Serum BUN, creatinine, and electrolytes
Urinalysis, with measurement of ketones, and microalbuminuria if testing is available
Urine culture if microscopic abnormality
Other cultures as appropriate
Thyroid function tests (TSH and FT4)
EKG

Based on the American Diabetes Association Clinical Practice Recommendations, 1997, and The American Association of Clinical Endocrinologists Guidelines for Management of Diabetes, 1995.

Microalbuminuria and Proteinuria. Normal albumin secretion from the kidneys ranges from 2.5-30 mg/24 hr. Microalbuminuria may detect early changes in renal function. This can be measured by several methods, including 24-hour urine, a "spot" urine specimen with albumin–creatinine ratio calculated, and urine microalbumin dipstick. Routine urine dipsticks do not detect albumin until significant proteinuria occurs. Diabetic patients with a urine albumin excretion rate of 30-300 mg/24 hrs are considered as having microalbuminura, whereas proteinuria is defined as urine albumin >300 mg/24 hr. Detection of microalbuminuria is important, as it can herald the onset of diabetic renal disease. It underscores the need for control of all factors affecting renal function.

History and Physical Examination

Since diabetes causes such vast systemic complications, a detailed history and physical exam during initial evalutaion is necessary to optimize treatment. Pertinent patient history specific to diabetes is listed in Table 39–12.

Physical exam should include data specific to the diabetic patient (Table 39–13).

Management

A multidisciplinary team approach is vital to the successful management of the hospitalized diabetic patient. This team should include an endocrinologist, primary-care providers, staff nurses, registered dietician, diabetes educator, social worker, and other consultants as needed. It is important to have all members of the team assembled upon admission to the hospital. This seems a basic point, but all too often goes neglected, especially when diabetes is not the focus of attention on admission. One recent study (Koproski, Pretto, &

TABLE 39–12. Pertinent History for the Diabetic Patient

What is the patient's chief complaint?
How long has the patient had diabetes?
What diabetes medications has patient used in the past?
What are the patient's current medications? If patient is on insulin, ask specifically about type(s), amount, and time(s) of administration. (See Table 39–19 for specific drugs affecting glucose control.)
Does the patient monitor blood glucose? How often? What type of blood glucose monitor does the patient have? Does patient have the most recent blood glucose values available?
Has the HgbA1C level been followed? What are the most recent levels?
How did the diabetes present at diagnosis? (e.g., polyuria, polydipsia, polyphagia, unexplained weight loss or gain)
Is there a family history of diabetes or other endocrine problems?
Does the patient have a history of gestational diabetes? Delivery of an infant weight > 9 lb? Toxemia? Stillbirth?
Are there currently signs/symptoms of hypo- or hyperglycemia? (e.g., polyuria, polydipsia, blurred vision)
Has the patient gained or lost weight recently?
What is the patient's nutritional status? Does the patient follow a specific diabetes diet, including snacks (for those patients taking insulin)?
Has the patient ever been hospitalized or undergone surgery? Any hospitalizations or emergency room visits for diabetes or its complications, such as hypoglycemia, diabetic ketoacidosis (DKA), or infection?
Does the patient have a history of hypoglycemic unawareness?
Are there any risk factors for diabetic complications—hypertension, history of smoking, lipid abnormalities?
Are there any symptoms of diabetic complications—ophthalmologic (retinopathy), neuropathy, nephropathy, vascular (cardiovascular, cerebrovascular, peripheral vascular), sexual dysfunction, and infections?
What type of diabetes education has the patient received in the past?
Are there any lifestyle or economic factors that influence management?

Poretsky, 1997) showed that diabetes team intervention appears to reduce hospital length of stay, improve glycemic control, and reduce the rate of recurrent hospitalization. Necessary education and adjustments to diabetes therapy by appropriate team members should begin early in the hospitalization to prevent unnecessary hospital days and to afford a timely discharge.

TABLE 39–13. The Physical Examination of the Diabetic Patient

Height and weight measurements
Vital signs, including orthostatic measurements
Assessment of hydration status—skin turgor, mucous membranes
Ophthalmoscopic exam
Thyroid palpation
Cardiac exam
Evaluation of pulses
Careful foot inspection
Skin exam—lipohypertrophy or lipoatrophy at previous insulin injection sites? Any rashes, breakdown, wounds, signs of infection?
Complete neurologic exam, with attention to reflexes, and vibratory, pinprick and light-touch sensations

Management issues will be discussed in two sections. The first covers basic diabetes management, with emphasis on the hospitalized patient. The second covers management of acute and chronic complications.

Management goals for the treatment of diabetes depend on the type of diabetes. Goals of treatment for type 1 and type 2 are listed in Table 39–14.

Education

One of the most important and underappreciated aspects of diabetes care is patient education. Many hospitals employ diabetes educators for this purpose. Prior to discharge from the hospital, a patient should receive education regarding the following:

- Weight management
- Nutrition principles and specific diet instructions
- Self-blood glucose monitoring (SBGM)
- Appropriate exercise
- Medications, including appropriate administration times and techniques

TABLE 39–14. Biochemical Indices of Metabolic Control in Diabetes

Type 1 Diabetes—level of treatment:
- Minimal (unacceptable under all normal circumstances)
  - -HbgA1C 11-13%
  - -Many self-monitored blood glucose (SMBG) values >300 mg/dL
  - -Intermittent ketonuria
  - -Mean blood glucose level >300 mg/dL
- Average (improvement should be attempted if the patient's clinical and personal situations permit)
  - -HbgA1C 8-9%
  - -Premeal SMBG 160-200 mg/dL
  - -Rare ketonuria
  - -Mean blood glucose level 160-240 mg/dL
- Intensive (desired, if possible to achieve without significant serious side effects)
  - -HbgA1C 6-7%
  - -Premeal SMBG 80-120 mg/dL
  - -Bedtime SMBG 100-140 mg/dL
  - -Essentially no ketonuria
  - -Mean blood glucose level 120-160 mg/dL

Type 2 Diabetes—suggested biochemical indices of metabolic control:
- Unacceptable
  - -Fasting blood glucose >200 mg/dL
  - -Postprandial blood glucose >235 mg/dL
  - -HbgA1C >9.0
- Improvement should be attempted
  - -Fasting blood glucose 140-200 mg/dL
  - -Postprandial blood glucose 180-235 mg/dL
  - -HgbA1C 7.5-9.0
- Acceptable
  - -Fasting blood glucose 80-140 mg/dL
  - -Postprandial blood glucose 100-180 mg/dL
  - -HgbA1C 6.4-7.8

Adapted with permission from Lebovitz. (1994). (pp. 1–2).

- Signs/symptoms of hypo- and hyperglycemia and treatment for each
- Sick-day rules
- Individualized goals of therapy, including limits of acceptable blood sugars and when to call the health-care practitioner

Diet

For the patient who is able to eat, an appropriate American Diabetes Association diet (or other diet as deemed appropriate by a registered dietician) should be ordered. To calculate caloric needs, one must first know the desired body weight (DBW) of the patient. Tables 39–15 and 39–16 show calculation of DBW and maintenance calories, respectively.

When a hospitalized diabetic patient is newly diagnosed, requires significant dietary changes, or needs review of current nutrition principles, a registered dietician should be consulted. Table 39–17 lists nutrition recommendations for people with diabetes. Refer to the section on surgery and procedures for management of the NPO patient.

Exercise

A carefully crafted exercise plan is an important part of outpatient management for most people with diabetes. Vigorous physical exercise is rarely part of the inpatient regimen, and thus is not discussed in detail here. However, a few points are important for the patient who participates in physical activity during hospitalization.

In nondiabetic individuals who exercise, plasma glucose levels remain fairly stable because of the body's ability to regulate increased glucose uptake by exercising muscles, and increased hepatic glucose production through the balancing of insulin and counterregulatory hormones—catecholamines, glucagon, growth hormone, and cortisol (Peragallo-Dittko et al., 1993). In diabetic individuals who are insulin-dependent, hypoglycemia is a major concern, since exogenous insulin may enhance glucose uptake in exercising muscle. This also may occur in individuals on sulfonylureas. Hypoglycemia may occur during exercise or several to many hours afterward.

In individuals with hyperglycemia and ketosis, exercise may exacerbate both. Because their insulin level in this case is too low, unopposed glucoregulatory hormones increase plasma glucose, free fatty acids, and ketones.

Hyperglycemia may occur with exercise in well-controlled diabetics, probably due to sympathetic stimulation (Peragallo-Dittko et al., 1993). One must also avoid precipitation or exacerbation of cardiovascular disease in a population at increased risk for angina, myocardial infarction, arrhythmia, or sudden death.

Benefits of exercise include lower blood glucose, improved insulin sensitivity, lower HgbA1C levels, improved lipid levels, cardiovascular conditioning, improvement in mild–moderate hypertension, and weight reduction (Horton, 1994). For those hospitalized patients who are considered for physical activitiy, the following guidelines may be of benefit:

- Avoid exercise in those with significant cardiovascular disease, retinopathy, or foot problems.
- Obtain an exercise stress test for patients >35 years old prior to initiating an exercise program.
- Begin exercise 60 to 90 minutes after a meal.
- Avoid exercise when insulin action is likely to be at its peak.
- Monitor blood glucose before and after exercise. Do not initiate exercise if blood glucose <60 mg/dL.
- Eat snacks as recommended by health-care provider. Consider this if the blood glucose is low before or after exercise, or if exercise occurs more than 2 hours after a meal.

Blood-Glucose Monitoring

Ideally, blood glucose should be monitored by fingerstick four times daily (before meals and at bedtime): (1) in the newly diagnosed diabetic, (2) during acute illness, (3) when

TABLE 39–16. Guidelines for Calculating Calorie Requirements

Age	Calorie Requirements
0–12 yr	1000 cal for 1st yr + 100 cal/yr over age 1 yr
12–15 yr	
Female	1500–2000 cal + cal/yr over age 12 yr
Male	2000–2500 cal + 200 cal/yr over age 12 yr
15–20 yr	
Female	13–15 cal/lb (29–33 kcal/kg) DBW
Male	15–18 cal/lb (33–40 kcal/kg) DBW
Adults	
Physically active	14–16 cal/lb (31–35 kcal/kg) DBW
Moderately active	12–14 cal/lb (26–31 kcal/kg) DBW
Sedentary	10–12 cal/lb (22–26 kcal/kg) DBW
Sedentary >55 yr, obese, and/or inactive	10 cal/lb (22 kcal/kg) DBW
Pregnancy	
DBW prepregnancy	$13.6\ cal \cdot lb^{-1} \cdot day^{-1}$ ($30\ cal \cdot kg^{-1} \cdot day^{-1}$)
>120% DBW prepregnancy	$10.9\ cal \cdot lb^{-1} \cdot day^{-1}$ ($24\ cal \cdot kg^{-1} \cdot day^{-1}$)
<90% DBW prepregnancy	$16.3–18.2\ cal \cdot lb^{-1} \cdot day^{-1}$ ($36–40\ cal \cdot kg^{-1} \cdot day^{-1}$)
Lactation	15–17 cal/lb (33–37 kcal/kg) DBW

DBW, desirable body weight.
2- to 4-lb weight gain; calories may be reduced slightly if obese, with early excessive weight gain, or with sedentary life-style.
Reprinted with permission from Daly. (1994). (p. 109).

TABLE 39–15. Estimation of Desirable Body Weight

Build	Women	Men
Small	−10%	−10%
Medium	100 lb for 1st 5 ft of height; 5 lb/inch for each inch >5 ft	106 lb for 1st 5 ft of height; 6 lb/inch for each inch >5 ft
Large	+10%	+10%

Consult growth grids for desirable body weight of children.
Reprinted with permission from Daly. (1994). (p. 98).

TABLE 39–17. Nutrition Recommendations for People with Diabetes

Calories • Sufficient to achieve and maintain reasonable body weight
Carbohydrates • Percentage of calories from carbohydrates can vary (many recommend 50% of calories/day) • Base amount on eating habits and glucose and lipid goals
Protein • Should be 10–20% of total caloric intake/day • With onset of nephropathy, restrict protein to adult recommended dietary allowance (0.8 gm/kg/day)
Fat • <10% of kcal/day from saturated fat • Percentage of calories from total fat can vary (many recommend <35% kcal/day) • Dietary cholesterol is <300 mg/day
Fiber • Same as general public (20–35 gm/day)
Alternative Sweeteners • Nutritive sweeteners (fructose, corn sweeteners, honey, hydrogenated starch hydrolysate) and nonnutritive sweeteners (aspartame, acesulfame K, saccharin) may be used in moderate amounts
Sodium • Avoid excessive amount (>400mg/single serving, >800mg/meal, >3000mg/day) • <2400mg/day for people with hypertension

Adapted with permission from Daly. (1994). (p. 109).

adjusting insulin therapy or oral medications, and (4) when the patient receives intensive insulin therapy. It is helpful to obtain a 3:00 A.M. fingerstick–blood glucose when there is a danger of nighttime hypoglycemia, such as when presupper NPH insulin dosage is increased. This intensive monitoring, called self–blood-glucose monitoring (SBGM), should be done for as long as necessary once discharged. If this is difficult for compliance reasons, patients may be instructed to check blood glucose at home one to two times daily, rotating times they test. For example, someone on fixed-dose BID Regular and NPH insulin may check glucose one day in the A.M. before breakfast and in the P.M. before dinner, the next day in the A.M. before breakfast and P.M. before bedtime, and the next day in the A.M. before breakfast and in the P.M. before lunch. Always ask patients to record these blood-glucose values. It is helpful if they bring these values with them if hospitalization is planned.

Some situations for hospitalized patients require changes from the usual monitoring times. For the patient who is NPO, blood glucose levels may be checked every 6 hours, with sliding-scale regular insulin coverage every 6 hours. Intravenous dextrose (D5W) should be administered. Refer to the section on enteral and parenteral nutrition for more on monitoring blood glucose in special situations.

Medication

Sulfonylureas. These oral hypoglycemic agents work by stimulating insulin release from the beta cells. It is generally felt that sulfonylureas have extrapancreatic effects—namely, reduced hepatic glucose production, increased cellular insulin receptors, and increased efficiency of insulin secretion (Lebovitz, 1994), although this point is controversial (Molitch, 1995).

Sulfonylureas should be started after diet therapy fails. Those who typically show good response to these agents are patients over 30 years of age who are normal weight or obese, with hyperglycemia <5 years, and are willing to maintain diet therapy. Individuals who have a fasting plasma glucose >250 mg/dL usually do not respond so well to oral therapy, and may require insulin for stabilization (Lebovitz, 1994). Sulfonylureas are contraindicated: (1) in pregnancy, (2) in patients with significant kidney or liver disease (because of reduced clearance and subsequent predisposition to hypoglycemia), (3) during acute illness or surgery, and (4) in patients with insulin deficiency (IDDM).

Second-generation sulfonylureas (glyburide, glipizide, and glimepiride) are the agents of choice in this category because of fewer side effects, a higher therapeutic index than first-generation agents, and lower effective dose (Maratos-Flier, 1995). The major side effect is hypoglycemia. Other side effects include nausea, vomiting, skin reactions, and hematologic reactions. Extreme care should be used in selecting an agent for elderly patients, in whom there is typically a 30 to 50% decrease in renal function and, therefore, a danger of profound hypoglycemia (Lun, 1993). Chlorpropamide should be avoided due to its long half-life of 72 hours. Table 39–18 lists all oral antidiabetic agents.

Initiate therapy using the lowest possible dose. Where possible, these agents should be administered 30 minutes before eating, to allow for an adequate plasma concentration of drug at the time the meal is eaten. Adjustments to dosing should be made every 4 to 7 days. Take into account the other medications that the patient takes, since a considerable number of drugs cause hypo- or hyperglycemia (Table 39–19).

Biguanides. Metformin (Glucophage) is the only biguanide approved in the United States for use as an antidiabetic agent for type 2 diabetics. Other biguanides have been associated with lactic acidosis, but the risk with appropriate administration of metformin is very small—0 to 0.084 cases/1000 patients (Bailey, 1992). Its mechanism of action is unclear, but it appears principally to decrease hepatic glucose production, and enhance insulin action in the peripheral tissues. It may also decrease gastrointestinal absorption of glucose. It does not stimulate insulin secretion, and, therefore, when used as monotherapy should not cause hypoglycemia. Treatment can be associated with a small

TABLE 39–18. Oral Antidiabetic Agents

Oral Antidiabetic Agent Type	Drug	Recommended Dosage	Half-life	Onset/ Duration	Comments
First-Generation Sulfonylureas	Tolbutamide (Orinase)	500–3000 mg/d in 2–3 divided doses	5.6 hr	Onset: 1 hr Duration: 6–12 hr	Limited clinical utility for all first-generation sulfonylureas
	Aceto-hexamide (Dymelor)	250–1500 mg/d in 2–3 divided doses	5 hr	Onset: 1 hr Duration: 10–14 hr	
	Tolazamide (Tolinase)	100–1000 mg/d in single or 2 divided doses	7 hr	Onset: 4–6 hr Duration: 10–14 hr	
	Chlorpropamide (Diabenese)	100–500 mg/d in single dose	35 hr	Onset: 1 hr Duration: 72 hr	Caution in kidney patients and elderly. May cause disulfiram-like reactions with alcohol, hyponatremia
Second-Generation Sulfonylureas	Glyburide (DiaBeta, Micronase, Glynase)	1.25–20 mg/d in single or 2 divided doses Glynase prestab: 0.75–12 mg/d in single or 2 divided doses	Biphasic Approx 10 hr	Onset: 1 hr Peak: 4 hr Duration: 24 hr	Increase in increments of 2.5 mg weekly Glynase prestab-increase in increments of 1.5 mg weekly
	Glipizide (Glucotrol, Glucatrol XL)	2.5–40 mg/d in single to 2 divided doses. Doses >15 mg should be given in divided doses XL: 5–20 mg/d in single dose	2–4 hr	Onset: 1 hr Peak: 1–3 hr Duration: 12–16 hr	Start at 2.5–5 mg Increase in increments of 2.5–5 mg every 3–5 days XL: increase by 5 mg every 1–2 weeks
	Glimepiride (Amaryl)	1–4 mg/d in single dose		Onset: 1 hr Peak: 2–3 hr Duration: 24 hr	Start at 1–2 mg Increase 1–2 mg every 1–2 weeks up to max 8 mg Take 30 min before first main meal daily
Biguanide	Metformin (Glucophage)	500–2500 mg/d in 2–3 divided doses	6 hr	Onset: 1 hr Peak: 2 hr Duration: 24 hr	Take with meals Hold for creatinine >1.4 in females and >1.5 in males Hold 48 hr pre-procedures Increase in increments on 1 tablet/week
Alpha-Glucosidase Inhibitor	Acarbose (Precose)	Pts <60 kg: 75–150 mg/d in 3 divided doses Pts >60 kg: 75–300 mg/d in 3 divided doses	2 hr	Onset: 30 min Peak: 1 hr Duration: no studies available on enzyme inhibition	Take with first bite of meals Increase by 25–50 mg every 4–8 wks based on 1hr postprandial glucose levels
Thiazolidinedione	Troglitazone (Rezulin)	200–600 mg/d	16–34 hr	Onset: Peak: 2–3 hr Duration:	Take with food. Increase by 200 mg every 2–4 weeks

weight loss (several kilograms). Studies have shown metformin decreases cholesterol and triglyceride levels (Barzilai, 1995).

Metformin is useful in treating the syndrome of insulin resistance, and is particularly useful in treating obese type 2 patients. It may be used alone or in combination with sulfonylureas. It is contraindicated in patients who have a potential to develop lactic acidosis, such as those with liver disease, kidney disease, alcoholism, and cardiopulmonary insufficiency. Therefore it should not be used when the serum creatinine is greater than 1.4 mg/dL in females and greater than 1.5 mg/dL in males. Metformin is absolutely contraindicated in pregnancy.

In the acute setting, metformin must be held 48 hours before surgery or procedures that increase risk of kidney or liver impairment, such as when contrast dye is to be given. It is restarted when the danger of acute illness and potential for lactic acidosis diminishes (many times a judgment call, but usually at least 48 hours postprocedure).

Side effects are mostly gastrointestinal: nausea, vomiting, abdominal discomfort, and diarrhea. This occurs in approximately 20% of all patients, and is usually transient,

TABLE 39–19. Drugs Associated with Hypoglycemia and Hyperglycemia

Drug	Mechanism of Action	Clinical Significance
Drugs Associated with Hypoglycemia: Mechanisms of Action and Relative Clinical Significance		
Alcohol	Impairs gluconeogenesis and increases insulin secretion	+++
Anabolic steroids	Unknown	+
Beta-adrenergic antagonists	Inhibit glycogenolysis; attenuate signs and symptoms of hypoglycemia	++
Dicumarol	Inhibits hepatic clearance of tolbutamide (Orinase) and chlorpropamide (Diabinese)	++
Chloramphenicol (Chloromycetin)	May inhibit metabolism of sulfonylureas	++
Chloroquine (Aralen)	Unknown	++
Clofibrate (Atromid-S)	Unknown	+
Disopyramide (Norpace)	Unknown	++
Pentamidine isethionate (NebuPent, Pentam 300)	Causes cytolytic response in pancreas accompanied by release of insulin	+++
Phenylbutazone (Azolid, Butazolidin)	Reduces clearance of sulfonylureas	++
Salicylates	Increase insulin secretion and sensitivity; may alter pharmacokinetic disposition of sulfonylureas	++
Sulfonamides	Alter clearance of sulfonylureas	+
Drugs Associated with Hyperglycemia: Mechanisms of Action and Relative Clinical Significance		
Alcohol	Chronic ingestion increases metabolism of tolbutamide (Orinase)	+
Asparginase (Elspar)	May be related to inhibition of insulin synthesis	++ (diabetic ketoacidosis has been reported)
Beta-adrenergic antagonists	Inhibit insulin secretion	++
Calcium channel antagonists	Inhibit insulin secretion	+/–
Combination oral contraceptives	Unknown	++
Diazoxide (Hyperstat IV, Proglycem)	Inhibits insulin secretion	+++
Diuretics	May be related to hypokalemia	++
Glucocorticoids	Increase gluconeogenesis; depress insulin action	+++
Glycerol	Unknown	++ (hyperglycemic hyperosmolar nonketotic coma has been reported)
Lithium salts (Eskalith, Lithane, Lithobid)	May decrease insulin secretion	+
Niacin	Unknown	++
Pentamidine isethionate (NebuPent, Pentam 300)	Promotes pancreatic toxicity	+++
Phenytoin sodium (Dilantin)	Inhibits insulin secretion	++
Rifampin (Rifadin, Rimactane)	Enhances metabolism of tolbutamide	+
Sympathomimetics	Increase glycogenolysis and gluconeogenesis	++

Reprinted with permission from White, Hartman & Campbell. (1993).

subsiding within weeks of initiation. For this reason, administering with meals and at the lowest possible dose can minimize these gastrointestinal effects. Metformin is started at 500 mg BID. Dosage adjustment may be made at weekly intervals. Refer to Table 39–18 for dosage range.

Thiazolidinediones. Troglitazone (Rezulin) has been approved as an antidiabetic agent for type 2 diabetes either as monotherapy, or in combination with insulin or sulfonylureas. It belongs to a new class of drugs called thiazolidinediones. Troglitazone works by decreasing insulin resistance through reduction of hepatic glucose production, and by increasing glucose uptake by skeletal muscle, liver, and adipose tissue (Teter, 1997). Mechanism of action is felt to be facilitated through binding to peroxisome proliferator-activated receptors, regulating transcription of insulin-responsive genes necessary for glucose and lipid metabolism (Saltiel & Olefsky, 1996).

Recommended starting dose is 200 mg once daily with food, which increases absorption. Peak effects are seen within 2 to 3 hours, and half-life is 16 to 34 hours. Dosage may be increased in 200-mg increments in 2 to 4 weeks up to 600 mg once daily if there is no improvement in glycemic control (Teter, 1996). Current insulin dosage should be continued when troglitazone is started, and should be decreased by 10 to 25% when the fasting plasma glucose concentration falls below 120 mg/dL (Teter, 1996).

Troglitazone is excreted in the feces and only slightly in urine; therefore, adjustment for renal dysfunction is not necessary. Caution is advised in hepatic disease, since reversible elevations of AST and ALT have been found in 2.2% of patients (Teter, 1996). Troglitazone has an extremely favorable side effect profile and is generally well tolerated.

Alpha-Glucosidase Inhibitors. Acarbose (Precose) is approved as an antidiabetic agent for type 2 diabetes. Acarbose works by inhibiting intestinal brush border alpha-glucosidases that are required for breakdown of starches, dextrins, maltose, and sucrose into absorbable monosaccharides. This delays digestion and absorption of intestinal carbohydrates, and lowers postprandial serum insulin levels (Hollander et al., 1997).

Recommended starting dose is 25 mg three times daily with the first bite of a meal. Dosage may be increased every 4 to 8 weeks based on 1-hour postprandial blood glucose levels. Maximum dosage for patients <60 kg is 50 mg TID, and for patients >60 kg is 100 mg TID.

Mild to moderate hypoglycemia should be treated by oral glucose (dextrose) instead of sucrose (cane sugar) because acarbose inhibits absorption of sucrose. Severe hypoglycemia is treated with IV glucose or IM Glucagen.

Side effects are usually gastrointestinal. Acarbose may increase serum transaminases, and therefore it is recommended to check these levels every 3 months for the first year and periodically thereafter.

Insulin. The approach to giving insulin differs between type 1 and type 2 diabetes. As long as you understand the pathophysiological process behind diabetes, you will be able to guide the insulin therapy appropriately.

It is important to understand that insulin secretion in the nondiabetic individual has two characteristics. The first is that the pancreas produces a basal amount of insulin at all times. The second is that the pancreas secretes extra insulin in response to a carbohydrate load (i.e., after eating). This pattern should govern replacement therapy, and medication should mimic this normal physiologic insulin response (Fig. 39–7).

Human insulin or the newer insulin analogue lispro are the best choices for insulin replacement because they are the least antigenic. Table 39–20 gives a list of available insulins, along with drug duration and peak times.

Type 2 Diabetes. As you remember, type 2 diabetes is caused by the pancreas's inability to produce enough in-

TABLE 39–20. Types of Insulin

Insulin Type	Onset/Peak/Duration
Rapid-acting insulin	Onset: 15 min–1hr
Humalog (Lispro)	Peak: 30–90 min
	Duration: 4–6 hr
Short-acting insulin	Onset: 30 min
Human Regular	Peak: 2–5 hr
Humulin R	Duration: 5–8 hr
Novolin R	
Velosulin BR Human Insulin	
Animal Regular	
Regular Iletin I (beef/pork)	
Regular Iletin II, 100 units (pork)	
Regular Iletin II, 500 units (pork)	
Pruified Pork Regular Insulin	
Intermediate-acting insulin	Onset: 1–3 hr
Human	Peak: 6–12 hr
Humulin L (Lente)	Duration: 16–24 hr
Humulin N (NPH)	
Novolin L (Lente)	
Novolin N (NPH)	
Animal	
Iletin I NPH (beef/pork)	
Iletin I Lente (beef/pork)	
Lente (beef)	
NPH (beef)	
Iletin II Lente (pork)	
Iletin II NPH (pork)	
Purified Pork Lente	
Purified Pork NPH	
Long-acting insulin	Onset: 4–6 hr
Human	Peak: 8–20 hr
Humulin U	Duration: 24–28 hr
Animal	
Ultralente	
Fixed Combinations	Onset: 30 min
Human	Peak: 7–12 hr
Humulin 70/30	Duration: 16–24 hr
Novolin 70/30	
Humulin 50/50	

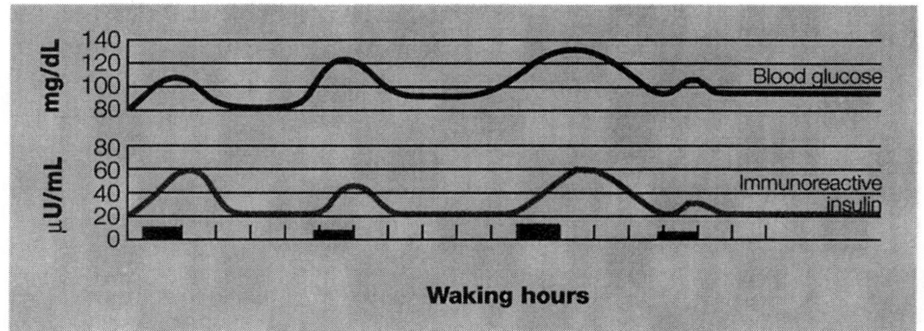

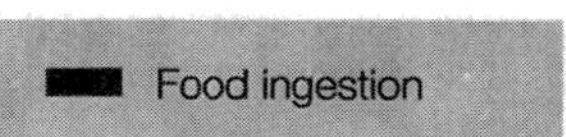

Figure 39–7. Patterns of blood glucose levels and immunoreactive insulin levels (insulin secretion) in person who does not have diabetes. *(From Beaser. [1993].)*

sulin to overcome insulin resistance. At least 25% of type 2 diabetics are unable to secrete enough insulin for diet and oral agents to be effective, and require exogenous insulin replacement (Beaser, 1992). Knowing when to give insulin in a type 2 diabetic patient is a major factor in achieving good glycemic control. (Refer to Table 39–3 for goals of therapy.) Several factors that are important for determining when to use insulin in the type 2 patient are:

- Does the patient remain hyperglycemic despite maximum dose of oral antidiabetic agents?
- Is this an acute, self-limiting event such as surgery or severe stress-induced hyperglycemia, or is oral antidiabetic therapy contraindicated, such as in pregnancy or renal disease?
- Is the patient allergic to oral antidiabetic agents, particularly sulfa-containing drugs?

Insulin therapy may be needed only temporarily to overcome glucose toxicity and regain blood-glucose control. Intensive insulin therapy may be needed to overcome insulin resistance.

Once glycemic control is attained, beta-cell function and peripheral glucose uptake may improve enough to decrease insulin requirements. In the patient with type 2 diabetes, when insulin requirements decrease to 0.3-0.4 units/kg/day, it is reasonable to consider switching to an oral agent (Skyler, 1997).

Mild diabetes (fasting blood glucose <140 mg/dL) is treated by diet and exercise. If this fails, an oral agent such as a sulfonylurea or metformin is used. Mild type 2 diabetics rarely need insulin.

Moderate diabetes (fasting blood glucose 140-200 mg/dL) is treated by pharmacologic therapy along with diet and exercise. Several approaches may be used. Often, only an oral antidiabetic agent is needed. Insulin therapy may also be used, and basal insulin therapy is usually enough. This means using intermediate or long-acting insulin to mimic the body's basal insulin secretion. Usual dosage is 0.3-0.6 units/kg/day. This may be done several ways in the hospitalized patient (Table 39–21)

Severe diabetes (fasting blood glucose >250 mg/dL) requires multiple insulin injections. Insulin dosage is usually between 0.5 and 1.2 units/kg/day. If the patient is very insulin resistant, they may require >1.5 units/kg/day. These patients require basal insulin coverage, and most require short-acting insulin (regular or lispro) for mealtime coverage (Table 39–22).

Very severe diabetes (fasting blood glucose >250-300 mg/dL) usually coincides with loss of beta-cell function and insulin deficiency. It is therefore treated like type I diabetes, and insulin therapy is covered in the next section.

Combination therapy is the choice of many practitioners. "BIDS" therapy (bedtime insulin–daytime sulfonylurea) is common, and was mentioned earlier. Others have used metformin with insulin in both types 1 and 2 diabetics, with the idea of decreasing hepatic glucose production and improving insulin action, thereby reducing insulin requirements. Study results have been mixed (Skyler, 1997). The sulfonylurea–metformin combination may be used when patients do not achieve desired glycemic control on maximum dose of a sulfonylurea agent. Studies are underway to determine effectiveness of acarbose–insulin and thiozolidinedione–insulin therapy (Skyler, 1997). One recent study reports that the acarbose–insulin combination therapy in type 1 diabetics demonstrated significantly decreased postprandial glucose and HgbA1C with no increase in the incidence of hypoglycemia (Hollander, Pi-Sunyer, & Coniff, 1997).

Type 1 Diabetes. Physiologic insulin replacement is extremely important in type 1 diabetes, since insulin-secreting capacity is gone. Replacement may be accomplished by what is termed either conventional or intensive insulin therapy. Refer to Table 39–14 for goals of therapy.

Dosing should begin at 0.5-1.0 units/kg/day. In a newly diagnosed type 1 diabetic, insulin requirements may decrease initially (<0.5 units/kg/day) because of the remission phase, or "honeymoon period." This is a period after initial diagnosis when beta cells continue to produce some insulin. The phase is variable in duration, but usually lasts several weeks.

"Conventional therapy" implies a two-shot regimen, or what is called a "split–mixed" regimen. This involves the mixture of intermediate-acting insulin and short-acting insulin twice daily—before breakfast and dinner (Fig. 39–8). A potential problem with this method is nighttime hypoglycemia (Hirsch & Hirsch, 1993). This problem is usually

TABLE 39–21. Possible Insulin Regimens in Type 2 Diabetic Patients with Moderate Diabetes

Bedtime intermediate-acting insulin (NPH or lente) to control basal insulin and reduce A.M. fasting plasma glucose, with endogenous insulin-controlling postprandial glucose levels
Daytime oral antidiabetic agent to control postprandial glucose levels, plus bedtime intermediate-acting insulin (NPH or lente) to control basal insulin and reduce fasting plasma glucose; this is called "bedtime insulin–daytime sulfonylurea" or "BIDS" therapy (Jarvinen et al., 1993 and Skyler, 1997).
Use of a long-acting insulin (ultralente) given before breakfast

TABLE 39–22. Possible Insulin Regimens in Type 2 Diabetic Patients with Severe Diabetes

Twice daily intermediate-acting insulin (NPH or lente) alone or with twice daily short-acting insulin (regular or lispro). Intermediate and short-acting insulins can be combined as a single injection. If the short-acting insulin chosen is regular, it should be given 30 minutes before meals. If lispro is selected, it is given with meals.
Daily long-acting insulin (ultralente) with or without a short-acting insulin (regular or lispro) at meals
Continuous insulin infusion

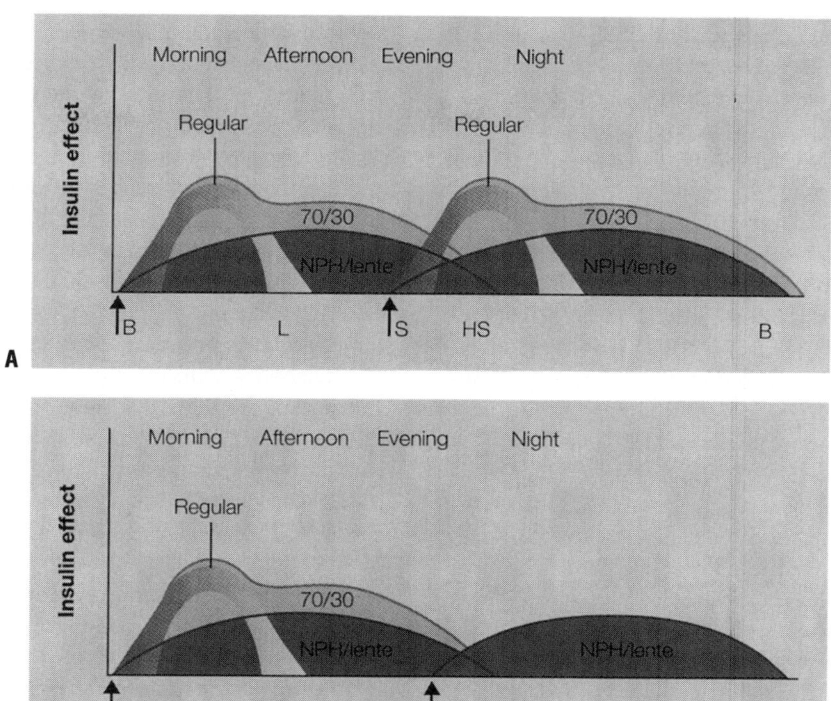

Figure 39–8. Commonly recommended regimens for insulin replacement in patients with type 2 diabetes. **A,** Pattern of insulin action for "split-mix" regimen of regular insulin plus intermediate insulin (NPH or lente) taken before breakfast and before supper. Pattern for 70/30 premixed insulin (70% NPH, 30% regular) is superimposed. **B,** Pattern for similar regimen that uses only intermediate insulin at bedtime instead of mixed dose before supper. B, breakfast; L, lunch; S, supper; HS, bedtime. Arrows indicate time of insulin administration. *(From Beaser. [1992].)*

corrected through use of a three-shot regimen, moving the evening intermediate-acting insulin to bedtime.

Intensive insulin therapy is meant to closely mimic physiologic insulin secretion. "Intensive" means three or four injections per day, or use of a continuous subcutaneous insulin pump. Obviously, this requires a patient who is motivated to monitor frequent blood glucose levels, adjust food intake, and give supplemental insulin as prescribed if the blood glucose is not within the desired range. Supplemental insulin is given by sliding scale or by carbohydrate counting.

The most typical method is the three-shot regimen of morning intermediate-acting and short-acting insulin, dinner short-acting insulin, and bedtime intermediate-acting insulin (Fig. 39–9). This regimen helps lower fasting plasma glucose, since intermediate-acting insulin given at bedtime continues to work throughout the night.

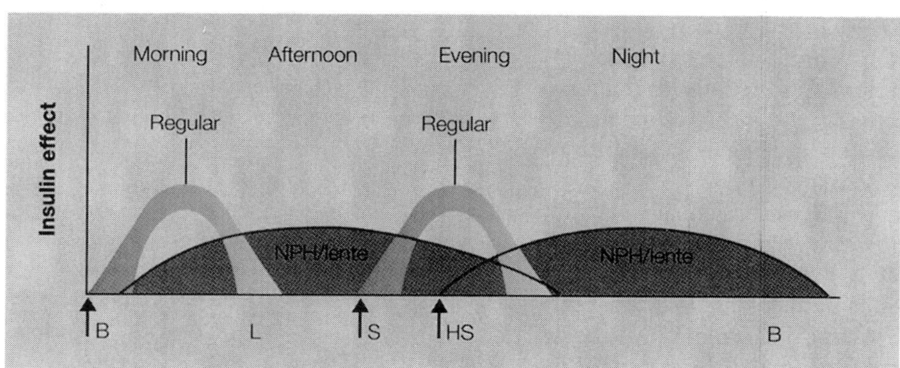

Figure 39–9. Pattern of insulin action in treatment regimen commonly used for patients with type 1 diabetes. Mix of regular and intermediate (NPH or lente) insulin is taken before breakfast, regular insulin alone is taken before supper, and intermediate insulin alone is taken at bedtime. B, breakfast; L, lunch; S, supper; HS, bedtime. Arrows indicate time of insulin administration. *(From Beaser. [1993].)*

The four-shot regimen (shown in Fig. 39–10 A and B) involves giving short-acting insulin before each meal (for postprandial insulin), and an intermediate-acting insulin before bedtime (for basal insulin). This offers the patient more flexibility with eating times, and well-educated patients are able to adjust insulin dosage to food intake. The patient must not delay eating, however, because of the risk of hyperglycemia once the short-acting insulin effect is gone.

Another four-shot regimen is to use short-acting insulin before meals and long-acting insulin at breakfast and dinner (for basal insulin) (Fig. 39–10B). This method allows flexibility in meal timing, but increases the risk of hypoglycemia in the evening when short-acting insulin may peak at the same time as the A.M. ultralente.

An alternative to mulitple daily injection therapy is continuous subcutaneous insulin injection (SCII) via an insulin pump that delivers short-acting insulin at basal rates of 0.5-1.0 units/hr and premeal bolus supplements for postprandial coverage (Fig. 39–11). Some studies have shown this method best at improving glycemic control, while others have shown no clear improvement (Hirsch & Hirsch, 1993). Disadvantages of the pump include the risk of diabetic ketoacidosis if insulin delivery is interrupted, hypoglycemic coma, and infection at injection site.

Perioperative Management

The complications of diabetes mellitus make perioperative management a challenge. There are major risks associated with anesthesia and surgery in this patient population (Table 39–23).

Diabetic patients requiring renal transplant or coronary artery bypass grafting have a greatly increased morbidity, and therefore require 30 to 50% more time in the hospital following major surgery than the nondiabetic (Gavin, 1992).

Due to the many risks mentioned, extraordinary care should be taken preoperatively to determine safety of anesthesia and surgery. Preoperative assessment should include identification of diabetes type, review of previous glycemic control, existence and degree of diabetes-related complications, and overall cardiovascular evaluation.

Patients on long-acting sulfonylureas (Chlorpropamide) should be switched to a shorter-acting agent (such as Glipizide) or insulin several days before the procedure. Those on long-acting insulin (ultralente) should be switched to intermediate acting (NPH or Lente) or short-acting (Regular) insulin several days before surgery. As previously mentioned, metformin should be discontinued 48 hours prior to surgery or any procedure using IV contrast dye.

Diabetics with poor glucose control (blood glucose > 240 mg/dL) should be admitted the day prior to surgery, if time permits, for stabilization of the blood glucose level. Due to the increasing practice of establishing simultaneous insulin and glucose infusions, rapid regulation of blood glucose levels can be achieved in situations where this was not feasible preoperatively.

The key to metabolic control is to maintain blood glucose in an acceptable range, generally considered 120-180 mg/dL. This involves a system of frequent blood glucose monitoring and insulin therapy/glucose infusion.

By definition, major surgery requires general anesthesia. Most oral agents are held on the morning of surgery (except in special cases like metformin, which is held for 48 hours in advance). For type 2 patients, many require insulin during this period, especially if the blood sugar is >180-200 mg/dL. If the patient is controlled on diet or oral agents alone, and has adequate control (fasting blood glucose <180 mg/dL or HgbA1C of 8-10%), intensive therapy may not be needed (Gavin, 1992). Even then, the blood glucose must be monitored and insulin given as needed per sliding scale every 4 to 6 hours.

The algorithm for estimating insulin dosage is as follows: One unit of insulin disposes an average of 8 gm of glucose, and decreases blood glucose by 50 mg/dL in a normal steady-state condition. D5W administered at 100 mL/hr delivers 5 gm of glucose. You must factor in stress and an

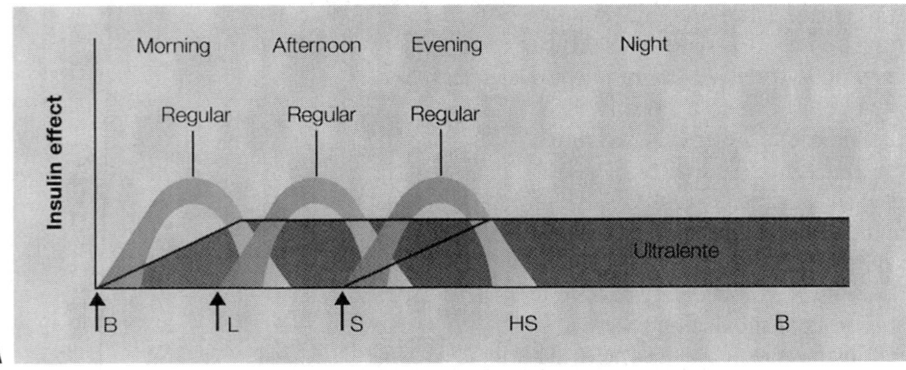

Figure 39–10. Two patterns of insulin action for multiple daily injection regimins of intensive insulin therapy in patients with type 1 diabetes. **A,** Ultralente insulin is taken twice a day, before breakfast and supper, and regular insulin is taken three times a day, before each meal.

(Continued)

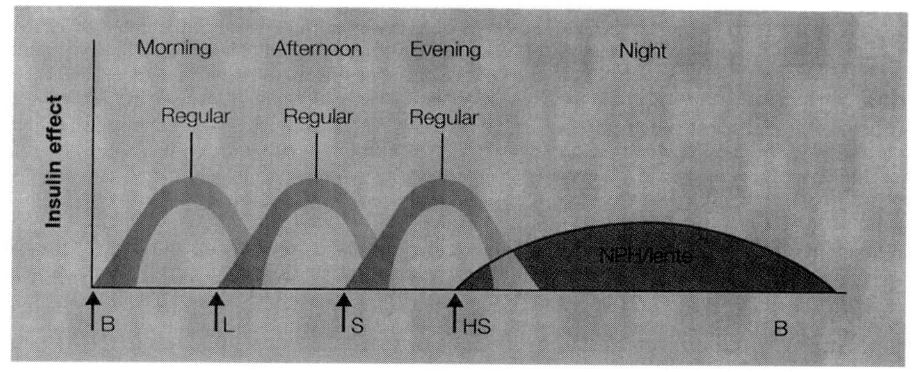

Figure 39–10. *(Continued)* **B,** Regimen of regular insulin taken before meals and intermediate insulin (NPH or lente) taken at bedtime. B, breakfast; L, lunch; S, supper; HS, bedtime. Arrows indicate time of insulin administration. *(From Beaser. [1993]).*

individual's condition to make appropriate adjustments based on this algorithm.

There are many ways to administer insulin during this period. The two most accepted ways will be covered in this text. The traditional method is to administer 30 to 50% of the intermediate-acting insulin on the morning of surgery, and infuse glucose (D5W) at a rate of 100 mL/hr. The major drawback with this method is that insulin absorption may be unpredictable, and hypoglycemia may result if surgery is significantly delayed.

A preferred but more intensive method is the use of separate insulin and glucose infusions. This is recommended for all patients with type 1 diabetes, insulin-treated patients with type 2 diabetics, and poorly controlled drug- or diet-treated patients with type 2 diabetes who are undergoing general anesthesia regardless of the length of the procedure (Arauz-Pacheco & Raskin, 1994).

It should be noted that insulin given intravenously has a half-life of 20 minutes, and discontinuation of the insulin drip may produce a rapid state of insulin deficiency and hyperglycemia. Also, insulin adheres to plastic IV tubing. To avoid this problem, the accepted practice is to run the first 50 mL of insulin infusion through the IV tubing before connecting it to the patient. Gavin (1992) lists guidelines for estimation of insulin dose based on the algorithm noted earlier (Table 39–24). Also shown is a guideline for perioperative diabetes management with an insulin drip (Table 39–25). This is meant as an example, and must be adjusted based on patient requirements and hospital practices. The dextrose-solution infusion rate should be evaluated hourly along with insulin-infusion rate, with appropriate adjustments to each made based on intraoperative glycemic monitoring.

For minor surgical procedures or diagnostic tests requiring NPO status, it is still desirable to use an insulin infusion for type 1 patients or type 2 patients requiring >50 units of insulin per day. If insulin infusion therapy is not possible, one half to two thirds the usual intermediate insulin dose may be given in the morning, with sliding scale regular insulin coverage every 4 to 6 hours based on blood glucose values. For type 2 diabetics requiring oral agents or insulin <50 units per day, medication may be held in the morning, with sliding scale coverage every 4 to 6 hours.

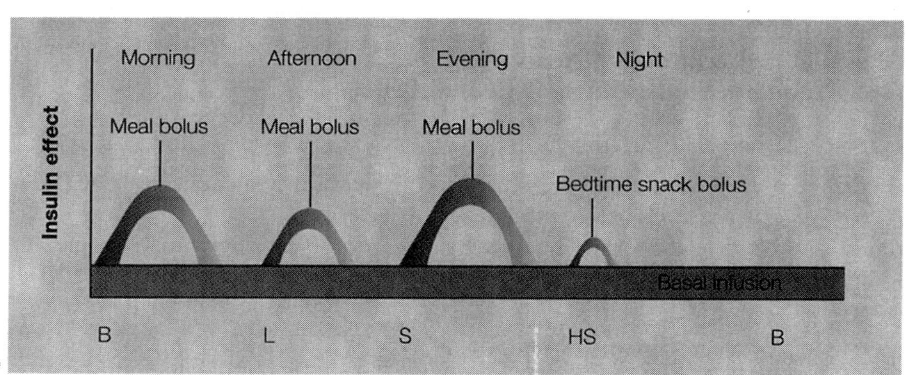

Figure 39–11. Pattern of insulin action for continuous subcutaneous insulin infusion by pump. A basal insulin level is provided, with incremental boluses at the time of meals and snacks. B, breakfast; L, lunch; S, supper; HS, bedtime. *(From Beaser. [1993].)*

TABLE 39–23. Challenges to Perioperative Management of the Diabetic Patient

- Severe hyperglycemia with or without ketosis may develop due to stress-induced release of counterregulatory hormones and inadequate insulin secretion.
- Marked dehydration may occur with hyperglycemia because of osmotic diuresis.
- Hypoglycemia may occur when insulin is given to fasting patients unless a source of carbohydrate is also given.
- Diabetic nephropathy may further complicate fluid and electrolyte management. Hyperkalemia and hypokalemia are particular problems, as well as the danger of developing acute renal failure.
- Hypoglycemia may occur without any symptoms in hypertensive diabetics receiving beta blockers.
- Autonomic neuropathy may cause profound hypotension and arrhythmia during induction of general and spinal anesthesia (Arauz-Pacheco & Raskin, 1994).
- Diabetic patients with atherosclerosis have a higher risk of postoperative myocardial infarction than the general population (Arauz-Pacheco & Raskin, 1994).
- Wound healing may be impaired in the presence of hyperglycemia (blood glucose >240 mg/dL) due to fibroblast and leukocyte dysfunction (Rosenberg, 1990). Protein catabolism, decreased circulation at peripheral sites, and inadequate nutritional status also play a role in delaying wound healing.
- Postoperative infections occur more frequently in patients with diabetes. This includes wound infections, urinary tract infections, pneumonia, and other systemic infections (Gavin, 1992).
- Thromboembolic events are more likely to occur in this population due to increased platelet aggregation.
- Nausea, vomiting, and aspiration are risks in the diabetic patients with gastroparesis due to autonomic neuropathy.

TABLE 39–24. Guidelines for Estimation of Insulin Dose[a]

- For insulin-treated diabetics (IDDM and NIDDM) or >50 U/day, selected regular insulin dose is 36 U/day.
  Example: for a blood glucose (BG) level of 141–180 mg/dL, administer 1.5 U/hour (36 U/day) according to algorithm.
- For patients treated with diet, oral agents, or insulin, <50 U/day, selected regular insulin dose is 24 U/day.
  Example: for BG of 141–180 mg/dL, administer 1.0 U/hour (24 U/day), algorithm should be modified.
- Anticipate further dose adjustments based on the following parameters:
  - Conditions associated with increased insulin needs:
    - Previous poor BG control (average fasting blood sugar >240 mg/dL, glycosylated hemoglobin >10%): selected dose × 1.5.
    - Obesity, hepatic disease: selected dose × 1.5.
    - Severe infection, steroid therapy: selected dose × 2.
  - Type of surgery:
    - General surgery: use selected dose.
    - Renal transplant: selected dose × 2.
    - Coronary artery bypass graft: selected dose × 3–5.

[a] Regular insulin infusion rate (U/hour) = dose ÷ 24.
IDDM = insulin-dependent diabetes mellitus; NIDDM = non–insulin-dependent diabetes mellitus.
Reprinted with permission from Gavin. (1992).

Postoperative Management

Following major surgery, the insulin and glucose infusions should be continued until the patient is able to eat solid foods without difficulty. The insulin infusion should be stopped one-half hour after the patient receives a regular insulin injection subcutaneously. Since the half-life of regular

TABLE 39–25. Guidelines for Perioperative Diabetes Management with an Insulin Drip

- Insulin: Regular (human) 25 U in 250 mL of normal saline (1 U/10 mL).
- Intravenous infusion of insulin: Flush 50 mL through line before connecting to patient. Piggyback insulin line to the perioperative maintenance fluid line.
- Perioperative maintenance fluid: Fluids must contain 5% dextrose (rate 100 mL/hour).
- Blood glucose (BG): Monitor hourly intraoperatively.

	Insulin	
BG (mg/dL)	***(U/hour)***	***(mL/hour)***
<80	0.0	0.0
81–100	0.5	5.0
101–140	1.0	10
141–180	1.5	15
181–220	2.0	20
221–260	2.5	25
261–300	3.0	30
301–340	4.0	40
>341	5.0	50

- BG <80 mg/dL): Stop insulin and administer intravenous bolus of 50% dextrose in water (25 mL). Once BG >80, restart insulin infusion. It may be necessary to modify the algorithm.
- Decreased insulin needs: Patients treated with diet or oral agents or <50 U insulin/day, endocrinologic deficiencies.
- Increased insulin needs: Obesity, sepsis, steroid therapy, renal transplant, coronary artery bypass.

Reprinted with permission from Gavin. (1992).

insulin given intravenously is 20 minutes, subcutaneous regular insulin is important in preventing insulin deficiency and the potential for ketosis. Ideally, the patient should receive premeal short-acting insulin and bedtime intermediate-acting insulin for the first 24 to 48 hours after resuming oral feeding, to ensure maximum flexibility should clinical conditions suddenly change. Fingerstick blood glucoses should be checked premeal, at bedtime, and at 3:00 A.M. during this transition period. When returning the type 1 patient to a more routine insulin regimen, the clinician may prescribe either a dose based on 80 to 100% of the previous day's requirements, or may place the patient back on his or her previous regimen, with minor adjustments based on the most recent glycemic control.

The type 2 patient may be returned to his or her original oral agent once the patient is tolerating solid food for 24 to 48 hours. Preprocedure dosage is usually resumed. Metformin should be restarted only when the danger of acute decompensation postoperatively has passed—at least 48 hours after surgery, and only then if the serum creatinine is less than 1.4 mg/dL in females and less than 1.5 mg/dL in males.

Management of Enteral and Parenteral Nutrition and Insulin Therapy. It is ideal to manage patients who receive the extra carbohydrate load of enteral nutrition with an insulin infusion. The standard tube-feeding formula delivers 12 to 16 gm of carbohydrate per hour. The insulin infusion rate should, for example, be 1 unit/hour for basal requirements + 2 units/hour for a continuous tube-feeding rate of 100 mL per hour (or 15 gm of carbohydrate) = 3 units per hour. This dose is calculated for the steady state, and should be individualized for each patient (refer to Table 39–24 on calculation of insulin requirements).

In most institutions, it is difficult to obtain hourly fingerstick blood glucoses, so insulin infusion may be unsafe. It is also acceptable to treat a diabetic on enteral nutrition with BID NPH insulin, with regular insulin coverage every 6 hours per sliding scale. Refer to Table 39–26 for guidelines for tube feeding and insulin administration.

Management of the patient receiving bolus tube feedings can be complex. If the bolus feedings are given at every 3-hour or every 6-hour intervals, then blood glucose should be checked before every feeding, and supplemental regular insulin given every 6 hours as needed per sliding scale. Again, this should be individualized. Every 3-hour or every 4-hour regular insulin coverage for bolus feedings is possible in carefully monitored situations, but should be discouraged due to the danger of possible accumulation/"stacking effect" of regular insulin given too frequently, and risk subsequent risk of hypoglycemia. Insulin action may be peaking from the previous dose when the next dose is given. If possible, diabetic patients should receive bolus feeds at 3- or 6-hour intervals rather than every 4 hours, so as to allow for more predictable blood sugar response and improved control in response to insulin adminstration at 6-hour intervals.

Management of blood glucose and total parenteral nutrition (TPN) should also be done with an insulin infusion. TPN solutions are typically 25% dextrose. A rate of 100 mL/hour, for example, would infuse 25 gm of carbohydrate per hour. This would require an insulin drip of 2 to 3 units per hour. Alternate means to control blood glucose are (1) to place insulin directly in the TPN bag or (2) to give subcutaneous regular insulin every 6 hours per sliding scale, as well as BID NPH insulin if needed. The method of adding

TABLE 39–26. Guidelines for Tube Feeding (TF) Insulin-Treated Diabetes Patients

Standard formula (240 mL): 30–40 g carbohydrate
Thus, 100 mL/hour TF = 12–16 g carbohydrate/hour
Insulin dose based on previous regimen, degree of stress, and rate of TF.

A. Insulin drip (70 kg = IBW)

	Rate
Basal needs (modify for stress etc.)	1 U/hour
Continuous TF @ 100 mL/hour (15 g)	2 U/hour
Actual dose	3 U/hour (72 U/day)

Adjust dose according to customized algorithm

B. NPH subcutaneously twice daily (total dose = 72 U)

Administered 24 U of NPH twice per day (2/3) (+) regular subcutaneously (1/3) twice per day (same times)

Blood glucose (mg/dL)	Regular (U)
<180	0
180–220	6
221–260	8
261–300	10
>300	12

Modify NPH dose as per use of supplemental regular insulin from previous day

TF = tube feeding; IBW = ideal body weight.
Reprinted with permission from Gavin. (1992).

regular insulin to the TPN bag is calculated as follows: (1) give supplemental regular insulin every 6 hours by sliding scale for the first 24 to 48 hours, (2) calculate the total number of units given over 24 hours, (3) add two thirds of this calculated dose to the TPN bag, and (4) give regular insulin supplements per sliding scale every 6 hours.

Problems Specific to Hospitalized Diabetic Patients

Several simple management issues may require attention when attempting glycemic control in the hospitalized patient. First, timing of meals and snacks is important. It is common for meals and snacks to be delayed, resulting in the increased risk of hypoglycemia in the patient who has received antidiabetic medication. Timing between insulin administration and meal consumption must be considered, and is especially important in those patients on intensive insulin therapy.

Second, hospital diet orders may not match the caloric intake of the home diet. As mentioned earlier, taking a diet history on admission serves several purposes. If the hospital does not include snacks as part of the diabetic diet order, these must be specified (especially bedtime snack).

Third, insulin absorption may be erratic due to fluid shifts, hemodynamic changes, and changes in blood flow to the subcutaneous tissue in the acutely ill patient (Hirsch, Paauw, & Brunzell, 1995). Counterregulatory stress response may increase insulin requirements. Narcotic administration may decrease gut absorption of food, and further complicate medication effectiveness, especially in the case of diabetic gastroparesis.

Pancreas and Islet Cell Transplantation

Successful pancreas transplantation has been shown to improve quality of life in diabetics by eliminating the need for exogenous insulin, frequent fingerstick blood glucose monitoring, and extreme dietary restrictions (American Diabetes Association, 1997). Almost 7000 pancreas transplants have been reported to the International Pancreas Transplant Registry from 1966 to 1994 (Sutherland, 1996). Approximately 85% of those transplants were in diabetic renal allograft recipients (Sutherland et al., 1994). The Pancreas Transplant Registry reports a success rate (insulin-independence for >one year) of over 75% for pancreas transplants performed with a simultaneous kidney transplant, and over 50% when performed as a solitary organ transplant (Sutherland et al., 1994).

Bladder-drained solitary pancreas transplants with good HLA matches have reportedly shown success rates over 70%. With bladder-drained solitary pancreas transplants, urine amylase can be used to monitor for rejection. A decrease could indicate declining graft function, with the need for treatment or graft biopsy. Episodes of rejection in kidney–pancreas transplant recipients may be easier to detect and treat, since treatment of kidney rejection usually helps to treat rejection of the pancreas, although independent monitoring of both graft functions is recommended since isolated organ rejection may occur in a small percentage of patients (Sutherland et al., 1994).

At present, the American Diabetes Association [ADA] (1997) recommends pancreas–kidney transplantation for type 1 diabetic patients with end-stage renal disease, providing they: (1) meet medical criteria for kidney transplantation, (2) have clinical problems with exogenous insulin therapy, and (3) do not have surgical risk for the dual-transplant procedure. The ADA recommends pancreas-only transplantation for type 1 diabetics without evidence of renal failure, providing they also have: (1) a history of frequent acute severe metabolic complications requiring medical attention, (2) clinical and emotional problems with exogenous insulin therapy that are so severe as to be incapacitating, and (3) consistent failure of other therapeutic approaches to ameliorate the situation.

Risks of pancreas–kidney transplantation include a higher rejection rate and longer hospitalizations than kidney transplant only, higher readmission rate than with kidney transplant only, and side effects of immunosuppression (ADA, 1992). Pancreas-only transplantation risks include the side effects of lifelong immunosuppressive therapy to prevent graft rejection and recurrence of autoimmune insulinitis that would result in beta-cell destruction. Because of the severity of some of these side effects, pancreas-only transplantation should only be considered in those patients with an unacceptable quality of life.

Pancreas transplantation has repeatedly been shown not to reverse existing microvascular complications of diabetes (Molitch, 1995), although there are reports that some of the secondary complications of diabetes may be prevented (Sutherland, 1996). For example, neuropathy and early nephropathy may be favorably influenced by pancreas transplantation (Sutherland, 1996). There are no reports yet that pancreas transplantation increases life expectancy.

Islet-Cell Transplantation

Islet-cell transplantation has not had the success rate of pancreas transplantation. The International Islet Transplant Registry reported 240 islet allografts from 1970 to 1994, 230 of which were done in type 1 diabetics (Sutherland, 1996). Of these, only 20 were able to remain insulin independent for at least 1 week posttransplant. The lack of success at present is felt to be due to immunosuppressive agents given posttransplant which are in themselves diabetogenic, and the reduced beta-cell mass that occurs with organ dispersal and islet purification (Sutherland, 1996).

Kenyon et al. (1996) found, however, that even in the absence of complete insulin independence, excellent glycemic control can be observed in islet allograft recipients with partial graft function. In fact, the long-term glycemic control was better than those undergoing intensive insulin therapy in the Diabetes Control and Complications Trial (The Diabetes Control and Complications Trial Research Group, 1993). It is hoped that newer immunosuppressant and immunologic therapies will increase the success rates of islet-cell transplantation. The ultimate goal would be to perform islet-cell transplantation early in the course of diabetes, before the onset of chronic complications, and in such a way that continuous immunosuppression would not be needed (Kenyon et al., 1996).

Acute Complications of Diabetes

If inadequately treated, hyperglycemia may progress to serious metabolic complications of diabetic ketoacidosis (DKA) or hyperosmolar nonketotic coma (HHNK). Hypoglycemia is a common complication of diabetes therapy, with the potential for serious consequences. These conditions are medical emergencies and require prompt action.

Diabetic Ketoacidosis

Diabetic ketoacidosis (DKA) is a state of uncontrolled diabetes mellitus in which there is hyperglycemia (usually >300 mg/dL), acidosis—a significant lowering of arterial blood pH (<7.3), and an elevation of total blood ketone body concentration (beta–hydroxybutyrate plus acetoacetate) (Alberti, 1995). It occurs in 2 to 5% of type I diabetic patients per year, and DKA-related deaths occur in 1 to 10% of patients, depending on treatment circumstances and locale (Genuth, 1994).

Pathophysiology. DKA is caused by either an absolute or relative insulin deficiency. In type 1 diabetes it can be seen as the initial presentation or subsequently, when exogenous insulin administration is omitted. Relative insulin deficiency can result when a precipitating factor such as sepsis, trauma, illness, or other extreme body stressor produces a state of high insulin resistence. Counterregulatory hormones are implicated here, as they antagonize the effects of insulin.

In both absolute or relative insulin deficiency, counterregulatory hormones (glucagon, epinephrine, growth hormone, and cortisol) are produced at an excessive rate, stimulating ketone body formation and gluconeogenesis. Without insulin to keep the fatty acids inside the fat cells (as the lipid component of triglycerides), fatty acids are released into the blood and attach to albumin. These fatty acids are the precursors for ketoacid production (Fleckman, 1993). Massive osmotic diuresis occurs from serum glucose levels above the renal threshold (>200 mg/dL) and glucose spills into the urine. Glucose pulls water and sodium with it and ketoacids are excreted in urine with sodium and potassium salts, creating severe electrolyte loss.

Laboratory and Diagnostic Tests. Diagnosis is based on the presence of hyperglycemia (glucose >300 mg/dL), metabolic acidosis (blood pH <7.3), and positive serum or urine ketones. Laboratory and diagnostic tests should be performed to confirm the diagnosis and to identify possible precipitating causes. These include: serum glucose, electrolytes, BUN and creatinine, urine and serum ketones, complete blood count with differential, arterial blood gas, electrocardiogram, chest x-ray, beta-HCG (human chorionic gonadotrophin) level in women of childbearing age, and appropriate cultures.

The history must focus on recent events, including infection, illness, and noncompliance with insulin therapy. The most common cause of DKA is infection, most often urinary tract infection or pneumonia (Fleckman, 1993). Subtle infections such as sinus, dental, and perirectal abscesses are also fairly common (Fleckman, 1991). Other causes such as myocardial infarction and pregnancy should be ruled out. Rare causes of DKA include Cushing's disease and acromegaly, which elevate counterregulatory hormones.

Table 39–27 lists typical signs and symptoms in patients presenting with DKA.

Management. Most patients are initially treated in the intensive care unit or in a setting where they can be constantly monitored. The major therapeutic interventions include fluid replacement, insulin administration, and potassium replacement. Certain calculations are important for diagnosis and management of DKA. See Table 39–28.

Serum Osmolality. Calculation of serum osmolality is important for evaluating mental status changes. A clinically significant hyperosmolar state potentially exists when serum osmolality exceeds 320 mOsm/kg.

Serum Sodium. Serum sodium is corrected for the degree of hyperglycemia to assess fluid volume deficit. Elevated corrected sodium indicates greater free-water deficit and the need for more isotonic replacement fluid to prevent hypotension when insulin is given.

Anion Gap. The anion gap is the calculation obtained by subtracting measured anions (chloride and bicarbonate) from measured cations (sodium). A normal anion gap is 6-10 mEq/L. The anion gap is elevated in DKA (>12 mEq/L) due to the presence of unmeasured anions, including ketoacids.

Fluid. It is estimated that most patients with DKA have lost 4 to 8 liters of fluid (Fleckman, 1991). Usually, one liter of

TABLE 39–27. Signs and Symptoms of Diabetic Ketoacidosis (DKA)

Altered mental status due to hyperosmolality and central nervous system acidosis
Hyperventilation (from mild tachypnea to Kussmaul respirations)
"Fruity" or acetone breath
Decreased skin turgor and dry mucous membranes
Hypotension
Tachycardia
Nausea and vomiting
Abdominal pain similar to acute surgical abdomen pain
Fever

TABLE 39–28. Useful Calculations

(A) *Calculation of effective serum osmolality*

$$2\,[Na^+ + K^+] + \frac{[\text{glucose in mg/dL}]}{18}$$

(B) *Correction of serum sodium*

$$\text{Corrected } Na^+ = [Na^+] + 1.6 \times \frac{[\text{glucose in mg/dL}] - 100}{100}$$

(C) *Calculation of the anion gap*

$[Na^+] - [Cl^- + HCO_3^-]$

(D) *Evaluation for pure metabolic acidosis*

Pco_2 = The last two numbers of the pH

$Pco_2 = 1.5\,[\text{serum } HCO_3^-] + 8 \pm 2$

(A), Effective serum osmolality correlates with mental status abnormalities. BUN diffuses freely into cells and does not contribute to *effective* serum osmolality. (B), Corrected serum sodium assists in estimation of free water deficits. (C), A falling anion gap indicates successful therapy. (D), A lower than predicted Pco_2 indicates respiratory alkalosis and may be a clue to sepsis.

Reprinted with permission from Fleckman. (1993).

isotonic fluid (normal saline) is given over the first 30 to 60 minutes, followed by a second liter of normal saline (NS) over the ensuing hour. If the patient is hypotensive or has an estimated fluid loss in excess of 10%, another liter of NS may be given over the following hour. Bladder catheterization should be performed in most cases, so that fluid replacement can be better managed. Fluid is then changed to half-isotonic solutions, such as ½NS, and given at a rate of 250-500 mL/hr for the next few hours. When the blood glucose level decreases to 250 mg/dL, fluids are changed to a dextrose-containing solution such as D5 ½NS. This allows continuation of insulin therapy to control ketoacidosis while preventing hypoglycemia. In the average patient, fluids are usually replete after 12 to 24 hours (Genuth, 1994).

Insulin. Only regular insulin should be used. A continuous insulin infusion should be started at a rate of 0.1 unit/kg/hr. Fingerstick blood glucose levels should be monitored hourly, and the insulin infusion rate doubled every 1 to 2 hours if there has not been a drop of at least 50-100 mg/dL in the blood glucose or if there is no improvement in the anion gap and pH (Fleckman, 1993). Insulin infusion rate may be decreased once the blood glucose is <250 mg/dL and the anion gap and pH have improved. Insulin infusion is usually continued until the patient is able to tolerate food. Regular insulin 4 to 10 units SC should be given one-half hour before the insulin infusion is stopped to keep a steady insulin dose available and prevent recurrence of ketoacidosis (Genuth, 1994).

Potassium. Potassium replacement requires perhaps the most attention, since rapid shifts occur once insulin is given. It is estimated that the average potassium deficit is approximately 5 mEq/kg body weight (Genuth, 1994). Upon presentation, serum potassium is usually normal or elevated despite total body potassium depletion due to diuresis. This is due to a pH-related extracellular shift. An EKG may help establish the presence of life-threatening hyperkalemia (widened QRS complexes, peaked T waves). Once insulin is given, potassium shifts from the extracellular fluid back into the intracellular spaces, dramatically decreasing serum potassium levels. Without potassium repletion there is a significant danger of hypokalemia. Because of this, potassium should be given from the onset of therapy, as long as urine output has been demonstrated and life-threatening hyperkalemia has been ruled out. Fleckman (1993) recommends 40 mEq over one hour for potassium <3 mEq/L; 30 mEq over 1 hour for serum potassium <4 mEq/L; and 20 mEq over 1 hour for serum potassium <5 mEq/L. Higher doses of potassium should be given in larger volumes of intravenous fluid rates, not to exceed 40 mEq/hr.

Bicarbonate. Bicarbonate is not given for DKA routinely because of the secondary risk of hypokalemia. However, in the case of severe acidosis (arterial blood pH <7.0 or bicarbonate level <5.0 mEq/L) or hyperkalemia (serum potassium >6.5 mEq/L), bicarbonate may be given at a dose of 50-200 mEq in 250-1000 mL ½NS over 30 to 60 minutes (Genuth, 1994).

Phosphate. Phosphate is depleted with osmotic diuresis, appearing normal on initial test, but rapidly falling when insulin is given. Effects of replacement remain unclear, since clinical effects of hypophosphatemia are rarely seen (Genuth, 1994). It is given if CNS deterioration, cardiac dysfunction, hemolysis, or rhabdomyolysis follow a decrease in serum phosphate once insulin is given. Dosage is small—usually 1-2 mM phosphate/kg body weight intravenously over 6 to 12 hours.

Magnesium. As with phosphate, magnesium replacement is rarely given unless cardiac arrhythmias occur not associated with hypokalemia. Replacement dose is 10-20 mEq magnesium sulfate intravenously over 30 to 60 minutes (Genuth, 1994).

Table 39–29 lists essential components of initial monitoring of the patient during therapy.

Hyperglycemic Hyperosmolar Nonketotic Syndrome

Hyperglycemic hyperosmolar nonketotic (HHNK) syndrome is characterized by hyperglycemia (blood glucose often >600 mg/dL), hyperosmolality (serum osmolality >320 mOsm/kg), and typically the absence of ketosis. Statistically, it is responsible for approximately 1/1000 hospital admissions (Genuth, 1994), occurring mostly in adults over 50 years old who have type 2 diabetes. Interestingly, 35% of patients presenting with HHNK are previously undiagnosed diabetics. Infection is the most common precipitating event, occurring in 32 to 60% of all cases (Lorber, 1995).

TABLE 39–29. Components to Be Monitored Initially in Diabetic Ketoacidosis (DKA)

Vital signs hourly
Mental status assessment hourly
Glucose every 1-2 hours by fingerstick
Serum electrolytes initially, then every 1-2 hours until stabilized
Arterial blood gas hourly until the pH>7.0, then only if the patient is not improving
Hourly intake and output; monitor urine for ketones
Consider monitoring central venous pressure

TABLE 39–31. Signs and Symptoms of HHNK

Poor skin turgor; dry mucous membranes
Altered mental status
Focal neurologic signs, such as seizures, aphasia, bilateral hypo- or hyperreflexia, hemiparesis, positive Babinski sign, nystagmus, hemianopsia, acute quadriplegia, and dysphagia; these signs are often so similar to cerebrovascular accident that investigation for stroke and treatment for HHNK must be done simultaneously until the metabolic status stabilizes and final neurologic status can be determined.
Tachycardia
Normal respiratory rate and blood pressure, unless underlying cause is infection; sepsis may cause hypotension, tachypnea, and fever.
Nausea, vomiting, and abdominal distention and pain

Pathophysiology. This syndrome results from a degree of relative insulin deficiency that may impair glucose utilization and encourage hepatic glucose production, but not such deficiency as to produce lipolysis and ketoacid production (as in DKA). Also, there is less production of counterregulatory hormones, and thus less stimulation of ketoacid production. HHNK syndrome is often precipitated by dehydration from varying causes (Table 39–30).

Usually polyuria and polydipsia occur for days to weeks before the syndrome presents. Elderly people are particularly susceptible because of impaired thirst mechanism and renal function (with decreased renal excretion of glucose). The resultant dehydration can be profound, greater than in DKA, with both intracellular and extracellular fluid loss from osmotic diuresis. Average fluid loss may range from 9 to 12 liters (Clement & Torrens, 1995). If left untreated, the patient develops hypovolemia, shock, coma, and death. Mortality ranges from 12 to 42% (Genuth, 1994).

History and Physical Findings. History must include a careful evaluation of possible precipitating factors. Signs and symptoms of HHNK are described in Table 39–31.

Laboratory and Diagnostic Tests. Diagnosis is established following presentation with a clinical picture of dehydration and altered mental status. Laboratory findings are serum blood glucose >600 mg/dL (although the typical presentation is >1000 mg/dL) and serum osmolality >320m Osm/kg. Other laboratory abnormalities may include elevated BUN, creatinine, triglycerides, and white blood count.

TABLE 39–30. Causes of Dehydration in HHNK

Infection, particularly pneumonia and urinary tract infections
Cerebrovascular event
Myocardial infarction
Pancreatitis
Uremia with nausea and vomiting
Procedures that increase osmotic load, such as dextrose-containing fluids and TPN
Diuretics, both thiazide and loop
Medications that inhibit secretion or action of insulin, such as propranolol, phenytoin, cimetidine, and corticosteroids (Lorber, 1995)

Management. Upon presentation, fingerstick and serum glucose, electrolytes, BUN, creatinine, complete blood count with differential, arterial blood gas, urinalysis, EKG, chest x-ray, and appropriate cultures should be checked. If appropriate, blood and urine cultures should be obtained.

Treatment is similar to that for DKA. The priority is fluid replacement because of the severity of intracellular dehydration and hyperosmolality. As outlined by Genuth (1994), the first objective is to raise circulating volume. One liter of NS should be infused over the first 30 minutes. If the patient then is still hypotensive, a second liter of NS should be infused over the ensuing 30 to 60 minutes. After that, fluid should be switched to ½NS at approximately 500 mL/hr. As in DKA, when blood glucose reaches 250 mg/dL, fluid should be switched to D5 ½NS. If the serum sodium level is >150 meq/L at this point, fluid should be D5 0.2%NS.

Insulin is given only when adequate fluid replacement has begun. If it is given without adequate replacement, there is a danger of fluid shifts of 2 to 3 liters out of the extracellular space and resultant hypovolemia (Lorber, 1995). A continuous insulin infusion should be started at a rate of 0.1 unit/kg/hr, as in DKA. Blood glucose levels are monitored hourly, with a desired fall of 100 mg/dL/hr. If the fall in glucose exceeds 200 mg/dL/hr, the insulin infusion rate may be halved. Once the serum glucose level has reached 250 mg/dL, the infusion rate may be decreased to 1 to 2 units per hour. Subcutaneous regular insulin should be given 30 minutes before discontinuing the insulin infusion. The infusion may be stopped once HHNK has resolved.

Potassium is needed as in DKA, although at more cautious dosing probably because of less acidosis and vomiting. Rates should be 10-20 mEq/hr (Genuth, 1994). Phosphate and magnesium repletion is the same as in DKA, and is only given for severe loss with clinical signs and symptoms.

Blood glucose monitoring follows a schedule much like in DKA. Empiric antibiotic coverage should be considered when infection is suspected given the prevalence of infection in patients with HHNK.

Complications of HHNK include hypovolemia with shock, acute kidney failure secondary to hypovolemia and acute tubular necrosis, acute respiratory distress syndrome (ARDS), thromboembolism, and disseminated intravascular coagulation (DIC).

Hypoglycemia

Hypoglycemia is defined as blood glucose <40 mg/dL, accompanied by CNS symptoms that respond to glucose administration (Comi, 1993). Blood glucose levels <70 mg/dL may produce symptoms, and should receive attention to avoid severe hypoglycemia. In the diabetic patient, hypoglycemia may be caused by (1) variable absorption at the insulin injection site, (2) an error in insulin administration, (3) delayed or missed meals, (4) decreased carbohydrate intake, (5) exercise, (6) alcohol consumption, (7) medication (such as a beta blocker), or (8) delayed gastric emptying due to gastroparesis. Additionally, insulin needs may vary with the menstrual cycle in women with diabetes. The rapid fall in progesterone at the onset of menses may cause decreased insulin requirement resulting in hypoglycemia.

In the hospitalized diabetic patient, it is important to recognize and treat hypoglycemia quickly. Patients may exhibit any of the signs or symptoms of hypoglycemia listed in Table 39–32.

If the hypoglycemic patient is alert enough to take oral food, 10 to 15 gm of a carbohydrate source should be given. This is equivalent to 2 to 3 glucose tablets, 4 to 6 oz of milk, 4 to 6 oz of orange juice, or 4 to 6 oz of regular cola. It takes approximately 5 gm of glucose to raise the blood glucose concentration by 50 mg/dL (Santiago, Levandoski, & Bubb, 1994). With severe hypoglycemia and CNS symptoms, 1 mg of glucagon IM or SC may be administered or 50% glucose solution (D50) IV 20 to 50 mL (1/2-1 ampule). Since glucagon may cause nausea and vomiting, D50 might be preferred if rapid IV access is available. Blood glucose should be monitored every 15 to 30 minutes until stable, then at 30- to 60-minute intervals until it is determined that the danger of repeat hypoglycemia is over. The tendency is to overtreat hypoglycemia, thereby creating subsequent hyperglycemia.

TABLE 39–32. Neurologic Changes Associated with Hypoglycemia

Neurogenic	Neuroglycopenic
Diaphoresis	Headache
Tremor	Confusion
Palpitations	Slurred speech
Anxiety	Abnormal or inappropriate behavior
Pallor	Loss of coordination
	Seizures
	Loss of consciousness

Chronic Complications of Diabetes

Long-term diabetes often results in chronic complications encompassing multiple-organ systems. Microvascular complications involve damage to the vascular endothelium of the eye (retinopathy), kidney (nephropathy), and nerves (neuropathy). Atherosclerotic-related complications—such as coronary artery disease, cerebrovascular disease, and peripheral vascular disease—are termed macrovascular complications. A brief discussion of the common complications follows.

Chronic complications appear to be related to the duration of diabetes and the degree of long-term hyperglycemia. The results of the Diabetes Control and Complications Trial (DCCT), a 10-year study in type 1 diabetes, showed that intensive insulin therapy (three or four injections per day or continuous subcutaneous insulin infusion) with lowering of HgbA1C from 9.0% to 7.2% over 6 to 10 years decreased the development of retinopathy by 76%, neuropathy by 69%, and microalbuminuria by 34%. In cases where complications were present at the beginning of the study, intensive therapy and improved glycemic control were associated with: (1) a decreased risk of the progression of existing retinopathy to conditions requiring laser therapy in 56% of trial subjects, (2) a decreased risk of progression of microalbuminuria to significant proteinuria in 56% of trial subjects, and (3) a decreased risk of clinical neuropathy at 5 years in 57% of trial subjects (The Diabetes Control and Complications Trial Research Group, 1993).

Retinopathy

Diabetic retinopathy occurs in both type 1 and type 2 diabetes. It is the leading cause of new onset blindness in persons ages 20 to 74 (American Diabetes Association, 1997). After 20 years of diabetes, almost all type 1 diabetics and >60% of type 2 diabetics have some evidence of retinopathy (American Diabetes Association, 1997). In type 1 diabetics, retinopathy usually does not appear in the first 5 years after diagnosis of diabetes, and rarely before puberty (Nathan, 1993). In type 2 diabetics, retinopathy may appear at the time of diagnosis, since this form of diabetes may be present for years before it is diagnosed.

The course of retinopathy begins with dot hemorrhages, microaneurysms, and "hard exudates," which are yellowish-appearing lipid deposits leaked from retinal vessels. This is termed background or mild nonproliferative diabetic retinopathy (NPDR). Moderate NPDR is characterized by increased retinal hemorrhages and microaneurysms, and development of microvascular changes, such as neovascularization and cotton-wool spots (or "soft exudates") caused by infarct of the retinal capillaries (Aiello & Cavallerano, 1994). Severe NPDR is characterized by severe hemorrhages and microaneurysms, as well as venous beading.

The disease may then progress to proliferative diabetic retinopathy (PDR), with increased risk of permanent visual loss. It is characterized by neovascularization on or within one disc diameter of the optic disc, and preretinal fibrous tissue proliferation. The new vessels rupture easily, causing preretinal and vitreous hemorrhages (Aiello & Cavallerano, 1994). Of special note in hospitalized patients is the fact that PDR is a relative contraindication to thrombolytic therapy.

Diabetic macular edema may occur at any stage of retinopathy and causes moderate visual loss. Diabetics are more prone to other ocular complications, such as cataracts and glaucoma.

The primary treatment for diabetic retinopathy and macular edema is laser photocoagulation, which may prevent visual loss in many patients. The 1997 American Diabetes Association retinopathy screening recommendations are listed in Table 39–33.

Nephropathy

Diabetic nephropathy is the leading cause of end-stage renal failure (ESRD) in the United States (DeFronzo, 1994). Historically, clinical nephropathy develops in type 1 diabetes 15 to 20 years after diagnosis, and 30 to 40% of these patients progress to ESRD. In type 2 diabetes, clinical evidence of nephropathy usually appears 5 to 10 years after diagnosis, and 3 to 5% progress to ESRD (Haas, 1993). As with retinopathy, however, nephropathy may be present at diagnosis of type 2 diabetes, since kidney damage may begin at the onset of diabetes, while the disease remains subclinical and undiagnosed.

Microalbuminuria is defined as 30-300 mg/day of albumin excretion and is the first sign of renal disease. If untreated, it will likely progress to ESRD. Good glycemic control and early intervention are keys in treatment strategy. Treatment interventions include control of hypertension and use of ACE inhibitors. Many clinicians prescribe them even if the patient is normotensive. ACE inhibitors have been shown to: (1) decrease peripheral vascular resistance, (2) slow glomerular hypertrophy, (3) slow the rate of decrease in glomerular filtration rate, (4) improve insulin sensitivity, and (5) improve the serum lipid profile (DeFronzo, 1994).

Development of proteinuria, defined as >500 mg protein per liter or >300 mg of albumin per 24 hours, typically precedes nephrotic syndrome and ESRD by 5 to 10 years (Nathan, 1993). Once proteinuria has developed, good glycemic control will not slow the progression of the nephropathy.

TABLE 39–33. American Diabetes Association Retinopathy Screening Guidelines

- Yearly dilated opthalmoscopic exam for type I diabetics beginning 5 years after onset of diabetes
- Dilated opthalmoscopic exam for type II diabetics on diagnosis, and yearly
- Fundus photography can be useful in documenting retinal changes over time

The pathology of nephropathy begins with renal hypertrophy and expansion of glomeruli. This leads to thickening of the glomerular basement membrane and arteriosclerosis. With advancing nephropathy, glomeruli become sclerosed. At end-stage, there is diffuse glomerulosclerosis with few functioning filtration units.

Because early intervention slows progression of the disease, the ADA (1997) recommends that a routine urinalysis be performed yearly on diabetics. If positive for protein, screening for microalbuminuria should be done. Many diabetologists feel that routine dipstick is not sensitive enough to detect microalbuminuria in a treatable stage, and recommend at least yearly performance of a microalbumin screen (i.e., ratio of microalbumin to creatinine on a spot urine) or 24-hour urine for protein.

Studies suggesting benefits from dietary restriction of protein in delaying the progression from early nephropathy are intriguing but to date inconclusive. It is felt that protein should be restricted to 0.8 gm/kg/day in patients with overt nephropathy (ADA, 1997). When the GFR begins to decline, it is recommended that protein intake be further reduced to 0.6 gm/kg/day. As individual situations vary, it is wise to plan dietary changes with a registered dietician.

Neuropathy

Within 5 to 10 years from the onset of diabetes, most patients show slowed motor and sensory nerve conduction on electrophysiologic studies (The DCCT Research Group, 1988), and nearly 60% of diabetics have symptoms (Haas, 1993). Although the etiology of diabetic neuropathy is not completely understood, it is felt that hyperglycemia alters cellular metabolism, which ultimately results in impaired nerve conduction and nerve axonal transport. Ischemia from vascular disease may further decrease nerve function (Pfeifer, 1994).

There are several types of neuropathies. The most common is distal symmetric sensorimotor neuropathy, demonstrated on physical exam initially as decreased vibratory sensation in the toes and loss of ankle reflexes. This may progress to complete anesthesia of the feet and lower legs. Light touch and pinprick sensation may also be lost. The same sensory loss may occur in the hands, creating the "glove and stocking" distribution pattern. Inability to sense temperature differences occurs; paresthesias of the feet can progress to total numbness. Symptoms may be mild to severe and disabling, especially at night, and can greatly affect quality of life.

Entrapment neuropathies are a type of focal neuropathy, and may result from increased susceptibility of nerves to external pressure, such as in carpal tunnel syndrome. Another entrapment neuropathy involves loss of nerve fibers for proprioception leading to pressure spots on the foot (Clement, 1995). This leads to callus formation that is susceptible to ulceration and infection.

Other forms of focal neuropathy may occur as well. Mononeuropathies develop suddenly, with sharp, stabbing pains, and generally resolve spontaneously over weeks to months. They commonly affect cranial nerves III, IV, VI, and VII, as well as thoracic nerves 4 through 12. Radiculopathy pain (from T4 through T12 nerve involvement) may mimic gastrointestinal or chest pain. Plexopathy is a focal neuropathy involving the brachial, lumbar, or sacral nerves.

Autonomic neuropathy is a diffuse neuropathy impairing both sympathetic and parasympathetic nerves, with far-reaching effects. It may involve the cardiovascular system, causing orthostatic hypotension, dizziness, and syncope. A cardiac denervation syndrome may occur, with fixed heart rates of 80 to 90 beats per minute, unchanged by exercise, sleep, or stress (Haas, 1993). These patients are at higher risk for anesthesia-induced arrhythmia. Loss of nerve function may also result in silent myocardial infarction, as patients are unable to experience anginal pain. In the patient with autonomic dysfunction and uncontrolled diabetes, hyperglycemia may produce osmotic diuresis, fluid loss, and further potential for hypotension.

Treatment of cardiovascular complications of autonomic neuropathy includes educating the patient to change positions slowly. A cardiac evaluation is advised before beginning an exercise program. Hypoglycemia should be avoided, as it increases oxygen demand on the heart. Hyperglycemia should be also be avoided to prevent osmotic diuresis.

Autonomic neuropathy affecting the gastrointestinal system presents as (1) gastroparesis (gastric slowing), with symptoms of early satiety, bloating, nausea, vomiting; (2) malabsorption, with resulting constipation or diarrhea, weight loss; and (3) fecal incontinence. Erratic blood glucose levels often result from unpredictable and variable nurient absorption. Treatment may include eating small, frequent meals and careful blood glucose monitoring, as well as treatment of the individual symptoms.

In the genitourinary system, autonomic neuropathy may cause bladder hypotonicity and potential for recurrent urinary tract infections due to urine stasis. Patients should be educated regarding the signs/symptoms of urinary tract infections. A bladder retraining program may be necessary. In men, erectile dysfunction and retrograde ejaculation may occur.

Hypoglycemic unawareness is the reduced ability to sense low blood glucose levels. It is caused by autonomic neuropathy involving the adrenal medulla. It can be extremely dangerous because patients are left without the usual neurogenic warning signs when hypoglycemia ensues, thereby increasing the risk of severe hypoglycemia. Patients should monitor blood glucose often (at least four times daily), and both patients and family members learn emergency treatment of hypoglycemia. Patients with hypoglycemic unawareness are not candidates for intensive glycemic control; therefore, target blood glucose range should be relaxed slightly to reduce the potential for hypoglycemia.

Other manifestations of autonomic neuropathy are sudomotor dysfunction and dark vision. With sudomotor dysfunction, sympathetic nerve dysfunction impairs the body's ability to regulate core temperature. Longer nerves are preferentially affected before shorter nerves. Therefore, lack of sweating (anhidrosis) occurs in the lower extremities, while compensatory hyperhydrosis occurs in the upper body, exhibited by excessive perspiration on the trunk and face. Dark vision occurs due to the inability of the pupil to adapt size to changes in light. Pupil size decreases, and thus patients have poor dark adaptation.

Macrovascular Complications

Atherosclerosis—in the form of coronary artery disease (CAD), peripheral vascular disease and cerebrovascular disease—accounts for approximately 80% of total diabetic mortality (Garber, 1994). Of these, 75% of diabetes-associated deaths are due to CAD. Seventy-seven percent of hospital admissions for diabetes complications are due to CAD. Coronary artery disease tends to be more severe in diabetic patients, and occurs at a younger age and in more females than in the general population. Many diabetics also have other risk factors that contribute to progression of macrovascular disease, such as hypertension, hyperlipidemia, hyperinsulinemia (in type 2 patients), and obesity. Tobacco use further increases this risk.

Treatment of macrovascular complications does not differ from recommendations for the general population. Reduction of risk factors should begin at diagnosis. This includes control of hypertension and hyperlipidemia, smoking cessation, and weight reduction. There should be a low threshold for cardiac work-up if ischemia is suspected, even if symptoms are somewhat atypical. In the diabetic patient, establishing glycemic control often yields a reduction of hypertriglyceridemia. Further discussion of hyperlipidemia is discussed in Chapter 29.

Diabetic Foot Infections

The topic of diabetic foot infections merits discussion, since recent data show these infections to be the cause of 20% of all hospitalizations in North America. If foot infections occur in conjunction with peripheral vascular disease, there is a greater risk that the patient will need lower extremity amputation. Data shows that one-half to two-thirds of all lower extremity amputations in the United States occur in diabetics, with >50,000 amputations in diabetics per year (Frykberg & Veves, 1996).

Neuropathy, peripheral vascular disease, and immunopathy all play roles in placing the diabetic at risk for foot infection. Table 39–34 lists the major risk factors for diabetic foot infection, and lists the pathophysiologic processes contributing to each risk factor.

Three to five organisms are typically cultured from moderate to severe diabetic foot wounds, most commonly aerobic gram-positive cocci including *Staphylococcus aureus*, coagulase-negative *staphylococci,* and group B *strep-*

TABLE 39–34. Major Risk Factors for Diabetic Foot Infection

Neuropathy	Vascular Disease	Immunopathy
Peripheral sensory "glove and stocking" distribution sensory deficits—negative symptoms paresthesias—positive symptoms Motor neuropathy Muscle weakness, atrophy "intrinsic minus" foot Footdrop Structural deformity Autonomic neuropathy Sympathetic failure Abnormal thermoregulatory responses Arteriovenous shunting Impaired maximal hyperemia Venous oxygenation Anhidrosis Dry skin, fissuring	Macrovascular Premature atherosclerosis Iliac and SFA disease Trifurcation disease characteristic Foot vessels spared Microvascular Capillary basement membrane thickening Altered nutrient exchange No "small vessel disease" Medial arterial calcification Medial smooth muscle atrophy	Abnormal host response Neutrophil dysfunction: Impaired chemotaxis Impaired phagocytosis Impaired bacterial killing

Reprinted with permission from Frykberg & Veves. (1996).

tococci (Frykberg & Veves, 1996). Wound culture should preferably be obtained from deep tissue at the base of the ulcer.

Foot infections are classified according to severity. Mild, or nonlimb threatening, infections are superficial, with <2 cm cellulitis and no signs of bone or joint involvement or systemic toxicity. Limb-threatening ulcers exhibit >2 cm cellulitis, with possible bone (osteomyelitis) or joint (septic arthritis) involvement, lymphangitis, and signs of systemic toxicity. Hyperglycemia is common.

Guidelines for the management of mild infection are listed in Table 39–35.

The patient with limb-threatening infection requires immediate hospitalization. Components of the management plan for diabetic patients with limb-threatening infections are provided in Table 39–36.

Follow-Up

Upon discharge, patients should be given parameters for calling their practitioners. This must be tailored to the individual patient, but a general example for the insulin-dependent diabetic would be as follows:

TABLE 39–35. Management of Mild Infections in Diabetic Patients

No weight-bearing on affected foot
Culture and sensitivities
Broad-spectrum oral antibiotics
Debridement and local dressings
Podiatric evaluation with frequent follow-up
Modified footwear
Education of patient for proper foot care principles

- Monitor blood glucose four times daily—before meals and at bedtime. Record.
- Call your practitioner for a blood glucose <60 or >400 once, or consistently <100 or >200.

A follow-up appointment should be arranged with the patient's practitioner(s) to encourage compliance and continued monitoring of blood glucose control.

▶ ADRENAL DISORDERS

Each of the two adrenal glands weighs 3 to 5 grams, and sits just above the upper tip of the kidneys. Normal size is

TABLE 39–36. Management Plan for the Diabetic Patient with a Limb-Threatening Infection

Bed rest
Podiatric consultation
Culture and sensitivities
Broad-spectrum intravenous antibiotics
Surgical debridement, drainage, and other procedures such as open amputation
Dressing changes
Podiatric appliances and footwear
Endocrine consult
Glycemic control, often requiring increased doses of insulin
Possible vascular surgery consult for evaluation of peripheral vascular disease and to assess the need for revascularization or amputation
Tests to determine bone or joint involvement; plain x-rays are not definitive; MRI or bone scan are felt to be best (consult with hospital radiologist)
Other consultations as needed, such as Infectious Disease and Orthopedic Surgery

about 2 inches in width at the widest point. The adrenal glands receive arterial blood from the aorta and renal arteries. The right adrenal drains into the inferior vena cava and the left into the left renal vein (Fig. 39–12).

There are two distinct endocrine tissues in each adrenal gland. The adrenal cortex is the outer layer, consisting of 80% of the gland. The cortex produces several types of steroid hormones. The adrenal medulla is the inner layer, consisting of the remaining 20% of the gland. The medulla produces catecholamines.

This section will address two of the more common adrenal disorders that the acute care nurse practitioner may encounter with hospitalized patients. Cushing's syndrome and Addison's disease involve inappropriate glucocorticoid secretion, an adrenal cortex dysfunction. Pheochromocytoma, a disorder involving catechoamine-secreting tumors, is also seen in the hospitalized patient, although is uncommon. This disorder is discussed in Chapter 30.

Cushing's Syndrome

Cushing's syndrome is the name applied to the condition of glucocorticoid excess. Cushing's "disease" refers to adrenal glucocorticoid excess when caused by pituitary secretion of ACTH.

Pathophysiology

Cortisol and other glucocorticoids are produced by the adrenal cortex. They increase gluconeogenesis and glycogen synthesis, inhibit protein synthesis, increase protein breakdown, and stimulate lypolysis. They are also antiinflammatory and immunosuppressive. Glucocorticoids enhance vascular reactivity, thereby maintaining blood pressure. Cortisol (hydrocortisone) is the major endogenous glucocorticoid.

Under normal circumstances, cortisol secretion is influenced by the feedback control loop of the hypothalamic–pituitary–adrenal axis. Circadian cycles and stress influence higher nerve centers which stimulate the hypothalamus to produce coticotropin-releasing hormone, which stimulates the anterior pituitary to produce ACTH. This in turn stimulates the adrenal gland to produce cortisol. Figure 39–13 shows this feedback control loop in detail.

Cushing's syndrome may be caused by exogenous glucocorticoids, such as those taken for treatment of autoimmune and inflammatory disorders, or by exogenous ACTH. Endogenous Cushing's syndrome has several etiologies. First, Cushing's disease is caused by pituitary hypersecretion of ACTH due to a benign pituitary adenoma. This accounts for 70% of all endogenous cases. Second, ectopic production of ACTH may occur due to malignant tumors, primarily in the lungs, or slow-growing carcinoid tumors (15% of all endogenous cases). Third, adrenal tumors, both benign and malignant, may cause excessive glucocorticoid production (15% of all endogenous cases).

Most patients with Cushing's disease are women (80%), ages 20 to 40 (Samuels, 1995). Ectopic ACTH syndrome is more common in men, and occurs usually between ages 40 and 60.

History and Physical Examination

The history should include assessment of current medical problems, neuropsychiatric disorders, alcohol history, and medications. Physical and mental stress, as well as depression and alcoholism, can cause mild hypercortisolemia (i.e., pseudo-Cushing's), and need to be screened. Exogenous glucocorticoid use must also be identified. Signs and symptoms of cortisol excess are listed as follows:

- Body habitus—central (truncal) obesity, moon facies, supraclavicular fat pad, and buffalo hump
- Muscle wasting—weakness, fatigue

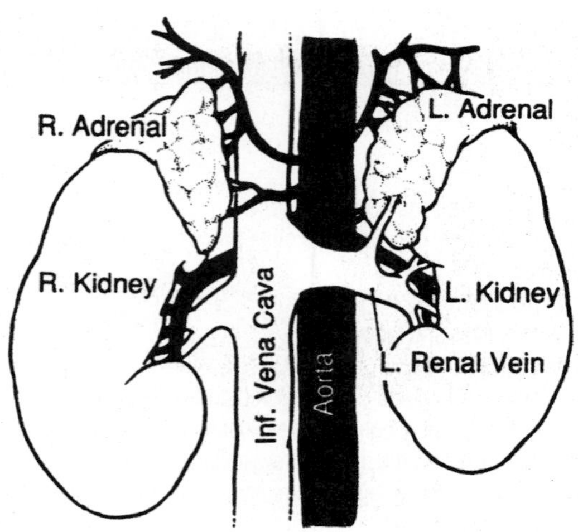

Figure 39–12. Gross anatomy of the adrenal glands. *(From Greenspan. [1997].)*

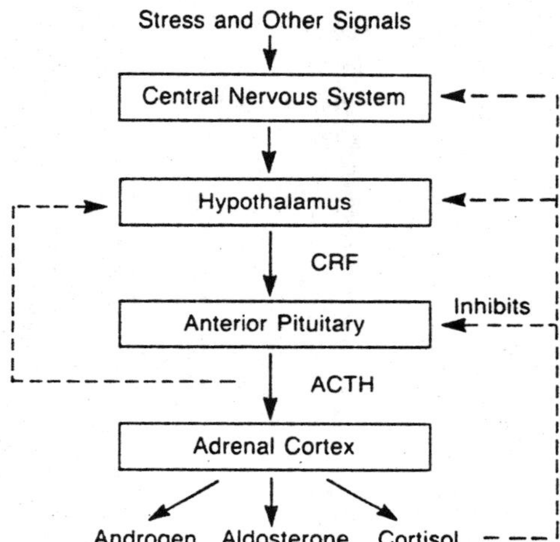

Figure 39–13. Mechanism for regulation of glucocorticoid secretion. *(From Greenspan. [1997].)*

- Skin changes—thinning of skin; ecchymosis; violaceous striae of abdomen, thighs, and axillae
- Cardiovascular—hypertension, atherosclerosis, congestive heart failure, and edema
- Hypogonadism and irregular menses
- Opportunistic infections and poor wound healing
- Osteoporosis and fractures
- Psychiatric disturbances—depression, emotional lability, sleep disturbances, impaired memory
- If due to pituitary tumor, may see headache, visual field disturbance, and hypopituitarism
- If due to ACTH excess, may see hyperpigmentation
- If androgen excess present also, may see hirsutism, acne, or virilization in females

Laboratory and Diagnostic Tests

The sequence of diagnosis is as follows: (1) establish the diagnosis of hypercortisolism, (2) distinguish ACTH-dependant hypercortisolism from adrenal neoplasm, and then (3) distinguish Cushing's disease from an ectopic ACTH-producing tumor (Fitzgerald, 1992).

The most useful test in determining Cushing's syndrome is the 24-hour urine collection for urinary free cortisol (Findling & Doppman, 1994). In most patients with endogenous Cushing's syndrome, 24-hour urinary free cortisol is >100 mcg/24 hr. Normal is usually <50 mcg/24 hr, depending on the test method used.

Another method for determining cortisol secretion is the low-dose overnight 1 mg dexamethasone suppression test. The patient is given 1 mg of dexamethasone po at 11 P.M., and a plasma cortisol level is drawn at 8 A.M.. Normal response is suppression of plasma cortisol to < 3-5 mcg/dL. Patients with Cushing's syndrome will not have suppression of cortisol production. False–negatives may be due to the occasional intermittent nature of hypercortisolism, or Cushing's disease (pituitary ACTH-dependent). False–positives may occur due to (1) drugs that accelerate dexamethasone metabolism (phenytoin, phenobarbital, rifampin), (2) estrogen therapy or tamoxifen, or (3) endogenous depression (Findling & Doppman, 1994).

The next step is to determine whether the hypercortisolism is ACTH-dependent or ACTH-independent. This may be determined by plasma ACTH levels via immunoradiometric assays. Although there are some difficulties with false–low levels, a general guideline for interpretation is as follows. An undetectable or very low ACTH level in a patient with hypercortisolism suggests adrenal tumor. A normal or slightly elevated ACTH level is suggestive of pituitary adenoma. A markedly elevated ACTH level may indicate ectopic secretion of ACTH.

If the plasma ACTH levels are low or undetectable, an adrenal source of hypercortisolism is pursued. An adrenal MRI is done to search for an adrenal tumor.

Some endocrinologists will choose to further distinguish between a pituitary and ectopic source of ACTH by performing further biochemical diagnostic tests. The following tests are usually done if the ACTH level is >10 pg/mL: (1) the high-dose dexamethasone suppression test, (2) the 8-mg overnight dexamethasone suppression test, or (3) the CRH (corticotropin releasing hormone) test (Meier & Biller, 1997).

A high-resolution MRI of the pituitary may be done once an ACTH-dependent Cushing's syndrome is diagnosed in order to screen for an adenoma. Since 10 to 20% of the normal population have incidental tumors of the pituitary or adrenal glands (most <6 mm in size), many centers accept the presence of a macroadenoma (>0.8-1 cm) as evidence for Cushing's disease (Meier & Biller, 1997).

A more accurate test is inferior petrosal sinus sampling (IPSS) for ACTH levels. Most centers consider this test to be essential in all patients without an unequivocal lesion demonstrated in the biochemical testing (Meier & Biller, 1997). IPSS is done by inserting catheters into the femoral veins and threading them simultaneously into the petrosal sinuses. If ACTH samples in the sinuses are >2.5 higher than the peripheral samples, there is a strong indication of a pituitary source of ACTH production. This sampling is best performed by skilled radiologists.

If the ACTH levels are similar, further search for a carcinoid tumor (an ectopic source of ACTH) begins. Chest, abdomen, and pelvis CT scans or MRIs are usually done. Neck imaging may be helpful if the patient has medullary thyroid cancer.

Management

Treatment depends on cause. An endocrine referral is appropriate for proper test interpretation and further diagnostic testing.

Cushing's disease is treated by transsphenoidal microadenectomy. This technique is 95% successful for first-time treatment (Loriaux, 1991). An immediate repeat procedure usually cures 50% of those who fail the first time. Radiation therapy is an option for failed cases, as well as bilateral adrenalectomy. Patients are given hydrocortisone for 6 to 18 months postoperatively to treat the adrenal insufficiency that develops. Treatment for ectopic ACTH-secreting tumor is surgical ablation. Treatment for adrenal carcinoma and benign adrenal adenomas is also surgical ablation.

Medical treatment is not as successful as surgery in Cushing's syndrome, and is accompanied by significant medication side effects (Miller & Crapo, 1993). Currently, drugs such as mitotane, metyrapone, aminoglutethimide, ketoconazole, and RU-486 are used for medical management. Reasons for medical therapy are (1) to correct metabolic abnormalities before surgery, (2) to palliate surgically noncurable disease, and (3) to achieve remission pharmacologically in patients who would not benefit from surgery.

Follow-Up

Patients should be advised to follow-up with their endocrinologist upon discharge in order to monitor progress with glucocorticoid replacement. For the patient with bilateral adrenalectomy, the patient must be educated on the need for life-long corticosteroid and mineralocorticoid replacement. Patients should be instructed on signs/symptoms of adrenal insufficiency.

Addison's Disease

Addison's disease is defined as hypofunction of the adrenal cortex. It occurs in 1 out of 100,000 people, and equally among men and women of all age groups (Corrigan, 1989).

Pathophysiology

Adrenal insufficiency is caused by either dysfunction of the adrenal cortex (primary adrenal insufficiency), or inadequate ACTH secretion (secondary adrenal insuffiency). In primary adrenal insufficiency, more than 90% of the adrenal cortex function must be impaired before signs and symptoms develop. Destruction of the adrenal gland may also produce mineralcorticoid defiency (including aldosterone).

The most common cause is autoimmune adrenalitis, either of the adrenal gland itself or associated with a polyglandular autoimmune syndrome. Other causes include surgical removal of the adrenal gland, infection (tuberculosis, AIDS, and fungal), bilateral adrenal hemorrhage from anticoagulants or sepsis, or metastasis into the adrenal gland. Some medications given in high doses may cause adrenal insufficiency by reducing circulating levels of adrenal steroids, such as ketoconazole, aminoglutethimide, and rifampin (Jones, 1995).

Secondary adrenal insufficiency is caused by a deficiency of ACTH associated with panhypopituitarism from disease involving the hypothalamic–pituitary axis or with use of exogenous steroids.

History and Physical Examination

The patient should be questioned about the following symptoms of adrenal insufficiency: weakness, fatigue, anorexia, nausea, vomiting, diarrhea, abdominal pain, orthostatic hypotension, arthralgias and myalgias, psychiatric disorder (from memory loss to psychosis), and salt-craving.

Physical examination should focus on the following signs: weight loss, hyperpigmentation (seen with primary adrenal insufficiency), vitiligo (seen in 10-20% of patients with autoimmune adrenalitis), hypotension (seen in both primary and secondary adrenal insufficiency), and decreased pubic and axillary hair and amenorrhea in women due to loss of adrenal androgen secretion. Hyperpigmentation may be generalized or localized on such areas as knees, elbows, creases of hands, or mucous membranes.

Laboratory and Diagnostic Tests

Hyponatremia and hyperkalemia occur as a result of aldosterone deficiency and is seen in primary adrenal insufficiency. Serum chloride and bicarbonate may also be reduced. Prerenal azotemia may be seen in primary adrenal insuffiency due to volume depletion. Hypercalcemia occurs in 10 to 20% of patients (Williams & Dluhy, 1991). TSH level may be elevated. EKG may show nonspecific changes. There may also be a normochromic anemia, eosinophilia, and leukocytosis on CBC. Hypoglycemia may be seen in secondary adrenal insufficiency.

Diagnosis is made based on administration of a short or rapid ACTH (cosyntropin) stimulation test. This will show whether the adrenals are able to secrete cortisol in response to administration of ACTH. The procedure for the rapid ACTH stimulation test is as follows:

1. A baseline plasma cortisol is drawn.
2. A synthetic form of ACTH, cosyntropin 250 mcg, is given IM or IV.
3. Plasma cortisol levels are drawn 30 and 60 minutes after the initial injection.

Posttest levels that are <18 mcg/dL are abnormal, and thus indicative of adrenal insufficiency. Also, an increment increase of <8 mcg/dL above baseline are considered abnormal, unless the person already has an elevated cortisol in response to illness. The response may also be blunted if there is a cortisol-binding deficiency, such as in liver disease, nephrotic syndrome, and multiple myeloma.

Other tests may be performed to determine the cause of adrenal insufficiency. A long ACTH stimulation test may be performed by infusing cosyntropin IV over 48 to 72 hours, and plasma cortisol and urinary 17-hydroxycorticosterone measured serially. Patients with primary adrenal insufficiency will show an insufficient increase in these levels, whereas those with secondary adrenal insufficiency will have adequate cortisol response over a 2- to 3-day period.

Plasma ACTH levels may be measured before and after ACTH administration. A low level signals secondary adrenal insufficiency, while a high level signals primary adrenal insufficiency. Some endocrinologists perform other tests, such as the CRH stimulation test or the insulin tolerance test.

Management

An endocrine consult should be maintained. A rapid ACTH stimulation test may be performed by the nurse practitioner to further aid in diagnosis.

Steroid hormone replacement in physiologic dosage is the mainstay of therapy. Hydrocortisone is the drug of choice, and is given in a dosage range of 15-40 mg/day in divided doses. A typical dose is 20 mg QAM, 10 mg QPM. Prednisone (2.5-7.5 mg daily) or dexamethasone (0.25-0.75 mg daily) may be another alternative steroid replacement choice.

During times of stress—such as febrile illness, trauma, and surgical or diagnostic procedure—stress-dose steroids should be given in order to prevent adrenal crisis, which can be fatal. Doubling or tripling the glucocorticoid dose may be fine for mild or moderate infections, but for more major stressors such as surgery with general anesthesia, hydrocortisone 100 mg every 6 hours should be given. Stress-dose steroids may be tapered over 1 to 2 days after the stress is resolved.

Fludrocortisone (Florinef) is the drug used for aldosterone replacement in primary adrenal insufficiency. It is given in a daily dose of 0.05 to 0.2 mg daily. Mineralocorticoid production in secondary adrenal insufficiency is usually preserved, so replacement is not needed in most cases.

Hospitalized patients in adrenal crisis should be treated emergently for hypotension and potential hypoglycemia with D5W and 0.9% NS solution IV. Plasma cortisol and ACTH levels should be drawn, and replacement with hydrocortisone 100 mg IV every 6 hours begun. (Some endocrinologists may replace initially with dexamethasone.) At this replacement dose, hydrocortisone has enough mineralocorticoid effect that this is not needed. Once the patient is stabilized, an investigation of precipitating cause should begin. Stress-dose steroids should then be tapered to maintenance dose over 1 to 3 days after stress is resolved. Electrolytes should be monitored.

For those patients who have been treated with exogenous steroids for nonadrenal disorders for long periods, taper should be done gradually. For some, recovery of the complete pituitary–adrenal axis may take 6 to 12 months.

Follow-Up

Prior to discharge, the patient should, if possible, be instructed in parenteral self-administration of steroids, and should be given instructions to carry medical identification. The patient should be educated regarding signs and symptoms of adrenal insufficiency, and told to call his or her health-care provider at the onset of illness or infection. Discharge instructions should advise patients to take steroids with food.

REFERENCES

Aiello, L. M. & Cavallerano, J. D. (1994). Ocular complications. In L. E. Lebovitz (Ed.), *Therapy for diabetes mellitus and related disorders* (2nd ed.). (pp. 235–248). Alexandria, VA: American Diabetes Association.

Alberti, K. (1995). Diabetic acidosis, hyperosmolar coma, and lactic acidosis. In K. L. Becker (Ed.), *Principles and practice of endocrinology and metabolism* (2nd ed.). (pp. 1316–1329). Philadelphia: J. B. Lippincott.

American Association of Clinical Endocrinologists. (1995). AACE Guidelines for the Evaluation and Treatment of Hyperthyroidism and Hypothyroidism (on-line). Available at web site: http://www.aace.com/guidelines/index.html

American Association of Clinical Endocrinologists. (1995). AACE Guidelines for the Management of Diabetes Mellitus (on-line). Available at web site: http://www.aace.com/guidelines/index.html

American Association of Clinical Endocrinologists. (1996). AACE Clinical Practice Guidelines for the Diagnosis and Management of Thyroid Nodules (on-line). Available at web site: http://www.aace.com/guidelines/index.html

American Diabetes Association. (1992). Pancreas transplantation for patients with diabetes mellitus. *Diabetes Care, 15*(11), 1668–1672.

American Diabetes Association. (1996). *Diabetes 1996: Vital Statistics*. Alexandria, VA: American Diabetes Association.

American Diabetes Association. (1997). American Diabetes Association: Clinical practice recommendations 1997. *Diabetes Care, 20* (Supple. 1).

Arauz-Pacheco, C. & Raskin, P. (1994). Surgery and Anesthesia. In L. E. Lebovitz (Ed.), *Therapy for diabetes mellitus and related disorders* (2nd ed.). (pp. 156–163). Alexandria, VA: American Diabetes Association.

Bailey, C. J. (1992). Biguanides and NIDDM. *Diabetes Care, 15*(6), 755–772.

Bartalena, L., Brogioni, S., Grasso, L., Bogazzi, F., Burelli, A., & Martino, E. (1996). Treatment of amiodarone-induced thyrotoxicosis, a difficult challenge: Results of a prospective study. *Journal of Clinical Endocrinology and Metabolism, 81* (8), 2930–2933.

Barzilai, N. (1995). Clinical use of metformin in the United States. *Diabetes Spectrum, 8* (4), 194–197.

Beaser, R. S. (1992). Fine-tuning insulin therapy. *Postgraduate Medicine, 91*(4), 323–330.

Becker, C. (1985). Hypothyroidism and atherosclerotic heart disease: Pathogenesis, medical management, and the role of coronary artery bypass surgery. *Endocrine Reviews, 6* (3), 432–440.

Bianco, C. M. (1996). Diabetes insipidus. Your role in managing this multifacted disease. *American Journal of Nursing, 96* (8), 30–31.

Brent, G. A. & Hershman, J. M. (1986). Thyroxine therapy in patients with severe nonthyroidal illnesses and low serum thyroxine concentration. *Journal of Clinical Endocrinology and Metabolism, 63,* 1–8.

Burch, H. B. & Wartofsky, L. (1993). Life-threatening thyrotoxicosis. *Endocrinology and Metabolism Clinics of North America, 22* (2), 263–277.

Burman, K. (1995). Hyperthyroidism. In K. L. Becker (Ed.), *Principles and practice of endocrinology and metabolism* (2nd ed.). (pp. 367–385). Philadelphia: J. B. Lippincott.

Burmeister, L. A. (1995). Reverse T3 does not reliably differentiate hypothyroid sick syndrome from euthyroid sick syndrome. *Thyroid, 5,* 435–442.

Chopra, I. (1997). Euthyroid sick syndrome: Is it a misnomer? *Journal of Clinical Endocrinology and Metabolism, 82* (2), 329–334.

Clement, S. (1995a). Chronic complications of diabetes mellitus. In M. T. McDermott (Ed.), *Endocrine Secrets* (pp. 20–28). Philadelphia: Hanley & Belfus.

Clement, S. (1995b). Diabetes mellitus. In M. T. McDermott (Ed.), *Endocrine Secrets* (pp. 1–12). Philadelphia: Hanley & Belfus.

Clement, S. & Torrens, J. I. (1995). Acute complications of diabetes mellitus. In M. T. McDermott (Ed.), *Endocrine Secrets* (pp. 13–19). Philadelphia: Hanley & Belfus.

Coffland, F. I. (1993). Thyroid-induced cardiac disorders. *Critical Care Nurse, 13* (3), 25–30.

Comi, R. J. (1993). Approach to acute hypoglycemia. *Endocrinology and Metabolism Clinics of North America, 22* (2), 246–262.

Corrigan, E. K. (1989). *Addison's disease* (NIH Publication No. 90-3054). Bethesda, MD: Office of Health Research Reports.

Daly, A. (1994). In L. E. Lebovitz (Ed.), *Therapy for diabetes mellitus and related disorders* (2nd ed.). (pp. 95–101). Alexandra, VA: American Diabetes Association.

DeFronzo, R. A. (1994). Nephropathy. In L. E. Lebovitz (Ed.), *Therapy for diabetes mellitus and related disorders* (2nd ed.), (pp. 256–269). Alexandria, VA: American Diabetes Association.

The Diabetes Control and Complications Trial (DCCT) Research Group. (1988). Factors in development of diabetic neuropathy: Baseline analysis of neuropathy in feasibility phase of diabetes control and complications trial. *Diabetes, 37,* 476–481.

The Diabetes Control and Complications Trial (DCCT) Research Group. (1993). The effect of intensive treatment of diabetes on the development and progression of long-term complications in insulin-dependent diabetes mellitus. *The New England Journal of Medicine, 329* (14), 977–986.

Dillman, W. H. (1996). The thyroid. In J. C. Bennett & F. Plum (Eds.), *Cecil textbook of medicine* (20th ed.). (pp. 1227–1245). Philadelphia: W. B. Saunders.

Dong, B. J., Hauck, W. W., Gambertoglio, J. G., Gee, L., White, J. R., Bubp, J. L., & Greenspan, F. S. (1997). Bioequivalence of generic and brand-name levothyroxine products in the treatment of hypothyroidism. *Journal of the American Medical Association, 277* (15), 1205–1213.

Drucker, D. J. & Burrow, G. N. (1985). Cardiovascular surgery in the hypothyroid patient. *Archives of Internal Medicine, 145,* 1585–1587.

Expert Committee on the Diagnosis and Classification of Diabetes Mellitus. (1997). Report of the expert committee on the diagnosis and classification of diabetes mellitus. *Diabetes Care, 20* (7), 1183–1197.

Fain, J. A. (1993). National trends in diabetes. *Nursing Clinics of North America, 28* (1), 1–7.

Findling, J. W. & Doppman, J. L. (1994). Biochemical and radiologic diagnosis of Cushing's syndrome. *Endocrinology and Metabolism Clinics of North America, 23* (3), 511–536.

Fitzgerald, P. (1992). *Handbook of clinical endocrinology* (2nd ed.). Norwalk, CT: Appleton & Lange.

Fleckman, A. M. (1991). Diabetic ketoacidosis. *Practical Diabetology, 10* (3), 1–8.

Fleckman, A. M. (1993). Diabetic ketoacidosis. *Endocrinology and Metabolism Clinics of North America, 22* (2), 181–207.

Foster, D. W. (1991). Diabetes mellitus. In J. D. Wilson, E. Braunwald, K. J. Isselbacher, R. G. Petersdorf, J. B. Martin, A. S. Fauci, & R. K. Root (Eds.), *Harrison's principles of internal medicine* (12th ed.). (pp. 1739–1759). New York: McGraw-Hill.

Frykberg, R. G. & Veves, A. (1996). Diabetic foot infections. *Diabetes/Metabolism Reviews, 12* (3), 255–270.

Garber, A. L. (1994). Myocardial infarction. In H. E. Lebovitz (Ed.), *Therapy for diabetes mellitus and related disorders* (2nd ed.). (pp. 337–340). Alexandria, VA: American Diabetes Association.

Gavin, L. A. (1992). Perioperative management of the diabetic patient. *Endocrinology and Metabolism Clinics of North America, 21* (2), 457–473.

Genuth, S. (1994). Diabetic ketoacidosis and hyperosmolar hyperglycemic nonketotic syndrome in adults. In H. G. Lebovitz (Ed.), *Therapy for diabetes mellitus and related disorders* (2nd ed.). (pp. 66–76). Alexandria, VA: American Diabetes Association.

Greenspan, F. S. (1997). The thyroid gland. In F. S. Greenspan & G. J. Strewler (Eds.), *Basic & clinical endocrinology* (5th ed.) (pp. 192–262). Stamford, CT: Appleton & Lange.

Haas, L. B. (1993). Chronic complications of diabetes mellitus. *Nursing Clinics of North America, 28* (1), 71–85.

Haugen, B. R. & Ridgway, E. C. (1995). Hypothyroidism. In M. T. McDermott (Ed.), *Endocrine secrets* (pp. 175–177). Philadelphia: Hanley & Belfus.

Hirsch, I. B. & Farkas-Hirsch, R. (1993). Type I diabetes and insulin therapy. *Nursing Clinics of North America, 28* (1), 9–23.

Hirsch, I. B., Paauw, D. S., & Brunzell, J. (1995). Inpatient management of adults with diabetes. *Diabetes Care, 18* (6), 870–878.

Hollander, Pi-Sunyer, X. & Coniff, R. F. (1997). Acarbose in the treatment of type I diabetes. *Diabetes Care, 20* (3), 248–253.

Horton, E. S. (1994). Exercise. In H. E. Lebovitz (Ed.), *Therapy for diabetes mellitus and related disorders* (2nd ed.). (pp. 107–115). Alexandria, VA: American Diabetes Association.

Jones, R. E. (1995). Adrenal insufficiency. In M. T. McDermott (Ed.), *Endocrine Secrets* (pp. 156–160). Philadelphia: Hanley & Belfus.

Kenyon, N. S., Alejandro, R., Mintz, D. H., & Ricordi, C. (1996). Islet cell transplantation: Beyond the paradigms. *Diabetes/Metabolism Reviews, 12* (4), 361–370.

Koproski, J., Pretto, Z., Poretsky, L. (1997). Effects of an intervention by a diabetes team in hospitalized patients with diabetes. *Diabetes Care, 20* (10), 1553–1555.

Kovacs, L. & Robertson, G. L. (1992). Syndrome of inappropriate antidiuresis. *Endocrinology and Metabolism Clinics of North America, 21* (4), 859–875.

Lasswell, W. J. & Burman, K. D. (1995). Hyperthyroidism. In M. T. McDermott (Ed.), *Endocrine Secrets* (pp. 171–174). Philadelphia: Hanley & Belfus.

Lebovitz, L. E. (1994). Sulfonylurea drugs. In L. E. Lebovitz (Ed.), *Therapy for diabetes mellitus and related disorders* (2nd ed.). (pp. 116–123). Alexandria, VA: American Diabetes Association.

Lorber, D. L. (1995). Nonketotic hypertonicity in diabetes mellitus. *Medical Clinics of North America, 79* (1), 39–52.

Loriaux, D. L. (1991). The treatment of Cushing's syndrome and adrenal cancer. *Endocrinology and Metabolism Clinics of North America, 20* (4), 767–771.

Lun, W. S. (1993). Use of oral hypoglycemic agents in the elderly. *Practical Diabetology,* 10–13.

Mandel, S. J., Brent, G. A., & Larsen, P. R. (1993). Levothyroxine therapy in patients with thyroid disease. *Annals of Internal Medicine, 119* (6), 492–502.

Maratos-Flier, E. (1995). Oral agents for the treatment of type II diabetes mellitus. In K. L. Becker (Ed.), *Principles and practice of endocrinology and metabolism* (2nd ed.). (pp. 1235–1237). Philadelphia: J. B. Lippincott.

Meier, C. A. & Biller, M. K. (1997). Clinical and biochemical evaluation of Cushing's syndrome. *Endocrinology and Metabolism Clinics of North America, 26* (4), 741–762.

Miller, J. W. & Crapo, L. (1993). The medical treatment of Cushing's syndrome. *Endocrine Reviews, 14* (4), 443–458.

Molitch, M. E. (Ed.). (1995). *Medical knowledge self-assessment program in the subspecialty of endocrinology and metabolism.* Philadelphia: American College of Physicians.

Nathan, D. M. (1993). Long-term complication of diabetes mellitus. *The New England Journal of Medicine, 328* (23), 1676–1685.

National Diabetes Data Group. (1979). Classification and diagnosis of diabetes mellitus and other categories of glucose intolerance. *Diabetes, 28,* 1039–1057.

Peragallo-Dittko, V., Godley, K, & Meyer, J. (Eds.). (1993). *A Core Curriculum for Diabetes Education* (10th ed.). Chicago: American Association of Diabetes Educators and the AADE Education and Research Foundation.

Pfeifer, M. A. (1994). Painful or insensitive lower extremity. In J. E. Lebovitz (Ed.), *Therapy for diabetes mellitus and related disorders* (2nd ed.). (pp. 279–282). Alexandria, VA: American Diabetes Association.

Rhoades, R. & Pflanzer, R. (Eds.). (1992). *Human physiology* (2nd ed.). Orlando, FL: Saunders College Publishing.

Robertson, G. L. (1995). Diabetes insipidus. *Endocrinology and Metabolism Clinics of North America, 24* (3), 549–572.

Roman, S. H. & Harris, M. I. (1997). Management of diabetes mellitus from a public health perspective. *Endocrinology and Metabolism Clinics of North America, 26* (3), 443–474.

Rosenberg, C. (1990). Wound healing in the patient with diabetes mellitus. *Nursing Clinics of North America, 25* (1), 247–261.

Safrit, H. F. (1992). Thyroid disorders. In P. A. Fitzgerald, (Ed.), *Handbook of clinical endocrinology* (2nd ed.). (pp. 156–226). Norwalk, CT: Appleton & Lange.

Saltiel, R. & Olefsky, J. (1996). Thiazolidinediones in the treatment of insulin resistance and type II diabetes. *Diabetes, 45* (12) 1661–1669.

Samuels, M. H. (1995). Cushing's syndrome. In M. T. McDermott (Ed.). (pp. 116–121). *Endocrine secrets.* Philadelphia: Hanley & Belfus.

Santiago, J. V., Levandoski, L. A., & Bubb, J. (1994). Hypoglycemia. In H. E. Lebovitz (Ed.), *Therapy for diabetes mellitus and related disorders* (2nd ed.). (pp. 170–177). Alexandria, VA: American Diabetes Association.

Sarkar, S. D. & Becker, D. V. (1995). Thyroid uptake and imaging. In K. L. Becker (Ed.), *Principles and practice of endocrinology and metabolism* (2nd ed.). (pp. 307–313). Philadelphia: J. B. Lippincott.

Schilling, J. S. (1997). Hyperthyroidism: Diagnosis and management of Graves' disease. *The Nurse Practitioner, 22* (6), 72–95.

Shapiro, L. E. & Surks, M. I. (1995). Hypothyroidism. In K. L. Becker (Ed.), *Principles and practice of endocrinology and metabolism* (2nd ed.). (pp. 404–412). Philadelphia: J. B. Lippincott.

Singer, P. A., Cooper, D. S., Daniels, G. H., Ladenson, P. W., Greenspan, F. S., Levy, E. G., Braverman, L. E., Clark, O. H., McDougall, I. R., Ain, K. V., & Dortman, S. G. (1996). Treatment guidelines for patients with thyroid nodules and well-differentiated thyroid cancer. *Archives of Internal Medicine, 156* (19), 2165–2172.

Skyler, J. S. (1997). Insulin therapy in type II diabetes: Who needs it, how much of it, and for how long? *Postgraduate Medicine, 101* (2), 85–96.

Slag, M. F., Morley, J. E., Elson, M. K., Crowson, T. W., Nettle, F. Q., & Shafer, R. B. (1981). Hypothyroxinemia in critically ill patients as a predictor of high mortality. *Journal of the American Medical Association, 245,* 43–45.

Smallridge, R. C. (1992). Metabolic and anatomic thyroid emergencies: A review. *Critical Care Medicine, 20* (2), 276–291.

Smallridge, R. C. (1995). Thyroid function tests. In K. L. Becker (Ed.), *Principles and practice of endocrinology and metabolism* (2nd ed.). (pp. 299–306). Philadelphia: J. B. Lippincott.

Streff, M. M. & Pachucki-Hyde, L. C. (1996). Management of the patient with thyroid disease. *Nursing Clinics of North America, 31* (4), 779–796.

Sutherland, D. E. R. (1996). Pancreas and islet cell transplantation: Now and then. *Transplantation Proceedings, 28* (4), 2131–2133.

Sutherland, D. E. R, Gruessner, R. W. G., et al. (1994). Results with renal transplants after previous solitary pancreas transplants. *Transplantation Proceedings, 26* (2), 448–449.

Teter, M. L. (1997). Troglitzaone: A new class of oral antihyperglycemic for the treatment of type II diabetes. *The Nurse Practitioner, 22* (7), 119–121.

Wartofsky, L. (1996). Treatment options for hyperthyroidism. *Hospital Practice, 31* (9), 69–83.

Wartofsky, L. & Ahmann, A. J. (1995). The thyroid nodule. In K. L. Becker (Ed.), *Principles and practice of endocrinology and metabolism* (2nd ed.). (pp. 345–353). Philadelphia: J. B. Lippincott.

White, J. R., Hartman, J., & Campbell, R. K. (1993). Drug interaction in diabetic patients. The risk of losing glycemic control. *Postgraduate Medicine, 93* (3), 131–139.

Williams, G. H. & Dluhy, R. G. (1991). Diseases of the adrenal cortex. In J. D. Wilson, E. Braunwald, K. J. Isselbacher, R. G. Petersdorf, J. B. Martin, A. S. Fauci, & R. K. Root (Eds.), *Harrison's principles of internal medicine* (12th ed.). (pp. 1713–1735). New York: McGraw-Hill.

Yki-Jarvinen, H., Kauppila, M., Kujansuu, E., Lahti, J., Marjanen, T., Niskanen, L., Rajala, S., Ryysy, L., Salo, S., Seppala, P., Tulokas, T., Viikari, J., Karjalainen, J., & Taskinen, M. (1992). Comparison of insulin regimens in patients with non-insulin-dependent diabetes mellitus. *The New England Journal of Medicine, 327* (20), 1426–1433.

40

Neurological Problems

Catherine Borkowski-Benoit

Caring for patients with neurologic disease presents significant challenges to the acute care nurse practitioner. The caregiver must be able not only to manage the patient's medical problems, but must also assist the patient to manage the human responses to an often devastating illness or injury at a personal, family, and community level (Keane & Richmond, 1993). An exhaustive review of normal neuroanatomy and physiology is beyond the scope of this chapter, but a brief overview is included to highlight the areas most relevant to clinical practice. Discussion of the most common neurological problems likely to be encountered by the acute care nurse practitioner follows.

▶ OVERVIEW OF NEUROANATOMY AND PHYSIOLOGY

Cells of the Nervous System

The nervous system is made up of two types of cells: neurons and neuroglia. The neuron is the basic anatomical and functional unit of the nervous system. Neurons have the ability to generate and transmit impulses and influence other neurons, muscle cells, and glandular cells by transmitting nerve impulses to them. The three major components of a neuron include the cell body, a single axon (which carries nerve impulses to other neurons or to end organs), and several dendrites (which receive nerve impulses from the axons of other neurons and conduct impulses toward the cell body).

Neuroglia cells, or glial cells, provide structural support, protection, and nourishment to neurons. Comprising 40% of the brain and spinal cord mass, they are five to ten times more prevalent than neurons. There are six types of neuroglia cells in the nervous system, each having a particular function (Table 40–1). These cells are the origins of most primary central nervous system (CNS) tumors.

Physiology of Nerve Impulse Conduction

The initiation of a nerve impulse involves the generation of an action potential. Action potentials travel along the axon and are transmitted across the synapse (the junction between nerve cells) by a chemical interaction involving neurotransmitters. When the neuron is in a resting state, the intracellular space carries a negative electric charge relative to

TABLE 40–1. Types of Neuroglia Cells

Microglia	Phagocytic function; remove the waste products of neurons
Oligodendrocytes	Produce the myelin sheath of the axon (which acts as an insulator for the conduction of impulses) in the CNS
Astrocytes	Provide nutrition for neurons; form a structural support between capillaries and neurons; form part of the blood–brain barrier
Ependyma	Line the ventricular system; aid the production of cerebrospinal fluid (CSF)
Schwann Cells	Form the myelin sheath around axons in the peripheral nervous system (PNS)
Satellite Cells	Support neuron cell bodies within ganglia of the PNS

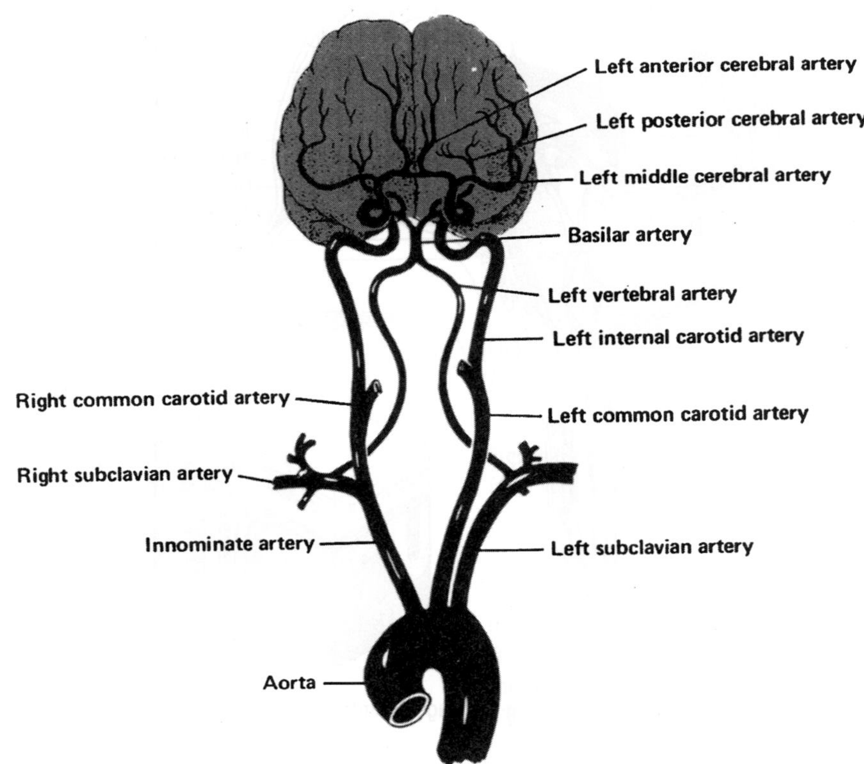

Figure 40–7. Arteries in the neck and the cerebral arteries. *(From Burrell. [1992]. [p. 840].)*

or cranial surgery. Patients may develop temperature elevations in the range of 105° to 107°F without exhibiting diurnal variation or sweating. These "central fevers" are often resistant to conventional treatment with Tylenol or other antipyretics.

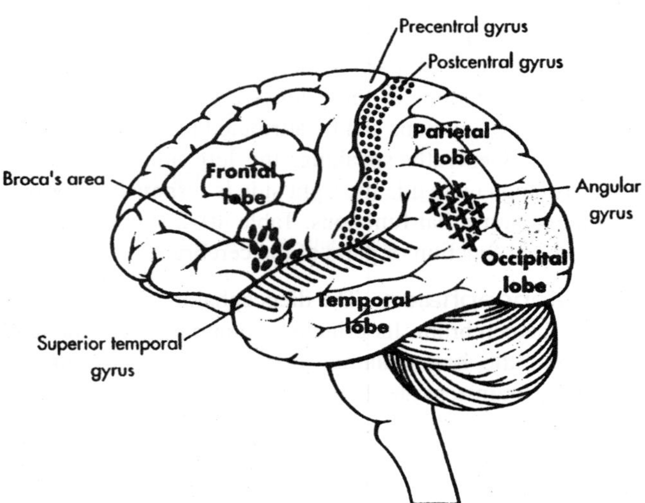

Figure 40–8. Major lobes and areas of the brain. *(Used with permission from Lewis, Collier, & Heitkemper. [1996].)*

The basal ganglia is composed of a group of structures located deep within the cerebral hemispheres. These structures function to modulate the initiation, execution, and completion of voluntary and automatic movements associated with skeletal activity, particularly in the hands and the lower extremities (i.e., swinging of the arms while walking). Examples of basal ganglia dysfunction include Parkinson's disease and drug-induced syndromes such as Tardive dyskinesias.

The Cerebellum. The cerebellum is involved in regulating muscle synergy throughout the body by interpreting incoming sensory information and providing corrective feedback after this information is evaluated. Principle cerebellar functions are listed in Table 40–4.

The Brainstem. The brainstem includes the midbrain, the pons, and the medulla. Ascending and descending fibers pass through the brainstem going to and from the cerebrum and cerebellum. The origins of cranial nerves III through XII also emanate from the brainstem (Fig. 40–10). Respiratory, vasomotor, and cardiac functions are regulated by the medulla. The reticular activating system (RAS) is a diffuse system that extends through the brainstem to the cerebral cortex. The RAS is a regulatory system controlling the sleep–wake cycle, arousal, and consciousness.

TABLE 40–2. Location and Function of Parts of the Cerebrum

Part	Location	Function
Cortical areas		
Motor		
Primary	Precentral gyrus	Controls initiation of movement on opposite side of body
Supplemental	Anterior to precentral gyrus	Facilitates proximal muscle activity, including activity for stance and gait, and spontaneous movement and coordination
Sensory		
Somatic	Postcentral gyrus	Registers body sensations from opposite side of body
Visual	Occipital lobe	Registers visual images
Auditory	Superior temporal gyrus	Registers auditory input
Association areas	Parietal lobe	Integrates somatic and special sensory inputs
	Posterior temporal lobe	Integrates visual and auditory inputs for language comprehension
	Anterior temporal lobe	Integrates past experiences
	Anterior frontal lobe	Controls higher-order processes (i.e., judgment, insight, reasoning)
Language		
Comprehension	Angular gyrus	Integrates auditory language (understanding of spoken word)
Expression	Broca's area	Regulates verbal expression
Basal Ganglia	Near lateral ventricles of both cerebral hemispheres	Controls and facilitates learned and automatic movements
Thalamus	Below basal ganglia	Relays sensory and motor inputs to cortex and other parts of cerebrum
Hypothalamus	Below thalamus	Regulates endocrine and autonomic functions (i.e., feeding, sleeping)
Limbic system	Lateral to hypothalamus	Influences affective (emotional) behavior and basic drives such as feeding and sexual behavior

From Lewis, Collier, & Heitkemph. (1996).

The Cranial Nerves. Twelve pairs of cranial nerves are part of the peripheral nervous system. The nerves are numbered in the order in which their nuclei connect to the cerebral hemispheres and the brainstem. Cranial nerves I and II attach to the cerebral hemispheres, while III through XII attach to the brainstem. The functions of the cranial nerves most relevant to clinical practice are summarized in Table 40–5.

The Spinal Cord

Continuous with the brainstem, the spinal cord is a cylindrical mass of nervous tissue encased within the vertebral column. Thirty-one pairs of spinal nerves exit from the cord: 8 cervical, 12 thoracic, 5 lumbar, 5 sacral, and 1 coccygeal (Fig. 40–11). Each spinal nerve has a posterior root and an anterior root. The posterior root contains the sensory fibers that transmit impulses from skin segments called dermatomes. The motor root carries impulses from the spinal cord via the peripheral nerve to the muscles.

A cross section of the cord reveals gray matter that is centrally located in the shape of an "H" surrounded by white matter. The gray matter contains the cell bodies and neuronal projections, and the white matter contains the axons of the descending motor fibers and the ascending sensory fibers, some of which are myelinated.

Motor Pathways. Descending tracts carry impulses responsible for muscle movement. The corticospinal (pyra-

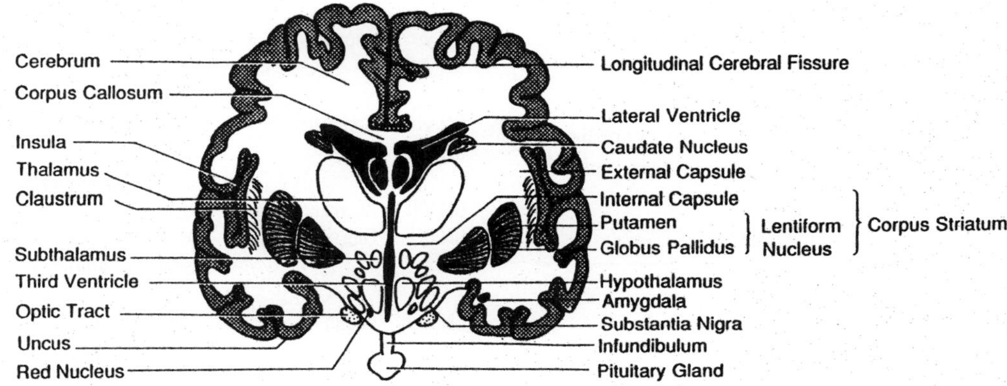

Figure 40–9. The diencephalon. *(From Burrell. [1992]. [p. 843].)*

TABLE 40–3. Functions of the Hypothalamus

Temperature control by monitoring the temperature of blood that flows through the hypothalamus and appropriately affecting sweat glands, peripheral blood vessels, and muscles
Water metabolism through the regulation of antidiuretic hormone (ADH)
Control of secretions from the pituitary, i.e., growth hormone and follicle-stimulating hormone
Involvement with the autonomic nervous system to regulate visceral and somatic activities
Control of appetite
Involvement in the regulation of the sleep–wake cycle
Control of the thirst center

midal tract) carries impulses for voluntary movement from the motor cortex in the brain to the peripheral nerves. These tracts cross in the brainstem. The extrapyramidal system includes motor pathways in the cerebral cortex, the brainstem, the basal ganglia, and the spinal cord. It works to maintain muscle tone and coordinate some automatic activities such as walking. Last, the cerebellar system receives both sensory and motor information. This system coordinates muscular activity, helps to control posture, and maintains equilibrium (Fig. 40–12).

Sensory Pathways. Ascending tracts carry sensory information from the skin, muscles, joints, viscera, and blood vessels to higher levels in the CNS for interpretation. The spinothalamic tracts transmit pain, temperature, and crude touch impulses. Fibers from these tracts cross to the opposite side of the spinal cord within one or two spinal segments from their point of entry into the cord. The posterior columns carry information of proprioception and vibratory sense. Impulses ascend the cord uncrossed until reaching the area of decussation or crossing in the medulla. They are then sent to the thalamus.

The Autonomic Nervous System. Part of the peripheral nervous system, the autonomic nervous system (ANS) governs the activities of the viscera, including the functions of cardiac muscle, smooth (involuntary muscle), and glands. The two major subdivisions of the ANS include the sympathetic and parasympathetic systems. These two systems function together to maintain a stable internal environment for the body. Primarily a motor system, the ANS consists of preganglionic and postganglionic nerves.

In the sympathetic nervous system, the preganglionic cell bodies are located in the thoracolumbar area, specifi-

TABLE 40–4. Principle Cerebellar Functions

Control of fine movement
Control of coordination of movement
Control of balance
Coordination of the action of muscle groups
Maintenance of feedback loops to correct movement

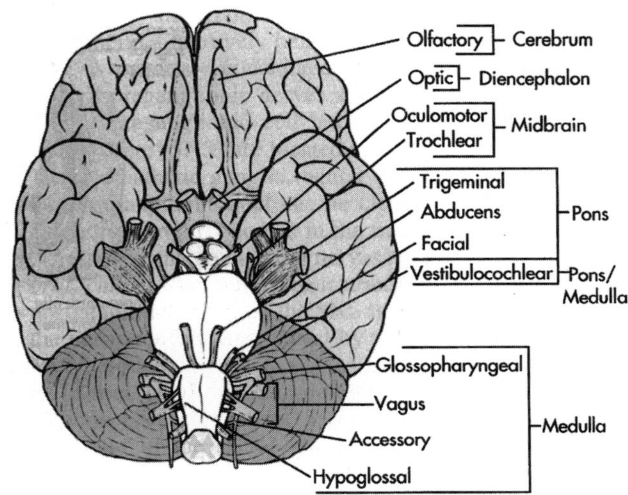

Figure 40–10. The cranial nerves and their sites of origin in the brainstem. *(Used with permission from Lewis, Collier, & Heitkemper. [1996].)*

cally from T1 to L2. The postganglionic neurons lie close to the spinal column along the vertebral bodies. The major neurotransmitter released by the postganglionic fibers of the sympathetic nervous system is norepinephrine. Acetylcholine is the neurotransmitter most commonly released by the preganglionic fibers. Activated during situations of stress, the sympathetic system is also termed the "fight or flight" system. Sympathetic stimulation causes blood pressure and heart rate to increase and vasoconstriction of blood vessels to occur.

The cranio–sacral area houses the preganglionic cell

TABLE 40–5. The Cranial Nerves

CN I	Olfactory	Sense of smell
CN II	Optic	Vision
CN III	Oculomotor	Elevation of the upper eyelid, pupillary constriction, and the majority of the extraocular movements
CN IV	Trochlear	Movement of the eye in the downward, outward direction
CN V	Trigeminal	Motor: muscles responsible for jaw clenching Sensory: the face
CN VI	Abducens	Lateral deviation of the eye
CN VII	Facial	Motor: muscles of the face Sensory: anterior two-thirds of the tongue
CN VIII	Acoustic	Hearing and balance
CN IX	Glossopharyngeal	Motor: pharynx Sensory: eardrum, pharynx, and posterior tongue
CN X	Vagus	Motor: palate, pharynx, and larynx Sensory: pharynx and larynx
CN XI	Spinal Accessory	Moves the large muscles of the neck
CN XII	Hypoglossal	Moves the tongue

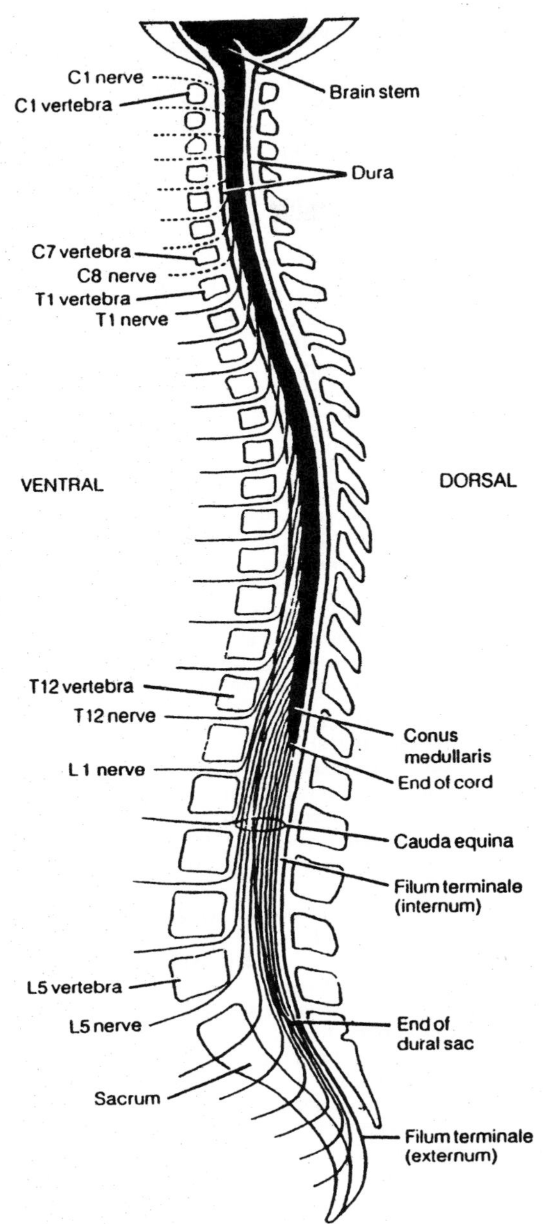

Figure 40–11. The spinal cord lying within the vertebral column. *(From Burrell. [1992]. [p. 847].)*

bodies for the parasympathetic nervous system. Acetylcholine is the neurotransmitter released at both the preganglionic and postganglionic sites. Parasympathetic system stimulation produces activities of normal body maintenance (e.g., gastrointestinal activity).

▶ SEIZURE DISORDERS

Epilepsy is a paroxysmal syndrome characterized by recurrent episodes in which there is a disturbance in skeletal motor function, sensation, autonomic visceral function, behavior, or consciousness (Hickey, 1994). Each year, 125,000 individuals in the United States are diagnosed with epilepsy (Hauser & Hesdorffer, 1990). Although epilepsy may start at any age, the incidence is highest in children under 2 years of age and in adults over 65 years of age. Males are more commonly affected than females and the incidence is higher in black populations and socially disadvantaged communities.

The etiology of epilepsy is multifactorial. History of severe head trauma, central nervous system infection, stroke, or structural lesion (i.e., a brain tumor) are among the most clearly established factors associated with the onset of recurrent seizures in adults. Epilepsy may occur in families; however, the role of heredity as a factor is less significant than environmental and acquired influences. With some patients, epilepsy is deemed idiopathic, or without identifiable cause.

Pathophysiology

Seizures occur due to aberrant electrical activity from a nidus of abnormally hyperactive or hypersensitive neurons that form an epileptogenic focus. The focus can be thought of as an autonomous group of neurons that fire large numbers of paroxysmal discharges, often in bursts. The factors that cause this firing are not clear. Any stimulus that causes the cell membrane of the neuron to depolarize induces a tendency to spontaneously fire. The focus is often associated with an area of gliosis or scarring in the brain tissue. The scarring is thought to disrupt the normal chemical and structural environment of the neurons, making abnormal firing more likely. Repetitive firing from an epileptic focus can produce permanent changes in neuron excitability. This effect, called kindling, has important implications for good seizure control in patients with epilepsy. The longer a patient remains poorly controlled, the less likely it is that the seizures will be easily controlled in the future.

History and Physical Findings

A careful history is a major cornerstone in the diagnosis of epilepsy. Important information to obtain includes family history and history regarding the mother's pregnancy, the birth process, and childhood development. In addition, history of previous illnesses, head injury, child abuse, and encephalopathic illnesses should be sought. The adult who presents with new onset of seizures should be questioned regarding a history of old strokes, congenital anomalies, and neoplasm (particularly melanoma and cancer of the breast, lung, colon, and kidney).

If the patient has an established diagnosis of epilepsy, a detailed seizure history should be obtained and may provide valuable information regarding the site of the epileptic focus. This should include information regarding precipitating factors and antecedent events, as well as a description of a typical seizure's onset, duration, frequency, and postictal state. If the patient is unable to provide a clear account

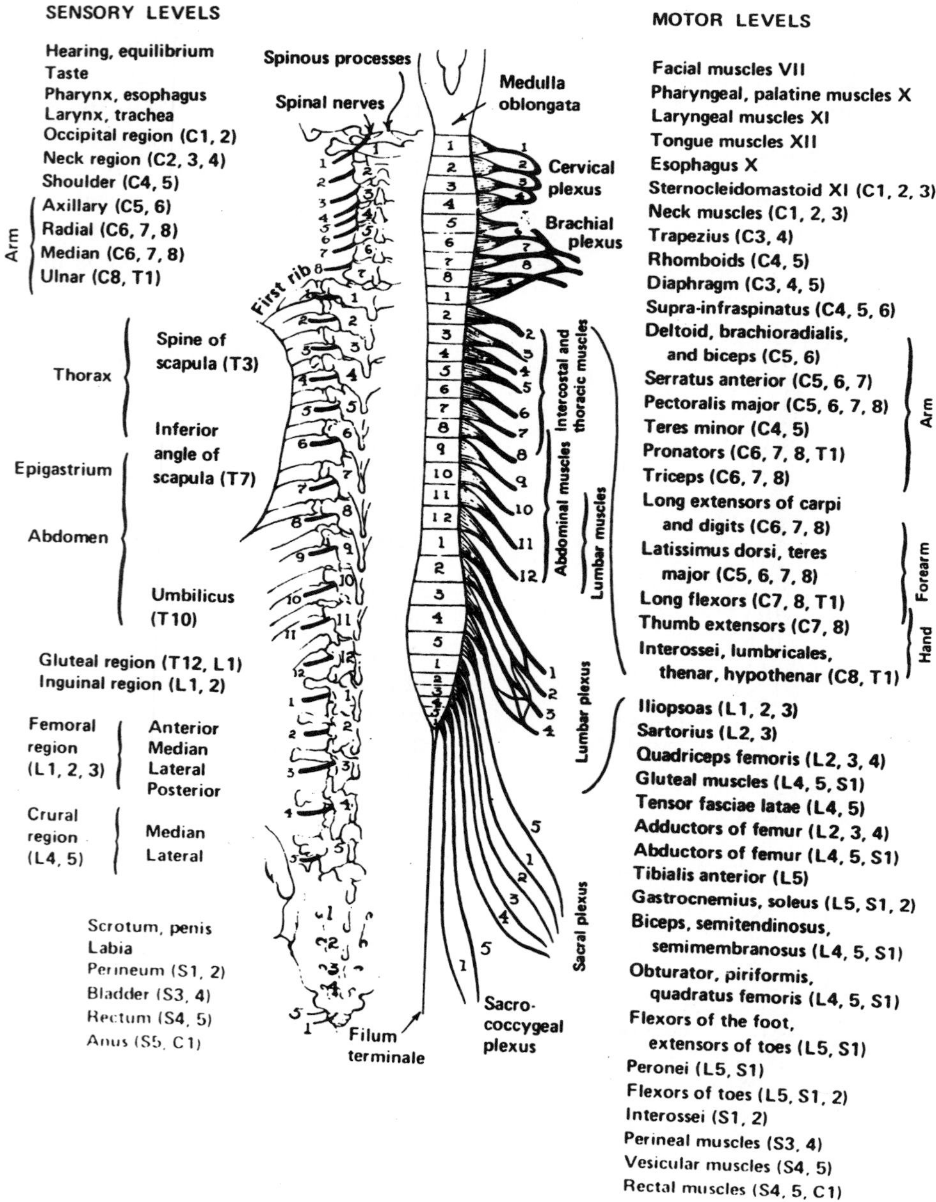

Figure 40–12. Spinal cord and spinal roots. *(From Burrell. [1992]. [p. 848].)*

of his or her seizures, this information should be obtained from a reliable observer who has witnessed the events.

The physical and neurological exams should be carried out with special reference to any signs of localized neurologic abnormality. These would include disorders of thought processes or memory, motor weakness, sensory disturbance, or reflex abnormalities.

Classification of the Epilepsies

Clinical manifestations of a seizure vary depending on the site of the electrical disturbance. In spite of this variability, the ability to classify epileptic events is an important step in determining an appropriate treatment plan. The International Classification of Epileptic Seizures is a practical system based on the clinical nature of the onset of the seizure (Table 40–6).

Partial seizures are those that originate from a particular focal region of the brain. These events are classified primarily on whether consciousness is impaired during the seizure. Simple partial seizures result in no impairment in consciousness, whereas complex partial seizures involve impairment in consciousness or awareness of the environment. In addition, automatisms or abberations in behavior are frequently seen. Common examples of automatisms include facial grimacing, lip-smacking, and picking at clothing.

Generalized seizures are characterized by bihemispheric

TABLE 40–6. The International Classification of Epileptic Seizures

I. Partial (focal, local) seizures
  A. Simple partial seizures (consciousness not impaired)
    1. Motor (abnormal movement of an arm, leg, or both; Jacksonian march)
    2. Somatosensory or special sensory (gustatory, olfactory, auditory)
    3. Autonomic (tachycardia, respiration, flushing)
    4. Psychic (déjà vu, fearful feeling)
  B. Complex partial seizures (with impairment of consciousness)
    1. Beginning as simple partial seizure and progressing to impairment of consciousness
      a. No other symptoms
      b. Motor, somatosensory, special sensory, autonomic, or psychic symptoms
      c. Automatisms
    2. With impairment of consciousness at onset
      a. No other symptoms
      b. Motor, somatosensory, special sensory, autonomic, or psychic symptoms
      c. Automatisms
  C. Partial seizures evolving to secondarily generalized seizures
    1. Simple partial leads to generalized seizures
    2. Complex partial leads to generalized seizures
    3. Simple partial leads to complex partial leads to generalized seizures
II. Generalized seizures (convulsive or nonconvulsive, all associated with loss of consciousness)
  A. Absence (petit mal)
    Onset in childhood; approximately 50% ending in adolescence and 50% supplanted by tonic–clonic
    Symptoms include altered awareness or attention and blank stare, may include eye blinking lasting 5–30 s
    Can be mistaken as learning disabilities or behavior problems if unrecognized
  B. Myoclonic
    Characterized by short, abrupt muscular contractions of arms, legs, and/or torso
    Symptoms include symmetrical or asymmetrical, synchronous or asynchronous single or multiple jerks; possible brief loss of consciousness
  C. Clonic
    Symptoms include muscle contraction and relaxation usually lasting several minutes
    Distinct phases may not be easily observable
  D. Tonic
    Symptoms include an abrupt increase in muscle tone (contraction), loss of consciousness and autonomic signs, lasting from 30 s to several minutes
  E. Tonic–clonic (grand mal)
    Tonic—may begin with a shrill cry caused by secondary expulsion of air due to abrupt closure of the epiglottis; rigidity, opisthotonos, extension of arms and legs; jaw may snap shut; temporary (up to 1 min); cessation of respiration; nonreactive, dilated pupils; decreased heart rate
    Clonic—begins suddenly and ends gradually, characterized by quick, bilateral, severe jerking movements; stertorous respirations; autonomic symptoms; lasts 2–5 min
    Postictal—muscle flaccidity; gradual return of consciousness; amnesia related to the seizure; patient may need 0.5–1 h of sleep
  F. Atonic
    Characterized by abrupt loss of muscle tone followed by postictal confusion; injury likely if seizure uncontrolled
III. Unclassified epileptic seizures—cannot be classified because of inadequate or incomplete data; include some neonatal seizures, e.g., rhythmic eye movements, chewing, and swimming movements

From Santilli. (1996).

involvement from the start of the event. Impairment in consciousness may be the first clinical indication of the event, followed by bilateral motor manifestations. The tonic–clonic seizure, one of the most common types of generalized events, is characterized by a loss of consciousness followed by a tonic contraction of the musculature (tonic phase) causing the patient to fall to the ground. Apnea and cyanosis are commonly noted. The clonic phase follows, manifested by rhythmic muscle contractions and hyperventilation. In the postictal phase, the patient complains of muscle soreness and fatigue and may sleep for several hours. There is generally no memory of the event.

Laboratory and Diagnostic Tests

The electroencephalogram (EEG), a recording of the electrical activity of the brain, is a pivotal tool in the diagnosis and treatment of epilepsy. The recording is accomplished by affixing 21 electrodes to the scalp with a paste-like substance. Recordings are taken at rest, after hyperventilation, with photic stimulation, and during sleep. Wave types vary with activity and specific stimulation.

Classification of brain waves is based on the number of cycles per second (cps). EEG interpretation involves looking at four frequency bands: delta rhythms, theta rhythms, alpha rhythms, and beta rhythms. EEG abnormalities include epileptiform activities, slowing of normal rhythms, abnormalities of amplitude, or disorders of age-specific patterns. A neurologist skilled in the interpretation of EEGs can provide helpful assistance when attempting to corrolate these findings to a clinical situation.

A normal EEG, however, does not exclude epilepsy. Only a small percentage of patients with epilepsy have abnormal EEGs the first time the test is done. Therefore, the EEG must be reviewed and interpreted along with other subjective and objective data.

If routine EEG fails to disclose abnormalities, a variety of additional techniques are available. Simultaneous EEG and video monitoring offers the ability to correlate the patient's behavior during the clinical event with electrographic changes on the EEG. Activation procedures such as photic stimulation, hyperventilation, and sleep deprivation are sometimes helpful in provoking abnormalities. In some situations, special recording methods such as nasopharyngeal or sphenoidal leads are used to record abnormalities in the temporal lobes. Intensive monitoring, using prolonged video and EEG monitoring, may be necessary to provide a definitive diagnosis in a small percentage of patients.

To rule out the presence of a structural abnormality (i.e., strokes, tumors) contributing to seizures, imaging studies such as computerized tomography (CT), magnetic resonance imaging (MRI), and positron emission tomography (PET) are used. Neuropsychological evaluation is also a useful component in the diagnostic process. Cognitive abilities, memory, concentration, and personality assessments all provide valuable information regarding higher cortical functions.

Laboratory data including CBC, serum electrolytes, calcium and phosphate, liver function tests (AST/SGOT, total bilirubin, and alkaline phosphatase), BUN, creatinine, and blood glucose should be obtained to establish a baseline and to determine any contribution of metabolic factors to the occurrence of seizures. Laboratory studies are also important for identifying liver and bone marrow function abnormalities related to the use of antiepileptic drugs (AEDs). An elevation in liver function parameters is often seen in patients receiving AEDs.

Management

In approximately 70% of patients, epilepsy is controlled with AEDs. More than half of these individuals are completely controlled, while 20 to 30% report improvement in seizure frequency. In the remaining patients, seizures are intractable (Hauser & Hesdorffer, 1990). The primary goal of AED therapy is to obtain maximum control of seizures with minimal medications and side effects. Choosing an appropriate medication involves the assessment of a variety of factors. The type of seizure is a key consideration, as some AEDs are better suited for the treatment of particular types of seizures. Table 40–7 highlights commonly used AEDs and the seizure types for which they are often prescribed. Since 1993, three more AEDs have been approved by the FDA. Felbamate (Felbatol) and Gabapentin (Neurontin) have been shown to be effective in the treatment of complex partial seizures. Lamotrigine (Lamictal) has been efficatious in the treatment of a variety of epilepsy types.

Lifestyle factors are also important when choosing a medication. If the patient is going to be compliant with the medication regimen, he or she must understand and accept the need to take medication. The dosing schedule of the

TABLE 40–7. Antiepileptic Medications

Generic Name	Trade Name	Therapeutic Dosage	Therapeutic AED Level	Seizure Type	Common Side Effects
Carbamazepine	Tegretol	10–15 mg/kg/day Half-life: 9–19 h	4–12 μg/mL	Secondary tonic–clonic Complex partial Simplex partial	Lethargy, dizziness, ataxia, behavioral changes, blurred or double vision, aplastic anemia
Clonazepam	Klonopin	0.05–0.20 mg/kg/day Half-life: 18–20 h	20–80 μg/mL	Absence Myoclonic	Drowsiness, slurred speech, double vision, behavior changes, increased salivation
Divalporex sodium, Valproate	Depakote Depakene	20–60 mg/kg/day Half-life: 6–18 h	50–150 μg/mL	Myoclonic Absence, tonic–clonic, mixed seizure types	Hair loss, tremor, elevated liver enzymes, irregular menses, increased appetite, nausea and vomiting (not as common with Depakote)
Ethosuximide	Zarontin	15–35 mg/kg/day Half-life: 24–72 h	40–100 μg/mL	Absence	GI upset, loss of appetite, headache, lethargy, behavior changes, dizziness
Phenobarbital	Luminal	4–6 mg/kg/day Half-life: 53–104 h	10–40 μg/mL	Tonic–clonic	Changes in sleep pattern, drowsiness, excitability, irritability, cognitive impairment
Phenytoin	Dilantin	5–10 mg/kg/day Half-life: 7–22 h	10–25 μg/mL	Tonic–clonic Complex partial Simple partial	Nystagmus, blurred or double vision, gingival hyperplasia, ataxia, skin rash, folate deficiency
Primidone	Mysoline	12–25 mg/kg/day Half-life: 3–12 h	5–12 μg/mL	Tonic–clonic Complex partial Simple partial	Drowsiness, hyperactivity in children, ataxia, behavior changes

Adapted with permission from Santilli. (1996).

medication must also be reasonable when compared with the patient's lifestyle. If the patient will be more compliant with once or twice daily dosing, then an attempt should be made to prescribe a medication that can safely be dosed once or twice daily.

Following introduction of an AED, careful monitoring of blood levels must take place. It is important to remember, however, to treat the patient rather than the blood level. Although each medication has a prescribed therapeutic range, patients often find their own range within which seizures are well controlled. When more than one medication is in use, drug interactions may change the blood levels. More frequent blood-level monitoring must take place in these situations. Likewise, patients with intercurrent illnesses (i.e., influenza or other viral illnesses) may require more frequent monitoring as absorption of AEDs may be impaired.

If prescribed medications do not offer good control of seizures, additional medications can be added. However, this should be done one medication at a time so that efficacy and side effects can be carefully monitored. The more medications the patient is taking, the greater the risk of drug interaction and toxicity. Patients should be reevaluated frequently during medication changes.

In addition to careful medication management, patients must be taught which factors precipitate seizures. Sleep deprivation and the use of alcohol and recreational drugs can promote seizures. The effect these situations have on the individual patient should be reviewed and discussed.

Approximately 20% of patients treated with AEDs continue to have seizures or experience serious side effects from medications despite appropriate managment (Hauser & Hesdorffer, 1990). For some of these patients with medically refractory epilepsy, surgery is an option. Individuals who benefit most from surgery are those whose seizures originate from a clearly defined, unilateral focus. In these situations, cortical excisions can be done without producing serious neurologic deficits, and with reasonable expectation that seizures will come under better control or be eliminated. Corpus callosotomy and hemispherectomy are other procedures that can be offered in specific cases where cortical excision would not be efficacious. Hemispherectomy is offered only to patients with congential hemiplegia or a history of Rosausser's encephalitis.

Evaluation and Follow-Up

Because epilepsy is a chronic illness, lifetime management with medications is often necessary. Patients need to have a clear understanding of their medications, as well as how to manage issues such as missed doses and the dosing of medications during intercurrent illnesses. They also need to learn the importance of, and know how to arrange for, blood-level monitoring.

Family members should be told what to do during and after a seizure. They should be reminded that it is not necessary for the patient to be seen by a health-care professional after a single seizure, unless the seizure is prolonged and there is concern about status epilepticus or complications or injuries associated with the seizure.

Like other chronic diseases, epilepsy can have an impact on many aspects of daily living. Patients face the challenge of living and adjusting to the personal limitations imposed by the illness. In addition to careful medical management, they often need assistance with employment, educational, and financial issues. This support can be provided by local social workers and resource specialists. The local chapter of the Epilepsy Foundation of America (EFA) is also a valuable resource for patients and families.

▶ TIA AND STROKE

A transient ischemic attack (TIA) refers to a neurologic deficit that is transient or lasts less than 24 hours with complete recovery of symptoms. The goal of treatment following TIA is to prevent the developement of a thrombotic stroke. A daily regimen of aspirin is often prescribed for its antiplatelet benefits. An assessment for and counseling regarding stroke risk factors should also be done. In situations where the deficit completely disappears after a period of 24 hours or longer, the term "reversible ischemic neurologic deficit" (RIND) is used.

A stroke is characterized by the sudden or very rapid development of neurologic symptoms that result from disease of the blood vessels that supply the brain. The term "stroke" is used commonly in clinical practice in reference to persistance of neurologic deficit for longer than 24 hours. This type of event is caused by several different pathologic processes.

Pathophysiology

Stroke can be classified as either ischemic or hemorrhagic based on the underlying pathology. Ischemic strokes include embolic and thrombotic events. Primary intracerebral hemorrhage and subarachnoid hemorrhage are the two major types of hemorrhagic events (Adams & Victor, 1993).

Cerebral embolism, the second most common cause of stroke, results in necrosis and edema of the area supplied by the involved vessel (Whisnant, 1990). The heart is the major source of embolic material. Cardiac situations that contribute to cerebral embolization include atrial fibrillation, valvular disease, prosthetic valves, myocardial infarction (MI), rheumatic heart disease, and bacterial endocarditis. Atherosclerotic plaques from extracranial vessels are another, less common source of emboli.

Primary thrombotic occlusion is the most common cause of cerebral infarction and often occurs in a vessel partially occluded by atherosclerosis. Thrombotic events are commonly associated with conditions that accelerate atherosclerosis, including hypertension and diabetes mellitus (Whisnant, 1990).

Intracerebral hemorrhage can occur spontaneously in patients with hypertension, amyloid angiopathy, or atherosclerosis. Degenerative changes in the walls of the arteries are seen with these conditions, resulting in rupture and hemorrhage. Hemorrhages that occur as a result of hypertension usually involve the small penetrating arteries in locations such as the putamen, thalamus, pons, and cerebellum. Amyloid angiopathy is associated with lobar hemorrhages that tend to be multiple and recurrent.

Subarachnoid hemorrhage usually occurs as the result of a ruptured sacular aneurysm or an arteriovenous malformation (AVM). Rupture of a micotic aneurysm that occurs as a result of septic embolism is another rare cause. An aneurysm represents a defect in the arterial wall that commonly occurs at the site of arterial bifurcation or branching. An AVM represents a tangle of arteries and veins that often extends from the surface into the brain parenchyma, causing a combined intracerebral and subarachnoid hemorrhage at time of rupture.

History and Physical Findings

Past medical history is important in the process of predicting which patients are at risk for stroke. Hypertension, heart disease, smoking, alcohol consumption, diabetes, and hypercholesterolemia clearly are factors that put patients at increased risk. Other factors include high-grade carotid stenosis, atrial fibrillation, previous stroke or TIA, and recent anterior MI. Antiphospholipid antibodies such as lupus anticoagulant and anticardiolipin antibodies also may increase the risk of stroke.

The manifestations of stroke are variable, depending on the anatomic site of the lesion, the size of the lesion, and the presence of collateral circulation. Symptoms can include motor and sensory deficits, communication deficits or aphasias, affective and intelluctual deficits, and spatial–perceptual alterations. Anterior cerebral artery occlusion, for example, causes paralysis of the contralateral foot and leg, impaired gait, and abulia (inability to perform acts voluntarily or make decisions). Sensory impairment is noted in the areas of motor weakness. Occlusion of vessels in the posterior circulation (i.e., the vertebral artery) cause symptoms of staggering gait and ataxia, nystagmus, clumsiness, dysphagia, and dysarthria.

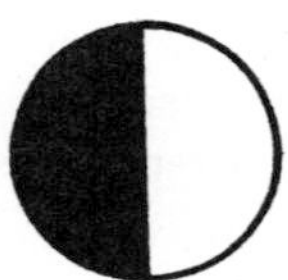
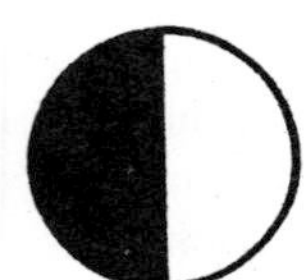

Figure 40–13. Left homonymous hemianopsia (right optic tract). A lesion of the optic tract interrupts fibers originating on the same side of both eyes. Visual loss in the eyes is therefore similar (homonymous) and involves half of each field (hemianopyia). *(Used with permission from Bates. [1983].)*

Embolic strokes tend to produce symptoms that begin suddenly, with a maximum deficit occurring at the onset (Whisnant, 1990). If the embolism resolves, however, symptoms can improve markedly. Middle cerebral artery occlusions are commonly embolic. When the entire distribution of the artery is affected, the resulting symptoms include contralateral hemiparesis, contralateral homonymous hemianopia (blindness in the corresponding halves of the visual fields of both eyes, Fig. 40–13), and aphasia with left-hemisphere involvement.

Conversely, thrombotic events are characterized by an erratic progression of symptoms over hours or days. Neurologic deficits can fluctuate or change in a step-wise fashion sometimes referred to as a "stroke in evolution." Thrombotic strokes are commonly preceeded by TIAs, as these transient events are likely related to microemboli breaking off from atherosclerotic plaques in the extracranial arteries (Feinberg, 1994).

With hemorrhagic events, the sudden onset of severe headache is generally the presenting symptom. Patients may describe this headache as the worst they have ever experienced. There may be loss of consciousness and progression to coma in situations of significant hemorrhage. Other signs include meningeal irritation and nuccal rigidity. The events often occur during episodes of physical exertion.

Laboratory and Diagnostic Tests

Careful history, physical, and neurologic examinations often provide a fairly accurate clinical impression of stroke. To plan an appropriate course of therapy, however, it is imperative to distinguish a hemorrhagic event from infarction. The CT scan is the primary diagnostic tool because it easily identifies acute hemorrhage. Repeat CT scanning is often performed to evaluate the size of the infarct and the effectiveness of treatment, as infarcts are often not visible on CT scan for 48 to 72 hours.

MRI is more accurate than CT scanning in detecting early cerebral infarct, but is less sensitive in identifying acute hemorrhage. It is therefore not useful as an emergency diagnostic tool. MR angiography is a valuable, noninvasive technique of imaging cerebral vessels. Conventional angiography, however, is a more definitive test and is necessary at times, particularly when surgery is planned.

Evaluation of the carotid circulation is also an important part of a stroke work-up, particularly when an ischemic event occurs. Carotid ultrasound and Doppler evaluation can provide accurate information regarding vascular disease at the carotid bifurcation. Evaluation of some of the intracranial arteries can be accomplished with transcranial Doppler. This technique is particularly helpful when evaluating vasospasm following subarachnoid hemorrhage.

When searching for a cardiac source of emboli, transesophageal echocardiography (TEE) is particularly accurate in the detection of mural thrombi, valvular vegetations, and embolic sources in the great vessels (i.e., ulcerated plaques). TEE is also very sensative in the detection of patent foramen ovale when paradoxical embolism is suspected. Holter monitoring may provide information regarding unsuspected episodes of atrial fibrillation when no other source of embolism is found.

Management

Stroke is a preventable disease. The priority of therapy, therefore, is prevention, both in the patient who is at risk for infarction and for the patient who has already had a stroke. Patients with known risk factors need to be closely monitored and managed with regard to their risks. The prophylactic use of warfarin (Coumadin) in patients with atrial fibrillation has been shown to be highly effective in reducing stroke and death (Matchar, McCrory, Barnett, & Feussner, 1994). It is used, however, with some risk. For patients who are not candidates for coumadin treatment, aspirin is recommended. Although it is less effective, it is less risky than anticoagulation. In patients with a history of TIAs or minor stroke, both aspirin and ticlopidine reduce the risk of stroke (Harbison, 1992). Aspirin should be used first, but in patients who either do not tolerate or respond to aspirin, ticlopidine can be used.

For patients with known carotid stenosis, carotid endarterectomy has now been shown to be superior to medical management in symptomatic patients with lesions of 70% or greater (NACENT, 1991). When stenosis is less than 30%, the surgery worsens outcomes. Patients with symptomatic intermediate (30-70%) stenosis, studies are still underway.

Treatment options following acute stroke depend on the etiology of the event. Goals of acute management, regardless of etiology, include prevention of further neurologic deficit and lessening of disability. Rapidly reestablishing reperfusion is the primary goal in the treatment of acute ischemic stroke. Treatment with thrombolytic agents (tPA) has shown particular promise in working toward this goal. Pilot studies have shown that prompt intravenous or selective intraartrial administration can reestablish perfusion after carotid and vertebrobasilar artery thromboses (Hacke, 1994). Success is influenced by thrombus age, composition, site of occlusion, and status of collateral circulation. Patient outcomes measured at the 3-month point show a higher proportion of patients who were treated with tPA had minimal or no disability (NINDS Stroke rt-PA Stroke Study Group, 1995). It is important to remember, however, that the use of thrombolytic therapy increases the incidence of intracerebral hemorrhage which ultimately yields poorer outcomes.

Anticoagulants such as heparin and coumadin have frequently been used for treatment of acute ischemic stroke (TOAST). Currently, this use is being reassessed in a large, multicenter study treating acute stroke with a safer, fractionated form or low molecular weight heparin (LMWH). Given by intravenous infusion or subcutaneous injection, coagulation studies during LMWH treatment do not need to be serially monitored. Thus far, results indicate improved outcome for patients only at 6 months, with no improvement at the 10-day or 3-month monitoring intervals. The study was completed in December 1997 (Kay et al., 1995).

Ancrod (Arvin) is a serine protease that produces effective defibrinogenation without interfering with other coagulation factors or platelet turnover and causes no serious bleeding. It has been widely used in peripheral vascular disease and deep vein thrombosis (Bell, 1984). One small randomized multicenter study using one week of intravenous ancrod therapy showed a trend toward functional improvement (Sherman, Barbour, Levy et al., 1994).

Antiplatelet agents such as aspirin and ticlopidine have demonstrated effectiveness in prevention of stroke, and may be used as an alternative therapy in stroke patients for whom heparin is contradindicated. Their use as a confirmed therapy in improving stroke outcome continues to be an open issue.

Treatment of the patient following an intracerebral hemorrhage involves careful management of blood pressure and control of cerebral edema. Steroids have not been shown to be effective with this population. Osmotic diuretics such as Mannitol are transiently beneficial when attempting to reduce brain swelling. In situations where hemorrhage is precipitated by a clotting abnormality, as in the case of anticoagulant therapy, appropriate treatment of the coagulopathy should be instituted. Surgical evacuation of a hematoma, if it is in an accessible location, may be a life-saving measure, particularly if signs of herniation begin to emerge.

Treatment following subarachnoid hemorrhage secondary to aneurysmal rupture involves careful medical management in preparation for possible surgical intervention. Key issues include avoidance of hypertension, management of cerebral edema, and treatment of vasospasm. Generally noted to occur between 2 and 10 days posthemorrhage, vasospasm is the result of the release of vasoactive agents such as serotonin and catecholamines. The resultant spasming of the vessels in the area of hemorrhage often cause drowsiness and worsening of neurologic signs. Treatment consists primarily of volume expansion to increase cerebral perfusion and the administration of calcium-channel blockers such as nimodipine to decrease vasospasm. Timing of surgical intervention is largely dependent on the neurologic condition of the patient. Early surgery (within the first 24-48 hours posthemorrhage) virtually eliminates the risk of a second, often fatal hemorrhage.

Follow-Up

Care of the stroke patient involves complex medical management during the acute phase. Once the patient has stabilized neurologically, the focus turns to the task of adaptation to the neurologic deficit. Issues of risk-factor modification for prevention of recurrent stroke need to be addressed. Patients and families need assistance during the transition from acute care hospital to rehabilitation setting, and later into the community. The National Stroke Association and the American Heart Association can provide valuable information, resources, and referral services to ease these transitions.

▶ BRAIN TUMORS

Approximately 35,000 adult Americans develop new brain tumors each year (Mahaley, Mettlin, Natarajan, Laws, & Peace, 1989). Males are more likely to be affected than females, and incidence among whites is higher than blacks. Incidence rises with age up to 65 years, with the exception of a peak during childhood for primary tumors.

Brain tumors can be classified as either primary or metastatic. Glioblastoma multiforme is the most common histological type of primary tumor, followed by meningioma and astrocytoma. Metastatic tumors most frequently originate from the lung, breast, genitourinary tract, and gastrointestinal tract. Table 40–8 outlines the pathological classification of CNS tumors, according to the World Health Organization (Zulch, 1986).

Sixteen percent of patients with primary brain tumors have a family history of cancer (Mahaley, Mettlin, Natarajan, Laws & Peace, 1989). Some genetic disorders, such as neurofibromatosis and tuberous sclerosis, are associated with brain tumors. Exposure to environmental factors has been poorly corrolated to the development of brain tumors.

TABLE 40–8. Outline of the Pathological Classification of Central Nervous System Tumors, According to the World Health Organization

- Tumors of neuroepithelial tissue (including glial, neuronal, poorly differentiated, embryonal, and pineal-cell tumors)
  - Astrocytic tumors
  - Oligodendrogliomas
  - Ependymal and choroid-plexus tumors
  - Pineal-cell tumors
  - Neuronal tumors
  - Poorly differentiated and embryonal tumors
    - Glioblastomas
    - Medulloblastomas
  - Medulloepitheliomas
  - Primitive polar spongioblastomas
  - Gliomatosis cerebri
- Tumors of nerve-sheath cells
- Tumors of the meninges and related tissue
- Primary malignant lymphomas
- Tumors of blood-vessel origin
- Germ-cell tumors
- Other malformative tumors and tumor-like lesions
- Vascular malformations
- Tumors of the anterior pituitary
- Local extensions from regional tumors
- Metastic tumors
- Unclassified tumors

From Zulch. (1986).

Pathophysiology

Primary brain tumors originate from the various cells and structures found within the brain. Metastatic brain tumors originate from their primary tumor of origin, commonly in the lung, breast, gastrointestinal tract, or genitourinary tract.

Basic concepts of oncogenesis, or the development of tumors, can be applied to primary brain tumors (Maxwell & Black, 1988). Oncogenes are present in all cells of the body, but typically are either not active or are very tightly regulated by promoters or supressors. Any change in this regulation can lead to the development of a tumor. Oncogenes work by stimulating or promoting cell mitosis. Thus, anything that serves to either stimulate the promoter or inhibit the suppressor ultimately increases the activity of the oncogene (Klein, 1987). Astrocytomas and medulloblastomas are examples of tumors that may develop as a result of a promoter stimulating an oncogene (Bigner & Vogelstein, 1990). Retinoblastomas, osteosarcomas, and meningiomas are examples of tumors that occur as a result of the deletion of a supressor on a particular chromosome (Benedict, Murphree, Banerjee, Spina, Sparkes, & Sparkes, 1983). This theory raises the possibility of using gene therapy to treat these tumors.

Another aspect of tumor development is the fact that many malignant tumors induce angiogenesis or the formation of new blood vessels (Folkman & Klagsbrun, 1987). This is thought to occur as a means of promoting tumor growth by increasing nutrient supply. Malignant astrocytomas are an example of tumors that stimulate angiogenesis. In addition, these tumors secrete factors that increase vascular permiability. This accounts for the surrounding edema that often accompanies both benign and malignant tumors.

Also, some tumors secrete immunosuppressive substances that interfere with the body's natural ability to fight tumor-cell growth (Bullard, Gillespie, Mahaley, & Bigner, 1986). Again, this is seen with astrocytomas. Examples of these substances include prostaglandins and a glioblastoma-derived T-cell supressive factor.

History and Physical Findings

Brain tumors present a variety of clinical pictures, depending largely on their type and location. Common symptoms include headache, seizures, and/or progressive neurological deficit. Headache is more frequently reported with tumors that produce ventricular obstruction and hydrocephalus (i.e., ependymomas, hemangioblastomas, and medulloblastomas). Seizures are commonly seen with mixed gliomas and oligodendrogliomas. Progressive neurological deficits are often seen with invasive, destructive tumors such as glioblastoma multiforme.

Laboratory and Diagnostic Tests

Neurodiagnostic studies, particularly MRI, have revolutionized imaging of brain tumors. Tumor location and volume can be accurately measured, as well as location in relation to critical structures, including blood vessels. Gadolinium, the MRI contrast agent, helps differentiate between the borders of tumor and edema. MRI angiography can assist in distinguishing vascular masses from tumor.

Management

Most brain tumors cause edema in the surrounding brain parenchyma. The use of high-dose corticosteroids can help reduce this edema, thereby lowering intracranial pressure and temporarily improving focal deficits. Improvement in neurologic function is usually noted within 24 to 48 hours of beginning therapy. Although use of a variety of steroids has been documented, Dexamethasone is most widely used to treat cerebral edema because of its relatively low mineralocorticoid (salt-retaining) effects. Standard dose at initiation of therapy is 4 to 6 mg q.i.d. Side effects are the same as those that are seen in other groups of patients using steroids. Following the completion of definitive therapy (radiation therapy or surgery), steroids can be slowly tapered and discontinued. Patients with incompletely treated tumors, however, may continue to experience cerebral edema and neurologic deterioration when the dosage is decreased. Frequently, patients with malignant primary or metastatic tumors use steroids chronically to maintain some degree of neurologic function during the last months of their lives.

In situations where intracranial hypertension becomes life threatening, osmotic agents such as Mannitol can acutely lower intracranial pressure by reducing brain water. Prescribed in the usual dose of 1 g/kg (approximately 250 cc of a 20% solution in an average adult), Mannitol can reduce intracranial pressure by 30 to 60% for a duration of 2 to 4 hours. Small doses can be administered every few hours thereafter as needed to control intracranial pressure. It is useful, however, for only a short time until more definitive treatment can be instituted.

Surgery continues to be the most common treatment modality for all types of brain tumors. It not only provides positive histologic information for diagnosis, but also offers the possibility of an improvement in neurologic function and even of cure. As with all surgical procedures, operative risk is involved. One of the major considerations is the location of the tumor. If located in a surgically inaccessible area (i.e., in the region of the brainstem, hypothalamus, or third ventricle), the removal of even benign tumors may be impossible. On the other hand, location in a relatively silent area (i.e., anterior frontal or temporal lobe), a large resection can be performed with relatively little postoperative deficit.

Improved technology in the operating room has vastly improved the effectiveness of tumor resection. The use of the microscope and intraoperative magnification, advanced stereotactic and ultrasound technology, and the intraoperative monitoring of evoked responses all significantly improve the outcome and reduce the morbidity and mortality of brain tumor surgery.

Radiation therapy has a significant role not only in the treatment of histologically malignant tumors of the brain, but also in the treatment of benign tumors such as meningiomas and pituitary adenomas. Although malignant gliomas are not radiosensitive, data reveals that whole brain postoperative radiation therapy significantly lengthens survival in affected patients. The usual treatment regimen is 5500 to 6000 cGy delivered over a 5- to 6-week period. In attempts to spare as much normal brain as possible from the adverse effects of radiation, part of the dose is delivered to the whole brain and an additional dose of cone-down radiation is delivered to the tumor bed. Steroids should be continued throughout the course of therapy, as radiation often causes an increase in cerebral edema.

Brachytherapy, the stereotactic implantation of interstitial radionuclide sources into the tumor, has had a positive effect on median survival in patients with glioblastomas. Other noninvasive stereotactic radiosurgical methods that have been used with some success include the modified linear accelerator with stereotactic guidance, the gamma knife, and the proton beam.

Although chemotherapy has a beneficial effect in the treatment of brain tumors in some patients, the number of available agents is surprisingly small. For malignant gliomas in adults, carmustine (BCNU), lomustine (CCNU), cisplatin, and procarbazine are the drugs of choice. Lymphomas and medulloblastomas have shown good response with Methotrexate. The side effects associated with the use of these drugs are significant; therefore, they are often best tolerated in the young patient with minimal neurologic deficit.

Follow-Up

The management of the patient with a brain tumor spans a variety of treatment modalities, circumstances, and situations. Overall goals for the long term include maximizing neurologic function, insuring that the patient is free from pain, and preparing the patient for the long-term implications of his or her illness with respect to prognosis.

The responses of the patient and family are influenced by a variety of factors, including type of tumor, grade, and location. The Karnofsky Performance Scale (Table 40–9) (Bender, Yasko & Strohl, 1996), a widely used scale to quantify the functional status of cancer patients, is often helpful in tracking the patient's quality of life over a period of time.

TABLE 40–9. Karnofsky Performance Scale

100	Normal; no complaints; no evidence of disease
90	Ability to carry on normal activity; minor signs or symptoms of disease
80	Normal activity with effort; some signs or symptoms of disease
70	Ability to care for self; inability to carry on normal activity or do active work
60	Occasional assistance necessary but ability to care for most needs
50	Considerable assistance and frequent medical care necessary
40	Disabled; special care and assistance necessary
30	Severely disabled; indication for hospitalization although death not imminent
20	Very sick; hospitalization necessary; active supportive treatment necessary
10	Moribund; fatal processes progressing rapidly
0	Dead

From Lewis, Collier, & Heitkemper. (1996).

▶ CENTRAL NERVOUS SYSTEM INFECTIONS

Infections of the CNS can conveniently be divided into the following categories: (1) infections of the meninges and CSF or meningitis, (2) infections of the brain parenchyma or encephalitis, and (3) parameningeal infections, or infections that occur in and around the meninges.

Although the nervous system is well insulated from systemic infections, organisms causing CNS infection usually gain entry by one of four major routes. The bloodstream is the most common portal of entry. Other routes include direct implantation (i.e., via lumbar puncture or ventriculoperitoneal shunt), local extension of an established infection (i.e., frontal sinusitis), or via the peripheral nervous system (i.e., herpes simplex or rabies).

Bacterial Meningitis

The common causal organisms associated with bacterial meningitis change with the age of the patient. In neonates, group B *streptococci, E coli,* and *L Monocytogenes* are the common sources. *Neisseria meningitidis* and *streptococcus pneumoniae* are the leading causes of childhood meningitis. Adults are most often infected with *Streptococccus pneumoniae* and *neisseria meningitidis* (Richardson, 1996). Meningococcal infections are among the most virulent and typically involve a fulminating infection with overwhelming septicemia (meningococcemia).

Pathophysiology

Bacterial meningitis is an inflammation of the leptomeninges that results from entry of organisms into the subarachnoid space. The presence of the bacteria in the CSF induces the release of cytokines that set off an inflammatory process. This process involves the influx of leukocytes into the subarachnoid space and results in cerebral edema and increased intracranial pressure with resultant neurologic changes. Other factors such as oxygen-free radicals and excitatory amino acids that are released during the inflammatory response can contribute directly to neuronal cell death (Tuomanen, 1995). Fibrotic changes of the arachnoid layer can cause fibrosis and scarring to occur. Adhesions in the subarachnoid space can interfere with the normal circulation and absorption of CSF.

History and Physical Findings

Adults with bacterial meningitis usually present with headache, fever, neck stiffness, and altered consciousness (Durand, Calderwood, Weber et al., 1993). Kernig's and Brudzinski's signs, commonly described signs of meningeal irritation, are present in only half of adult patients (Tunkel & Scheld, 1995). The presence of a petechial or purpuric rash is indicative of meningococcal disease. Seizures occur in approximately 20% of patients. Coma, usually indicative of a poor prognosis, occurs in 5 to 10% of patients (McGillicuddy & Hoff, 1992).

Complications of bacterial meningitis can cause a variety of neurologic deficits. Cranial nerve dysfunctions are common. Papilledema and blindness may occur as the result of optic nerve compression. Loss of corneal reflexes and facial nerve palsies can also occur. Vestibulocochlear nerve irritation can cause vertigo, tinnitus, and deafness. Noncommunicating hydrocephalus is sometimes noted as a result of exudate-causing adhesions that prevent the normal flow and absorption of CSF. Deterioration in neurologic function may be an indication of worsening of the infection.

Laboratory and Diagnostic Tests

Definitive diagnosis and identification of the infecting organism can be made only by examination of the CSF (Fig. 40–14). There is urgency in performing a lumbar puncture to obtain a CSF sample before beginning treatment with antibiotics, as the patient is often acutely ill and can quickly progress to coma and death if left untreated. The obtained sample is purulent and turbid, with a low glucose and elevated protein. Polymorphonuclear (PMN) cells are the predominant white blood cell type present in the CSF. Diagnosis requires the isolation of an organism by gram stain and culture.

Other routine tests to be obtained in all patients with presumptive bacterial meningitis include CBC with differential, serum electrolytes, BUN, creatinine, and urinalysis. Blood, sputum, and nasopharyngeal cultures are obtained in attempts to identify the causative organism. MRI or CT scan of the head is often helpful when searching for a parameningeal focus of infection.

Management

Patients with bacterial meningitis are acutely ill and require intensive care unit managment. The patient without significant alteration in mental status complains of severe headache.

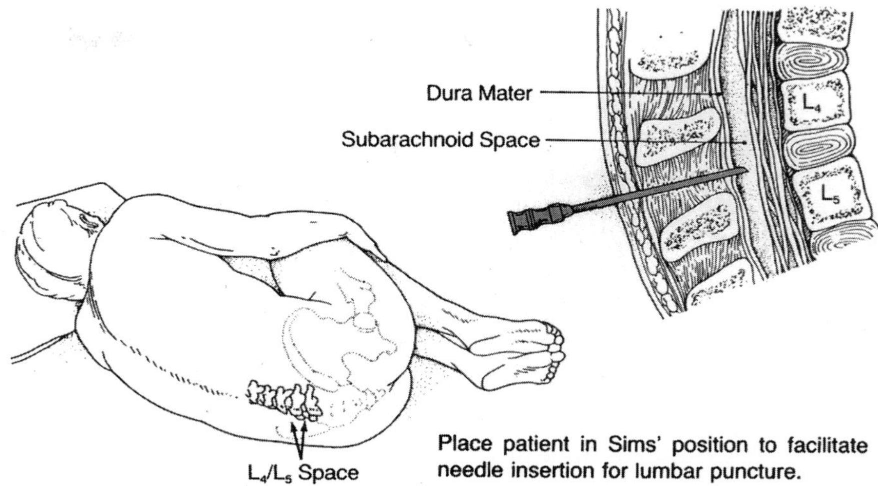

Figure 40–14. Position for lumbar puncture. *(From Burrell. [1992]. [p. 875].)*

Changes in level of consciousness occur with increased intracranial pressure. Volume status is a concern because of the likely presence of cerebral edema. Unless hypotension is a problem, the patient is kept mildly fluid-restricted.

Antibiotics remain the cornerstone of treatment. The initial dose is often given immediately following lumbar puncture, before results of gram stain and culture are available. The choice of antibiotics is therefore directed toward the likely pathogen for the patient's age group. Third-generation cephalosporins (i.e., cefotaxime or ceftriaxone) are widely used for initial treatment. Once the infecting organism has been identified and drug sensitivities have been determined, appropriate changes in antibiotic regimen can be made. Patients are generally hospitalized for the entire course of intravenous antibiotic therapy.

Patients with meningococcal disease are infectious anc can spread the organism to others by respiratory route until they have been on antibiotics for 24 hours. Therefore, it is recommended that family and household members be treated with prophylactic antibiotics. Hospital staff should practice principles of respiratory isolation when caring for the patient.

The use of steroids in the treatment of adults with bacterial meningitis has not been proven to be efficatious. With infants and children, however, the early administration of Dexamethasone has been shown to reduce the risk of hearing loss and other neurologic sequelae (Lebel, Freij, Syrogiannopoulos et al., 1988).

Viral Meningitis

The most common viral groups that infect the subarachnoid space and the leptomeninges are mumps, coxsackievirus, and echovirus. Other potential agents include herpes viruses, arthropod-borne viruses, and human immunodeficiency virus (HIV).

History and Physical Findings

Clinical symptoms noted with viral meningitis are similar to those seen with bacterial meningitis, but the course is generally less fulminant. Neurologic signs are mild, and may include lethargy, irritability, mild drowsiness, and minor reflex changes. The duration of the illness is usually 10 to 14 days; significant sequelae are rare. A careful history may reveal evidence of a viral illness in a family member or other close contact of the patient.

Laboratory and Diagnostic Tests

CSF findings in viral meningitis are markedly different than those found in bacterial illness. There is generally lymphocytic rather than neutrophil pleocytosis, protein elevation is only moderate, and the glucose content is nearly always normal in contrast to the reduced CSF glucose content in bacterial meningitis. For diagnostic purposes, it is important to verify that the CSF is actually free of bacteria or a fungal agent responsible for the infection.

Management

There is no known treatment for viral meningitis. Management is purely supportive, with emphasis on the control of head and neck pain and fever. Hospitalization and isolation are not necessary. The illness is self-limiting, with none of the life-threatening complications seen in its bacterial counterpart.

Viral Encephalitis

Encephalitis is an acute inflammation of the brain that is usually caused by a virus. The CNS can be infected by many different viruses, some of them endemic to certain geographical areas and associated with certain seasons of the year. Commonly, encephalitis is preceded by a primary infection elsewhere in the body. Herpes simplex and rabies are two exceptions in which the virus enters the CNS ascends along the peripheral nerve.

Mumps, herpes simplex virus 1 (HSV-1), and arboviruses (i.e., eastern equine encephalitis) are the most frequent etiologic agents associated with the disease. Encephalitis caused by mumps is benign except in rare instances. Herpes simplex is the most common cause of encephalitis in the United States, and is associated with a high incidence of residual deficits. The infection is characterized by destructive lesions in the inferior frontal and temporal lobes. The mortality rate is 10 to 40% (Whitley, 1990).

Arboviruses have a variable course and prognosis. Eastern equine encephalitis is the most severe with a mortality rate of 70 to 90%. Western equine encephalitis and St. Louis encephalitis are more benign diseases with much lower mortality rates.

History and Physical Findings

Manifestations of encephalitis are similar to those of meningitis, but usually have a more gradual onset. Headache, high fever, seizures, neck stiffness, and changes in level of consciousness may be noted. In herpes simplex encephalitis, personality changes, memory loss, and aphasia may be seen secondary to frontal and temporal lobe involvement.

Laboratory and Diagnostic Tests

Diagnosis is based on clinical findings as well as CSF analysis. The CSF is usually colorless, with a slightly elevated pressure. The WBC count is elevated with increased lymphocytes. CSF protein is also elevated while glucose is normal.

The work-up of herpes simplex encephalitis also includes CT or MRI. These studies show inflammation and edema in the regions of the frontal or temporal lobes. EEG shows characteristic periodic sharp-wave activity temporally on a background of focal or diffuse slowing. Brain biopsy provides definitive diagnosis.

Management

The general management of the patient with viral encephalitis focuses on supportive and symptomatic care. Control of fever and headache are important goals to achieve for the comfort of the patient. Osmotic diuretics may be used to control cerebral edema. Anticonvulsants are sometimes given for seizure prophylaxis. In cases of confirmed or highly suspected herpes simplex encephalitis, acyclovir is administered intravenously.

Brain Abscess

Brain abscess is caused by one of several mechanisms. Most commonly, they occur as a result of direct extension of a primary infection of the middle ear, mastoid, or sinus. Direct introduction of bacteria following head injury or intracranial surgery, however, can also occur. Some cases are also the result of hematogenous spread from a distant site of infection. The most commonly identified infecting organisms include *Streptococcus, Staphylococcus,* and *Bacteroides* species (Mampalam & Rosenblum, 1988).

Pathophysiology

Brain abscess formation involves two stages. The first stage is one of diffuse cerebritis in which a poorly marginated area is associated with edema and destruction of brain tissue. At this stage, successful treatment involves the use of antibiotics alone; surgical intervention is not indicated. During the second stage, usually occuring from 4 to 9 days from the onset of symptoms, the center of the infection becomes a semiliquid mass of pus and necrotic brain tissue. Gradually, encapsulation occurs and a free abscess forms. The abscess can be of variable size and shape, but most often occurs in the white matter. Daughter abscesses may form surrounding the major abscess.

History and Physical Findings

Brain abscesses most commonly present with a progression of focal neurologic signs, headache, and mental status changes. Flulike symptoms and fever are present in only about half of patients. Focal or generalized seizures may occur. Depending on the size of the abscess, signs of increased intracranial pressure may also be present.

Laboratory and Diagnostic Tests

Blood work reveals peripheral leukocytosis in only about half of patients. Erythrocyte sedimentation rate (ESR) is usually elevated. MRI and CT scans are reliable in localizing the presence of an abscess. A characteristic "ring enhancing" lesion seen on these studies is specific for brain abscess (Fig. 40–15). Definitive diagnosis, however, is often made only at surgery. Diagnostic work-up also includes the search for parameningeal infections. Skull X-rays or CT scan with bone windows provide information regarding the involvement of the mastoids or sinuses.

Management

Treatment of brain abscesses involves the use of antibiotics, as well as surgical intervention for drainage, either by needle aspiration or total excision. Antibiotic therapy alone may be used in selected patients; however, abscesses larger than 3 cm are generally refractory to medical therapy alone (Mampalam & Rosenblum, 1988). For patients at risk for increased intracranial pressure, immediate surgery is necessary to reduce mass effect.

Antibiotics are started preoperatively, with the choice of drug determined by the likely source of the infection. Recommended empiric therapy includes penicillin or ampicillin for a suspected source of sinusitis. For otitis media or mastoiditis, ceftriaxone, penicillin, and ampicillin are used. Oxacillin and ceftriaxone are recommended for posttraumatic and postsurgical abscesses. When gram stain and culture results are obtained, antibiotic therapy can be adjusted appropriately.

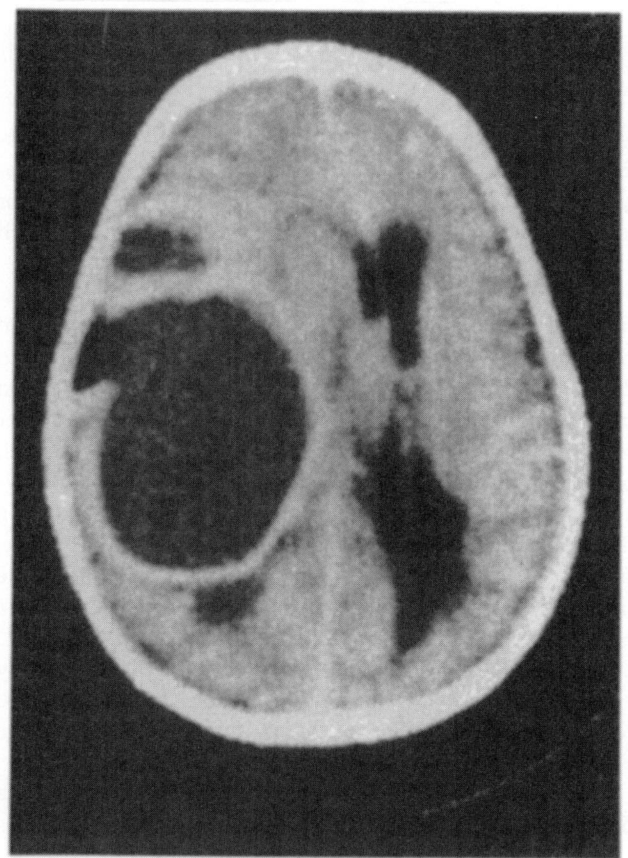

Figure 40–15. CT of right parietal abscess in patient with chronic otitis media. *(From Burrell. [1992]. [p. 1001].)*

HIV Infection of the Nervous System

The nervous system is a major target for the human immunodeficiency virus (HIV). One half to two thirds of patients with AIDS are affected with neurologic disease, most often in the late stages of their illness (McGuire & So, 1994). Neurologic involvement may be in the form of primary HIV infection, or as secondary complications due to opportunistic infections.

Primary HIV Infection

HIV enters the nervous system early in the course of the disease. The initial CNS infection is usually asymptomatic; however, in 10% of patients, neurologic disease may be the first manifestation of HIV (Perlstein & Ake, 1987). Patients may present with an acute encephalopathy that is represented by symptoms of confusion, memory loss, and mood disturbance. Other common acute processes include aseptic meningits, cranial neuropathies (particularly Bell's palsy), and ascending or transverse myelitis.

Chronic infection associated with HIV is most commonly represented in the form of AIDS dementia complex. Patients often present with a constellation of cognitive, behavioral, and motor impairments that can initially be mistaken for depression. These symptoms relate to the presence of small nodules of inflammatory microglial cells in both gray and white matter, focal and diffuse demyelination, and spongy changes in the spinal cord. Cortical atrophy and ventricular enlargement are noted on neuroimaging studies. HIV-associated myelopathy, peripheral neuropathies, and lumbosacral polyradiculopathy are other commonly noted processes related to chronic HIV infection.

Treatment consists of anti-HIV chemotherapy, primarily with azidothymidine (AZT). Clear benefits have been noted in the treatment of children with AIDS encephalopathy. Some benefit has been demonstrated with adults in the area of cognitive function (McGuire & So, 1994).

Opportunistic Infections of the CNS

Patients with AIDS are at increased risk for infection of the CNS with toxoplasmosis, cryptoccus, tuberculosis, herpes simplex, herpes zoster, cytomegalovirus (CMV), and progressive multifocal leukoencephalopathy (PML). Treatment is the same as in nonimmunosuppressed individuals, although the course of therapy is often prolonged.

Toxoplasmosis is the most common opportunistic infection to cause encephalitis or focal intracerebral lesions and occurs in as high as 40% of patients with AIDS (Luft & Remington, 1988).

Treatment commonly consists of a combination of pyrimethamine, sulfadiazine, and leucovorin. Mortality rates are noted to be as high as 80%, with a relapse rate after initial treatment of 60% (Porter & Sande, 1992).

Cryptococcal meningitis occurs in approximately 10% of patients with AIDS and is treated with Amphotericin B. Tuberculosis is treated with the typical first-line drugs of Isoniazid, Rifampin, Pyrazinamide, and Ethambutol. As was previously discussed, herpes simplex encephalitis is treated with intravenous acyclovir. The viral encephalitis caused by CMV is treated with the antivirals Ganciclovir (DHPG) and Foscarnet. There is no known treatment for PML.

Follow-Up

Patients with central nervous system infections may be left with a broad range of sequelae following their illness. Deficits may include dementia, seizures, hearing loss, hemiplegia, and hydrocephalus. Vision, cognitive skills, hearing, and motor abilities should be assessed with appropriate referral made as indicated. Many patients require ongoing follow-up long after their antibiotic or medical regimens have been completed.

▶ MULTIPLE SCLEROSIS

Multiple sclerosis (MS) is a chronic, progressive disease that is characterized by demyelination in the CNS. Predominantly occurring in caucasion persons, MS affects women more often than men. The usual age of onset is between 15 and 50 years.

The cause of MS is unknown. One theory suggests that some environmental factor, possibly a group of viruses, acts early in life to initiate the disease process in patients who may be genetically susceptible. The susceptibility of MS seems to be inherited. A child or a first-degree relative of a person with MS has a 20- to 50-fold increased risk for developing the disease themselves (Sadovnick & Baird, 1988). Environmental factors also affect the development of the disease. Previous studies have documented an increased prevalence of MS progressing north or south of the equator (Sadownick & Ebers, 1993).

Pathophysiology

In MS, an inflammatory demyelinating process occurs that is thought to be triggered by a virus. Activated T-cells enter the CNS and, in conjunction with astrocytes, disturb the blood–brain barrier promoting the entry of other immune mediators into the CNS. These factors damage oligodendrocytes (the cells that produce myelin) and cause demyelination. This process, occurring in multiple areas of the CNS, results in sclerosis, or plaque formation.

MS is characterized by periods of disability (exacerbation) alternating with periods of recovery (remission). In early stages, the myelin sheath is damaged during the exacerbation, but the nerve fiber remains intact and impulse transmission continues. The patient complains of symptoms, but remains functional. The disease then progresses to a state of remission, as a result of healing of the demyelinated areas by sclerotic tissue. In later stages of the disease, the myelin sheath is totally destroyed and is replaced by hard, sclerotic plaques. Axonal damage occurs, resulting in permanent loss of function.

History and Physical findings

The onset of MS is often gradual and insidious, with symptoms sometimes manifested (in retrospect) months or years before actual diagnosis. The course of the disease is also variable. To be consistent with a diagnosis of MS, symptom involvement must occur in one of the following patterns:

- *Relapsing–recurring multiple sclerosis:* Two or more exacerbations, separated by one month or more and lasting more than 24 hours without subsequent recovery.
- *Secondary progressive multiple sclerosis:* A clinical history of clearly defined exacerbations and remissions with or without complete recovery followed by slow progression of signs and symptoms over a period of at least 6 months.
- *Primary progressive multiple sclerosis:* Slow or stepwise progression of signs and symptoms over a period of at least 6 months (Brod, Lindsey, & Wolinsky, 1996).

The diagnosis of MS is a clinical one, based on neurologic abnormalities indicative of CNS dysfunction. The history and neurological exam must show evidence of involvement of two or more parts of the CNS. The deficits or involvement may not be attributable to a single lesion, such as a brain tumor.

Symptoms include motor, sensory, and cerebellar dysfunction, but may vary considerably from patient to patient because of the varied distribution of the disease process in the CNS. Common symptoms include spasticity; intention tremor; motor weakness; numbness, tingling, and other paresthesias; blurred vision; nystagmus; ataxia; and bowel, bladder, and sexual dysfunction. Urinary problems are variable. Some patients experience urinary retention due to a flaccid (hypotonic) bladder. Others complain of urgency, frequency, and dribbling or incontinence due to a spastic (hypertonic) bladder. The remaining patients have a mixture of retention and emptying problems.

Relapses or worsening in symptoms are precipitated by a variety of factors. Physical and emotional trauma or stress, fatigue, infection, and cold or humid weather are among the events that trigger exacerbations in some patients.

Women with MS who become pregnant often note a decreased number of exacerbations during pregnancy. This is thought to occur due to the hormonal changes on the immune system. During the postpartum period, however, exacerbations may occur with increased frequency (Abramsky, 1994).

Psychiatric complications include depression, euphoria, emotional lability, and psychosis. Understandably, reactive depression can occur as a result of the diagnosis or due to increasing disability. Euphoria is often noted late in the course of the disease, and is thought to be a result of generalized intellectual deterioration and extensive cerebral demyelination. Psychosis, which occurs rarely, is usually the result of the use of high-dose corticosteriods for treatment of acute exacerbations.

Laboratory and Diagnostic Tests

Adjuncts to the clinical diagnosis of MS include MRI, evoked potentials, and CSF analysis. MRI has become an important tool in diagnosis, as well as an excellent measure of disease severity and progression. Characteristic white-matter lesions are evident throughout the brain and spinal cord in affected patients (Fig. 40–16). These lesions actually correlate weakly with clinical status as MRI has the ability to detect areas of demyelination that have no obvious clinical correlate.

Evoked potentials often demonstate abnormalities that may not be clinically evident. Visual-evoked potentials are abnormal in 75 to 97% of patients with MS; somatosen-

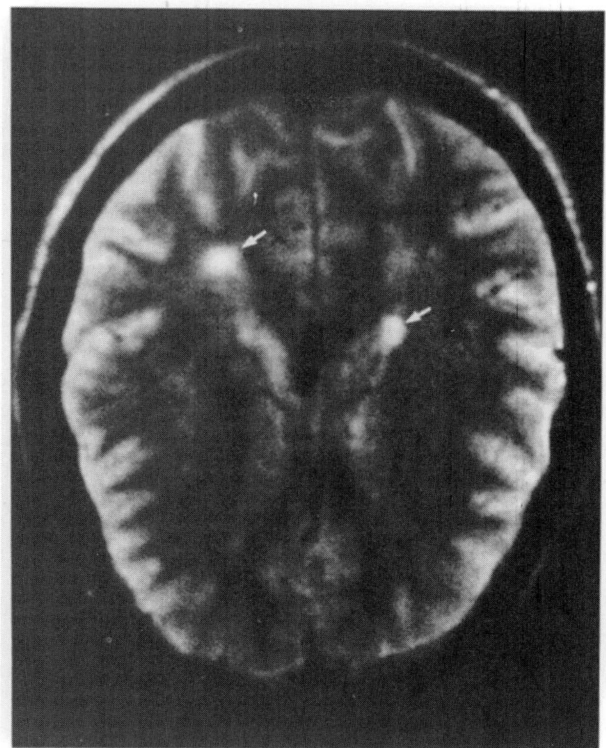

Figure 40–16. MRI of brain demonstrating two plaques (*Arrows*) of multiple sclerosis in white matter. *(From Burrell. [1992]. [p. 1048].)*

sory-evoked potentials are abnormal in 72 to 87% of patients; and brainstem auditory-evoked responses are abnormal in 50 to 70% of patients with MS (Brod, Lindsey, & Wolinsky, 1996).

CSF analysis reveals an increase in oligoclonal immunoglobulin G Oligoclonal bands may be detected by CSF electrophoresis. This finding, however, is not specific to MS alone.

Management

Therapeutic management of the patient with MS is aimed at treating and preventing the progression of the disease and providing symptomatic relief. Interferon beta-1b (Betaseron) and interferon beta-1a (Avonex) are two immunomodulators that have been shown to positively impact the course of the disease in patients with relapsing–remitting MS. One study reports that the use of Betaseron can decrease relapses by 30% and decrease the development of new lesions as assessed by serial MRIs (IFNB Multiple Sclerosis Study Group, 1993).

Administered by subcutaneous injection every other day, Betaseron should be used continuously if tolerated well, and should be stopped only for intolerable side effects or recurrence of the disease at a rate equal to or greater than the initial presentation. Fatigue and systemic flulike symptoms may be severe enough for patients to consider stopping the drug. Although these symptoms are more prominent on the first day after injection, and generally persist for only the first one to three months of therapy, they may be severe enough to require routine premedication with Tylenol or a nonsteroidal antiinflammatory medication.

Other noted side effects include depression, anxiety, confusion, neutropenia, and elevation of liver transaminases. CBC with differential and blood chemistries including liver enzymes and platelet count should be drawn prior to the onset of therapy and at 3-month intervals while taking the drug.

Other immunosupressive agents including Imuran, Cytoxan, cyclosporine, and cyclophosphamide have been shown to produce some beneficial effect in patients with MS. The side effects of their use, however, must be weighed against the potential benefit of treatment.

Acute exacerbations or relapses of MS have been shown to respond favorably to the administration of intravenous methylprednisolone. More than 85% of patients experience improvement in neurological status within three to five days after treatment is initiated (Wolinsky, 1993). The medication is administered intravenously at a dosage of 250 to 500 mg every 12 hours for 3 to 7 days. This is followed by oral prednisone at a dose of 60 to 80 mg daily for 7 days. The prednisone is then tapered by 10 mg every 4 days over a 1-month period.

As with all steroids, the use of methylprednisolone is not without side effect. Patients may complain of fluid retention, gastric irritation, restlessness, anxiety, and insomnia. Psychosis has been observed in a small number of patients. Infection and sepsis are rare complications.

Symptomatic therapies can significantly improve the quality of life for patients with MS. Baclofen is often used to control spasticity. Ditropan may be helpful for patients with urinary urgency, while patients with urinary retention may benefit from an intermittent self-catheterization program. Fatigue, a common symptom experienced by the patient with MS, may improve with the use of amantadine or Prozac.

Follow-Up

Long-term management of the MS patient is aimed at keeping the patient active and maximally functional. The patient and family need information regarding the avoidance of factors that precipitate exacerbations, as well as a plan for management during periods of relapse. Strategies to maximize self care in the face of increasing neurologic deficits should be investigated. Patients with neurologic deficits are likely to benefit from the involvement of an outpatient or home-care physical or occupational therapist. The National Multiple Sclerosis Society and its local chapters can serve as valuable resources for patients and families.

PARKINSON'S DISEASE

Parkinson's disease is a movement disorder of unknown cause that results in damage of the dopamine-producing cells in the substantia nigra. This leads to a depletion of dopamine in the basal ganglia, resulting in the characteristic symptoms or classic triad of Parkinson's disease: bradykinesia or slowness of movement, increased muscle tone, and resting tremor.

It is estimated that in the United States, there are approximately 40,000 new patients diagnosed each year. The disease is one of older and late adulthood, with the first symptoms most often occurring after 50 years of age. Men and women are equally affected. Although there is no culture preference, the disease rarely occurs in African-Americans.

Pathophysiology

It is first important to differentiate between parkinsonism and Parkinson's disease. Parkinsonism is a syndrome characterized by bradykinesia, rigidity, and tremor. It has a variety of known causes including head trauma, exposure to neurotoxins (MPTP), and chemical and drug intoxication. The degenerative or idiopathic form of parkinsonism is the form commonly referred to as Parkinson's disease.

The pathophysiology of Parkinson's disease involves the degeneration of the dopamine-producing cells in the substantia nigra. A neurotransmitter important in the functioning of the extrapyramidal system, dopamine is present along with acetylcholine in balanced amounts in the basal ganglia. A lack of dopamine leads to parkinsonlike symptoms.

History and Physical Findings

As with many degenerative diseases of the nervous system, symptom development is gradual and insidious. Initially, patients may experience a mild tremor that is more pronounced at rest and is aggravated with emotional stress or concentration. The tremor disappears with complete muscle relaxation and sleep, and is often described as "pill-rolling" because of the characteristic motions of the thumb and forefinger.

As the disease progresses, the muscle rigidity and bradykinesia become more pronounced. Abnormal muscle tone is referred to as cog-wheel or lead-pipe rigidity because of its jerky quality when the extremity is passively ranged. Bradykinesia affects not only voluntary but automatic movements as well. These include blinking, swinging the arms when walking, swallowing saliva, self-expression with facial movements, and minor movements to adjust posture. This lack of automatic movement accounts for some of the secondary symptoms of Parkinson's disease, including masked facies, drooling, shuffling gait (often called festination), and stooped posture. Other secondary manifestations include the development of a monotonic voice and complaints of generalized weakness, muscle fatigue, constipation, and dysphagia.

While the majority of patients do not experience cognitive impairments, dementia can occur in up to 40% of individuals (Calne, 1995). This is an important point of assessment—patients with dementia are at higher risk for experiencing acute confusion or other adverse side effects when treated with medication.

Laboratory and Diagnostic Tests

There are no specific laboratory or diagnostic tests for Parkinson's disease. Diagnosis is based on history and physical exam alone, with particular attention paid to the presence of at least two of the three characteristics of the classic triad: bradykinesia, muscle rigidity, and tremor.

Management

The goal of pharmacologic management is to correct the imbalance of neurotransmitters in the CNS. Levodopa (in combination with carbidopa as Sinemet) is often the first drug of choice in the treatment of Parkinson's disease. A precursor to dopamine, levodopa is converted to dopamine in the basal ganglia. However, almost 99% of levodopa is metabolized peripherally before crossing the blood–brain barrier. Carbidopa, the second component in the drug Sinemet, increases the amount of levodopa available within the CNS. Symptoms respond to treatment with Sinemet in about 80% of patients with Parkinson's disease. There is, however, a decline in benefit from levodopa after the first several years of use.

Adverse effects associated with levodopa use include nausea, vomiting, and orthostasis. An additional side effect associated with prolonged use of levodopa is the development of the "on–off phenomenon." Occurring in approximately 50% of patients who are treated for 5 years or more, the effect is characterized by periods of severe akinesia, hypotonia, and apprehension that begin and end abruptly and can last for 30 minutes to several hours. This effect can be lessened by dosing levodopa on a every 2-hour basis.

A variety of other medications have proven to be effective in the treatment of Parkinson's disease. Bromocriptine (Parlodel) is a dopamine-receptor agonist that activates dopamine receptors. When used as an adjuvant drug along with Sinemet, it can lower the need for levodopa by as much as 30%. Selegiline (Eldepryl), an MAO inhibitor, is sometimes used in combination with Sinemet. As MAO is the degredative enzyme for dopamine, the use of Eldepryl causes levels of dopamine to increase. Anticholinergics (cogentin, artane) are useful in relieving tremor, particularly early in the course of the disease. The antiviral agent amantadine (Symmetrel) is helpful in reducing signs of rigidity and akinesia by increasing endogenous dopamine release at the nerve terminal.

Some patients are candidates for surgical treatment of Parkinson's disease. Pallidotomy, or lesioning into the globus pallidus, is one stereotactic procedure that is performed on patients who fail to show improvement in their symptoms with conventional drug therapy. Although the procedure was developed in the 1950s, the intervention is seeing a resurgence with advances in contemporary technology. The best candidate for surgery is the patient with advanced Parkinson's disease who still responds to levodopa therapy but whose symptoms are not sufficiently controlled by medication. Recent studies indicate that postoperative patients can expect a marked improvement in all three of the classic symptoms of Parkinson's disease (Laitinen, Bergenheim, & Hariz, 1992).

Follow-Up

Patients with Parkinson's disease need routine medical follow-up to assess for the effectiveness of their medications and the presence of medication-related side effects. Table 40–10 offers a classification of severity of Parkinson's disease that is useful in tracking the progression of the disease.

In addition, involvement with speech, occupational, and physical therapists assists the patient to maximize functional status and maintain independence in activities of daily living for as long as possible.

TABLE 40–10 Classification of the Severity of Parkinson's Disease

Stage	Clinical Symptoms
1	Unilateral
2	Bilateral
3	Bilateral plus postural reflexes
4	Requires aids because of stage 3
5	Bedridden because of stage 3

From Hoehn & Yahr. (1967).

▶ MYASTHENIA GRAVIS

Myasthenia gravis (MG) is a chronic, progressive disease of the neuromuscular junction that is marked by weakness and progressive fatigue. The peak age of onset is between 20 and 30 years. Up to the age of 40, women are affected two to three times as frequently as men; after age 40, the incidence is equal.

Pathophysiology

MG is thought to be caused by an autoimmune process in which antibodies cause destruction of the acetylcholine receptor sites at the neuromuscular junction. Because acetylcholine molecules are not able to attach and stimulate the muscle, contraction of the muscle is incomplete. Consequently, the patient experiences muscle fatigue and weakness. Antiacetylcholine receptor antibodies are detectable in the serum of 70 to 85% of patients with MG (Lewis, Collier & Heitkemper, 1996). The thymus gland, which is involved in supplying T-lymphocytes for cellular immunity, often shows proliferative changes in the patient with MG. Thymic hyperplasia has been noted in 80% of patients while 10% have thymic tumors (Adams & Victor, 1985).

History and Physical Findings

The chief complaint of patients with MG is easy fatigueability of skeletal muscles with activity. Muscle fatigue is less of a problem in the morning and becomes more prominent as the day progresses. Periods of rest temporarily restore strength. As the disease progresses, muscle fatigue is noted earlier in the day and with less exertion.

The muscles of the eyes and face, and muscles involved in speech and mastication, are involved early in the course of the disease. Ocular myasthenia is a form of the disease that involves only the eye muscles. Ptosis and diplopia are common symptoms, as are complaints of chewing and swallowing difficulties. Patients may find that it is more difficult to eat after talking and that their voice fades and becomes nasal the longer they are involved in conversation. The muscles of the neck, shoulder girdle, and hips are less frequently involved. In advanced cases, however, all muscles are weakened including the diaphragm, abdominal, and intercostal muscles, and external sphincters of the bladder and bowel. There is generally no sensory involvement and reflexes are normal.

The actual course of the disease is variable, but is generally characterized by periods of exacerbation and remission. Exacerbations can be triggered by secondary illness, pregnancy, surgery, and emotional stress. Osserman's (1958) clinical classification scale identifies several general groups that are helpful when choosing therapeutic options and predicting the course of the disease (Table 40–11).

An exacerbation of symptoms or an acute weakening, called a crisis, has two etiologies. Myasthenic crisis occurs as a result of the natural worsening of the disease, or due to changes in dosing or absorption of medications. Cholinergic crisis results from overdosage of anticholinesterase medications (neostigmine, mestinon).

The patient in crisis experiences increased skeletal muscle weakness, ptosis, and worsening of bulbar and respiratory signs. Airway maintenance is a priority of management, and intubation is often necessary. Once a secure airway is established, diagnosis of the origin of the crisis can proceed.

Laboratory and Diagnostic Tests

The Tensilon test, useful in evaluating crisis, is also the cornerstone of initial diagnosis. Performed only in an area where clinical support and emergency medications and equipment are available, the test involves infusion of a

TABLE 40–11 Osserman's Clinical Classification Scale for Myasthenia Gravis

Group I	Ocular myasthenia . . . involves ocular muscles only causing symptoms of ptosis and diplopia. No mortality; high incidence of spontaneous remission
Group IIA	Mild generalized myasthenia with ocular symptoms . . . usually responds well to medication and has low mortality rate
Group IIB	Moderately severe generalized myasthenia with mild bulbar and ocular involvment . . . doesn't respond as well to medications; restricts activities of daily living; low mortality rate
Group III	Acute severe myasthenia, with bulbar and respiratory complications . . . rapid deterioration, frequent crises and high mortality rate
Group IV	Late severe myasthenia . . . develops from other groups after 2 years; severe respiratory and bulbar involvement; responds poorly to meds, high mortality rate

From Osserman. (1958).

small dose of Tensilon (2 mg). The patient is observed for signs of improvement in skeletal muscle strength, as well as for the adverse effect of respiratory compromise. Atropine, the antidote, should be available if needed. If no severe effects occur, an additional 8 mg of Tensilon is infused and the patient is observed for clinical improvement.

If the patient is alert and cooperative, the Tensilon (edrophonium) test is a highly reliable method of distinguishing between myasthenic and cholinergic crisis. Intravenous administration of Tensilon should cause transient improvement in symptoms when given to the patient in myasthenic crisis. The patient in cholinergic crisis either fails to improve or shows worsening of symptoms. In addition, patients in cholinergic crisis may experience increased salivation, nausea and vomiting, diarrhea, and increased bronchial secretions.

Other valuable studies include EMG and acetylcholine receptor antibody assay. EMG shows a pattern that is pathognomonic for myasthenia gravis. Fifty percent of patients with ocular myasthenia and 80 to 90% of patients with generalized myasthenia have elevated levels of acetylcholine receptor antibody. Evaluation of the thymus by CT scan identifies the presence of thymoma. Thymic hyperplasia is not so easily diagnosed by CT.

Management

Four general methods of treatment are currently available for MG: treatment with anticholinesterase agents, immunosuppression with steroids and cytotoxic drugs, thymectomy, and plasma exchange.

Anticholinesterase therapy is the initial treatment of choice in all cases of MG. These drugs inhibit the breakdown of acetylcholine and allow its accumulation at the synapse. Prostigmin and mestinon are two commonly prescribed anticholinesterase agents. Side effects associated with their use include increased parasympathetic activity such as diarrhea, nausea, vomiting, incontinence, bradycardia, hypotension, and pupillary constriction. A typical starting dose of mestinon is 60 mg every 4 hours. Patients should be instructed to observe and document their response to therapy so that appropriate changes can be made in dosing.

High-dose corticosteroid therapy, often using Prednisone in doses of 60-100 mg/day, is indicated in treatment of most patients with MG unless there is major contraindication. Used in conjunction with anticholinesterase agents, steroids are also valuable when attempting to improve the patient's condition prior to thymectomy. Greater than 90% of patients have been shown to benefit from the use of steroids (Engel, 1976), although their use is not without consequence. Drawbacks include generalized immunosuppression and the risk of relapse of symptoms as a result of withdrawal or reduction in dose.

Cyclosporine in sufficiently high doses has been shown to induce significant improvement in some aspects of myasthenic weakness. This may, in part, be due to the reduction in the mean titers of antibody to the acetylcholine receptor. Unfortunately, improvement does not persist when the drug is withdrawn.

Surgical therapy in the form of thymectomy offers a marked improvement in symptoms in selected patients with MG. Ideal candidates are young patients, early in the course of their disease for whom anticholinesterase agents do not produce optimum improvement with a minimum of side effects. As many as 90% of selected patients experience a remission or sustained improvement in their symptoms for as long as 5 years following thymectomy (Mathew, Cuschieri, & Tankel, 1992).

Plasmapheresis has been shown to be an effective treatment when used in conjunction with anticholinesterase agents and immunosuppressives. The antibodies that cause MG are essentially plasmapheresed out of the system, resulting in improvement in symptoms that, in the best of circumstances, can last for months. Repeat exchanges are often necessary to maintain improvement.

Follow-Up

Patients with MG are faced with the challenge of living with a chronic neurologic disease that invariably impacts on daily living. In addition to a potentially restrictive medical regimen, they need to be educated regarding the importance of planning activities of daily living to avoid fatigue. They also need to be educated regarding the potential adverse reactions to specific drugs, as well as how to handle crisis situations.

▶ AMYOTROPHIC LATERAL SCLEROSIS

Amyotrophic lateral sclerosis (ALS), also known as Lou Gehrig disease, is a progressive, degenerative neuromuscular disease characterized by destruction of motor cells in the anterior gray horns of the spinal cord as well as degeneration of the pyramidal tracts. Its etiology is unknown, but it is most commonly recognized by atrophy, weakness, spasticity, and a total lack of sensory involvement. Males are more often affected than females. The onset is usually during middle age and, although the rate of disease progression is somewhat variable, 50% of people die within 2 to 5 years of the onset of symptoms; 20% live for 5 years; and 10% live for 10 years. A few individuals have been reported to survive as long as 20 years (Mitsumoto, 1994).

Pathophysiology

The most common form of motor system disease, ALS is characterized by degeneration and death of anterior horn cells of the spinal cord, the motor nuclei of the brainstem (especially the nuclei of cranial nerves VII [facial] and XII [hypoglossal]), the pyramidal or corticospinal tracts, and the precentral cells of the frontal lobe of the brain. Involvement of the upper motor neurons (or the brain and the spinal cord) results in spasticity and motor weakness. The involvement of lower motor neurons (or the peripheral nerves) causes flaccidity and muscle atrophy. Cognitive and sensory function as well as vision and hearing are preserved.

History and Physical Findings

ALS is diagnosed primarily on the basis of history and neurological examination. Patients most often present with complaints of weakness and clumsiness of their upper extremities, as well as fatigue or a feeling of heaviness involving their lower extremities. If the frontal lobe cells are involved, emotional lability may be noted.

Physical examination reveals muscle wasting and atrophy commonly involving the intrinsic muscles of the hands, as well as the shoulder and upper arm muscles. Muscle spasticity, fasciculations, hyperreflexia, and motor weakness are also observed. Brainstem or bulbar involvement is evidenced by atrophy of the tongue and depressed gag and swallow reflexes. If the disease has progressed to the point of respiratory involvement, the patient often complains of dyspnea. In advanced stages, speech is difficult to understand, and chewing, swallowing, and managing secretions become progressively more difficult. Death typically occurs as a result of aspiration or infection leading to respiratory failure.

Laboratory and Diagnostic tests

There is no single definitive test to confirm the diagnosis of ALS. Currently, the diagnosis remains one of exclusion, where problems such as spinal cord compression that mimic the symptoms of ALS are ruled out. Commonly ordered studies in the diagnostic process include MRI to rule out cord compression and electrophysiology studies (EMG/NCV). The EMG demonstrates fibrillations, which are indicative of denervation. Blood creatinine phosphokinase (CPK) levels are also elevated.

Management

General Management

There is no known treatment to cure or arrest the progression of ALS. Management is essentially symptomatic, aimed at optimizing the patient's condition, thus enabling him or her to remain as independent as possible. Progressive physical limitations obviate the benefit of early involvement with physical and occupational therapists. Assistive devices such as a cane, walker, or splints might preserve independence with ADLs for a longer period of time. Speech therapy is also helpful in educating the patient with bulbar involvement about techniques in voice projection.

Respiratory Management

Eventually, all respiratory parameters worsen with ALS. Respiratory muscle fatigue and diaphragmatic failure contribute to this slowly progressive decline in pulmonary function by putting the patient at increased risk for atelectasis and pneumonia. Physical signs of respiratory failure are not reliable indicators of the progression of the disease, as they often remain within normal range until the terminal stages. Forced vital capacity (FVC) is generally accepted to be the best measure of pulmonary function to follow throughout the course of the illness (Shiffman & Belsh, 1993). FVC should therefore be measured on a routine basis as part of the ongoing assessment of the patient. As the disease progresses, there is often a sharp drop in FVC in the 6 months prior to death. FVC measurements of less than 50% of predicted suggest an increased likelihood of respiratory arrest.

As swallowing function deteriorates along with respiratory function, the patient is at increasing risk for aspiration. Patients and families need to learn ways to prevent aspiration, e.g., sitting fully erect and flexing the neck slightly when eating, and elevating the head of the bed with blocks. If aspiration is apparent despite these measures (or if silent aspiration is confirmed by swallowing study), percutaneous esophagogastrostomy (PEG) should be considered. If a PEG is in place, the patient should sit or lie with the head of the bed elevated after being fed.

When the FVC drops below one liter, noninvasive ventilation should be considered (Sherman & Paz, 1994). Bimodal passive airway pressure (BIPAP) involves the use of a nasal mask and nasal pillows to deliver pressure during patient inspiration. Inspiration is augmented with positive pressure and expiration is passive. Patients using BIPAP report symptomatic relief of dyspnea, improvement in fatigue, improved appetite, and improved sense of well-being. A discussion of code status and the options of tracheostomy and long-term ventilation should take place well before the terminal decline in pulmonary status.

Nutritional Management

Dysphagia, tongue atrophy, and bulbar weakness combine to have a significant effect on the nutritional status of the patient with advanced ALS. Slowie et al., (1983) found that 70% of 20 randomly selected ambulatory ALS patients ingested fewer calories than the recommended daily allowance (RDA) using the 24-hour dietary recall method. Weight loss is due not only to reduction in calorie intake, but also to an increased resting energy expenditure due to an increased effort at respiration.

All patients benefit from consultation with a nutritionist. Potential topics of education include proper swallowing techniques, selection of foods of the proper consistency to avoid choking and aspiration, and information regarding the proper amounts of protein and calories for optimal nutrition. When weight loss exceeds 5% of normal body weight or if symptomatic dysphagia occurs, PEG placement for delivery of enteral nutrition should be considered. Patients receiving PEG feedings maintain body weight, which in turn has a significant effect on survival time (Mazzini et al., 1995).

Medication Management

In 1996, the Food and Drug Administration made riluzole available for the treatment of ALS. The use of this medication is based on the theory that excitotoxic damage to motor neurons plays a role in the development of ALS (Choi, 1988). Experimental models have suggested that glutamate excitotoxicity can damage motor neurons and excessive concentrations of glutamate are present in the blood and CSF of patients with ALS. Glutamate transport is impaired in motor control areas of the brain and spinal cord in ALS patients because of a defect in transport proteins. Riluzole inhibits the release of glutamate and reduces neuronal damage in these experiemental models (Rothstein & Kuncl, 1995). Clinical trials of riluzole have shown a statistically significant benefit in prolonging the life of patients with ALS. Recommended dosing of riluzole is 50 mg bid. The drug is generally well tolerated. Regular monitoring of liver function is suggested.

Follow-Up

Patients with ALS and their families need ongoing follow-up and care up to and including the terminal phase of illness. Realistic information about status is necessary to ground the discussion of how best to manage the final stages of this debilitating, fatal disease.

REFERENCES

Abramsky, O. (1994). Pregnancy and multiple sclerosis. *Annals of Neurology, 36,* S38.

Adams, R. & Victor, M. (1993). *Principles of neurology* (5 ed.). New York: McGraw-Hill.

Bates, B. (1983). *A guide to physical assessment* (3rd ed.). Philadelphia: J. B. Lippincott.

Bell, W. (1984). Defibrinogenation with Arvin in thrombotic disorders. In S. Sherry & A. Scriabine (Eds.), *Platelets and thrombosis* (p. 272). Baltimore: Baltimore University Press.

Bender, C., Yasko, J., & Strohl, R. (1996). Nursing role in the management of cancer. In S. Lewis, I. Collier, & M. Heitkemper (Eds.), *Medical–surgical nursing: Assessment and management of clinical problems* (pp. 261–315). St. Louis: Mosby.

Benedict, W., Murphree, A., Banerjee, A., Spina, C., Sparkes, M., & Sparkes, R. (1983). Patient with 13 chromosome deletion: Evidence that the retinoblastoma gene is a recessive cancer gene. *Science, 219,* 973–975.

Bigner, S. & Vogelstein, B. (1990). Cytogenetics and molecular genetics of malignant gliomas and medulloblastoma. *Brain Pathology, 1,* 12–18.

Brod, S., Lindsey, W., & Wolinsky, J. (1996). Multiple sclerosis: Clinical presentation, diagnosis and treatment. *American Family Physician, 54* (4), 1301–1311.

Bullard, D., Gillespie, G., Mahaley, M., & Bigner, D. (1986). Immunobiology of human gliomas. *Seminars in Oncology, 13,* 94–109.

Burrell, L. (1992). *Adult nursing in hospital and community settings.* (p. 838). Norwalk, CT: Appleton & Lange.

Calne, D. (1995). Diagnosis and treatment of Parkinson's disease. *Hospital Practice, 30,* 83–88.

Choi, D. (1988). Glutamate neurotoxicity and disease of the nervous system. *Neuron, 1,* 623–634.

Durand, M., Calderwood S., & Weber, D. et al. (1993). Acute bacterial meningitis in adults: A review of 493 episodes. *New England Journal of Medicine, 328,* 21–28.

Engel, W. (1976). Myasthenia gravis, corticosteroids, and anticholinesterases. *Annals of the New York Academic Society, 274,* 623–630.

Feinberg, W. (1994). Guidelines for the management of transient ischemic attacks. *Heart Disease and Stroke, 3,* 275.

Folkman, J. & Klagsbrun, M. (1987). Angiogenic factors. *Science, 235,* 442–447.

Hacke, W. (1994). Thrombolytic therapy in acute ischemic stroke: An update. *Fibrinolysis, 8,* 216–220.

Harbison, J. (1992). Ticlopidine versus aspirin for the prevention of recurrent stroke. Analysis of patients with minor stroke from the Ticlopidine Aspirin Stroke Study Group. *Stroke, 23,* 1723–1727.

Hauser W. & Hesdorffer, D. (1990). *Epilepsy: Frequency, causes and consequences.* New York: Demos Publications.

Hickey, J. (1994). *The clinical practice of neurological and neurosurgical nursing* (3rd ed.). Philadelphia: J. B. Lippincott.

Hoehn, M. & Yahr, M. (1967). Parkinsonism: Onset, progression, and mortality. *Neurology, 17,* 427–432.

IFNB Multiple Sclerosis Study Group (1993). Interferon beta-1b is effective in relapsing–remitting multiple sclerosis. I. Clinical results of a multicenter, randomized, double-blind, placebo-controlled trial. *Neurology, 43,* 655–661.

Kay, R., Wong, K., Yu, Y., Chan, Y., Tsoi, T., Ahuja, A., Chan, F., Fong, K., Law, C., Wong, A., et al. (1995). *New England Journal of Medicine, 333,* 1588–1593.

Keane, A. & Richmond, T. (1993). Tertiary nurse practitioners. *Image: The Journal of Nursing Scholarship, 25,* 281–284.

Klein, G. (1987). The approaching era of the tumor supressor genes. *Science, 238,* 1539–1545.

Laitinen, L., Bergenheim, A., & Hariz, M. (1992). Leksell's posteroventral pallidotomy in the treatment of Parkinson's disease. *Journal of Neurosurgery, 76,* 53–61.

Lebel, M., Freij, B., Syrogiannopoulos, G., et al. (1988). Dexamethasone therapy for bacterial meningitis: Results of two double-blind, placebo-controlled trials. *New England Journal of Medicine, 319,* 964–971.

Lewis, S., Collier, I., & Heitkemper, M. (1996). *Medical-surgical nursing, assessment and management of clinical problems* (4th ed.). St. Louis: Mosby.

Luft, B. & Remington, J. (1988). AIDS commentary: Toxoplasmic encephalitis. *Journal of Infectious Disease, 157,* 1–6.

Mahaley, M., Mettlin, C., Natarajan, N., Laws, E., & Peace, B. (1989). National survey of patterns of care for brain-tumor patients. *Journal of Neurosurgery, 71,* 826–836.

Mampalam, T. & Rosenblum, M. (1988). Trends in the management of bacterial brain abscesses: A review of 102 cases over 17 years. *Neurosurgery, 23* (4), 451–458.

Matchar, D., McCrory, D., Barnett, H., & Feussner, J. (1994). Medical treatment for stroke prevention. *Annals of Internal Medicine, 121* (1), 41–53.

Mathew, P., Cuschieri, R., & Tankel, H. (1992). Outcome after thymectomy for myasthenia gravis: A retrospective review. *Scottish Medical Journal, 37* (4), 103.

Maxwell, M. & Black, P. (1988). Oncogenes, growth factors and brain tumors. In P. Kornblith & M. Walker (Eds.), *Advances in neuro-oncology* (pp. 159–176). Mount Kisco, NY: Futura.

Mazzini, L., Corra, T., Zaccala, M., Mora, G., Del Piano, M., & Galante, M. (1995). Percutaneous endoscopic gastrostomy and enteral nutrition in amyotrophic lateral sclerosis. *Journal of Neurology, 242,* 695–698.

McGillicuddy, J. & Hoff, J. (1992). Infections of the central nervous system. In A. Crockard, R. Hayward & J. Hoff (Eds.), *Neurosurgery: the scientific basis of clinical practice* (2nd ed.) vol. 2) Boston: Blackwell Scientific Publications.

McGuire, D. & So, Y. (1994). Neurologic dysfunction in HIV: Intracranial disorders. In P. Cohen, M. Sande, & P. Volberding (Eds.), *AIDS Knowledge Base.* Boston: Little, Brown.

Mitsumoto, H. (1994). Classification and clinical features of amyotrophic lateral sclerosis. In H. Mitsumoto & F. Norris (Eds.), *Amyotrophic Lateral Sclerosis. A Comprehensive Guide to Management.* New York: Demos Publications.

NACENT Collaborators (1991). Beneficial effects of carotid endarterectomy in symptomatic patients with high-grade carotid stenosis. *New England Journal of Medicine, 325,* 445–451.

NINDS Stroke rt-PA Stroke Study Group (1995). Tissue plasminogen activator for acute ischemic stroke. *New England Journal of Medicine, 333,* 1581–1587.

Osserman, K. (1958). *Myasthenia gravis.* New York: Grune and Stratton.

Perlstein & Ake. (1987). AIDS. Impact on neuroscience nursing practice. *Journal of Neuroscience Nursing, 19* (6), 300–304.

Porter, S. & Sande, M. (1992). Toxoplasmosis of the central nervous system in acquired immunodeficiency syndrome. *New England Journal of Medicine, 327,* 1643–1648.

Richardson, M. (1996). Bacterial meningitis. *British Journal of Hospital Medicine, 55* (ll), 685–688.

Rothstein, J. & Kuncl, R. (1995). Neuroprotective strategies in a model of chronic glutamate-mediated motor neuron toxicity. *Journal of Neurochemistry, 65,* 643–651.

Sadovnick, A. & Baird, P. (1988). The familial nature of multiple sclerosis: Age-corrected empiric recurrence risks for children and siblings of patients. *Neurology, 38,* 990–991.

Sadownick, A. & Ebers, G. (1993). Epidemiology of multiple sclerosis: A critical overview. *Canadian Journal of Neurological Science, 20,* 17–29.

Santilli, N. (ed.). (1996). Managing seizure disorders. Philadelphia: Lippincott-Raven.

Sherman, D., Barbour, P., Levy, D., et al. (1994). Ancrod for the treatment of acute ischemic brain infarction. *Stroke, 25,* 1755–1759.

Sherman, M. & Paz, H. (1994). Review of respiratory care of the patient with amyotrophic lateral sclerosis. *Respiration, 61,* 61–67.

Shiffman, P. & Belsh, J. (1993). Pulmonary function at diagnosis of amyotrophic lateral sclerosis. Rate of deterioration. *Chest, 103,* 508–513.

Slowie, L., Paige, M., & Antel, J. (1983). Nutritional considerations in the management of patients with amyotrophic lateral sclerosis (ALS). *Journal of the American Dietetic Association, 83,* 44–47.

Tunkel, A. & Scheld, W. (1995). Acute bacterial meningitis. *Lancet, 346,* 1675–1680.

Tuomanen, E. (1995). Mediators of inflammation and the treatment of bacterial meningitis. *Current Opinions in Infectious Disease, 8,* 218–223.

Whisnant, J. (1990). Classification of cerebrovascular disease. *Stroke, 21,* 637–642.

Whitley, R. (1990). Viral encephalitis. *New England Journal of Medicine, 323,* 242–249.

Wolinsky, J. (1993). Multiple sclerosis. *Current Neurology, 13,* 167–174.

Zulch, K. (1986). *Brain tumors: Their biology and pathology* (3rd ed.). Berlin, Germany: Springer-Verlag.

41

Gastrointestinal Problems

Judy Cavanaugh
Ellen Schmidt
Linda M. Lord

Gastrointestinal (GI) problems are ubiquitous in the acute care setting. This chapter first addresses commonly encountered GI symptoms—diarrhea, constipation, nausea, and vomiting. Specific disorders of the upper GI tract, pancreas, liver, gallbladder, and bowel are covered. Finally, because of their particular clinical importance, enteral access devices are discussed in detail.

▶ GASTROINTESTINAL SYMPTOMS

Diarrhea

Pathophysiology

Diarrhea is the rapid evacuation of excessive amounts of unformed stool. Although there is no universal definition of diarrhea, the most clinically practical definitions involve both stool frequency and consistency. A common definition is three or more liquid stools per day (Bliss, Guenter, & Settle, 1992). The usual abnormality of diarrhea is ineffective absorption of water and electrolytes in the colon. Distention from the retained fluid then stimulates propulsive contractions. Diarrhea can be secretory, exudative, or osmotic in nature; or due to abnormal bowel motility or fecal impaction.

Secretory diarrhea is due to active intestinal secretion of fluid and electrolytes into the bowel lumen. Causes include cholera, parasites, bacterial infections, viruses, antibiotic therapy, bacterial overgrowth, laxatives, intestinal resections, Zollinger–Ellison (ZE) syndrome, bowel carcinomas, or hyperthyroidism. The diarrhea generally continues, even when no enteral nutrition is being given. Exudative diarrheas can be caused by bacillary dysentary (Shigella) and inflammatory bowel diseases, such as Crohn's disease and ulcerative colitis.

Osmotic diarrhea is caused by poorly absorbable or osmotically active solutes that encourage the movement of fluid into the bowel lumen. Causes include nutritional fluids or medications with high osmolalities, bile acid malabsorption, lactose intolerance, or pancreatic/biliary disease. The diarrhea usually ceases when the nutrients or medications are stopped, bile acid malabsorption is treated with cholestyramine, or appropriate pancreatic enzymes are administered.

Altered bowel motility can occur postvagotomy or postgastrectomy and with diabetes, hyperthyroidism, scleroderma, irritable bowel syndrome, ileocecal valve resection, and in some partially obstructive carcinomas. In altered bowel motility, diarrhea may alternate with constipation. Fecal impaction itself can be manifested by the leakage of some liquid stool around the retained solidified stool.

History and Physical Findings

A full history includes definition of normal bowel habits and when the deviation from normal occurred. It should be noted whether the patient is receiving any medications known to cause diarrhea. These include antibiotics, sorbitol-containing liquids, lactulose, mannitol, and magnesium-containing antacids and laxatives. If the patient is receiving enteral tube feedings, the formula type, administration schedule, location of nutrient delivery, and possibility of formula contamination need to be addressed. Stool frequency, consistency, color, volume, presence of bright or dark blood, and appearance of undigested food particles, mucus, or fat should be noted. The patient should be assessed for fever that may accompany an infectious source or inflammatory bowel disease. The abdomen should be examined for any masses or tenderness. A rectal exam or proctoscopy can be helpful to assess for inflamed tissue or an obstructing lesion.

Prolonged diarrhea can lead to dehydration and electrolyte/metabolic abnormalities (particularly hypokalemia and acidosis). Therefore, the patient's urinary output, stool volume, pulse and respiratory rate, orthostatic blood pressure, and mucus membrane/skin turgor evaluation need to be obtained. Zinc deficiency may also develop and can cause continued diarrhea, rashes, taste changes, poor wound healing, and immunosuppression.

Laboratory and Diagnostic Tests

In patients with diarrheal stool that is bloody or positive for occult blood, infectious disease, inflammatory bowel disease, ischemic bowel, and carcinoma must be considered. At least two to three stool cultures on subsequent days should be obtained for *Clostridium difficile* toxin in patients who have been on antibiotic therapy within two weeks prior to the onset of diarrhea (Aronsson, Mollby, & Nord, 1984). A microscopic inspection of fecal smears for abundant polymorphonuclear leukocytes can indicate an invasive inflammatory process involving the colon. These processes include ulcerative colitis, *C difficile* colitis, and Shigella or Campylobacter infections. Stool should be sent for ova and parasites in those patients who live in endemic areas, especially if peripheral blood smears show eosinophilia. If bacterial enterocolitis is a possibility, stool and rectal swabs can be cultured for routine bacterial pathogens such as Campylobacter, Salmonella, Shigella and *Escherichia coli,* preferably before antibiotic therapy is started. Stool specimens should be evaluated for Cryptosporidium in immunocompromised patients, including patients with AIDS.

In suspected lactose intolerance, a breath hydrogen test or lactose intolerance test may be performed. In high-volume diarrhea after extensive bowel resections or with pancreatic or biliary disease, a 24- to 72-hour stool collection for fecal fat can be sent to determine malabsorption. Patients are usually on a high-fat diet at this time. Bile acid malabsorption may occur after iliectomy and, in place of diagnostic testing, a trial of cholestyramine may be used to see if diarrhea lessens. Thyroid-stimulating hormone and a free T4 level may be drawn if hyperthyroidism is possible. If laxative abuse is suspected, a comprehensive urine laxative screen or a sodium hydroxide test on the stool to detect the presence of phenolphthalein-containing laxatives can be performed.

In diarrhea that persists, an abdominal film, barium enema, and upper GI series with a small bowel follow-through should be considered. Endoscopic examination and intestinal biopsies may need to be done if pseudomembranous colitis, a viral infection, inflammatory bowel disease, or carcinoma is suspected.

Altered laboratory values that usually point to dehydration, in the absence of kidney disease, are an elevated urine specific gravity, an elevated blood urea nitrogen, and hypernatremia/hyperchloremia. Low serum potassium and carbon dioxide levels indicate hypokalemic acidosis due to stool losses. If diarrhea is prolonged, a serum zinc level should be obtained and supplemental zinc initiated.

Management

Primary emphasis is on fluid resuscitation prior to any diagnostic studies. Replacement fluid may be either in the form of an oral rehydration solution or isotonic intravenous therapy that contains potassium and some sodium, chloride and bicarbonate, citrate, or acetate. Intravenous solutions must be used when oral solutions are not tolerated or when dehydration is severe. Signs and symptoms of severe dehydration include tachycardia, hypotension, decreased urine output, and cold extremities. Response to therapy is best assessed by a return of urine output of at least 0.5 to 1 mL/kg/hour.

Treatment is then aimed at the etiology of the diarrhea. If diarrhea is associated with medications, alternate medications should be considered. If a stool is positive for *C difficile* toxin or if protoscopy reveals pseudomembraneous colitis, treatment entails administration of metronidazole or vancomycin enterally. Other bacterial pathogens (Salmonella, Shigella, Campylobacter and *E coli*) are treated with the appropriate antibiotic, which commonly entails the quinolones such as ciprofloxin or norfloxacin. With viral infections due to immunosuppression, the underlying disease will determine treatment. Antiretroviral therapy should be given with HIV-infected patients. In transplant or cancer patients, immunosuppressive therapy or chemotherapy can be decreased but this may risk graft rejection or cancer spread.

Patients undergoing extensive bowel resections may need to be treated temporarily with total parenteral nutrition, but some enteral nutrition should be initiated early to maintain gut health (Lord, 1995) and improve the intestinal remnant's absorptive capacity (Levy, Frileux, Sandrucci, et al., 1988). In patients with watery diarrhea associated with ZE syndrome or vasoactive intestinal peptide tumors (VIPomas) where the tumor is not found, symptomatic treatment with octreotide may be used to treat the diarrhea. If retained stool is discovered on rectal exam or abdominal film, treatment usually entails fecal disimpaction and, if needed, enema administration until it clears (see the section on constipation). If a carcinoma, inflammatory bowel disease, ZE syndrome, or pancreatic/biliary disease is diagnosed, treatment revolves around the primary disease. Dietary manipulations and the use of pancreatic enzymes may be useful in pancreatic diseases. In documented lactose intolerance, lactase capsules or tablets may be tried with meals, lactase liquid may be added to milk, and lactose-free dairy products are available. Zinc deficiency may be treated with zinc supplements in the form of zinc sulfate capsules or zinc acetate.

If the onset of diarrhea correlates with the administration of enteral tube feedings, several issues should be explored before the feedings are stopped. The formula should be checked for contamination (examine formula for curdling, check to see that the formula is hanging at room temperature no longer than recommended manufacturer hang times, that clean technique is used for preparation, and that unused formula is being stored properly).

Look at the administration schedule and the location of nutrient delivery. If small bowel feedings are being administered, the initial infusion rate should be continuous. If needed, the rate can be slowly increased to 12 to 16 hours per day continuous infusion cycle, as tolerated. Gastric feedings can accommodate a variety of feeding schedules, although each feeding should infuse over at least 20 minutes to avoid nausea and vomiting. In critically ill patients, both gastric and small bowel feedings are generally started at a continuous rate and advanced to goal volume, as tolerated. Both isotonic and hypertonic formulas may begin at full strength, but it's prudent to begin at low rates (especially in the small bowel), advancing the rate every 8 to 12 hours until the goal volume is achieved. Formulas should be checked for lactose content in those patients who are lactose intolerant, although most formulas are lactose-free. If the tube feeding administration schedule is appropriate and formula contamination is ruled out, the feedings can be discontinued for 24 hours to see if the diarrhea ceases. If the diarrhea stops, the feeding formula may be the cause and reinitiating tube feedings at a low, continuous rate with a slower advancement schedule may be better tolerated.

If diarrhea persists and infectious etiologies have either been excluded or treated, antidiarrheal medications may be given. Infectious sources of diarrhea must be ruled out before administering antimotility agents, as keeping pathogenic organisms in the bowel can cause intestinal distention and prolong the disease process. Nonprescription medications are encouraged initially and include bulk-forming agents, adsorbents, antimotility agents, and antisecretory agents. Bulk-forming agents, such as pectin, provide bulk to the stool by absorbing water and making the stool more formed. Adsorbents, such as kaolin and activated attapulgite or charcoal, are thought to reduce diarrhea by absorbing the pathogenic bacteria, viruses, and toxins in the intestine. Loperimide (Imodium) is an over-the-counter antimotility agent that delays intestinal transit by acting on the intestinal smooth muscle to inhibit peristalsis. Bismuth preparations, such as Pepto-Bismol, are antisecretory agents that may be useful for viral or traveler's diarrhea (enterotoxigenic *E coli*). Narcotic prescription medications may be needed occasionally and include antimotility agents such as diphenoxylate HCl with atropine sulfate (Lomotil), codeine phosphate, and tincture of opium.

Follow-Up

In patients with persistent diarrhea or inflammatory bowel disease (IBD), a gastroenterologist should be consulted for further work-up with endoscopy or a barium study as appropriate. Steroid therapy is generally begun on patients with IBD. If the diarrhea resolves, be sure that the patient is having regular bowel movements to avoid constipation.

Constipation/Obstipation

Pathophysiology

Ingested foods generally reach the colon by 2 to 6 hours. Water is absorbed in the cecum and ascending colon. Most of the ingested material that is not absorbed takes several days for evacuation. Defecation occurs when the rectosigmoid junction relaxes and peristaltic intestinal waves propel the contents of the left colon and sigmoid into the rectum. Dilation of the internal sphincter creates the feeling of tenesmus. Constipation results when there is a persistent delay in discharge of fecal contents compared with usual bowel habits or incomplete evacuation. Many times, this results in straining and pain with defecation and passage of small, firm stools. Constipation can be due to the lack of fiber or water in the diet, metabolic/endocrine disorders (diabetes, hypothyroidism, uremia, hypercalcemia/hypokalemia), drugs (morphine, codeine, atropine, aluminum-containing antacids, calcium-containing supplements, calcium channel blockers, bile acid binders), smooth muscle disorders (scleroderma or amyloidosis), irritable bowel syndrome, neurogenic disorders (multiple sclerosis, Hirschsprung disease, spinal cord injuries/tumors, tabes dorsalis), volvulus, anal spasm (fissures, proctitis, hemorrhoids), intestinal tumors, or obstruction caused by masses/adhesions outside the intestine. Obstipation occurs when there is no evacuation of feces and no flatus, suggesting total intestinal obstruction.

History and Physical Findings

History taking should include fiber and fluid intake, nausea or vomiting, narcotic use, laxative use, intake of potassium-wasting medications (diuretics) or other causes for hypokalemia, ingestion of aluminum-containing antacids or calcium-containing supplements, previous surgeries (adhesions/stricture), and evidence for intestinal transit or neurogenic disorders. Normal bowel patterns need to be assessed along with when the deviations from normal occurred. The presence or absence of flatus should be noted. Stool size, color, and caliber as well as the presence of bright or dark blood, undigested food particles, or mucus should be recorded. Constipation or obstipation may be accompanied by back or hip pain, headache, and tachycardia. If not treated, anal ulcers, fissures, hemorrhoids, colonic diverticuli, sigmoid volvulus, or perforated viscus can develop. A rectal exam can reveal retained stool, anal spasm, rectal prolapse, hemorrhoids, or rectal masses.

Laboratory and Diagnostic Tests

Serum levels of potassium, calcium, and glucose should be obtained to check for abnormalities that would alter motility (hypokalemia, hypercalcemia, or hyperglycemia). A free T4 level and thyroid-stimulating hormone should be drawn if hypothyroidism is suspected. An abdominal film is useful to determine if there is an impaction or obstruction. A barium enema, sigmoidoscopy, or colonoscopy will diagnose some intestinal obstructions, tumors, volvulus, diverticular strictures, and proctitis. If no structural abnormality, disease process, or medication is identified as the cause for the constipation and it does not respond to fluid and fiber supplementation, a colonic transit study can be performed. This involves a radiographic film of the abdomen 5 days after the ingestion of radiopaque markers to determine delayed transit. If more than 20% of the markers are retained, the location of the markers can determine the location of decreased transit or obstruction. Slow progression of the radiopaque markers to the distal colon indicates dysfunction in colonic transit time. Anorectal dysfunction or outlet obstruction is identified when the markers are retained in the rectosigmoid region. Anal manometry is performed at times to check for any element of sensory dysfunction that may be genetic or have diminished with aging.

Management

Treatment of retained stool entails the administration of osmotic agents, laxatives, suppositories, or enemas until the stool is cleared. Manual fecal disimpaction can also be tried. Promotility agents are usually given to patients who have bowel motility disorders.

If fiber or fluid intake is insufficient, high-fiber foods or medicinal fiber supplements along with increased fluid intake are encouraged. The beneficial effects of fiber on elimination are most likely due to bowel distention from the undigested fiber and associated water along with increased bacterial mass. This produces larger, softer stools that are easier to eliminate. Fiber intake should be gradually increased, as colonic gas formation and subsequent gas pains can occur as the intestinal flora adapts. A goal of at least 30 gms of fiber per day is encouraged. Fiber is contraindicated in patients with intestinal pseudo-obstructions, smooth muscle disorders, or gastrointestinal stenosis or obstructions. In patients with spinal cord injuries, a bowel rehabilitation program generally includes the intake of at least 30 grams of fiber per day and a bisacodyl or glycerol suppository every other day along with digital stimulation.

In patients with laboratory values indicating potassium, calcium, thyroid, or glucose abnormalities, the underlying etiology needs to be investigated and treated.

Osmotic agents (magnesium salts, sodium phosphate, sorbitol, glycerol, or lactulose) pull water into the bowel lumen, increasing the water content of the stool which encourages movement of fecal material through the colon. Although these agents are generally safe, long-term use of magnesium salts can increase the serum magnesium to toxic levels and likewise sodium phosphate can increase serum sodium and phosphorus levels, especially in patients with renal insufficiency. Laxatives have a prokinetic effect, increase intestinal secretions, and decrease intestinal absorption. Stimulating laxatives (bisacodyl, cascara, senna, phenolphthalein) should only be used occasionally if needed and discouraged as a chronic measure to prevent constipation, as this can lead to dependency of the agent for defecation. In addition, laxative abuse can produce colonic nerve damage, fecal incontinence in the elderly, secondary steatorrhea, osteomalacia, and hyperaldosteronism. Mineral oil, an emollient, interferes with the absorption of fat-soluble vitamins and aspiration of this substance in high-risk patients can cause a lipoid pneumonia.

When patients have difficulty defecating, they should be told to breathe regularly to prevent the Valsalva's maneuver. Holding one's breath while straining creates a positive intrathoracic pressure, impeding venous return to the right atrium. It also causes increased vagal tone that can lead to bradycardia and syncope. The Crede maneuver, manual pressure and gentle rubbing on the abdomen, may be helpful to mobilize the retained stool.

Follow-Up

The patient should be followed until there is return of regular bowel movements without the excessive use of laxatives or enemas.

Nausea and Vomiting

Pathophysiology

Most body areas contain afferent pathways that lead to the medulla oblongata and can trigger vomiting. Sympathetic afferent pathways stemming from gastrointestinal distention can also induce vomiting. Vomiting begins when both the somatic and visceral efferent pathways cause diaphragmatic contraction, glottis and pyloric closure, and stomach relaxation. This is followed by peristaltic contractions from the stomach, and abdominal, diaphragmatic, and intercostal contractions. Any stomach contents are then discharged upward out the mouth. Common causes are gastroparesis, gastrointestinal distention and obstruction, drug and chemical effects, pathogenic bacteria and viruses, gastric neoplasms, hepatitis, pancreatitis, pregnancy, motion sickness, myocardial infarction, radiation treatments, uremia, acidosis, and mineral abnormalities (hypercalcemia, hyper- or hypomagnesemia). When oxygen delivery is decreased to the medulla oblongata—such as during shock, vascular occlusion, or increased intracranial pressure—vomiting can occur. In some cases the contents may be aspirated down the bronchial tree and cause aspiration pneumonia. Persistent, forceful vomiting can cause a Mallory–Weiss tear or Borhaave's syndrome (rupture of the distal esophagus).

History and Physical Findings

When vomiting occurs, history taking should include whether it is preceded by nausea, when the vomiting began, any precipitating or relieving factors, the frequency, and if it is sudden, projectile, or persistent. The color and volume of the vomitus is important to note. Clear or greenish vomitus that may have undigested food particles represents stomach contents, bright yellow vomitus represents bile or upper intestinal contents, and dark brown vomitus with a feculent odor is associated with lower intestinal contents or a prolonged bowel obstruction. Previous abdominal surgery raises the possibility of adhesive disease. All medications should be reviewed carefully for possibility of nausea and vomiting side effects.

Physical examination should include abdominal auscultation and a neurologic assessment. Listen for a succussion splash and high-pitched rushes or tinkles that can indicate a gastric outlet obstruction. Metabolic disturbances associated with diabetes, adrenal insufficiency, and uremia can cause nausea and vomiting. Pathogenic bacteria and viral causes of vomiting are assessed through history taking for the possibility of ingesting spoiled or contaminated foods or exposure to viral infections.

Laboratory and Diagnostic Tests

Persistent vomiting can cause dehydration, a hypochloremic alkalosis, and hyponatremia. As sodium and hydrogen ions are depleted, the kidneys excrete potassium in exchange for sodium, leading to hypokalemia.

If vomiting occurs immediately postprandially, causes include a pyloric or high intestinal obstruction or gastroparesis which can be diagnosed by a barium swallow, gastritis or gastric neoplasms that can be seen during a gastroscopy, or uremia. Projectile vomitus without preceding nausea can be caused by pyloric stenosis or stimulation to the medulla oblongata trigger zone from drugs/chemicals, radiation, or uremia. If a drug/chemical is suspected as initiating the vomitus, blood levels can be obtained or the drug/chemical can be stopped to see if the vomiting ceases. Elevated amylase and lipase concentrations are consistent with pancreatitis due to alcohol or gallstones. A pregnancy test should be considered in women of child-bearing age. A CT scan of the head should be done if the neurologic exam is suggestive of increased intracranial pressure. Lower intestinal obstructions or gastrocolic fistulas can cause feculent vomitus that can be diagnosed by a barium swallow or contrast enema.

Management

Initially, the patient should be rehydrated, realizing that there may be potassium and chloride deficits. In persistent vomiting, intravenous fluids containing sodium chloride and potassium chloride should be administered to treat dehydration and correct electrolyte abnormalities. Severe dehydration is manifested by tachycardia, hypotension, decreased urine output, and cold extremities. Intravenous fluids should be administered until there is a return of urine output of at least 0.5-1 mL/kg/hour. A large-bore nasogastric tube allows decompression and drainage of the stomach and is therapeutic in partial bowel obstruction.

The underlying cause, if known, should be treated in order to stop the vomiting. Any altered serum magnesium or calcium levels should be treated appropriately. An H2 blocker (cimetidine, famotidine, nizatidine, ranitidine) or proton pump inhibitor (lansoprozole, omeprazole) may be given for gastritis or pyloric spasm.

An antiemetic drug can be tried if an intestinal obstruction is ruled out. Chlorpromazine, perphenazine, and prochlorperazine are phenothiazines that block dopamine receptors in the chemoreceptor trigger zone of the brain. They also have a sedative effect and patients may exhibit extrapyramidal symptoms with higher dosages. Antihistamines, such as diphenhydramine, hydroxyzine, and promethazine, have antimuscarinic, sedative, and H1 blocking effects that make them effective antiemetics. These are appropriate for vertigo and motion sickness. Dronabinol, which contains the active ingredient cannabis, is a central sympathomimetic that binds to cannabinoid receptors in the central nervous system. It also has an appetite-stimulating effect. Dronabinol may be used with highly emetogenic cancer drugs or for treatment in AIDS patients with nausea, anorexia, and weight loss. Ondansetron HCl and granisetron are selective 5HT3 receptor antagonists that can be used for prevention of nausea and vomiting associated with chemotherapy and postoperatively (ondansetron HCl). The administration of a prokinetic agent, such as metoclopramide or cisapride, and small, frequent meals may be tried in patients with disturbances in gastric motility.

Follow-Up

A surgical consultation should be obtained for bowel obstructions and a gastroenterology consult for any chronic problems with gastrointestinal motility.

▶ PROBLEMS OF THE UPPER GASTROINTESTINAL TRACT

Gastroesophageal Reflux Disease

Pathophysiology

Gastroesophageal reflux disease (GERD) is defined as reflux of gastric or duodenal contents into the esophagus. The idea that esophagitis is related to reflux emerged in 1935. During the following two decades, gastroesophageal reflux was believed to be related primarily to anatomic factors, namely the presence of a hiatal hernia. This has been refuted in more recent studies.

The cause of reflux disease is multifactorial. Transient relaxations of the lower esophageal spinchter, decreased peristalsis, or delayed gastric emptying are factors thought to be contributory. The lower esophageal sphincter (LES) controls the pressure barrier between the stomach and esophagus. This sphincter is an area of smooth muscle regulated by neural, pharmocologic, and hormonal mechanisms. High basal resting LES tone is conferred by its intraabdominal position, vagus nerve input, and alphaadrenergic stimulation. Metoclopramide, pentobarbital, histamines, and antacids also increase LES tone. The hormone gastrin increases resting tone while estrogens, progesterone, glucagon, secretin, and cholecystokinin all decrease resting tone. Medications that decrease resting tone include anticholinergics, theophylline, meperidine, and calcium channel blockers. Eating fatty foods, smoking, and use of alcohol also decrease LES tone. During pregnancy, reflux is often worsened due to circulating estrogens and progesterones that decrease LES tone, not necessarily associated with increased intraabdominal pressure.

Normal LES pressure ranges from 12 to 30 mm Hg. There is wide variation in interpretation of pressures, but generally pressures less than 6 mm Hg are compatible with reflux and pressures greater than 20 mm Hg are sufficient enough to prevent reflux. Other factors that contribute to reflux include delayed gastric emptying and impaired esophageal clearance. Previous abdominal surgery at or near the gastroesophageal junction, such as vagotomy for peptic ulcer disease, may predispose the patient to reflux disease. A diagnosis of Raynaud's disease may be related to a diagnosis of scleroderma. Patients with scleroderma may have dysmotility syndromes in which reflux esophagitis can occur. Diabetic patients may have gastroparesis that could predispose them to reflux and heartburn. In patients who experience dysphagia and/or weight loss, esophagitis and/or stricture possibly due to malignancy must be ruled out.

History and Physical Findings

GERD is characterized by heartburn or esophageal mucosal damage. The symptoms of heartburn are often described as intermittent retrosternal burning sensations often exacerbated after a large meal, or recumbency, or occasionally by bending over.

A careful history is critical to the work-up of GERD. The patient should be asked detailed questions regarding factors that stimulate reflux. Information regarding food intake, medications, previous abdominal surgery, and presence of Raynaud's disease, scleroderma, diabetes, and peptic ulcer disease (PUD) should also be elicited. In addition, the patient should be questioned about any recent weight loss or dysphagia.

On physical examination, blood pressure and heart rate and rhythm should be evaluated to exclude cardiac disease. Palpation of the abdomen should be performed to exclude epigastric mass. Finally, a rectal examination should be performed and the stool should be tested for occult blood.

Laboratory and Diagnostic Tests

Barium swallow is widely used for reflux but has a sensitivity as low as 25%. Endoscopy is superior to a barium swallow because it allows direct visualization of the mucosa and biopsies, if necessary. The majority of patients with GERD, however, do not need endoscopy initially. If a patient has dysphagia, unexplained recent significant weight loss, occult bleeding, or an epigastric mass, Barrett's esophagitis should be excluded immediately by an upper endoscopy.

Management

For many patients, lifestyle modifications should be made and include: decreased intake of fatty foods; weight reduction; avoidance of bowel straining; elevation of the head of the bed with 6-inch blocks; and avoidance of cigarettes, alcohol, coffee, and large meals. Medications that lower sphincter tone should be minimized, and over-the-counter antacids can be used. If these measures do not completely resolve the reflux, a short trial (approximately 6 weeks) of H2 blockers may be used. If, after several weeks, there is still no improvement in symptoms, an upper endoscopy is warranted. After endoscopy documenting erosive esophagitis despite lifesyle modifications and H2 blockers, some patients may be given a trial of omeprazole or be referred for surgical intervention. Patients with symptoms despite treatment with omeprazole, such as diabetics and patients with scleroderma, may benefit from a prokinetic agent. The first-line choice is the drug metroproclopramide, which raises LES and promotes gastric emptying.

Surgical intervention is usually reserved for patients with obvious stricture, tumor, or bleeding, and patients who are refractory to medical management. Also evidence of marked esophagitis and dysplasia with Barrett's esophagitis constitute indications for a surgical procedure. Surgical treatment involves gastric wrapping to improve LES function, repair of hiatal hernia, or resection.

Follow-Up

Patients on H2 blockers should be monitored every 4 to 6 months after the initial trial period. If symptoms are stable, this interval may be increased. Endoscopy should be considered for a baseline evaluation of esophageal and gastric mucosa after one year of therapy or sooner if symptoms warrant. Successful management of this disease relies heavily on patient education and cooperation. Giving patients a thorough explanation of factors that either contribute to or prevent reflux will help provide long-term control.

Hiatal Hernia

Approximately 80% of all patients with significant GERD have a sliding hiatal hernia. A sliding hiatal hernia consists of displacement of the cardioesophageal junction upward into the posterior mediastinium, exposing the LES to a negative intrathoracic pressure. In a paraesophageal hernia all or part of the stomach is herniated into the thoracic cavity, while the gastroesophageal junction remains below the diaphragm. As a result, esophageal reflux is not common. Rarely, these hernias may occur in conjunction with a sliding hiatal hernia. Less than 10% of hiatal hernias are classified as paraesophageal.

As in the work-up of GERD, a careful history from the patient is indicated. Patients with reflux may report regurgitation into the throat and mouth, called "water brash," especially while lying down. Nausea and vomiting due to a hernia is relatively uncommon in adults. Chronic aspiration resulting from reflux may be the cause of pulmonary symptoms such as wheezing and dyspnea in both adults and children. Of note, infants who present with vomiting and failure to thrive should be evaluated for the presence of a hiatal hernia. Recent studies have indicated that having a certain amount (2-3 cm) of intraabdominal esophagus is necessary for optimal esophageal function and LES tone and peristaltic clearing of acid is impaired in patients with a hiatal hernia (Altorki, 1989).

Diagnosis of a hiatal hernia is made by evidence of herniation on a barium swallow. Rarely are changes in the esophageal mucosa visible on x-ray. In patients with concurrent diseases such as angina, cholelithiasis, diverticulitis, and PUD, special testing such as motility studies and/or PH monitoring may be indicated to discern the cause of symptoms.

Esophageal motility studies document LES pressure and esophageal peristalsis. Lack of peristalsis may suggest scleroderma or achalasia. Prolonged PH monitoring is the most sensitive way to determine abnormal reflux. An esophageal probe measures PH continuously over a 24-hour period and stores it in a small recorder. A relationship between symptoms and reflux can be determined. Many of these studies have shown that most patients have reflux at night.

Approximately 50% of patients with sliding hiatal hernias do not need surgical intervention. Conservative management of reflux is usually successful (see the section on GERD). For medically compliant patients without improvement, anti-reflux surgery can be done either transabdominally or transthoracically. The most effective procedure is the Nissen fundoplication. This operation totally surrounds the distal esophagus with the adjacent gastric fundus so that the gastroesophageal spinchter passes through a short tunnel of stomach. Approximately 90% of patients have lasting relief after the operation.

Paraesophageal hernias may cause complications even without associated symptoms and should be repaired. A frequent complication includes hemorrhage due to venous congestion and erosion of the stomach mucosa. Obstruction at the GE junction due to torsion of the stomach can occur. In a paraesophageal hernia, unlike a sliding hernia, other organs such as the spleen and large intestines may also herniate into the thoracic cavity. Long-term results of surgical repair are excellent.

The usual postoperative follow-up of a patient after a Nissen fundoplication is a visit at 2 weeks. The patient is usually sent home with a soft diet. At the 2-week follow-up, if the diet has been tolerated it can be advanced to regular. The patient is seen again at 1 month and discharged if tolerating the diet without difficulty.

Peptic Ulcer Disease

Pathophysiology

Approximately 2% of the adult population in the United States is affected by PUD, and 5 to 10% of the population have the disease at some point in their lifetime. Men are affected three times more often than women. Duodenal ulcers are ten times more common in younger patients than gastric ulcers, but in older age groups their occurrence is equal. The incidence of PUD has declined to below half of what it was 20 years ago.

Peptic ulcers are caused when vulnerable epithelium (often at or near mucosal transition zones) are exposed to gastric acid and pepsin. When the term "peptic ulcer disease" was first used, the most important factor was thought to be the peptic activity in gastric juice. Since then, excessive acid production has been implicated as the causative agent. Excess acid production is the hallmark of duodenal ulcer disease. Pepsin secretion is also elevated in duodenal ulcer disease. Gastric acid production is usually normal in patients with gastric ulcers; however, it is axiomatic that if gastric secretions contain no acid, a benign peptic ulcer cannot be present. Appreciation of the role of acid secretion on the development of ulcers has led to emphasis on therapy with antacids and H2 blocking agents as the mainstay of medical management and to operations that reduce acid secretion as the major surgical approach (Way, 1991).

Impairment of mucosal defense mechanisms also plays an important role in the development of ulcers. Mucosal integrity is governed by mucus secretion, mucosal blood flow, bicarbonate production, and cellular repair mechanisms. Mucus and bicarbonate protect the mucosa from acid and pepsin by maintaining a neutral PH and aqueous environment at the surface of the gastric epithelium. Prostaglandins are linked to mucus production and secretion, bicarbonate secretion, and repair of the mucosal barrier.

Stress, smoking, medications, and heredity have been implicated in the development of ulcer disease. Studies have shown a higher incidence of chronic stress in ulcer patients than in controls and an increase in acid production in response to stress (Goroll, 1995). Epidemiologic studies have shown that smokers develop ulcers twice as frequently as nonsmokers (Goroll, 1995). The risk of developing an ulcer in a steroid-dependent patient is about double that of a patient not on steroids, but the incidence of PUD in patients on steroids is only 2% (Goroll, 1995). A relationship between aspirin and other nonsteroidal antiinflammatory agents (NSAIDs) and gastric ulcers exists. This is thought to be partly related to inhibition of prostaglandin synthesis by these medications. Heredity does play a role in PUD. Increased gastrin release and pepsin secretion related to meal stimulation have been found to be hereditary traits among ulcer patients and their families.

Duodenal Ulcers. Approximately 95% of duodenal ulcers commonly occur in the duodenal bulb, within 2 cm of the pylorus. Excess acid production in duodenal ulcer patients is often related to an increased number of parietal and chief cell masses and responses to food and hormonal stimulation. Other factors known to increase patient susceptibility to duodenal ulcers include: blood type O and the presence of helicobactor pylori infection, often documented by cultures taken at time of endoscopy or blood testing.

Gastric Ulcers. Gastric ulcers are commonly separated into three types. Type I ulcers are most common and often found in patients with no duodenal ulcer disease. These ulcers are often associated with the presence of *Helicobacter pylori* infection. Type II ulcers are located near the pylorus and often occur in association with duodenal ulcers. Type III ulcers occur in the antrum of the stomach and are often associated with chronic use of aspirin or nonsteroidal anti-inflammatory agents.

Stress Ulcers. Stress ulcers occur following a physiologically stressful illness. The four major causes associated with the development of these ulcers include sepsis, shock, burns, and central nervous system (CNS) tumors or trauma. Ulcers that occur in the setting of sepsis, shock, or burns are called Curlings ulcers. These are caused by decreased mucosal resistance likely due to ischemia, circulating toxins, and decreased gastric mucosal blood flow. Cushings ulcers associated with CNS tumors or trauma are caused by increased gastric acid secretion, and are more prone to perforation than Curlings ulcers. The discovery of a stress ulcer almost always stems from an episode of acute bleeding.

History and Physical Findings

Epigastric pain, usually described as aching, gnawing or burning, is often the presenting symptom of duodenal ulcers. The pain is usually relieved by food or antacids. If the pain is chronic, the diagnosis of a duodenal ulcer is often made after exclusion of other possible sources such as cholelithiasis, pancreatitis, or GERD. Patients should also have a stool guaiac recorded.

The principal symptom is epigastic pain relieved by food or antacids as in duodenal ulcers. Compared with duodenal ulcers, the pain in a gastric ulcer tends to appear earlier after eating, often within thirty minutes. Vomiting and anorexia are more common with a gastric ulcer. Overlap of symptoms between gastric and duodenal ulcers is common; therefore, accurate diagnosis must be made by x-ray or endoscopy.

Hemorrhage is usually the first manifestation of a stress ulcer. Pain rarely occurs prior to bleeding.

Laboratory and Diagnostic Tests

Test selection should be individualized for each patient. Patients with recurrent disease should have endoscopy versus x-ray to rule out *H pylori* infection or gastric cancer. To determine ulcer location and appropriate treatment, endoscopy is warranted, especially in patients over 40 years of age where there is a greater risk of gastric cancer.

Patients with severe duodenal ulcer disease refractory to medical management, those with recurrent ulcer especially after surgical treatment, and patients with hyperparathyroidism or other endocrine tumors should have a fasting serum gastrin level to determine the presence or absence of a gastrinoma (Zollinger–Ellison [ZE] syndrome). ZE syndrome is an uncommon cause of PUD.

Management

Medical treatment of PUD includes avoidance of aspirin, nonsteroidals, regular nutritious meals, prescription of an H2 blocker, and treatment of *H pylori*. For duodenal ulcers, continue full-dose therapy for 4 weeks; if symptoms are resolved, switch to maintenance therapy (half dose) for another 4 to 8 weeks to avoid relapse. If symptoms persist, continue therapy.

With gastric ulcers, continue full treatment for 6 to 8 weeks or until symptoms resolve, whichever is longer; then switch to maintenance for another 4 to 8 weeks. For patients refractory to initial therapy after 4 weeks, switch to omeprazole. The safety of long-term use of this drug is unknown, so therapy should be no longer than 8 to 12 weeks (Goroll, May & Mulley, 1995). Carafate may also be used to stimulate mucous production and decrease peptic activity in gastric juice. Endoscopy should be repeated to evaluate symptoms refractory to medical management after 6 to 8 weeks.

Treatment of *H pylori* consists of either double- or triple-agent therapy. The first reported therapy to cure *H pylori* infection consisted of a 14-day course of tetracycline, bismuth, and metronidazole. This regimen was found to have an eradication rate between 77% and 82%. In a recent review of the world literature, bismuth triple therapy achieved an 89.2% eradication rate in more than 2000 patients. Dual therapy is an attractive treatment option because of its simplicity and improved compliance. The combination of clarithromycin and either a proton pump inhibitor or ranitidine bismuth citrate have yielded eradication rates in the range of 64 to 84%. Two dual therapies have been approved by the FDA: (1) omeprazole (40 mg qd) and clarithromycin (500 mg tid) and (2) ranitidine bismuth citrate (400 mg bid) and clarithromycin (500 mg tid). Dual therapy is generally better tolerated than triple therapy, although, dual therapy is destined to be replaced by a proton pump inhibitor-based triple therapy in the future. This regimen consists of proton pump inhibitor and two antibiotics. This therapy has consistently achieved eradication rates exceeding 85%. The optimal duration of this therapy has yet to be determined.

Acute bleeding should be managed appropriately (see the section on UGI bleeding) and endoscopy performed early (within 24 hours) in most cases. Approximately 75% of patients are successfully managed by medical care alone. Rebleeding while hospitalized is associated with a mortality rate of around 30%. Many instances of rebleeding occur within 2 days of the original bleed. Early surgical intervention is indicated for rebleeding. Approximately 10% of patients with a bleeding ulcer require emergency surgery. The usual surgical procedure is pyloroplasty and vagotomy.

Selection criteria for surgical versus medical therapy depends upon baseline medical condition and the rate of bleeding. Bleeding recurs within 5 years for a third of all peptic ulcer patients. Elective surgery should be recommended for patients who had chronic symptoms preceding the bleed or those with large duodenal ulcers. When bleeding is minor, the first manifestation of disease and/or caused by medications such as aspirin, medical treatment is usually successful therapy. Surgical treatment usually entails an antrectomy (removal of the distal half of the stomach) and vagotomy (resection of a 1-2 cm segment of each vagal trunk). This often results in delayed gastric emptying.

Treatment of stress ulcers consists of management of bleeding (see the section on UGI bleeding) and endoscopy. All patients with sepsis, shock, or burns should be placed on prophylactic H2 blockers upon admission. Ulcers that occur in patients on H2 blockers usually need surgical treatment. The utilization of gastric artery infusions of vasopressin to control bleeding and avoid surgery in the critically ill patient has also been shown to be effective.

Complications

Duodenal and Gastric Ulcers. Possible complications from a duodenal or gastric ulcer include obstruction, perforation, or bleeding. Obstructing ulcers usually cause persistent symptoms of pain combined with recent emesis. Weight loss may also be present. Initial treatment for an obstructing duodenal ulcer includes hospitalization, NPO, IV fluids, H2 blockers, and NG tube decompression of the stomach. Endoscopy should be done to rule out an obstructing neoplasm. After 48 to 72 hours if the patient is clinically improved, liquids may be started and advanced to solid food. If the patient is not better or can only tolerate liquids, surgical intervention is indicated. Two-thirds of patients with acute obstruction fail to improve with medical therapy and require an operation. Many patients eventually require an operation even if they recover with medical therapy initially.

Duodenal ulcers can perforate anteriorly or posteriorly. Ulcers that perforate posteriorly often present with bleeding because they erode into a branch of the gastroduodenal artery. Anterior perforations usually do not present with bleeding since there are no major blood vessels that lie on the anterior surface of the duodenum. They are generally diagnosed by the demonstration of free air in the peritoneal cavity on x-ray. Perforated ulcers are managed surgically. Definite surgical repair should not be done if there is overwhelming sepsis and/or other coexisting serious medical problems until these are better controlled.

Patients who present with combined perforation and bleeding usually have two ulcers known as "kissing ulcer." Ulcers presenting in the second portion of the duodenum (postbulbar ulcers) bleed frequently, although ulcers in this area are less common. Endoscopic therapy to control bleeding ulcers has been shown to be effective. The indications for this treatment include active bleeding at the time of endoscopy and presence of a visible vessel. Methods used include cautery of the vessel with a heater probe or injection into the ulcer of epinephrine or a sclerosing agent. If initial treatment fails, repeat treatment may succeed. Patient status should be closely monitored and surgical intervention is necessary with repeat endoscopic failure.

Bleeding from a duodenal ulcer can be sudden and massive with hematemesis and shock or chronic and occult with progressive weakness due to anemia. Peptic ulcers are the most common cause of massive GI bleeding. Treatment consists of management of bleeding (see the section on UGI bleeding) and endoscopy.

Follow-Up

Follow-up in nonoperative patients should include rescope and rebiopsy at 6 weeks. For operative patients the follow-up should be at approximately 2 weeks and then monthly for those patients who need B_{12} shots depending upon how much stomach was resected. If the patient has had two thirds or greater of the stomach removed, monthly B_{12} shots will be needed for life to prevent the development of pernicious anemia.

Gastric Cancer

Gastric cancer occurs rarely under the age of 40 and men are two times more likely than women to develop it. Current incidence in the U.S. is 10 new cases per 100,000 of population per year. Gastric cancers are almost always adenocarcinomas. Squamous-cell tumors of the proximal stomach are extensions from esophageal tumors. Extension of gastric tumors occurs by intramural spread, extraluminal growth, and lymphatic metastases. The majority of patients have metastases when first diagnosed.

Patients with gastric cancer often report symptoms of vague abdominal fullness that may have been present for some time, but have recently worsened. Anorexia and weight loss are common; vomiting and dysphagia may also be present. Physical exam should include a rectal exam with guaiac to detect occult bleeding and abdominal exam to document palpable abdominal masses. Evidence of distant metastases may be demonstrated by the presence of Virchow's node, which is an enlarged supraclavicular lymph node, on the left side (Fig. 41–1).

Endoscopy and biopsy are essential for patients suspected of a gastric cancer. Abdominal CT scan is also

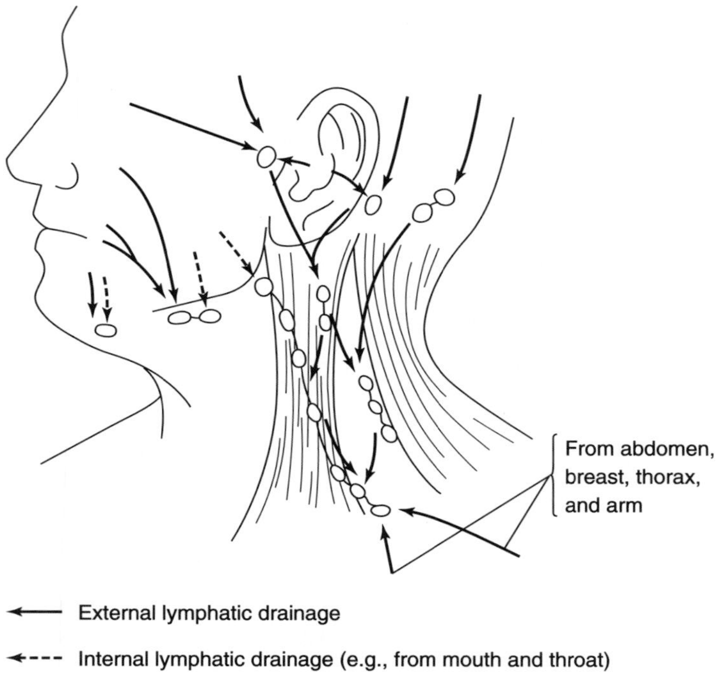

Figure 41–1. Virchow's node.

needed to evaluate for the presence of metastatic disease and resectability of the tumor.

Surgical resection is the only curative treatment for gastric cancer. Resection of tumors in the proximal stomach often includes splenectomy because splenic lymph nodes are often a primary site of metastases. Patients undergoing total or subtotal gastrectomy need monthly vitamin B_{12} replacement for life to prevent pernicious anemia. There is no proven regimen of adjunct therapy for treatment of gastric cancer. In advanced cases, clinical trials may be entered for treatment with experimental agents. The overall 5-year survival of gastric cancer is approximately 12%.

Patients should be followed at monthly intervals when they receive B_{12} shots and/or more frequently for management of diet and/or pain control if not managed by a medical oncologist.

Duodenal Tumors

Primary duodenal tumors occur rarely. Malignant duodenal tumors most often are lymphomas, leiomyosarcomas, and/or adenocarcinomas. They occur most frequently in the second portion of the duodenum. Presentation often includes pain, obstruction, bleeding, obstructive jaundice, and presence of an abdominal mass. Tumors are usually diagnosed by endoscopy and are often missed on barium x-ray studies.

Management of these tumors is resection. Pancreaticoduodenectomy, or Whipple procedure, is often necessary due to the proximity of the duodenum to the pancreas. Unresectable lesions are treated with radiation and chemotherapy. The 5-year survival rate after resection is approximately 30%. The overall 5-year survival rate is lower, at about 18%.

Gastrointestinal Bleeding

Pathophysiology

Gastrointestinal bleeding may result from diseases along the entire gastrointestinal tract. Upper gastrointestinal (UGI) bleeding is one of the most common indications for hospital admission. UGI bleeding sources include the esophagus, stomach, and duodenum. Lower GI bleeding originates distally including the terminal ileum, colon, and rectum. The major factors that determine therapy and diagnosis are the rate and volume of bleeding. Approximately 75% of patients will stop bleeding spontaneously.

Hematemesis is the vomiting of blood; usually this represents UGI bleeding proximal to the ligament of Treitz. The presence of blood clots reflects massive bleeding, while "coffee-ground" vomitus indicates a slower rate of bleeding with retention of hematin. Melena (black, tarry stools) usually reflects a UGI source. Hematochezia (passage of clots or blood per rectum) reflects a LGI source. Red or black stools can also be associated with the ingestion of food dye substances or iron. Only 50 mL of blood is necessary to produce melena. After 1000 mL of blood, melena persists for 5 days. A guaiac-positive stool may persist for 3 weeks following hematemesis or melena.

UGI bleeding is a frequent cause of hospital admission

and inpatient morbidity and mortality. The incidences and causes of UGI bleeding in a given area vary according to the incidence of peptic ulcer disease, alcoholism, use of NSAIDs, and the elderly. Lesions that present with UGI bleeding include peptic ulceration and acute mucosal lesions, such as gastritis, erosions, esophagogastirc varices, reflux esophagitis, Mallory–Weiss tears, and gastric neoplasms.

Peptic ulceration is a common cause of UGI bleeding. A history of recurrent dyspepsia, usually nocturnal and relieved with antacids or meals, is suggestive. Hemorrhage from a duodenal ulcer is four times more common than gastric ulcer bleeding. Bleeding is the presenting problem in 15% of patients and 10 to 15% of all duodenal ulcer patients will have an episode of brisk hemorrhage.

Acute mucosal lesions make up one third of all UGI bleeding sources. Stress ulceration and bleeding are probably caused by decreased gastric blood flow that is secondary to splanchnic vasoconstriction. UGI bleeding has been described in one third of patients with septicemia. Eight key risk factors for stress bleeding have been documented: multiple systems trauma, hypotension, respiratory failure, renal failure, sepsis, jaundice, recent surgery, and burns.

Esophagogastric varices are a common cause of bleeding in patients with cirrhosis, accounting for 50 to 75% of their UGI bleeding. Hiatal hernias are a cause of occult chronic blood loss. Mallory–Weiss tears of the esophagogastric mucosa are replaced in 5 to 10% of UGI bleeding sources usually with vomiting or retching. Other less common sources of UGI bleeding include gastric neoplasms (including leiomyoma, leiomyosarcoma, adenocarcinona, lymphoma, and leukemia), gastroduodenal polyps, angiomas, aortoenteric fistula, duodenal diverticula with prolapsed mucosa, vascular ectasia, and hematobilia.

Lesions below the ligament of Treitz that bleed are considered LGI sources. The majority of the lesions arise from the colon and include diverticula, angiodysplastic lesions, cancers, inflammatory bowel disease (IBD), and hemorrhoids. Many diseases may cause lower gastrointestinal (GI) bleeding. Causes of lower GI bleeding include diverticulosis, AV malformations, and colon cancer. Inflammatory bowel disease can cause bleeding especially in younger patients. In older patients, bowel ischemia may be the cause, especially if there are risk factors for emboli such as atrial fibrillation.

The small intestine is a rare source of bleeding. The small intestine sources are usually neoplastic, inflammatory, or diverticular. The most common causes of jejunal and ileal bleeding are Meckel's diverticulum (a true congenital diverticulum usually located within two feet of the ileocecal valve). Other causes are intussusception and regional enteritis. Bleeding lesions in the small intestine are very rare and include hereditary hemorrhagic telangiectasia (Rendu–Osler–Weber syndrome).

Colonic bleeding is commonly caused by carcinoma, diverticula, vascular ectasia, colitis, and polyps. Polyps are usually located in a position that causes rectal and anal bleeding usually seen as unaltered blood on the stool surface, hemorrhoids, fissures, and proctitis. The familial disorder of Peutz–Jeghers syndrome, a diffuse gastrointestinal polyposis and mucocutaneous pigmentation, is another rare cause of bleeding.

Polyps, cecal ulceration, sarcomas, lymphomas, leukemia, hematologic disorders, cystomegalovirus infection, and ischemic syndromes are all rare causes of colonic bleeding. Anorectal sources include hemorrhoids, fistulas, fissures, and proctitis. The presence of these lesions does not rule out a proximal source for the blood loss, and a careful evaluation of the LGI tract is essential.

History and Physical Findings

In obtaining the patient's history, an accurate description of the bleeding episode and nature of the stool should be obtained. Melena (black, tarry stools) is a result of upper GI bleeding. Conversion of red blood to darker black stool is related to the time it has been in the intestine. The black color and characteristic odor of melenotic stool results from bacterial digestion during passage through the intestines. Hemotochezia is the passage of clots or bright red blood per rectum (BRBPR) and is usually the result of bleeding from the colon, rectum, or anus. BRBPR from an upper GI source quickly leads to shock. Melena without hematemesis generally means the cause is beyond the pylorus, as does hematochezia (unaltered blood). Occult blood can be caused by as little as 10 cc of blood. This is usually detected by a stool guaiac test.

GI bleeding can also present with hematemesis, which is bloody vomitus, and is usually indicative of an upper GI source. Bright red blood suggests current, active bleeding while "coffee ground" emesis results when the blood has been in the stomach for a period of time and exposed to gastric acid. GI bleeding without hematemesis generally means the cause is beyond the pylorus, as does hematochezia (unaltered blood).

The amount of bleeding also needs to be assessed. Bleeding associated with carcinoma is not usually massive. Melena is usually seen with right colon cancer, but may be too subtle to detect. Diverticula and arterial venous malformations (AVM) are the most common causes of massive rectal bleeding. Bleeding from diverticulitis is usually mild to moderate. Ulcerative colitis may be accompanied by mild to moderate bleeding or massive hemorrhage.

Family history requires inquiry regarding a history of familial polyposis; drug ingestion also should be investigated. Patient history regarding previous episodes of bleeding and the cause, medications (especially nonsteroidal use), presence of ulcer disease, alcohol use, and previous abdominal or vascular surgery should be documented.

An abdominal exam to rule out abdominal mass and possible tumor is important. The skin and mucosal surfaces require examination for hemorrhagic telangiectasias, the lesions of Rendu–Osler–Weber syndrome or Peutz–Jeghers syndrome. Abdominal exam reveals a mass, tumor, or intussusception and accompanied by a quiet right lower quadrant. Rectal exam may be diagnostic for tumors, polyps, and anal lesions and to rule out palpable mass or hemorrhoid. Occult blood loss can be caused by as little as 10 cc of blood and is usually detected by a stool guaiac test.

Laboratory and Diagnostic Tests

All patients should have a large-bore NG tube inserted to determine if bleeding is from the upper or lower GI tract. If the NG aspirate is bilious, the bleeding is most likely a lower GI source. Return of blood or "coffee ground" drainage is compatible with an upper GI source. Upper and/or lower endoscopy should be performed within 24 hours to determine the source of bleeding. An upper GI series with small bowel follow-through should be done if endoscopy is nondiagnostic. In patients with known varices, endoscopy is mandatory because a significant amount may be bleeding from a nonvariceal source. If the patient is not actively bleeding, colonoscopy may be helpful.

Use of angiography for selected patients may be useful if the other studies are nondiagnostic. Patients with bright red blood per rectum should also have bedside anoscopy to rule out an anal source of bleeding. Angiography or a 99mTC-labeled erythrocyte imaging is helpful in localizing active bleeding. Barium enema with air contrast is a reliable accurate method of diagnosing colonic lesions but should not be performed before angiography.

If no source of bleeding can be determined with colonoscopy, a small bowel lesion may be the source. This is uncommon and often requires intraoperative endoscopy to pinpoint the lesion.

Management

Initial care of the patient presenting with GI bleeding includes evaluation of circulatory status, establishment of an adequate airway ensuring oxygenation and ventilation, and volume replacement, if necessary. These measures should be undertaken prior to any diagnostic testing. In an uncomplicated bleeding patient, replacement of circulatory volume should be done with an isotonic fluid (lactated ringers) and/or blood transfusion, as needed. Inotropic (increased cardiac activity) and/or vasoconstrictive agents are contraindicated and detrimental because they cause peripheral vasoconstriction with resultant cellular hypoxia. To accomplish rapid adequate volume replacement, insertion of at least two large-bore IV catheters is necessary. The most important initial assessment of volume status is urine output, which should be measured every 1 hour via a Foley catheter.

Endoscopic therapy such as cauterization and/or injection of bleeding ulcers or varices may be helpful in the control of bleeding. Serial hematocrtits (every 4-6 hours) and frequent monitoring of blood pressure, pulse, urine output, and volume of NG drainage and/or bloody stools should be done. During an ongoing diagnostic work-up, the decision for surgical intervention depends on the rate and duration of bleeding rather than the specific cause. The patient's clinical status must be considered. Patients who present with hypotension and the need for 4 units or more of blood to achieve and maintain circulatory stability usually require early surgical intervention. Patients who are age 60 or older have less tolerance of ongoing blood loss before cardiac, pulmonary, or renal complications occur.

Approximately 85% of patients stop bleeding within several hours of admission to the hospital (Way, 1991). Rebleeding that occurs within 2 days often requires surgical intervention. Rebleeding is most common in patients with varices, ulcers, anemia, or shock. Esophagitis and/or gastritis can cause large amounts of bleeding. These conditions usually respond to supportive treatment and medical management with H2 blockers.

Patients with portal venous hypertension from alcoholic cirrhosis develop esophageal varices. Endoscopic injection and sclerosis of varices or banding may be used in the management of these patients. A TIPS procedure (transjugular intrahepatic portasystemic shunt) to reduce portal hypertension and therefore decrease blood flow through the varices can be used in patients with esophageal varicies. This procedure allows for stabilization of the patient who is a candidate for liver transplantation, the only definitive cure of cirrhosis. The underlying cause of liver failure must be corrected also. Isolated gastric varices are usually the result of splenic vein thrombosis resulting in sinistral or left-sided portal hypertenson. Splenectomy is indicated for resolution.

A Mallory–Weiss tear, which is a partial thickness tear of the distal esophageal mucosa that usually heals without surgical intervention, is an uncommon cause of UGI bleeding. AV malformations of the stomach can occur and need surgical repair. Patients who have had previous aortic surgery are at risk for an aortoduodenal fistula caused by erosion of the proximal suture line into the duodenum. This cause of bleeding is difficult to diagnose and carries a high mortality.

▶ PROBLEMS OF THE PANCREAS

The pancreas is located in the retroperitoneum of the upper abdomen. It is usually divided into three anatomic areas: the head, body, and tail. The pancreas has exocrine and endocrine functions. Exocrine function is secretion of 1 to 2 liters per day of a solution containing digestive enzymes. Pancreatic enzymes are synthesized, stored, and released by the acinar cells of the gland. Amylase and lipase are stored and secreted in active forms. The endocrine function of the pancreas includes release of insulin after a meal and release of glucagon during periods of fasting. Insulin is formed in the beta cells and glucagon is formed in the alpha cells of the pancreas.

Pancreatitis

Pathophysiology

Pancreatitis is an inflammatory disease caused by activation, secretion, and autodigestion of the pancreas by its own enzymes. Pancreatitis is usually classified as acute or chronic. In acute pancreatitis there is sudden upper abdomenal pain, nausea and vomiting, and increased serum amylase. Chronic pancreatitis is defined by chronic pain and exocrine or endocrine insufficiency. Many patients being treated for chronic pancreatitis become addicted to narcotics. Pancreatic cancer occurs more frequently in the setting of chronic pancreatitis. Patients with chronic pancreatitis can have attacks of acute pancreatitis. The most common causes of pancreatitis include gallstone disease or alcoholism. Other causes include trauma, hypercalcemia, and hyperlipidemia.

Approximately 40% of acute pancreatitis episodes are caused by gallstones. The etiology is most likely transient obstruction of the ampulla of Vater and pancreatic duct by a gallstone.

Alcoholic pancreatitis accounts for 40% of the cases of pancreatitis in the U.S (Way, 1991). Usually alcohol abuse has been present for 6 years or more prior to the initial attack. Often signs of chronic pancreatitis can be detected microscopically even with the first attack. Direct and indirect effects of alcohol are responsible for pancreatitis. In research studies, alcohol has been shown to produce ultra structural changes in acinar cells. Administration of alcohol also stimulates pancreatic secretion and induces spasm of the sphincter of Oddi. This results in partial ductal obstruction coupled with increased secretion. Even with avoidance of further alcohol, parenchymal damage continues to occur due to ductal obstruction and fibrosis.

Hypercalcemia is also associated with acute pancreatitis. Increased calcium is thought to facilitate development of calculi in the ducts resulting in obstruction. Occasionally hyperlipidemia appears transiently in some patients during an attack of acute pancreatitis. In other patients with primary hyperlipidemia, especially those with elevated LDLs, pancreatitis may be a direct consequence of this disease. Diet control may reduce the occurrence of future attacks of pancreatitis. Direct trauma, either from surgical injury or external abdominal impact, can also cause chronic pancreatitis. Idiopathic acute and chronic pancreatitis accounts for approximately 15% of cases. Drug-induced acute pancreatitis may be more common than suspected. Common drugs involved include oral contraceptives, diuretics, and tetracyclines.

Pancreatitis can be edematous or hemorrhagic. Edematous pancreatitis is inflammation of the glandular tissue and surrounding retroperitoneal structures surrounding a small focus of parenchymal necrosis. Hemorrhagic pancreatitis is associated with more complications and a higher mortality rate.

History and Physical Findings

The diagnosis of acute pancreatitis is often made on the basis of clinical exam. Patients usually present with nausea and vomiting and an acute occurrence of epigastric pain often radiating to the back. Severe cases of pancreatitis may present with symptoms of shock. Patients may present with jaundice related to biliary obstruction from inflammation. Chronic pancreatitis may cause abdominal pain, diabetes mellitus, malabsorption, or be asymptomatic. Physical findings usually include epigastric abdominal tenderness with decreased or absent bowel sounds, and—depending on the severity of the pancreatitis—dehydration, tachycardia, and/or hypotension may be present. Temperature may be elevated. Evidence on chest x-ray of pleural effusion especially on the left may be present. If an abdominal mass is palpable, it could represent a swollen pancreas (due to inflammation), pseudocyst, or abscess.

Laboratory and Diagnostic Tests

The patient's hematocrit may be elevated due to dehydration and the white blood cell count may be mildly elevated. WBC greater than 12,000/uL is unusual without abscess. Liver function studies should be normal but an elevation in the bilirubin may suggest gallstone pancreatitis. Serum amylase usually rises to more than 2.5 times normal levels (normal <60) within 6 hours of the onset of acute pancreatitis. Values greater than 1000 IU/dL are usually associated with gallstone pancreatitis. Lower values are more common in alcoholic pancreatitis. Abdominal x-ray is usually abnormal in about two thirds of cases. The most common finding is an isolated segment of small bowel that is dialated. Chest x-ray may reveal pleural effusion especiallly on the left. CT scan should be obtained on any patient who is not showing signs of clinical improvement at 48 hours. Findings may include phelgmon, pancreatic pseudocyst, necrosis, or abscess. Abdominal ultrasound may demonstrate gallstones and should be obtained if gallstone pancreatitis is suspected. In patients with jaundice and gallstones on ultrasound, both surgical and GI consults should be obtained for possible endoscopic retrograde cholangiopancreatography (ERCP) to evaluate the common bile duct and clear any stones prior to a laproscopic cholecystectomy. These techniques allow patients with gallstone pancreatitis and jaundice to be treated with minimal invasiveness and hospital stays.

Management

Treatment of acute pancreatitis includes NPO status, NG tube (if vomiting is present), and IV fluids. Hypoxemia may also be present and severe enough to require ventilation therapy. Parenteral nutrition should be started for any patient unable to eat for 1 week. Endoscopic retrieval of an impacted gallstone to resolve the pancreatitis followed by laparoscopic cholecystectomy is an accepted practice for treatment of gallstone pancreatitis. Patients frequently require surgical treatment consisting of debridement of necrotic tissue, gallbladder removal, and drainage of infection to attain clinical improvement.

Complications of acute pancreatitis include pseudocyst formation, abscess, and GI bleeding from adjacent inflamed stomach or duodenum. Bowel obstruction from involvement with inflammatory process may also occur. Pancreatic pseudocyst formation is a common complication of pancreatitis and usually occurs at 2 to 3 weeks. A pseudocyst is an encapsulated collection of fluid located within or adjacent to the pancreas. A pseudocyst has no epithelial lining. The etiology of a pseudocyst is ductal destruction by pancreatitis or trauma. Complications of a pseudocyst include rupture, gastric outlet obstruction, jaundice, or hemorrhage into the cyst. Treatment of a pseudocyst that is enlarging or has been present for greater than 6 weeks is necessary. Treatment is surgical and consists of an internal drainage procedure, as debris in pseudocyst drainage will not drain through a catheter. External drainage with percutaneous catheters may be appropriate for critically ill patients with large collections for temporization and/or shrinkage of very large pseudocysts. Pancreatic abscess formation follows secondary bacterial contamination of necrotic pancreatic debris. Surgical drainage is usually required as abscesses are often multiloculated and unable to be drained adequately percutaneously.

Medical treatment of chronic pancreatitis includes abstinence from alcohol, replacement of pancreatic enzymes if malabsorption and steatorrhea are present, and oral agents or insulin for diabetic control. The value of surgical treatment in patients with chronic pancreatitis is primarily to relieve intractable pain. Surgical treatment consists of a procedure to facilitate drainage of pancreatic secretions and removal of diseased pancreas. Treatment is usually successful in patients with familial pancreatitis, but less so in patients with alcoholic pancreatitis.

Ranson's criteria is often used for prognosis in patients with acute pancreatitis. The higher number of criteria present coincide with a higher mortality rate. Initial criteria include: age over 55; WBC greater than 16,000; blood glucose greater than 200; serum LDH greater than 350; and SGOT greater than 250. Criteria developing during the first 48 hours include a decrease in HCT by greater than 10%; BUN rise greater than 8 mg/dL; serum CA++ less than 8 mg/dL; arterial PO_2 less than 60 mm Hg; base deficit less than 4 meq/L; and estimated fluid sequestration greater than 600 mL. Presence of 0 to 2 criteria equal a 2% mortality rate; 3 to 4 criteria equal a 15% rate; 5 to 6 criteria equal a 40% rate; and 7 to 8 criteria equal a 100% mortality rate.

Pancreatic Cancer

Pancreatic cancer is the third leading cause of death from cancer in 35 to 55-year-old men. Approximately 25,000 new cases of pancreatic cancer are diagnosed each year, with the peak occurring in the 1950s and 1960s. The majority of patients have tumors in the head of the pancreas. About 80% of the tumors are ductal adenocarcinomas; the remainder are islet cell tumors and cystadenocarcinomas. Risk factors associated with the development of pancreatic cancer are cigarette smoking, increased consumption of dietary fat, previous gastrectomy, and race. In the United States pancreatic cancer is more prevalent in blacks than whites. Patients with pancreatic cancer often present with metastatic disease because symptoms occur late in the disease process and are usually vague.

Patients often present with weight loss, abdominal fullness or pain, and obstructive jaundice. Back pain is also present in some patients. Sudden onset of diabetes mellitus may also be a manifestation of pancreatic cancer.

Abdominal CT usually demonstrates a mass most often located in the head of the pancreas. Needle biopsy may be done under CT guidance to obtain celullar information.

Treatment of pancreatic cancer is surgical, if possible. Patients who are nonresectable often benefit from nonsurgical placement of biliary stents to relieve biliary obstruction and jaundice. Patients with peri-ampullary neoplasms, common bile duct tumors, or duodenal tumors often present with many of the same symptoms as pancreatic cancer. Treatment of these lesions is also resection.

Overall survival is poor for patients with pancreatic cancer. Survival rates are approximately 30% at 2 years and only 10% at 5 years (Way, 1991). Postoperative radiation for resectable patients is indicated to prevent local recurrence.

Other Pancreatic Problems

Cystic lesions of the pancreas can also present with many of the same symptoms as pancreatic cancer. Many mucinous cystadenomas evolve into cystadenocarcinomas over time; therefore, surgical removal is usually recommended. Complete excision of a cystadenocarcinoma has a better survival rate than pancreatic ductal cancer with a 70% 5-year survival.

Islet cell tumors of the pancreas are either nonfunctioning or functioning, malignant or nonmalignant. Most often these tumors are functioning and benign. Insulinomas are the most common functional tumors seen; approximately 75% are solitary and benign. Insulinomas arise from the beta cells and produce increased amounts of insulin and symptoms of hypoglycemia. Approximately 10% are malignant with metastatic disease present at the time of diagnosis. The other 15% are manifestations of multifocal pancreatic disease, such as islet cell hyperplasia, and are also benign. Surgical resection of these may be done by enucleation, if possible, or pancreatic resection. Intraoperative ultrasound is often used to detect nonpalpable tumors. Nonfunctional islet cell tumors are usually malignant. Metastatic disease is often present at the time of diagnosis. Treatment of these tumors is surgical resection, if possible.

▶ PROBLEMS OF THE LIVER

The liver is one of the largest organs in the body and represents approximately 2% of total body weight. Liver function includes formation of bile by hepatocytes, formation of glycogen and proteins, and filtration of the bloodstream. The liver also synthesizes fibrinogen and prothrombin essential for clotting. Two common diseases of the liver that often lead to further complications are cirrhosis and hepatitis.

Cirrhosis

Cirrhosis is an irreversible state of chronic liver disease. Currently, it is the third leading cause of death in men in their 50s. Cirrhosis can be caused by alcoholism, postnecrotic cirrhosis that develops insidiously over the years from subclinical chronic active hepatitis, or, more rarely, primary biliary cirrhosis. Approximately 15% of alcoholics develop cirrhosis (Way, 1991). Primary biliary cirrhosis is characterized by obstructive jaundice with hyperlipidemia and pruritis with no obstruction of large bile ducts. Ascites is present late in the course of the illness. The first liver function test to become abnormal is the prothrombin time (PT). The PT is prolonged due to the short serum half life of the factors that determine prothrombin time. The half life of these proteins can be as short as seven days (Goroll, May, & Mulley, 1995). Diagnosis is made by needle biopsy of the liver. The clinical course of a patient with cirrhosis depends upon the severity of the disease.

Cirrhosis often causes portal hypertension and encephalopathy. These conditions lead to varices, ascites, hypersplenism, and coma. Management of ascites includes dietary salt restrictions and diuretic therapy with spironalactone. Patients who have refractory ascites despite these measures may need therapeutic paracentesis. Removal of more than 2 liters of fluid at a time is not recommended due to the possibility of intravascular volume depletion. Paracentesis is a temporizing measure. Patients with incapacitating ascites may benefit from the placement of a peritovenous shunt. Results with these shunts are variable as they are associated with high rates of complications including infection and coagulopathies. TIPS can successfully control ascites.

Encephalopathy is due to intestinally derived toxic substances that escape hepatic detoxification due to hepatocellular dysfunction and portasystemic shunting. Elevation of blood ammonia levels often correlates with hepatic encephalopathy. Treatment, on an ambulatory basis, includes correction of fluid and electrolyte imbalances, discontinuation or restriction of any medications metabolized by the liver, and restriction of dietary protein intake to 30 to 40 grams per day. Specific therapy for encephalopathy is with lactulose, a synthetic, nonabsorbable disaccharide that is metabolized to organic acids by enteric bacteria, causing an osmotic catharsis. Lactulose also suppresses the growth of ammonia-forming bacteria in favor of lactose-fermenting organisms.

Coagulopathy related to cirrhosis results from reductions in vitamin K dependent clotting factors (II, VII, IX, and X) due to decreased heptic protein synthesis and increased plasma proteolytic activity. Malnutrition resulting in decreased absorption of vitamin K and hypersplenism resulting in thrombocytopenia may also be contributory. An increased prothrombin time may respond to vitamin K 10 mg IM for 3 days. However, in the absence of bleeding, measures to correct coagulation factors are not generally indicated.

Esophageal varices are common in patients with cirrhosis due to the portal hypertension. Bleeding varices occur in 20 to 30% of all cirrhotic patients. Management of bleeding varices includes supportive measures as with any other GI bleed (see the section on UGI bleeding). In addition, IV administration of vasopressin may be used to decrease portal venous pressure. Endoscopic sclerotherapy or banding is the initial treatment of choice. Operative shunts for treatment of varices by lowering the portal hypertension carry high morbidity and mortality. The TIPS procedure is now the procedure of choice to lower portal pressure without major abdominal surgery. This is often used as a temporizing measure to allow for resuscitation and as a bridge to the definitive cure for cirrhosis—transplantation. Any patient who has abstained from alcohol for 6 months would be considered for a liver transplant. Patients with hypersplenism that is causing early satiety and pain can be evaluated for splenectomy.

Hepatitis

Hepatitis is a viral disease with five different types: A, B, C, D, and E. The symptoms of hepatitis may include loss of appetite, nausea, fever, local tenderness in RUQ, and liver enlargement. Jaundice may also be present. The patient often has elevated LFTs that may be abnormal for 3 to 6 months.

Hepatitis A is shed in the stool and transmission occurs mainly by the fecal–oral route. Prior exposure is manifested by the presence of an antibody to hepatitis A which confers lifelong immunity. Hepatitis A is self-limited and does not lead to chronic hepatitis. Hepatitis A has an incubation period of approximately 30 days from the time of exposure to the onset of symptoms.

Hepatitis B is usually spread through infected blood, but the virus has also been found in saliva, semen, vaginal secretions, and breast milk. The incubation of hepatitis B is approximately 12 weeks. The antigen is usually gone by 6 months; presence after this time is considered chronic infection. Many patients with chronic hepatitis do not present with an acute episode. Many are not symptomatic, although some patients can be classified as having chronic active hepatitis. In chronic patients, hepatitis B antigen (HBeAg) is the product of the gene that codes for the virus core and its presence signifies a state of high virus replication. These patients are at risk for significant liver injury and high infectivity.

Hepatitis C was first recognized in transfusion recipients. However, with current screening tests, the risk of obtaining hepatitis C after a transfusion is negligible. Hepatitis C has a mean incubation period of 7 weeks. Approximately 50% of patients who contract hepatitis C progress to chronic infection and liver injury.

Hepatitis D is caused by a defective RNA virus that requires coinfection by hepatitis B (a DNA virus) to support its replication. Infection with hepatitis D occurs either simultaneously with hepatitis B or is superimposed on hepatitis B. The incubation period is similar to hepatitis B. The outcome of simultaneous acute hepatitis B and hepatitis D infection is similar to the outcome of hepatitis B alone. Patients with chronic hepatitis B infection who sustain a superimposed hepatitis D infection may progress to severe fulminant hepatitis or convert a chronic hepatitis to a chronic active hepatitis.

Hepatitis E is a disease that is prevalent in underdeveloped countries and transmitted by the fecal–oral route. It has a mean incubation period of approximately 40 days. The clinical course is similar to that of hepatitis A, although there is a slightly higher incidence of fulminant disease. This disease is self-limited and does not progress to chronic disease.

Fulminant hepatitis is characterized by a sudden onset of high fever, nausea and vomiting, chills, jaundice, convulsions, shock, and coma. Death usually occurs within 10 days.

Precautions such as avoiding intimate contact and careful handwashing after contact with the hepatitis patient are necessary to avoid transmission of the virus in all forms of hepatitis. In cases of hepatitis A, household contacts and small groups with a same source outbreak should be given immune globulin prophylaxis. Routine immunoprophylaxis is not necessary for casual contacts at work or school. Preexposure prophylaxis is recommended for travel to underdeveloped countries where hepatitis A is endemic. Prophylaxis of hepatitis B is accomplished by administration of hepatitis B vaccine. The duration of protection after vaccine is not known, although new exposures are thought to trigger a new immune response; therefore, boosters are not recommended for immunocompetent patients. In patients with immune compromise, boosters are recommended every 5 to 7 years. For postexposure prophylaxis, administration of a combination of hepatitis B immune globulin and hepatitis B vaccine is recommended. These should be given as soon as possible after exposure. An example is in the delivery room for babies born to mothers with chronic active hepatitis, or active hepatitis B during the third trimester of pregnancy. There is no vaccine for hepatitis C and immune globulins are of no proven benefit to prevent or attenuate the disease, although some sources recommend a single injection of IG for exposure to hepatitis C. Prevention of hepatitis D is achieved by prevention of hepatitis B. There is no vaccine for hepatitis E and immunoprophylaxis is not known to prevent or attenuate the disease.

As there is no carrier state of hepatitis A, a follow-up visit should be made 2 to 3 weeks after the onset to reevaluate liver function and patient status. In hepatitis B infection, patients should be followed monthly to determine antigen clearance from serum. If the antigen is present beyond 6 months, the hepatitis is considered a chronic infection. Patients with hepatitis C infection should be followed monthly for liver function studies and referred to a gastroenterologist for possible liver biopsy to rule out cirrhosis if liver function worsens. Patients with chronic hepatitis C on liver biopsy should be offered treatment with alpha interferon. In June 1998, the FDA approved ribavirin in combination with interferon for patients who do not respond to initial therapy or relapse after therapy is completed. In December 1998, the FDA approved Rebetron combination therapy with ribaviron and interferon for treatment of chronic hepatitis C in patients with compensated liver disease previously untreated (Hubbard, 1998). Patients with hepatitis D infection should be followed as those with hepatitis B. As in hepatitis A, hepatitis E patients can be seen at 2 to 3 weeks following resolution of symptoms for an evaluation of status and liver function.

Liver Tumors

Primary hepatic cancer is uncommon in the United States, though the incidence is high in parts of Asia and Africa. The etiologic factors are environmental or cultural in these areas as people in the United States of similar racial backgrounds are at only slighter greater risk than caucasians of developing hepatoma. Approximately 9000 cases each year are diagnosed in the United States, mostly in patients over age 50, although cases do occur in children. Chronic hepatitis B infection is the main etiologic factor worldwide. Cirrhosis from any cause is also associated with an increased risk. Staple foods in Africa such as ground nuts and grain contain certain fungus metabolites called aflatoxins. These have been shown experimentally to be capable of producing liver tumors.

Hepatomas constitute approximately 80% of primary hepatic cancers. In 70% of patients, tumor has already metastasized outside the liver at diagnosis. Cholangiocarcinomas represent approximately 15% of primary liver cancers. Extrahepatic metastases are also often found at the time of diagnosis.

Symptoms of a liver tumor may include RUQ pain and weight loss. A patient with known cirrhosis may experience deterioration characterized by an increase in hepatic failure, bleeding varices, and/or ascites. History of hepatitis B infection or aflatoxin ingestion are important history points.

Serum bilirubin and liver function tests may be elevated but are difficult to interpret in the cirrhotic patient. Alfa–feto protein levels are often elevated in the patient with hepatoma. Abdominal ultrasound and/or abdominal CT scan demonstrate hepatomas in 80% of patients. CT angio is often used to define lesions and determine resectability.

Surgical resection is the only possibility of cure. Criteria for resection include: confinement of tumor to the liver with no extrahepatic extension, excision will completely remove tumor, and, if excision requires lobectomy, that the remaining liver is healthy and has sufficient reserve to take over liver function. Generally, cirrhotic patients have insufficient reserve to survive lobectomy. Only about 25% of patients with primary live tumors are candidates for resection. The 5-year survival for patients after curative resection is about 30%. Many patients with unresectable lesions die within 1 year of diagnosis. Patients who are unresectable may be considered for transplantation.

Metastatic Liver Lesions

Metastatic liver lesions are much more common than primary tumors of the liver. Cancers of the breast, lung, pancreas, stomach, colon, kidney, ovary, and uterus are responsible for approximately 75% of metastatic tumors (Way, 1991).

Patients often present with weight loss, fatigue, and anorexia. RUQ pain, ascites, and jaundice are also common. Abdominal CT is often diagnostic of liver metastases.

Treatment options vary with the amount and size of lesions present. Single lesions amenable to resection are often treated in this way. However, many patients who present with liver disease after their original diagnosis and treatment commonly present with more than one lesion. A combination of resection and/or cyrosurgery and/or chemotherapy are possible treatment options in the patient with more than one lesion. Cryosurgery is the cryoablation or freezing of tumors not amenable to resection due to either location and/or size. Infusion of chemotherapy directly into the liver is also used for treatment. The chemotherapy is delivered via a surgically implanted hepatic artery pump. Prognosis varies with the amount of liver involvement by tumor. Patients with extensive hepatic replacement by tumor usually survive only a few months, contrasted by a 2- to 5-year survival for patients with solitary lesions.

Benign Tumors

Hemangiomas

Benign tumors of the liver also occur as do hepatic cysts. Hemangiomas are the most common benign hepatic tumor. The liver is a frequent site after skin and mucous membranes. Women are affected in a 6:1 ratio as compared with men.

Patients who have large hemangiomas (>4 cm) usually present with abdominal pain and/or a palpable mass. Many are found incidentally on CT of the abdomen or at laparotomy. Surgical excision is indicated in patients who are symptomatic.

Hepatic Adenomas

Hepatic adenomas occur almost exclusively in women and are related to oral contraceptives. Approximately 50% of patients are symptomatic. Many present with RUQ pain and/or acute hemorrhage due to rupture of the adenoma. Symptomatic patients usually have a palpable mass.

Patients with an acute bleed require emergent surgical resection. Adenomas may regress with discontinuation of oral contraceptives; therefore, tumors less than 6 cm may be managed expectantly. Tumors that enlarge or are greater than 6 cm should be removed due to the possibility of rupture and the progression to malignancy has been observed. Most patients recover fully from surgery and recurrence is rare.

Focal Nodular Hyperplasia

Focal nodular hyperplasia (FNH) is a benign lesion with no malignant potential. It is found in women more often than men by a 2:1 ratio. There is some evidence that exogenous estrogen may influence growth of the lesion. Most patients with FNH are asymptomatic. Patients who are symptomatic with right upper quadrant abdominal pain are candidates for surgical resection.

Hepatic Cysts

Hepatic cysts are usually solitary unilocular lesions that are asymptomatic. Large cysts may present as an abdominal mass associated with abdominal pain. Most cysts can be unroofed, at times laparoscopically. Solitary cysts lined with cuboidal epithelium are classified as cystadenomas and should be resected as they are premalignant. Patients with polycystic liver disease who have abdominal pain may benefit from surgical drainage of larger cysts or partial resection.

Hepatic Abcesses

Hepatic abscesses may originate from bacterial, parasitic, or fungal sources. The presence of a single abscess versus multiple abscesses is seen equally. Single abscesses affect the right lobe more frequently than the left and often develop in patients with diabetes. Multiple abscesses are often distributed throughout both lobes. In many patients, the development of a hepatic abscess follows a suppurative process elsewhere in the body. Often, they are due to direct spread from a biliary source such as the gallbladder. Abdominal infections such as appendicitis or diverticulitis may spread and involve the liver. Other sources may be from bacterial endocarditis, renal infection, pneumonia, or dental abscess. In approximately 10 to 15% of cases, no source can be found. These abscesses are referred to as cryptogenic.

Patients may present with symptoms such as malaise and fatigue followed by fever and often epigastric or RUQ pain. Fever may include high spikes up to 40-41°C. Presence of jaundice is usually a bad prognostic sign. Elevated WBC is commonly seen, usually over 15,000/uL. Abdominal CT is used for diagnosis and treatment by guiding percutaneous drainage.

Treatment also includes prompt administration of IV antibiotics with broad-spectrum agents narrowed when culture results are obtained. Surgical drainage is indicated when catheter drainage fails or is inadequate. A solitary liver abscess is associated with a 10% mortality rate.

Liver Transplantation

Liver transplantation was first successfully performed on a human in 1963 by Dr. Thomas Starzl. Since then, the indications for transplant have rapidly increased. The most common diseases for which transplant in adults is indicated include: chronic active hepatitis, autoimmune hepatitis, alcoholic cirrhosis, primary biliary cirrhosis, and sclerosing cholangitis. Another indication is Wilson's disease, a hereditary disease in which a decrease in a glycoprotein to which copper attaches causes an accumulation of copper in various organs including the liver, producing cirrhosis and liver failure.

Another indication for transplant includes Budd–Chiari syndrome, a rare disorder that results from obstruction of hepatic venous outflow. Most cases are caused by spontaneous thrombosis of the hepatic veins often associated with polycythemia vera or use of oral contraceptives. Many patients are improved with side-to-side portacaval shunt or TIPS. Some patients may have an idiopathic stenosis of the vena cava. Most patients with this stenosis have active hepatitis B. Hemochromatosis is a disease of iron metabolism in which iron accumulates in body tissues, and liver dysfunction and failure occur. The most common indication for transplant in children is extrahepatic biliary atresia.

Current contraindications to liver transplantation include active substance abuse, positive HIV status, and evidence of irreversible CNS disease. It is not a requirement that liver size and blood type of the donor match the recipient. Liver size may be modified to fit the recipient. Donor livers may be preserved up to 36 hours with current methods. This longer time period allows for greater use of available donor livers. One donor liver may be able to provide tissue for transplantation into two patients. However, the results with this are not as successful as with transplantation of an unaltered graft. The practice of living related donors in which a segment of liver is removed and transplanted continues to expand.

▶ PROBLEMS OF THE GALLBLADDER

Cholelithiasis and Chronic Cholecystitis

Cholelithiasis is the presence of stones in the gallbladder. The most common form of symptomatic gallbladder disease is chronic cholecystitis. Biliary colic caused by obstruction of the cystic duct, usually from an impacted gallstone, contributes to inflammation and scarring of the gallbladder.

Patients often present with an acute onset of abdominal pain located either in the RUQ or epigastric area. In many cases, the pain radiates to the back. The onset of pain may be related to eating a fatty meal. Nausea and/or vomiting may also occur.

Patients with these symptoms should be evaluated by abdominal ultrasound. An EKG and chest x-ray should also be obtained to rule out any cardiac disease. If the ultrasound is nondiagnostic, an upper GI should be done to rule out other possible causes of pain such as an ulcer.

Laparoscopic cholecystectomy is recommended for the patient with biliary colic. Gallbladder removal resolves symptoms in approximately 95% of patients. The other important reason to do a cholecystectomy is to avoid migration of stones into the common bile duct (CBD). Stones that lodge in the CBD can cause serious problems, namely obstruction and resultant jaundice and/or infection. Abdominal exploration and opening the duct surgically to remove stones may be avoided by early cholecystectomy. Currently, the accepted practice for treatment of cholelithiasis with biliary colic and CBD stones is to first have the gastroenterologist perform an ERCP to remove the ductal stones and then take the patient to surgery for gallbladder removal. Conversely, if stones are found in the duct during a laproscopic removal, the patient may undergo stone removal by ERCP after surgery.

Acute Cholecystitis

Most often acute cholecystitis results from a gallstone impacted in the neck of the gallbladder that is obstructing the cystic duct. This causes the gallbladder to become inflamed and distended, causing abdominal pain. Most attacks resolve spontaneously but it is possible that they will progress to an infectious process. Approximately 5% of cases of acute cholecystitis occur without gallstones present. This is called acalculous cholecystitis. Bile stasis from prolonged fasting, such as with patients who are NPO on hyperalimentation, may also cause acalculous cholecystitis.

Patients present with the same pain that they have had with biliary colic; however, in acute cholecystitis the pain does not improve and is associated with abdominal tenderness. Usually a low-grade fever is also present.

The WBC count is often elevated to the range of approximately 15,000/uL. Abdominal ultrasound should be done to evaluate the gallbladder and common bile duct. If stones are not present, a HIDA scan can be done to evaluate the gallbladder. If the gallbladder is not seen, the test is positive and most likely represents acalculous cholecystitis.

Treatment of acute cholecystitis includes NPO status, IV fluids, and antibiotics. Usually cephalosporins are used. If patients improve rapidly with these measures, they may be discharged and return electively for cholecystectomy. If patient's do not improve, they often require surgery during the same admission. If the patient's medical condition is unstable, drainage of the gallbladder with a cholecystostomy tube may be done as a temporizing measure until the patient is able to tolerate surgery.

The major complications of acute cholecystitis include perforation, gangrene, and empyema. The incidence of perforation is around 10%. This can occur as early as a few days after the onset of cholecystitis or as late as several weeks. A high fever and sepsis is seen with empyema as the gallbladder contains frank pus. Gangrenous cholecystitis often leads to free perforation of the gallbladder. This occurs in a small number of patients, approximately 1 to 2%.

Cholangitis

Cholangitis is infection of the bile ducts, often due to obstruction of bile flow. Patients present with abdominal pain, fever, and possibly jaundice.

Most cases of cholangitis can be successfully treated with IV antibiotics. Suppurative cholangitis refers to presence of sepsis often superceding biliary symptoms. This constitutes an emergency and requires surgical or endoscopic drainage. After control of infection, the source of biliary obstruction must be resolved.

Gallbladder Cancer

This is an uncommon tumor seen mostly in elderly patients. It is often associated with gallstones and occurs in women by a 2:1 ratio. Most primary tumors of the gallbladder are adenocarcinomas and have spread by the time of surgery, although it is possible to discover an incidental tumor after cholecystectomy where the lesion is confined to the gallbladder and completely excised. Obstruction of the duct by tumor may produce acute cholecystitis. Other patients may present with jaundice and/or cholangitis. The prognosis of gallbladder carcinoma is poor. Most patients do not survive past 1 year after diagnosis as there is no proven adjunctive therapy.

▶ PROBLEMS OF THE BOWEL

Anatomy and Physiology

Small Bowel

The small intestine consists of the duodenum (20 cm), jejunum (100-110 cm), and ileum (150-160 cm). The small bowel is attached by the mesentery, which carries vascular supply and lymphatic drainage. The mesentery courses from the left of the L2 to the right of the S1 joint. The blood supply to the jejunum and ileum is via the superior mesenteric artery (SMA). Innervation is sympathetic and parasympathetic which affect secretion and motility. The small bowel is responsible for digestion and absorption of fat, protein, carbohydrates, water, and electrolytes (water, bile, gastric, salivary, and intestinal fluids average 10 liters per day). The small bowel absorbs 90% of the 9 liters of fluid that pass into the duodenum per day. The small bowel also releases a variety of hormones into the blood, for example, secretin, cholecystokinin, and other peptides. The small bowel mucosa serves as a barrier against pathogens entering the blood.

Large Bowel

The colon and rectum make up 20% of the GI tract (3-5 feet), extending from the ileum to the rectum. The cecum, ascending colon, and hepatic flexure comprise the right colon; the distal transverse colon, splenic flexure, descending colon, and rectosigmoid comprise the left colon. The ascending and descending colons are fixed in the retroperitoneal space. The transverse and sigmoid colons are suspended in the peritoneal cavity by their mesocolons. The caliber of the lumen is greatest at the cecum. The colon wall has four layers: mucosa, submucosa, muscularis, and serosa. The wall of the colon is so thin that it becomes markedly distended when obstructed.

The rectum is about 15 cm in length. The anal canal, which measures 4 cm, begins at the terminal rectum and passes through the levator ani muscles. It is surrounded by an inferior and exterior sphincter mechanism. The internal sphincter is an involuntary muscle and is contracted at rest. The external sphincter is voluntary and is a specialized continuation of the levator muscles of the pelvic floor. The dentate line is the true mucocutaneous junction located 1.0 to 1.5 cm above the anal verge. The superior mesenteric artery (SMA) supplies the colon to the splenic flexure; the inferior mesenteric artery (IMA) to mid-rectum; and branches of the internal ileac artery supply the distal rectum and anus.

The colon is more than a receptacle and conduit for the end products of digestion. Average uptake of the large bowel is 1500 cc per day, but it can absorb up to 5000 cc per day. Six hundred mL of flatus is normally expelled per day. There are normally 200 cc of gas in the intestinal tract and the amount of detectable gas is seldom increased in patients who complain of bloating and distention. The large bowel has several functions: absorbs sodium, chloride, and water; secretes potassium, bicarbonate, and mucus; is the site of digestion of certain carbohydrates and proteins; and provides the environment for the bacterial production of vitamin K.

Intestinal Transit

The stomach empties in 3 to 4 hours. Digested food reaches the ileocecal valve by 2 to 3 hours, completing passage in 9 hours. Mass peristaltic waves (gastrocolic reflex) occur after meals and propel the bolus from the hepatic flexure onward. Defecation occurs when peristaltic waves, accompanied by relaxation of the rectosigmoid junction, propel the contents of the left or descending and sigmoid colon into the rectum. The major portion of digested material requires several days for evacuation.

Diagnostic Features of Bowel Problems

When the colon is the source of pathological process, there is an alteration in GI function. The patient may report a change in the caliber of stool, diarrhea, constipation, obstipation, hematochezia, melena, rectal tensesmus (cramping pains with straining or incomplete evacuation), and/or urgency. The exam should include: a pelvic exam (in woman), a digital/rectal exam, visualization and palpation of the abdomen, noting any masses, malnutrition, stigmata of portal hypertension, and a stool exam for blood.

The biochemical baseline should be established, nutritional status assessed, and liver function tests (LFT) and carcinogenic embryonic antigen (CEA) obtained, which if elevated could indicate a neoplastic process. Diagnostic studies should include anoscopy, which requires an anoscope, rigid sigmoidoscopy, flexible sigmoidoscopy, or colonoscopy. Other useful diagnostic studies include barium enema, abdominal flatplate, and small bowel follow-through.

Bowel Obstruction

Pathophysiology

Bowel obstruction is defined as the interference with normal progression of intestinal contents and is one of the most common surgical emergencies. Bowel obstruction is most common in adults over 50, but can occur at any age. Three quarters of all bowel obstructions occur in the small bowel and only one quarter in the large bowel. Mechanical blockage, which can be partial or complete, results from an intraluminal obstruction such as tumor, gallstones, or extraluminal compression such as adhesions (the most common cause) or hemorrhage. Paralytic ileus is not a true obstruction, but loss of organized peristalsis.

History and Physical Findings

Simple mechanical obstruction of the small bowel is accompanied by accumulation of fluid and gas proximal to the obstruction producing distention of the intestine and resulting in four primary clinical manifestations. The first is abdominal pain. This is initially a severe cramping pain with hyperperistalsis. Then, after a short time the pain subsides, the patient feels well, alternating with crampy episodes. These attacks usually occur every 4 to 5 minutes. The pain is diffuse and felt across the upper abdomen in a high obstruction and at the umbilicus in a lower ileal obstruction. If distention continues, this colicky pain may stop and the patient may have generalized abdominal discomfort. Crampy pain followed shortly by explosive diarrhea often signifies a partial obstruction. If there is no quiescent period and the pain is severe and constant, this could indicate strangulation.

Vomiting is the second manifestation and occurs immediately after obstruction. In a high obstruction, vomiting is copious and frequent and may decompress the obstruction. With a low obstruction the vomitus is thick, dark, and malodorous (feculent) from stagnation and bacterial effect. Reflex vomiting does not usually accompany colon obstruction and may not occur at all if the ileocecal valve is competent because the small bowel does not distend.

The third manifestation is failure to pass gas or feces (obstipation), although if the obstruction is high in the jejunum, gas and feces may pass through. Fourth, abdominal distention is a result of a longstanding obstruction. In a high, small bowel obstruction there may be no generalized distention.

The physical exam in the case of a simple mechanical small obstruction yields few signs in the first 24 hours. The vital signs are normal, and dehydration and distention are not marked. If the patient appears ill during this period, strangulated obstruction is more probable. Auscultation of the abdomen is of great value. The abdomen is quiet except during attacks of colicky pain, then loud and high-pitched metallic sounds in rushes or bursts are heard. A completely quiet abdomen can mean strangulated bowel or gangrenous bowel. Palpation reveals muscle guarding during colicky pain and slight tenderness between attacks. A mass or localized tenderness usually indicates strangulation. The patient appears seriously ill 48 to 72 hours after the obstruction. There is marked dehydration, abdominal distention, and vital signs become increasingly more abnormal; shock occurs in late simple obstruction.

Laboratory and Diagnostic Testing

The loss of large amounts of isotonic extracellular fluid into the intestine is responsible for altered lab findings. The body responds to the sudden volume decrease by antidiuresis and renal sodium retention. The hematocrit rises in proportion to the fluid loss. Sodium, potassium, and chloride concentrations in the plasma change little. Acid–base changes (pH and carbon dioxide levels) are minimal. There is an increase in the BUN secondary to decreased urine flow. When urine is produced, the specific gravity is often 1.025 to 1.030, with mild proteinuria. If untreated, sodium-free water restores the acute loss of extracellular volume with a decrease plasma, sodium, and chloride concentration. The urine output increases slowly and potassium is excreted. The hematocrit then begins to drop. Metabolic acidosis often occurs. Respiratory acidosis can also occur if distention of the abdomen is enough to elevate the diaphragm.

The white blood cell count rises slightly with simple mechanical obstruction to about 15,000 per mm^3 with a shift to the left. An increase to 20,000 per mm^3 with marked polymorphonucleic cells (PMN) suggests strangulation (not a sensitive indicator), and the white count can increase to

40 to 60 per mm^3, which suggests mesenteric vascular occlusion. The serum amylase may also rise, confusing the picture. Amylase enters the blood by regurgitation from the pancreas because of back pressure from the duodenum.

The radiological findings are most diagnostic. These should be performed within the first hour. Supine and upright position plane films of the abdomen (without contrast medium), posterior, anterior, and lateral views of the chest (if the patient can sit up; left lateral decubitus films if the patient must remain supine) are the most important initial films. Gas fluid levels are the most important criteria in the x-ray diagnosis of intestinal obstructions. In normal adults on plane films, gas is visible in the colon and stomach. Small bowel gas is rarely visible due to rapid transit time. If the normal progression of intestinal content is altered, gas collects with retained fluid and produces gas fluid levels best seen on the upright abdominal film. This is highly suggestive of intestinal obstruction, including ileus, but can also be seen in severe constipation.

Barium enema is another useful diagnostic tool. If the clinical presentation and plane abdominal films suggest colon obstruction, barium enema helps determine the type and location of obstruction. It can also be helpful if the gas distribution on the plane films is not clear. Barium enema in this situation does pose some risk. An inflamed lesion, such as diverticulitis or appendicitis, can be perforated and a partial obstruction can be connected to a complete obstruction. Another useful diagnostic tool is an intravenous pyelogram (IVP). This may be indicated to look for ureteral calculi, often responsible for a paralytic ileus. An upper GI is used to differentiate postoperative ileus from mechanical obstruction. If some contrast medium, either barium or gastrographin, passes through the gastrointestinal tract, the diagnosis of ileus is more likely. Computerized tomography (CT) scanning of the abdomen is becoming the test of choice in demonstrating small bowel obstruction. This is most helpful when extra luminal abnormalities are suspected or when prompt intervention is required (Schwartz, 1998).

Large bowel obstruction usually does not strangulate, except with a volvulus. Principally a storage organ, the large bowel has a relatively minor absorptive and secretory function. Fluid and electrolyte sequestration progresses more slowly. Large bowel obstructions are most dangerous when distention is progressive. This then causes a closed loop, if the ileocecal valve is competent, the colon can then rupture, usually at the cecum because that is the largest diameter and the tension is related to the diameter.

Initial symptoms of a large obstruction are abdominal pain, vomiting, and obstipation followed by abdominal distention, severe colicky pain with hyperperistalsis and quiescent periods. This is similar to simple mechanical bowel obstruction and small bowel obstruction.

Management

The management of both simple mechanical bowel obstruction and large bowel obstruction is fluid and electrolyte therapy, decompression of the bowel, and surgical intervention timed appropriately. All patients should be operated on, except those in the immediate postoperative phase. Simple mechanical obstruction of less than 24 hours' duration requires minimal preoperative preparation. Patients with simple mechanical bowel obstruction greater than 24 hours require preparation prior to operation by repleting fluid and electrolytes. These patients should have central venous catheters placed to measure the central venous pressure. As long as the central venous pressure remains below 10 to 12 cm of water, the replacement should be rapid. When there is a sudden rise in central venous pressure, the endpoint of volume replacement is reached.

An indwelling bladder catheter to more accurately measure urine output and a nasogastric tube for bowel decompression should also be inserted. To determine the amount the fluid volume needed to replete the loss, an initial hematocrit should be assessed. If this value is 55, for example, there has been approximately 40% loss of plasma in extracellular fluid volume. This helps you calculate the amount of fluid required to replace the loss. The solution used should be lactate ringers and 5% dextrose and water in equal proportions; if gastric loss is excessive, then use normal saline solution. When the patient's urinary output increases, potassium then should be added and antibiotics should also be given. The goal is to normalize the electrolyte concentration and acid–base balance by the time the volume deficit has been repaired.

Strangulation requires emergent operation with vigorous fluid and electrolyte preparation, antibiotics, and nasogastric tube suction. Intestinal decompression is obtained by intubating the gastrointestinal system. Two types of tubes are used. First, the short tube for gastric aspiration. This is usually a LeVeen sump tube that prevents further intestinal distention by removing all air swallowed and empties the stomach, preventing aspiration during removal of stomach contents. The second tube, the long tube, also is used for aspiration, this time of the small intestine. These tubes, the Miller–Abbott as an example, have an aspiration lumen and a mercury-containing balloon at the end. The patient lies on the right side with his or her heels elevated so gravity pulls the tube into the small intestine through the pylorus aiding in decompression of the small intestine.

There are four types of obstruction that require emergent surgery: (1) strangulation, due to the risk of sepsis; (2) closed-loop obstruction, due to risk of strangulation; (3) colon obstruction, because this can progress to a closed-loop obstruction; and (4) simple mechanical obstruction. If surgery is performed within the first 24 hours, there is essentially no mortality. The surgical procedures done are divided into five categories: (1) procedures not requiring opening of the bowel (lysis of adhesion, reduction of incarcerated hernia); (2) an enterotomy for removal of obturation obstruction (gallstones); (3) resection of the obstructing lesion or strangulated bowel with primary anastomosis; (4)

bypassing an obstruction; and (5) forming a cutaneous stoma above the obstruction (colostomy, cecostomy).

Postoperative management is essentially the same as preoperative: fluids, electrolyte replacement, antibiotics, and gastrointestinal decompression. This is more difficult in the postoperative intestinal obstruction because of the large volume of sequestrated isotonic third-space fluid. The patient usually begins to mobilize these fluids on approximately the third postoperative day and the intravenous fluid therapy must be given carefully during this period. Sodium and potassium levels must be kept in the normal range (low levels can prolong paralysis of the gastrointestinal tract). Gastrointestinal decompression must be maintained for approximately 5 or 6 days, until bowel function resumes.

Ileus

An ileus is paralysis or inhibition of the intestinal muscle function due to neural, humoral, or metabolic factors. Ileus can be divided into three categories. The adynamic ileus is diminished or absent motility because of inhibition of the neuromuscular apparatus, which occurs after every abdominal operation. Each segment of gastrointestinal tract regains function differently. The small bowel motility returns in approximately 24 hours; gastric motility in approximately 48 hours; and colonic motility in approximately 3 to 5 days. If the ileus persists postoperatively, it can become a clinical problem. Other causes of adynamic ileus are intraperitoneal inflammation (such as appendicitis or acute pancreatitis), pathological conditions (such as ureteral calculi or fracture of the spine), thoracic problems (such as pneumonia or fractured ribs), and systemic causes (such as hypokalemia, hyponatremia, and toxemia). Drugs can also cause an adynamic ileus. Some common drugs are morphine, propantheline, antacids, anticoagulants, phenothiazines and ganglionic blocking agents.

The second type of ileus is a spastic ileus. This is uncommon and defined as uncoordinated hyperactivity of the intestine as seen in heavy metal poisoning and uremia. The third type of ileus is the ileus of vascular occlusion. The bowel wall is incapable of coordinated motility because it is dying from ischemia.

With the postoperative adynamic ileus, the patient remains disinterested in food and surroundings beyond postoperative day three or four. On exam, the abdomen is distended, tympanic with occasional bowel sounds.

Laboratory values are needed to determine the cause, which can include anemia, sepsis, hyponatremia, hypokalemia, and hypoosmolarity. Radiological testing, such as abdominal plane films, can help distinguish between an ileus and mechanical obstruction. If these are not conclusive, a small bowel follow-through is obtained using oral contrast medium, which should reach the cecum in approximately 4 hours. If a stationary column of contrast medium is seen in 4 hours, there is a complete obstruction.

Treatment of ileus is accomplished by treating the primary source (correcting fluid electrolyte derangements, draining an abscess). The abdominal distention should be treated by gastrointestinal intubation.

Inflammatory Bowel Disease

Crohn's Disease

Crohn's disease is a chronic granulomatous disease of the alimentary tract. This is characterized by spontaneous remissions and acute exacerbation. The peak onset is from the teens to age 30. Small bowel only is involved in 30%, ileocolitis occurs in about 55%, and the colon only is involved in about 15%.

Typically, the patient is a young adult with a long history of chronic abdominal pain and diarrhea. The diagnosis is often delayed, on a 3-year average, because of the vague symptoms. Abdominal pain over the years progresses to persistent dull, aching pain and is most prominent in the lower abdomen. It is often crampy and symptomatic, increasing over time. Diarrhea usually occurs every 3 to 5 days and rarely contains mucous, pus, or blood. Intermittently explosive diarrhea is associated with meals and is frequently nocturnal. Weight loss ensues. One third of the patients complain of fever, loss of strength, and easy fatigability. Perianal disease is also associated with Crohn's disease and may be the only presenting feature (fissure, fistula, stricture, abscess). Extraintestinal manifestations of Crohn's disease are arthritis, arthralgia, uveitis, iritis, hepatitis, pericholangitis, erythema nodosum, and pyoderma gangrenosum.

The diagnosis is confirmed by barium x-ray studies of the small bowel. Radiographic enteroclysis shows a nodular contour and narrowing of the bowel lumen with sinus clefts and linear ulcers. Clinical symptoms and response to drug therapy do not correlate with x-ray features of Crohn's disease. There is no need to repeat these studies, unless exacerbation occurs and a stricture is suspected or for pre- or postoperative evaluation.

Treatment is adjusted for presentation. Frequently, there is a presentation of acute intestinal obstruction, usually produced by intense edema and inflammation of the bowel wall, although complete obstruction is uncommon. Intravenous fluids, nasogastric suction, and medication are initiated; usually treatment is symptomatic followed by remissions and exacerbation. The goals are to relieve abdominal pain, control the diarrhea, correct nutritional deficiencies, and treat infection. Sulfasalazine is an intraluminal antibiotic and has some beneficial effects. Corticosteroids can also be helpful with acute exacerbations of ileitis.

Possible immunologic abnormalities with Crohn's have been studied and azathioprine and 6-mercaptopurine have been shown to be helpful (Schwartz, 1994). Diet had little effect. Most patients with Crohn's disease require operation during the course of their illness. The site of Crohn's disease is a prognostic indicator. Ileocolitis has the highest rate of recurrence after resection; permanent cure is a rare event. Operative complications include obstruction, abscess, fistula, free perforation, urologic complications, hemorrhage, cancer, perianal disease, and growth retardation. Optimum treatment of these complications is surgical resection of the involved segment with restored intestinal continuity. There is a high rate of recurrence after an operation, usually in small bowel proximal to the ileocecal valve. Crohn's disease often burns out with advancing age.

Ulcerative Colitis

Ulcerative colitis is a nonspecific inflammatory bowel disease of the large intestine. It affects both sexes and occurs at all ages. The onset is usually between the second and fourth decades. The cause is unknown.

Clinical manifestations are characterized by remissions and exacerbations. They range from inactive to fulminant disease and the rectum is usually involved. The patient can present with minimally bloody stools, diarrhea, or sudden onset with bleeding, tenesmus, crampy abdominal pain, fever, and explosive diarrhea. The basic symptoms are usually bleeding per rectum and diarrhea (the amount of bleeding is related to the amount of diseased mucosa). Diarrhea occurs every 1 to 2 hours and is nocturnal. The diarrhea is often only blood and mucous. Massive hemorrhage though is uncommon.

On physical exam, the findings are nonspecific and depend on the severity of the disease. The patient may present with abdominal pain and tenderness. The patient may be seen with distention and fever, tachycardia, and an elevated white blood cell count, which is indicative of toxic megacolon.

Diagnosis must be made by endoscopy; proctoscopy may be enough to diagnose Crohn's disease, though, because the disease is always in the rectum. Total colonoscopy and barium enema should not be done in an acute episode due to the risk of perforation. The mucosa can appear with minimal edema and friability to severe ulceration with edema and bleeding. There is always a loss of normal vascular supply when there is edema. After recovery from an acute attack, the total colonoscopy is done to determine the extent of the disease with multiple biopsies taken. Barium enema, although less sensitive, can be diagnostic in determining the extent of the disease and serves as a baseline. The differential diagnosis of ulcerative colitis is made when the disease is seen as continuous starting in the upper anal canal and spreading proximally. Crohn's disease reveals patchy areas with areas of normal mucosa. Infectious diarrheal diseases, infective colitis caused by Campylobacter, gonococcal proctitis, schegelis salmonella, and clostridium must be distinguished.

The medical management of longstanding active ulcerative colitis with bleeding and diarrhea requires treatment of the symptoms. These patients are frequently anemic, hyponatremic, and show weight loss and vitamin deficiency. Occasionally, they require hospitalization for resuscitation. Cortisone enemas are used empirically for symptomatic proctitis and proctosigmoiditis. 5-Aminosalicylic acid also helps by acting on the lumen of the colon and inhibiting the inflammatory process. Sulfasalazine standard is also standard treatment as a conjugate of 5-aminosalcylic acid and sulfapyridine (Azulfidine 1 gram increased to 4 grams per day). Side effects occur in approximately 10% of the patients who develop nausea, vomiting, stomach upset, rash, and headache. Therapeutic response may take 3 to 4 weeks.

Fulminate colitis requires IV hydrocortisone 100 mg q 8 h. Less severe disease is treated with Prednisone 40 mg to 60 mg per day, tapering over several weeks to 20 mg or less. Response should be evident within 1 week. Long-term use of steroids has not been proven to prevent relapse. Hourly diarrhea is common with acute ulcerative colitis and antidiarrheal drugs are helpful such as diphenoxylate (Lomotil) and loperamide (Imodium). Surgical therapy is indicated when the disease has cutaneous or systemic manifestations, severe mucosal dysplasia, cancer is evident, or if the disease has been present for greater than 10 years. The operation consists of total proctocolectomy with an ileostomy or a pouch procedure and an ileoanal anastomosis.

With ulcerative colitis, fatty infiltration of the liver is seen in 40 to 50% of the patients and with accompanying cirrhosis in 2 to 5%. Controlling the primary disease decreases fatty infiltration, but this is irreversible if it has progressed to cirrhosis. Primary scerlosing cholangitis can also occur and is a progressive disease presenting with obstruction and jaundice and is not reversible.

As with Crohn's disease, ulcerative colitis patients can present with arthritis, usually at the knees, ankles, and wrists. Symptoms of bile duct cancer, erythema nodosum, pyoderma gangrenosum, apthus ulcers, uveitis, episcleritis, iritis, and conjunctivitis usually improve when the bowel disease improves.

The most serious complication from inflammatory bowel disease is colon or rectal cancer. There is an increased risk with prolonged ulcerative colitis. If the total large bowel is involved and if the duration of the disease has been greater than 10 years with persistent inflammation, patients require follow-up with colonoscopy every 6 to 12 months. Biopsies must be done and if severe dysplasia is present on repeat biopsies, total proctocolectomy should be considered.

Diverticular Disease

Diverticulosis. Diverticular disease describes a clinical spectrum. Diverticulosis refers to the presence of diverticula, without inflammation. Colonic diverticula occur where the main blood vessels pass to supply the colonic mucosa, a point of weakness, the teniae coli. Diverticulosis is most common in the sigmoid colon, although it can occur anywhere. Depletion of dietary fibers is suspected to be responsible for the development of colonic diverticular disease. Diverticulosis requires no treatment. Diverticular hemorrhage, although uncommon, can cause massive colonic bleeding.

Diverticulitis. Diverticulitis denotes infection associated with diverticula. Diverticula readily fill with colonic contents which causes inflammation. If the obstructing plug remains, the inflammation spreads and gives rise to intramural fistulas and perforation of a single diverticulum, the initiating event in diverticulitis. The infectious process is usually pericolic in nature. The infection is the result of a perforation of a diverticulum and then to estravasation of feces from the lumen to the serosal surface of the colon. In most cases, the body's natural defenses confine the infection. If the fecal contamination is significant or if the patient's response to infection is compromised, abscess formation or peritonitis can occur.

Clinical presentation is similar to appendicitis, often called "left-sided appendicitis." Patients with acute diverticulitis usually complain of left lower quadrant abdominal pain and may radiate to the left suprapubic area or back. Constipation or occasionally diarrhea may be noted (symptoms may be similar to irritable bowel symptoms). Fever and chills are not unusual. If the inflammation is adjacent to the bladder, frequency or urgency of urination may be present. Rectal bleeding is rare in the presence of diverticulitis. Most signs and symptoms are a result of inflammation around the diverticula, which leads to acute diverticulitis, perforation, abscess, and fistula formation or stenosis.

On physical exam the most common finding is tenderness over the left lower abdomen. If the inflammation present is considerable, a poorly circumscribed area of induration may be palpated in this region. A tender mass is suggestive of an abscess (more likely) or localized phlegmon. The small bowel may be involved in the inflammatory process, leading to an ileus or partial obstruction. Abdominal distention is seen here. Rectal examination may demonstrate pelvic tenderness and a pelvic abscess may be palpated. This may also be felt on vaginal examination.

Often the diagnosis of diverticulitis is made on clinical grounds and abdominal flat plate. If there is doubt, three tests can be considered: computed tomography (CT) of the abdomen, ultrasonography, or contrast enema. CT scan is the test of choice because it can show a thickened colonic wall, inflammation, and associated abscess, fistulas, and obstruction. Gentle radiographic enema should be obtained if perforation is suspected. Barium enema, laxatives, and colonoscopy should not be done until the acute episode has subsided to avoid perforation. The most obvious change in the colon is the thickening of the circular muscle wall, which makes the lumen look corrugated. These clefts in the muscle are responsible for the sawtooth signs seen on barium x-ray studies.

The treatment usually requires hospital admission. In nonoperative therapy the patient is placed on a clear liquid diet, unless signs of an ileus or bowel obstruction are present. Broad spectrum antibiotics should be used; morphine and codeine should be avoided. Meperidine may be used as needed. As soon as the fever is gone and there is no evidence of bowel obstruction, regular diet and a bulk-producing agent, such as psyllium, should be started to prevent hypersegmentation of the sigmoid bowel. When fever is gone, a contrast x-ray with gastrographin enema may be obtained. On x-ray, it is sometimes difficult to distinguish between diverticulitis and carcinoma. Films are suggested of carcinoma if there is involvement of a long segment of bowel, there is bowel spasm, presence of diverticula elsewhere in the bowel, or if there are tapered ends in the bowel segments. Surgical therapy of diverticulitis is reserved for complications, for those patients who respond to medical therapy, for recurrent episodes of acute diverticulitis, or if carcinoma cannot be excluded.

Seventy percent of patients who recover from one uncomplicated episode of diverticulitis have no recurrence. If the patient suffers recurrent attacks of diverticulitis, surgical treatment should be considered usually 4 to 6 weeks later, when the inflammation has resolved.

There are several complications of diverticulitis. Perforation of a diverticulm that is not localized and causes generalized fecal peritonitis is rare, but requires surgical intervention. The diseased segment of the bowel is resected and a celiotomy is done. The distal segment of bowel is sutured or stapled closed. This is called Hartmann's operation. If the peritonitis is so severe that the perforated segment cannot be resected, then the diversion of feces with a completely diverting colostomy is constructed proximal to the perforation.

Diverticular abscess can also occur as a result of perforation. An important advance in the treatment of diverticulitis has been the development of percutaneous drainage of abdominal abscesses. An elective resection can then be carried out. If percutaneous drainage is not possible, it is necessary to perform a Hartmann's operation.

A fistula between the sigmoid colon and other organs, including bladder, small intestine, vagina, and skin is a frequent complication of diverticulitis. A sigmoid-vesicle fistula is seldom a cause for emergency surgical treatment. Before operative therapy, the cause of the fistula must be confirmed and then the diseased segment of the colon containing the site of perforation is excised.

Carcinoma of the Colon and Rectum

Carcinoma of the colon and rectum is the most common carcinoma of the gastrointestinal tract. The etiology is unknown. Hereditary factors have been implicated in a small percent of patients. Dietary factors, however, are of significance. Diets high in animal fat and low on fiber have been cited as factors influencing rectal and colon carcinoma. Diets high in fiber are theorized to decrease colonic transit time and therefore decrease contact time of carcinogens. Half of the large bowel carcinomas of patients with strong family histories occur before the age of 40, compared with the general population at the age of 65. Almost all of colon and rectal carcinomas are adenocarcinomas.

Colon and rectal carcinoma populations can be divided into two groups: high risk and low risk. High risk indicates a family history of cancer, particularly colorectal cancer; cancer of the prostate and bladder in men; cancer of the cervix, uterus, ovary, and breast in women; and those patients with a family history of colorectal polyps or endometrial carcinoma. Colonic work-up should be done at age 40 for these patients and every 3 or 5 years following. The low-risk population is defined as patients with no signs or symptoms and no known risk factors. Mass screening for occult blood is the most practical detection mechanism for this population.

Symptoms of colon and rectal carcinoma are nonspecific. The first sign or symptom may be change in bowel habits or rectal bleeding (this does not necessarily mean an early lesion). Abdominal pain, bloating, constipation, and diarrhea are caused by partial bowel obstruction, usually seen with advanced carcinoma. This is most common in the carcinoma of the rectosigmoid colon. Rectal colon cancer presents with tenesmus, an incomplete evacuation of the bowel. Cancer of the right and transverse colon frequently presents with weakness and anemia. With rectal bleeding, blood can be bright or dark, and with or without clots. Noticeable blood usually indicates a left-sided lesion; right or transverse lesions present with occult blood. Cardiac patients presenting with these symptoms may also have angina or heart failure secondary to the anemia. Weight loss and decreased appetite are usually signs of advanced carcinoma. Septicemia is rare but can occur. Streptococcus bovis bacteremia is suggestive of colorectal carcinoma. Early detection is the only way to improve cure.

Routine digital exam is often diagnostic in the case of rectal cancer. Characteristic findings are hard, rough, and irregular surface. Straining brings the higher lesion to the fingertip. Proctoscopy has little place in diagnosing colon cancer because of the limited examination it allows. Flexible sigmoidoscopy permits visualization of the rectum, sigmoid colon, and often the descending colon and mucosa. If used with barium enema, this is an acceptable exam of the large bowel.

Colonoscopy is the most accurate and complete examination of the large bowel. Ninety percent of colonoscopists can reach the cecum, which allows direct visualization of the lesion and also allows biopsy. Colonoscopy should also be considered complementary with a barium enema study for complete work-up that would rule out synchronous lesions and polyps. Barium enema studies with air contrast are often diagnostic. A good study demonstrates a lesion 1 cm or larger or an apple-core lesion that is characteristic of a large lesion. Chest x-ray should be obtained to rule out pulmonary metastasis. An intravenous pyelogram is also obtained if there are signs of obstructive uropathy or abnormal renal function. CT scan for liver metastasis is only obtained with abnormal LFTs or in increasing carcinoembryonic antigen (CEA). This is a glycoprotein antigen produced by large bowel carcinoma. It is nonspecific. Smoking, pancreatitis, and ulcerative colitis may also increase levels. It is not so valuable a screening test, but if the CEA level is abnormal preoperatively with large bowel carcinoma, the level increases with recurrence or a metastasis and is therefore a useful follow-up mechanism.

Standard therapy for colorectal carcinoma is surgical excision. Radiation and/or chemotherapy is often used with surgical excision. Preoperative bowel preparation is required for all colorectal carcinoma operations. A complete mechanical clearance of the bowel is done to decrease the endogenous bacteria in the bowel lumen to help prevent wound infection and intraabdominal abscess. Most often whole-gut lavage with polyethylene glycol electrolyte solution is used. This way, the patient may have a regular meal until the morning before the operation. The patient then drinks the 4-liter solution at a rate of 250 cc every 10 minutes, which should clear the diarrheal effluent in 3 to 10 hours. Preoperative prophylactic nonabsorbable antibiotics also have been shown to reduce the infection rate. A second-generation cephalosporin is often used and continued postoperatively for two doses.

With intraperitoneal colon cancer, the primary objective is to remove the primary tumor, along with the surrounding soft tissues and lymphatics. The length of the bowel resected is dependent on the blood vessels supplying the segment involved with cancer, because the lymphatics accompany the arterial supply in the colon. For carcinoma of the right colon, a right hemicolectomy is done with 10 to 12 cm of terminal ileum. The ileum is then anastomosed to the left transverse colon using either sutures or stapling technique. Cancer of the hepatic flexure is resected with an extended right hemicolectomy. For carcinoma of the splenic flexure, the left transverse or descending colon is taken. For carcinoma of the descending colon, a left hemicolectomy is done. A sigmoid colectomy is performed for carcinoma of the sigmoid and rectosigmoid colon.

For rectal carcinoma, there are three main procedures performed: (1) an anterior resection of the colorectum, and an anastomosis above the anterior peritoneal reflection (10 cm); (2) a low anterior resection with the anastomosis below the level of the anterior perineal reflection (5 cm); and (3) an abdominal perineal resection. Abdominal perineal resection is removal of the colorectum and the anal canal and the sigmoid colon is brought out as a permanent colostomy. This procedure is generally used for lesions within 5 cm of the anal verge.

Appendix

Pathophysiology

Obstruction of the lumen is the dominant factor in acute appendicitis. Fecalith (a hard mass consisting of inspissated feces) is the usual cause of the appendiceal obstruction, although hypertrophy of the lymphoid tissue can also obstruct the lumen, as can vegetable and fruit seeds, inspissated barium from previous x-rays studies, and intestinal worms. Following the occlusion of a lumen, a close-loop obstruction is produced. The appendix continues to secrete and rapidly causes distention. Also causing distention is the rapid multiplication of resident bacteria. The capacity of the appendix is only about 0.1 mL.

Appendicitis can present at any age, but is most common in the second and third decades. The male to female ratio is 2:1 between the ages of 15 and 25; after that it is 1:1.

History and Physical Findings

This distention stimulates nerve fibers (visceral afferent pain fibers) producing vague, dull, diffuse pain. Vascular congestion also occurs secondary to distention and can cause reflux, nausea, and vomiting. The pain worsens as does the inflammatory response, shifting the pain to the right lower quadrant. The patient develops fever, leukocytosis, and tachycardia. Because of the distention, vascular compromise, and bacterial invasion, the appendix will then perforate. Some episodes of acute appendicitis, though, subside spontaneously.

Clinical manifestations are not specific for a given disease, but are specific for disturbance of a physiologic function or functions. The identical picture can result from a wide variety of acute processes within or near the peritoneal cavity that produce the same alterations of function as acute appendicitis.

The presenting symptoms of appendicitis are primarily abdominal pain. Initially the pain is diffuse, usually in the lower epigastrium or umbilical region. The patient describes it as steady and moderately severe, occasionally with pain and cramping. In 1 to 12 hours (usually 4 to 6 hours), the pain localizes to the right lower quadrant. Some patients experience right lower quadrant pain as the initial symptom. Anatomic location of the appendix vary and this can cause a different locus of pain. Anorexia is also usually present. Seventy-five percent of patients vomit, usually once or twice. If vomiting precedes the pain, the diagnosis of appendicitis should be questioned. Most people report obstipation before the abdominal pain and that having a bowel movement would relieve the pain. Some patients, usually children, experience diarrhea.

With uncomplicated appendicitis, vital signs are usually unchanged. Temperature elevation is usually only 1 degree. The pulse rate may be elevated slightly and the patient usually prefers to lie supine with the thighs drawn up, especially the right side. Any motion increases the pain and the patient moves slowly. Tenderness is often maximal at or near a point in the right lower quadrant known as McBurney's point (between an inch and a half to two inches from the anterior spinous process of the ileum on a straight line drawn from the process to the umbilicus). Rebound tenderness is also usually present maximally in this region and is indicative of peritoneal irritation. Rosivig's sign, pain in the right lower quadrant when pressure is exerted in the left lower quadrant with palpation, is another indication of peritoneal irritation. Some patients experience cutaneous hyperesthesias in the area supplied by the spinal nerve on the right at T10, T11, and T12. This can be elicited by gently picking up the skin between the forefinger and thumb. Early on, the patient may demonstrate voluntary guarding with palpation; this can progress to involuntary or true reflux rigidity. Signs of localized muscle irritation may also be present. The psoas sign is an indication of irritation near that muscle. The patient lies on his or her left side, and the examiner slowly extends the right thigh which stretches the ileopsoas muscle. This is positive if extension produces pain. A positive obturator sign is produced by passive internal rotation of the flexed right thigh with the patient supine. This hypogastric pain indicates irritation of the obturator or internus muscle.

Laboratory and Diagnostic Testing

Moderate leukocytosis ranging from 10,000 to 18,000 per mm^3 with a moderate polypmorphonucleaic nuclear cell (PMN) predominance indicates uncomplicated acute appendicitis. If the appendix is perforated, white cell counts are higher than 18,000 per mm^3 or if there is an extreme shift to the left. Radiography is used only when the diagnosis cannot be made by history and physical examination. Plane films of the abdomen often show a distended loop of small bowel in the right lower quadrant. A radiopaque fecalith in the right lower quadrant is nearly always associated with appendicitis. Barium enema studies can also be helpful when done gently. A nonfilling appendix and mass effect on the cecum or terminal ileum are findings of appendicitis. Chest films sometimes are necessary to rule out disease of the right lower lobe lung field. The lesion here would irritate nerves at T10, T11, and T12, and may simulate appendicitis.

Management

Ideally, the appendix should be removed before rupture to prevent complications. Appendicitis cannot be treated with antibiotics because of its obstructive etiology. For a ruptured appendix, with or without abscess, the patient should be prepared for surgery and given intravenous fluids and antibiotics. Some believe that treating the abscess and delaying the appendectomy for 6 weeks to 3 months should be the treatment course.

▶ ENTERAL ACCESS DEVICES

Choosing the Enteral Access Device

Gastric Versus Small Bowel Devices

Gastric devices are more common than small bowel devices, because they are generally easier to insert and can accommodate all feeding schedules. Gastric feedings can be administered as a bolus or intermittent drip, freeing the patient from the tube-feeding administration set for most of the day. However, these devices are only appropriate for those patients who have adequate gastric emptying and intact gag and cough reflexes.

Small bowel devices are recommended when gastric emptying is delayed such as during the early postoperative or posttrauma course, when nasogastric tube output is high, and during periods of emesis. In these cases, patients may need temporary decompression and drainage of the stomach with a gastric device while feeding distally in the small bowel. Patients with any compromise in glottic closure or cough reflex are candidates for small bowel devices to minimize aspiration risk. This includes ventilated or obtunded patients. In addition, small bowel devices may be considered with gastric outlet obstruction, significant gastroesophageal reflux disease, and upper gastrointestinal fistulas. Jejunostomy tubes are appropriate after extensive upper gastrointestinal surgery such as esophagectomy, pancreaticoduodenectomy, or total gastrectomy. Figure 41–2 shows placements for enteral access.

Short-Term Versus Long-Term Devices

Nasoenteric feeding tubes are short-term devices used when enteral tube feedings are needed for no more than 8 to 12 weeks. If tube feedings are needed after this period of time, a long-term device such as a gastrostomy or jejunostomy should be inserted to avoid sinusitis, erosion of the nasal septum or esophagus, or distal esophageal stricture. A long-term device is also used when it is too risky to insert a nasoenteric feeding tube such as with oropharyngeal surgeries; nasal fractures or bleeds; and esophageal varices, strictures, or fistulas. A cervical pharyngostomy may be performed for small-bore feeding-tube placement when nasal or oropharyngeal surgery prohibits the insertion of a nasally placed tube.

Nasoenteric Tube Insertion and Detection of Tube Position

Nasoenteric feeding tube insertion is usually a bedside procedure and can be performed by registered nurses or nurse practitioners who are properly trained (Figs. 41–3 and 41–4). Measurement of minimum tube length needed for gastric placement is estimated by adding the distance of the tube from the tip of the nose to an earlobe to the bottom of the xiphoid process. Small bowel placement in an adult requires at least 40 inches of tubing or more. For small bowel feedings, the tube tip should be inserted to the ligament of Treitz or jejunum to prevent reflux of the feeding formula (Gutske, Varma, & Soergel, 1970) or migration of the tube itself back into the stomach.

Nasal passage can be facilitated by asking the patient which nostril is easier to breathe from or looking in each nostril and selecting the larger one. Neosynephrine nosedrops may aid placement in patients with a boggy mucosa. The tube tip should be lubricated and then guided down the natural curvature of the nasal vault to the esophagus. At this point the patient's head should be bent forward and, if possible, the patient should be asked to swallow while the practitioner directs the feeding tube posteriorly. If the patient has a hyperactive gag reflux, a topical anesthetic sprayed at the back of the throat may aid tube placement.

When the tube tip is in far enough for gastric position, it should be checked. Auscultation of insufflated air is not a reliable method to detect tube-tip location (Metheny, McSweeney, & Wehrle, 1990; Neumann & Meyer, 1995), although the tube tip is probably in the esophagus or mouth if the air eructates through the mouth. Also, if air is insufflated easily through the feeding tube, the tube is probably not kinked. Aspiration of fluid through the tube, on the other hand, can give some information as to tube-tip location. Using a 60-mL syringe, insufflate 30 mL of air through

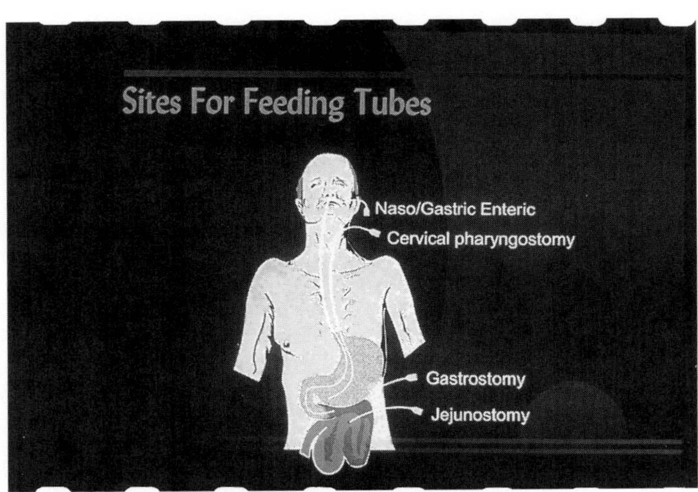

Figure 41–2. Placements for enteral access.

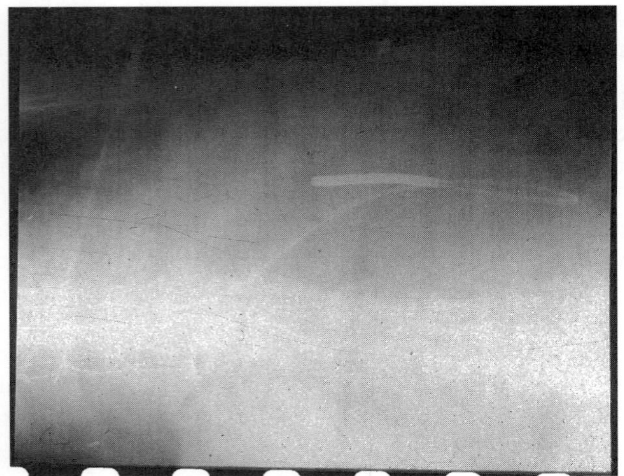

Figure 41–3. Radiographic film of a nasoenteric feeding tube placed into the stomach.

the tube, then attempt aspiration (Methany, Reed, & Wiersema, 1993). Gastric aspirates tend to be cloudy and green, tan, off-white, or brown. Intestinal aspirates are generally distinctly clear and yellow or bile-colored. Unfortunately, respiratory aspirates can be pale yellow, serous, off-white, or tan, and appear similar to gastric aspirates (Methany, Reed, & Bergland, 1994). However, if at least 15 to 20 mL of fluid can be retrieved by aspiration, the tube tip is probably not in the lung as lung fluid tends to dissipate.

In addition to visualizing the aspirate, pH paper testing can further predict tube-tip location. If the pH is highly acidic, less than or equal to 4, gastric placement is usually assured (Neumann & Meyer, 1995). The pH of the small intestine rises to 6 or more and respiratory pH is usually more alkaline with a pH over 7. However, gastric pH can rise with antacids, H2 receptor antagonists (Methany et al., 1993), enteral tube-feeding formulas, and reflux of intestinal bile (Fuchs & DeMeester, 1990). No current method for tube-tip location can replace a radiographic film, but the visualization and pH paper testing of aspirates can offer some useful information prior to obtaining the radiographic film or advancing the feeding tube further into the small bowel. A tracheally intubated patient offers no guarantee against feeding-tube insertion into the lung.

Many successful bedside techniques for small bowel placement of feeding tubes have been described. The following techniques require an experienced practitioner and have a reported success rate of 87 to 93%: bending the distal end of the stylet 30 to 45 degrees with rotation of the tube during insertion (Davis, Sun, & Dalton, 1994; Thurlow, 1986; Zaloga, 1991), gastric insufflation (Schultz, Santanello, Monk, et al., 1993; Ugo, Mohler, & Wilson, 1992), or the feel of decreased resistance at the pylorus followed by small bowel motility "pull" (Caufield, Page, & Pestana, 1991). Some of these techniques involve right lateral decubitus positioning (Shultz et al., 1993; Thurlow, 1986; Ugo et al., 1992; Zaloga, 1991). These methods take an average of 15 to 40 minutes to accomplish. Another method requiring preinsertion metoclopramide and an unweighted feeding tube uses no special bedside insertion technique, takes an average of 5 minutes to perform, and has a success rate of about 90% (Lord, Weiser-Maimone, Pulhamus, et al., 1993). If bedside techniques are unsuccessful, feedings tubes can be placed into the small bowel under fluoroscopy or endoscopy. However, these methods require special equipment, are more costly, and often involve scheduling delays.

Enteral Device Care and Treatment of Problems

Monitoring Enteral Device Position

All nasoenteric feeding tubes or long-term devices should be monitored to detect any migration of the device inward or outward. Some devices have numerical markings that

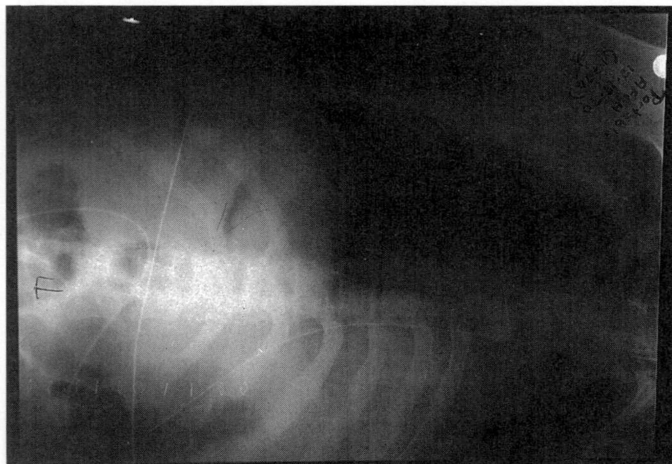

Figure 41–4. Radiographic film of a nasoenteric feeding tube placed into the small bowel.

serve as a reference for tube location, but if not, the site of entry into the nares or stoma tract should be marked with tape or indelible ink.

Enteral Device Malposition and Treatment

Inward migration of a nasogastric feeding tube into the small bowel may lead to diarrhea if the feeding infusion rate is rapid. In addition, some medications, such as sulcrafate or antacids, require gastric administration. The malpositioned tube should be partially pulled back and secured. On the other hand, migration of a small bowel feeding tube into a stomach that has delayed emptying may lead to high feeding residuals, vomiting, and potential aspiration. In this case, the tube must be removed and a new tube inserted as far as possible into the small bowel. Nasoenteric feeding tubes can be secured to the nose or cheek with tape or transparent physiologic dressings; however, this may not be adequate in confused or young patients. A nasal bridle can be inserted around the nasal septum with the ends tied together outside the nose. A nasal bridle can either be a small-bore tube (Forlaw, Chernoff, & Guenter, 1990) or umbilical tape (Popovich, Lockrem, & Zivot, 1996). The nasoenteric feeding tube is then attached to the nasal bridle with a clamp or sutures. If the patient pulls the tube, the nasal bridle prevents it from being dislodged.

Gastrostomy and jejunostomy device position should also be monitored closely. Inward migration of a gastrostomy device and balloon can block off the pyloric channel and cause vomiting. This can be prevented by gently pulling the device outward and securing the external disc at about 1/4-inch leeway from the skin. If an external disc is not available, the tube needs to be sutured or taped into position. Leakage of formula or gastrointestinal contents may occur when the gastrostomy or jejunostomy device has migrated outward into the stoma tract. The tube needs to be reinserted and secured. If the device contains an internal balloon, the water content in the balloon should be aspirated to see if the volume is adequate. An appropriate amount of water should be reinstilled into the balloon to keep the device positioned. If the water aspirated is less than the amount originally instilled, the balloon may have a leak and a replacement gastrostomy device needs to be inserted (Fig. 41–5).

Pain occurring during feedings may be caused by device migration outward into the peritoneal space and probably requires radiographic evaluation for repositioning. If a gastrostomy or jejunostomy tube has completely dislodged out of a mature stoma tract, the same tube should be immediately reinserted until it can be replaced with a new device. These tracts can close off within hours. Early dislodgement of a percutaneous gastrostomy tube before an adhesion has formed between the stomach and abdominal wall can lead to peritonitis and is therefore a medical emergency. These patients often require surgical exploration.

Maintaining Enteral Device Patency

In order to keep enteral devices patent, they should be flushed regularly with water and a pump used when feeding infusion rates are slow. In order to prevent tube rupture, a pressure no greater than 40 p.s.i. should be reached with a syringe or infusion pump. Syringe sizes of at least 30 mL for gastrostomy tubes and 60 mL for nasoenteric or jejunostomy tubes should be used for fluid flushes. At least a 20 to 30 mL water flush is recommended every four hours with continuous feedings and before and after intermittent feedings and medications (Scanlan & Frisch, 1992). Solutions with an acidic pH can precipitate the protein in enteral formulas and cause clogging. Therefore, acidic fluids such as cranberry juice should not be used as tube irrigants (Methany, Eisenberg, & McSweeney, 1988; Wilson & Haynes-Johnson, 1988). In addition, enteral devices should be flushed with water before and after checking for gastric residuals to avoid gastric acid precipitation of proteins (Powell, Marcuard, Farrior, et al., 1993).

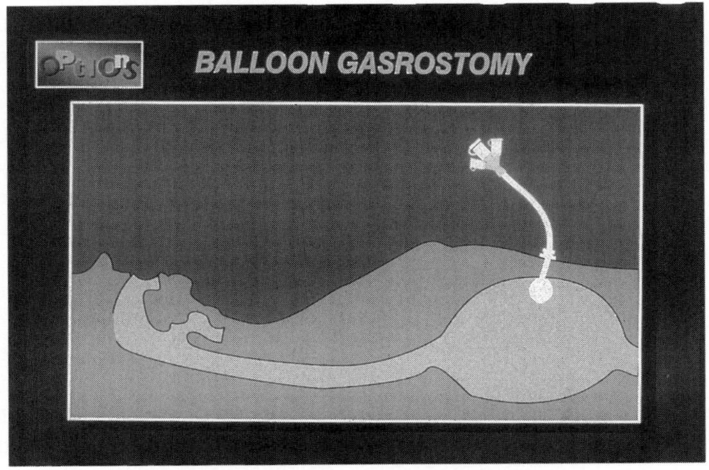

Figure 41–5. Ballon gastrostomy.

The risk of clogging is affected by the type of enteral access, feeding-formula composition, bacterial contamination of the feeding formula, and medication instillation. Enteral-device clogging is more frequent with nasoenteric feeding tubes and jejunostomies tubes compared with gastrostomy tubes due to their longer length and smaller internal diameters. Feeding formulas that are calorically dense or contain fiber are more viscous and therefore more prone to clogging enteral devices. Bacterial contamination of a feeding formula can occur by not utilizing clean technique during formula preparation or hanging a formula at room temperature longer than the manufacturer's recommended hang times. Medications may be given through enteral devices, but must be done carefully. Liquid forms of medication should be administered when possible. Thick syrups and bulk-forming agents should be avoided. Solid tablets that are crushed into a fine powder and adequately dissolved in water can be given (Scanlan & Frisch, 1992) as long as they are not enteric-coated or sustained-release. Medications should be given separately to avoid precipitation and at least a 5-mL water flush administered between each one.

Salvaging a Clogged Enteral Access Device

As soon as a clogged tube is discovered, the declogging process should begin to improve the chances of success (Mateo, 1994). Initially, a syringe of warm water is used to aspirate, then irrigate the tube. Water has been found to be just as effective as carbonated beverages and proteolytic agents like papain (meat tenderizer) (Marcuard, Stegall, & Trogdon, 1989). If a syringe of warm water does not dislodge the clog, a solution of pancrealipase activated with sodium bicarbonate is useful (Marcuard & Stegall, 1990). The following steps are common to the syringe method of declogging an enteral access device:

1. Attach a 30 mL to 60 mL syringe to the end of the enteral device and aspirate as much fluid as possible. Discard the fluid.
2. Fill the syringe with 5 mL of warm water and attach it to the end of the enteral device. Instill the water under manual pressure for one minute. A back-and-forth motion of the plunger may also be used to help detach the clog.
3. Leave the water in the device and clamp it for 5 to 15 minutes.
4. Refill the syringe with 5 mL of warm water and try to aspirate or flush the device.
5. If the device remains clogged, repeat this procedure substituting a pancrealipase–sodium bicarbonate solution in step 2. (**Note:** A pancrealipase–sodium bicarbonate solution may be made by mixing one crushed Viokase tablet or 1 teaspoon Viokase powder with one crushed 325-mg nonenteric-coated sodium bicarbonate tablet or 1/8 teaspoon baking soda dissolved in 5 mL warm water.)

Manufacturers have developed mechanical devices for declogging that include small-diameter hollow catheters and plastic decloggers that are inserted into the clogged enteral device. Practitioners attempting to employ these mechanical devices should be educated as to their use. The french size and length of the enteral device must be obtained so that the appropriate mechanical device can be obtained. The mechanical device is then measured so as not to exceed the length of the enteral device. This is to prevent breakage of the enteral device. Small-diameter hollow catheters allow the instillation of the declogging solution directly proximate to the clog. Plastic decloggers have threaded ends and mechanically break up the clog with a twisting motion. There is an enteral feeding tube declogging kit marketed that combines the use of a small-diameter hollow catheter and a patented "enzyme cocktail" and buffer system, "Clog Zapper" by Corpak Medsystems.

Management of Gastrostomy and Jejunostomy Insertion Sites

Immediately after insertion of gastrostomies and jejunostomies, a dry sterile dressing is usually applied. This may be removed after 24 hours and the site left open to air. A solution of half-strength peroxide may be used to remove any dried-up drainage around the site but is irritating to healing tissue. The insertion site may be gently cleansed daily with soap and water, followed by a water rinse (Kundz, 1992). A cotton-tip applicator can be useful for cleaning around any external discs.

Complications

Pressure Necrosis

When skin breakdown is noted at the insertion site, the distance between any internal and external discs needs to be assessed. There should be about a 1/4-inch leeway between the skin and external disc when the patient is in the sitting position. If the discs are too tight, the external disc needs to be gently pulled outward. The external disc needs to be adjusted periodically in patients who are gaining weight or otherwise undergoing changes in their abdominal girth size.

Infection

A topical antibiotic ointment may be indicated if there's evidence of increasing site redness, excoriation, firmness, warmth, and purulent drainage. Systemic antibiotics may be necessary if these symptoms are accompanied by a fever unattributed to any other source, but this is rare. A fungal overgrowth may occur with topical antibiotic use, which manifests as a maculopapular rash. In this case, the site should be kept as dry as possible, and an antifungal cream or powder applied. Fungal rashes may also occur in areas where there is persistent skin moisture, which is why the site should be left open to air. Culturing of the exit site is inappropriate as there is always contamination. Attempts to eradicate these organisms lead to selection of resistant bacteria.

Granulation Tissue

The formation of granulation tissue around gastrostomy and jejunostomy sites is a common occurrence in active patients. It appears as raised, shiny, beefy-red tissue and emerges from around the insertion site. Granulation tissue is formed from rapid epithelialization, excess movement, or trapped moisture. Gastric contents may leak from the stoma site until the granulation tissue is eliminated. Treatment entails the topical application of silver nitrate sticks, 2 to 3 times per week for 2 to 3 weeks as needed. The access device should be securely positioned to prevent movement and the site kept clean and dry.

Removal of Gastrostomies and Jejunostomies

Most gastrostomies have either an internal balloon that is deflated prior to removal or an internal disc or mushroom made of flexible plastic that somewhat deforms as the device is pulled outward. Percutaneous endoscopic gastrostomies should not be removed for at least three weeks after insertion because the internal balloon or disc holds it in position. If the tract is not properly healed, the stomach may separate from the peritoneum and gastric contents can leak internally requiring surgical repair. With open gastrostomy or jejunostomy tubes, the stomach or intestine is sutured to the abdominal wall and they, therefore, can be removed safely at any time. The practitioner secures the skin surrounding the device with the fingers of one hand and firmly pulls the device outward with the other hand. This is a quick, but painful procedure and a topical anesthetic is often used. Premedication with an analgesic and sedative can be used with devices that contain a plastic internal disc, as these are more difficult to remove. If the internal disc is too large to deform, cutting the external portion of the gastrostomy tube should be discouraged. If the internal disc is allowed to pass through the bowel, it may not pass through the ileocecal valve and then require surgical removal. A few gastrostomy devices require endoscopic removal. Jejunostomy tubes generally are easier to remove as no internal disc or balloon holds them in place. After removal of the enteral device, the site is covered with a sterile gauze for about 24 hours while the tract closes.

REFERENCES

Aronsson, B., Mollby, R., & Nord, C. E. (1984). Diagnosis and epidemiology of *Clostridium difficile* enterocolitis in Sweden. *Journal of Antimicrobial Chemotherapy, 14* (suppl), 85–95.

Bliss, D. Z., Guenter, P. A., & Settle, R. G. (1992). Defining and reporting diarrhea in tube-fed patients—What a mess! *American Journal of Clinical Nutrition, 55,* 753–759.

Caufield, K. A., Page, C. P., & Pestana, C. (1991). Technique for intraduodenal placement of transnasal enteral feeding catheters. *Nutrition Clinical Practitioner, 6,* 23–26.

Davis, T. J., Sun, D., & Dalton, M. L. (1994). A modified technique for bedside placement of nasoduodenal feeding tubes. *Journal of the American College of Surgeons, 178,* 407–409.

Forlaw, L., Chernoff, R., & Guenter, P. (1990). Enteral delivery systems. In J. Rombeau, M. Caldwell (Eds.), *Clinical nutrition: Enteral and tube feeding* (pp. 179–182). Philadelphia: W. B. Saunders.

Fuchs, K. & DeMeester, T. (1990). Intragastric pH pattern analysis in patients with duodenogastric reflux. *Digestive Diseases 8,* (suppl 1), 54–59.

Goroll, A. H., May, L. A., & Mulley, A. G. (1995). Gastrointestinal problems. *Primary Care Medicine.* Philadelphia: J. B. Lippincott.

Gutske, R. F., Varma, R. R., & Soergel, K. H. (1970). Gastric reflux during perfusion of the proximal small bowel. *Gastroenterology, 59,* 890–895.

Hubbard, P. (1998). Hepatitis C. *The American Journal for Nurse Practitioners, 2* (11), 17–31.

Illig, K. A. & Cowles-Husser, W. (1996). Biliary tract, peptic ulcer disease, and jaundice. In K. A. Illig & W. C. Husser (Eds.), *The Rochester Manual: Practical Patient Care.* New Jersey: Laennec Publishing.

Kundz, J. (1992). Nursing implications for patients with a percutaneous endoscopic gastrostomy or jejunostomy. *Gastrointestinal Endoscopy Clinics of North America, 2,* 207–213.

Levy, E., Frileux, P., Sandrucci, S., et al. (1988). Continuous enteral nutrition during the early adaptive stages of the short bowel syndrome. *British Journal of Surgery, 75,* 549–553.

Liang, B. A., Fendrick, A. M., & Chey, W. D. Approach to the patient with Helicobacter pylori-associated epigastric pain. *Hospital Physician, 2198,* 36–44.

Lord, L. M. & Sax, H. S. (1994). The role of the gut in critical illness. *AACN Clinical Issues, 5* (10), 450–458.

Lord, L. M., Weiser-Maimone, A., Pulhamus, M., et al. (1993). Comparison of weighted vs. unweighted enteral feeding tubes for efficacy of transpyloric intubation. *JPEN, 17,* 271–273.

Marcuard, S. P., Stegall, K. L., & Trogdon, S. (1989). Clearing obstructed feeding tubes. *JPEN, 13,* 81–83.

Marcuard, S. P. & Stegall, K. L. (1990). Unclogging feeding tubes with pancreatic enzyme. *JPEN, 14,* 198–200.

Mateo, M. A. (1994). Maintaining patency of enteral feeding tubes. *The Online Journal of Knowledge Synthesis for Nursing, 1,* 1–13.

Methany, N., Eisenberg, P., & McSweeney, M. (1988). Effect of feeding tube properties and three irrigants on clogging rates. *Nursing Research, 37,* 165–169.

Metheny, N., McSweeney, M., & Wehrle, M. A. (1990). Effectiveness of the ausculatory method in predicting feeding tube location. *Nursing Research, 39,* 262–267.

Methany, N., Reed, L., & Bergland, B. (1994). Visual characteristics of aspirates from feeding tubes as a method for predicting tube location. *Nursing Research, 43,* 282–287.

Methany, N., Reed, L. & Wiersema, L. (1993). Effectiveness of pH measurements in predicting feeding tube placement: An update. *Nursing Research, 42,* 324–331.

Neumann, M. J. & Meyer, C. T. (1995). Hold that x-ray: Aspirate pH and auscultation prove enteral tube placement. *Journal of Clinical Gastroenterology, 20,* 293–295.

Popovich, M. J., Lockrem, J. D., & Zivot, J. B. (1996). Nasal bridle revisited: An improvement in the technique to prevent unintentional removal of small-bore nasoenteric feeding tubes. *Critical Care Medicine, 24,* 429–431.

Powell, K. S., Marcuard S. P., Farrior, E. S., et al. (1993). Aspirating gastric residuals causes occlusion of small-bore feeding tubes. *JPEN, 17,* 243–246.

Scanlan, M. & Frisch, S. (1992). Nasoduodenal feeding tubes: Prevention of occlusion. *Journal of Neuroscience Nursing, 24,* 256–259.

Schultz, M. A., Santanello, S. A., Monk, J., et al. (1993). An improved method for transpyloric placement of nasoenteric feeding tubes. *International Surgery, 78,* 79–82.

Schwartz, S. I., Shires G. T., & Spencer, F. C. (1994). Liver. *Principles of Surgery.* New York: McGraw-Hill.

Thurlow, P. M. (1986). Bedside enteral feeding tube placement into duodenum and jejunum. *JPEN, 10,* 104–105.

Ugo, P. J., Mohler, P. A., & Wilson, G. L. (1992). Bedside postpyloric placement of weighted feeding tubes. *Nutrition Clinical Practititioner, 7, 284–287.*

Way, L. (1991.) Stomach and duodenum, liver, biliary tract, pancreas. In L. W. Way (Ed.) *Current surgical diagnosis and treatment.* Norwalk, CT: Appleton & Lange.

Wilson, M. F. & Haynes-Johnson V. (1988). Cranberry juice or water? A comparison of feeding-tube irrigants. *Nutritional Support Services, 37,* 165–169.

Zaloga, G. P. (1991). Bedside method for placing small bowel feeding tubes in critically ill patients. *Chest, 100,* 1643–1646.

42

Renal Problems

Kathleen M. Powers
Mildred Lam

Patients with renal or urinary tract disease are commonly encountered in both acute care settings and in outpatient areas. The chief complaint of a patient with renal disease may be initially attributed to disease in another organ system. For example, a patient who presents with edema may be thought to have cardiac failure; only after investigation, however, is nephrotic syndrome diagnosed. On the other hand, a chief complaint that relates to the kidneys or urinary tract may be a sign of multisystem disease. For instance, a patient with hematuria may have metastatic carcinoma.

This chapter begins with a brief review of renal and urinary tract anatomy and physiology. The major portion of the chapter is devoted to five common renal syndromes: urinary tract infection, hematuria, proteinuria (including nephrotic syndrome), acute renal failure, and chronic renal failure.

▶ RENAL ANATOMY AND PHYSIOLOGY

Anatomy of the Kidney

The kidneys are located in the retroperitoneal space on either side of the aorta and vena cava. Each kidney weighs approximately 125 gm; but together, these organs, which together account for less than 0.5% of body weight, receive about 20% of cardiac output.

Each kidney is connected to the aorta by a renal artery and to the inferior vena cava by a renal vein. The main renal artery branches into several segmental arteries, which then progressively branch within the kidney itself into lobar, arcuate, and interlobular arteries. Interlobular arteries, which are located in the cortical (outer) zone of the kidney, give rise to afferent arterioles, each of which supplies a glomerulus and its nephron.

The kidney is covered by a thin layer called Glisson's capsule, which contains many nerve fibers. Acute stretching of the renal capsule causes exquisite pain. Such pain may occur, for instance, in acute obstruction of a ureter by a kidney stone, in subcapsular accumulation of a traumatic perinephric hematoma, or in acute pyelonephritis with generalized edema of the kidney. Renal parenchyma consists of two zones: cortical (outer) and medullary (inner). The outer or cortical zone contains all of the glomeruli, while the medullary zone contains tubules, loops of Henle, and collecting ducts.

The basic functional unit of the kidney is the nephron; each kidney contains approximately 1 million nephrons. Each nephron has several parts (Fig. 42–1). The afferent arteriole (which arises from an interlobular artery) enters Bowman's space and branches into a glomerular capillary network, which then coalesces into an efferent arteriole. Bowman's capsule, a layer of parietal epithelium that surrounds the glomerular capillaries and their associated cells, is contiguous with the proximal tubule of the nephron. The tubular portion of the nephron consists of the proximal convoluted and proximal straight tubules; the thin descending, thin ascending, and thick ascending limbs of the loop of Henle; the distal convoluted tubule; and the collecting duct, which drains into the renal calyces.

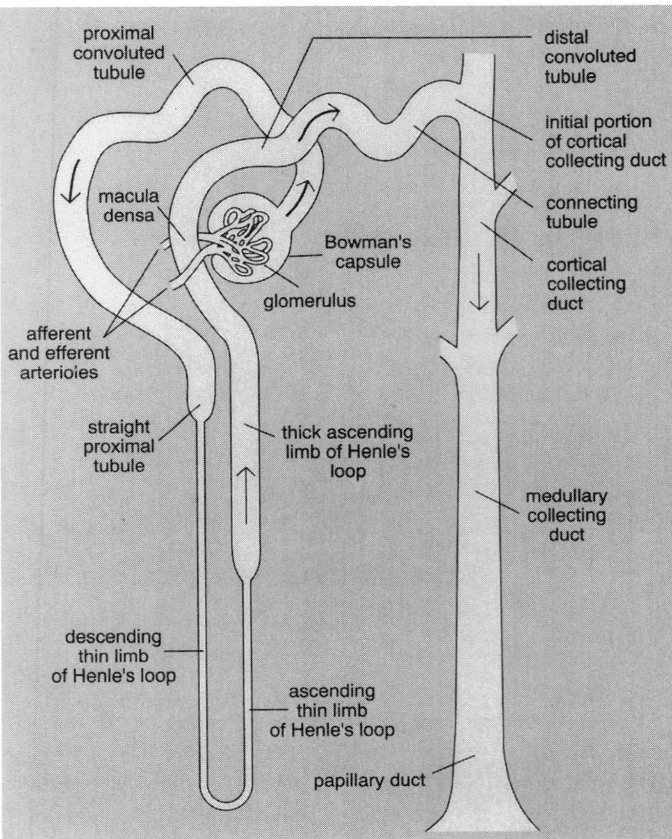

Figure 42–1. Parts of the nephron: afferent and efferent arterioles, glomerulus, proximal convoluted tubule, loop of Henle, distal convoluted tubule, and collecting duct. Blood enters the afferent arteriole and flows through glomerular capillaries to form a plasma ultrafiltrate which enters the proximal tubule. As it travels through the convoluted tubules, loop of Henle, and collecting duct, the ultrafiltrate is gradually transformed into urine. *(Used with permission from Vander. [1995].)*

Blood enters the nephron through afferent arteriole, traverses the glomerular capillary network, and exits the glomerulus through the efferent arteriole. As blood travels through the glomerular capillaries, a fraction of the plasma component (about 20%) is filtered through the glomerular filtration barrier, forming an ultrafiltrate that enters Bowman's space. From there, the ultrafiltrate flows into the proximal tubule and begins its trip through the proximal tubule, loop of Henle, distal tubule, and collecting duct, undergoing transformation from plasma ultrafiltrate into urine.

Urine exits from the collecting ducts and papillae into the collecting system, which consists of calyces, renal pelvis, and ureter for each kidney. Urine flows down the ureters, is stored in the urinary bladder, and ultimately is excreted via the urethra (Fig. 42–2).

Basic Renal Physiology

There are several functions of the kidney. The best-known function is an excretory one: the kidney helps the body eliminate toxic products of normal metabolism. Equally important, however, is the kidney's role in the regulation of both extracellular fluid volume (ECFV) and plasma osmolality (P_{osm}). ECFV is maintained constant through the regulation of renal sodium excretion, while P_{osm} is maintained through regulation of water excretion. A third function of the kidney is to regulate the composition of the extracellular fluid with respect to certain ions, notably potassium, calcium, magnesium, and phosphate. The kidney also plays an important role in maintaining the body's acid–base balance. Finally, the kidney serves as an endocrine organ, producing several important hormones or autacoids such as renin, erythropoietin, vitamin D metabolites, and prostaglandins. Each of the major functions of the kidney is discussed in more detail later; first, however, a discussion of basic renal processes is necessary.

Basic Renal Processes

Three basic processes transform blood that enters the kidney into urine: filtration, reabsorption, and secretion.

Filtration is the process by which blood entering afferent arterioles is transformed into a plasma ultrafiltrate. Blood must pass through the glomerular filtration barrier, which has three layers: the fenestrated glomerular capillary

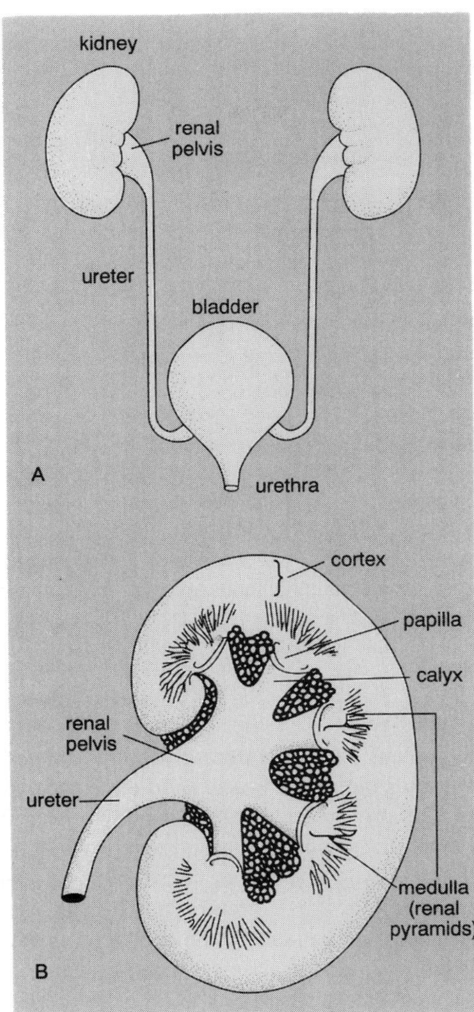

Figure 42–2. A, The urinary collecting system: calyces, renal pelvis, ureters, bladder, and urethra. **B,** Sagittal section of a kidney: all glomeruli are located in the **cortex.** After traversing proximal tubules, loops of Henle, and distal tubules, tubular fluid flows into the **collecting ducts,** which are located in the **medullary pyramids.** Multiple collecting ducts converge to form a **papilla,** from which urine empties into a **calyx. Calyces** converge into the **renal pelvis,** which funnels into the **ureter.** *(Used with permission from Vander. [1995].)*

endothelium, the basement membrane itself (a mucopolysaccharide-rich, highly negatively charged layer), and the foot processes, or extensions, of the epithelial cells that cover the glomerular capillaries (Fig. 42–3). This three-layered barrier normally does not permit the passage of larger elements such as blood cells and protein molecules. Generally substances of molecular weight >50,000 daltons are unable to pass the filtration barrier, especially if they are negatively charged (e.g., albumin, which has a molecular weight of 69,000 and is highly anionic). Substances that are able to pass freely through the filtration barrier include water, creatinine, urea, sodium, potassium, chloride, bicarbonate, and a host of electrolytes and small molecules. These form an ultrafiltrate of plasma, which collects in Bowman's space and begins its journey down the proximal tubule, where it undergoes further alteration by the remaining two processes.

Glomerular filtration rate (GFR) can be calculated from a 24-hour urine sample by the following formula:

$$\text{GFR} = \text{creatinine clearance} = \frac{U_{cr} \times V}{P_{cr}}$$

where U_{cr} is the urinary concentration of creatinine in mg/dL, P_{cr} is the plasma concentration of creatinine in mg/dL, and V is the urine flow rate in mL/min. Normal GFR ranges from 100 to 150 mL/min.

Reabsorption is the process by which ions and molecules in the filtrate are returned to the circulation instead of being excreted in urine. It is an energy-requiring process, generally powered by the enzyme Na^+-K^+ATPase, an ATP-splitting enzyme located in the renal tubular cells. The process of tubular reabsorption occurs mainly in the proximal tubular cells, but takes place to a lesser extent in the loop of Henle and distal tubular cells. Each day reabsorption salvages thousands of mEq of sodium, chloride, bicarbonate, and other ions, as well as nearly 200 liters of water, which would otherwise be lost in the urine.

Secretion is the process by which tubular cells can extract a substance from the circulation and add it to what has been filtered by the glomeruli. The major cation that undergoes tubular secretion in the normal state is potassium. Like reabsorption, tubular secretion is an energy-requiring process and allows transport of ions and molecules from the peritubular capillaries, through tubular cells, and into the lumen of the nephron, ultimately resulting in their excretion in the urine. Tubular secretion of ions allows enhanced excretion of potassium, hydrogen ion, and a multitude of other organic acids and bases. Excretion of these substances would otherwise be limited to what could enter the tubular lumen by glomerular filtration alone.

Normal renal blood flow is 1000 to 1200 mL/min. Of the blood that enters the kidney, approximately 55% is plasma, and of the plasma fraction, about 20% is filtered through the glomerular basement membrane and enters the proximal tubule. Normal glomerular filtration rate is thus 100 to 150 mL/min, or 150 to 180 L/day.

Glomerular filtrate contains approximately 150 to 180 liters of water, 25,000 mEq of sodium, and 4300 mEq of bicarbonate per day. Tubular reabsorption returns over 99% of filtered water, sodium, and bicarbonate into the circulation, preventing these precious substances from being lost in the urine. We excrete less than 1% of the vast amount of these substances that are filtered by the glomeruli.

Figure 42–4 illustrates the segments of the nephron where reabsorption and secretion of sodium, potassium, and water take place.

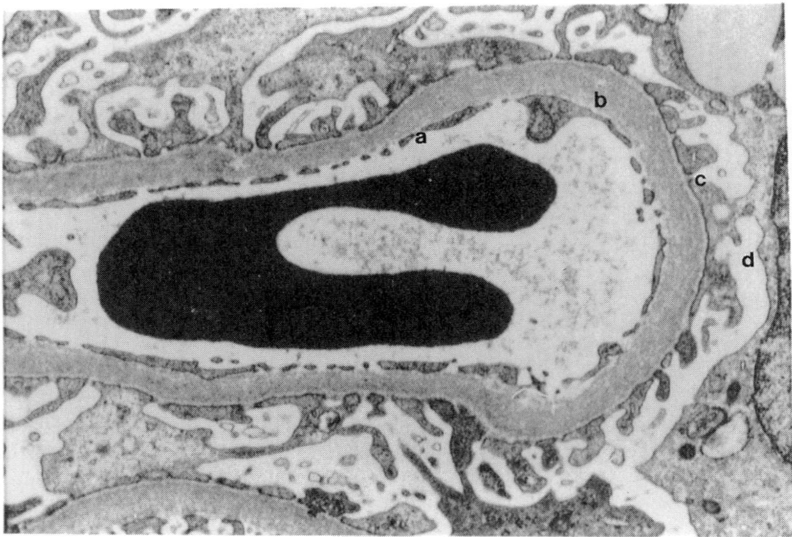

Figure 42–3. A single glomerular capillary loop containing a red blood cell in its lumen and demonstrating the layers of the glomerular filtration barrier: fenestrated capillary endothelium (A), glomerular basement membrane (B), epithelial cell foot processes (C). Plasma traverses the glomerular barrier from the endothelial (lumen) to the epithelial side, forming an ultrafiltrate which enters Bowman's space (D) and is collected into the proximal convoluted tubule. *(x6400; Courtesy of Benjamin Sturgill, MD.)*

Functions of the Kidney

Excretion of Metabolic Waste Products. The kidney is the organ primarily responsible for removing certain waste products of metabolism from the body—in particular, urea, a product of protein metabolism, and creatinine, a product of muscle metabolism. Each of these small molecules is freely filtered at the glomerulus and thus passes from the circulation into the renal tubules. A portion of filtered urea is reabsorbed by the renal tubules, but approximately 50% is ultimately excreted by the nephron. Filtered creatinine is not reabsorbed, but is secreted in small amounts by the tubules. Thus, although the tubular handling of these two substances differs, each reaches the urine primarily by means of glomerular filtration. In addition to these two major metabolic waste products, there are countless others that are excreted from the body primarily by the kidney. However, because the blood levels of both urea and creatinine are easily measured, these two substances are used as markers for the excretory function of the kidney. Blood levels of urea and creatinine rise in proportion to decreases in glomerular filtration rate, and their measurement thus provides a simple way of estimating renal function.

Regulation of Extracellular Volume and Osmolality. The kidney maintains a constant extracellular fluid volume (ECFV) and plasma osmolality (P_{osm}). ECFV

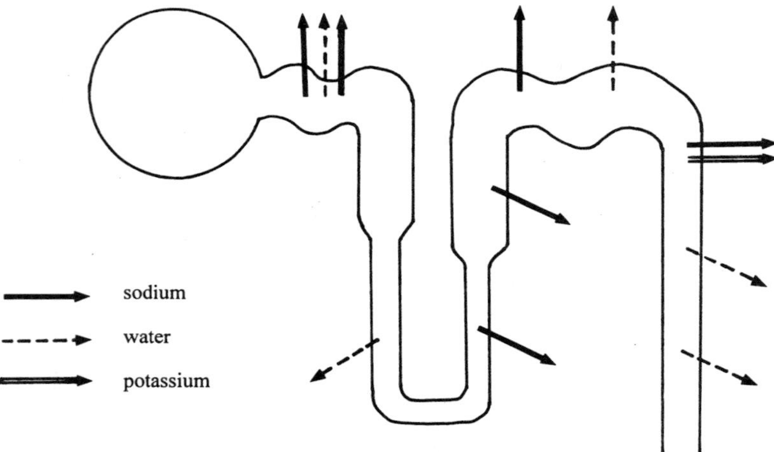

Figure 42–4. Sites of renal tubular reabsorption and/or secretion of sodium, potassium, and water.

is regulated primarily through renal reabsorption and excretion of sodium, while P_{osm} is regulated through renal reabsorption and excretion of water. Renal tubular reabsorption of sodium and water is influenced by a number of factors. A major factor is intravascular volume, which is detected by stretch receptors, or baroreceptors, located in the cardiac atria and some of the great vessels, as well as in the renal afferent arterioles. Other factors affecting the kidney's reabsorption of sodium and water include neural factors such as sympathetic nervous system activity, and hormones such as angiotensin (made in the general circulation), aldosterone (made in the adrenal cortex), and antidiuretic hormone (released by the pituitary gland).

Regulation of Extracellular Fluid Composition. The kidney also plays a role in regulating the blood concentrations of numerous ions, including potassium, calcium, phosphate, and magnesium. Maintenance of plasma concentrations of these ions within a very narrow range is crucial for normal cardiac and neuromuscular function. The regulation of these substances is achieved through a combination of glomerular filtration, tubular reabsorption, and tubular secretion.

Regulation of Acid–Base Balance. Normal metabolism of a typical Western diet results in the generation of approximately 1 mEq/kg/day of hydrogen ion, which must be excreted to prevent development of a life-threatening acidosis. The kidney plays a major role in the excretion of this daily acid load. Renal tubular reabsorption of filtered bicarbonate ion is an important part of this function, since loss of bicarbonate in the urine would cause acidosis. Additionally, the renal tubules are responsible for excretion of H+ in buffered forms, known as titratable acids and ammonium.

Secretion of Hormones and Autacoids. Although the kidney is not usually thought of as an endocrine organ, it does play a role in the functioning of several endocrine systems. The renal afferent arterioles synthesize and release renin, which helps to regulate sodium and water balance. The proximal tubules generate erythropoietin, a hormone that stimulates the bone marrow to produce red blood cells. The kidney also synthesizes a number of metabolites of vitamin D, which plays a major role in normal bone formation and remodeling. The kidney also produces a number of autacoids (substances that are made and used within the same organ), the most important of which are prostaglandins. Prostaglandins affect renal sodium and water handling and thus are important in the normal regulation of extracellular fluid volume and plasma osmolality.

▶ COMMON CLINICAL SYNDROMES

Urinary Tract Infection

Urinary tract infection (UTI) is one of the most common problems seen in outpatient practice. As many as 30% of women with acute urinary tract infections and significant bacteriuria have involvement of the renal parenchyma. Acute cystitis is an infection of the bladder; acute urethritis or acute urethral syndrome involves only the urethra. Acute pyelonephritis is an infection involving the kidney parenchyma and renal pelvis and is caused by ascent of the offending organism from the bladder via the ureters to the kidneys. Bacteria can then enter the renal parenchyma via the renal pelvis and can produce scarring and/or abscesses.

In general, gram-negative bacteria are more commonly seen, although gram-positive organisms (*Enterococcus faecalis* and *Staph aureus*) are occasionally present. In uncomplicated acute infections the most common pathogen is *E coli,* whereas chronic infections are often associated with more unusual pathogens. Approximately 30% of patients with dysuria and pyuria have negative urine cultures; in these patients, acute urethral syndrome caused by agents such as *Chlamydia trachomatis, Neisseria gonorrheae,* or herpes simplex virus should be considered.

History and Physical Findings

Signs and symptoms of a lower UTI (cystitis or urethritis) include dysuria, urgency, frequency, and suprapubic or low back pain. The patient may also describe cloudy or bloody urine. Acute prostatitis is often associated with dysuria, dyspareunia, and pain in the low back, testicular, or perineal area. With acute pyelonephritis, fever, chills, flank (costovertebral angle [CVA]) pain and tenderness, nausea, vomiting, and tachycardia can be seen.

Laboratory and Diagnostic Tests

A dipstick test for pyuria (which measures leukocyte esterase produced by neutrophil granules) has a negative predictive value of >90% and positive predictive value of 50% (Wallach, 1996). For dipstick detection of white blood cells, the sensitivity ranges from 100% for >50 white blood cells/high-power field (WBCs/hpf) to 44% for 6-12 WBCs/hpf. For detection of bacteria, the sensitivity is 73% for large numbers and 46% for moderate numbers of organisms. On microscopic exam the finding of one or more bacteria per oil-immersion field in an unspun urine specimen or the finding of many (>10 and especially >20) bacteria/hpf of the centrifuged sediment correlates well with quantitative cultures of more than 10^5/mL organisms. White blood cell casts are generally indicative of pyelonephritis. Renal tubular epithelial casts suggest the presence of acute tubular necrosis with acute renal failure. Squamous epithelial cells are indicative of contamination, since these originate from the urethra or vagina.

Urine culture should be obtained in any patient with acute pyelonephritis or recurrent lower-tract infection. Routine ordering of a urine culture, especially in a female patient with a first-time uncomplicated cystitis, remains a controversial issue.

Complete blood count (CBC) may reveal a mild leukocytosis even with lower urinary tract infection. A marked leukocytosis, especially with a left shift, suggests acute pyleonephritis.

Radiologic imaging of the urinary tract is not indicated in females with an uncomplicated episode of cystitis or pyelonephritis. However, a male with a urinary tract infection (lower or upper) should be carefully investigated for the presence of a urinary tract abnormality. In males, therefore, and in females with recurrent UTIs or complicated cases of pyelonephritis (persistent fever or flank pain, frequent recurrence, infection with resistant organisms), an intravenous pyelogram, renal ultrasound exam, or computed tomographic (CT) scan may be helpful in identifying an abscess, kidney stone, hydronephrosis, or other urinary tract anomaly.

Management

Many UTIs resolve spontaneously, without antibiotic therapy. Nevertheless, treatment of UTIs is advisable to relieve symptoms and to prevent ascending infections that lead to pyelonephritis. Furthermore, renal parenchymal infections that are inadequately treated can result in progressive loss of renal function. Although first or uncomplicated UTIs may be treated empirically, it is important to obtain a urine culture and sensitivities in cases of recurrent infection, where unusual or resistant organisms may be the cause. If acute urethral syndrome is considered, specific cultures for the etiologic agents listed earlier should be obtained.

An uncomplicated lower UTI may be treated with a single dose of trimethoprim-sulfamethoxazole, 160/800 mg, two tablets; however, such treatment is only about 85% effective. Better results are obtained with a 3-day course of trimethoprim-sulfa or cephalexin, 250 to 500 mg every 6 hours, ciprofloxacin 250 to 500 mg every 12 hours, ofloxacin 200 mg every 12 hours, or norfloxacin 400 mg every 12 hours. Acute prostatitis generally responds well to treatment as for cystitis, with trimethoprim-sulfa, a cephalosporin, or a quinolone.

Acute urethral syndrome caused by chlamydia organisms do not respond to standard antibiotic therapy; 7 days of doxycycline 100 mg twice daily is the treatment of choice. Azithromycin, erythromycin, and ofloxacin are alternative antibiotics for treatment of nongonococcal urethritis.

Acute pyelonephritis requires a lengthier regimen that should be administered intravenously until the patient has been afebrile for at least 24 hours. A typical regimen for uncomplicated pyelonephritis is ampicillin 1 gram IV every 6 hours and gentamicin 1 mg/kg IV every 8 hours initially; then oral amoxicillin/clavulanic acid 500 mg every 8 hours to complete a 14-day course. Alternative regimens for patients with pyelonephritis who are not septic and who are able to tolerate oral fluids and medications are: trimethoprim-sulfamethoxazole 160/800 mg every 12 hours for 14 days, ciprofloxacin 750 mg every 12 hours for 14 days, or ofloxacin 200 to 300 mg every 12 hours for 14 days. For patients with pyelonephritis, urine cultures should be repeated 2 to 3 weeks following completion of the treatment course.

Males with either an upper or lower tract UTI, and females with recurrent UTIs should be referred to a urologist or nephrologist for further work-up. A female with more than two UTIs in a 6-month period may be considered for one of several antibiotic regimens: continuous (or thrice-weekly) prophylaxis, postcoital prophylaxis, or patient-initiated treatment.

Hematuria

Hematuria is defined as the presence of an abnormal number of red blood cells (RBCs) in the urine. Less than 3% of normal people have >3 RBCs/hpf. A single episode of hematuria does not necessarily require a full evaluation, since hematuria may occur with a bacterial or viral infection, exercise, or trauma. However, if there is recurrent gross hematuria or a persistent finding of >3 RBCs/hpf on urinalysis, the patient should have a complete work-up to find the source of hematuria.

History and Physical Findings

Evaluation of hematuria begins with a thorough history and physical. Pinpointing exactly when the hematuria takes place can provide important clues as to its cause. For instance, hematuria is found in approximately 18% of people after strenuous exercise and is commonly found in women after sexual intercourse. Identifying the phase of micturition during which hematuria occurs may help lead to the localization of the disease. For example, initial hematuria (i.e., initially present and clearing by end of urination) is often associated with an anterior urethral cause; terminal hematuria (occurring only at the end of the stream) implies bladder neck or prostatic urethral involvement; and total hematuria (present throughout micturition) suggests the bladder or upper urinary tract (including kidney) as the possible source of bleeding. Symptoms associated with hematuria are important: dysuria, fever, CVA tenderness, and renal colic should all be explored. Current medications, illnesses, and significant past medical history can play an important role in identifying the cause of hematuria. For example, patients with sickle cell trait/disease or analgesic abuse may develop papillary necrosis; antibiotics can cause interstitial nephritis; and cyclophosphamide can cause hemorrhagic cystitis. The most common causes of hematuria are listed in Table 42–1.

Laboratory and Diagnostic Tests

The most important elements in the diagnostic work-up of hematuria follow.

Urinalysis. Gross hematuria is easily detected by the human eye. Note urine color, odor, and appearance. The pres-

TABLE 42–1. Common Causes of Hematuria

Pseudohematuria
- Foods (e.g., beets, blackberries, and rhubarb)
- Medications (e.g., rifampin, phenytoin, phenolphthalein)
- Pigmenturia (e.g., hemoglobin, myoglobin, porphyria)
- Vaginal bleeding
- Oxidizing contaminants (e.g., povidone, hypochlorite, bacterial peroxidases)

Glomerular diseases
- IgA nephropathy
- Goodpasture's syndrome
- Membranoproliferative glomerulonephritis
- Postinfectious glomerulonephritis
- Collagen–vascular diseases (e.g., systemic lupus, polyarteritis nodosa)
- Hemolytic–uremic syndrome

Hereditary diseases
- Hereditary nephritis (Alport's)
- Polycystic kidney disease
- Medullary sponge kidney
- Sickle cell disease or trait

Urinary tract infections
- Urethritis
- Cystitis
- Prostatitis
- Pyelonephritis

Other causes
- Malignancy (kidney, ureters, bladder, prostate)
- Renal infarction
- Trauma
- Schistosomiasis
- AV malformation or varices
- Kidney stones
- Coagulopathy
- Hypercalciuria

ence of clots essentially rules out glomerular diseases, although small stringy clots may be seen in upper tract disease and large thick clots suggest bladder disease. On microscopic examination, the number of RBCs does not correlate with the significance of the causative lesion; a simple cystitis may cause gross hematuria, while a renal-cell carcinoma may result in only a few RBCs/hpf. Size and shape of RBCs should be noted: distorted, heterogeneous RBCs are more likely to be glomerular in origin. RBC casts or hemoglobin casts also indicate glomerular origin but if such casts are not present, glomerular disease is certainly not ruled out. WBC casts suggest infection of the renal parenchyma (pyelonephritis).

Radiologic Imaging Studies. These are determined by the suspected disease process and location of the lesion, which are in turn based upon the history, physical examination, and careful examination of the urine sediment. A urologic evaluation including ultrasound, CT scan, IVP, and cystoscopy is often indicated to exclude lower urinary-tract causes of hematuria. An algorithm for the diagnostic workup of hematuria is given in Table 42–2.

Proteinuria

Proteinuria is not, itself, a disease. Rather, it is a clinical indication that significant renal disease may exist. Proteinuria may indicate serious underlying renal or systemic disease or it can be idiopathic. As part of a standard urinalysis, it can be found in up to 9% of people presenting for a routine physical. The urine dipstick is the most common test used to detect the presence of proteinuria. Since the dipstick method can be affected by many factors (e.g., concentration, medications, urine pH), a 24-hour urine is the only reliable way to measure amount of proteinuria. In healthy adults there should be less than 150 mg of protein in a 24-hour urine collection. Proteinuria is considered significant when >300 mg/24 hr is found. Protein excretion of greater than 1 g/24 hr necessitates a work-up for renal parenchymal disease; excretion of > 3 gm/24 hr is referred to as "nephrotic-range" proteinuria and usually indicates glomerular disease. Causes of nonnephrotic range proteinuria include strenuous exercise, fever, congestive heart failure, orthostatic (postural) proteinuria, and tubulo–interstitial or vascular disease.

Table 42–3 lists common causes of nephrotic-range proteinuria.

TABLE 42–2. Workup of Hematuria Detected by Urine Dipstick

Urine Sediment Findings	Associated Conditions	Workup	Specific Disease Examples
Negative	Hemoglobinuria, myoglobinuria, dilute urine	Repeat urinalysis	
RBCs	Coagulopathy, disease of ureters or calyces	IVP, ultrasound, CT scan, cytology	Calculi, papillary necrosis, polycystic disease, GU trauma, neoplasm, sickle cell disease, parasites
RBCs and WBCs	Disease of lower GU tract	Urine culture, cytology, cystoscopy, ultrasound	GU tract infection, reflux, GU tract malignancy
RBCs and WBC casts	Interstitial disease	Urine culture, lymph node biopsy	Drug reaction, pyelonephritis, endocarditis, embolic disease, TB, sarcoidosis
RBC casts, hemoglobin casts, dysmorphic RBCs	Glomerular disease	ANA, ASO titer, C3/C4, HBsAg, renal biopsy	Hypertension, diabetes, glomerulonephritis (e.g., immune-complex or postinfectious), drug reaction

TABLE 42–3. Common Causes of Nephrotic-Range Proteinuria

Primary Glomerular Disorders	Minimal change disease, proliferative glomerulonephritis, IgA nephropathy, focal segmental glomerulosclerosis, membranoproliferative glomerulonephritis (not associated with extrarenal or systemic disease)
Autoimmune	Systemic lupus, Goodpasture's syndrome, Wegener's granulomatosis, rhematoid arthritis, polyarteritis nodosa
Neoplastic	Multiple myeloma, leukemia, lymphoma, Hodgkin's disease
Infectious	HIV infection, hepatitis, syphilis, endocarditis, postinfectious glomerulonephritis
Toxins/Drugs	NSAIDs, heroin, penicillamine, gold
Miscellaneous	Preeclampsia, eclampsia, amyloidosis, renovascular hypertension

History and Physical Findings

Signs and symptoms associated with proteinuria, especially nephrotic syndrome, include: generalized weakness and fatigue; edema and weeping of edema fluid through the skin; pleural effusions; and ascites.

While proteinuria itself causes minimal symptoms, the underlying cause of the proteinuria (such as systemic lupus, diabetes, or malignancy) may have prominent clinical manifestations. In addition, longstanding heavy proteinuria may result in certain complications. These include hyperlipidemia and hypercoagulability, which are discussed further in the section on management of proteinuria.

Laboratory and Diagnostic Studies

The diagnostic workup of proteinuria includes spot urine protein/creatinine ratio, 24-hour urine and creatinine clearance, serum VDRL and cryoglobulins, hepatitis panel, HIV antibodies, collagen vascular screen, renal ultrasound, and biopsy. Spot urine protein:creatinine ratio is obtained from a spot (untimed) urine sample. The ratio of protein to creatinine concentrations (in mg/dL) provides a rough estimate of the 24-hour urine protein excretion. A protein:creatinine ratio of >3.5 correlates with a 24-hour urine protein excretion of >3 gm (i.e., nephrotic-range proteinuria). Twenty-four hour urine protein and creatinine clearance provide the best quantitative measurement of urinary protein excretion and glomerular filtration rate.

Nephrotic syndrome may have an infectious etiology. The VDRL—positive in patients with a history of syphilis—may identify the cause of nephrotic syndrome as being due to syphilis, but may also be a clue to the presence of collagen–vascular disease. Serum cryoglobulins may be present in hepatitis C and a variety of collagen–vascular diseases. A hepatitis panel is useful in diagnosing hepatitis B and C, which may be associated with glomerular lesions that cause nephrotic syndrome. HIV antibody titers should be checked. HIV nephropathy may cause nephrotic syndrome, as may several opportunistic infections that affect immunocompromised patients.

The collagen–vascular screen includes the ANA, C3, C4, and ESR, which may be abnormal in patients with various autoimmune disorders. A variety of autoimmune diseases and vasculitides may manifest with nephrotic syndrome.

Renal ultrasound is used to document the size and texture of the kidneys and may provide important clues to the cause of nephrotic syndrome. Large kidneys are seen with diabetes, HIV nephropathy, amyloidosis, and infiltrative malignancies. Small, echogenic kidneys suggest chronic glomerulonephritis.

Percutaneous renal biopsy allows a specific diagnosis of the underlying renal disease to be made. Knowing the exact cause of proteinuria allows the clinician to: (1) determine treatment plan, (2) determine the prognosis of the disease, and (3) inform the patient whether the underlying disease is likely to recur following renal transplantation.

Figures 42–5 and 42–6 give algorithms for the diagnostic work-up of proteinuria.

An important part of the workup of proteinuria is a careful urine sediment examination. Figure 42–7 gives

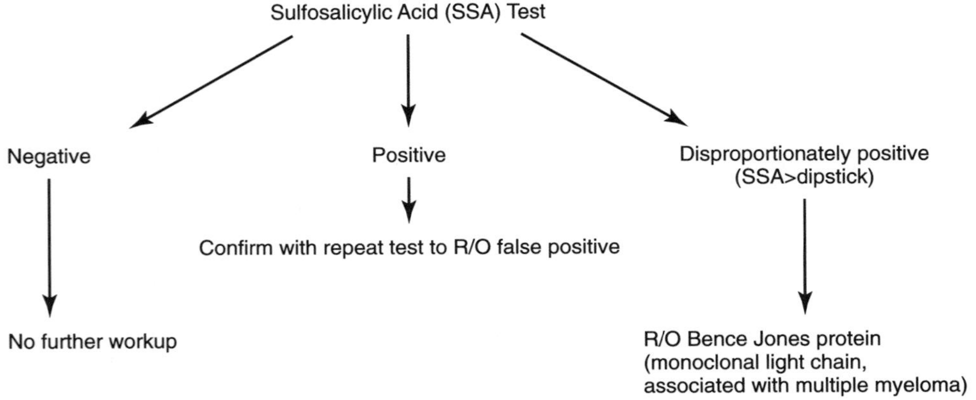

Figure 42–5. Algorithm for the initial workup of proteinuria detected by urine dipstick.

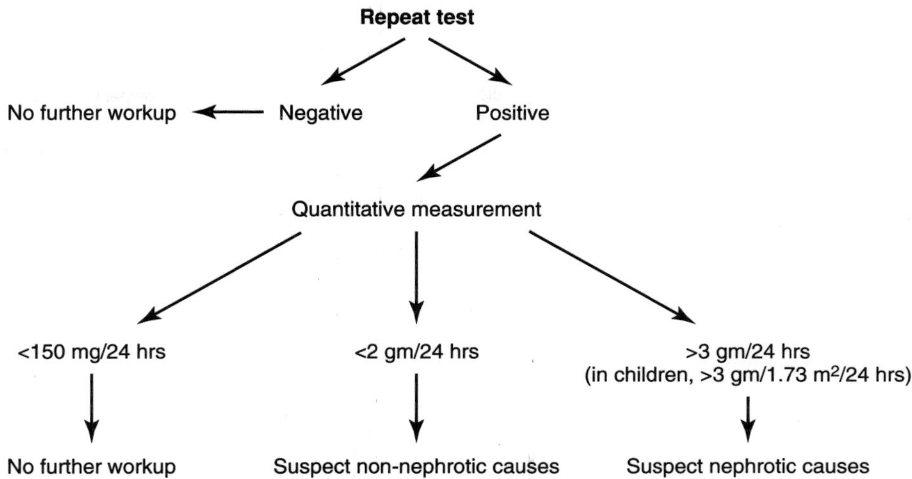

Figure 42–6. Algorithm for the further diagnostic workup of proteinuria detected by urine dipstick.

broad categories of urine sediment findings encountered in the workup of proteinuria, and examples of diseases associated with each.

Management

Standard treatments for proteinuria include the use of dietary protein restriction, angiotensin-converting enzyme (ACE) inhibitors, lipid therapy, anticoagulation, and diuretics. Protein loss, hypoalbuminemia, hyperlipidemia, and hypercoagulability are complications of chronic nephrotic syndrome. Accurate diagnosis and aggressive treatment are necessary to prevent the devastating effects of these disorders.

Since protein loss leads to hypoalbuminemia, various means of decreasing urinary protein loss have been investigated. Mild dietary protein restriction of about 0.8 gm/kg/24 hr is often recommended for patients with nephrotic syndrome. This may decrease intraglomerular capillary pressure and, thereby, decrease proteinuria. Angiotensin-converting enzyme (ACE) inhibitors (e.g., lisinopril, enalapril, benazepril) are also helpful in reducing protein loss by reducing glomerular capillary pressure.

Hypoalbuminemia decreases plasma oncotic pressure, resulting in a shift of intravascular plasma fluid into the interstitial space and resulting in peripheral edema and ascites. Gentle diuresis with loop diuretics and metolazone or hydrochlorothiazide may be effective in maintaining serum albumin levels. Nutritional support is also necessary to support hepatic protein synthesis.

Hyperlipidemia can be found in nephrotic patients because of increased lipoprotein production by the liver. Both dietary and pharmacologic therapy is usually required to treat this complication, which can otherwise result in accelerated atherosclerosis.

Patients with nephrotic syndrome often have decreased blood levels of antithrombin III and other proteins that usually regulate clotting. Patients are at greater risk for peripheral venous thrombosis, renal vein thrombosis, and pulmonary embolism. Treatment for such thromboses is intravenous standard heparin or subcutaneous low–molecular-weight heparin (enoxaparin) in the acute phase, followed by 6 to 12 months of oral warfarin (Coumadin) therapy.

Proteinuria <2 gm/24 hr (benign sediment)
Orthostatic proteinuria, early renal disease, tubulointerstitial disease (e.g., drug reaction)

Nephritic sediment (RBC casts)
Post-infectious glomerulonephritis, hereditary nephritis, IgA nephropathy

Nephrotic sediment (>3 gm/24 hr; oval fat bodies, fatty casts)
Primary glomerular disease (minimal change, membranous, focal segmental glomerulosclerosis) diabetic nephropathy, amyloidosis

Broad, waxy or granular casts (+ nephrotic proteinuria)
Advanced renal disease

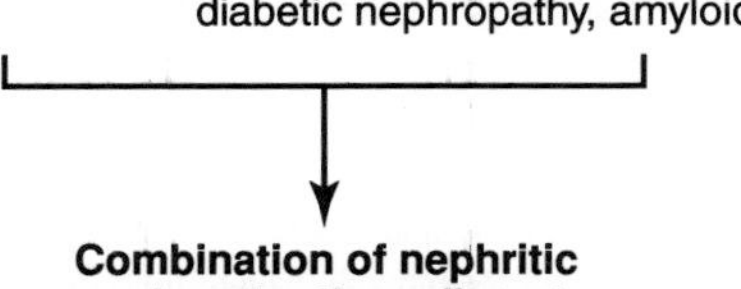

Figure 42–7. Urine sediment findings encountered in the workup of proteinuria, and examples of diseases associated with each.

In addition to these general therapeutic measures, specific treatment is available for some causes of nephrotic syndrome. These are entirely determined by the underlying cause of the proteinuria. For example, minimal change disease usually responds well to a 4- to 8-week course of prednisone. Membranous glomerulopathy has a more variable response and often requires a longer course of treatment. Lupus nephritis is generally treated with cyclophosphamide (usually administered IV monthly for 6-12 months) in combination with prednisone. Thrombotic thrombocytopenic purpura and hemolytic uremic syndrome respond, if at all, to such measures as plasma exchange and administration of intravenous immunoglobulin. Some types of nephrotic syndrome, such as those caused by IgA nephropathy and focal segmental glomerulosclerosis, do not respond well or predictably to any known therapy. Thus it is important to identify the cause of nephrotic syndrome in a given patient by doing appropriate serologic tests and/or a renal biopsy. The information gained from these diagnostic studies can then help to determine the most appropriate type of therapy.

Acute Renal Failure

Acute renal failure (ARF) is defined as a rise in blood urea nitrogen (BUN) and serum creatinine levels occurring over a period of days to weeks. ARF develops in approximately 5% of hospitalized patients. Despite technological advances, such as hemodialysis and continuous renal replacement therapy, the mortality associated with this disorder remains very high (30-60%). It is important to recognize and treat ARF promptly, since recognition of reversible causes may shorten the duration of the renal failure, and judicious management may help prevent or minimize the metabolic and other complications of this condition.

Pathophysiology

There are numerous causes of ARF, but the most common is acute tubular necrosis (ATN), in which renal tubules are damaged and become detached from their underlying basement membrane. Although new tubular epithelial cells eventually grow and replace the destroyed ones, the process of recovery usually takes several days to weeks.

There are two causes of ATN: toxins and ischemia. A few of the more common insults that can damage the renal tubular epithelium are listed in Table 42–4.

Although ATN is the most common cause of ARF, there are several other categories of renal disease that produce an acute rise in BUN and serum creatinine.

Acute Glomerulonephritis. Diseases that affect the glomeruli can result in inflammatory changes, deposition of immune complexes, and occlusion of glomerular capillary loops, resulting in a decrease in glomerular filtration rate. Examples of diseases that produce acute glomerulonephritis include systemic lupus erythematosus and other collagen–vascular diseases, Goodpasture's syndrome (crescentic glomerulonephritis with pulmonary hemorrhage), hemolytic–uremic syndrome, and poststreptococcal glomerulonephritis.

Acute Interstitial Nephritis. Conditions that evoke an inflammatory reaction in the renal tubules and interstitial tissue can result in acute renal failure. The interstitium may be damaged by the use of semisynthetic penicillins (e.g.,

TABLE 42–4. Most Common Causes of Acute Tubular Necrosis (ATN)

Toxic Causes of ATN

Intravenous contrast dye: These hypersomotic, iodinated compounds are potentially damaging to tubular cells, especially in patients who are diabetic, are severely dehydrated, or have underlying renal insufficiency. Contrast dyes that can cause ATN include those used in intravenous pyelograms (IVPs), computed tomographic (CT) scans, coronary angiography, arteriography, and venography. However, the intravenous contrast material used in nuclear isotope scans, ventilation/perfusion scans, and magnetic resonance imaging (MRI) scans does not cause renal tubular damage.

Antibiotics: Especially aminoglycosides (gentamicin, tobramycin, amikacin), acyclovir, polymyxin, and amphotericin B.

Heavy metals: Especially arsenic, lead, mercury, and platinum.

Ethylene glycol: Commonly known as antifreeze, this compound is sometimes used by alcoholics to obtain a "buzz" similar to that from ethanol; it is also ingested in suicide attempts. It is an extremely toxic substance, and consumption of even small amounts may cause severe metabolic acidosis, irreversible neurologic damage, and acute renal failure.

Other toxins: Including fungicides, pesticides, carbon tetrachloride.

Ischemic Causes of ATN

Severe volume depletion, hemorrhage, hypotension, or shock: These conditions may result in a transient severe decrease in blood flow to the kidney, causing ischemic damage to the sensitive renal tubules. Examples are hemorrhagic, cardiogenic, and septic shock.

Trauma, major surgery: These can be associated with periods of hypotension or with excessive unrecognized fluid losses, resulting in ischemia to the renal tubules.

Rhabdomyolysis: Massive breakdown of skeletal muscle occurs (e.g., secondary to crush injury, electrical shock, heat stroke, or ingestion of various toxins), resulting in release of myoglobin into the circulation. Often associated with severe fluid losses, rhabdomyolysis is usually accompanied by severe vasoconstriction, with a decrease in blood flow to the kidney. There is also some degree of toxic injury which occurs, since myoglobin itself can damage the renal tubules.

Hemolysis: With massive hemolysis, such as occurs in a transfusion reaction, intense vasoconstriction occurs, resulting in a decrease in blood flow to the kidney and consequent tubular necrosis.

nafcillin) or nonsteroidal antiinflammatory drugs, or by deposition of calcium or uric acid (usually in association with marked hypercalcemia or hyperuricemia).

Major Vessel Disease. Occlusion of the renal arteries by thrombi or emboli may result in acute renal failure. A less common cause to be considered in this category is aortic dissection involving both renal arteries.

Urinary Tract Obstruction. Obstruction to the flow of urine may occur at any level of the urinary tract. The ureters may be occluded by stones, clots, tumor, or fibrotic bands. Obstruction at the level of the bladder or bladder neck may occur because of tumor or prostatic hypertrophy. The urethra may be obstructed by fibrosis or congenital malformation. Any obstructive process may cause hydronephrosis (dilation of the collecting system), with backpressure on the renal tubules and resultant kidney damage.

Although a rise in BUN and serum creatinine most commonly signify the presence of acute renal failure, it is important to recognize the presence of prerenal azotemia (*azo* = nitrogen, *emia* = blood), a condition in which the BUN increases despite relatively normal functioning of the kidneys. Two major mechanisms for development of prerenal azotemia are excessive urea production and increased renal tubular urea reabsorption.

Excessive Urea Production. Since urea is a metabolic product of protein, any condition in which muscle, blood, or protein breakdown occurs can produce prerenal azotemia. Catabolic states (e.g., in postoperative or septic patients), administration of high-dose steroids, and breakdown of large amounts of blood in the GI tract or a hematoma (e.g., in a hip cavity following hip fracture or surgery) can produce large amounts of urea, temporarily exceeding the kidneys' ability to excrete it and thereby causing a rise in the BUN.

Increased Renal Tubular Urea Reabsorption. Normally, about 50% of the urea filtered by the glomeruli is reabsorbed by the renal tubules and returned to the circulation instead of being excreted in the urine. Under certain conditions, especially volume depletion and edema-forming states (congestive heart failure, cirrhosis and ascites, nephrotic syndrome), renal tubular reabsorption increases and a greater-than-normal amount of urea is returned to the blood, resulting in an increase in BUN.

Although not specifically a cause of prerenal azotemia, diabetic ketoacidosis can cause a spurious elevation in serum creatinine. This occurs because the ketoacids generated in diabetic acidosis are falsely measured as creatinine by the auto-analyzer method that is used in most clinical laboratories. An apparent rise in serum creatinine seen in acute diabetic ketoacidosis does not necessarily mean, therefore, that the patient is in acute renal failure; some of the measured creatinine may actually represent ketoacids rather than creatinine. A more comprehensive list of the causes of acute renal failure is given in Table 42–5.

History and Physical Findings

The workup of a patient with an elevated BUN and serum creatinine begins with a good history and physical examination. One should be alert for a history or physical signs consistent with known causes of ARF: Is there any recent history of excessive fluid loss (e.g., diarrhea) or hemorrhage? Has there been a documented hypotensive episode? Has the patient been exposed to any known nephrotoxins such as radiographic contrast dye, aminoglycosides, nonsteroidal antiinflammatory drugs, or antifreeze? Is there any history of a condition that might predispose to urinary tract obstruction (e.g., benign prostatic hypertrophy, metastatic colon carcinoma)? Are there any physical signs of dehydration, edema-forming states, cancer, collagen–vascular disease, or prostatic hypertrophy?

It is also important to establish the patient's baseline renal function if possible; differential diagnosis, diagnostic workup, and therapeutic management differ for patients with ATN and chronic renal failure. Consider, for example, a patient who presents with a serum creatinine of 7 mg/dL. If one establishes that the creatinine was 1.0 mg/dL 2 weeks ago, one may consider diagnostic possibilities such as NSAID toxicity, urinary tract obstruction due to malignancy, and acute lupus nephritis. It is appropriate to do an extensive diagnostic workup, including many serologic tests and a renal biopsy, and to initiate dialysis within the next few days. On the other hand, if one discovers that the patient had a serum creatinine of 6 mg/dL 3 months ago, one should consider diagnoses such as diabetic nephropathy, hypertensive renal disease, or a chronic, progressive glomerulonephritis. A diagnostic workup is unlikely to reveal a reversible cause of renal failure, and immediate initiation of dialysis is unnecessary in the face of slowly progressive disease.

Laboratory and Diagnostic Tests

Laboratory studies obtained in patients with ARF serve several purposes: they provide clues as the etiology of the renal failure, help to distinguish prerenal azotemia from actual renal failure, establish whether the patient has acute or chronic renal failure, and indicate the severity of the metabolic abnormalities that the patient suffers as a consequence of the renal failure, thus allowing one to plan for appropriate treatment (including dialysis). Basic studies include serum chemistry profile (including serum calcium, uric acid, and liver enzymes), complete blood count, urinalysis, urinary indices, and renal ultrasound.

Complete blood count may reveal unsuspected leukocytosis (e.g., from sepsis or leukemia) or thrombocytopenia. The hematocrit is also useful, since ARF is usually associated with a relatively normal hematocrit. Chronic renal failure is usually accompanied by a gradual decrease in erythropoietin synthesis by the kidneys and, therefore, a chronic, progressive (but normocytic) anemia.

Urinalysis may reveal such clues as multiple renal tubular epithelial cells (sloughed from necrotic tubules in ATN), red blood cell casts (seen in acute glomerulonephri-

TABLE 42–5. Causes of Acute Renal Failure

Prerenal Azotemia
- Volume depletion
  - Hemorrhage
  - Gastrointestinal losses
  - Sweating
  - Diuretic use/abuse
  - Burns
- Edema-forming states
  - Congestive heart failure
  - Cirrhosis and ascites, hepatorenal syndrome
  - Nephrotic syndrome
- Catabolic states
  - Sepsis
  - Postoperative state
  - Steroid use
  - Tetracycline use
- Breakdown of blood in the GI tract, resorption of hematoma

Drugs and Toxins
- Heavy metals: arsenic, mercury, lead, platinum
- Carbon tetrachloride and other organic solvents
- Ethylene glycol
- Pesticides and fungicides
- X-ray contrast dye
- Antibiotics: aminoglycosides, amphotericin B, penicillins, sulfonamides, tetracycline, rifampin
- Other drugs: nonsteroidal antiinflammatory agents, methoxyflurane, furosemide, EDTA

Ischemic Disorders
- Major trauma, surgery
- Massive hemorrhage, severe volume depletion
- Pancreatitis
- Shock (septic, cardiogenic, hemorrhagic)
- Rhabdomyolysis
- Hemolysis, transfusion reaction

Glomerular and Vascular Diseases
- Postinfectious glomerulonephritis
- Collagen–vascular diseases: systemic lupus erythematosus, scleroderma, polyarteritis nodosa
- Henoch–Schonlein purpura
- Bacterial endocarditis
- Goodpasture's syndrome, crescentic glomerulonephritis
- Wegener's granulomatosis
- Malignant hypertension
- Hemolytic–uremic syndrome, thrombotic thrombocytopenic purpura

Interstitial and Tubular Diseases
- Interstitial nephritis due to infection, drugs, hypercalcemia, oxalate deposition, multiple myeloma
- Pyelonephritis
- Papillary necrosis
- Radiation nephritis

Major Vessel Diseases
- Renal artery thrombosis, embolism, or stenosis
- Renal vein or inferior vena cava thrombosis
- Dissecting aneurysm with renal artery involvement

Urinary Tract Obstruction
- Urethral: stenosis or stricture; posterior urethral valves
- Bladder neck: prostatic hypertrophy or carcinoma, bladder carcinoma; functional obstruction (secondary to neuropathy or drugs)
- Ureteral:
  - ureteral–pelvic junction stricture
  - intraureteral: stones, clots, tumor, trauma, foreign bodies
  - extraureteral: endometriosis, malignancy, fibrosis, accidental ligation

tis), and oxalate crystals (formed in acute ethylene glycol toxicity). Heavy proteinuria (3-4+ by dipstick) also strongly suggests preexisting renal disease (e.g., diabetic nephropathy or any of a number of chronic glomerulonephritides), since ATN is associated only with mild proteinuria.

Urinary indices are obtained from a simultaneous chemistry panel and spot urine chemistries. These indices (Table 42–6) are primarily useful in distinguishing prerenal azotemia from ATN. Note that these urinary indices are of limited use in patients who have received diuretics within the past 24 hours, who have underlying chronic renal insufficiency, and who are not oliguric (i.e. whose urine output exceeds 400 mL/day).

Renal sonographic examination is a simple, noninvasive examination that can help to rule out urinary tract obstruction and hydronephrosis. It can also reveal whether the kidneys are normal in size and texture (as in ATN), or small and dense (as in chronic disease that results in fibrosis and shrinkage of the kidneys).

Management

Judicious management can help to prevent or at least minimize the metabolic and hemodynamic disturbances that often accompany ARF. Since ATN lasts, on average, from several days to two weeks, appropriate and careful management can delay or prevent the need for dialysis.

The cornerstone of the management of ATN is dietary restriction. Restriction of dietary sodium, potassium, protein, and fluid can help to minimize the azotemia, acidosis, hyperkalemia, and fluid overload that tend to occur with ATN. A typical "renal failure diet" is: 2 gm Na^+, 60 mEq K^+, 60 gm protein, 1000 cc fluid. If the patient has "nonoliguric" ATN (i.e., produces >400 cc/day of urine), the daily fluid allowance can be much more liberal.

TABLE 42–6. Urinary Diagnostic Indices[a]

	Prerenal	ATN
BUN/creat	> 20	10–20
U_{Na+}	< 20	> 40 meq/L
U/P creatinine	> 40	< 20
Fractional excretion of Na^+ (FENa)	< 1	> 2%

$$FENa = \frac{U_{Na+} P_{cr} \times 100\%}{P_{Na+} U_{cr}}$$

[a] U_{Na+} and P_{Na+} = urine and plasma (or serum) Na^+ concentration in mEq/L; U_{cr} and P_{cr} = urine and plasma (or serum) creatinine concentration in mg/dL.

Medical Therapy. Even with the most stringent dietary restrictions, patients with ATN may become hyperkalemic. If serum K^+ concentration rises above 5.5 mEq/L, particularly if it rises toward 7.0 mEq/L, urgent treatment of hyperkalemia is required. Table 42–7 lists the acute treatments of hyperkalemia.

The purposes of insulin, sodium bicarbonate, albuterol, and calcium gluconate in the emergent treatment of hyperkalemia are to drive K^+ intracellularly. Although a temporizing measure, treatment with these agents may be lifesaving until the hyperkalemia can be treated definitively. Glucose and insulin should be administered simultaneously to prevent hypoglycemia. Calcium gluconate has the most rapid onset of action and should be used when signs of advanced cardiac toxicity associated with hyperkalemia are present (i.e., QRS widening or ventricular arrhythmias by EKG).

Unlike the temporizing measures described above, sodium polystyrene resin (Kayexalate) binds K^+ in the GI tract and allows it to be excreted from the body. Each gram of Kayexalate binds 1 mEq of K^+. Although the resin usually takes 1 to 2 hours to work, it is a useful adjunct to the more rapidly acting agents listed in Table 42–7.

Various other pharmacological interventions have been studied in ATN; unfortunately, most have shown no definite benefit. Diuretics are often employed at the onset of ATN, in an effort to increase the urine output and thus make the patient's fluid and electrolyte status easier to manage. An increase in urine output can sometimes be demonstrated with a moderate dose of a loop diuretic (e.g., furosemide 40-120 mg IV, or bumetanide 1-4 mg IV). However, repeated diuretic doses should not be tried if there is no response, since they only add to the patient's fluid intake and may cause toxicity (e.g., deafness) if high doses accumulate. Other medications that have been used in an attempt to prevent ATN or to shorten its course include calcium-channel blockers, pentoxifylline (Trental), atrial natriuretic peptide, and low-dose (<5 μg/kg/min) dopamine. While there is experimental evidence to support the use of these agents, clinical trials have not demonstrated any consistent benefit (except for the use of calcium-channel blockers in renal transplantation). This is partly because, in real life, the insults that cause ATN cannot be anticipated and medications cannot therefore be given prophylactically. In addition, the side effects of these medications must be considered (e.g., cardiac arrhythmias and digital necrosis from dopamine; hypotension from atrial natriuretic peptide).

TABLE 42–7. Treatment of Hyperkalemia

Agent	Dosage
Emergency/Acute Treatment	
Glucose and insulin	D_{50} 50 mL IVP and regular insulin 10 U IVP
Sodium bicarbonate	1 ampule (44 mEq) IVP
Albuterol	2–4 puffs
Calcium gluconate	1 ampule
Nonemergent Treatment	
Sodium polystyrene (Kayexalate)	30 gm PO/NGT/PR

One additional pharmacologic intervention that may hold some promise for the future is the administration of renal growth factors such as epidermal growth factor. Levels of these naturally occurring factors have been found to be increased in kidneys that are recovering from ATN. Studies are currently underway to determine whether administration of these growth factors can speed regeneration of renal tubules damaged by ATN and shorten the clinical course of the disorder.

Even with careful medical management, approximately 80% of patients with oliguric renal failure and 60% with nonoliguric ATN ultimately require some form of renal replacement therapy to correct fluid and metabolic derangements. This can take several forms, as listed here.

Hemodialysis. The patient's blood is pumped at a rapid rate (300-400 ml/min) through a hollow-fiber dialyzer that consists of thousands of capillaries, each of which is made of a synthetic semipermeable material. The microscopic holes in the capillary walls (as in real capillaries) allow the passage of water, electrolytes, and small molecules, but not of blood cells or proteins. Bathing the outsides of the capillaries is a solution called dialysate. Dialysate contains "normal" concentrations of substances that do not need to be altered (e.g., sodium, chloride, calcium), but lacks substances that one wishes to remove from the patient's blood (e.g., urea, creatinine, phosphate). As blood flows through the dialyzer capillaries and dialysate flows around them, urea and creatinine diffuse from the patient's blood into the dialysate, which is continuously discarded. Meanwhile, sodium and chloride concentrations do not change because there is no gradient for their diffusion. At the same time, plasma and its constituents (electrolytes, but not proteins or blood cells) can be pulled through the capillary membranes by applying a negative pressure, or partial vacuum to the outside of the capillaries. This allows excess fluid to be removed from the patient and discarded with the dialysate.

Performance of hemodialysis requires insertion of a dual-lumen catheter into either the femoral, internal jugular, or subclavian vein. Complications of insertion include bleeding and accidental puncture of an artery or a lung.

Continuous Arteriovenous or Venovenous Hemofiltration. The principle of this technique is similar to that of dialysis, except that the patient's blood moves very slowly through the hollow-fiber device. In continuous arteriovenous or venovenous hemofiltration (CAVH or CVVH), separate arterial and venous catheters are inserted into the patient's femoral artery and vein; the difference in pressure between the two vessels causes fluid to flow through the tubing between them. In CVVH, a dual-lumen venous catheter is employed, and a pump moves blood slowly through the tubing. In either case, blood continuously enters the hemofilter, where it flows through hollow capillary fibers. As it does so, plasma leaks through the holes in the capillary walls. The microscopic drops of plasma that seep out of the capillaries are collected in tubing and drain into a bag, where the volume can be measured. Since this technique allows fluid removal slowly and continuously over a 24-hour period, the volume shifts are much better tolerated than with hemodialysis, where several liters of fluid may be rapidly removed in 3 to 4 hours. With CAVH/CVVH, the removal of plasma itself results in no change in serum concentrations of BUN, creatinine, or electrolytes. However, because of the large amount of plasma removal occurring in a 24-hour period, the plasma can be continuously replaced with a plasma substitute that *lacks* substances that need to be removed from the patient's blood. By continuously removing plasma and replacing it with a urea- and creatinine-free plasma substitute, one can then accomplish the same end as with hemodialysis: lowering blood levels of toxic substances. In both CAVH and CVVH, the removal of toxic metabolites can be further enhanced by the addition of a dialysate. The processes of CAVH, CVVH, CAVH-D, and CVVH-D are illustrated in Figure 42–8.

The relative indications for initiating renal replacement therapy are listed in Table 42–8. These are *relative* indications and, depending on the circumstances, do not nec-

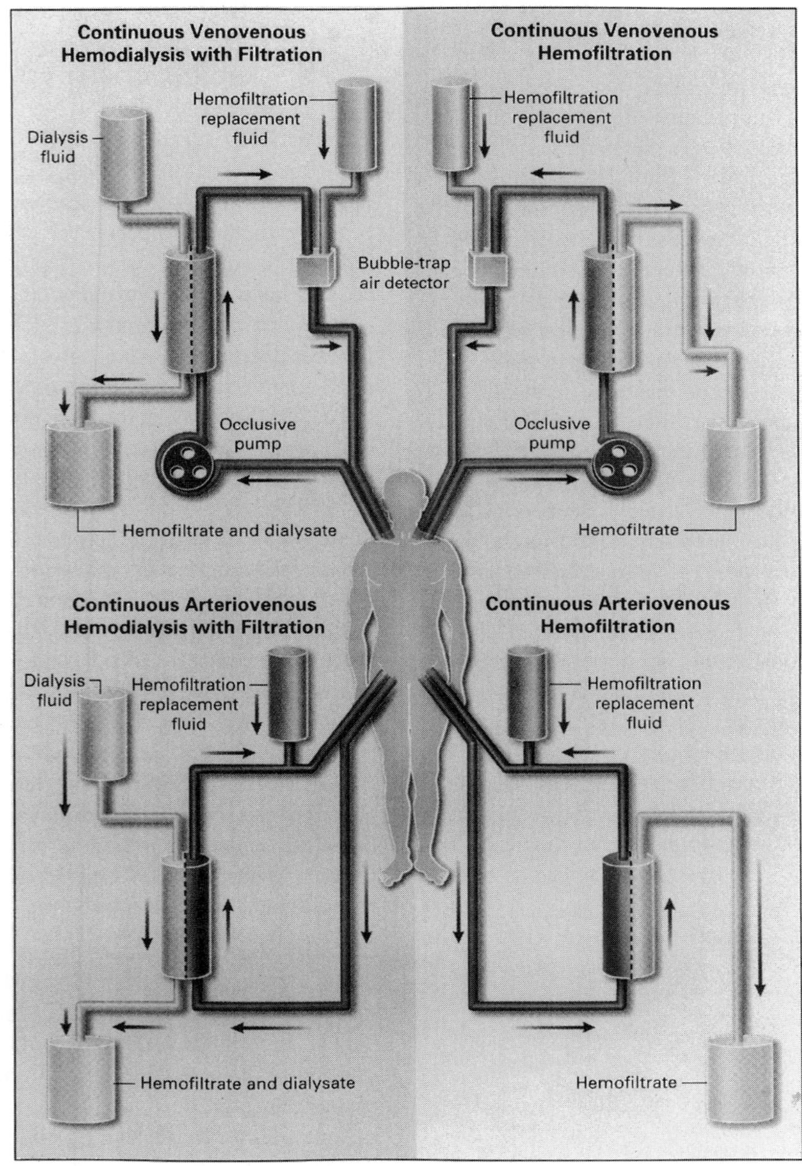

Figure 42–8. Modes of continuous renal replacement therapy: venovenous hemofiltration with and without dialysis; arteriovenous hemofiltration with and without dialysis. *(Used with permission from Forni & Hilton. [1997].)*

TABLE 42–8. Indications for Initiation of Dialysis in Acute Renal Failure

BUN >100 mg/dL, serum creatinine >10 mg/dL
Serum K^+ >6.0 mEq/L despite medical management
Serum bicarbonate <10 mEq/L, arterial pH <7.20
Fluid overload
Uremic symptoms: nausea/vomiting, lethargy, muscle twitching, seizures
Pericarditis

From Kean, Alexander, Bailie, et al. (1996). p. 568.

essarily mean that dialysis must be initiated on an emergency basis. However, several of these abnormalities tend to occur simultaneously. For instance, patients often become nauseated, fluid-overloaded, and hyperkalemic as the BUN approaches 100 mg/dL and the serum creatinine approaches 10 mg/dL.

The course of ATN typically includes an oliguric phase (urine output <400 cc/day) lasting from several days to several weeks. This is sometimes followed by a polyuric phase lasting 2 to 4 days in which urine output is greater than normal, often several liters/day. A gradual return to normal renal function follows, with BUN and serum creatinine falling to baseline levels over the next few days to weeks. Subtle abnormalities of renal function (such as inability to concentrate the urine maximally when dehydrated) may persist for up to a year.

The overall mortality of ATN remains approximately 50 to 70% despite the advances of modern medicine and technology. Factors that predict a higher mortality include: older age of the patient, multisystem failure, severe infection, and extensive burns. Careful management of patients' fluid and electrolyte abnormalities, preservation of hemodynamic stability, and treatment of coexisting conditions remain the major aims of therapy in patients with ATN.

Chronic Renal Failure

Chronic renal failure (CRF) exists when there has been significant damage to the renal parenchyma resulting in decreased glomerular filtration rate (GFR). Irrespective of the cause of the damage, when the serum creatinine exceeds 2.0 mg/dL eventual progression to end-stage renal disease (ESRD) is likely.

Serum creatinine, rather than blood urea nitrogen (BUN), is used to estimate GFR. Since approximately 50% of filtered urea is reabsorbed, BUN does not provide a reliable estimation of GFR. BUN can also be affected by GI bleeding, tissue trauma, corticosteroids, tetracyclines, diet, liver disease, and sickle cell anemia. On the other hand, creatinine is filtered, not reabsorbed, and minimally secreted by the renal tubules. Since almost all creatinine in the urine represents filtered creatinine, serum creatinine is proportional to GFR. A rise in serum creatinine from 1.0 to 2.0 mg/dL, therefore, reflects a decrease in renal function of approximately 50%. GFR may be estimated using the Cockcroft–Gault formula:

$$\textit{Males:}\ \text{GFR} = \frac{(140 - \text{age}) \times (\text{lean body weight in kg})}{(\text{serum cr}) \times 72}$$

Females:

$$\text{GFR} = \left(\frac{(140 - \text{age}) \times (\text{lean body weight in kg})}{(\text{serum cr}) \times 72}\right) \times 0.85$$

Most institutions use creatinine clearance as a more accurate method of estimating GFR. The formula for calculating creatinine clearance, in mL/min, is:

$$C_{cr} = \frac{[\text{Urine}_{cr}] \times (\text{volume of urine per 24 hours})}{[\text{Serum}_{cr}] \times 1440}$$

Normal ranges: *males:* 97-137 mL/min/1.73m^2
females: 88-128 mL/min/1.73m^2

These values decline with increasing age. A properly collected sample should contain 15 to 20 mg creatinine/kg body weight/24 hr for males and 10 to 15 mg creatinine/kg body weight/24 hr for females.

The incidence of ESRD continues to grow in the United States, with the most recent figures from the United States Renal Data System (USRDS) showing that 69,000 people developed ESRD in 1995 compared with 41,000 in 1989. The total number of living patients who received renal replacement therapy as of December 1995 was 257,266 including those who had undergone renal transplantion. As of December 1996, the most common cause of ESRD continues to be diabetes, which accounts for 40% of cases with ESRD; hypertension accounts for 26%; primary glomerulonephritis, 12%; and other conditions, 22%. Table 42–9 gives the major causes of chronic renal failure.

History and Physical Findings

Since the development of chronic renal failure generally occurs over years and even decades, nearly every organ system can be affected. Patients may appear chronically ill and complain of being weak and fatigued. These symptoms can be attributed to the anemia of chronic renal disease, as well as to the insidious accumulation of a variety of uremic toxins. Patients may develop weight loss, stating that "food doesn't taste the same" and often complaining of a metallic taste in their mouths.

Most patients remain asymptomatic until their creatinine clearance drops below 10 to 15 mL/min, at which time they are considered to have ESRD. Patients often blame their underlying disease (e.g., diabetes) for their fatigue, sleep disturbances, malaise, weakness, and GI complaints. They may not notice a change in the amount of urine they produce, or in fact may have noticed an increase in urine output (due to inability to concentrate their urine). Patients are frequently perplexed when told that their kidneys have failed. It is important to reinforce with them that it is the

TABLE 42–9. Major Causes of Chronic Renal Failure

Glomerulopathies
Primary glomerular diseases
Focal segmental glomerulosclerosis
Membranous glomerulopathy
Membranoproliferative glomerulonephritis
Crescentic glomerulonephritis
IgA nephropathy
Systemic diseases
Diabetes
Collagen–vascular diseases
Malignancy
Postinfectious glomerulonephritis
Amyloidosis
Sickle cell nephropathy
Heroin abuse
Hereditary diseases
Alport's syndrome
Polycystic kidney disease (PKD)
Medullary cystic disease
Oxalosis
Fabry's disease
Vascular diseases
Hypertensive nephrosclerosis
Arteriolosclerosis
Renal artery stenosis
Obstructive disorders
Congenital (e.g., posterior urethral valves, urethral web)
Prostatic disease (hypertrophy or neoplasm)
Nephrolithiasis
Retroperitoneal or urinary tract tumor
Tubulointerstitial diseases
Drug hypersensitivity
Analgesic nephropathy
Reflux/chronic pyelonephritis
Heavy metals
Idiopathic

quality and not the quantity of urine that determines their kidneys' capacity to excrete waste products.

A number of other systems may be affected by the development of chronic renal failure, producing a variety of symptoms and physical findings. Patients may complain of diffuse pruritus, chronic nonhealing sores, and easy bruising. The skin may be dry and excoriated, and may have a yellowish cast because of the retention of urinary pigments in the bloodstream (giving rise to the name "uremia," literally "urine in the blood"). Pale conjunctivae and decreased visual acuity may be present. Patients may complain of a feeling of "sand in the eyes," associated with the finding of injected sclerae. These abnormalities are due to elevation of the serum phosphate and calcium–phosphate product, with subsequent deposition of microscopic calcium–phosphate deposits in the conjunctivae. Pulmonary involvement in chronic renal failure may be manifested by the development of pulmonary edema, with patients complaining of dyspnea, orthopnea, and even hemoptysis, in association with typical findings of pleural effusions and rales. Cardiovascular manifestations are also frequent and may include hypertension, congestive heart failure symptoms, angina, and even pericarditis. Gastrointestinal symptoms of uremia include anorexia, nausea, vomiting, and hiccups. Nonspecific genitourinary symptoms include polyuria, nocturia (due to inability to concentrate the urine normally in response to fluid deprivation), and impotence or decreased libido. Neuromuscular symptoms include decreased muscle strength, restless legs, or cramps. Patients may develop a variety of neurologic manifestations, including asterixis, seizures, lethargy, inability to concentrate, irritability, peripheral neuropathy, and myoclonic twitching.

Laboratory and Diagnostic Tests

Every effort should be made to determine the cause of renal failure, since many disorders are partially or wholly reversible. Examples of such disorders are renal artery stenosis and obstructive uropathy.

Urinalysis, serum chemistry panel, complete blood count, iron studies, parathyroid levels, and renal imaging studies should be performed on patients with newly diagnosed chronic renal failure (especially ESRD). Urinalysis may reveal proteinuria, hematuria, pyuria, granular, and cellular casts, depending on the etiology and stage of underlying renal disease. BUN and creatinine are generally proportionally increased (in approximately a 10:1 ratio). Serum sodium may be decreased, particularly if the patient is fluid-overloaded. Serum potassium is generally normal as long as the patient maintains urine output, but may be elevated in the very late stages of uremia. Serum bicarbonate is generally decreased, and a moderate anion gap (up to 20 mEq/L) may be present. Typically, serum calcium is decreased (because of abnormalities in production of vitamin D metabolites by the kidney), while serum phosphate is increased. Serum magnesium, amylase, and creatine phosphokinase (CPK) may be mildly increased; however, marked elevations in the latter two should raise the suspicion of a superimposed condition such as pancreatitis or rhabdomyolysis.

Normochromic normocytic anemia is usually present and is generally proportional to the degree of azotemia, representing a decrease in erythropoietin synthesis by the ailing kidneys. White blood cell and platelet counts are generally within normal limits, although platelet aggregation may be affected (as manifested by an abnormally long template bleeding time). Serum iron, ferritin, and transferrin saturation are usually within normal limits. Nevertheless, they should always be obtained in ESRD patients to rule out underlying iron deficiency prior to starting erythropoietin.

Serum parathyroid hormone (PTH) is usually elevated, particularly if chronic renal failure has been present for several years. A baseline level should be obtained in ESRD patients prior to initiating therapy with calcitriol.

The finding of small kidneys (<10 cm in length) on renal imaging studies, particularly in association with increased echogenicity, supports the diagnosis of longstanding, irreversible renal failure. Large, cystic kidneys suggest the diagnosis of adult autosomal dominant polycystic kidney disease (PKD). Enlarged kidneys may also be found in amyloidosis, infiltration with leukemia or lymphoma, and HIV nephropathy.

Management

Once a patient's serum creatinine reaches approximately 3.0 mg/dL, creatinine clearance is sufficiently decreased that any further small decrease in renal function can markedly increase the serum creatinine. Many extrinsic factors affect the course and/or rate of decline of the disease process. It is important that patients discuss all medications with the renal team, since many commonly used medicines can affect serum creatinine (e.g., trimethoprim-sulfa [Bactrim], cimetidine, and NSAIDs). Other factors affecting the course of the disease are infection, blood pressure, volume depletion, and radiographic contrast dye.

Diet. Diet plays an important role in the treatment of chronic renal disease. Each dialysis center and renal clinic is staffed with a renal nutritionist who evaluates each patient's nutritional needs and counsels the patient about protein, salt, fluid, potassium, and phosphorus intake. The patient's mode of renal replacement therapy also has an impact on the type of diet restrictions he or she must follow (e.g., peritoneal dialysis patients have a much more liberal diet and increased fluid allowance).

Medications. Upon starting dialysis, each ESRD patient should bring all medications that have been previously prescribed, and these medications should be reviewed for further use. Once dialysis is initiated, the need for many medications is decreased. Antihypertensive and diuretic requirements normally decrease with fluid removal, and insulin requirements often decrease as renal failure progresses, even before initation of dialysis.

Standard medications that are added for management of ESRD are listed in Table 42–10.

Calcium carbonate or calcium acetate should be taken exactly at mealtimes. Additionally, the doses should be proportional to the size of the meal. When serum phosphate is markedly elevated, such that the product of the serum calcium (in mg/dL) and serum phosphate (in mg/dL) exceeds 70, aluminum hydroxide is used as a phosphate binder instead.

Patients with chronic renal failure usually have impaired ability to synthesize 1,25$(OH)_2$ vitamin D_3, the active metabolite of vitamin D_3. As a result they develop hypocalcemia and secondary hyperparathyroidism, which can lead to increased bone resorption and disordered bone formation. The synthetic form of 1,25$(OH)_2$ vitamin D_3, known as calcitriol or Calcijex, can be administered intravenously at the time of dialysis to prevent, retard, or even reverse disturbances in calcium and phosphate regulation and the bone disease suffered by many dialysis patients.

TABLE 42–10. Medical Therapy in End-Stage Renal Disease

Drug	Purpose
Renal multivitamin	Water-soluble vitamins (especially B and C) and folate are lost in dialysis
Iron supplements	Supplements blood loss from hemodialysis and frequent blood draws
Calcium carbonate or calcium acetate	Important for binding phosphorus in the GI tract
Stool softeners (e.g., docusate sodium)	Compensates for the constipation induced by phosphate binders and dietary fluid restriction; laxatives may be needed occasionally
Medications typically administered during dialysis:	
Recombinant human erythropoietin	Initiated when the hematocrit falls below 30% to stimulate red blood cell production; the initial dose is 25-50 units/kg, up to 100 units/kg with close monitoring of blood pressure (BP) and hematocrit
Calcitriol (Calcijex)	To treat hypocalcemia and secondary hyperparathyroidism due to chronic renal failure

Calcitriol can also be administered as an oral form, Rocaltrol, although this is not as effective as the intravenous form.

▶ RENAL REPLACEMENT THERAPY

Renal replacement therapy teaching should begin when a patient's serum creatinine reaches approximately 5 mg/dL. The options of peritoneal dialysis, hemodialysis, and transplantation should all be discussed. The decision of which mode of therapy is to be used should be left to the patient unless there are preexisting conditions that would not allow for use of one of the modalities. For example, multiple abdominal surgeries may make peritoneal dialysis impossible; age and cardiac status can affect the patient's suitability for renal transplantation; severe blood vessel disease may make it difficult or impossible to construct a vascular access for hemodialysis.

Chronic Dialysis Access Options

For a patient to undergo hemodialysis, a reliable vascular access of sufficient size to support a blood flow of 350 to 400 mL/min must be constructed or surgically inserted. The following are some of the common options.

Arteriovenous Fistula

Arteriovenous fistula (AVF) is the preferred vascular access, and current recommendations for the management of ESRD suggest that an attempt be made to provide an AVF for as many patients as possible. Support for use of AVF as an access comes from the USRDS data, which show that AVF accesses last longer and provide better clearances than synthetic grafts. An AVF is created by the surgical anastomosis of an artery and vein, most commonly the radial artery with the cephalic vein. This form of access takes approximately 1 month to mature after construction. A functioning fistula has a palpable thrill and a bruit by auscultation.

Arteriovenous Graft

When the vascular surgeon determines that the patient's own blood vessels are inadequate to develop an AVF, a polytetrafluoroethylene (PTFE, or Gore–Tex) graft is used to form a conduit from artery to vein (usually in either the forearm or upper arm). An AV graft takes approximately 4 to 6 weeks after construction to mature; a thrill and bruit should be present over a functioning graft.

PermCath

When the previous two options are not available or practical, a PermCath may be used. This is a cuffed soft flexible Silastic dual-lumen catheter that is placed surgically into the internal jugular or subclavian vein, and tunneled in the subcutaneous tissue to exit on the anterior chest wall. PermCaths are often used in patients with refractory access problems, as well as in patients who have comorbid illnesses and whose survival is expected to be less than a year.

Peritoneal Dialysis Catheter

A peritoneal dialysis (PD) catheter, such as the Tenckhoff catheter is, on average, 25 to 30 cm long with either single or dual cuffs. It may be either straight or curled. Approximately 15 cm of the catheter floats freely in the abdominal cavity and 5 to 10 cm is tunneled through the abdominal wall. The remaining length is used to connect with the dialysate tubing.

Complications of Vascular Access

Prevention of, or early intervention in, access complications is important in maintaining a chronic dialysis access device. Patients and staff are taught to feel for a thrill (palpable buzz) daily in a patient's AVF or AV graft. If there is no palpable thrill, patients are instructed to seek attention immediately in an emergency room or dialysis clinic. Thrombosis of a graft (signified by absence of a thrill or bruit) usually requires surgical intervention within 2 to 4 days. After this time the chances of successful surgical declotting decrease considerably. Many centers also use urokinase infusion as a method for medical declotting.

Stenosis of a graft, generally occurring at the venous anastomosis, often presents with a swollen extremity or, in the case of subclavian vein stenosis, facial swelling. Interventional radiology plays an important role in the treatment of stenosis. Balloon angioplasty is normally attempted with >50% stenosis and has been quite successful. Angiographic placement of expandable metallic stents (Wallstents) within areas of stenosis has also been used with some success.

Infection is another common complication of chronic dialysis access. Infections are treated aggressively both in vascular accesses, where life-threatening sepsis can occur, and in peritoneal dialysis catheters, where infection can lead to bacterial or fungal peritonitis and sepsis. Broad spectrum antibiotics are used; these include vancomycin, gentamicin, third-generation cephalosporins, and occasionally rifampin, fluconazole, or amphotericin B.

Another complication of hemodialysis vascular access devices is "steal" syndrome, in which blood normally supplying the hand is shunted through a fistula or graft, resulting in ischemic hand pain and formation of digital ischemic ulcers. Other complications include air embolism, wall pseudoaneurysm, carpal tunnel syndrome, and seroma formation.

Renal Replacement Modalities

Hemodialysis

Hemodialysis is the movement of water and solutes from a patient's blood across a semipermeable membrane into an electrolyte solution called dialysate. The movement of solutes occurs through two mechanisms: diffusion and ultrafiltration. Diffusion is the movement of solutes in random motion down a concentration gradient, through a porous membrane. Diffusion may be limited by the size of the solute particles and of the membrane pores. Ultrafiltration is the process by which water and solutes are driven by hydrostatic pressure through the porous membrane. Dialyzers, or semipermeable membrane devices, are produced by many medical manufacturing companies. The composition of these dialyzers and their clearances vary from one dialyzer to another; so it is important to know the composition, surface area, and urea clearance to choose a dialyzer that is correct for a particular patient.

Hemodialysis is usually initiated when a patient's serum creatinine clearance falls to <10 ml/min and/or symptoms of uremia develop. Relative criteria for initiation of dialysis include symptomatic azotemia (e.g., nausea/vomiting, fatigue, muscle twitching, dyspnea). Absolute criteria for dialysis include hyperkalemia, pulmonary edema, intractable acidosis, mental status changes (especially lethargy or seizures), and pericarditis.

Since patients with chronic failure have maintained high levels of toxins over a long period of time, rapid removal of those toxins can cause dialysis disequilibrium, seizures, hypotension, and/or arrhythmias. The initial dialysis session should be relatively short, for example, 2 hours at low blood flow rates (approximately 200 mL/min). Potassium and calcium concentrations in the dialysate are prescribed in accordance with predialysis bloodwork (e.g., more severe hyperkalemia warrants a lower concentration of potassium in the dialysate). The length of the dialysis treatment should increase by 30 min/day and the rate of blood flow by 50 mL/min per day until the patient has reached 4 hours with a blood flow of 400 mL/min. At that time, the patient can be placed on a regular dialysis schedule of 3 weekly sessions.

Problems and Complications of Hemodialysis. Hypotension is the most common problem encountered in hemodialysis. It can be related to the patient's target (or "dry") weight, cardiac status, or antihypertensive therapy. Management should include frequent evaluation of target weight, with appropriate adjustment if the patient has actually gained tissue weight. A baseline cardiac work-up may be warranted to exclude underlying cardiac disease, since many dialysis patients have left ventricular hypertrophy secondary to chronic anemia, hypertension, or atherosclerotic disease. The patient's antihypertensive medications should also be reviewed. Patients' antihypertensive medication requirements often decrease sharply with initiation of dialysis, since hypertension in ESRD is often volume-related; thus, treatment of dialysis-induced hypotension may be as simple as having the patient omit taking antihypertensive drugs prior to dialysis.

Muscle cramps are another common complication. These occur when patients gain an excessive amout of fluid weight (>1 kg/day) between dialyses, and removal of a large amount of fluid is attempted during a relatively short dialysis session. Patients should be admonished to adhere to their fluid restriction so that they gain no more than 2 to 3 kg between dialysis sessions. Administration of a small amount of mannitol or hypertonic saline, or increasing the sodium concentration in the dialysate, may help relieve cramps; but the resultant increase in plasma osmolality may increase the patient's thirst.

Arrhythmias and chest pain can occur during dialysis for many reasons. Hyperkalemia or hypokalemia are frequently the cause of arrhythmias. A check of serum potassium midway through dialysis and an appropriate adjustment in dialysate K^+ concentration can correct the problem. Hypotension can cause arrhythmias or chest pain; management includes close observation and administration of small amounts of intravenous fluid or albumin. The dialysis blood flow rate should be decreased to 200 mL/min, or even stopped, during evaluation of arrhythmia or chest pain. If EKG changes are present, or if chest pain is persistent, the patient should be taken off dialysis and a repeat EKG obtained. Emergent cardiac evaluation and/or admission should follow. At the very least, a stress test should be obtained as soon as possible, and cardiac evaluation is strongly suggested.

Anemia is a common problem in patients receiving hemodialysis. This is multifactorial, although the major contributing factor is a deficiency of erythropoietin (which is synthesized by fibroblasts adjacent to renal proximal tubular cells). Another factor is that red cell survival is shortened in dialysis patients, both because of the uremic environment in which the cells circulate and because of hemolysis as cells flow through the hollow fibers of the dialyzer. In addition, there is loss of red cells during the return of the patient's blood from the dialysis tubing back to the patient at the end of dialysis, as well as the loss of blood from frequent venipunctures for laboratory tests. Many dialysis patients are therefore iron-depleted. Close observation of iron stores and careful regulation of erythropoietin dose can correct most anemias. If anemia is unresponsive to this therapy, further evaluation of the cause is warranted. Anemia can be caused by acute or slow GI bleed, PTH or aluminum bone disease, infection, or a chronic inflammatory process.

Peritoneal Dialysis

Peritoneal dialysis is accomplished by infusing dialysate solution (dextrose-containing electrolyte solution) into the peritoneal cavity and allowing it to dwell there for several hours. Diffusion and ultrafiltration take place in peritoneal dialysis much as in hemodialysis, using the peritoneal membrane instead of a synthetic dialyzer membrane. The patient's blood perfuses the capillaries of the peritoneal membrane, which acts as the semipermeable membrane across which molecules diffuse. Substances removed from the patient's blood by diffusion are then discarded when the dialysate is drained from the peritoneal cavity periodically. CAPD (continuous ambulatory peritoneal dialysis) is the most common form of peritoneal dialysis and consists of four to five daily exchanges each containing 1 to 3 liters of dialysate. Each exchange dwells for 4 to 5 hours in the peritoneal cavity and is drained out just before the next exchange. Dialysate normally takes about 20 minutes to drain out; prolonged drain time can be an indication that the peritoneal membrane is scarred, that the catheter is malpositioned, or that the patient is constipated. The type of dialysate solution used determines the amount of ultrafiltration: higher glucose concentrations result in higher ultrafiltration rates and more fluid removal.

Complications of Peritoneal Dialysis. Tunnel infections, occurring along the subcutaneous tract of the PD catheter, are a common problem in peritoneal dialysis.

TABLE 42–11. Suggested Initial Therapy of Peritonitis in CAPD Patients

Criteria for diagnosis

Positive peritoneal fluid culture, *or*

2 of 3 signs: cloudy drainage, abdominal pain, peritoneal fluid WBC count >100/mL with >50% neutrophils

Initial Treatment of Peritonitis

1. Cefazolin, 500 mg/L loading dose, then 125 mg/L in each exchange; or 15 mg/kg in one exchange/day (19 mg/kg if patient's urine output is >500 mL/day).
2. Gentamicin, 0.6 mg/kg (ideal body weight) IP in one exchange/day. Loading dose is required only if patient's urine output is >500 mL/day or if patient appears septic: loading dose = 1.5-2.0 mg/kg.
3. Cefazolin and gentamicin may be safely mixed in the same dialysate bag.

Courtesy of Karl Koenig, MD.

Suggested Follow-Up Theory of Peritonitis Based on Culture Results

Gram positive organisms on culture

Enterococcus	Staph aureus	Other Gram positives
Stop cephalosporin; add ampicillin 125 mg/L; continue aminoglycoside; treat x 14 days.	Stop aminoglycoside; continue cephalosporin; add rifampin 600 mg po qd; treat x 21 days.	Stop aminoglycoside; continue cephalosporin; treat x 14 days.

If no improvement in 48 hrs, reculture and re-evaluate

Gram negative organisms on culture

Single Gram negative	Pseudomonas, xanthomonas	Multiple organisms and/or anaerobes
Adjust antibiotics according to sensitivities; treat x 14 days.	Continue aminoglycosides with each exchange; stop cephalosporin; add agent with anti-pseudomonas or anti-xanthomonas activity*; treat x 21 days.	Consider surgical intervention; add metronidazole 500 mg IV or po q8hrs; treat x 21 days.

If no clinical improvement after 48 hrs: repeat cell count, cultures, and Gram stain. If culture positive, remove catheter.

If no clinical improvement after 48 hrs and exit site infection present, remove catheter.

* ceftazidime 125 mg/L IP
piperacillin 4 gm q 12h IV (adults), 150 mg/kg q12h IV (children)
ciprofloxacin 500 mg bid po (avoid in children)
aztreonam 1000 mg/L loading; then 250 mg/L IP
imipenem 500 mg/L loading; then 200 mg/L IP
trimethoprim/sulfa 320/1600 mg po q 1–2 days
aminoglycosides 6–8 mg/L IP in each exchange

Figure 42–9. Suggested antimicrobial therapy of peritonitis in CAPD patients. *(Adapted from Keane, Alaxander, Bailie, et al. [1996]. [pp. 562, 564].)*

Signs indicating infection are tenderness, drainage, and/or redness at the catheter insertion site. Treatment with antibiotics is necessary (Table 42–11). Peritonitis should be suspected when the patient presents with abdominal pain, fever, and/or cloudy dialysate. A sample of peritoneal fluid (effluent) should be sent for cell count and differential, Gram stain, and culture. Early treatment is advisable to avoid sepsis and permanent scarring of the peritoneal membrane with subsequent decrease in efficiency of dialysis. Treatment should be started empirically while culture results are pending. Several algorithms for empiric therapy are given in Figure 42–9.

REFERENCES

Alkhunaizi, A. M. & Schrier, R. W. (1996). Management of acute renal failure: New perspectives. *American Journal of Kidney Diseases, 28,* 315–328.

Chan, L. & Alfrey, A. C. (1997). Chronic renal failure: Manifestations and pathogenesis. In R. W. Schrier (Ed.), *Renal and electrolyte disorders* (5th ed.). (pp. 507–543). Philadelphia: Lippincott-Raven.

Daugirdas, J. T. & Ing, T. S. (1994). *Handbook of dialysis* (2nd ed.). Boston: Little, Brown.

Fauci, A. S. et al. (Eds.). (1998). *Harrison's principles of internal medicine* (14th ed.). New York: McGraw-Hill.

Forni, L. G. & Hilton, P. J. (1997). Continuous hemofiltration in the treatment of acute renal failure. *New England Journal of Medicine, 336,* 1306.

Kaysen, G. A. (1997). Proteinuria and the nephrotic syndrome. In R. W. Schrier (Ed.), *Renal and electrolyte disorders* (5th ed.). (pp. 640–684). Philadelphia: Lippincott-Raven.

Keane, W. F., Alexander, S. R., Bailie, G. R., et al. (1996). Peritoneal dialysis-related peritonitis treatment recommendations: 1996 update. *Peritoneal Dialysis International, 16,* 557–573.

Rose, B. D. (1987). *Pathophysiology of renal disease* (2nd ed.). New York: McGraw-Hill.

Stamm, W. E. & Hooton, T. M. (1993). Management of urinary tract infections in adults. *New England Journal of Medicine, 329,* 1328–1334.

Sutton, J. M. (1990). Evaluation of hematuria in adults. *Journal of the American Medical Association, 263,* 2475–2480.

Thadhani, R., Pascual, M., & Bonventre, J. V. (1996). Acute renal failure. *New England Journal of Medicine, 334,* 1448–1460.

Vander, A. J. (1995). *Renal physiology.* New York: McGraw-Hill.

Wallach, J. (1996). *Interpretation of diagnostic tests.* Boston: Little, Brown.

Yaqoob, M. M., Alkhunaizi, A. M., Edelstein, C. L., et al. (1997). Acute renal failure: Pathogenesis, diagnosis, and management. In R. W. Schrier (Ed.). (pp. 449–506). *Renal and electrolyte disorders* (5th ed.). Philadelphia: Lippincott-Raven.

43

Genitourinary Problems

Milton Coll

A reasonable understanding of urology is necessary for all clinically active personnel. Urology seems small in focus, but all experienced providers recognize the pervasiveness of the field. This chapter identifies several frequently occurring situations that present in both the inpatient and outpatient clinical settings. Presentation, history and physical exam, evaluation, and management are covered. At the end of the chapter are several urologic emergency situations that all providers must be able to recognize.

▶ GROSS HEMATURIA

The first clinical situation is the evaluation of the adult patient with gross hematuria. The history must begin with gender and age. Young women are more likely to have lower tract infections while older men are more at risk for prostatic and bladder neoplasms. The history should also include where in the stream the bleeding occurred. Although not always a reliable indicator, initial gross hematuria that clears early in the stream suggests bleeding distal to the sphincter mechanism, that is, prostatic or urethral. Total, midstream, and terminal hematuria suggests bladder or upper tract pathology. If clots are present and are long and thin, a renal or ureteral site should be considered. Short, thick clots are more often seen with urethral, prostatic, or bladder lesions.

Was the bleeding painful or painless? If painful, was there discomfort in the flank or abdomen, or was it primarily suprapubic, urethral, or meatal, suggesting a lower tract etiology? Upper tract discomfort can have many causes including pyelonephritis, trauma, tumor, stones, or vascular events (i.e., bleeding arteriovenous malformations/varicosities) with clot colic. Lower tract symptoms, especially if associated with other irritative and obstructive voiding symptoms, suggest a juxtavesical process such as a distal ureteral stone or tumor, pelvic organ inflammation near the bladder, or a prostatic lesion.

Gross hematuria associated with painful lower tract symptoms can also be caused by intravesical processes including cystitis, transitional cell cancer, and bladder stones. Prostatic and urethral pathology including BPH with bleeding, cancer of the prostate, urethral strictures, and tumors can similarly cause painful lower tract bleeding.

Painless bleeding suggests a more ominous etiology, but can also be due to benign processes including vascular lesions, stones, and infection. It is important also to determine if there is a history of trauma, including iatrogenic manipulation (i.e., catheters, GU, or GYN surgery) and blunt or penetrating injury.

Does the patient take anticoagulants? Overanticoagulated patients with gross hematuria require evaluation as the majority have clinically significant pathology that was unmasked by the anticoagulation. A prior familial or personal history of urolithiasis, sickle cell disease, or bleeding diatheses is clearly significant. TB exposure and other risk factors for papillary necrosis (i.e., diabetes, obstruction, phenacetin use, cirrhosis, pyelonephritis, and renal vein thrombosis) likewise are important clues to determine the etiology of gross hematuria.

Similarly, occupations and exposures should be considered. Smokers and employees in the petroleum and

the ureteral stones with or without an internal catheter (J2 stent) or ureteroscopy. ESWL also is the usual first line of treatment for visible stones in the proximal two thirds of the ureter. The stone-free rate increases if the stone can be pushed up into the renal pelvis. J2 catheters are usually required for this manipulation to unobstruct renal units, and to prevent fragments resulting from lithotripsy of large renal pelvic stones from later obstructing the ureter.

ESWL of the upper urinary tract is felt to be safe and not associated with any long-term, clinically significant complications. The treatment depends on being able to visualize the stones by fluoroscopy or ultrasound. Technology has advanced significantly and the most modern spark gap-generated devices are clearly superior and associated with the lowest retreatment rates yet.

Contraindications to ESWL monotherapy include very large stones that would produce large obstructing fragments, uncorrected bleeding diatheses, untreated obstructive uropathy (i.e., without a stent), untreated urinary infection, and pregnancy.

Stones in the distal ureter are best removed under direct vision via the ureteroscope. More proximal stones are more difficult to manipulate ureteroscopically. Therefore, the decision to approach these stones endoscopically should depend on the availability of necessary technology (i.e., laser, EHL, or ultrasonic lithotriptors) and the surgeon's comfort level with the technique.

If a patient has a large renal pelvic stone (i.e., greater than 2 cm), percutaneous nephrostolithotripsy (PCNL) should be considered primarily. This technique requires that a percutaneous nephrostomy catheter be strategically placed into the kidney, and a tract dilated to allow passage of a nephroscope into the collecting system. Direct vision ultrasonic, laser, or electrohydraulic lithotripsy with extraction of fragments can then be performed. Occasionally, one must combine PCNL with ESWL for complete removal of stone fragments.

There are still indications for open surgery. A large ureteral stone not successfully treated by ESWL and unreachable to the ureteroscope is best managed by ureterolithotomy. Large misshapen renal pelves secondary to chronic obstruction with stones should have open surgery to tailor and correct drainage from the kidney and simultaneous stone extraction. Most modern urologists, however, make every effort to first manage stones by the minimally invasive techniques described earlier.

Prevention

Once the stone has passed or been removed, attention turns to prevention. The stone must be analyzed: 75 to 80% of stones in the United States are composed of calcium oxalate or calcium phosphate; 10 to 15% are made of uric acid; 5% are struvite or infection stones; and, finally, only 1% is composed of cystine (an inherited homozygous recessive disorder).

All patients must increase their water intake enough to assure urinary volumes of 2½ to 3 liters per day. If the patient has just had his or her first stone or if his or her most recent was greater than a year ago, increasing urinary volume may be all that is necessary to prevent a recurrence for many years. However, if a patient forms more than one stone per year, or presents with multiple stones, a full metabolic evaluation is in order. This work-up includes blood samples for calcium, phosphate, uric acid, creatinine, and intact PTH (usually associated with calcium phosphate stone formers). Twenty-four–hour urine collections should be obtained on the patient's usual diet and studied for volume, calcium, phosphate, oxalate, uric acid, and citrate.

Most recurrent calcium oxalate stone formers have hyperabsorptive hypercaliuria and these collections may well be unremarkable. However, after an oral calcium challenge, repeat 24-hour urinary calcium excretion is above normal. Prevention of more stones, then, consists of increasing water intake and strenuously decreasing dietary calcium. If still not successful, sodium cellulose phosphate (a nonabsorbable ion exchange resin) may be used.

About one third of recurrent calcium oxalate stone formers leak calcium into the urine even on low-calcium diets. This can be demonstrated by the 24-hour collection after a calcium fast. They are best treated by increasing fluid intake and adding thiazide diuretics which increase distal tubular absorption of calcium.

Interestingly, on occasion one cannot identify hypercalciuria despite frequent calcium oxalate stone recurrences. A good portion of these patients have decreased 24-hour urine collections for citrate (an inhibitor) and are treated by exogenous potassium citrate.

Secondary hyperoxaluria from inflammatory bowel disease or malabsorption following bowel resection or bypass results in frequent calcium oxalate stone recurrences. These patients typically cannot absorb their fatty acids leaving the oxalate unbound and then hyperabsorbed. Occasionally, bypassed bowel must be reinstated.

Recurrent uric acid stone formers again must be encouraged to increase their water intake and to follow a low-purine diet. These patients typically maintain an acidic urinary pH without the normal periodic alkalinization that should occur during the day. The soluability of uric acid is less at an acidic pH. Prevention efforts therefore usually include alkalinization of the urine (sodium bicarbonate, sodium citrate, or potassium citrate). Those patients with continued recurrences are usually next treated with Allopurinol to prevent uric acid formation.

Struvite or triple phosphate stones usually result from chronic infection with or without foreign bodies and stasis. Efforts therefore must be made to eliminate the source of infection.

Finally, cystine stones are fortunately rare as they often can be nearly unmanageable. These patients can produce stones at an alarming rate (i.e., 5-15 per day). Treatment depends on increasing fluid intake and alkalinizing urine to a pH of nearly 8.0. It is often necessary to add chelating agents (Thiola, Penicillamine) to make the excreted cystine more soluble in urine and decrease the frequency of recurrences.

▶ URINARY TRACT INFECTIONS

Community-acquired urinary infections (UTI) are usually caused by common gram-negative organisms, with *E coli* responsible for about 85% of cases. The usual source of the pathogen is the patient's bowel flora.

History and Physical Findings

UTI symptoms can vary from nonexistent to overwhelming. The majority of patients describe lower tract irritative voiding symptoms including frequency, urgency, dysuria, and a sensation of incomplete emptying. Patients also note suprapubic and vaginal pressure and pain. Some note such extreme lower tract discomfort as to develop acute urinary retention.

It is most important to note upper tract symptoms, specifically flank pain, fever, and chills as this alters your approach to the evaluation and treatment of infection. If the patient reports symptoms suggesting pyelonephritis, the infection is by definition complicated and requires more involved evaluation and treatment.

The work-up must begin with a careful history. Did the patient have childhood infections or infection complicating pregnancies as might occur with congenital problems including vesicoureteral reflux? Is the patient an infrequent voider, and thereby allows long periods of urinary stasis in the bladder? Has she had a recent hormonal change (i.e., menarche or menopause) that could affect the normal vaginal flora? Does she take tub or bubble baths or use feminine products (including spermicidal creams) that may cause a chemical vaginitis affecting the normal vaginal floral barrier? Does she wipe from the back to front drawing pathogens anteriorly? Is there a problem with incontinence of stool or urine or constipation? Is there an association with sexual intercourse? Finally, is there any other history of significance including diabetes, stone disease, urologic surgery, or neuropathy?

Physical exam should include careful abdominal exam evaluating for flank tenderness and bladder distention. A neurologic exam should be included, which may discover neuropathy and ultimately a neurogenic bladder.

Laboratory and Diagnostic Tests

An ultrasound of the kidneys and cystoscopy should be done to evaluate the complicated UTI. Cystoscopy examines the bladder for a large postvoid residual, and for evidence of a refluxing orifice, ectopic orifice, ureterocele, fistula, and stones should be performed. If any irregularities are discovered, an IVU or voiding cystourethrogram (to rule out reflux) should be done.

Management

Uncomplicated UTI

The majority of patients who develop urinary tract infections are women, and they usually get the uncomplicated variety. Along with typical irritative voiding symptoms, these patients can also have gross hematuria. The majority do not have flank pain, fever, or chills. Those who do or who have had repeated infections with the same organism (relapsing infections) or frequent reinfections with different organisms have a more complicated situation and require more aggressive evaluation.

The usual patient who presents is a young female with her first infection or who has had less than two per year. Her symptoms are from the lower tract. They always respond quickly and completely to a short course of oral antibiotics. They recur infrequently with no more than two per year. If a culture is obtained, the organism is usually *E coli* or Proteus. Symptoms usually resolve after a 3-day course of a broad spectrum antibiotic (e.g., Macrodantin, Septra, or a flouroquinolone). A culture is not necessary unless the symptoms do not quickly resolve. A repeat urinalysis should be done one to two weeks after treatment and, if unremarkable, no further evaluation is indicated.

Often a patient reinfects within a few days of completion of initial therapy. Then, one must determine whether the initial infection was truly eradicated by the antibiotic. A urine culture and sensitivity are then necessary. If, according to the urine culture, the organism should have been eradicated, one then becomes concerned about underlying pathology that prevented clearance of infection. Similarly, patients who initially clear and then reinfect within a few weeks to months, or those who have relapsing infections (with the same organism), have reason to be concerned. These patients have not yet become septic, but have a more complicated clinical picture.

If there is an association with sexual relations ("honeymoon cystitis"), then one antibiotic tablet after intercourse indefinitely can be very effective. Patients still get infected, but the symptoms are more tolerable and of shorter duration.

Often the evaluation does not identify any underlying pathology and the patient and provider are always reassured. The patient should then be instructed to keep a supply of antibiotics at home and self-treat as needed with no more than a few days of treatment at a time to minimize symptoms. If the patient develops upper tract, symptoms or fever, then reevaluation is in order in case pathology was initially missed.

Complicated UTI

All men with urinary infection, regardless of age, are considered complicated. They require a full evaluation including an upper tract imaging study (IVU or ultrasound), cystoscopy, and possibly a urinary flow rate determination. Younger men are more likely to be infected due to stricture disease or stones, while infections in older men are usually due to bladder outlet obstruction by an enlarged prostate. Prostatitis should also be considered in both age groups.

Occasionally, patients with uncomplicated UTIs continue to reinfect frequently, despite a negative work-up and self-treatment. Suppressive therapy should then be instituted with a single antibiotic tablet per day (e.g., flouroquinolone, 1/2 Septra DS, or 50 mg Macrodantin) for 6 months. If symptomatic infections recur, self treatment or suppression can be reinstated.

Urinary tract infections associated with pyelonephritis are clearly more worrisome. An exhaustive evaluation must be performed before one can accept that no serious underlying pathology exists. Clearly, an IVU, cystoscopy, and probably voiding cystourethrogram are needed. Long-term suppressive therapy has to be considered early if recurrent pyelonephritis occurred and no other treatable pathology could be discovered.

On occasion, patients present with asymptomatic bacteriuria. These patients usually are elderly women who are unaware of symptoms. They, too, should receive the same evaluation as any patient with a complicated infection. If no pathology is discovered, no treatment is indicated. These patients should be followed periodically especially if their infection was with a urea-splitting organism that can quickly produce a stone. Therefore, a KUB or ultrasound annually is recommended.

Patients with indwelling catheters are always colonized by bacteria. Chronic exposure to antibiotics should be avoided as the bacteriuria will not resolve while the foreign body is present. The exposure will select resistant organisms. Patients should only be treated for short periods of time if septic. Every effort should be made to avoid indwelling foreign bodies, if possible.

UROLOGIC EMERGENCIES

Obstruction

As mentioned in the discussion of stones, the scenario of infection behind obstruction is frequent and can be life threatening. When a patient is admitted with the diagnosis of an obstructed ureter or kidney (i.e., congenital, stricture, stone, etc.), one must recognize if there is also sepsis. With high-grade renal obstruction, the kidney cannot drain and, therefore, decreases renal blood flow by preglomerular vasoconstriction. Antibiotics administered cannot get into the obstructed collecting system from the bloodstream and cannot reach the infected static urine. The situation resembles a deep abscess.

All patients with obstructed upper tracts and sepsis must have immediate drainage either by an externally draining ureteral catheter or by percutaneous nephrostomy. This occurs relatively frequently and results in catastrophe if the provider does not recognize the significance of sepsis with obstruction.

Also, all urologists have at some point or another been fooled by renal colic. Patients are not infrequently wrongly admitted with this diagnosis. Careful exam is, therefore, always indicated. One must keep an open mind, especially if the history and exam are not completely consistent with the diagnosis. One must know the differential diagnosis for intra- and retroperitoneal pathology (e.g., rupturing abdominal aortic aneurysm, perforated viscus, penetrating ulcers, diverticulitis, etc.). Obtain the definitive tests early (i.e., IVU) and quickly proceed to the next study (i.e., CT) if obstruction is not confirmed. Always remember that there may be a serious nonurologic explanation for the presentation.

Fournier's Gangrene

Fournier's gangrene is rapidly progressing necrotizing fasciitis of the genitalia. Patients are usually diabetic and frequently immunocompromised. The involved organisms are usually mixed aerobic and anaerobic gram-positive cocci, gram-negative rods, and anaerobes including *Bacteroides* and *Clostridia*. The organisms gain entry to the subcutaneous tissue via trauma to the local area, extension from a urinary tract infection, or extension from perianal or retroperitoneal sites. Once infection occurs, the organisms cause liquefactive necrosis of the tissue that spreads quickly. The involved planes usually limit the infection to the perineum and anterior abdominal wall. Overwhelming tissue destruction and death can occur within only a few hours.

The initial lesion is a red plaque that resembles cellulitis. Patients usually have fever and appear more ill than is otherwise expected. The tissue adjacent to the plaque becomes edematous and may appear "doughy" and bleached. After a brief time the reddened central lesion may develop a blister containing yellow or purpuric fluid strongly suggesting necrosis. There may be crepitance in the subcutaneous tissue from gas-forming organisms.

Unless the diagnosis is suspected and early antibiotics and extreme debridement initiated, the patient develops a fulminating fasciitis and dies. Therefore, all providers must recognize the significance of genitalial cellulitis, especially with the presence of sepsis, blisters, and crepitance.

Neurologic Impairment

Advanced prostate cancer metastasizes to bone. When a patient is admitted with acute lower extremity neuropathy or sudden bowel and bladder incontinence and has a history or exam consistent with prostatic cancer, one must consider spinal cord metastases with compression. This is a true emergency requiring steroids and radiation or neurosurgical decompression if one hopes to salvage or restore neurological function. Therefore, beware of the older male patient with acute neurologic loss.

44

Infectious Diseases

Janet M. Hines
Neil O. Fishman
Stephanie Green

▶ CRITICAL CONCEPTS OF INFECTIOUS DISEASES

In the appropriate management of infectious diseases, the following four concepts should be kept in mind:

- The clinician must be able to distinguish between colonization and infectious disease.
- The culture *cannot* distinguish between colonization and infectious disease.
- Narrowest antibiotic coverage is best.
- Treatment may require drainage, not just antibiotics.

Colonization Versus Infectious Disease

Under normal conditions, the body is *colonized* with multitudes of microorganisms—bacteria, fungi, and viruses. The body's defenses, namely, the skin (a physical barrier) and the immune system (with both specific and nonspecific components), are normally in equilibrium with the defenses microorganisms use. These microorganisms can sustain themselves without causing any harm to the host: no tissue is destroyed, and no nutrients are stolen. However, when the homeostasis is disrupted, disease may occur. An important example of this concept illustrates both the harmful effects of antibiotics, and the need to be parsimonious when using antibiotics. When a woman takes cephalexin (Keflex) for cellulitis, for example, any organism that is susceptible to the antibiotic is killed. This includes organisms colonizing the vaginal epithelium, like viridans streptococci, and some *E coli, Proteus,* and *Hemophilus* species. Organisms not susceptible to the cephalexin, like *Candida,* also normally exist in the vagina in small numbers. After the susceptible organisms are killed or reduced in number by the cephalexin, *Candida* doesn't have to compete with them for nutrients or space. They multiply and "overgrow." Without competing organisms to restrain their growth, they can cause tissue damage as they compete with and use the body for nutrients. The result is vaginal candidiasis, with itching, irritation, and discharge.

Vaginal candidiasis is an example of how the "dose," or absolute number of organisms, produces disease. Infectious disease can also result when the skin or mucous membrane integrity is disrupted. A traumatic wound may become infected by *Staphylococcus aureus*, which often colonizes the skin. Disease may also result when the organism is *virulent* (it possesses characteristics that allow it to cause disease, despite a low *inoculum,* or number of organisms). An example of a virulent organism is *Shigella,* which only requires between 10 and 100 organisms to cause severe diarrhea. *Salmonella,* by contrast, requires perhaps 10,000 to 100,000 organisms.

It is useful to be aware of the organisms found colonizing different sites of the body (known as *normal microbial flora*). These organisms are the most likely to cause disease in those sites when there is an abnormally high number of organisms, or the skin or mucosal integrity is disrupted. Table 44–1 shows normal microbial flora for important sites. Interestingly, the colonization patterns change

TABLE 44–1. Normal Microbial Flora

	Gram-Positive	Gram-Negative
Skin	Coagulase negative staph *Staphylococcus aureus* *Corynebacterium* spp. ("diphtheroids")	Enteric GNRs (*E coli,* Proteus, Klebsiella)—more likely to be found in the groin area
Mouth	Viridans streptococci Anaerobes	*Hemophilus* spp.
Colon	*Enterococcus* spp. *Streptococcus* spp. *Lactobacillus* spp.	Enteric GNRs Anaerobes
Vagina	*Streptococcus* spp. *Lactobacillus* spp.	Enteric GNRs Anaerobes

Key: GNRs = gram-negative rods; spp. = species (plural)

in the setting of the stress associated with acute disease or hospitalization. Soon after the onset of debility, a patient can be colonized with gram-negative rods on the body surface, particularly in the oral cavity and around the genital and rectal area.

Limits of the Culture

Because infections can be caused by the organisms that normally colonize the body, culture data must be interpreted with care. The culture cannot distinguish between colonization and infectious disease. For example, a patient recovering from abdominal surgery may develop a cough. A sputum specimen may show gram-negative rods on the gram stain and *E coli* on culture. But, if there are no white cells in the specimen, and certainly if there is no infiltrate on the chest x-ray, the finding likely represents colonization. (Culture interpretation is discussed in more detail in the microbiology section.) To properly interpret the culture, the clinician must also consider the gram stain, the manner of obtaining the culture, and certainly the entire clinical picture.

The Manner of Obtaining the Culture

In this postoperative patient, for example, *E coli* from an expectorated sputum specimen may reflect either oropharyngeal colonization or the agent causing pneumonia. *E coli* from a protected brush specimen obtained by bronchoscopy in the affected segment of lung is much more likely to represent the agent causing pneumonia than it is colonization of the oral cavity.

The Gram Stain

The organism reported on culture is more likely a pathogen *if* it is present on the gram stain in high numbers, particularly if there are relatively high numbers of WBCs on the stain. A predominance of epithelial cells in the gram stain argues against the specimen being representative of the site of infection. If the organism isolated in culture is absent on gram stain, it suggests it is present in a very small quantity. This finding, by itself, does not necessarily argue against the organism's causing disease. It is best to refer to the proportion of WBCs to epithelial cells, as well as to the virulence of the organism, in attempting to determine whether it is responsible. For example, coagulase negative staph from a cutaneous abscess with no WBCs is not likely to be the causative pathogen.

Antibiotic Coverage

Use of antibiotics encourages resistance among any organism that is exposed to them by "selective pressure." Any environmental pressure exerted upon an organism (like the presence of an antibiotic) kills those organisms that are *susceptible* to it, though organisms that are *resistant* to the antibiotic survive. There is enough genetic variability in many microorganisms that organisms resistant to almost any antibiotic (or other environmental pressure) exist within the flora. Thus, resistant organisms are "selected" and, consequently, they predominate in the flora that exists in a person after treatment with antibiotics. Therefore, to prevent the development of resistance, the antibiotic chosen must have activity *only* against the narrowest spectrum of organisms.

Half of hospitalized patients on antibiotics do not receive the most appropriate antibiotic. Therefore, there are increased health-care costs and adverse drug reactions, in addition to the development of resistance. Vancomycin-resistant enterococci (VRE), methicillin-resistant *S aureus* (MRSA), multidrug-resistant coagulase negative staphylococci, and penicillin-resistant pneumococci are among the most important multidrug-resistant pathogens.

Drainage

Pus must be drained. Antibiotic levels are generally not sufficient to eradicate organisms that are harbored at the center of an abscess. "Drainage" may entail something as simple as warm compresses to facilitate healing of a skin abscess (furuncle), or as complex as open laparotomy to drain loculated areas of pus within the abdomen after a ruptured appendix.

▶ A PRIMER ON MICROBIOLOGY

Clinicians may encounter a bewildering array of microorganisms in the hospital environment. Knowledge of their classification is essential to management of the infections they cause.

Definitions

Infection is the presence of microorganisms within the body. *Disease* occurs when the infecting microorganisms cause tissue damage or dysfunction. *Virulence* means the ability of an organism to cause disease. An avirulent organism is one that causes little harm, and may in fact live in *symbiosis* with the host (in other words, they both live off the same nutrients, but do not compete with each other). *Commensals,* or *colonizers,* are organisms that live in certain well-defined areas (or *niches*) of the body, and do not cause disease. These are generally avirulent organisms, but as mentioned earlier, if present in high enough quantities, they could cause disease.

Bacteria

Most disease we encounter is caused by bacteria. These organisms are smaller than red blood cells, and the subcellular machinery they use is different from that of humans. Antibiotics take advantage of this fact, so that they preferentially injure the bacteria while leaving the human cells generally intact. Different bacteria have different ecological niches, meaning that some organisms thrive in 98° moist environments, such as the GI tract, while others prefer the cooler, dryer surface of the skin.

Bacteria are generally divided into gram-positive and gram-negative based on the way they take up gram stain (Table 44–2). The way they take up stain depends on their structure, and the structure also determines how they behave, so that it is useful from a functional standpoint to divide microorganisms into gram-positive and gram-negative. Because not all bacteria can be classified easily based on their appearance by gram stain, there are other groups of bacteria: anaerobes (which can be either gram-positive or gram-negative), mycobacteria, rickettsiae, spirochetes, and higher bacteria (Table 44–3).

Gram-Positive Cocci

Staphylococcus aureus normally inhabits the skin a small percentage of the time, but it can be a persistent and invasive organism under the right circumstances. When *S aureus* is found in a culture obtained from a sterile site, it should always be treated as a pathogen, not a contaminant, since it is such a virulent organism. It tends to form abscesses, and sticks to prosthetic material easily. Often it requires a longer duration of treatment than other bacteria. Diabetics and those with renal failure are particularly predisposed to infection with *S aureus.*

Coagulase negative staphylococci are related to *S aureus* in their structure and the fact that they colonize the skin. They are, however, much less virulent. This is a group of multiple different species (best known is *S epidermidis*), which are named coagulase negative staphylococci because

TABLE 44–3. Other Classifications of Bacteria

Anaerobes	
Gram-Positive	*Clostridium difficile* and other *Clostridium* spp. *Peptococcus* *Peptostreptococcus* Anaerobic *Streptococci* *Propionibacterium acnes*
Gram-Negative	*Bacteroides fragilis* Other *Bacteroides* spp. *Prevotella* spp.
Others	
Mycobacteria	*Mycobacteria tuberculosis* *Mycobacteria avium-intracellulare* complex (MAC) Other *Mycobacteria* spp.
Rickettsiae	*Rickettsia rickettsiae* (rocky mountain spotted fever) Other *Rickettsia* spp. *Ehrlichia* spp.
Spirochetes	*Treponema pallidum* (agent of syphilis) *Borrelia burgdorferi* (agent of Lyme disease)
Higher Bacteria	*Mycoplasma pneumoniae* *Chlamydia* spp.

TABLE 44–2. Classification of Bacteria by Gram Stain

Gram-Positive Bacteria		Gram-Negative Bacteria	
Gram-Positive Cocci	***Gram-Positive Rods***	***Gram-Negative Cocci***	***Gram-Negative Rods***
Staphylococcus aureus Coagulase negative staphylococci *Streptococcus pyogenes* (Group A beta-hemolytic strep) *Streptococcus pneumoniae* Viridans steptococci *Enterococcus* spp.	*Corynebacterium diphtheriae* Other *Corynebacterium spp.* (diphtheroids) *Listeria monocytogenes* *Bacillus* spp.	*Neisseria meningitidis* *Neisseria gonorrheae* *Moraxella catarrhalis*	*Enterobacteriaciae*[a] *Vibrio cholerae* Other *Vibrio* spp. *Campylobacter spp.* *Helocobacter pylori* *Salmonella* spp. *Shigella* spp. *Pseudomonas* spp. *Acinetobacter* spp. *Hemophilus* spp. *Legionella* spp.

Key: spp. = species (plural)
[a]*Enterobacteriaciae:* a family of bacteria that includes: *Escherichia coli, Proteus* spp., *Enterobacter* spp., *Klebsiella pneumoniae, Citrobacter* spp., *Serratia* spp., *Morganella* spp., and *Providencia* spp.

the coagulase reaction distinguishes between them from *S aureus* (which is coagulase positive). When encountered in clinical specimens, they most often represent contaminants. In patients with indwelling prosthetic devices (such as prosthetic heart valves or central venous catheters), they may cause true infection when isolated from a site that is normally sterile (such as the bloodstream). Though they are relatively avirulent, they tend to be resistant to antibiotics, and it is not at all uncommon to find coagulase negative staphylococci that are sensitive only to vancomycin.

Streptococcus pyogenes (Group A beta-hemolytic strep) causes strep throat. For unclear reasons, a small percentage of people infected with this organism develop either rheumatic fever or glomerulonephritis several weeks later. Treatment of strep throat with a prolonged course of penicillin (either 10 days of oral penicillin or an injection of intramuscular benzathine penicillin) is recommended to prevent rheumatic fever. Treatment does not seem to lower the risk of glomerulonephritis.

It is worth mentioning here that the designation "group A beta-hemolytic" is sometimes used by microbiology labs to identify *S pyogenes.* There are over 100 species of streptococci, and they can be classified serologically (using antibodies, and divided into groups A, B, C, etc.), by hemolytic pattern (alpha [incomplete hemolysis of the agar]; beta [complete hemolysis]; and gamma [no hemolysis]), or by biochemical means. Preliminary culture reports often only identify strep by its hemolytic pattern or serologic group. Since these organisms behave differently, these preliminary reports can be acted upon when this is considered.

Group B strep (*S agalactiae*) tends to cause infection in diabetics or the elderly; Groups C, F, and G strep all behave like group A strep, but are much less common and should not cause rheumatic fever. Group D strep organisms (*S bovis*) are important because of the strong association between endocarditis caused by this organism and gastrointestinal tract malignancy. If such a condition is identified, therefore, the GI tract should be explored for occult tumor.

Other groups are not so important. To make things more confusing, not all strep fit into such groups. In general, if a strep can be categorized as a group (i.e., a group designated by a letter of the alphabet), it is beta hemolytic. (Group D are not beta hemolytic, though.) Viridans streptococci and pneumococci are alpha hemolytic. Enterococci can have any hemolytic pattern, but are most commonly gamma hemolytic.

Streptococcus pneumoniae is the most common bacterial cause of pneumonia and may cause meningitis in adults. It is a colonizer of the oropharynx, so finding pneumococcus in the sputum is not always indicative of pneumococcal pneumonia. The specimen should be accompanied by plenty of white blood cells and very few epithelial cells to indicate that the specimen was obtained from the lungs rather than the oropharynx or nasopharynx.

Enterococci are normally found in the gastrointestinal tract. In the hospitalized patient, enterococci can colonize the skin. The enterococcus is not a very virulent organism, but it is rather hearty and difficult to kill. It usually requires two antibiotics used together for synergy, and also requires a more prolonged period of treatment to eradicate the infection. Enterococcus becomes easily antibiotic resistant; vancomycin-resistant enterococcus is a particularly feared pathogen, and in some cases may be resistant to all known drugs. In such cases the question becomes whether to treat, rather than with what agent, and infectious disease consultation is warranted.

Viridans streptococci, like the coagulase negative staph, are similar to each other. Specifically, they colonize the mouth (most commonly) as well as occasionally the gastrointestinal tract and the skin. They are the most common cause of endocarditis, probably because they are able to stick to abnormal surfaces of the endothelium of the heart valves. They have less importance elsewhere, although they can rarely cause infectious disease at almost any site. They tend to be susceptible to penicillin alone or in combination with an aminoglycoside.

Table 44–4 demonstrates how the *Streptococcus* species are differentiated from one another.

TABLE 44–4. Differentiation of the Most Common *Streptococcus* Species

Species	Group (defined by reaction with antibodies)	Hemolytic pattern	Comments
Streptococcus pyogenes	Group A	Beta hemolytic	The only Group A strep is *S pyogenes*
Streptococcus agalactiae	Group B	Beta hemolytic	The only Group B strep is *S agalactiae*
Viridans streptococci	Nongroupable	Alpha hemolytic (rarely beta)	Species include: *S sanguis* *S mutans* *S mitis* *S salivarius* *S anginosus* *S intermedius*
Streptococcus pneumoniae (pneumococcus)	Nongroupable	Alpha hemolytic	
Enterococci	Some are Group D	Alpha or gamma hemolytic (occ. beta)	

Gram-Positive Rods

Corynebacterium diphtheria is the causative agent of diphtheria, a pharyngeal infection characterized by a necrotic gray membrane covering the posterior pharynx. If untreated with antitoxin, respiratory failure develops. It is extremely uncommon in the postvaccination era, but important to mention here in that it is the origin of the word *diphtheroids,* which are organisms that resemble, but do not cause, diphtheria.

Other *Corynebacterium* species (diphtheroids) colonize the skin, and are essentially avirulent. Except for prosthetic devices and in extremely debilitated patients, diphtheroids almost never cause disease. They are, however, commonly isolated from clinical specimens. In such cases they should be viewed as contaminants.

Like diphtheroids, *Bacillus* species also colonize the skin, are relatively avirulent, and are most commonly encountered as contaminants in clinical specimens.

Most commonly seen in the elderly, diabetics, or immunosuppressed patients, *Listeria monocytogenes* can cause meningitis or sepsis. It can be very serious infection in pregnancy. It does not colonize the body, so, when found in cultures it should be considered a pathogen.

Gram-Negative Cocci

Neisseria meningitidis (*N meningitidis*) can cause meningitis or sepsis. It is a colonizer of the oropharynx in about 15% of the population at any given time. Occasionally, it is reported as an isolate from a throat culture (though it is not a cause of pharyngitis) and does not require treatment. When a case of meningococcal meningitis is identified, the issue of prophylaxis of close contacts often comes up. Because the disease can be so devastating, even those with minimal contact feel the need to take antibiotic prophylaxis. In actuality, only those who had intimate contact (family, roommate, sexual partners) should receive prophylaxis. Health-care workers do not need prophylaxis unless mouth-to-mouth resuscitation has been performed, as long as standard precautions are followed.

Infection with *Neisseria gonorrheae,* the causative agent of gonorrhea, presents as a urethral or cervical discharge. It may cause a syndrome known as disseminated gonococcal infection, in which the organism may cause a vasculitic rash or a monoarticular arthritis. It is usually associated with gonococcal bacteremia.

Moraxella catarrhalis, formerly known as *Branhamella catarrhalis,* behaves similarly to *Hemophilus influenzae,* but is much less likely to cause disseminated or serious infection. It most commonly is an agent responsible for bronchitis, sinusitis, or otitis media.

Gram-Negative Rods

Enterobacteriaciae include many organisms (as listed in Table 44–2), that behave similarly. They normally colonize the gastrointestinal tract, but cause trouble when they are found in other body sites (urine, lungs, etc.). In the hospitalized patient, they can also colonize the skin, particularly dependent areas (like the lower back, which can be particularly problematic in a patient recovering from spine surgery). They are virulent enough to form abscesses under the right conditions, but should also be recognized as possible contaminants due to their ubiquitous presence in the hospitalized patient. They can acquire resistance to antibiotics, so treatment must be based on the susceptibility pattern.

Salmonella spp. are an important cause of diarrhea and can also cause bacteremia in patients with HIV or sickle cell disease. Interestingly, reptiles may be a source of *Salmonella,* and generally shouldn't be kept as pets by the immunocompromised.

Shigella spp. represent another important cause of diarrhea. It is notable that the infectious dose of *Shigella* is small—only 10 to 100 organisms are required to cause disease, compared with the 10,000 to 100,000 required for *Salmonella* or *Campylobacter.* Thus, it is easy to catch when around a source. It is not a common cause of extraintestinal disease, though the diarrhea it causes can be quite severe.

Another cause of diarrhea, *Campylobacter* spp. are much more common in the United States than the *Vibrio* species. The resultant diarrhea may be bloody or watery, and is characteristically (though not exclusively) "crampy." A gram stain of the stool shows the organism's characteristic gull-wing shape. Rarely, it may cause bacteremia, though it grows so slowly that it sometimes is identified only after the diarrheal episode resolves. If such occurs, treatment is only necessary if the patient remains ill or is otherwise debilitated.

Vibrio cholerae, while only rarely encountered in the United States, is the prototypical cause of watery diarrhea (cholera). It has been isolated in shellfish in the Gulf of Mexico, but is much more common in South America or Asia. If it is suspected in someone who has recently returned from such an area, the microbiology laboratory should be notified, as special culture techniques are required. It can be acquired through eating contaminated food or contact of a patient infected with *V cholerae.*

Other *Vibrio* spp. (*V parahemolyticus, V vulnificus,* etc.) are, like the agent of cholera, potential causes of diarrhea. Unlike cholera, however, they can be found in the United States (particularly the Gulf Coast and the mid-Atlantic) and they (more commonly, in fact) cause bloody diarrhea (which *V cholerae* never does). Suspect these organisms in the patient with diarrhea who gives a history of recent shellfish ingestion. The microbiology lab should be notified of your suspicions.

The discovery of the role of *Helicobacter pylori* in peptic ulcer disease has revolutionized its treatment. Currently, there is ample evidence to implicate *H pylori* in most cases of peptic ulcer disease. It is still important to establish its presence prior to treatment, which usually entails clarithromycin, metronidazole, and omeprazole.

Pseudomonas is a commonly encountered agent of the hospital environment. It is normally found in water supplies and earth, and is found as a colonizer of a healthy human only in unusual circumstances. It is quite virulent, causing bacteremia, abscesses, and infection of almost any organ, particularly those that are exposed to indwelling devices. It easily acquires antibiotic resistance and, as such, can be quite difficult to treat.

Acinetobacter acts like a close cousin to *Pseudomonas,* though it seems not to be quite so virulent. It is found in the same environmental sources, and easily acquires antibiotic resistance.

Hemophilus spp. are important causes of pneumonia, meningitis, bronchitis, otitis media, and sinusitis. *Hemophilus influenzae* is not so common since the advent of the vaccine for children. Adults, especially those who smoke, may still be infected by *H flu* (particularly the kind without a capsule, which was not included in the vaccine).

Legionella was virtually unheard of until the 1976 outbreak at the Legionnaires' convention in Philadelphia. Since then, it has been recognized as another important cause of pneumonia, particularly in elderly, hospitalized, or debilitated patients. Though it is commonly referred to as an "atypical" pathogen, it actually presents more like *Strep pneumoniae* (the classic "typical" cause of pneumonia). It is difficult to culture, except in an experienced laboratory, and the lab must be notified of your suspicion so they can use the proper media. Urine legionella antigen is not so sensitive for *Legionella,* but it may add to the overall specificity of the work-up since it is specific.

Anaerobes

The term *anaerobes,* when used clinically, refers to organisms that do not thrive in an oxygen-enriched environment. In conditions that involve their site of colonization, they should be considered potential pathogens. These organisms include *Clostridium* spp., *Peptostreptococcus* spp., anaerobic streptococci, *Actinomyces* spp. and *Propionibacterium* spp. (which are gram-positive), as well as *Bacteroides* spp., *Porphyromonas* spp., *Prevotella* spp., and *Fusobacterium* spp., which are gram-negative. *Clostridium difficile, C tetani* (the agent of tetanus), and *C botulinum* (the agent of botulism) are usually excluded from clinical consideration of anaerobes, since they produce distinct clinical syndromes that, when considered, are easily recognized. Anaerobes are normally found in the gastrointestinal tract, particularly the colon, as well as the mouth (in crevices between the teeth and gums), and the vagina.

Clostridium difficile (*C difficile*) is also an anaerobe that colonizes the gut when antibiotics eradicate some or all of the normal flora in the gut. In some cases, it may be the predominant organism seen, and under the right circumstances, toxin is produced. Diarrhea or frank colitis results. Diagnosis is tricky. It is important to understand that just because the organism or the toxin is detected does not mean that treatment is indicated. Only the syndrome of diarrhea requires treatment. It is also important to note that the suspicion of *C difficile* infection (based on diarrhea in the setting of recent or present antibiotic administration) is enough to justify empiric treatment. The sensitivity and specificity of the test are not sufficient to markedly alter a clinical impression. The first choice for treatment is oral metronidazole (Flagyl). Oral vancomycin is a second alternative, but is discouraged because of the fear of inducing vancomycin resistance among enterococci in the gut (though the development of resistance is probably more complicated). Intravenous metronidazole is less effective because it does not reach the gut lumen in acceptable concentrations.

Mycobacteria

Mycobacteria tuberculosis is the causative organism in tuberculosis (TB). The most common clinical presentation of TB is a chronic pneumonia that is manifest by a productive cough and fever with constitutional symptoms (such as weight loss). The duration of illness at the time of presentation is *generally* at least two weeks. Because of its contagious nature, recognition of this syndrome (a subacute illness with cough and constitutional symptoms) is extremely important in identifying who should be placed in respiratory isolation (see infection control section). Treatment of the organism requires multiple drugs given simultaneously for several months. It should be reported to the local public health authorities.

In general, other mycobacteria are much less virulent than *M tuberculosis.* However, in certain situations (not always the immunocompromised), they can cause disease, most commonly in the lungs or the skin. Consultation with the appropriate specialist (infectious disease, pulmonary, or dermatology) is warranted.

Fungi

Fungi have a more advanced cell structure than do bacteria. Antifungal antibiotics target a substance in the fungal cell wall that is neither present in humans nor bacteria.

Candida spp. colonize multiple sites on the body, particularly the mouth, lower gastrointestinal tract, and vagina. The organism load increases in the presence of general debility or immune compromise, as well as in the setting of antibiotic administration, since the natural flora in these areas is altered. In such settings, it may cause thrush (white plaques on a red base on the oral mucosa) or vaginal candidiasis. *Candida* may cause bloodstream infection in neutropenics, those with indwelling central venous catheters, diabetics, and those who have undergone abdominal surgery. The finding of *Candida* in the bloodstream should never be considered a contaminant. Since the advent of fluconazole, treatment of *Candida* bloodstream infections has been much easier, though it is important to remember that some species of *Candida* are resistant to fluconazole: *C krusei* is completely resistant, and *C parapsilosis* and *C glabrata* are more difficult to treat (i.e., they may require higher doses) than are *C albicans* and *C tropicalis.*

Aspergillus is an environmental pathogen, meaning that it may be found on inanimate surfaces, both inside and outside the hospital. It most commonly preys on immune compromised patients (most classically neutropenics), causing a progressive pneumonia, an invasive sinusitis, or systemic infection. It is difficult to diagnose, and should be suspected in the neutropenic patient who has fever without a clear source that persists despite appropriate empiric antibacterial agents. Treatment is likewise difficult, and requires much higher doses of amphotericin B than used for *Candida. Aspergillus* is occasionally found as a colonizer in the airways, but if there is any doubt about its pathogenicity, infectious disease or pulmonary consultation should be sought.

Mucor is one of the most feared fungi, as it attacks the sinuses and facial tissue relentlessly. Antifungal therapy when used alone is generally ineffective, so extensive debridement is necessary. The unusual patient who survives is generally disfigured from the infection and the surgical debridement. It preys on diabetics and occasionally those with cell-mediated immune deficiencies.

Viruses

Viruses are so small they do not carry much of their own machinery. Since they depend on the host (human) cell's machinery, safe treatment of these infections is difficult.

Herpes Simplex 1 and 2

Herpes simplex types 1 and 2 infections are extremely common. They, like the other members of the Herpesvirus family (which also includes varicella zoster virus, Epstein–Barr virus, and cytomegalovirus), are most commonly symptomatic during the initial infection, but remain latent within the body for life. Most other viruses (like influenza, rhinovirus, etc.) are eradicated from the body after a period of days or weeks. Herpes simplex type 1 usually infects the oral area, and herpes simplex type 2 usually infects the genital area; however, there are exceptions to this tendency. The initial infection, whether it be type 1 or 2, is characterized by painful vesicles on a red base, which rapidly ulcerate. The primary infection may be asymptomatic, and often viral shedding may occur without symptoms. When a patient is acutely ill or immunocompromised, a symptomatic recurrence may occur. The vesicular or crusted lesion at the vermilion border of the lip is easy to recognize. However, the genitals should be examined when a patient has a fever without a clear source, and is unable to complain of the pain and tingling that commonly precede the lesions. Contact isolation is sufficient to prevent transmission.

Varicella Zoster

Varicella zoster, the virus that causes chicken pox, is important to consider in the hospital setting. Shingles, or herpes zoster, is a condition in which this virus reactivates from its latent state. Shingles will manifest as vesicles on a red base along a dermatome. Though they resemble those described for herpes simplex, the zoster vesicles will generally be in different stages of evolution (all the herpes simplex vesicles appear to be at the same stage), and the herpes simplex vesicles do not have a dermatomal distribution. About 10% of the adult population should be considered susceptible to varicella infection. Thus, when a case of shingles (or the rare case of chicken pox in the adult population) occurs, the patient should be placed in respiratory isolation. Health-care workers who have had chicken pox, or who have had positive varicella titers, may enter the room without a mask.

Treatment for shingles with acyclovir will accelerate healing of the rash and reduce the acute pain. Postherpetic neuralgia is still a very significant problem; studies examining corticosteroid therapy have been controversial.

Cytomegalovirus

This virus also commonly infects people in childhood, such that only about 25% of the adult population is at risk for infection. When infection occurs in childhood, it resembles a mild cold. When it occurs in adulthood, it may look like mononucleosis, with fever, fatigue, and swollen lymph nodes. It may reactivate and cause disease in the immunocompromised, particularly HIV infected patients with advanced disease and transplant patients. Standard isolation is sufficient to protect from new infection, as the virus is found in the secretions of someone with a reactivation or an acute infection. Acquisition in the hospital is not common. It is much more likely to happen in situations that resemble day-care settings, in which secretions abound and gloves are not worn in each instance of contact with secretions. Acute infection poses the greatest risk to seronegative immunocompromised patients mentioned earlier, as well as to pregnant women who are not already seropositive.

Measles Virus

In the post-vaccine era, measles is extremely rare. Cases continue to occur, however, so a high index of suspicion is required to prevent transmission. Measles should be considered in anyone with conjunctivitis and coryza, followed by a rash. The measles rash is maculopapular, becoming confluent, and characteristically begins on the face, spreads to the trunk, and finally to the palms and soles. A patient presenting with fever, a generalized maculopapular rash, and either cough, conjunctivitis, or coryza, should be immediately placed in respiratory isolation until it can be determined with certainty whether measles is present. Serologic testing and/or viral culture (depending on the microbiology lab's capability) generally should be done to confirm the diagnosis. Such a situation is generally reportable to the local health department (in addition, certainly, to the hospital Infection Control department).

Respiratory Viruses

This group of viruses—*Influenza, Adenovirus, Parainfluenza, Respiratory Syncytial Virus*—is implicated not only in upper respiratory illness, but also in community-acquired pneumonia. It is difficult to reliably differentiate its clinical presentation from bacterial causes. In most cases, a patient is said to have a viral community-acquired pneumonia when the sputum cultures do not reveal a typical bacterial pathogen. Influenza and adenovirus are the most likely pathogens in normal hosts. When a patient is not responding to treatment for community-acquired pathogens, culture of the sputum for viruses can be useful, particularly in the immunocompromised. When a virus is revealed to be the pathogen, antibacterial therapy and its associated toxicities can be eliminated.

Parasites

Very few parasites should be mentioned in a text on acute care of inpatients, since history of travel to an indigenous area is rare. This section will only discuss parasites for which recent travel is not necessary for acquisition.

Giardia lamblia

This agent causes diarrhea. It accounts for 5 to 10% of cases of diarrhea in the United States, depending on the region. It should be suspected in a patient with diarrhea who gives a history of exposure to cold water, though interpersonal transmission also happens, so such a history is not always readily detectable. There are no reliably occurring characteristics about the diarrhea itself, though it may be associated with a prolonged duration of illness, malabsorption, and weight loss. Flatulence and belching are said to be common, and fever less common. The diagnosis is made by sending the stool for examination for ova and parasites. Some labs have immunofluorescent assays strictly for giardia. Treatment is with metronidazole, though failures and relapses may occur.

Pneumocystis carinii

Pneumocystis carinii pneumonia (PCP) is most commonly seen in patients with HIV who have CD4 counts below 200. It presents as a subacute, relatively slowly progressive respiratory illness with cough and dyspnea, most commonly with fever. Hypoxia may occur early in the illness, though as the infection advances, hypoxia may be profound, requiring intubation and associated with ARDS. Interestingly, in non-HIV patients immunosuppressed with malignancy, PCP presents much more rapidly, and most commonly after taper of steroids. Since HIV risk factors or the HIV diagnosis itself is not always disclosed, PCP should be considered in any patient with fever and interstitial infiltrates. Diagnosis is by sputum examination for the organism. Because the cough is generally nonproductive, sputum induction or bronchoscopy is frequently necessary. Treatment is by high doses of trimethoprim–sulfamethoxazole. If the partial pressure of oxygen (pO_2) is less than 70, steroids should be added. Such a maneuver saw a dramatic improvement in mortality from PCP in the early part of the HIV era.

▶ USE OF THE MICROBIOLOGY LABORATORY

Specimen Collection

Proper collection of the specimen is perhaps the most important indicator of the ultimate usefulness of microbiologic studies. Once in the microbiology laboratory, there are few reliable clues as to whether organisms isolated are the pathogens or represent colonizing flora in an area around the site. Some guidelines to specimen collection follow.

The specimen collected should represent the disease process. In other words, a urine culture that is not obtained as a clean catch may mislead by suggesting that colonizing organisms normally found in the perineum are pathogenic. Insertion of a swab into a sinus tract draining pus is tempting, but should be avoided because it is likely that skin colonizers have recognized the area as another site to colonize and flourish. The tissue (more precisely, the bone) at the base of the tract should be biopsied instead.

Additionally, the area surrounding the site of suspected infection should be cleaned aseptically so that colonizing flora are not mistakenly obtained and do not then confuse the issue.

A sufficient quantity should be obtained. Sufficient is anything more than what is on a swab. In other words, don't swab an abscess; rather, aspirate the pus. It is a misconception that a swab is sufficient or desired by the microbiology laboratory. In actuality, it is the least efficient in terms of amount of material obtained. In fact, its material can also be toxic to fungi and mycobacteria. It should only be used for obtaining specimens from mucous membranes, and then special attention should be paid to whether the *correct* swab is being used. For example, some swab materials are toxic to viruses or to chlamydia. Generally, when such organisms are sought they require transport media to be available at the bedside for immediate inoculation. It should be confirmed with the microbiology lab that the proper swab accompanies such transport media. In cases other than mucous membranes, tissue itself should be obtained. The tissue most likely to yield the organism is the tissue that is intact, but just adjacent to a collection of pus. If tissue cannot be obtained, however, pus should be obtained. If the specimen is difficult to obtain (i.e., requires surgery or an invasive procedure to obtain it), then as much as possible should be sent to the microbiology lab. It is also worth noting that whenever a biopsy is being obtained, if infection is even a remote possibility, it should be sent to the microbiology laboratory in addition to surgical pathology. It is much easier for the pathologist to get more tissue from the micro lab than vice versa: formalinized tissue is essentially useless for microbiologic exam.

The specimen should be placed into the proper transport system and delivered promptly to the lab. As mentioned earlier, actual tissue adjacent to the pus collection should be obtained if at all possible. Such tissue can be placed into a sterile specimen cup without any accompanying media, if it is to go to the microbiology lab promptly. If it requires overnight transit, transport media should be used. If pus is obtained, it can likewise be placed into a sterile specimen container. Alternatively, it can be left in the syringe if the needle is removed and replaced with an airtight hub. Specimens for fastidious (hard to culture) organisms may require specific transport media; such organisms are listed in Table 44–5. Anaerobic organisms in particular may require such media; however, if the specimen is solid or a significant amount of liquid, conditions within the specimen remain hospitable for anaerobes; if the specimen is transported quickly, no specific transport media may be needed.

The specimen should be obtained prior to the administration of antimicrobial agents. While it is still vastly preferable to obtain a specimen *after* antibiotic treatment rather than not at all, every effort should be made to obtain the specimen first.

The lab should be warned about any potential laboratory hazards. Any specimen that is contagious from person to person is also hazardous to the laboratory staff if proper precautions are not taken (for example, specimens suspected of having TB are worked with under a hood). Whenever such a situation is encountered, the micro lab should be notified. However, some specimens are hazards to lab workers when they are not a hazard on the floor. One reason this occurs is that the culture system serves to *amplify* the number of organisms, so that the inoculum encountered in the microbiology laboratory is high enough to cause disease. Another reason for a lab hazard is that the process of culturing makes the organism enter into a stage of the life cycle that (a) would not be encountered in the patient (thus

TABLE 44–5. Obtaining Specimens for Particular Sites

Condition	Site/Specimen	Collection Device	Organisms	Miscellaneous
Strep throat	Tonsils and tonsillar fossae	Cotton-tipped swab collection device	*S pyogenes* (Group A beta-hemolytic strep)	In general, other bacteria isolated from this site are not clinically relevant
Bacterial pneumonia	Expectorated sputum intubated patient: tracheal aspirate or bronchial washings	Sterile screw-capped jar	*S pneumoniae* *L pneumophila* *H influenzae* many others	Elicit deep cough; patient should not expectorate saliva or nasal secretions for collection; not acceptable for anaerobic culture
Pulmonary tuberculosis	Three early A.M. specimens, expectorated	Sterile screw-capped jar	*M tuberculosis*	5–10 cc required for proper yield
Viral pneumonia	Nasopharyngeal swab/aspirate	Calcium alginate-tipped wire swab, or aspiration with a bulb syringe	Influenza A, B, C Parainfluenza 1.2.3 Adenovirus RSV	
Sinusitis	Endoscopically obtained specimen from affected sites	ENT consultation	Multiple	
Urinary tract infection	Clean catch midstream urine, or straight catheterization	Sterile screw-capped jar	Enterobacteriaciae	Send promptly (under 2 hr) or refrigerate
Bacteremia, fungemia	Blood from site disinfected by iodine and alcohol	Blood culture vials (multiple types, institution specific)	Most bacterial species *Candida* species	20–30 cc required per set
Mycobacteremia, fungemia (some)	Blood, as above	Lysis-centrifuation tube; biphasic bottle	*M avium-intracellulare* Dimorphic fungi	20–30 cc required per set
Catheters	2″ of catheter tip	Sterile screw-capped jar	Multiple	Collect aseptically; only vascular catheters are acceptable (i.e., not foley catheters)
Soft tissue (abscess)	Tissue at periphery of abscess, or pus—as much as possible	Sterile screw-capped jar, syringe capped with rubber stopper (not needle), or swab collection device	Multiple	

making the patient noninfectious), and (b) is infectious. Such a situation occurs with the so-called dimorphic fungi (*Histoplasma, Blastomyces,* and *Coccidioides*).

A guideline to obtaining specimens for particular sites is included in Table 44–5.

Identification of Organisms

The microbiology laboratory identifies organisms by microscopic examination, culture, or a number of other techniques using antibodies or DNA probes.

Microscopic Examination

Specimens are stained directly from specimens obtained from otherwise sterile body sites, to allow for preliminary identification of organisms. They can also be used to help distinguish colonization from disease. In other words, a sputum specimen may have many gram-negative rods, but if there are few or no white blood cells in the specimen, the bacteria likely represent colonization. One final use of a stain is identification of certain viruses, particularly herpes simplex or herpes zoster, by DFA (direct fluorescent antibody staining). Table 44–6 lists the steps in preparing a Gram stain.

Culture

Culture is the only definitive way to identify an organism. Culture of an otherwise sterile body fluid is straightforward, in that the only task is to provide all the nutrients that the suspected pathogen may need. Culture of sites that are not sterile—for example, the stool—requires the ability to differentiate between pathogens and commensals. Antibiotics can be impregnated into the media to kill the commensals and allow the pathogen to survive. More often, only some of the commensals are eliminated, and other tests must be used to differentiate the pathogen from the commensals. Such tests usually take advantage of a unique biochemical trait of the pathogen. For example, *E coli* O157:H7, the pathogen of enterohemorrhagic diarrhea associated with hemolytic–uremic syndrome, is differentiated from other *E coli* (which are predominant commensals in the stool) by the fact that the former do not metabolize sorbitol. Colonies that do metabolize sorbitol produce a biochemical end-product that is pigmented, thus nonpigmented colonies are selected to further test as *E coli* O157:H7.

While awaiting identification of an organism, it is often helpful to discuss the work-up with the microbiology laboratory technician. Not only can clues be ascertained about the organism's identity, but the certainty of a preliminary diagnosis can also be discussed.

TABLE 44–6. Preparation of a Slide for Gram Staining

1. A clean glass slide should be labeled to indicate onto which side of the slide the specimen is placed. The name of the patient or the patient number should also be on the slide.
2. The specimen should be dropped onto the slide, or rolled onto it if obtained by a swab. There should be varying degrees of thickness of the specimen (if it is too thick, it is uninterpretable).
3. Air drying is sufficient, yet inefficient. If a flame is used, the specimen should be very briefly passed through the flame so as not to burn the specimen.
4. Flood the slide with crystal violet; rinse off with tap water after 30–60 seconds.
5. Flood the slide with gram's Iodine; rinse off with tap water after 30–60 seconds.
6. Carefully drip acetone–alcohol decolorizer onto the slide until the fluid coming off of the slide has no color to it.
7. Flood the slide with safranin or fuchsin; rinse off with tap water after 30–60 seconds.
8. Allow the slide to air dry; examine under oil immersion (1000×).
9. Interpretation of gram-stained slides for clinical purposes should only be done with ample experience; the expiration date should be checked prior to use, and control slides should be stained weekly, with the results recorded, to ensure quality control.
10. Of note, if a specimen is to be placed onto a slide for staining and interpretation elsewhere (as for a DFA for herpes viruses), steps 1 and 2 should be followed, with the additional comment that it is essential that there is positive identification of the patient on the slide (name or medical record number and date).

Use of Serology

It is important to recognize that antibody responses to different infections are variable. For example, in acute CMV infection, the IgM antibody may remain elevated for up to a year, and the IgG may disappear after only a few months. Thus, the presence of IgM and IgG does not indicate the timing of infection reliably. Moreover, there are technical concerns with each assay that prevent generalizations about the sensitivity and specificity of a test. It is best to only rely upon serology to detect those infections for which serologic means is well-studied, and for which positive and negative results have consistent implications. The most important point, as is applicable to any test, is that it is more likely to be truly positive in situations in which the pretest probability (the clinical impression) for the disease in question is high. The common infections that are relatively reliable as diagnosed by serology are listed in Table 44–7.

Susceptibility Testing

Susceptibility testing does not need to be performed on every isolate. For example, Group A strep is essentially universally susceptible to penicillin. Reference labs will periodically check susceptibilities on such organisms to ensure that they remain susceptible. Susceptibilities should be performed on any meaningful clinical isolate (i.e., isolated in sufficient quantities to suggest they are responsible for dis-

TABLE 44–7. Common Infections Reliably Diagnosed by Serology

HIV-1, HIV-2
Epstein–Barr virus
Hepatitis A, B, C, D, E viruses
Measles, mumps, rubella

ease) for which the susceptibility is generally unpredictable. It is much more difficult to perform susceptibilities on organisms that grow slowly or have difficult growth requirements, like anaerobes, mycobacteria, or fungi.

Because the goal of susceptibility testing is to predict the likelihood of success with an antimicrobial treatment regimen, the result should be used as a guide to assist with the choice of an antibiotic. In other words, a "susceptible" result means that under ordinary conditions (i.e., those that allow sufficient serum levels of the drug), the infection is very likely to be effectively treated. "Resistant" means that it is unlikely the infection will be effectively treated; however, it is not unusual for a patient to begin to respond to a drug to which the organism is subsequently found to be resistant. The clinician then faces the dilemma of changing therapy in the face of improvement, or continuation of therapy despite *in vitro* testing that suggests the drug will not work. In most cases, the clinical scenario rules; in other words, other factors that go into improvement, like effective drainage may have supervened. However, it is not so clear if this is the correct approach in patients who are recovering from a life-threatening infection, and infectious disease consultation is warranted.

▶ PHARMACOLOGY OF ANTIBIOTICS

Principles of Therapy

Using the conceptual approach to therapy, there are 5 primary interventions (Kim & Gallis, 1989):

- Careful observation without antibiotics
- Preventive/prophylactic therapy
- Empiric therapy for a suspected but unproven infection
- Therapeutic trial with antimicrobials
- Specific therapy for a documented infection.

Each approach has both beneficial effects and specific limitations. To complicate matters, optimal therapy or the duration of treatment is not known for many infections. Complex clinical situations arise that may require multiple antibiotics, with a broader spectrum of activity. This can contribute to the escalating problem of antibiotic resistance, as well as to increased toxicity. It is important, however, to identify whether an infection is really present.

Any antibiotic can be toxic. For example, a previously healthy 32-year-old woman was treated with penicillin for a sore throat. After three doses she began to develop a desquamating rash and was hospitalized. She developed a deep vein thrombosis of the left lower extremity on the second hospital day, and also had a massive pulmonary embolism (PE) despite adequate anticoagulation. She had an inferior wall myocardial infarction while recovering from the PE. Findings on cardiac catheterization were consistent with a coronary artery vasculitis. The patient was felt to have an allergic vasculitis secondary to penicillin, and responded to steroids. Thus, use of any antibiotic must be justified.

Tables 44–8 through 44–10 list important considerations in antibiotic therapy. Please confirm all doses with those recommended by the manufacturer in the product insert.

Among the adverse reactions that can develop on antibiotics, some are predictable based on the class of drug, and others are entirely unpreventable. Immunologic reactions, particularly the Type I (immediate type hypersensitivity reaction, IgE mediated), cannot be predicted unless the patient has a history of a similar reaction in the past. In such a case the drug, if given at all, should be given only after consultation with specialists in infectious disease and allergy/immunology. Type I reactions are most common with the penicillins but can occur with any drug at all. It is important to note that reactions (whether type I or not) to penicillin can also occur when the same patient is administered cephalosporins: there is about a 10% chance of cross-reactivity in such cases.

Dosing in Renal Insufficiency

As with many drugs, dosing of antibiotics often must be adjusted for renal insufficiency. Whether the dose or the interval should be adjusted is a property of each drug, and should be attended to when adjusting doses.

Vancomycin Dosing

The patient's ideal body weight (IBW) should be calculated by the following formula:

Male: 50.0 kg + (2.3 × inches over 5 ft)
Female: 45.5 kg + (2.3 × inches over 5 ft)

The creatinine clearance (CrCl) should then be calculated according to the following formula:

Male: (140 – age) × IBW (kg)/[72 × serum creatinine]
Female: 0.85 × CrCl for male

Dose vancomycin depending on the creatinine clearance:

CrCl > 50 ml/min:	1 gm IV q12
CrCl < 50 ml/min:	1 gm IV q24
Hemodialysis:	1 gm every 7 days

Gentamicin Dosing

Once-daily dosing of aminoglycosides may be less toxic than traditional dosing. It should not be used on neutropenic patients; those being treated for suspected or documented endocarditis; those with cystic fibrosis, cirrhosis, ascites, or myasthenia gravis; pregnant women; dialysis patients; those being treated for staphylococcal or enterococcal infections when the aminoglycoside is used for synergy; or patients in acute renal failure.

The creatinine clearance should be calculated as cited earlier under vancomycin dosing. If the patient is obese (>20% IBW), take 40% of excess weight and add it to the IBW. Obese patient dosing weight is 0.4 × (ABW – IBW) +

TABLE 44–8. Classification of Antimicrobial Agents

Penicillins	Generic Name	Brand Name	Usual Dose
Penicillins	Penicillin V	Various	250–500 mg tid-qid
	Penicillin G	Various	Various
	Procaine penicillin	Duracillin	Various
	Benzathine penicillin G	Bicillin	600,000–1.2 MU once, or once a week
Aminopenicillins	Amoxicillin	Various	250–500 mg tid
	Ampicillin	Omnipen	250–500 mg q6 po 150–200 mg/kg/d IV
	Amoxicillin–clavulanate	Augmentin	500 po bid to 875 po bid
	Ampicillin–sulbactam	Unasyn	1.5–3.0 gm IV q6h
Antipseudomona 1 penicillins	Mezlocillin	Mezlin	3 gm IV q4h
	Piperacillin	Pipracil	3–4 gm IV q4–6h
	Piperacillin–tazobactam	Zosyn	3.375 gm IV q6h
	Ticarcillin	Ticar	3 gm IV q6h
	Ticarcillin–clavulanate	Timentin	3.1gm IV q4–6h
Beta-lactamase inhibiting penicillins	Nafcillin	Unipen, Nafcil	1–2 gm IV q4
	Dicloxacillin	Dynapen	250–500 mg po q6
	Cloxacillin	Tegopen, Cloxapen	250–500 po q6
	Oxacillin	Prostaphlin	1–2 gm IV q4
Related Antibiotics			
Carbapenems	Imipenem/cilastatin	Primaxin	500 mg IV q6
	Meropenem	Merrem	500 mg to 1 gm IV q8
Monobactams	Aztreonam	Azactam	1–2 gm IV q8
Cephalosporins			
1st generation, oral	Cephalexin	Keflex, various others	250–500 mg po q6
	Cephradine	various	250–500 mg po q6h
	Cefadroxil	Duracef	500 mg to 1 gm po q12
1st generation, IV	Cefazolin	Ancef, Kefzol	250–500 mg po q8
	Cephapirin	Cefadyl	500 mg to 1 gm po q6h
2nd generation, po	Cefuroxime axetil	Ceftin	250–500 mg po q12h
	Cefprozil	Cefzil	250–500 mg po q12
	Cefaclor	Ceclor	250–500 mg po q8h
	Loracarbef	Lorabid	400 mg po q12
2nd generation, IV	Cefuroxime	Zinacef, Kefurox	750 mg to 1.5 gm IV q8h
	Cefamandole	Mandol	500 mg q6–2 gm IV q4
	Cefotetan	Cefotan	1–3 gm IV q12
	Cefoxitin	Mefoxin	1 gm q8–2 gm q4
	Cefmetazole	Zefazone	2 gm IV q6–12
3rd generation, po	Cefixime	Suprax	200–400 po q12–24
	Cefpodoxime proxetil	Vantin	100–200 mg po q12
	Ceftibuten	Cedex	400 mg po qd
3rd generation, IV	Cefotaxime	Claforan	1 gm q8–2 gm q4 IV
	Cefoperazone	Cefobid	2 gm q12–4 gm q6 IV
	Ceftazidime	Fortaz, Tazicef, Taxidime	1–2 gm IV q8–12
	Ceftizoxime	Cefizox	1 gm q12–4 gm q8 IV
	Ceftriaxone	Rocephin	500 mg q12–2 gm qd IV
4th generation, IV	Cefepime	Maxipime	1–2 gm IV q12
Aminoglycosides			
IV	Gentamicin	Garamycin	ONCE DAILY: 5.1 mg/kg IV peak serum level: 16–24 mcg/mL trough serum level: undetectable TRADITIONAL DOSING: 2 mg/kg load, then 1.7 mg/kg q8h peak: 4–10 mcg/mL trough: 1–2 mcg/mL
	Tobramycin	Nebcin	As for Gentamicin
	Kanamycin	Kantrex	ONCE DAILY: 15 mg/kg IV peak: 56–64 mcg/mL

(Continued)

TABLE 44–8. Classification of Antimicrobial Agents *(Continued)*

	Kanamycin *(Contd.)*		trough: undetectable TRADITIONAL DOSING: 7.5 mg/kg q12 peak: 15–30 mcg/mL trough: 5–10 mcg/mL
	Amikacin	Amikin	As for Kanamycin
	Netilmicin	Netromycin	ONCE DAILY: 6.5 mg/kg IV peak: 22–30 mcg/mL trough: undetectable TRADITIONAL DOSING: 2.0 mg/kg load, then 2.0 mg/kg q8 peak: 4–10 mcg/mL trough: 1–2 mcg/mL
	Streptomycin	Various	7.5 mg/kg q12 (max 2 gm qd)
	Spectinomycin	Trobicin	2 gm IM (gonorrhea)
po	Neomycin	Various	Various
Miscellaneous Classes and Antibiotics			
Macrolides	Erythromycin	Various	250–500 mg po q6h 500 mg to 1 gm po q6 IV
	Azithromycin	Zithromax	po: 500 po qd × 1 day, then 250 po qd d.2–5 IV: 500 IV qd
	Clarithromycin	Biaxin	500 mg po q12
Tetracyclines	Tetracycline	Various	250–500 mg po q6 500 mg to 1 gm IV q12
	Doxycycline	Various	100 mg po q12 100 mg IV q12
	Minocycline	Minocin	100 mg po q12
Fluoroquinolones	Ciprofloxacin	Cipro	250–750 mg po q12 200–400 mg IV Q12
	Ofloxacin	Floxin	200–400 mg po or IV q12
	Levofloxacin	Levaquin	250–500 mg po or IV qd
Sulfonamides	Trimethoprim–Sulfamethoxazole	Bactrim, Septra	1 double-strength (DS) or 2 single-strength (SS) tablets po bid 8–10 mg/kg/d of trimethoprim component, divided q6–8h
Miscellaneous	Clindamycin	Cleocin	150–450 mg po q6h 300–900 mg IV q8h
	Metronidazole	Flagyl	250–500 mg po q6h 250–500 mg IV q8h
	Chloramphenicol	Chloromycetin	50 mg/kg IV, divided q6h
	Vancomycin	Vancocin	500 mg to 1.5 mg IV q12 125 mg po q6h

IBW, where ABW is actual body weight. The dose of aminoglycosides should be rounded to the nearest 50 mg. A serum BUN and creatinine should be obtained at least every 2 days, and a random level of the aminoglycoside should be obtained 8 to 14 hours before the next dose. Assistance with dosing should be sought with the hospital's pharmacokinetics service, if available, or pharmacist. See Table 44–11 for aminoglycoside dosing in renal insufficiency.

▶ MANAGEMENT, AS GUIDED BY THE SUSPECTED SITE OF INFECTION

In general, management of infectious disease cases can be considered by the site of infection. Following is a description of the presentations of infection at the site, appropriate work-up of infection at each site, including the steps required to establish the diagnosis, the suspected pathogens, antimicrobial management, and other management.

Central Nervous System Infections

Meningitis

Meningitis is an infection of the tissues lining the brain and/or spinal cord. Acute meningitis most often presents with a severe headache and fever. It is important to note that headache and fever are very nonspecific, and much more often represent a "viral syndrome," such as influenza. The diagnosis of meningitis is based on the presence of meningismus, or a neck that resists passive flexion. In such

TABLE 44–9. Common Adverse Drug Reactions

Reaction	Drug Class	Comments
Gastrointestinal upset	Penicillins	
	Cephalosporins	
	Macrolides	
	Metronidazole	
	Sulfonamides	
	Fluoroquinolones	
CNS dysfunction	Fluoroquinolones	Especially in elderly patients, patients with underlying CNS abnormalities
	Minocycline	Vestibular dysfunction
Bone marrow suppression	Chloramphenicol	All cell lines
	Sulfonamides	
	Beta-lactams (esp. nafcillin)	Leukopenia
	Vancomycin	
	Penicillins	Thrombocytopenia
Nephrotoxicity	Aminoglycosides	
	Amphotericin	
	Sulfonamides	
Ototoxicity	Aminoglycosides	
	Vancomycin	
	Erythromycin	
Pseudocholelithiasis (gallbladder sludge)	Ceftriaxone	
Seizures	Beta-lactams, particularly Imipenem	Decrease the seizure threshold
Disulfiram reaction	Some cephalosporins	
	Metronidazole	
	Chloramphenicol	
Hemolysis due to G6PD deficiency	Sulfonamides	
	Dapsone	
	Nitrofurantoin	
	Primaquine	
"Red man" syndrome	Vancomycin	
Hepatotoxicity	Erythromycin (primarily cholestasis)	
	Sulfonamides	
	Amoxicillin–clavulanate	
	Oxacillin	
	Isonaizid	
	Rifamycin	
Neuropathy	Metronidazole	
	Isoniazid	
Metallic taste	Metronidazole	
Photosensitivity	Tetracyclines	
Vitamin K deficiency	All antibiotics	
C difficile infection	All antibiotics, particularly ampicillin, clindamycin	
Serum sickness reaction	Cefaclor	
	Loracarbef	
Platelet dysfunction	Some cephalosporins, Ticarcillin	
Failure of oral contraceptives	Penicillins (particularly ampicillin, piperacillin, ticarcillin, mezlocillin)	
	Doxycycline	
	Rifamycins	

a case, the patient's head is lifted by the examiner, without assistance from the patient. Such a finding also distinguishes true meningismus from the muscular stiffness that may accompany a benign viral syndrome. Other findings that suggest meningitis include photophobia (light causes pain in the eyes), and more dramatically, confusion or seizures.

Meningitis is an infectious disease emergency. This is because the cranium is an enclosed space, and the infection and inflammation that ensue displace space, and then may

TABLE 44–10. Important Drug–Drug Interactions

Effect	Drug
Increased PT on oral anticoagulants	Some cephalosporins Metronidazole Sulfonamides Trimethroprim
Decreased PT on oral anticoagulants	Rifamycins
Increased cyclosporin levels	Macrolides
Decreased cyclosporin levels	Sulfonamides
Increased theophylline	Ciprofloxacin Enoxacin Norfloxacin
Cardiac arrhythmias with terfenadine, astemizole, or cisapride	Macrolides Azoles
Increased effect of neuromuscular blocking agents	Clindamycin Aminoglycosides Macrolides[a] Quinolones[a] Tetracyclines[a]
Decreased seizure threshold	Imipenem with ganciclovir Beta-lactams with beta-lactams

[a] The stated effect is rare; the drug may be used with caution.

TABLE 44–11. Aminoglyoside Dosing in Renal Insufficiency

Aminoglycoside	Creatinine Clearance	Dose
Gentamicin/tobramycin	>50 ml/min	5 mg/kg/24h
	30–49 ml/min	5 mg/kg/36h
	20–29 ml/min	5 mg/kg/48h
Amikacin	>40 ml/min	15 mg/kg/24h
	30–39 ml/min	15 mg/kg/36h
	20–29 ml/min	15 mg/kg/48h

cause brain damage. *Treatment must be initiated as soon as possible.* By convention, treatment should be initiated 30 minutes after the patient hits the door, whether the work-up is complete or not.

Diagnosis. Because the treatment must be initiated so rapidly, attempts at diagnosis must be efficient. Lumbar puncture (LP) is the most helpful test, but (1) it requires expertise, and sometimes it is technically difficult (particularly in the elderly patient with degenerative changes in the spine that distort the normal architecture); and (2) in rare cases, it may result in herniation of the brain through the foramen magnum. This latter results from the presence of a block in the flow of the spinal fluid, usually at the level of the fourth ventricle. This may be caused by mass effect. Examination is not helpful in definitively establishing whether it is safe to perform lumbar puncture; however, a normal exam in a host not likely to have brain masses is sufficient to say that the LP can be performed. In the presence of cranial nerve abnormalities, lateralizing defects, or papilledema, the brain should be imaged prior to LP. The most efficient imaging modality is CT of the brain without contrast; its sensitivity suffers somewhat, but whether to proceed to other imaging modalities is dependent upon the suspicion of the presence of a mass.

Cerebrospinal fluid obtained by lumbar puncture should be evaluated both chemically and sent for cell count and culture. Findings suggestive of bacterial versus other infections are presented in Table 44–12.

Fluid should always be examined by gram stain and cultured for bacteria. If these studies are negative, the decision whether to continue to treat for bacterial pathogens, consider other pathogens requiring treatment, or dismiss the presentation as a case of viral meningitis, will depend on the CSF findings as mentioned earlier.

Treatment. Empiric treatment for acute meningitis in the adult generally consists of a third-generation cephalosporin, such as ceftriaxone or cefotaxime, which crosses the blood–brain barrier. In the elderly, in diabetics, and in any hosts who are at risk for a cell-mediated immune defect, ampicillin is added in order to cover *Listeria.*

If cultures are positive, the coverage may be tailored appropriately, based on the expected or actual susceptibilities. Treatment should generally be continued for 10 to 14 days. Treatment for meningitis is delineated in Table 44–13.

Other Elements of Management. When meningococcal meningitis is diagnosed, the issue of prophylaxis of close contacts inevitably surfaces. Because meningococcal meningitis is renowned for its fulminant course in otherwise vigorously healthy young people, panic ensues among anyone who remotely contacted the individual diagnosed, and many will request prophylaxis. Because meningococcus is transmitted by respiratory droplets rather than aerosols, which travel further than aerosols, prophylaxis is recommended *only* for close contacts. Generally prophylaxis is

TABLE 44–12. Laboratory and Diagnostic Tests That Differentiate Bacterial Versus Other Infectious Organisms

	Bacterial	Viral	Fungal	Tuberculous
Opening pressure	>18 cm H_2O	Normal	Varied	Varied
WBC	1000–5000	100–1000	100–500	100–500
Type cell predominant	Neutrophil	Lymphocyte (though may be neutrophil early)	Varied	Lymphocyte (though may be neutrophil early)
Protein	Elevated	Normal	Varied	Increased
Glucose	Markedly decreased (<40)	Normal	Decreased	Decreased

TABLE 44–13. Treatment of Meningitis

Clinical Setting	Empiric Rx	Likely Pathogens	Definitive Rx	Dosage Regimen	Duration
Meningitis community-acquired 18–50-yr-old	Ceftriaxone + vancomycin[a]	*S pneumoniae*	If MIC <=0.1: penicillin G	12–20 mu/d IV in 6 divided doses	10–14 d
			If MIC >0.1: ceftriaxone	2 gm IV q12h	
		N meningitidis	Ceftriaxone	2 gm IV q12h	
		H influenzae	Ceftriaxone	2 gm IV q12h	
Meningitis community-acquired 50+ yr-old	Ampicillin + ceftriaxone +/– vancomycin	As above	As above	As above	10–14 d
		Listeria monocytogenes[b]	Ampicillin +/– gentamicin	2 gm IV q4h consult pharmaco-kinetics	
		Pseudomonas aeruginosa	Cefepime or ceftazidime	2 gm IV q8h	
		Other gram-negative rods	Ceftriaxone	2 gm IV q12h	
Postsurgical	Cefepime + vancomycin	*S aureus*	Nafcillin[c] ± intraventricular vancomycin	2 gm IV q4h	14 d
		Coagulase negative staphylococcus	Vancomycin ± intraventricular vancomycin		
		Pseudomonas aeruginosa	Cefepime or ceftazidime ± intraventricular gentamicin	2 gm IV q8h	
		Other gram-negative rods	Ceftriaxone[d]	2 gm IV q12h	

[a] Several cases of ceftriaxone resistant pneumoccoci have been reported.
[b] Risk factors for *L monocytogenes:* age > 50 years, HIV and other immunosuppressive states, pregnancy.
[c] If beta-lactam allergy, use trimethoprim/sulfamethoxazole; if MRSA, use vancomycin.
[d] If organism is ceftriaxone susceptible.

recommended for household or intimate contacts who had more than 4 hours of contact within the past week. It is also recommended for those who may have been exposed directly to secretions (such as in kissing, or those who administer mouth-to-mouth resuscitation, or performance of nasopharyngeal suction or intubation without a mask).

Regarding treatment of the patient with acute meningitis, care should be taken not to volume overload the patient, as increased intracranial pressure can result. Seizures should be treated aggressively. Use of steroids is controversial; when used, they should be administered as soon as possible—ideally, before the administration of antibiotics. It is postulated that minimization of the inflammation may minimize morbidity.

Endovascular Infections

Endovascular infections include endocarditis, septic thrombophlebitis, and central line-associated infections. They are considered together because they share a common site, the vascular system, which gives these infections certain shared properties. Specifically, when infection is established in the endovascular system (the internal surface of the heart or the blood vessels), it is difficult to eradicate. Treatment can often require several weeks of intravenous antibiotics.

Pathophysiologically, infection begins when the endothelium (which is the lining of the arteries, veins, or the heart) is damaged. Sterile clot forms at the site of the damage. Bacteria that may be present within the bloodstream find it easy to attach to such a damaged site. (Parenthetically, transient bacteremia is common after microtrauma to blood vessels in certain areas. It often results after brushing the teeth or bowel movements.) Because the clot continues to grow, once bacteria attach, they are protected from the elements of the bloodstream that normally fight off infection (antibodies, phagocytes, and complement). The bacteria have all the nutrients they need within the clot, and as they thrive, they multiply and continuously seed the bloodstream with more bacteria. (Thus arises the concept that endovascular infections are associated with the continuous presence of bacteremia, as manifested by persistently positive blood cultures.)

All of the manifestations of endocarditis result from any combination or all of the etiologies listed in Table 44–14.

Endocarditis

Endocarditis is an infection of the lining of the heart (endocardium), most commonly the valves. People with abnormal heart valves are predisposed to endocarditis. Age-related degenerative changes and mitral valve prolapse have replaced rheumatic valvular disease as the most important reasons for endocarditis. Also important are congenital valvular disease and having a history of past infective endocarditis. The most common etiologies of endocarditis are listed in Table 44–15.

Symptoms. The patient who presents with endocarditis often has a number of very nonspecific complaints. Often it is only when these symptoms are considered altogether that they are recognized as representing endocarditis. Fever is the most common manifestation. It is important to note that

TABLE 44–14. Manifestations of Endocarditis

Local effects of the infection in the valve or heart tissue itself	Valvular insufficiency may result in congestive heart failure Myocardial abscess may present as failure of antibiotic therapy, or less commonly as interruption of the conduction system (with consequent arrhythmias)
Embolization of clot (infected or uninfected) to distant sites	Stroke (particularly in the distribution of the middle cerebral artery) Pulmonary emboli (when the right side of the heart is involved) Coronary artery emboli (with resultant myocardial infarction and myocarditis) Often embolization is clinically silent
Persistent bacteremia	Infection at distant sites (e.g., pneumonia or meningitis)
Reaction of the immune system to the continuous presence of infection	Splenomegaly, petechiae, and glomerulonephritis Normochromic normocytic anemia Elevated erythrocyte sedimentation rate
Others	The constitutional symptoms (e.g., weight loss, malaise, fatigue, and anorexia) Musculoskeletal symptoms (e.g., arthralgias, myalgias, and low back pain)

From Weinstein & Schlesinger. (1974).

in a patient with no other localizing complaints, the fever is usually present for an unusual length of time (a matter of days or even weeks). This length of time helps distinguish it from most undifferentiated viral syndromes. There is nothing specific about the fever pattern or the height of the fever. Fever is almost invariably present in patients with endocarditis; however, it may not be present in the elderly, or those with liver, renal, or heart failure. In addition to fever, the patient with endocarditis notably complains of other constitutional symptoms (malaise, fatigue, anorexia, weight loss). Arthralgias and myalgias, particularly in the lower back, are often present. An important picture to recognize is the patient complaining of low back pain and incidentally mentioned constitutional symptoms. Symptoms referable to the cardiac system (such as dyspnea or palpitations) tend, though not exclusively, to occur later in the disease.

TABLE 44–15. Etiologies of Endocarditis

Agent	Percentage of Cases
Viridans streptococci	30–40%
Enterococci	5–18%
Other streptococci	15–25%
Staphylococcus aureus	10–27%
Coagulase negative staphylcocci	1–3%
Gram-negative rods	1.5–13%
Fungi	2–4%
Miscellaneous bacteria	<5%
Mixed infections	1–2%
"Culture negative"	<5–24%

From Scheld & Sande. (1995).

Signs. The clinical manifestations of endocarditis reflect either persistent bacteremia (with infection in distant sites, usually causing vascular damage) or persistent antigenemia (with stimulation of the immune system). Such findings are:

- *Fever:* As mentioned earlier, the pattern is not specific for endocarditis.
- *Murmur:* A murmur is not necessary for the diagnosis, but most cases will have a murmur. More specific for the diagnosis of endocarditis is a new murmur or a changing murmur. However, new or changing murmurs are found in less than 10% of cases of endocarditis. Moreover, interobserver and intraobserver variability often occurs, despite the convention of grading murmur intensity as I to VI, so the new or changing murmur may not always be a reliable finding.
- *"Embolic manifestations":* This term generally encompasses all of the skin manifestations seen in endocarditis. This includes the presence of petechiae, Osler's nodes, Janeway lesions, and splinter hemorrhages. Petechiae often occur in crops, or groups, in one area of the body at a time, particularly on the mucous membranes. Osler's nodes and Janeway lesions are time-honored descriptions of two different phenomena that are often confused. Osler's nodes are painful purplish nodules located on the pads of the fingers or the thenar eminence. Janeway lesions are hemorrhagic macules on the palms and soles. Finally, splinter hemorrhages (linear hemorrhages in the nailbeds that parallel the axis of the digit) suggest the presence of endocarditis. They are located in the proximal aspect of the nailbeds; those found in the distal nailbeds are more likely to be related to minor trauma and are not related to endocarditis.
- *Splenomegaly* is a manifestation of emboli or of the reaction of the immune system to the persistent infection.
- *Stroke* occurs as a result of either septic emboli or rupture of a mycotic aneurysm. Emboli to the brain generally result in an infarct in the distribution of the middle cerebral artery. A mycotic aneurysm is a weakness in the wall of a cerebral vessel due to infection invading the blood vessel itself. Because the vessel becomes weak, the wall ruptures and intracerebral hemorrhage results. If anticoagulation is anticipated, exclusion of the possibility of bleeding is necessary by CT of the head.
- A normal renal sediment tends to argue against endocarditis, as the kidney is often affected by infection, infarction, or glomerulonephritis.

Diagnosis. The diagnosis of endocarditis requires a high degree of clinical suspicion to put all the various nonspecific findings into a picture that suggests endocarditis. When endocarditis is suspected, *blood cultures* should be obtained from at least two separate sites. The reason for separate sites is that an organism isolated from cultures obtained from two separate sites is more likely to represent true bacteremia than contamination. Since endocarditis is sometimes caused by organisms that colonize the skin, this distinction is of utmost importance. The amount of time that should elapse between blood cultures is not so important in diagnosing endocarditis, unless one is trying to establish the presence of continuous (as opposed to intermittent) bacteremia. Drawing the blood cultures hours apart supports continuous bacteremia, which suggests endocarditis. Conversely, if the patient is sick enough to require urgent treatment, the blood cultures should be drawn as soon as possible (though still from different sites) to allow culture of the blood in the absence of antibiotics. The single most important factor contributing to the yield of blood cultures is the *volume* of blood drawn. However, there is a point of diminishing returns: three sets of blood cultures (20 cc per set, or 10 cc per bottle) is optimal. The yield does not increase appreciably with more than three sets drawn (Weinstein et al., 1983).

Echocardiography is important in establishing the diagnosis of endocarditis, though it should not be the sole criterion for making the diagnosis. It is important to note that a negative study does not exclude the presence of endocarditis. Also, the technical quality of the study should be considered in interpreting the result; in other words, a negative study in an obese patient ultimately adds little to the information.

In the absence of pathologic examination of tissue (valve surgery or autopsy), the diagnosis of endocarditis depends on the sum of all clinical data, which may still be rather unclear. Thus, it is important to make use of time off antibiotics to help establish the diagnosis, if at all possible. In other words, an outpatient with a fever but no localizing signs should *never* be placed on empiric antibiotics. If the patient is sick enough to require antibiotics, blood cultures should always be obtained prior to initiation of antibiotics.

Treatment. Treatment of endocarditis is initially empiric, and generally includes antibiotics active against the skin flora. It is additionally important to realize that when the patient is clinically stable, antibiotics need not be started emergently. In other words, observation off of antibiotics may help to establish the diagnosis. Infectious disease consultation is entirely appropriate in such a circumstance.

Definitive treatment is tailored to the organism; once isolated, an organism suspected in causing endocarditis is subjected to more testing than are most other lab isolates. Namely, susceptibility testing is essential for most organisms, and guides the treatment for most staphylococci and gram-negative rods. A special susceptibility test known as the minimum inhibitory concentrations (MIC), performed on viridans streptococci, is important in deciding the treatment and treatment duration. Guidelines for treatment are included in Tables 44–16 and 44–17.

Empiric and definitive treatment of some of the more common causes of endocarditis are listed in Table 44–16.

Other Aspects of Management. Surgery is occasionally necessary in the management of endocarditis. The widely accepted Dinubile criteria are listed in Table 44–17.

"Culture negative endocarditis" is important to mention in that as specifically defined, it is generally caused by organisms not easily cultured by most bacterial culture systems. The most likely such organisms are *Hemophilus* spp., *Actinobacillus actinomycetemcomitans, Cardiobacterium hominis, Eikenella corrodens,* and *Kingella kingae,* together referred to by the HACEK acronym. Of course, a more common reason for cultures to be falsely negative is prior administration of antibiotics when there is no established etiology for a fever.

Another consideration in the appropriate management of endocarditis is prevention of endocarditis. Antibiotics should be used responsibly to minimize the likelihood of the development of resistance in the community. Tables 44–18 and 44–19 include the most recent AHA guidelines. (Dajani et al., 1997 and Wilson et al., 1995).

Septic Thrombophlebitis

Septic thrombophlebitis differs from endocarditis in that it usually develops in the venous system in an area whose endothelium is abnormal due to the presence of an indwelling device. It may occur in either peripheral (superficial septic thrombophlebitis) or central veins. Its presentation usually is that of a fever without a clear source in a hospitalized patient with indwelling devices. Bacteremia that does not clear despite removal of vascular catheters points to septic thrombophlebitis. Generally, if peripheral venous catheter sites are indurated or red, they are likely to be the source. In the case of septic thrombophlebitis affecting the central veins, there may be edema and erythema in the extremity distal to the catheter. The diagnosis is made by physical examination and the finding of positive blood cultures. Surgical exploration establishes the diagnosis in the case of superficial septic thrombophlebitis, and is necessary for treatment. In the case of central vein septic thrombophlebitis, diagnosis is established by imaging the central veins (usually the brachiocephalic, subclavian, and superior and inferior venae cavae). Such imaging usually requires the characterization of the flow in the affected vessels, so either an ultrasound or a magnetic resonance scan with angiography is necessary. Ultrasound is generally used first. Treatment of superficial septic thrombophlebitis requires surgical removal of the involved vein. Septic thrombophlebitis of the great veins interestingly usually responds to removal of the catheter, administration of antibiotics specific for the of-

TABLE 44–16. Empiric and Definitive Treatment of Endocarditis

Clinical Setting	Empiric Treatment	Likely Pathogens	Definitive Treatment	Dosage Regimen	Duration
Native valve	Vancomycin + gentamicin[a]	*S aureus*	Nafcillin[b] + gentamicin	Nafcillin: 2 gm IV q4h	4—6 weeks
				Gentamicin (peak concentration 3–4 mcg/mL)	3 days only
		Viridans streptococci, MIC<0.1[c]	Penicillin G	12–18 mu/day IV in 6 divided doses	4 weeks
			OR		
			Penicillin G + gentamicin	Penicillin G: 12–18 mu/day IV in 6 divided doses	2 weeks
				Gentamicin (peak concentration 3–4 mcg/mL)	2 weeks
		Viridans streptococci MIC 0.1–0.5[c,d]	Penicillin G + gentamicin	Penicillin G: 18 mu/d IV in 6 divided doses	4 weeks
				Gentamicin (peak concentration 3–4 mcg/mL)	2–4 weeks
		Viridans streptococci MIC >0.5	Penicillin G + gentamicin	18–30 mu/d IV in 6 divided doses	4–6 weeks
				Gentamicin (peak concentration 3–4 mcg/mL)	4–6 weeks
		S pneumoniae	Penicillin G[e]	20 mu/d in 6 divided doses	4–6 weeks
		Enterococcus spp.[f]	Ampicillin + gentamicin	2 gm IV q4 h	4–6 weeks
				Gentamicin (peak concentration 3–4 mcg/mL)	4–6 weeks
Prosthetic valve[g]	Vancomycin + gentamicin	*S aureus*	As above[b] +/– rifampin	600 mg po q12 h	6 weeks[h]
		Coagulase negative staphylococcus	Vancomycin + gentamicin + rifampin[i]	(see "Vancomycin Dosing" and "Gentamicin Dosing")	6 weeks
				Gentamicin (peak concentration 3–4 mcg/mL)	2 weeks
				Rifampin: 600 mg po q12h	4 weeks

[a] For subacute bacterial endocarditis or chronic endocarditis, can await cultures if patient clinically stable.
[b] If beta-lactam allergy or MRSA, use vancomycin.
[c] Alternative: ceftriaxone 2 gm IV/IM q24h × 4 to 6 weeks.
[d] Or, if organism is nutritionally deficient.
[e] Up to 12% of isolates penicillin resistant; obtain MICs.
[f] Review susceptibilities: 30% of isolates are multidrug resistant; penicillin G 18–30 mu/d can be substituted for ampicillin if microorganism susceptible.
[g] Surgery usually required.
[h] May require subsequent oral therapy.
[i] Rifampin should not be added to the regimen unless the organism is shown to be susceptible to both vancomycin and gentamicin.

fending organism, and heparinization. In some cases, thrombolysis is considered. Treatment should be continued at least 2 to 3 weeks, but depends on the organism and the rapidity of response to treatment. Infectious disease consultation is warranted.

TABLE 44–17. Criteria for Surgical Intervention in Endocarditis

Hemodynamic decompensation
Emboli (cerebral, coronary, peripheral)
Extravalvular myocardial invasion (abscess, pericarditis)
Extravalvular foreign body
"Resistant" infection
In vitro resistance to bactericidal antibiotics (for example, enterococci resistant to vancomycin, ampicillin, and aminoglycosides) inability to achieve adequate serum or tissue levels persistent bacteremia or fungemia despite appropriate treatment highly virulent organisms
"Large" vegetations (though this remains controversial)
Prosthetic valves

From Dinubile, (1982).

Central Line-Associated Infection

Such infections are quite common in the hospitalized, particularly the intensified, patient. The presentation is usually one of a fever without a readily identifiable source. Occasionally there is tenderness or erythema around the line insertion or tunnel site. In the absence of another source for the fever, the line is assumed the source, even if there are no local signs of infection. In such a case, the line should be removed, with the tip aseptically sent for culture. A new line may initially be placed in the same site. Some operators prefer to change the initial line by inserting a new line over a wire inserted into the same site. While such a practice is not ideal, realistically, intensified patients may have few sites to spare. A fresh stick is clearly optimal, and should be used when the patient will only require the central line for a few more days. If the line is changed over a wire, it is important to change the line to a *new* site if (1) the blood culture or tip culture is positive, or (2) the fever does not remit. Management of infection in semipermanent

TABLE 44–18. Antimicrobial Prophylaxis for the Prevention of Bacterial Endocarditis in Patients with Underlying Cardiac Conditions[a,b]

Clinical Considerations	Endocarditis Prophylaxis Recommended	Endocarditis Prophylaxis Not Recommended
Cardiac conditions	*High-risk category* prosthetic cardiac valves (including bioprosthetic and homograft valves) Previous bacterial endocarditis Complex cyanotic congenital heart disease (e.g., single ventricle states, transposition of the great arteries, tetralogy of Fallot) Surgically constructed systemic pulmonary shunts or conduits *Moderate-risk category* most other congenital cardiac malformations (other than above and below) Acquired valvular dysfunction (e.g., rheumatic heart disease) Hypertrophic cardiomyopathy Mitral valve prolapse with valvular regurgitiation and/or thickened leaflets[a]	*Negligible risk category* (no greater risk than the general population) Isolated secundum atrial septal defect Surgical repair of atrial septal defect, or patent ductus arteriosus (without residual beyond 6 months) Previous coronary artery bypass graft surgery Mitral valve prolapse without valvular regurgitation[a,c] Physiologic, functional, or innocent heart murmurs[a] Previous Kawasaki disease without valvular dysfunction Previous rheumatic fever without valvular dysfunction Cardiac pacemakers and implanted defibrillators
Dental procedures	Dental extractions Periodontal procedures including surgery, scaling and root planing, probing, and recall maintenance Dental implant placement and reimplantation of avulsed teeth Endodontic (root canal) instrumentation or surgery only beyond the apex Subgingival placement of antibiotic fibers or strips Initial placement of orthodontic bands but not brackets Intraligamentary local anesthetic injections Prophylactic cleaning of teeth or implants where bleeding is anticipated	Restorative dentistry[d] (operative and prosthodontic) with or without retraction cord[e] Injection of local intraoral anesthetic (except intraligamentary injections) Shedding of primary teeth
Respiratory tract	Tonsillectomy and/or adenoidectomy Surgical operations that involve respiratory mucosa Bronchoscopy with a rigid bronchoscope	Tympanostomy tube insertion Endotracheal intubation Bronchoscopy with a flexible bronchoscope, with or without biopsy[f]
Gastrointestinal tract	Sclerotherapy for esophageal varices[g] Esophageal stricture dilation[g] Endoscopic retrograde cholangiography with biliary obstruction[g] Biliary tract surgery[g] Surgical operations that involve intestinal mucosa[g]	Transesophageal echocardiography[f] Endoscopy with or without gastrointestinal biopsy[f]
Genitourinary tract	Prostatic surgery Cystoscopy Urethral dilation	Vaginal hysterectomy[f] Vaginal delivery[f] Cesarean section In the absence of infection for urethral catheterization, uterine dilation and curettage, therapeutic abortion, sterilization procedures, or insertion or removal of intrauterine devices
Other		Cardiac catheterization, including balloon angioplasty Implanted cardiac pacemakers, implanted defibrillators, and coronary stents Incision or biopsy of surgically scrubbed skin Circumcision

[a]Recommendations of the American Heart Association, (1997). Refer to the article for a complete discussion about the topic. (Dajani, 1997.)
[b]This table lists select procedures but is not meant to be all-inclusive.
[c]Individuals with mitral valve prolapse with thickening and/or redundancy, especially men >45 years, may have increased risk of endocarditis.
[d]This includes restoration of decayed teeth (filling cavities) and replacement of missing teeth.
[e]Clinical judgment may indicate antibiotic use in selected circumstances that may create significant bleeding.
[f]Prophylaxis is optional for high-risk patients.
[g]Prophylaxis is recommended for high-risk patients; optional for medium-risk patients.

TABLE 44–19. Antimicrobial Prophylaxis for the Prevention of Bacterial Endocarditis in Patients with Underlying Cardiac Conditions[a]

Situation	Drug	Dosage Regimen
Dental/oral/upper respiratory/esophageal procedures		
Standard general prophylaxis	Amoxicillin	2 gm po 1 hour before procedure
Unable to take oral medications	Ampicillin	2 gm IM or IV within 30 minutes before procedure
Allergic to penicillin	Clindamycin OR	600 mg po 1 hour before procedure
	Cephalexin[b] OR	2 gm po 1 hour before procedure
	Azithromycin or clarithromycin	500 mg po 1 hour before procedure
Allergic to penicillin and unable to take oral medications	Clindamycin OR	600 mg IV within 30 minutes before procedure
	Cefazolin[b]	1 gm IM or IV within 30 minutes before procedure
Genitourinary/gastrointestinal procedures (excluding esophageal)		
High-risk patients	Ampicillin + gentamicin	Ampicillin 2 gm IM/IV + gentamicin 1.5 mg/kg (not to exceed 120 mg) within 30 minutes before starting the procedure; THEN Ampicillin 1 gm IM/IV or amoxicillin 1 gm po 6 hours later
High-risk patients allergic to ampicillin/amoxicillin	Vancomycin + gentamicin	Vancomycin 1 gm (infused over 90 minutes) plus gentamicin 1.5 mg/kg IV (not to exceed 120 mg); infusions should be completed within 30 minutes of starting procedure
Moderate-risk patients	Amoxicillin or ampicillin	Amoxicillin 2 gm po 1 hour before starting procedure OR Ampicillin 2 gm IM/IV within 30 minutes of starting procedure
Moderate-risk patients allergic to ampicillin/amoxicillin	Vancomycin	Vancomycin 1 gm (infused over 90 minutes); infusion should be completed within 30 minutes of starting procedure

[a]Recommendations of the American Heart Association, (1997). Refer to article for a complete discussion about the topic. (Dajani, 1997.)

[b]Cephalosporins should not be used in individuals with immediate-type hypersensitivity reactions (urticaria, angioedema, or anaphylaxis to penicillins).

catheters (Hickman, Perma-cath) requires infectious disease consultation unless the line is to be removed.

Pneumonia and Other Respiratory Tract Infections

Pneumonia is one of the most common infections encountered in the community, being the most likely reason a patient is hospitalized with an infection. Classic symptoms include cough productive of green or bloody sputum, fever, chills, rigor, and occasionally shortness of breath. Signs include rales and other signs of consolidation; occasionally asymmetrically diminished respiratory excursion is found. Classic symptoms and signs are, however, not the rule. More commonly the diagnosis rests upon the chest x-ray, where infiltrates are the *sine qua non* of pneumonia.

Since not all respiratory infections are pneumonia, it is important to differentiate pneumonia from sinusitis, bronchitis, and the nonspecific syndrome designated "upper respiratory infection" (URI). Sinusitis may also be associated with a productive "cough," though this cough is actually made of secretions draining from the sinus cavity. Acute sinusitis is characteristically associated with the sensation of congestion, though it is occasionally associated with asymmetric tenderness of the face overlying the maxillary or frontal sinuses. Chronic sinusitis is also associated with congestion, but not necessarily with tenderness. It is important to note that the chest x-ray should be normal in sinusitis.

The chest x-ray should also be normal in bronchitis. Since there are no easily performed definitive tests for bronchitis, it is said to be a "diagnosis of exclusion." The reason to distinguish between pneumonia and bronchitis is that infections of the bronchial tubes are much more likely to be viral. Moreover, the "drainage" of bronchitis is easier than that of pneumonia: whereas the bronchial tree is made of fairly well-conducting tubes, the lung itself acts like a sponge. Thus antibiotics are not indicated in most cases of bronchitis. In smokers and those with chronic lung disease, however, drainage is impaired, so antibiotics are indicated. It is also important to note that purulent sputum alone, without fever or signs of consolidation, is not necessarily an indication for antibiotics.

Pneumonia is also one of the most common infections encountered in hospitalized patients, though it does not have the classic appearance of community-acquired pneumonia. (It is designated nosocomial pneumonia when it occurs more than 48 hours after admission to the hospital.)

The presentations of community-acquired and hospital-acquired (nosocomial) pneumonia are different because their presentations generally reflect the underlying competence of the lung to mobilize secretions. Community-acquired pneumonia affects people who have normal lung function and normal immunity. The hospitalized patient with pneumonia generally is debilitated or intubated. The patient does not mobilize secretions or aerate the alveoli as efficiently as he or she should; nor can an effective cough be generated.

Therefore, the patient with community-acquired pneumonia is more likely to have the rales, egophony, and sputum production that are classically associated with pneumonia. Nosocomial pneumonia can be caused by organisms that are relatively weak, or avirulent. Virulent organisms may cause both types of pneumonia.

Pneumococci are the most common cause of community-acquired pneumonia. The prevalence of drug resistance among pneumococci has been steadily increasing in the last few years. About one third of strains of *S pneumoniae* are resistant to penicillin, though there is marked geographic variation and some areas have as much as 50%. Infectious disease consultation is warranted in assistance with the management of pneumonia or meningitis caused by high-level-resistant pneumococci.

Diagnosis

The first step in establishing the diagnosis is performance of a chest x-ray, which in the case of pneumonia will show an infiltrate. Unfortunately, the radiographic finding of an infiltrate is not specific for infection: it is commonly said that such a finding may represent blood, water, or pus (infarction, pulmonary edema—cardiogenic or ARDS—or pneumonia). Occasionally such an infiltrate may instead be atelectasis, which should have a different radiographic pattern, though the distinction between atelectasis and infiltrate is sometimes quite difficult. In such cases, excluding other causes may be necessary (i.e., determination of signs of CHF by exam, or the presence of hypoxia to support the diagnosis of ARDS). Therefore, the chest x-ray is at best an imprecise measure of the presence of pneumonia.

As in any infection, culture of affected body fluids is essential for diagnosis. In otherwise healthy patients, sputum production can be copious and easily mobilized, leading to the microbiologic diagnosis of the pneumonia in most cases. In the debilitated patient, sputum production may be scant, so that induction of sputum by respiratory therapy or bronchoscopy may be necessary to make the diagnosis. To complicate matters more, the mechanically ventilated patient may produce large amounts of secretions simply in response to the presence of a foreign body (the endotracheal tube). Thus, when the sputum is obtained, the relative proportions of white blood cells to respiratory epithelial cells should be examined. If there is a preponderance of WBCs (different institutions have different criteria), the sputum is more likely to represent infection of the lung parenchyma. Most important to remember in the challenge of diagnosing pneumonia is that the overall presentation should be evaluated. For example, consider a ventilated patient with fever and an infiltrate that the radiologist reads as "pneumonia vs. atelectasis." The sputum reveals moderate WBCs, moderate epithelial cells, and moderate gram-negative rods. The patient who develops increasing oxygen requirements (in absence of other cardiorespiratory causes for hypoxia) is more likely to have pneumonia. The patient who is successfully weaning from the ventilator probably does not have significant infection; the sputum findings likely represent secretions related to the presence of the tube and colonization by a gram-negative rod.

Regarding the collection of sputum, its prognostic value is related to the manner in which it was collected. The sputum should be expectorated from the lungs. Saliva is not helpful, nor are secretions from the upper airways, which may be similar to sputum in their gross appearance. If the patient is incapable of expectorating sputum, induction of sputum or bronchoscopy with protected specimen brush are effective alternatives, though not easily performed.

Finally, it is helpful to realize that oral flora are often the organisms that cause pneumonia, particularly in the nosocomial setting (in which the pathogenesis is aspiration). Thus the same organisms may be seen in both a sputum specimen contaminated with oral flora and one that is representative of the pathogen causing pneumonia. The way to tell the difference depends on (1) the proportion of WBCs to epithelial cells, and (2) the clinical presentation. Microbiology laboratories at different institutions use different criteria, but in general, >25 WBCs per low-power field suggests that the specimen was obtained from the lungs rather than the upper airways. More than 25 epithelial cells per low-power field suggests contamination from the upper respiratory tract. A specimen with <10 WBCs per low-power field is unlikely to reflect a pulmonary parenchymal process.

Treatment

The lack of precision in establishing the diagnosis of pneumonia in the hospitalized patient should be recognized. Thus, in many cases, nosocomial pneumonia is treated according to empiric guidelines. Empiric and definitive treatment are discussed in Table 44–20. Dosages should be confirmed by referring to the manufacturers' product insert for each agent. No therapy is indicated for otherwise healthy adults with bronchitis. Smokers and those with chronic obstructive lung disease may be treated for acute bacterial exacerbation of chronic bronchitis with 5 to 10 days of antibiotics. The choice is based on cost (trimethoprim-sulfa or doxycycline) or drug allergies, as it is not clear if other antibiotics indicated for such an exacerbation have a significant advantage. Other choices include amoxicillin–clavulanate, an oral cephalosporin, azithromycin or clarithromycin, or the newer fluoroquinolones (ofloxacin, levofloxacin, sparfloxacin, trovafloxacin, or grepafloxacin).

Urinary Tract Infection

Urinary tract infection (UTI) is important because of the frequency of its occurrence (40% of all nosocomial infections), and the fact that diagnosis is, unfortunately, not straightforward.

There is a spectrum of syndromes of infection of the

TABLE 44–20. Empiric and Definitive Therapy for Pneumonia and Other Respiratory Infections

Clinical Setting	Empiric Treatment	Likely Pathogens	Definitive Treatment	Duration
Community-Acquired Pneumonia				
Without comorbidity[a] and <60 years of age	Azithromycin + penicillin G	*Strep pneumoniae*	Penicillin G[b,c] 1.5 mu IV q4h	7–14 days[d]
		Mycoplasma spp. or *Legionella* spp.	Azithromycin 500 mg IV q24h (change to po within 48 hours)	5 days[f]
		Chlamydia pneumoniae	Doxycycline 100 mg IV q12h	10–14 days[d]
With comorbidity[a], multilobar involvement, >60 years of age or gram-negative bacilli on sputum gram stain	Levofloxacin[e]	As above	As above	10–14 days
		H influenzae	TMP–SMX 8–10 mg/kg/d TMP, in 3–4 divided doses	
		Legionella spp.	Azithromycin 500 mg IV q24h (change to po within 48h)	5 days
Transplant recipient (on cyclosporin A or tacrolimus)	Levofloxacin[e]	*Strep pneumoniae*	Penicillin G[b,c] 600,000 units IV q6h	14–21 days[d]
		H influenzae *Mycoplasma* spp. *Chlamydia pneumoniae* *Legionella* spp.	Levofloxacin 500 mg IV q24	10–14 days[d]
Aspiration Pneumonia				
Outpatient acquired	Penicillin G + metronidazole	Oral flora	Penicillin G, 10–12 mu IV qd in 4 divided doses, + metronidazole 500 IV/po q12h OR Clindamycin 600 IV q8h	10–14 days[g]
Nosocomial (includes nursing home)	Ampicillin/sulbactam + gentamicin[c]	Oral flora	Amp–sulbactam 1/5 gm IV q6h + gentamicin (see "Gentamicin Dosing")	
		Enteric gram-negative rods	TMP–SMX 8–10 mg/kg/d in 3–4 divided doses + metronidazole 500 IV/po q12h	
		P aeruginosa	Piperacillin 3 gm IV q6h + gentamicin (see "Gentamicin Dosing")	
		S aureus	Nafcillin[h] 2 gm IV q4–6h or cefazolin[i] 500 mg IV q8h	

[a] Comorbidities: COPD, ESRD, liver disease, RR>30/min, SBP<90 mm Hg, DBP<60 mm Hg, Pao_2<60 mm Hg or $Paco_2$>50 mm Hg.
[b] If beta-lactam allergy: azithromycin 500 mg IV q24 h; switch to oral therapy within 48 hours.
[c] Review susceptibilities: *S pneumoniae* resistance ranges from 2.4–6%.
[d] Should switch to oral therapy once clinical improvement occurs.
[e] If *P aeruginosa* a consideration (ANC<500 or resident of chronic care facility), add tobramycin.
[f] Note: The duration we recommend is based on European studies demonstrating adequate therapy after a 5-day course. The manufacturer's product information recommends 10 days.
[g] Can switch to oral therapy once improvement occurs.
[h] If penicillin allergy, use clindamycin or trimethoprim/sulfamethoxazole; if MRSA, use vancomycin.
[i] If critically ill, expanded spectrum coverage may be warranted. Possibilities include imipenem or meropenem, piperacillin–tazobactam, or trovafloxacin.

urinary tract, from simple cystitis (manifest as burning with urination and urinary frequency), to acute pyelonephritis (commonly manifest as fever with unilateral flank tenderness). Most UTIs in the population at-large occur in otherwise healthy women with normal urinary tracts. A smaller but still significant percentage occur in older men with urethral obstruction due to prostatic hypertrophy. In the hospital, UTI is the most common nosocomial infection, but usually occurs in patients with indwelling urethral catheters or after urinary tract procedures.

It is important to recognize that indwelling urinary catheters, if left in long enough, will ultimately be associated with bacteriuria—which is not the same as UTI (it represents colonization). Virtually all patients with catheters in place for 30 days will have bacteriuria (Warren et al., 1982). It is important to realize, however, that the presence of bacteriuria without symptoms does not by itself merit treatment. In fact, once colonization is established, in most cases it is benign—with no symptoms—and resolves with removal of the catheter. Occasionally, however, indwelling catheterization can result in local complications (cystitis, prostatitis, epididymo–orchitis) or bloodstream infections, which has significant mortality associated with it. It is not yet possible to predict when such complications will occur, so often bacteriuria and asymptomatic infection are overtreated.

The hospitalized patient with a UTI is unlikely to present with the typical symptoms (urinary frequency, dysuria, suprapubic pressure, or flank pain), and more often simply manifests a fever. As explained earlier, fever in the hospitalized patient merits evaluation of all possible sites of infection; exclusion of possible sources depends on the epidemiologic likelihood of that source causing infection in that patient, as well as the risk associated with dismissing a site prematurely.

Diagnosis

The urinary tract is evaluated for infection by inspecting the urine. However, there are no urine findings that are pathognomonic for urinary tract infection. A finding of pyuria is only predictive of UTI in a patient whose prior probability for UTI is relatively high (see chapter on positive/negative predictive values). In other words, pyuria found on a urinalysis on a patient with no symptoms should not necessarily be acted upon—whether to act upon it would depend on the reason for obtaining the urinalysis. If preop, while pyuria may not be terribly predictive for UTI, it may be worth the risk of antibiotic treatment to treat to prevent the risk of bacteremia.

In a noncatheterized patient, finding more than 5 to 10 white cells per high-power field suggests infection. A gram stain of uncentrifuged urine is helpful, in that if more than one organism per oil-immersion field is found, it is also suggestive of infection. Generally, micro labs will report urine gram stains semiquantitatively (rare, few, moderate, many). It is helpful to know what your microbiology laboratory does. Urine dipsticks usually test for leukocyte esterase and nitrite. They are both good tests in the setting of a patient for whom there is a reasonable likelihood of infection. Leukocyte esterase tests for WBCs (generally a positive result when there are more than 10 WBCs per high-power field); false-negatives are more likely than false-positives. Nitrite tests for the presence of bacteria, and similarly is more likely to produce false-negative than false-positive results.

Urine culture should never be obtained without urinalysis. Although bladder urine is normally sterile, it may easily become contaminated when passed through the urethra or through a catheter (even a newly inserted catheter). Thus, when organisms grow from the urine, the microbiology lab normally quantifies the amount of growth, resulting in a statistical discrimination between infection and colonization (in other words, someone with 10^5/mL *E coli* is more likely to have UTI than is someone with 10^3/mL *E coli,* who probably simply has colonization.

Diagnosis of UTI in a patient with an indwelling catheter should involve collection of the urine from a sampling port on the catheter itself; such a specimen correlates with urine obtained by suprapubic aspiration in 90% of cases (Bergquist et al., 1980). Such a specimen is more likely to be reliable when obtained from a catheter that has not yet had the chance to acquire a biofilm that might facilitate colonization of the catheter lumen (i.e., in place for less than a week). While quantitation of growth in urine obtained by clean catch is well-studied, such studies have not been done in specimens obtained from indwelling urinary catheters. It is generally accepted, but by no means proven, that any growth more than 10^2/mL is accepted as evidence for urinary tract infection in the right clinical circumstance in patients with indwelling urinary catheters.

Of note, the symptoms or signs of UTI in combination with fever and/or upper tract findings (i.e., costovertebral angle tenderness) argue for pyelonephritis. Pyelonephritis is a reason to hospitalize elderly patients and some adult patients; all patients should be treated for 14 days at a minimum.

Treatment

Treatment of UTI is usually guided by culture results in the hospital setting. In the outpatient setting, symptoms are generally treated without obtaining a culture, provided the patient has no underlying immune deficiency or debility, and a normal urinary tract. In the hospitalized patient, when the culture result is not obtainable (i.e., urine culture leaked in transit), empiric treatment must be undertaken. Such treatment is guided by the most likely organisms to colonize the periurethral area, and the resistance profiles seen in the hospital (Table 44–21). Dosages should be confirmed by referring to the manufacturer's product insert for each agent.

TABLE 44–21. Empiric and Definitive Therapy for UTIs

Clinical Setting	Empiric Treatment	Likely Pathogens	Definitive Treatment	Duration
Urinary Tract Infection				
Uncomplicated	TMP–SMX	Enteric gram-negative rods	TMP–SMX 160 mg/800 mg (1 double strength tablet) po bid	3 days
		Coagulase negative staphylococci (*S saprophyticus*)		
		Enterococcus spp.[a]	Amoxicillin 250 mg po q8h	
Complicated	Ampicillin[b] +/– gentamicin[c]	Enteric gram-negative rods	TMP–SMX 8–10 mg/kg/d TMP IV/po in 3–4 divided doses	14 days
		Enterococcus spp.[a]	Amoxicillin 500 mg po q8h +/– gentamicin (peak concentration 3–4 mcg/mL)	
		P aeruginosa	Piperacillin 3 gm IV q6h +/– gentamicin (see "Gentamicin Dosing")	
		C albicans	Fluconazole 100 mg po qd	5 days
Prostatitis				
Acute, <35 years old	Cefixime + doxycycline	*N gonorrheae*	Same as empiric cefixime 400 mg po once	One dose only
		C trachomatis[d]	Doxycycline 100 mg po bid	14 days
Acute, >35 years old	TMP–SMX	Enteric gram-negative rods	TMP–SMX 160 mg/800 mg (1 double strength tablet) po bid	2 weeks
Chronic	Levofloxacin	Enteric gram-negative rods	Levofloxacin 500 mg po qd	4 weeks[e]
		Enterococcus spp.[f]	Amoxicillin 500 mg po q8h	3 months

[a] Review susceptibilities: 30% of isolates multidrug resistant.
[b] Ampicillin dose = 1 gm IV q6h.
[c] Consider use of piperacillin + gentamicin for antimicrobial coverage against *Pseudomonas aeruginosa* for immunocompromised patients, residents of chronic care facilities, and nosocomial infections.
[d] Always treat for *Chlamydia trachomatis,* even if not isolated, due to high coinfection rate.
[e] May require longer duration of therapy.
[f] Review susceptibilities: 30% of isolates are multidrug resistant.

Prevention

Guidelines for prevention of infection have been established by the Centers for Disease Control and Prevention (Wong & Hooton, 1982), which mainly focus on aseptic management of the urinary catheter. However, most important is to avoid catheterization in the first place. According to Wong & Hooton (1982), indications for catheterization include: (1) relief of urinary tract obstruction; (2) neurogenic bladder or other conditions associated with urinary retention; (3) when needed for urologic procedures; and (4) for the determination of urine output in otherwise critically ill patients.

Other Aspects of Management

Candiduria is not an uncommon finding in the hospitalized patient. Generally it represents colonization, but because it can progress to invasive infection, it should not be ignored. If the patient is otherwise asymptomatic, the catheter should be removed or replaced. If colonization then persists, whether to treat it with amphotericin bladder washings or to watch the patient is controversial and has not been adequately studied. Our approach has generally been to treat with systemic therapy (fluconazole) if: (1) there are other sites that are colonized, such as the respiratory tract; (2) there is evidence of upper tract involvement; or (3) the patient is at risk for invasive disease (immunocompromised, diabetes mellitus, presence of central lines, or history of recent abdominal surgery). Upper tract involvement is investigated when there is fever or other signs of dysfunction of the urinary tract; an imaging study of the upper tract (ultrasound or CT scan) can be done. If these conditions are not present, we tend to observe the patient rather than use amphotericin bladder washings.

Skin, Wound, and Soft Tissue Infections

Infections of the skin are not uncommon in hospitalized patients, in part due to the surgical procedures and indwelling devices that invade the skin, but also due to the decreased integrity of the skin in debilitated patients.

Cellulitis

Cellulitis presents most commonly as a relatively rapidly spreading area of erythema, generally in the site of preceding trauma or break in the skin integrity (though often such a break in skin integrity is not clinically apparent). Such infections may be problematic in anyone with venous or lym-

TABLE 44–25. Treatment of Patients with Sepsis

Clinical Setting	Empiric Treatment	Likely Pathogens	Definitive Treatment	Duration
Without Obvious Source				
Unknown source	TMP–SMX 8–10 mg/kg/d TMP IV in 3–4 divided doses + gentamicin see dosing table	Gram-positive cocci Gram-negative rods[j]	Based on culture results	Depends on clinical setting
If *P aeruginosa* suspected[a]	Piperacillin 3–4 gm IV q6h OR cefepime/ceftazidime 2 gm IV q8h + tobramycin see dosing table			
If *B fragilis* possible	Add metronidazole 500 mg IV q12h			
If IV catheter in place and patient critically ill[b]	Add vancomycin see dosing table			
Intravenous drug use	Vancomycin + gentamicin[c]	Gram-positive cocci (including MRSA) Gram-negative rods	Based on culture results	Depends on clinical setting
Catheter related[d]	Cefazolin[e,f] 1 gm IV q8h + gentamicin	*S aureus*	Cefazolin[f] OR nafcillin[f] 2 gm IV q4–6h	14 days (if catheter removed)[g] OR 4 weeks (if catheter not removed)
		Coagulase-negative staphylococci	Vancomycin (see dosing table)	
		Enteric gram-negative rods[j]	TMP–SMX 8–10 mg/kg/d TMP IV in 3–4 divided doses	
		P aeruginosa[j]	Piperacillin 3–4 gm IV q6h + gentamicin (see dosing table)	
		C albicans	Fluconazole 400 mg IV q24h (switch to po as soon as clinical improvement occurs) OR amphotericin B 0.5 mg/kg/d IV	
Intraabdominal source	Ampicillin–sulbactam + gentamicin	Polymicrobial	Based on culture results	
Pneumonia Related: See Pneumonia Section				
Urosepsis: normal host	Ampicillin[h] 2 gm IV q6h + gentamicin	Enteric gram-negative rods[j] *Enterococcus*[j] spp.	TMP–SMX 8–10 mg/kg/d TMP IV in 3–4 divided doses Ampicillin 2 gm IV q6h + gentamicin then amoxicillin 500 po q8h	14 days total[i]
Immunocompromised host, chronic care facility resident, anatomic abnormality, or gram-negative rods on gram stain	Piperacillin 3 gm IV q6h OR cefepime/ceftazidime 2 mg IV q8 + gentamicin	Same as above + *P aeruginosa*	Piperacillin 3 gm IV q6h + gentamicin then levofloxacin 500 po q24h	

[a] For example, necrotic skin lesions (ecthyma gangrenosum), burns, necrotizing or nosocomial pneumonias, nosocomial empyemas, etc.
[b] This is a clinical decision; guidelines include hemodynamic instability or evidence of serious infection.
[c] If patient has septic physiology, use tobramycin instead of gentamicin.
[d] Optimal treatment requires prompt removal of the catheter.
[e] If patient hemodynamically unstable, consider using vancomycin instead of cefazolin.
[f] Use vancomycin if MRSA or penicillin allergy.
[g] May want to follow with 14 days of oral therapy.
[h] Ampicillin dose = 2gm iv q6h.
[i] Can switch to oral therapy after clinical improvement occurs.
[j] Review susceptibilities.

TABLE 44–26. Noninfectious Causes of Fever

Type of Etiology	Specific Examples	Making the Diagnosis
Malignancy	Hodgkin's disease	Imaging and biopsy
	Non-Hodgkin's lymphoma	Imaging and biopsy
	Leukemia	Imaging and biopsy
	Renal cell carcinoma	Imaging and biopsy
	Hepatoma	Imaging and biopsy
	Atrial myxoma	Echocardiogram
Autoimmune diseases	Systemic lupus erythematosis	AMA, clinical criteria
	Still's disease	Clinical criteria
	Polymyalgia rheumatica/temporal arteritis	Clinical criteria, biopsy
	Polyarteritis nodosa	Clinical, biopsy
	Erythema multiforme	Distinct rash, biopsy
Hypersensitivity reactions	Drug fever	Discontinuation of drug, with rechallenge
	Hypersensitivity vasculitis	Biopsy
	Serum sickness	Clinical
	Rheumatic fever	Jones criteria
Granulomatous diseases	Inflammatory bowel disease	Biopsy
	Sarcoidosis	Biopsy

Treatment

Drainage is the most important aspect of treatment; otherwise, antibiotics generally are appropriate for abdominal organisms. Empiric treatment is trimethoprin-sulfamethoxazole and metromidazole, but should be adjusted according to susceptibilities.

Important Noninfectious Causes of Fever

Any evaluation of fever must take into account the possibility of several noninfectious conditions that may cause fever. These diagnoses should be considered in parallel to the infectious differential diagnosis. In other words, they should not necessarily be considered a diagnosis of exclusion, as some noninfectious causes of fever may be life-threatening. In ordering the differential of noninfectious causes of fever, the patient's epidemiologic risks should be taken into account, just as they are with infectious causes of fever.

The classic "fever of unknown origin" (FUO) definition usually does not apply to the patient who is hospitalized for another reason and then develops a fever in the hospital. The most common causes of classic FUO in adults are infection, neoplasm, and collagen vascular disease, followed by a number of miscellaneous causes. The most important causes of noninfectious FUO are listed in Table 44–26. An excellent discussion of fever can be found in "Fever of Unknown Origin" (Gelfand & Wolff, 1995).

The hospitalized patient may be less likely to have the conditions shown in Table 44–26, simply because he or she is more likely to have fever as a result of procedures and conditions that occur by virtue of the hospitalization. Fever in a patient with a central line in place should always be considered to come from the line, unless there is strong evidence for another cause. However, it is possible for a fever to resolve simply after removal of the line. In such a case, if the line culture and blood cultures are negative, and the patient otherwise continues to improve, then antibiotics need not be given. Such a case *may* be due to a reaction to the catheter material or to the presence of clot while the line was in place, but since such cases do not appear to need antibiotics, it may be considered noninfectious.

Pancreatitis, cholecystitis (both with and without stones), and the presence of a large hematoma are conditions that may cause fever, and may be found on abdominal CT scan.

Drugs are an important cause of fever. The most likely agents are penicillins, sulfonamides, procainamide, and amphotericin.

Finally, gout may be precipitated in the hospital but go unnoticed when the physical exam excludes the extremities, and particularly when the patient cannot complain of pain.

REFERENCES

Ad Hoc Committee of the Committee on Trauma, National Research Council Division of Medical Sciences. (1964). Postoperative wound infections: The influence of ultraviolet irradiation of the operating room and various other factors. *Annals of Surgery, 160* (2).

Bergquist, D. et al. (1980). The relevance of urinary sampling methods in patients with indwelling Foley catheters. *British Journal of Urology, 52,* 92.

Classen, D. C., Evans, R. S., Pestonick, S. L., et al. (1992). The timing of prophylactic administration of antibiotics and the risk of surgical wound infection. *New England Journal of Medicine,* 326, 281–286.

Culver, D. H. et al. (1991). Surgical wound infection rates by wound class, operative procedure, and patient risk index. *American Journal of Medicine, 91* (Suppl. 3B), 1525–1575.

Dajani, A. S. et al. (1997). Prevention of bacterial endocarditis: Recommendations by the American Heart Association. *JAMA, 277,* 1794–1801.

Dinubile, M. J. (1982). Surgery in active endocarditis. *Annals of Internal Medicine, 96,* 650.

Gelfand, J. A. & Wolff, S. M. (1995). Fever of unknown origin. In G. L. Mandell, J. E. Bennett, & R. Dolin (Eds.), *Mandell, Douglas and Bennett's Principles and Practices of Infectious Diseases,* (4th ed.). New York: Chruchill Livingstone.

Haley, R. W. et al. (1985). Identifying patients at high risk of surgical wound infection: A simple multivariate index of patient susceptibility and wound contamination. *American Journal of Epidemiology, 121,* 206–215.

Kernodle, D. S. & Kaiser, A. B. (1995). Postoperative infections and antimicrobial prophylaxis. In G. L. Mandell, J. E. Bennett, & R. Dolan (Eds.), *Mandell, Douglas and Bennett's Principles and Practices of Infectious Diseases* (4th ed.), (pp. 2742–2756). New York: Churchill Livingstone.

Kim, J. H. & Gallis, H. A. (1989). Observations on spiraling empiricism: Its causes, allure, and perils with particular reference to antibiotic therapy. *American Journal of Medicine, 87,* 201–206.

Scheld, W. M. & Sande, M. A. (1995). Endocarditis and intravascular infections. In G. L. Mandell, J. E. Bennett, & R. Dolin (Eds.), *Mandell, Douglas and Bennett's Principles and Practices of Infectious Diseases* (4th ed.). New York: Chruchill Livingstone.

Warren, J. W. et al. (1982). A prospective microbiologic study of bacteriuria in patients with chronic indwelling urethral catheters. *Journal of Infectious Diseases, 146,* 719–723.

Weinstein, L. & Schlesinger, J. J. (1974). Pathoanatomic, pathophysiologic, and clinical correlations in endocarditis (first of two parts). *New England Journal of Medicine, 291,* 832.

Weinstein, M. P. et al. (1983). Clinical significance of positive blood cultures: A comprehensive analysis of 500 episodes of bacteremia and fungemia in adults. *Review of Infective Disease, 5,* 35.

Wilson, W. R. et al. (1995). Antibiotic treatment of adults with infective endocarditis due to Streptococci, Enterococci, Staphylococci, and HACEK microorganisms. *JAMA, 274,* 1706–1713.

Wong, E. S. & Hooton, T. M. (1982). Guidelines for the prevention of catheter-associated urinary tract infections. *Infection Control,* 2, 125.

45

Breast Problems

Margaret Levy

▶ ANATOMY AND PHYSIOLOGY

Structurally, the breast is a skin appendage; functionally, it is a modified sweat gland. The breast consists of skin, subcutaneous tissue, and breast tissue. Breast tissue is composed of connective tissue (stroma) and glandular tissue (parenchyma). The parenchyma is divided into 15 to 20 lobes, each of which is made up of 20 to 40 lobules. Each lobule contains 10 to 100 tuboalveolar secretory units, which are the functional elements of the breast. An elaborate duct system connects the secretory units and eventually converges under the nipple/areola complex into excretory ducts and sinuses. An average of 12 to 15 excretory ducts drain the entire breast (Fig. 45–1). The breast is invested between two layers of fascia: the superficial pectoral fascia (immediately beneath the dermis) and the deep pectoral fascia (which lines the pectoralis major and serratus anterior muscles). Connecting the two layers of fascia and helping to support the weight of the breast are connective tissue bands, the suspensory ligaments of Cooper. The weight and size of the breast in the adult female is determined by the amount of fat accumulated in the connective tissue between the lobules. This fatty deposition begins at puberty.

The nipple and its surrounding areola are more darkly pigmented than the breast skin. The pigmentation darkens during pregnancy. The lactiferous ducts that converge beneath the nipple are surrounded by smooth muscle, which involuntarily contracts during suckling. On the surface of the areola are 8 to 10 often visible nodules representing superficial projections of Montgomery's glands. These are specialized sebaceous glands. Adjacent to these may be miniature ducts that drain tiny accessory mammary glands. The ducts open into small sinuses on the areola. Milk may eject from these as well as the nipple during lactation (Haagensen, 1986).

The arterial supply of the breast is derived from the internal thoracic, axillary, and intercostal arteries. Venous drainage is much more anatomically variable, but generally follows the arteries. Approximately 3% of the lymph from the breast flows into the internal mammary chain, the rest into the axillary nodes (Osborne, 1987). The regional nodal basins are the axillary, infraclavicular, supraclavicular, and cervical nodes.

The skin of the upper half of the breast is innervated by the third and fourth branches of the cervical plexus. The skin of the lower breast is innervated by the thoracic intercostal nerves. Within the breast, there are no major sensory or motor nerves. Within the axilla, the major motor nerves that define the surgical anatomy are the long thoracic nerve of Bell (which supplies the serratus anterior) and the thoracodorsal nerve (which supplies the latissimus dorsi). The intercostobrachial nerve plexus traverses the axilla. It supplies sensation to the upper inner arm and axillary area.

The breast is physiologically active from puberty to menopause, always ready to serve its sole purpose—to produce, store, and secrete milk. It is important to recognize, however, that in modern society, there are also psychosocial issues that influence a woman's breast-protective response. The fear of breast loss (which often prohibits women from seeking necessary medical attention) is, thus, both instinctive and cultural.

Normal physiologic changes that occur during the

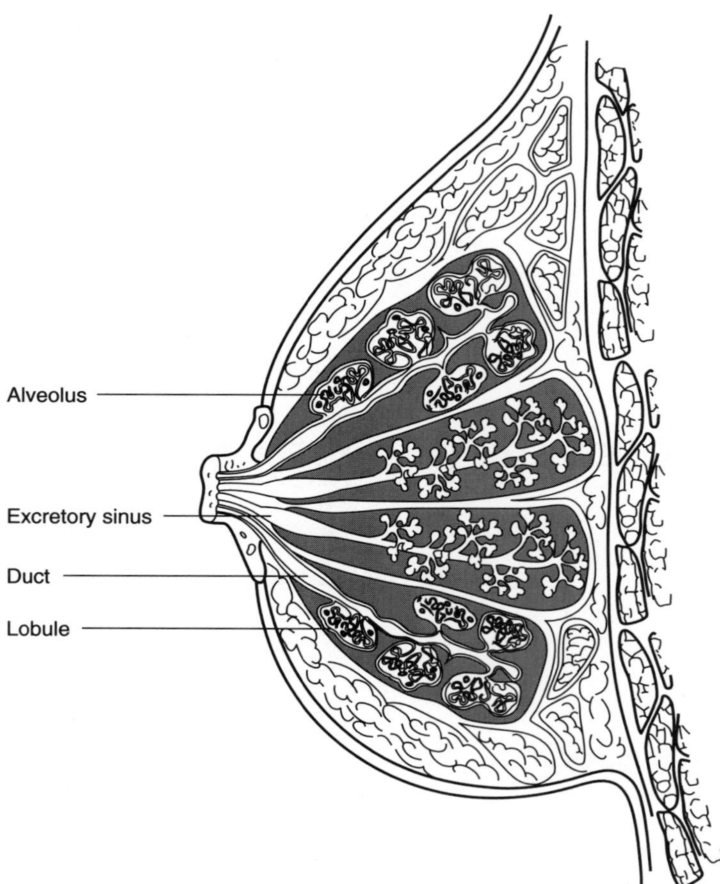

Figure 45–1. Internal anatomy of the breast. *(Used with permission from Greenfield. [1993].)*

menstrual cycle are hormonally driven, as are the changes that occur during pregnancy and lactation. Histologic changes in normal breast tissue are controlled by circulating sex-steroid hormones that bind to receptors in the breast. During the follicular phase of the menstrual cycle, estrogen levels increase. Estrogen stimulates breast epithelial proliferation. When ovulation occurs, estrogen stimulation peaks. Thereafter, luteal progesterone secretion peaks, which results in further changes in breast epithelium. In the two weeks between ovulation and menses, mammary ducts dilate and alveolar cells secrete lipid drops. There is both intraluminal fluid secretion and extraluminal fluid accumulation within the lobules. Blood flow also increases. This explains the premenstrual breast fullness and discomfort that many women experience. Once menstruation ensues and circulating levels of the stimulating hormones decline, breast tissue edema resolves.

During pregnancy, prolactin secretion increases progressively. Prolactin (a pituitary hormone), placental lactogen, chorionic gonadotropin, and progesterone prepare the breast for lactation. All of the breast elements—ducts, lobules, and alveoli—are stimulated during pregnancy. Mammary epithelial proliferation marks the first half of pregnancy, while the second half is characterized by colostrum accumulation in the alveoli, hypertrophy of the myoepithelial cells, and continued epithelial proliferation. After parturition, placental lactogen, estrogen, and progesterone levels fall abruptly, while prolactin levels do not. Growth hormone, insulin, and cortisol create the hormonal milieu necessary for prolactin-induced milk production. Desquamated epithelial cells, the basic component of colostrum, are secreted into the ducts and alveoli. Lactoglobulin, lactalbumin, fatty acids, and fat-soluble vitamins combine to make colostrum nutritionally and immunologically valuable to the newborn infant. Colostrum usually gives way to milk 24 hours after parturition. Another hormone, oxytocin, is secreted by the pituitary in response to suckling and other neural impulses. Oxytocin causes the myoepithelial cells to contract and eject milk from the alveoli into the lactiferous ducts and sinuses, the "milk let-down" reflex.

Normal breast changes occur with menopause because of glandular atrophy. Although a few lobules always remain, the breasts of aged women are composed largely of fat, stroma, and ducts. With the atrophy of the lobules and supporting elements, the breasts may become ptotic. Clinical examination becomes easier.

▶ HISTORY AND PHYSICAL FINDINGS

A focused medical history to assess risk factors should include previous history of breast problems, previous history of cancer, family history of breast, ovarian or colon cancer, reproductive history (age of menarche, age at menopause, age of delivery of first term and subsequent pregnancies), lactational history, hormonal history (e.g., use of birth control pills, fertility drugs, replacement therapy), current medications, and social history. The patient should be questioned about any breast symptoms (mass, pain, change in appearance, or nipple problems).

With the patient seated in front of the examiner, the breasts are inspected for symmetry. The skin is examined for erythema, edema, dimpling, retraction, ulceration, lesions, or visible masses. The nipples and areolae are viewed to look for symmetry, inversion, crusting, or lesions. (Hoogstraten & Burn,1989). The regional lymph nodes are palpated. In the absence of clinically obvious breast cancer, a palpable node generally represents benign adenopathy and is a common occurrence. With the patient supine, the breasts are palpated bimanually with the arm down at the side and again with the arm placed over the head. The breast tissue is compressed gently against the chest wall in a continual radially directed pattern. Note any masses, gross cysts, tenderness, thickenings, asymmetry, or architectural distortion. The nipples should be tested for discharge.

For descriptive purposes, each breast is divided into four quadrants: upper outer, upper inner, lower outer, and lower inner. Abnormalities are described and localized by radiants and distance from the nipple (e.g., 2 cm mass in LUOQ, 2 o'clock, 3 cm from nipple; smooth, mobile, firm). Any abnormality should be documented, and appropriate diagnostic tests, referrals, and follow-up recommendations are discussed and recorded. A normal exam should prompt a breast-monitoring program appropriate for a patient's age and risk-factor analysis.

▶ DIAGNOSTIC AND INTERVENTIONAL BREAST IMAGING

Mammography

Currently, the most effective method available for the early detection of breast cancer is mammography. Breast cancer is the most common nonskin cancer in women in the United States. In 1996, approximately 184,000 new cases were diagnosed and 44,000 women died as a result of the disease. Finally, within the last decade of the twentieth century, we are seeing a slight decline in the breast cancer death rate, despite the increasing incidence. It is believed that mammography is responsible for both statistics. With increasing use of screening mammography, more cancers are being diagnosed. Because this results in earlier diagnosis, more women are being cured. Screening mammography guidelines are, however, a continued source of controversy. Table 45–1 lists general screening guidelines. A large part of the controversy, unfortunately, relates to the cost of screening and the interventions that may result from that screening. Most breast specialists recommend annual mammography for all women over the age of 50 because the incidence of breast cancer is age related. Yet once a woman reaches 65, despite the increasing risk for developing breast cancer with advancing age, screening mammography is only covered every other year. Data from numerous clinical trials indicate that annual screening mammography in patients between the ages of 50 and 80 can reduce breast cancer mortality by as much as one third.

The question of how often to screen younger women is even more controversial. Recent data (Cody, 1995) suggest that screening mammography is as effective in early diagnosis for patients under 50 as it is in those over 50. Compared with women whose initial diagnosis was made clinically (palpable mass), mammographically diagnosed cancers are smaller, lymph nodes are more often negative, and histologic findings are more likely to show *in situ* or microinvasive disease. Each of these is associated with a better prognosis than clinically detected cancers. Although the diagnostic accuracy of mammography is compromised by the normal dense fibroglandular pattern seen in many premenopausal breasts, no other modality has been found superior for diagnosing early-stage breast cancer.

The arguments against screening mammography as mentioned earlier are usually related to cost. The efficiency of a preventive health program is judged by its cost per life year gained and mammography gives less good value than other activities. Further, screening mammography is said to increase the number of "unnecessary" biopsies. An unnecessary biopsy is always defined retrospectively as a biopsy that is negative for malignancy. Removing a lesion and proving that it is histologically benign is a necessary intervention with a good result. Certainly, improving the diagnostic accuracy of mammography and developing other noninvasive technologies for diagnosing breast cancer should be areas of intense research activity.

Using the age of 50 as a starting point for annual mammography is based on the median age of menopause and the sharp rise in the curve in terms of the incidence of breast cancer after menopause. Given the wide variation in age of normal and surgical menopause, and the wide use of

TABLE 45–1. Breast Screening for Asymptomatic Women by Age

Age	Breast Self-Examination	Clinical Examination	Mammography
18–35	Monthly	Yearly	Baseline age 35
35–50	Monthly	Yearly	Q 1–2 years
Over 50	Monthly	Yearly	Yearly

hormonal replacement therapy, it would be preferable to be able to prescribe screening mammography more selectively, based on the information derived from an individual patient's mammogram. For example, obese breasts, even in a 30-year-old woman, are mammographically lucent and thus easy to read. Women with large, pendulous breasts that are difficult to examine clinically may benefit from yearly mammography beginning at age 30. On the other hand, some postmenopausal women have extremely radiodense breasts that significantly diminish the sensitivity of mammography. These patients may benefit more from a combination of clinical exam, ultrasonography, and periodic mammography. Using risk-factor analysis, clinical examination, and the baseline mammogram, the health-care provider should prescribe an appropriate breast-monitoring program suited to the patient's individual needs.

A standard screening mammogram includes two projections of each breast: the medial lateral oblique view and the cranial caudal view. If necessary, for diagnostic purposes, additional views are added, such as straight or 90-degree medial lateral, exaggerated cranial caudal, spot compression, and magnification views. Each of these can provide the radiologist with additional information that adds to the accuracy of the basic mammogram in diagnosing breast pathology. Ultrasonography may be needed to further characterize a lesion. The primary-care provider, who usually does not see, and certainly is not trained to interpret, mammograms must rely upon the radiologist's reports. The recommendations provided by the radiologist should be followed. Obviously, the primary-care provider must have complete confidence in the radiologist and the facility at which the mammogram was performed. A missed lesion has serious medical and legal implications. Although a delay in diagnosis of several months is generally not associated with any change in prognosis, staging, or treatment options, a lesion missed on a mammogram often results in a delay in diagnosis of 1 to 2 years (the time until the next routine mammogram). To insure the highest quality for mammography, these guidelines may be useful:

1. Refer to a high-volume facility, preferably one that has a radiologist who specializes in breast imaging.
2. Obtain feedback from patients about the facility.
3. Obtain feedback from breast specialists about the technical quality and accuracy of the films and reports.
4. Maintain communication with the radiologist; verbal and/or typed reports should be available in a timely manner. Is the prescribing health-care provider immediately informed of positive findings?
5. When additional imaging is needed after the baseline mammogram, how is the patient informed and scheduled for these studies? Does the radiologist speak with or examine her when a problem is found?
6. How is the patient informed of the results of the mammogram?

The radiologist's report:

1. Should be clear, concise, and complete.
2. Should state in which breast is the lesion, and if it is seen in both views.
3. Recommendations should be precise and specific.
4. Current films should be compared with previous films (most recent, previous, and oldest).
5. Lesion should be described by size, contour (shape and margins), and location.
6. Lesion should be rated (benign, indeterminate, or malignant).
7. If biopsy, clinical correlation, additional views, sonography, or short-interval follow-up is recommended, be certain that the patient is informed. Take the responsibility to phone the patient and document this. Make sure you receive a report indicating that whatever was recommended has been done. A written reminder to the patient about follow-up is optimal.

Ultrasonography

While mammography is used for both breast-cancer screening and diagnosis, breast ultrasonography is currently used only for diagnosis, either as a complement to physical examination to further characterize a palpable mass, or to further characterize a mammographically detected lesion. In this regard, it is very useful in obviating the need for biopsy. Mammography and palpation cannot distinguish between a cystic or solid lesion, whereas ultrasonography has that capability. Subclinical cysts (those that are initially found on mammography) and asymptomatic palpable cysts require no intervention once confirmed by sonography. Noncystic masses can be further characterized and—in experienced hands—can be as reliable as mammography in predicting whether a lesion is benign or malignant. Sonography can be used to facilitate procedures, including needle/guide wire placement for excisional biopsy, core needle biopsy, and cyst aspiration. There are a few indications for whole-breast screening using sonography: to detect suspected leaks from silicone implants; to evaluate high-risk patients with extremely homogeneous tissue density on mammography; and to exclude multicentric malignancy when the primary lesion is discovered by sonography.

Magnetic Resonance Imaging

Breast magnetic resonance imaging (MRI) has few clinical applications at the present time; it has been used as a modality to evaluate breast implants for intracapsular or extracapsular rupture. MRI in the evaluation of breast cancer requires administration of intravenous contrast. The identification of otherwise unsuspected multifocal cancer seems to be its primary utility, although sonography is probably as accurate and is less costly.

Interventional Breast Radiology

There are invasive and minimally invasive techniques for localization and biopsy of nonpalpable breast lesions. The invasive or surgical procedure has been used for over 30 years. With this technique, a localizing needle and guide wire apparatus is inserted into or in close proximity of a lesion using mammographic or ultrasound guidance. Using the end of the needle as the focal point, the surgeon is able to excise the area of interest and a small amount of surrounding breast tissue through a 1- to 2-inch cosmetically placed incision. The procedure is done in the outpatient setting with local anesthesia that can be supplemented with intravenous sedation to maximize patient comfort. The success rate is over 95%.

Newer techniques enable occult lesions to be biopsied percutaneously rather than surgically. This is accomplished with ultrasound or with a specifically designed mammography table that allows lesions to be identified stereoscopically for precise localization. This equipment is costly and requires a trained technician, but it offers these obvious advantages to the patient: it is almost painless, almost scarless, and can be less costly than a traditional biopsy. In experienced hands, it has the same success rate as needle-localized excision biopsies.

The indication for stereotactic-core needle biopsy is a nonpalpable mammographically detected lesion for which histologic diagnosis is required. The breast is suspended through an aperture with the patient lying prone on the table. With mammographic imaging, the lesion is localized in x, y, and z coordinates using the principle of parallax shift ("stereo views"). An automated large caliber biopsy gun is used to obtain multiple core specimens (Burbank, 1996). The technique is rapidly advancing but is not yet available in all areas of the country. It should be performed in an appropriate setting, such as a multidisciplinary breast center, by a radiologist or surgeon with a high level of experience in breast care, and with a pathologist who is experienced in diagnosing lesions based on core specimens. The larger the core, the greater the diagnostic accuracy. Currently, multiple cores (at least six) using 14-gauge needles are recommended.

Ultrasound guided-core and fine-needle biopsies have the advantage of being office-based procedures; the equipment is less costly, portable, smaller; and because it is done in real-time, preprocedure positioning that requires a trained technician is not necessary. Accuracy is improved with the patient seated and the breast immobilized and partially compressed with paddles similar to those used for mammography.

Currently, the technology is available to allow a radiologist or surgeon to completely core out a lesion percutaneously using a specially designed instrument call a mammotome (Burbank, 1996). This device can be used with both stereotactic and sonographic equipment. In the future, it may supplant the need for lumpectomy in the treatment of breast cancer. The "ABBI" system, which combines stereotactic principles with semiinvasive surgery, is not recommended, offering no real advantage over either technique. Digital mammography and computer-assisted diagnosis are under development. There may be a time in the not too distant future when a woman will carry all of her mammograms on a wallet-sized key card.

▶ CLINICAL BREAST PROBLEMS

Breast Masses

A breast lump that is discovered by a patient or found during a clinical exam requires immediate attention. The practitioner must be astute to this common clinical problem. Regardless of the patient's age and other risk factors, the priority of the management plan is to rule in or rule out cancer. This does not mean that every lump requires an immediate biopsy, but it does require careful, well-documented clinical decision making.

A smooth, well-circumscribed mass in a premenopausal woman is usually a benign cyst (which is fluid filled) or fibroadenoma (which is solid). To differentiate these, the history may be helpful. A cyst is more common and more likely to be acute and painful. Women develop symptomatic breast cysts most frequently in the third decade of life. Fibroadenoma is the most common solid breast tumor in women from ages 16 to 25. The mass is usually painless, three dimensional, and very mobile. There is no exogenous cause, and there seems to be a genetic predisposition. Fibroadenomas are estrogen responsive and may enlarge during pregnancy. Multiple fibroadenomas (which may be bilateral) are quite common.

Any primary health-care provider should be familiar with the technique of fine-needle aspiration (FNA). This technique provides the most rapid, cost-effective way of differentiating and diagnosing these lesions. The skin over the mass is sterilized with alcohol. A small amount (1 cc) of local anesthesia can be injected into the subcutis, but most patients can tolerate the aspiration without anesthesia. The mass is stabilized with the thumb and index finger of the nondominant hand. Using a 10-cc syringe and a 20-gauge needle, the needle punctures the skin and enters the mass. If fluid is noted in the hub of the needle, continue to decompress until the mass is no longer felt (Fig. 45–2). Remove the needle, cap the syringe, and send the fluid to an experienced cytologist for evaluation. Typical cyst fluid varies from translucent straw color or light green to turbid gray or dark green. A patient who has a grossly bloody cyst should be referred to a specialist for surgical biopsy. Occasionally,

Figure 45–3. Typical appearance of cyst on ultrasound.

between the ages of 25 and 50. Histopathologically, it probably exists in 90% of women (Love et al., 1982).

The etiology of cystic mastopathy has eluded investigators for decades. A neurohormonal imbalance is the most likely common denominator, but the precise mechanism is hotly debated. Since estrogen stimulates duct epithelial development and progesterone causes lobular–alveolar proliferation, an imbalance of these hormones has been implicated. In animal models, large doses of estrogen induces epithelial proliferation and cyst formation. Although estrogen, estradiol, and progesterone levels can be measured in human beings during different phases of the menstrual cycle, there is no conclusive evidence that women with cyclical breast pain and nodularity have abnormal or higher levels of these hormones than nonsymptomatic women. It may be that the ratio of estrogen to progesterone creates the hormonal milieu necessary for pathologic breast change. Prolactin has been implicated by some in causing mastalgia (Peters et al., 1984). This is probably not uniformly true, but explains why bromocriptine (a prolactin inhibitor and dopamine agonist) helps some women and not others. Another puzzling question is why some women with multiple cysts, large or small, have no breast discomfort at all, while other women whose breasts contain no documented cysts are very symptomatic.

Benign breast pain is a clinical problem that can be classified as follows:

- Mild: premenstrual tenderness that does not interfere with normal activities of daily living
- Moderate: localized or diffuse tenderness, may begin at ovulation and intensify until menstruation begins; associated with sleep interference and exercise discomfort
- Severe: continuous (no relation to menstrual cycle); restricts normal activities of daily living

This classification is useful as a guide to management. Mild mastalgia usually is well tolerated and no specific treatment is needed. Moderate breast pain often responds to premenstrual diuretics, nonsteroidal antiinflammatories, salt and caffeine restriction, and vitamin E supplements (400-1000 units daily) (Minton et al., 1979). Severe mastodynia requires more aggressive treatment, such as bromocriptine (Durning & Sellwood, 1982). Some women improve using oral contraceptives, while in some, the pill can cause breast pain. Tamoxifen has been successfully used to treat chronic breast pain, but clinical trials have not established its efficacy in this regard. The most effective drug for the most severe cases appears to be danocrine, an androgen derivative. Patients who require drug therapy should be treated by a breast specialist. Dosages must be titrated and patients must be carefully monitored for response, side effects, and toxicity. In extremely rare instances, subcutaneous mastectomy is indicated to control breast pain.

The histopathology of fibrocystic breast disorder (Table 45–4) is important because it defines a subset of women who are at increased risk for developing breast cancer (Proppe, 1984). Only those women with histologically proven hyperplasia should be considered at increased risk. The most significant risk is conferred by ductal or lobular hyperplasia with atypia (five times greater than in women who have not had a breast biopsy) (Winchester, 1986). It is important to note that the severity of clinical symptoms has no correlation to histopathology.

Although symptomatic fibrocystic disorder generally resolves after menopause, patients on hormonal replacement therapy may continue or begin to experience mastalgia. It may be necessary to modify the treatment, or in some cases, to discontinue it. Any newly appearing or unusual breast symptom in postmenopausal patients warrants investigation.

Nipple Discharge

Bilateral, elicited nipple secretion is not unusual and is rarely a sign of significant breast pathology. With stimulation, many women produce a discharge that may be clear, gray, brown, yellow, green, black, or milky. No specific treatment is required for a physiologic discharge. A spontaneous nipple discharge is clinically significant. When associated with a mass, a unilateral, uniductal, bloody, sticky, or clear/watery discharge is suspicious of breast cancer. The same type of discharge without an associated mass is more likely to be due to an intraductal papilloma or to duct ectasia. The discharge should be tested for occult blood. A sample may be smeared on a glass slide. Cytologic evaluation of the discharge may demonstrate exfoliated malignant or benign papillary cells, but the latter does not rule out the need for surgical consultation. Imaging studies should begin with mammography, and may include contrast ductography (galactography). This technique involves cannulation of a dilated duct, introduction of contrast material, and mammography. This may demonstrate an intraductal lesion,

TABLE 45–4. Histologic Classification of Benign Breast Lesions

Cystic changes
- Macrocysts
- Microcysts
- Duct ectasia (plasma cell mastitis)

Fibrous changes
- Stromal fibrosis
- Fibroadenoma
- Involutional changes
- Sclerosing adenosis

Hyperplastic changes
- Proliferation of duct epithelium, including intraductal papillomatosis
- Lobular hyperplasia
- Proliferation of ductules, including blunt duct adenosis
- Ductal hyperplasia with atypia
- Lobular hyperplasia with atypia

but cannot distinguish between a benign and malignant one. Ultrasonography is of limited use in the evaluation of the subareolar ductal lumen (McSweeney-Kossoff, 1992). Papillomas are usually too small to be detected by this technique with standard equipment. Surgical treatment is usually indicated for unilateral, uniductal, spontaneous nipple discharge. The technique entails identification of the discharging duct through a small periareolar incision, and excision of the involved duct with a surrounding rim of breast tissue. Prior to closing the incision, a stimulation test to check for residual discharge determines if further duct exploration is necessary.

The most common cause of a bloody or serosanguinous nipple discharge is an intraductal papilloma; the least common cause is carcinoma. The frequency of carcinoma as a cause of nipple discharge increases with age. Duct ectasia and fibrocystic changes also cause this type of discharge, but more commonly the discharge due to these etiologies is multiductal and nonbloody. A bloody nipple discharge may occur during pregnancy (Haagensen, 1986). It usually begins during the middle or last trimester, and may persist for several weeks after delivery (or longer if the patient is breast feeding). No treatment is required.

Galactorrhea, a spontaneous usually bilateral milky discharge, is not associated with breast pathology per se, but is usually caused by an endocrine disorder relating to elevated prolactin secretion. When evaluating a patient with a nipple discharge, the medical and social history should include a complete list of medications. Marijuana, oral contraceptives, phenothiazine, methyldopa, some antihypertensives and antidepressants, among others, have been associated with galactorrhea. Milk secretion may be a symptom of thyroid disease. Trauma to the chest wall, including surgical trauma, can result in pituitary stimulation of prolactin secretion. More commonly, hyperprolactinemia is caused by a pituitary adenoma (Kleinberg et al., 1977).

The work-up of galactorrhea should include serum prolactin levels and thyroid function tests. Abnormal results should prompt a referral to an endocrinologist. Hyperprolactinemia is further elucidated by computerized tomography of the pituitary fossa and visual field measurements. Bromocriptine therapy may be indicated. Only in rare cases is neurosurgical intervention required.

Breast Infections

Skin and soft tissue infections can occur anywhere on the body, with the breast being no exception. Like any integumentary infection, clinical signs and symptoms include pain, redness, warmth, tenderness, and swelling. The vast majority of breast infections occur in the postpartum period or during lactation. Milk is an excellent culture medium for bacteria, and natural ingress is through the nipple. Thus, although *staphlococcus aureus* is the most common causal organism, any oral flora, as related to suckling, can be found. Antibiotics should be prescribed empirically; cephalexin is the drug of choice; clarithromycin can be used for patients who are not able to take cephalosporins. Warm compresses and analgesics are helpful. If tolerable, nursing should be continued. Lactational mastitis may progress to an abscess. If the abscess is small and superficial, needle aspiration may be the only additional treatment needed. Most breast abscesses, however, require surgical drainage.

In nonlactating patients, breast infections are uncommon. It behooves the practitioner to be alert to the possibility of inflammatory breast cancer. If suspected, surgical consultation should not be delayed. If inflammatory breast cancer has been ruled out, antibiotics should be prescribed as described earlier, and continued until symptoms resolve. Nonbacterial mastitis does not respond to antibiotics and requires only symptomatic treatment (dry heat and NSAIDs). The most common cause of breast abscess in nonlactating women is an infected cyst. Treatment consists of aspiration or surgical drainage.

A class of breast infections that is often clinically challenging is the chronic subareolar abscess. This manifests itself as a small tender periareolar mass with overlying erythema, sometimes associated with nipple retraction and/or nipple discharge. When a dilated, ectactic subareolar terminal duct becomes obstructed with inspissated material, bacterial contamination can result in a pocket of infection. Antibiotics and simple surgical drainage are inadequate treatment for this condition and will result in an indolent, recurring infection. Surgery that removes the involved ducts and surrounding breast tissue is curative. In women who may become pregnant in the future, care should be taken to remove only the diseased ducts. Otherwise, the nipple should be disconnected and the central duct system excised. Numbness of the nipple is a common postoperative sequela.

A Montgomery's gland abscess is similar to an infected epidermal inclusion cyst in presentation and treatment. Mondor's syndrome presents as a tender, cordlike thickening, usually located in the upper outer quadrant or lateral aspect of the breast. It represents a superficial phlebitis of the lateral thoracic or thoracoepigastric vein. The inflammation only occasionally causes erythema of the overlying skin; more often, one may see retraction of the skin along the course of the vein that appears as a groove or furrow particularly when the arm is raised above the head. The condition is benign and self-resolving. Symptomatic relief can be achieved with NSAIDs and/or dry heat. Full recovery can be expected within 3 to 8 weeks

Breast Problems in the Male

Gynecomastia is the abnormal development of breast tissue in the male breast. It presents clinically as a unilateral or bilateral subareolar breast mass that is firm, rubbery, and diskoid. A more generalized breast enlargement or hypertrophy is usually due to fat deposition. Work-up includes a careful history and physical exam. If an organic cause is suspected, further testing should be appropriately targeted. Mammography and/or sonography may help distinguish between this condition and breast malignancy. Surgical consultation is appropriate.

The condition may be idiopathic, drug induced, hormonal, or organic. Gynecomastia is not uncommon during puberty as a transient condition. If it persists for more than 1 year and it becomes the source of anxiety or embarrassment, the patient may need surgical intervention; the procedure of choice is a subcutaneous mastectomy. Elderly men may develop gynecomastia when testosterone levels decline. No treatment is required. Breast hypertrophy may result from developmental abnormalities of the genito-urinary tract, such as Klinefelter's syndrome and testicular feminization. Testicular tumors are another known cause, as is liver disease. Drugs known to cause breast hypertrophy are numerous and include phenothiazine, digoxin, cimetidine, marijuana, and tricyclic antidepressants. The condition may resolve when the drug is discontinued or the underlying cause is treated.

Male breast cancer comprises less than 1% of all reported cases of breast cancer in this country. A middle-aged male with a hard, painless breast mass, nipple retraction, or a bloody discharge should be referred to a surgeon immediately. A breast mass occurring in a position that is other than subareolar is suspicious.

Surgical treatment of breast cancer in males entails a modified radical mastectomy. Postoperative radiation adds no survival benefit. Adjuvant chemotherapy is used on the same theoretical basis as it is in women, although no randomized controlled clinical trials have been done because the number of male breast cancer patients is small. Stage for stage, the prognosis is probably similar to that of females. Because axillary node metastases are more commonly found in males at the time of primary treatment, however, the overall prognosis is worse for men. An interesting difference in breast cancer between men and women is that estrogen receptors are positive more often in males (approximately 85%) (Donegan & Redlich, 1996).

Breast Masses in Children

Breast masses are rare in the pediatric population. The majority of prepubertal "masses" are actually due to early breast-bud development, for which surgical intervention is contraindicated. Clinically, this presents as a unilateral subareolar mass that is small, rubbery, and sometimes tender. In young girls, prepubertal cysts and fibroadenomas can be distinguished with ultrasonography and fine-needle aspiration. In boys, as mentioned earlier, gynecomastia is the most common finding. Breast abscesses can be readily diagnosed. Primary breast cancer is extremely rare in children; metastatic cancer presenting as a breast mass is more common. In a reported series of 74 children who presented with breast masses obtained over a 14-year period, four were due to metastatic cancer from a distant primary site (West et al., 1995).

Breast Cancer

Ductal Carcinoma In Situ

The term "ductal carcinoma *in situ*" (DCIS) describes a heterogeneous group of cancers in which the tumor cells are confined within the ducts. The unifying feature is that there has been no invasion of tumor cells across the basement membrane into the surrounding breast stroma. The histologic subtypes are cribiform, papillary, micropapillary, solid, and comedo. The comedo subtype is associated with the greatest malignant potential (Talamonti, 1996).

There has been almost a threefold increase in the proportion of breast cancers classified as DCIS in the past 15 years, probably due to the increased utilization of screening mammography. About one quarter of all cancers detected by mammography are DCIS. The most frequent mammographic presentation is a cluster of microcalcifications without a mass.

The treatment of DCIS evolved significantly during the last decade. Previously, simple mastectomy was the standard therapy. It offers virtually 100% cure when DCIS is not associated with microinvasive breast cancer. The dilemma faced by experts in the field had been that we could offer women with early-stage invasive breast cancer the option of breast conservation with rates of survival and recurrence equivalent to those patients who had undergone mastectomy, yet women with noninvasive (and thus less aggressive) breast cancer could not be offered this choice; that is, until quite recently. In a recent NSABP trial (B17), women treated with lumpectomy alone were compared with women who underwent lumpectomy followed by standard radiotherapy. Adding radiation reduced the local recurrence rate from 16.4% to 7% (Fisher et al., 1993). About half of the local recurrences are invasive carcinoma (Hermann et al., 1992). Other studies continue to show the effectiveness of excisional biopsy combined with radiotherapy in treating DCIS, and this is now the standard of care as an alternative to mastectomy for many women.

As we learn more about the biological behavior of DCIS, the rate of local recurrence will be reduced still further. We hope to identify those women who are at increased risk for local recurrence, and thus would derive greater benefit from mastectomy as the initial primary treatment. Currently, women in this category are those with tumors larger than 4 cm, those with multicentric disease, and women in whom histologically clear margins cannot be achieved with a reasonable cosmetic result.

Tumor histology is also a factor; patients with extensive high-grade comedo necrosis are at increased risk for developing both local recurrence and invasive cancer. For this group of patients, the outside parameter of tumor size for breast conservation is 2.5 cm (Hermann et al., 1992). We also are collecting data to define another subgroup of women—those for whom lumpectomy without radiotherapy is adequate treatment. Currently, it may be appropriate to offer this option to women whose tumors are less than 1 cm in diameter with clear excisional margins and no histologic evidence of comedo necrosis. This is particularly applicable to women of an advanced age or those who have a limited life expectancy.

Lobular Carcinoma In Situ

Lobular carcinoma *in situ* (LCIS) is not a clinically detectable lesion. The diagnosis is made incidentally when tissue is removed for a palpable or mammographically detected lesion. On sectioning, LCIS may be identified as an incidental finding in the surrounding breast tissue. Although the significance and treatment of LCIS remains controversial, there is a greater understanding of its behavior because of several major studies. The largest series of patients was followed for 47 years. Eighteen percent of the patients with biopsy-identified LCIS eventually developed invasive breast cancer, 50% in the ipsilateral and 50% in the contralateral breast (Haagensen et al., 1978). It appears that unlike DCIS, LCIS is not a pre-invasive lesion that progresses to invasive breast cancer if left untreated. Rather, the thinking today is that LCIS is a histologic marker denoting an increased susceptibility to invasive cancer that is unrelated to the site of the lobular neoplasm, and the cancer is usually not of lobular origin.

LCIS is diagnosed most commonly in premenopausal women and it is bilateral in 25%. Multicentricity is a frequent observation. Women with LCIS have a lifetime risk of developing invasive breast cancer that is about ten times that of the normal population. The vast majority of women (approximately 75%) with LCIS never develop breast cancer. This paradox has important treatment implications. (Goldschmidt & Victor, 1996). In the past, just as for DCIS, simple mastectomy was the standard treatment. Many surgeons also performed a "mirror image" contralateral breast biopsy at the same time. With our current knowledge of LCIS, this treatment approach has become outdated. To protect a patient with LCIS from developing breast cancer in the future, bilateral mastectomies would be required. This aggressive surgery, however, is offered only to a highly selected small number of patients; for example, those with LCIS and a strong family history of breast cancer, or those patients whose diagnosis causes undue cancer phobia. All patients with LCIS should be followed by a breast specialist and the decision regarding prophylactic mastectomy should be made collaboratively with a full understanding of the risks and benefits. Currently, the preferred management strategy for patients with LCIS entails monthly breast self-examination, semiannual clinical examination, and annual mammography.

Invasive Breast Cancer

Breast cancer will soon exceed lung cancer as the leading cause of cancer deaths in American women. It is the leading cause of death for women ages 40 to 55. Between 1950 and 1990, the annual incidence of breast cancer increased by 52% (White et al., 1996). Fortunately, the mortality rate remained almost level during that same period. Only recently has there been a slight downward trend in mortality rates. The lifetime risk of a woman developing breast cancer based on actuarial calculations is 1 in 8. Figure 45–4 provides an algorithm for diagnosis and treatment.

Histology. In the breast, epithelial cells line ducts, acini, and lobules. Breast cancer can develop in any of these sites. As discussed previously, when malignant epithelial cells remain within the confinement of the basement membrane, the cancer is defined as *in situ.* When the tumor invades beyond the basement membrane, infiltrating or invasive cancer exists (Shousha, 1989). The most frequent histologic subtype, comprising approximately 75% of all invasive tumors, is ductal. The gross and microscopic features of these tumors are quite variable. The biologic behavior is equally variable, but is somewhat related to histologic features. This type of cancer usually presents clinically as a hard, gritty poorly defined breast mass or mammographically as a spiculated mass (Fig. 45–5).

The second most common histologic subtype is invasive lobular carcinoma, comprising approximately 15%. Clinically, it is important to note that unlike other invasive breast cancers, lobular carcinoma often presents as a vague thickening or ill-defined mass; it is much less clinically dis-

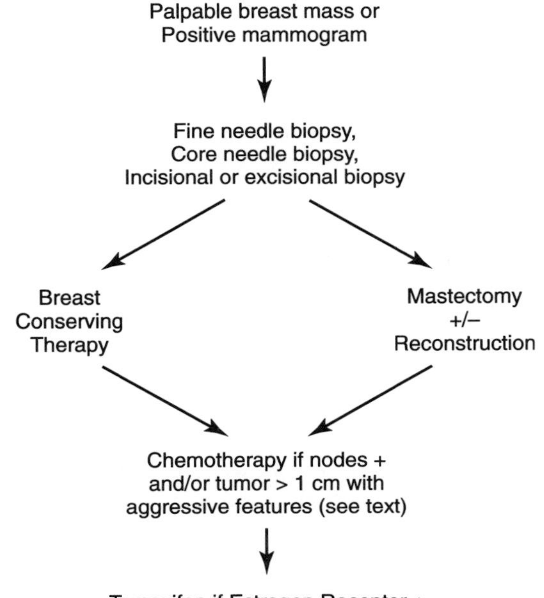

Figure 45–4. Algorithm for diagnosis and treatment of breast cancer.

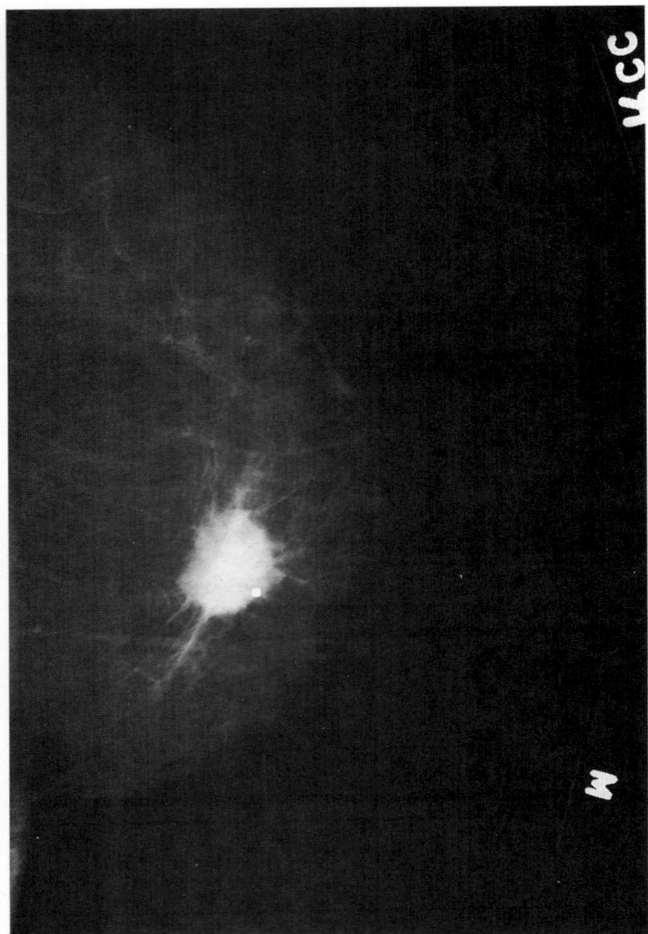

Figure 45–5. Typical appearance of invasive ductal carcinoma on mammogram.

tinct than ductal carcinoma. Further, it may result in a falsely negative mammogram. It is more often bilateral and multifocal than other subtypes. Treatment is similar to that of invasive ductal carcinoma once multicentricity has been ruled out. Breast-conserving treatment may be more challenging because it is sometimes difficult to obtain histologically clear margins during surgery. Approximately 5% of invasive breast cancers are medullary. These tumors are clinically distinct by virtue of the soft but well-defined character of the palpable tumor. Histologically, they are distinguished by a marked lymphoid infiltration. Although medullary carcinoma tends to occur in younger women, the prognosis is better than for invasive ductal carcinoma and treatment is the same. Other histologic subtypes include tubular, mucinous, papillary, colloid, secretory (juvenile), apocrine, and adenoid cystic.

The most common nonepithelial breast carcinomas are sarcomas (arising from mesenchymal tissue) and lymphomas. Cystosarcoma phyllodes is a breast neoplasm with variable biologic behavior. It is most often clinically mistaken for a giant fibroadenoma from which it may originate. Phyllodes tumors are usually benign. Treatment requires surgical excision followed by an extended period of follow-up due to the possibility of local recurrence. Malignant cystosarcomas are characterized by rapid growth and large size. Total mastectomy is the treatment because of the likelihood of rapid recurrence. Lymph-node dissection is not required because these tumors spread hematogenously, not via the lymphatics. The breast is occasionally the site of metastatic tumor from a distant primary site.

Paget's disease is a form of breast cancer with important clinical implications. The diagnosis is frequently missed, although its manifestation often causes the patient to seek medical attention. The most common symptom is a change in the nipple: redness, roughness, or erosion. Paget's disease is most often mistaken for eczema or dermatitis of the nipple/areola complex. Erosions that involve the areola and adjacent skin are not due to Paget's disease, however, and a dermatologic consultation is appropriate. Conversely, any patient with an area of redness, roughness, thickening, or erosion of the nipple should be referred to a surgeon for biopsy. Although in the past, mastectomy was uniformly recommended for treatment, breast conservation can be offered to women with a confined lesion. Despite the need to remove the nipple/areola complex and central portion of the breast, a reasonable cosmesis can be obtained. Breast irradiation is required postoperatively. Unfortunately, there are cases in which the breast neoplasm is found in an area remote from the nipple, or it may not be clinically or mammographically detectable at all. In these cases, a mastectomy remains the most appropriate treatment, and with thorough histopathologic sectioning, the primary tumor is usually found.

Risk Factors. As mentioned earlier, some histologically identifiable lesions are associated with an increased risk for developing invasive breast cancer. Certainly, ductal carcinoma *in situ* is recognized as such a lesion, which if left untreated confers a very high likelihood of progressing to invasive cancer. Lobular carcinoma *in situ* is a marker for increased risk, unrelated to the site of origin. Any woman who has had a biopsy finding of atypical ductal or atypical lobular hyperplasia is considered to be four to five times more likely to develop breast cancer than the average woman. Some breast pathologists place proliferative changes (florid hyperplasia without atypia, papillomatosis, sclerosing adenosis) in a "slightly increased risk" histologic category (Page, 1996).

It is now recognized that approximately 5 to 10% of breast cancers are attributable to inheritance of a high-risk susceptibility gene that is autosomal dominant. About 15 to 25% of breast cancers occur in woman with a family history of breast cancer in a first-degree relative; thus, half of these are random or due to an as-yet-unknown gene mutation. The mutated BRCA1 gene is responsible for about

45% of hereditary early-onset breast cancers. The median age of onset is 45 years. Female carriers of the mutated gene have an 87% lifetime risk of developing breast cancer. The gene also confers increased risk for developing ovarian, colon, and (in males) prostate cancer. The mutated BRCA2 gene is found in 40% of hereditary early-onset breast cancer patients. A third type of inherited breast cancer (about 7% of the identified genetically linked group) is due to a mutated autosomal recessive gene for ataxia–telangiectasia (Radford & Zehnbauer, 1996). Until genetic testing for breast cancer has wide clinical acceptance and availability, any woman with a first-degree relative (mother, daughter, sister) with breast cancer should be considered at increased risk. At greatest risk are those whose progenitors have had premenopausal bilateral breast cancer.

Because the incidence of breast cancer increases exponentially during the postmenopausal period, and because 85 to 90% of cases are among women with no family history, age is the most important risk factor (Goldschmidt & Victor, 1996). Certainly, any woman previously treated for breast cancer is at an increased risk for subsequent breast cancer. There are several minor risk factors that include: nulliparity or first full-term pregnancy after age 30, caucasian race (higher incidence in Hawaiian women and Ashkenazi Jewish women), prior exposure to radiation, early menarche (before 12), and late menopause (after 55). There is conflicting data regarding obesity, high-fat diet, excess alcohol consumption, and cigarette smoking in relation to breast-cancer risk. More controversial, and still unresolved, is the role of exogenous estrogen in breast carcinogenesis. Reports in the literature are contradictory. The inconsistency itself is important because it indicates that the link, if any, is not strong. Numerous studies on estrogen replacement therapy and breast cancer risk have not given us the answers our patients need. If we assume a small increased risk that may increase with advancing age and prolonged use, the risk should be weighed against the known benefits and assessed for each individual patient based on family history, personal medical history, overall health-care concerns, lifestyle, and patient preference. The use of oral contraceptives has also been cited as a possible risk factor, but there is currently no conclusive evidence to support this hypothesis.

Health-care providers must play an active role in counseling women about their breast-cancer risk so that appropriate monitoring programs can be individualized. Genetic testing for breast cancer raises ethical challenges, as yet unresolved. At this time, we do not know who should be tested, and moreover, what are the implications and impact of the test results on patients and their families. It is important for the practitioner to remain informed about medical advances, the available preventive strategies, current standards of monitoring and treatment, and to have access to appropriate expertise.

Currently, the options for patients considered at high risk are: regular mammography and clinical examination, bilateral prophylactic mastectomy, or the preventive use of Tamoxifen (recently approved for this use after a national clinical trial demonstrated a decreased incidence of breast cancer in high-risk women taking the drug) (Hiatt, 1995). Annual mammography in a woman who has a significant family risk of breast cancer (a first-degree relative who had premenopausal breast cancer, or two first-degree relatives of any age with breast, ovarian, or colon cancer) should begin screening ten years before the age of onset in the relative, or at the age of 30, whichever comes first. Any woman who has had breast, colon, endometrial, or ovarian cancer should be similarly screened. Women in these two groups should be offered genetic counseling and should be followed regularly by a breast specialist who can counsel the patient regarding ongoing prevention trials, surgical options, and be available to cope with the psychosocial impact of the management strategies.

Staging. In the United States, the most widely used system for staging breast cancer is based on the TNM (tumor size, nodal involvement, metastatic disease) classification system that is summarized in Table 45–5. Staging has both prognostic and treatment implications. Overall, the 5-year disease-free survival rate for Stage I breast cancer is 80%, whereas for Stage IV it is 0 (August & Sondak, 1993). Tumor size and axillary node status are highly significant predictors of outcome. Patients with positive nodes are at in-

TABLE 45–5. Breast-Cancer Staging

I	=	T1/N0
II	=	T0/N1 T2/N0 T1/N1 T2/N1
IIIA	=	T0/N2 T2/N2 T3/N1 T1/N2 T3/N0 T3/N2
IIIB	=	Any T/N3; Any T4
I, II, III	=	No evidence of distant metastasis (M0)
IV	=	Any T/Any N with distant metastasis (M1)
T0	=	No evidence primary tumor
Tis	=	*In situ* cancer
T1	=	Tumor 2 cm or less
T2	=	Tumor 2–5 cm
T3	=	Tumor > 5 cm
T4	=	Tumor extends to skin or chest wall
Presurgical Node Staging		
N0	=	No palpable ipsilateral axillary nodes
N1	=	Palpable but movable axillary nodes
N2	=	Fixed axillary nodes
N3	=	Palpable regional nodes or arm edema
Surgical Node Staging		
N0	=	Histologically negative axillary nodes
N1	=	Microscopic axillary nodal involvement
N2	=	Gross axillary nodal involvement—fixed or matted
N3	=	Histologically positive regional nodes (beyond axilla)

T = tumor size
N = nodal involvement (clinical or surgical)
M = metastatic disease (M0 or M1)

creased risk for developing distant metastases. The number of involved nodes correlates directly with the risk of recurrent disease and overall survival (Bookman et al., 1991). In addition to the clinical examination, the staging work-up of all patients with newly diagnosed breast cancer should include: bilateral mammography (if not already done), chest x-ray, complete blood count, bone scan, and liver functions tests. These are done because breast cancer usually metastasizes to the bone (or bone marrow), lung (or pleura), and/or liver. Serum markers are not yet available for breast cancer staging, screening, or follow-up. There is intense research activity to find tumor-related factors that may add to our ability to predict relapse (local recurrence or systemic metastatic disease) and thus to define subgroups of women who may benefit from chemotherapy and other forms of treatment.

As mentioned earlier, tumor histology has some bearing on prognosis. Other tumor factors—such as histologic grade, rate of mitoses, the presence of blood vessel or lymphatic invasion, DNA ploidy, S-phase, and protease cathepsin levels—each seem to impact on prognosis, but none have been clinically as useful as tumor size and axillary node status. Growth factor receptors, oncogenes, and genetic alterations each are currently being investigated as potential prognostic indicators. Hormonal receptor status (estrogen and progesterone receptors) is important both for prognosis and treatment. Patients with estrogen receptor-positive tumors have a better prognosis. Patient age has long been thought to influence prognosis, but recent studies have resulted in conflicting data. There seems, however, to be mounting evidence that, stage for stage, patients younger than age 35 at the time of diagnosis have a poorer prognosis than older women (Bonnie et al., 1995).

Treatment. Today, breast cancer is treated by a team of health-care providers including surgeons, medical and radiation oncologists, nurses, social workers, and physical therapists. Fortunately, with increased awareness and increasing utilization of mammography, most patients can be provided with both medical and surgical treatment options. It should be emphasized, however, that not every patient is a candidate for breast-conserving treatment (BCT) and not every patient can be cured. Breast-conserving treatment is defined as local tumor control ("lumpectomy") followed by a course of radiotherapy that lasts approximately six weeks. Until noninvasive methods are available that enable us to diagnose lymphatic metastases, axillary node dissection is necessary for most patients to complete accurate staging and significantly decrease the risk for later axillary recurrence. In patients for whom chemotherapy is contraindicated, or for those whose axillary node status will not affect treatment, axillary node dissection is not required if the nodes are clinically negative, but the axilla should be included in the radiation field. Breast-cancer treatment is summarized in Table 45–6; surgical methods are illustrated in Figure 45–6.

TABLE 45–6. Breast Cancer Therapy

Breast Surgery
Extended (supraradical) mastectomy
Radical mastectomy
Modified radical mastectomy
Total mastectomy
Quadrantectomy (partial mastectomy)
Wide excision (lumpectomy)
Lymph Nodes
Complete axillary node dissection (levels 1, 2, 3)
Low axillary dissection (levels 1 and 2)
Sentinel node biopsy
Radiotherapy
Breast, regional nodes, tumor boost
Breast, axillary nodes, tumor boost
Breast, tumor
Chest wall
Systemic Therapy
Neoadjuvant chemotherapy
Adjuvant chemotherapy
Hormonal therapy (e.g., Tamoxifen)
Bone-marrow transplant or stem-cell rescue
Future Modalities
Gene therapy
Immunotherapy
Chemoprevention
Stereotactic and other nonsurgical tumor-ablative techniques

Radical mastectomy is reserved for those patients whose tumors involve the pectoralis major muscle. The modified version of this operation had become the standard of care for breast cancer until the early 1980s. A modified radical mastectomy removes the breast, axillary lymph nodes, and pectoralis minor muscle. An even less radical version of this procedure, the most commonly performed mastectomy for breast cancer today, preserves the pectoralis minor. For those women who choose the procedure, or for those women in whom BCT is contraindicated (as discussed later in this section), the option of breast reconstruction should be explored in consultation with a plastic surgeon. For a woman who has a choice between BCT and mastectomy, it is only her psychosocial issues that should influence her decision because there is no difference in outcome (local control and disease-free survival) between the two in treating early-stage breast cancer. The risk of local recurrence (4-10% over ten years) after BCT seems to depend primarily on achieving histologically negative margins at the time of lumpectomy or reexcision (Smith et al., 1995). An extensive intraductal component (more than 25% of the tumor) also has a negative impact on local control. BCT is not an appropriate choice for treating locally advanced breast carcinoma. BCT is contraindicated in women with tumors larger than 4 cm, for patients with inflammatory breast cancer, and for patients with documented collagen–vascular disease. For women in whom cosmesis is not a factor and for women without access to a radiation treat-

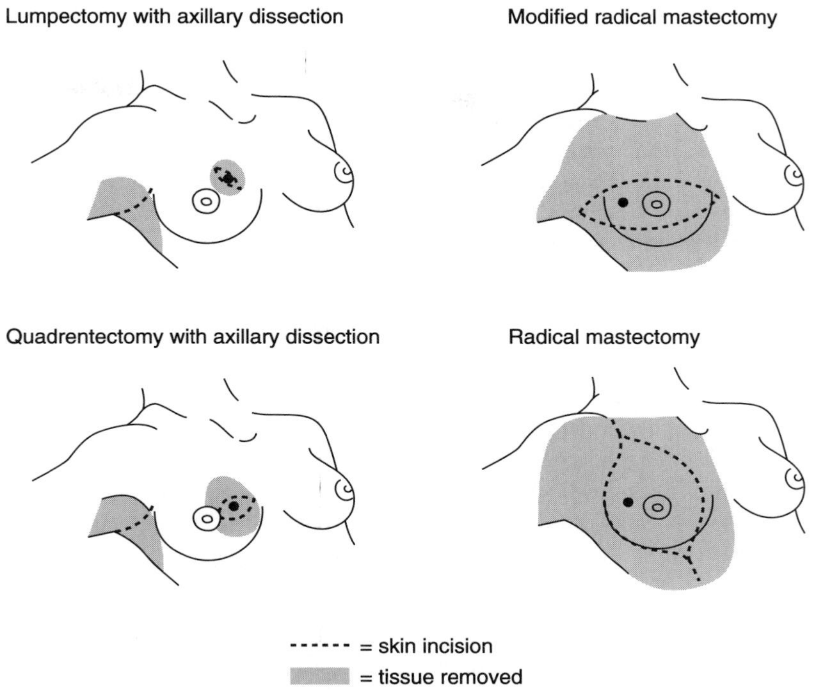

Figure 45–6. Surgical treatment of breast cancer.

ment facility, mastectomy is the preferred treatment. Radiation is contraindicated during pregnancy.

We are now learning that tumor size at initial presentation may not preclude BCT. Several researchers have been exploring the concept of preoperative "down staging" using neoadjuvant (induction) chemotherapy. The patient receives several cycles of chemotherapy and, if the tumor responds and shrinks to an appropriate size, BCT can be used (Perez, 1996). Early local recurrences are a potential drawback; outcome data will be important in evaluating this new modality.

A lumpectomy should remove the tumor and a margin of normal breast tissue surrounding the tumor. The margins must be examined microscopically and some women may require additional surgery to achieve histologically clear margins. Clear margins are critical for minimizing the risk of local recurrence. Patients, particularly those who are small breasted, should be willing to accept moderate asymmetry or deformity if their desire is breast conservation. It may otherwise be appropriate to select mastectomy with reconstruction as an alternative strategy.

An axillary lymph node dissection to remove the level 1 and level 2 nodes is usually performed through a separate incision under the arm. As part of the general trend toward the "less is better" concept, several researchers have developed a technique to distinguish between node–negative and node–positive patients by removing a single "sentinel" node. By injecting the breast tumor or biopsy bed with dye or radioactive marker, the sentinel node absorbs the substance and is, thus, identifiable by the surgeon. If this node is histologically negative for metastatic tumor on frozen section, a formal axillary dissection is not required. It should be emphasized that when performed by experienced surgeons, level 1 and/or level 2 axillary dissections have little negative impact on morbidity or cosmesis.

After the patient has recovered from the surgery in 2 to 3 weeks, radiotherapy is instituted. The standard regimen is a total of 4500 to 5000 cGy to the breast, with an additional boost of 1000 to 1600 cGy to the tumor bed. The treatments are divided over a 6-week period. In experienced hands, side effects should be minimal. During treatment, the patient may experience a "sunburn" over the breast; later, she may notice a darkening and/or thickening of the skin. Radiation therapy is also indicated for patients with inflammatory breast cancer, locally advanced disease, and chest wall recurrence after mastectomy.

Anyone who has had an axillary lymph node dissection is at risk for developing lymphedema of the homolateral upper extremity. Clinically, lymphedema manifests as swelling of the fingers, hand, forearm, upper arm, or entire arm. In the era of more radical breast surgery, lymphedema was a more common complication. Now, approximately 4% of patients develop this problem. It can occur immediately postoperatively, after several months, after several years, or even 20 years after cancer therapy. The cause is unknown, and treatment is difficult.

Lymphedema, however, can be avoided with patient education and compliance. Patients should have no external sources of pressure applied to the arm—this includes blood pressure cuffs, tourniquets (no blood draws or IV lines), binding clothing, tight jewelry, and so on. Patients should avoid even minor injuries (bruises, cuts, sunburn, insect bites, pet scratches) to the arm by wearing protective gloves or clothing when appropriate. Strenuous lifting and/or carrying heavy objects, extremes of temperature, and cutting of cuticles are also to be avoided. Patients may resume their traditional deodorant and underarm shaving with an electric razor once the incision has healed. A low-fat, low-salt diet is recommended.

Any increase in the girth of the arm should prompt a visit with the surgeon and a consultation with a physical therapist who is familiar with lymphedema care. Any sign of infection of the extremity should be aggressively treated. Established lymphedema is treated with physical therapy, elastic or pneumatic compression devices, and diuretics. Surgical intervention is rarely necessary.

Adjuvant Therapy. As with many aspects of breast-cancer treatment, controversies abound regarding the indications and parameters for chemotherapy. The rationale for adjuvant chemotherapy for early-stage breast cancer is based on accumulated data from previous and ongoing clinical trials. Systemic therapy is administered to eradicate microscopic metastatic disease before it becomes clinically detectable. Breast cancer is often very sensitive to chemotherapy. There are several standard multidrug regimens commonly used in clinical practice, and newer drugs that may be more effective and less toxic are being developed. Chemotherapy seems to be more effective in premenopausal patients, whereas hormonal therapy seems to be more effective in postmenopausal patients. This may relate to the observation that hormonal receptors are more often positive in postmenopausal patients. There is general agreement that patients with small (less than 1 cm) tumors and negative axillary nodes regardless of menopausal status do not require chemotherapy. Premenopausal patients with positive nodes, regardless of tumor size, are treated with combination multidrug chemotherapy. Similarly postmenopausal patients whose tumors are estrogen receptor (ER) negative benefit from chemotherapy, with improvement in survival and local control compared with women who are not treated. Postmenopausal ER positive patients do as well with Tamoxifen therapy given for 5 years. There is general agreement that patients with T2 tumors (or larger) benefit from chemotherapy regardless of node or receptor status. Tamoxifen is added if the tumor is ER positive. Most protocols call for between 6 and 12 months of chemotherapy administered in cycles. Any Stage III patient requires aggressive chemotherapy, such as induction chemotherapy or high-dose chemotherapy with peripheral blood stem-cell transplantation commonly known as "stem cell rescue." This method is replacing autologous bone marrow transplantation because of its lower morbidity and lower cost. It is another area of very active clinical investigation. Another area of study is the timing of chemotherapy to determine if it is advantageous to treat patients preoperatively, postoperatively but prior to radiotherapy, or after radiotherapy. Results in patients undergoing BCT point toward lower systemic recurrence rates when chemotherapy is given before radiation. Local recurrence rates, however, are higher in these women (Recht et al., 1996).

The limiting factors and toxicities of systemic chemotherapy in addition to bone marrow suppression (leukopenia, thrombocytopenia) include weight alterations, hair loss, nausea/vomiting, and amenorrhea. Tamoxifen may induce hot flashes, vaginal discharge, weight gain, phlebitis, nausea, and/or retinopathy. Gynecologic monitoring is required in all patients on Tamoxifen who have not had a hysterectomy because it increases the risk for endometrial cancer (Balch et al., 1993).

Inflammatory Breast Cancer. The acute-care provider has an important role in diagnosing inflammatory breast cancer (IBC), the most life threatening form of breast cancer. Although its clinical presentation is characteristic, it is often confused with other inflammatory conditions of the breast. Recognizing IBC is critical, and it should be considered an urgent problem that requires immediate attention. If untreated, it is rapidly progressive and uniformly fatal; survival is measured in months. With aggressive multimodal therapy, we are now achieving local control and remissions of two years or more.

The diagnosis of IBC is based on the following signs and symptoms: erythema of one third or more of the breast skin with overlying warmth, peau d'orange (orange peal) appearance of the skin secondary to skin edema, and enlargement and/or induration of the breast with ill-defined thickening or diffuse lesions within the breast (Gradishar, 1996). Mammographically, a discrete lesion is not seen, but diffuse density with skin thickening is the most common finding. When these clinical features are present, fine-needle or core-needle biopsy confirms the presence of malignancy, and treatment can be instituted based on the clinical presentation and cytologic or histologic confirmation. Some oncologists may still prefer an incisional biopsy to include a segment of skin because the presence of tumor cells in the dermal lymphatics is pathognomonic of IBC.

Induction chemotherapy with multiple drugs is the initial treatment, and usually includes an anthracycline (doxorubicin or epirubicin). After maximum clinical response is observed, mastectomy is still the preferred surgical treatment, which is followed by radiotherapy. High-dose chemotherapy is being used in clinical trials, but its efficacy in treating IBC has not been established.

Locally Advanced Breast Cancer

Locally advanced breast cancer is usually clinically obvious. The term includes most Stage III tumors. A patient with any one of the following features is included in this category: tumors larger than 5 cm, involvement of the overlying skin (e.g., satellite skin nodules), fixation to the chest wall muscles, axillary nodes that are matted and/or multiple, or involvement of any other regional nodes (infraclavicular, supraclavicular, cervical). It represents 10 to 15% of all patients at the time of initial diagnosis. By utilizing the same multimodal approach to treatment as described above for IBC, rates of disease-free survival have improved considerably.

Metastatic and Recurrent Breast Cancer

It is often the primary-care provider who first becomes alerted to the clinical manifestations of metastatic breast cancer. The preferential sites of distant metastases are bone, lung, and liver. Central nervous system metastases are less common. Skeletal metastases present in several ways: pain, hypercalcemia, impending or pathologic fractures, spinal cord compression, and spinal instability (Blamery, 1986). These should be easily recognized. Treatment includes orthopedic intervention and pain management, localized radiation and, chemotherapy and/or hormonal therapy. Acute hypercalcemia requires controlled hydration and calcium-lowering agents such as calcitonin or mithramycin. The development of lung or pleural metastatic disease is often manifested clinically by breathing problems. Treatment is both symptomatic (such as thoracentesis for a pleural effusion) and systemic.

Metastases to the liver become clinically evident with weight loss, jaundice, ascites, and/or abdominal pain. Central nervous system metastases are best palliated with radiation. Steroids are given to decrease intracranial pressure. Patients with widespread metastatic disease may benefit from endocrine manipulation (e.g., oophorectomy, adrenalectomy, hypophysectomy) combined with multidrug chemotherapy. Terminal care is aimed at pain control and emotional support.

Locally Recurrent Breast Cancer

Chest-wall recurrence after mastectomy is the site of first failure in less than 10% of patients, but it is an ominous prelude to distant metastatic disease in most. Local excision (if possible) followed by chest-wall radiation is often effective for local control. The role of systemic chemotherapy is uncertain. Patients who develop recurrent breast cancer after BCT should be treated with completion mastectomy. The role of excisional therapy for the purposes of prolonged breast conservation is under investigation. Regional node recurrence is rare; treatment includes radiation to the entire node basin and is usually followed by chemotherapy; results are poor and long-term survival is unlikely.

Recommendations for Following Breast-Cancer Patients

Patients who have been treated for breast cancer require life-long follow-up because breast cancer can recur many years after the primary treatment. Strategies for managing patients after treatment have evolved in recent years in a search for appropriate, cost-effective screening modalities. There is also some debate about who should be providing this ongoing care: the primary-care provider, the surgeon, the medical oncologist, the radiation oncologist, or all of them. For whomever has the responsibility, at a minimum in the first posttreatment year, quarterly clinical follow-up is needed. Thereafter, annual mammography should be reinstated and semiannual clinical examination may alternate among the treatment team members. Patients at high risk for recurrence and patients on ongoing treatment protocols should continue under the care of their medical oncologists. Patients on Tamoxifen who have not had a hysterectomy should be examined by their gynecologists every 6 months. Data show that routine follow-up bone and liver scans do not improve survival or influence health-related quality of life (G.M.O. Investigators, 1994). Yearly complete blood counts, liver function tests (alkaline phosphatase at a minimum), and chest x-rays are, however, recommended. There are no serum tumor markers (such as CEA and CA15-3) that are useful for monitoring patients to detect subclinical metastatic breast cancer.

An ongoing relationship with the treatment team members is not only important for diagnosing recurrent breast cancer, detecting contralateral breast cancer, managing sequalae of both the disease and the treatment, but it also can be of benefit to the patient in terms of restoring self-confidence and a sense of well-being. It is equally important that patients who are at the end of their lives due to terminal illness do not become abandoned by the health-care providers with whom they established a trusting relationship.

Nurse practitioners have a key role in the diagnosis and management of all major and minor breast disorders. In a unique way, nurse practitioners also can provide information and psychosocial support to help women work through very sensitive issues. Nurse practitioners should consider taking a lead in breast-cancer research in areas such as prevention, risk factors, screening/early detection, diagnosis, treatment, and rehabilitation (Dow, 1996). Nurse practitioners can lead the way in educating women about breast-cancer and educating breast-cancer patients before, during, and after treatment. Helping women deal with the side effects of treatment is another important arena. After treatment, follow-up assessment is a vital activity for the nurse practitioner, as is running breast-cancer support groups for patients and their families. The trend toward nurse practitioners in oncology is increasing. Patient care, case management, activism, advocacy, and research all benefit from participation and leadership by nurse practitioners.

REFERENCES

August, D. A. & Sondak, V. K. (1993). Breast. In L. J. Greenfield, M. W. Mulholland, K. T. Oldham, & G. B. Zelenock (Eds.), *Surgery, scientific principles and practice,* (pp. 1235–1285). Philadelphia: J. B. Lippincott.

Balch, C. M., Singletary, S. E., & Bland, K. I. (1993). Clinical decision-making in early breast cancer. *Annals of Surgery, 217* (3), 207–225.

Blamery, R. W. (1986). *Complications in the management of breast cancer,* (p. 166). East Sussex, England: Bailliere Tindall.

Bonnie, P., Romain, S., Charpin, C., Tubiana, N., Martin, P. M., & Piana, L. (1995). Age as a prognostic factor in breast cancer: Relationship to pathology and biologic features. *International Journal of Cancer, 62,* 138–144.

Bookman, M. A., Goldstein, L. J., & Scher, R. M. (1991). Medical management of early stage breast cancer. In C. M. Haskell (Ed.), *Current problems in cancer,* (pp. 160–232). St. Louis: Mosby.

Burbank, F. (1996). Stereotactic breast biopsy: Its history, its present and its future. *American Surgeon, 62,* 128–150.

Cody III, H. S. (1995). The impact of mammography in 1096 consecutive patients with breast cancer, 1979-1993: Equal value for patients younger and older than age 50 years. *Cancer, 76,* 1579–1584.

Donegan, W. L. & Redlich, P. N. (1996). Breast cancer in men. *Surgical Clinics of North America, 76* (2), 343–363.

Dow, K. H. (1996). *Contemporary issues in breast cancer,* (p. 275). London: Jones and Bartlett.

Durning, P. & Sellwood, R. A. (1982). Bromocriptine in severe cyclical breast pain. *British Journal of Surgery, 69,* 248.

Fisher, B., Constantino, J., & Redmond, C. (1993). Lumpectomy compared with lumpectomy with radiation therapy for treatment of intraductal breast cancer. *New England Journal of Medicine, 328,* 1581–1586.

G.M.O. Investigators impact of follow-up testing on survival and health-related quality of life in breast cancer patients. (1994). *Journal of the American Medical Association, 271* (20), 1587–1592.

Goldschmidt, R. & Victor, T. (1996). Lobular carcinoma *in situ* of the breast. *Seminars in Surgical Oncology, 12,* 314–320.

Gradishar, W. J. (1996). Inflammatory breast cancer: The evolution of mulitmodal treatment strategies. *Seminars in Surgical Oncology, 12,* 352–363.

Greenfield, L. J. (1993). In L. J. Greenfield, M. W. Mulholland, K. T. Oldham., & G. B. Zelenock (Eds.), *Surgery, scientific principles and practices.* Philadelphia: J. B. Lippincott.

Haagensen, C. D. (1986). *Diseases of the Breast* (3rd ed.). (pp. 14, 62). Philadelphia: W. B. Saunders.

Haagensen, C. D., Lane, N., Lattes, R., & Bodian, C. (1978). Lobular neoplasia (so-called lobular carcinoma *in situ*) of the breast. *Cancer, 42,* 737–769.

Harris, J. R. (1987). Breast disease. Philadelphia: J. B. Lippincott.

Hermann, G., Schwartz, I., & Tartter, P. (1992). *Nonpalpable breast cancer: Diagnosis and management,* (pp. 98–101). New York: Igaku-Shoin.

Hiatt, R. A. (1995). Ethics and economics of genetic testing for breast cancer. In B. A. Stoll (Ed.), *Reducing breast cancer risk in women,* (pp. 55–65). The Netherlands: Kluwer Academic Publisher.

Hoogstraten, B. & Burn, I. (1989). Diagnosis of breast cancer. In B. Hoogstraten, I. Burn, & H. J. G. Bloom (Eds.), *Breast Cancer,* (pp. 57–68). London: Springer–Verlag.

Kleinberg, D. L., Noel, G. L., & Frantz, A. G. (1977). Galactorrhea. *New England Journal of Medicine, 296,* 589–600.

Love, S. M., Gelman, R. S., & Silen, W. (1982). Fibrocystic "disease" of the breast—a nondisease? *New England Journal of Medicine, 307,* 1010–1014.

McSweeney-Kossoff, M. (1992). Clinical role of breast ultrasonography (Monograph). *The Female Patient, 17,* 130–135.

Minton, J. B., Foecking, M. S., Webster, D. J. T., & Matthews, R. H. (1979). Caffeine, cyclic nucleotides, and breast disease. *Surgery, 86,* 105–109.

Osborne, M. (1987). Breast development and anatomy. In J. R. Harris (Ed.), *Breast diseases,* (p. 4). Philadelphia: J. B. Lippincott.

Page, D. L. (1996). The woman at high risk for breast cancer: Importance of hyperplasia. *Surgical Clinics of North America, 76* (2), 221–230.

Perez, C. A. (1996). Neoadjuvant chemotherapy and breast conserving therapy for tumors larger than 3 cm. *Breast Diseases, 6* (4), 350–353.

Peters, F., Schuth, W., & Scheurich, B. (1984). Serum prolactin levels in patients with fibrocystic breast disease. *Obstetrics and Gyndcology, 64,* 381.

Proppe, K. H. (1984). Pathology and epidemiology of benign breast changes (Monograph). *The Fibrocystic Breast: A Multidisciplinary Approach,* 6–8.

Radford, D. M. & Zehnbauer, B. A. (1996). Inherited breast cancer. *Surgical Clinics of North America, 76* (2), 205–220.

Recht, A., Come, R. A., Henderson, I. C., Gelman, R. S., Silver, B., Hayes, D. F., Shulman, L. N., & Harris, J. R. (1996). The sequencing of chemotherapy and radiation therapy after conservative surgery for early stage breast cancer. *New England Journal of Medicine, 334,* 1356–1361.

Shousha, S. (1989). Histology of breast carcinoma and related conditions. In B. Hoogstraten, I. Burn, & H. J. G. Bloom (Eds.), *Brease Cancer,* (pp. 13–44). London: Springer–Verlag.

Smith, M. C., Nowelsk, W., Zdeblick, M. J., Jeffrey, S., Carlson, R. W., Stockdale, F. E., & Goffinet, D. R. (1995). The importance of lumpectomy surgical margin status in long term results of breast conservation. *Cancer, 76,* 259–267.

Talamonti, M. S. (1996). Management of ductal carcinoma *in situ. Seminars in Surgical Oncology, 12,* 300–313.

West, K. W., Rescorla, F. J., Scherer III, L. R., & Grossfeld, J. L. (1995). Symptomatic breast masses in the pediatric population. *Journal of Pediatric Surgery, 30,* 182–187.

White, G. L., Griffith, C. J., Nensteil, R. O., & Dyess, D. L. (1996). Breast cancer: Reducing mortality through early detection. *Clinical Reviews,* 77–102.

Winchester, D. P. (1986). The relationship of fibrocystic disease to breast cancer. *American College of Surgeons Bulletin, 71,* 29–31.

46

Hematologic Problems

Carina Knowlton Moravec

▶ BLOOD FORMATION

Anatomy and Physiology

The major functions of blood include nutrition, oxygenation, cleansing of wastes, and defense against microbes (Babior & Stossel, 1990). Over half of the blood volume is composed of plasma. Plasma is mainly water and serves as a transport medium for ions, proteins (such as immunoglobulins and the coagulation proteins), hormones, and end products of metabolism. The other half of the blood volume consists of the formed elements which include red blood cells (erythrocytes), white blood cells (leukocytes), and platelets.

Hematopoietic Cells

Hematopoiesis, or the production of blood cells, occurs primarily in the bone marrow. The liver, spleen, lymph nodes, and thymus are involved in hematopoiesis during embryonic life, but after birth extramedullary (outside the bone marrow) hematopoiesis only occurs during abnormal circumstances, and then mainly in the liver and spleen. The pluripotent hematopoietic stem cell resides mainly in the bone marrow and in small amounts in the peripheral blood. It is the source of the three types of blood cells: erythrocytes, leukocytes, and platelets.

The stem cell is an immature (undifferentiated) cell that has the capacity to reproduce itself and to mature (differentiate) into any one of the different types of blood cells. As the stem cell divides and matures, it differentiates into one of two committed cell lines: lymphoid or myeloid. The committed lymphoid cells eventually mature into T lymphocytes or B lymphocytes. The committed myeloid stem cell develops into a *colony-forming unit–granulocyte, erythrocyte, macrophage, megakaryocyte* (CFU–GEMM) (Jandl, 1996). This colony-forming unit, in turn, has the potential to develop along discrete cell lines: the erythroid line (leading to the formation of red cells), the granulocyte–monocyte line (leading to the formation of the phagocytic white cells, eosinophils, and basophils), and the megakaryocytic line (leading to the formation of platelets). As the various types of blood cells mature, they are released into the peripheral circulation. Figure 46–1 shows a model for hematopoietic cell differentiation and the growth factors involved at the various stages of differentiation.

Regulation of Hematopoiesis

Because blood cells have a limited life span, they need to be replaced constantly. Generally, production and destruction rates are balanced in a steady state, but depending on environmental stimuli, such as bleeding or infection, various cells may be produced in larger-than-normal quantities. Production of each of these cell lines is regulated by cytokines that influence the rate of growth and differentiation of the stem cells in the marrow. Cytokines are proteins that are produced by cells of the immune system and that regulate the immune response. Some examples of cytokines are granulocyte–macrophage colony-stimulating factor (GM–CSF), which stimulates the growth of granulocytes and macrophages, and interleukin-3 (IL-3), which stimulates the stem cell.

Red Blood Cells. All tissues of the body require a steady supply of oxygen in order to survive. Red blood cells (RBCs) take up oxygen in the lungs, transport it, and de-

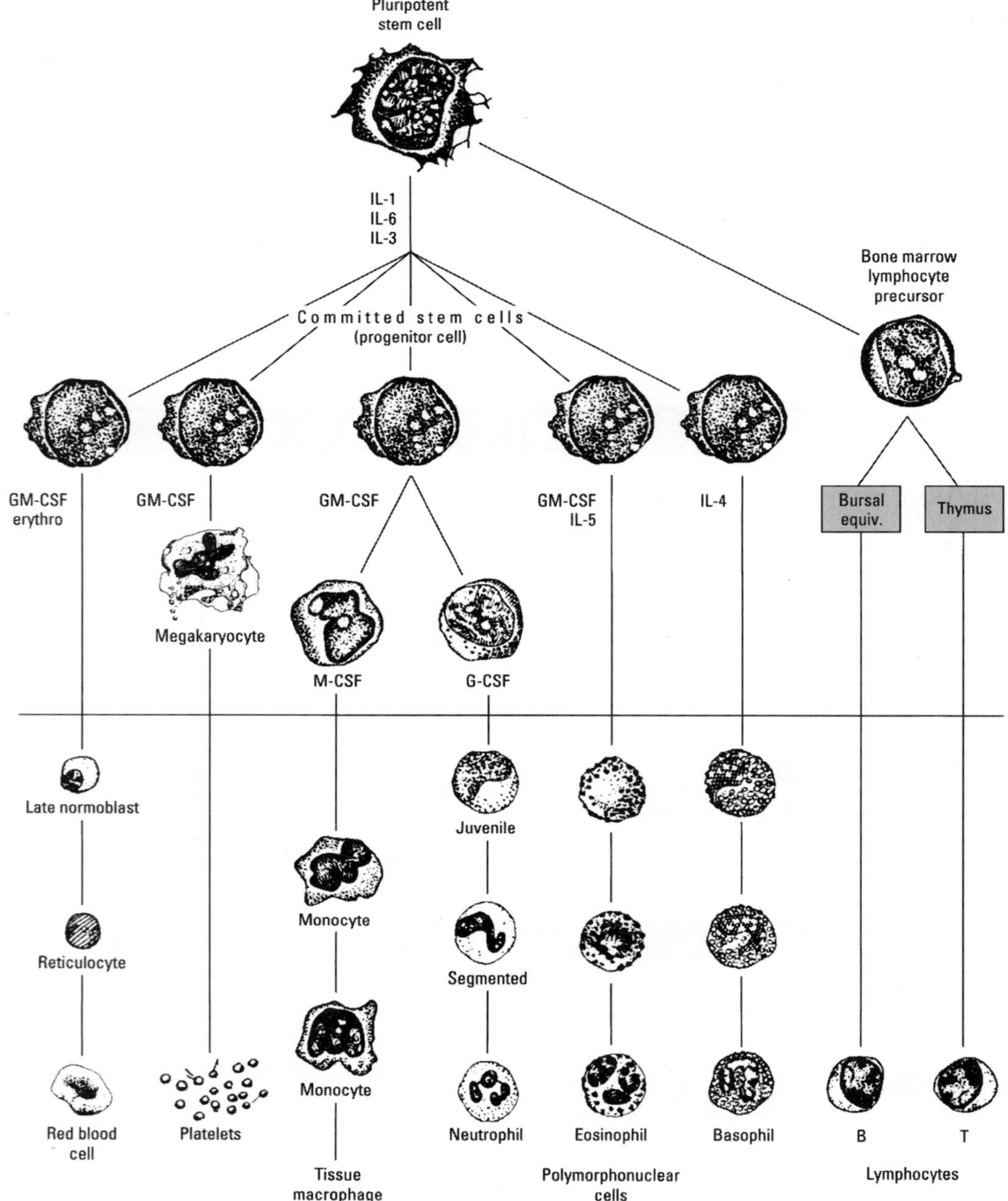

Figure 46–1. Hematopoiesis. *(Copyright 1985. Amgen Inc. All rights reserved. Amgen Inc. 1840 DeHavilland Drive, Thousand Oaks, California 91320-1789.)*

liver it to the tissues. The number of RBCs is crucial. If the number of RBCs is too low (anemia), the oxygen-carrying capacity is compromised, whereas too many RBCs (polycythemia) increases the viscosity to the blood and thus slows blood flow to the tissues. The rate of red-cell production is primarily controlled by erythropoietin, produced mainly by the kidneys and influenced by the oxygen content of the blood as sensed by the juxtaglomerular apparatus in the kidneys. RBC production is increased at times of blood loss, at high altitude, and in pulmonary diseases that affect the transport of oxygen from the lungs to the blood. RBCs survive approximately 4 months, at which time they are disposed of by the spleen.

The mature RBC is a biconcave disc filled with hemoglobin. The heme section is the oxygen-transporting portion. Oxygen diffuses from the lungs into the alveolar capillary, and as the RBC passes through the lungs, oxygen binds to the four sites in the heme region. The oxygen-binding properties of heme allow the RBC to fill up with oxygen in the lungs and then release it at the tissue level, as demonstrated by the oxygen–hemoglobin dissociation curve. Iron is an essential component of the hemoglobin molecule. Iron deficiency results in anemia from failure to synthesize hemoglobin, thus compromising oxygen transport. In addition to its oxygen-carrying function, hemoglobin can also bind to hydrogen, acting as a minor acid buffer.

White Blood Cells. White blood cells (WBCs), all of which defend against microbes or other foreign proteins, can be divided into two major categories: phagocytes and lymphocytes. The primary role of phagocytes is to localize and kill invading microorganisms. The primary role of lymphocytes is to initiate and carry out immune responses, including the manufacture of antibodies.

Phagocytes perform their role primarily in the tissues, where they travel to the site of inflammation (chemotaxis) and kill microbes by engulfing them (phagocytosis). Many substances, including complement fragments and bacterial products, stimulate this chemotactic migration. Phagocytic cells are divided into two subgroups: granulocytes and monocytes. The granulocytes include neutrophils, basophils, and eosinophils. Neutrophils are produced daily in huge numbers. Their main function is to find and kill bacteria, especially resident microorganisms such as staphylococci and gram-negative enteric flora (Jandl, 1996). They also play an important role in acute inflammatory processes. Neutrophils are the first phagocytic cells to appear at the site of acute inflammation (Cotran et al., 1989). During severe inflammatory reactions, neutrophils cause additional damage to surrounding tissues by releasing proteolytic enzymes and oxygen-free radicals. This process is thought to occur, for example, in the adult respiratory distress syndrome.

Eosinophils develop in the marrow along the same maturation steps as do neutrophils but they make up only about 4% of a normal WBC count. Eosinophils play a defensive role against parasites and in allergic reactions.

Basophils account for only 0.5 to 1% of the total WBC count. The role of the basophil is not well clarified, but they are known to play a part in immediate hypersensitivity reactions. Basophils release histamine when stimulated, which in turn results in the signs and symptoms of allergic reaction such as rhinitis, bronchospasm, urticaria, angioedema, and anaphylaxis (Babior & Stossel, 1990).

Monocytes constitute 4 to 8% of the total WBC count. Within 24 to 36 hours of entering the circulation, they migrate out to the tissues where they undergo further maturation into macrophages and make up the monocyte–macrophage system, also called the *reticuloendothelial system* (RES). Hepatic Kupffer cells, alveolar macrophages, and peritoneal macrophages are examples of tissue macrophages (Jandl, 1996). In the bloodstream monocytes have similar functions as the neutrophil, to find and kill microorganisms and are important in killing bacteria, protozoa, cells infected with viruses, and tumor cells. In addition, monocytes and macrophages play a crucial role in recognizing foreign antigens and presenting them to lymphocytes, thus stimulating the immune response. Macrophages also secrete biologically active products, including cytokines that modulate immune responses (e.g., GM–CSF), enzymes that can degrade connective tissue, and chemotactic factors (Cotran et al., 1989; Newcombe, 1993).

Lymphocytes are essential components of the immune system. They recognize and are instrumental in the elimination of foreign proteins, pathogens, and tumor cells. Lymphocytes control the intensity and specificity of the immune response (Paraskevas & Foerster, 1993). There are two general types of lymphocytes: T lymphocytes (T cells), which provide cell-mediated immunity, and B lymphocytes (B cells), which produce the antibodies of humoral immunity. As with the other cells already described, stem–cell differentiation of lymphocytes occurs in the bone marrow. During fetal life, some lymphocytes migrate to the thymus gland and mature into T-cells. It is in the thymus that T-cells learn to differentiate self from non-self. There are four major subsets of T-cells: helper T cells, suppressor T-cells, cytotoxic T-cells, and memory T-cells. Cell-mediated activities are of great importance in delayed hypersensitivity reactions; graft rejection; graft-versus-host disease (GVHD); and in defense against fungal, protozoal, and most viral infections. T cells also regulate immune activities through the secretion of lymphokines.

B lymphocytes mature into cells that respond to stimulation from foreign proteins by differentiating into memory cells and plasma cells. The plasma cells in turn produce specific antibodies that inactivate or destroy foreign proteins and pathogens.

Memory B and T cells impart immunological memory. These cells respond to repeated exposures to specific antigens with greater efficiency than during the first exposure. This memory provides the rationale for vaccinations (Babior & Stossel, 1990). Natural killer (NK) cells, another subset of lymphocytes, kill tumor cells and cells infected by viruses by lysing them. Thus, they play an important role in tumor surveillance.

The activities of phagocytes and immune cells overlap in numerous mutually beneficial ways. For example, immune cells often participate in chronic inflammatory reactions. Conversely, engulfment of foreign protein by macrophages is a preparatory step leading to antibody production.

Platelets. Platelets are small cell fragments that are produced by the disintegration of megakaryocytes in the bone marrow. Under normal circumstances, platelets circulate in the bloodstream for approximately 10 days. Their production is regulated by thrombopoietin, interleukin-3 (IL-3), and granulocyte–macrophage colony-stimulating factor (GM–CSF) (Babior & Stossel, 1990). The primary functions of platelets include the formation of a cellular plug that temporarily arrests bleeding and the contribution of substances essential to the coagulation process.

Anemias

Anemia is a low red-cell mass that results in the inability of the blood to supply adequate amounts of oxygen to the tissues of the body because of low hemoglobin levels.

Pathophysiology

Anemia is due to excessive blood loss, inadequate production, or excessive destruction of red cells. Inadequate production can be due to the failure of the stem cell to manufacture red cells, or there may be a failure of all three cell lines leading to pancytopenia such as in aplastic anemia or the myelodysplastic syndromes. Aplastic anemia is characterized by cellular depletion and fatty replacement of the bone marrow, resulting in decreased production of erythrocytes, leukocytes, and platelets, causing pancytopenia. Aplastic anemia can have multiple causes, including drugs, chemicals, irradiation, infections, and immune dysfunction. In megaloblastic anemia, the marrow may produce sufficient erythrocyte colony-forming units (CFU–Es) but the cells fail to mature and divide, accumulating in the marrow as dead and dying cells. Abnormal hemoglobin synthesis with normal DNA synthesis and normal maturation of the cells is manifested in the hypochromic anemias, such as iron deficiency, anemia of chronic disease, the thalassemias, and sideroblastic disorders.

Excessive destruction can be due to primary disorders of red-cell membranes, secondary disorders of red-cell membranes, immunohemolytic anemias, Heinz body hemolytic anemias, glycolytic defects, hemoglobinopathies, splenomegaly, or generalized disease.

History and Physical Findings

Many of the manifestations of anemia are similar and are related to the rate of onset, the hemoglobin level, degree of reduction in blood volume, and the adequacy of the cardio–pulmonary system to compensate (Jandl, 1996). Moderate anemia usually does not produce many symptoms, especially if the onset has been gradual. However, patients with significant cardiovascular or pulmonary disease may develop symptoms early. The initial compensations involve the cardiovascular system and include increased cardiac output, heart rate, and stroke volume. A systolic flow murmur may be heard. This high-output response may be described by the patient as thumping palpitations, buzzing in the head, high-pitched tinnitus, dizziness, and postural faintness or syncope. Reduced perfusion to the skin causes pallor of the tarsal conjunctivae, nail beds, and palmar creases, as well as lack of blanching of the nail beds with pressure. Other symptoms may include exertional dyspnea, muscle weakness, headache, or lethargy. Visual changes and shortness of breath at rest are indicative of more severe anemia. Severe anemia or a more moderate anemia coupled with significant cardio–pulmonary disease can result in high-output congestive heart failure, angina, claudication, or myocardial infarction. Respiratory failure is often associated with pulmonary edema and is difficult to treat. Transfusions should be infused very slowly in these patients to avoid life-threatening cardiac failure.

The patient should be asked about any abnormal blood loss, change in bowel habits, melena, aspirin use, family history of anemia, history of malignancies, symptoms of infections, presence of chronic inflammatory process, number of pregnancies, pica, dysphagia, lead exposure, dietary iron intake, menstrual blood loss, gastric resection, changes in nails, and glossitis. The physical exam should include checking for glossitis, cheilitis, splenomegaly, rectal mass, guaiac positive stools, pelvic mass, signs of chronic infections, inflammatory disorders, and signs of malignancy.

Glossitis, cheilitis, koilonychia (a disorder of the nails, where they become thin and concave from side to side), and esophageal web formation are commonly found with severe iron-deficiency anemia.

A history of gastric surgery, diet that includes raw fish, symptoms of terminal ileal disease, vitiligo, hypothyroidism, steatorrhea, chronic nitrous oxide abuse, or glossitis is more indicative of B_{12} deficiency. Vegetarians who avoid eating eggs and dairy products as well as meat may develop B_{12} deficiency. Patients with B_{12} deficiency are often severely anemic by the time of diagnosis as the anemia is usually asymptomatic because it develops slowly. The classic symptoms are sore tongue, and numbness and tingling of the extremities. The neuropathy generally involves symmetrical paresthesias in the hands and feet, which can progress to ataxia from loss of vibratory and position sense. This occurs from degeneration of the posterior columns of the spinal cord. Mild memory loss, irritability, depression, and psychosis can also occur as a result of B_{12} deficiency. The most common cause of B_{12} deficiency in the United States is an autoimmune deficiency called *pernicious anemia.* In this disorder, autoantibodies are produced against gastric parietal cells as well as intrinsic factor. It is diagnosed by achlorhydria after histamine stimulation. It is also often accompanied by other autoimmune disorders such as thyroid disease, rheumatoid arthritis, diabetes mellitus, or vitiligo. A second common cause of B_{12} deficiency is gastric achlorhydria alone in the elderly, which results in the inability to absorb vitamin B_{12}.

A history of alcoholism, poor nutrition, pregnancy, blood dyscrasias, chronic hemolytic anemia, sprue, severe psoriasis, and anticonvulsant therapy is more indicative of folate deficiency. Patients with folate deficiency may also develop psychosis and depression, but do not develop neuropathies.

Aplastic anemia often presents insidiously because the decrease in marrow production of the blood-forming elements is generally gradual. Patients not only manifest signs of anemia, but also of leukopenia and thrombocytopenia, such as frequent and persistent infections, and bleeding.

Laboratory and Diagnostic Tests

The most important test in the evaluation of anemia is the complete blood count (CBC), reticulocyte count, and the microscopic examination of the peripheral blood smear. Other confirmatory and diagnostic tests may be performed once a differential diagnosis is formed. The diagnostic criteria for anemia are a decreased hemoglobin (Hgb), hematocrit (Hct), or RBC count. Mild anemia is defined as a Hgb less than 12 g/dL in menstruating women, less than 11 g/dL in pregnant women, and less than 13 g/dL in men. Moderate anemia is defined as a Hgb of 7 to 10 g/dL, and severe anemia is a Hgb less than 7 g/dL (Glassman, 1997). The patient's intravascular volume status should be taken into account when analyzing these results. If the patient is dehydrated, the degree of anemia may be worse than what the Hct indicates. If the patient is volume overloaded, the dilutional affect will lower the Hct without a change in the actual number, production, or loss of RBCs.

The peripheral smear and the red-cell indices, mean corpuscular volume (MCV), and mean corpuscular hemoglobin concentration (MCHC) should be evaluated next. The red-cell distribution (RDW) is a measure of the homogeneity of the RBC population. It is elevated in deficiency states such as iron, folate, and vitamin B_{12} deficiency and when there is a marked reticulocytosis. It is useful in differentiating thalassemia (normal RDW) from nutritional deficiency. It is important not only to identify the type of anemia, but to also identify the etiology of the anemia in order to target treatment appropriately. Table 46–1 lists various anemias, categorized by red-cell morphology, and Figure 46–2 presents an algorithmic approach to the differential diagnosis of anemias by red-cell indices.

Microcytic Hypochromic Anemias (MCV <82, MCHC <32). These are small, pale cells. The most common cause is iron deficiency, thus serum iron, total iron binding capacity (TIBC), ferritin, and the percent of iron saturation should be measured. The most sensitive of all these tests in differentiating among iron deficiency, anemia of chronic disease, sideroblastic anemia, and hemoglobinopathies is the serum ferritin. Elevated TIBC, a ferritin less than 10 ng/mL, and percent saturation less than 10% indicate iron deficiency. Iron deficiency can be due to decreased dietary intake of iron, impaired absorption from malabsorption syndromes or gastrectomy, or increased requirements such as during periods of rapid growth, blood loss, or pregnancy.

Decreased TIBC, high ferritin, low iron, and normal percent saturation is more indicative of the anemia of chronic disease (ACD). This is associated with acute or chronic infections, malignancies, or inflammatory disorders. If ACD is diagnosed, the investigation should focus on finding a cause.

TABLE 46–1. Differential Diagnosis of Anemia by Red-Cell Morphology

Microcytic (MCV 50–82; MCHC 24–32)	1. Iron deficiency a. Chronic blood loss b. Inadequate intake c. Inadequate absorption d. Excess demand 2. Hemoglobinopathies a. Sickle cell anemia b. Thalassemias 3. Sideroblastic anemias 4. Chronic disease
Normocytic-Normochromic (MCV 82–92; MCHC 32–36)	1. Hemorrhage 2. Hemolysis 3. Aplastic anemia, pure red-cell aplasia 4. Marrow inflitrations 5. Hypothyroidism 6. Chronic disease 7. Chronic renal failure 8. Cirrhosis 9. Early iron deficiency
Macrocytic (MCV > 100; MCHC 32–36)	1. B_{12} deficiencies 2. Folic acid deficiencies 3. Antimetabolites 4. Accelerated erythropoiesis (acute hemolysis, hemorrhage) 5. Increased membrane surface area (liver disease) 6. Aplastic anemia

Adapted by permission from Goroll & Mulley. (1987). (p. 384).

High or normal iron levels, normal TIBC and percent saturation, with a high ferritin suggests hemoglobinopathy. Hemoglobin electropheresis can help make the diagnosis of hemoglobinopathy. Thalassemia minor is a common, inherited defect in globulin synthesis. The diagnosis of β-thalassemia-minor is confirmed by elevated levels of hemoglobin A_2 and/or hemoglobin F by hemoglobin electrophoresis.

Normochromic Normocytic Anemias. These anemias are classified according to the response of the marrow. Thus a reticulocyte count should be checked. If the reticulocyte count (a measure of new red blood cell production in the marrow) is high, it indicates hemolysis or hemorrhage. If hemorrhage is ruled out, check the bilirubin, haptoglobin, LDH, and a direct Coomb's test. Check for splenomegaly. If the direct Coomb's test is positive, check an indirect Coomb's. A positive indirect Coomb's indicates either a warm autoimmune hemolytic anemia or a transfusion reaction. A warm autoimmune hemolytic anemia may be due to malignancy, collagen–vascular disease, infection, medications such as quinidine, penicillin, methyldopa, and cephalosporins, or it could be idiopathic. A negative indirect Coomb's could indicate either a warm or, less commonly, a cold autoimmune hemolytic anemia. This less common au-

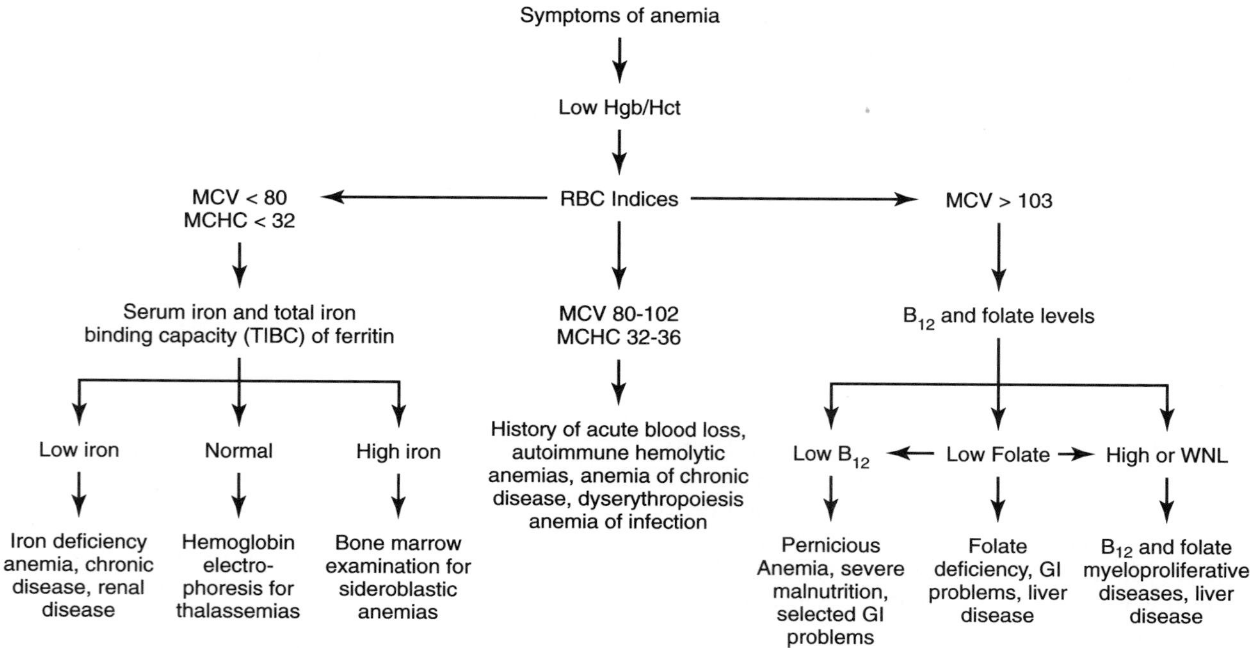

Figure 46–2. Differential diagnosis of anemia by red cell indices. *(Adapted with permission from Glassman. [1997]. [p. 75].)*

toimmune hemolytic anemia may be due to infectious mononucleosis, mycoplasma, malignancies, tertiary syphilis, or it may be idiopathic.

If the reticulocyte count is not elevated, as it should be in response to the anemia, the cause could either be a dilutional anemia or marrow underproduction. Inadequate marrow production could be due to chronic diseases such as renal failure, myxedema, Addison's disease, or alcoholic liver disease. If the peripheral smear shows many teardrop and fragmented cells, a marrow aspiration and biopsy should be performed.

A very low reticulocyte count coupled with pancytopenia suggests aplastic anemia, and a marrow biopsy should be obtained.

Macrocytic Anemia (MCV > 98). Many of these patients have folate and/or vitamin B_{12} deficiency, and some will have liver disease (Goroll & Mulley, 1987). Cigarette smoking, aplastic anemia, and refractory anemia also cause elevations in the MCV. The higher the MCV, the more likely that the cause is folate or B_{12} deficiency or refractory anemia. Red cell distribution width (RDW), a measure of the homogeneity of the red-cell population, is generally elevated in folate and vitamin B_{12} deficiency. These deficiencies are also often associated with macrocytosis, which is diagnosed by the presence of hypersegmented polymorphonuclear white cells, oval macrocytes, and nuclear–cytoplasmic dissociation on the blood smear. B_{12} and folate levels should be measured but can be affected by recent dietary intake and antibiotic treatment. The diagnosis of these deficiencies may also be made by a therapeutic trial of folate or B_{12}, but not simultaneously. Small doses of either vitamin should be used. If the reticulocyte count increases within 10 days, the deficiency is known. If the diagnosis of vitamin B_{12} deficiency is made, the Shilling test is done to distinguish between malabsorption and a deficiency due to lack of intrinsic factor. Marrow studies are usually not required, but if performed, a marrow aspiration as well as biopsy should be obtained. Thyroid function tests can determine whether there is an associated hypothyroidism.

Hemolytic Anemias. Failure of erythropoiesis in the bone marrow results in a drop in the hemoglobin of approximately 1 gm per week. A drop of more than 1 gram a week is indicative of bleeding or hemolysis. The most common tests performed if hemolytic anemia is in the differential are: serum haptoglobin, erythrocyte lactate dehydrogenase (LDH), indirect bilirubin, and the Coomb's test. If hemolysis is present, serum haptoglobin becomes saturated with the hemoglobin from hemolysis, does not bind to radioactive hemoglobin, and is low or absent. Neither LDH nor indirect bilirubin are specific for hemolytic anemia as they can both be elevated by other disorders such as megaloblastic anemia, and liver dysfunction. LDH can be elevated by numerous other factors as well. Spherocytes or microspherocytes on the blood smear are indicative of hemolytic anemia. Schistocytes or helmet cells on the blood smear are indicative of an intravascular hemolysis from vasculitis such as occurs in disseminated intravascular coagulation, thrombotic thrombocytopenic purpura (TTP), hemolytic–uremic syndrome (HUS), or malignant hypertension. Figure 46–3 is a chart of abnormal cell morphology. The Coomb's test is

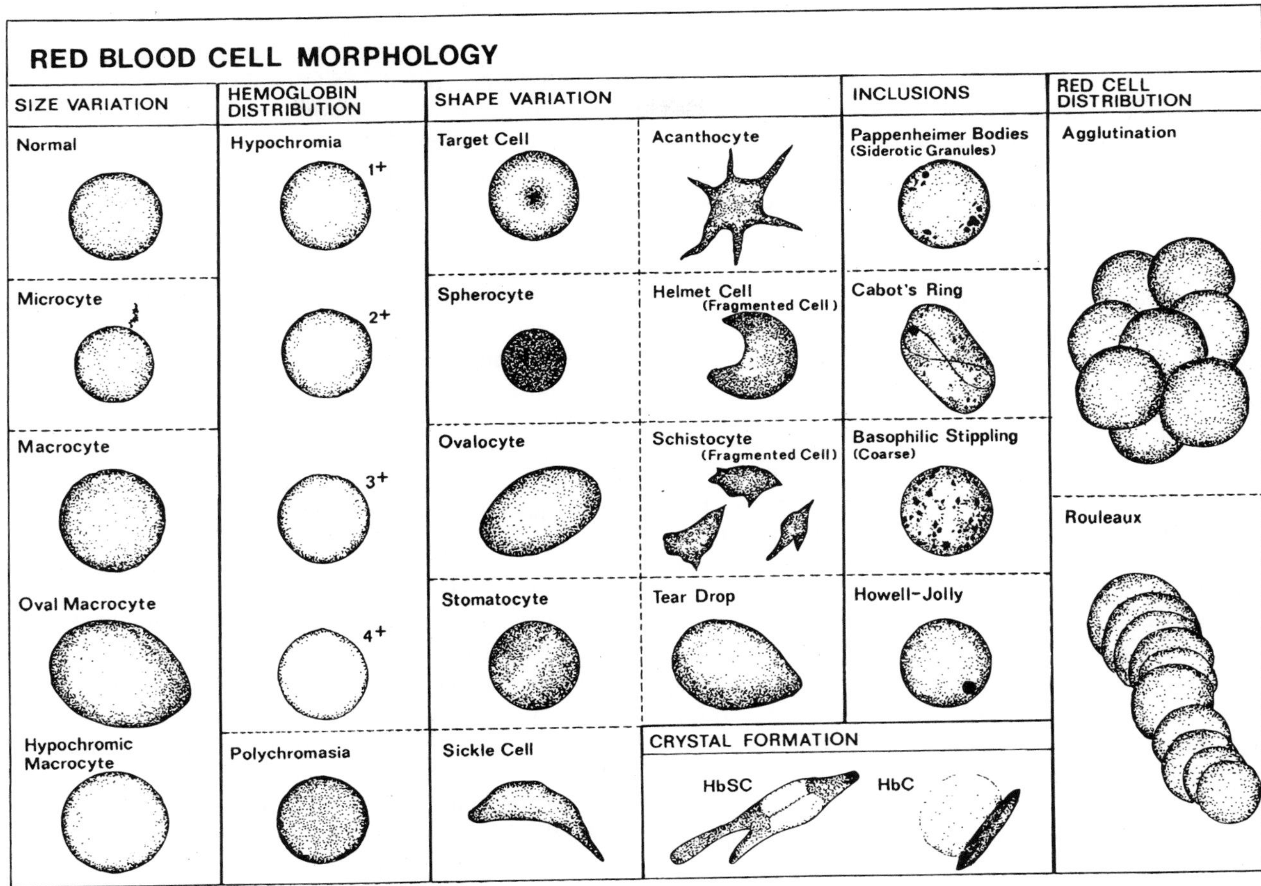

Figure 46–3. Red blood cell morphology. *(Used with permission from Harmening, [Ed.]. [1997]. [p. 82].)*

used to determine whether autoimmune hemolytic anemia is present. A positive direct Coomb's is indicative of autoimmune hemolytic anemia. A complement-only positive Coomb's test is indicative of the presence of a cold-reacting IgM that is not present on erythrocytes at core body temperatures. When the direct Coomb's test is positive for IgG and complement but no C'3d is present, autoimmunity is probably not the cause of the hemolysis. A positive direct Coomb's to IgG alone or with complement is present in warm-mediated autoimmune hemolytic anemia and results in destruction of red cells by the spleen. A positive indirect Coomb's causes difficulties with cross-matching for blood transfusions, but is not useful for diagnostic purposes. If the MCHC is nonartificially elevated, hereditary spherocytosis, the most common inherited abnormality of the erythrocyte membrane, is present.

A sudden drop in the hematocrit, without obvious bleeding, in a patient with underlying hemolytic anemia indicates problems with marrow function. An appropriate response to anemia is an elevated reticulocyte count. If this is low or decreasing, it is important to examine the marrow to determine the cause of marrow failure. Possible causes include advancing chronic renal failure with a relative reduction in erythropoietin production, folate or iron deficiency, acute infections, parvovirus infection of the marrow, or drug suppression of the marrow.

Patients with paroxysmal nocturnal hemoglobinuria (PNH) generally have an elevated reticulocyte count, normal erythrocyte morphology, negative direct Coomb's test, absent haptoglobin, absent bone marrow iron, and excessive iron in the urine. Flow cytometry helps establish the diagnosis.

Pyruvate kinase deficiency and glucose-6-phosphate dehydrogenase (G-6PD) deficiency also cause hemolytic anemia. Pyruvate kinase deficiency causes severe hemolytic anemia and is almost always diagnosed in childhood. G-6PD deficiency is a genetic trait that protects the individual from death if infected with malaria. It is more common in African-American men (present in approximately 10%) but also occurs in the general population. This disorder causes episodic hemolysis. The more severe, but less common Mediterranean form causes chronic hemolysis. Certain medications, such as primaquine and Dapsone, can induce a hemolytic anemia in individuals with this deficiency. G-6PD can be easily identified and measured in the laboratory.

Aplastic Anemia. The CBC in aplastic anemia shows not only anemia, but also leukopenia and thrombocytopenia. The anemia is generally normochromic and normocytic. The reticulocyte count is low, indicative of the lack of marrow response to the anemia. A bone-marrow aspirate and biopsy should be performed if pancytopenia is present. The marrow will be markedly hypocellular and the marrow space will be occupied by fat. All degrees of aplastic anemia can be seen, ranging from mild to severe and imminently life-threatening. Severe aplastic anemia is defined as a granulocyte count less than 500, a platelet count less than 20,000, and a reticulocyte count less than 0.1%.

Management

Management of iron deficiency anemia involves iron supplementation, usually orally. Treatment is imperative if the patient is symptomatic and has underlying cardiac or pulmonary dysfunction as well, the anemia is moderately severe (Hgb less than 8 g/dL), the patient is pregnant, the patient has had a subtotal gastrectomy or gastrojejunostomy, has menorrhagia, or is recovering from megaloblastic anemia. Ferrous sulfate is the best absorbed form of oral supplementation. The optimal dose is 300 mg ferrous sulfate, or 60 mg of elemental iron, three to four times a day. If ferrous gluconate is used, the dose should be 600 mg, or 70 mg elemental iron, three to four times a day. Iron is best absorbed on an empty stomach. Concurrent administration of vitamin C may enhance absorption. The most common side effects are constipation, diarrhea, nausea, and abdominal discomfort. The degree of gastrointestinal upset is related more to the amount of iron than to the preparation. Slow-release preparations, which are used to reduce the side effects, often are poorly absorbed. Parenteral iron is rarely indicated, and is only used if the patient does not respond, is not absorbing the iron, or is intolerant of all oral preparations. Side effects are many and can be life-threatening. The effect of treatment is apparent within in 10 days. However, it may take several weeks for the Hgb to return to normal and several months for iron stores to be restored.

The anemia of chronic disease does not respond to iron or vitamin supplementation. If the hemoglobin falls below 7 gm/dL, packed red blood cell transfusions may be indicated. Supplemental iron is also not useful in patients with β-thalassemia-minor.

Vitamin B_{12} deficiency is treated with parenteral vitamin administration. Initial treatment is with 100 to 1000 (μg IM daily for up to 2 weeks, then twice a week for a month, then once a month, generally for life. Folic acid deficiency is generally treated with oral dosing of 1 to 2 mg per day. Four to 5 weeks of treatment is generally sufficient.

Warm autoimmune hemolytic anemia is acutely treated with steroids. Once the hemolysis has been controlled, treatment of the underlying disorder should begin. Lymphoma, leukemia, and, occasionally, solid tumors are associated with this type of hemolytic anemia. Once control of the underlying disorder is obtained, the steroids are tapered slowly, over 2 to 3 months. Serial hematocrit, reticulocyte count, and direct Coomb's testing is performed to evaluate response. Splenectomy is helpful in some patients. Cold antibody-mediated autoimmune hemolytic anemia is rarely severe enough to be life-threatening.

All possible offending medications and chemical exposures should be removed in the patient with aplastic anemia. Patients with moderate to severe anemia may be treated with androgens. Allogeneic marrow or stem-cell transplantation is the treatment of choice for severe aplastic anemia and a major transplant center should be contacted at diagnosis to provide consultation regarding how to maximize the patient's chance for a successful transplant. Unfortunately, many individuals do not have a properly matched donor. Some of these patients respond to treatment with antithymocyte globulin (ATG), cyclosporine, steroids, and growth factors.

Follow-Up

The patient should be educated on the cause of the anemia, how the treatment works, and management of side effects to ensure compliance. Repeat CBCs should be done at a frequency determined by the degree of anemia and the cause. For example, anemia of chronic disease can be followed according to changes in symptoms; vitamin B_{12} deficiency can be reevaluated within 2 to 4 weeks of starting treatment and then less frequently if a response is established. Anemia that does not respond to treatment or for which a clear cause was not found, should be worked up further, including a marrow aspiration and biopsy.

The most common cause of death from PNH is thrombosis in the mesenteric veins, hepatic veins, and venous sinuses of the brain. Some patients with PNH eventually develop myelodysplastic syndrome that can evolve into acute leukemia, thus should continue to be evaluated periodically. Patients with autoimmune hemolytic anemias may die from either uncontrolled hemolysis, the underlying secondary disorder, or pulmonary emboli.

Patients who have received steroid treatment for warm hemolytic anemia are at risk for infections, hyperglycemia, avascular necrosis of the weight-bearing joints, and all the other complications of steroid therapy, thus should be watched carefully.

Sickle Cell Anemia

Pathophysiology

Sickle cell disease consists of a group of genetic disorders characterized by a predominance of hemoglobin S (HbS) (Charache, et al., 1991). In the United States they are found predominantly in African-Americans and Hispanics from the Caribbean, Central America, and parts of South America.

The type of hemoglobin produced by an individual is determined by the two beta globin genes located on the

11th chromosome and the four alpha globin genes located on the 16th chromosome. Sickle cell anemia is found in those who are homozygous for the sickle beta globin gene (βS). Because the alpha genes are located on a different chromosome, these patients can have two different problems with hemoglobin production: sickle cell anemia as well as alpha globin gene abnormality, the most common being alpha thalassemia. Sickle cell trait is found in those who have a normal beta globin gene and a βS globin gene. The result is normal production of hemoglobin A and S with a predominance of hemoglobin A. The red cells in these individuals only sickle under unusual circumstances such as marked hypoxia.

The two cardinal features of sickle cell disorders are chronic hemolytic anemia and vaso-occlusion resulting in ischemic tissue injury. The hemolytic anemia is caused by abnormal properties of hemoglobin S or by repeated sickling and unsickling, which produces irreversible red cell membrane changes and erythrocyte destruction. The hemolytic anemia begins insidiously, generally during the first 3 months of life, although it can begin as early as at 6 weeks of life.

Sickled red cells tend to clump and thus produce vascular obstruction, leading tissue hypoxia. The organs most commonly affected are those with venous sinuses where blood flow is slow and oxygen tension and pH are low, such as the spleen, kidneys, and bone marrow or those areas with a limited supply of arterial blood such as the eyes and head of the femur. However, other sites can be affected as well. Vaso-occlusive crises can start as early as 6 to 12 months of age. Splenomegaly generally develops by about 6 months of life as the spleen is the major site of hemolysis in early life. The spleen is eventually destroyed by infarctions due to vascular occlusion. Fulminant sepsis with pneumococcus and other encapsulated bacteria is a leading cause of death in children due to this functional asplenia that develops early in life.

History and Physical Findings

The manifestations of sickle cell anemia can be broadly classified into chronic constitutional problems and acute episodes of pain and tissue damage (Jandl, 1996). Chronic hemolytic anemia generally begins insidiously around 3 months of age and is fully manifested by moderate to severe anemia by about 9 months of age. Bacterial infection is the leading cause of death at all ages.

Acute episodes of musculoskeletal pain are the most prevalent symptomatic manifestations of sickle cell anemia and account for most of the hospital admissions (Jandl, 1996; Shapiro & Ballas, 1994). They are caused by occlusions in the microcirculation and most commonly affect the lumbar spine, abdomen, and femurs, but can also occur in any extremity, chest, or head. Although most attacks are unpredictable and a cause is not readily evident, certain events such as acidosis, hypoxia, and dehydration are known to trigger crises. Infection is the most common triggering event in children. The pain of these crises can be excruciating. The frequency and severity varies from individual to individual. Some attacks are mild or moderate in intensity and may only last a few hours, where as others are excruciatingly painful and last 5 to 7 days. The average rate of occurrence is 0.8 episodes per patient-year in patients with sickle cell anemia (Platt et al., 1991). The number of painful episodes per year is a measure of clinical severity and correlates with early death in patients with sickle cell anemia who are over 20 years of age (Platt et al., 1991).

The earliest manifestation of sickle cell anemia is generally the hand–foot syndrome, characterized by dactylitis in which the small bones of the hands and feet are damaged by microinfarctions caused by a marginal blood supply to rapidly growing bones. It is generally first seen between the ages of 3 and 20 months and is manifested by low-grade fever, pain, and swelling of the hands and feet. Radiological changes develop within 1 to 2 weeks and are generally reversible. The hand–foot syndrome does not usually recur but bone or joint crises occur sporadically throughout life in most adults and older children. On physical exam there is tenderness and swelling over the sites of infarction. Fever, local warmth, and erythema are uncommon. Salmonella osteomyelitis should always be in the differential when patients complain of bone and joint pain, particularly if fever, local warmth, and erythema are present. Osteomyelitis usually involves severe multiple lesions in the long bones, and spreads to other bones if not treated with antibiotics. Aseptic necrosis of the femoral heads is common by young adulthood. It is the major cause of crippling in adult patients. Aseptic necrosis of the humeral heads also occurs and causes only mild to moderate pain in most patients, but some require surgery for severe pain.

Abdominal crises are often difficult to distinguish from cholecystitis, hepatic crises, and renal or intestinal colic. The diagnosis of painful crisis is one of exclusion, aided by the history. The patient's usual hemoglobin level does not change or only worsens slightly during a crisis. In sickle crisis, bowel tones are generally present and neutrophils on the blood smear do not appear toxic. Often the patients themselves can help distinguish a sickle crisis from an acute abdomen crisis requiring surgical intervention.

Hepatomegaly occurs early in life but significant hepatic damage occurs gradually and is not manifested until adulthood. A hepatic crisis usually presents with acute right upper quadrant pain, acute painful enlargement of the liver, fever, and moderately severe jaundice that resolves spontaneously in five to ten days. Each episode of hepatic crisis damages the liver. Intrahepatic cholestasis presents with severe right upper quadrant pain, hepatomegaly, and severe enough liver failure to cause hepatic encephalopathy, and shock. The serum bilirubin can climb as high as 100 to 300 mg/dL. This is usually a terminal event.

Cholelithiasis is common. Cholecystitis occurs in about

10 to 15% of patients with gallstones. It can be difficult to distinguish between cholecystitis and abdominal crises. Cholecystectomy is recommended if there is any doubt about the presence of acute cholecystitis.

Renal tubular dysfunction is common with loss of the ability of renal tubules to concentrate or dilute urine. Hematuria is common. Renal failure and the nephrotic syndrome occur from sludging of sickled cells. About 40% of men with sickle cell anemia develop intermittent priapism, caused by nonthrombotic obstruction by sickled cells. The attacks usually resolve spontaneously. Attacks lasting more than 24 hours frequently result in impotence.

Neurovascular complications occur in 6 to 25% of patients with sickle cell anemia. Nearly 9% of children with sickle cell anemia will develop a hemiparetic stroke during the first decade of life (Powars, 1994). Seizures, transient ischemic attacks (TIAs), and strokes occur as a result of vascular occlusion by sickled cells. Those children who have suffered one stroke generally have recurrent strokes, resulting in permanent motor disabilities and IQs less than 70. Neurovascular episodes in older adolescents and adults are generally manifested as intracranial hemorrhage associated with an approximately 50% mortality. Long-term transfusion therapy is 90% effective in preventing recurrent stroke after the initial cerebral vascular accident (Wang et al., 1991). Without transfusion therapy, strokes generally recur within 3 years in over half the patients (Vichinsky, 1994).

Leg ulcers over the malleoli and distal leg are common after the age of 5. They tend to erode and spread as long as the patient remains ambulatory and are very slow to heal. The most serious ocular complications of sickle cell anemia are proliferative and nonproliferative retinopathy that can eventually lead to blindness. The development of glaucoma is often triggered by ocular trauma.

Pulmonary crises present with fever, cough, pleural pain, pulmonary infiltrates, and leukocytosis. They are caused by microvascular occlusion. Bacterial pneumonia is the most common cause of pulmonary crises in children. Infiltrates may involve several lobes and are slow to resolve. Pulmonary artery occlusions and myocardial hemosiderosis along with a high cardiac output state combine to put tremendous stress on the heart. The rib cage is often enlarged in the antero–posterior dimension due to cardiac dilatation, and is called the "hoop-shaped chest." Pulmonary hypertension eventually leads to cor pulmonale in older patients.

Children with sickle cell anemia have growth delays, particularly evident in late childhood and adolescence. They also have developmental delays and slow sexual maturation, which can be a source of great psychological conflict but is amenable to therapeutic intervention.

Chronic hemolytic anemia is a feature of sickle cell anemia. Infections can cause aplastic crises. Folate depletion can cause megaloblastic crises. Splenic sequestration crises present with sudden onset of anemia below baseline levels, a painfully enlarged spleen, and hypovolemic shock; death can occur shortly after.

Laboratory and Diagnostic Tests

The diagnosis of sickle cell disease is based on quantitative hemoglobin electrophoresis. If 80% or more hemoglobin S is found in association with another abnormal hemoglobin, and no hemoglobin A, no further testing is needed. However, if only one abnormal hemoglobin is found, it can be difficult to distinguish between sickle cell anemia and some of the sickle beta thalassemia syndromes. Electrophoresis patterns are similar in sickle cell anemia, the sickle beta thalassemias, and hemoglobin S in association with the hereditary persistence of fetal hemoglobin syndrome. Measurement of HbA_2 and HbF may help in providing a definitive diagnosis. Sickle cell disease should not be made from either a sickle-cell preparation or solubility test. Neither of these tests are reliable in distinguishing sickle cell anemia from sickle cell trait. A history of painful crises, hemolytic anemia, and irreversibly sickled cells on the blood smear also help to secure the diagnosis. Hemoglobin electrophoresis and measurement of the minor hemoglobins A_2 and F in other family members may also assist in making a final diagnosis. Molecular biology can be used for a definitive diagnosis, but it is usually unnecessary to go to this level of testing.

Sickle cell screening at birth has been shown to effectively reduce morbidity and mortality, as the first manifestation of the disease is potentially fatal pneumococcal sepsis or splenic sequestration. Definitive diagnostic testing with hemoglobin electrophoresis should follow a positive screening test.

At the initial exam, the patient should have a complete blood count (CBC), reticulocyte count, and hemoglobin electrophoresis. Urinalysis, liver function tests, BUN, creatinine, electrolytes, and chest x-rays should also be obtained. Other tests that may be useful depending on the symptoms include: arterial blood gases, pulmonary function tests, ECG, imaging studies done to detect the presence of gallstones, and MRI of the femoral heads or humeral heads to determine if the patient has avascular necrosis.

Hemolytic anemia is chronically present in individuals with sickle cell anemia. The white count is generally about twice normal. The white count may rise even higher during a painful crisis episode. It may be difficult to distinguish a painful crisis involving the abdomen from a surgical emergency from the changes in the blood counts.

Hyperkalemic, hyperchloremic metabolic acidosis, results from the loss of concentrating ability of the kidneys. Hematuria is a common problem caused by papillary necrosis.

MRI is superior to CT scanning as a diagnostic tool for suspected intracerebral hemorrhage. Endoscopic retrograde cholangiography is the best method to make the diagnosis of cholecystitis. MRI with T_2 weighted imaging is best for early diagnosis of bone or joint crises as well as in differentiating acute bone infarction from acute osteomyelitis as changes usually do not develop until after the pain of bone or joint crisis resolves.

Management

Initial treatment of sickle cell anemia diagnosed at birth is twice daily oral penicillin as prophylaxis against pneumococcal organisms. The leading cause of death in children with sickle cell anemia is pneumococcal sepsis. Education about the disease for the parents should begin at time of diagnosis and continued throughout all the complications and manifestations of the disease.

Painful crises are the most common, disabling, and demoralizing complications of sickle cell anemia (Shapiro & Ballas, 1994). Codeine preparations are sufficient for mild to moderate pain, but hydromorphone, morphine, or oxycodone is needed to manage the more severe painful episodes. Ketorolac may also be useful for severe, but not intolerable pain. Morphine is the drug of choice for acute painful episodes that last more than 24 hours. As a last resort, anesthesia with fentanyl and other similar anesthetics may be necessary. Acupuncture, transcutaneous stimulation, and hypnosis have also been used for chronic pain. Exchange transfusions are used for anemic crises, late-stage pregnancy, major surgery, and any life-threatening complications of sickle cell anemia. The acute chest syndrome is best managed aggressively with exchange transfusions and antibiotic treatment of pneumonias. Splenic sequestration crisis is managed with immediate blood transfusions to improve blood volume. Splenectomy is recommended for survivors.

Osteomyelitis is treated with antibiotics. Hip arthroplasty can be performed but has a high failure rate by 5 years. Hip replacement is often also unsuccessful. Leg ulcers are best managed by bed rest with the legs elevated and compresses with cleansing oxidants for several days to several weeks. Also used are: debridement; topical antibiotics; absorbent, porous dressings; and collagen matrix wrappings. Skin grafting may be necessary. Transfusions to keep the HbS proportion of cells below 50% have also been found to be beneficial. Bed rest is imperative for healing.

The defect in renal tubule concentrating ability can be reversed with blood transfusions in children, but this is ineffective in adults. Hematuria is often severe enough to require blood transfusions. Protracted hematuria is best managed conservatively. Frank renal failure is managed with dialysis. Renal transplantation is an option, but the outcome is often poor. Persistent priapism is managed with sedation, analgesia, local cooling, transfusion, exchange transfusion, and hydration.

The most effective approach to management of proliferative retinopathy has been laser photocoagulation.

Hydroxyurea has been demonstrated to have a beneficial effect on 75 to 80% of patients by increasing the level of fetal hemoglobin (HbF). The presence of HbF appears to have a sparing effect on sickled erythrocytes; Rodgers (1997) recommends 10 to 25 mg/kg daily as the optimal dose. The use of hydroxyurea has also been shown to have a beneficial effect by reducing episodes of painful crises, acute chest syndrome, and the need for blood transfusions. Long-term follow-up is still necessary to determine the long-term safety of this treatment (Vichinsky & Lubin, 1994). Although treatment with hydroxyurea shows promise, major sickle cell-related complications can occur with HbF levels above 20%.

Research is currently ongoing in the area of genetic engineering with the ultimate goal being to replace the defective gene causing sickle cell anemia. Allogeneic marrow transplantation is also being investigated as a possible treatment for this disease (Walters et al., 1996).

Follow-Up

The leading causes of death in adults with sickle cell anemia are cardiopulmonary disease such as acute chest syndrome or chronic lung disease, chronic renal failure, stroke, and infections. Some patients with sickle cell lead full lives, reaching 60 or 70 years of age. Not only must patients be evaluated on a regular basis for physical changes, but also for the effect that this chronic debilitating disease is having on their quality of life. Adding to the stress is the unpredictable nature of the disease. These factors adversely affect school and work attendance and require appropriate counseling.

Leukemias

Cancer is the second most common cause of death among children and adults. It accounts for approximately 10% of all deaths in the 1 to 14 age group and 23% of all deaths in adults. Leukemia is the most common childhood malignancy (Parker, Tong, Bolden, & Wingo, 1997).

The primary problem in leukemia is the neoplastic, uncontrolled clonal proliferation of one type of hematopoietic cell (e.g., lymphocyte, granulocyte, monocyte, or erythrocyte) or a precursor of one of these cells. This uncontrolled proliferation can occur at any point during the maturation of the hematopoietic cell. For example, in acute lymphoblastic leukemia, an immature lymphoblast escapes the normal constraints of cell division and maturation and begins to clone multiple copies of itself at an immature stage. Normally, the cell would divide and mature in a predictable fashion. As a result of the massive proliferation of these cells in the marrow, other cell lines—such as erythrocytes, thrombocytes, and neutrophils—do not develop, resulting in anemia, neutropenia, and thrombocytopenia. In addition, the leukemic cells do not function normally, resulting in an immune-compromised state. Leukemic cells can infiltrate the bone marrow, the blood, and various other body tissues, such as tonsils, lymph nodes, spleen, kidneys, gingivae, skin, testes, and the central nervous system (CNS).

Leukemias are generally classified into four types: acute or chronic and lymphoid or myeloid in origin. The terms "acute" and "chronic" refer to the rapidity of onset and progression of the disease as well as the maturity of the cell line involved. Acute leukemias involve undifferentiated or immature cells and are rapid in onset and progression. Untreated, a patient with acute leukemia may have a life expectancy of only days to months. However, acute leukemias are responsive to conventional chemotherapy and patients can have long-term disease-free survival with treatment. Conversely, the chronic leukemias have a gradual onset and prolonged clinical course. Life expectancy may be greater than 10 years in some cases. Although the chronic leukemias can be easily controlled with conventional chemotherapy, cure is rare and conventional chemotherapy typically does not change life expectancy. Leukemias are also classified according to the cellular origin of the proliferating cells (i.e., lymphoid or myeloid). Thus, leukemias are classified into four major types:

- Acute lymphoblastic leukemia (ALL)
- Acute myelogenous leukemia (AML)
- Chronic myelogenous leukemia (CML)
- Chronic lymphocytic leukemia (CLL)

Acute Lymphoblastic Leukemia

Acute leukemia is the most common childhood malignancy. Approximately 2000 cases are reported in the United States annually. Seventy-five percent of these cases are acute lymphoblastic leukemia (ALL). The peak incidence of ALL is from 2 to 6 years of age. It is more common in boys than girls.

Thirty years ago the disease was uniformly fatal; now more than 50% of children who present with ALL are alive 5 years after the initial diagnosis. Recent advances in molecular, cytogenetic, and immunologic areas have demonstrated the heterogeneity of the disease. This has led to changes in the way leukemias are identified and treated.

History and Physical Findings. The clinical presentation of ALL is often sudden. Symptoms are generally present for a only a few weeks prior to diagnosis. The signs and symptoms reflect infiltration of the bone marrow with leukemic lymphoblasts as well as *extramedullary* (outside the bone marrow) spread of the disease. Reduction in the number of normal hematopoietic precursors produces the typical symptoms of fever, pallor, petechiae, and bruising.

Neutropenia results in fever, night sweats, and infections. Thrombocytopenia results in petechiae, purpura, retinal hemorrhages, and bleeding. Anemia results in fatigue, malaise, pallor, anorexia, and weight loss. In older adults, anemia can present as dyspnea, angina, and dizziness. As a result of neutropenia and anemia, infection and hemorrhage are present in one third of patients at diagnosis.

Leukemic cells can invade other organs or sites besides the bone marrow. This is termed extramedullary disease and can result in lymphadenopathy, splenomegaly, and hepatomegaly. Extramedullary disease is more common in ALL than in acute myelogenous leukemia (AML). Infiltration of the periosteum and bone is common. The resulting bone pain and arthralgias are more common in children than in adults. A thymic mass can be found on a chest x-ray in 15% of adults with ALL.

CNS disease is rare at diagnosis, occurring in only 5-10% of adults at diagnosis and 3% of children, but it is a common site of relapse. Patients with CNS involvement generally present with headache and papilledema from increased intracranial pressure without focal neurologic signs. Leukemic infiltration or hemorrhages can be seen on the fundoscopic exam.

The work-up includes a physical exam to determine the degree of extramedullary spread and rule out infections. The patient should be examined for the presence or absence of lymphadenopathy, hepatomegaly, splenomegaly, or painless testicular swelling indicating possible extramedullary disease. Potential sites of infection such as the lungs, oropharynx, and perianal area should be examined. The patient should also be examined for signs of hemorrhage, and a full neurologic exam including the optic fundi should be performed.

Laboratory and Diagnostic Tests. ALL is diagnosed through the examination of the blood and marrow. A complete blood count (CBC) including differential; bone marrow aspirate with biopsy; blood chemistries including renal and hepatic function, uric acid, and electrolytes; coagulation studies; and a chest x-ray should be performed in a patient who is suspected of having leukemia. Typically patients have anemia, thrombocytopenia, neutropenia, and leukocytosis. About one-third of patients have a hemoglobin of less than 8 g/dL at diagnosis (Hoelzer, 1996). More than half of patients have platelet counts less than 50,000/uL at diagnosis. Neutropenia is variable at diagnosis. Only 20% of patients have granulocyte counts less than 500/uL. Twenty-seven percent of patients have a low WBC (less than 5,000/uL), and approximately 50% of patients have a normal or high WBC (> 10,000/uL). A small number of patients, 16%, have a marked leukocytosis (> 100,000/uL) at diagnosis.

A bone marrow aspiration (BMA) and biopsy must be performed to diagnose most types of leukemia, especially the acute leukemias. In ALL, more than 25% of cells on BMA must be lymphoblasts. The leukemic cells are evaluated for morphology, with special cytochemical stains, immunophenotyping, biochemical studies, cytogenetic analysis, and molecular analysis. These tests are done to determine whether the patient has acute lymphoblastic or acute myelogenous leukemia and to subclassify each case of ALL. An accurate diagnosis is crucial because it will determine the choice of chemotherapy agents. If a patient with ALL is treated with agents for AML, the disease will not respond but the patient can still suffer serious side effects from the treatment, further delaying appropriate treatment. The differential also includes chronic myelogenous leukemia in blast crisis, the leukemic phase of non-Hodgkin's lymphoma, and viral infections.

Possible laboratory findings include hyperuricemia, which can lead to uric acid nephropathy and renal failure. Calcium, potassium, phosphate, and clotting studies may be abnormal as well. LDH is generally markedly elevated in ALL.

A chest x-ray is performed to determine whether or not there is any mediastinal involvement. A lumbar puncture (LP) is performed to rule out CNS disease. Generally, patients receive intrathecal methotrexate starting with the first LP.

Morphologic Classification. The FAB (French–American–British Cooperative Group) classification is the standard classification for ALL. It is based on the morphologic appearance of the leukemic cell. ALL is classified into three categories:

- **L1:** Eighty to 85% of all pediatric cases and approximately 30% of adult cases of ALL are of the L1 type. This subtype is associated with the best prognosis in children.
- **L2:** The most common adult ALL. Only 15% of childhood cases are L2.
- **L3:** The least common ALL. The cells are morphologically identical to those of Burkitt's lymphoma, generally a B-cell ALL. L3 carries the worst prognosis.

Cytochemistry. Cytochemical evaluations are performed to further clarify the question of whether the patient has acute lymphoblastic or acute myelogenous leukemia, and thus to guide treatment. The *sudan black reaction* and *myeloperoxidase* stains must be negative in ALL. The *periodic acid–Schiff reaction* will reveal clumpy positivity (except in L3) but many AML cells will also be positive. *Chloroacetate esterase* is negative in ALL. Blast cells of > 90% of patients with ALL contain the enzyme *terminal deoxynucleotidyl transferase (TdT).* This is not present in mature normal lymphocytes. It is also rarely present in AML and thus helps to further differentiate ALL from AML. T3 leukemias often stain positively with oil red O.

Immunobiology. Immunobiology is the study of the antigens that are expressed on the cell surface. These tests are performed to subclassify the leukemic clone and thus help to guide treatment. They also provide information for determining prognosis. Eighty percent of ALL arises from B cells. Most of these cells express the common ALL antigen or CALLA (the CD10 antigen) as well as other B-cell antigens (CD19 and CD20).

Infants with ALL have a uniformly poor prognosis. They have lymphoblasts that arise from a relatively less differentiated B-cell precursor.

Fifteen to 20% of ALL cases arise from the T-cell lineage. They express antigens such as CD5 and CD7. The subclassification of T-cell ALL into early, intermediate, or mature thymocyte types is based on the expression of various T-cell differentiation antigens.

A very small percentage of ALL cases lack either B-cell or T-cell features and are termed null-cell ALL. Sometimes antigens normally found on myeloid cells can be expressed by either T- or B-cell lymphoblasts. These are termed myeloid antigen positive ALL and are a type of hybrid leukemias. There are two different types of hybrid leukemias:

- Biphenotypic leukemia consists of clones of a single neoplastic cell that coexpresses both myeloid and lymphoid features.
- Bilineage leukemia consists of two distinct subpopulations of leukemia cells. Each cell expresses either myeloid or lymphoid features.

AML with lymphocyte surface markers has a better prognosis with higher rates of complete remission (CR), a longer time to treatment failure, and better overall survival. However, AML with positive TdT markers (ALL markers) have lower CR rates, less durable remissions, and worse survival rates. Studies of myeloid–antigen positive ALL are inconsistent. Some studies show that this disease carries a poor prognosis with lower CR rates, but other studies are not in agreement.

Cytogenetics. Cytogenetics is the study of the chromosomes inside the cell. Chromosomal abnormalities are a common finding in leukemias. These abnormalities serve as markers for the disease. Recent data shows that some cytogenetic changes may actually be leukemogenic. They also provide the most clinically useful approach to subclassifying the acute leukemias. Thus, cytogenetic studies provide a more accurate determination of prognosis and can help to guide treatment. The best results are obtained from marrow aspirations. In addition to standard cytogenetic studies, fluorescenct *in situ* hybridization (FISH) is a newer technique that can demonstrate abnormalities when cytogenetic results are normal (Sandberg & Chen, 1996).

Numerical chromosomal changes (*aneuploidy*) occur more frequently in ALL than in AML. The most common chromosome number within the cell is called the *modal number.* Leukemic cells are termed *hypodiploid* when the mode is less than 46 chromosomes and *hyperdiploid* when the mode is greater than 46 chromosomes. Patients with high hyperdiploid leukemic cells (>50 chromosomes) have a longer median survival. *Pseudodiploidy* is the state of having 46 chromosomes but with an abnormal karyotype or arrangement of the chromosomes. Hypodiploidy and pseudodiploidy are associated with poor prognosis (Sandberg & Chen, 1996).

The Philadelphia chromosome is a balanced translocation of chromosomes 9 and 22, generally written as t(9;22). Six percent of children and 17% of adults with ALL are Philadelphia chromosome positive (Ph+). These patients generally have the L2 morphology, respond well to induction chemotherapy but have short CRs, and little chance of cure with conventional chemotherapy (Sandberg & Chen, 1996).

Another common cytogenetic abnormality in ALL is the translocation of material between chromosomes 4 and 11, occurring in 5% of ALL patients. Most cases tend to be L1 or L2. Patients with this cytogenetic abnormality are generally young females, often have splenomegaly, CNS disease at diagnosis, and a high WBC (>40,000) at diagnosis. The prognosis is poor.

The t(8;14) translocation is also seen in ALL. It occurs in L3 type ALL but was first identified in patients with Burkitt's lymphoma. In fact L3 ALL and Burkitt's may well be different manifestations of the same disease. This group of patients has a high incidence of CNS disease at diagnosis and has a poor prognosis (Sandberg & Chen, 1996).

Prognostic Indicators. Most centers rank patients according to prognostic indicators. Those with poor-risk disease are treated with more aggressive, intensive treatments. Thus, the ability to accurately determine the prognosis allows the practitioner to target treatment with more accuracy.

Poor prognostic indicators include a high white blood cell (WBC) count at diagnosis (> 50,000 in children; > 30,000 in adults), mediastinal mass, age > 40, those who are very young (< 2 years of age, especially < 1 year of age) and those > 10 years of age, the presence of the Philadelphia chromosome t(9;22), other cytogenetic abnormalities such as t(4;11), t(8;14), L3 morphology, null, T-cell, or B-cell phenotype, expression of myeloid surface antigens (mixed lineage), CNS disease, and a prolonged induction phase (> 28 days) prior to achieving a complete remission (Borson & Loeb, 1994; Hoelzer, 1996). Hyperdiploidy or the specific cytogenetic abnormality of combined trisomy 4 and 10 are good prognostic indicators.

Management. The goals of treatment for ALL are to control bone marrow and systemic disease, prevent relapse, and restore normal hematopoiesis. The four major phases are induction, CNS prevention, consolidation, and maintenance therapy. The goal of induction therapy is to reduce the leukemic burden below the level of detection, which is approximately less than 10^8 or 10^9 malignant cells. It is generally assumed that there are a substantial number of leukemic cells that persist undetected, leading to relapse within weeks or months if no further therapy is given. This is the rationale for the use of postremission therapies.

Induction Therapy. Allopurinol 150 to 600 mg orally should be started on all patients 12 to 48 hours prior to starting antileukemic therapy and continued for 2 to 3 days to prevent uric acid nephropathy. Dose is based on size and tumor bulk. The goal of induction chemotherapy is to induce a complete remission (CR). Children with ALL can achieve a CR approximately 90% of the time with a combination of vincristine, prednisone, and L-asparaginase. Daunorubicin is often added for patients with a poor prognosis to improve long-term survival (McKenna & Baehner, 1996). For higher risk groups, cyclophosphamide is sometimes used as a fifth drug.

Vincristine and prednisone with the addition of various other chemotherapy agents are used for adult ALL. The agents commonly added to the vincristine–prednisone combination are Adriamycin, cyclophosphamide, daunorubicin, L-asparaginase, cytosine arabinoside, mercaptopurine, and methotrexate. The median CR rate in several large studies using combinations of the above agents ranges from 64 to 85%. Over 33% of these become long-term disease-free survivors with a range of 3 to 18 years (Hoelzer, 1996). Mortality during induction chemotherapy varies from 3% in children to 20% in those over 60 years of age.

CNS Prophylaxis. CNS disease is uncommon at diagnosis but common as a site for relapse. Without prophylaxis, 30 to 50% of adults and 59 to 67% of children will develop CNS disease. It is easier to prevent CNS disease than it is to treat it. Once CNS relapse has occurred, it is likely to occur again despite treatment. In patients with good prognostic indicators intrathecal MTX (IT–MTX) alone or IT–MTX with Ara-C and hydrocortisone (triple therapy) are used to prevent CNS relapse. IT–MTX can be administered via lumbar puncture or through an implanted Ommaya reservoir. In patients with a poor prognosis, craniospinal or cranial radiation plus IT–MTX are used. Small children with immature nervous systems have a higher incidence of CNS toxicity with craniospinal radiation.

Consolidation. Consolidation (or intensification) is used in virtually all postremission regimens and consists of high-dose chemotherapy shortly after achievement of a CR with agents that are unlikely to be cross-resistant with the initial induction regimen. A few regimens use the same agents that were used for induction. Consolidation has been shown to increase the length of disease-free survival (DFS) in adults and in high-risk children. It is not clear that consolidation improves outcomes in low-risk children.

Maintenance Therapy. Maintenance therapy for ALL consists of lower dose chemotherapy agents. The standard regimen for children is daily oral mercaptopurine, weekly or twice-weekly MTX, and monthly pulses of vincristine and prednisone (McKenna & Baehner, 1996). It is generally continued for 2.5 to 3 years. Some studies are showing that in a subset of children with good-risk ALL, even a shorter period of maintenance therapy may be sufficient. In adults, maintenance therapy consists of a similar regimen for 2 years. Other agents such as daunorubicin, Adriamycin, cytosine arabinoside, actinomycin D, and teniposide have been added to determine if long-term DFS can be improved. What is clear from these studies is that the omission of maintenance therapy in adults reduces DFS duration. Maintenance therapy is generally well tolerated.

Follow-up

Relapse. More than half of adult patients relapse, most within 2 years of achieving a CR. Most relapse in the bone marrow (BM). Patients with isolated *extramedullary* relapse have a high risk for BM relapse and should be treated with systemic therapy as well as local treatment. High dose Ara-C in combination with L-aspara-ginase, m-amsacrine, idarubicin, or mitoxantrone produces remissions in an average 50 to 60% of adult patients with relapsed or refractory ALL (Hoelzer, 1996). Most of these patients eventually relapse again with a 5-year survival rate of only 5%. The best results in adults who have relapsed is a bone marrow transplant (BMT) while in second remission, with a 26% leukemia-free survival (LFS) at 3 years. Adults who have poor-risk ALL (e.g., Ph+) have only a 10-25% LFS at 5 years with conventional chemotherapy. Thus, they may benefit from a BMT in first remission where survival averages 46% at 3 years.

Approximately 20% of children relapse following the cessation of therapy. The first year carries the highest risk for relapse. The long-term LFS rate in those children who are retreated is 30% (McKenna & Baehner, 1996). Children who relapse within one year of discontinuing maintenance therapy or while on maintenance therapy have a poor prognosis and benefit from a BMT in second remission. Those who relapse more than a year after discontinuation of maintenance chemotherapy have a chance for cure if treated aggressively with conventional chemotherapy.

The testes are a major site of extramedullary relapse in males. Bilateral wedge biopsies are performed to confirm the relapse. If the biopsy is positive, the patient should receive a minimum of 2400 cGy to both testes as well as intensified systemic therapy.

CNS relapse occurs in approximately 5 to 10% of children with ALL. Therapy depends on the type of CNS prophylaxis they already received. Those who only received IT therapy should be put into remission with IT therapy. Craniospinal radiation is then used to increase the duration of remission. In those patients who have already received cranial radiation, IT therapy or intraventricular therapy alone and intraventricular therapy with low-dose craniospinal radiation has been used.

Marrow Transplantation. There are three types of donors for marrow transplantation. Allogeneic donors are HLA (human leukocyte antigen) compatible. They can be relatives or unrelated donors. Unrelated donors are matched with patients through various marrow registries. Autologous transplantation involves the use of a patient's own stem cells collected and frozen prior to high-dose chemotherapy with or without radiation. The use of an identical twin as the marrow or stem cell donor is termed syngeneic. One major toxicity of allogeneic transplants is graft versus host disease (GVHD). GVHD is the reaction of the newly transplanted immune system to its new host, the patient. In its acute form it is mainly manifested in the skin, gastrointestinal (GI) tract, and the liver. In the skin, it can vary from a mild skin rash to desquamation of the skin. In the GI tract it can manifest as nausea, vomiting, and mild to severe diarrhea. In the liver, GVHD manifests as mild to severe liver dysfunction. A patient can develop one-, two-, or three-system GVHD. GVHD is rare in syngeneic transplants and should not, by definition, occur in autologous transplants. There is, however, a reaction similar to GVHD seen in autologous transplants. It is termed auto-GVHD and tends to be less severe and present somewhat differently with more involvement of the GI tract and skin and less liver involvement.

Late Toxicities. Cranial radiation can have a significant effect on IQ scores and neuropsychological function, especially in children under 6 years of age at diagnosis (McKenna & Baehner, 1996). In this study, the most significant deficits were in the areas of verbal learning and verbal memory. Intrathecal therapy alone does not cause impairment in test scores. In addition, children who receive craniospinal radiation have significant reductions in growth. If treated promptly, these children respond to growth hormone replacement.

The use of anthracyclines, such as daunomycin, to improve LFS can cause cardiac dysfunction if used in large doses. Alkylating agents, such as cyclophosphamide, are associated with sterility and secondary malignancies. Epipodophyllotoxins, such as etoposide and tenoposide, are also associated with secondary malignancies.

Acute Myelogenous Leukemia

Acute myelogenous leukemia (AML) represents approximately 15 to 20% of the acute leukemia cases in childhood and approximately 80% of acute leukemia in adults.

Pathophysiology. The leukemic clone in AML can develop at any point during the maturation of the myeloid stem cell, early progenitor cell (CFU–GEMM) or in one of the immature precursors (erythroblast, myeloblast, monoblast, or megakaryoblast).

History and Physical Findings. The median age at diagnosis of AML is approximately 60 years of age. As with ALL, antecedent symptoms are brief in duration. The most common presenting symptoms are pallor, fatigue, bleeding, or fever. One third of patients will present with bruising or hemorrhage. One quarter will present with a serious infection. Gingival hypertrophy or *leukemia cutis* (infiltration of the leukemia into the skin) occurs in approximately half of patients with monocytic leukemia. Splenomegaly and hepatomegaly are not common in adults and occur in less than 25%, but occur in approximately half of children. Lymphadenopathy, bone pain, and arthralgias are less common with AML (20%) than with ALL (Weinstein, 1996). Respiratory distress can be present at diagnosis but is generally due to infection. AML is not always limited to the marrow or peripheral blood, as other organ systems may develop leukemic infiltrates. Rarely, a patient will develop a mass of leukemic cells, called a granulocytic sarcoma or chloroma in the skin, sternum, ribs, orbit, or spinal cord as well as other tissues.

Laboratory and Diagnostic Tests. The diagnosis of AML is based on a careful history and physical exam in conjunction with peripheral blood and bone marrow examinations. The diagnosis of AML is established when 30% or more of all nucleated marrow cells are blasts. The aspiration is stained and a battery of histochemical reactions are applied to facilitate the diagnosis of AML versus ALL and the FAB subclassification. The aspirate is also sent for immunophenotyping and cytogenetic studies.

Peripheral blood studies must include a CBC with the differential. The total WBC is elevated in one third of patients, but very high WBCs, greater than 100,000/μl, are uncommon, occurring in less than 10% of adults and 20% of children. *Leukostasis* is the intravascular clumping of blasts leading to hemorrhage and infection. It is uncommon but does occur more frequently in AML than in ALL. It generally does not occur with white counts less than 100,000/μl. The presenting signs and symptoms of leukostasis are somnolence, seizures, stroke, or severe dyspnea, tachypnea and hypoxemia. "Cotton wool" spots due to retinal ischemia can sometimes be seen on funduscopic exam in patients with a very high white count. Peripheral blasts are present in 85 to 90% of patients. The ANC is almost always depressed, < 1500 in half of the patients at diagnosis. If a fever is present, it is important to conduct a thorough search for a focus of infection. Common sites of infection include: mouth, sinusitis, otitis, pharyngitis, pneumonia, peri-rectal abscess, and hemorrhoids. A baseline chest x-ray should be obtained, regardless of symptomatology.

Moderate anemia is common and is typically normocytic. If severe, anemia can cause cardiac dysfunction, such as murmurs, CHF, and dysrhythmias. The platelet count is typically less than 100,000/μl and often less than 20,000/μl. Thrombocytopenia can cause petechiae as well as internal bleeding and should be evaluated during the physical exam.

Other peripheral blood studies such as the LDH, electrolytes, uric acid, creatinine, BUN, and lysozyme should be performed as well. The uric acid is often mildly to moderately elevated. LDH may be elevated, but not so often as in ALL. Coagulation studies including plasma fibrinogen should also be done if the patient has any signs of bleeding or if there is suspicion that the patient has the M3 subtype (acute promyelocytic leukemia).

HLA typing of patients less than 65 years of age and family members is often performed at diagnosis so that this information is available if a marrow transplant is considered in the future or if the patient needs HLA-matched platelets.

CNS involvement and cranial neuropathies are rare at diagnosis. It is more common in children, with a 5 to 20% incidence overall and a higher incidence in those with the M4 or M5 subtypes. In adults, the cerebrospinal fluid is examined in symptomatic patients and those with the M4Eo subtype. The risk of bleeding is reduced but not eliminated if the platelet count is over 50,000/μl when the lumbar puncture is performed.

Classification and Staging

MORPHOLOGIC CLASSIFICATION. AML is a heterogeneous disease. It is subclassified by morphologic appearance in 8 subtypes according to the French–American–British (FAB) classification (Table 46–2). Morphology and cytochemistry are often sufficient to differentiate AML from ALL. In those rare cases where the diagnosis is difficult, immunohistochemistry—which is the use of monoclonal antibodies that recognize B-cell antigens (ALL), T-cell antigens (ALL) or myeloid antigens (AML)—is usually sufficient to accurately diagnose these cases.

CYTOCHEMICAL EVALUATIONS. Myeloid cells stain sudan black positive and myeloperoxidase positive.

CYTOGENETICS. Clonal chromosomal abnormalities can be detected in most cases of AML. Cytogenetic analyses should be performed on every newly diagnosed patient prior to the initiation of therapy because the cytogenetic abnormality serves as a marker for the disease and because certain cytogenetic abnormalities are prognostic indicators and can thus help guide treatment. Translocation of t(8;21) is associated with the M2 subtype. Translocation of t(15;17) is pathognomonic of the M3 subtype or acute promyelocytic leukemia (APL). Inversion (16) or t(16;16) is associated with M4Eo (acute myelomonocytic leukemia with abnormal eosinophils). Rearrangements of 11q (long arm of chromosome 11), generally t(9;11) are associated with M5. Rearrangements of 3q are associated with M2, M4, or M6 subtypes.

TABLE 46–2. French–American–British (FAB) Sub-Classification of AML

M0	AML lacking myeloid differentiation. Sometimes resembles lymphoblasts of L2 (ALL) subtype. Requires immunohistochemical staining for diagnosis.
M1	Acute myeloblastic leukemia without maturation; large poorly differentiated myeloblasts.
M2	Acute myeloblastic leukemia with maturation. Auer rods are often visible.
M3	Acute promyelocytic leukemia; associated with DIC.
M4	Acute myelomonocytic leukemia.
M5	Acute monocytic leukemia.
M6	Erythroleukemia.
M7	Megakaryoblastic leukemia.

Prognostic Indicators. Good prognostic indicators include age (children between the ages of 3 and 10), and the chromosomal abnormalities t(8;21) and inv(16). The M2 subtype with the translocation of t(8;21) is associated with the most favorable prognosis in adults. These patients have high rates of CR (85-100%) and many are cured with conventional chemotherapy. The M3 subtype or acute promyelocytic leukemia (APL) and the translocation of t(15;17) is also associated a good prognosis. M4Eo (acute myelomonocytic leukemia with abnormal eosinophils) and inversion (16) or t(16;16) is also associated with a high rate of CR and good outcomes.

Poor prognostic indicators include age (children less than 1 year of age), a high WBC at diagnosis (greater than 20,000/μl and particularly over 100,000/μl), deletions of chromosomes 5 and 7, trisomy 8, antecedent hematologic disorders, particularly myelodysplastic syndrome (MDS), myeloproliferative disease, or leukemia following chemotherapy or radiation for other malignant or nonmalignant diseases. M5 and rearrangements of 11q (long arm of chromosome 11), generally t(9;11), is usually a disease of children or young adults who have skin or gum infiltration with leukemia cells and short remissions. AML with abnormal thrombopoiesis and rearrangements of 3q generally results in an increased platelet count (over 1,000,000/μl) and a poor prognosis. Most cases are M2, M4, or M6 subtypes. AML with bone marrow basophilia and the translocation t(6;9) is generally a disease of young adults and carries a poor prognosis.

Management. Chemotherapy for AML is generally divided into two stages: induction chemotherapy followed by consolidation therapy. Allogeneic or autologous marrow transplantation may follow in patients younger than 65. Refer to the treatment of ALL for a discussion of the rationale for the different stages of treatment. Allopurinol 150 to 600 mg orally should be started on all patients 12 to 48 hours prior to starting antileukemic therapy and continued for 2 to 3 days to prevent uric acid nephropathy. Dose is based on size and tumor bulk.

Induction. The basic induction regimen for AML has not changed significantly for the past 15 to 20 years. The most important factor in determining survival is the attainment of a CR. This may seem obvious, but it is mentioned because AML remissions are harder to attain and require more intensive regimens than in ALL. The standard agents used in AML induction regimens are daunorubicin (DNR) (45-60 mg/m^2/day for 3 days) and cytarabine (ara-C) (100-200 mg/m^2 for 7 days). This combination results in a CR for 40-85% of adults less than 60 years of age, and a lower CR rate for those older than 60. Idarubicin (12 mg/m^2/day) plus ara-C appears to be effective as well. This combination induced a higher CR rate and longer CR duration than ara-C and DNR, especially in younger adults or those with an initial WBC greater than 50,000/μl.

Nearly all patients treated with these regimens will experience total alopecia and profound bone marrow hypoplasia. Most will develop moderately severe nausea and vomiting, mild to moderate stomatitis, esophagitis, and diarrhea; about half will develop hepatic toxicity.

Other agents have been added or substituted in an effort to increase remissions and improve survival. However, these changes have not added significantly to the long-term survival with AML mainly because as the aggressiveness of the regimen increases, so do toxicities that may preclude further therapy. For example, substituting doxorubicin for daunorubicin results in greater gastrointestinal toxicity. Substituting mitoxantrone for daunorubicin does not change outcome. Using high-dose cytarabine alone (1-3 gm/m^2 every 12 hours for 6 days) has not improved CR rates except in a small subset of patients who have CD34 positive cells. However, neurologic toxicity in the form of cerebellar dysfunction is increased with this regimen. Older adults have a greater than 30% risk of dying from regimen-related toxicities (RRT) than younger patients, whereas young adults die of refractory disease more often than older patients.

Many patients do not achieve a CR with the initial induction attempt. A repeat bone marrow aspiration 1 to 2 weeks following treatment can help determine effect of treatment and may identify those patients who might benefit from immediate reinduction.

Post-remission Therapy. Intensive, early consolidation treatment in AML appears to improve survival compared with either maintenance or late intensification therapies. High-dose ara-C (3 g/m^2 BID) appears more effective than standard-dose ara-C for maintaining longer remissions. Also, receiving more than one course of high-dose consolidation may result in longer remission duration. The addition of potentially noncross-resistant drugs to high-dose ara-C—such as amsacrine, etoposide, cyclophosphamide, or mitoxantrone with diaziquone—have yielded encouraging early results.

Allogeneic bone marrow transplantation (BMT) is often considered during first remission for high-risk patients. BMT offers a lower relapse rate but this is offset by a higher mortality rate due to regimen-related toxicity. The disease-free survival following allogeneic BMT in first CR ranges from 40 to 60% in adults and 48 to 66% at 5 years in children (Weinstein, 1996). Allogeneic BMT is the only regimen likely to cure a patient with refractory AML or one who relapses within 6 months of achieving a CR.

Autologous BMT offers a much lower treatment-related mortality (no GVHD, no immunosuppressive drugs) but relapse is greater. The increased relapse rate is thought to be due to the lack of the graft-versus-leukemia (GVL) effect or possible contamination of stored marrow with undetected leukemia cells.

The inability to receive postremission therapy because

of toxicities leads to early relapse. Examples of toxicities that could prevent timely administration of postremission therapies include bacterial or fungal infections that occur following treatment with induction therapy, poor performance status, poor nutritional status, or hepatitis.

CNS Prophylaxis. There is a lower frequency of CNS disease in AML than in ALL. The frequency of CNS disease in children who do not receive CNS prophylaxis is 20% (Weinstein, 1996). In adults, the frequency of CNS disease is 1 to 5%. Children with the M4 and M5 subtypes and adults with the M4Eo subtype are at the highest risk of CNS relapse. Every child with AML should undergo an LP to determine if CNS disease is present. There is controversy, however, as to when this LP should be performed. There is concern that the LP could introduce blasts into the CNS, thus establishing CNS disease. Often the initial diagnostic LP is performed after blasts have been cleared from the peripheral blood. Intrathecal therapy with methotrexate or cytosine arabinoside (ara-C) is effective in clearing the CNS. In adults, the cerebrospinal fluid (CSF) is examined in symptomatic patients and those with the M4Eo subtype. The risk of bleeding is reduced but not eliminated if the platelet count is over 50,000/μl when the lumbar puncture is performed.

Common Disease-Related Complications. It is important to be aware that the two major causes of mortality during induction are infections and hemorrhage. Some of the more common complications of treatment other than pancytopenia and those described above include typhlitis, renal failure, and granulocytic sarcomas (chloromas) (Cheson, 1995). Typhlitis or neutropenic enterocolitis presents as severe abdominal pain in the neutropenic patient. The pain can also be accompanied by bloody diarrhea, absent bowel sounds, rebound tenderness, and fever. Radiographs of the abdomen may show a soft tissue mass in the right lower quadrant, a dilated colon, or pericecal edema. A barium enema may show a mass in the cecum. The etiology is unclear but is likely due to *Clostridium septicum.* Stool cultures should be performed and, if positive, treated appropriately.

Renal failure occurs secondary to uric acid nephropathy, nephrotoxic drugs, sepsis, and renal infiltration by leukemic cells. Granulocytic sarcomas are composed of granulocytic precursors. They tend to occur near neural structures, in bone and periosteum, as well as in soft tissue, lymph nodes, skin, breasts, ovaries, and the gastrointestinal tract. The appearance of these tumors may antedate overt AML by months to years. They generally respond to radiation and to chemotherapy.

Patients with acute promyelocytic leukemia (APL) have a high rate of CR, and many are cured of their disease. However, virtually all patients with APL have clinical or subclinical disseminated intravascular coagulation (DIC) at diagnosis. Chemotherapy often exacerbates this problem, but the underlying disease must be controlled in order to control the DIC. The bleeding associated with DIC is treated with fresh frozen plasma to replete clotting factors, fibrinogen if the fibrinogen is low, and platelets if the patient has thrombocytopenia. Heparin is used if there is evidence that small vessels are clotting, but is only used after treatment with chemotherapy is underway. The APL cell can be induced to differentiate into mature granulocytes with all-trans-retinoic acid (ATRA), a naturally occurring metabolite of vitamin A (Wiernik, Gallagher & Tallman, 1996). Many patients can achieve a complete remission with ATRA. Since these remissions are short, ATRA treatment is generally followed by standard induction chemotherapy. This, then, is often followed by two consolidation courses of an anthracycline-based regimen.

Patients with acute monocytic (M5) leukemia frequently have involvement of the gums, skin, and central nervous system.

Follow-Up. Follow-up and evaluation of patients who have had treatment for AML include monitoring for signs of relapse and the management of toxicities due to the chemotherapy regimen. It includes periodic CBCs to monitor for possible relapse and awareness of the complications listed below.

Relapse. It is much more difficult to attain a second remission following relapse with AML than with ALL. Because the results of marrow transplantation done in early first relapse and in second remission are similar, allogeneic marrow transplant in early relapse should be considered if a suitable donor is readily available.

Some newer chemotherapy agents show promise in relapsed or refractory AML. They include idarubicin, topotecan, carboplatin, tiazofurin, diaziquone, and 2-chlorodeoxyadenosine (2-CDA). High-dose ara-C with or without an additional agent such as L-asparaginase, mitoxantrone, etoposide, fludarabine, aclarubicin, daunorubicin, or amsacrine appears to be the most effective agent. Interleukin-2 is being investigated for induction therapy in patients with minimal residual disease.

Other Causes of Morbidity and Mortality. Although relapse of the leukemia is the most common cause of death in children with AML, infections are a major cause of mortality as well. Patients with AML are immune compromised from the disease invading the marrow, from treatment-related granulocytopenia as well as cellular and humoral immune suppression, and from immunosuppressants to prevent and treat GVHD following marrow transplant. They are susceptible to bacterial, fungal, viral, and parasitic infections.

Patients with AML are also susceptible to hemorrhage due to low platelet counts. Generally, patients receive platelet transfusions when the platelet count falls below 15,000-20,000/μl, or higher if there are clinical signs of bleeding.

Growth and development and sexual maturation are generally normal in children treated with conventional chemotherapy. However, there can be problems with gonadal failure and short stature following marrow transplantation. As with ALL, learning disabilities can develop following CNS treatment or prophylaxis with cranial radiation.

Chronic Myelogenous Leukemia

Pathophysiology. Chronic myelogenous leukemia (CML) is a myeloproliferative disorder characterized by the neoplastic, clonal proliferation of pluripotent stem cells. The fact that it is a disease of the stem cells is significant as it renders the disease incurable unless treated with marrow transplantation, which destroys the stem cell. The etiology is unknown but the incidence is greater in individuals with known radiation exposure.

There are three phases of CML: chronic phase, accelerated phase, and blast crisis. Most patients are diagnosed in chronic phase (CML–CP). This phase can last 3 to 5 years.

History and Physical Findings. The median age at diagnosis with CML is 50 years of age. However, the age range is wide, ranging from 15 to 80 years. Patients generally present with fatigue, malaise, headache, fever, chills, weight loss, left upper quadrant (LUQ) fullness, or early satiety. Splenomegaly is a common finding, causing some of the presenting complaints such as LUQ fullness and early satiety. Approximately 20 to 40% of patients have no symptoms, however, and the disease is diagnosed during routine physical exams on these patients.

Laboratory and Diagnostic Findings. Diagnosis is based on peripheral blood and bone marrow examinations. Peripheral blood studies must include a CBC with the differential. A high white blood cell count is common at diagnosis. Sixty percent of patients have a WBC greater than 100,000/μl. Anemia is common due to crowding out of erythrocyte precursors in the marrow by white cells. Thrombocytosis is common. Leukocyte alkaline phosphatase (LAP) is low or absent.

Cytogenetic (chromosomal) studies on the marrow are crucial as part of the diagnostic work-up of this disease. Translocation of chromosomes 9 and 22, written as t(9;22), is found in over 95% of patients with CML, and is termed the Philadelphia chromosome. The result of this translocation is a new fusion gene called *BCR/abl,* and is thought to be the cause of CML. It can be identified by the polymerase chain reaction (PCR) technique performed on either peripheral blood or marrow cells. Even patients with CML who do not have the Philadelphia chromosome are generally positive for the BCR/abl gene. Those patients with presumed CML who are Philadelphia chromosome negative and who are negative for the BCR/abl gene probably have some other disorder such as myelodysplastic syndrome, a myeloproliferative disorder, or chronic myelomonocytic leukemia (CMML).

In chronic phase, the marrow has less than 30% immature cells and the peripheral blood has less than 20%. The average WBC is 225,000/μl at diagnosis with a range of 20,000 to 600,000/μl and less than 5% myeloblasts. Basophils and eosinophils generally number less than 5%. The platelet count is over 450,000/μl in 50% of patients and over 1,000,000/μl in 25%. The LDH and the uric acid are often elevated.

Accelerated phase (CML–AP) occurs at a median of four years after diagnosis, but some patients are diagnosed in accelerated phase. It is heralded by the onset of new fevers, weight loss, and difficulty in controlling the WBC with chemotherapy. The marrow exam shows increasing blasts, as does the peripheral blood smear. Some patients develop extramedullary blastic infiltrates. These extramedullary tumors can precede the development of blast crisis, are caused by the accumulation of blast cells, and manifest as lymph node enlargement, osteolytic bone lesions, cutaneous infiltration, and epidural tumors with cord compression. Progressive anemia, reticulin-positive myelofibrosis, progressive splenomegaly, basophilia, and thrombocytopenia or thrombocytosis are characteristic of the accelerated phase. A marrow exam will often show additional chromosomal abnormalities. The accelerated phase usually lasts from 3 to 9 months before progressing to blast crisis (Canellos, 1996).

More than 80% of patients with CML die in blast crisis (CML–BC). It can occur at any time, but on average occurs 3 to 5 years following diagnosis. Five percent of patients present in BC. Patients present with fevers, night sweats, splenic pain, bone pain, weakness, fatigue, malaise, easy bruisability, nausea, anorexia, splenomegaly, and hepatomegaly. The hematologic exam looks like that of an acute leukemia. Most patients (60%) present with a myeloid blast crisis while 20 to 33% develop a lymphoid blast crisis. The hemoglobin is low, usually less than 10 g/dL. The WBC is elevated, generally greater than 50,000/μl, and can be high enough to cause leukostasis in the CNS resulting in multifocal bleeding, in the lungs (leading to dyspnea and hypoxemia), and in other organ systems. The platelet count is usually less than 100,000/μl. Hemorrhage can occur in the retina, skin, or mucous membranes. Diagnostic criteria are not firm, but generally there should be at least 30% blasts in the marrow for a diagnosis of blast crisis. Seventy to 80% of patients in blast crisis have additional chromosomal abnormalities that often develop 3 to 6 months prior to the development of blast crisis. CML–BC is one of the most refractory hematologic diseases. It lasts 2 to 6 months, eventually leading to death, even with treatment.

Management. Hydroxyurea (Hydrea) is the most common initial treatment for CML. It is a palliative, not curative treatment and is used to control the WBC and symptoms. Sixty to 80% of patients in chronic phase will respond within days. The usual dose is 500 mg to 2 gm/m^2 per day. To avoid excessive myelosuppression, the WBC should be targeted to greater than 10,000/µl with a normal hemoglobin and spleen size (Canellos, 1996). Side effects are mild and include myelosuppression and minor skin changes. Unfortunately, Hydrea does not change the natural history of the disease; thus the average time to the development of AP and BC is unchanged by this agent.

The use of interferon alpha (IF-() can result in the loss of the Philadelphia chromosome (CR) in a small percentage of patients. Thaler et al. (1996) reported complete hematologic remissions in 39% and major cytogenetic responses in 13% of a group of 74 patients with CML treated with IF-α. Even though the CR rate is low, this is the first treatment other than marrow transplantation that may be potentially curative. It takes months to see a hematologic response, and 6 to 12 months to see a cytogenetic response. Hehlmann et al. (1997) reviewed four studies looking at the survival advantage of interferon over hydroxyurea and busulfan. It is clear that interferon is superior to busulfan in prolonging survival. The survival advantage of interferon over hydroxyurea ranged from 10 to 20 months. This is an important question as the side effects of interferon are significant and many patients stop treatment because they find them intolerable. Common side effects are fever, chills, malaise, myalgias, fatigue, and headache which generally resolve a few weeks into treatment. However, prolonged treatment with IF-α can cause additional problems including abnormal liver function, nausea, diarrhea, proteinuria, hair thinning, hemolysis, hypothyroidism, neurological toxicities, depression, and psychosis. The usual dose is 5 million units/m^2 per day, subcutaneously. This is adjusted according to side effects and WBC.

Busulfan was used in the past but is rarely used now for the palliative treatment of CML. However, it is used as part of many conditioning regimens prior to marrow or peripheral blood stem-cell transplantation.

Allogeneic BMT is currently considered the only curative treatment for CML. The best results are achieved in chronic phase and within one year of diagnosis. If the transplant is performed in chronic phase, from a matched allogeneic donor, the long-term survival is approximately 50 to 70%. If it is performed in accelerated phase, the survival is approximately 30%; and in blast crisis, it is only 10 to 20%, mainly due to the increased incidence of relapse when the transplant is performed in advanced disease. Follow-up evaluation posttransplant includes a periodic marrow examination for the BCR/abl transcript. The return of this gene postmarrow transplant predicts relapse (Radich et al., 1995).

Once the patient progresses to AP the response to chemotherapeutic agents is poor and most patients progress to blast crisis. The treatment for blast crisis resembles that for acute leukemia. Ara-C is used for myeloid BC. The response is poor with only 20 to 30% of patients converting back to the chronic phase. Survival is only 2 to 12 months, even for responders, as they tend to develop blast crisis again. Vincristine and prednisone with or without an anthracycline and ara-C are used for lymphoid BC. The response is better with 40 to 70% converting back to the chronic phase.

Chronic Lymphocytic Leukemia

Pathophysiology. Chronic lymphocytic leukemia (CLL) is a monoclonal malignant proliferation of small lymphocytes that initially accumulate in the marrow and peripheral blood, and then in lymph nodes, liver, and spleen as the disease progresses. This accumulation results in enlargement of these organs and decreased marrow function (Deisseroth et al., 1997). Ninety-five percent are of B-cell origin. The disease generally progresses slowly, with a natural history measured in years. Thirty percent of the leukemias in the United States are CLL.

A small number of patients (3-10%) develop Richter's syndrome which manifests as a conversion to an aggressive lymphoma characterized by fevers, weight loss, decreased absolute lymphocyte count (ALC), bulky disease, and extranodal involvement. The response to treatment is poor and the median survival after transformation is 4 months. On rare occasion, acute leukemia (ALL) develops in patients with CLL.

History and Physical Findings. The diagnosis of CLL is based on the history, physical exam, peripheral blood counts, lymphocyte morphology, marrow evaluation, immunophenotyping of lymphocytes, and staining for light chains. Patients are often asymptomatic and the diagnosis is incidental with the finding of an elevated ALC on a routine CBC. If the patient is symptomatic, the symptoms are generally nonspecific with enlarged cervical, axillary, or inguinal nodes being the most common presenting complaint. On exam, the characteristic finding is lymphadenopathy that becomes more prominent as the disease progresses (O'Brien et al., 1996). Some patients have hepatomegaly or splenomegaly and complain of left upper quadrant discomfort and early satiety. Eventually, most patients develop splenomegaly as the disease progresses. The following are uncommon at diagnosis, but do occur in a small percentage of patients: fever, sweats, weight loss (B symptoms), serious infections, anemia, thrombocytopenia, immune neutropenia, and an exaggerated reaction to insect bites. More than 90% of patients are over 50 years of age at diagnosis.

Infections are common in patients with CLL because most (50-70%) have hypogammaglobulinemia as well as B-cell and T-cell dysfunction. Decreases in IgM usually precede deficiencies in IgG and IgA (Deisseroth et al., 1997). Upper and lower respiratory infections are the most common, but skin, soft tissue, and urinary tract infections as well as sepsis also occur. Because many of these infections can be life-threatening, it is recommended that patients receive IV immunoglobulin (IVIg) replacement monthly if the patient is hypogammaglobulinemic or has a history of one or more major bacterial infections. Some patients develop autoimmune hemolytic anemia (15%) or autoimmune thrombocytopenia. Patients with CLL have an increased risk for developing other malignancies such as skin or colon cancer, lymphomas, or multiple myeloma.

Laboratory and Diagnostic Tests. Lymphocyte counts can range from 5,000 to 500,000/µl. Hyperviscosity, however, is uncommon. The minimum criteria for the diagnosis of CLL include a persistent lymphocytosis greater than 5000/µl with marrow involvement (O'Brien et al., 1996). The majority of CLL is of B-cell origin (B-CLL). These cells have a characteristic morphological appearance. Immunophenotyping of lymphocytes is required for diagnosis and will typically show a weak expression of the membrane-bound immunoglobulins IgM +/– IgD and express B-cell antigens such as CD19, CD20, CD21, and CD5 as well as HLA-DR (Deisseroth et al., 1997). Either kappa or lambda light chains may be present. Surface immunoglobulin (sIg) has low cell surface density expression (O'Brien et al., 1996). If an unusual phenotype is found or the morphological appearance is atypical, a lymph node biopsy for histologic evaluation may be necessary.

Ultrasound examination of the abdomen, chest x-rays, CT of the abdomen, CT of the chest, bone marrow aspiration, and a marrow biopsy may also be necessary to aid in the diagnosis and establishing the extent of disease. Thirty to 50% of patients have chromosomal abnormalities when cytogenetic studies are performed. The most common cytogenetic abnormalities involve chromosomes 12 and 14. Those without cytogenetic abnormalities have a better survival risk.

Classification and Staging. The Rai and Binet staging are the most commonly used to classify this leukemia and are used to identify different risk categories (Deisseroth et al., 1997). These classifications assist in determining when to begin treatment and the aggressiveness of the treatment. Most clinical trials in the United States use the Rai staging system, whereas the European trials use the Binet staging system. Table 46–3 lists the criteria in both of these staging systems.

Management. Most patients with CLL do not require immediate treatment, as many patients live for long periods without therapeutic intervention. Patients diagnosed at Rai stage 0 have approximately a 60% or greater chance of living more than 20 years. Conventional treatment for CLL does not cure the disease nor does it prolong survival in patients with early-stage disease. The median survival is 4 to 6 years, despite advances in treatment. Survival correlates strongly with Rai and Binet stages (Deisseroth et al., 1997). Indications for treatment include Rai stage III or IV or Binet stage C at diagnosis because anemia and thrombocytopenia are predictive of a poor outcome. Disease-related symptoms (fever, night sweats, weight loss), progressive bone marrow failure (anemia, thrombocytopenia), autoimmune thrombocytopenia, hemolytic anemia, granulocytopenia, massive splenomegaly, bulky lymphoid disease, progressive leukocytosis with lymphocyte doubling time less than every 6 months, and increased frequency of bacterial, fungal, and viral infections are all indications for treatment as well.

Allopurinol is used to decrease the incidence of uric acid nephropathy in patients with large tumor burdens. Chemotherapeutic agents used as first-line treatment include fludarabine and the alkylators chlorambucil or cyclophosphamide. Chlorambucil combined with prednisone results in response rates of 64 to 74% (Deisseroth et al., 1997). Cyclophosphamide is often combined with vincristine and prednisone in the CVP regimen, resulting in a response rate of 44 to 77%. Fludarabine alone has been shown to result in a 75% CR rate in previously untreated patients (Deisseroth et al., 1997). Combination chemother-

TABLE 46–3. Rai and Binet Staging Systems for Chronic Lymphocytic Leukemia

Stage	Lymphocytosi	Lymphadenopathy	Hepatomegaly or Splenomegaly	Hemoglobin (g/dL)	Platelets ($\times 10^3/\mu L$)
Rai System					
0	+	–	–	≥11	≥100
I	+	+	–	≥11	≥100
II	+	±	+	≥11	≥100
III	+	±	±	<11	≥100
IV	+	±	±	Any	<100
Binet System					
A	+	± (<3 lymphatic groups[a] positive)	±	≥10	≥100
B	+	± (≥3 lymphatic groups[a] positive)	±	≥10	≥100
C	+	±	±	<10	<100

[a] Cervical, axillary, inguinal nodes; liver; and spleen are each considered one group whether unilateral or bilateral.

From Deisseroth, Kantarjian, Andreeff, et al. (1997). (p. 2323).

apy using COP (cyclophosphamide, vincristine, and prednisone), CHOP (cyclophosphamide, doxorubicin, vincristine, and prednisone), and CAP (cyclophosphamide, doxorubicin, and prednisone) among others have been used for CLL with varying results. The use of maintenance therapy has been studied extensively (Wilhelm et al., 1997). Chlorambucil has shown favorable results as a maintenance agent.

Other chemotherapeutic agents have been used for CLL as well with some promising results: 2-chlorodeoxyadenosine (2-cda), deoxycoformycin, interferon alfa, interleukin-2, leustatin, and pentostatin. Fludarabine and 2-chlorodeoxyadenosine (2-CDA) both have shown responses in patients who fail to respond to first-line drugs. The major toxicity with these two agents are myelosuppression, immunosuppression, and infections. Autologous and allogeneic hematopoietic transplants have been used in patients with aggressive disease. The role of these modalities remain to be clarified, but they may be curative or may increase disease-free survival in some patients.

Follow-Up. Individuals with CLL should have regular CBCs to assist in determining the tempo of disease, when to begin treatment, and the effectiveness of treatment. The frequency of these tests should be determined by the stage of disease, tempo of the disease, chemotherapy agent, and any complications the patient may be experiencing such as frequent infections. It is crucial to keep in mind that infectious problems are common and are a leading cause of death in these patients. Following treatment with chemotherapy, the presence of minimal residual disease can be detected through immunophenotyping. The co-expression of CD19, CD20, CD21, or CD24 with CD5 is a useful marker for minimal residual disease.

Myelodysplastic Syndromes

Pathophysiology

Myelodysplastic syndromes (MDS) are a group of clonal disorders characterized by one or more peripheral cytopenias, hypercellular bone marrow, ineffective myelopoiesis, morphologic changes of dyserythropoiesis, and abnormal granulopoiesis and megakaryocytes (Cheson, 1995). A defect is thought to occur at the stem-cell level, leading to alteration in the control of proliferation and differentiation. MDS was previously referred to as preleukemia, smoldering leukemia, sideroblastic anemia, RAEB, or oligoblastic leukemia. The etiology is unknown in most cases of *de novo* MDS. Exposure to ionizing radiation or some chemicals, particularly benzene, has been linked to the development of MDS. Therapy-induced MDS, also referred to as secondary MDS, is known to occur following chemotherapy treatment of breast, lung, ovarian, and gastrointestinal cancers, Hodgkin's disease, non-Hodgkin's lymphomas, seminoma, multiple myeloma, polycythemia vera, CLL, as well as nonmalignant conditions. The highest risk is seen following treatment with alkylating agents, nitrosureas, and procarbazine. Risk increases with increasing cumulative doses of these agents. Radiation therapy alone, without chemotherapy, carries the lowest risk of secondary MDS/AML. Death from MDS is generally due to bleeding or infection. Approximately 20 to 40% of MDS cases evolve to acute leukemia (Third MIC Cooperative Group, 1988).

MDS is generally subclassified by morphologic criteria using the French–American–British (FAB) Morphology Group classification system.

Refractory Anemia. Anemia (hemoglobin < 11 g/dL) is the primary problem in refractory anemia (RA) with variable amounts of dyserythropoiesis, dysgranulopoiesis, or megakaryopoiesis. The marrow is normocellular or hypercellular. Marrow blasts number less than 5%. Approximately 36% of patients with MDS fall into this subtype according to a large multivariate analysis performed by Greenberg et al., (1997).

Refractory Anemia with Ringed Sideroblasts. Also called acquired sideroblastic anemia, refractory anemia with ringed sideroblasts (RARS) is similar to refractory anemia except for the presence of more than 15% ringed sideroblasts in the marrow. Dysgranulopoiesis and dysmegakaryopoiesis are not present in true RARS. Approximately 15% of patients newly diagnosed with MDS fall into this category (Greenberg et al., 1997).

Refractory Anemia with Excess Blasts. In refractory anemia with excess blasts (RAEB), cytopenias of two or more marrow elements are present. The peripheral blood has abnormalities in all three cell lines. Dysgranulopoiesis is common and more pronounced. The marrow is hypercellular with dyspoiesis of all three lines and occasionally ringed sideroblasts. Five to less than 20% blasts are found in the marrow. Approximately 26% of patients with MDS have RAEB (Greenberg et al., 1997).

Chronic Myelomonocytic Leukemia. In chronic myelomonocytic leukemia (CMML) there is peripheral absolute monocytosis greater than $>1 \times 10^9$/L. This is associated with proliferation of monocytes in the marrow. There is a variable degree of trilineage dysplasia. Approximately 15% of cases with newly diagnosed MDS fall into this category (Greenberg et al., 1997).

RAEB in Transformation. The diagnosis of RAEB in transformation (RAEB-t) is based on the finding of cytopenias with lab features that fit none of the above nor do they fit frank AML. Peripheral blasts number greater than 5%; marrow blasts number between 21% and 30%. Approximately 8% of patients with newly diagnosed MDS fall into this category (Greenberg et al., 1997).

AML. Transformation to AML is based on typical findings in the marrow including greater than 30% blasts. Risk factors for transformation to AML include FAB classification, percentage of marrow blasts, cytogenetic pattern, and number of cytopenias (Greenberg et al., 1997). Approximately 30% of patients with MDS die with leukemia (Greenberg et al., 1997). Indicators predictive of evolution to AML include the FAB classification, percentage of marrow blasts, cytogenetic pattern, and number of cytopenias (Greenberg et al., 1997).

Data from the Greenberg analysis show a poorer prognosis for patients with RAEB or RAEB-t, those with marrow blasts greater than 10%, those with two or three cytopenias, and those patients with complex cytogenetic abnormalities or chromosome 7 abnormalities (Greenberg et al., 1997).

History and Physical Findings

At diagnosis patients present with a variety of symptoms indicative of marrow dysfunction. As with frank acute leukemia, symptoms are characteristic of the marrow lines that are affected, but generally include signs of anemia: fatigue, weakness, pallor, exertional dyspnea, easy fatiguability, angina, and cardiac failure. Many patients have years of marginal anemia that may or may not be responsive to iron therapy prior to diagnosis. As the disease progresses, signs and symptoms of thrombocytopenia also develop, including easy bruising and hemorrhages. Infections and fever become more common as the myeloid line is affected. Physical findings are nonspecific. Ten to 40% of patients have hepatic or splenic enlargement.

Laboratory and Diagnostic Tests

The diagnosis of MDS is based on history and the results of peripheral blood and bone marrow examinations. The marrow has characteristic abnormalities that involve one or more of the cell lines. The peripheral blood shows variable degrees of cytopenias, depending on the FAB classification. One of the most predictive lab values is the initial platelet count, with thrombocytopenia predicting a poor outcome.

Cytogenetics. Nearly 80% of patients with MDS have abnormal chromosome studies. The most common involve chromosomes 5, 7, or 8. Unlike AML, there does not appear to be a link between particular cytogenetic abnormalities and specific FAB subtypes of MDS (Silverman, 1997). The finding of multiple, complex abnormalities is associated with a poor prognosis. Deletions of the long arm of chromosomes 20 [del(20q)] or 5 [del(5q)], deletion of the Y chromosome (-Y), or normal karyotypes carry a better prognosis (Greenberg et al., 1997). Patients with chromosome 5 or 7 abnormalities, or both, combined with other abnormalities have a poor prognosis.

Management

Many treatment strategies have been used for MDS. Most have been ineffective. Some have significant toxicity without improvement in outcome. Vitamins, particularly vitamin B_{12}, and folic acid have been used empirically, but are ineffective in treating the anemia or in prolonging survival. Hormonal therapy such as glucocorticoids have resulted in transient increases in blood counts, but again, survival is not improved. Androgens are minimally effective. Growth factors such as GM–CSF, G–CSF, and ethythropoietin have some effect on blood counts, but do not change the course of the disease. Aggressive chemotherapy with daunorubicin and cytosine arabinoside (Ara-C), fludarabine and Ara-C, or high-dose Ara-C alone can induce remissions in some patients. Chemotherapy agents, such as 5-azacytidine, and ATRA, that induce differentiation, have shown some promise, but results are inconsistent. Allogeneic marrow or peripheral blood transplantation appears to be the only form of curative therapy, resulting in a disease-free survival of 25 to 70% (Appelbaum, 1995). The rate of disease-free survival depends on the subclassification of the disease at time of transplant. Transplantation performed in the RA stage results in the higher survival rates, whereas if it is performed in the RAEB stage or beyond, the risk of relapse is higher. The optimal timing of marrow transplantation is unknown. The decision is based on the stage of disease, with more advanced stages providing less time to progression to acute leukemia and with that, a worse prognosis for long-term survival posttransplant. The tempo and progression of the disease is also considered in the decision-making, as is the frequency of infections and blood and platelet transfusions. The International Prognostic Scoring System (IPSS) for MDS may also be useful in determining when to transplant (Greenberg et al., 1997). Median survival posttransplant is longer in patients who do not have excess blasts, have been diagnosed a short period of time, and are less than 40 years of age.

Because of age and other factors, many patients are only able to receive supportive care consisting of blood product transfusions and antibiotics, but not treatment that changes the course of the disease. Regardless of the ineffectiveness of supportive care in changing the natural history of the disease, it is crucial as many patients die of infections or hemorrhage before they ever transform to AML.

Follow-Up

The worst prognosis is in patients with RAEB or RAEB-t, greater than 10% marrow blasts, and two to three cytopenias, and in patients with complex cytogenetic abnormalities or chromosome 7 abnormalities (Greenberg et al., 1997). Patients should be evaluated on a regular basis with physical exams and CBCs to follow the progression of the disease, evaluate for the presence of any complications such as infections or bleeding, and to determine when to transfuse with blood or platelets. Because the only curative treatment is allogeneic marrow or peripheral blood transplantation, this should be discussed with patients under 65 years of age. If this is a viable option, arrangements should be made to HLA-type the patient and family members. If there are no appropriately matched family members, a search for an unrelated donor takes an average of 4 to 6 months.

Non-Hodgkin's Lymphomas

Non-Hodgkin's lymphomas (NHL) are groups of malignancies of the lymphoid system. They are caused by uncontrolled growth and proliferation of lymphocytes. Generally, the lymph nodes are involved but extranodal (outside the lymph node) involvement is also common. There are several types of non-Hodgkin's lymphomas. They arise from B-, T-, pre-B-, pre-T-, and null-cells and at various stages of cell differentiation. Most NHL are of B-cell origin. The disease becomes blood-borne early in the process and thus can spread to distant sites easily. This is in contrast to Hodgkin's disease which spreads in an orderly fashion from one lymphoid region to adjacent regions.

The major risk factors associated with the development of NHL are immune deficiencies, either congenital (such as Wiskott–Aldrich syndrome and X-linked lymphoproliferative syndrome) or acquired (such as HIV infection and the human T-cell leukemia/lymphoma virus type I [HTLV-I]). The incidence increases with age from childhood to age 80 (Vose et al., 1996). NHL in children behave differently from the disease in adults. Children have a tendency for early dissemination and disease is found in the CNS and peripheral blood more frequently.

Pathophysiology

Accurate identification of the various subtypes is essential to predict prognosis and to select the most effective treatment. NHL are categorized by grade (classification) and by stage of the disease. The grade or classification is the more important factor in determining treatment.

Classification. Several classifications are used for lymphoma; none are perfect. The classification used should aid the practitioner in making decisions such as when to begin treatment, determining prognosis, whether the goal of treatment should be cure or palliation, and which regimen is likely to be the most effective. The Rappaport system is the oldest, but in the United States has mainly been replaced by the Working Formulation which is based on the histologic appearance of the cell (see Table 46–4). The Working Classification, however, does not include the newer advances in immunologic and genetic studies. The Revised European–American Classification of Lymphoid–Neoplasms (REAL) is the newest classification in use and may be used more frequently in the near future, as it uses morphologic, immunologic, and genetic techniques to better classify tumors into well-defined disease entities (Harris et al., 1994). It can be confusing to have several classifications in use concurrently. In clinical practice it is important to understand what the diagnosis assigned by the pathologist means and what system is being used to classify the tumor. Various tables are available to interconvert the classifications (Harris et al., 1994). Table 46–5 lists the disease entities included in the REAL Classification, and Table 46–6 compares the REAL Classification with the Working Formulation. The discussion on the various lymphomas, diagnosis, and treatment will be based on the Working Formulation, as this is the more commonly used classification for determining treatment and prognosis in the United States at this time.

TABLE 46–4. Working Formulation Classification of Non-Hodgkin's Lymphoma

Low Grade (Indolent)

A. Malignant lymphoma, small lymphocytic
- consistent with chronic lymphocytic leukemia
- plasmacytoid

B. Malignant lymphoma, follicular, predominantly small cleaved cell
- diffuse areas
- sclerosis

C. Malignant lymphoma, follicular mixed, small cleaved and large cell
- diffuse areas
- sclerosis

Intermediate Grade

D. Malignant lymphoma, follicular, predominantly large cell
- diffuse areas
- sclerosis

E. Malignant lymphoma, diffuse, small cleaved cell

F. Malignant lymphoma, diffuse mixed, small and large cell
- sclerosis
- epithelioid cell component

G. Malignant lymphoma, diffuse large cell
- cleaved cell
- noncleaved cell
- sclerosis

High Grade

H. Malignant lymphoma, large cell, immunoblastic
- plasmacytoid
- clear cell
- polymorphous
- epithelioid cell component

I. Malignant lymphoma, lymphoblastic
- convoluted cell
- nonconvoluted cell

J. Malignant lymphoma, small noncleaved cell
- Burkitt's
- follicular areas

Adapted from DeVita, Jaffe, & Hellman. (1985). (p. 1634). Used with permission.

Indolent (Low-Grade) Lymphomas. Indolent or low-grade lymphoma is a favorable diagnosis. There is often a relatively long natural history. Because of its indolent nature, patients may live with the slow-growing disease for years. However, it is not generally considered curable by conventional treatment methods.

Small lymphocytic lymphoma is the tissue manifestation of the B-lymphocyte proliferation seen in CLL. Richter's transformation is the development of a diffuse large-cell lymphoma in a patient with a history of chronic lymphocytic leukemia or a low-grade well-differentiated lymphoma. This is clinically and histologically a more aggressive disease than the usual large-cell lymphoma and carries a poor prognosis.

TABLE 46–5. List of Lymphoid Neoplasms Recognized by the International Lymphoma Study Group (REAL Classification)

B-Cell Neoplasms

I. Precursor B-cell neoplasm: Precursor B-lymphoblastic leukemia/lymphoma

II. Peripheral B-cell neoplasms
   1. B-cell chronic lymphocytic leukemia/prolymphocytic leukemia/small lymphocytic lymphoma
   2. Lymphoplasmacytoid lymphoma/immunocytoma
   3. Mantle cell lymphoma
   4. Follicle center lymphoma, follicular
      - Provisional cytologic grades: I (small cell), II (mixed small and large cell), III (large cell)
      - Provisional subtype: diffuse, predominantly small cell type
   5. Marginal zone B-cell lymphoma
      - Extranodal (MALT-type +/– monocytoid B cells)
      - Provisional subtype: Nodal (+/– monocytoid B cells)
   6. Provisional entity: splenic marginal zone lymphoma (+/– villous lymphocytes)
   7. Hairy cell leukemia
   8. Plasmacytoma/plasma cell myeloma
   9. Diffuse large B-cell lymphoma
      - Subtype: Primary mediastinal (thymic) B-cell lymphoma
   10. Burkitt's lymphoma
   11. Provisional entity: High-grade B-cell lymphoma, Burkitt-like

T-cell and Putative NK-Cell Neoplasms

I. Precursor T-cell neoplasm: Precursor T-lymphoblastic lymphoma/leukemia

II. Peripheral T-cell and NK-cell neoplasms
   1. T-cell chronic lymphocytic leukemia/prolymphocytic leukemia
   2. Large granular lymphocyte leukemia (LGL)
      - T-cell type
      - NK-cell type
   3. Mycosis fungoides/Sezary syndrome
   4. Peripheral T-cell lymphomas, unspecified
      - Provisional cytologic categories: medium-sized cell, mixed medium and large cell, large cell, lymphoepithelioid cell
      - Provisional subtype: Hepatosplenic $\gamma\delta$ T-cell lymphoma
      - Provisional subtype: Subcutaneous panniculitic T-cell lymphoma
   5. Angioimmunoblastic T-cell lymphoma (AILD)
   6. Angiocentric lymphoma
   7. Intestinal T-cell lymphoma (+/– enteropathy associated)
   8. Adult T-cell lymphoma/leukemia (ATL/L)
   9. Anaplastic large cell lymphoma (ALCL), CD30+, T-, and null-cell types
   10. Provisional entity: Anaplastic large-cell lymphoma, Hodgkin's-like

Hodgkin's Disease

I. Lymphocyte predominance
II. Nodular sclerosis
III. Mixed cellularity
IV. Lymphocyte depletion
V. Provisional entity: Lymphocyte-rich classical HD

Used with permission from Harris, Jaffe, Stein, et al. (1994). (p. 1362).

Aggressive (Intermediate- or High-Grade) Lymphomas. These are unfavorable, rapidly progressive, and fatal in a short period of time without treatment. Newer treatment strategies have resulted in long-term disease-free survival (cure) in about 50% of patients. Burkitt's lymphoma is a specific, aggressive subtype of small noncleaved cell, high-grade NHL. The type seen in the United States is associated with the t(8;14) translocation and is rarely associated with the Epstein–Barr virus (EBV). Most common sites of involvement with Burkitt's are the abdomen, gastrointestinal tract, and bone marrow. Burkitt's requires multiagent treatment, including CNS prophylaxis.

HIV-related lymphomas are usually high-grade B-cell lymphomas of the small noncleaved cell type or the large-cell immunoblastic type. They generally involve multiple lymph nodes as well as extranodal sites such as the gastrointestinal tract, bone, and the CNS.

Lymphoblastic Lymphoma. Lymphoblastic lymphoma tends to behave like T-cell acute lymphocytic leukemia (ALL) with early dissemination and frequent metastases to the CNS. Treatment is similar to that for poor-prognosis ALL. Patients commonly present with a mediastinal mass, which can cause superior vena cava syndrome, pericardial effusions, cardiac tamponade, or pleural effusions. It is primarily seen in adolescent males.

History and Physical Findings

The history and physical exam should pay special attention to symptoms such as weight loss, fevers, night sweats, and pruritis, which are signs of more extensive disease. The exam should include all lymph node areas, including a careful abdominal exam to evaluate for the presence of masses. Signs and symptoms of NHL result from infiltration of various organs and tissues, pressure on various organs and tissues as the lymphadenopathy increases, and quantitative and functional deficits in normal cells. The following are common presenting signs and symptoms.

Lymphatic System. Often patients present with enlarged lymph nodes in the cervical, axillary, and/or inguinal regions that are unresponsive to antibiotics, particulary those with nodular lymphomas. These nodes tend to be hard, rubbery, and generally painless.

Gastrointestinal System. Patients can present with loss of appetite or weight loss, nausea and vomiting, indigestion, abdominal pain, or bloating. Splenomegaly is a common finding in patients with nodular lymphomas. Involvement of the GI tract is more commonly seen in diffuse lymphomas. Large abdominal tumors may indicate Burkitt's lymphoma.

Neurological System. Pressure or pain in the lower back, extending down the legs, can indicate tumor mass in the spinal cord area. Headache can indicate CNS involvement, as can double vision which is seen more often in the high-grade lymphomas.

TABLE 46–6. Comparison of the REAL Classification and the Working Formulation

	B-Cell Neoplasms	T-Cell Neoplasms
Indolent	B-cell chronic lymphocytic lymphoma/small lymphocytic lymphoma	Lymphoblastic lymphoma (most cases)
	Lymphoplasmacytoid	Adult T-cell leukemia/lymphoma, chronic and smoldering types
	Follicle center, follicular (grades I, II)	*Mycosis fungoides*
	Marginal zone/MALT	
	Splenic marginal zone	
	Hairy cell leukemia	
	Plasmacytoma/myeloma	
Moderately aggressive	B-cell prolymphocytic leukemia	T-cell chronic lymphocytic lymphoma/prolymphocytic leukemia
	Mantle cell	Adult T-cell leukemia/lymphoma, chronic type
	Follicle center, grade III	Angiocentric, some cases
		Angioimmunoblastic
Aggressive	*Diffuse large B-cell*	Large granular lymphocytic, aggressive NK type
		Peripheral T-cell, unspecified
		Angiocentric, some cases
		Intestinal T-cell
		Adult T-cell leukemia/lymphoma, acute and lymphomatous types
		Anaplastic large cell
Highly aggressive	Precursor B-lymphoblastic	Precursor T-lymphoblastic
	Burkitt's	
	High-grade B-cell, Burkitt-like	

Note: Entities in italics are those most likely to be encountered in Western adult patients.
From Grogan, Miller, & Fisher. (1997). (p. 836).

General. Patients may complain of fatigue, a flu-like syndrome, infections, or generalized aching. B symptoms (fever, night sweats, weight loss) generally indicate more extensive disease. Pruritis, bone pain, coughing, or abnormal pressure/congestion in the face, neck, and upper chest can also be presenting symptoms. Marrow involvement with signs and symptoms of pancytopenia is more frequent in patients with nodular lymphomas.

Other. Involvement of the GI tract, testes, thyroid, skin, breast, central nervous system, or bone is more common in diffuse lymphomas. Endemic Burkitt's lymphoma often presents with large tumors involving the abdomen and the bones of the jaw.

Laboratory and Diagnostic Tests

Lymph-node biopsy of the largest and most accessible node is the first step in the diagnostic process. Several tests are performed on the tissue to assist in the classification of the tumor. Immunophenotyping of the tumor by flow cytometry or immunohistochemistry characterizes the lymphoma by determining which immunological markers are present on the surface of the cell. Flow cytometry uses a semiautomated instrument that measures antibodies on a large number of cells. Immunohistochemistry is a technique of antibody staining on microscope slides. Cytogenetic studies determine whether there are any chromosomal abnormalities in the lymphoma cells, some of which are associated with particular classifications of NHL and assist in the diagnosis. These techniques help differentiate between lymphoma and a reactive lesion or lymphoma and an undifferentiated carcinoma. If immunophenotyping studies are unable to assign lineage, immunoglobulin and T-cell gene rearrangement studies are performed. These techniques use electrophoresis to assess clonality, thus determine if a given proliferation is malignant, and assign lineage (T-cell versus B-cell).

Cytogenesis. Seventy to 80% of non-Hodgkin's lymphomas are of B-cell origin. Some can be of T-cell origin. The lymphomas of T-cell origin can activate macrophages throughout the body, destroying normal blood cells. Their prognosis is worse than for B-cell lymphomas

Chromosomal Abnormalities. Over 90% of patients with NHL have chromosomal abnormalities. These abnormalities are markers for the disease. They correlate with the histologic, immunologic, and clinical features of the disease but do not generally guide treatment options.

The t(14;18) translocation is strongly associated with follicular lymphomas and some diffuse large-cell lymphomas. This cytogenetic abnormality results in the overproduction of the bcl-2 protein in tumor cells. Polymerase chain reaction (PCR) tests can detect bone marrow disease in patients with this chromosomal abnormality. The bcl-2 gene rearrangement gene may be associated with shorter disease-free survival. The t(8;14) translocation is strongly associated with Burkitt's lymphoma. The t(11;14) translocation is strongly associated with mantle cell lymphoma.

Staging. Staging of the lymphoma is useful in determining prognosis and guiding treatment (Table 46–7). Once a

TABLE 46–7. Staging of NHL

Stage I	Involvement of a single lymph node region or single extralymphatic organ
Stage II	Involvement of two or more lymph node regions or extralymphatic sites on the same side of the diaphragm
Stage III	Involvement of lymph node regions or extralymphatic organs or sites on both sides of the diaphragm
Stage IV	Diffuse or disseminated involvement of more than one extralymphatic[a] organ with or without associated lymph node involvement. Involvement of the bone marrow confers stage IV disease.
Constitutional Symptoms	
Type A	Asymptomatic
Type B	Fevers, night sweats, and weight loss greater than 10% of body weight

[a] Extralymphatic sites of involvement can include bone marrow, liver, gastrointestinal tract, spleen, bone, and less commonly, lung, thyroid, testes and the central nervous system.

TABLE 46–8. Staging Procedures for Non-Hodgkin's Lymphomas

Initial Studies

Confirmed histologic diagnosis
History and physical examination
Laboratory analysis

- Complete blood count, platelet count
- Renal function studies
- Calcium, uric acid, LDH
- Liver function studies

Chest x-ray
CT scan of chest, abdomen, and pelvis
Bone marrow biopsy

Additional Studies (as needed)

Bone scan
Ultrasonography
^{67}Ga scan
Gastrointestinal evaluation if primary tumor is in Waldeyer's ring
CT scan of brain (if neurological symptoms are present)
MRI of spine or myelogram (if neurological symptoms are present)
Lumbar puncture (high-grade NHL or symptoms present)
Cytologic examination of effusions (if present)

Additional

Polymerase chain reaction analysis (PCR)
Flow cytometry/immunophenotyping of peripheral blood and/or marrow
Immunohistochemistry analysis
Flow cytometry for DNA analysis
Cytogenetic analysis of lymph node, blood, or marrow

Staging of NHL is based on history, physical examination, and the tests described in this table.
Adapted by permission from Wiernik, Canellos, Dutcher, & Kyle. (1996). (p. 909).

histologic grade is assigned, the patient can be staged by determining how extensive the disease is. Staging is based on history, physical examination, and tests described in Table 46–8.

Baseline peripheral blood studies include CBC with differential, LDH, hepatic function, renal function, calcium, and uric acid. Radiographic studies include chest x-ray and chest CT to look for mediastinal lymphadenopathy which is common in lymphoblastic lymphoma, a disease of older children. Abdominal and pelvic CTs are done to determine the extent of disease in the abdomen. Other studies may be required depending on symptoms and include sonography, bone scan, and MRI of bone and head. Bilateral bone marrow aspirates and biopsies are performed to rule out marrow involvement. Lumbar puncture is used to evaluate for presence of CNS disease if the patient is at high risk, such as those patients with high-grade lymphoma, primary paranasal sinus disease, testicular disease, and bone marrow involvement. Extralymphatic sites of involvement can include bone marrow, liver, gastrointestinal tract, spleen, bone, and—less commonly—lung, thyroid, testes, and the central nervous system.

Management

Treatment strategies depend on the grade or histologic subtype, stage, age, and performance status. In NHL, as compared with Hodgkin's disease, the grade of the disease determines treatment more than does stage of disease.

Asymptomatic patients with indolent (low-grade) lymphomas may not need systemic treatment for several years after diagnosis. Large lymph nodes in one or two areas can be treated with local radiation with follow-up every 2 to 3 months; systemic therapy should be initiated before the disease spreads so much that there is compression of organs or the bone marrow is totally involved with disease.

Patients with follicular mixed, small- and large-cleaved cell, and large-cell lymphoma generally need systemic treatment sooner than other indolent lymphoma patients. This is probably due to the combination of cells; the large cell is likely a replicative cell and small-cell lymphoma tends to metastasize to multiple organs.

Stage I and II Indolent (Low-Grade) Lymphomas. As discussed earlier, the low-grade lymphomas often have a relatively long natural history. Radiation therapy seems to offer the best prolonged disease-free survival (MacManus & Hoppe, 1997). Because the relapse rate is high, however, research is ongoing investigating the use of adjuvant chemotherapy and biological response modifiers such as alpha-interferon and monoclonal antibodies.

Stage III and IV Indolent (Low-Grade) Lymphomas. Many forms of therapy result in 60 to 75% complete remission (CR); however, they are not durable remissions. Second and subsequent CRs are possible but each subsequent CR is generally shorter.

Oral alkylating agents are used for patients with minimal tumor burden who wish to avoid toxicity. Chlorambucil 0.1-0.2 mg/kg/day, orally, and cyclophosphamide 1.5-2.5 mg/kg/day, orally, are the agents commonly used. Response is slow, however, and it may take years to achieve a CR.

Toxicity is minimal but there is potential for secondary AML with prolonged use of alkylating agents.

Combination chemotherapy is preferable for patients with a high tumor burden, rapid tumor growth, or extensive marrow involvement as the response is faster than with oral alkylating agents. The most commonly used combinations include CVP (cyclophosphamide, vincristine, prednisone, every 21 days for a minimum of 6 cycles or 2 cycles following achievement of a CR) and C-MOPP (cyclophosphamide, vincristine, procarbazine, prednisone, every 28 days) (Fisher, 1995).

Total nodal irradiation is useful in patients with stage III disease. Newer agents such as anti-CD20 monoclonal antibody (IDEC), fludarabine, and 2-chloro-2'-deoxyadenosine (CdA) may be alternatives for low-grade lymphomas. It is not known yet what the long-term effects are. Interferon has been used as a maintenance agent and seems to produce prolonged disease-free survival (DFS) in patients with indolent lymphomas, a high tumor burden, and a more aggressive disease. High-dose chemotherapy and total body irradiation followed by autologous bone marrow transplant (ABMT) has shown high rates of initial response. Follow-up is still too short to know whether these patients are cured.

Stage I or II Aggressive (High- or Intermediate-Grade) Lymphomas. Combination chemotherapy and local radiation is the standard of treatment for stage I or II aggressive lymphomas since most of these patients tend to have microscopic dissemination of disease at diagnosis. If CR is achieved and sustained beyond 2 years, the likelihood of being cured is high. One of the oldest and most commonly used combination chemotherapy regimens is CHOP. It consists of cyclophosphamide 750 mg/m^2 IV on day 1, adriamycin 50 mg/m^2 IV on day 1, vincristine 1.4 mg/m^2 IV on day 1, and prednisone 100 mg orally, daily, for 5 days. (See Table 46–13, p. 1117.) This regimen is repeated every 21 days for eight cycles. The toxicity of this regimen is generally not very severe and includes nausea, vomiting, hair loss, and moderate leukopenia. Some patients receive local radiation after completing chemotherapy for local control of disease.

Stage III or IV Aggressive (High- or Intermediate-Grade) Lymphomas. Combination chemotherapy is the treatment of choice for stage III or IV aggressive lymphomas. First-generation drug combinations include CVP and CHOP, described earlier. Thirty percent of patients treated with CHOP achieved durable CRs. Second-generation agents were developed in the 1970s in an attempt to improve the percentage and duration of CRs. These include: m-BACOD (bleomycin, adriamycin, cyclophosphamide, vincristine, prednisone, plus methotrexate with leucovorin rescue) and COP-BLAM. The dose-limiting toxicity with these regimens tends to be myelosuppression. Other common toxicities include nausea, vomiting, alopecia, and neurotoxicity. Patients should have a CBC, blood chemistries, history and physical exam, and tumor measurements at monthly intervals while undergoing treatment. Most relapses occur in the first year, but later relapses also occur.

The newer, third-generation regimens include: ProMACE/cytaBOM (prednisone, doxorubicin, cyclophosphamide, and etoposide, followed by cytarabine, bleomycin, vincristine and methotrexate with leucovorin rescue); MACOP-B (methotrexate with leucovorin rescue, doxorubicin, cyclophosphamide, vincristine, prednisone, and bleomycin); Pro-MACE-MOPP (prednisone, methotrexate, adriamycin, cyclophosphamide, and etoposide, alternating with nitrogen mustard, vincristine, procarbazine, and prednisone); LNH-80; and COP-BLAM III. A study conducted by the Southwest Oncology Group (SWOG) and the Eastern Cooperative Oncology Group (ECOG) showed that there was no difference in partial or complete responses between CHOP versus m-BACOD versus ProMACE-CytaBOM versus MACOP-B (Fisher, 1993). Overall, there was a 44% DFS rate at 3 years. However, the regimen-related mortality for the four regimens was higher for the newer regimens: CHOP: 1%; ProMACE-CytaBOM: 3%; m-BACOD: 5%; and MACOP-B: 6%. Thus, there is no clear indication that any of the newer regimens offer an advantage over CHOP.

Some patients present with oncologic emergencies such as superior vena cava syndrome, pleural effusions, spinal cord compression, and sepsis. Superior vena cava syndrome is caused from the rapid growth of the lymphadenopathy compressing the superior vena cava, impeding the return of blood to the heart. Prompt chemotherapy, followed by local radiation, is indicated. Lymphatic obstruction, or direct pleuropulmonary involvement by the lymphoma, can cause pleural effusions. This can be treated with radiation, systemic or local chemotherapy. Spinal cord compression can occur at presentation or during treatment. Local radiation and corticosteroids are the most common treatment. Emergency laminectomy and corticosteroids, followed by radiation, are also used. Hyperuricemia with renal dysfunction can be seen while the patient is going through treatment, especially with large tumor burdens. Allopurinol, hydration, and sometimes alkalization of the urine can help prevent the nephropathy sometimes seen with hyperuricemia.

Follow-Up

Frequency of follow-up evaluations depends on the tempo of the disease, treatment regimens, and symptomatology. During treatment, the patient may need to be seen daily, if necessary. Following treatment, the interval is gradually increased as signs and symptoms of toxicity improve. Restaging is often done just prior to the end of the treatment regimen. If disease is still present, other treatment modalities such as marrow transplantation may need to be employed. Because recurrence of disease is common, new or persistent symptoms should be evaluated for this possibility.

Low-Grade Lymphomas. Most low-grade lymphomas respond to chemotherapy but eventually the disease becomes refractory. One third evolves into a diffuse aggressive lymphoma which tends to respond to treatments for diffuse lymphomas. Most patients with low-grade lymphomas live with recurrent disease. Median survival following diagnosis is 6 years. The median disease-free interval following completion of therapy is only 17 months. The 5-year survival is 80%, whereas the 10-year survival is 30 to 50%. Patients with recurrent low-grade lymphoma may benefit from high-dose treatment with hematopoietic transplantation if they had a brief first or second remission with chemotherapy and/or if they attained only PRs with second-line or subsequent chemotherapy but are still drug-sensitive (Horning, 1997).

Aggressive Lymphomas. Poor prognostic factors for the aggressive lymphomas include: age greater than 60, stage III or IV disease, two or more extranodal sites (tumor bulk), poor performance status, and an elevated LDH. Low-risk patients have none or one poor-risk factor. Low-intermediate risk patients have two poor-risk factors. High-intermediate risk patients have three poor-risk factors. High-risk patients have four or five poor-risk factors.

More than half (55-65%) of patients with advanced-stage intermediate- or high-grade NHL will either be refractory to treatment or relapse after treatment with chemotherapy. Once relapse occurs, the only chance of cure is with an autologous or allogeneic hematopoietic transplant. Autologous BMT offers a 10 to 70% prolonged disease-free survival. Best results are in patients who responded well to the initial chemotherapy and who undergo transplant with no or minimal residual disease. Various preparative regimens with and without total body irradiation (TBI) may be used.

A number of regimens such as DHAP (dexamethasone, high-dose cytosine arabinoside, and cisplatin), ESHAP (etoposide, solumedrol, high-dose ara-C, and cisplatin), and MINE-ESHAP (mesna, ifosfamide, mitoxantrone, and etoposide, followed by ESHAP) have been utilized as salvage regimens. They may produce overall response rates of 30 to 69%, with the MINE-ESHAP regimen currently yielding the best responses (Rodriguez-Monge & Cabanillas, 1997). However, they do not offer a realistic probability of cure. DHAP and ESHAP are often used prior to ABMT to reduce tumor bulk, and thus improve long-term survival.

As the results of treatment in non-Hodgkin's lymphoma in children have improved, it has become evident that there are potential long-term complications that influence the quality of life as these children mature. The most significant complications include impaired gonadal function, late cardiac failure from anthracyclines, the risk of secondary malignancies, particularly with the use of alkylating agents, and the psychological impact of having survived a life-threatening illness.

Hodgkin's Disease

Hodgkin's disease (HD) is one of the few malignancies whose natural history has been favorably altered by modern diagnosis and therapy.

Pathophysiology

Signs and symptoms of Hodgkin's disease result from infiltration of various organs and tissues, pressure on various organs and tissues as the lymphadenopathy increases, and quantitative and functional deficits in normal cells. Many complications are oncologic emergencies, such as superior vena cava syndrome, pleural effusions, spinal cord compression, and sepsis such as described earlier with NHL.

History and Physical Findings

Hodgkin's disease occurs at any age. There is a bimodal distribution with one peak at 20 to 29 years. The most common histology in this age range is nodular sclerosis. There is a second peak at greater than 60 years of age, which is often lymphocyte-depleted histology.

The history and physical exam should pay special attention to symptoms such as weight loss, fevers, night sweats, and pruritis. Less than half of patients have these B symptoms, but they are indicative of more extensive disease. Also investigate for the presence of alcohol-induced pain, a family history of Hodgkin's disease, history of immunosuppressive illness, history of previous cancer, and history of previous chemotherapy or radiation therapy. The exam should include all lymph node areas, including a careful abdominal exam to evaluate for the presence of masses, hepatomegaly, splenomegaly, Waldeyer's ring inspection, and bony tenderness. The most common initial finding is asymptomatic supraclavicular or cervical lymphadenopathy. However, the pattern of involvement at presentation is dependent on the histologic subgroup (Bonadonna et al., 1996). Most patients with lymphocytic predominance (LP) present with localized disease in the upper cervical nodes. Patients with lymphocyte depleted (LD) histology tend to present with abdominal node involvement as well as extranodal extension. When HD is found below the diaphragm, it is generally widely disseminated. Those with nodular sclerosis (NS) histology tend to present with supradiaphragmatic disease and mediastinal node involvement. This is seen as a large asymptomatic anterior mediastinal mass on x-ray. Superior vena cava obstruction is rare in HD. Those with mixed cellularity (MC) generally present with either upper torso disease or with lymphoma on both sides of the diaphragm without regional predilection. Spread of the disease is generally to contiguous nodes, unlike NHL where there is usually an earlier blood-borne dissemination and more widespread metastasis. Although commonly cited, generalized pruritis and alcohol-induced pain in sites of lymphadenopathy are rare presenting symptoms. Patients are often anergic.

Laboratory and Diagnostic Tests

An adequate biopsy of more than one intact node should be reviewed by an experienced hematopathologist for the presence of Reed–Sternberg (RS) cells, RS cell precursors, host inflammatory cells, and cells appearing in response to cytokines liberated by RS cells. Reed–Sternberg cells are giant cells with a symmetrical, mirror-image nucleus that gives the cell an "owl eye" appearance. The lacunar cell, a variant of the RS cell, is seen in nodular sclerosis HD. Biopsy of inguinal lymph nodes should be avoided if other peripheral nodes are easily accessible.

Histologic Types of HD

1. Nodular sclerosis HD (NSHD) is the most frequent histological type with 80% of cases showing this histology. It is more common in young females and carries a good prognosis.
2. Mixed cellularity HD (MCHD) is less common, comprising 10 to 15% of cases. The prognosis is worse and tends to be more advanced at diagnosis. It is more common in patients greater than 40 years of age. It is often confused with NHL and other lymphomas.
3. Lymphocyte-predominant HD (LPHD) occurs in approximately 5% of cases. It is more common in young males. There is often an indolent history with excellent responses to any treatment. It can progress to large-cell NHL or lymphocytic depletion.
4. Lymphocyte depleted HD (LDHD) is rare. It is associated with advanced disease at diagnosis and behaves aggressively. Patients often present with subdiaphragmatic disease and bone marrow involvement. It may be confused with large-cell lymphoma.

Immunophenotyping shows the presence of CD15 and CD30 and the absence of CD45. The presence of chromosomal translocations are common, but there is no consistent cytogenetic abnormality.

Laboratory and Diagnostic Imaging. Laboratory tests include a CBC because hematologic abnormalities such as leukocytosis, lymphopenia, and eosinophilia are associated with advanced disease. The ESR is elevated in more advanced disease. Chemistries include liver function tests, LDH, uric acid, serum copper, and calcium.

Chest x-ray and CT of the chest are done to evaluate mediastinal adenopathy, extension of adenopathy into surrounding tissues, and to determine the bulk of the disease which is important for prognostic determination. CT scanning of the abdomen is used to assess dissemination to abdominal nodes (stage III) or extranodal involvement (stage IV). Bipedal lymphangiography is the most accurate tool for the assessment of low paraaortic and paracaval node involvement. As compared with NHL, Hodgkin's disease rarely involves Waldeyer's ring, the epitrochlear, popliteal or mesenteric nodes, intestinal lymphoid tissue, the testicles, peripheral blood, or the CNS. Thus, routine scans of these sites are not usually necessary, unless the patient presents with symptoms suggestive of involvement in these areas. Gallium (^{67}Ga) scanning can be used when other tests are inconclusive and for detecting residual disease at the end of therapy. It is most useful in evaluating nodal involvement above the diaphragm.

Bilateral bone marrow biopsies (not aspirations) from the posterior iliac crests are useful in determining marrow involvement, particularly if there is disease above and below the diaphragm, bony lesions, or an elevated serum alkaline phosphatase. A needle or surgical biopsy of suspicious sites may be done if the results would alter treatment. If effusions are present, the fluid should be sent for cytological evaluation.

Staging laparotomy has nearly been abandoned in HD and should only be performed if finding occult disease below the diaphragm would change the treatment plan. In general, staging laparotomy is not performed if the staging already shows the patient will benefit from combined systemic and local treatment (i.e., chemotherapy and radiation). Table 46–9 shows decision-making guidelines on the use of staging laparotomy.

Staging. The Ann Arbor Staging criteria for Hodgkin's disease was revised in 1989 (and renamed Cotswold's) to reflect the use of CT scanning and is described in Table 46–10. The stage at diagnosis helps determine prognosis and guide treatment.

TABLE 46–9. Decision-Making for Staging Laparotomy

Staging laparotomy should be performed on	1. Patients with clinical stage (CS) IA, IIA, and IIIA when radiation alone is being considered because 20-31% of patients with disease above the diaphragm at diagnosis will have microscopic disease in the abdomen (Bonadonna et al., 1996)
Staging laparotomy is not required for those patients with	1. Clear clinical stage IIIB or IV disease who are scheduled for chemotherapy 2. A bulky mediastinal mass (> 1/3 diameter of thorax) who are already slated to receive combined treatment 3. Isolated high cervical or non-bulky mediastinal involvement and lymphocyte-predominant or nodular sclerosing HD who may be managed with subtotal nodal radiation alone 4. Four or more involved sites above the diaphragm (require systemic therapy) 5. Females <26 years of age with NSHD and are asymptomatic with only one site above diaphragm

Adapted with permission from Mathai & Robinson. (1994). (p. 150).

TABLE 46–10. The Cotswold's Staging Classification[a] for Hodgkin's Disease

Stage	Features
I	Involvement of single lymph node region or lymph structure
II	Involvement of two or more lymph node sites on the same side of diaphragm; the number of sites should be indicated by subscript (e.g., II_3)
III	Involvement of lymph node regions on both sides of diaphragm
III_1	With or without splenic, hilar, celiac, or portal node involvement
III_2	Paraaortic, iliac, mesenteric node involvement
IV	Diffuse or disseminated involvement of one or more extra-nodal organs or tissues, with or without associated lymph node involvement
A	No symptoms
B	Fever, night sweats, unexplained weight loss >10% body weight
X	Bulky disease with a mass >10 cm or widening of the mediastinum by more than 1/3
E	Involvement of a single extranodal site contiguous or proximal to a known nodal site
CS	Clinical stage
PS	Pathologic (postlaparotomy) stage

[a] The Ann Arbor Staging Criteria for Hodgkin's Disease was revised in 1989 and named the Cotswold's Staging Classification for Hodgkin's Disease to reflect the use of CT scanning. The stage at diagnosis helps determine prognosis and guide treatment.

Adapted by permission from Wiernik, Canellos, Dutcher, & Kyle (Eds.). (1996). (p. 865).

TABLE 46–11. Recommended Treatment Modalities by Stage of Disease

Stage	Recommended Treatment Modality
IA/IIA No bulky mediastinal disease	Subtotal nodal radiation (40–44 Gy to involved areas, 35 Gy to uninvolved areas)
IB/IIB	Combination chemotherapy (3–6 cycles) followed by subtotal nodal radiation If PS IB or IIB, stages by laparotomy, total nodal radiation may be used
I and II, A and B with bulky mediastinal disease	Combined chemotherapy, followed by radiation
IIIA	Combination chemotherapy followed by low-dose radiation or moderate-dose radiation sandwiched by combination chemotherapy If minimal laparotomy-defined stage IIIA: subtotal or total nodal radiation
IIIB	Combination chemotherapy followed by local or total nodal radiation
IV	Combination chemotherapy with low-dose radiation to sites of bulky adenopathy

There are three main treatment strategies for Hodgkin's Disease: radiation therapy alone, combination chemotherapy alone, and combined modality treatment (chemotherapy plus radiation). Thus the goal is to tailor the therapy to eradicate the disease but at the same time to limit the intensity to avoid lethal toxicity.

Prognostic Factors. Unfavorable prognostic indicators for HD include the number of initial disease sites, tumor mass, systemic B symptoms, incomplete response or relapse within 12 months of chemotherapy, age greater than 60 years, male gender, lymphocyte-depleted histology, performance status, elevated LDH with elevated ESR, and low hematocrit at diagnosis.

Management

There are three main treatment strategies for HD: radiation therapy alone, combination chemotherapy alone, and combined modality treatment (chemotherapy plus radiation). Approximately one third of patients with HD die without evidence of disease. A large number of these die of complications from the therapy. Thus the goal is to tailor the therapy to eradicate the disease but at the same time to limit the intensity to avoid lethal toxicity. Table 46–11 describes recommended treatment modalities as determined by stage of disease.

Stage IA to IIA without Bulky Mediastinal Disease. Subtotal nodal irradiation alone is indicated in patients with pathologic stage I or II, A or B after laparotomy with limited disease above the diaphragm and as well as those with LP or NS histology, younger than 40 years of age, and erythro–sedimentation rate (ESR) less than 70. The 10-year disease-free survival (DFS) is 70 to 80% with this strategy (Bonadonna et al., 1996). Inverted Y-field radiation supplemented with radiation to the supraclavicular and mediastinal node chains is used for the rare patient with PS IA or IIA below the diaphragm.

Stage IB or IIB without Bulky Mediastinal Disease. Combined modality treatment with three to six cycles of combination chemotherapy plus involved-field radiation or total nodal radiation results in approximately 85% DFS at 10 years.

Stage I or II, A or B, with Bulky Mediastinal Disease. Combination chemotherapy generally precedes radiation because the bulky disease can often be shrunk down successfully with chemotherapy, thus limiting the size of the radiation field. The 10-year DFS is greater than 80%.

Stage IIIA. Limited stage IIIA disease can be treated with subtotal or total nodal radiation alone, with survival similar to that of the stage IIA patients. When the disease is more extensive, involving the retroperitoneal nodes, a commonly used regimen uses total nodal irradiation followed by six cycles of MOPP, ABVD, or MOPP/ABVD chemotherapy. Some patients are treated with a "sandwich" approach, using two to four cycles of combination chemotherapy, followed by 30 to 35 Gy of radiation, finished with two or three more cycles of chemotherapy. ABVD chemotherapy appears to have better results than MOPP in these patients. Another approach is to administer alternating combination chemotherapy such as MOPP/ABVD, followed by low-dose radiation

(25 Gy) to areas of bulky involvement. Table 46–12 lists common combination chemotherapy regimens used in the treatment of Hodgkin's disease. Table 46–13 lists doses and toxicities of major antineoplastic agents used in lymphoma.

Stage IIIB. The treatment most often used is four to six cycles of ABVD chemotherapy, followed by involved-field or total nodal radiation. Six cycles of MOPP/ABVD or two cycles following complete remission is also commonly used. Low-dose (25 Gy) radiation can be administered to areas of bulky disease.

Stage IVA and B. A minimum of six cycles or two cycles beyond complete remission of MOPP/ABVD or ABVD is commonly used. Low-dose radiation to the areas of bulky involvement may improve results.

Radiation Fields Commonly Used in the Treatment of HD

1. Subtotal nodal or lymphoid radiation: mantle and spade fields; used for stages IA, IIA, and pathologic stage IIB.
2. Total nodal or lymphoid radiation: mantle and inverted-Y fields; used for stages IIB and IIIA.
3. Involved field radiation: only for sites of known disease; used in combination with chemotherapy.

The most common immediate side effects from the chemotherapy regimens used for the treatment of HD include marrow suppression, nausea and vomiting, oral mucositis, and alopecia. Procarbazine in MOPP produces an MAO-inhibitor-like effect and patients should be warned to avoid the foods and medications that potentiate hypertension with this class of drugs. Vincristine and vinblastine can both produce peripheral neuropathy, although it is much more common with vincristine than with vinblastine. Vinorelbine can also produce mild peripheral neuropathy. Hemolytic anemia can be seen with advanced disease. Combination chemotherapy is the best way to manage this complication, although if the patient is receiving radiation alone, corticosteroids may be used.

TABLE 46–12. Common Combination Chemotherapy Regimens

Regimen	Description
ABVD (nonalkylating)	Doxorubicin, bleomycin, vinblastine, dacarbazine; the "gold standard" for HD treatment Toxicities: less leukemogenic than MOPP, sterility not seen
MOPP (alkylating)	Nitrogen mustard, vincristine, procarbazine, prednisone Toxicities: marrow (dose-limiting), sterility, secondary myelodysplasia and AML
MOPP-ABV ("hybrid")	Nitrogen mustard, vincristine, procarbazine, prednisone, doxorubicin, bleomycin, vinblastine
ChlVPP (alkylating)	Chlorambucil, vinblastine, procarbazine, prednisone
VBM (nonalkylating)	Vinblastine, bleomycin, methotrexate
MOPP-ABVD	Alternating monthly cycles
EVA (nonalkylating)	Etoposide, vinblastine, doxorubicin (effective in MOPP-resistant patients)
MVPP (alkylating)	Mustargen, vinblastine, procarbazine, prednisolone

Follow-Up

Response to therapy should be evaluated near the completion of therapy. This evaluation should be based on clinical and laboratory findings as well as reimaging areas known to have disease at diagnosis. It is important to note that residual radiographic abnormalities following irradiation to an area may persist for months to years following treatment and represent necrosis or fibrosis rather than disease. However, if abnormalities persist following chemotherapy alone, they may represent residual disease. Serial imaging tests such as MRI, CT scanning, and gallium scanning may help determine whether the area is improving or progressing. Suspicious lesions should be biopsied.

Following therapy, patients should be seen every 2 to 3 months during the first and second year, every 4 months in the third year, every 6 months in the fourth and fifth years, and annually thereafter. Follow-up studies should focus on known sites of disease at diagnosis. Patients who are disease-free for over 10 years after treatment may be considered cured. Most relapses occur within the first 3 to 4 years after therapy.

Long-term complications are common and should be assessed regularly. Common complications include hypothyroidism in 10 to 20% of patients who receive mantle radiation. Sterility occurs following pelvic radiation and in men who received MOPP. Oral contraception during treatment may reduce the incidence of ovarian failure. Pneumonitis can occur following mantle radiation. Lung fibrosis occurs in 10 to 15% of patients who receive more than 200 mg/m^2 of bleomycin. Cardiac failure and cardiomegaly can develop if Adriamycin is used, particularly if a cumulative dose of more than 550 mg/m^2 is used or in combination with radiation to the chest. Mediastinal radiation can lead to pericarditis, pericardial effusions, premature coronary artery disease, and myocardial fibrosis. Avascular necrosis of femoral heads, knees, or ankles—and less commonly of the upper extremity joints—can develop following prolonged use of prednisone such as with MOPP. Cell-mediated immunity is depressed for years following treatment with MOPP and/or radiation and predisposes patients to serious infections as well as secondary neoplasms. Secondary leukemias may develop following treatment for HD. The highest risk of acute leukemia seems to be in patients who received MOPP chemotherapy plus radiation. Nearly 11% of these patients develop AML within twelve years of treatment. The risk is 2 to 6% if chemotherapy alone is used. The use of ABVD does not seem to substantially increase the risk of secondary malignancies. NHL, epithelial tumors, and sarcomas have also been linked to HD treatment.

TABLE 46–13. Dose and Toxicity of Major Antineoplastic Agents for Lymphomas

Class	Dose[a] (mg/m2)	Dose Frequency	Acute Toxicity: Leukocyte	Acute Toxicity: Platelet	Acute Toxicity: Nausea and Vomiting	Other Toxicity
Tubulin Binding Agents						
Paclitaxel	130–250 IV	q 3 wk	Marked	Moderate	Mild	Anaphylactoid response, sensory neuropathy, alopecia
Vincristine	1–1.4 IV	q wk	Mild	Mild	Mild	Distal neuropathy, inappropriate ADH
Vinblastine	6 IV	q wk	Marked	Moderate-Marked	Mild	Mucositis
Topoisomerase II Inhibitors						
Etoposide	100–200 IV	q 3–4 wk	Moderate	Mild	Mild	Mucositis
Mitoxantrone	12–14 IV	q 3–4 wk	Marked	Moderate	Mild	Cholestasis, cardiac
Doxorubicin	25–75 IV	q 3–4 wk	Marked	Marked	Moderate	Alopecia, cardiomyopathy
Idarubicin	10–15 IV	q 3–4 wk	Marked	Marked	Moderate	Alopecia, mucositis, cardiomyopathy
Antimetabolites						
Methotrexate	100–400 IV	q 3–4 wk	Moderate-marked	Moderate	Mild	Stomatitis
Cytarabine (cytosine arabinoside)	300–4000 IV	q 3–4 wk	Marked	Marked	Moderate	Cholestasis, mucositis, neurotoxicity
Deoxycoformycin	4 IV	q 1–2 wk	Mild	Mild	Mild	Neurotoxicity (at high doses), conjunctivitis
2-Chloro-2′-deoxyadenosine	4 IV	qd × 7	Mild	Moderate	Mild	Immune suppression
Fludarabine	20–25 IV	qd × 5	Moderate-marked	Mild	Mild	Neurotoxicity, stomatitis, hepatitis
Alkylating Agents						
Cyclophosphamide	350–1500 IV	q 3–4 wk	Marked	Mild	Moderate	Cystitis, pulmonary fibrosis, water retention
Ifosfamide	1000 IV	qd × 5 with mesna	Moderate-marked	Moderate	Mild	Nephrotoxicity, cystitis, neurotoxicity
Mechlorethamine	6 IV	q 2–4 wk	Marked	Moderate	Moderate	Leukemia
Chlorambucil	1–3 po	qd	Moderate	Moderate	Mild	Leukemia
Dacarbazine	150 IV	qd × 5	Mild	Mild	Marked	Flu-like syndrome, venoocclusive disease
Procarbazine	100 po	qd × 7–14 d	Moderate	Moderate	Mild	Sensitivity to amines, sterility, leukemia
CCNU	100–150 po	q 4 wk	Marked	Marked	Moderate	Leukemia, pulmonary fibrosis, renal failure
Miscellaneous						
Bleomycin	5–10 IV	q 2–4 wk	Rare	Rare	Mild	Skin, pulmonary fibrosis, fever, hypersensitivity reactions
Cisplatin	50–100 IV	q 3–4 wk	Mild	Moderate	Severe	Renal failure, Mg^{2+} wasting, peripheral neuropathy, anemia

[a] Doses per cycle are typical of those used in combination regimens, but appropriate modification must be made depending on other drugs used, organ dysfunction, and other considerations.

Adapted by permission from Wilson & Chabner. (1998).

Children with HD have the added problem of impaired growth, impaired sexual maturation due to gonadal failure, and relatively longer period to develop secondary malignancies. ABVD, MOPP/ABVD, or COP (cyclophosphamide, vincristine, and procarbazine)/ABVD for six monthly cycles, followed by low-dose radiation has been highly successful for children with HD who have not yet attained full growth. The problems of impaired growth and development are lower with these combined modality treatments than with the standard adult combination chemotherapy regimens.

Relapse. If relapse of disease occurs after primary treatment with radiation therapy, most clinicians treat with systemic chemotherapy. Failure to respond to primary treatment with radiation therapy should be followed by systemic chemotherapy, preferably Adriamycin-containing regimen, such as ABVD. Patients who relapse more than 1 year after achieving a CR can be retreated with the initial chemotherapy regimen. However, patients who relapse less than 1 year after completing chemotherapy or whose disease progresses during chemotherapy treatment show signs of drug resistance and should be treated with a noncross-resistant regimen. Regimens for patients resistant to MOPP and ABVD generally contain etoposide, lomustine, or vinorelbine.

High-dose chemotherapy with or without radiation followed by autologous stem-cell transplant is another salvage therapy. The response rate depends on the initial response and the timing of relapse and ranges from 15 to 30% DFS in patients who are refractory to initial treatment and up to 80% in patients who relapse more than 12 months after achieving a CR (Bonadonna et al., 1996).

Multiple Myeloma

Pathophysiology

Multiple myeloma (MM) is one of the plasma-cell dyscrasias. It is characterized by uncontrolled malignant proliferation of plasma cells in the bone marrow or tissues. In most cases these malignant cells make an excess amount of monoclonal immunoglobulin (IgG, IgA, IgD, IgE) or kappa or lambda light chains. The malignant transformation occurs in the pre-B cell population or perhaps as early as the stem-cell level. IL-6 is the major myeloma growth factor thought to be essential for myeloma-cell proliferation. Because of this, IL-6 and its receptor are a target for treatments aimed at blocking myeloma-cell proliferation. The failure of natural killer cells and T-cells to regulate B-cells may also be a factor in the development of MM. Other cytokines can suppress normal immunoglobulin production, leading to infections.

History and Physical Findings

Myeloma can present at almost any age, but the incidence rises with age. The mean age at diagnosis is 60 years. It is more common in men and in African-Americans. The clinical manifestations of myeloma are related to tumor growth and the associated bone destruction, effects of the paraprotein in the serum or the kidney with proteinuria and renal disease, marrow infiltration, leading to marrow failure, and immunosuppression caused by hypogammaglobulinemia (Joshua & Gibson, 1996). Bone pain is the most common presenting symptom. Bone pain should not be ignored, as it may be the site of a pathologic fracture. Lytic bone lesions due to tumor infiltration with active dissolution of bone and are generally found in the axial skeleton and proximal ends of the long bones. Compression fractures of the vertebral bodies or myeloma infiltration of the vertebrae or pelvic bones cause back pain. Carefully palpate and percuss the spine to determine if there are specific areas of spinal tenderness. Extradural plasmacytomas or direct extension of a vertebral tumor into the spinal canal can lead to spinal cord compression, a medical emergency. Once paraplegia develops as a result of spinal cord compression, it is usually not reversible. Pathologic fractures of ribs are often caused by coughing due to respiratory tract infections. Punched-out lytic lesions are often seen in the skull with MRI. Cranial plasmacytomas can sometimes be palpated. Hypercalcemia is usually associated with extensive bone destruction and can become a medical emergency if not detected early. Myeloma cells can invade the pleura, causing pleuritic symptoms.

As multiple myeloma develops, monoclonal proteins (M-proteins) are released into the circulation. They cause a variety of problems, including hyperviscosity, a decreased anion gap, and increased plasma volume with pseudohyponatremia. The clinical presentation of hyperviscosity syndrome includes blurred vision, lassitude, confusion, obtundation, and loss of consciousness, and constitutes an indication for immediate plasmapheresis. Hemorrhage from a hyperviscosity-associated coagulopathy can also be seen. M-proteins can have antibody activity against red cells, clotting factors, and immunoglobulins. The M-proteins are thought to be causative agents in the peripheral neuropathies seen in myeloma.

Anemia is common and is thought to be multifactorial. Likely causes include marrow infiltration, renal dysfunction, and anemia of chronic disease. Pancytopenia can occur with advanced disease infiltrating the marrow.

Recurrent infections cause significant morbidity and mortality. Pneumococcal pneumonia is common. The most widely accepted causes of this increased susceptibility to infections are thought to be depression of normal immunoglobulin synthesis and an impaired response to antigens.

Approximately 50% of patients with MM develop renal dysfunction. More than a quarter of patients have renal failure at diagnosis. Deposition of Bence Jones proteins (immunoglobulin light chains) in the proximal tubules and hypercalcemia are thought to be the major culprits. Dehydration, uric acid nephropathy, infection, and amyloidosis also contribute to renal dysfunction.

Laboratory and Diagnostic Tests

Laboratory tests should include CBC with differential, renal function tests, LDH, calcium, uric acid, C-reactive protein (CRP), β-2 microglobulin, electrophoresis to detect the presence of monoclonal proteins in the serum (SPEP) and Bence Jones proteins in the urine (UPEP), and serum quantitative immunoglobulin. Immunofixation is used to investigate the abnormal bands detected by electrophoresis. It is important to determine the presence, type, and amount of monoclonal protein in the serum and urine. A large monoclonal peak (greater than 3 g/dL) and/or large amounts of Bence Jones proteins in the urine, along with reduced levels of other immunoglobulins, are usually indicative of MM. A 24-hour urine for creatinine clearance and total urine protein should be collected if the renal function is abnormal or Bence Jones proteins are present in the urine.

MRI is the preferable imaging technique to determine the presence of lytic lesions. Special attention should be given to all areas of bone pain or tenderness that are weight-bearing to identify or rule out pathologic fractures.

Marrow biopsy and aspiration should be done to determine the extent of marrow involvement. Generally, a plasmacytosis greater than 10% is present.

The three minimum criteria for the diagnosis of multiple myeloma as recommended by the Chronic Leukemia and Myeloma Task Force of the National Cancer Institute are: (1) the presence of monoclonal globulin with, (2) plasmacytosis of more than 5% on either bone marrow aspirate or tissue biopsy, and (3) osteolytic lesions unexplained by other causes (Joshua & Gibson, 1996).

Staging is based on the Durie–Salmon staging system and is one tool in determining prognosis (see Table 46–14).

Prognosis. Prognostic factors include the intrinsic proliferative capacity of the myeloma clone, tumor mass, renal function, and host-tumor interactions. The intrinsic proliferative capacity of the myeloma clone is measured by the plasma cell labeling index (PCLI), the serum thymidine kinase (STK) level, and the morphologic appearance of the cell. The most commonly used indicators of tumor mass are the β2 microglobulin and the staging system described earlier.

TABLE 46–14. Durie–Salmon Staging Criteria

Stage	Criteria	Median Survival
I Low Tumor Mass	All of the following: Hemoglobin > 10 g/dL Normal serum calcium Normal bone structure or solitary plasmacytoma on radiologic evaluation Low M component: IgG < 5 g/dL; IgA < 3 g/dL Bence Jones < 4 g/24-hour urine collection	
II Intermediate Tumor Mass	Findings do not fit either stage I or stage III	
III High Tumor Mass	One or more of the following: Hemoglobin <8.5 g/dL Calcium >12 mg/dL Extensive skeletal destruction and major fractures High M component: IgG > 7 g/dL; IgA > 5 g/dL Bence Jones > g/24-hour urine collection	
	Subclassifications	
A	Relatively normal renal function with creatinine < 2.0 mg/dL	
B	Abnormal renal function with creatinine ≥ 2.0 mg/dL	

Note: Staging of multiple myeloma is based on the Durie–Salmon staging system and is one tool in determining prognosis.
Adapted by permission from Greip & Kyle. (1996). (p. 538).

Management

Multiple myeloma is both chemotherapy and radiotherapy sensitive. The first major decision regarding treatment is when to begin. Patients in stage I, typically a smoldering myeloma, do not seem to benefit from early treatment and it can be delayed until the disease begins to show signs of progression with results similar to those of patients with symptomatic myeloma that are treated at presentation. Patients with solitary plasmacytomas of the bone respond well to local radiation with a usual dose of 40 to 50 Gy. Radiation is also used to alleviate bony pain, particularly those with vertebral column involvement and for pathologic fractures after fixation.

Patients who have more advanced disease, with hypercalcemia, myeloma-induced renal dysfunction, severe anemia, and recurrent infections in the setting of hypogammaglobulinemia, benefit from immediate treatment with chemotherapy. This is followed by local radiation if bony lesions are present. Standard treatment consists of melphalan and prednisone. However, because melphalan is excreted by the kidneys, it presents a problem for patients with renal failure. The dose must be adjusted for renal function. This regimen can be marrow suppressive in older patients. Cyclophosphamide also has good activity against myeloma. It has myelotoxicity, and can cause hemorrhagic cystitis. Vincristine is used in several of the myeloma regimens but its value as an active agent against myeloma is doubtful.

Combination therapy appears to have an advantage over single-agent chemotherapy. Commonly used regimens are VAD (vincristine, adriamycin, dexamethasone), VBMCP (vincristine, BCNU, melphalan, cyclophosphamide, prednisone), VMCP/VBAP (vincristine, melphalan, cyclophosphamide, prednisone alternating with vincristine, BCNU, adriamycin, prednisone), ABCM (adriamycin, BCNU, cyclophosphamide, melphalan), and PCAB (prednisone, cyclophosphamide, Adriamycin, BCNU).

The achievement of the plateau phase, a period of tumor quiescence in which the malignant clone appears dormant, is linked to survival. The plateau phase is defined as three to six months of clinical stability, stable paraprotein levels, and transfusion independence. Once patients achieve this plateau phase, continued chemotherapy does not appear to be of benefit; rather, continued treatment with alkylating agents can increase the likelihood of secondary leukemia. Interferon-α (IFN-α) appears to have activity in myeloma and has been used with chemotherapy in alternating regimens, following attainment of CR, and as a salvage regimen in patients who do not respond to alkylators. It has been found to prolong the response duration when used as a maintenance agent following chemotherapy, but it has not been shown to improve survival.

Unfortunately, none of these treatments are curative at conventional doses. Fewer than 5% of patients with MM survive to 10 years. The only curative regimen appears to be allogeneic marrow or stem-cell transplantation with a 30 to 34% DFS at 4 to 5 years (Joshua & Gibson, 1996). However, it is unclear when allogeneic transplantation should be performed: at diagnosis, after achieving the plateau phase, or at the earliest signs of progression. Autologous transplants are less toxic and the remission rate can be high depending on the pretransplant regimen. However, the relapse rate is higher than with allogeneic transplants.

Treatments currently under investigation include monoclonal antibodies against IL-6, the use of purged autologous marrow, positive selection of stem cells during autologous peripheral blood stem cell collections, and the use of modulating agents against multidrug resistance.

Follow-Up

Few patients are cured of multiple myeloma; thus, progression of disease and its complications are common. Some of the common problems encountered as the disease progresses include lytic bone lesions with pathological fractures, hypercalcemia, hyperviscosity, cryoglobulinemia, renal failure, infections, marrow failure, and anemia.

The axial skeleton is particularly prone to destruction by lytic bone lesions. Any complaints of pain should prompt a thorough investigation for fractures or for lytic lesions that have the potential for pathologic fractures. Epidural cord compression from vertebral fractures is a potential medical emergency that can lead to paralysis if not treated promptly. Pain management is crucial as bony lesions and fractures are quite painful until treated or surgically stabilized. Bisphosphonates may reduce the risk of fractures and hypercalcemia.

Approximately 50% of patients will develop hypercalcemia at some time during the course of their disease. The manifestations of hypercalcemia include polyuria, thirst, constipation, lethargy, clouding of consciousness, nausea, and vomiting. The measured calcium level should be corrected for the level of serum albumin. Patients with significant hypercalcemia should be vigorously hydrated with intravenous fluids and given loop diuretics to enhance calcium excretion. Avoid dyazide diuretics. High-dose corticosteroids and bisphosphonates are very effective in reducing high calcium levels.

Anemia is common. Many patients respond to erythropoietin, particularly early in the disease process. If there is no response, red-cell transfusions may be necessary.

Renal failure in multiple myeloma has multiple causes, described earlier. The only effective treatment is control of the disease with chemotherapy, which can also be renal toxic. Renal function must be monitored closely.

Infections are common, particularly sinusitis and pneumonia. *Streptococcus pneumoniae* and *staphylococcus aureus* are the most common pathogens. Intravenous immunoglobulin is recommended in those patients who are severely hypogammaglobulinemic.

Plasma exchange is the treatment of choice for hyperviscosity, repeated as frequently as needed.

▶ BLOOD COAGULATION

Anatomy and Physiology

The normal hemostatic system is designed to protect against bleeding from injured blood vessels. Hemostasis is usually accomplished by a combination of three sequential and interrelated processes involving blood vessels, platelets, and coagulation proteins. This complex system is highly regulated to ensure that clotting occurs only at a site of injury and only as long as the integrity of the vessel is compromised. The clotting processes are balanced by the complex mechanism of fibrinolysis, which breaks down clots and maintains or reestablishes blood flow once the vessel injury has healed. The balance between these two mechanisms and their activators and inhibitors is vital. An imbalance in one direction results in excessive bleeding, whereas an imbalance in the other direction results in excessive clotting. The following section presents the normal sequence of coagulation and fibrinolysis, as well as selected bleeding disorders.

Vascular Phase

The vascular phase refers to several instantaneous compensatory responses that occur when a vessel is injured. The initial vascular reaction to injury is constriction of vascular smooth muscle that limits blood loss. Contraction of precapillary sphincters may control capillary bleeding. Blood loss is also controlled by the apposition of surrounding tissues and by increased pressure of interstitial fluid as blood leaks from the vessel into the interstitium.

Platelet Phase

The platelet phase refers to the formation of a soft mass of aggregated platelets that provides a temporary patch over the injured, bleeding vessel. Almost immediately after vascular injury, platelets begin to adhere to the exposed subendothelial basement membrane and collagen fibers (Jandl, 1996). Adherent platelets release adenosine diphosphate (ADP), which causes platelets to change from their normal shape into a spherical form with pseudopods, become sticky, and aggregate, thus increasing the size of the platelet plug. ADP and collagen trigger arachidonic acid formation which is required for the formation of thromboxane A_2, a substance that induces further platelet aggregation. Ultimately, aggregated platelets plug the injured vessel. The dual processes of vascular constriction and platelet plug formation are responsible for initial hemostasis in minor injuries. Activated platelets in turn activate the clotting cascade.

Coagulation Phase

The final phase of hemostasis is the formation of a fibrin clot. The coagulation process is most commonly viewed as a series of enzymatic reactions in which clotting factors are sequentially activated and is known as the clotting cascade. The clotting factors are all present in the circulating blood in their inactive form until a stimulus for clot formation occurs. Twelve different substances have been identified as major clotting factors. All of the clotting factors except factor VIII are produced by the liver. Four of the clotting factors require the presence of vitamin K for their production: factors II (prothrombin), VII, IX, and X. Calcium is required for most of the reactions of the clotting cascade.

The coagulation process can be initiated by two different pathways: the extrinsic mechanism, the rapid tissue-derived pathway; and the intrinsic mechanism, the slower, more complex, surface-mediated set of reactions. The pathways are known to interact *in vivo* and in all probability synergize each other's activities. Both pathways must be intact for normal hemostasis to occur. Both extrinsic and intrinsic mechanisms eventually lead to the activation of factor X, with the remaining steps of the coagulation sequence being identical. The sequence of the coagulation process is shown in Figure 46–4. A schematic view of primary hemostasis is shown in Figure 46–5.

Differentiation between the two pathways is helpful in isolating and understanding pathologic mechanisms, medication actions, and coagulation tests. The function of the extrinsic pathway is tested in the laboratory by the prothrombin time (PT). Because the intrinsic pathway involves a greater number of interactions, coagulation initiated by this process proceeds more slowly than that initiated by the extrinsic pathway. The function of the intrinsic pathway is commonly analyzed by the partial thromboplastin time (PTT).

The final common sequence results in a loose web of fibers that is capable of stopping the bleeding in small and medium-sized arteries and veins. Plasminogen and other components of the fibrinolytic mechanism are incorporated into the fibrin clot as it solidifies.

Coagulation is regulated by three major mechanisms: the elimination of activated clotting factors, protease inhibitors which inhibit coagulation, and the destruction of the fibrin clot. Activated clotting factors are rapidly cleared by the liver, a protective mechanism that prevents activated clotting factors in the circulation from starting clots in inappropriate sites. They are also inactivated by antithrombin III and the protein C–protein S system. Antithrombin III is the major inhibitor of thrombin and factor Xa. Heparin anticoagulation works through its interaction with antithrombin III. Individuals with an inherited deficiency of antithrombin III are prone to develop venous thromboembolism. Protein C neutralizes factors V and VIII with the help of an accelerator, protein S. The fibrinolytic system, described in more detail below, degrades the fibrin clot. Finally, endothelial cells regulate coagulation by a number of activities, including synthesis of a prostaglandin and an enzyme that inhibit platelet function.

Fibrinolysis

The removal of clots when the vessel injury has healed is as important as the formation of the clot itself. The process of fibrinolysis maintains or reestablishes blood flow. Of the numerous mechanisms known to result in fibrinolysis, the

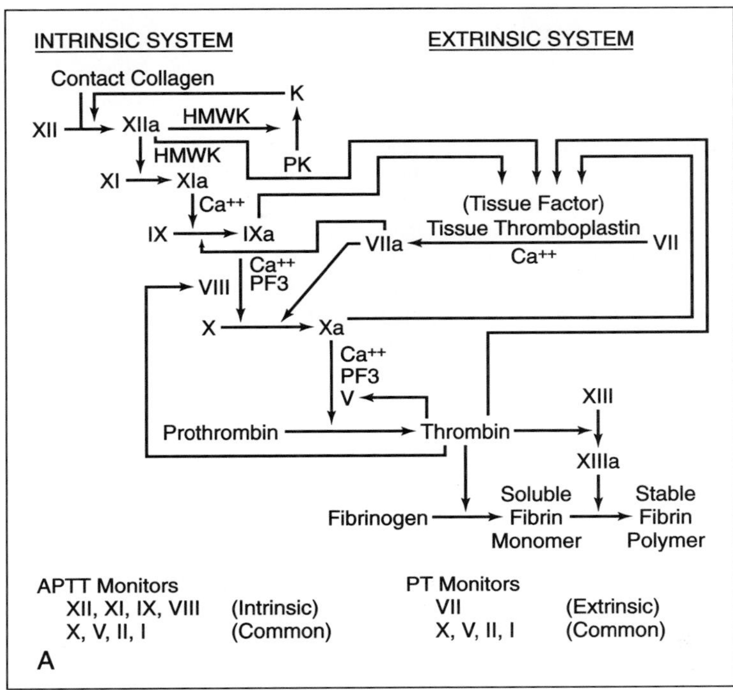

Figure 46–4. The intrinsic and extrinsic pathways of the "cascade" theory of coagulation. *(By permission from Harmening & Lemery. [1997]. [p. 495].)*

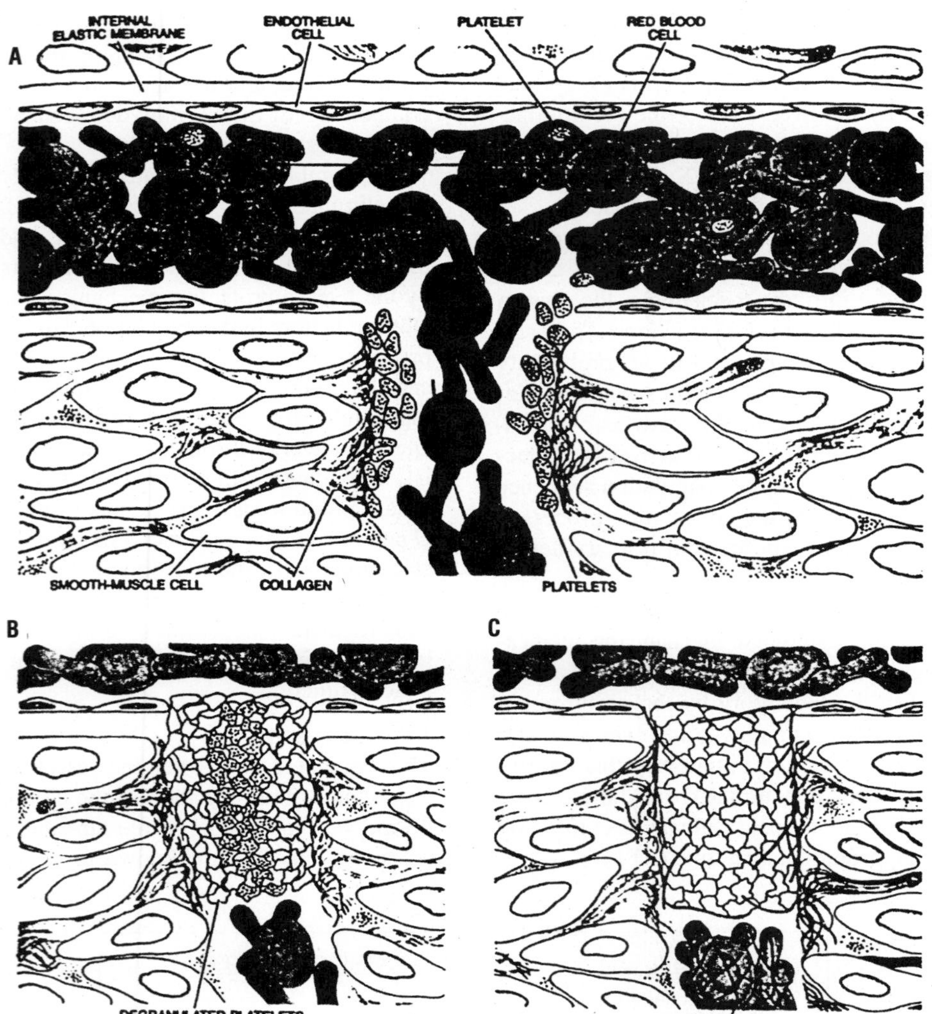

Figure 46–5. Schematic review of primary hemostasis and formation of the platelet plug. As blood begins to flow out through a gap in the vessel wall, platelets in the presence of vWF adhere to collagen fibrils in the subendothelium **(A)**. Exposure to subendothelial agonists causes platelet shape changes and adhesion, upregulation of fibrinogen receptors, and initiation of the arachidonate and phosphoinositide secretory and signaling pathways. Secretion of platelet granules causes other passing platelets to adhere to the sticky first layer, building up a loose platelet plug **(B)**. Meanwhile, prothrombinase and tenase (Xase) complexes form and convert prothrombin to thrombin. Thrombin binds to its receptors and converts both plasma and platelet-bound fibrinogen into fibrin strands **(C)**, after which thrombin receptors are internalized. These strands form a meshwork that consolidates the platelet plug and draws the platelets into a firm, if temporary, seal. *(From Zucker. [1980]. Copyright 1980 by Scientific American, Inc. All rights reserved.)*

process mediated by plasmin is considered to be of greatest significance. Plasmin is found only in minute quantities in plasma, but its precursor, plasminogen, is normally abundant. Plasminogen is believed to be synthesized by the liver. Fibrinolysis is controlled by the complex interplay of substances that activate plasminogen with substances that prevent its activation. The best known activator is tissue plasminogen activator (tPA). Under normal circumstances, the balance is in favor of those substances that prevent activation, thus favoring clot stability. A schematic diagram of the fibrinolytic mechanism is shown in Figure 46–6.

Fragments of the fibrin clot, known as fibrin degradation products (FDPs), are released into the circulation as the clot is broken down. Fibrin degradation products are potent inhibitors of coagulation, which act by binding to thrombin, and by interfering with the binding of fibrin threads to form the fibrin clot. Generally, fibrin degradation products are present in such small numbers that their anticoagulant effect is not clinically important. However, the level of FDPs rises in circumstances that involve massive coagulation and fibrinolysis such as occurs with disseminated intravascular coagulation (DIC) and in fact is a marker for this disorder.

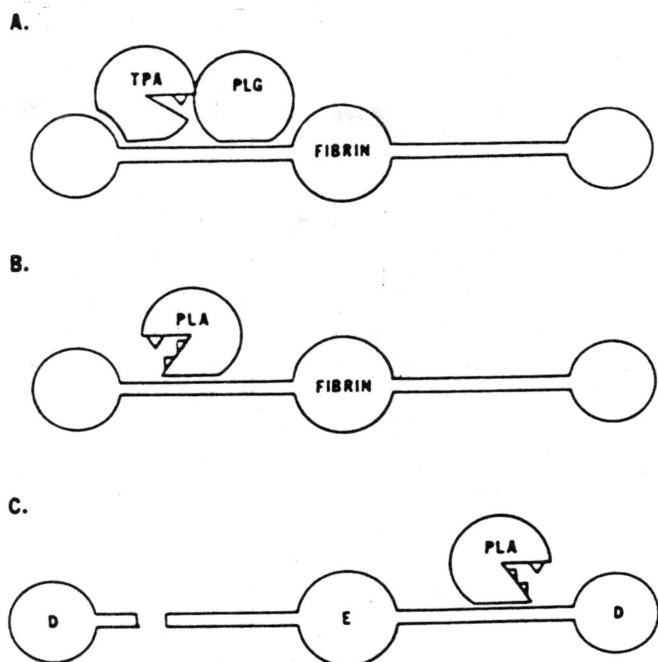

Figure 46–6. Schematic diagram of the fibrinolytic system. **A,** Both tissue plasminogen activator (TPA), derived from endothlial cells, and plasminogen (PLG) are incorporated into the matrix of a fibrin clot. In the presence of fibrin, which functions as a cofactor, TPA rapidly activates plasminogen to plasmin (PLA). **B** and **C,** Plasmin then degrades the fibrin monomer, releasing the fibrin degradation products D and E. Plasmin can be inhibited by α_2-antiplasmin, which is also present in the clot matrix, but this depends on the same binding site involved in the interaction of plasmin and fibrin. Thus, as long as the plasmin remains bound to fibrin, it will remain active. *(Brandt. [1985].)*

Bleeding Disorders

Abnormal bleeding occurs when the intricate relationship between the various elements in the hemostatic system is disturbed. Numerous defects in the hemostatic system are possible. Furthermore, many drugs inhibit hemostasis as the intended drug action or as a side effect. Bleeding disorders are usually categorized as vascular, platelet, or coagulation abnormalities. They are listed in Table 46–15. In each, bleeding is the primary manifestation.

The bleeding may be minor, such as petechiae and easy bruising of the skin, or major, with massive hemorrhage. If bleeding is spontaneous or occurs for a prolonged period of time following trauma or surgery, suspect an abnormality in the hemostatic system. Delayed, prolonged bleeding or significant deep tissue bleeding, such as muscle and soft tissue hematomas, or hemarthroses, suggests a coagulation cascade abnormality. Skin and mucosal bleeding, such as petechiae and purpura, suggest platelet problems, either quantitative or qualitative. Ecchymoses, especially in different stages of healing, can indicate either a platelet or coagulation factor abnormality. Oozing or bleeding from old puncture sites or wounds may indicate problems with platelets, inadequate coagulation factors, and increased fibrinolytic activity as is seen in DIC. The initial screening tests should include the PT, INR, PTT, and platelet count. If these tests are normal, measure the bleeding time, which is a measure of platelet function. Table 46–16 campares several common causes of bleeding disorders by their associated laboratory abnormalities. The remainder of this chapter will discuss some common defects in platelet and clotting factor abnormalities.

Thrombocytopenia

Pathophysiology. Thrombocytopenia is defined as a platelet count of less than 150,000/mm^3. Spontaneous bleeding can occur when the platelet count falls below 10,000/mm^3. Bleeding is likely if invasive procedures are performed at platelet counts lower than 50,000/mm^3 or if surgery is performed at platelet counts lower than 80,000/mm^3.

History and Physical Findings. The history should include a thorough drug history, including recent chemotherapy, and a history of recent transfusions. Ask about recent episodes of hemorrhage that required transfusions. Look for splenomegaly and petechiae on the physical exam.

Laboratory and Diagnostic Tests. The work-up of severe thrombocytopenia should include a marrow aspiration and biopsy to evaluate marrow function. A decreased number of megakaryocytes in the marrow indicates a lower-than-normal production of platelets. This could be due to medications such as gold, sulfonamides, ethanol, and thiazides. Viral infections such as cytomegalovirus, influenza,

TABLE 46–15. Disorders of Hemostasis

I. Platelet disorders
  A. Quantitative platelet disorders
    1. Thrombocytopenia
      a. Diminished or defective platelet production
        i. Inherited (Fanconi syndrome, amegakaryocytic thrombocytopenia, hereditary thrombocytopenia)
        ii. Acquired (aplastic anemia, marrow inflitration, ionizing radiation, myelosuppressive drugs, megakaryocytic aplasia, viral infections, drugs (alcohol, thiazide diuretics), nutritional deficiencies (vitamin B_{12}, folic acid)
      b. Nonimmune platelet destruction
        Thrombotic thrombocytopenic purpura-hemolytic-uremic syndrome (TTP-HUS), pregnancy, infection, Kasabach-Merritt syndrome, drug-induced, venomous snake bites, acute respiratory distress syndrome (ARDS), severe burns, cardiopulmonary bypass, severe aortic stenosis
      c. Immune platelet destruction
        Idiopathic thrombocytopenic purpura (ITP), HIV infection, cyclic thrombocytopenia, drug-induced, heparin-induced, posttransfusion purpura
      d. Platelet sequestration
        Hypersplenism, hypothermia
      e. Loss of platelets due to massive transfusion
      f. Pseudothrombocytopenia
    2. Thrombocytosis
      a. Primary
        Essential thrombocythemia, other myeloproliferative disorders
      b. Secondary (reactive)
        Malignant disease, inflammatory disorders, acute blood loss, iron deficiency, hemolytic anemia, splenectomy, response to drugs, response to exercise, recovery from thrombocytopenia, prematurity, vitamin E deficiency in infants
  B. Qualitative platelet disorders
    1. Inherited
      a. Glycoprotein (GP) abnormalities
        Glanzmann thrombasthenia, Bernard-Soulier syndrome, pseudo-von Willebrand disease, Wiskott-Aldrich syndrome,
      b. Granule abnormalities
        storage pool deficiencies, gray platelet syndrome
      c. Abnormalities of platelet coagulant activity
      d. Abnormalities of signal transduction and secretion
        Defects in arachidonic acid metabolism, thromboxane
        A2 sensitivity, calcium mobilization, and calcium responsiveness
    2. Acquired
      Uremia, antiplatelet antibodies, cardiopulmonary bypass, myeloproliferative disorders, dysproteinemias, drug-induced, liver disease, DIC, Bartter syndrome
II. Vascular disorders
  A. Nonpalpable purpura
    1. Increased transmural pressure gradient
      Valsalva, coughing, vomiting, childbirth, weightlifting, suction purpura, venous stasis high altitude
    2. Decreased integrity of microcirculation
      Senile purpura, glucocorticoid excess, vitamin C dificiency, Ehlers-Danlos syndrome, pseudoxanthoma elasticum, amyloid inflitration of blood vessels, MELAS syndrome (mitochondrial encephalopathy, lactic acidosis, and strokes)
    3. Trauma
      Physical injuries, ultraviolet radiation (sunburn, solar purpura), infectious (bacterial, fungal, viral, parasitic), embolic (infectious organisms, atheroemboli, fat emboli, tumor emboli, calciphylaxis), neoplastic, allergic and/or inflammatory (serum sickness, pigmented purpuric eruptions, contact dermatitis, dysproteinemias, pyoderma gangrenosum, visceral inflammatory disease), toxic chemicals, thrombotic (disseminated intravascular coagulation, coumarin skin necrosis, heparin-associated skin necrosis, protein C or S deficiency, purpura fulminans, paroxysmal nocturnal hemoglobulinuria (PNH), antiphospholipid antibody syndrome, drug related
    4. Unknown (psychogenic purpura, familial Mediterranean fever)
  B. Palpable purpura
    1. Cutaneous vasculitis (Henoch-Schonlein purpura, acute hemorrhagic edema of infancy, collagen vascular disease, systemic vasculitis, hypersensitivity vasculitis, drug-induced vasculitis, infectious vasculitis, paraneoplastic vasculitis)
    2. Dysproteinemias (Cryoglobulenemia, hyperglobulinemic pupura of Waldenstrom, cryofibrinogemenia, lambda light chain vasculopathy)
    3. Primary cutaneous diseases
    4. Papular-purpuric "gloves and socks" syndrome
  C. Disorders with telangiectasia ("petechial" cherry angiomata, Osler-Weber-Rendu disease, CREST syndrome, chronic actinic telangiectasia, chronic liver disease, AIDS-associated telangiectasia, pregnancy-associated telangiectasia, ataxia telangiectasia)
  D. Kaposi sarcoma

(Continued)

TABLE 46–15. Disorders of Hemostasis *(Continued)*

- E. Fabry disease
- F. Extramedullary hematopoiesis
- G. Angioma serpiginosum

III. Disorders of blood coagulation
- A. Congenital
  1. Abnormalities of plasma factors involved in fibrin formation
     a. Deficient or defective synthesis of specific factors (fibrinogen, prothrombin, factors V and VII to XIII)
     b. Deficiency of factors giving abnormal laboratory tests but not clinically significant (factor XII, prekallikrein, high-molecular-weight kininogen
  2. Abnormalities of plasma factors involved in platelet function and in fibrin formation (von Willebrand's disease)
  3. Hereditary multiple factor deficiency syndromes
- B. Acquired vitamin K deficiency, liver disease, amyloidosis, nephrotic syndrome, Gaucher disease, circulating anticoagulants (factor specific immunoglobulins, lupus-type anticoagulant, nonimmunoglobulin inhibitors) defibrination syndromes (disseminated intravascular coagulation, hyperfibrinolysis)

IV. Thrombosis

Adapted from Williams. (1995). (pp. 1279–1280).

mononucleosis, measles (including measles vaccination), dengue fever, and Thai hemorrhagic fever can also result in decreased thrombopoiesis. Aplastic anemia causes marrow failure and involves the other cell lines, leading to anemia and leukopenia along with thrombocytopenia, commonly referred to as pancytopenia. Marrow infiltration by a malignant clone such as in leukemia, lymphoma, myelodysplastic syndrome, myelofibrosis, and metastatic carcinomas affects the ability of the marrow to function normally, and thus affects platelet, red cell, and white cell counts.

If the marrow shows a normal or increased number of megakaryocytes in the presence of thrombocytopenia, the blood smear should be examined for the presence of fragmented red cells, indicating hemolysis. The presence of schistocytes indicates the possibility of a clostridial infection, DIC, thrombotic thrombocytopenic purpura (TTP), hemolytic uremic syndrome (HUS), or destruction by a prosthetic heart valve. Helmet cells on the blood smear are more indicative of G6PD deficiency or pulmonary emboli.

Alloantibodies can be produced when a patient is re-

TABLE 46–16. The Presumptive Diagnosis of Common Bleeding Disorders by the "Primary" Screening Tests

Platelet Count	Bleeding Time	Partial Thromboplastin Time	Prothrombin Time	"Presumptive" Diagnosis	Common Causes: Hereditary	Common Causes: Aquired
Decreased	Prolonged	Normal	Normal	Thrombocytopenia	Aldrich syndrome; others	ITP; drugs; other secondary forms[a]
Normal	Prolonged	Prolonged	Normal	von Willebrand's disease	—	Disseminated lupus erythematosus; inhibitors of VIII_{ag}
Normal or increased	Prolonged	Normal	Normal	Disorder of platelet function	Thrombasthenia; deficient release reaction	Drugs; uremia; dysproteinemias; thrombocythemia
Normal	Normal	Prolonged	Normal	Coagulation abnormality in intrinsic pathway	Hemophilia A or B; deficiency of prekallikrein, HMW kininogen, Passovoy factor, factors XI and XII	Inhibitors of factor VIII_c and of lupus type
Normal[b]	Normal[b]	Prolonged	Prolonged	Coagulation abnormality in common or multiple pathways	Deficiency of factors V, X, prothrombin or fibrinogen; dysfibrinogenemias	Liver disease; vitamin K deficiency; intravascular coagulation; fibrinogenolysis; heparin
Normal	Normal	Normal	Prolonged	Coagulation abnormality in extrinsic pathway	Deficiency of factor VII	—
Normal	Normal	Normal	Normal	—	Deficiency of factor XIII; hereditary telangiectasia	Allergic purpura; scurvy; drugs; autoerythrocyte sensitization

[a] ITP, idiopathic thrombocytopenia purpura.
[b] May be abnormal in acquired disorders that also produce deficiencies of multiple coagulation factors.
Lee, Bithell, Foerster, et al. (ed). (1993). (p. 1315).

ceiving frequent platelet transfusions, resulting in refractoriness to platelet transfusions. Autoantibodies can destroy platelets as they are being produced. Some drugs such as quinidine, quinine, sulfonamides, antithymocyte globulin (ATG), and heparin can result in the development of antiplatelet antibodies. These antibodies can be identified and quantified by special tests. Heparin can induce platelet aggregation as well as antiplatelet antibodies.

Platelets can be destroyed by nonimmune mechanisms such as pulmonary artery catheters, subacute bacterial endocarditis, prosthetic heart valves, severe valvular stenosis, and extracorporeal circulation such as cardiopulmonary bypass. They can be consumed more rapidly than they are produced by concurrent problems such as renal transplant rejection, sepsis, malignant hypertension, toxemia of pregnancy, the hemolytic uremic syndrome (HUS), disseminated intravascular coagulation (DIC), thrombotic thrombocytopenic purpura (TTP), and primary pulmonary hypertension. HUS is characterized by hemolytic anemia, thrombocytopenia, and acute renal failure. TTP is characterized by microangiopathic hemolytic anemia, thrombocytopenia, fluctuating neurological abnormalities, acute renal failure, and fever. The pathological characteristic of TTP is the presence of hyaline microthrombi composed of platelets and fibrin that occlude arterioles and capillaries in multiple organs.

If there is no hemolysis, splenomegaly should be ruled out. Normally, 70 percent of the platelet pool is in the circulation and 30 percent is in the spleen. In splenomegaly, up to 80% of the platelet pool may be sequestered in the spleen.

If the marrow production is normal, or greater than normal, there is no hemolysis on the blood smear, and the spleen is normal in size, platelet destruction due to immune or nonimmune mechanisms is the likely culprit. Some autoimmune diseases such as rheumatoid arthritis, Grave's disease, Hashimoto's thyroiditis, and myasthenia gravis are associated with platelet antibodies and result in thrombocytopenia. Idiopathic throbocytopenic purpura (ITP) is an immune-mediated phenomenon that is often associated with a recent history of a viral illness. It does not cause hemolysis, a fact that helps distinguish it from TTP. The blood smear in ITP shows platelets that are normal in size and normal red and white blood cell morphology. Marrow evaluation is not necessary to diagnose ITP, but may be necessary to rule out other disorders causing thrombocytopenia.

Management. If the patient is thrombocytopenic, any nonessential medication that is known to affect marrow production or platelet destruction should be discontinued. If a viral etiology is suspected, there are some effective antiviral treatments available such as Ganciclovir for cytomegalovirus (CMV) and amantadine for Influenza A. However, the thrombocytopenia may develop weeks after the viral illness, making viral treatment of questionable utility. The treatments of choice for severe aplastic anemia, the leukemias and the lymphomas were described earlier in this chapter. Metastatic carcinoma that is affecting marrow function requires systemic treatment if it is responsive to chemotherapy, unless the patient is in the terminal stages. If the patient is found to have splenomegaly, treating the cause will generally reduce the size of the spleen and thus improve platelet counts. In severe or unresponsive cases, it may be necessary to perform a splenectomy.

ITP often is self-limited in children. From 30 to 70% of children recover without intervention within a few weeks (George et al., 1996). Children with platelet counts over 30,000 generally do not need hospitalization or treatment if they are asymptomatic or only have minor purpura (George et al., 1996). Adults with platelet counts less than 20,000 with bleeding should be hospitalized. If the platelet count in a child is less than 20,000 with bleeding or less than 10,000 with minor bleeding, treatment is necessary. Treatment is also necessary for adult-onset ITP when the platelet count is less than 20,000 and in those with platelet counts less than 50,000 who have significant bleeding or risk of bleeding. Prednisone is the initial treatment of choice. Commonly used regimens include: 1 to 2 mg/kg per day for 21 days in adults or children, 60 mg/m^2 per day (children), or 4 mg/kg per day (children) for 7 days followed by a tapering dose until day 21 (George et al., 1996). The use of high-dose dexamethasone has shown some promise. Intravenous immunoglobulin (IVIg) can also be used as a first-line treatment in severe thrombocytopenia with life-threatening bleeding. Splenectomy can also be effective in carefully selected patients (George et al., 1996). TTP is treated with plasma exchange and high-dose steroids.

Platelet transfusions are indicated only when the platelet count falls below 10,000-15,000/mm^3, thus reducing the number of platelet antigens the patient is exposed to and the incidence of developing alloantibodies. However, if bleeding develops at this level or if an invasive procedure is anticipated, the platelet count should be kept higher with transfusions. Surgery can often be conducted safely with platelet counts higher than 80,000/mm^3. Patients with thrombocytopenia from an autoimmune process should only receive platelets if actually bleeding. Those with platelet alloimmunization due to previous platelet transfusions often respond better to human leukocyte antigen (HLA)-matched platelets.

Follow-Up. Follow-up is dependent on the cause of thrombocytopenia. For example, ITP in children often resolves within 4 to 6 weeks, whereas in adults, it may be a chronic problem, requiring frequent platelet counts and treatment. Thrombocytopenia due to drugs should be monitored until platelet counts return to normal. This may take a few weeks with most medications. Platelet counts should be remeasured if new bleeding episodes occur.

Normal Platelet Count with Prolonged Bleeding Time

Pathophysiology. The bleeding time measures the time to formation of a platelet plug and is not affected by clotting factors. It is abnormally prolonged in thrombocytopenia and with platelet dysfunction. The problem can be congenital with impaired adhesion or aggregation, abnormal platelet factor III, or agranular platelets. It is beyond the scope of this chapter to discuss the congenital problems. Acquired problems with platelet function include uremia, which is thought to be due to a dialyzable inhibitor of platelet function. Medication-induced platelet dysfunction is the most common cause of platelet dysfunction, with salicylates and nonsteroidal antiinflammatory drugs (NSAIDs) being the most common offenders. Aspirin exerts its effects for the life-time of the platelets present at time of ingestion by inhibiting thromboxane A2 synthesis. NSAIDs exert their effect only until the drug is metabolized and excreted. Other drugs that can affect platelet function include some anesthetics, carbenicillin, dextran, plasma expanders, dipyridamole, ethanol, and sulfinpyrazone. Liver disease can also affect platelet function.

History and Physical Findings. As described earlier, a history of previous bleeding, family history, and a drug history are crucial in the evaluation of bleeding. Skin and mucosal bleeding, such as petechiae and purpura, suggest platelet problems. Ecchymoses can indicate either a platelet or coagulation factor abnormality.

Laboratory and Diagnostic Tests. A normal PT, PTT, and platelet count combined with a prolonged bleeding time indicates a problem with platelet function.

Management. All nonessential drugs that have the potential to affect platelet function should be discontinued. Avoid invasive procedures if the drug was ingested in the previous 48 hours, or until the bleeding time has normalized to avoid excessive bleeding.

Follow-Up. The bleeding time should be monitored until it normalizes or becomes stable.

Coagulation Factor Disorders (Prolonged PT and PTT)

The PT measures the function of the extrinsic pathway and thus tests for the presence of factors I, II, V, VII, & X. If the PT is prolonged in isolation, without other abnormalities in coagulation tests, a likely cause is early liver dysfunction which will eventually evolve into prolongation of both the PT and the PTT. Because factor VII has the shortest half-life of all the coagulation factors, early problems with synthesis of the coagulation factors can manifest as isolated factor VII deficiency and isolated prolongation of the PT. However, because factor VII deficiency can be a rare hereditary autosomal dominant trait, the history should include questions regarding family history of abnormal bleeding.

The PTT measures the function of the intrinsic pathway and thus tests for the presence of factors VIII, IX, XI, and XII. Deficiencies of factors VIII, IX, and XI account for the majority of factor deficiencies. The differential diagnosis of isolated prolongation of the PTT includes: circulating anticoagulant; von Willebrand's disease; hemophilia A and B; congenital deficiency of factors XI and XII; congenital deficiency of Fletcher, Passovoy and Fitzgerald Factors; or heparin therapy. It is not in the scope of this chapter to discuss these abnormalities in detail.

Pathophysiology. Prolonged PT and PTT indicates an abnormality in both pathways or in the common pathway. The most common causes are vitamin K deficiency, severe liver disease, heparin therapy, or vitamin K antagonists such as coumadin. Vitamin K is a fat-soluble vitamin produced by the normal gut flora. Vitamin K-dependent coagulation factors are synthesized in the liver. Malabsorption, oral antibiotics, oral anticoagulants, and parenteral hyperalimentation not supplemented with vitamin K can all affect the manufacture, absorption, or action of vitamin K, resulting in the decreased synthesis of these factors.

Circulating antibodies to specific clotting factors, DIC, and congenital fibrinogen disorders can also result in prolongation of the PT and the PTT, but will not be discussed here.

History and Physical Findings. The history should include previous problems with bleeding, a family history, and a drug history. Delayed, prolonged bleeding or significant deep tissue bleeding, such as muscle and soft tissue hematomas, and hemarthroses, suggest a coagulation cascade abnormality. Ecchymoses indicate problems with inadequate coagulation factors, or platelets.

Laboratory and Diagnostic Tests. Antibodies to specific clotting factors can be measured if their presence is suspected. The presence of these antibodies rarely causes significant bleeding. Thrombocytopenia will be present if DIC is the cause of the bleeding. If liver disease is the cause, other liver function tests will be abnormal, as defects in the manufacture of the clotting factors generally occurs with severe liver disease. Fibrinogen levels can be measured to determine whether the defect is one of a congenital fibrinogen disorder.

Management. Treatment is aimed at the specific problem. Patients who are on total parenteral nutrition (TPN) should receive vitamin K weekly to prevent clotting factor abnormalities. Parenteral vitamin K administration takes approximately 4 to 24 hours to show some improvement in the PT and PTT. If the patient is actively bleeding, administration of fresh frozen plasma—which contains all the clotting factors—can restore hemostasis. The treatment of liver dysfunction is aimed at the cause but includes the same management for active bleeding. Coumadin overdose is treated with parenteral vitamin K and with fresh frozen

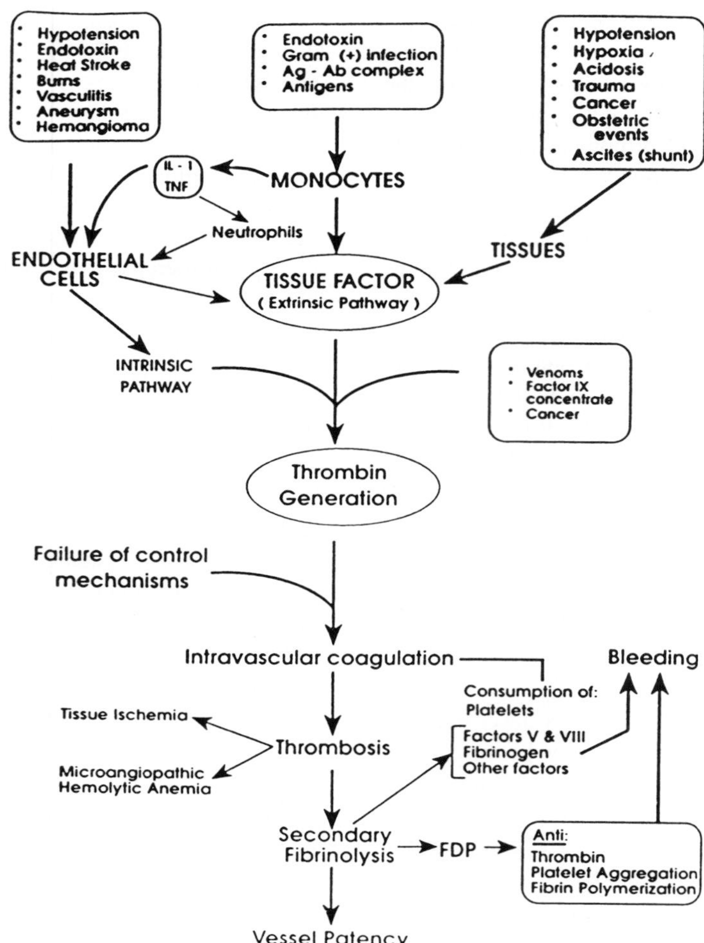

Figure 46–7. Main initiation pathways of DIC and its consequences. Triggers (shown in boxes) can activate (1) the extrinsic coagulation system by tissue factor expressed on cell surfaces; (2) the intrinsic coagulation system by causing injury to endothelial cells; (3) coagulation factors, e.g., factor X by cancer cells, factor II by snake venoms. All of these lead to thrombin generation that in the presence of failure of the control mechanisms results in intravascular coagulation. This in turn, can lead to thrombosis (that may be minimized by triggering secondary fibrinolysis) and to consumption of platelets, fibrinogen, and other coagulant factors. Bleeding can be caused by depletion of these essential hemostatic components; by the anticoagulant effects of fibrinogen/fibrin degradation products; and by further depletion of fibrinogen, factor V, and factor VIII by plasmin if generated in excess by the secondary fibrinolysis or if uninhibited due to diminished antiplasmin levels.

plasma if the patient is actively bleeding. Protamine is administered in cases of heparin overdose.

Follow-Up. The PT and PTT should be measured frequently until normalized or within therapeutic levels.

Combined Disorders

Prolonged PT and PTT with thrombocytopenia is generally caused by DIC, dilutional coagulopathy, or severe liver disease. Severe hepatic dysfunction results in decreased synthesis of all the coagulation factors except the von Willebrand factor. The liver normally clears activated coagulation factors and, in severe liver disease, they accumulate resulting in the tendency to develop DIC. Thrombocytopenia occurs because of the effects of alcohol on the marrow as well as splenomegaly, which is often present.

Dilutional coagulopathy results from large infusions of stored bank blood, or crystalloid solutions. Treatment is geared toward replacement of coagulation factors with fresh frozen plasma (FFP). A rule of thumb is to use one unit of FFP for every five units of bank blood. Platelets are transfused as needed. Cryoprecipitate can be used if the fibrinogen level is less than 100.

Disseminated Intravascular Coagulation. Disseminated intravascular coagulation (DIC) is a pathological syndrome resulting in the indiscriminate formation of fibrin clots throughout all or most of the microvasculature. Paradoxically, diffuse bleeding results and is generally the hallmark sign as clotting factors and platelets are consumed during the widespread coagulation.

Pathophysiology. Inappropriate coagulation results from the introduction of thromboplastic substances into the bloodstream. These thromboplastic substances stimulate clotting despite the lack of actual bleeding. Tissue thromboplastin is released into the circulation by damaged cells in individuals with massive burns, injuries, and systemic infections, particularly gram-negative sepsis. About 50% of patients with DIC have obstetric problems, whereas another 33% have cancer (Kumar et al., 1992). The fetus, placenta, and the amniotic fluid contain thromboplastic substances that are released into the maternal circulation during obstetrical complications such as abruptio placenta and amniotic fluid embolism. Certain malignant tumors release small amounts of thromboplastic material into the circulation, particularly when the disease is disseminated. The most critical time for the development of DIC is during initial treatment with chemotherapy, because the tumor cells are dying and releasing massive amounts of thromboplastic into the circulation. Some malignancies can present with DIC, particularly acute promyelocytic leukemia (APL). Figure 46–7 illustrates various factors that can initiate DIC. Table 46–17 lists these and other disorders associated with DIC.

The two major consequences of DIC are bleeding and organ ischemia (Fig. 46–8). Widespread deposition of fibrin clots in the microcirculation leads to ischemia in organs such as the kidney, liver, brain, and eyes. RBCs are damaged as they pass through the fibrin strands. These damaged RBCs are called schistocytes (refer to Fig. 46–3). As the

TABLE 46–17. Major Disorders Associated with DIC

Obstetric Complications
Abruptio placentae
Retained dead fetus
Septic abortion
Amniotic fluid embolism
Toxemia
Infections
Gram-negative sepsis
Meningococcemia
Rocky Mountain spotted fever
Histoplasmosis
Aspergillosis
Malaria
Neoplasms
Carcinomas of pancreas, prostate, lung, and stomach
Acute promyelocytic leukemia
Massive Tissue Injury
Traumatic
Burns
Extensive surgery
Miscellaneous
Acute intravascular hemolysis, snakebite, giant hemangioma, shock, heat stroke, vasculitis, aortic aneurysm, liver disease

DIC = disseminated intravascular coagulation.
From Cotran, Kumar, & Robbins. (1994). (p. 624).

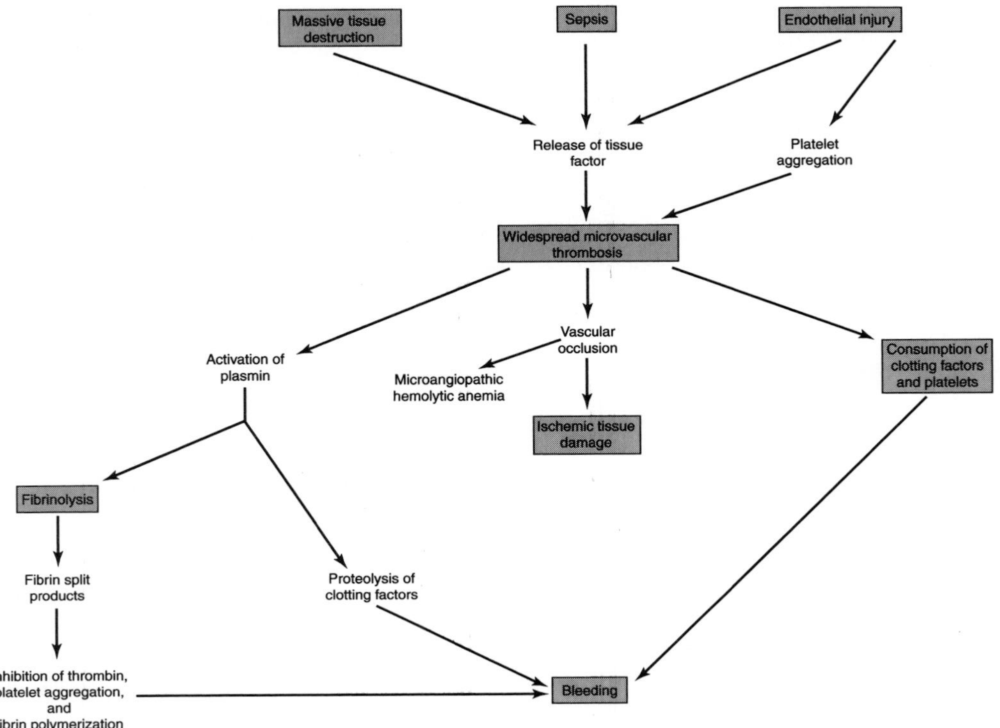

Figure 46–8. Pathophysiology of disseminated intravascular coagulation (DIC). *(From Cotran, Kumar, & Robbins. [1994]. [p. 625].)*

disseminated clotting continues, circulating platelets and clotting factors are consumed, and bleeding ensues. Fibrinolysis is activated as a result of the widespread clotting, yielding abnormally large amounts of circulating fibrin degradation products (FDPs). In these large numbers, FDPs aggravate bleeding because they inhibit platelet aggregation, act as anticoagulants, and impair fibrin polymerization. FDPs are also thought to increase capillary permeability and may contribute to the development of the adult respiratory distress syndrome (ARDS).

History and Physical Findings. Patients who have undergone extracorporeal circulation or thoracic surgery, or who have developed septic shock, hypoxemia, or hypoperfusion, are at risk for the development of DIC. Also at risk are those individuals who have had recent obstetrical complications, as listed earlier, or massive trauma. These patient should be observed closely for signs of bleeding. DIC can occur in a chronic or acute form. The chronic form is more subtle and easily goes unrecognized. The acute form tends to be more severe and sudden in onset. Clinical manifestations range in severity from prolonged bleeding from a venipuncture site to spontaneous massive hemorrhage. In massive hemorrhage, bleeding occurs from mucous membranes, sites of injury (including venipuncture and injections sites, and surgical wounds), and any orifice. Deep-tissue bleeding may also occur. Petechiae, purpura, and ecchymoses are common. Table 46–18 lists various types of bleeding that may be found on physical exam. In addition, prolonged bleeding from wounds or needle-puncture sites, occult blood in body excreta or excretions (emesis, feces, urine), or bleeding from mucous membranes may signal the development of DIC. In chronic DIC, thrombosis is the most common symptom. Recurrent thrombophlebitis is the most common manifestation of chronic DIC. The definitive diagnosis of DIC depends on laboratory tests.

Laboratory and Diagnostic Tests. Multiple coagulation test abnormalities are found in DIC. These include prolonged prothrombin time (PT), partial thromboplastin time (PTT), and thrombin time (TT); decreased fibrinogen and platelet counts; increased FDPs; and the presence of schistocytes on the blood smear. Decreased levels of factors II, V, VIII, and X are also found, but are not commonly measured. Table 46–19 lists the laboratory abnormalities associated with DIC.

Management. DIC always occurs as the result of some other underlying abnormality, thus the treatment of DIC is directed toward the underlying disorder. For example, infection requires the use of antibiotics. Fetal demise or a retained placenta requires the removal of the uterine contents. General support measures, such as fluid and blood replacement, and maintenance of adequate oxygenation and tissue perfusion are essential. The bleeding may be slowed by giving the patient transfusions of platelets, fresh frozen plasma (which contains all the clotting factors), and cryoprecipitate (for factors V and VIII and fibrinogen replacement). The use of heparin is controversial. As a potent anticoagulant, it inactivates the massive intravascular clotting, and thus, inhibits consumption of the coagulation factors. However, it promotes bleeding. Some patients, such as those with acute promyelocytic leukemia (APL), often respond well to the use of heparin if it is initiated when coagulation tests are just beginning to become abnormal. These patients should have the above-mentioned coagulation studies checked prior to starting and at least once a day while undergoing chemotherapy. Heparin, used in this manner, may prevent the consumption of platelets and clotting factors. However, it is probably inappropriate to use heparin in the face of active bleeding. If heparin is used, platelets and clotting factors may still need to be administered, if low, to prevent bleeding.

As stated earlier, the symptoms of DIC occur on a spectrum, from subclinical to massive hemorrhage. All patients with DIC should be monitored for bleeding, and all body excreta should be tested for occult blood. Vital signs should be monitored frequently, depending on the severity of symptoms and on the other underlying process. Large ecchymoses can form due to frequent blood pressure (BP) measurements. Consider inserting an arterial line for BP monitoring if this occurs. Be observant for signs of internal

TABLE 46–18. Physical Findings in Bleeding Disorders

Finding	Description	Probable Cause
Petechiae	Small capillary hemorrhages Flat, 1 mm–3 mm in diameter, do not blanch with pressure, deep red or reddish purple in color Most common in dependent areas	Vessel or platelet abnormalities, disseminated intravascular coagulation (DIC)
Purpura	Petechiae that have grown together to form a larger lesion	Vessel or platelet abnormalities, DIC
Ecchymoses (bruises)	Larger macular areas, blue-black initially, fading to brownish-green, then yellow Due to blood in the subcutaneous tissues and skin	Usually from veins. Common with disorders of platelet and vessels as well as coagulation defects, DIC
Hemarthrosis	Hemorrhage into synovial joints May have no external evidence of bleeding, only complaints of severe joint pain	Severe hereditary coagulation disorders or DIC

Bithell, T. C. (1993). (p. 1302).

TABLE 46–19. Laboratory Tests in DIC

Manifestation	Acute DIC	Chronic DIC
Clinical	Usually hemorrhagic	None or thrombotic
Screening tests		
PT, PTT	Usually prolonged	Normal
Platelets	Usually decreased	Normal or slightly decreased
Fibrinogen	Usually decreased, but may be normal	Usually normal
Confirmatory tests		
Fibrin monomer	Positive; can be negative, if severe	Positive
FDP	Strongly positive, usually >40 μg/ml	Positive, >40 μg/ml
D dimer	Positive	Positive
Other assays		
Thrombin time	Normal or abnormal	Usually normal
Factor assays	Decreased V, VIII	Normal V, VIII
Antithrombin III	May be low	Usually normal

PT, prothrombin time; *PTT,* partial thromboplastin time; *FDP,* fibrin degradation products.
Schmaier. (1991). (p. 480).

bleeding, such as flank pain, painful or swollen joints, decreased level of consciousness (LOC), or headache. If IV or arterial punctures must be performed, direct pressure will need to be applied for longer than usual to achieve hemostasis. Avoid intramuscular or subcutaneous injections. Avoid the use of salicylates or nonsteroidal antiinflammatory drugs that affect platelet function.

Follow-Up. Coagulation tests should be performed daily or more often until normalized. The prognosis of DIC varies markedly, depending on the underlying cause and the amount of intravascular clotting. DIC may cease spontaneously, or it may respond to prompt and aggressive treatment. Residual dysfunction of affected organ systems such as the kidneys, eyes, etc., can occur. In other cases, the organ ischemia and bleeding lead to death.

Heparin-Induced Thrombocytopenia

Pathophysiology. The incidence of heparin-induced thrombocytopenia (HIT) is as high as 8 to 15% (Harmening & Lemery, 1997). In a few patients, spontaneous platelet aggregation occurs on first exposure to heparin. In most patients thrombocytopenia develops after 6 to 10 days of heparin therapy. Type I is generally a mild thrombocytopenia that occurs shortly after heparin exposure. Type II is more severe and occurs later during the course of heparin therapy. The mechanism is thought to be the development of IgG antibodies specifically targeted at the compound formed between heparin and platelet factor IV (Aster, 1995). These antibodies also react with endothelial cells on vessel walls that are coated with platelet factor IV. Activation of these antibodies appears to be more common in patients treated with unfractionated heparin than in patients treated with low-molecular weight heparin.

History and Physical Findings. The key to diagnosing HIT is to maintain a high index of suspicion for all patients receiving heparin. If new thromboses or unexplained heparin resistance develops, consider HIT and obtain a platelet count (Chong, 1995). The length of time the patient has been on heparin will help determine which type of thrombocytopenia the patient has. In Type I, which occurs early, patients bleed very little. In Type II, which occurs later during the course of therapy, the bleeding may be life-threatening. Venous and arterial thromboses can occur simultaneously with HIT and do not resolve until the heparin is discontinued. Common arterial thromboses include stroke, myocardial infarction, and end-organ dysfunction such as renal failure (Chong, 1995). Common venous thromboses include extensive deep vein thromboses, often complicated by recurrent pulmonary emboli. DIC occurs occasionally.

Laboratory and Diagnostic Findings. Obtaining a platelet count twice a week once the patient has been on four days or more of heparin may help in detecting HIT early. Thrombocytopenia varies in severity, being more severe and life-threatening in Type II HIT. The diagnosis of HIT is based on the following criteria: thrombocytopenia occurring during heparin therapy, exclusion of other causes of thrombocytopenia (infection, other drugs, autoimmune thrombocytopenia), resolution of thrombocytopenia after discontinuing heparin, and detection of heparin-dependent platelet antibodies in the serum by an *in vitro* test (Chong, 1995).

Management. Patients with Type II heparin-induced thrombocytopenia must have the heparin discontinued for the platelet count to normalize. Coumadin may be substituted. However, as it takes 3 to 5 days to achieve a full effect from coumadin, other antithrombotic drugs, such as low molecular-weight heparinoid (Orgaran), should be used. Once an antibody response has developed to unfractionated heparin, low-molecular weight heparin should be avoided. If the patient has proximal deep vein thromboses and thus is at high risk for pulmonary emboli (PE), a Greenfield filter may prevent pulmonary emboli. Patients with Type I HIT may not require treatment as they are often asymptomatic and their mild thrombocytopenia usually resolves without discontinuing heparin.

Follow-Up. It generally takes 5 to 7 days for the platelet count to return to normal once the heparin is discontinued. The patient should continue to be observed carefully, as venous and arterial thrombosis, as described earlier, is often associated with Type II HIT. Reinitiation of heparin, including low molecular-weight heparin, generally results in thrombocytopenia again and should be avoided. The mortality rate of Type II is as high as 20% (Harmening & Lemery, 1997).

The Hypercoagulable State

Hypercoagulable states include a number of poorly defined abnormalities that are thought to be associated with hyperactivity of the coagulation system and/or the development of thromboembolic events (Bertina, 1997). They can be associated with decreased protein C, antithrombin III, plasminogen, and/or thrombocytosis as well as clinical conditions such as malignancies, pregnancy, or postoperative states (Marlar, 1994). Hereditary thrombotic state includes protein C and protein S deficiencies, and antithrombin III deficiency, among others. The lupus anticoagulant is an autoimmune disorder in which autoantibodies develop against phospholipid membranes (Marlar, 1994).

Pathophysiology

The most important inhibitor to coagulation is antithrombin III (AT-III) (Canton, 1997). It can be activated by heparin and the heparin sulfates. Even in small doses, heparin converts AT-III from a slow, relatively ineffective inhibitor to a fast, effective one.

The protein C (PC) system is a natural anticoagulant mechanism. Protein S is a cofactor in this system which enhances protein C function. Protein C is synthesized by hepatocytes, and is vitamin K-dependent. Once it is activated by thrombin, it degrades factors VIIIa and Va, two of the major cofactors involved in thrombin generation.

Congenital or acquired changes in coagulation or fibrinolysis have been associated with an increased risk of thrombosis. Type I deficiency is a quantitative deficiency and is due to reduced synthesis of a normal protein. Type II is a qualitative deficiency, making the protein nonfunctional.

History and Physical Findings

Anyone under the age of 40 who presents with recurrent thrombosis should be evaluated for hereditary defects of proteins C and S, the serpin family, and the fibrinolytic system. Individuals with AT-III deficiency generally present with deep venous thrombosis (DVT), often complicated by pulmonary emboli, although arterial thrombosis also occurs. The thrombotic episodes are usually linked to a triggering event such as surgery, bed rest, pregnancy, or oral contraceptives.

Heterozygous deficiency of protein C is also associated with DVT or pulmonary emboli, as well as warfarin-induced skin necrosis, generally occurring prior to age 40. Homozygous protein C deficiency is rare and is associated with purpura fulminans and DIC in the newborn infant. Protein S deficiency is associated with DVT, but can also present with cerebral arterial thrombosis. The differential diagnosis should be kept broad, however, as venous thrombosis may also be the presenting sign of malignancy in an otherwise healthy individual. The most common clotting abnormalities associated with malignancy are elevation of fibrin degradation products (FDPs), and an increase or decrease in fibrinogen, and factors V and VIII, as well as other factors.

Laboratory and Diagnostic Tests

The following tests should be performed when a patient is suspected of having a thrombotic disorder: protein C functional and antigenic assay, protein S total and free antigenic assay, functional assay for AT-III, fibrinogen (clot-based assay), plasminogen (functional assay), LA test, APA, PAI-1 and TPA, TPA-PAI-1 complexes.

Protein C deficiencies should be identified with a functional assay; then an immunologic assay is used to distinguish between Type I and Type II. In Type I deficiency the plasma concentration is low in all three assays (Aiach et al., 1997). Type II deficiencies are best identified by coagulation assays.

Management

Intravenous heparin, followed by long-term warfarin therapy, is the treatment of choice for most patients with DVT. Low molecular-weight heparin is easier to administer than standard heparin and does not require frequent monitoring.

Follow-Up

Protime (PT) and the international normalized ratio (INR) are used to monitor warfarin therapy. Partial thromboplastin time (PTT) is used to monitor heparin therapy. Low molecular-weight heparin produces a more predictable anticoagulation compared with standard heparin, making frequent laboratory monitoring unnecessary.

REFERENCES

Aiach, M., Borgel, D., Gaussem, P., et al. (1997). Protein C and protein S deficiencies. *Seminars in Hematology, 34* (3), 205–217.

Aster, R. H. (1995). Heparin-induced thrombocytopenia and thrombosis. *New England Journal of Medicine, 332* (20).

Appelbaum, F. R. (1995). Allogeneic bone marrow transplantation for treatment of malignancy. In J. S. MacDonald, D. G. Haller, & R. J. Mayer (Eds.), *Manual of oncologic therapeutics* (3rd ed.). (pp. 489–494). Philadelphia: J. B. Lippincott.

Babior, B. M. & Stossel, T. P. (1990). *Hematology: A pathophysiological approach* (2nd ed.). New York: Churchill Livingstone.

Bertina, R. M. (1997). Introduction: hypercoagulable states. *Seminars in Hematology, 34* (3), 167–70.

Bithell, T. C. (1993). The diagnostic approach to the bleeding disorders. In G. R. Lee, T. C. Bithell, J. Foerster, et al., (eds). Wintrobe's Clinical Hematology, (9th Ed.) Philadelphia: Lea and Febiger.

Bonadonna, G., Santoro, A., & Wiernik, P. H. (1996). Diagnosis and treatment of Hodgkin's disease. In P. H. Wiernik, G. P. Canellos, J. P. Dutcher, & R. A. Kyle (Eds.), *Neoplastic diseases of the blood,* (pp. 863–892). New York: Churchill Livingstone.

Borson, R. & Loeb, V. (1994). Acute and chronic leukemias in adults. *CA: A Cancer Journal for Clinicians, 44* (6), 323–352.

Brandt, J. T. (1985). Current concepts of coagulation. *Clinical Obstetrics Gynecology, 28,* 13.

Brittinger, G., Hellriegel, K. -P., & Hiddemann, W. (1997). Chronic lymphocytic leukemia and hairy-cell leukemia—diagnosis and treatment: Results of a consensus meeting of the German CLL Co-operative Group. *Leukemia, 11* (Suppl. 2), S1–3.

Canellos, G. P. (1996). Diagnosis and treatment of chronic granulocytic leukemia. In P. H. Wiernick, G. P. Canellos, J. P. Dutcher, & R. A. Kyle (Eds.), *Neoplastic diseases of the blood,* (pp. 65–79). New York: Churchill Livingstone.

Canton, M. M. (1997). Introduction to thrombosis and anticoagulant therapy. In D. M. Harmening, (Ed.), *Clinical hematology and fundamentals of hemostasis* (3rd ed.). (pp. 566–584). Philadelphia: F. A. Davis Company.

Charache, S., Lubin, B., & Reid, C. D. (Eds.). (1991). *Management and therapy of sickle cell disease.* U.S. Department of Health and Human Services: Public Health Service, National Institutes of Health, NIH Publication No. 91-2117.

Cheson, B. D. (1995). Acute leukemias. In J. S. Macdonald, D. G. Haller, & R. J. Mayer (Eds.), *Manual of oncologic therapeutics,* (3rd ed.). (pp. 271–281). Philadelphia: J. B. Lippincott.

Chielsa, B. E. (1997). Morphologic changes associated with disease. In D. M. Harmening (Ed.), *Clinical hematology and fundamentals of hemostasis* (3rd ed.). Philadelphia: F. A. Davis Company.

Chong, B. H. (1995). Heparin-induced thrombocytopenia. *British journal of haematology, 89,* 431–439.

Cotran, R. S., Kumar, V., & Robbins, S. L. (1989). *Pathologic basis of disease* (4th ed.). Philadelphia: W. B. Saunders.

Cotran, R. S., Kumar, V., & Robbins, S. L. (1994). In S. L. Robbins (Ed.). *Pathologic basis of disease,* (5th ed.). (p. 625). Philadelphia: W. B. Saunders.

Deisseroth, A. B., Kantarjian, H., Andreeff, M., et al., (1997). Chronic leukemias. In V. T. DeVita, S. Hellman, & S. A. Rosenberg (Eds.), *Cancer: principles and practice of oncology* (5th ed.). Philadelphia: Lippincott-Raven.

DeVita, V. T., Jaffe, E. S, & Hellman, S. (1985). Hodgkin's disease and the non-Hodgkin's lymphomas. In V. T. DeVita, S. Hellman, & S. A. Rosenberg (Eds.), *Cancer: Principles and practice of oncology,* (2nd ed.). (p. 1634). Philadelphia: J. B. Lippincott.

Fisher, R. I., Gaynor, E. R, Dahlberg, S., et al. (1993). Comparison of a standard regimen (CHOP) with three intensive chemotherapy regimens for advanced non-Hodgkin's lymphoma. *New England Journal of Medicine, 328,* 1002–1006.

Fisher, R. I. (1995). Non-Hodgkin's lymphoma. In J. S. Macdonald, D. G. Haller, & R. J. Mayer (Eds.), *Manual of oncologic therapeutics* (3rd ed.). (pp. 294–299). Philadelphia: J. B. Lippincott.

George, J. N., Woolf, S. H., Raskob, G. E., et al. (1996). Idiopathic thrombocytopenic purpura: A practice guideline developed by explicit methods for the American Society of Hematology. *Blood, 88* (1), 3–40.

Glassman, A. B. (1997). Anemia: Diagnosis, and clinical considerations. In D. M. Harmening (Ed.), *Clinical hematology and fundamentals of hemostasis,* (3rd Ed.). (pp. 71–79). Philadelphia: F. A. Davis Company.

Goroll, H. A. & Mulley, A. G. (1987). Evaluation of anemia. In H. A. Goroll, L. A. May, and A. G. Mulley (Eds.), *Primary care medicine.* Philadelphia: J. B. Lippincott.

Greenberg, P., Cox, C., LeBeau, M. M., et al. (1997). International scoring system for evaluating prognosis in myelodysplastic syndromes. *Blood, 89* (6), 2079–2088.

Greipp, P. R. & Kyle, R. A. (1996). Staging, kinetics, and prognosis of multiple myeloma. In P. H. Wiernik, G. P. Canellos, J. P. Dutcher, & R. A. Kyle (Eds.), *Neoplastic diseases of the blood,* (pp. 537–557). New York: Churchill Livingstone.

Grogan, T. M., Miller, T. P., & Fisher, R. I. (1997). A Southwest Oncology Group perspective on the Revised European–American lymphoma classification. *Hematology/Oncology Clinics of North America, 11* (5), 819–846.

Harris, N. L., Jaffe, E. S., Stein, H., et al. (1994). A revised European–American classification of lymphoid neoplasms: A proposal from the International Lymphoma Study Group. *Blood, 84* (5), 1361–1392.

Harmening, D. M. & Lemery, L. D. (1997). An overview of hemostatic mechanism, platelet structure and function, and extrinsic and intrinsic systems. In D. M. Harmening (Ed.), *Clinical hematology and fundamentals of hemostasis* (3rd ed.). Philadelphia: F. A. Davis Company.

Hehlmann, R., Willer, A., Heimpel, H., et al. (1997). Randomized studies with interferon in chronic myelogenous leukemia (CML) and comparative molecular aspects. *Leukemia, 11* (Suppl 3), 506–511.

Hoelzer, D. F. (1996). Diagnosis and treatment of adult acute lymphocytic leukemia. In P. H. Wiernik, G. P. Canellos, J. P. Dutcher, & R. A. Kyle (Eds.), *Neoplastic diseases of the blood,* (pp. 295–319). New York: Churchill Livingstone.

Horning, S. J. (1997). High-dose therapy and transplantation for low-grade lymphoma. *Hematology/Oncology Clinics of North America, 11* (5), 919–935.

Jandl, J. H. (1996). *Blood: Textbook of hematology,* (2nd ed.). Boston: Little, Brown.

Joshua, D. E. & Gibson, J. (1996). Diagnosis and treatment of multiple myeloma. In P. H. Wiernik, G. P. Canellos, J. P. Dutcher, & R. A. Kyle (Eds.), *Neoplastic diseases of the blood,* (pp. 561–583). New York: Churchill Livingstone.

Kumar, V., Cotran, R. S., & Robbins, S. L. (1992). *Basic pathology* (5th ed.). Philadelphia: W. B. Saunders.

Lee, G. R., Bithell, T. C., Foerster, J., et al. (1993). *Wintrobe's clinical hematology,* (9th ed.). Philadelphia: Lea & Febiger.

Lin, A. Y. & Li, F. P. (1996). Etiology and epidemiology of chronic leukemias. In P. H. Wiernik, G. P. Canellos, J. P. Dutcher, & R. A. Kyle (Eds.), *Neoplastic diseases of the blood,* (pp. 9–20). New York: Churchill Livingstone.

Marlar, R. A. (1994). The hypercoagulable state. In M. E. Wood & P. A. Bunn (Eds.), *Hematology/Oncology secrets.* Philadelphia: Hanley & Belfus.

MacManus, M. P. & Hoppe, R. T. (1997). Overview of treatment of localized low-grade lymphomas. *Hematology/Oncology Clinics of North America, 11* (5), 901–918.

Mathai, G. & Robinson, W. A. (1994). Hodgkin's disease. In M. E. Wood & P. A. Bunn (Eds.), *Hematology/Oncology secrets,* (p 150). Philadelphia: Hanley & Belfus, Inc.

McKenna, S. M. & Baehner, R. L. (1996). Diagnosis and treatment of childhood acute lymphoblastic leukemia. In P. H. Wiernik, G. P. Canellos, J. P. Dutcher, & R. A. Kyle (Eds.), *Neoplastic diseases of the blood,* (pp. 271–294). New York: Churchill Livingstone.

Morrison, V. A. (1994). Chronic leukemias. *CA: Cancer Journal for Clinicians, 44* (6), 353–377.

Newcombe, D. S. (1993). Monocytes and macrophages. In J. L. Spivak & E. R. Eichner (Eds.), *The Fundamentals of Clinical Hematology,* (3rd ed.). Baltimore: Johns Hopkins University Press.

O'Brien, S. & Keating, M. J. (1996). Diagnosis and treatment of chronic lymphocytic leukemia. In P. H. Wiemick, G. P. Canellos, J. P. Dutcher, & R. A. Kyle (Eds.), *Neoplastic diseases of the blood,* (pp. 107–122). New York: Churchill Livingstone.

Paraskevas, F. & Foerster, J. (1993). The lymphocytes. In R. G. Lee, T. C. Bithell, J. Foerster, et al. (Eds.), *Wintrobe's clinical hematology,* (9th ed.). Philadelphia: Lea & Febiger.

Parker, S. L., Tong, T., Bolden, S., & Wingo, P. A. (1997). Cancer statistics, 1997. *CA: Cancer Journal for Clinicians, 47* (5), 5–27.

Platt, O. S., Thorington, B. D., Brambilla, D. J., et al. (1991). Pain in sickle cell disease: Rates and risk factors. *New England Journal of Medicine, 325* (1), 11–16.

Powars, D. P. (1994). Natural history of disease: The first two decades. In S. H. Embury, R. P. Hebbel, N. Mohandas, & M. H. Steinberg (Eds.), *Sickle cell disease: Basic principles and clinical practice.* Philadelphia: Raven Press.

Radich, J. P., Gehly, G., Gooley, T., et al. (1995). Polymerase chain reaction detection of the BCR-ABL fusion transcript after allogeneic marrow transplantation for chronic myeloid leukemia: Results and implications in 346 patients. *Blood, 85* (9): 2632–2638.

Rodgers, G. P. (1997). Overview of pathophysiology and rationale for treatment of sickle cell anemia. *Seminars in Hematology, 34* (3), Suppl 3, 2–7.

Rodriguez-Monge, E. J. & Cabanillas, F. (1997). Long-term follow-up of platinum-based lymphoma salvage regimens. *Hematology/Oncology Clinics of North America, 11* (5), 937–947.

Rothstein, G. (1993). Origin and development of the blood and blood-forming tissues. In R. G. Lee, T. C. Bithell, J. Foerster, et al. (Eds.), *Wintrobe's clinical hematology,* (9th ed.). Philadelphia: Lea & Febiger.

Saito, H. (1991). Normal hemostatic mechanisms. In O. D. Ratnoff & C. D. Forbes (Eds.), *Disorders of hemostasis,* (2nd ed.). Philadelphia: W. B. Saunders.

Sandberg, A. A. & Chen, Z. (1996). Cytogenetics of acute leukemia. In P. H. Wiernik, G. P. Canellos, J. P. Dutcher, & R. A. Kyle (Eds.), *Neoplastic diseases of the blood,* (pp. 249–269). New York: Churchill Livingstone.

Schmaier, A.H. (1991). Laboratory studies in dissemination intravascular coagulation and activated coagulation. In J. Koepke (Ed.), *Practical laboratory hematology.* New York: Churchhill Livingstone.

Seligsohn, U. (1995). Disseminated intravascular coagulation. In E. Beutler, M. A. Lichtman, B. S. Coller, & T. J. Kipps (Eds.), *Williams hematology* (5th ed.). (p. 1498). New York: McGraw-Hill.

Shapiro, B. S. & Ballas, S. K. (1994). The acute painful episode. In S. H. Embury, R. P. Hebbel, N. Mohandas, & M. H. Steinberg (Eds.), *Sickle cell disease: Basic principles and clinical practice,* (pp. 531–543). Philadelphia: Raven Press.

Silverman, L. R. (1997). Myelodysplastic syndrome. In J. F. Holland, R. C. Blast, D. L. Morton, et al. (Eds.), *Cancer medicine,* (pp. 2593–2615). Baltimore: Williams & Wilkins.

Thaler, J., Gastl, G., Fluckinger, T., et al. (1996). Interferon alpha-2c therapy of patients with chronic myelogenous leukemia: Long-term results of a multicenter phase-II study. *Annals of Hematology, 72* (6), 349–355.

Third MIC Cooperative Group (1988). Recommendations for a morphologic, immunologic, and cytogenetic (MIC) working classification of the primary and therapy related myelodysplastic disorders. *Cancer Genet Cytogenet, 23* (1), 88.

Tuzuner, N. N. & Bennett, J. M. (1996). Classification of the acute leukemias: Cytochemical and morphologic considerations. In P. H. Wiernik, G. P. Canellos, J. P. Dutcher, & R. A. Kyle (Eds.), *Neoplastic diseases of the blood,* (pp. 191–209). New York: Churchill Livingstone.

Vichinsky, E. P. (1994). Transfusion therapy. In S. H. Embury, R. P. Hebbel, N. Mohandas, & M. H. Steinberg (Eds.), *Sickle cell disease: Basic principles and clinical practice.* Philadelphia: Raven Press.

Vichinsky, E. P. & Lubin, B. H. (1994). A cautionary note regarding hydroxyurea in sickle cell disease. *Blood, 83* (4), 1124–1128.

Vose, J. M., Bierman, P. J., & Armitage, J. O. (1996). Diagnosis and treatment of non-Hodgkin's lymphoma of adults. In P. H. Wiernik, G. P. Canellos, J. P. Dutcher, & R. A. Kyle (Eds.), *Neoplastic diseases of the blood,* (pp. 907–924). New York: Churchill Livingstone.

Walters, M. C., Patience, M., Leisenring, W., et al. (1996). Bone marrow transplantation for sickle cell disease. *New England Journal of Medicine, 335,* 369–376.

Wang, W. C., Kovnar, E. H., Tonkin, I. L., et al. (1991). High risk of recurrent stroke after discontinuance of five to twelve years of transfusion therapy in patients with sickle cell disease. *The Journal of Pediatrics, 118* (3), 377–382.

Weinstein, H. J. (1996). Diagnosis and treatment of childhood acute myelocytic leukemia. In P. H. Wiernik, G. P. Canellos, J. P. Dutcher, & R. A. Kyle (Eds.), *Neoplastic diseases of the blood,* (pp. 321–330). New York: Churchill Livingstone.

Wiernik, P. H., Gallagher, R. E., & Tallman, M. S. (1996). Diagnosis and treatment of acute promyelocytic leukemia. In P. H. Wiernik, G. P. Canellos, J. P. Dutcher, and R. A. Kyle (Eds.), *Neoplastic diseases of the blood,* (pp. 353–380). New York: Churchill Livingstone.

Wilhelm, M., Tony, H.-P., Rueckle-Lanz, H., et al. (1997). First line therapy of advanced chronic lymphocytic leukemia. *Leukemia, 11* (Suppl. 2), S14–S18.

Williams, W. J. (1995). Classification and clinical manifestations of disorders of hemostasis. in E. Beutler, M. A. Lichtman, B. S. Coller, & T. J. Kipps (Eds.), *Williams hematology,* (5th ed.). (pp 1279–1280). New York: McGraw-Hill.

Wilson, W. H. & Chabner, B. A. (1998). Principles of chemotherapy for lymphomas. In G. P. Canellos, T. A. Lister, & J. L. Sklar (Eds). *The lymphomas.* Philadelphia: W. B. Saunders.

Yardumian, D. A., Mackie, I. J., & Machin, S. J. (1986). Laboratory investigation of platelet function: A review of methodology. *Journal of Clinical Pathology, 39,* 701.

Zucker, M. B. (1980). The functioning of blood platelets. *Scientific American, 242* (6), 86.

47

Immunologic Problems

Debra Tribett

NORMAL IMMUNE ANATOMY AND PHYSIOLOGY

The human body is continually exposed to an ever-changing environment of microorganisms. The normal immune system provides a physical barrier and a protective chemical response to protect the body's internal environment from invasion from foreign microorganisms. The normal function of the immune system may be impaired congenitally; by therapeutic interventions such as, surgery, invasive diagnostic procedures, medications; or by trauma. When caring for hospitalized patients, the acute care nurse practitioner (ACNP) is faced with a situation where multiple aspects of the patient's immune system may be compromised. Understanding the normal immune system response is critical to the anticipation of potential situations of immunocompromise, implementing measures to support normal immune function, and for intervention with therapies to manipulate immune response.

The immune system has the ability to recognize self from nonself. Foreign substances such as microorganisms, cells, or tissues from other people trigger an immune response that attempts to eliminate the nonself from the body. The term *antigen* is often used to refer to the agent that can trigger an immune response. The immune system can distinguish between a vast number of molecules and will respond or not respond to each individually with great specificity. A memory of an encounter with an antigen is part of the immune response, so as to protect the body with a more rapid and vigorous response if the specific antigen is encountered in the future.

The first line of immune system defense is an intact epithelial surface barrier with normal secretion production. This mechanical barrier serves to prevent entry or remove microorganisms soon after contact with body surfaces. Collectively the skin, eye, respiratory tract, gastrointestinal tract, and genitourinary tract form this barrier. The normal human body has an endogenous bacterial flora on these surfaces that competes with potential pathogens to prevent deeper penetration of the pathogens. Coupled with the characteristics of surface secretions (acid pH, lysosymes, secretory IgA), flushing actions of body fluids (tearing, ciliated mucosa, voiding urine), and intact function of protective reflexes (sneezing, coughing, swallowing), an effective barrier between internal and external environments is maintained.

The second line of defense is a nonspecific defense called the inflammatory response. Phagocytic white blood cells (WBC) produced by the bone marrow circulate within the cardiovascular and lymphatic systems awaiting activation. Five subgroups of WBCs exist in the body: neutrophils, monocytes, eosinophils, basophils, and lymphocytes. Only neutrophils, monocytes, and eosinophils are involved in the nonspecific defense of the body.

First responders are the polymorphonuclear leukocytes or mature segmented neutrophils that attempt to phagocytize the invading antigen by engulfing it and releasing toxic enzymes contained within the cell to kill the antigen. Neutrophils respond within minutes to an antigen and live for only a few hours in the tissues performing their duty. Dying in the process, their remains and that of the foreign antigen are commonly referred to as "pus." A constant supply of new neutrophils from the bone marrow is necessary to replace this component of the immune response. In times of increased demand for neutrophils, bands (the immature form of neutrophils) are released into the bloodstream. Eosinophils are the type of WBC that respond to parasitic antigens. They are fewer in number than other phagocytic cells and are also involved in allergic responses of the immune system.

Monocytes are larger phagocytic cells released by the bone marrow. They circulate briefly within the vascular system for about one day. They settle in the tissues throughout the body and mature into cells called macrophages. Tissue macrophages live for months until activated to perform their phagocytic functions. This may be in response to an invading microorganism or as part of the body's scavenger system to remove senescent or damaged cells. Macrophages are highly metabolic and produce numerous cytokines that influence the activity and growth of other cells.

Cytokines are peptides that may act on the cells producing them, on other cells nearby, or on cells remote from the site of their synthesis. Examples of cytokines produced by macrophages are interleukin-1 (IL-1), tumor necrosis factor (TNF), and interleukin-6 (IL-6). Cytokines can paradoxically induce injury to host-tissue during the normal defense against microorganisms. Both IL-1 and TNF are cytokines that can induce a febrile response in the host.

A form of WBC called a *natural killer* (NK) cell is a subtype of lymphocyte. The NK cell is nonphagocytic but is able to attack and destroy certain viral infected or tumor cells by other means. The actions of these cells are a part of the nonspecific natural immune response.

A series of chemical reactions involving more than 25 plasma proteins collectively referred to as complement activation is another of the components of the second-level nonspecific immune response. A cascade reaction may be triggered by bacterial products or when the third-level specific immune response has formed an immune complex of antibody and antigen. The resulting antimicrobial effects from complement activation include lysis of cells, opsonization, and generation of peptide fragments, which help to regulate inflammatory and immune responses.

A highly selective third level of immune response involves the humoral- and cell-mediated processes of the lymphocytes. Lymphocytes are WBC produced in the bone marrow and are differentiated into T and B varieties. The B-lymphocyte precursor cells stay in the bone marrow, whereas T-lymphocyte precursor cells migrate to the thymus gland where they are differentiated into CD_4 helper/inducer cells and CD_8 suppresser/cytotoxic cells. The ratio of T-helper to T-suppresser cells is normally 2:1. After maturation the B and T cells migrate to the peripheral lymphoid tissues, such as the lymph nodes and spleen. The virgin lymphocytes carry surface receptors that enable them to bind with antigens. If the virgin lymphocytes do not become activated, they die within a few days. When activated, they survive and proliferate, yielding clones of cells that may undergo further cycles of activation and proliferation. The B lymphocytes are responsible for humoral antibody response and T lymphocytes are responsible for cell-mediated immunity. A normal immune response involves a complex cooperative stimulation of both cell types.

To trigger the specific immune response, an antigen must be processed by an antigen-presenting cell (APC). Macrophages function as an APC by capturing a minute amount of antigen and displaying it to the antigen-specific CD_4 helper T lymphocyte for recognition. The CD_4 helper T lymphocyte plays a pivotal role in the orchestration of the specific immune response. The T-helper cell becomes activated and begins to release cytokines such as interleukin-2 (IL-2), which communicate chemically with other lymphocytes to activate them. The proliferation of activated lymphocytes carry out the functions of inactivation and elimination of the antigen.

Some B lymphocytes interact directly with a specific antigen through antigen receptors and become activated. Activation of B lymphocytes is also stimulated by the T-helper lymphocyte. Clonal proliferation of the activated B cell occurs with generation into plasma cells which secrete immunoglobulins (Ig) or antibodies. Antibodies travel through tissue fluids to seek out the specific antigen that triggered their production. There are different classes of immunoglobulins: IgA, IgM, IgG, IgD, and IgE. The B cells of submucosal lymphoid tissue produce IgA. In the primary response to an antigen, IgM is produced by plasma cells. The most abundant immunoglobulin is IgG, produced during the secondary humoral response of plasma cells. Although its physiological function is yet unknown, IgD is found on the surface of B lymphocytes. Only minute amounts of IgE are normally found in the serum but it plays a key role in allergic responses to antigens. When IgE binds to an antigen, it reacts with mast cells and basophils which release mediators responsible for the acute reactions associated with allergic response. Not all activated B cells differentiate into Ig-producing plasma cells. Instead, they revert to a resting state and become memory B lymphocytes of the specific antigen exposure. Future exposure to a previous antigen encounter triggers a more rapid antibody response from memory B lymphocytes to protect the host.

The T lymphocyte killer/suppresser cells have a different antigen receptor than the T-helper cells. They respond by killing the antigen-bearing cell. They play an important role in the immune defense against viruses, intracellular bacteria, and in immune surveillance against malignancy. The differentiation of this cell line is in response to antigen recognition and exposure to IL-2.

Both helper and killer T cells develop memory cells that persist to protect the host from future antigen exposure. A second challenge by an antigen evokes a more rapid and efficient immune response. These memory cells may persist for years after an initial antigen exposure.

The human body is protected by a complex defense network and, as a result, very few of the numerous microorganisms to which it is exposed produce disease. The ability of a microorganism to produce disease is determined by its virulence and the condition of the host's immune defense. In the acute care setting today, the virulence of microorganisms is increasing and more patients with compromised immune defenses are present. This creates challenges for the ACNP in preventing and treating infection in a variety of patient situations. This is particularly evident in patients infected with the human immunodeficiency virus (HIV).

▶ HUMAN IMMUNODEFICIENCY VIRUS

Pathophysiology

The human immunodeficiency virus (HIV) is a single-stranded RNA virus of the retrovirus family. The virus was identified in 1983–1984 and was previously known as human T lymphotrophic virus type III (HTLV-III), lymph–adenopathy-associated virus (LAV), and AIDS-related virus (ARV). There are two subtypes of HIV. The more prevalent type in the United States, Europe, Australia, and central Africa is HIV-1. The HIV-2 strain is found in west Africa, parts of Europe, and less commonly elsewhere. Prior to the identification of the virus, its devastating effects were evident in patients and were first reported in 1981. The term *acquired immune deficiency syndrome* (AIDS) was coined in 1981 to describe the condition of patients who would later be determined to be in the late stages of HIV infection.

This virus gains entry into the human body via sexual contact, parenteral transmission, and vertical transmission from mother to child. Infected blood and body fluids such as semen, cervicovaginal secretions, and breast milk are the primary vehicles for virus transmission. Sexual practices that result in trauma (anal intercourse), the presence of ulcerative genital lesions, or other sexually transmitted diseases facilitate viral entry past normal epithelial barriers. Parenteral transmission can occur when needles and syringes contaminated with HIV-infected blood are shared by intravenous drug users or when health-care workers suffer an accidental needlestick injury. Prior to 1985 in this country and currently in many parts of the developing world, HIV-infected blood or blood-product transfusions are sources for parenteral transmission. Mothers infected with HIV may transmit the virus during or after birth and through breastfeeding to their infants. Recipients of transplanted organs or tissues prior to the availability of HIV testing are another group who may have inadvertently been infected with the virus.

Once the virus has breached the first-line epithelial defenses, it has an attraction to cells that express the CD_4 surface molecule. This includes the T-helper lymphocyte as well as monocytes/macrophages, microglial cells, and Langerhans' cells. Infection of the CD_4 cells causes damage to normal immune system function. These HIV-infected cells are destroyed as the virus uses the cell's own DNA to replicate itself. It is estimated that the number of CD_4 cells destroyed in a day approximates 10^9. Eventually the body is unable to replace the lost cells. The loss of T-helper CD_4 cells results in a reversal of the helper/suppresser ratio. An average decline in the CD_4 cell count of 50/mm^3 per year is the natural course of HIV infection. The monocyte/macrophage cell is also a target for HIV virus. These cells are a reservoir for HIV in the body and their function may become abnormal.

Once HIV is present in the body there is a typical burst of viremia. The body responds with an immune response and a subsequent level of equilibrium or a "set point" of viral replication is attained about six months after infection that varies from person to person. The HIV has an ability to replicate at high levels with an estimated turnover of 10 billion virons a day for many years (Ho et al., 1995). The set point established determines the natural progression of disease. Higher levels of viral burden ($>10^5$ copies of virus/mL) are associated with a relatively rapid course of HIV infection, whereas, those with a lower level ($<10^4$ copies of virus/mL) demonstrate a relatively slow progression of the disease. However, the natural course of HIV infection has been dramatically altered since the introduction of antiretroviral agents called protease inhibitors (PI) in 1996.

As a natural consequence of RNA viral replication, mutation of the viral genome occurs. These mutations occur irrespective of the presence of antiretroviral drugs. The pathogenesis of immune function due to HIV infection is incompletely understood. It is likely through the collective dysfunction of APC such as macrophages and the depletion of CD_4 T-helper lymphocytes.

In most cases, antibody to HIV appears within 2-8 weeks after infection with IgM production preceding that of IgG. Antibodies to the various HIV viral proteins do not appear simultaneously. In some instances it may be as long as 3 months after infection before antibody is detectable. It is during this window of time between infection and antibody detection that a screening test for HIV using the enzyme-linked immunosorbent assay (ELISA) may be negative even though a person is infected with HIV.

The destruction of CD_4 T lymphocytes results in the hallmark of HIV disease, defective cell-mediated immunity. The rate of cell destruction varies from patient to patient. In untreated adults in the United States, the time between infection with HIV and the development of AIDS is a median of 10 years. During this time the patient is generally asymptomatic. The level of CD_4 count defined as AIDS is 200 cells/mL (CDC, 1993). Defective cell-mediated immunity increases the likelihood for opportunistic infection from viruses, slow-growing bacteria, fungi, and development of malignancy. The level of CD_4 T-lymphocyte count associated with development of these problems has been identified (Table 47–1). This association is the basis for institution of medication prophylaxis against opportunistic infection in asymptomatic patients. Unfortunately, no effective prophylaxis is yet available for malignancy.

Abnormalities in B-lymphocyte responses are also present in HIV infection. Increases in IgG are a consequence of polyclonal B-cell activation resulting in hypergammaglobulinemia. Autoantibodies directed against the body's own erythrocytes, platelets, neutrophils, lymphocytes, and myelin have been demonstrated in patients with HIV infection. Clinical thrombocytopenia and peripheral neuropathy are HIV-associated problems associated with this abnormal autoimmune response. Although B-lymphocyte production of antibody to HIV occurs, there is no evidence that the antibody to HIV produced has a protective role.

Early in HIV disease antibody response to vaccines can be formed. A decrease in this ability has been documented in advanced HIV disease. There is controversy over the ability of vaccines to produce disease-specific antibody in HIV-positive patients and the effect of vaccines on HIV viral load. Some, but not all, studies have shown an increase in HIV viral load for weeks to months following vaccine administration in individuals with preserved CD_4 cell counts.

History and Physical Findings

Human immunodeficiency virus is believed to infect approximately one million people in the United States. Patients at any point on the spectrum of HIV disease may access the health-care system for problems unrelated to or directly as a result of their HIV disease. The ACNP may provide care to patients episodically in emergency departments and acute care inpatient settings. It is important for the ACNP to identify the high-risk patient for HIV in order to offer testing, to identify signs and symptoms associated with acute HIV infection, or to detect evidence of immunocompromise in the patient with full-blown AIDS.

Many risks for HIV infection can be identified when obtaining a history from a patient. High-risk groups for HIV include men who have sex with men, intravenous drug users, recipients of blood product or blood transfusions prior to 1985, transplant recipients, and sexual partners of a high-risk group. Children of infected mothers have a 10 to 50% chance for HIV infection. Recent trends from 1992 to 1996 reveal that non-Hispanic black men, Hispanic men, and non-Hispanic black women who had heterosexual risk exposures account for increasing proportions of reported cases of AIDS (CDC, 1997b). Occupational exposure must also be considered for patients who are health-care providers or work in areas where regular or accidental exposure to blood and body secretions occur.

TABLE 47–1. T-Lymphocyte Counts Associated with Opportunistic Infections

CD_4 T-Lymphocyte Count	Opportunistic Infection
> 500/µL	Mycobacterium tuberculosis
< 200/µL	Pneumocystis carinii pneumonia
< 100/µL	Toxoplasma gondii
< 50/µL	Mycobacterium avium complex
	Cytomegalovirus
	Fungal infection (Candida species, Cryptococcus neoformans)

The risk for HIV/AIDS is worldwide, therefore the ACNP must be aware of the prevalence of HIV infection in foreign countries. When assessing risk factors for HIV in the immigrant patient, it is important to remember that women are infected almost as often as men. In third-world developing countries, particularly in sub-Saharan Africa, heterosexual transmission is responsible for the majority of cases. Treatment for HIV infection is not available to the majority of AIDS patients throughout the world. Industrialized nations of western Europe, North America, Australia, and New Zealand have more access to newly available drug therapy for HIV.

The ACNP could encounter a patient with acute HIV infection. A mononucleosis-like syndrome develops approximately 3 to 6 weeks after initial infection in 50 to 70% of patients with primary HIV infection (Pantaleo, Graziosi, & Fauci, 1993). The patient may present with signs and symptoms including fever, lymphadenopathy, pharyngitis, maculopapular rash, hepatosplenomegaly, diarrhea, myalgia, weight loss of 10 pounds, and a variety of neurological symptoms. These symptoms persist for 1 to 3 weeks and spontaneously resolve.

Signs and symptoms of HIV infection may be absent for up to ten years after the initial infection. When symptoms begin, they may be nonspecific or attributable to other diseases. When HIV disease is advanced, signs and symptoms of AIDS-defining illness—severe, persisting constitutional decline, opportunistic infection, or malignancy—may cause the patient to seek medical care. The combination of complaints in the situation of a patient at high risk for HIV infection should prompt a thorough evaluation by the ACNP. Symptoms that may prompt an undiagnosed HIV patient to seek health care are listed in Table 47–2.

When performing a physical exam on any patient, the ACNP should be aware of the physical findings that might be suggestive of HIV-related disease. The physical examination of the HIV-positive patient may be totally within normal limits or demonstrate any finding characteristic of any non–HIV-related disease that could be seen in an adult population. If oral candidiasis or oral hairy leukoplakia is detected in a patient without an apparent cause, it may be an early manifestation of HIV disease. Testing for HIV would be indicated. In patients with advanced HIV disease,

TABLE 47–2. Symptoms Prompting Undiagnosed HIV-Infected Person to Seek Care

Generalized Complaints	Fever/chills occurring for ≥ 4 weeks Night sweats Unexplained weight loss Malaise/fatigue Persistent swollen glands
Respiratory	Cough—productive or nonproductive Shortness of breath on exertion or at rest
Gastrointestinal	Anorexia Nausea Vomiting Chronic diarrhea Mouth sores Bleeding gums Nonpainful oral lesions Painful or difficult swallowing Abdominal pain
Neurological	Visual disturbances Difficulty concentrating Memory loss Personality change Headaches Pain or abnormal sensations in lower extremities
Musculoskeletal	Joint pain Muscle ache
Genitourinary	Urethral discharge, burning Vaginal discharge, burning, itching Lesions on genitalia or rectum
Skin	Rash Extreme dryness, itching New onset lesions

weight loss, decrease in body fat and muscle mass, temporal wasting, and a cachexic appearance are seen.

During examination of the skin many abnormalities may be observed that are linked to HIV disease. Seborrheic dermatitis particularly of the glabella and nasolabial folds and generalized folliculitis from an eosinophilic or bacterial etiology are common dermatologic manifestations in patients with HIV infection. Herpes zoster or "shingles" may occur in immunocompromised HIV patients. Generalized molluscum contagiosum versus localized areas on the genitalia may occur in patients with advanced HIV infection. Kaposi's sarcoma lesions may occur early in HIV disease. Petechiae are seen in patients with HIV-associated thrombocytopenia.

The chief complaint of patients presenting to the acute care setting may also increase the suspicion of the presence of HIV-related disease. This is particularly the case when the history of the patient includes risk factors for exposure to HIV. Infection with HIV must be considered as an etiology or contributing factor when evaluating patients with general symptoms of fever, cough, shortness of breath, diarrhea, or genital complaints.

The insidious development over 1 to 4 weeks of a combination of symptoms (fever, nonproductive cough, dyspnea on exertion, fatigue) coupled with nonspecific physical findings of tachypnea and crackles can lead to different diagnoses. In a patient not known to have HIV infection, this presentation could be attributed to bronchitis, community-acquired pneumonia, or a flu-like illness. However, in a patient known or suspected to be HIV positive with CD_4 counts of less than 200/mm^3, *pneumocystis carinii* pneumonia (PCP) is likely.

Bacterial pneumonia is a frequent pulmonary disorder in HIV-infected patients. The most frequent bacterial source is *Streptococus pneumoniae.* The patient may present with classic symptoms of pneumococcal pneumonia, such as fever, dyspnea, productive cough with purulent or rusty-colored sputum, pleuritic chest pain, chills, and myalgia. Symptoms are usually more dramatic and develop over 2 to 14 days. However, it is still possible for bacterial pneumonia to present atypically, more like a case of PCP.

Chronic diarrhea may present in over half of patients during the course of HIV disease. The etiology of diarrhea may be related to medication side effects, infection with enteric pathogens, food intolerances, motility disorders, malignancy (Kaposi's sarcoma, lymphoma), HIV enteropathy, or unknown causes. Malnutrition secondary to diarrhea contributes to severe weight loss. The term *HIV wasting syndrome* includes patients with chronic diarrhea and loss of > 10% of baseline body weight and is an AIDS-defining disease. Differentiation of diarrhea of small bowel etiology versus colonic etiology may be determined from the patient history. Small bowel diarrhea is associated with large volume and urgency. Patients with colonic diarrhea have tenesmus, incontinence, and urgency.

When examining patients for complaints associated with possible sexually transmitted disease, HIV should be considered in the differential diagnosis list. Transmission of HIV is facilitated by the presence of other genital ulcerations or infections. Patients with HIV disease may present with condyloma acuminatum, an outbreak of genital herpes simplex, primary syphilis chancre, molluscum contagiosum, or urethral discharge suggestive of gonorrhea or chlamydia. Female patients may present with vulvovaginal candidiasis or pelvic inflammatory disease, particularly if associated with tubo–ovarian abscess. Cervical dysplasia and invasive cervical cancer are also seen in women with AIDS.

Laboratory and Diagnostic Tests

HIV Detection

The initial screening test for HIV infection is the HIV enzyme-linked immunosorbant assay (ELISA). This serologic test is currently used to detect antibodies to HIV-1. If the test is performed early after infection with HIV (within the first 12 weeks), prior to the development of detectable antibody, this test can give false–negative results. The ELISA is both highly sensitive (>99%) and highly specific (>99% in high-risk populations). The ELISA test for HIV-1 can usually detect HIV-2 infection. However, the sensitivity for HIV-2 is unacceptably low. Therefore, blood banks should routinely screen for both HIV-1 and HIV-2. A repeatedly positive ELISA is confirmed by the Western Blot. Because of its high sensitivity, a negative ELISA does not routinely warrant a Western Blot test. A positive ELISA and confirmatory Western Blot mean that that patient is infected with HIV and therefore contagious. This test is used to confirm a diagnosis of HIV. Testing for HIV should be performed when high incidence of clinical suspicion for HIV exists based on patient history and risk factors for exposure.

Prior to the development of antibody, HIV antigen can be detected in the peripheral blood mononuclear cells and plasma by the qualitative polymerase chain reaction or PCR. This test is not usually performed as a screening test due to its expense. It is used for clarification of indeterminate results of ELISA and Western Blot testing. If HIV is detected with this test, infection has occurred.

HIV Quantification

Quantitative measurement of plasma HIV RNA or plasma viral load can be performed by three commercially available assays: reverse transcriptase polymerase chain reaction (RT-PCR), ultrasensitive branch chain DNA (bDNA), and nucleic acid sequence-based amplification (NASBA) methods. Values may be undetectable (<400–500 copies/mL depending on the assay chosen) if the patient is receiving effective therapy against HIV. Upper levels may be detected in hundreds of thousands to over a million of virons/mL in patients with advanced disease. Quantity of HIV in the plasma is the best available surrogate marker of HIV-1 disease progression: high levels indicate a poor prognosis and reduced levels indicate improved prognosis (Mellors et al., 1996). The results of viral load testing are now used to guide therapy for HIV. The detection of even moderate HIV in the plasma appear to reflect very active HIV replication in lymphoid tissue (Carpenter et al., 1997). The measurable plasma viral load reflects the balance between viral production and clearance.

Viral load testing should be performed at baseline when HIV infection is confirmed then again in 2 to 4 weeks. Based on the level detected, antiretroviral medications may be recommended to be started. If medications are begun, viral load testing should be repeated in 3 to 4 weeks to determine a therapeutic clinical response. The ideal target level of HIV RNA after initiation of treatment is undetectable but an acceptable target is < 5000 copies/mL. A decrease in viral load of >0.5 log is indicative of antiviral activity. Retesting should be performed about every 3 to 4 months. If levels return to or are within 0.3 to 0.5 log of the pretreatment value, a treatment failure is suggested and a change in therapy should be considered. The HIV RNA should be determined using the same assay (bDNA, RT-PCR, NASBA) for every sample from the patient. The viral load should not be checked within a month of acute illness or immunization as these situations can cause transient increases in viral load.

The measurement of the absolute CD_4 T-lymphocyte count is used to detect depletion of this cell line by HIV. The CDC has classified HIV infection based on absolute CD_4 count and clinical manifestation of conditions associated with HIV infection (Table 47–3). A count of 200 cells/μL meets the definition of AIDS. The level of CD_4 cells is also used as an indicator for initiation of prophylactic medication for opportunistic infections. When antiretroviral medication is used, a rise in CD_4 cell count may occur. It is currently unknown if this increase in CD_4 cells provide antiinfective protection to the patient comparable with that afforded to a patient whose count never declined below the current level (CDC, 1997b). However, a continued decline in the CD_4 is associated with immune system decline and is usually associated with a rising viral load. An increasingly reported phenomenon in patients receiving antiretroviral therapy is a discordance between CD_4 cell count and viral load. In this situation, the viral load returns to or near pretreatment levels while the CD_4 count remains substantially above the pretreatment level. The pathophysiology of this phenomenon is not known, but it is clear that HIV replication leads to disease progression (Carpenter et al., 1997). Therefore, a treatment change should be considered in this clinical situation.

HIV Resistance

During active HIV replication, mutations occur frequently in the gene sequences of the virus. Antiviral drugs can inhibit viral growth but impose selective pressure for the development of resistance. The emergence of resistance even to combination drug therapy is apparent when quantitative measurement of HIV increases and CD_4 counts decrease. New commercial testing for genotyping of patient HIV isolates to identify mutations (codons) of the HIV reverse transcriptase gene are available. Single or multiple locations of mutation may indicate resistance to a single drug or multiple drugs. This type of testing is at present very expensive and is not standard of care at this time. When used clinically, it is reserved for use in situations where the patient has received multiple antiretroviral drugs over the course of the disease and treatment failure is evident. Genotyping may help select a drug combination that will suppress viral load. Proponents of this type of testing foresee its use prior to institution of drug therapy to identify preexisting drug resistance of the HIV-causing disease in an individual patient.

Initial Laboratory Evaluation of the Patient with HIV

Other laboratory tests should be obtained in the initial evaluation of HIV-positive patients and periodically during treatment to monitor for side effects of medications and disease

TABLE 47–3. 1993 Revised CDC AIDS Surveillance Case Definitions for Adolescents and Adults

CD_4 Cell Categories	Clinical Category A: Asymptomatic, PGL, or Acute HIV Infection	Clinical Category B: (Non-A or C Conditions)	Clinical Category C: AIDS Indicator Conditions
≥ 500/mm³ (≥ 29%)	A1	B1	C1
200–499/mm³ (14–28%)	A2	B2	C2
<200/mm³ (<14%)	A3	B3	C3

Clinical Category A Conditions
- Asymptomatic HIV infection
- Persistent generalized lymphadenopathy (PGL)
- Acute primary HIV infection with accompanying illness or history of acute infection

Clinical Category B Conditions
- Bacillary angiomatosis
- Candidiasis, oropharyngeal (thrush)
- Candidiasis, vulvovaginal persistent, frequent, or poorly responsive to therapy
- Cervical dysplasia (moderate or severe)/cervical cancer in situ
- Constitutional symptoms, such as fever (38.5°C) or diarrhea lasting > 1 month
- Oral hairy leukoplakia
- Herpes zoster (shingles) involving at least two distinct episodes or > one dermatome
- Idiopathic thrombocytopenia purpura
- Listeriosis
- Pelvic inflammatory disease, particularly if complicated by tubo–ovarian abscess
- Peripheral neuropathy

Clinical Category C Conditions
- Candidiasis of esophagus, bronchi, trachea, or lungs
- Invasive cervical cancer
- Coccidioidomycosis, disseminated or extrapulmonary
- Cryptococcosis, extrapulmonary
- Cryptosporidiosis, chronic intestinal (>1 month duration)
- Cytomegalovirus disease (other than liver, spleen, or nodes)
- Cytomegalovirus retinitis with loss of vision
- HIV-related encephalopathy
- Herpes simplex: chronic ulcers > 1 month duration, bronchitis, pneumonitis, or esophagitis
- Histoplasmosis, disseminated or extrapulmonary
- Isosporiasis, chronic intestinal > 1 month duration
- Kaposi's sarcoma
- Lymphoma: Burkitt's, immunoblastic, or primary of the brain
- *Mycobacterium avium* complex or *M kansasii* disseminated or extrapulmonary
- *M. tuburculosis,* any site pulmonary or extrapulmonary
- *Mycobacterium,* other species or unidentified species disseminated or extrapulmonary
- *Pneumocystis carinii* pneumonia
- Recurrent pneumonia
- Progressive multifocal leukoencephalopathy
- Recurrent salmonellosis sepsis
- Toxoplasmosis of the brain
- HIV wasting syndrome

manifestations. A complete blood count with differential is performed to detect anemia, neutropenia, and/or thrombocytopenia. Anemia with elevated MCH may be caused by antiretroviral therapy such as zidovudine.

A serum chemistry panel is advocated as part of the initial laboratory evaluation because of the high incidence of concurrent illness. It also serves as a basis of comparison for monitoring for side effects caused by antiretroviral or prophylactic medications. Liver transaminases and bilirubin may be elevated due to underlying liver disease or from administration of medications.

Hepatitis serology is performed to identify preexisting infection and should include hepatitis B surface antigen (HBsAg) and antibody to hepatitis B core antigen. Hepatitis C is frequently seen in patients with HIV and can be determined by the presence of antibody to hepatitis C virus (anti-HCV).

Serology for toxoplasmosis IgG is determined to identify past exposure to this infection. As the CD_4 cell count declines to below 100 cells/μL, reactivation of this organism may occur in the patient with positive toxoplasmosis serology and AIDS.

Serology for CMV is suggested for patients with HIV who are not at such high risk for CMV that seropositivity can be assumed. The majority of male homosexual, intravenous drug user, and hemophiliac patients are seropositive for CMV. A patient with positive serology for CMV may have a reactivation of this virus when the immune system is severely compromised.

Screening for syphilis should be performed with a VDRL or RPR study. Between 25 to 30% of HIV-positive patients have positive serology for syphilis. A positive result should be confirmed by a FTA-ABS. Detection of primary infection or inadequately treated past infection is important in the HIV patient. Syphilis has been described with fulminant presentation, rapid progression, and failure of standard penicillin therapy in patients with HIV disease.

A chest radiograph should be obtained as a baseline study for future comparison. It also may detect asymptomatic lung infection or other lesions.

All patients should have a tuberculin skin test with a standard Mantoux test. A response of ≥ 5 mm is considered a positive result in a patient with HIV infection. A positive PPD should be evaluated with a chest radiograph for determination of active pulmonary disease. Based on the clinical situation, drug therapy should be prescribed for TB prophylaxis or disease treatment.

Female patients should have a gynecological exam with a cervical PAP smear. A high rate of cervical dysplasia with rapid progression to carcinoma occurs in HIV-infected women. Abnormal PAP smears should be followed up with colposcopy and possible biopsy.

Laboratory Monitoring of Medication Side Effects

Once antiretroviral therapy and/or prophylactic medications are implemented in the care of the patient with HIV, laboratory assessment for toxicities or side effects of the medications is indicated. Generally, a CBC with differential, a basic metabolic panel, triglycerides, and a hepatic panel picks up the most anticipated side effects of antiretroviral medications. If pancreatitis is suspected, amylase and lipase testing is helpful in detecting this side effect of medications or overindulgence of alcohol. For patients with complaints of myalgia, obtaining a CPK or aldolase may help in the detection of myositis. In acutely ill patients a close watch on creatinine and BUN to determine deterioration in renal function is necessary. Dosages of medications may need to be reduced if renal insufficiency or failure is detected.

Laboratory Diagnosis of Specific HIV-Related Problems

Laboratory testing of a patient with known HIV and fever would include testing similar to that of any patient with a fever: complete blood count with differential, serum chemistry panel, urinalysis and urine culture, standard blood cultures, and a chest radiograph. The CD_4 count of the individual with HIV is important to determine the risk for opportunistic infection. If the CD_4 count is < 200 cells/mm^3 a special blood culture for mycobacteria and a serum cryptococcal antigen would be additional appropriate tests. The blood culture for mycobacteria routinely take 3 to 8 weeks to obtain results due to the slow growth of the organism. Empiric therapy may be started in a symptomatic high-risk patient prior to obtaining the final results.

If the HIV patient has a fever with localized signs and symptoms suggestive of a pulmonary problem, pulse oximetry, arterial blood gases, and routine sputum gram stain and culture should be obtained. Additional special sputum specimens for acid fast bacilli and induced sputum for *pneumocystis carinii* would be indicated and are important to identify opportunistic organisms that commonly cause pulmonary infections in this patient population. An elevated serum lactic dehydrogenase is present in over 90% of patients with PCP. When a diagnosis cannot be made by less invasive testing, a bronchoscopy with brochioalveolar lavage may be necessary to obtain secretions for laboratory analysis.

Diarrhea is a common problem that may be related to side effects of medication or lactose intolerance. Diarrhea lasting more than five days should be evaluated for infectious etiologies. The initial limited evaluation of a patient with HIV should include stool analysis for specific bowel pathogens. Three stools specimens should be sent for examination for ova and parasites. A stool culture for enteric bacterial pathogens, an acid fast stain, and assessment for the presence of fecal leukocytes should be performed. If the patient has been taking prophylactic antibiotics to prevent opportunistic infections, a specimen for *clostridium difficile* toxin would be indicated. Blood cultures should also be obtained. If the source of diarrhea cannot be discerned by a limited evaluation, endoscopic evaluation with a flexible sigmoidoscopy or colonoscopy with ileoscopy should be performed. In a patient with a history and physical exam suggestive of small bowel disease, an esophagogastroduodenoscopy with small bowel biopsies and duodenal aspiration may be performed.

Treatment

Antiretroviral Therapy

Treatment for patients with HIV involves the use of antiretroviral drugs to reduce viral replication, prophylactic use of medication against opportunistic infections, and treatment for specific infections or malignancies that develop during the course of HIV disease. Recent research and the availability of new drugs have changed the recommendations and treatment options for HIV disease. The information in this chapter on antiretroviral therapy for HIV infection reflect the updated recommendations from the International AIDS Society—USA Panel (Carpenter et al., 1997).

These recommendations specify therapy for patients with HIV RNA levels greater than 5000 to 10,000 copies/mL regardless of CD_4 cell counts. In particular, symptomatic patients and patients with CD_4 counts in the range of 350 to 500 cells/mL when HIV RNA assays are not available should also receive therapy.

Therapy should be considered for any patients with HIV disease and detectable plasma HIV RNA who request therapy and are willing to make a lifelong commitment of compliance to drug-therapy regimens. Institution of drug therapy might be safely deferred in patients with low plasma HIV RNA and high CD_4 cell counts with close monitoring of these values every 3 to 6 months to detect changes indicative of deterioration.

Current FDA-approved antiretroviral drugs are listed in Table 47–4. Three categories of antiretroviral agents are available: nucleoside analog reverse transcriptase inhibitors (NRTI), protease inhibitors (PI), and nonnucleoside reverse transcriptase inhibitors (NNRTI). The nucleoside analogs or NRTIs inhibit HIV reverse transcriptase by slowing or preventing formation of DNA copies of HIV in infected cells. The PI category of drugs prevent cleavage of protein precursors essential for HIV maturation, infection of new cells, and viral replication. The introduction of this category of drugs has made a major impact on the clinical improvement and prolonged survival of HIV patients. The NNRTI drugs also inhibit reverse transcriptase through a different mechanism with different toxicity and resistance patterns than the NRTI drugs.

The preferred initial regimen of drug therapy is a potent three-drug combination sometimes referred to as a "cocktail" or as highly active antiretroviral therapy (HAART).

TABLE 47–4. Antiretroviral Therapy

Class/Drug	Usual Daily Dose	Common Side Effects	Monitoring
Nucleoside Analogues—Nucleoside reverse transcriptase inhibitors (NRTI)			
Retrovir, zidovudine (AZT)	300 mg BID	Anemia, neutropenia, nausea, malaise, headache, insomnia	CBC with differential
Videx, didanosine (DDI)	> 60 kg 200 mg BID < 60 kg 125 mg BID	Peripheral neuropathy, pancreatitis, dry mouth, hepatitis	CBC with differential, aminotransferases, amylase, triglycerides, periodic neurologic exam
Hivid, zalcitabine (ddC)	0.75 mg TID	Peripheral neuropathy, apthous ulcers, hepatitis pancreatitis	Aminotransferases, amylase, to periodic neurologic exam
Epivir, lamivudine (3TC)	150 mg BID	Rash, peripheral neuropathy	Monthly neurologic exam
Zerit, stavudine (d4T)	>60 kg 40 mg BID <60 kg 30 mg BID	Peripheral neuropathy, pancreatitis, hepatitis	Aminotransferases, amylase, to periodic neurologic exam
Combivir (zidovudine + lamivudine)	300 mg zidovudine + 150 mg lamivudine in one pill BID	Same as taking the two drugs individually	
Nonnucleoside Reverse Transcriptase Inhibitors (NNRTI)			
Viramune, nevirapine	200 mg QD for 2 weeks; then 200 mg BID	Rash, hepatitis	Transaminases
Rescriptor, delavirdine	400 mg TID	Rash	
Protease Inhibitors (PI)			Hyperglycemia, new onset diabetes mellitus
Invirase, saquinavir Fortovase saquinavir in gel cap formula	600 mg TID with food 1200 mg TID	Nausea, abdominal pain, diarrhea, headache	Aminotransferases, triglycerides, cholesterol
Norvir, ritonavir	Day 1 300 mg BID Days 2–3 400 mg BID Day 4 500 mg BID Then 600 mg BID	Nausea, vomiting, diarrhea, circumoral and peripheral paresthesias, asthenia, ↑ cholesterol, ↑ triglycerides	Aminotransferases, triglycerides, cholesterol
Crixivan, indinavir	800 mg TID on an empty stomach; drink 48 oz fluids QD	Kidney stones, Asymptomatic ↑ indirect bilirubin	Aminotransferases, bilirubin, triglycerides, cholesterol
Viracept, nelfinavir	750 mg TID with food	Nausea, diarrhea, asthenia, rash	Aminotransferases, triglycerides, cholesterol

This regimen includes two NRTI drugs and one PI drug. The primary alternative regimen for patients in whom use of protease inhibitors are not practical or tolerated would include two NRTI drugs and one NNRTI drug. In circumstances where neither of these regimens are possible, initiation of two NRTI drugs is preferable to no therapy at all for patients at high risk for short-term disease progression.

Prior to the initiation of HAART, the health-care provider and patient must discuss the advantages and disadvantages of these regimens. The patient must be willing to make a commitment to strict adherence to a sometimes complex schedule of taking medications that are expensive and with possible toxic side effects. Noncompliance with medication dosing (skipping doses or starting and stopping drugs frequently) can result in rapid virus replication and development of HIV resistance to drug therapy. Past medical history of the patient must be considered when selecting the combination of drugs and drug dosages included in triple-drug regimens. Common side effects of each drug must be considered when prescribing therapy to patients with preexisting conditions. For example, a patient with a history of kidney stones may not be a candidate for receiving Crixivan® which carries a reported incidence of kidney stones as a side effect.

Access to medications may also be a limiting factor to the drug therapy selected. All of these drugs are expensive. The lack of health-care coverage for prescription medications limits options available to patients. Although programs are available from pharmaceutical companies for indigent patients, they cannot be relied upon for unlimited patient support. State-based programs vary widely in their coverage of medications, budgets, formulary, and eligibility requirements. Outside of the United States, particularly in third-world countries, drug availability may be nonexistent.

The indications for changing an existing antiretroviral regimen include treatment failure, toxicity or intolerance of a drug, noncompliance to a regimen, or the current use of monotherapy or dual-therapy regimens. Research-based absolute criteria for treatment failure are not currently available. Generally, a patient who has previously reached an undetectable HIV RNA concentration using a specific drug combination would be considered for a therapy change if HIV RNA rises to greater than 2000 to 5000 copies/mL. In a patient situation where a significant drop in HIV RNA occurred, but not to undetectable levels, a confirmed increase to greater than 5000 to 10,000 copies/mL should indicate a treatment change. Other indications for treatment failure include a lack of initial decline in HIV RNA levels, a rise in HIV RNA to pretreatment levels, continued decline in CD_4 cell count, or evidence of clinical disease progression. A thorough assessment for other causes for the rise in HIV viral load must be considered before drug therapies are altered. The limited numbers of alternative drug choices poses a dilemma in the practical application of these guidelines in patients who do not have favorable or sustained response to HAART.

If drug toxicity occurs, the suspected drug should be discontinued until the toxic effect is resolved. If at all possible, the dose of the PI component of HAART should be continued to minimize the development of drug resistance. If it is not clear which drug is the offending agent, all three drugs should be stopped briefly. A decision to replace one or all drugs must be made on an individual patient basis, influenced by availability of alternative drugs.

Patients receiving dual NRTI or monotherapy should be evaluated for signs of treatment failure before changing the regimen. If HIV RNA levels are undetectable, the patient could be safely followed for signs of increasing viral load before changing the regimen. If the viral load is greater than 5000 to 10,000 copies/mL, alternative drug therapy should be instituted. The patient who falls in the intermediate range of 400 to 5000 copies/mL should be monitored for a confirmed rising trend in plasma HIV RNA, at which time therapy should be altered.

Clinical trials for several new antiretroviral drugs are currently underway. The pharmaceutical companies also make these new, non-FDA approved agents available to patients who have failed existing approved therapies. The ACNP may encounter a patient with HIV who is participating in such a trial or receiving compassionate use of a new medication. Adverse drug interactions and suspected side effects of experimental agents are events that must be watched for closely and well documented for patients participating in clinical trials. At this time, Glaxo-Wellcome is studying a NRTI drug 1592U89 (abacavir). Adefovir (Preveon) is a drug in a new class of agents call nucleotides under development by Gilead. DuPont–Merck has a new once-a-day NNRTI drug called efavirenz (Sustiva) before the FDA for New Drug Approval (NDA).

Because of the complexity of HAART and the possible drug interactions with other medications, patients must receive adequate education to ensure compliance with the regimen selected. The regimen should take into account the patient's lifestyle as well as the interactions and side effects of the drugs. For example, a drug requiring refrigeration such as ritonivir would not be an appropriate selection for a homeless person. Individualized teaching regarding the selected regimen is necessary. For some patients, a written schedule surrounding their normal activities of daily living may be needed to transition from a hospital schedule of controlled dosing. Written materials must be available in each patient's language and for patients who are illiterate. Management of anticipated side effects must also be addressed prior to discharge. Linking the patient with resources for follow-up should be arranged as part of discharge planning. Nurse case managers and nurse practitioner colleagues in the community are excellent resources for patients with medication management questions or problems.

Treatment of Occupational Exposure to HIV

Treatment of health-care providers who have suffered occupational exposure to HIV-infected blood with antiretroviral medication has been recommended by the CDC. Categories of risk include high risk (injury that involves a large volume of blood and a high titer of HIV), increased risk (injury that involves either a large volume of blood or high titer of HIV), and no increased risk (injury involves neither a large volume of blood nor a high titer of HIV). Skin exposures are considered at increased risk if a high titer of HIV, prolonged contact, extensive area is exposed, or if a compromise of skin integrity is present. Therapy includes a combination of two or more agents depending on the assessment of risk of the exposure (Table 47–5). After counseling the employee and obtaining verbal informed consent, treatment should be initiated within one hour of exposure and continued for a period of four weeks. Dosages of antiretroviral agents are the same as when prescribing for an HIV-infected patient.

Opportunistic Infection Prevention

Also in 1997, the U.S. Public Health Service (USPHS) and the Infectious Diseases Society of America (IDSA) published updated guidelines for the prevention of opportunistic infection in patients with HIV. Opportunistic infections cause significant morbidity and mortality for patients with HIV. Use of prophylactic medications and HAART have decreased the incidence of opportunistic infection in HIV patients in the United States.

The patient education responsibilities of the ACNP can be integrated into the prevention of opportunistic infection efforts when caring for HIV-infected patients. Advising patients concerning the prevention of exposure to opportunistic pathogens is an important component of infection prevention. General areas for patient education include potential for exposure from: sexual contact, environment and occupation, pets, food and water, and travel. All patients should be assessed for their existing knowledge in these areas and provided with information individualized to their situations. For example, a homeless female with AIDS with a history of IV drug use living in a crowded shelter would have different risks from a gay businessman newly diagnosed with HIV who travels frequently for business out of the United States to third-world countries. Patient education is an ongoing aspect of care. Opportunities in the acute care area may be limited based on the condition of the patient and the amount of time for the encounter. Referral to health-care providers who are experienced in care of HIV-infected persons should be established for all HIV-positive patients as part of discharge planning. Care provided by physicians with more experience with HIV is associated with lower risk of death (Kitahata et al., 1996) for this patient population.

Primary prophylaxis is defined as the use of medication to prevent the occurance of an opportunistic infection. The level of CD_4 is used to determine the risk for opportunistic infection. (Refer to Table 48–1.) Secondary prophylaxis is the use of medication to prevent a reoccurrence after a documented opportunistic infection episode. Prior to the use of HAART, patients usually did not have large rises in CD_4 cell counts. Patients who have responded favorably to HAART with rises in CD_4 counts to greater than 200/mL may not have regeneration of clones of cells that provide protection against specific opportunistic infection. Until clinical studies provide a clear answer, the USPHS/IDSA recommends initiating and continuing prophylaxis based on the lowest documented CD_4 cell count.

The first opportunistic infection associated with AIDS was identified as PCP. Since use of primary and secondary prophylaxis against PCP and with increased longevity of patients with AIDS, many other opportunistic infections may occur as the patient survives but the immune system becomes more suppressed.

Prophylaxis for PCP should be instituted for patients with a CD_4 count of <200/mL or those with oropharngeal

TABLE 47–5. CDC Recommendations for Occupational Postexposure Antiretroviral Prophylactic Treatment

Type of Exposure	Source Material	Prophylactic Treatment	Drug Regimen
Percutaneous	Blood		
	highest risk	Recommended	Retrovir, Epivir, and Crixivan
	increased risk	Recommended	Retrovir, Epivir, and Crixivan
	no increased risk	Offer	Retrovir and Epivir
	Body fluids		
	bloody or infectious	Offer	Retrovir and Epivir
	other body fluids	Not offer	
Mucous membrane	Blood	Offer	Retrovir, Epivir ± Crixivan
	Infectious fluid	Offer	Retrovir and Epivir
	Other body fluid	Not offer	
Skin (increased risk)	Blood	Offer	Retrovir, Epivir ± Crixivan
	Infectious fluid	Offer	Retrovir and Epivir
	Other body fluid	Not offer	

candidiasis or unexplained fever lasting 2 or more weeks. Trimethoprim-sulfamethoxazole (TMP-SMZ) at a dose of one double strength tablet orally every day is the treatment of choice for PCP prophylaxis. This inexpensive drug is also the first choice for prophylaxis against *toxoplasma gondii* for patients with IgG antibody to this organism and a CD_4 count < 100/mL. An alternative oral drug regimen for both organisms includes dapsone 50 mg daily, with pyrimethamine 50 mg and leucovorin 25 mg weekly.

When the patient reaches a CD_4 count of < 50/mL, prophylaxis against *mycobacterium avium* complex (MAC) should begin. Either oral clarithromycin 500 mg BID or azithromycin 1200 mg q week are effective first-choice agents. Oral rifabutin 300 mg daily is an alternative, but many drug interactions occur with this agent and must be considered before it is prescribed.

If an HIV-infected person has a tuberculin skin test reaction of > 5 mm and exclusion of active tuberculosis, had a prior positive skin test result without treatment, or had recent contact with an active case of tuberculosis, there is a strong recommendation to receive a 12-month course of prophylactic therapy to prevent active disease. The drug isoniazide (INH) in an oral dose of 300 mg daily in combination with 50 mg of pyridoxine is prescribed. In situations where observed twice-weekly therapy is chosen, the INH dose is increased to 900 mg with the same pyridoxine dose. An alternative oral therapy is 600 mg of rifampin daily. When exposure to mulidrug resistant TB is likely, the choice of prophylactic agents for the patient should be made after consultation with local public health authorities.

Immunizations are also a part of disease prophylaxis in patients with HIV. Pneumococcal vaccine 0.5 mL is strongly recommended to be administered via intramuscular injection to all patients regardless of CD_4 count. If 5 years have passed since the administration of this vaccine, a second dose is optional. It is generally recommended that all patients susceptible to hepatitis B (anti-HBc negative) should receive the series of three vaccines for prevention of hepatitis B virus infection. Annual influenza vaccination before influenza season is generally recommended for HIV-infected patients using either whole or split virus vaccine 0.5 mL intramuscularly. Alternative oral antiviral agents for influenza, amantadine, and rimantidine exist for the prophylaxis of influenza but require BID dosing.

Primary prophylaxis is not generally recommended for most patients for the following organisms: *candida* species, *cryptococcus neoformans, histoplasma capsulatum,* and cytomegalovirus (CMV). Prophylaxis may be considered in unusual circumstances. The high cost of medications, effectiveness of oral agents, drug toxicities and interactions, and/or the development of drug resistance are rationale for not using routine primary prophylaxis for these infections. Until data from prospective controlled trials indicate otherwise, patients with advanced HIV disease should be monitored closely for the development of these opportunistic infections so that treatment can be initiated promptly if acute infection occurs.

After chemotherapy for an acute episode of opportunistic infection in the HIV-infected adult, prophylaxis against recurrence of the disease is recommended for life as the standard of care. For PCP one double strength TMP-SMZ daily is the first choice, with alternative regimens including a combination of dapsone, pyrimethamine, and leucovorin.

When encephalitis due to *toxoplasma gondii* has been documented, sulfadiazine 500 to 1000 mg QID plus pyrimethamine 25 to 75 mg daily and leucovorin 10 mg daily are the first choice. An alternative therapy for sulfa-allergic patients substitutes clindamycin 300 to 450 mg every 6 to 8 hours and is combined with pyrimethamine and leucovorin.

Documented disseminated disease attributed to MAC requires a multidrug regimen. Oral clarithromycin 500 mg is administered BID along with one or more of the following drugs: ethambutol 15 mg/kg once daily and/or rifabutin 300 mg once daily. An acceptable alternative for clarithromycin is azithromycin 500 mg combined with either ethambutol or rifabutin, or both drugs.

Cytomegalovirus infection with end-organ disease is often treated with intravenous (IV) medication: ganciclovir 5-6 mg/kg IV for 5-7 days/week, foscarnet 90-120 mg/kg IV daily, or cidofovir 5 mg/kg IV every other week. Ganciclovir is the only drug available in an oral form requiring 1000 mg TID. For CMV retinitis, ganciclovir in a sustained-release intraocular implant may be placed every 6 to 9 months. All of these agents have been shown to be first choices by randomized controlled trials providing strong evidence for efficacy and benefit. Choice of agent must be made based on toxicities of the drugs in a given patient and the site of CMV infection.

Daily oral dosing of fluconazole 200 mg is the first choice for documented infection with *cryptococcus neoformans.* Higher dose (400 mg daily) fluconazole is used for documented disease caused by *coccidioides immitis.* Oral itraconazole 200 mg BID is recommended after documented disease with *histoplasma capsulatum.* Itraconazole may be substituted as an alternate therapy in place of fluconazole. Fluconazole may be used for an alternative oral therapy to itraconazole. Amphotericin B by using intermittent IV dosing can be substituted in all three infections.

Only if patients are troubled with frequent or severe episodes of herpes simplex infections or *candida* infection in the oropharynx, vagina, or esophagus is daily therapy recommended. Oral acyclovir 400 mg BID or 200 mg TID are regimens that can be used for herpes suppression. Fluconazole in oral doses between 100 to 200 mg daily is effective against recurrent *candida* infections.

Treatment of Acute Pulmonary Infections

The preferred therapy for acute PCP is TMP-SMZ. The usual adult dose in less symptomatic patients is two double-strength tablets every 8 hours for 21 days. Those who are more seriously ill or cannot tolerate oral medications receive parenteral therapy of 15 mg TMP/kg/day. Patients with more severe PCP with a $PaO_2 < 70$ mm Hg should receive prednisone therapy. A dose of 40 mg orally should precede the first TMP-SMX by 15 to 20 minutes and be given BID for 5 days. The dose is decreased to 40 mg daily for 5 days and then continued at 20 mg per day for the remaining 11 days of therapy. Many HIV patients develop an allergic rash reaction to TMP-SMZ. Alternative regimens include oral or IV clindamycin and primaquine or IV pentamidine isethionate.

Bacterial pneumonias should be treated with an antibiotic appropriate to the isolated organism. Pneumococcal pneumonia, the most common bacterial lung infection in patients with HIV, may be treated with ceftriaxone 2 gm IV daily or cefotaxime 2 gm IV every 8 hours. Erythromycin or vancomycin IV may be used as alternative therapies.

If acute respiratory failure develops in patients with HIV and pnuemonia, medical management and nursing care should follow the same protective strategies for any patient with acute diffuse lung injury. It is important to maintain adequate hydration, avoiding overhydration which may result in pulmonary edema and worsening hypoxemia. Administration of supplemental oxygen is usually required. Intubation and mechanical ventilation may be necessary to provide adequate oxygenation. Aggressive therapies should be used if based on the patient's directives for such measures.

Treatment of Diarrhea

While awaiting a diagnosis of specific etiology for diarrhea in the patient with HIV, empiric therapy is not advocated. Supportive therapy to prevent dehydration and to maintain nutrition are indicated. Oral dietary supplements can be used to increase caloric intake. Lactose-free or low-fat diets may reduce malabsorption symptoms. Parenteral electrolytes, fluids, and alimentation are necessary if the patient is unable to tolerate oral food and fluids. Antimotility agents such as loperamide or diphenoxylate may be helpful in patients when diarrhea is not associated with bloody stool, presence of fecal leukocytes, or abdominal cramping. If an enteric pathogen is identified, specific antimicrobial therapy is indicated.

Follow-Up

Today, HIV infection is considered a chronic manageable disease. With the advances in antiretroviral therapy and prophylaxis against opportunistic infection, a patient who is compliant with complex medication regimens and lifestyle modifications can live for many years after HIV infection is diagnosed. Even patients meeting the criteria for AIDS have experienced dramatic improvements in their conditions in response to PI drugs. Because of its dynamic state and complex regimens, the ongoing care of patients with HIV disease should be managed by health-care providers experienced with care of the HIV patient. Newly diagnosed patients should be referred to an infectious disease specialist, a multidisciplinary clinic specializing in HIV patient care, or a physician experienced with HIV disease. Survival of patients with AIDS is significantly associated with the experience of the primary-care physician (Kitahata et al., 1996). Linking the patient with an experienced health-care provider prior to discharge can facilitate continuity of care.

Depending on the condition of the patient with HIV and disease manifestations, other specialists may be called upon for consultation regarding a specific problem. A pulmonologist may be needed to perform a diagnostic bronchoscopy or to manage a critically ill patient requiring mechanical ventilation. A gastroenterologist may need to perform endoscopic examiniations in a patient with chronic or severe diarrhea. A neurologist may be called upon to evaluate a patient with complex abnormal neurological findings. The pharmacist may be consulted when a drug regimen involving multiple agents is initiated or modified. A dietician may be needed to assist in planning a diet for wasting patients with food intolerances.

Prior to discharge from an acute care facility, an initial assessment of patient resources is essential to identify areas where ongoing support is or will be needed. A social services consult is particularly helpful in the situation when a patient with HIV has limited financial reserves or lacks in-

TABLE 47–6. Suggested Patient Education Topics for Patients with HIV Infection

1. Counseling on prevention of HIV transmission to others	Safer sex practices Household contacts Blood and body fluid contact situations Risk behaviors related to IV drug use Pregnancy issues
2. Explanation of anticipated course of HIV treatment	Monitoring viral load Monitoring CD_4 counts Monitoring for opportunistic infection
3. Avoidance of opportunistic infection	Sexual Environmental Occupational Pet-related Food and water Travel-related
4. Opportunistic infections	Prophylactic medications Signs, symptoms, and seeking health care
5. Counseling on general wellness and health maintenance	Diet Exercise Smoking cessation Alcohol use Routine eye exams and retinal exams Gynecological exam with PAP smear
6. Antiretroviral therapy	Treatment options Compliance with regimen Side effects and their management Monitoring therapy for effectiveness

surance coverage for obtaining medications. Establishing a source for medication to ensure uninterrupted supply is crucial for the success of antiretroviral therapy. Referral to substance abuse programs may also be needed for patients with abuse of drugs and/or alcohol. Assistance with the paperwork required for state or local programs for the indigent patient or social security disability is often a need.

Home-health agencies or long-term care facilities may be required for the more debilitated patient with AIDS. Meal delivery to the home may also be a need after discharge. In some cases, hospice care may be needed for those with end-stage disease.

Length of stay as an inpatient in today's acute care facilities is limited and there is inadequate time to cover all the areas of patient education needed for patients with a new diagnosis of HIV or AIDS. Priority topics include methods to prevent the spread of HIV infection to other household members, sexual contacts, or through recreational drug use. If medications have been initiated, the patient, family, and/or significant other needs to be clear on dose, frequency, special circumstances associated with taking the pills, and potential dangerous side effects or drug interactions specific to their individualized multidrug regimen. Other general areas for patient education of a newly diagnosed patient with HIV are included in Table 47–6. The receptiveness of the patient and time constraints of the encounter dictate how much patient education is realistic during hospitalization.

The potential psychosocial needs of patients with HIV disease are as enormous as their physiological needs. Coming to accept a diagnosis of HIV takes time. Disclosure of a new diagnosis of HIV to a sexual partner is a threatening situation where the patient may need considerable help and support during and after such an interaction. Many patients with HIV infection may have little family support during their illness. Often friends, coworkers, or neighbors are not privy to the patient's diagnosis, so the patient may feel isolated and alone. Spiritual needs of the patient must not be overlooked in the psychosocial assessment and plan of care.

The ACNP can play a major role in the diagnosis and treatment of HIV disease in the acute care setting today. The focus of the ACNP practice is on stabilization of acute illness and restoration of the patient to maximal health potential. Caring for the hospitalized patient with HIV infection is a perfect example of a patient population in need of the skills and knowledge of the ACNP.

REFERENCES

Bartlett, J. G. (1996). *The Johns Hopkins Hospital 1996 Guide to Medical Care of Patients with HIV Infection.* Baltimore: Williams & Wilkens.

Bartlett, J. G. & Feinberg, J. (1996). Management of opportunistic infections in patients with HIV infection: Update. *Infectious Diseases in Clinical Practice, 4,* 267–276.

Carpenter, C. J., Fischl, M. A., Hammer, S. M., Hirsch, M. S., Jacobsen, D. M., Katzenstein, D. A., Montaner, J. S. G., Richman, D. D., Saag, M. S., Schooley, R. T., Thompson, M. A., Vella, S., Yeni, P. G., & Volberding, P. A. (1997). Antiretroviral therapy for HIV infection in 1997 updated recommendations of the International AIDS Society—USA panel. *Journal of the American Medical Association, 277,* 1962–1969.

Centers for Disease Control. (1992). 1993 revised classification system for HIV infection and expanded surveillance case definition for AIDS among adolescents and adults. *Morbidity and Mortality Weekly Report, 41,* 1–19.

Centers for Disease Control. (1996a). Update: Provisional public health service recommendations for chemoprophylaxis after occupational exposure to HIV. *Morbidity and Mortality Weekly Report, 45,* 468–472.

Centers for Disease Control. (1996b). Ten leading nationally notifiable infectious diseases—United States, 1995. *Morbidity and Mortality Weekly Report, 45,* 883–884.

Centers for Disease Control. (1996c). *HIV/AIDS Surveillance Report,* 8.

Centers for Disease Control. (1997a). Update: Trends in AIDS incidence, deaths, and prevalence—United States, 1996. *Morbidity and Mortality Weekly Report, 46,* 165–173.

Centers for Disease Control. (1997b). USPHS/IDSA guidelines for the prevention of opportunistic infections in persons infected with human immunodeficiency virus. *Morbidity and Mortality Weekly Report, 46,* 1–46.

Condra, J. H. & Emini, E. A. (1997). Preventing HIV-1 drug resistance. *Science & Medicine, 4* (1), 2–11.

Crowe, S. & Mills, J. (1997). Virus infections of the immune system. In. D. P. Sites, A. I. Terr, & T. G. Parslow (Eds.), *Medical immunology* (9th ed.). (pp. 748–765). Stamford, CT: Appleton & Lange.

Drugs for HIV infection. (1997). *The Medical Letter, 39,* 111–116.

Greenspan, D. & Greenspan, J. S. (1996). HIV-related oral disease. *Lancet, 348,* 729–733.

Ho, D. D., Neumann, A. U., Perelson, A. S., et al. (1995). Rapid turnover of plasma virions and CD4 lymphocytes in HIV-1 infection. *Nature, 373,* 123–125.

Ho, D. D. (1996). Viral counts in HIV infection. *Science, 272,* 1124–1125.

Kitahata, M. M., Koepsell, T. D., Deyo, R. A., Maxwell, C. L., Dodge, W. T., & Wagner, E. H. (1996). Physicians' experience with the acquired immunodeficiency syndrome as a factor in patients' survival. *New England Journal of Medicine, 334,* 701–706.

Klaus, B. D. (1996). Applying viral load measurements to HIV care. *Nurse Practitioner, 21,* 102–104.

Klaus, B. D. & Grodesky, M. J. (1997). Prophylaxis of HIV-associated opportunistic infections: 1997 recommendations. *Nurse Practitioner, 22,* 69–79.

Leibowitz, R. E., Tatarakis, J., & Delgado, J. (1995). HIV infection/AIDS and critical care. *Critical Care Nursing Clinics of North America, 7,* 651–659.

Masur, H., Whitcup, S. M., Cartwright, C., Polis, M., & Nussenblatt, R. (1996). Advances in the management of AIDS-related cytomegalovirus retinitis. *Annals of Internal Medicine, 125,* 126–145.

Mellors, J. W., Rinaldo, C. R., Gupta, P., White, R. M., Todd, J. A., & Kingsley, L. A. (1996). Prognosis in HIV-1 infection predicted by the quantity of virus in plasma. *Science, 272,* 1167–1170.

Pantaleo, G., Graziosi, C., & Fauci, A. S. (1993). The immunopathogenesis of human immunodeficiency virus infection. *New England Journal of Medicine, 328,* 327–335.

Saag, M. S., Holodniy, M., Kuritzkes, D. R., O'Brien, W. A., Coombs, R. W., Poscher, M. E., Jacobsen, D. M., Shaw, G. M., Richman, D. D., & Volberding, P. A. (1996). HIV viral load markers in clinical practice. *Nature Medicine, 2,* 625–629.

Tribett, D. (1995). Human immunodeficiency virus (HIV) and acquired immunodeficiency syndrome (AIDS). In N. A. Urban, K. K. Greenlee, J. M. Krumberger, & C. Winkelman (Eds.), *Guideline for critical care nursing.* (pp. 574–586) St. Louis: Mosby.

Tschachler, E., Bergstresser, P. R., & Stingl, G. (1996). HIV-related skin disease. *Lancet, 348,* 659–663.

Wheeler, D. A. (1997). Human immunodeficiency virus in the health care setting. *Occupational Medicine: State of the Art Reviews, 12,* 741–756.

Zuccotti, G. & Sepkowitz, K. A. (1995). Evaluation of fever in HIV-infected patients: A CD_4-based approach. *The AIDS Reader, 5* (4), 190–197.

48

Rheumatic Problems

Joanne Sandberg-Cook
Susan Hoch

Rheumatic diseases are extremely common in the United States, causing disability in 37 million Americans. Two thirds of those affected are women. Arthritis, the most common problem in this diverse group of disorders, is the leading health problem in people over the age of 50 and the most common cause for visits to health-care providers in the population above the age of 65 (Hannan, 1997). There are over 100 different conditions classified as rheumatic diseases. The costs are enormous. Medical costs alone are estimated at $72.3 billion; lost wages account for another $77.1 billion (Hannan, 1997). The chronic, incurable nature of these diseases makes the patient vulnerable to the lure of unproven therapies costing many more billions of dollars. Rheumatic diseases cause pain, immobility, joint destruction, weakened bones, and damage to internal organs that can affect functional independence and shorten life span.

Rheumatic diseases can be classified in many ways Because joint pain is common to virtually all of the rheumatic diseases, a simple classification starts with the number of joints involved. Single-joint symptoms (monoarticular arthritis) constitute a common presentation of infection, trauma, tumor, or crystal-induced diseases.

Multiple-joint symptoms (polyarticular arthritis) can be further subdivided into inflammatory polyarthritis, degenerative polyarthritis, and metabolic polyarthritis. Rheumatoid arthritis, systemic lupus erythematosis, systemic sclerosis (scleroderma), vasculitis, transient viral syndromes, and sero-negative spondyloarthropathies—which also cause back pain and deformity—are examples of rheumatic diseases. Osteoarthritis, the most common rheumatic disease, can involve many small and large joints including the spine and present as a monoarticular or polyarticular process. Polyarticular gout, calcium pyrophosphate disease (pseudogout), amyloidosis, and osteoporosis are all examples of metabolic diseases that feature frank arthritis or musculoskeletal pain as part of the symptom complex.

Extraarticular disorders can also cause joint pain. These include bursitis, tendinitis, cysts, and regional pain syndromes such as fibromyalgia, chronic fatigue syndrome, and reflex sympathetic dystrophy. Carpal tunnel syndrome and other nerve entrapment syndromes can be seen as isolated problems or as complications of intraarticular disorders. Infectious diseases including sexually transmitted diseases, Lyme disease, and other bacterial and viral syndromes should not be overlooked.

Classification of all these diseases is difficult because the cause of many is unknown. A detailed classification is available from the American College of Rheumatology and published in the *Primer on the Rheumatic Diseases.*

▶ MONOARTHRITIS

One of the most common and challenging problems in rheumatology is presented by the patient with an acute monoarthritis. Information from history and physical exam may be helpful in directing you toward likely possibilities but ultimately arthrocentesis and examination of joint fluid is the most direct diagnostic procedure.

History and Physical Findings

A history of trauma may suggest fracture, internal derangement, or hemarthrosis. Previous similar episodes of acute painful monoarthritis, particularly of the lower extremities, suggest a crystal synovitis. The presence of fever, chills, rash, diarrhea, or tick bites may be important clues to Lyme disease. Risk factors such as sexual history, immunodeficiency, and intravenous drug use should be elicited. Preexisting osteoarthritis may acutely exacerbate or a patient with rheumatoid arthritis may now have developed a septic joint. In the case of a prosthetic joint, infection is always a concern.

On physical examination, care should be taken to evaluate whether the involved joint is truly arthritic or whether the process is periarticular or cellulitic. Often, it can be quite difficult to distinguish between a cellulitis and a septic arthritis. Patients with an acute bursitis present with swelling and pain around the joint but careful examination reveals that the range of motion of the joint remains intact. Limited range of motion nearly always suggests true joint involvement.

The examiner should try to perform a complete physical examination on the patient with monoarthritis as there may be other diagnostic clues present. In gonococcal arthritis, pustular skin lesions may be noted. Small patches of psoriasis in the umbilical area or gluteal fold or nail pitting may suggest psoriatic arthritis Conjunctival injection might suggest Reiter's disease. Other joints may be found to be abnormal pointing to more longstanding disease. Tophi on the ears or over the olecranon bursae or Achilles tendon suggest an acute exacerbation of chronic tophacous gout.

The algorithm in Figure 48–1 offers a simple approach to the evaluation of an acute monoarthritis. Particularly in the emergency room setting, x-ray may be helpful to exclude fracture, tumor, ischemic necrosis, or preexisting joint disease. In the setting of an acute monoarthritis, plain x-ray is likely to show only soft tissue swelling and possibly a joint effusion.

Laboratory and Diagnostic Tests

The most critical and direct step, then, is to determine the nature of the joint effusion by arthrocentesis. Arthrocentesis should be performed in all patients with a monoarthritis to exclude infectious causes, to diagnosis a crystal-induced arthritis, and to distinguish between inflammatory and noninflammatory joint disease. Arthrocentesis is an office procedure that can be done with minimal discomfort to the patient. The approach to individual joints is beyond the scope of this chapter and the reader is referred to any standard rheumatology textbook.

There are very few situations in which diagnostic arthrocentesis is contraindicated. If untreated cellulitis or suspected cellulitis is present, the risk of introducing an organism into the joint is high. Patients with known bleeding disorders, including those that are anticoagulated, are at risk of developing a hemarthrosis if tapped. However, if the clinical situation requires diagnostic arthrocentesis, the use of a small-gauge needle in the hands of a skilled individual increases the safety factor for these patients.

The general approach begins with the identification of anatomic landmarks. The proposed point of entry is marked and the area cleansed with povidine–iodine and allowed to dry. With judicious use of local anesthetic, the procedure need not be painful. The area around the proposed point of entry can be sprayed with a topical anesthetic such as Fluori–Methane (dichlorofluoromethane15%/trichloromonofluoromethane 15%) until the patient notes a burning or freezing sensation and the skin blanches. Alternatively, local subcutaneous anesthesia with 1 to 2% xylocaine can be used alone or in addition to the topical spray. Using appropriate sterile technique, a 20 to 21-gauge needle attached to a 5 to 10-cc syringe is introduced into the joint. Only a small amount of fluid is necessary for a diagnostic tap but removal of as much fluid as possible may improve the patient's comfort.

Arthrocentesis is also used therapeutically. In acute gout, removal of crystal-laden synovial fluid may decrease joint inflammation. In septic arthritis, the daily drainage of inflammatory joint fluid may decrease cartilage damage as well as indicate the success or failure of the patient's systemic antibiotic treatment.

Injection of corticosteroid into the joint is appropriate only when a diagnosis has been made and sepsis is ruled out. Intraarticular steroids provide rapid relief of pain and inflammation with minimal systemic side effects.

As shown in Figure 48–1, normal joint fluid is clear, transparent, and quite viscous. (One should be able to read print through the fluid.) A drop of fluid placed under a plain light microscope should reveal few white blood cells, most of them mononuclear in nature. The white blood cell count should be less than 200 mm^3 with less than 25% polymorphonuclear leukocytes. Under compensated polarized microscopy, there should be no visible crystals. Knowing the characteristics of the joint fluid, a differential diagnosis can be established as seen in Figure 48–1.

If inflammatory or purulent fluid is aspirated, it is essential to try to distinguish a septic arthritis from an acute crystal-induced synovitis from other causes of an inflammatory arthritis because of the different implications for management and treatment. The two immediate crucial tests here are the observation under compensated polarized light microscopy for crystals and the gram stain. While acute gouty arthritis and a septic arthritis have been rarely reported to coexist in the same joint (Baer et al., 1986), the finding of intracellular crystals of either monosodium urate in acute gouty arthritis or calcium pyrophosphate in acute pseudogout would establish a diagnosis of a crystal-induced monoarthritis and direct subsequent treatment. A gram-

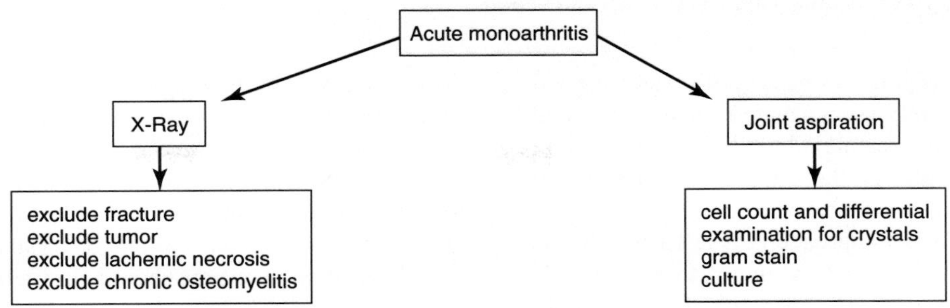

Types of Joint effusions

Criteria	Normal	Non-inflammatory	Inflammatory	Purulent	Hemorrhagic
1. volume	< 3.5 ml	often > 3.5 ml	often > 3.5 ml	> 3.5 ml	> 3.5 ml
2. color	clear	xanthochromic	xanthochromic to white	depends on organism	bloody
3. clarity	transparent	transparent	translucent to opaque	opaque	bloody
4. viscosity	high	high	low	variable	like blood
5. mucin clot	firm	firm	friable	friable	
6. clot	no	occasional	often	often	
7. WBC(mm3)	< 200	200-2000	2000-100,000 (20,000 average)	> 50,000	blood
8. % polys	< 25%	< 25%	> 75%	> 75%	blood
9. culture	Neg	Neg	Neg	Pos or Neg	Neg

Differential Diagnosis of Joint Effusions

Non-inflammatory	Inflammatory	Purulent	Hemorrhagic
Osteoarthritis Trauma Osteochondritis Avascular necrosis SLE Amyloidosis Chronic crystal synovitis	Rheumatoid arthritis Reiter's syndrome Acute crystal synovitis Psoriatic arthritis Enteropathic arthritis Lyme Disease Viral arthritis Rheumatic fever Infectious arthritis bacterial tuberculosis fungal	Bacterial infection Acute gout	Trauma Fracture Blood dyscrasia Charcot joint Pigmented villonodular synovitis Tumor

Aspiration of Inflammatory or Purulent Fluid from Monoarthritis

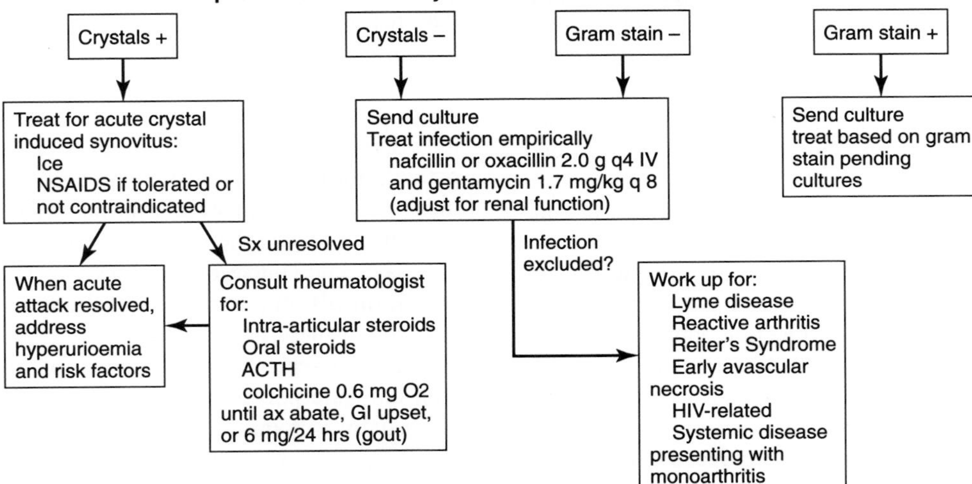

Figure 48–1. Differential diagnosis and management of acute monoarthritis. *(From Baker & Schumacher. [1993]. [pp. 164–187]; Emmerson. [1996]. [pp. 445–451].)*

stained slide showing polynuclear neutrophils with ingested gram-positive or more rarely gram-negative organisms would allow for initial antibiotic treatment based on the gram stain while awaiting the results of the culture of the synovial fluid.

Many times, this initial approach fails to clearly differentiate the cause of the inflammatory monoarthritis; crystals are not found and the gram stain is negative. In this setting, it is incumbent to treat infection empirically. Antibiotics are chosen to cover both gram-positive and gram-negative organisms even though the majority of septic joints are caused by gram-positive bacteria. A reasonable initial approach would be nafcillin or oxacillin 2 grams every 4 hours intravenously with gentamycin 1.7 mg/kg every 8 hours adjusted for the patient's renal function. The Figure 48–1 algorithm addresses this approach.

A relatively common problem in the hospital setting is the patient who is already receiving antibiotics and is then noted to have a swollen joint. Arthrocentesis yields an inflammatory joint effusion and synovial fluid gram stain and culture are negative. Yet the patient may have a septic arthritis. If crystal-induced arthritis can be excluded, it is prudent to treat the patient as if he or she had a proven septic arthritis with daily joint aspiration until the effusion is resolved and continued antibiotic therapy for 4 to 6 weeks.

Another frequently encountered clinical problem is the differential diagnosis of monoarthritis in the patient with overlying cellulitis. Aspiration of a joint through an area of cellulitis in a patient not receiving antibiotics is not recommended due to the risk of introducing infection into the joint. In this situation, it is prudent to obtain blood cultures and to culture the leading edge of the cellulitis and initiate antibiotic therapy. The joint can then be aspirated subsequently and if an inflammatory joint fluid is obtained, gram stain may still be helpful although a culture may not be. Nuclear medicine studies may also be helpful in distinguishing cellulitis from underlying bone or joint involvement. Using a bone-reacting isotope, such as technicium 99M oxidronate, and looking at delayed uptake, joint or bone involvement can be distinguished from the increased blood flow initially seen in cellulitis. Tagged white blood cell scans can also be useful.

Gonococcal arthritis is an important diagnosis to consider in a patient with a monoarthritis. Often the patient reports a migratory polyarthritis or tendinitis prior to the development of the monoarthritis. Women tend to present with disseminated gonococcal infection more often than men, often a week or so after menses. Gram stain and culture of the affected joint may not yield the organism. Careful observation for the characteristic skin lesions and appropriate pharyngeal, cervical, urethral, and rectal cultures may be diagnostic, if done.

In communities where Lyme disease is endemic, it is not uncommon to see untreated Lyme disease present as an acute monoarthritis. History of a tick bite, exposure to deer, skin lesion, aseptic meningitis, or heart block may be helpful clues and serology is usually diagnostic.

Finally, many systemic diseases including Reiter's syndrome, inflammatory bowel disease, and HIV infection may present as a monoarthritis Careful history and physical examination, exclusion of septic or crystal-induced arthritis, and observation over time should clarify the diagnosis.

▶ POLYARTHRITIS

The approach to the patient with polyarthritis differs from the approach to monoarthritis. While infection and crystal synovitis are included in the differential diagnosis of polyarthritis, for the most part, you are trying to determine whether the patient has joint involvement or whether the complaint emanates from periarticular structures or muscle. Figure 48–2 presents an algorithm to help in this decision-making process.

History and Physical Findings

First, you must distinguish whether the patient has a true arthritis. Is the patient complaining of diffuse joint pain or tenderness? Is there joint swelling? Is there erythema overlying the joint? In contrast, are the complaints those of muscle tenderness; are they localized to a pattern of specific tender points that might suggest fibromyalgia?

If there is joint swelling, the next step is to observe the nature of the swelling. Is there heat or erythema or discoloration of the skin over the involved joints? Does the swelling seem hard or bony? Is there palpable thickening—or bogginess—of the normally thin synovium? Hard bony enlargement suggests primary or secondary osteoarthritis; warmth, erythema, and boggy swelling are indicative of inflammation.

The next thing to consider is the pattern of joint involvement. Asymmetric involvement of small joints and the spine suggest a possible spondylarthropathy such as Reiter's disease, ankylosing spondylitis, or psoriatic or enteropathic arthritis. In contrast, symmetric small-joint involvement suggests rheumatoid arthritis, systemic lupus erythematosus, or related rheumatic diseases.

The time course of the illness is important. Early hepatitis, rubella, or parvovirus infection can mimic rheumatic disease but these processes tend to be self limited. Serum-sicknesslike reactions to a variety of agents can present with an acute polyarthritis as well as other symptoms but are usually self limiting. Where the polyarthritis has persisted for 6 weeks or more, the likelihood is very high that you are dealing with one of the established rheumatic diseases, such as rheumatoid arthritis, systemic lupus erythematosus, and mixed connective tissue disease, for which there are specific criteria for the diagnosis. Careful history

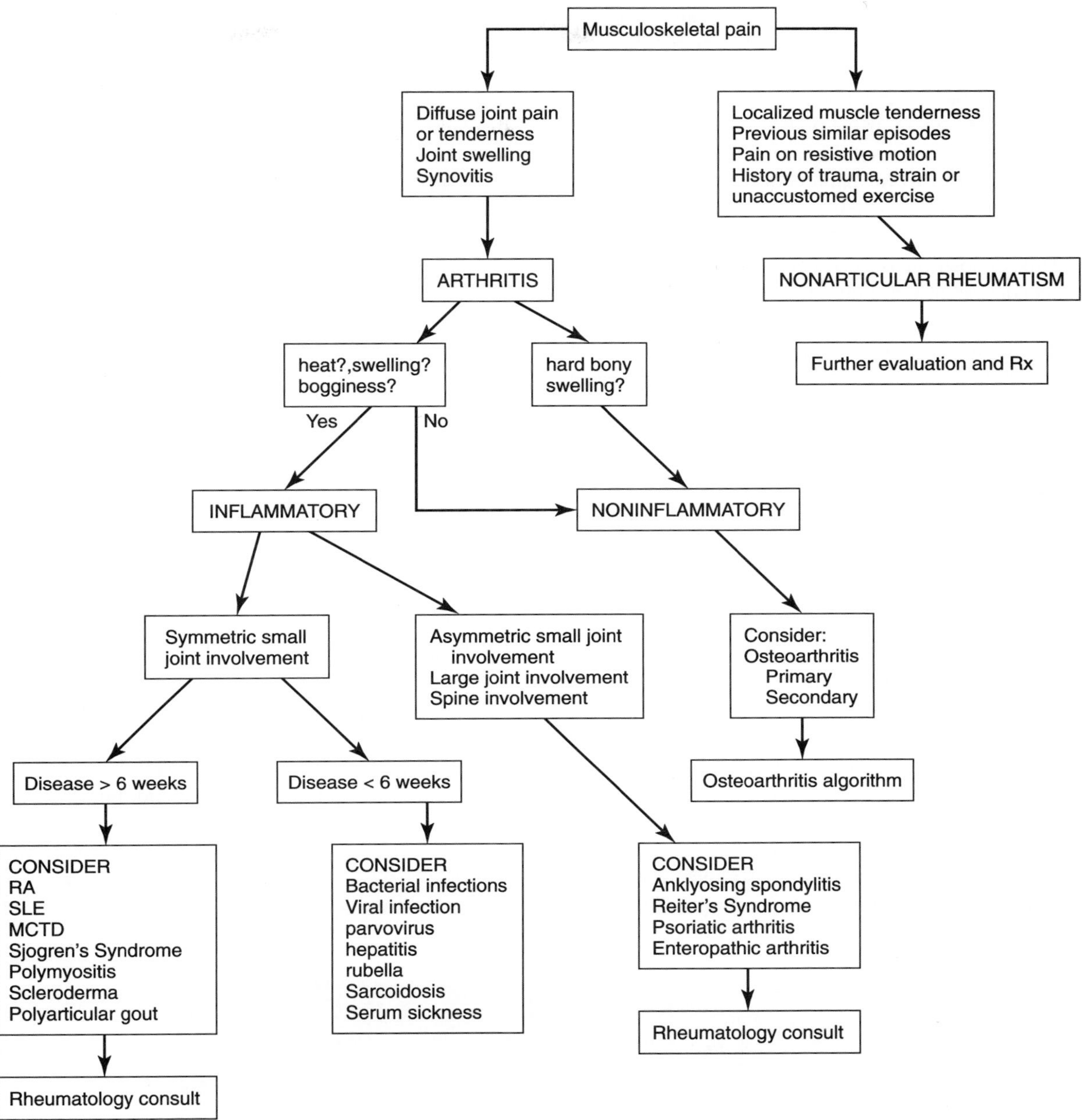

Figure 48–2. Differential diagnosis of polyarthritis. *(From Pinais. [1994]. [pp. 769–774]; Rheumatology Disorders. [1979]; Sergent. [1993]. [pp. 381–388].)*

and physical examination should clarify the diagnosis. Mention should be made of the patient with polyarticular gout which, in its chronic phase, has been too often confused with rheumatoid arthritis. The finding of tophi on physical exam and the characteristic x-ray appearance of gouty erosions associated with a high uric acid level should be diagnostic.

SELECTED MAJOR RHEUMATIC DISEASES

Gout

Since the identification of monosodium urate crystals in synovial fluid 35 years ago (McCarty & Hollander, 1961), it has become apparent that crystal deposition can be associated with both inflammatory and degenerative changes. These rheumatic syndromes are a common problem, particularly in older patients, and often in the setting of other acute disease. Fortunately, if the acute attack is recognized early, appropriate and successful treatment can be initiated.

Acute gouty arthritis (or bursitis or tenosynovitis) is an acute inflammatory arthritis that results from the tissue deposition of crystals of monosodium urate monohydrate (MSU). This deposition occurs because the extracellular fluid is supersaturated with urate. Hyperuricemia is defined as a value of serum or plasma urate acid greater than two standard deviations above the mean corrected for the sex of the patient. While hyperuricemia is associated with gout, it is not necessary for the development of gout.

A typical case is described here. A 60-year-old woman is admitted for evaluation of irregular heartbeat. She is found to be in atrial fibrillation and congestive heart failure and is treated with digitalis, furosemide, and warfarin. Four days after admission, the congestive heart failure is improving but she is awakened at 4 A.M. with the acute onset of severe pain and swelling in her right great toe. The pain is so intense that she is unable to bear the weight of the bedcovers and she cannot walk. She has never had similar pain. Examination shows that the right great toe is diffusely swollen, erythematous, and somewhat shiny.

Clinically, this is most likely acute gout although a septic arthritis or other acute monoarthritis should be considered. The abrupt onset of severe inflammation, usually at night and involving a lower extremity suggests acute gout. Local cooling of the extremity presumably causes local supersaturation and precipitation of monosodium urate crystals with subsequent accumulation of neutrophils. The MSU crystals trigger the release of various mediators from neutrophils (proteases, free radicals, and leukotrienes), resulting in inflammation. The first MTP joint is characteristically involved in 75% of cases but other joints may be involved (Fig. 48–3). Polyarticular involvement can be seen. The abrupt onset and severity of the signs and symptoms are the clinical clues. If the attack is not treated, it gradually subsides over 7 to 10 days, often with peeling of the skin over the joint.

Laboratory and Diagnostic Tests

Under light microscopy, characteristic needle-shaped crystals are diagnostic. Only one drop is needed for diagnosis. After performing arthrocentesis, place one drop of joint fluid on a clean glass slide and cover immediately with a clean cover slip. Crystals can be seen under an ordinary light microscope. Under compensated polarized microscopy, however (Fig. 48–4), they exhibit negative birefringence. That is, when the long axis of the crystal is parallel to the slow vibration of light through the compensator, the crystals appear a bright yellow. As the axis of polarized light is rotated so that the long axis of the crystal is perpendicular to the direction of the light, the crystal appears blue. In acute gout, crystals are seen within polymorphonuclear neutrophils.

Treatment

The treatment of acute gout depends to a great extent on comorbid conditions (Emmerson, 1996). One hundred years ago, colchicine, which works by inhibiting phagocytosis of MSU crystals through its effect on microtubules, was the only available treatment. Despite gastrointestinal upset and diarrhea, due to its narrow therapeutic window, it was effective in reducing joint inflammation within 48 hours.

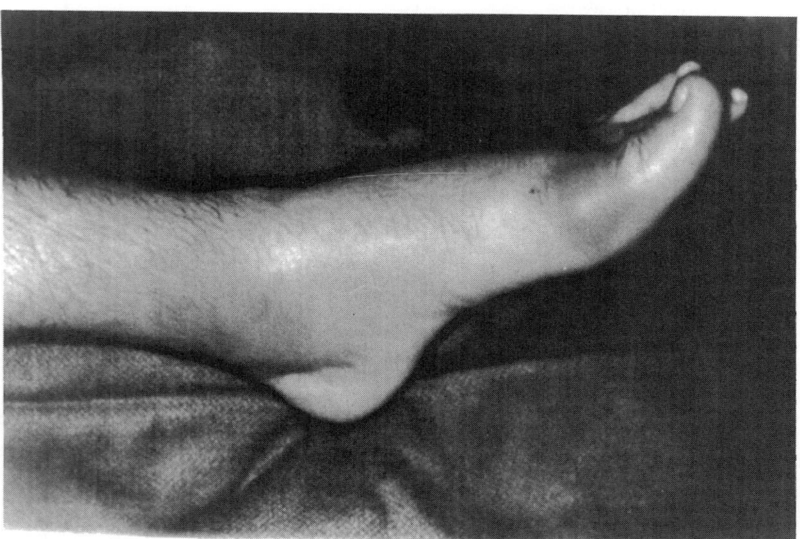

Figure 48–3. Gout: podagra. The base of the big toe and the ankle are red, swollen and painful. *(Reprinted from the Clinical Slide Collection on the Rheumatic Diseases, Copyright 1991, 1995. Used with permission of the American College of Rheumatology.)*

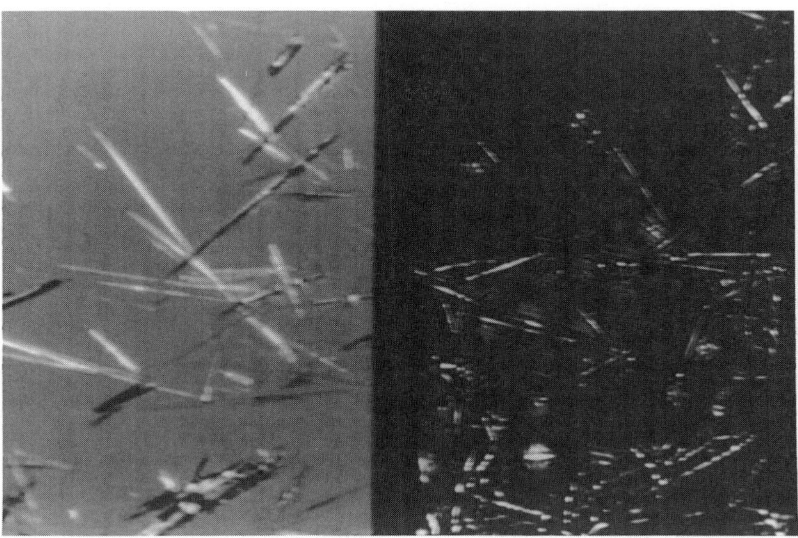

Figure 48–4. Gout: urate crystals (polarized and ordinary light microscopy). When urate crystals are viewed under high-power compensated light microscopy they are strongly negatively birefringent. *(Reprinted from the Clinical Slide Collection on the Rheumatic Diseases, Copyright 1991, 1995. Used with permission of the American College of Rheumatology.)*

Colchicine can be dangerous in patients who are elderly or frail and cannot tolerate diarrhea and in those with hepatic and/or renal insufficiency. While colchicine can also be given intravenously, additional toxicity—including bone marrow suppression and extravasation with tissue necrosis—can occur.

In the office, nonsteroidal antiinflammatory drugs (NSAIDs) can reduce the pain and inflammation in acute gouty arthritis. Indomethacin in doses of 150 to 300 mg, qd in divided doses, naproxen 100 to 1500 mg, qd in divided doses, and other NSAIDs can be used to terminate an attack in 1 to 3 days. Unfortunately, in the hospitalized fragile elderly patient with acute gout, NSAIDs may pose considerable risk particularly if there is renal dysfunction, congestive heart failure, anticoagulant therapy, past or current peptic ulcer disease, or gastrointestinal bleeding.

In patients with significant comorbidities, corticosteroid treatment with either intraarticular or systemic corticosteroids can be helpful. In the patient with a single involved joint, intraarticular injection of corticosteroids produces rapid reduction in pain and inflammation in 1 to 24 hours with minimal side effects. Joint infection is rare, although, occasionally, the patient may experience a postinjection flare of inflammation.

For the patient with acute polyarticular gout, treatment with systemic corticosteroids can be quite effective. Oral prednisone at a dose of 30 to 50 mg/day or intravenous methylprednisolone 40 to 80 mg/day with gradual tapering over 7 to 10 days works well. Resolution is prompt and, with a long tapering schedule, rebound attacks rarely occur. ACTH therapy has also been used; however, it can present problems with the dependence of therapeutic efficacy on the sensitivity of the adrenal cortex and can cause side effects of hypokalemia and fluid retention due to excess mineralocorticoid release.

In addition to acute gout, patients with longstanding hyperuricemia may present with chronic tophaceous gout. On occasion, small hand joint involvement can be confused with rheumatoid arthritis; however, observation of tophaceous deposits on the pinna of the ear (Fig. 48–5), over the olecranon bursa, and over the Achilles tendon should suggest the diagnosis unless the inexperienced examiner has confused them with nodules. Aspiration of a chalky white material containing masses of needle-shaped negatively birefringent crystals under compensated polarized microscopy is diagnosed. Radiographically the erosions of gout can be distinguished from those of rheumatoid arthritis.

Hyperuricemia results either because of overproduction of urate or from decreased urinary secretion. Causes of overproduction of uric acid include ethanol ingestion, increased intake from a high-purine diet, overproduction from enzyme deficiency of HGPRT or other enzymes, and excessive cell turnover as in various myeloproliferative disorders and psoriasis. Decreased urinary excretion of uric acid is seen in patients with renal insufficiency from intrinsic renal disease. Diuretics reduce renal excretion of uric acid, as do other drugs such as low-dose salicylates, pyrazinamide, ethambutol, and niacin. Dehydration, starvation, and ketosis can contribute to decreased urinary excretion. Ethanol also contributes to hyperuricemia by decreasing excretion.

The issue of treatment of hyperuricemia is always raised when a patient is found to have acute gout. While gout can be prevented either by correction of the cause of hyperuricemia or by prescribing medications that alter uric

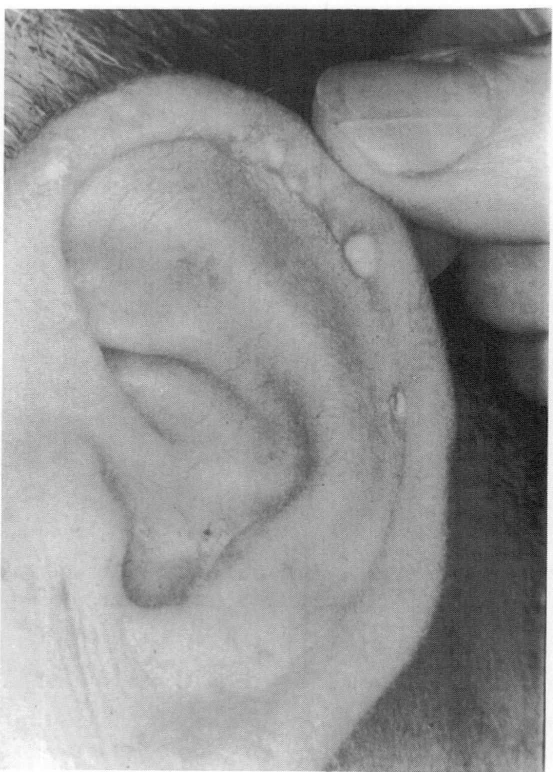

Figure 48–5. Gout: tophi, ear. Small tophi on the helix of the ear have a typical whitish appearance as a result of urate deposition. *(Reprinted from the Clinical Slide Collection on the Rheumatic Diseases, Copyright 1991, 1995. Used with permission of the American College of Rheumatology.)*

acid metabolism, there is no role for the immediate treatment of hyperuricemia at the time of the acute gouty attack.

Identification and modification of factors contributing to hyperuricemia may allow the serum urate level to fall considerably. However, if the patient has had recurrent gout and particularly if there is evidence of tophaceous gout, the patient requires treatment for hyperuricemia. Dietary habits should be elicited and use of alcohol discouraged. A low-purine diet can be discussed if dietary factors seem to be contributing to gouty attacks. There are two types of drugs available to lower uric acid levels; uricosuric drugs (such as probenecid or sulfinpyrazone) and xanthine oxidase inhibitors (such as allopurinol). Evaluation of the 24-hour urine excretion of uric acid is helpful in deciding on uric acid-lowering therapy. If the urine uric acid level is high, uricosuric drugs should not be used. Additionally, they are contraindicated in patients with a history of renal stones or with renal insufficiency. In that case, allopurinol should be used. Often, an attack of acute gout may follow the institution of uric acid-lowering therapy apparently due to sudden change in the serum uric acid concentration. To prevent this, treatment with low-dose prophylactic colchicine at a dose of 0.6 mg once or twice a day should be started at the same time the uric acid-lowering agent is begun. Therapy should be started with a low dose and gradually increased.

Acute Calcium Pyrophosphate Dihydrate Crystal Deposition Disease

Acute calcium pyrophosphate dihydrate (CPPD) crystal deposition disease looks very much like gout, so much so that it is called pseudogout. Like gout, it usually presents as an acute monoarthritis in a middle-aged or elderly adult. The knee is the most common joint involved, but other large joints such as the wrist, shoulder, and ankle can be involved as can small joints of the hand, the first MTP (pseudopodagra), and others. The clinical setting is often the same with occurrence several days after surgery or other illness. As in acute gout, pain is severe, develops rapidly, the skin is warm and red, and the joint is very tender.

Laboratory and Diagnostic Tests

Diagnosis is made by arthrocentesis of the joint and identification of characteristic crystals. CPPD crystals are more difficult to see than MSU crystals. They are rhomboidal rather than needle-shaped and described as weakly positively birefringent. Sometimes, it is helpful to ask the laboratory to spin down the synovial fluid to concentrate the crystals in the sediment. Again, as in gout, crystals should be seen within polymorphonuclear leukocytes.

In addition to acute pseudogout, deposition of CPPD crystals can produce a chronic pyrophosphate arthropathy. This condition is often seen in elderly women with or without a history of acute attacks and involves knees, shoulders, elbows, wrists, hips, and ankles. X-rays show the presence of chondocalcinosis, resulting from deposition of CPPD crystals in articular cartilage. Several types of rheumatic disease have been described in these patients including an inflammatory arthritis and a rare severely destructive arthropathy.

The finding of CPPD crystal deposition should stimulate the practitioner to look for associated metabolic conditions including hyperparathyroidism, hemochromatosis, gout, hypophosphatasia, hypomagnesemia, and Wilson's disease. Hypothyroidism and ochronosis may be associated. Diagnostic laboratory screening may be helpful.

Treatment

Acute pseudogout is treated similarly to acute gout, with NSAIDs, if tolerated, or with intraarticular or systemic steroids. Colchicine 0.6 mg bid to tid may be helpful. Chronic pyrophosphate arthropathy is treated similarly to osteoarthritis with the use of analgesics, non-steroidal antiinflammatory drugs, joint injection, physical therapy, and surgery.

Rheumatoid Arthritis

Rheumatoid arthritis (RA) is defined as a chronic, systemic, inflammatory disease of unknown etiology causing erosive synovitis of small and large joints as well as potentially life-threatening nonarticular manifestations The American College of Rheumatology's recently revised criteria for the diagnosis of RA includes: (1) morning stiffness lasting more than 1 hour, (2) arthritis in three or more joint areas, (3) symmetric arthritis of the hand joints, (4) rheumatoid nodules, (5) the presence of rheumatoid factor, and (6) radiographic changes consistent with the diagnosis (American College of Rheumatology, 1996).

Rheumatoid arthritis affects 1 to 2% of the adult population with prevalence increasing with age. There is a 2.5 to 1 female-to-male prevalence. The etiolgy is thought to be an autoimmune reaction to many different antigenic agents in a genetically susceptible individual. Endocrine, metabolic, nutritional, hormonal, and psychosocial factors have all been studied. Infectious agents, including bacteria and viruses, remain primary suspects. These includes retroviruses, Epstein–Barr, and herpes viruses. Definitive proof of an infectious cause of RA has not been identified.

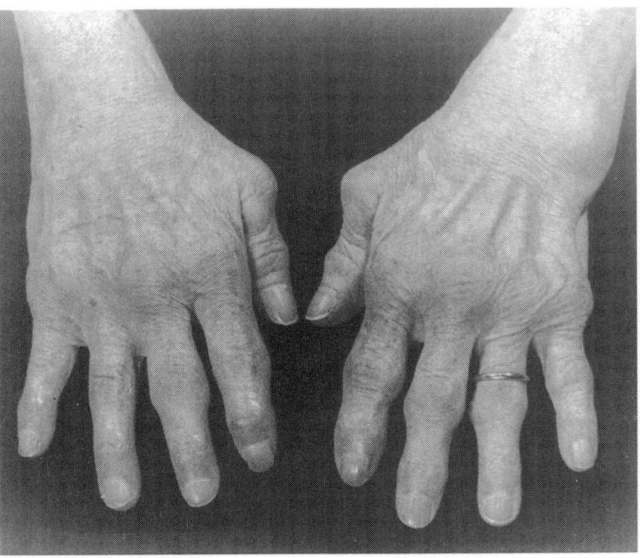

Figure 48–6. Rheumatoid arthritis involving the dips showing small muscle wasting, prominent ulnar styloid, and swelling of the DIPs and PIPs. *(Reprinted from the Slide Atlas of Rheumatology, Rheumatoid Arthritis of the Hands and Feet. Used with permission of Paul A Dieppe, BSc, MB, BS, MRCP.)*

Pathophysiology

The pathology of RA is characterized by microvascular injury to synovial cells that triggers an inflammatory response. The inflammation causes a hypertrophic, edematous synovium and production of inflammatory synovial fluid. The resultant proliferation of granulation tissue (pannus) eventually leads to joint destruction. The disease is chronic with a waxing and waning course which usually persists for the lifetime of the individual, although spontaneous remissions without recurrance are reported (Wilder, 1993).

History and Physical Findings

The clinical manifestations of RA typically develop insidiously but explosive onset with symptoms developing over several days or even hours is reported. RA is a systemic disease; patients often complain of fatigue, malaise, weight loss, diffuse myalgia, and low-grade fever. Pain, swelling, erythema, and heat symmetrically involving the small joints of the hands and feet is typical (Fig. 48–6). Eventually, severe ulnar deviation at the MCP joints may occur (Fig. 48–7). Wrists, elbows, shoulders, cervical spine, hips, and knees are often involved. RA never involves the lower back. Morning stiffness lasting more than one hour and often much of the day is common. Pain and stiffness that worsens with rest and improves with activity is usual.

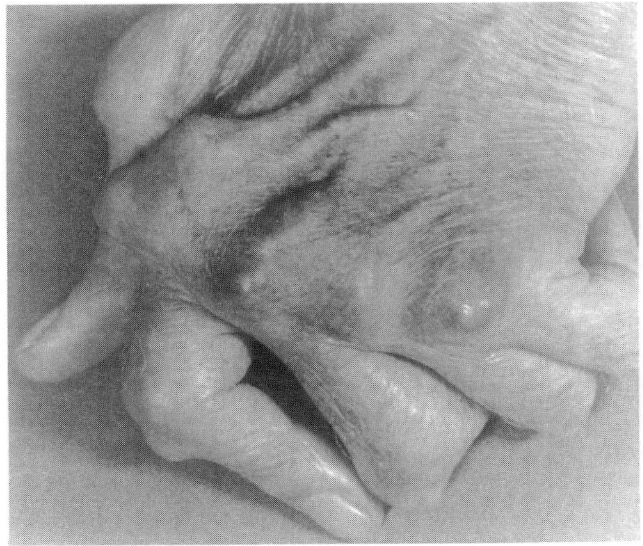

Figure 48–7. Severe deformity in advanced rheumatoid arthritis of the hand showing muscle wasting, subluxation and ulnar deviation of the MCPs, flexion deformity of the PIPs, "Z" deformity of the thumb, and rheumatoid nodules on tendons. *(Reprinted from the Slide Atlas of Rheumatology, Rheumatoid Arthritis of the Hands and Feet. Used with permission of Paul A Dieppe, BSc, MB, BS, MRCP.)*

Extraarticular Manifestations. Subcutaneous nodules at pressure points (olecranon, extensor surface of the forearm, ischial tuberosity) are noted in up to 30% of patients (Fig. 48–8). Rheumatoid factor (RF) is present in virtually all patients with rheumatoid nodules. Other skin lesions seen in RA include the vasculitic lesions of palpable purpura and splinter hemmorhages around the nail beds. Palmer erythema is commonly seen.

Respiratory manifestations include inflammation of the cricoarytenoid joint, causing stridor and respiratory dis-

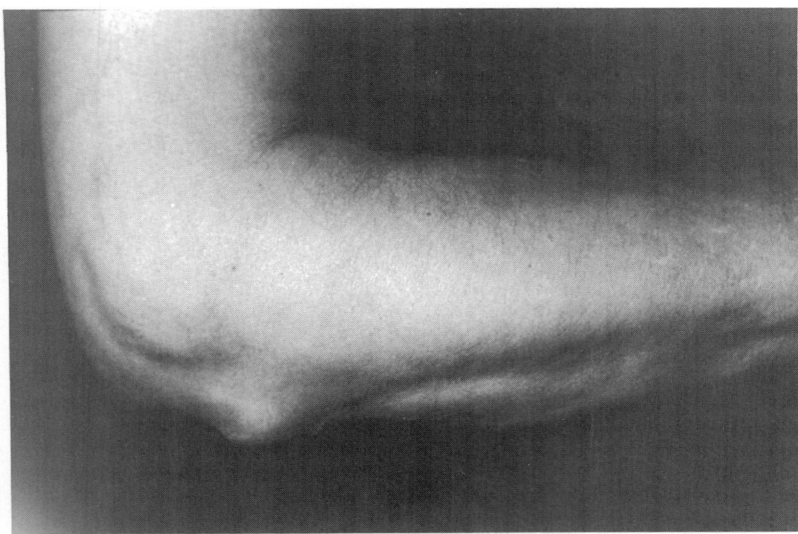

Figure 48–8. Rheumatoid arthritis: subcutaneous nodule, olecranon. A large subcutaneous nodule located on the extensor surface of the forearm near the elbow. *(Reprinted from the Clinical Slide Collection on the Rheumatic Diseases, Copyright 1991, 1995. Used with permission of the American College of Rheumatology.)*

tress. Interstitional lung disease, pulmonary nodules, and pleuritis can also be seen in patients with more severe disease. Cardiac manifestations are rare and include nodules involving the myocardium and valves, conduction abnormalities, aortitis, and pericarditis (Anderson, 1993). Neurologic complications can result from erosion of the odontoid with instability of the cervical spine and cord compression. The slow development of progressive paresthesias and motor weakness with hyperactive reflexes and the presence of a Babinski sign should alert the clinician to an impending cord compression. Entrapment neuropathies including carpal tunnel syndrome are seen in RA and may be an early manifestation.

Laboratory and Diagnostic Tests

Rheumatoid arthritis is a clinical diagnosis. Laboratory testing is used only to support the clinical diagnosis. The most commonly used tests are not specific to rheumatoid arthritis and should be ordered only when a strong clinical suspicion exists. The erythrocyte sedimentation rate (ESR) is elevated in the presence of inflammatory diseases, malignant tumors, and infectious disease. In RA, elevation of the ESR varies with the degree of inflammation and can be used as a guide to treatment. Rheumatoid factor (RF) is present in 80 to 85% of patients with RA. In addition to rheumatoid arthritis, RF can be found with many other inflammatory diseases including systemic lupus erythematosis (SLE), Sjogren's syndrome, systemic sclerosis, hepatic cirrhosis, and sarcoidosis, as well as such infections as bacterial endocarditis, tuberculosis, and mononucleosis (Callegari & Williams, 1995). The presence of rheumatoid factor in a patient with other manifestations of RA can confirm the diagnosis and high titers may indicate more aggressive disease. A negative test, however, does not rule out RA as a diagnosis. Other laboratory abnormalities seen in RA include hypochromic–microcytic anemia which meets the criteria of anemia of chronic disease, thrombocytosis, and eosinophilia. Antinuclear antibodies (ANA) in significant titers are positive in up to 50% of patients with RA (versus in 95% of those patients with SLE) (Anderson, 1993).

X-rays should always be obtained in those situations where exclusion of a fracture is imperative. X-rays in early RA may show soft-tissue swelling but joint damage does not become apparent for several years, making x-ray a low-yield procedure for early diagnosis. Later in the course of the disease, x-rays may be helpful in determining the effectiveness of treatment and/or assessing the extent of erosive change (Fig. 48–9).

Management

The treatment of rheumatoid arthritis has several goals. The relief of pain, the alleviation of joint inflammation, the maintainence and/or restoration of joint function, and the prevention of bone and cartilage destruction are the traditional goals of treatment. In the past, rheumatologists used a pyramid approach to treatment with the basic program of education, conservation of energy, joint protection, and pain-relieving or antiinflammatory medications. In this model, the so-called disease-modifying medications are reserved for later stages of the disease or when more conservative approaches have failed. In recent years, clinicians have begun to use more aggressive treatment regimes with multiple medications earlier in the course of the disease in an effort to interrupt the complicated effects of inflammation before permanent damage is done (Fig. 48–10). After the disease is brought into remission, medications are

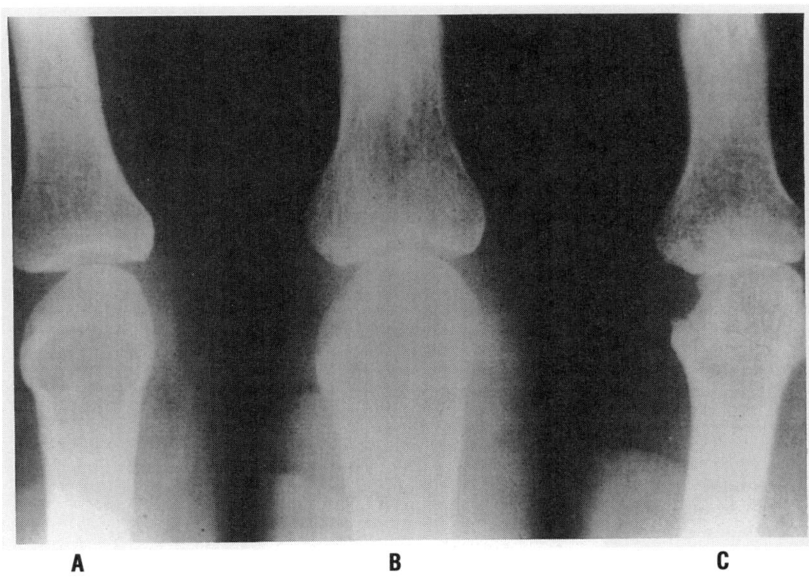

Figure 48–9. Rheumatoid arthritis: progressive metacarpophalangeal erosion. Note the progressive changes beginning with **(A)** soft tissue swelling followed by **(B)** thinning of the radial side of the cortex and minimal joint space narrowing to **(C)** a marginal erosion appearing on the radial aspect of the MCP head. *(Reprinted from the Clinical Slide Collection on the Rheumatic Diseases, Copyright 1991, 1995. Used with permission of the American College of Rheumatology.)*

slowly withdrawn while nonmedical approaches including, physical and occupational therapy, education and counseling are continued (McCarty, 1993).

Patients are often frightened and depressed after receiving a diagnosis of RA. They need to know that RA is a lifelong, chronic disease for which there is control but no cure, with a small chance of spontaneous remission within the first 2 years of disease. Patients need to understand that treatment often takes weeks to months to provide relief. Many patients become discouraged because of this and change physicians frequently or fall victim to the allure of unproven remedies and promises of cure with unconventional therapies. Careful explanation of the physiology of the disease and how it causes joint pain and destruction must be offered to patients as a basis for understanding the rationale of suggested treatment regimes. Emotional support is vital.

RA causes multiple symptoms and often disabling fatigue. A modified activity program that includes periods of rest interspersed with periods of activity can help the patient during disease flares. Bed rest is seldom needed and contributes to deconditioning. Splinting of an acutely inflammed joint allows for complete rest of a single joint without immobilizing the patient. Protecting joints by learning alternate ways of performing tasks is often recommended and taught by occupational therapists.

Exercise is used to maintain joint range of motion and muscle strength. This is achieved with a combination of isotonic and isometric exercises. After the inflammation has subsided, strength training and aerobic conditioning may be initiated as tolerated by the patient and under the supervision of a physical therapist. Water-based exercise programs are very useful and are frequently available as group activity through local YMCA programs or at health clubs. The application of ice and/or heat may provide relief to patients during intensely painful episodes.

The patient with RA may require other orthopedic supports such as shoe orthotics, neck collars, canes, crutches, and walkers to provide ambulatory support. Other functional equipment to facilitate activities of daily living (ADLs)—such as raised toilet seats, dressing devices, and kitchen aids—are available. The occupational therapist should be consulted early in the course of the disease to assess the patient's ability to perform ADLs and to provide assistive devices and education as needed.

Drug Therapy. The goal of drug therapy is to suppress inflammation early in the course of the disease in an attempt to avoid the largely irreversible tissue damage and functional loss that can develop if inflammation is not controlled. Aspirin in large doses or nonsteroidal antiinflammatory drugs are the mainstay of early and ongoing therapy. Their effect is quick and they are generally well tolerated. GI side effects can often be controlled with the administration of these agents with food. Hypersensitivity reactions can occur, but are rare. Hepatic and renal toxicity are uncommon, but should be monitored. The selection of an NSAID is based on many factors including cost, previous experience of both the patient and the clinician, duration of action of the drug, and the complexity of the dosing regime (Table 48–1). As with all drugs, elderly patients should be started on lower doses, with increases made slowly.

Slow-acting antirheumatic drugs (SAARDs) are those drugs occasionally referred to as disease-modifying anti-

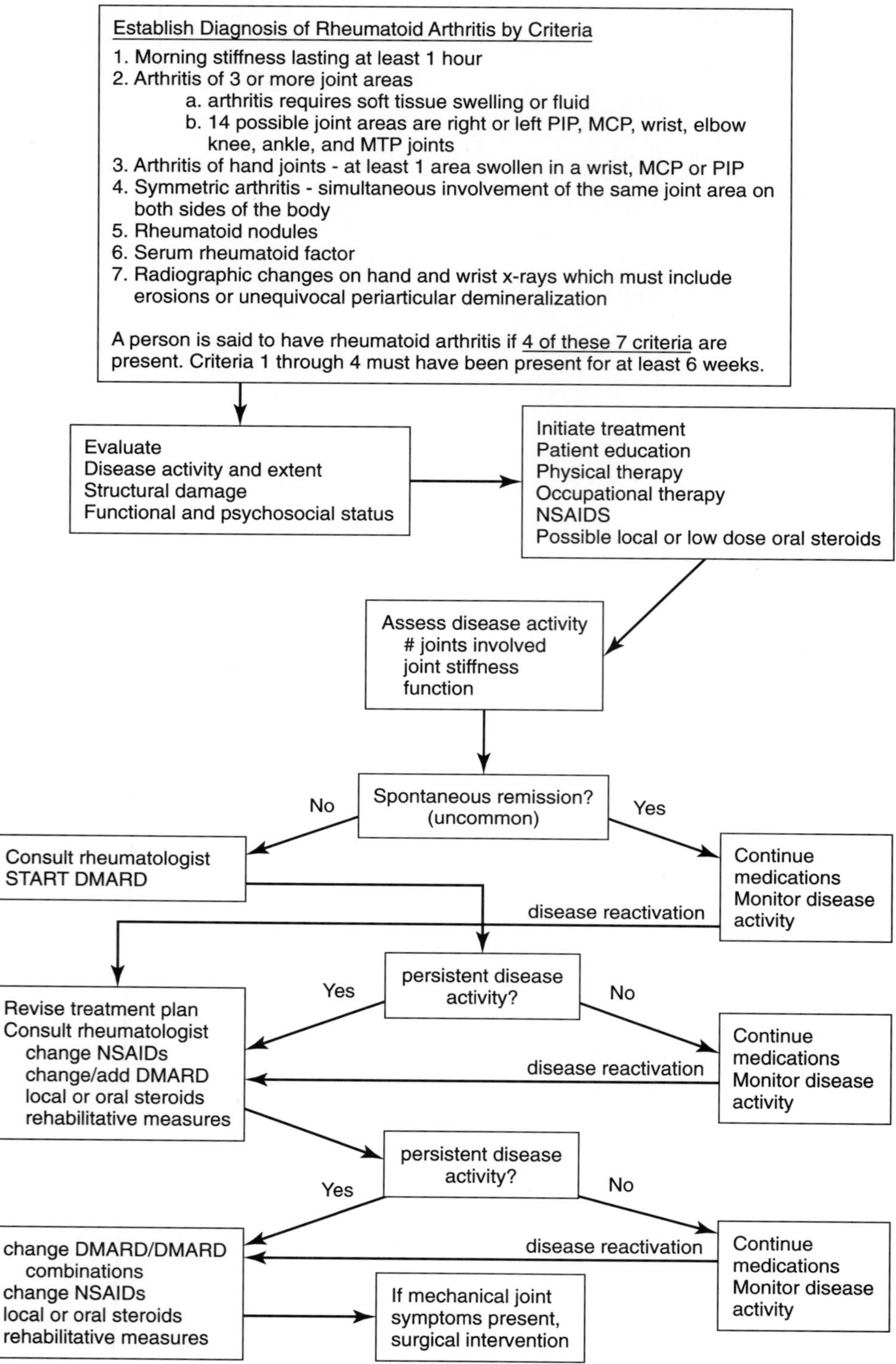

Figure 48–10. Medical management of rheumatoid arthritis. *(From American College of Rheumatology Ad Hoc Committee. [1996]. [pp. 713–722]; Arnett et al. [1988]. [pp. 315–324].)*

TABLE 48–1. Table of Nonsteroidal Antiinflammatory Drugs (NSAIDs)

Generic	Brand Name	Dose Range (mg/day)	Dose Interval	Comments
Salicylates				
Acetylsalicylic acid	Aspirin	1000–6000	qid	
Nonacetylated salicylates[a]				
Choline magnesium trisalicylate	Trilisate	1500–3000	bid to tid	Liquid available Salicylate levels available
Salicylsalicylic acid	Disalcid	1500–3000	bid to tid	Salicylate levels available
	Salflex	1500–3000	bid to tid	Salicylate levels available
Short Serum Half Life NSAIDs				
Diclofenac potassium	Cataflam	100–200	bid to tid	Liver function abnormalities
Diclofenac sodium	Voltaran	100–200	bid to tid	Liver function abnormalities
Fenoprofen calcium	Nalfon	1200–3200	tid to qid	Acute interstitial nephritis
Flurbiprofen	Ansaid	100–300	bid to qid	
Ibuprofen	Motrin	1200–3200	tid to qid	Liquid available
Ketoprofen	Orudis	150–300	tid to qid	
	Oruvail	150–300	qd	
Meclofenamate sodium	Meolomen	200–400	tid to qid	Higher incidence of diarrhea
Tolmetin sodium	Tolectin	800–1800	tid	Pediatric approval for JRA
Long Serum Half Life NSAIDs				
Diflunisal	Dolobid	500–1500	bid	A derivative of salicylate but not metabolized to salicylate
Indomethaoin	Indocin	50–200	bid to tid	Efficacy in ankylosing spondylitis and gout
Nabumetone	Relafen	1000–2000	qd to bid	Nonacidic pro-drug undergoes hepatic transformation to active acidic metabolite Liver function abnormalities Use with care in liver disease
Naproxen sodium	Naprosyn	750–1500	bid	Liquid available Pediatric approval for JRA
Oxaprozin	Daypro	600–1200	qd	
Piroxioam	Feldene	20	qd	
Sulindac	Clinoril	300–400	bid	May have a lower incidence of prostaglandin-mediated renal effects

Doses are given as mg/day and should be divided by the dose interval when prescribing.

[a] Nonacetylated salicylates have decreased effects on platelets, gastric mucosa, and prostaglandin-mediated renal function as compared to acetylsalicylic acid. They are generally considered safe in aspirin-sensitive asthma.

Reprinted from Snyderman and Hayes. (1997).

rheumatic drugs (DMARDs) (Table 48–2). The actual potential of these drugs to modify or change the course of the disease is controversial. When to start these medications and in which order depends on the experience and practice setting of the clinician. A consensus of practicing rheumatologists has yielded the following guidelines (Jain & Lipsky, 1997).

For mild and/or early RA, the initial DMARD tried is hydroxychloroquine in doses of 200 to 400 mgs per day. Hydroxychloroquine is well studied and is of proven efficacy over many years of use. This is a well-tolerated agent, which rarely causes ocular toxicity. Most rheumatologists recommend a biannual eye examination.

Low-dose weekly methotrexate has become the most commonly used DMARD in recent years. It is well tolerated and effective at controlling symptoms. Doses range from 7.5 to 25 mg weekly orally or by injection. Side effects include stomatitis, GI toxicity, increased incidence of rheumatoid nodules, and cytopenias. Methotrexate has been associated with hepatic toxicity, although the actual incidence of serious liver disease is low. The American College of Rheumatology has recommended baseline liver function studies and monitoring of LFTs including serum albumin every 4 to 8 weeks. Pretreatment liver biopsies and/or biopsies at 5- and 10-year intervals do not appear to be cost justified (Jain & Lipsky, 1987). Pneumonitis is reported and is a potentially serious side effect. Methotrexate is well tolerated by older patients. Given the overall safety and effectiveness of methotrexate, it has become the drug of choice in patients with aggressive rheumatoid arthritis.

Gold compounds have been used in the treatment of rheumatoid arthritis for many years. Oral preparations are generally well tolerated and moderately effective but diarrhea is common and they seem to lose efficacy over time (Jain & Lipsky, 1997). Parenteral gold is felt to be an effective SAARD although the frequency of side effects including rash, stomatitis, proteinuria, thrombocytopenia, and leukopenia limits its usefulness as a long-term agent.

TABLE 48–2. Slow-Acting Antirheumatic Drugs

Agent	Dose	Potential Adverse Effects[a]	% of Patients Who Discontinue Treatment Owing to Toxicity
Hydroxychloroquine	200–400 mg po qd	GI, cutaneous, retinopathy	3–8
Methotrexate	7.5–(25–30) mg po once a week (can be given IM)	GI, mucocutaneous, cytopenias, elevation LFTs, cirrhosis, pneumonitis	10–35
Auranofin	3–6 mg po qd	GI toxicity more common than with injectable gold	10
Injectable gold	Initial dose 10 mg, 25 mg 2nd week, then 50 mg IM per week	Dermatitis, stomatitis, cytopenia (thrombocytopenia most common), proteinuria/nephrotic syndrome, pneumonitis	30
Sulfasalazine	Start at 500–1000 mg and increase to 2–3 g po qd	GI, mucocutaneous, CNS disturbance (such as headache, irritability, and dizziness), cytopenia, elevation of LFTs	20–30
d-Penicillamine	125–250 mg qd, then increase up to 750 mg–1 g qd	Rash, stomatitis, GI, dysgeusia, cytopenia, proteinuria/ nephrotic syndrome, autoimmune disease	20–50
Cyclosporine	Start at 2.5 mg/kg/d then increase up to 5 mg/kg/d po	Nephrotoxicity (acute and/or chronic), hypertension, GI, neurotoxicity, gingival hyperplasia, hypertrichosis	15–30
Azathioprine	Start 0.5–1 mg/kg/d then increase up to 2.5 mg/kg/d po	GI, stomatitis, cytopenia, drug fever, hepatitis, pancreatitis, oncogenicity	15–30
Cyclophosphamide	50–100 mg/d po (up to 2.5 mg/kg/d)	GI, alopecia, cytopenia, increased risk of infection, bladder toxicity, drug-induced infertility, oncogenicity	—

[a] The list of adverse effects is an overview—the information is not all-inclusive.
GI = Gastrointestinal; LFTs = liver function tests; CNS = central nervous system.
From Jain & Lipsky. (1997). (pp. 63–64).
Reprinted from Snyderman and Hayes. (1997).

Sulfasalazine, with doses in the 2-3 gm/day range, has also been of demonstrated value in the treatment of RA. Side effects are most common early in the treatment course and include GI toxicities, rashes, stomatitis, and LFT elevations. Bone marrow suppression is a rare but potentially fatal side effect and regular monitoring is recommended.

D-penicillamine also has a long experience base in the treatment of RA but is less frequently used as a first choice due to potentially serious side effects These include bone marrow suppression, proteinuria, and nephrotic syndrome. Rarely, autoimmune syndromes including lupus, Goodpasture's syndrome and myasthenia gravis, are seen.

Cyclosporine has been shown to suppress activity in RA at about the same level as parenteral gold or methotrexate. The most serious adverse effect is both acute and chronic renal failure which may be exacerbated by the concurrent use of NSAIDs. Hypertension, GI toxicity, and neurotoxicity have been reported.

Other agents used in the treatment of RA include the more toxic azathioprine and cyclophosphamide, but these agents are reserved for patients with severe disease or, in the case of cyclophosphamide, in patients with vasculitis (Jain & Lipsky, 1997). There is empiric evidence to suggest that the use of these drugs is associated with a marked decrease in inflammation that is sustained over time and remission is not uncommon. Close clinical and laboratory monitoring for side effects is essential.

There is considerable interest in the use of tetracyclines, particularly minocycline for the treatment of RA. Studies have found good tolerance and efficacy, particularly in early disease. The mode of action is unknown but minocycline has antimicrobial, antiinflammatory, and immunomodulatory effects. Dosages of 100 mg by mouth twice daily seem to be effective without significant side effects (O'Dell, Haire, et al., Palmer, 1997).

Clinicians are now using combinations of two or more SAARDs in lower doses with some reported success but more study is needed (Table 48–3).

Glucocorticoids have both antiinflammatory and immunosuppressant effects but no ability to change the course of the disease. The long-term adverse affects of steroids are well-known, making these agents less desirable as routine treatment for RA. These can include cutaneous atrophy, cataracts, glucose intolerance, myopathies, and osteoporosis. Steroids are routinely used for life-threatening complications of RA such as vasculitis or rheumatoid lung disease. Low-dose steroids (10 mg or less) are frequently used as a bridge to provide relief while waiting for SAARDs to begin working. The goal, in this instance, is to use the lowest effective dose and to taper and discontinue as soon as possible. Intraarticular injections of steroids can be helpful when one or two joints flare, causing pain or disability. Intraarticular steroids should never be administered if there is any suspicion of joint infection.

Current investigational therapies are in clinical trials. These include biologicals, including T-cell directed therapies, targeted against specific components of the immune system. There are efforts to induce tolerance to arthritogenic

TABLE 48–3. Review of Some Trials Evaluating Combination Therapy

Combination	Ref	Design	Duration	Results	Side Effects	Comments
HCQ/MTX	149	Double-blind, placebo-controlled	6 mo	Benefit	Slight increase	HCQ + MTX > HCQ
HCQ/D-PCN	12	Controlled, double-blind	24 mo	No benefit	No increase	D-PCN > HCQ + D-PCN
CQ/D-PCN	54	Randomized	12 mo	No benefit	Increased	
Gold/HCQ	130	Double-blind, placebo-controlled	12 mo	Benefit	Increased	Gold + HCQ > Gold
	117	Double-blind, placebo-controlled	6 mo	No benefit	No increase	Suboptimal response to GST
Gold/CsA	4	Pilot study	6 mo	Benefit	No increase	Suboptimal response to GST
SSZ/Gold	37	Open study	12 mo	Benefit	"Well tolerated"	Background SSZ
SSZ/D-PCN	37	Open study	12 mo	Benefit	"Well tolerated"	Background SSZ
	147	Open study	6 mo	Benefit	Increased	
MTX/CQ	43	Placebo-controlled	6 mo	Slight benefit	Increased	
MTX/AUF	165	Randomized, double-blind	48 wk	No benefit	Slight increase	
MTX/SSZ	137	Observational	24 mo	Benefit	No increase	4 patients
	57	Open study	24 wk	Benefit	No increase	SSZ-resistant RA
MTX/HCQ/SSZ	108	Double-blind, placebo-controlled	24 mo	Benefit	"Well tolerated"	MTX + HCQ + SSZ > MTX or HCQ + SSZ
	109	Open study	—	Benefit	—	Suboptimal response to SAARD
MTX/AZA	168	Double-blind	48 wk	No benefit	No increase	
MTX/AZA/HCQ	85	Open study	18 mo	Benefit	"Well tolerated"	Refractory RA
	96	Observational study	1–18 y	Benefit	"Low toxicity"	
MTX/CsA	4	Pilot study	6 mo	Benefit	No increase	Suboptimal response to MTX
	151	Randomized, double-blind	6 mo	Benefit	No significant increase	Suboptimal response to MTX
CYP/AZA/HCQ	95	Observational study	5–60 mo	Benefit	Increased (malignancy)	Refractory RA

HCQ = hydroxychloroquine; MTX = methotrexate; D-PCN = d-penicillamine; CQ = chloroquine; CsA = cyclosporine; SSZ = sulfasalazine; AUF = auranofin; CYP = cyclophosphamide; GST = injectable gold; RA = rheumatoid arthritis; SAARD = slow-acting antirheumatic drugs

From Jain & Lipsky. (1997). (pp. 63–64).

antigens using monoclonal antibodies, vaccination, oral administration of antigen, and to develop newer immunosuppressants and immunomodulators (Jain & Lipsky, 1997).

The American College of Rheumatology (1996) suggests that referral to a rheumatologist may be helpful when RA presents with significant pain, stiffness, or swelling requiring immediate aggressive therapy. Other indications for referral may include disease that which does not respond to NSAIDs within 3 to 4 months, functional deterioration affecting quality of life, or rapid disease progression. Certainly those patients experiencing life-threatening disease complications, including cardiac, pulmonary, opthalmic, or vasculitic involvement, should be referred to a rheumatologist.

Rheumatoid arthritis is relatively common and as such is seen frequently in hospitalized patients. The nurse practitioner should be familiar with this disease, including the extarticular manifestations, the need for ongoing therapy, and the ways in which current therapy may interfere with unrelated treatment regimes. Patients with RA commonly present for orthopedic surgery including joint replacement, and medical management of disease must continue throughout the pre- and postoperative periods in order to maintain optimal control. Preoperative cervical spine films identify those patients who may be at risk of cervical subluxation if the neck is hyperextended during intubation. The patient with RA may be more susceptible to joint infection, especially if immunosuppressed and/or suffering with erosive joint disease. Serious drug side effects can occur and must be considered in any patient who presents with acute medical illness such as GI bleeding, blood dyscrasias, and renal or liver dysfunction. Pain-control issues, the need for additional assistance with ADLs, adjustment, and vocational issues may be present and require referral to rehabilitation and counseling professionals.

The optimal approach to the patient with RA remains controversial as the disease is so variable, the cause is unknown, and the outcomes are uncertain. Only persistent research and the experience of millions of patients with this devastating disease will provide us with better, safer treatments and, hopefully, one day, cure.

Systemic Lupus Erythematosus

One of the most enigmatic rheumatic diseases that the nurse practitioner may encounter is systemic lupus erythematosus (SLE). A useful definition of lupus is that it is a chronic inflammatory multisystem disease that may affect the skin, joints, kidneys, central nervous system, and other organs. The diagnosis of lupus is made using well-established criteria published by the American College of Rheumatology (Tan, Cohen et al., 1982). For a diagnosis of SLE to be made, 4 of the 11 criteria, as seen in Table 48–4, must be present either simultaneously or serially.

Lupus has a predilection for women in their reproductive years (ages 15–35), possibly due to hormonal effects.

The incidence of SLE has been estimated to be higher among black and Asian women in the United States. Prevalence figures range from 4 to 250 cases per 100,000 population (Tan, Cohen et al., 1982). Genetic factors are suspected, given the approximately 25% concordance found among identical twins. In addition, up to 12% of relatives of SLE patients themselves have SLE.

History and Physical Findings

It is important to realize that patients with SLE may present in any of a number of seemingly unrelated ways. This could include: sudden renal failure, acute psychosis, pancytopenia, pleuropericarditis, photosensitive rash, seizures, or arthritis. The most common initial presentation (55% of patients) is a nonspecific arthritis or arthralgia. Unlike rheumatoid arthritis, the arthritis of SLE is rarely erosive. Skin involvement is seen at presentation in 20% of patients and nephritis in only 5%. Ultimately, arthritis is the most common symptom seen in SLE with over 90% having some joint manifestations. Skin is involved in approximately 70%; the kidneys in 50%; and central nervous system involvement is relatively rare with only 15% having psychosis or seizure. Nonspecific complaints of fatigue, fever, weight loss, and malaise tend to be quite common but are not diagnostic (Tan, Cohen et al., 1982).

The classic "butterfly rash" seen in approximately 70% of patients with SLE consists of a fixed erythema over the bridge of the nose and cheeks sparing the nasolabial folds. This lesion may be accentuated by fever and the patient may look flushed. It does not result in scarring. In contrast, the lesions of discoid SLE, which is seen in up to 25% of patients, often scar. These lesions are raised erythematous patches with keratotic scaling. Follicular plugging is common and often central scarring, telangiectasia and atrophy of the skin result. Pigmentary disturbances of postinflammatory hypo- or hyperpigmentation are commonly noted and may present cosmetic problems in more darkly pigmented individuals. Discoid lesions are commonly found on the face, neck, pinna, and scalp. Photosensitivity is another dermatologic manifestation of and criterion for SLE despite the fact that not all patients with SLE develop rash after exposure to sunlight. A variety of rashes can be seen, including bullous and urticarial lesions.

TABLE 48–4. Criteria for the Diagnosis of Systemic Lupus Erythematosus (SLE)

1. Malar rash	
2. Discoid rash	
3. Photosensitivity	
4. Oral or nasopharyngeal ulcers	
5. Arthritis	
6. Serositis (pleuritic or pericarditis)	
7. Renal disorder—persistent proteinuria or cellular casts	
8. Neurologic disorder—seizures or psychosis	
9. Hematologic disorder—either	Hemolytic anemia
	OR
	Leukopenia (<4000/mm^3)
	OR
	Lymphopenia (<1500/mm^3)
	OR
	Thrombocytopenia (<100,000/mm^3)
10. Immunologic disorder:	LE cells
	OR
	Antibodies to ds DNA
	OR
	Antibodies to Smith antigen
	OR
	False–Positive serologic test for syphilis
11. Positive antinuclear antibody (ANA) test	

Tan, Cohen, Fries, et al. (1982).

While serositis is a diagnostic criteria for SLE, it is important to recognize that there are a number of other pulmonary and cardiac manifestations that can be associated with SLE. Both acute lupus pneumonitis and more chronic lupus pneumonitis can be seen. In the acutely ill patient, severe pulmonary hemorrhage can occur. Other patients may develop insidious onset of shortness of breath with clinical and pathologic features of pulmonary fibrosis. Secondary pulmonary hypertension can be seen in SLE although it is more commonly associated with either mixed connective tissue disease or scleroderma. Pulmonary embolism must always be considered in the differential diagnosis of chest pain, shortness of breath, or hemoptysis in SLE. Many patients have anticardiolipin antibodies and a propensity for thrombosis. In addition to pericarditis, other cardiac manifestations, including valvular heart disease, have been noted in patients with SLE. Echocardigraphic studies have documented that valvular involvement is more common than previously described. This suggests that SLE patients may be at increased risk for bacterial endocarditis. Many rheumatologists recommend that patients with SLE take prophylactic antibiotics for surgical or dental work. In acute SLE, myocarditis can often be associated with acute pericarditis. In more longstanding SLE, it has become evident that premature atherosclerosis and coronary artery disease are now part of the natural history of SLE. Many factors may contribute to this, including immune complex formation in coronary arteries, hypertension, lipid abnormalities, and glucocorticoid effects.

Hematologic abnormalities are commonly seen in patients with SLE. A classical hemolytic anemia with a positive direct Coombs test is seen in a minority of patients. Many patients also have a normochromic, normocytic anemia that is multifactorial due to suppression of bone marrow by disease or by medications, increased GI blood loss from antiinflammatory medications, and concomitant iron deficiency. Leukopenia is characteristic of acute SLE with approximately 20% of patients having white blood counts of less than 4000/mm^3. During active disease, lymphopenia defined as a lymphocyte count of less than 1500/mm^3 on at least two occasions is often seen. A high white blood count in SLE raises the spectre of infection or suggests recent high-dose corticosteroids. Mild thrombocytopenia is quite common in SLE; rarely are platelet counts of less than 50, 000 noted. SLE can present as isolated idiopathic thrombocytopenic purpura with the rest of the criteria for SLE developing years later. The association of immune thrombocytopenia and autoimmune hemolytic anemia (so-called Evans' syndrome) can be seen in SLE.

Clinical evidence of renal involvement is seen ultimately in 50% of patients. The most common renal finding is proteinuria, which can be seen at any time in the disease process. Hematuria, pyuria, and the presence of cellular casts can be observed. Renal insufficiency tends to develop in more longstanding disease, but patients can present with explosive acute renal failure. While patients with SLE may have normal kidneys by light microscopy, immunofluorescence and electron microscopy almost always identify deposits of immunoglobulin or complement proteins. Focal glomerulonephritis is seen in a minority of patients, perhaps 15%. Diffuse proliferative glomerulonephritis is unfortunately more common with involvement of more than 50% of glomeruli. Another small minority of the lupus population has purely membranous glomerulonephritis characterized by thickening of the glomerular basement membrane by deposits of immunoglobulin and complement with little cellular proliferation noted. Patients may also have renal involvement in the form of interstitial and tubular nephritis (Tan, Cohen et al., 1982).

A wide variety of neurologic manifestations can be seen in patients with SLE. Seizures occur in approximately 15% of patients and are one of the neurologic criteria for diagnosis. However, other signs of impairment of the nervous system can be encountered and include peripheral neuropathies, stroke, chorea, organic brain syndromes, transverse myelitis, aseptic meningitis, and even coma. Migraine headache is said to occur with a threefold incidence in patients with SLE. In addition to psychosis, the other neurologic criteria for the diagnosis of SLE, a variety of neuropsychiatric manifestations including cognitive disorders, depression, and affective disorders are seen.

Two other lupus-related syndromes should be mentioned. Drug-induced lupus is a syndrome in which a drug produces an illness that looks clinically and immunologically quite similar to SLE. While there are a number of agents that have been reported to produce drug-induced SLE, the antiarrhythmic drug procainamide and the antihypertensive drug hydralazine are most frequently reported. Other drugs that have been associated with drug-induced SLE include isoniazid, quinidine, propylthiouracil, dilantin, trimethadione, chlorpromazine, and D-penicillamine. In the case of procainamide and hydralazine-induced lupus, individuals who are slow acetylators appear to be at higher risk. The disease begins after the patient has been on the medication for several months; cumulative dosage, older age, and female sex may be additional risk factors. HLA-DR4 has been associated with procainamide- and hydralazine-induced lupus. Rash, fever, polyarthritis, pleuropericarditis, and pulmonary lesions are frequently seen in drug-induced lupus but renal or psychiatric disease are rare. High titer antinuclear antibody is usually present; however, antibody to double-stranded DNA and low complement levels are not seen. In over 90% of patients with drug-induced lupus, antibody to histone is present.

Another lupus-related syndrome is the antiphospholipid antibody syndrome. When it is associated with SLE, it is considered secondary. In addition, there is a primary antiphospholipid antibody syndrome where the patient does not meet criteria for SLE but has antibodies reactive with phospholipids. These patients can present to the obstetrician with recurrent fetal loss, to the neurologist with stroke, to the internist with deep vein thrombophlebitis, and/or pulmonary embolism. On examination, livido reticularis may be noted on the skin. The laboratory may reveal thrombocytopenia. These patients may have a false–positive test for syphilis, either RPR or VDRL, indicating the presence of antibody reactive with phospholipid. Anticardiolipin antibodies as measured by ELISA assay may be positive. The partial thromboplastin time or PTT may be prolonged indicating the presence of what has been termed a lupus anticoagulant. These patients often benefit from anticoagulation with aspirin, heparin, or coumadin, depending on the clinical setting.

Laboratory and Diagnostic Tests

The immunologic criteria often represent an important clue to the diagnosis of SLE in a patient with a puzzling multisystem disease. The discovery of the LE cell by Hargraves (Hargraves, Richmond & Morton, 1948) provided the initial key to our understanding of the role of autoantibodies in this disease and was widely used for diagnosis until its use was superseded by the development of the antinuclear antibody test or ANA (Friou, 1957). Unfortunately, the antinuclear antibody test is not specific for the diagnosis of SLE. While 99% of patients with SLE have a positive ANA test during their illness, there are many other conditions that can also yield a positive ANA. Figure 48–11 provides a framework for evaluating the positive ANA test result.

It is important to remember that the antinuclear antibody test is an indirect immunofluorescence test in which the patient's serum is allowed to bind to a cell substrate. If the patient's serum contains antibodies that react with cellular antigens, the antibodies in the patient's sera then bind to the cells. If the slide is developed with a fluorescent labeled antibody to human antibody, a pattern of bound human antibody is noted. The laboratory reports both a titer of antibody based on the highest dilution at which fluorescence was noted to be present. The higher the titer, the more antibody is present and, generally, the more likely it is to be a significant and meaningful test result. The laboratory also

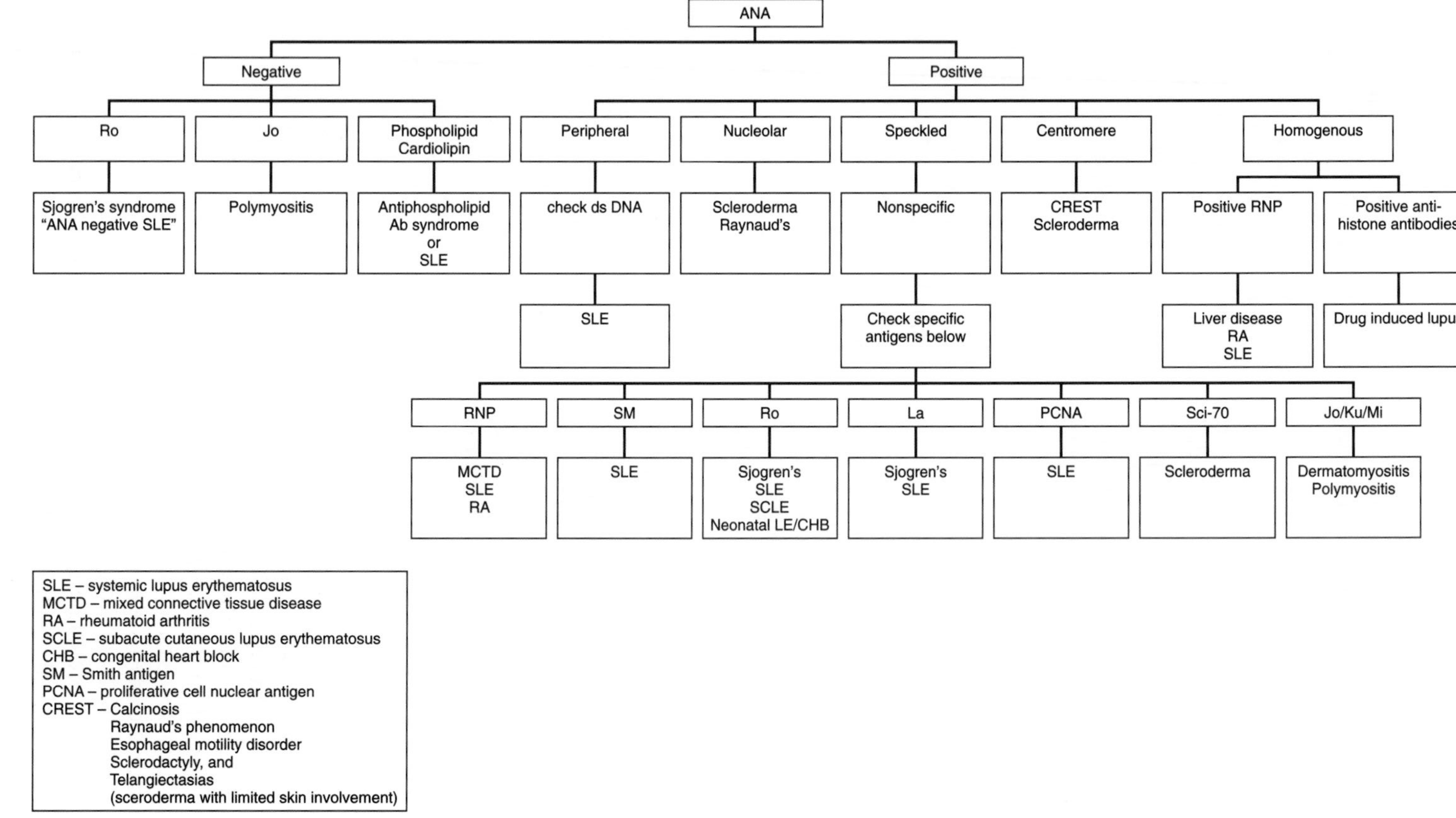

Figure 48–11. Interpretation of the fluorescent ANA test. *(From Craft & Hardin. [1993]. [pp. 164–187].)*

describes the pattern of stained fluorescence as peripheral, nucleolar, speckled, homogeneous, and centromeric. As seen in Figure 48–11, different patterns are associated with different cellular antigens and some convey disease specificity. The presence of a peripheral pattern signals that antibodies are binding to double-stranded DNA located along the nuclear membrane. This pattern and the presence of antibody to double-stranded DNA is specific for SLE. The other SLE-specific antigen, the Smith antigen or Sm, gives a speckled pattern of fluorescence (Friou, 1957).

Rheumatologists often are asked to consult on a patient in whom a positive ANA test has been found. In reviewing records, it is sometimes difficult to ascertain why the test was ordered. When ordering an ANA, try to decide what you are looking for and how this test might help you in your differential diagnosis. Knowing what the pattern of fluorescence is and looking further for antibodies to specific autoantigens may allow you to clarify whether a serious autoimmune situation is present. This test cannot be interpreted on its own but must be correlated with the patient's clinical features.

Management

The treatment of SLE requires a comprehensive approach, and rheumatology consultation is mandatory, both in confirming the diagnosis and in initiating treatment. Like any other chronic disease, patient education and knowledge play a vital role in improving outcome. Support groups and information from the Arthritis Foundation and the Lupus Foundation can be helpful in assisting patients in understanding this complex illness. It is important to monitor the patient for changes in disease activity every 3 to 6 months. Early on, renal disease or other life-threatening manifestations may not have declared themselves. The laboratory can assist in the identification of patients who have developed worrisome renal, hematologic, or serologic involvement. While not all patients with SLE are photosensitive, photoprotection with sunscreens containing UV light-blocking chemicals with a sun protection factor (SPF) of at least 15 or greater should be used. Local steroid creams are helpful for resolution of discoid lesions. In patients with mild symptoms, nonsteroidal antiinflammatory drugs are useful. Antimalarial drugs such as hydroxychloroquine have had a role in the treatment of skin manifestations of SLE. More recently a controlled trial of hydroxychloroquine in patients on steroids with stable lupus showed a reduction in serious flares in the group given hydroxychloroquine (The Canadian Hydroxychloroquine Study Group, 1991).

More severe disease manifestations require the addition of corticosteroids; by and large, most patients with SLE improve with steroid treatment. The doses of steroids that have been used are highly variable. For control of severe disease, initial therapy is usually either high-dose daily prednisone in the range for 1 to 2 mg/kg/day or 40 to 100 mg or so called "pulse therapy" of up to 100 mg of methylprednisolone intravenously for 3 days followed by 40 to 60 mg prednisone daily. Tapering of steroids by no more than 5 to 10% weekly is initiated when disease activity is clinically controlled. For severe manifestations of SLE, such as diffuse proliferative glomerulonephritis and varieties of central nervous system lupus, treatment with cytotoxic drugs such as cyclophosphamide is often initiated both to control disease activity and to allow for reduction of potential steroid toxicity, so-called "steroid sparing." By and large the intensity of treatment is related to the severity of involvement.

Other concerns for the management of SLE include a recognition that infection is a major cause of morbidity and mortality in treated disease. Patients should receive influenza and pneumococcal immunizations. As previously mentioned, many rheumatologists recommend antibiotic prophylaxis for surgical and dental procedures.

Pregnancy is a major issue for the patient with SLE. In general, lupus flares—particularly renal and hematologic—are probably increased in pregnancy. Women with SLE are more likely to have pregnancies complicated by hypertension, hyperglycemia, and diabetes. Increased fetal loss as well as increased preterm births and intrauterine growth retardation is reported. Rarely, maternal antibodies may cross the placenta producing the so-called neonatal lupus syndrome characterized by cutaneous lupus and congenital heart block.

SLE can present two challenges for the nurse practitioner: (1) in identifying the presence of this acute disease and (2) in managing it on a long-term basis. Survival has improved greatly for the patient with SLE and, as this happens, new problems are developing. There is little data on the safety of postmenopausal estrogen replacement in SLE, but studies are being done. The predisposition to accelerated atherogenesis in SLE means that more women with SLE in their 40s and 50s will present with coronary artery disease. There is also concern about a potential excess of lymphoma and other malignacies in SLE patients treated with cytotoxic drugs.

Vasculitis

The vasculitic syndromes are a number of relatively rare diseases characterized by inflammation of blood vessel walls resulting pathologically in structural injury and necrosis and clinically in manifestations of tissue and organ ischemia. These syndromes can be characterized in a number of ways, by the size of the vessels involved, by the pathology of the inflammatory process, and by whether they are considered primary or secondary. From the clinical perspective of the nurse practitioner, these are often the mystery patients, those with an unexplained systemic illness with cardinal symptoms and signs of organ system ischemia. These patients present with a bewildering array of problems. Fevers, night sweats, and weight loss suggest a malignancy.

There are arthralgias, myalgias, and possibly arthritis. Patients may have renal insufficiency or abdominal pain and GI bleeding or acute stroke or foot drop suggesting mononeuritis multiplex. Careful examination of the patient's skin may reveal signs of diffuse vascular insufficiency, livedo reticularis, or evidence of local necrosis and gangrene with skin infarction.

The vasculitic syndromes tend to be relatively rare, and data on disease incidence is imprecise. Giant-cell arteritis appears to be the most common primary vasculitic syndrome, with an estimated incidence of 15 to 30 per 100,000 followed by polyarteritis nodosa, Henoch–Schonlein purpura, and hypersensitivity angiitis. Wegener's granulomatosis, Takayasu's arteritis, Kawasaki syndrome, and Churg Strauss tend to be quite rare.

Pathophysiology

There are a number of different pathogenetic mechanisms for vascular damage in vasculitic syndromes. In some vasculitic syndromes—for example, the secondary vasculitis seen in systemic lupus erythematosus—immune complex formation and subsequent vessel formation lead to vascular injury. Granuloma formation is seen in Wegener's granulomatosis. Giant-cell formation is characteristic of giant cell (temporal arteritis). Antibodies to endothelial cell and endothelial cell antigens may play a role in some vasculitic syndromes. There is evidence for induction and up regulation of leukocyte and endothelial cell adhesion molecules. In addition, various cytokines appear to be involved in the induction of the immune response and its amplification. Other molecules whose role in pathogenesis of vasculitis is the subject of current investigation include endothelin, produced in greater amounts by damaged endothelial cells and endothelial derived relaxing factor (EDRF).

Vasculitic syndromes can be considered primary or secondary. The various primary vasculitic syndromes represent unique clinical syndromes of unknown cause and their nomenclature has recently been standardized by the Chapel Hill Consensus Conference (Jennette et al., 1994). The causes of secondary vasculitis include infection-related vasculitis (hepatitis B, hepatitis C, HIV), vasculitis secondary to other defined connective tissue disease such as rheumatoid arthritis or systemic lupus erythematosus, drug hypersensitivity-related vasculitis, vasculitis secondary to cryoglobulins, malignancy-related vasculitis, and the syndrome of hypocomplementemic urticarial vasculitis.

Giant-Cell Arteritis

Pathophysiology. Giant-cell arteritis (GCA) is a systemic arteritis of unknown etiology affecting large- and medium-sized arteries. Pathologically there is a characteristic lymphocytic and plasma cell infiltration of the vessels with the formation of multinuclear giant cells. Giant-cell arteritis is seen almost exclusively in people over age 60 with a female preponderance. Temporal artery involvement is common, but the term "giant-cell arteritis" is preferred because other large arteries beside the temporal artery may be involved. One feature of giant-cell arteritis is a myalgic syndrome called polymyalgia rheumatica (PMR), a clinical syndrome characterized by the usually acute onset of muscle pain and stiffness in the shoulder and pelvic girdle region associated with an elevated sedimentation rate and by a clinical response to low doses of corticosteroids. Whether GCA or PMR are manifestations of one disease process with variability of phenotypic expression or whether they are different processes with overlapping manifestations is uncertain. What is clear is that many patients, but not all, with GCA have myalgic complaints and that patients presenting with clinical signs of PMR may have an associated giant-cell arteritis. In addition to the symptoms of PMR, patients with giant-cell arteritis often have local manifestations of temporal headache, scalp tenderness or (rarely) scalp necrosis, jaw claudication, and, unfortunately visual loss due to an anterior ischemic optic neuropathy. Nonspecific symptoms of fever, anorexia, weight loss, and malaise may be present. The laboratory shows a mild anemia, often abnormal liver function tests, and an elevated sedimentation rate. Diagnosis of PMR is a clinical one; diagnosis of giant-cell arteritis is a pathologic one. Of patients with giant-cell arteritis with temporal artery symptoms, more than 90% have a pathognemonic abnormal temporal artery biopsy whereas among patients with polymyalgia–rheumatica symptoms only, less than 50% have a positive biopsy.

Management. Corticosteroids remain the initial drug of choice for the treatment of both PMR and GCA. Patients with PMR have an almost miraculous rapid response to low doses of corticosteroid in the range of 10 to 15 mg of prednisone daily. In fact, failure to improve within several days at this dosage should make one doubt the diagnosis and consider other possibilities such as occult malignancy, multiple myeloma, thyroid disease, rheumatoid arthritis, or infection. For treatment of giant-cell arteritis with visual or vascular complications, dosages of prednisone of 60 mg daily should be begun. As disease activity comes under control, the dosage of prednisone is tapered by 5 mg weekly initially and then by no more than 10% of the dose per week. Patients often require treatment for 2 to 5 years. Recently, methotrexate has begun to be used as a steroid-sparing agent.

Polyarteritis Nodosa

Pathophysiology. Polyarteritis nodosa (PAN) is defined (Jennette et al., 1994) as a necrotizing arteritis of medium and small arteries. Patients present with a variety of symptoms including weight loss, fever, peripheral neuropathy, myalgias, arthralgias, palpable purpura, hypertension, heart failure, and abdominal pain. The pathology of PAN is a focal segmental necrotizing vasculitis. The artery is infiltrated by primarily polymorphonuclear neutrophils;

there is fibrinoid necrosis of the media. Characteristically there is coexistence of active and healed or healing vascular lesions in the same tissues. With the destruction of the integrity of the vessel wall, microaneurysms develop. The diagnosis is made by biopsy showing the classical lesion or by arteriography demonstrating microaneurysms as well as narrowing of involved vessels. Hepatitis B surface antigen is found in less than 33% of patients with PAN.

Management. Treatment of polyarteritis nodosa has been revolutionized by the use of prednisone and cyclophosphamide. The standard treatment regimen has been to use cyclophosphamide approximately 2 mg/kg/day. However, side effects from daily cyclophosphamide have included hemorrhagic cystitis, bladder cancer, bone marrow suppression, and ovarian failure. More recently, pulse cyclophosphamide may be just as effective and may be less toxic for the patient. In hepatitis B-related polyarteritis nodosa, use of steroids and cyclophosphamide may allow the hepatitis B virus to replicate. Protocols involving interferon alpha and vidarabine may be more effective for this group of patients.

Patients with a microscopic form of polyarteritis nodosa involving arterioles, venules, or capillaries have been separated out from those with polyarteritis nodosa. These patients differ from those with classical PAN by the association of rapidly progressive glomerulonephritis and pulmonary involvement. A rare subtype of PAN, Churg–Strauss syndrome is characterized by eosinophilia, asthma, and necrotizing vasculitis.

Wegener's Granulomatosis

Pathophysiology. Wegener's granulomatosis is a form of granulomatous vasculitis involving the upper and lower airway and kidney. The ACR criteria for the diagnosis include nasal or oral inflammation with bloody nasal discharge or oral ulcers, abnormal chest x-ray with nodules, fixed infiltrates or cavities, abnormal urinary sediment with RBC or RBC casts, and evidence of granulomatous inflammation on biopsy. Two of four criteria are required for biopsy. The characteristic pathology is a triad of vasculitis, necrosis, and granulomas often with multinucleated giant cells.

A characteristic antibody, the antineutrophil cytoplasmic antibody (ANCA) has been found to be highly specific for Wegener's granulomatosis (van der Woude et al., 1985). Further studies have shown that this antibody recognizes a serine proteinase called proteinase 3 (PR-3). These antibodies are almost always present in active disease. *In vitro,* ANCA appear to enhance neutrophil activation and may adhere to endothelial cells suggesting a possible pathogenetic role in Wegener's.

Management. Standard treatment of Wegener's has been with prednisone and oral cyclophosphamide. More recent studies have looked at protocols using methotrexate, pulse cyclophosphamide, and cyclosporin.

Takayasu's Arteritis

Takayasu's arteritis is an idiopathic large vessel giant-cell arteritis of unknown etiology with a predilection for women of reproductive age. This disease occurs with excess incidence in women of Asian background. The clinical symptoms with Takayasu's arteritis vary from completely asymptomatic patients who are incidentally found to have unequal blood pressures or bruits to young women presenting with catastrophic events such as stroke, congestive heart failure, or, rarely, ruptured aortic aneurysm. The diagnosis is a clinical one; the sedimentation rate is used to assess disease activity. Angiography is the standard for detection of diseased vessel involvement. Glucocorticoids are the mainstay of treatment of the inflammatory phase; methotrexate and cyclophosphamide have been used in addition. Other important modalities are control of hypertension, use of antiplatelet agents, and surgery for stenotic lesions.

Henoch–Schonlein Purpura

Pathophysiology. Henoch–Schonlein purpura is a small-vessel vasculitis affecting primarily skin and vessels of the gastrointestinal tract and kidney. It is seen primarily in children, often after a viral upper respiratory infection. The pathology is similar to that of PAN. In some patients, deposits of IgA can be demonstrated on immunofluorescence.

Henoch–Schonlein purpura is a syndrome occuring in previously healthy 5 to 15-year olds characterized by palpable purpura, arthritis, abdominal pain, and renal dysfunction. There are no laboratory tests specific to the syndrome. Most cases are self limited with a good prognosis; however, 5% of patients progress to renal failure. Treatment is supportive. Steroids are usually not required and are unhelpful in renal disease (White, 1993).

Conditions that Mimic Vasculitis Syndromes

Finally, no discussion of vasculitic syndromes would be complete without mention of some of the common conditions that can mimic vasculitis. The patient with atheromatous emboli can present with purpuric skin lesions, renal failure, fever, or abdominal pain. Here the diagnosis is made on biopsy by finding a characteristic cholesterol cleft in the vessel wall. The patient with atrial myxoma presents with embolic lesions that may look like vasculitis. Patients with various thrombotic states may develop signs and symptoms of tissue ischemia. This is quite commonly seen in patients with the primary antiphopspholipid syndrome but may also been seen in patients with TTP, antithrombin III deficiency, and protein C and protein S deficiencies. Subacute bacterial endocarditis is another condition to consider in the setting of peripheral emboli, fever, and elevated sedimentation rate. A variety of neoplastic diseases can mimic vasculitis or can have an associated vasculitis. Pyoderma gangrenosum can be confused with a vasculitic ulcer, so biopsy here is helpful in making this diagnosis. Calciphylaxis is a rare syndrome of progressive ischemic necrosis occurring in the setting of end-stage renal disease associated with hyperparathyroidism caused by progressive vascular calcification.

▶ SERONEGATIVE SPONDYLOARTHROPATHIES

Pathophysiology

The seronegative spondyloarthropathies are a related group of rheumatoid factor negative, ANA negative diseases characterized by inflammatory asymmetrical oligoarthritis, and inflammatory spinal involvement. They are traditionally associated with a predictable group of extraarticular manifestations including skin, ocular, and GI manifestations. Cardiac involvement is reported but uncommon. Clinical diseases that fall within this category are ankylosing spondylitis, Reiter's syndrome, psoriatic arthritis, and arthritis associated with inflammatory bowel disease. The etiology or pathogenesis of these disorders is poorly understood but there is a strong association with the histocompatibility antigen HLA-B27, which is positive in 6 to 8% of the caucasian population. Conversely, HLA-B27 is positive in 90% of patients with ankylosing spondylosis (AS), in 60 to 80% of patients with Reiter's syndrome, and 50% of patients with psoriatic arthritis who also have spondylitis (Osial, Cash, & Eisenbeis, 1993). The significance of this relationship is unclear. Other factors known to be associated with this group of diseases include an inflammatory response to specific infections including *Chlamydia, Yersinia,* and *Salmonella.* This sterile inflammatory response to an infection remote from the joint is often referred to as reactive arthritis and is felt to be the pathogenesis of Reiter's syndrome as well as of the arthritis associated with inflammatory bowel disease.

Ankylosing Spondylitis

History and Physical Findings

Ankylosing spondylitis (AS) is a chronic, systemic inflammatory disorder with sacroiliac joint inflammation as its earliest distinguishing sign. Peripheral small-joint involvement is uncommon, but the hips and shoulders are commonly involved. Clinical manifestations often begin in adolescence or early adulthood, and the disease is three times more common in men. Women seem to develop the disease later than men and generally experience milder courses. The most common and often initial sign is low back pain and stiffness of insidious onset, not associated with injury. Patients often experience pain and inflammation at attachment points including heels, pelvis, buttocks, hips, and shoulders (enthesopathy). When this inflammatory reaction occurs along the spinal ligaments, bony spurs called syndesmophytes form leading to the characteristic "bamboo spine" seen in classic AS. The back pain in AS is relieved by activity and worsened by rest. Nights and early mornings are the worst times for these patients and they often get up and exercise in the night before they are able to go back to sleep. Physical signs may be minimal in the early stages, but there is often limitation in the motion of the lumber spine. There is a gradual loss of lumber lordosis and a gradual loss of chest expansion due to the involvement of the costovertebral joints. Typical deformity develops after 10 or more years and can progress to spinal fusion in a flexed position severe enough to interfere with the patient's field of vision.

Extrarticular Manifestations. Extrarticular manifestations that can be seen include acute iritis, which occurs sometime during the course of the disease in 25 to 30% of patients. Cardiac involvement is rare but potentially serious. The risk of cardiac involvement increases with age and disease duration. Ascending aortitis, aortic valve incompetence, and conduction abnormalities are the most commonly seen abnormalities. Neurologic complications can occur as a result of spinal deformity, spinal fractures, or dislocation. Fractures most often occur in the cervical spine and can cause quadraplegia. Progressive cauda equina syndrome is seen in longstanding AS and results in pain, incontinence, and sensory loss (Khan, 1990).

Laboratory and Diagnostic Tests

There is no single diagnostic test that is pathgnomonic of AS. HLA-B27 is occasionally used as an aid to diagnosis but is expensive and often not available away from academic centers. Most patients can be diagnosed on the basis of history and physical examination. X-ray changes typical of AS, including ankylosis of the SI joints and the "bamboo" spine, are late findings. Sacroileitis is the most common finding in early disease. Hip involvement shows up as concentric joint space narrowing with osteophyte formation (Khan, 1990).

Management

All patients with AS need ongoing supportive education regarding their disease in order to improve compliance with complicated, lifelong regimes. Nonsteroidal antiinflammatories, especially indomethacin, have been used to alleviate the pain and inflammation of AS. Second-line agents have been tried with varied success. Sulfasalazine, 2 to 3 grams a day, has been found to be effective in alleviating symptoms for many patients. Oral steroids have no long-term value because of their potential for serious side effects, although pulse IV steroids have been used in the past. Perhaps the single most important treatment in AS is a physical therapy program that emphasizes spinal-extension and chest-expansion exercises. These exercises, in addition to maintaining and enhancing mobility, encourage the patient to maintain an upright posture as the disease progresses. The most beneficial overall exercise is swimming.

Reiter's Syndrome/Reactive Arthritis

Reiter's syndrome was originally described in 1916 as a clinical triad consisting of arthritis, nongonococcal urethritis, and conjunctivitis following an episode of dysentary. Incomplete Reiter's, an oligoarthritis without the associated urethritis or conjunctivitis, was subsequently recognized to follow veneral infections, especially *Chlamydia trachomatis,* as well as dysenteries caused by *Yersinia, Salmonella, Shigella,* and *Campylobacter* (Osial et al., 1993). Up to 70% are HLA-B27 positive.

History and Physical Findings

Typically, the patient is a young adult who presents with an acute arthritis, assymetrically involving weight-bearing joints, especially knees or ankles. The inflammation and joint effusion can be impressive. Inflammation can involve tendon insertion sites (enthesopathy) and cause pain at the heel, Achilles tendon, and low back. Arthritis of the small joints of the hands or feet can appear as a "sausage digit" (Fig. 48–12). In classic Reiter's, the arthritis typically appears one to three weeks after the urethritis or diarrhea; 40% of patients many develop conjunctivitis. The triad may not be present simultaneously, making the diagnosis more elusive. Frequently patients may not even remember the diarrheal illness that precipitated the syndrome. Skin involvement can include shallow, painless ulcers of the glans penis called balanitis circinata which is seen in up to 25% of patients with post *Chlamydia* and post *Shigella* Reiter's (Fan & Yu, 1993). The classic rash associated with Reiter's (keratoderma blenorrhagia) involves the palms and soles, begins as clear vesicles, and progresses to keratotic nodules (Fig. 48–13). This rash looks exactly like pustular psoriasis and is treated with medium-intensity topical steroid preparations.

Laboratory and Diagnostic Tests

Diagnosis of Reiter's syndrome is almost always based on history and physical examination. An x-ray finding of sacroiliitis in a patient with an asymmetrical arthritis may help to confirm the diagnosis. No specific laboratory finding is diagnostic but a urethral swab or cervical brushings looking for *Chlamydia* is recommended. Nonspecific inflammatory tests, such as the erythrocyte sedimentation rate and C-reative protein, may demonstrate significant inflammation and may normalize as the symptoms subside. Reiter's syndrome was the first rheumatic disease known to be associated with HIV infection.

Management

Nonsteroidal antiinflammatory drugs are the first-line agents used for relief of symptoms. Indomethacin or naproxen are effective for many patients but can cause significant GI toxicity and should be taken with food. Sulfasalazine at 2–3 grams a day has been shown to be effective in controlling the symptoms of Reiter's. There is ongoing debate as to the effectiveness of long-term antibiotic therapy given the association between Reiter's and infection. All trials to date have been inconclusive, but this remains an area of interest to researchers. Methotrexate has been used in the treatment of Reiter's with some success (Creemers et al., 1994). The usual dose of Methotrexate is 7.5 to 25 mg po weekly and improvement is seen within 6 weeks of initiation of therapy.

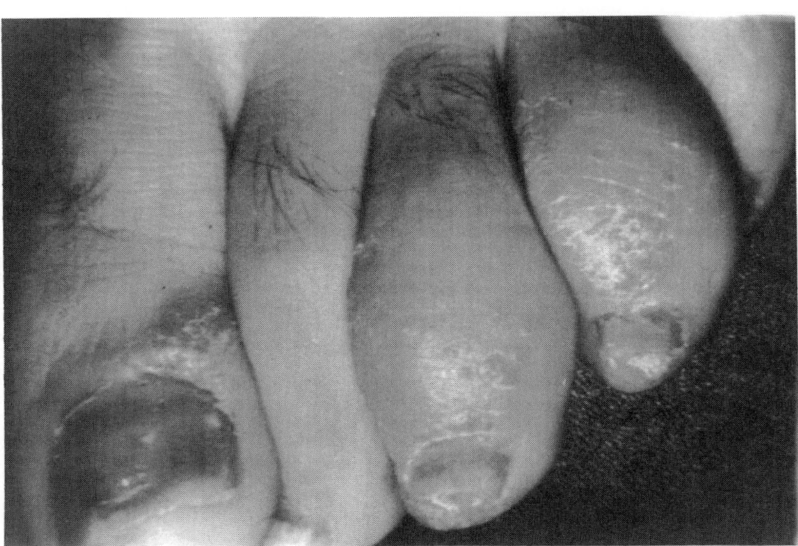

Figure 48–12. Sausage digit and rash. The "sausage" shape of these toes is caused by marked soft tissue swelling. This finding is seen in both fingers and toes. *(Reprinted from the Clinical Slide Collection on the Rheumatic Diseases, Copyright 1991, 1995. Used with permission of the American College of Rheumatology.)*

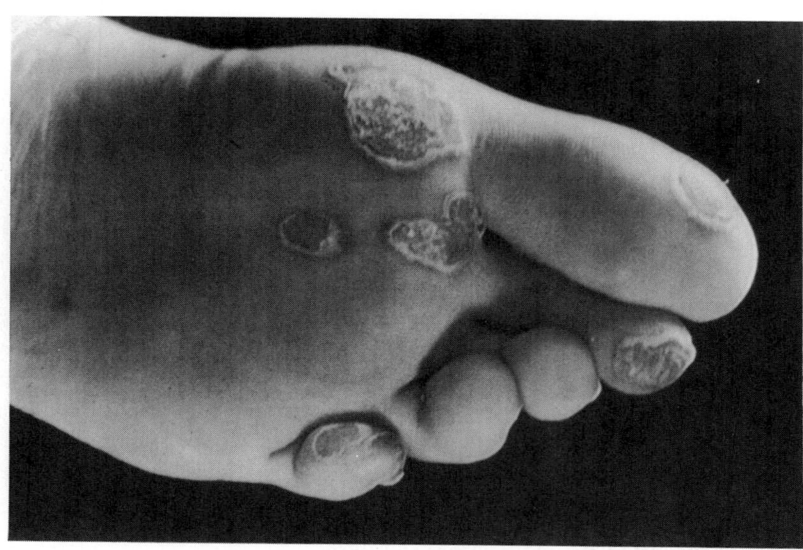

Figure 48–13. Reiter's syndrome: keratoderma blennorrhagica. Discreet, scaly, and plaquelike lesions resemble psoriasis. *(Reprinted from the Clinical Slide Collection on the Rheumatic Diseases, Copyright 1991, 1995. Used with permission of the American College of Rheumatology.)*

Although the prevalence of side effects is low, they can be serious and include liver toxicity, anemia, leukopenia, and pulmonary fibrosis. Routine monitoring of CBCs and liver enzymes is imperative. Reiter's seen in association with HIV should not be treated with immunosuppressant drugs such as methotrexate as this increases the risk of opportunistic infection in these patients.

Inflammatory Bowel Diseases

Inflammatory bowel diseases, including Crohn's disease and ulcerative colitis, have long been known to be associated with the spondyloarthropathies. Arthritis can occur in as many as 17 to 20% of patients with inflammatory bowel disease with the highest prevalence in Crohn's (Mielants & Veys, 1990). Sacroiliac involvement is not uncommon and may be indistinguishable from AS. An association with HLA-B27 is seen.

Polyarthritis is seen in a large percentage of patients who have undergone intestinal bypass surgery for morbid obesity. Symptoms can develop 2 to 30 months after surgery. The arthritis is symmetrical, polyarticular, and migratory. Most cases are transient and there is no joint deformity or erosive disease. Nonsteroidal antiinflammatory medications are usually sufficient to control the arthritis, but occasionally oral antibiotics are used (Mielants & Veys, 1990).

Psoriatic Arthritis

Pathophysiology

Psoriatic arthritis is simply defined as inflammatory seronegative arthritis associated with psoriasis. The absence of rheumatoid factor and the identification of specific subsets help to distinguish psoriatic arthritis from rheumatoid arthritis. Of the patients with psoriasis, 5 to 7% develop arthritis. The proportion goes up with more severe psoriasis. There is a strong correlation with HLA-B27 as well as other genetic markers (Ruzicka, 1996).

The pattern of joint involvement varies widely. Classification by Moll and Wright in 1973 defines five distinct types of psoriatic arthritis based on patterns of joint involvement:

1. Asymmetrical oligoarticular arthritis primarily involving proximal and distal interphalangeal joints of the hands and feet (Fig. 48–14); digital attachment arthritis results in the classic "sausage digit" (refer to Fig. 48–12); the knee and hip joints are often involved.
2. Distal interphalangeal involvement only.
3. Mutilating osteolysis of the involved phalanges with severe deformities and bone resorption of the distal ends of the phalanges.
4. Symmetrical polyarthritis similar to rheumatoid arthritis; this is usually rheumatoid factor negative and can run a milder course.
5. Spinal form occuring in 5 to 40% of patients with psoriatic arthritis including saroiliitis and the development of spinal fusion which is reminiscent of ankylosing spondilitis.

This classification has been simplified but the basic categories hold true and are useful as aids to diagnosis.

Laboratory and Diagnostic Tests

There is no definitive laboratory test for the diagnosis of psoriatic arthritis. Inflammatory tests such as the erythrocyte sedimentation rate and C-reactive protein may be ele-

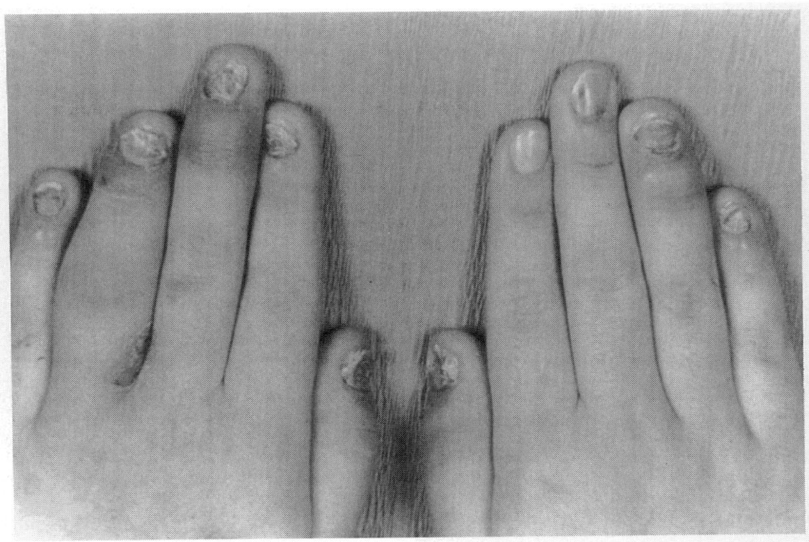

Figure 48–14. Psoriatic arthritis: nail dystrophy and arthritis. Punctate pitting of the nails is a common finding in patients with psoriatic arthritis. *(Reprinted from the Clinical Slide Collection on the Rheumatic Diseases, Copyright 1991, 1995. Used with permission of the American College of Rheumatology.)*

vated. The diagnosis is a clinical one based on characteristic skin and nail changes and patterns of joint involvement (see previous discussion). Usually the skin changes occur before joint involvement, but, in a small percentage of patients, the arthritis may be the presenting sign. If psoriatic arthritis is suspected, all patients should be examined carefully for small, easily missed psoriatic patches in the scalp, intergluteal fold, or perineal region.

X-rays may demonstrate the classic "pencil in cup" deformity of the distal interphalangeal joints (Fig. 48–15), and massive bony resorption with telescoping fingers may be late radiographic findings. Spinal involvement may be represented by saroiliitis or fusion. Spinal involvement, when it occurs, is similiar to AS, but is less predictable.

Management

Treatment for psoriatic arthritis has been disappointing. Many antiarthritic therapies do not influence skin lesions

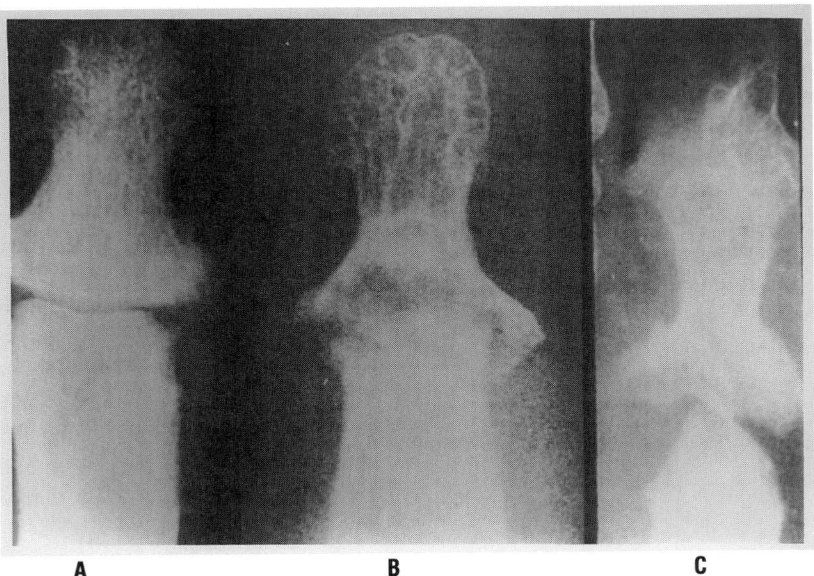

A B C

Figure 48–15. Psoriatic arthritis: progressive joint changes (Roentgenograms). Progressive changes seen in these interphalangeal joints beginning with **(A)** mild soft tissue swelling, narrowing of the joint space, and erosion of adjacent condyles progressing to **(B)** greater bone loss to **(C)** further loss of bone and tapering to a "pencil-in-cup" appearance. (*Reprinted from the Clinical Slide Collection on the Rheumatic Diseases, Copyright 1991, 1995. Used with permission of the American College of Rheumatology.)*

and some may actually exacerbate the psoriasis (NSAIDs, gold, plaquenil). Conversely, suppression of the skin disease may be important in controlling the arthritis although this, too, is uncertain. Patients with severe skin involvement should be referred to a dermatologist. Topical treatments with steroid and tar preparations are commonly prescribed. Oral psoralen with UV-A radiation (PUVA) can be helpful. Topical Tacrolimus (FK 506) shows promise (Ruzicka, 1996).

Nonsteroidal antiinflammatories can help with joint and back pain and are commonly prescribed. Both indomethacin and naproxen have proven beneficial. Methotrexate is the only established second-line drug that seems to benefit both the skin and joint disease. Generally doses in the 5 to 25 mg range given po once per week have been effective in producing remission in many patients. Methotrexate is limited by its potential liver and lung toxicity. Routine monitoring of CBCs and liver enzymes is imperative. Methotrexate is potentially teratogenic; women of childbearing age should be carefully counseled and be using reliable methods of birth control. Cyclosporine A has recently been shown to have significant antipsoriatic effect. In addition, reductions in joint pain and inflammation as well as reduction in the use of NSAIDs has been reported. Doses of 1.5 to 6 mg per day for 8 weeks or more are required. Renal toxicity is a concern, and patients should be monitored frequently for renal toxicity and hypertension throughout the course of treatment (Winchester, 1995). Currently, methotrexate and cyclosporine should be considered the drugs of choice for moderate to severe psoriatic arthritis.

Evaluation and Follow-Up

Nurse practitioners caring for these patients must be sensitive to pain-control issues as well as the need for additional assistance with ADLs. Referral to such rehabilitation services as physical therapy or occupational therapy may be helpful. A dermatologic consult may be needed to assist with complicated skin involvement. Referral to rheumatology is appropriate if the diagnosis is in doubt or if current therapy is ineffective or causing unacceptable side effects. Second-line agents can cause major organ toxicity and need to be monitored carefully. The association of these diseases with HIV is well described, making obtaining a history of possible risk factors for HIV important for both diagnostic and therapeutic reasons. These syndromes may have overlapping etiologies and a better understanding of the diseases may lead to the development of more satisfactory treatments.

▶ OSTEOPOROSIS

Pathophysiology

The skeleton consists of a collagenous matrix impregnated with and surrounded by calcium phosphate salts. It serves both structural and homeostatic functions, providing protection for internal organs and serving as a reservoir for the calcium and phosphate needed for cellular function. Normal bone integrity is maintained by a dynamic balance between bone formation and breakdown. Metabolic bone diseases are manifested by bone pain and fractures secondary to generalized abnormalities of bone tissue caused by either an abnormal rate of bone resorption or an abnormality in the process of bone formation. Bone loss can be accelerated in a number of ways. Immobilization for several weeks results in rapid bone resorption. Chronic diseases, including renal or hepatic failure, Cushing's disease, hyperparathyroidism, inflammatory arthritis, and hypercalcemia, can all lead to osteoporosis. Deficiencies in vitamin D and calcium as well as eating disorders that may lead to these deficiencies are certainly contributing causes. The American diet is typically low in calcium, which is particularly worrisome in the diets of children and adolescents as this is when peak bone mass is formed.

Osteoporosis, the most common of all metabolic bone diseases, is defined by the World Health Organization as a bone mineral density 2.5 standard deviations or more below the mean bone density of gender-matched young normal persons. It is characterized by decreased bone mineral density (osteopenia) and ultimately fractures. Twenty-five million Americans suffer from osteoporosis; 80% of these are women. Most osteoporotic fractures occur in the vertebrae, hip, and forearm. The incidence of hip fracture increases exponentially after age 50 in women and age 60 in men. At age 55, a woman has a 40% risk of a bony fracture. One third of all caucasian women over the age of 80 will have a hip fracture. Following a hip fracture, 10 to 20% of patients die within 6 months. Half of those who survive are unable to walk without assistance and one fourth require long-term care. Ten billion dollars a year are spent on treatment of hip fracture and this is expected to rise to $60 billion by the year 2020 (Gambert, 1996).

History and Physical Findings

Vertebral compression fractures are often associated with acute back pain and disability. The prevalence of compression fractures is about 20% in postmenopausal women (Asch, 1996). These fractures can occur spontaneously or result from minimal trauma such as sneezing, coughing, or bending. These fractures can be asymptomatic and account for loss of height, kyphosis, and skeletal deformity. The most commonly fractured vertebrae are the lower thoracic and upper lumbar. Acute vertebral fracture can be quite painful and patients present themselves to nurse practitioners in offices and emergency rooms for pain management and assistance with activities of daily living.

Risk Factors

Many risk factors have been identified (Table 48–5). The three leading risk factors are age, female gender, and a family history of osteoporosis. Osteoporosis is a disease affect-

TABLE 48–5. Factors That Contribute to the Development of Osteoporosis

Failure to achieve peak bone mass
Genetic factors
Ethnic origin
Low calcium intake
Sedentary lifestyle
Intercurrent illness
Common conditions that contribute to bone loss
Advancing age
Female sex
Nulliparity
Fair skin
Short stature
Slender body build
Early menopause
Intercurrent illness
Cigarette smoking
Sedentary lifestyle
Possibly genetic factors and low calcium intake
Malignant diseases
Carcinoma metastatic to bone
Multiple myeloma
Endocrine and metabolic diseases
Cushing's syndrome
Hypercalciuria
Hyperparathyroidism
Hyperthyroidism
Hypogonadism
Nutritional disorders
Alcoholism
Anorexia nervosa
Malabsorption
Osteomalacia
Drugs
Anticonvulsants
Furosemide (Lasix)
Glucocorticoids
Tetracyclines
Thyroid hormone in excessive doses
Other conditions
Primary biliary cirrhosis
Severe liver disease
Renal failure

ing 58% of those between the ages of 70 and 79 years and 84% of those 80 years and older (Asch, 1996). In women, estrogen helps to maximize peak bone mass and maintains it until menopause when the rate of bone loss is quite rapid for approximately 6 years. Late onset of menarche, amenorrhea, or early menopause can reduce peak bone mass. The risk of osteoporosis in female athletes who may be anorexic or amenorrheic due to reduced body fat is high. Primary prevention strategies and careful patient education is imperative. Small, thin women have a lower peak bone mass which increases risk for osteoporosis. Most people are unaware of a family history of osteoporosis but can often recall details such as the presence of kyphosis or hip fracture in a close relative.

Patients with rheumatic diseases as well as asthma, COPD, cystic fibrosis, and others are often on corticosteroids for greater than 6 months putting them at high risk for bone loss and subsequent fracture. The skeletal risk of these drugs appears to be both dose and duration dependent. The greatest bone loss happens in the first 6 months of therapy. Predisone doses as low as 7.5 mg per day cause significant bone loss. Every-other-day dosing does not appear to alter the risk. It has been estimated that one fourth of these patients sustain an osteoporotic fracture The American College of Rheumatology recommends the following interventions for the prevention and treatment of glucocorticoid-induced osteoporosis (ACR, 1996):

1. Bone density measurements in all patients who appear likely to be taking corticosteroids long term.
2. Begin preventative strategies including calcium, vitamin D, sex hormone replacement, and weight-bearing exercises programs as instructed by a physical therapist. Careful patient education regarding modifiable risk factors. Balance and gait evaluations, postural training, and back-extension exercises should be emphasized.
3. Bisphosphonates and calcitonin are reserved for those patients who sustain a fracture in spite of primary prevention strategies. Calcitonin is often used for its analgesic properties during the acute phase of the fracture with the drug gradually tapered. The use of bisphosphonates is not recommended in premenopausal women or men under 50, as the long-term side effects are unknown.
4. Follow-up bone density mass in 6 to 12 months to measure efficacy of therapeutic intervention.

Laboratory and Diagnostic Tests

The quality of bone helps to determine whether it will fracture. For a fracture to occur, the bone architecture must be altered and (usually) the patient must sustain at least mild trauma. Not all fractures can be prevented, but the risk of fracture can be measured and appropriate preventative strategies prescribed. The development of dual-energy x-ray absorptiometry (DEXA) make it possible to accurately measure the bone mineral density (BMD) in the lumber spine, the femoral neck, and the forearm with minimal radiation exposure. By measuring the BMD at all three sites, one is able to assess the density of both cortical and trabecular bone. Trabecular bone (mostly spine) is lost as a result of estrogen deficiency and long-term steroid use. Cortical bone loss occurs with calcium balance disorders. If measurement must be confined to only one area, probably the hip is best as it is composed of both trabecular and cortical bone.

DEXA scores have been standardized to allow comparisons between patients and matched controls. This is recorded as grams per square centimeter and converted into standard deviations (SD) with the mean either a gender-matched normal adult population or gender- and age-matched control population. Osteoporosis is defined as a reading 2.5 standard deviations below the young adult population mean (T score). If the reading is –1.0 to –2.5 SD, the diagnosis is osteopenia, which reflects bone loss without substantial fracture risk. When the score is –2.0 standard deviations below age-matched controls (Z score) without adequate explanation, secondary causes of osteoporosis must be ruled out (Asch, 1996) (Fig. 48–16). Secondary causes are present in about 10% of those with osteoporosis and include hyperparathyroidism, renal disease malabsorption, multiple myeloma, and alcoholism.

Although BMD measurement is currently the best predictor of fracture risk, it is far from perfect. Accurate reading can be complicated by severe degenerative disease, previous compression fractures, prior back surgeries, and aortic calcification—all of which make bone appear more dense than it actually is. This can be avoided by measuring at the forearm, although this is a more limited measurement. BMD measurement is indicated whenever the outcome of the test will affect treatment decisions. The AACE recommends BMD in the following settings (AACE Guidelines, 1996):

1. Risk assessment in perimenopausal or postmenopausal women who are willing to try currently available interventions.
2. Patients on long-term glucocorticoid therapy who are candidates for preventative therapies.
3. Patients with asymptomatic primary hyperparathyroidism in whom skeletal loss would result in parathyroidectomy.
4. Patients undergoing treatment for osteoporosis to monitor therapeutic response.

Management and Prevention

Osteoporosis is a disease in which prevention and treatment merge as the approach to both are currently similar. Treatment decisions need to be individualized based on the patient's age, life expectancy, lifestyle, activity level, ability to comply with recommendations, risk of falling, or other fracture risk. The first step is risk reduction with the elimination of those factors that contribute to loss of bone density, including dose reduction or elimination of drugs that may be a factor, smoking and alcohol cessation, and correction of metabolic abnormalities.

Primary prevention strategies should be emphasized as early as possible starting with calcium and vitamin D recommendations in childhood and adolescence. Adequate calcium and vitamin D are necessary for the formation of peak bone stock, and their need continues throughout life—with supplements necessary in the diets of the elderly. For postmenopausal women, as well as those on long-term glucosteroids, a daily intake of 1500 mg of elemental calcium and 800 IU of vitamin D is recommended. Regular weight-bearing exercise is fundamental as it enhances the development of bone in children and adolescents and slows the rate of bone loss in the elderly. A structured program of aerobic and strength-training programs can be useful even in the frail elderly. Preventing falls, especially in the elderly, is of primary importance in preventing fractures. Assuring the

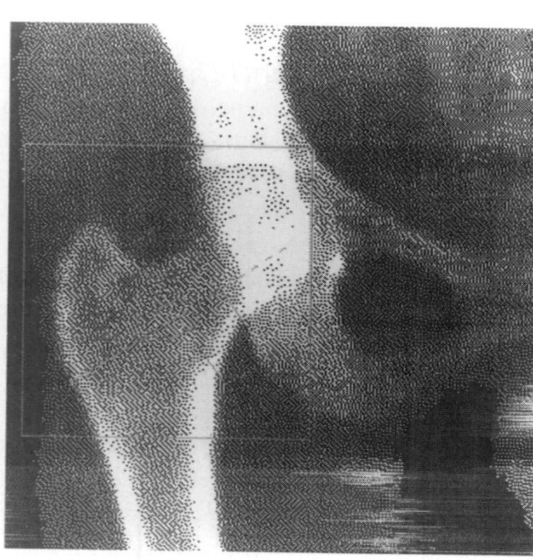

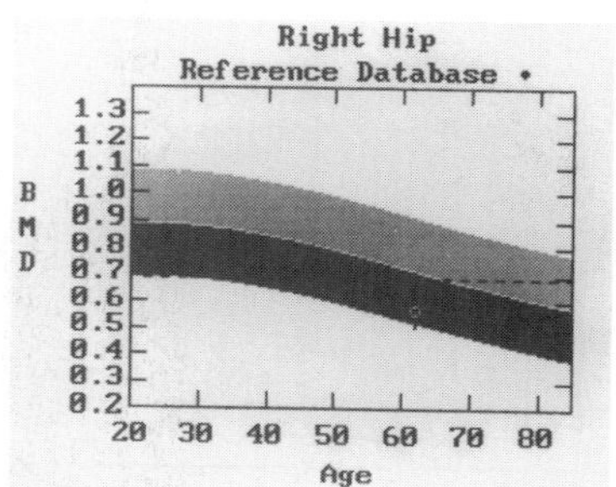

BMD(Neck[R]) = 0.561 g/cm²

Region	BMD	T		Z	
Neck	0.561	-3.34 (22.0)	63%	-1.59	78%
Troch	0.472	-2.77 (30.0)	65%	-1.63	76%
Inter	0.719	-3.06 (29.0)	63%	-1.95	73%
TOTAL	0.588	-3.23 (28.0)	60%	-2.05	70%
Ward's	0.571	-2.05 (20.0)	72%	+0.51	111%

• Age and sex matched
T = peak bone mass
Z = age matched TK 10/25/91

Figure 48–16. DEXA reading showing osteoporosis including both T and Z scores.

safety of the physical environment, wearing proper shoes, and using ambulatory assistive devices as well as reconditioning through exercise can be helpful. Limiting the use of drugs that may cause dizziness, loss of balance, orthostasis, confusion, or disorientation is recommended.

Hormone replacement remains in the first line of defense against osteoporosis and is a critical part of treatment programs whenever possible. Postmenopausal women without contraindications should be considered for estrogen replacement therapy (ERT). Progestin should be administered concomitantly in women who have not undergone hysterectomy. Estrogen has been shown to prevent bone loss by 50% in this group (Asch, 1996). Even in older women, estrogen increases bone mineral density in the spine by several percentage points after 1 to 2 years of therapy (Asch, 1996). ERT also relieves the symptoms of urogenital atrophy, may be cardioprotective, and may decrease the symptoms of Alzheimer's disease. Current data recommends 0.625 mg/day of estrogen to prevent and treat osteoporosis. Estrogen administered by any route produces effects on the skeleton. Side effects, including breast tenderness and the return of menstrual bleeding, often limit compliance. A possible increase in the size of gallstones may occur. The risk of both uterine and breast cancer appears to be minimally increased in women taking ERT.

Bisphosphonates have been shown to be effective in inhibiting bone resorption and therefore are currently used to prevent osteoporotic fractures. There are three bisphosphonates available in the United States: (1) etidronate has been used over the longest time and has well-demonstrated efficacy in both the prevention and treatment of osteoporosis as well as the treatment of Paget's disease; (2) pamidronate has also been shown to be effective in the secondary prevention of glucocorticoid osteoporosis; and (3) alendronate has recently been approved for the prevention and treatment of steroid-induced and postmenopausal osteoporosis and has been shown to increase vertebral bone mass by about 8% over 3 years and to decrease the incidence of fracture by 59% (Liberman et al., 1995). The usual dosage is 10 mg daily on an empty stomach, although a 5-mg dose has been released specifically for prevention of osteoporosis. Alendronate is poorly absorbed and can cause upper GI distress and even esophageal ulceration. Other bisphosphonates are in clinical trials with efforts directed at improving absorption of these substances.

Salmon calcitonin used parenterally has been available for two decades for the treatment of osteoporosis and hypercalcemia. The requirement for daily or alternate-day injections limited its use for the long-term treatment of osteoporosis but it was and is commonly used during the acute phase of vertebral compression fractures for its analgesic property at doses of 100 IU/day or every other day. The recent development of a nasal spray delivery system, 200 IU/day, makes this a more viable option for both short- and long-term treatment and fracture prevention. The data shows a 3 to 5% increase in vertebral bone density over three years (Asch, 1996). This preparation is virtually free of side effects and generally well tolerated, although expensive.

Recently, there is interest in alternatives to true estrogens for the treatment of postmenopausal women. Compounds that produce the beneficial effects of estrogen without stimulating endometrial or breast tissue are being studied. Other androgenic compounds with estrogenic activity are being evaluated. Some endocrinologists have considered parathyroid hormone as a possible treatment for osteoporosis (Lindsay, 1996). The use of fluoride to increase bone mass has been evaluated for some time. Initially, the required dose was poorly tolerated by patients and expensive. Currently, slow-release, enteric-coated preparations are available and well tolerated. The effect on vertebral bone mass remains controversial with conflicting studies. The status of fluoride remains undecided.

REFERENCES

AACE Clinical Practice Guidelines for the Prevention and Treatment of Postmenopausal Osteoporosis. (1996). *Endocrine Practice, 2* (2), 157–169.

American College of Rheumatology Guidelines of Rheumatology Referral. (1996). American College of Rheumatology.

American College of Rheumatology. Clinical Slide Collection on the Rheumatic Diseases, 1991, 1995.

American College of Rheumatology Ad Hoc Committee on Clinical Guidelines. (1995). Guidelines for the Management of Rheumatoid Arthritis. *Arthritis Rheum, 30,* 713–722.

Anderson, R. (1993). Rheumatoid arthritis, clinical features and laboratory. In *Primer on the Rheumatic Diseases* (10th Ed.). (pp. 90–96). Arthritis Foundation.

Arnett, F. C., et al. (1987). The American Rheumatism Association 1987 Revised Criteria for the Classification of Rheumatoid Arthritis. *Arthritis Rheum. 31,* 315–324.

Asch, E. (1996). Management of osteoporosis in elderly women. *Long Term Care Forum, 6* (4), 6–8.

Baer, P. A., Tenenbaum, J., Fam, A. G., et al. (1986). Coexistent septic and crystal arthritis. Report of 4 cases and literature review. *Journal of Rheumatology, 13,* 604–607.

Baker, D. G. & Schumacher, H. R. (1993). Acute Monoarthritis. *NEJM, 329,* 1013–1020.

Borigini, M. J. & Paulus, H. E. (1995). Rheumatoid arthritis. In Weisman, M. H. & Weinblatt, M. E. (Eds.)., *Treatment of the Rheumatic Diseases.* Philadelphia: W. B. Saunders, pp. 31–51.

Callegari, P. E. & Williams, W. (1995). Laboratory tests for rheumatic diseases. *Post Graduate Medicine, 97* (4), 65–74.

Canadian Hydroxychloroquine Study Group. (1991). A randomized study of the effect of withdrawing hydroxychloroquine sulfate in systemic lupus erythematosus. *New England Journal of Medicine, 324,* 150.

Craft, J. & Hardin J. A. (1993). Antinuclear Antibodies. In Kelly, W. N. et al. (Eds.). *Textbook of rheumatology* (4th ed.). Philadelphia: W. B. Saunders, (pp. 164–187).

Creemers, M., Piet, L. C. M., van Riel, M. J., et al. (1994). Second line treatment in sero-negative spondyloarthropathies. *Seminars in Arthritis and Rheumatism, 24* (2), 71–81.

Emmerson, B. T. (1996). The management of gout. *New England Journal of Medicine, 334,* 445–451.

Fan, P. T. & Yu, D. T. (1993). Reiter's syndrome. In *Primer on the Rheumatic Diseases* (12th Ed.). (pp. 158–160). Arthritis Foundation.

Friou, G. J. (1957). Clinical application of lupus serum nucleoprotein reaction using fluorescent antibody technique. *Journal of Clinical Investigations, 36,* 890.

Gambert, S. (1996). The high cost of osteoporosis in elderly women. *Long Term Care Forum, 6* (4), 2.

Hannan, M. T. (1997). Epidemiologic perspectives on women and arthritis: An overview. *Arthritis Care and Research, 9* (8), 424–433.

Hargraves, M. M., Richmond, H. & Morton, R. (1948). Presentation of two bone marrow elements: The "tart" cell and the "L. E. cell." *Proc. Staff Meet. Mayo Clinic, 23,* 25.

Jain, R. & Lipsky, P. (1997). Treatment of rheumatoid arthritis. *Medical Clinics of North America, 81* (1), 57–84.

Jennette, J. C., Falk, R. J., Andrassy, K., et al. (1994). Nomenclature of systemic vasculitides. Proposal of an international consensus conference. *Arthritis and Rheumatism, 37,* 187–192.

Khan, M. A. (Ed). (1990). Ankylosing spondylitis and related spondyloarthropaties. *Spine: State of the Art Reviews.* (pp. 497–688). Phildelphia: Hanley and Belfus.

Lawrence, R. C., Hochberg, M. C., Kelsey, J. L., et al. (1989). Estimates of the prevalence of selected arthritic and musculoskeletal diseases in the United States. *Journal of Rheumatology, 14,* 427.

Liberman, U., Weiss, S., Broll, J., et al. (1995). Effect of oral alendronate on bone mineral density and the incidence of fracture in postmenopausal osteoporosis. *New England Journal of Medicine, 333* (22), 1438–1444.

Lindsay, R. (1996). Treatment of osteoporosis, the gold standard, now and in the future. Presented at the American College of Rheumatology 1996 National Scientific Meeting.

McCarty, D. J. (1993). Treatment of rheumatoid arthritis. *Arthritis and Allied Conditions* (12th Ed.). Philadelphia: Lea and Febiger. (pp. 877–885).

McCarty, D. J., & Hollander, J. L. (1961). Identification of urate crystals in gouty synovial fluid. *Annals of Internal Medicine, 54,* 452–460.

Mielants, H. & Veys, E. M. (1990). The gut in the spondyloarthropathies. *Journal of Rheumatology, 17,* 7–10.

O'Dell, J. R., Haire, C. E., Palmer, W., et al. (1997). Treatment of early rheumatoid arthritis with minocycline or placebo: Results of a randomized, double blind, placebo-controlled trial. *Arthritis and Rheumatism, 40* (5), 842–848.

Osial, T., Cash, J., & Eisenbeis, C. H. (1993). Arthritis associated syndromes. *Primary Care, 20* (4), 857–882.

Pinals, R. S. (1994). Polyarthritis and Fever. *NEJM.* 330, 769–774.

Recommendations for the Prevention and Treatment of Glucocorticoid induced Osteoporosis. (1996). *Arthritis and Rheumatism, 39* (11), 1791–1801.

Rheumatologic Disorders: An Office Guide to Differential Diagnosis. Syntex Laboratories Inc. Issue 10, June 1979.

Ruzicka, T. (1996). Psoriatic arthritis. *Archives of Dermatology, 132,* 213–219.

Sergent, J. S. (1993). Polyarticular Arthritis. Chapter 23 in Kelley, W. N. *Textbook of rheumatology,* (4th ed.). Philadelphia: W. B. Saunders, (pp. 381–388).

Snyderman & Hayes. (1997). Non-steroidal anti-inflammatory drugs. *Medical Clinics of North America, Advances in Rheumatology, 1.*

Tan, E. M., Cohen, A. S., Fries, J. F., et al. (1982). Special article: The revised criteria for the classification of systemic lupus erythematosus. *Arthritis and Rheumatism, 25,* 1271–1277.

van der Woude, F. J., Rasmussen, N.. Lobatto, S., et al. (1985). Autoantibodies against neutrophils and monocytes: Tool for diagnosis and marker of disease activity in Wegener's granulomatosis. *Lancet, 1,* 425.

White, P. (1993). Other pediatric rheumatic diseases. *Primer on the Rheumatic Diseases* (12th Ed.). (pp. 176–178). Arthritis Foundation.

Wilder, R. L. (1993). Rheumatoid arthritis. In R. Schumacher (Ed.), *Primer on the Rheumatic Diseases* (10th Ed.). (pp. 86–89). Arthritis Foundation.

Winchester, R. (1995). Psoriatic arthritis. *Dermatologic Clinics, 13* (4), 779–792.

49

Eye Problems

Mary Zemyan Polito
Joseph R. Polito

▶ ANATOMY AND PHYSIOLOGY

The eye is the specialized, sensory organ that transmits visual information to the brain via the optic nerve (CN II). Cranial nerves III (oculomotor), IV (trochlear), and VI (abducens) supply the four rectus and the two oblique eye muscles, the levator palpebrae, and autonomic innervation.

External Structures

Lymphatics from the lateral conjunctiva drain to the preauricular nodes just anterior to the tragus of the ear. The nasal conjunctival lymphatics drain to the submandibular nodes. These are important routes for the spread of infections and tumors.

The eyelids are composed of skin, conjunctiva, and striated and smooth muscle. The tarsus is the dense, fibrous plate that forms the framework of the lid. The lid distributes tears over the surface of the eye, limits the amount of light entering, and protects the anterior surface of the globe.

The lacrimal gland is located in the upper outer wall of the anterior orbit. The gland produces tears that flow over the cornea and drain via the puncta into the lacrimal sac and nasolacrimal duct to the nasal meatus. Tears serve as protection with their flushing action and natural antimicrobial components.

Meibomian and zeiss glands are sebaceous glands of the eyelid margins that produce meibum, an important ingredient in preserving the normal tear film on the surface of the eye.

The globe is composed of three layers: (1) the outer fibrous layer comprises the cornea anteriorly and the sclera posteriorly; (2) the middle layer consists of the choroid posteriorly and the ciliary body and iris anteriorly; and (3) the innermost layer is the retina.

The conjunctiva is a clear, vascular membrane that covers the anterior half of the sclera (the bulbar conjunctiva) and the lids (palpebral conjunctiva). It serves as a protective barrier to microbial invasion.

The sclera, a tough, white covering of approximately the posterior five-sixths of the globe, is continuous anteriorly with the cornea and posteriorly with the external sheath of the optic nerve. It is the structure that appears as the "white of the eye." It physically supports the internal structures of the eye and, with the cornea, maintains the structural integrity of the globe. The episclera is a thin layer of tissue composed of collagen (which is contiguous with the sclera) and vessels (which are contiguous with the ciliary circulation).

The cornea is the clear, avascular, transparent anterior one sixth of the globe. It forms the front of the anterior chamber and has sensory innervation primarily for pain. It serves as protection as well as for most of refraction. The cornea is composed of several layers including the epithelium, stroma, and endothelium.

Internal Structures

The iris is the circular, pigmented smooth muscle posterior to the cornea and is the most anterior portion of the vascular layer of the eye. The pupil is an opening in the iris that controls the amount of light reaching the retina by dilating and constricting in response to changes in light intensity and to autonomic stimuli. (See Plate 1 in color section.)

The lens is a transparent, biconvex body situated between the posterior chamber and the vitreous through which light rays are focused onto the retina. Images are focused onto the retina by contraction or relaxation of the ciliary body to change the thickness of the highly elastic lens (when focusing from far distance to near the process is called accommodation).

The zonular apparatus is the suspensory structure of the lens. It functions in conjunction with the ciliary body in accommodation. The ciliary body also functions to form the aqueous fluid of the eye.

The vitreous is the transparent, colorless mass of soft, gelatinous material filling the eyeball behind the lens. It plays an important role in maintaining the form of the eye.

Schlemm's Canal is a circular channel at the junction of the sclera and cornea through which aqueous humor leaves the eye.

The retina is the innermost layer of the eye. It transforms light energy into electrical impulses and transmits them via the optic nerve to the brain. Two landmarks of the retina include the optic disc (where the optic nerve enters the eye, together with the central retinal artery and vein) and the macula. The macula is the site of central vision and color perception. The fovea is an area of 1.5-mm diameter in the center of the macula responsible for the fine acuity of central vision (Color Plate 3).

Light energy that reaches the retina is transformed into electrical impulses that are transmitted via the optic nerve, passing through the optic canal along with the ophthalmic artery, vein, and autonomic innervation of the eye. The optic nerves converge at the optic chiasm, located just superior to the pituitary gland. A hemidecussation occurs in the chiasm so that all visual information to both eyes from the right visual space is transmitted to the left cerebral cortex, and vice versa. The optic tracts begin at the posterior aspect of the chiasm and terminate in the lateral geniculate bodies. From there, the optic radiations supply the occipital (visual) cortex.

Emmetropia is the condition of the normal eye when light rays are focused exactly on the retina and vision is perfect. Myopia (nearsightedness) occurs when images are focused in front of the retina rather than on it, causing blurred vision. In hyperopia (farsightedness), images are focused behind the retina. Astigmatism can be defined as a visual defect in which the unequal curvature of one or more refractive surfaces of the eye, usually the cornea, prevents light rays from focusing clearly at one point on the retina.

▶ OPHTHALMOLOGIC ASSESSMENT

A few key points about the ophthalmologic assessment should be noted prior to patient evaluation.

1. Include in the history, information about corrective lenses, contacts (include wearing schedule and cleaning practices), ophthalmic medications, ocular conditions, injury, systemic diseases (which may have ocular manifestations), and systemic symptoms attributable to ophthalmic disease (such as headache, nausea, and vomiting caused by acute angle-closure glaucoma).
2. The visual acuity (VA) is the most important part of the exam and should never be excluded. Visual acuity testing should be deferred in very few cases, such as in chemical exposure to the eye. In this case, copious irrigation is warranted before attempting VA.
3. VA testing should always be done with and without the patient's corrective lenses. If the patient's corrective lenses are not available, the pinhole occluder should be used. It gives a reasonable estimate of the best corrected VA. (A pinhole corrects refractive errors by permitting only the central light rays to enter the eye to reach the fovea, avoiding peripheral distortion.)
4. Patients who are unable to read any letters on a vision chart should still have their VA tested and recorded as to their ability to count fingers at the maximal distance from the eye (for example, "CF at 3 feet"), recognize hand motion (HM), perceive light and the direction from which it is projected (LP with proj.), perceive light but not the direction (LP without proj.), or unable to see light at all (NLP). Testing the affected eye first may prevent the patient from remembering letters of the visual chart.
5. Check patients for the presence of contact lenses. Funduscopic exam is easier with the contacts in place, but the lenses should be removed to use drops (especially fluorescein which can permanently stain lenses), conduct the ocular physical exam, and to treat.
6. Dilation of the pupil allows for a better funduscopic evaluation, but should be performed with caution. An acute angle-closure glaucoma attack can be precipitated with the use of mydriatic and cycloplegic agents, especially in those with a personal or family history of acute closed-angle glaucoma, those with shallow anterior chambers, and those being treated with systemic atropine. Pupil dilation can cause some older style, iris-plane lens implants (from cataract surgery) to become displaced, causing serious complications. The pupils should not be dilated if serial neurologic exams are to be performed. Always document pupil dilation done with pharmacologic agents in the medical record so that future examinations are not misleading. The use of cycloplegics and some mydriatics will cause the loss of accommodation and proper patient education will be required regarding driving, operating machin-

ery, reading, etc. If an ophthalmology referral has been made, it is best to defer dilation until the patient is seen by the ophthalmologist.

7. Corneal staining is the procedure used to detect irregularities of the corneal surface. It is done by wetting sterile fluorescein paper with sterile saline or topical anesthetic and then touching it to the surface of the lower conjunctival sac (sterile fluorescein drops are also available). The patient should be directed to blink to spread the stain over the corneal surface. A penlight with a cobalt blue filter is then used to examine the surface. The affected area(s) will absorb more of the dye and is easily visualized. If no area of irregularity exists, a uniform film of dye covers the cornea.
8. General warning signs include decreased VA; circumcorneal injection; corneal edema; corneal staining; pupils with abnormal size, shape, or reaction to light; abnormal intraocular pressure; muscle paresis; elevation of retina on fundus exam; and papilledema.
9. General warning symptoms include altered or decreased vision, ocular pain, photophobia, light flashes, double vision, visual field loss, and metamorphopsia.
10. Eye conditions that warrant referral to an ophthalmologist include those listed in Table 49–1.

▶ THE RED EYE

The red eye is a common problem in the acute care setting (Table 49–2). The most common cause is conjunctivitis, which is usually benign, though other causes such as glaucoma can threaten sight. A few key points should be noted before discussion of the red eye.

1. A red eye associated with reduced visual acuity (VA) or a red eye associated with pain (as opposed to a foreign body sensation) usually indicates a problem requiring referral to an ophthalmologist.
2. Visual acuity is normal at the onset of conjunctivitis. It can be greatly reduced due to acute angle-closure glaucoma, uveitis, and keratitis.
3. With adequate illumination the examiner can usually see corneal clouding associated with acute angle-closure glaucoma, corneal ulceration, and keratitis.
4. Conjunctivitis is a diffuse superficial injection of the vessels overlying the sclera. The vessels can be mobilized by the examiner using the edge of the lower lid or a cotton-tipped applicator. This is in contrast to scleritis, a much less common but more serious condition, which is an inflammation of deeper vessels causing a bluish–red hue. In this case the injected vessels are immobile and there is more pain.
5. Hyperemia of the vessels surrounding the cornea (circumcorneal or perilimbal injection) is indicative of more serious conditions such as uveitis, keratitis, and glaucoma.
6. A red eye with pain and a mid-dilated, fixed (nonreactive to light) pupil is strong evidence for acute angle-closure glaucoma, requiring immediate referral to an ophthalmologist. Nausea, vomiting, and headache may accompany the ocular findings.
7. Bacterial conjunctivitis is usually bilateral, affecting the eyes equally, while viral conjunctivitis can present unilaterally or bilaterally with one eye more affected than the fellow eye. VA is normal in both.
8. Photophobia is a finding in keratitis and in iritis. In iritis, light directed into the unaffected eye will often cause pain in the affected eye. This is not usually seen in keratitis.
9. Topical steroids should be used only in conjunction with proper slit-lamp examination. They can cause a number of serious side effects. For example, topical steroids inappropriately used in a herpes simplex viral keratitis can lead to viral proliferation and subsequent sight-threatening complications. Long-term steroid use can also cause corneal clouding, increased intraocular pressure, and cataracts.
10. When selecting a topical ophthalmic antibiotic preparation without culture results, the practitioner should consider the most likely causative organisms, the history of and circumstances sur-

TABLE 49–1. Eye Conditions That Warrant Referral to an Ophthalmologist

Acute vision loss
Retinal detachment
Acute glaucoma attack
Central retinal artery or vein occlusion
Endophthalmitis
Herpetic corneal lesion, and corneal ulcers or abrasions that do not heal within 48 hours
Iritis/uveitis
Orbital cellulitis
Hyphema (blood in the anterior chamber)
Penetrating trauma
Chemical or alkali burn
Abnormal eye movements
Macular degeneration
Diabetic or hypertensive retinopathy
Irregular pupil (size, shape, or reaction to light)
Papilledema
Acute proptosis
Any condition the examiner is uncomfortable diagnosing and treating

TABLE 49–2. Red Eye

	Bacterial	Viral	Allergic	Acute ACG	Iritis
Onset	Several days	Several days	1–2 days	Usually 2–3 hours	1–2 days
Hyperemia	Severe	Mild	Diffuse	Circumcorneal	Circumcorneal; bluish–red hue and diffuse
Affected eye	Bilateral	Either, but one eye usually worse	Bilateral if both exposed to allergen	Usually unilateral	Usually unilateral
Discharge	Mucopurulent; heavy neutrophils	Watery, monocytes	Watery, stringy	Watery	Watery
Pain	Gritty	Gritty	Gritty	Moderate to severe	Moderate, dull eye pain
Cornea	Clear	Clear	Clear	Cloudy	Precipitates
Pupil	Normal	Normal	Normal	Mid-dilated oval, fixed	Constricted
Vision	Normal	Normal	Normal	Significantly reduced	Reduced
Age	Any, but usually children and immunocompromised	Any	Any	Usually over 40 years old	Usually young adult (15–25)
Systemic symptoms	No	Possible URI symptoms	No	Nausea, vomiting, possible prostration	Usually none
Miscellaneous	Epidemic school or work	Preauricular node; public pool use; epidemic	Hay fever or ocular irritant	Family history of ACG More common hyperopic	Photophobia common

rounding the injury or infection, and bacterial prevalence in the geographic area. Topical antibiotics should not be used indiscriminately since almost all topical ophthalmic antibiotics can cause local irritation and allergic reactions. A broad-spectrum antibiotic can cause a superinfection. Nevertheless, the benefit of ocular antibiotics in the presence of infection almost always outweighs the risk of adverse effects. Prophylactic use is indicated when there is a clear likelihood of the development of infection. Cultures should be obtained in cases not responding to therapy.

11. Anesthetic eyedrops should never be prescribed to a patient. These agents are for diagnostic purposes only. They inhibit the reepithelialization of the cornea and inappropriate use may lead to corneal deterioration and perforation. In addition, there is a high possibility of the patient unknowingly reinjuring an anesthetized eye. Oral analgesics and topical nonsteroidal antiinflammatory agents should be used to control pain in corneal abrasions.

Conjunctivitis

Conjunctivitis is an inflammation of the mucous membrane that covers the anterior ocular sclera (the bulbar conjunctiva) and the inner surfaces of the lids (the palpebral conjunctiva). Common signs and symptoms include hyperemia (greater at the periphery than at the corneal limbus), discharge, itching, burning, and foreign body sensation. There may be increased tearing. Edema of the conjunctiva (chemosis) can cause lid swelling (pinguecula; a benign, yellowish triangular thickening of the bulbar conjunctiva that can sometimes be found on routine examination is not chemosis). Pupil reactivity to light is normal and the cornea is clear. No foreign bodies or abrasions should be present. Classification of the various forms of conjunctivitis is most commonly based on etiology: bacterial, viral, allergic, fungal, chemical, and parasitic. Careful handwashing and proper hygiene are important to prevent the spread of infection to others. Tubes of ointment and unused contents of drop bottles should be discarded at the end of treatment to avoid the risk of using contaminated material in the future. Contact lens wearers should be instructed to discontinue contact lens use until the conjunctivitis is resolved. Often broad-spectrum topical antibiotics are prescribed. Mild infections can be treated with bacitracin, erythromycin, or combinations of bacitracin/polymixin B, and bacitracin/neomycin/polymixin B. Sulfacetamide is a popular first-line antibiotic but there are a growing number of resistant organisms. The aminoglycosides (e.g., gentamycin and tobramycin) and the quinolones (ciprofloxacin, norfloxacin, and ofloxacin) should be reserved for resistant conjunctival infections or when pseudomonas coverage is necessary. Neomycin-containing solutions should be avoided because of the hypersensitivity reactions that can occur in a significant number of patients.

Acute Bacterial Conjunctivitis

Acute bacterial conjunctivitis begins unilaterally with the fellow eye becoming involved within one to two days. Symptoms include irritation, tearing, and mucopurulent discharge. The patient may note that the eyelids are stuck together upon awakening. Crusting is usually obvious on lid margins and lashes. The visual acuity is normal. Lymphadenopathy is minimal or absent. The corneas are clear with a bright corneal light reflex. Subconjunctival hemorrhage may be present. Pathogens most commonly associated with acute bacterial conjunctivitis include staphylococcus aureus, streptococcus pneumoniae, and *H influenza.* Acute bacterial conjunctivitis is easily transmitted by direct contact.

Diagnosis is usually made by history and physical findings. Cultures are required in severe or refractory cases that do not respond to treatment within 2 to 3 days. Other causes of red eye must be excluded (as discussed in this section).

Most cases of acute bacterial conjunctivitis resolve promptly with antibiotic therapy. If treatment is based on clinical characteristics alone, a broad-spectrum topical ophthalmic antibacterial preparation (e.g., 10% sulfacetamide) should be chosen. Antibiotic therapy is discontinued when the inflammatory process has resolved. Drops are instilled every 2 to 4 hours and can be used in combination with an ophthalmic antibiotic ointment used before sleep.

Antibiotic ointments alone can be used on an every 4- to 6-hour basis. Lid scrubs and warm compresses are helpful to remove mattering on the lids, especially if there is an associated blepharitis. The lid scrubs and compresses are *essential* in the treatment of chronic bacterial conjunctivitis. Eye cosmetics should be discarded; they are likely contaminated. Patients should be reevaluated within 48 hours if the condition is not improving, sooner if worsening; otherwise, within 7 to 10 days if the condition is not fully resolved.

Neonatal Conjunctivitis

Purulent bacterial conjunctivitis is an uncommon, acute, severe form of conjunctivitis that is usually caused by Neisseria gonorrhea. It occurs in neonates as a result of vaginal delivery in an infected mother and in adults from direct contact with individuals with gonococcal urethritis or pelvic inflammatory disease. The course is rapidly progressive with marked swelling of the eye, severe chemosis, and redness of the lids. The exudate can initially be serous, becoming purulent and copious. In infants the purulent conjunctivitis is usually bilateral but usually affects the adults unilaterally.

Corneal perforation can occur; therefore, treatment must be aggressive and requires prompt ophthalmic consultation. Topical antibiotics alone are inadequate. Pathogen-specific parenteral antibiotics are necessary and close follow-up by an ophthalmologist is essential. Frequent irrigation is also necessary in removing copious secretions. Mothers of affected neonates and sexual partners must also be treated.

Viral Conjunctivitis

It can be difficult to distinguish between bacterial and viral conjunctivitis based on history and physical exam. Viral conjunctivitis is more common during the summer and may be related to changes in sunlight and temperatures. They often produce more tearing, watery discharge, and preauricular adenopathy. It often begins unilaterally with the initial eye often being more affected than the fellow eye. Additional viral symptoms such as fever, myalgia, rhinorrhea, and cough are often present. Routine cultures are negative; however, topical antibiotics are generally recommended in cases of nonspecific conjunctivitis.

Adenoviruses. Adenoviruses are classified by serotypes using a numbering system. Dawson & Sheppard (1992) discuss adenovirus types 2, 3, 6, and 7 as causes of pharyngeal conjunctival fever (PCF), one of the more benign viral infections. This is usually a self-limiting disease characterized by fever, pharyngitis, cervical adenitis, and a nonpurulent conjunctivitis. It is unilateral in onset and occurs most frequently in children and young adults. Fecal excretion of the virus can continue for weeks, which may account for some epidemics of PCF associated with poorly chlorinated swimming pools. Treatment consists of cool compresses and topical antibiotics to prevent secondary infection. Patients must be reevaluated if symptoms do not improve within 7 to 10 days.

Epidemic keratoconjunctivitis (EKC) is usually caused by adenovirus type 8 but other serotypes have been reported. This is an acute, more aggressive form of conjunctivitis not associated with respiratory symptoms. It is unilateral at onset and associated with preauricular adenopathy. Symptoms in the fellow eye may be delayed and much less severe. This form of viral conjunctivitis involves the cornea resulting in eye pain, photophobia, foreign body sensation, and decreased vision. Corneal findings can include punctate surface defects that stain with fluorescein. The virus is extremely contagious. It can remain infectious on equipment for long periods. Materials exposed to infected patients should be completely cleansed or sterilized. Thorough handwashing in both clinical and home settings is important. Unit-dose drop vials are preferred in clinical settings.

Management is supportive and may include cool compresses, astringent drops, and cycloplegics. In patients with marked reduction of VA, topical corticosteroids are used. Patients should be followed by an ophthalmologist.

Allergic Conjunctivitis

Ocular allergy is a frequent cause of conjunctivitis. Diffuse or patchy bilateral redness, chemosis, and watering are typical. Allergic conjunctivitis is usually distinguished by its itching, seasonal association, and recurrence. The etiology can often be determined by history and can include allergy to topical medications, contact lens solutions, eye makeup, hay fever, and seasonal allergy.

Treatment begins with avoidance of the allergen, if

possible. Cool compresses, topical vasoconstrictors, and antihistamines are helpful in mild cases. More aggressive forms may require the use of ocular mast-cell stabilizers, nonsteroidal antiinflammatory agents, and even short-term topical steroids. Follow-up is carried out on an as-needed basis.

Chlamydial Conjunctivitis

Chlamydial conjunctivitis occurs in neonates through vaginal delivery in an infected mother and is also transmitted venerally in sexually active adults. These infections are often only mildly symptomatic and are not associated with any specific signs or symptoms. They can include preauricular adenopathy, lid edema, chemosis, and mucopurulent discharge. Systemic antibiotics for the treatment of chlamydia are used as well as topical antibiotics to treat secondary ocular infection.

Iritis

Inflammation confined to the iris (the anterior portion of the uveal tract) is the form of uveitis termed iritis. Iritis can be associated with many disease processes but often a cause cannot be determined. It can be acute or chronic but this section will be limited to the acute form. Iritis can progress to serious complications including glaucoma and blindness.

Iritis most commonly occurs in young adults. It presents with ocular pain, redness, photophobia, blurred vision, and tearing. These symptoms occur in the absence of a discharge, trauma, or foreign body. There are many conditions associated with iritis including autoimmune diseases such as juvenile rheumatoid arthritis, ankylosing spondylitis, inflammatory bowel disease, Reiter's syndrome, and sarcoidosis. Infectious diseases such as syphilis, Lyme disease, and tuberculosis are also possible causes of iritis. A thorough review of systems can help uncover these etiologies.

On exam there is a ciliary flush present with a diffuse hyperemia. The pupil may be small and irregular secondary to synechiae (adhesions) which can develop between the iris and cornea or lens. Slit-lamp exam is necessary to confirm the diagnosis by identifying inflammatory cells in the anterior chamber, protein leakage into aqueous fluid (flare), and possible precipitates of white blood cells adhering to the endothelial surface of the cornea.

The goal of treatment is to decrease the inflammation and pain. Cycloplegics prevent formation of synechiae and control pain. The use of topical corticosteroids is essential to decrease inflammation. Caution must be used when using topical steroids as mentioned previously (see item 9 in the section "Red Eye"). Injections of periocular steroids may be necessary in severe cases. Therapy is usually tapered gradually depending on the amount of clinical response. An acute episode of iritis takes several weeks to resolve.

Episcleritis

A nonspecific inflammation of the episcleral vessels, episcleritis is fairly common. Generally it is a disease of young adults (20-50 years old). The etiology can be associated with systemic diseases such as rheumatoid arthritis as well as stress, poor nutrition, or fatigue. Usually it is self-limiting but systemic evaluation is indicated, particularly when the episcleritis is recurrent.

The associated redness is usually unilateral and often distributed in quadrants. Pain or discomfort and edema may also be present. Examination should be directed at ruling out other causes of a red eye.

Due to the self-limiting nature, there may be no treatment indicated. The clinical course may be shortened with the use of topical steroidal and nonsteroidal antiinflammatory agents. Antimetabolites can be used in severe cases.

Scleritis

Scleritis is a serious, rare, autoimmune response that can result in the destruction of scleral tissue. It is more common in females. Underlying causes include various systemic diseases such as rheumatiod arthritis, systemic lupus erythematosus, herpetic disease, syphilis, tuberculosis, and gout.

Patients complain of pain, decreased vision, and globe tenderness. There is a diffuse inflammation that appears bluish–red and the involved vessels are immobile.

Scleritis can be a sight-threatening condition and requires referral to an ophthalmologist. Some mild cases may require little treatment. More serious forms may need cycloplegics, topical steroids, and systemic antiinflammatories, steroids, and antimetabolites.

Keratitis

A generalized term meaning inflammation of the cornea, keratitis has many possible causes including infectious, degenerative, toxic, allergic and traumatic. A careful history will help to reveal possible etiologies. A detailed discussion is not possible in this text but it is important to recognize serious corneal signs that require referral. They include lack of corneal clarity or corneal light reflex, corneal staining (especially without a known cause), circumcorneal injection, decreased visual acuity, and corneal lesions.

Note: A pterygium is a triangular fold of growing tissue extending onto the cornea from the sclera. Although a pterygium can grow over the cornea and interfere with vision, it is a nonurgent condition. Surgical treatment to remove the membrane is usually delayed until the vision is threatened since they tend to recur aggressively.

Herpes Simplex Viral Keratitis

Primary herpes simplex viral (HSV) infection occurs in children. It is often transmitted by contact with mouth sores. Additionally, a significant number of neonates born with HSV infection have ocular involvement. Some complications of neonatal HSV include corneal inflammation and ulceration, chorioretinitis, and optic neuritis. Because of the high association between neonatal ocular HSV and systemic infection, infants should have a full evaluation.

In adults, HSV infections are most commonly a reactivation of an earlier self-limiting conjunctivitis that the patient may or may not recall. Factors that may trigger this reactivation include stress, immunosuppression, fever, ultraviolet light exposure, trauma, and menstruation.

The keratitis caused by HSV is most frequently limited to the corneal epithelium, but can progress to chronic corneal inflammation, vascularization, scarring, and loss of vision. The condition is usually unilateral with foreign body sensation, tearing, pain, photophobia, and limbal injection. Multiple recurrences occur in a significant number of cases and can result in corneal anesthesia, ulceration, and scarring.

The diagnosis can be confirmed by the characteristic branching dendritic pattern seen on the cornea with fluorescein staining (Color Plate 4). Specimens can be obtained by scraping or swabbing for culture. Topical antiviral drops in addition to epithelial debridement by an ophthalmologist are the mainstays of treatment. Early treatment of this type usually leads to resolution within 2 to 3 weeks. Topical steroids can allow the virus to proliferate resulting in further penetration of the corneal tissue and subsequent sight-threatening complications. They are contraindicated in the treatment of a red eye if a diagnosis of dendritic ulcer has not been ruled out.

HSV is best managed by an ophthalmologist who will see the patient 2 to 3 days after the initial visit and then as necessary for several weeks.

Herpes Zoster Ophthalmicus

Herpes zoster ophthalmicus (HZO) is caused by the varicella–zoster virus and is caused by reactivation of a latent virus in which the ophthalmic division of the trigeminal nerve is affected after a prior episode of chicken pox.

Prodromal symptoms of herpes zoster infection include headache, malaise, cutaneous hyperesthesia, fever, and chills. Eruption of the vesicles then follows. Postherpetic neuralgia can persist for years after the lesions have healed. Ophthalmic findings vary. The lids may be affected with watery vesicles and may be swollen closed initially. Conjunctival hyperemia is common. Corneal involvement occurs in many patients with herpes zoster infection. Sight-threatening complications such as uveitis, scleritis, keratitis, optic neuritis, and secondary glaucoma can all occur and produce their respective signs and symptoms. These can include decreased vision, pain, photophobia, altered pupillary light reaction, elevated intraocular pressure, and corneal clouding.

Systemic antivirals (e.g., acyclovir and famcyclovir) are effective in decreasing the severity of the disease. Topical antivirals are ineffective in zoster keratitis, while corticosteroids are indicated for keratitis or uveitis. Cycloplegics should be used to manage photophobia and uveitis. Patients may require oral analgesics, including narcotics.

The cutaneous lesions of zoster heal within 3 weeks whereas ocular involvement can persist for weeks to months. Patients with HZO should be followed by an ophthalmologist.

Glaucoma

Glaucoma is a common cause of blindness in the United States especially among African-Americans. It often goes undiagnosed until significant, permanent visual loss occurs. Glaucoma is a multifactor optic neuropathy associated with a characteristic loss of optic nerve fibers. Most glaucoma patients will repeatedly have an intraocular pressure (IOP) greater than 21 mm Hg in the course of the disease. Because there is great individual variation in the susceptibility of the optic nerve to the IOP, there is no fixed numerical designation that confirms the diagnosis. Quigley (1993) notes that at screenings, 50% of patients with open-angle glaucoma will have pressures below 22 mm Hg. A significant number of all glaucoma patients may have IOP readings consistently below 22 mm Hg.

Types of glaucoma include primary open-angle, primary angle-closure, secondary, and congenital glaucomas. Ninety percent of primary glaucoma is of the open-angle type. Other risk factors in addition to IOP include race, age, and family history of open-angle glaucoma, especially in a sibling. Glaucoma is more prevalent in African-Americans. The prevalence of glaucoma increases dramatically with age.

Examination can reveal an increased IOP, an enlarged cup to disc ratio, asymmetry between the two optic discs, an area of focal hemorrhage, disc notching, and visual field defects. The central VA by Snellen chart remains normal until the advanced stages. Direct ophthalmoscopy through dilated pupils using the red free (green light) is a good way to evaluate the optic disc. The structures and abnormalities that are red in the fundus will appear black. This will sharpen the contrast of structures (and vessels as well as hemorrhages) and aid in evaluation. Any of the disc changes found on routine exam should signal the practitioner to evaluate further for glaucoma. Due to the elusive nature of the disease, acute care nurse practitioners can play an important role in the detection of undiagnosed glaucoma. Associated glaucoma findings or family history of glaucoma may be detected during examinations and appropriate referrals can be made at that time. Accurate diagnosis requires a complete ophthalmic exam including stereoscopic visualization of the optic nerve, accurate IOP measurement, gonioscopy (a method to view outflow structures), and visual field testing.

Treatment is directed at lowering IOP to a value that is deemed unlikely to cause further optic nerve damage. This is accomplished with the use of topical medications, systemic medications, laser therapy, and filtering surgery. It is important to continue a patient's glaucoma medications (unless contraindicated) upon admission to the hospital.

Topically applied glaucoma medications are used to decrease the amount of aqueous production or increase aqueous outflow. Many of the medications used, especially beta blockers, act on the autonomic nervous system and have systemic side effects (e.g., cardiopulmonary, mental, and visual symptoms) that can manifest as systemic illness in these patients.

Acute Angle-Closure Glaucoma

Angle-closure glaucoma occurs when there is a closure of the anterior chamber angle caused by a blockage in the flow of aqueous through the pupil from the posterior to the anterior chamber. Acute angle-closure glaucoma is an emergency and can lead to permanent visual loss in a matter of hours.

Signs and symptoms may include moderate to severe ocular pain, head or browache, nausea, vomiting, blurred or loss of vision, and colored halos around lights. Acute attacks can be precipitated by medications that cause pupil dilation (e.g., sinus decongestants, psychotropics, scopolamine). Factors that predispose to acute angle-closure glaucoma include patients with shallow anterior chambers, hyperopic (farsighted) patients, and those with a family history of angle-closure glaucoma.

Examination may reveal conjunctival injection particularly in the limbal area, a cloudy cornea, mid-dilated pupil, decreased VA, and increased IOP (Color Plate 5). Referral to the ophthalmologist should be made and emergency treatment initiated as soon as possible. Definitive therapy for angle-closure glaucoma is surgical. However, medical therapy is used first to lower the IOP and allow for clearing of the cornea. Medical therapy includes topical alpha–adrenergic agonists, beta–adrenergic blockers, and miotics such as pilocarpine. Carbonic anhydrase inhibitors can also be administered systemically or topically as well as systemic hyperosmotic agents.

Corneal Abrasion

A corneal abrasion is a loss of or damage to the surface epithelium of the cornea. If located centrally, involving the visual axis, an abrasion interferes with the light refraction of the cornea, causing decreased VA. Corneal abrasions can be serious because they can lead to complications such as infection, corneal ulceration, iritis, and recurrent erosions of the cornea.

The mechanism of injury provided by the history is important. For example, a fingernail injury may be superficial but can cause a corneal infection through contamination. Corneal abrasions from tree branches or other plant material can lead to fungal keratitis. Abrasions from projectiles, especially sharp, metallic foreign bodies, are able to penetrate or even perforate the cornea which can lead to an endophthalmitis or other internal trauma, and should be referred to the ophthalmologist.

Topical anesthesia is required to do an adequate examination of a patient with corneal abrasion due to the severe pain usually present. The diagnosis is usually made by history and the presence of the abrasion as seen with fluorescein staining. Additionally, one must rule out the presence of a foreign body which may have caused the abrasion and then been retained in the lid, conjunctiva, or cornea itself.

Other associated signs and symptoms include lacrimation, photophobia, foreign body sensation, blepharospasm, lid swelling, circumcorneal injection, diffuse conjunctival injection, and decreased VA. The examiner should ask about a history of prior trauma since recurrent erosions may be the cause. Other conditions can mimic corneal abrasion such as keratitis associated with ultraviolet light exposure, including sunlamps, welding, and sun exposure without adequate protection. These conditions tend to be bilateral. Herpes simplex virus often presents as an acute painful, red eye associated with fluorescein staining, which needs to be differentiated from corneal abrasion. Bacterial ulcers, especially in contact lens wearers, can also present in this manner.

Examination is carried out with anesthetic eyedrops and fluorescein staining. In suspected corneal perforation, a wound leak can be detected by observing fluorescein flow from the area of the wound (Seidel test). If fluorescein stain is unavailable, a central corneal abrasion can be detected as a decreased corneal light reflex. The cornea, conjunctiva, and eyelids, including eversion of the upper lids, must be checked thoroughly to rule out any retained foreign body. Slit-lamp exam is necessary if any doubt exists about a foreign body entering the eye or about the depth of the abrasion. These cases should be referred to the ophthalmologist.

Corneal abrasions are a source of significant pain and should be treated with oral analgesics. Topical analgesics, as mentioned previously, are never prescribed to the patient (see item 11 [p. 1184] in "The Red Eye" section). Cycloplegics can be prescribed to control pain and photophobia secondary to spasm of the iris and ciliary body. Use of cycloplegics are generally contraindicated in patients with head injury (due to neurological exams) and those at risk of acute closed-angle glaucoma (see item 6 [p. 1182] in the "Ophthalmologic Assessment" regarding pupil dilation). Whether or not pressure patching improves healing remains unclear. Topical antibiotic drops or ointment are used as prophylaxis against infection. Artificial tears can also be used to moisten the eye as necessary for added comfort.

The patient should be reevaluated in 1 to 2 days at which time most uncomplicated corneal abrasions will have healed. Remember to reinforce the importance of eye protection to avoid future trauma.

Corneal Ulcers

A corneal ulcer is a pathologic loss of the surface of the cornea due to progressive erosion and necrosis of the tissue. Ulcers usually occur secondary to another cause such as foreign body, blepharitis, infection, use of contact lens, and a number of other associated ocular phenomena.

Unilateral presentation is common. Signs and symptoms include conjunctival injection particularly at the limbal area, a grayish oval lesion on the cornea usually near the limbus, staining with fluorescein, pain, and decreased visual acuity. This should not be confused with a benign yellow–white ring-shaped deposit in the peripheral cornea known as corneal arcus (Color Plate 6).

Treatment focuses on the primary cause. Frequent (every 30-60 minutes) use of broad-spectrum topical antibiotic drops is indicated. Ulcers due to contact lens use require antibiotic coverage for pseudomonas. Close follow-up is necessary since such infections can lead to rapid destruction of corneal tissue. Complications can be serious and include secondary iritis, glaucoma, permanent corneal scarring, hypopyon (pus cells in the anterior chamber), and corneal perforation. Most corneal ulcers should resolve in about 48 hours; however, all ulcers are best followed by an ophthalmologist.

Blepharitis

An inflammatory condition of the eyelids, blepharitis is poorly understood. Pathologic components to the condition include abnormalities of the meibomian glands and their lipid secretions, staphylococcal infection, tear film abnormalities, seborrhea, and rosacea.

Patients complain of burning, itching, photophobia, and an irritating sandy, gritty feeling that is worse in the morning. Examination reveals crusting scales on the anterior lid margins, hyperemia of the lid margins, and mild to moderate conjunctival hyperemia. In chronic cases, thickening of lid margins, thinning or loss of lashes, and misdirected lashes (trichiasis) may become evident.

Complications can lead to corneal involvement including scarring and vascularization. The examiner must rule out other corneal and conjunctival conditions that may coexist with blepharitis. Blepharitis can be especially refractory in nursing home patients, debilitated patients, and in patients with Parkinson's disease.

Since there is no cure, treatment is long term and aimed at control. It is important for the patient to be aware of the chronic nature of blepharitis. Warm compresses and lid hygiene are the most important elements of therapy. They reduce the lid debris and bacteria. The patient must be instructed to cleanse the base of the lashes and lid margins, not just the skin of the eyelids. A dilute solution of baby shampoo or a commercially available eye solution should be used. Artificial tears and ointments can be helpful. Topical bacitracin and erythromycin are first-line antibiotic agents. Gentamycin, tobramycin, and ciprofloxacin can be used in problem cases. Oral tetracycline is used for rosacea. At times, topical steroids and oral antibiotics are needed. Lid hygiene and avoiding makeup and creams at lid margins need to be continued indefinitely. Follow-up should be with an ophthalmologist as necessary.

Hordeolum

An infection of a sebaceous gland of the eyelid, a hordeolum is often referred to as a sty. If a gland of Zeis is infected, an external hordeolum results and is located in line with the base of the eyelashes. If a meibomian gland is infected, an internal hordeolum results several millimeters in from the lid margin.

Symptoms include pain and tenderness of the affected lid. Examination reveals generalized lid swelling early in the development or a nodular swelling later. Internal hordeola have a redness in the area of the meibomian gland when the lid is everted. These cases may have a mucopurulent discharge when gentle pressure is applied over the gland.

The infection is usually caused by staphylococcus aureus but topical antibiotics are poorly effective. Hordeolum can be associated with staphylococcus blepharitis. It may be differentiated from a chalazion in that the latter is often painless. Internal hordeola can lead to chalazia development.

Treatment consists mostly of warm compresses every 4 to 6 hours. Follow-up is on an as-needed basis. Oral antibiotics may be necessary in difficult cases. Incision and drainage is reserved for treatment failures.

Chalazion

A chalazion is a chronic, sterile lipo-granulomatous inflammation of a blocked meibomian gland. It presents as a firm nodule within the eyelid, several millimeters from the lid margin. Patients usually report a painless lump of the affected lid generally developing over several days or weeks. Initially it may start as a diffuse swelling with some discomfort but soon forms an immobile nodule. Chalazia are associated with hordeola and blepharitis.

Treatment consists of warm compresses and digital gland massage. Incision and drainage may be necessary if not resolved within several weeks. Antibiotics are ineffective.

Subconjunctival Hemorrhage

A subconjunctival hemorrhage occurs with the rupture of a fragile conjunctival vessel. It obscures the sclera with a bright red bloodstain. There is no pain and vision remains unaffected. There is sometimes a history of injury or disease, but subconjunctival hemorrhages usually occur following bouts of coughing, straining, vomiting, or they may occur spontaneously. Less commonly they can be associated with uncontrolled hypertension or coagulopathies and these should be considered in recurrent cases. The eye should be carefully examined to rule out other diagnoses such as retained foreign body. Management is supportive and includes cool compresses to reduce the initial bleeding by vasoconstriction. Resolution occurs in 1 to 3 weeks. Restrictions of the patient's daily activities are not necessary.

▶ ALTERED VISION

Cataract

A cataract is the loss of transparency of the lens. Although related to aging, cataracts can also be associated with systemic disease (e.g., diabetes mellitus), trauma, long-term ultraviolet light exposure, genetics, and medications (e.g., corticosteroids). Symptoms vary from patient to patient and can depend on the size and location of the opacity as well as individual tolerance to the decrease in vision that the opacity creates. A small or peripheral opacity can produce minor symptoms, whereas dense or centrally located cataracts can cause marked loss of vision (Color Plate 7). Usually the visual loss occurs over a period of months to years. The glare that patients experience in sunlight may be a chief complaint. There can also be blurring, monocular double vision, and changes in color perception. The opacity can be seen with direct ophthalmoscopy as a white or cloudy area just posterior to the pupillary opening. Using the direct ophthalmoscope at a distance of one to two feet can also reveal a diminished red reflex due to lens opacity.

Treatment is surgical removal of the lens. It is usually done on an outpatient basis with local anesthesia. Recovery is relatively brief. Depending on the type of procedure, patients may be back to most of their daily activities within days. The most widely used surgical technique is to remove the lens nucleus and cortex and leave the posterior lens capsule in place (extracapsular extraction). It is in this anatomic location that the intraocular lens is usually implanted. The remaining capsule can later develop an opacity (secondary cataract) with the symptoms of a primary cataract. These secondary cataracts are treated in an office or at an outpatient facility with laser therapy. For the small number of patients who do not receive implants, glasses or contact lenses are used to correct the refractive error caused by the loss of the crystalline lens.

Hypermaturity of a lens exists when a cataract of long standing (densely white) progresses to leaking protein, which may result in a secondary (phacolytic) glaucoma. Swelling of the lens can cause the anterior chamber to become shallow and produce an acute angle-closure glaucoma attack (phacomorphic glaucoma). These will present as an acute red eye.

Cataract removal is one of the most successful of operations but still carries some risk of complications, including infection, intraocular hemorrhage, corneal damage, retinal detachment, and glaucoma.

Retinal Detachment

A retinal detachment is the separation of the neurosensory retina from the underlying pigment epithelium (its blood supply). Detachment can be caused by a break in the retina, by traction on the retina, or by leakage of fluid beneath the retina. Vision is lost in the involved area of detachment as long as it remains detached. This is an urgent condition that requires prompt ophthalmologic evaluation to prevent permanent visual loss.

Most detachments occur spontaneously and are more common with myopia (nearsightedness), other retinal diseases (e.g., diabetic retinopathy), previous cataract surgery, trauma, and tumors.

Patients may notice a sudden onset of floating spots (floaters), flashes of light (photopsia), or a visual field defect (often described as a "curtain" coming across their visual field). Reduced VA suggests macular involvement. There is no pain. Funduscopic exam with indirect ophthalmoscopy is required to detect breaks and detachments in the peripheral retina. In some cases, an associated vitreous hemorrhage may obscure visualization of retinal details. Differential diagnoses include vitreous hemorrhage, vitreous detachment, retinal vascular occlusion, ophthalmic migraine, and tumor.

Surgical reattachment can be accomplished with a variety of procedures and is usually scheduled within 1 or 2 days of the diagnosis.

Vitreous Floaters

Small opacities in the vitreous compartment of the eye are called *floaters.* Vitreous floaters can be associated with aging and myopia. Patients often describe "floating spots" or "specks" moving across their visual field (Color Plate 8). Floaters can be seen using a plus (black) lens on the ophthalmoscope while viewing the red reflex at a distance of 6 to 12 inches. Vitreous floaters may be a symptom of a small vitreous hemorrhage and in a minority of patients, retinal tear or detachment. Warning signs of a retinal tear or detachment are floaters associated with flashes of light, a sudden occurrence or great increase in the number of floaters (especially if they appear after recent eye surgery), or a change to large, diffuse floaters. Patients with these symptoms should be urgently evaluated by an ophthalmologist.

Diabetic Retinopathy

Diabetic retinopathy is a pathologic condition of the retina caused by microvascular damage associated with diabetes. It is a leading cause of blindness in the United States.

Although the exact pathogenesis is not fully understood, many pathologic changes occur to contribute to the poor retinal oxygenation that leads to retinopathy and blindness. One of the earliest changes is the loss of retinal capillary cells called pericytes. The vessel walls are unstable with the loss of these cells, leading to abnormalities in blood flow. Microaneurysms (capillary wall dilitations) develop and can rupture leading to intraretinal hemorrhages. Plasma leaks into the neurosensory retina and appears as hard exudates (small glistening yellow-white spots with defined borders) on funduscopic exam. This fluid can accumulate and cause macular edema (pale raised area in the macular region) with associated decreased vision. As diabetic retinopathy advances, the hypoxia leads to ischemic microinfarctions producing cotton-wool spots or soft exudates (white areas with feathery indistinct borders indicative of nerve fiber layer infarctions). When large areas of the retina are involved, leading to hypoperfusion, new vessels form. This vessel formation, neovascularization, involves the development of new, weak vasculature arising from the retina or optic disc that can extend into the vitreous cavity (proliferative retinopathy) and lead to severe hemorrhage or scarring in the involved areas. Persistent neovascularization leads to the formation of networks of fibrotic tissue that contracts and can cause traction retinal detachments. A sudden loss of vision can occur at any time during these late developments.

Diabetic retinopathy is classified into two categories: nonproliferative and proliferative, based on eye examination findings. The earliest changes of the nonproliferative category are often referred to as background diabetic retinopathy and includes fundus abnormalities within the neurosensory retina (Color Plate 9). Features are microaneurysms, dot and blot hemorrhages (round or oval shaped), hard exudates, and macular edema. Usually the examiner first sees venous dilatation and small red dots (microaneurysms). The hard exudates can be found around microaneurysms or areas of retinal edema. These exudates can reabsorb over months to years. Patients may not have a noticeable change in their visual acuity until the macula becomes involved. Background retinopathy may stay stable or advance slowly over many years.

The later developments in nonproliferative diabetic retinopathy are often referred to as preproliferative diabetic retinopathy. In addition to all the findings of background retinopathy, preproliferative diabetic retinopathy includes intraretinal microvascular abnormalities or IRMAs (irregularly dilated capillaries located within the retinal plane), cotton-wool spots (soft exudates), arteriolar narrowing, and capillary nonperfusion as seen on fluorescein angiography. These preproliferative changes indicate high risk for progression to proliferative diabetic retinopathy which causes severe visual loss.

Proliferative diabetic retinopathy is the presence of neovascularization which can cause retinal detachment and vitreous hemorrhage. When these complications occur, vision can be severely and permanently decreased. Blurred vision, sudden loss of vision, black spots, cobwebs, or flashing lights are all indications for an ophthalmology referral.

Direct ophthalmoscopy examination (using the hand-held ophthalmoscope) is often inadequate to evaluate for diabetic retinopathy due to its narrow field of view and two dimensionality. It is, therefore, imperative that all diabetic patients have regular eye examinations by an ophthalmologist. The American Diabetic Association (1992) recommends that patients with type I diabetes who have been diagnosed for 5 years should have a baseline examination. Patients with type II diabetes should have an examination at the time of the initial diagnoses of diabetes. Both groups should have annual exams thereafter and more often if indicated. Additionally, since retinopathy can progress rapidly during pregnancy, women with insulin-dependent diabetes should have ophthalmic care before a planned pregnancy with the additional ophthalmic exams beginning in the first trimester. Prompt referral to an ophthalmologist is imperative to initiate early, sight-preserving treatment. Evaluation by an ophthalmologist includes slit-lamp examination, indirect ophthalmoscopy (which provides a binocular, stereoscopic view of the posterior and peripheral retina, requiring specialized ophthalmic equipment), and fluorescein angiogram with fundus photography.

Treatment of diabetic retinopathy includes laser therapy (photocoagulation) (Color Plate 10), vitrectomy, and retinal reattachment procedures. Optimal medical management of diabetes, hypertension, and smoking cessation will greatly benefit the patient's prognosis, retinal and otherwise.

Hypertensive Retinopathy

Although there are numerous pathophysiologic retinal changes associated with hypertension, most patients are asymptomatic. The retinal signs, however, can provide important information about the presence, prognosis, and complications of hypertension.

Generalized narrowing of arterioles occurs with persistently elevated blood pressure. A relationship exists between the degree of narrowing and height of diastolic pressure. The walls of the retinal arterioles thicken with degenerative changes and there is a breakdown of the blood–retinal barrier with vessel leakage. Eventually, signs of ischemia and infarction become evident.

Narrowing of the retinal vessels can be difficult to assess. When using a visual comparison between retinal arterioles and veins, a common guideline is that the width of the artery is approximately two thirds to three fourths that of the corresponding vein. The degree of narrowing is graded I to IV with grade IV being narrowest.

Arteriolarsclerosis occurs as a compensatory process in response to persistently elevated pressure. Uniform distribution of the characteristic changes are usually seen throughout the body; therefore, the ophthalmic evaluation is a fair reflection of the general state of the arteriolar circulation. Generalized retinal arteriolarsclerosis is graded I to IV based on the severity of the thickening of the vessel wall (intensity of the color change) and arteriolovenular crossing characteristics (grade IV being worst). It is in this grading system that we find descriptions such as "copper-wiring" (copper luster/color of arterioles) and the more advanced change in color, "silver-wiring."

There are additional retinal changes associated with hypertensive retinopathy. Focal constriction is a localized narrowing of the arteriole with an abrupt decrease then increase in apparent width. Arteriolovenous crossings phenomena include an apparent compression of the vein or a deflection in the course of the vein. "Nicking" refers to zones of venous concealment of these arteriolovenous crossings. Flame-shaped hemorrhages or less common blot-like hemorrhages can be detected as well as microaneurysms, cotton-wool patches (soft exudates as described in the section on "Diabetic Retinopathy"), and edema. A "macular star" is the radial distribution of hard exudates that are elongated and oblique around the macula. Disc edema is a finding in malignant hypertension. Early findings can resolve with control of the hypertension.

Other diseases may cause these retinal findings. They include diabetes mellitus, vasculitis, cardiopulmonary insufficiency, blood dyscrasias, and causes of secondary hypertension.

Complications of hypertensive retinopathy include retinal detachment, macular and optic disc edema, and retinal artery or vein occlusion. All can cause significant and permanent vision loss.

Management focuses on controlling the hypertension. Collaboration between the ophthalmologist and the practitioner managing the hypertension will enhance the full evaluation of the patient and improve their management.

Central Retinal Artery Occlusion

A blockage of the central retinal artery causes a sudden, painless loss of vision within seconds to minutes. Some conditions associated with occlusion are cardiac valve disease, coronary artery disease, atherosclerosis, coagulopathies, giant-cell arteritis, hypertension, intravenous drug abuse, and complications from procedures such as cardiac catheterization, cardiac surgery, and arteriography.

Funduscopic examination shows a diffusely edematous, gray–white retina with a characteristic "cherry-red spot" at the macula (the visualization of the blood supply to the macula which does not come from the central retinal artery). Occasionally the visual acuity remains good but usually it is poor with the patient only being able to count fingers at close range or detect hand motion. There is a poor pupillary reaction to direct light but a normal consensual response (light into the unaffected eye will produce a normal response in both eyes).

Differential diagnoses to consider are retinal detachment, vitreous hemorrhage, retinal vein occlusion, trauma, and optic neuritis.

Central retinal artery occlusion is an ophthalmic emergency. Rapid referral to an ophthalmologist is imperative to increase the chances of restoring vision and preventing complications. Digital massage of the globe may force the embolus to a smaller branch. Vasodilation may relieve retinal artery spasm and is done by having the patient breathe into a paper bag or inhale carbogen (a mixture of 5% carbon dioxide and 95% oxygen). Efforts to lower the intraocular pressure include medications (e.g., oral acetazolamide and topical beta blockers) and anterior chamber paracentesis. Despite these efforts, the prognosis for restoring vision is poor.

The cause of the occlusion requires a careful systemic investigation including carotid ultrasonography and echocardiogram to determine a possible source of emboli and underlying disease.

Giant-cell arteritis (also known as temporal arteritis) must be excluded in older patients with sudden painless loss of vision. Giant-cell arteritis is an inflammatory disease of large and medium arteries. Although it is an uncommon cause of central retinal artery occlusion, it can affect the fellow eye and can leave the patient totally blind. An immediate erythrocyte sedimentation rate should be done in all cases of suspected central retinal artery occlusion to help rule out giant-cell arteritis.

Signs and symptoms of giant-cell arteritis may be fever, malaise, and weight loss over several weeks, headache, jaw claudication, and absence of direct light response in the affected eye. The fundus shows a pale, ischemic, edematous disc, cotton wool spots, and small hemorrhages. The erythrocyte sedimentation rate will be elevated in nearly all cases. Temporal artery biopsy must be done to confirm the diagnosis of giant-cell arteritis even if the sedimentation rate is normal. In the case of biopsy-confirmed giant-cell arteritis, systemic steroids must be given in large doses to prevent involvement of the other eye.

Central Retinal Vein Occlusion

The significant visual loss of central retinal vein occlusion usually occurs over a period of several hours. Found most often in the elderly, predisposing factors include glaucoma, blood dyscrasias, elevated hematocrit, diabetes mellitus, and hypertension.

Funduscopic evaluation reveals marked retinal flame-shaped hemorrhages in all quadrants in cases of central occlusion or hemorrhages of one quadrant in the case of a branch occlusion. Cotton-wool spots and edema of the optic disc and retina are also evident (Color Plate 11).

Diagnosis is usually made by funduscopic exam, but tests to rule out glaucoma are essential. Fluorescein angiography is usually warranted to determine the state of circulation.

The target of treatment is the associated disorder (e.g., hypertension, glaucoma). Close postocclusive monitoring is essential since secondary glaucoma occurs in a significant number of patients. Vitreous hemorrhage and retinal detachment are also possible complications. Laser therapy may be necessary to treat or prevent these complications.

Ocular Symptoms Associated with Migraine

Headache is a common complaint presenting to the healthcare practitioner. Simple headache can be due to eyestrain caused by an uncorrected refractive error, use of an incorrect glasses prescription, or unusually increased reading demands.

Migraine and its variants are disorders that can include ophthalmologic and neurologic signs and symptoms. Migraine consists of many syndromes including common migraine, classic migraine, complicated migraine, cluster headache, and migraine equivalents. The precise mechanism by which migraines occur is not known; however, vascular constriction and subsequent dilation play a role.

Classic and common migraines share many generalized features. They can occur at any age in men and women. There is usually a family history. Common migraine is characterized by a throbbing, generalized headache. It can be associated with autonomic nervous system symptoms, most notably nausea. Classic migraine usually includes a prodromal visual sensation (aura) preceding the headache. The visual symptoms typically begin near the center of the visual field as a gray or blank area (scotoma) with poorly defined borders. The area then slowly expands with bright zigzag lines (scintillations) appearing at the limits. The scintillations then typically move to the peripheral visual field. This usually occurs over a period of 10 to 20 minutes.

Complicated migraine includes associated neurologic phenomenon that are usually transient but can on rare occasion be permanent. One rare variety of complicated migraine is ophthalmoplegic headache which is associated with ocular nerve palsies and paralysis of one or more extraocular muscles. Retinal migraine is a transient or permanent monocular visual disturbance associated with a migraine episode. Migraine-equivalent refers to symptoms believed to result from migraine but that do not include typical symptoms of classic or common migraine.

Age-Related Macular Degeneration

Age-related macular degeneration (AMD), previously known as senile macular degeneration, is an atrophy or degeneration of the macula. The cause is unknown, but is associated with aging. It can be classified into two forms. Atrophic macular degeneration (nonexudative or "dry") is characterized by drusen (an accumulation of cellular debris between the layers of the retina resulting in pale yellow spots in the macular region) and a disruption of the retinal pigmented epithelium (Color Plate 12). This disruption can be seen with the direct ophthalmoscope as variations in the pigmentation of the central macular region. Vision in this stage may be unaffected but the practitioner may see the drusen on routine examinations. In exudative macular degeneration ("wet" form), there is eventual formation of an exudative elevation involving neovascularization and/or hemorrhages. Eventually this elevated area can leave a distinct scar that is seen as a pale, disciform lesion. In this form the patient may complain of slow or sudden painless loss of central vision or a distortion of vision.

Careful study of the macula is often required to detect early stages of the exudative form, which is treatable in some cases with laser photocoagulation to limit the extent of the resulting scotoma. Angiography can differentiate between wet and dry forms, and treatable versus nontreatable lesions.

There is essentially no treatment for dry AMD, but treatment of the complicating neovascularization can preserve vision. Low-vision counseling and visual aids for low vision can be very helpful to the patient. Although patients with AMD are often legally blind, they do usually retain useful peripheral and color vision. They should be advised that they will not become completely blind nor become unable to care for themselves. Patients should be followed by an ophthalmologist.

Amaurosis Fugax

Amaurosis fugax (fleeting blindness) is a unilateral transient loss of vision. It usually occurs over a few seconds to minutes and lasts from 1 to 5 minutes. Vision can return in 10 to 30 minutes. The most common cause is microemboli (fibrin–platelet aggregates) originating from the carotid arteries, especially the extracranial internal carotid. A carotid bruit may be audible. If the microembolus does not disaggregate, permanent visual defects can occur. The diagnoses is usually made by history. A cardiovascular evaluation is warranted.

▶ ABNORMAL PUPILS

Examination of the pupils is an essential part of the ophthalmic assessment. Features to be noted include pupillary size, shape, and reaction to light and accommodation. Testing of the pupillary light response should be done in dim illumination with the patient looking into the distance. The normal pupil responds to light with a brisk constriction followed by a slight increase in size to assume a relatively constant diameter. To test pupillary reaction to accommodation, the patient should look at the examiner's finger at a distance and then follow it as the examiner moves the finger toward the patient's nose. The pupils should constrict as the finger moves closer. Reaction to light without accommodation is termed light-near dissociation and is present in several diseases including syphilis.

It is important to note that a significant portion of the normal population will have up to one millimeter difference in pupil size from time to time. Also, pupil size, shape, and reaction can be altered due to prior ocular disease, ocular surgery, or trauma.

Horner's Syndrome

Horner's syndrome is a dysfunction in the sympathetic innervation to pupillary reaction producing eyelid ptosis and a miotic pupil that reacts equally to light and accommodation. There may also be an associated facial anhydrosis with Horner's syndrome. The difference in pupil size between the eyes is greater in dim light than in bright light. A relative afferent defect is not present. Horner's syndrome is seen with lesions along the lengthy sympathetic pathway such as stroke, tumor, aneurysm, and herpes zoster. The syndrome can occur in isolation or can be congenital. Sudden onset of Horner's syndrome necessitates immediate ophthalmology referral.

Relative Afferent Pupillary Defect

A relative afferent pupillary defect (Marcus–Gunn pupil) is present when the optic nerve is damaged. It is not seen when visual loss is due to conditions of the cornea, lens, vitreous, macula, or refractive state of the eye nor in amblyopia. To test for a relative afferent pupillary defect (RAPD), a light source should be moved from eye to eye. Patients with RAPD have pupillary constriction of both eyes when the light shines in the normal eye. But when the light swings to the abnormal eye, both pupils will dilate (because the abnormal eye does not perceive the light so well). Patients with normal pupillary light reflexes will show no change in the sizes of the pupils. Pathology of the optic nerve distal to the optic chiasm is the usual cause of RAPD.

Hippus is a physiologic change in the pupil size in reaction to light, especially more common in younger patients, which can make the detection of a weak RAPD difficult, but usually, a RAPD is obvious.

A fixed dilated pupil can indicate serious neurological disease such as a compressive lesion or trauma. However, pharmacologic dilation of the pupil, either accidental or factitious, must be ruled out. Pilocarpine 1% will not constrict a pharmacologically dilated pupil; however, it will constrict a dilated pupil due to compression. There is no relative afferent pupillary defect in a pharmacologically dilated pupil. Be aware of the numerous systemic medications that can also affect pupillary sizes.

▶ EMERGENCIES

Trauma and Foreign Bodies

Most trauma cases will need referral to an ophthalmologist. Nurse practitioners will need to be able to evaluate the urgency of the referral and stabilize the patient's condition.

All cases of trauma require a complete history and detailed examination. Usually an ophthalmology referral is necessary. The mechanism of injury is important to determine as well as the material of any foreign bodies. Often injuries are grouped as low- and high-velocity injuries or lacerating and blunt. A small piece of glass or nonreactive metal within the orbit is better tolerated than vegetative material (i.e., wood) which is more likely to cause inflammation and infection.

Some injuries that appear minor can be very serious and vice versa. For example, minor corneal abrasions can be extremely painful whereas a sight-threatening perforating foreign body (as when a patient has been hammering metal surface on metal surface) may feel only as a slight foreign body sensation followed by mild discomfort.

The initial exam of a patient with orbital trauma should include vital signs and a brief systemic review. It should be followed by visual acuity testing (which cannot be overemphasized) and a detailed ocular assessment of pupils, anterior segment, intraocular pressure, and fundus. Include next the orbital area, eyelids, and extraocular muscles. It is important to rule out a ruptured globe and determine injury to adjacent vital structures as an emergency consultation with an ophthalmologist or neurologist may be necessary. This must be done prior to repair of eyelid trauma. The pupil must be dilated for adequate ophthalmoscopic examination.

When examining the globe, great care must be taken not to apply additional pressure when retracting the lids. A safe way to open the lids is to place your fingers on the upper and lower bony margins of the orbit and pull the eyelids back. This should avoid compression. If a ruptured globe is suspected, a "no-touch" assessment is best. Rupture should be suspected in cases when the globe is deformed, the pupil is irregular, subconjunctival hemorrhage is marked, or the anterior chamber is shallow. Use of drops in this case should be avoided and the eye covered with a protective shield (not patched) until evaluated by an ophthalmologist. The patient should be stabilized and procedures taken to prepare the patient for possible surgery.

Always maintain a high index of suspicion for the presence of a foreign body in any trauma case, especially in children. Many trauma patients are unaware of or afraid to report the activity that caused the trauma. Corneal and conjunctival foreign bodies should be removed under slit-lamp magnification using topical anesthesia and a 21-gauge hypodermic needle. The accompanying rust ring is usually easier to remove 24 to 48 hours later, after the use of antibiotic drops. This procedure requires caution so as not to cause further damage. Organic foreign bodies are difficult to detect and may cause inflammatory and infectious complications.

Penetrating orbital trauma is potentially a life-threatening injury. Massive eyelid edema in the presence of a "minor injury" could be due to a cerebrospinal leak. Look also for rhinorrhea as an additional indication. Exophthalmos suggests damage to the orbital roof and is a sign not to be missed. Significant orbital trauma should be suspected in the presence of a traumatic subconjunctival hemorrhage that extends backwards so that the posterior border of the hemorrhage is not visible. Trauma to the orbital area can cause retrobulbar hemorrhages which may be responsible for an acute proptosis. (Proptosis without a history of trauma may be due to Graves' disease, unilateral tumor, cavernous sinus syndrome, and inflammatory disorders.)

CT scanning is useful to image the bones of the orbit in trauma. MRI is excellent for soft-tissue detail but would be contraindicated in the case of suspected magnetic intraocular or intraorbital foreign body due to the potential of migration.

Any trauma case that presents with a vague history or under suspicious circumstances should alert the practitioner to possible physical abuse. Some ocular injuries that occur with physical abuse include periorbital ecchymosis and edema, lid laceration, subconjunctival hemorrhage, corneal scarring or edema, hyphema, strabismus, vitreous hemorrhage and detachment, and retinal hemorrhages and detachments. Patients with a history of prior abuse or trauma may report a visual loss months after the incident. These cases of visual loss are usually due to a retinal detachment from a prior undiagnosed retinal tear.

During the recovery phase of accidental eye injury, patient education should include the use of protective eyewear, especially for industrial purposes and sports (particularly racquetball and hockey). Polycarbonate lenses are much stronger than standard plastic lenses. Protective lenses are necessary for patients who are monocular.

Hyphema

Hyphema is the presence of blood in the anterior chamber. It is mostly caused by blunt trauma but can be associated with surgery, vascular abnormalities, clotting disorders, and neoplasms. The blood can be visualized with direct ophthalmoscopy or even a penlight. The blood is visible behind the cornea, anterior to the pupil and iris (the anterior chamber).

Determining when the injury occurred is important to identify the possible period of rebleeding. A thorough history should also include questions about ocular diseases, eye surgery, blood dyscrasias, and drugs that can affect coagulation.

A complete eye exam by an ophthalmologist is necessary to rule out scleral ruptures, foreign bodies, and injury to other ocular structures.

In most cases the condition resolves without serious sequelae but complications including increased intraocular pressure, optic atrophy, and corneal blood staining can occur. Rebleeding is a major concern and usually occurs before the seventh day following the injury. Preventing or minimizing rebleeding and controlling secondary glaucoma are the main goals of treatment.

The patient should have the head of the bed elevated 30 degrees and the eye protected with a shield until seen by the ophthalmologist. Medical treatment is somewhat controversial and may vary with different ophthalmologists. Occasionally, surgery is necessary if the intraocular pressure cannot be controlled or if corneal blood staining occurs.

Endophthalmitis

Endophthalmitis is an infection of the internal structures of the eye. Generally it develops several days after ocular surgery or trauma, progresses rapidly, and is an ocular emergency.

The eye is injected and a hypopyon (white blood cells in the anterior chamber) is present. There is usually some loss of vision and the patient complains of pain. An atypical presentation can occur with symptoms appearing weeks to months after the incident and may have little associated pain. Rarely, symptoms can occur without a history of eye surgery and can be associated with malignancy, intravenous drug abuse, or distant infections in debilitated or immunosuppressed patients.

The causative organism is determined by intraocular culture obtained in the operating room. Intravitreal, systemic, and subconjunctival antimicrobial agents are used. Hospitalization and close follow-up by an ophthalmologist are required.

Orbital Cellulitis

Orbital cellulitis is usually caused by the same organisms that cause acute sinusitis, including pneumococci, streptococci, and staphlococci. It frequently arises from bacterial infection of the sinuses spreading through the orbital venous system or orbital walls. Orbital cellulitis may also be associated with penetrating trauma, dacryocystitis, periorbital skin infection, dental work, and systemic diseases. Clinical manifestations include swelling and redness of the eyelids, proptosis with decreased motility, chemosis, fever, and malaise. More severe involvement can include pain and visual loss as well. Acute visual loss is often due to an orbital abscess that must be treated as an emergency and surgically drained.

Patients with orbital cellulitis usually require hospitalization and the use of high-dose intravenous antibiotic therapy with coverage for penicillin-resistant, gram-negative, and anaerobic organisms. Specific antibiotic therapy is determined by cultures of direct aspirates of the abscess, sinus, or nasopharynx. Orbital cellulitis, as well as any infection around the orbital area, can lead to serious life-threatening complications due to the close anatomical proximity of the brain. Some complications can include posterior extension causing cavernous sinus thrombosis, meningitis, or brain abscess.

Cellulitis occurring anterior to the orbital septum is termed preseptal or periorbital cellulitis. It is characterized by lid edema, discomfort, and erythema. Most cases of preorbital cellulitis respond well to systemic antibiotics.

▶ HUMAN IMMUNODEFICIENCY VIRUS INFECTION

Ocular involvement is a common feature of human immunodeficiency virus (HIV) infection and can be easily overlooked by the practitioner. It usually manifests as retinal vascular disease, opportunistic infections of the retina and cornea, and malignancies affecting the ocular area.

Externally, a Kaposi's sarcoma may be noted in the lids or conjunctiva. This is a vascular tumor that appears on the conjunctiva as a red mass and can be confused with a subconjunctival hemorrhage. It is often present posterior to the lower lid, which must be retracted for adequate examination. On the skin of the eyelids, the lesion appears as a purple nodule or plaque. Such lesions may be the first sign of HIV infection. Herpes zoster ophthalmicus in a younger patient may also indicate HIV infection. If either of these conditions is found on routine exam, it would warrant further evaluation for HIV infection. Ophthalmic treatment for Kaposi's sarcoma lesions is not indicated as they do not interfere with vision or cause discomfort (for treatment of HZO, see the section on "The Red Eye"). Other external diseases seen in HIV infection include conjunctival microvascular disease, HSV keratitis, and molluscum contagiosum.

Retinitis is also a frequent problem associated with HIV infection. The cytomegalovirus is a common retinitis pathogen but other opportunistic pathogens have also been isolated. Retinitis can cause blindness due to optic nerve involvement and retinal detachment. Initially an asymptomatic lesion may be found on routine funduscopic examination. These lesions include cotton wool spots, retinal hemorrhages, microaneurysms, and retinal swelling. Disk edema may also be noted due to invasion of the pathogen or tumor. There may be photopsia, floaters, and decreased visual acuity. The areas of necrosis cause a visual field defect and their progression can be monitored by serial visual field testing. A variety of medications have met with limited results in treating this condition.

It is important for HIV-infected patients to be followed by an ophthalmologist in an attempt to preserve vision, especially as the CD4+ T-lymphocyte levels fall.

REFERENCES

American College of Physicians, American Diabetes Association, American Academy of Ophthalmology. (1992). Screening guidelines for diabetic retinopathy. Clinical Guideline. *Ophthalmology, 99,* 1626–1628.

Dawson, C. R. & Sheppard, J. D. (1992). Follicular conjunctivitis. In W. Tasman & E. Jaeger (Series Eds.) and I. R. Schwab (Section Ed.), *Duane's clinical ophthalmology: Vol. 4. External diseases and the uvea.* (Revised ed., Ch. 7, pp. 1–8). Philadelphia: J. B. Lippincott.

Quigley, H. A. (1993). Open-angle glaucoma. *New England Journal of Medicine, 328* (15), 1097–1106.

50

Head and Neck Problems

Daniel G. Deschler
Kathleen A. Walsh

▶ ANATOMY AND PHYSIOLOGY OF THE HEAD AND NECK

Ear

External Ear

The external ear is composed of the auricle (pinna) (Fig. 50–1), the external auditory canal, and the tympanic membrane. The outer skin lining of the external auditory canal contains hair follicles, cerumen glands, and sebaceous glands. Cerumen is created by the secretions of these glands and together with the hair follicles, the ear canal is cleansed of foreign matter.

The tympanic membrane (TM) serves as a partition between the external ear and the middle ear. A fibrous annulus encircles the TM and attaches it to the temporal bone. The superior portion of the TM, the pars flaccida, is thinly constructed as compared with the other portions of the eardrum, making it more prone to retraction with negative pressure. The normal tympanic membrane has a translucent pearl-color appearance. The structures of the middle ear can usually be visualized with use of the otoscope.

Middle Ear

The middle ear (tympanic cavity) is the air-filled space between the tympanic membrane and the inner ear located within the petrous segment of the temporal bone continuous with the mastoid bone. The eustachian tube, ossicles, and the oval and round windows comprise the middle ear (Fig. 50–2).

The eustachian tube is located anteriorly and leads medially and downward to the nasopharynx, joining the middle ear with the nasopharynx. This specialized tube allows air to travel between the two, equalizing pressure across the eardrum. Changes in external air pressure causes the eardrum to retract; conversely, if middle ear pressure is greater, the eardrum bulges. Abrupt change of pressure at the tympanic membrane can cause rupture of the membrane. The act of swallowing opens the eustachian tube, thereby, equalizing this sudden alteration.

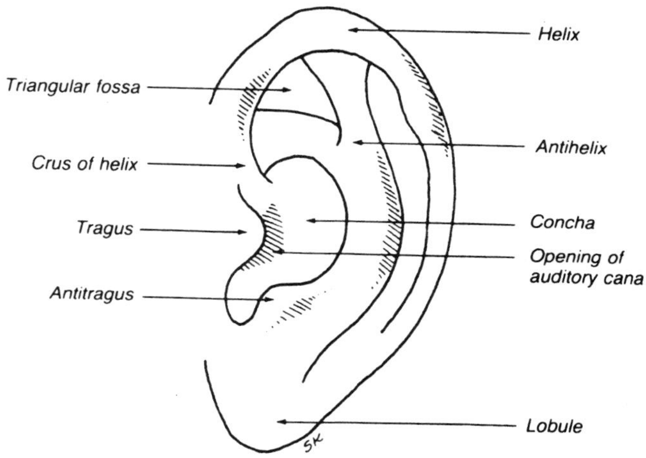

Figure 50–1. Lateral view of auricle. *(Used with permission from Lucente & Sobol. [1996].)*

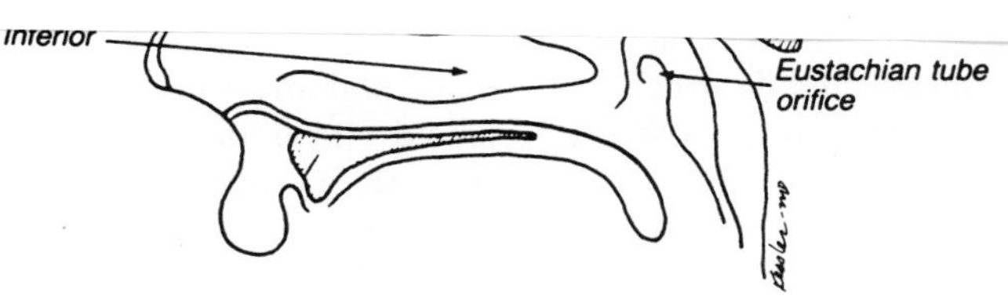

Figure 50–4. Lateral wall of nasal cavity. *(Used with permission from Lucente, Sorvino, & Slavit. [1993].)*

The oral cavity extends from the skin-vermilion border of the lips to the junction of the hard and soft palates. It contains the lips, cheeks, alveolar ridges, anterior two-thirds of the tongue, floor of mouth, retromolar trigone, and hard palate.

Lips and Cheeks

The buccal mucosa is the inner membrane lining of the lips and cheeks. The buccinator muscle at the lateral walls of

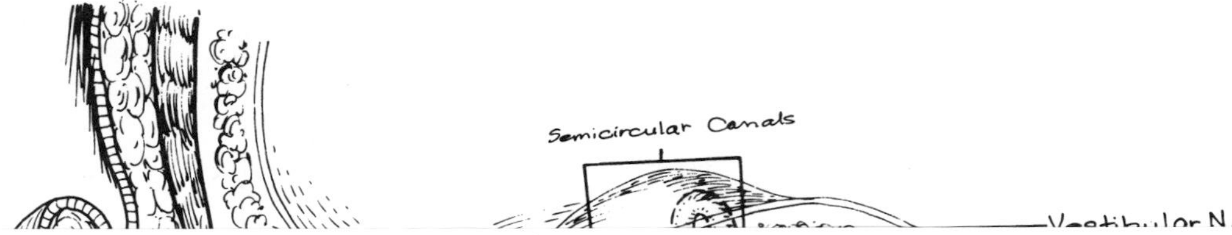

the oral cavity control the movement and position of food in the mouth. The opening of the parotid gland, called *Stenson's duct,* is located within the mucosa opposite the upper second molar.

Teeth and Gums

The teeth are situated in sockets along the alveolar processes of the mandible and maxillae. The alveolar ridges are overlaid by the gingivae. Permanent dentition of an adult usually consists of 32 teeth.

Tongue

Several muscles constitute the tongue and are divided into the extrinsic and intrinsic groups situated on both sides of the tongue. The extrinsic muscles aid in the movement of the tongue, form the floor of the mouth, and maintain tongue position. The intrinsic muscles originate within the tongue, changing its shape for speech and positioning of food for swallowing. The paired hypoglossal nerves (CN XII) innervate the tongue.

The tongue has a dorsal and ventral surface. The dorsal anterior two-thirds of the tongue are covered with filiform and fungiform papillae. The circumvallate papillae are larger in size and found at the posterior surface, in an inverted V-shape formation. The ability to discriminate taste sensations is initiated by the position of these papillae as they contain the taste receptors on the tongue. Taste buds also exist on the palate, hypophamyx, and esophagus. The line of circumvallate papillae divides the oral tongue from the base of the tongue, which is in the oropharynx. The lingual tonsil, a collection of lymphoid tissue, is situated at the posterior midline of the tongue.

Hard and Soft Palates

The hard palate constructs the anterior two thirds of the roof of the mouth. The palatine and superior maxillary bones form the hard palate which is lined with a thick mucous membrane. The posterior one third of the roof of the mouth, the soft palate, partitions the oropharynx and nasopharynx and from its midline hangs the uvula. The act of swallowing moves the soft palate upward, closing the nasopharynx to food and fluids.

Pharynx

The pharynx extends from the base of the skull to the esophagus and larynx and is formed by the superior, middle, and inferior constrictor muscles. The pharynx is divided into three regions: nasopharynx, oropharynx, and hypopharynx.

Nasopharynx

The nasopharynx's anterior border is the posterior nasal opening (the choana). The eustachian tube opening is located at the lateral wall. Situated at the posterior superior wall of the nasopharynx are the adenoids (pharyngeal tonsils). The superior surface of the soft palate defines the inferior wall of the nasopharynx.

Oropharynx

The oropharynx is in continuation with the oral cavity anteriorly and extends superiorly from the plane of the hard palate to the plane of the hyoid bone inferiorly. The tonsil and tonsillar fossa, the faucial pillars, comprise the lateral wall of the oropharynx. The posterior wall of the oropharynx is composed of the posterior tonsil pillar and the narrow lateral and posterior pharyngeal walls.

Hypopharynx

The hypopharynx is the inferior extension of the oropharynx, from the epiglottis to the openings of the esophagus and larynx. The superior boundary is marked by the hyoid bone, base of tongue, and constrictor muscle. The piriform sinuses and larynx form the inferior border. Posteriorly, the superior constrictor muscle and vertebrae bound the hypopharynx space.

The pharyngeal portion of swallowing is orchestrated by the specialized constrictor muscles of the oropharynx and hypopharynx as well as the suprahyoid and infrahyoid muscles. There are three phases of swallowing: the oral stage, pharyngeal stage, and esophageal stage.

Larynx

The larynx is a tubular cartilaginous and muscular structure connecting the pharynx and trachea. It is located between the fourth and sixth cervical vertebrae; it is positioned at the level of the third vertebrae in the child. The hyoid bone is attached to the larynx by the thyrohyoid membrane and muscle. The larynx is composed of a framework of articulating cartilages. There are three unpaired cartilages: the thyroid, epiglottis, and circoid. The paired arytenoid, corniculate, and cuneiform cartilages complete the laryngeal framework (Fig. 50–5).

The thyroid cartilage, with its shield-shaped appearance, is connected superiorly to the hyoid bone and articulates inferiorly with the circoid cartilage. The superior margin of the thyroid cartilage is attached to the epiglottis, a leaflike cartilage with a superior border that moves freely preventing food entering into the trachea.

The circoid cartilage is the only complete circle in the larynx. This signet-shaped structure is narrow at its anterior border and broad posteriorly. It forms the base of the larynx. The superior border of the circoid cartilage articulates with the two bilateral symmetrical arytenoid cartilages. The corniculate cartilages are positioned above the arytenoids in the aryepiglottic folds and along—with the cuneiform cartilages—provide structure to the aryepiglottic folds.

The position of the arytenoid allows the cartilage to glide, tilt, and rotate. It is at the posterior aspect of the arytenoid (the muscular process) that the majority of the intrinsic muscles of the larynx are attached. The vocal process of the arytenoid is attached to the vocal ligament (true vocal cord).

The true vocal cords are mucosa-lined ligaments that

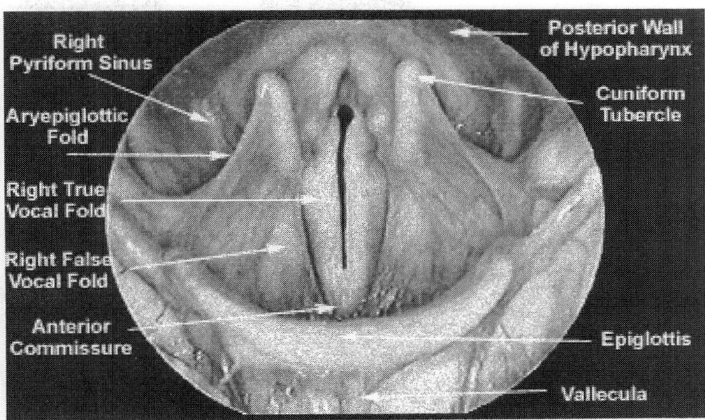

Figure 50–5. Structures of the larynx. *(Used with permission. Courtesy of Deschler, D. G. [1997].)*

stretch between the arytenoid and thyroid cartilages. Voice is produced with the adduction of the vocal cords. Abduction of the cords occurs during inspiration.

The false vocal cords (vestibular folds) are superior to the true cords. As their name implies, the false vocal cords do not normally contribute to phonation. The space separating the false and true cords is the laryngeal ventricle. The vestibule is the compartment above the false cords.

The laryngeal muscles are separated into intrinsic and extrinsic categories. The intrinsic muscles connect to the arytenoids and direct their pivotal position enabling fine-muscle control for vocal-cord movement. The extrinsic muscles are concerned with the total movement of the larynx and provide the support to adjacent structures of the neck.

The recurrent laryngeal nerve innervates the intrinsic muscles—specifically, opening action of the posterior cricoarytenoid muscle and closing action of the remaining muscles. The extrinsic muscles (particularly the cricothyroid) are innervated by the external branch of the superior laryngeal nerve. Sensation is provided by the internal branch of the superior laryngeal nerve which divides from the vagus nerve.

There are three general functions of the larynx. The ability to function as a conduit for air flow from the trachea upwards to the hypopharynx is the primary role of the larynx. It humidifies and filters incoming air. A second function of the larynx is to protect the trachea against aspiration. This protective mechanism is accomplished by the closure of the larynx during swallowing of food into the hypopharynx and esophagus. The recurrent laryngeal nerves direct this action. Speech production is the final and unique function of the human larynx.

Salivary Glands

Thousands of minor salivary glands are found within the oral cavity, oropharynx and larynx. There are three major paired salivary glands: the parotid, submandibular (Fig. 50–6), and sublingual glands. Largest of the three, the parotid gland is located in front of the ear, lying over the masseter muscle and beneath the ramus of the mandible. Its tail portion extends posterior and inferior to the angle of the mandible. The deep and superficial portions of the parotid gland are defined by the anatomic course of the facial nerve. This nerve divides into five principal branches (temporal, zygomatic, buccal, mandibular, and cervical).

At the anterior edge of the gland, the parotid (Stensen's) duct originates, crossing the masseter muscle and entering the buccinator muscle. It opens into the oral cavity opposite the upper second molar tooth.

The second largest of the salivary glands is the submandibular gland. This gland is situated at the floor of the mouth lying inferior and anterior to the angle of the mandible. Submandibular (Wharton's) ducts course between the gland itself and the hyoglossus muscle, terminating at the oral cavity adjacent to the frenulum and posterior to the lower incisor tooth.

Smallest of the major salivary glands is the sublingual gland. It is located beneath the submucosa of the floor of the mouth. Unlike the previous glands, the sublingual gland drains from numerous ducts at its superior surface into the oral cavity.

Saliva produced by the glands is controlled by the autonomic nerve system. Food within the mouth initiates the physical stimulation of saliva, while psychologic stimulation occurs by the sensory input of taste, smell, and even vision.

The daily production of saliva is estimated to be between 500 and 1500 cc of fluid (Jones, 1995; Sobol, 1993). The majority of this saliva originates from the parotid and submandibular glands.

Neck

Neck anatomy is approached by dividing the neck into triangles (Fig. 50–7) and describing the triangles' borders and their contents. It is this classification that assists the practitioner to evaluate a neck mass.

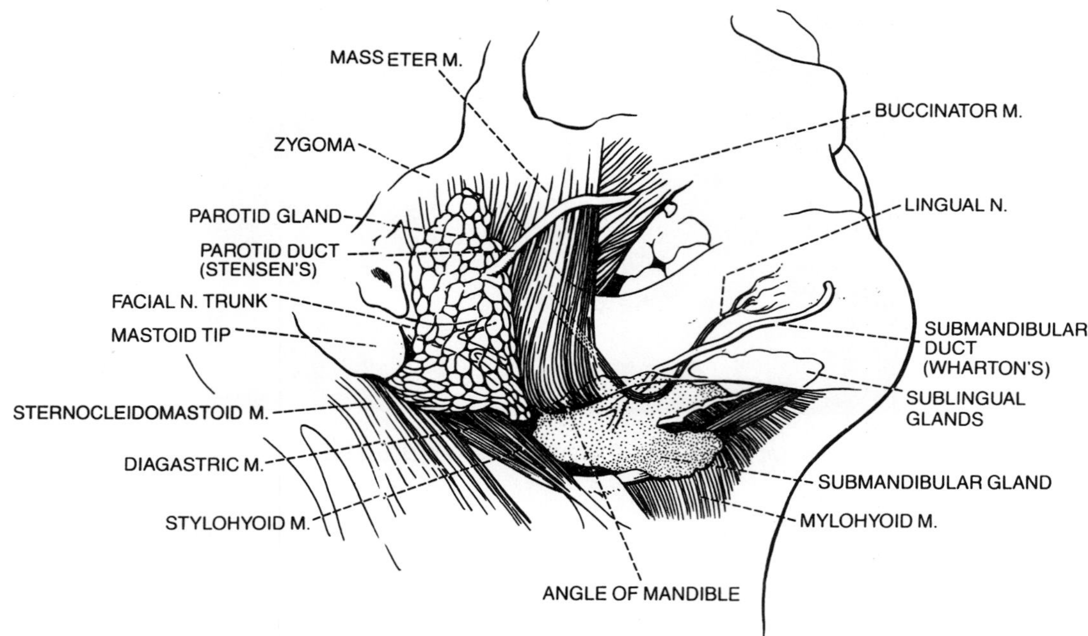

Figure 50–6. Anatomy of the parotid and submandibular glands. *(Used with permission from Wilson & Nadol. [1983].)*

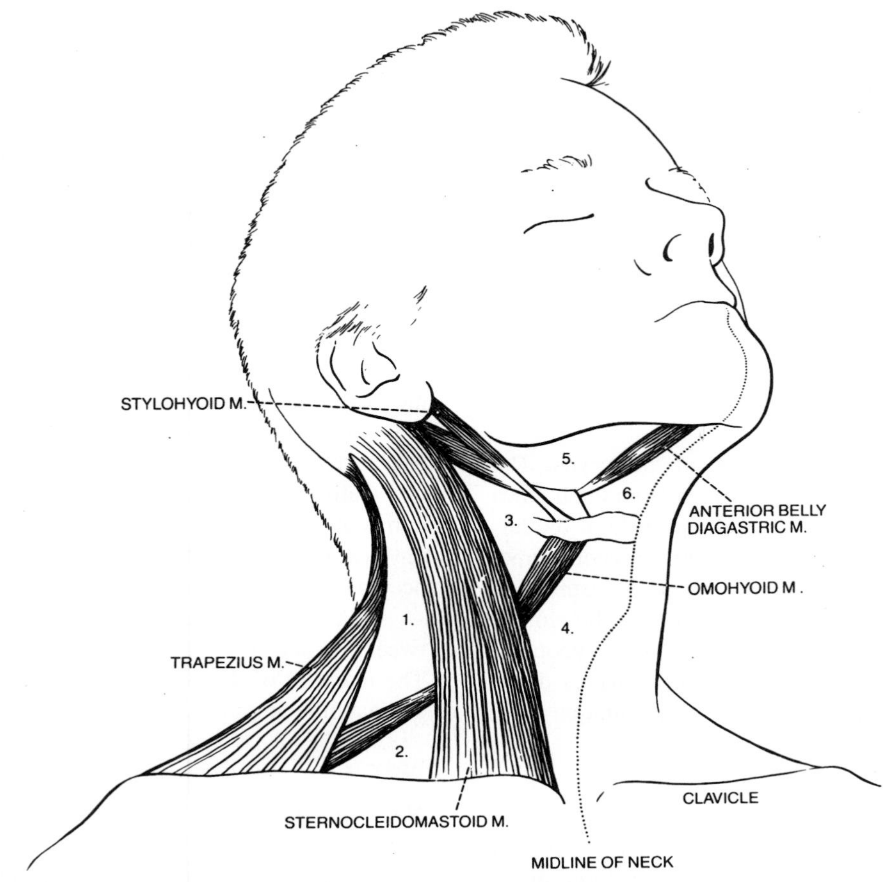

Figure 50–7. Anatomical triangles of the neck. *(Used with permission from Wilson & Nadol. [1983].)*

The anterior triangle is composed of the boundaries of the sternocleiodomastoid muscle posteriorly, the midline of the neck anteriorly, and the body of the mandible. The anterior triangle is further separated into the submandibular (digastric), carotid, muscular, and submental triangles.

The posterior triangle of the neck is outlined at its anterior edge by the sternocleiodomastoid muscle. The trapezius muscle is its posterior border and the clavicle forms the inferior border. The posterior triangle is divided into the occipital triangle and subclavian triangle.

Thyroid and Parathyroid Glands

The thyroid gland, largest of the endocrine glands, is composed of two lateral lobes linked by an isthmus that is located on the second, third, and fourth tracheal cartilages. The superior and inferior thyroid arteries supply blood to this exceptionally vascular structure. The recurrent laryngeal nerves are situated behind the lateral lobes of the thyroid in the tracheoesophageal grooves. This is of surgical importance because of the potential for nerve injury given their close proximity to the thyroid gland.

The thyroid gland consists of follicules that manufacture thyroid hormone. Also contained within this gland are parafollicular cells, producers of calcitonin.

The parathyroids are small bean-sized glands that lie along the posterior portion of the thyroid. There are usually two parathyroid glands at each thyroid lobe; however, the total number of parathyroids may vary from three to five. Parathormone (parathyroid hormone) is secreted by the parathyroid glands to maintain plasma calcium levels.

Further information regarding the physiology of the thyroid and parathyroid glands may be obtained by consulting an endocrinology text.

Trachea

The trachea connects the larynx to the bronchi of the lungs. The trachea is composed of 18 to 20 C-shaped cartilages. The posterior aspect of the trachea is absent of cartilage; rather, it is composed of soft tissue allowing for flexibility of the trachea and esophageal expansion.

The functions of the trachea are to filter, warm, and humidify incoming air. The lining of the trachea, consisting of a ciliated epithelium, contributes to the cleansing of the trachea, moving particles upward to the larynx or esophagus in order to be expectorated or swallowed.

Esophagus

The esophagus is a mucosally-lined muscular tube connecting the laryngopharynx above to the stomach below. Its length is approximately 25 cm from the cricopharyngeal area to the stomach. Skeletal muscle composes the upper one third of the esophagus, the middle third consists of skeletal and smooth muscle, and the lower third is completely smooth muscle. There are four layers of the esophageal wall: an outer longitudinal muscle, the muscularis propria, the submucosa, and the mucosa.

The cricopharyngeus muscle forms the pharyngoesophageal sphincter where muscular contraction directs food into the proximal esophagus. At the distal portion of the esophagus, the gastroesophageal sphincter allows food to enter into the stomach and then contracts to prevent reflux of food and gastric acid. Pressures within these two areas are higher than at other regions of the esophagus. Esophageal peristalsis—combined with changes in intraluminal pressure—aids in deglutition. Incompetence of the esophageal sphincters contributes to the development of reflux.

▶ DISORDERS OF THE HEAD AND NECK

Otologic Disorders

External Ear

Auricular Perichondritis. Auricular perichondritis usually results from trauma to the auricle such as insect bites, auricular hematomas, burns, frostbite, and lacerations (Davis & Powell, 1985). It may also be a complication of otitis externa. The usual causative agents are *Staphlococcus aureus* and strep species. *Pseudomonas aeruginosa* is also a frequently described organism (Graham, Lee, & Goldsmith, 1995). Symptoms include auricular swelling, warmth, pain, and fever. The physical findings may include inflamation and erythema of auricular skin; a pallid auricle is suggestive of severe frostbite. The use of oral anti-staph antibiotics such as Augmentin or a first-generation cephalosporin is suggested by Coppola & Yealy (1992) if the inflammation is contained to the ear and the patient is followed closely in the outpatient setting. Otherwise, intravenous antibiotics with similar coverage (i.e., Unasyn) is warranted to avoid progression to frank chondritis and cartilage loss. Outpatient antibiotics should continue for 10 to 14 days and correspond with the effective IV regimen. A thorough otologic exam is necessary to evaluate a possible temporal bone cause.

Auricular Hematoma. Auricular hematomas are usually caused by blunt trauma to the auricle, and are frequently seen in wrestlers (Schuller & Schleuning, 1994). The collection of blood between the perichondrium and auricular cartilage gives the ear a swollen purple appearance. It is necessary to drain the hematoma to prevent destruction of the cartilaginous support of the auricle, which may lead to the development of a "cauliflower ear."

Sterile aspiration of the auricular hematoma should be performed with a large-bore needle. If reaccumulation of the hematoma reoccurs or if aspiration is not effective, small incisions are made through the skin for drainage. Application of a pressure dressing or bolster dressing placed around the crevices of the pinna is necessary to prevent reaccumulation (Wilson & Nadol, 1983). The dressing should be left in place for 3 to 5 days and checked within 24 hours to assess for hematoma reformation. Antibiotics may be added to prevent infection and perichondritis.

External Otitis. External otitis, often called "swimmer's ear," is an infection of the external auditory canal (EAC) skin and may be acute or chronic. Water exposure, humid climates, trauma, absence of protective cerumen, and chronic middle ear disease are all risk factors (Bull, 1991). The patient may complain of mild to severe otolagia, otorrhea, and decreased hearing. On examination, exudative drainage and edema of the EAC are seen. *P aeruginosa* and *staph aureus* are two common organisms (Farrior, 1998).

Initial therapies involve suctioning and cleansing of the EAC; stopping instigating factors; and treating with local antibacterial, antiinflammatory, and analgesic agents. Cortisporin solution or suspension, containing neomycin, polysporin, and steroid, is effective, either directly placed in the ear canal or used with a gauze ear wick three or four times daily (Schuller & Schleuning, 1994). If infection appears to involve the surrounding tissues, then systemic antistaph antibiotics are recommended. Resistant cases may require culture and the use of appropriate aminoglycoside otic preparations (Farrior, 1998).

It is important to complete a thorough otoscopic exam, including pneumotoscopy, when the inflammation decreases to assess tympanic membrane (tm) status and possible middle ear pathology. Prophylatic care includes removal of appropriate instigating factors, periodic use of acidifying and drying agents, and manual drying with a hair dryer.

Chronic external otitis has less acute edema, but presents with a dry, crusted EAC and meatus. Cortisporin and steroid creams to the meatus can be tried. Fungal disease should be suspected. Therapy consists of frequent hygiene, acidification, and slow resolution (Farrior, 1998). Dermatologic referral after otolaryngological evaluation may be indicated in resistant cases.

Signs and symptoms of external otitis in diabetic patients should be taken seriously, and the patient should be expediently referred for evaluation of possible necrotizing external otitis.

Cerumen Impaction. Cerumen ("wax") impaction (CI) results from the failure of the normal cleaning mechanism of the external auditory canal (Fig. 50–8). Impaction of cerumen may occur due to a small or twisted EAC and abnormal cerumen. However, improper cleaning of the canal with the use of a cotton-tipped applicator is a major culprit in CI, pushing the cerumen medially (Zivic & King, 1993). Pain, hearing loss, itching, and otitis externa are symptoms of CI. Normal cerumen is tan–brown in color. A white–cheesy debris may indicate underlying infection. Cerumen removal can usually be performed by using softening agents such as Debrox (glycerine and peroxide) for 3 to 5 days prior to removal

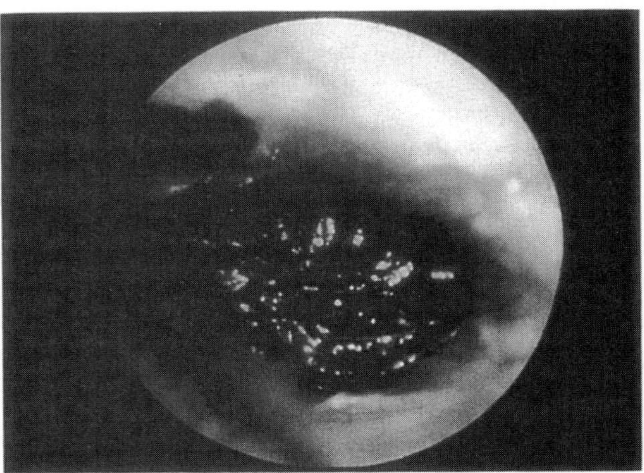

Figure 50–8. Cerumen in external ear canal. *(Used with permission from Sigler & Schuring. [1993].)*

(Fairbanks, 1996). Cerumenex is another choice but should be used for only the day prior to removal and can be more irritating. These agents should not be used if there exists a tympanic membrane (TM) perforation, external otitis, tympanostomy tube, or surgically created mastoid cavity. Irrigation as a method of removal should be avoided in these same instances. Ear irrigation is done with water at 37°C to avoid vertigo, and with the fluid introduced along the side of the canal toward the superior area of the TM. A curette or fine wire loop can be used for cerumen removal after immobilizing the head. Direct visualization is required and the instrument should go no further than 2 cm into the EAC. Hygiene in problematic cases may include periodic use of softening agents, and scheduled frequent cleaning by an otolaryngologist with the use of magnification.

Foreign Bodies. Cockroaches are the most commonly reported foreign body found in the EAC followed by beads and cotton as reported by Bressler & Shelton (1993). Mineral oil can be used to drown and immobilize the live insect allowing direct removal. Irrigation of the EAC should be avoided with organic substances, such as beans, as the introduction of water may expand the organic matter. Removal of a foreign body can be attempted with an earwax wire curette or a right-angle hook for those objects difficult to grasp. Extreme care should be taken during foreign body removal due to the risk of laceration of the EAC, otitis externa and tympanic membrane perforations, and facial nerve palsy (Bressler & Shelton, 1993). Referral to an otolaryngologist who will use a microscope may be required. In addition to an otoscopic exam, it is also important to document hearing prior to removal attempts. Audiometric evaluation should be ordered if there is a question of hearing loss or damage to the tympanic membrane.

Tumors of the External Ear. External ear tumors include exostoses, which are small benign bony growths covered by epithelium located near the tympanic membrane. They may occur as a result of frequent cold water swimming (Bull, 1991). Unless the slow-growing exostoses obstructs the ear canal, intervention is not necessary. Surgical excision is performed for removal.

Squamous-cell and basal-cell carcinoma are two common types of malignancies of the external ear. These tumors may arise from the skin surrounding the auricle, in the tragal area, or from the epithelium of the EAC. Symptoms may include ear drainage, hearing loss, and otolagia. Early recognition with biopsy performed are paramount to effective treatment.

Middle Ear

Otitis Media. Although acute otitis media (AOM) is one of the most-often diagnosed infections in childhood, with increasing age it becomes much less common (Celin, Bluestone, Stephenson, Yilmaz & Collins, 1991). Otitis media (Fig. 50–9) presents with complaints of unilateral otolagia, fever, hearing loss, vertigo, and otorrhea, which may be bloody. The patient may cite a history of recent upper respiratory infection. Examination of the ear reveals an inflamed, erythematous, bulging, and immobile tympanic membrane (TM). Normal landmarks are generally obscured. It is important to attempt pneumotoscopy to adequately assess mobility of the TM and presence/absence of effusion. Occasionally, spontaneous perforation occurs, which provides marked relief to the patient. Such TM perforations heal spontaneously in the vast majority of cases.

Cultures of middle ear aspirates in adults reveals a slightly different bacteriologic distribution than noted in children. Bluestone (1994) reports the *Haemophilus influenzae* pathogen is more prevalent in adults versus children, while *Streptococcus pneumoniae* infects greater numbers of children.

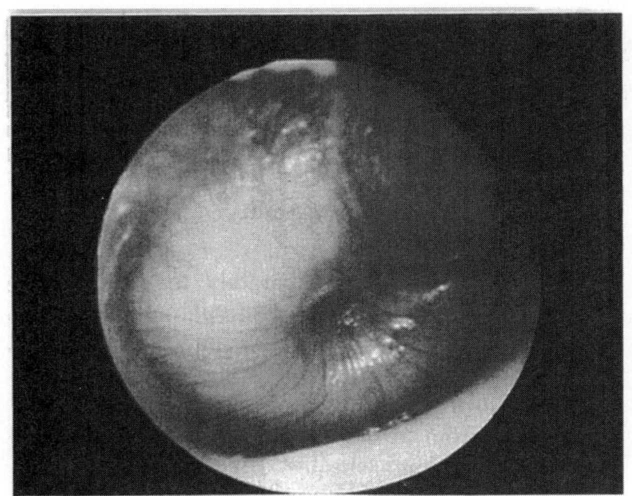

Figure 50–9. Acute otitis media. *(Used with permission from Sigler & Schuring. [1993].)*

Appropriate initial antibiotic therapy for adults may include Cefuroxime Axetil 250 mg for 10 to 14 days (Celin et al., 1991). Failures of initial therapy may then be treated with Augmentin 500 mg TID for 14 days. The infectious symptoms should respond within days to the antibiotic therapy. Patients are often left with a residual serous otitis media (SOM) after an episode of acute OM, which can take weeks to months to resolve.

Serous Otitis Media. Serous otitis media (SOM) is the result of eustachian tube dysfunction (ETD) which prevents adequate ventilation of the middle ear space resulting in negative pressure and fluid build-up. This may occur from infection such as an upper respiratory infection, be functional as in cleft palate patients—including those with submucosal clefts of the soft palate, or due to physical obstruction such as a soft tissue mass (Gold, Sperling, & Sobol, 1993).

Symptoms consist of vague discomfort, sense of fullness, tinnitus, crackling noises, and decreased hearing. Exam reveals an intact TM that has decreased mobility and air bubbles may be noted behind the TM. Patients are also unable to "pop" their ears with a valsalva maneuver, verifying ETD. The light reflex is generally not a helpful sign and more emphasis should be placed on mobility. Treatment consists of systemic decongestants (Sudafed 30-60 mg up to TID), local decongestants such as Afrin (2 puffs BID for up to and not beyond 4 days) (Sigler and Schuring, 1993), and limited autoinsufflation (ear popping). Antibiotics may be added (Amoxicillin or Bactrim) and given for up to 3 weeks to treat an underlying nasopharyngitis/adenoiditis. Serous otitis media may take weeks to months to resolve. It is important to consider a mass lesion, such as nasopharyngeal carcinoma, for unresolving cases with an atypical history.

Flying precautions should be suggested for patients with ETD and consist of (1) abstinence of alcohol before and during flight as it causes mucosal swelling, (2) use of Afrin prior to flight, and (3) use of Sudafed preceding and during flight.

Cholesteotoma. Cholesteotoma is the otologic condition in which keratinizing squamous epithelium (the normal lining of the EAC and external TM) grows in the confines of the middle ear and mastoid spaces, which are normally lined with mucosa. Progression leads to erosion of vital structures such as the ossicles, facial nerve canal, labyrinth, cochlea, and floor of the middle and posterior cranial fossae, because of expansive and enzymatic destruction (Graham, Lee, & Goldsmith, 1995; Pincus & Finazzo, 1993).

Two variants exist: (1) primary cholesteotomas, which are extremely rare, congenital anomalies that occur as a result of squamous epithelium behind an intact TM, and present as an opaque middle ear mass and conductive hearing loss; and (2) the secondary variation is more common and is the result of chronic middle ear disease and ETD (Weit,

Micco, & Bedoya, 1998). These cases present with a perforation or a retraction pocket (a thinned TM drawn into the middle ear by chronic negative pressure). Patients present with a conductive hearing loss and TM perforations that are draining or exuding keratinous debris.

Pneumotoscopy is helpful in differentiating perforations from retraction pockets—a retraction pocket snaps toward the examiner when the negative pressure in the middle ear is overcome. Management consists of referral to an otolaryngologist for possible surgical intervention before complications (bone and/or facial nerve erosion)occur.

Tympanic Membrane and Middle Ear Trauma. Injury to the tympanic membrane may be caused by direct or indirect trauma resulting in perforation of the thin-walled membrane (Fig. 50–10). Direct trauma is caused by a penetrating injury such as a Q-tip or hairpin used for cleaning the ear canal, or unskilled efforts to remove a foreign body. Indirect trauma may result from a slap to the auricle creating a sudden pressure, a welding injury with hot slag entering the ear, or blast injury. Sudden change in atmospheric pressure (barotrauma) caused by diving or rapid descent in an airplane can also cause TM perforation. A basilar or temporal skull fracture may tear the TM.

Bloody discharge from the ear or a visible laceration in the TM are two physical findings of middle ear trauma. The patient with a perforated TM complains of pain and hearing loss. It should be immediately assessed whether it is a conductive or sensorineural hearing loss using the Rinne and Weber tuning fork tests if audiometry is not available. If vestibular signs and symptoms of vertigo, nystagmus, and tinnitus are evident, a perilymphatic leak may be present suggesting inner ear injury requiring emergent treatment by an otolarngologist. The majority of uncomplicated TM perforations without infection will heal spontaneously (Sarti, Prager, & Lucente, 1993). A large perforation may require surgical repair.

Temporal Bone Fracture. Fractures of the skull base may involve the temporal bone. A longitudinal fracture parallels the longitudinal plane of the temporal bone while a transverse fracture transverses across it.

The longitudinal fracture occurring in approximately 80% of temporal bone fractures (Kmucha & Lee, 1995) results in dislocation of the tympanic ring and perforation of the TM leading to bleeding into the middle ear. Cerebrospinal fluid leaks and ossicular chain injury may occur. Facial nerve paralysis may be evident. Conductive hearing loss is common. Ecchymosis over the mastoid (Battle's sign) is typical of a longitudinal fracture.

Transverse fractures (approximately 20% of cases as reported by Kmucha & Lee, 1995) result from frontal or occipital trauma causing a transection of the internal acoustic canal and labyrinth fractures leading to severe or complete loss of auditory and vestibular function. Sensorineural loss is usually present. Damage to the facial nerve is seen in 40 to 50% of cases (Kmucha & Lee, 1995; Schuller & Schleuning, 1994). Otoscopic exam commonly reveals an intact TM with a hemotympanum present (Fig. 50–11), giving a bluish hue to the TM. Severe vertigo can occur with symptoms lasting for months. The patient may exhibit nystagmus.

A patient with a suspected temporal bone fracture should be thoroughly evaluated for other possible neurologic injuries (i.e., cervical spine). Determining the magnitude of injury to the ossicle chain, TM, the inner ear, the seventh cranial nerve, and possible cerebrospinal fluid

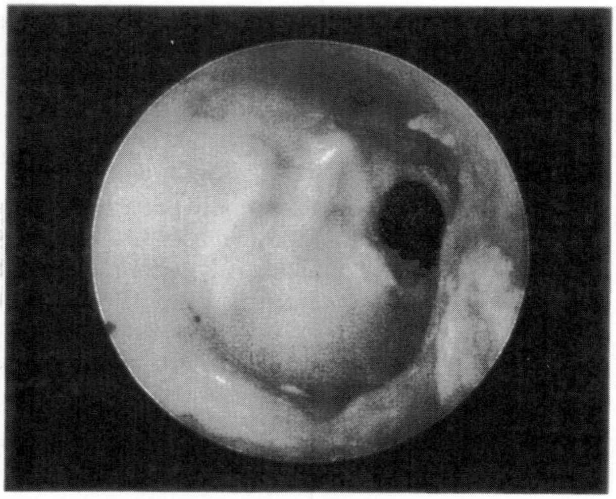

Figure 50–10. Tympanic membrane perforation. *(Used with permission from Sigler & Schuring. [1993].)*

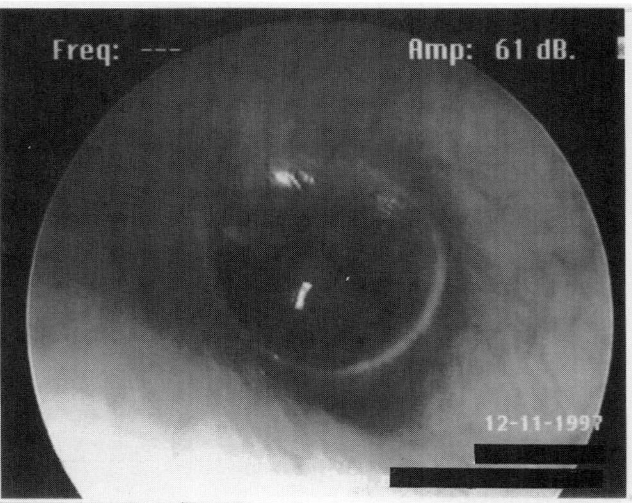

Figure 50–11. Hemotympanum (hemorrhagic exudation into the middle ear). *(Used with permission. Courtesy of Deschler, D. G. [1997].)*

(CSF) leak is paramount in the initial exam. An otoscope and tuning fork will greatly aid the practitioner in determining the status of the TM, ossicles, and middle ear space.

Plain films of the skull may not reveal temporal bone fractures; therefore, a CT scan of the temporal bones should be performed in the coronal and axial planes. Audiometry is useful in evaluating hearing loss.

Careful observation of the patient with specific regard to facial nerve functioning and CSF leak is essential in these cases. Surgery may be performed for persistent hearing loss postinjury and for exploration and repair of a transected facial nerve.

Tumors of the Middle Ear. The two types of middle ear tumors are glomus jugulare tumors and squamous-cell carcinoma. A glomus jugulare tumor is usually a benign tumor that arises from the jugular bulb. It may also begin in the middle ear and is labeled glomus tympanicum tumor. These tumors are highly vascular but slow growing. Expanding pressure leads to destruction of surrounding structures. The patient may complain of pulsatile tinnitus. Progressive conductive hearing loss occurs as the tumor grows. A bruit may be evident over the upper neck. Pulsation of the tumor increases with the pressure from a pneumatic otoscope. Manipulation of the ear canal and middle ear is to be avoided as the tumor has a propensity to hemorrhage profusely. Cranial nerves IX, X, XI, and XII may be affected at later stages of tumor growth. Metastasis to the lungs and cervical nodes has occurred (Graham, Lee, & Goldsmith, 1995). Carotid angiography reveals important diagnostic information; a CT scan with contrast and an MRI are also helpful in assessment of tumor extent. Treatment of a glomus tumor is surgical excision. Radiation therapy and tumor embolization are also considered.

Squamous-cell carcinoma of the middle ear may initially present with bleeding from the external auditory canal and conductive hearing loss. Severe otolagia and facial paralysis accompanied by sensorineural loss demonstrate inner ear involvement. A biopsy is performed to confirm the diagnosis of cancer. A patient with chronic otitis media or chronic otitis externa is at risk for squamous-cell carcinoma. The treatment consists of surgery for tumor ablation possibly involving a temporal bone resection.

TABLE 50–1. Etiologies of Hearing Loss

Conductive	Sensori-Neural
Cerumen impaction	Presbycusis
Acute otitis media	Noise-induced
Chronic otitis media	Drug toxicity
Serous otitis media	Meinere's syndrome
Otosclerosis	Acoustic neuroma
Injury to the tympanic membrane	Congenital (e.g., rubella, cytomegalovirus)
Cholesteatoma	Head trauma
Barotrauma	Central nervous system disease
Temporal bone fracture	Infection (e.g., meningitis, mumps)
Middle ear tumors	Metabolic disorders (e.g., diabetes, hypothyroidism, Paget's disease)
Ossicular discontinuity	

Inner Ear
Hearing Disorders

Hearing Loss. Hearing loss is classified as conductive, sensori-neural, or mixed. Conductive hearing loss is a failure of the external ear canal, the TM, or the ossicles to convey vibratory sound to the cochlea. Sensori-neural loss occurs because of damage to the cochlea, the acoustic nerve (CN VIII), and/or central auditory pathways. Both types of hearing loss have a multitude of etiologies and a thorough medical history is essential (Table 50–1).

A preliminary assessment of hearing loss is performed by the use of a tuning fork (Table 50–2).

Further assessment of hearing is accomplished by the use of an audiometer, an electronic device that provides the practitioner with the ability to assess pure tone, bone and air conduction, and speech thresholds. The audiometer creates pure tones with different frequencies and varying levels of intensity. Hearing is measured by decibels. The patient's ability to hear the tone at the lowest level is identified as the threshold. An audiogram graphically illustrates the hearing threshold level at every tested frequency for each ear. Testing for air conduction is by presenting tones through the earphones. The loudness and frequency are varied, thereby establishing a hearing threshold level (normal hearing level is a pure tone average of 20 decibels or less). Bone conduction is assessed by presenting tones through an oscillator placed on the mastoid bone. The tones are directly transmit-

TABLE 50–2. Tuning Fork Tests

	Weber	Rinne	Schwabach
Assessment	Determines whether a unilateral loss is sensori-neural or conductive	Compare bone conduction (BC) hearing with air conduction (AC)	Compare bone conduction of patient with normal hearing person
Placement of tuning fork	Midline of forehead	Initially at mastoid process, then lateral to ear canal	Mastoid
Normal	Tone heard equally in both ears	Positive AC tone louder at ear canal	Tone heard equally by patient and examiner
Conductive loss	Tone lateralized to affected ear	Negative BC Tone louder behind ear	Tone is heard longer by patient
Sensori-neural loss	Tone lateralized to better ear	Positive AC tone louder at ear canal	Tone is heard longer by examiner

ted through the bone, bypassing the middle ear structures and going directly to the cochlea. Deficient responses demonstrate abnormalities or impairment of the inner ear, cochlea, or acoustic nerve.

Audiometry brainstem response (ABR) is an electrophysiological study of the auditory pathways, further defining the site of a inner ear deficit (specifically at the level of the acoustic nerve midbrain or pons). ABR can be used for infants, young children, and patients unable to cooperate for a test. Malinoff (1993) presents a thorough description of audiology studies including interpretation of results.

It is important to differentiate between conductive and sensori-neural hearing losses; asymmetry between the right and left ears also determines possible/probable etiologies early in patient presentation. This early identification and subsequent referral to an otologist or neuro-otologist allows formulation of a treatment plan that may involve otologic surgery for an acoustic neuroma or cochlear implant for restoration of hearing.

Acoustic Neuroma. Acoustic neuroma is a benign tumor of the eighth cranial nerve usually arising from the vestibular portion of the nerve. Tumor growth may extend from the internal auditory canal into the cerebellopontine angle causing pressure on the surrounding cranial nerves.

Initial symptoms are ipsilateral tinnitus, vertigo, and ipsilateral sensori-neural hearing loss. With tumor extension, facial paralysis may result from compression of the facial nerves (CN VII) and, ultimately, signs and symptoms of an intracranial space-occupying lesion are evident.

The diagnosis of an acoustic tumor is determined by imaging studies, usually an MRI, demonstrating a mass in and widening of the internal auditory canal. Electronystagometry demonstrates a unilateral reduced or absent caloric response, while auditory brainstem response is abnormal. Surgery is the treatment of choice for removal of the acoustic tumor in most patients.

Vertigo/Dizziness. The complaint of vertigo or dizziness by a patient requires the practitioner to differentiate between the two entities. Dizziness is a general and subjective term used by the lay public to describe sensations of lightheadedness, weakness, unsteadiness, whirling motion, and syncope as well. Vertigo is described as the sensation of spinning or falling. It may be the patient or his or her environment that is spinning.

The diagnosis of vertigo is essentially obtained from the patient history. The patient should be queried concerning the timing, severity, duration, presence of associated aural and/or neurologic symptoms, and activity at the time of onset. It is also necessary to ascertain whether it is a peripheral (inner ear) or central (brainstem, cerebellum) disorder.

The Hallpike–Dix maneuver is used to distinguish benign peripheral positional vertigo from central positional vertigo. The patient is positioned quickly from sitting to supine with head (extended over the exam table) rotated first to the involved side, next rotated to the opposite side, and then straight forward for 30 seconds in each position. This exaggerated movement produces vertigo and nystagmus. McGee (1995) discusses the findings and features of the nystagmus (latency, adaptation, and fatigability) in establishing a diagnosis.

Treatment of vertigo is contingent on the etiology. Hart (1998) states an anatomic diagnosis (e.g., disorder of the inner ear) should be treated at the local site; for a physiologic disorder (e.g., vestibular system dysfunction) treat the system; and the cause treated for an etiologic diagnosis (e.g., diabetes mellitus).

Medications that are commonly used to treat vertigo include vestibular suppressants, anticholinergics, and antihistamines. Hart (1998) advocates the use of intravenous diazepam (5-20 mg initially, followed by IV infusion) for those individuals presenting to the emergency room with severe vertigo, titrating the dosage based upon its effect on the nystagmus and vertigo. Short-term use of benzodiazepines (2-10 mg four times daily for 2-3 weeks) is suggested to avoid addiction. Anticholinergics–Scopolamine patch may be useful as a prophylactic medication due to its delayed peak effects (McGee, 1995). Two of the more common antihistamines, meclizine (Antivert) and dimenhydrinate (Dramamine), are prescribed for extended treatment. Typical dosing for meclizine is 12.5-25 mg 3-4 times daily, while dimenhydrinate 50 mg, 1-2 tablets are taken every 4-6 hours (Hart, 1998; Sigler & Schuring, 1993).

Physical therapy is an important component of the treament plan for vertigo (especially for benign paroxysmal positional vertigo [BPPV]), as the vestibular system requires retraining to compensate for the dysequilibrium. Specific balance exercises are included in Hart's (1998) writings.

Vestibular Neuronitis. Vestibular neuronitis is a form of viral neuritis exclusively affecting the vestibular nerve, usually precipitated by a respiratory or an upper airway infection. The patient has an acute onset of vertigo with nausea, vomiting, and spontaneous nystagmus, demonstrating unilateral vestibular dysfunction without auditory symptoms. The imbalance experienced by the individual gradually diminishes over several weeks with resolution occurring in 6 to 12 weeks. Treatment consists of vestibular suppressants as described earlier.

Meniere's Disease. Meniere's disease is a disorder of the inner ear, distinguished by the triad of episodic attacks of debilitating vertigo, tinnitus, and sensori-neural hearing loss. The patient may experience these attacks in a random pattern, occurring numerous times a week, persisting from minutes to hours. The patient may also experience aural fullness. Severe nausea and vomiting can also occur.

The etiology of this disorder is related to changes in the endolymphatic system of the inner ear, consequently affecting the vestibular system. The presence of hydrops demonstrates an increase in endolymphic fluid resulting in a fluid overload status in the membranous labyrinth. The basis for this endolymphic fluid surplus is uncertain and may be associated with other disease processes (e.g. diabetes, hypothyroidism, hyperlipedemia) (Sobol & Guffin, 1993).

Meniere's disease is initially treated medically with the focus on reducing the endolymph fluid: restricted sodium intake (1500 mg/daily) and use of thiazide diuretics (hydrochlorothiazide 1 tablet twice daily) as suggested by Gantz & Gidley (1998). Vestibular suppressants, vasodilators, and specific labyrinth exercises may also be prescribed. The patient should be instructed to avoid alcohol, tobacco, and caffeine.

If conservative medical treatment is unsuccessful, referral to an otolaryngologist for surgical intervention should be discussed. Various surgical techniques such as labyrinthectomy, sac–vein decompression, vestibular neurectomy, and transtympanic aminoglycosides are explained in the literature (Gantz & Gidley, 1998; Wilson & Nadol, 1983).

Tinnitus. A patient who complains of noises heard in the ear or ringing of the ear may be suffering from tinnitus. It is important to realize tinnitus is a symptom, not a disease. Subjective tinnitus is defined as noise heard by the patient, but not by the observer. Objective tinnitus (less common) is sound heard by both. Description of the noises may include "ringing," "crickets chirping," or "buzzing." Determination of the classification of tinnitus allows specific orientation to assessment and treatment of the patient.

Schuller & Schleuning (1994) provide detailed causes of tinnitus. Numerous medical conditions have been identified as contributing to the development of subjective tinnitus; these include those of metabolic, neurologic, pharmacologic, and otologic origins (e.g., hyperlipedemia, skull fracture/head trauma, use of salicylates and NSAIDs, otosclerosis). Vascular disease such as arteriovenous malformations, carotid stenosis, and venous hum can be a direct cause of objective tinnitus. Palatomyoclonus and patulous eustachian tube are two mechanical sources of audible tinnitus.

Relief of tinnitus is provided by intervention directed at the underlying system disorder. Again, treatment of the vascular and mechanical abnormalities may reduce or eliminate the tinnitus, although options are limited. An audiogram should be performed as results may dictate further etiologic work-up. Various treatment plans have been recognized to assist the patient. Elimination of causative factors such as caffeine, smoking, and exposure to loud noise should be discussed. Medications need to be reevaluated, with reduced dosage or substitution attempted. Biofeedback, hypnosis, and electrostimulation may also be of benefit. Tinnitus maskers are used to deliver sound at the same frequency or tone to the affected ear(s), thus masking the noises heard by the individual. Amplification of sound by means of a hearing aid sometimes aids in alleviating tinnitus.

Ramsay–Hunt Syndrome. Ramsay–Hunt syndrome (herpes zoster oticus), a viral infection of the facial nerve ganglion, is characterized by herpetic vesicles of the ear, face and oral mucosa, profound ear pain, facial paralysis, sensori-neural hearing loss, and vertigo. At early stages of disease, all of these symptoms may not be present. The diagnosis is derived from clinical assessment of the patient, and increasing antibody titers to the herpes zoster virus substantiates the diagnosis. This painful viral infection may involve the facial nerve and other cranial nerves as well. Symptomatic treatment is provided with the use of Acyclovir, dosage 200 to 400 mg, five times daily, to lessen the duration of active infection (Adour, 1998). The use of corticosteroids as outlined by Adour are believed to alleviate pain and minimize postherpetic neuralgia and inflammation.

Nasal Disorders

Nasal Fractures

Fracture of the nasal bones happens more often than any other facial bone fractures. Nasal fractures vary from a single linear break, to several fractures causing greater deformity. The patient presents with a cosmetic disfigurement, more noticeable when the observer is behind and looking downward on the patient. Physical findings may reveal edema, periorbital ecchymosis, epistaxis, and possible septal hematoma. Nasal congestion/obstruction with pain and tenderness are frequent symptoms.

Schuller & Schleuning (1994) note that nasal x-rays are of little value in management of nasal trauma as damage to the cartilage of the nose is not apparent. The nasal septum needs to be clearly evaluated for possible hematoma. Subsequent treatment for a septal hematoma involves draining the collection of blood and packing the area to avoid further reaccumulation of blood. An untreated hematoma leads to infection, possible meninigitis and loss of septal cartilage with subsequent saddle nose deformity. A check for cerebrospinal fluid leak should be done by asking the patient if he or she had any clear discharge or bitter tasting from the nose or to the back of the throat after the injury. An ophthalmic examination should also be performed, especially if a nasoethmoid fracture is suspected.

Cosmetic deformity of the nose requires the fracture to be reduced. This may be done immediately postinjury. If edema obscures the assessment for deformity, the fracture may be reduced in a few days' time (Martini, Assael, & Har-El, 1993). Use of intranasal splints and packing are necessary to support the repair.

Epistaxis

Epistaxis is a common condition encountered by practitioners. Traditionally, it has been characterized as anterior or posterior. While this anatomic approach is useful, a practical way of approaching epistaxis is to define it in terms of (1) bleeding controllable by conservative measures and (2) that requiring referral and more invasive intervention.

The most common cause of epistaxis is trauma (e.g., nose picking) (Lucente, Sorvino, & Slavit, 1993). Other predisposing factors include cold weather, dry climates, exposure to chemicals (including recreational use of cocaine), septal deviations, and perforations. Bleeding/clotting abnormalities, hypertension, and nasopharyngeal cancer are other etiologies that require consideration in the appropriate environment (Sigler & Schuring, 1993).

Most nosebleeds occur from the anterior septum at Kiesselbach's Plexus, and cease with anterior pressure. These common bleeds are usually self-limited, but unfortunately recur often. Primary diagnosis consists of history for risk factors and physical exam with anterior rhinoscopy. If suspicious or actively bleeding areas are found, these can be cauterized with silver nitrate sticks. Anesthesia should first be given with 4% cocaine or lidocaine and neosynephrine on a cotton pledget placed against the area (Sigler & Schuring, 1993). All attempts at cautery should be guided and not done blindly. Opposing areas of one side of the nasal cavity should not be done simultaneously as synechiae may result, nor should opposite sides of the septum be done at the same time to avoid perforations.

Patient education concerning preventative measures focuses on maintaining a moist surface to aid healing and avoid crusting, which may lead to further bleeding. This can be done with daily application of an ointment (such as Vaseline or Bacitracin) applied to the septum and internal nares with a cotton applicator (Wurman, Sack, Flannery, & Lipsman, 1992). Humidification of the environment may also be helpful as well as use of saline sprays.

More profuse epistaxis without an easily identified source and multiple recurrent bleeding should be considered for referral. Such bleeding may require more active intervention ranging from anterior packing with Merocel sponges or gauze to consideration of arterial embolization or ligation.

Sinusitis

Sinusitis is defined as an inflammation of the paranasal sinus mucosa. Stafford (1993) has identified three forms: acute, subacute, and chronic. Acute sinusitis consists of symptoms and findings for less than one month, subacute lasts from 1 to 3 months, and chronic sinusitis is present for greater than 3 months.

The primary cause of sinusitis is obstruction of the sinus ostia leading to stasis and bacterial infection (Reilly, 1990). Factors predisposing to such obstruction include: viral rhinitis, polyps, tumors, septal deviation, foreign body, chronic inflammatory diseases, cystic fibrosis, and immunodeficiency.

Nasal discharge, cough, purulent nasal discharge, headache, and facial pain are the most common symptoms of acute sinusitis. Physical exam findings can be underwhelming with sinus transillumination being reliable only if it is significantly abnormal. Fever is actually uncommon. Williams & Simel (1993) concluded that maxillary toothache, poor response to nasal decongestants, abnormal transillumination, history of purulent nasal discharge, or such discharge noted on exam are most useful to practitioners. When all five are present, the likelihood of sinusitis rises sharply; when none are present, sinusitis is unlikely.

Screening sinus CT scan is the best diagnostic test (Chester, 1996). A standard sinus series can be useful but is limited in the assessment of the ethmoid sinuses and, reports Chester, is currently not significantly more inexpensive than limited sinus CT. An MRI scan is not indicated for sinus disease but is helpful for the evaluation of sinonasal tumor or intracranial complications of sinusitis (Reuler, Lucas, & Kumar, 1995).

Chronic sinusitis has a more insidious presentation and is more refractory to therapy. Chronic sinusitis is characterized by significant postnasal drip, reports of green or yellow foul drainage, vague complaints of facial pressure, headache, and congestion.

Treatment of sinusitis centers on antibiotic therapy. The most common organisms for community-acquired sinusitis are *Strep pneumoniae, H. flu,* anaerobes, *Moraxella catarrhalis, Staph aureus,* and gram-negative bacteria. *Moraxella* is more common in children and anaerobes are more common in chronic sinusitis (Reilly, 1990).

Stafford (1990) reports first-line therapy may begin with Amoxicillin 500 mg every 8 hours for 14 days. Bactrim DS is an excellent cost-effective alternative. Other options include azithromycin, clarithromycin, cefuroxime, amoxicillin–clavulanate. Cases with poor response or no clinincal improvement within a few days should be treated with the latter options (Ferguson, 1995).

Because chronic sinusitis is often the result of concomitant anaerobic infection, recommended antibiotic coverage is with amoxicillin–clavulanate or clindamycin, which should be administered for 4 to 6 weeks.

Adjunctive therapies for both acute and chronic sinusitis include nasal saline spray and steam inhalation which moisten inflamed mucosa. Nasal decongestants should be administered during acute sinusitis for no longer than 3 days as rebound congestion can occur. Pseudoephedrine and phenylephrine (systemic decongestants) should be prescribed cautiously as insominia can result. They are contraindicated in individuals with benign prostatic hypertrophy and hypertension. Steroid nasal sprays have been reported as an adjunctive therapy for decreasing sinus ostial inflammation; however, definite benefits have not been reported (Reuler, Lucas & Kumar, 1995; Richtsmeier, 1998).

Chronic sinusitis sufferers may benefit from an otolaryngology consultation for discussion of functional endoscopic sinus surgery (FESS). This surgery allows for selective removal of sinus disease. Chester (1996) reported that those individuals who failed medical therapy and subsequently underwent a FESS had a 91% rate of achieving good results.

Facial Fractures

Motor vehicle accidents and violence are two major causes of facial fractures as reported by Martini et al. (1993). Patients who have evidence of facial fractures/trauma must first be assessed for more serious injuries (airway obstruction, cervical spinal injury, and cerebral injury). Stabilization and repair of facial fractures are determined, after addressing life-threatening injuries. Referral to an otolaryngologist is essential to restoration of function and appearance of the injured patient.

Mandibular fractures usually result in the patient's inability to properly occlude the teeth. This may be accompanied by pain and trismus. Numbness of the chin and lower lip can occur as a result of injury to the inferior alveolar nerve. Immediate treatment incorporates the use of ice packs, antibiotics (especially if oral mucosa is torn), and analgesics. Repair of mandibular fracture involves immobilization of the bone by use of fixation devices, obtaining the goals of normal dental occlusion, and firm bony union of the fractured bone.

The zygomatic or malar bone determines the contour of a person's cheek, hence traumatic injury to the bone causes noticeable change in facial appearance. Normal convexity of the cheek is lost because of division of the zygomatic bone from the temporal, frontal, and nasal bones. Anesthesia of the cheek can occur due to damage to the infraorbital nerve. There may be evidence of a subconjunctival hemorrhage, diplopia, epistaxis, and drooping of the lateral canthus of the involved eye. Consultation with ophthalmology is necessary to rule out eye injury (e.g., detached retina or traumatized cornea). Again, treatment is symptomatic with repair of the zygomatic fracture by the surgeon after swelling has subsided.

Fractures of the midface region are classified according to the Le Fort system (Fig. 50–12). Absolute Le Fort fractures are rare. The Le Fort I fracture involves a transverse fracture line over the lower maxilla into the nasal cavity separating the lower maxilla from the facial skeleton. A Le Fort II fracture is described as a triangular fracture occurring through the infraorbital rim and nasal bone with the zygomatic bone remaining attached to the skull. The Le Fort III fracture, complete craniofacial disassociation, demonstrates separation of the nasal, maxilla and zygomatic bones from the cranium. Comminuted fractures of the midface produce a flattened face appearance.

Maxillary fractures result in profound facial edema and ecchymosis, distorting normal landmarks. Cerebrospinal fluid leaks and mild to severe epistaxis can occur. Malocclusion and an unstable maxilla are demonstrated by loose movement of the midface bones during palpation.

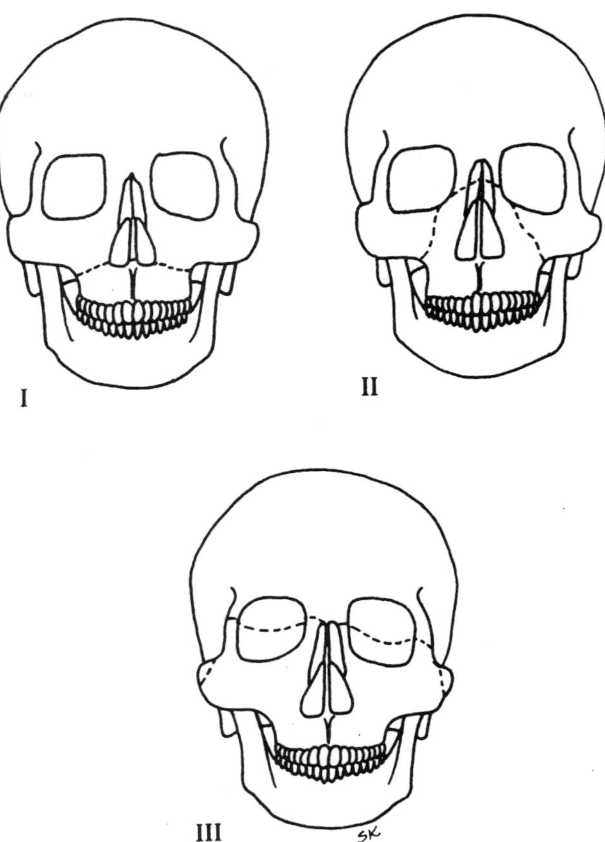

Figure 50–12. Le Fort classification of midfacial fractures. *(Used with permission from Lucente & Sobol [1993].)*

Repair of Le Fort fractures should be considered when the patient's medical condition is stable. The primary concern should be stabilization of the patient airway. Nasal intubation is contraindicated and enteral feeding tubes should not be placed nasally. Radiographic studies greatly aid the practitioner in assessing bony damage and devising a surgical plan for repair. Particular films that may be performed are sinus x-ray series, CT scan of head and facial bones (possibly including three-dimensional reformatting) (Lowlicht & Goodwin, 1995), and a panorex of the mandible.

Sleep Apnea

The patient with a presentation of sleep apnea may be unaware of his or her disturbance while the patient's partner has identified a problem, prompting intervention by the practitioner. Sleep apnea is defined as air-flow cessation due to an obstruction at the level of the nose and mouth for at least 10 seconds during sleep. The diagnosis is made if the apneic episodes happen more than 30 times in a 7-hour sleep period (Hausfeld, 1992; Sorvino & Salvit, 1993).

Two types of sleep apnea are identified: obstructive and central. Obstructive sleep apnea (OSA) may result from an upper airway narrowing or obstruction related to anatomical abnormalities or impaired function of the oropharyngeal and nasal structures. Central apnea is cessation of air flow secondary to absence of inspiratory effort. Mixed apnea is a combination of obstructive and central sleep pathologies.

Symptoms encountered with sleep apnea include daytime fatigue that may be so severe as to disturb normal activities, loud snoring, and difficulty in arousing from a sleeping state. Sexual impairment, morning headaches, and abnormal muscle activity during sleep can also occur. Obesity is a significant contributing factor in individuals with obstructive sleep apnea.

Diagnosis of OSA involves a thorough examination and history of the patient. Polysomnography testing assists in diagnosis by recording systemic measurements of oxygen saturation, respiratory effort, electroencephalography, electroculography, electrocardiogram, and nasal and oral air flow.

OSA management consists of medical and surgical therapies depending upon the severity of impairment. Avoidance of alcohol and weight reduction are discussed with the individual. Riley, Powell, Guilleminault, Clerk, & Troell (1995) conclude that although weight loss is an integral component of the treatment plan, it should not be considered as the singular or primary therapy for OSA.

Use of nasal continuous positive airway pressure (CPAP) or BiPAP may be used to deliver pressure to the airway, eliminating negative airway pressure formation, and thereby preventing upper airway obstruction. Results with CPAP are impressive. However, long-term compliance is a significant issue. Hausfeld (1992) reports a compliance rate of 50 to 60%, and Riley et al. (1995) less than 50% in their patient populations. Complaints of inconvenience, nasal irritation, claustrophobia, and sinusitis were cited by the researchers.

Dental devices and tongue-retaining devices that reposition either the mandible or tongue or elevate the soft palate are considerations for those with mild OSA. Surgical approaches involve efforts to circumvent or eliminate the upper airway obstruction and include tonsillectomy, uvulopalatopharyngoplasty (removal of the tonsils, anterior tonsillar pillar, and posterior 1-1.5 cm of the soft palate), septoplasty as well as tongue surgery. The success of the OSA surgery is variable with greater success in eliminating snoring.

Nasal, Paranasal Sinus Tumors

Benign Tumors. Nasal Polyps are the prolapsed lining of the nasal sinuses, usually the ethmoids. They may also occur from the nasal mucosa and turbinates. Nasal polyps present as watery, fleshy masses that are mobile to palpation. The etiology of the inflammatory polyps has not been clearly defined, although systemic allergy has been strongly implicated (Schuller & Schleuning, 1994). Benign inflammatory polyps are usually bilateral, although to varying degrees. Isolated unilateral polypoid masses require expedient referral to rule out serious entities such as inverted papilloma and carcinoma.

Marked polyps are nearly always associated with significant sinus disease, symptomatic or not, as they may obstruct the natural drainage path and outflow tracts of the sinuses. Some polyps may also be the result—not the cause—of chronic sinusitis. A triad of nasal polyps, aspirin sensitivity, and asthma has been reported in patients. Sigler & Schuring (1993) cite an estimated 8% of individuals with nasal polyps suffer from asthma and aspirin sensitivity. Symptoms usually consist of nasal obstruction, mouth breathing, hyponasal speech, and nasal fullness. A trial of nasal topical steroid (2 puffs daily of Vancenase, Nasoacort) for up to 1 month should be the first line of therapy. If significant sinus symptoms also exist, then a 3- to 4-week course of antibiotics may be added. A nasal polypectomy may be considered for definitive treatment.

Inverted Papilloma. An inverted papilloma may be similar to a nasal polyp; however, it is less opaque, with invaginations that intrude upon the supporting tissues of the nasal cavity. Described as a benign growth, it acts aggressively, spreading into surrounding structures. Approximately 10 to 13% of inverting papillomas develop into squamous-cell cancer (Feldman & Feldman, 1995). The patient may complain of nasal obstruction, rhinorrhea, and epistaxis. A CT scan may demonstrate bony erosion. Treatment involves a complete wide local excision of the papilloma to prevent recurrence.

Malignant Tumors. The majority of malignant tumors of the nasal cavity and paranasal sinuses are primarily squamous-cell cancers, followed by adenoid cystic carcinoma, adenocarcinoma, and melanomas. Risk factors for the development of these cancers include exposure to wood dust, nickel compounds, nitrosamines, and radium (Goodman, 1990; Sigler & Schuring, 1993). Textile and asbestos workers, snuff users, those involved with mustard gas, and petroleum refiners also have a high risk of tumor development (Goodman, 1990).

The patient may have initial symptoms of sinusitis, facial pain, nasal obstruction, discharge and epistaxis, and dysfunction of the cranial nerves. Physical assessment is aided by use of nasal speculum for visualization of the nasal cavity. Testing of cranial nerve function is an important diagnostic tool. Radiologic imaging with plain films, CT scan, and MRI is essential. The CT scan will demonstrate bony involvement and destruction, and soft-tissue involvement will be noted with an MRI. A definitive biopsy is required to plan treatment options.

The treatment of nasal and paranasal sinus cancers is dependent upon the tumor stage. Ohngren's line is a prognostic indicator used for maxillary sinus tumors (Sigler & Schuring, 1993). The line is drawn at a diagonal angle from the lateral canthus of the eye to the mandibular angle, separating the maxillary sinus into a posterosuperior suprastructure and an anteroinferior section. Tumors located superior to this line demonstrate a poorer prognosis because of the tumor's close adjacency to orbital contents as well as cribiform plate and infratemporal fossa. Surgery and radiation therapy as dual modalities are considered for malignant tumors.

Nasopharyngeal Tumors

Juvenile Nasopharyngeal Angiofibroma. Juvenile nasopharyngeal angiofibroma (JNA) is a benign tumor of the nasal cavity and nasopharynx occurring in preadolescent males. Typically they present with history of nasal obstruction and periodic nosebleeds. Angiography illustrates an extremely vascular mass, with possible extension of the mass into adjoining tissues. CT scan reveals bowing of posterior wall of maxillary sinus. Embolization of the vascular artery feeding into the JNA is recommended before surgical removal (Wilson & Nadol, 1983). Radiation therapy has also been used as an alternative to surgery.

Malignant Tumors of Nasopharynx. Nasopharyngeal carcinoma may present in any age group. There is a steady increase in incidence to ages 45 to 55 (Eisele, Clifford, & Johns, 1995). Goodman (1990) notes a male to female predominance of 3:1 exists. The Chinese population is at high risk. The most common presenting symptom is a progressive neck mass (Eisle, Clifford, & Johns, 1995; Wilson & Nadol, 1983), usually in the posterior triangle. Other presenting symptoms include epistaxis, pain, conductive hearing loss due to unilateral serous otitis media, and cranial nerve deficits in advanced cases.

Risk factors that are speculated for nasopharyngeal carcinoma involve smoking, exposure to cooking fumes, formaldehyde exposure, and herbal medicines. Yet, only Epistein–Barr virus and consumption of salted fish and other items high in nitrosamines and their breakdown products have been strongly and statistically linked as environmental risk factors (Eisele et al., 1995).

The diagnosis of cancer is made by biopsy of the nasopharynx. Imaging studies (MRI or CT) may reveal abnormal signals suggestive of tumor. Primary therapy consists of radiation therapy with surgery reserved for salvage. Early diagnosis and treatment are key to a favorable prognosis.

Oral Cavity, Oropharynx Disorders

Tongue

Examination of the tongue may demonstrate common normal findings that may concern an individual enough to seek medical attention. The following tongue disorders are commonly encountered in the practice setting and bear mention. Median rhomboid glossitis is distinguished by the absence of papillae at the midtongue, giving the appearance of a slick, red, smooth tongue surface. The patient is asymptomatic and treatment is not indicated. Geographic tongue (migratory glossitis) is characterized by varying areas of the tongue that lack filiform papillae and have a raised reddish margin. The duration of desquamation is variable as the areas may heal and then reappear in another area. It is of unknown etiology and the patient should be reassured that therapy is not necessary. Another tongue complaint is the hairy tongue; the elongated brown, black, or white papillae are discolored because of microorganisms. Burning or pain of the tongue may be noted by the individual. Although the etiology is uncertain, smoking, nutritional deficiencies, and poor oral hygiene have been linked to the development of hairy tongue. Aggressive dental hygiene composed of brushing the tongue with hydrogen peroxide several times a day may eliminate this unpleasant disorder.

Tongue Carcinoma. Cancer of the tongue is usually seen in older males; however, it is also seen in young males and females as a result of increasing numbers of tobacco and alcohol users. Poor dental/oral hygiene, smoking, chewing tobacco, and alcohol use are associated with squamous-cell carcinoma, the most common histology type of tongue cancer. Eisele et al. (1995) note the most prevalent site is the lateral border of the tongue; however, other areas may be involved. Early presenting signs and symptoms can include a painless ulceration or local thickening of the tongue. Otalgia, weight loss, dysphagia, and a palpable mass in the neck are signs of aggressive disease as decribed by Meyers and Meyers (1998). Tumor-spread to the cervical lymph nodes occurs in approximately 40% of tongue carcinomas (Eisele et al., 1995).

Treatment of tongue carcinoma is based upon tumor location, size, and the presence of metastatic involvement of neck lymph nodes. Radiation therapy and surgical resection are the two treatment modalities offered. Rehabilitation for speech and swallowing function is crucial for these patients.

Torus Palatinus and Torus Mandibularis

Torus palatinus and torus mandibularis are exostosis (benign bony growths), singular or multiple, located on the midline of the hard palate or mandible. They usually do not present any discomfort to the patient, and reassurance that it is not a malignant process should be communicated to the individual. Surgical excision is not necessary unless denture fitting is affected.

Ludwig's Angina

Ludwig's angina (LA) is an acute cellulitis originating at the floor of the mouth, involving the submandibular, submental, and sublingual spaces. *Streptococci* and anaerobes are two of the microorganisms often identified in this acute process. Edema of the oral cavity prompts excessive drooling and trismus, and the tongue is pushed posteriorly to create an obstructed airway. Etiologies linked to Ludwig's angina include dental infections and tooth extractions. Protection and maintenance of the patient's airway is of paramount concern and a tracheostomy may be necessary because of rapidly progressing edema. Incision and drainage of the abscess should be considered. A course of intravenous antibiotics with either penicillin or clindamycin should be given. Culture and sensitivity results will guide appropriate antibiotic therapy.

Tonsillitis

Tonsillitis is an inflammation of the palatine tonsils caused by either bacterial or viral microorganisms (Figs. 50–13 and 50–14). Beta–hemalytic *streptococcus* group A is the most commonly identified pathogen; *staphylcoccus aureus* and *H influenzae* have also been recognized (Fairbanks, 1996). The infection may either be acute or chronic in nature.

Symptoms include dysphagia, malaise, odynophagia, and referred otolagia. Pyrexia is present and may lead to febrile convulsions in young children. The tonsils are edematous and reddened; a yellow or white exudate may be present. Bilateral lymphadenopathy of the cervical nodes usually occurs.

There is much controversy regarding the need for and timing of a tonsillectomy and adenoidectomy. Differential diagnosis of diptheria, infectious mononucleosis, and scarlet fever, to name a few, should be considered as they have similar patient presentation. Many otolaryngologists utilize the following guidelines for determining surgery for tonsillitis: recurrent episodes of at least three a year for 3 years, five episodes each year for 2 years, seven or more episodes in 1 year, or 10 days absent from work or school in 1 year (Brodsky, 1998; Jones, 1995). Other indicators for tonsillectomy and adenoidectomy include obstructive sleep apnea, upper airway obstruction secondary to adenotonsillar hypertrophy, and peritonsillar abscess. Medical treatment is antibiotics, with pencillin (250-500 mg every 6 hours) being the drug of choice. Consider Augmentin (500 or 875 mg every 12 hours) or clindamycin (150-450 mg every 6 hours) for resistant pathogens.

Peritonsillar Abscess. A serious complication of tonsillitis is the development of a peritonsillar abscess (Quinsy). Pus formation between the tonsil capsule and its upper pole creates a bulge of the tonsil and edema of the anterior pillars, soft palate, and uvula. It is usually unilateral. The patient has extreme difficulty and pain with swallowing; referred otolagia and severe trismus may also result.

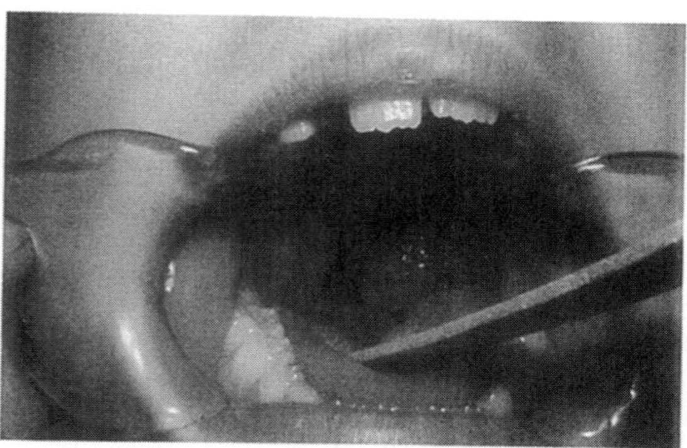

Figure 50–13. Enlarged tonsil. *(Used with permission from Sigler & Schuring. [1993].)*

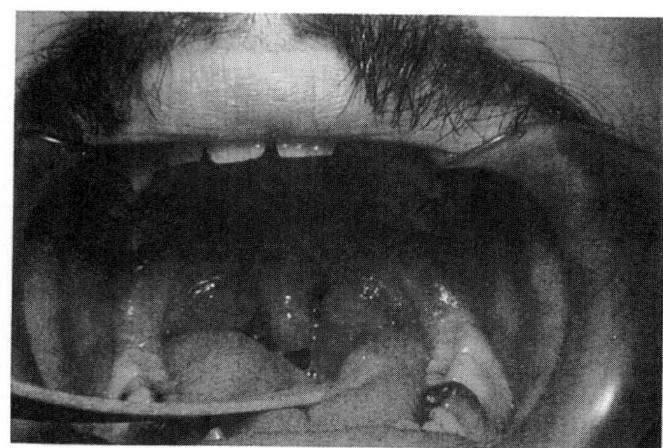

Figure 50–14. Chronic tonsillitis. *(Used with permission from Sigler & Schuring. [1993].)*

Treatment consists of immediate incision and drainage (I&D) of the abscess with concurrent administration of antibiotics (penicillin; if allergic, consider clindamycin). Studies evaluated by Savolainen, Jousimies-Somer, Makitie, & Ylikoski (1993) favored needle aspiration over I&D of the abscess with 80 to 90% effectiveness and less trauma to the patient. A tonsillectomy may also be undertaken at the immediate time or when the acute infection has been treated. Saltwater gargles and appropriate pain medication should also be part of the plan. Complications of a peritonsillar abscess include airway obstruction, dehydration, aspiration, deep neck abscess, jugular vein thrombosis, expanding mediastinitis, endocarditis, and glomerulonephritis (Epperly & Wood, 1990; Hall, 1990).

Pharyngitis. Pharyngitis, inflammation of the pharyngeal walls, may also extend to the tonsils, palate, and uvula. It is manifested by complaints of odynophagia (sore throat), dysphagia, malaise, and fever. Viral, bacterial, and fungal pathogens responsible include beta–hemolytic *streptococci, Neisseria gonorrhoeae,* and *Candida albicans.*

Physical fndings specific to pathogen type are well described by Bonilla & Bluestone (1995). They note that ulcerative lesions with nonexudative pharyngeal erythema implies a viral etiology (infectious mononucleosis should be ruled out). Streptococcal infections demonstrate tonsillar enlargement possibly with exudate, erythema, and petechiae at the soft palate. Creamy mucosal plaques on the pharynx are suggestive of fungal involvement.

Predisposing factors of smoking, recurrent sinusitis or tonsillitis, and gastroesophageal reflux may be identified during patient history. The winter season is the peak incidence for pharyngitis (Bonilla & Bluestone, 1995). The practitioner should be aware of the risk of rheumatic fever when diagnosing pharyngitis.

Cultures obtained of pharyngeal exudate distinguish streptococcal versus nonstreptococcal infections. A monospot test should be performed if infectious mononucleosis is suspected. The culture results dictate specific antibiotic coverage. Penicillin may begin empirically for a 7- to 10-day course. Those allergic to penicillin can be treated with cephalosporins or erythromycin. (It should be noted that copathogens may require broader coverage.) Biaxin (250-500 mg twice daily) and Lorabid (200-400 mg every 12 hours) are good choices but expensive. If a fungus is diagnosed, oral preparations such as nystatin, ketoconazole, and flucanzole can be used. Elimination of irritants and allergens, and proper treatment of underlying medical conditions are necessary in the management of pharyngitis. Analgesics, increased fluid intake, pharyngeal irrigations directed towards the posterior oropharynx, and humidification are adjunctive therapies.

Oropharyngeal Carcinoma. Cancer of the oropharynx includes the specific sites of tonsil, pharyngeal wall, soft palate, and base of tongue. The most common histology cell type is squamous-cell carcinoma (Eisele et al., 1995). Similar to oral cavity malignancies, oropharyngeal tumors are linked to smoking and alcohol consumption (Sigler & Schuring, 1993). These tumors tend to be large in size before they are identified as malignant. A unilateral tonsillar enlargement or ulceration may be the first indicator of oropharyngeal cancer. Dysphagia, globus sensation, and unilateral otolagia are typical physical complaints. Trismus may be apparent. Spread to regional lymph nodes in the neck is frequent with retropharyngeal and jugular nodes identified by Eisele et al. (1995) are common sites of involvement. CT and MRI scans provide the practitioner with crucial information for staging of the tumor and in formulating a treatment plan. Radiation therapy and surgical resection are the two therapies currently employed for oropharyngeal malignancies. Extensive reconstruction with pedicled flaps and microvascular tissue transfer is often required.

Zenker's Diverticulum. Zenker's diverticulum is the outpouching of the submucosa and mucosal layers of the hypopharynx. The etiology of this disorder focuses on the uncoordination of the cricopharyngeus muscle in relation to the inferior pharyngeal constrictor muscle. High intraluminal pressures at the level of the cricopharyngeus cause herniation of the mucosa.

Symptoms experienced by the individual are dysphagia, regurgitation of undigested food, and chronic aspiration usually occurring at night in a supine position. The diagnosis is confirmed by a barium swallow demonstrating a diverticulum at the neck (Schild & Snow, 1996). Esophagscopy may also be performed to rule out a malignancy, but extreme care is required as perforation of the sac can occur.

The age of the patient, the extent of dysphagia, and the size and location of the diverticula are key issues in determining the plan of treatment. Conservative medical management with antireflux medications (H2 blockers and proton pump inhibitors) and avoidance of postprandial reclining may be attempted prior to performing a surgical resection with excision of the sac for Zenker's diverticulum and a cricopharyngeal myotomy.

Laryngeal Disorders

Epiglottitis

Epiglottitis is an acute inflammation and localized infection of the supraglottic larynx, including the epiglottis, aryepiglottic folds, and arytenoids. *Haemophilus influenzae* type B is generally the causative pathogen (Wurtele, 1990); however, others have been identified. The incidence of this potentially life-threatening disorder in the adult population is 1/100,000 per annum (Carey, 1996). Due to the immmunization of children, the incidence has dramatically decreased in children during the past few years.

The adult patient with epiglottitis may exhibit severe dysphagia, odynophagia (pain with swallowing), a muffled ("hot potato") voice, and fever. These symptoms and the onset of dyspnea progressively worsen within in 48 to 72 hours, prompting emergent intervention as complete airway obstruction can result.

Physical examination of the individual reveals a bright red, edematous epiglottis causing obstruction of the pharynx at the tongue base. The most frequent physical findings reported by Fontanarosa, Polsky, & Goldman (1989) were anterior cervical adenopathy, mild respiratory distress, and excessive salivation. If the airway is stable, then indirect visualization is possible. Using a fiberoptic nasopharyngoscope will also provide safe visual assessment. Obtaining a lateral x-ray of the soft tissues of the neck is also warranted with widening of the epiglottis noted.

Appropriate emergency personnel (including the services of otolaryngology and anesthesiologist) and equipment need to be available as the presence of acute airway distress requires immediate action to stabilize the airway. Nasotrachial intubation, cricothyroidectomy, or tracheotomy may be needed. Close observation in an intensive care setting is recommended for the stable patient. The patient should be positioned with the head of the bed elevated. Inhaled mist via face mask or face tent and adequate hydration are important in treating epiglottis.

Blood cultures obtained during the initial diagnostic evaluation should guide antibiotic therapy. Broad-spectrum antibiotics Cefuroxime and Ampicillin/sulbactam are good choices against the influenza pathogen. Steroids may be considered to reduce edema and inflammation.

Resolution of epiglottis typically occurs within 3 to 5 days. Direct laryngoscopy showing a decrease of epiglottic edema will guide the timing of extubation. The patient should be instructed to follow-up with the involved otolaryngologist.

Acute Laryngitis

Most cases of acute laryngitis are caused by a viral infection of the upper respiratory tract. The resulting edema causes improper closure of the vocal cords, thereby producing hoarseness. This inflammation may also result in throat pain and difficulty in swallowing. Indirect laryngoscopy reveals vocal cords that are edematous and erythematous. Acute laryngitis is usually of short duration and management consists of avoidance of irritants (e.g., smoking), voice rest, and humidification. Whispering is discouraged as it causes strain at the vocal cord level. Soft speech is encouraged.

Chronic Laryngitis/Vocal Cord Nodules

An individual with hoarseness persisting more than a few weeks should be assessed for chronic laryngitis. It may result from excessive voice use as with singers or teachers, cigarette smoking, or chronic upper airway infection. Gastroesophageal reflux disease can also create laryngeal irritation. The voice is consistently hoarse and tires readily. The patient may complain of a sore throat with persistent throat clearing. Diffuse thickening of the cords with minimal to no erythema are present upon laryngoscopy exam.

Vocal cord nodules present as benign lesions at the junction of the anterior and middle thirds of the true vocal cords. Initially they may appear red, soft, and edematous, subsequently developing into white fibrous thick nodules. They are the result of repeated voice overuse, misuse, or abuse.

Treatment includes the previously mentioned therapies for acute laryngitis. Emphasis should be placed on the cessation of smoking if it is a predisposing factor. H2 blockers and antireflux medications are part of the medical management. Speech therapy is recommended for patients with improper voice production. Video stroboscopy of the larynx can further define specific areas of disease and assist the otolaryngologist and speech therapist in planning treatment. Surgical excision and laser therapy may be warranted for removal of vocal cord nodules if medical treatment is unsuccessful. Surgical intervention is only successful if the vocal misuse is addressed.

Laryngeal Trauma

Trauma to the larynx can occur as a result of blunt or penetrating injury to the anterior neck. Blunt injury may go unnoticed in the initial trauma evaluation as other more obvious injuries are treated. Assessment of the patient airway including the presence of hoarseness or stridor may indicate damage to the larynx. The patient may complain of dysphagia, odynophagia, neck pain, and dyspnea. Hemoptysis, stridor, and cough may also be evident.

Palpation of the neck should be exercised cautiously as further injury to the larynx and surrounding structures can happen. Edema and subcutaneous emphysema cause distortion of the neck, and the presence of crepitus and tenderness over the larynx strongly suggest a laryngeal fracture (Schaefer, 1998).

Indirect and direct laryngoscopy confirm the diagnosis of laryngeal trauma by revealing edema and ecchymosis. Cartilage fragments, bleeding, and lacerations may be evident. Radiographic films of the neck and chest should be undertaken to detail fractures, tracheal injury, hematoma, and pneumothorax. A CT scan can further differentiate a hyoid fracture, laryngeal fractures, and dislocation of thyroid and cricoid cartilages. Yet all evaluation is first dependent on airway stabilization.

Treatment of laryngeal trauma centers on stabilizing the patient's airway. If obstruction and distress are present, a tracheotomy is necessary. Further surgical intervention may also be required to repair fractures and lacerations. Schaefer (1998) provides a detailed protocol for acute laryngeal trauma containing surgical interventions. Medical management of the individual suffering from blunt soft-tissue injuries without fracture or airway obstruction should include humidified air, voice rest, bed rest with the head of bed elevated, and the administration of steroids. These measures decrease the laryngeal edema and slow the progression of subcutaneous emphysema and hematoma formation.

Vocal Cord Paralysis

Vocal cord paralysis (VCP) is a result of injury to the recurrent laryngeal nerve or vagus nerve that innervates the laryngeal muscles allowing for vocal cord movement. A common cause of VCP is direct trauma to the nerve during thyroid or cardiac surgery. Other etiologies are tumors of the skull base, thyroid gland, esophagus, and lung; viral infections; and degenerative neurological disorders. Terris, Arnstein, & Nguyen (1992) reviewed eight series of unilateral vocal cord paralysis and found over one third of the 1019 cases examined were related to neoplasms. However, there may be no identifiable cause deeming it as an idiopathic paralysis.

The individual presents with a breathy voice as a result of air escaping caused by inadequate closure of the glottis. Aspiration, especially of liquids, may occur. This may be severe in high vagal injuries as sensation is lost by denervation of the superior laryngeal nerve. If the paralysis is unilateral, the opposite vocal cord compensates by moving medially. Bilateral VCP poses the risk of airway obstruction and recurrent pneumonia secondary to chronic aspiration as the size of the airway is significantly diminished (Fig. 50–15).

The diagnosis of VCP is obtained by a thorough history taking and head and neck examination. Visualization of the vocal cords will show paralysis of the cord(s) (Fig. 50–16). A chest x-ray and CT/MRI scans of the head, neck, and chest may assist in the diagnosis. Consultation with an

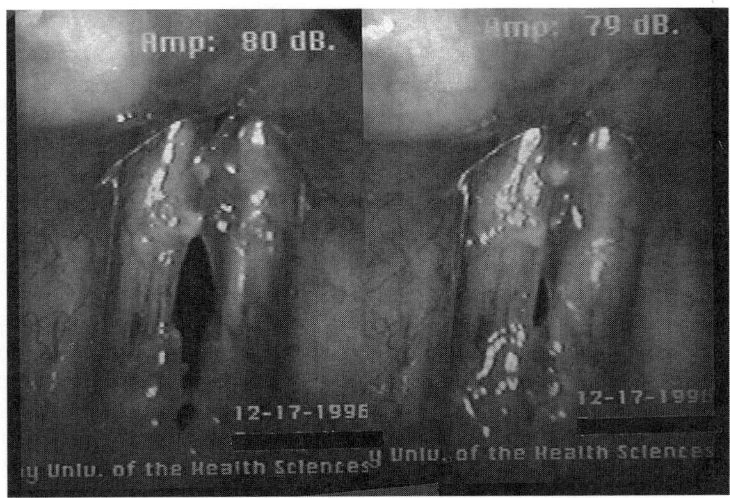

Figure 50–15. Diffuse thickening of bilateral vocal cords. This thickening may be a precursor to vocal cord nodules. *(Used with permission. Courtesy of Deschler, D. G. [1996].)*

otolaryngologist may lead to an endoscopic evaluation providing direct examination of the larynx, bronchioles, and esophagus. A videostroboscopy effectively demonstrating the asymmetry may also be undertaken to assess VCP.

Treatment of VCP is dependent on whether it is unilateral or bilateral, degree of symptoms, and etiology of loss. The individual with idiopathic VCP may be observed for up to one year prior to intervention, anticipating possible resolution. According to Hoffman, McCulloch, & Victoria (1998), voice therapy with a speech pathologist as a primary modality of treatment versus surgery is controversial. They do advocate speech therapy postsurgical repair and for those who are unable to undergo surgical intervention. Operative procedures for VCP include injection of the affected vocal cord with Teflon to augment the cord's mass, providing medialization. Another alternative is thyroplasty which provides direct medial movement of the paralyzed vocal cord. In cases of bilateral vocal cord paralysis, the emphasis is on protection and rehabilitation of the airway foremost, followed by definitive surgery for restoration of adequate voice.

Laryngeal Carcinoma

Cancers of the larynx account for approximately 2% of all malignancies (Goodman, 1990). Squamous-cell carcinoma is the most common cell type. Precipitating factors associated with laryngeal cancer include heavy cigarette smoking, excessive alcohol consumption, and exposure to

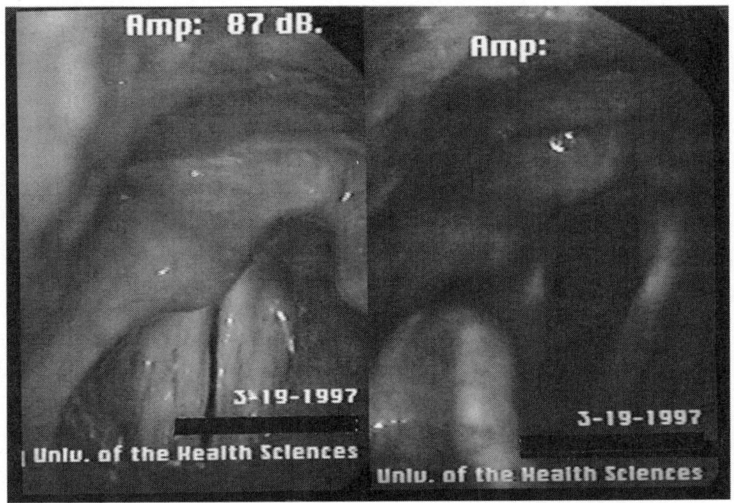

Figure 50–16. Right vocal cord paralysis. The right vocal cord (seen on the left side of the photo) is paralyzed. Note the decreased closure of the cord compared with the left cord. *(Used with permission. Courtesy of Deschler, D. G. [1997].)*

asbestos, wood dusts, and radiation (Gosselin, Gullane, & Irish, 1995).

The location of the tumor defines patient symptoms and determines the prognosis and management of the lesion. The supraglottic region is composed of the epiglottis, ventricular folds, arytenoid cartilages, and the aryepiglottic folds. This area has a rich lymphatic drainage system allowing early tumor spread to the neck. A supraglottic lesion may grow rather large before symptoms of dysphagia and odynophagia appear. If spread to the adjacent pharynx occurs, referred ear pain can be a frequent complaint.

Tumors of the glottic region—specifically, the true vocal cords and anterior commissure—tend to demonstrate early hoarseness or voice change. Metastasis occurs later because of lack of significant lymph drainage, allowing for improved prognosis of glottic cancer.

The subglottic area of the larynx (below the vocal cords) may produce less hoarseness; however, airway obstruction is of great concern. Bilateral neck lymph nodes are at high risk for tumor involvement from the subglottis.

Any individual with prolonged hoarseness (longer than 2 weeks) should be examined for suspicion of a laryngeal cancer. Palpation of the neck and larynx may reveal a mass or lymphadenopathy. Laryngeal exam by indirect laryngoscopy is required. Biopsy may be warranted. Radiographic imaging with a CT or MRI will further define location and possible extension of tumor. A chest x-ray is mandatory to assess for possible metastasis to the chest or a second primary tumor.

As stated earlier, staging of laryngeal carcinomas should direct therapy with the goals of tumor ablation for cure and restoration of function. Radiation therapy and surgery may each be considered as the primary modality of treatment for early glottic and supraglottic cancers. Subglottic cancers and advanced glottic/supraglottic cases will usually require more aggressive combined therapies (Sobol, Martini, & Har-El, 1993). Speech rehabilitation is important and achievable in this patient population and there has been great progress in providing the patient with functional speech.

Hypopharyngeal Carcinoma

Malignant tumors of the hypopharynx involve the pyriform fossa, posterior pharyngeal walls, and the postcricoid area of the larynx. The etiology and epidemiology are similar to oropharyngeal and laryngeal cancers. Because of the location of the tumor, the patient may manifest symptoms late in the disease process. Weight loss as a result of odynophangnia and dysphagia occurs. Voice changes become apparent and referred otolagia with locally advanced disease may present.

Diagnosis is achieved with endoscopic examination and biopsy. Combined therapy of radiation and surgery is usually contemplated early as Sobol et al. (1993) note the prognosis for hypopharyngeal carcinoma is poor as compared with laryngeal tumors.

Salivary Gland Disorders

Acute Sialoadenitis

Acute sialoadenitis is an acute inflammation of the submandibular or parotid gland leading to pain, overlying erythema, and swelling of the gland. Complaints of pain and tenderness, especially with eating, are common. Postsurgical, posttrauma, immunocompromised, and dehydrated patients have been identified to be at risk for developing acute sialoadenitis (Nadol, 1983b). It has also been associated with Sjorgen syndrome and has occurred as a result of radiation therapy and chemotherapy (Shemen, 1995). The common childhood disease of mumps is a viral infection of the parotid glands with bilateral involvment in up to 70% of incidents (Sobol, Lanza, & Har-El, 1993).

Staphylococcus aureus is the most frequent microorganism identified; however, other pathogens (*Mycobacterium tuberculosis* and *Streptococcus pneumoniae*) have been found in saliva cultures according (Shemen, 1995). Antibiotic therapy should be initiated promptly using an agent sensitive to gram-positive organisms. Ampicillin is a good choice with clindamycin or vancomycin considered for those allergic to penicillins.

Other therapies involve symptomatic and supportive actions such as warm compresses, use of sialogogues (substances increasing saliva production, such as lemon drops), good oral hygiene, and aggressive rehydration. Abscess formation can result from continued and progressive acute inflammation of the salivary glands requiring incision and drainage of the loculated areas of infection. Carroll & Wolf (1996) recommend excision of the gland for recurrent episodes of sialadenitis.

Sialolithiasis

Salivary calculi/sialolithiasis usually tend to develop in the submandibular gland followed by the parotid gland. Over 90% of cases of sialolithiasis involve the submandibular gland (Kretzschmar & Kretzschmar, 1996). The formation of calculi is a result of insipiated secretions obstructing the gland duct. This obstruction causes diminished salivary flow producing painful swelling of the gland, which worsens with eating. The patient may report extrusion of pieces of the calculi from the duct. Manual palpation of the salivary gland may reveal the presence of a stone or expression of pus. Sobol, Lanza, and Har-El (1996) report dental radiographic films may distinguish some stones; however, a CT scan is a more specific study.

Treatment of sialolithiasis consists of dilation of the duct and manual removal of the stone. For more difficult cases, surgical excision of the gland may be contemplated, dependent on the frequency of episodes and the patient's symptoms and discomfort.

Salivary Gland Tumors

Salivary gland neoplasms may be benign or malignant, with the parotid gland accounting for over 70% of all salivary tumors followed by the minor glands and the submandibular gland (Shemen, 1995). There is a greater chance of malignancy in the submandibular gland versus the parotid gland where benign lesions number 80 to 90% of all neoplasms (Kiener, 1992).

Fine-needle aspiration biopsy of the lesion may help determine tumor histology; however, it is not without risk to the facial nerve. The use of imaging scans provides valuable information regarding determination of cystic or solid mass, and possible lymph node involvement.

Two of the more common benign tumors are pleomorphic adenoma (benign mixed tumor) and papillary cystadenoma lymphomatosum (Warthin's tumor). They are slow growing, painless, nontender tumors that tend to arise in the posterior or tail of the parotid gland. Complete surgical excision of pleomorphic tumors with removal of a surrounding border of normal tissue is advocated, as there is a propensity for recurrence. Carroll & Wolf (1996) note recurrence rates averaging 30% with simple tumor removal. Excision of these tumors should be accomplished by a superficial parotidectomy and facial nerve dissection. Rare transformation of this tumor to an aggressive neoplasm similar to a malignancy is possible.

Papillary cystadenoma lymphomatosum usually affects elderly men and can present as bilateral multiple masses of the parotid tail. A nuclear medicine scan with Technetium isotope may demonstrate a bright area indicative of a Warthin's tumor. Surgical excision is generally the treatment of choice.

Malignant tumors of salivary glands have similar characteristics as benign lesions; however, because of the aggressive enlargement of the tumor, pain and facial nerve impairment may be evident. The most common malignancy (especially of the parotid gland) is the mucoepidermoid carcinoma with low- and high-grade histology types. According to Carroll & Wolf (1996), low grade is slow growing with neural invasion rare, while high-grade tumor shows more atypia. It behaves aggressively with spread to regional lymph nodes, and metastases to distant sites is not uncommon with the high-grade type. Facial nerve involvement may require sacrifice of nerve branches for total eradication of the parotid neoplasm.

Adenoid cystic carcinoma is the most common of minor salivary gland tumors. Perineural invasion can occur with pain and decreased sensation (hypesthesia) experienced, as well as facial spasm with possible facial nerve paralysis. Local recurrences and distant metastases may occur many years after initial diagnosis of adenoid cystic tumors and long-term survival is possible with systemic spread (Carroll & Wolf, 1996; Kiener, 1992).

Other salivary gland neoplasms include pleomorphic adenomas that have undergone malignant degeneration. Adenocarcinoma, acinic cell carcinoma, and lymphoma account for a smaller percentage of salivary tumors. Primary squamous-cell carcinoma of the parotid gland is infrequent, as metastatic lymph node involvement of the gland is more common and should be investigated. The treatment should involve dissection of the affected neck with the parotidectomy.

Treatment options for parotid gland tumors involve performing a superficial parotidectomy to avert facial nerve injury or a deep lobe complete parotidectomy for more involved tumor growth of benign or malignant cell type. Sacrifice of the facial nerve may be necessary because of tumor type and nerve involvement. Radiation therapy after a parotidectomy is performed for aggressive malignant neoplasms with lymph node involvement and recurrent benign lesions.

The prognosis of salivary gland tumor is dependent on histology and tumor grade. Parotid malignancies have better survival rates versus minor salivary gland tumors (Shemen, 1995).

Neck Masses

The patient who presents with a neck mass presents a diagnostic challenge to the practitioner. A thorough understanding of the anatomical structures of the neck is necessary to provide the framework for formulating and ultimately confirming a medical diagnosis. A review of the neck anatomy section presented earlier in this chapter is suggested.

A complete history and physical examination provide the basis for a working diagnosis. The age of the individual can also guide the practitioner in formulating a diagnosis, as benign lymphadenopathy is more common in children than adults (Moloy, 1992). The patient should be asked about his or her symptoms in a detailed and organized manner to avoid confusion regarding the patient complaint and presentation. Questions regarding previous or family history of cancer and use of alcohol, drugs, and smoking should be included in the initial assessment. Symptoms associated with malignant neck masses—including referred otolagia, change in voice, dysphagia, odynophagia, difficulty with breathing, and weight loss—also need to be explored.

The differential diagnosis of neck masses can be generally categorized as inflammatory, congenital, or neoplastic (benign and malignant). Location of the neck mass is crucial with regard to etiology. The more common disorders seen in an acute care setting will be presented as the list of possible diagnoses is quite extensive.

Inflammatory Process

Lymphadenopathy of the neck related to an acute inflammatory process may present as a painful, tender, erythematous mass that arises in a relatively short time. The cervical lymph nodes are typically affected. Bilateral involvement may also occur. An elevated temperature is not common, especially with children. Specific diagnoses include bacterial and viral infections (i.e., pharyngitis, mononucleosis, tuberculosis, cat scratch disease). Predominant microorganisms are *Staph auereus* and *Strep pyogenes* (Fairbanks, 1996). Antibiotic therapy can be initiated with supportive measures for pyrexia, pain management, and malaise.

Persistent cervical lymphadenopathy (with rubbery consistency to the nodes) lasting more than a few weeks may be a result of systemic disease such as toxoplasmos, tuberculosis, human immunodeficiency virus (HIV), and syphilis. Corresponding serologic and skin testing can be performed to establish the infectious agent. Histologic examination of the neck mass may also be required as is the case of sarcoidosis. (A chest x-ray with bilateral hilar adenopathy assists in this diagnosis.) The plan of care is based upon the disease process and associated symptoms.

Congenital Masses

Branchial cleft cysts, thyroglossal duct cysts, and dermoid cysts constitute the majority of congenital neck masses as noted by Moloy (1992). These anomalies differ in location and presentation, and may not manifest as a concern until adulthood.

Branchial cleft cysts are characterized as a cystic mass derived from incomplete embryologic development of the neck. These cysts are typically found at the anterior border of the sternocleidomastoid muscle; the auricular regions are less frequent sites (Lanza, Nash, Sobol, & Har-El, 1993). Infection of the cyst causes an increase in size and, if a fistula or sinus tract is involved, drainage at the neck may be evident. Treatment consists of antibiotic therapy. Incision and drainage of the cyst should be avoided. Lanza et al. (1993) state surgical excision with removal of any sinus tract as the favored plan, as these cysts are prone to cause recurrent infection.

Thyroglossal duct cysts, also a result of embryologic malformation, are located at the midline of the neck between the base of the tongue and the sternal notch. They may be palpable on bimanual examination. The act of swallowing causes the cyst to move in a vertical upward direction. Surgical removal of the cyst, accompanying duct, and a portion of the hyoid bone should be performed after any acute infection has been treated. A preoperative thyroid scan should be performed to assess location of thyroid tissue. Malignancy of the thyroglossal cyst duct is also a concern; papillary and squamous-cell carcinomas have been reported (Rowe, 1996).

Dermoid cysts usually appear at the submental region and at the midline of the neck. They may be cystic or solid upon palpation and are stationary with swallowing. Children typically present most often with a dermoid cyst and an excisional biopsy should be performed for its removal.

Neoplastic Masses

Benign. Benign tumors of the neck include lipomas and sebaceous cysts that are typically soft, spongy masses at the subcutaneous level and are nonadherent to other structures. Neck masses that originate from a neural source can cause symptoms of nerve compression along the neck or associated cranial nerve dysfunction. Neurofibromas, schwannomas, and neurilemmomas are difficult to diagnose prior to excision as noted by Schuller & Schleuning (1994) and resection of the involved nerve may be necessary.

Paraganliomas (previously described as glomus tumors) can develop from numerous sites of the head and neck region. A painless mass at the carotid bifurcation that is slow growing is suggestive of a carotid body tumor. An audible bruit may be appreciated. Vagal body tumors originate near the skull base adjacent to the inferior ganglion of the vagus. They may also be pulsatile. Vocal cord paralysis may be evident. Impairment of carotid blood flow can contribute to syncopal episodes.

Diagnostic work-up of a paraganglioma includes a CT scan or MRI with possible arteriography of both carotids, as Kmucha & Lee (1995) note there is a familial tendency of multiple tumors. The tumor size of paragangliomas may require embolization prior to definitive surgical resection. Recurrent cases may undergo further resection or radiation therapy may be considered. Malignant paragangliomas are rare.

Malignant. An isolated, firm neck mass discovered in an adult should be considered as a malignant metastatic lymph node until proven otherwise (Fig. 50–17). This general statement is based upon knowledge of the lymphatic system and correlation with primary sites of malignancy of the head and neck. The importance of a thorough head and neck examination coupled with detailed history taking (with an emphasis on social habits) is crucial to initiating

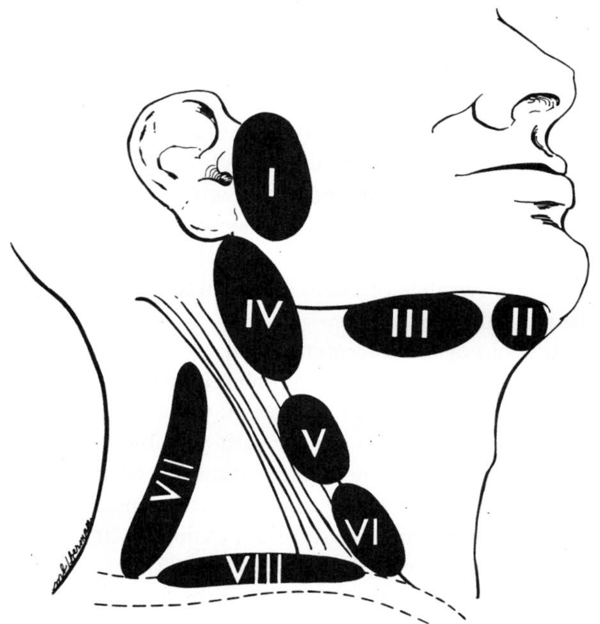

Figure 50–17. Major lymph node groups in the head and neck. *(Used with permission from American Academy of Otolaryngology, Head and Neck Surgery Foundation [1992].)*

appropriate management of the patient who presents with a neck mass.

A thorough work-up should be performed to assess for the possibility of concurrent disease, such as tuberculosis or cancer of the lung, breast, thyroid, or esophagus. The transplant population and those immunosuppressed may be at increased risk for development of cancer, possibly presenting with a neck mass.

Radiographic imaging with the use of a CT scan with contrast and/or MRI is extremely useful, demonstrating location and size of the mass and relationship to other structures of the head and neck. A chest x-ray should be completed in the preliminary work-up for a neck mass.

There should be no attempt to excise or biopsy a suspicious lymph node until a primary source is found, as seeding of the cancer cells may result with subsequent poor prognosis (Nadol, 1983a). Expedient referral to an otolaryngologist is recommended for a further detailed diagnostic work-up. This evaluation includes performing a panendoscopy, which enables the specialist to visualize the nasopharynx, oropharynx, larynx, bronchi, and esophagus. Biopsies can be obtained, the tumor properly staged, and appropriate therapy instigated. A fine-needle aspiration may also be useful.

Metastatic squamous-cell carcinoma is the most common cause of a malignant neck tumor in adults (Kmucha & Lee, 1995). Other histologic pathologies include adenocarcinoma, melanoma, lymphoma, and undifferentiated carcinoma.

All of these cancers—with the exception of lymphomas—are managed in a similar fashion. If a primary tumor site has been identified in the work-up, then the treatment plan is focused on tumor ablation. Surgical dissection of the neck is also advocated, allowing the neck mass to be removed in a composite fashion. Radiation therapy may be delivered to the primary site and involved areas of the neck as an adjunct to surgery or as primary therapy. An unknown primary tumor with involvement of neck lymph nodes requires a panendoscopy and biopsy of tonsil, nasopharynx, vallecula, piriform sinus, and vocal cord to rule out a primary site. The unknown neck tumor is treated by surgical dissection of the neck followed by radiation therapy.

Lymphomas of the neck are the most common malignant tumors in children (Lanza et al., 1993). Patients with acquired immunodeficiency syndrome (AIDS) are also at risk for lymphomas. As this is a disease of the lymphoid tissue, surgery beyond a biopsy of the neck for definitive diagnosis is not considered. Referral to a hematologist/oncologist for planning of radiation therapy and/or chemotherapy is necessary.

Neuroblastomas are a neurogenic soft-tissue tumor detected most often in children as metastasis from other body sites (Kmucha & Lee, 1995). However, the head and neck may be the primary site. It is an aggressive behaving malignancy with poor patient survival. Combined multimodality therapy of surgery, radiation therapy, and chemotherapy is considered in the treatment of neuroblastomas.

The causes of neck masses are numerous and a limited number of diagnoses have been presented in this chapter. Guidelines to follow include performing a complete head and neck examination, obtaining a thorough patient history, and ordering appropriate diagnostic laboratory blood tests and radiographic scans. Consultation with an otolaryngologist and a head-and-neck surgeon is always appropriate given the possibility of metastatic malignant disease.

Thyroid Disorders

Evaluation of the patient with a thyroid mass requires basic knowledge of common disorders of the thyroid, their associated signs and symptoms, and interpretation of diagnostic thyroid studies. It is beyond the scope of this chapter to present a complete discussion of thyroid function tests. The practitioner is advised to consult LoPresti's (1996) article detailing laboratory tests for thyroid disorders for a comprehensive review. Patient management may require a multispecialty approach with participation of an endocrinologist and head-and-neck surgeon.

Thyroid masses may be either benign or malignant. Females have a higher incidence of thyroid disease including cancer, according to Dobleman and Bumsted (1992). However, they note there is a greater chance of malignancy in males. An individual who has received radiation as a child is at higher risk for development of thyroid cancer.

Signs and symptoms of a thyroid mass are similar regardless of histology type. The patient may complain of a painless neck mass, dysphagia, hoarseness, odynophagia, and sensation of a lump in the throat. Symptoms of airway distress can occur if the mass extends into the retrosternal or intrathoracic regions causing tracheal compression. There may also be evidence of esophageal compression. Palpation of the gland may reveal a single mass or multiple nodules. Pain upon palpation is not common; however, inflammation of the gland may cause the patient to complain (Farwell & Braverman, 1996). A hard, firm thyroid nodule is suspicious for a malignancy, while soft cyst-like nodules are more representative of benign disease. Careful examination of the neck may reveal associated lymphadenopathy, increasing the likelihood of thyroid cancer.

The patient should be questioned and assessed regarding possible associated symptoms and signs of hypothyroidism and hyperthyroidism. The diagnostic evaluation of a thyroid mass includes appropriate blood tests. Subclinical cases of hypo- and hyperthyroidism may not demonstrate appreciable changes in serum levels of thyroid hormones (Sreenivas & Kadambi, 1995).

A fine-needle aspiration (FNA) biopsy of the thyroid mass may yield important cytologic histologic information as to whether a malignancy is present. The procedure is 80-90% accurate for histologic diagnosis when performed by experienced practitioners, claims Sobol, Lanza, & Har-El. (1993). The FNA may also reduce the size of the mass if it is cystic in origin.

The use of radionuclide thyroid scans with either radioactive iodine (iodine-123) or technetium pertechnetate (99m Tc) may aid in determining the size, appearance, and position of the mass. Most important, these scans demonstrate the gland's uptake of the radioactive material, thus ascertaining the function of the thyroid tissue.

A "hot" nodule shows increased uptake of the isotope and appears more solid on the scan. These hot nodules are usually hyperfunctioning, benign, and occur less commonly than cold nodules. A thyroid mass that does not show uptake of the isotope is termed a "cold" nodule, is hypofunctioning, and has a higher risk of being malignant. All cold nodules should not be considered malignant, as multiple cold nodules of the thyroid may suggest multinodular goiter.

Ultrasonography of the thyroid gland differentiates whether a mass is solid, cystic, or mixed. A solid or mixed mass is more indicative of a cancer versus a cystic lesion (Dobleman & Bumsted, 1992).

Thyroid Goiter

Thyroid goiter is a general term defining an enlarged thyroid gland. It may be uninodular or multinodular, possibly occurring at multiple sites in the gland. A common theory for nodular goiter development is the increase in thyroid tissue as a result of chronic stimulation of the thyroid stimulating hormone (TSH).

A toxic goiter produces excess thyroid hormone (separate from actions of the hypothalamic–pituitary system) that leads to hyperthyroidism. The development of nontoxic goiter is a result of inadequate production of the thyroid hormone and subsequent increase of TSH by the pituitary gland. Chronic TSH stimulation causing cellular changes in the gland may cause nontoxic goiter to progress to a toxic state.

The etiologies of toxic and nontoxic goiters with relation to the development of hypo- or hyperthyroidism are not fully described in this chapter; however, a general listing of causes of thyroid dysfunction is presented in Table 50–3.

Treatment planning for a thyroid goiter is based upon the results of the diagnostic studies performed and patient presentation. A patient with a toxic hyperthyroid nodule can be treated with antithyroid medication, radioactive iodine, or surgery. The risks and benefits of these therapies need to be fully discussed with the patient to ensure understanding and compliance of treatment.

Antithyroid medications prevent the synthesis of thyroid hormone; two of the most commonly used are propylthiouracil and methimazole. Adjustment of the drug dosage should be considered when euthyroidism is evident, usually in a 4- to 6-week period (Schilling, 1997). Beta blockers such as atenolol and propanolol may be given initially, especially for treatment of symptoms of palpitations and tachycardia.

Radioactive iodine (RAI) therapy may be offered to the patient who refuses surgery or is a poor operative candidate. A thyroid scan is performed to determine appropriate iodine administration and uptake and then an oral dose of radioactive iodine is given. Hypothyroidism is not an uncommon result; therefore, the patient should be educated for the possible need for thyroid replacement therapy. Pregnancy and breastfeeding are two contraindications of RAI therapy. Streff & Pachucki-Hyde (1996) stress women considering conception should be counseled to delay attempts until 6 months after RAI treatment.

The third option for hyperthyroidism/toxic goiter is surgery. A subtotal or near complete thyroidectomy may be performed for individuals who have either refused or failed RAI therapy or antithyroid medications, and women of childbearing age. Those patients with compressive symptoms and concerns regarding physical appearance are also candidates for thyroid surgery.

Nontoxic goiter as evidenced by euthyroid state and benign FNA results may be observed closely with periodic checks of serum TSH levels and palpation of the thyroid. Large or compressive multinodular goiters may require surgical excision.

Thyroiditis

There are various forms of thyroiditis, the inflammation of the thyroid gland. Table 50–4 gives a complete listing. The more commonly encountered disorders of Hashimoto's thyroiditis and subacute lymphocytic thyroiditis will be reviewed here.

Hashimoto's or chronic lymphocytic thyroiditis is the most common form of thyroid inflammation, typically occurring in women (Farwell & Braverman, 1996). Physical

TABLE 50–3. Related Causes of Thyroid Dysfunction

Hypothyroidism	Hyperthyroidism
Iodine deficiency	Graves' disease
Thyroidectomy	Toxic goiter
Hashimoto's thyroiditis	Thyroiditis
Antithyroid medications	Thyroid carcinoma
Radioactive iodine therapy	Amiodarone toxicity
Lithium	Pituitary gland tumors
Hypothalamic disorders	Iodine
Amiodarone toxicity	

TABLE 50–4. Inflammatory Thyroid Disorders

Chronic lymphocytic thyroiditis (Hashimoto)
Subacute granulomatous thyroiditis (de Quervain's disease)
Invasive fibrous thyroiditis (Reidel)
Subacute lymphocytic thyroiditis
Acute suppurative thyroiditis

examination may reveal a goiter that is nontender and firm. It does not usually cause pain. Symptoms of hypothyroidism may be present. High levels of antithyroid antibodies classify this as an autoimmune process. Thyroid hormone replacement therapy is indicated for hypothyroidism. Surgery may be indicated if there is a suspicion of cancer or if compression is evident.

Subacute lymphocytic thyroiditis may be episodic, or more frequently can occur in the postpartum period. A course of hyperthyroidism may be followed by a hypothyroid phase that is usually self-limiting. However, initiation of drug therapy for thyroid dysfunction may be required if the patient's symptoms are acute and protracted.

Benign Thyroid Neoplasm

The follicular adenoma, a benign tumor of the thyroid gland, is distinguished by its shape: round, firm, and encapsulated. The tumor is usually a lone nodule that is hypofunctioning. Pathological changes such as calcification, cystic degeneration, and hemorrhage may occur within the adenoma (Sobol, Lanza, & Har-El, 1993). Surgical removal may be necessary for a follicular adenoma.

Malignant Thyroid Neoplasms

Malignant tumors of the thyroid include follicular, papillary, medullary, and anaplastic carcinomas and lymphoma. A brief description of each cancer is presented to acquaint the practitioner. Refer to an endocrinology or pathology textbook for greater detail.

Follicular carcinoma is a well-differentiated carcinoma that is usually an encapsulated sole tumor. Metastases to the lungs and bone via a hematogenous route can occur.

Papillary cancer, another well-differentiated tumor, is multinodular, nonencapsulated, and the most commonly occurring thyroid malignancy. Sreenivas & Kadambi (1995) note tumor invasion to the lymph nodes and surrounding tissue is a negative prognostic factor. It affects more women than men. If the cancer is well-contained and discovered in its early stages, survival is greatly increased—with 20-year survival greater than 80% as noted by Sobol, Lanza, & Har-El, (1993).

The diagnosis of medullary thyroid carcinoma is validated by an elevated serum calcitonin; stimulation tests of pentagastrin and calcium are also helpful for early diagnosis. Obtaining a complete family history is crucial. There may be a pattern of autosomal dominant inheritancy with associated disorders of multiple endocrine neoplasms (MEN). Lymphatic and hematogenous metastasis demonstrate a poorer prognosis.

MENIIA is classified as medullary carcinoma, hyperplasia of the parathyroid, and pheochromocytoma. MENIIB includes medullary carcinoma, a marfan appearance, pheochromocytomas, multiple neuromas of the mucosa, and ganglioneuromatosis of the gastrointestinal tract.

Medullary carcinoma behaves aggressively, requiring prompt recognition and appropriate referral for surgical intervention with a total thyroidectomy recommended. Radioiodide therapy is not considered as this tumor does not take up the isotope.

Anaplastic carcinoma is an extremely aggressive malignant tumor of the thyroid gland found more typically in the older population. It accounts for less than 10% of malignant thyroid tumors (Hendrix, 1996). Rapid cell division leads to extensive involvement of surrounding structures and subsequent body metastases, possibly causing airway compromise and preventing curative tumor resection. Chemotherapy and radiation therapy may be offered to slow tumor growth. Care should be focused on palliative measures.

Treatment of thyroid cancers focuses on previously discussed therapies of surgery, RAI, and antithyroid medications. External radiation therapy and chemotherapy may also be employed. Tumor histology dictates the plan of care with specific regard to surgical intervention.

Parathyroid Disorders

Disorders of the parathyroid glands may be discovered by the onset and presence of hypoparathyroidism or hyperparathyroidism. The conditions associated with each are covered here as well as diagnostic studies for assessment of parathyroid function.

Hypoparathyroidism

Hypoparathyroidism may develop as a result of injury to the parathyroid gland or to its vascular system. The patient who has undergone thyroid surgery and/or neck exploration is at risk because of the difficulty in identifying the location of the parathyroid and the close association between the parathyroid and thyroid glands.

Symptoms of hypoparathyroidism—such as weakness, paresthesia of the extremities and perioral tissues, anxiety, and fatigue—are directly related to a decrease in ionized calcium. A positive Chvostek's sign (performed by tapping the facial nerve branches to demonstrate irritability) and a positive Trousseau's sign (using a blood pressure cuff or tourniquet to occlude the blood supply of the arm to lead to carpopedal spasm) confirm hypocalcemia.

Treatment of hypoparathyroidism is aimed at normalizing serum calcium levels by the emergent use of intravenous calcium gluconate and with subsequent administration of oral calcium and vitamin D supplements. Maintenance of serum phosphorus levels is also a focus. Long-term monitoring of serum calcium is necessary.

Hyperparathyroidism

There are essentially three types of hyperparathyroidism: primary, secondary, and tertiary as described by Aroesty & Har-El (1993). Excessive parathyroid hormone (PTH) secreted by the gland itself characterizes primary hyperparathyroidism. Secondary hyperparathyroidism is a result of hypocalcemia originating from another disease entity (e.g., renal failure) leading to an increased release of PTH. Tertiary hyperparathyroidism is a prolonged autonomous production of PTH by the parathyroid gland.

Primary hyperparathyroidism is the most common of parathyroid disorders and most frequent cause of hypercalcemia (Rice, 1996). The diagnosis is made by an elevated PTH assay level with associated hypercalcemia. Patient presentation is dependent upon the symptoms and effects of hypercalcemia. A thorough physical examination may reveal subtle physical findings.

The phrase "stones, bones and abdominal groans" appropriately describes this disorder. Symptoms of hyperparathyroidism may be multisystem involving the musculoskeletal (osteoporosis, muscle weakness, bone pain, and fractures), renal (polyuria, nephrolithasis), gastrointestinal (polydipsia, nausea), and neurological (fatigue, diminished or absent deep tendon reflexes, confusion).

Primary Hyperparathyroidism. The principal differential diagnoses of primary hyperparathyroidism are benign adenomas, primary hyperplasia, and parathyroid carcinomas. Benign adenomas of the parathyroid gland represent the majority of cases (Rude, 1996). Confirmation of the diagnosis is obtained by the biopsy results of normal histology of a second pair of parathyroid glands. Unilateral gland enlargement is more suggestive of an adenoma versus multiple glandular enlargement, which is indicative of hyperplasia. Of note, parathyroid hyperplasia is associated with multiple endocrine neoplasia (MEN) syndrome. Carcinoma of the pararthyroid is an uncommon occurrence—an estimated 1% of cases of hyperparathyroidism (Rice, 1996)—identified by higher calcium levels and surgical finding of an enlarged gland adhering to surrounding tissue.

Treatment of hyperparathyroidism is focused on the contributing factors associated with its development, whether it is of primary, secondary, or tertiary origin, and how it has affected the patient's metabolism. Complications of the disorder may determine the need for surgical intervention.

Surgery on the parathyroid glands can be complicated because of their small size and sometimes hidden location in the neck. Preoperative scanning with the use of a MRI or nuclear imaging studies (particularly a technetium Tc 99m sestamibi scan) can be helpful in determining location of the glands and ultimately reducing operative time for the patient.

The information contained in this chapter is by no means inclusive of all disorders of otolaryngology. It is hoped that a framework has been provided for the acute care nurse practitioner to perform an initial assessment and evaluation of individuals who present with a chief complaint or signs and symptoms of a head and neck disorder. Consultation and referral to an otolaryngologist and head-and-neck surgeon is prudent in all clinical situations that require advanced knowledge of head and neck anatomy and physiology, disorders of the region, and the ability to intervene surgically if necessary. Suggested resources are included to direct the practitioner to further resources in the specialty of otolaryngology and head-and-neck surgery.

SUGGESTED RESOURCES AND REFERENCES

1. American Academy of Otolaryngology—Head and Neck Surgery Foundation Inc., One Prince Street, Alexandria, VA 22314.
2. American Cancer Society, National Headquarters, 1599 Clifton Road, NE, Atlanta, GA 30329.
3. Society of Otorhinolaryngology and Head-Neck Nurses, Inc., 116 Canal Street, Suite A, New Smyrna Beach, FL 32168.
4. American Speech–Language–Hearing Association, 10801 Rockville Pike, Rockville, MD 20852.
5. National Institute on Deafness and Other Communication Disorders, 225 Haverford Avenue #1, Narberth, PA 19072.

REFERENCES

Adour, K. K. (1998). Idiopathic facial paralysis. In G. Gates (Ed.), *Current therapy in otolaryngology—head and neck surgery.* (pp. 96–98). St. Louis: Mosby.

American Academy of Otolaryngology, Head and Neck Surgery Foundation. (1992). Common problems of the head and neck region: A manual and guide for management of diseases and injuries in otolaryngology—head and neck surgery (p. 134). Philadelphia: W. B. Saunders.

Aroesty, J. H. & Har-El, G. (1993). Parathyroid disorders. In F. E. Lucente & S. M. Sobol (eds.), *Essentials of otolaryngology* (pp. 403–412). New York: Raven Press.

Bluestone, C. D. (1994). Otitis media. In G. Gates (Ed.), *Current therapy in otolaryngology—Head and neck surgery.* (pp. 11–15). St. Louis: Mosby.

Bonilla, J. A. & Bluestone, C. D. (1995). Pharyngitis: When is aggressive treatment warranted? *PostGraduate Medicine, 97,* 61–69.

Bressler, K. & Shelton, C. (1993). Ear foreign body removal: A review of 98 consecutive cases. *Laryngoscope, 103,* 367–370.

Brodsky, L. (1998). Tonsil and adenoid disorders. In G. Gates (Ed.), *Current therapy in otolaryngology—Head and neck surgery.* (pp. 414–421). St. Louis: Mosby.

Bull, P. D. (1991). *Lecture notes on diseases of the ear, nose and throat* (7th ed.). Oxford, England: Blackwell Scientific Publications.

Carey, M. J. (1996). Epiglottis in adults. *American Journal of Emergency Medicine, 14,* 421–424.

Carroll, W. R. & Wolf, G. T. (1996). In J. J. Ballenger & J. B. Snow, Jr. (Eds.), *Otorhinolarngology* (15th ed.). (pp. 390–400). Media, PA: Williams &Wilkins.

Celin, E. C., Bluestone, C. D., Stephenson, J., Yilmaz, H. M. & Collins, J. J. (1991). Bacteriology of acute otitis medis in adults. *JAMA, 266,* 2249–2252.

Chester, A. C. (1996). Chronic sinusitis. *American Family Physician, 53,* 877–887.

Coppola, M. & Yealy, D. M. (1992). Relapsing polychondritis: An unusual cause of painful auricular swelling. *Annals of Emergency Medicine, 22,* 81–85.

Davis, O. & Powell, W. (1985). Auricular perichondritis secondary to acupuncture. *Archives of Otolaryngology, 111,* 770–771.

Dobleman, T. J. & Bumsted, R. M. (1992). Management of the patient with a thyroid mass. In *Common problems of the head and neck region.* American Academy of Otolaryngology—Head and Neck Surgery Foundation. (pp. 151–166). (Rev. ed.). Philadelphia: W. B. Saunders.

Eisele, D. W., Clifford, A. R., & Johns, M. E. (1995). Carcinoma of the oral cavity and pharynx. In K. J. Lee (Ed.), *Essential otolaryngology: Head and neck surgery.* (6th ed.). (pp. 535–554). Norwalk, CT: Appleton & Lange.

Epperly, T. D. & Wood, T. C. (1990). New trends in the management of peritonsillar abscess. *American Family Physician, 42,* 102–112.

Fairbanks, D. N. F. (1996). *Pocket guide to antimicrobial therapy in otolaryngology—head and neck surgery.* Alexandria, VA: American Academy of Otolaryngology—Head and Neck Surgery Foundation.

Farrior, J. B. (1998). External otitis. In G. Gates (Ed.), *Current therapy in otolaryngology—Head and neck surgery.* (6th ed.). (pp. 1–4). St. Louis: Mosby.

Farwell, A. P. & Braverman, L. E. (1996). Inflammatory thyroid disorders. *Otolaryngologic Clinics of North America, 29* (4), 541–555.

Feldman, B. A. & Feldman, D. E. (1995). The nose and sinuses. In K. J. Lee (Ed.), *Essential otolaryngology: Head and neck surgery.* (6th ed.). (pp. 715–757). Norwalk, CT: Appleton & Lange.

Ferguson, B. F. (1995). Acute and chronic sinusitis. *Postgraduate Medicine, 97,* 45–57.

Fontanarosa, P. B., Polsky, S. S., & Goldman, G. E. (1989). Adult epiglottis. *Journal of Emergency Medicine, 7,* 223–231.

Gantz, B. J. & Gidley, P. W. (1998). Meniere's disease: Medical therapy. In G. Gates (Ed.), *Current therapy in otolaryngology—Head and neck surgery.* (6th ed.). (pp. 79–80). St. Louis: Mosby.

Gates, G. A. (1998). Current therapy in otolaryngology head and neck surgery (6th ed.). St. Louis: Mosby.

Gold, S. D., Sperling, N. M., & Sobol, S. M. (1993). Chronic hearing loss. In F. E. Lucente & S. M. Sobol (Eds.), *Essentials of Otolaryngology,* (pp. 77–92). New York: Raven Press.

Goodman, M. (1990). Head and neck cancer. In S. L. Guenwald, M. Hansen-Frogge, M. Goodman, & C. Henke Yarbro, (Eds.) *Cancer nursing principles and practice.* (2nd ed.). (pp. 889–928). Boston: Jones and Barlett Publishers.

Gosselin, B. J., Gullane, P. J., & Irish, J. C. (1995). Cancer of the larynx, paranasal sinuses, and temporal bone. In K. J. Lee (Ed.), *Essential otolaryngology: Head and neck surgery.* (6th ed.). (pp. 555–579). Norwalk, CT: Appleton & Lange.

Graham, M. D., Lee, K. J., & Goldsmith, M. M. (1995). Noninfectious disorders of the ear. In K. J. Lee (Ed.), *Essential otolaryngology: Head and neck surgery.* (6th ed.). (pp. 677–713). Norwalk, CT: Appleton & Lange.

Guida, R. A., Sorvino, D. W., & Sobol, S. M. (1993). Tonsillectomy and adenoidectomy. In F. E. Lucente & S. M. Sobol (Eds.), *Essentials of otolaryngology* (pp. 355–362). New York: Raven Press.

Hall, S. F. (1990). Peritonsillar abscess: The treatment options. *Journal of Otolaryngology, 19,* 226–229.

Hart, C. W. (1998). Vertigo. In G. Gates (Ed.), *Current therapy in otolaryngology—head and neck surgery.* (6th ed.). (pp. 62–66). St. Louis: Mosby.

Hausfeld, J. N. (1992). Snoring and sleep apnea syndrome. In *Common problems of the head and neck region.* American Academy of Otolaryngology—Head and Neck Surgery Foundation. (Rev. ed.). (pp. 85–96). Philadelphia: W. B. Saunders.

Hendrix, R. A. (1996). Diseases of the thyroid gland. In J. J. Ballenger & J. B. Snow, Jr. (Eds.), *Otorhinolarngology* (15th ed.). (pp. 401–416). Media, PA: Williams & Wilkins.

Hoffman, H. T., McCulloch, T. M., & Victoria, L. (1998). Laryngeal paralysis. In G. Gates (Ed.), *Current therapy in otolaryngology—Head and neck surgery.* (6th ed.). (pp. 446–452). St. Louis: Mosby.

Jones, K. M. (1995). The oral cavity, oropharynx, and hypolarynx. In K. J. Lee (Ed.), *Essential otolaryngology: Head and neck surgery.* (6th ed.). (pp. 461–479). Norwalk, CT: Appleton & Lange.

Kiener, D. J. (1992). Disorders of the salivary glands. In *Common problems of the head and neck region.* American Academy of Otolaryngology—Head and Neck Surgery Foundation. (Rev. ed.). (pp. 167–186). Philadelphia: W. B. Saunders.

Kmucha, S. T. & Lee, K. J. (1995). Highlights and pearls. In K. J. Lee (Ed.), *Essential otolaryngology: Head and neck surgery.* (6th ed.). (pp. 1087–1152). Norwalk, CT: Appleton & Lange.

Kretzschmar, J. L. & Kretzschmar, D. P. (1996). Common oral conditions. *American Family Physician, 54,* 225–234.

Lanza, J. T., Nash, M., Sobol, S. M., & Har-El, G. (1993). Neck masses. In F. E. Lucente & S. M. Sobol (Eds.), *Essentials of otolaryngology* (pp. 375–393). New York: Raven Press.

Lee, K. J. (1995). Essential otolaryngology (6th ed.). Norwalk, CT: Appleton & Lange.

LoPresti, J. S. (1996). Laboratory tests for thyroid disorders. *Otolaryngologic Clinics of North America, 29,* 557–575.

Lowlicht, R. A. & Goodwin, W. J., Jr. (1995). In K. J. Lee (Ed.), *Essential otolaryngology: Head and neck surgery.* (6th ed.). (pp. 839–856). Norwalk, CT: Appleton & Lange.

Lucente, F. E., Sorvino, D. W., & Slavit, D. H. (1993). Epistaxis. In F. E. Lucente & S. M. Sobol (Eds.), *Essentials of otolaryngology* (pp. 212–220). New York: Raven Press.

Malinoff, R. (1993). Audiology. In F. E. Lucente & S. M. Sobol (Eds.), *Essentials of otolaryngology* (Appendices). New York: Raven Press.

Martini, D. V., Assael, L. A., & Har-El, G. (1993). Bony facial trauma. In F. E. Lucente & S. M. Sobol (Eds.), *Essentials of otolaryngology* (pp. 413–425). New York: Raven Press.

McGee, S. R. (1995). Dizzy patients: Diagnosis and treatment. *Western Journal of Medicine, 162,* 37–42.

Moloy, P. J. (1992). How to (and how not to) manage the patient with a lump in the neck. In *Common problems of the head and neck region.* American Academy of Otolaryngology—Head and Neck Surgery Foundation. (Rev. Ed.). (pp. 129–151). Philadelphia: W. B. Saunders.

Myers, E. N. & Myers, J. N. (1998). Cancer of the anterior tongue. In G. Gates (Ed.), *Current therapy in otolaryngology—Head and neck surgery.* (pp. 262–265). St. Louis: Mosby.

Nadol, J. B., Jr. (1983a). Evaluation of neck masses. In W. R. Wilson & J. B. Nadol, Jr. (Eds.), *Quick reference to ear, nose, throat disorders* (pp. 237–254). Philadelphia: J. B. Lippincott.

Nadol, J. B. Jr. (1983b). Salivary gland disorders. In W. R. Wilson & J. B. Nadol, Jr. (Eds.), *Quick reference to ear, nose, throat disorders* (pp. 185–196). Philadelphia: J. B. Lippincott.

Pincus, R. L. & Finazzo, J. J. (1993). Ear drainage. In F. E. Lucente & S. M. Sobol (Eds.), *Essentials of otolaryngology* (pp. 113–120). New York: Raven Press.

Reilly, J. S. (1990). Sinusitis cycle. *Otolaryngology head and neck surgery, 103* (Suppl. Part 2), 856–861.

Reuler, J. B., Lucas, L. M., & Kumar, K. L. (1995). Sinusitis: A review for generalists. *Western Journal of Medicine, 163,* 40–48.

Rice, D. H. (1996). Surgery of the parathyroid glands. *Otolaryngologic Clinics of North America, 29* (4), 693–699.

Richtsmeier, W. J. (1998). Acute sinusitis. In G. Gates (Ed.), *Current therapy in otolaryngology—Head and neck surgery.* (pp. 348–353). St. Louis: Mosby.

Riley, R. W., Powell, N. B., Guilleminault, C., Clerk, A., & Troell, R. (1995). Obstructive sleep apnea. *Western Journal of Medicine, 162,* 143–148.

Rowe, L. D. (1996). Congential anomalies of head and neck. In J. J. Ballenger & J. B. Snow, Jr. (Eds.), *Otorhinolarngology* (15th ed.). (pp. 209–219). Media, PA: Williams & Wilkins.

Rude, R. K. (1996). Hyperparathyroidism. *Otolaryngologic Clinics of North America, 29* (4), 663–679.

Sarti, E. J., Prager, D. A., & Lucente, F. E. (1993). Ear trauma. In F. E. Lucente & S. M. Sobol (Eds.), *Essentials of otolaryngology* (pp. 139–144). New York: Raven Press.

Savolainen, S., Jousimies-Somer, H. R., Makitie, A. A., & Ylikoski, J. S. (1993). Peritonsillar abscess—Clinical and microbiologic aspects and treatment regimens. *Archives of Otolaryngology, Head Neck Surgery, 119,* 521–524.

Schaefer, S. D. (1998). Acute laryngeal trauma. In G. Gates (Ed.), *Current therapy in otolaryngology—Head and neck surgery.* (pp. 446–452). St. Louis: Mosby.

Schild, J. A. & Snow, J. B. (1996). Esophagology. In J. J. Ballenger & J. B. Snow, Jr. (Eds.), *Otorhinolarngology* (15th ed.). (pp. 1221–1223). Media, PA: Williams & Wilkins.

Schilling, J. (1997). Hyperthyroidism: Diagnosis and management of Graves' disease. *Nurse Practitioner, 22* (6), 72–92.

Schuller, D. E. & Schleuning II, A. J. (1994). *DeWeese and Saunders' otolaryngology—head and neck surgery* (8th ed.). St. Louis: Mosby.

Shemen, L. J. (1995). Salivary glands: Benign and malignant disease. In K. J. Lee (Ed.), *Essential Otolaryngology: Head and Neck Surgery.* (6th ed.). (pp. 505–533). Norwalk, CT: Appleton & Lange.

Sigler, B. A. & Schuring, L. T. (1993). *Ear, nose, throat disorders.* (p. 22). St. Louis: Mosby.

Sobol, S. M. (1993). Anatomy and physiology. In F. E. Lucente & S. M. Sobol (Eds.), *Essentials of otolaryngology,* (pp. 3–46). New York: Raven Press.

Sobol, S. M. & Guffin, T. N. (1993). Dizziness and vertigo. In F. E. Lucente & S. M. Sobol (Eds.), *Essentials of otolaryngology,* (pp. 144–153). New York: Raven Press.

Sobol, S. M., Lanza, J. T., & Har-El, G. (1993). Salivary gland enlargement. In F. E. Lucente & S. M. Sobol (Eds.), *Essentials of otolaryngology,* (pp. 278–294). New York: Raven Press.

Sobol, S. M., Lanza, J. T., & Har-El, G. (1993). Thyroid masses. In F. E. Lucente & S. M. Sobol (Eds.), *Essentials of otolaryngology* (pp. 394– 402). New York: Raven Press.

Sobol, S. M., Martini, D. V., & Har-El, G. (1993). Cancer of the head and neck. In F. E. Lucente & S. M. Sobol (Eds.), *Essentials of otolaryngology* (pp. 468–480). New York: Raven Press.

Sobol, S. M. (1996). In F. E. Lucente & S. M. Sobol (Eds.). *Essentials of otolaryngology* (3rd ed.). (pp. 4–13). Philadelphia: Lippincott-Raven.

Sorvino, D. W. & Slavit, D. H. (1993). Sleep disorders. In F. E. Lucente & S. M. Sobol (Eds.), *Essentials of otolaryngology* (pp. 229–240). New York: Raven Press.

Sreenivas, V. & Kadambi, P. (1995). Thyroid and parathyroid glands. In K. J. Lee (Ed.), *Essential otolaryngology: Head and neck surgery.* (6th ed.). (pp. 581– 610). Norwalk, CT: Appleton & Lange.

Stafford, C. T. (1990). The clinican's view of sinusitis. *Otolaryngology, Head and Neck Surgery, 108,* 807–812.

Streff, M. M. & Pachucki-Hyde, L. C. (1996). Management of the patient with thyroid disease. *Nursing Clinics of North America, 31* (4), 779–796.

Terris, D. J., Arnstein, D. P., & Nguyen, H. H. (1992). Contemporary evaluation of unilateral vocal cord paralysis. *Otolaryngology, Head and Neck Surgery, 107,* 84–90.

Wiet, R. J., Micco, A. G., & Bedoya, O. (1998). Cholesteatoma. In G. Gates (Ed.), *Current therapy in otolaryngology—Head and neck surgery.* (pp. 19–22). St. Louis: Mosby.

Williams, J. W. & Simel, D. L. (1993). Does this patient have sinusitis? *JAMA, 270,* 1242–1246.

Wilson, W. R. & Nadol, Jr. J. B. (1983). In W. R. Wilson & J. B. Nadol Jr. (Eds). *Quick reference to ear, nose, throat disorders.* Philadelphia: J. B. Lipincott Raven.

Wurman, L. H., Sack, J. G., Flannery, J. V., & Lipsman, R. A. (1992). The management of epistaxis. *American Journal of Otolaryngology, 13,* 193–209.

Wurtele, P. (1990). Acute epiglottis in children and adults: A large scale incidence study. *Otolaryngology, Head and Neck Surgery, 103,* 902–908.

Zivic, R. C. & King, S. (1993). Cerumen impaction management for clients of all ages. *Nurse Practitioner, 18,* 29–37.

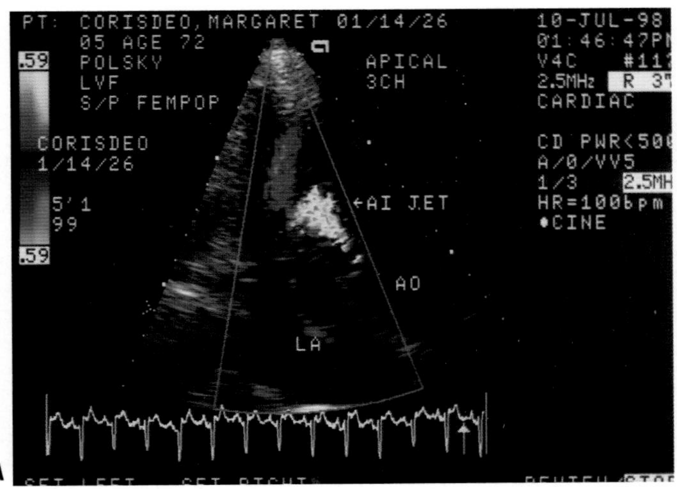

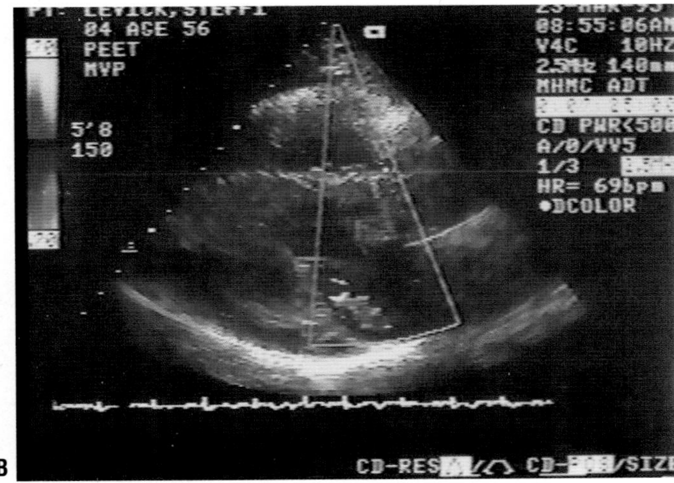

Color Plate 1. Color flow Doppler images of aortic and mitral regurgitation. **A,** Apical long-axis view showing mild aortic regurgitation (AR). **B,** Parasternal long-axis view showing mitral regurgitation (blue "flame").

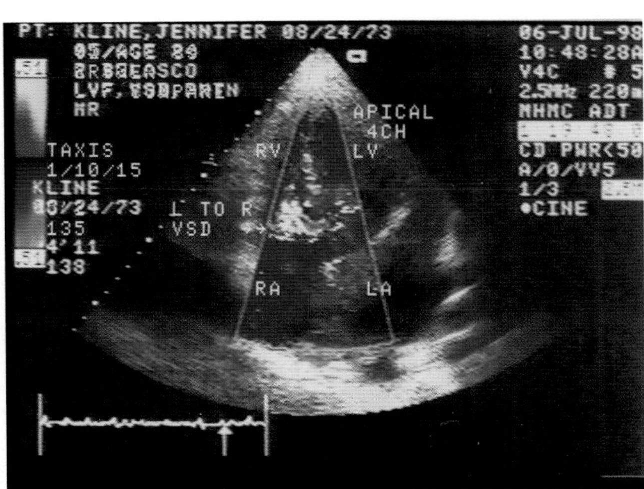

Color Plate 2. Apical four-chamber color Doppler view showing ventricular septal defect.

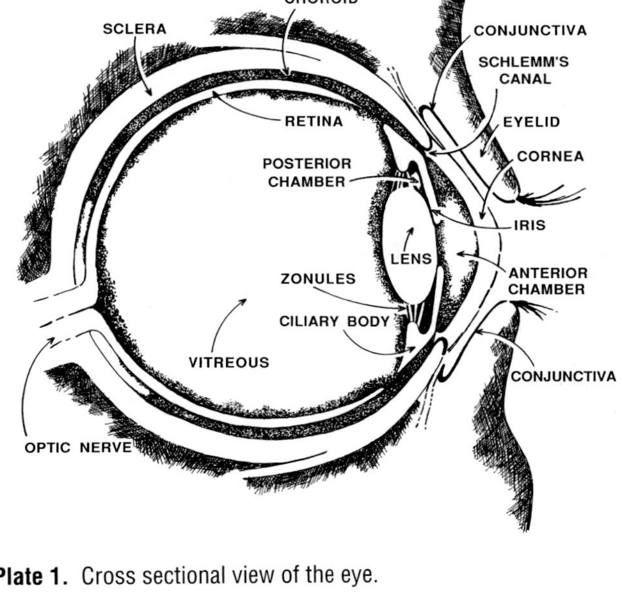

Plate 1. Cross sectional view of the eye.

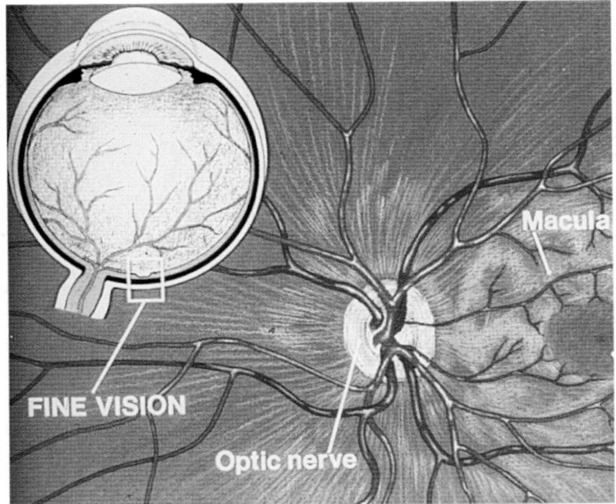

Color Plate 3. Normal retina, left eye. *(Courtesy American Academy of Ophthalmology.)*

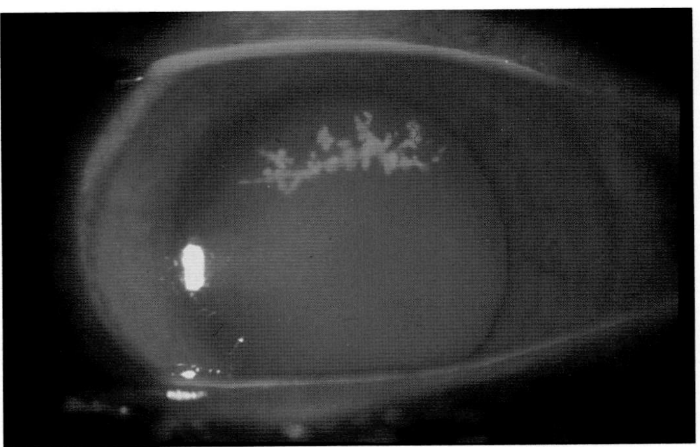

Color Plate 4. Multiple linear, branching ulcers of a herpetic ulcer (dendrites) detected by corneal staining with fluoroscein under cobalt blue light. *(Courtesy American Academy of Ophthalmology.)*

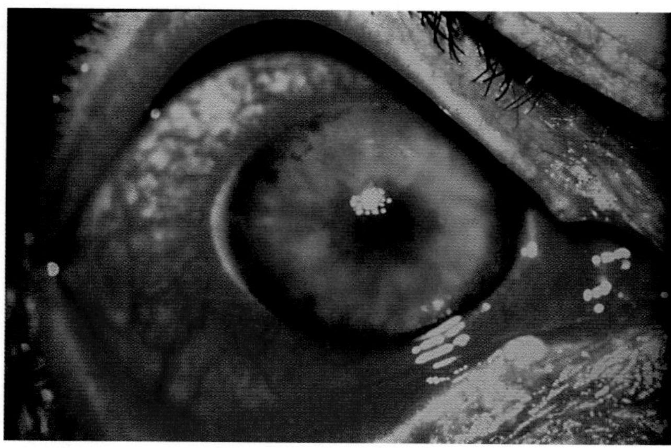

Color Plate 5. Glaucomatous eye. Note corneal edema (seen as corneal clouding), scattered corneal light reflex, and circumcorneal and peripheral injection. Pupil is constricted due to topical pilocarpine. *(Courtesy American Academy of Ophthalmology.)*

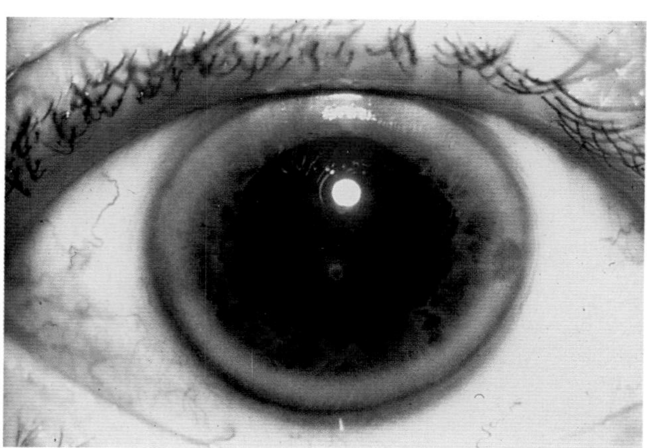

Color Plate 6. Corneal arcus (arcus senilis), a yellow-white ring-shaped deposit in the peripheral cornea. Note uninvolved clear area between the arcus and white sclera. *(Courtesy American Academy of Ophthalmology.)*

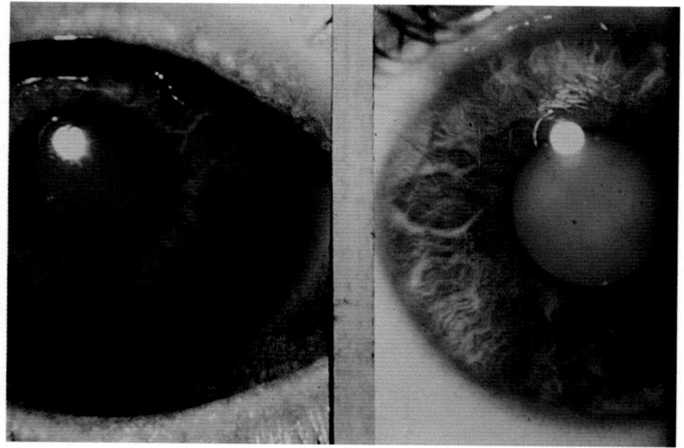

Color Plate 7. Cataract. The left is minimal compared to the dense cataract on the right. *(Courtesy American Academy of Ophthalmology.)*

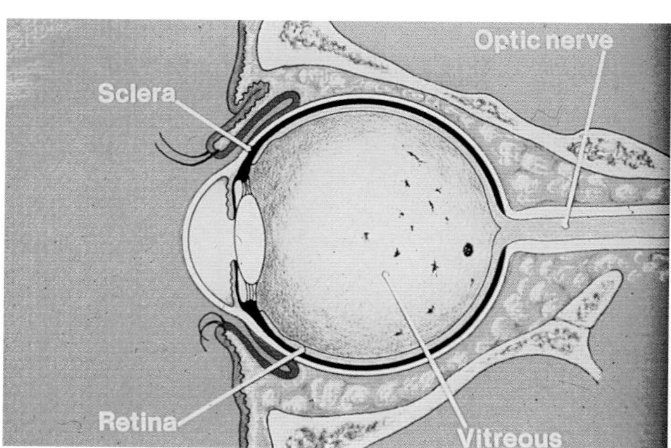

Color Plate 8. Diagram of floaters (specks) in the vitreous. *(Courtesy American Academy of Ophthalmology.)*

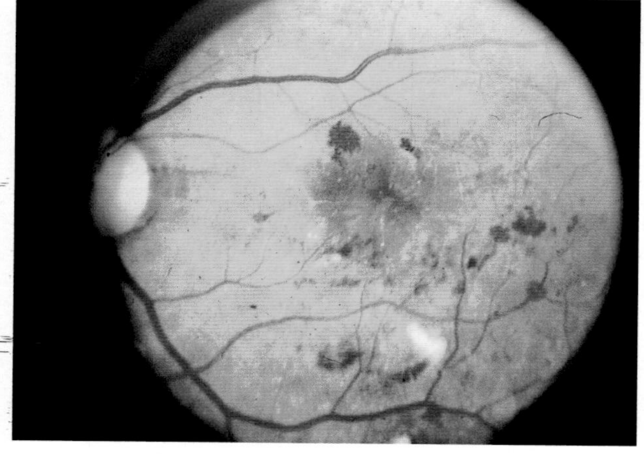

Color Plate 9. Nonproliferative diabetic retinopathy. Note multiple areas of dot and blot hemorrhages and hard exudate. *(Courtesy American Academy of Ophthalmology.)*

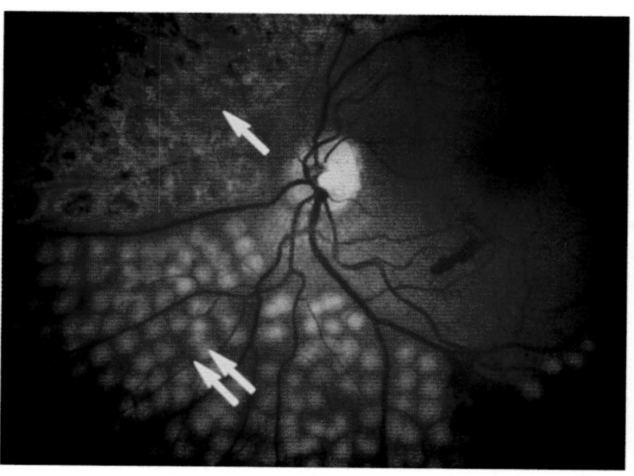

Color Plate 10. Panretinal photocoagulation (laser) scars in proliferative diabetic retinopathy. Old laser scars *(single arrow)* and new *(double arrow)* laser burns. *(Courtesy American Academy of Ophthalmology.)*

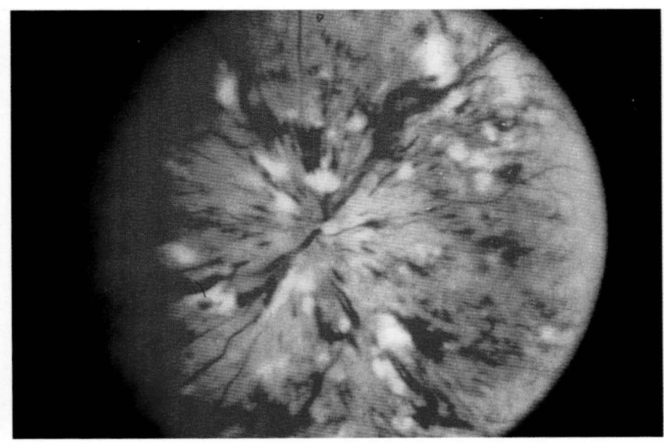

Color Plate 11. Central retinal vein occlusion. Note areas of hemorrhage, ishcemia, and diffuse retinal edema with obscuring of retinal detail. *(Courtesy American Academy of Ophthalmology.)*

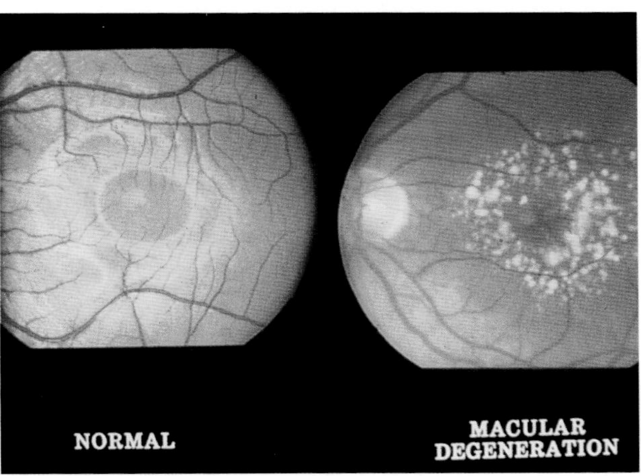

Color Plate 12. Age-related macular degeneration. Note areas of drusen and pigmentary changes of the macula. *(Courtesy American Academy of Ophthalmology.)*

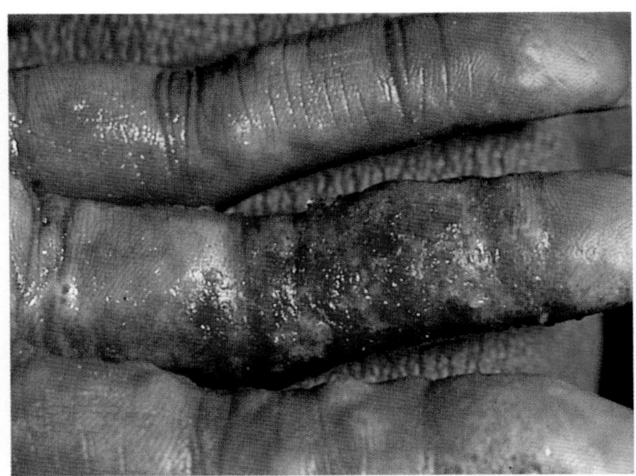

Color Plate 13. Acute eczema.

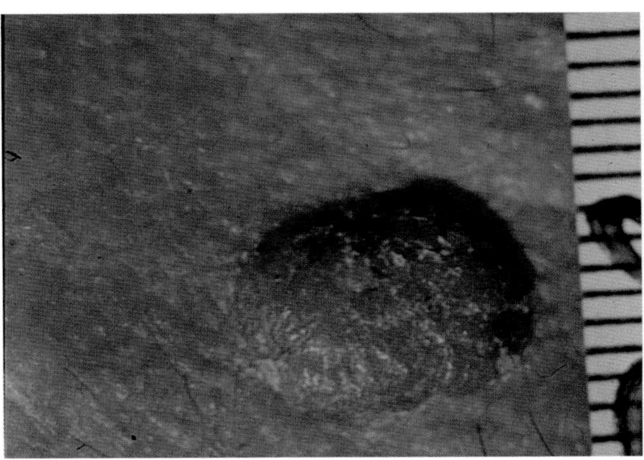

Color Plate 14. Lyme disease.

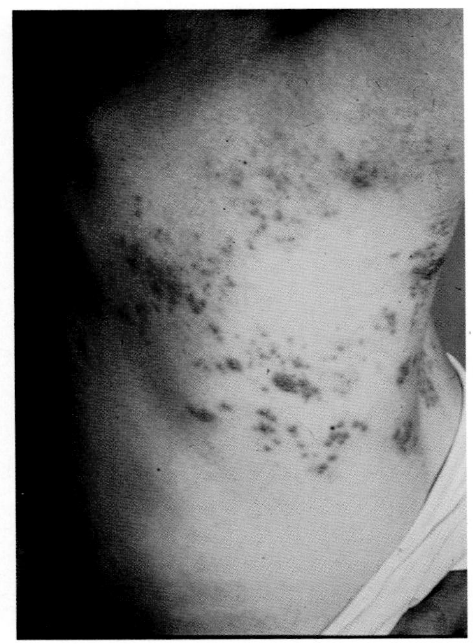

Color Plate 15. Herpes simplex.

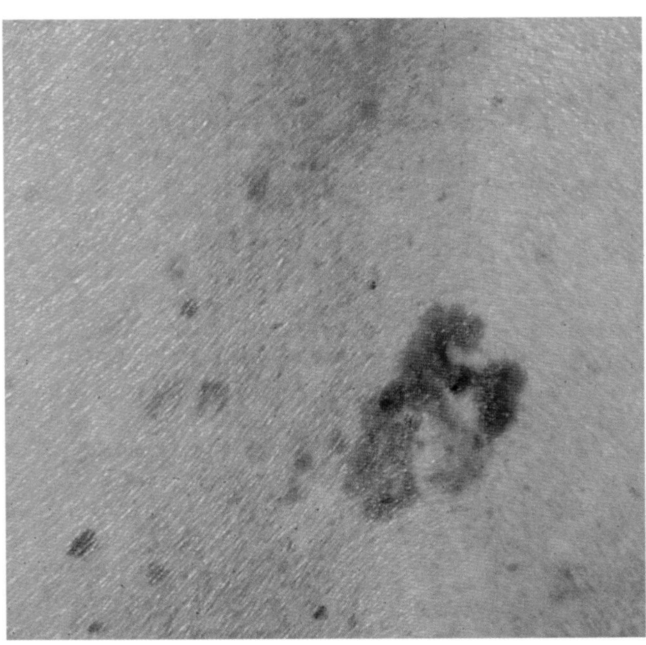

Color Plate 16. Varicella.

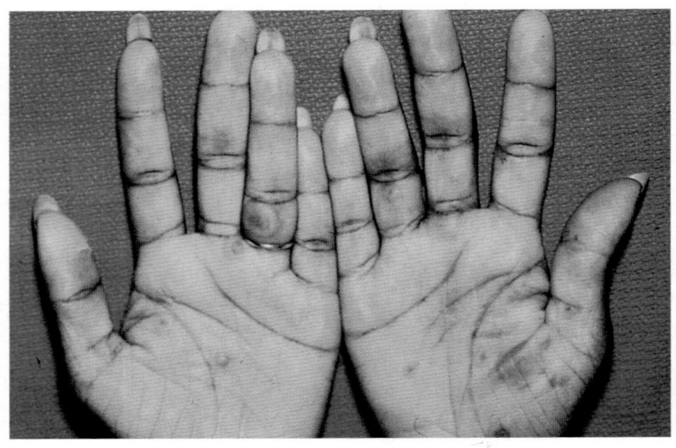

Color Plate 17. Targetoid lesions of erythema multiforme.

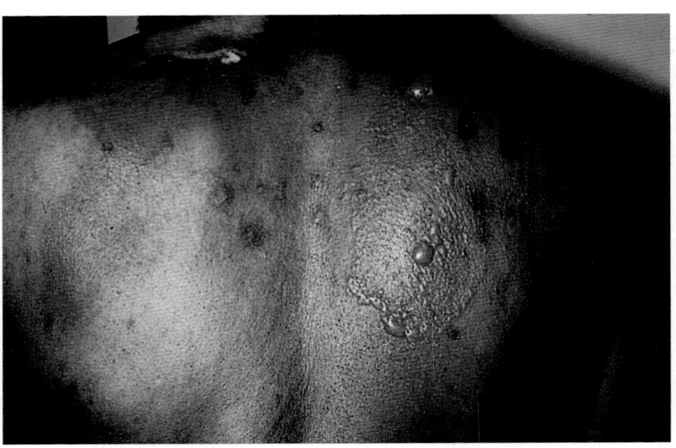

Color Plate 18. Toxic epidermal necrolysis.

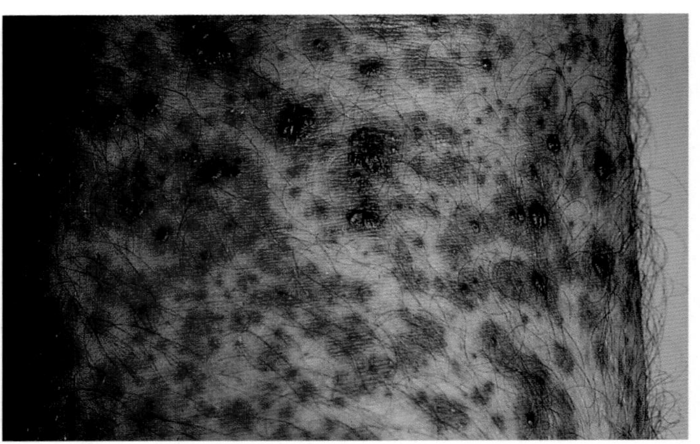

Color Plate 19. Vasculitis.

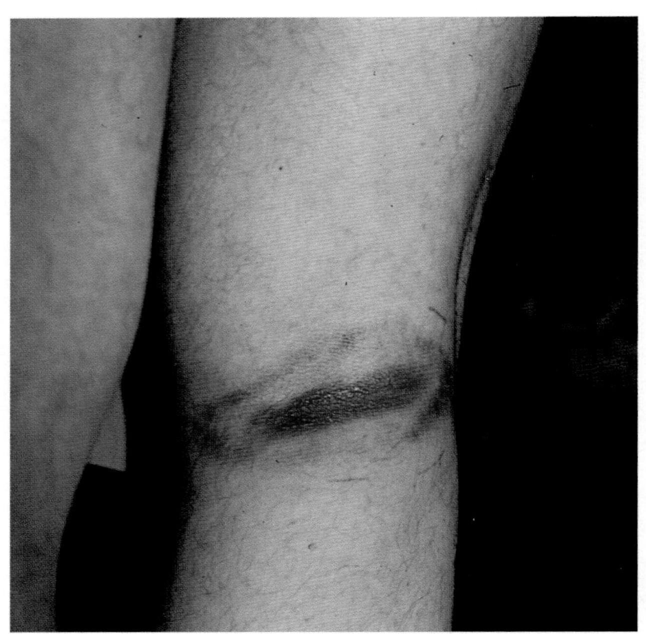

Color Plate 20. Seborrheic keratosis.

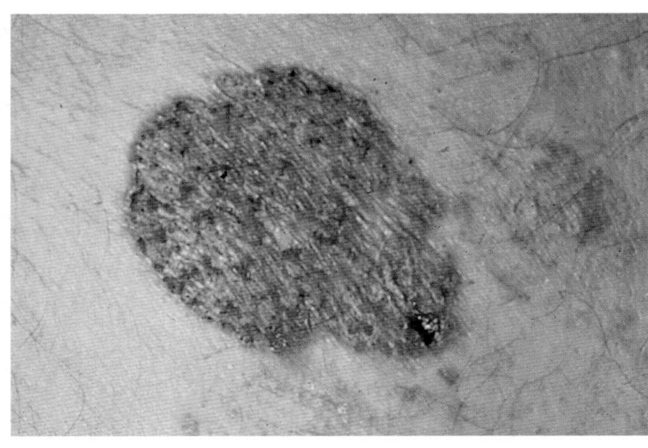

Color Plate 21. Bowenoid basal-cell carcinoma.

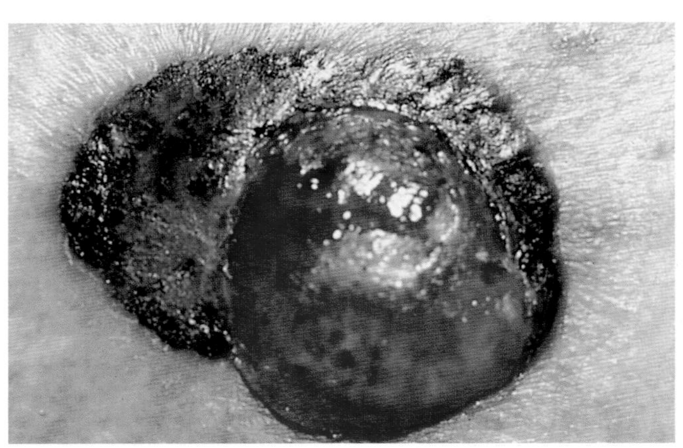

Color Plate 22. Superficial spreading melanoma.

51

Skin Problems

Marie Uberti-Benz

The skin is the largest and most accessible organ of the body. Real or perceived abnormalities of the skin are among the most frequent concerns brought by patients to healthcare providers. How well the skin functions and looks is of concern to everyone and all providers should be aware of the common, as well as serious, cutaneous maladies.

▸ COMMON SKIN PROBLEMS

Pruritus

Itch is an aggravating, poorly understood symptom that can range in intensity from minor annoyance to suicidal obsession. Most patients with pruritus do not openly excoriate their skin. Several cutaneous processes lead patients to dig and tear the affected areas, however, preferring the pain or discomfort of open scratches to incessant itching. Specifically, atopic dermatitis, scabies, and the itch of renal and liver diseases may have only the secondary signs of chronic excoriation as their chief manifestations.

All patients with pruritus should have a complete cutaneous examination. History should include a review of pertinent medical history, particularly for kidney, liver disease, or symptoms of a tumor such as weight loss; chronic and recent drug ingestion, washing habits, and topical exposures.

Xerosis

The most common cause of generalized pruritus is dry skin, otherwise known as "winter itch" or xerosis. Chronic xerosis is especially prevalent in atopics and in the general population as it ages. Low humidity, cold weather, frequent bathing, and "strong" concentrated or deodorant soaps all contribute to a scaly, dry, or "ashy" look to the skin.

Severe xerosis consisting of thick scale with exacerbation of skin lines is called ichthyosis. Ichthyosis, meaning "fishlike" scaling, can be hereditary or acquired. Acquired ichthyosis is important to distinguish from more modest dry skin as it can herald a systemic disorder such as gastric cancer, lymphoma, or sarcoidosis. Ask the patient, "How long has your skin been this dry?" If the answer is "all my life," a work-up for systemic disease may not be indicated.

The treatment of xerosis consists of changing bathing habits, protection from excessive environmental exposure, and the regular use of emollients. Bathing should be altered to relatively short, lukewarm showers using a fatted soap such as Dove, Tone, or Neutrogena. Application of an emollient while still damp discourages water evaporation from the skin surface. Vaseline remains the gold standard in emollient therapy, but aqueous preparations may be more cosmetically acceptable. Recently, the alpha hydroxy acids as a group, specifically lactic acid emollients (e.g., Lac-Hydrin), have demonstrated efficacy in improving xerotic skin, even to the point of allowing "skip days" without relapse.

Eczema/Atopic Dermatitis

Atopy is a group of related hypersensitivity disorders including asthma, hayfever, sinus problems, and eczema. They are related disorders of hyperirritability to environmental allergens such as dust, pollen, smoke, pet dander, molds and in the case of the skin, environmental changes or irritants. Many patients with eczema have a personal or family history of other atopic conditions.

Atopic dermatitis is frequently called the "itch that rashes" as the clinical changes occur only after pruritic skin is scratched or rubbed. *Acute eczema* is usually "wet," oozing or weeping with significant erythema (Color Plate 13). *Chronic eczema* is dry, thickened, or "lichenified" with exaggeration of skin markings, and often hyper- or hypo-pigmented.

Clinical manifestations of atopic dermatitis or eczema change with age. A classic manifestation of a "budding atopic" is a prominent infraorbital fold called a *Denny–Morgan line.* In later life, dark circles (allergic "shiners") may accompany this crease so that the patient complains of "always looking tired."

Newborns may experience difficult to treat diaper rash or overall dryness. Young children through early teenagers itch and scratch the antecubital and popliteal fossae, frequently developing characteristic lichenification of these areas. Widespread eczema is not uncommon in this group, with some children having itch severe enough to disrupt sleep.

The hands are the areas of most concern for older teenagers through middle adulthood. Generalized eczema becomes less common but the multitude of environmental assaults that nonatopic hand skin tolerates may lead to frequent bouts of both acute and chronic hand dermatitis. A particularly troublesome and idiopathic form of hand eczema is known as *dyshidrosis* which consists of small blisters along the sides of fingers. These blisters are often seasonal, with exacerbation in the spring months.

Atopic older adults develop focal dry, scaly patches called *nummular* eczema, superimposed on diffuse dry skin. These patches are more common on extensor surfaces, are often coin shaped, and may coexist with stasis dermatitis changes.

The management of atopic skin is a lifelong process and involves aggressive patient education. Parents of young children should be taught gentle skin-care techniques, including the use of mild soaps, emollients, and humidifiers in winter weather. Atopic children are prone to complications from common cutaneous infections such as *Staphylococcus aureus,* which colonizes broken atopic skin. Herpes simplex infections may become widespread (*Kaposi's varicelliform eruption*) and ordinary warts and molluscum are often harder to control.

Treatment may also involve intermittent use of topical, and occasionally systemic, steroids. The least potent steroid to control the dermatitis should be employed and overuse discouraged to prevent atrophic changes. About 15% of atopics develop a true exogenous or contact allergen and patch testing should be considered for recalcitrant cases.

Allergic Phenomenon

Cutaneous allergic reactions can be divided into (1) *contact,* meaning a reaction to a topical exogenous agent, and (2) *systemic,* meaning a reaction to an internal agent.

Contact Allergy

Contact allergies are widespread, the most common being to the rhus antigen known as poison ivy. Nearly everyone can be sensitized to poison ivy given sufficient exposure to the plant resin. Poison ivy can occur for the first time in childhood, particularly if children live or play in endemic areas, but may develop at any time later in life. The first reaction to poison ivy generally develops within 1 to 2 weeks of exposure but previously sensitized patients may break out within days or even hours.

The characteristic rash of poison ivy is a streaky erythematous, fixed urticarial eruption that progresses to small blisters or large bullae. Because the eruption breaks out over several days up to 2 weeks, patients often assume they are "spreading it" from leakage of blister fluid. Different areas of the skin break out at different rates, however, depending on how much antigen was applied to the skin and the thickness of the affected area. Facial, eyelid, and groin skin are substantially thinner than back or abdominal skin and can react to lower concentrations of antigen; thin skin is also prone to substantial swelling or edema.

Patients should be educated about the characteristic features of the poison ivy plant ("leaves of three, let them be") but should also be advised that the plant can take many forms, including vines and bushlike shapes. It is often intermingled with harmless vegetation such as English ivy. In addition, patients should be advised that the entire plant contains the rhus resin in stable form, including dead leaves and roots, and that fomites such as gardening or golf gear can retain the rhus chemical. Petting dogs that have run through patches of poison ivy can also trigger the rash in humans.

Treatment consists of alleviating the itch with judicious use of antihistamines and treating the blisters with soaks, baths, and drying solutions. Steroids can suppress the urticarial component of the rash, but do little once blisters are established. Localized areas respond to topical steroids but larger areas or those with vital areas such as the face or groin affected may require a short course of systemic steroids. Secondary infection or impetiginization with yellow oozing, honey-colored crusts, and surrounding cellulitis is not uncommon and may require topical or systemic antibiotics.

Other frequent causes of contact dermatitis include nickel, neosporin, and latex. Nickel is a frequent sensitizer—in men more commonly due to workplace exposure, and in women due to jewelry, particularly pierced ears. Once sensitized, patients may react to multiple metals, including gold, as many objects, especially jewelry, are alloys that contain nickel to harden them. Stainless steel is the exception, and is safe for nickel-sensitive patients.

Neosporin is a commonly applied topical antibiotic, found in many over-the-counter products, including first-aid creams. Chronic dermatitis—such as stasis dermatitis and leg ulcers in which patients may apply neosporin in a long-term, intermittent fashion—is associated with a relatively high degree of sensitization, up to 15% in some leg ulcer populations.

Latex, a natural rubber derivative, has caused many reactions in the last decade due to widespread use in condoms and rubber gloves. Health-care workers have the highest reaction rates to latex, with some studies indicating up to 7% of the workforce sensitized.

Most reactions to latex are of the delayed contact dermatitis type, with chronic hand eczema the most common manifestation. *Contact urticaria,* an immediate urticarial response, is not rare. These urticarial reactions can be life threatening, with even brief exposures such as during dental or gynecology procedures, producing potentially fatal angioedema and anaphylaxis. Nonlatex gloves are available, with some medical centers attempting to become "latex free."

Other relatively common contact allergens include paraphenelenediamine and some preservatives. Paraphenelenediamine is the active ingredient found in most permanent hair dye products available in the United States. It can cross react with sulfa products such as PABA.

Almost all topical products require chemical preservation. A small segment of the population may become sensitized to these widespread agents which include PABA, Quaternium 15, and formaldehyde releasers such as Imidazolidinyl urea.

Urticaria or Hives

Urticaria is a pruritic, transient swelling of the skin resulting from increased permeability of blood vessels. Urticaria is a reaction pattern, meaning a response to any number of different antigens including foods, drugs, and environmental agents such as insect bites, viruses, and systemic disease.

Most episodes of urticaria begin abruptly but resolve slowly over days or weeks. Each individual hive lasts up to twelve hours, with that site being resistant to new lesion development for a number of hours due to histamine depletion in that area, though recurring crops with different areas afflicted at different times are the norm. Swelling of the subcutaneous tissue is called *angioedema* and can be life threatening if a vital organ, such as the airway, is compromised.

The majority of patients with urticaria have hives over a limited time span and can identify the trigger as a food, such as nuts or shellfish, or a drug, such as penicillin or sulfonamides. However, a small subset of patients (up to 5%) have chronic urticaria with recurrent bouts over months or years, unassociated with any clear stimulus.

Rare patients with recurrent angioedema should be evaluated for a genetic defect of C1 esterase inhibitor deficiency or malfunction.

The treatment of urticaria requires stabilization of the patient who may be in respiratory distress due to laryngeal, tongue or lip edema, or with wheezing. Epinephrine, antihistamines, and steroids are useful for acute management, although it should be remembered that steroids take 24 to 48 hours to begin to work. Long-term control consists of minimizing trigger factors as well as avoidance of direct histamine releasers, particularly aspirin, nonsteroidal antiinflammatory agents, morphine, codeine, and Demerol. Patients should be advised that antihistamines prevent the next outbreak and do not control the present one; therefore, they must be taken on a regular schedule. Both traditional and newer, less sedating antihistamines are available, with difficult cases sometimes requiring a trial-and-error approach to determine which medication works best for the individual patient.

Acne

Acne is a common follicular disorder of impaction of the pores of facial and sometimes truncal skin, leading to bacterial overgrowth in the obstructed oil glands. Acne can begin as early as 10 or 11 years of age, becomes more common in mid to late teenage years but frequently persists into midlife, particularly in women. Acne begins on the forehead and nose in most patients and moves down the face with time. The chin and jaw, presumably containing the most hormonally reactive glands, are the sites of most lesions after adolescence. Significant prepubertal acne, or acne associated with menstrual irregularities, alopecia, or hirsutism, should trigger a search for an endocrine abnormality.

Blackheads and whiteheads are called comedones and are the primary lesions of acne. Each comedone represents an obstructed follicular orifice by cohesive cells lining the shaft. Secondary lesions of papules, pustules, and cysts result from disruption of the swollen blocked oil gland by lipid byproducts and bacterial overgrowth.

The first step in treatment consists of patient education. Scrubbing, overwashing in an attempt "to keep the face clean," and harsh soaps should be avoided and substituted with mild washing techniques.

There are three major classes of comedolytic agents: Benzoyl peroxide, Tretinoin (a vitamin A derivative), and hydroxy acids. Each beta hydroxy acid (or salicylic acid) requires proper use to avoid excessive irritation. Benzoyl peroxide is available over the counter and has the advantage of also being somewhat antibacterial, but may bleach clothing or towels and can trigger an allergic reaction in some individuals.

Tretinoin remains the gold standard for comedolytic activity. Choosing a concentration and base compatible with the patient's skin type can diminish irritancy. Patients who use Tretinoin should use photoprotection and those with darker pigmentation should be advised of a slight risk of hypopigmentation.

Both topical and oral antibiotics are useful in the long-term control of papulopustular acne. Topical preparations of erythromycin and clindamycin are available in a range of bases and delivery systems. Oral antibiotics—such as tetracycline, minocycline, doxycycline, and erythromycin—should be reserved for more severe or diffuse pustular disease.

Accutane is a synthetic retinoid, indicated for recalcitrant, scarring, cystic acne. It is associated with a potential for significant vitamin A toxic side effects including a ***high risk of severe birth defects if taken while a woman is pregnant.*** Women of childbearing age must have a negative pregnancy test before starting Accutane and use both oral and barrier contraception during therapy. The pregnancy test should be repeated at least monthly while on Accutane. The 20-week recommended course of Accutane can also trigger hypertriglyceridemia, as well as mucosal dryness, pseudotumor cerebri, and other reactions necessitating careful clinical and laboratory follow-up. However, the majority of severe cystic acne patients have near-complete resolution of their disease after one course of treatment. Therefore, this drug, if used cautiously, remains valuable in carefully selected cases.

Alopecia

Hair loss can be divided clinically into scarring and nonscarring processes.

Scarring Alopecia

Scarring alopecia involves loss or destruction of the hair bulbs. Local processes that gradually damage hair bulbs include hot combs, tight braiding such as corn braids in childhood, and inflammatory fungal infections. Tight braiding characteristically results in loss of the first few centimeters of the frontal hairline in women by their twenties and thirties.

Discoid lupus is a variant of systemic lupus that causes an inflammatory scarring reaction to antibodies deposited chiefly in the scalp, face, and ears. Early lesions are fixed urticarial or purple plaques; later lesions are centrally scarred with a burnt-out appearance of erythema, hypopigmentation, and hyperpigmentation. Treatment of early lesions with intralesional or topical high-potency steroids, plaquinil, and sun avoidance may prevent some areas of scarring and hair loss.

Nonscarring Alopecia

The three most common types of nonscarring hair loss include pattern hair loss, telogen defluvium (effluvium), and alopecia areata.

Pattern Hair Loss. Pattern hair loss, historically called *male pattern baldness,* is now recognized in both men and women. Pattern hair loss is hereditary and apparently requires sufficient unopposed male hormone to fully express the predisposition. Men frequently exhibit full expression of scalp hair loss about 20 years after puberty; women, about 20 years after menopause. The pattern differs in women, in that the loss occurs primarily as thinning over the top of the crown, whereas in men bitemporal recession significantly precedes more complete central crown hair loss.

Telogen Defluvium (Effluvium). Telogen defluvium (effluvium) is an enhanced turnover of the normal hair metabolism. At any one time, the normal scalp has about 90% of the hairs in the growing or anagen phase of development. Approximately 10% are in the resting or telogen phase. The telogen phase ends with the hair falling out, having an atrophic white tip or "club." In pregnancy, more hairs may be shunted into the growing or anagen phase; thus, women who are pregnant may truly have denser hair growth. However, at the end of pregnancy, those hairs that normally would have cycled into the resting phase do so, subsequently falling out almost simultaneously, with a sudden shedding of hair in the postpartum period. This phenomenon can also be seen with supplemental hormonal discontinuation, or after periods of medical illness or stress. In some individuals, telogen defluvium develops repeatedly, particularly seasonally in the fall months. Fortunately, the hair does revert to the growing phase. The hair density may not be as thick, however, as prior to the telogen episodes. Unexplained, prolonged telogen hair loss should precipitate a search for an underlying cause, such as anemia, thyroid disease, or malnutrition as in bulimia or anorexia.

Alopecia Areata. Alopecia areata is an autoimmune disorder of unknown etiology that characteristically produces sudden, asymptomatic bald areas. Alopecia areata may be familial and is associated with an endocrine disorder such as diabetes or thyroid disease in about 10% of cases. Alopecia areata affects only pigmented hair, leaving white hairs in place. The bald areas frequently spontaneously regrow the hair over a period of months; more severe cases result in alopecia totalis, implying total loss of scalp hair, and alopecia universalis, or the loss of all body hair including eyelashes.

Poor prognostic indicators for regrowth of hair include a diffuse pattern of nail pits, development of alopecia areata in childhood, and a pattern of alopecia about the ears, progressing around the scalp to more extensive involvement.

Multiple therapeutic modalities to reverse alopecia areata are discussed in the literature, with topical or intralesional steroids usually employed. Immunotherapy with a topical agent used to induce a counterallergic reaction remains experimental and must be carefully monitored.

Papulosquamous Disorders

This group of cutaneous lesions producing excess amount of scale often have distinguishing visual patterns, enabling clinical differentiation.

Psoriasis

Psoriasis is a common disorder of excessive epidermal turnover, resulting in thickened, scaly, erythematous plaques.

Psoriasis affects up to 2% of the population and is often familial with variable expression. Psoriasis can develop at any age, from infancy to the elder years, suggesting an environmental factor is needed to activate genetic expression.

The classical lesions of psoriasis are distributed on the extensor surfaces of the elbows, knees, buttocks, and scalp. Thick silvery plaques bleed when the scale is picked, known as the Auspitz sign. Highly active psoriasis may *koebnerize,* meaning those areas of trauma (i.e., from scratching), may lead to a psoriatic exacerbation.

There are several types of psoriasis that differ from this classical form of psoriasis.

Inverse Psoriasis. Inverse psoriasis affects the intertriginous areas with significantly less scale than classical psoriasis. These areas are shiny or dull red, mimicking candidiasis or intertrigo.

Psoriatic Nail Disease. Psoriatic nail disease forms "nail pits," "oil spots," or yellow subungual debris easily confused with onychomycosis.

Psoriatic Erythroderma. Psoriatic erythroderma consists of widespread involvement of the skin with diffuse thickened erythema and modest scale. Erythroderma can also be triggered by drug reactions and cutaneous lymphoma, and can result in death from high output cardiac failure and secondary infections.

Pustular Psoriasis. Pustular psoriasis can be localized or diffuse. Localized pustular psoriasis affects primarily the palms and soles with pustules, erythema, and scale. Recurrent crops of sterile pustules may be disabling and unaffected by conventional psoriatic treatments.

Generalized pustular psoriasis produces lakes of pus over large affected areas, with a significant risk of sepsis, hypocalcemia, and death. Pustular psoriasis may be precipitated by abrupt discontinuation of chronic systemic steroids used to control psoriasis, a practice that should be discouraged.

Treatment of psoriasis is varied and must be tailored to the individual patient. Localized areas can be controlled, at least initially, with topical steroids, but patients develop tachyphylaxis or the ability of the psoriatic skin to override the effect of the steroid. Potential steroid side effects include localized atrophy, telangiectasia, steroid acne, and adrenal suppression from ultrapotent steroids applied over large areas for prolonged periods of time. The risk of adrenal suppression is greater in children with a larger body surface area to mass ratio.

Steroid-sparing treatment modalities include topical tars, anthralin, and zinc. Many patients improve in the summer months, leading to success with ultraviolet B therapy in carefully controlled doses in some patients. The mechanism of UVB therapy is unclear. A topically applied vitamin D derivative, calcipotriol (Dovonex) is helpful in limited doses for approximately 70% of psoriatic patients.

More aggressive modalities for severe, disabling, or life-threatening psoriasis include methotrexate, PUVA, and actiretin.

Cummulative doses of methotrexate must be monitored to limit the risk of methotrexate-induced cirrhosis and fibrosis of the liver.

PUVA is a combination of Psoralen, a photosensitizing vegetable derivative, and ultraviolet A, a longer wavelength ultraviolet light. PUVA produces remission of psoriasis in some severe cases, but premature aging of the skin and enhanced risk of cutaneous tumors, including squamous-cell carcinoma and melanoma, severely limit PUVA's usefulness.

The aromatic vitamin A analog Acitretin has efficacy in treating resistant psoriasis but is teratogenic and can only be used in women past childbearing age. Acitretin has the potential for vitamin A toxic side effects including mucosal dryness, hyperlipidemia, and skeletal hyperostosis, and therefore only a tiny fraction of psoriasis patients are candidates for this class of drug.

Seborrheic Dermatitis

Seborrhea is considered a "cousin" to psoriasis in that it is also a condition of excess scale, but the scale is typically much less thick and is limited to the "seborrheic" areas. These areas include the scalp, ears, eyebrows, perinasal area, chest, and groin.

Seborrhea waxes and wanes over a lifetime and flares are frequently precipitated by stress and fatigue. Severe, resistant seborrhea can be seen in immunocompromised patients, particularly those with HIV infection, and in those with neurological disorders such as Parkinson's, mental illness, cerebral palsy, stroke, or head injury.

Treatment consists of gentle washing and the judicious use of topical steroids, with the least potent steroid that is effective always preferred. Tar and zinc shampoos are helpful in controlling the dandruff of scalp seborrhea. Topical ketoconozole, in cream and shampoo forms, has been useful as a steroid-sparing agent in relatively mild disease.

Lichen Planus

Lichen planus is a unique disorder consisting of pruritic, purple, polygonal papules usually distributed (at least initially) acrally on the flexor wrists and ankles. Lichen planus is subject to koebnerization, in that trauma or excoriations may precipitate new lesions. Histologically, there is a dense collection of lymphocytes at the dermal–epidermal junction, hence lesions mimicking lichen planus are called *lichenoid.* Lichen planus often affects the mucosal surfaces including the mouth, penis, and vulva, with a lacy-white reticulated pattern that can be confused with leukoplakia. Crops of lesions may develop over months, with episodes lasting months to years. Relapses are not uncommon.

Lichen planus is speculated to be a reaction pattern to unknown stimuli. Drugs, viruses (especially hepatitis B and C), and graft-versus-host disease have been implicated.

Therapy consists of alleviating the pruritus and using steroids judiciously. Topical steroid treatment of lichen planus is always preferable to systemic use. Patients should be instructed not to smoke, and close follow-up of mucosal surfaces is indicated to monitor for the potential development of squamous-cell carcinoma.

Pityriasis Rosea

Pityriasis rosea is a mildly pruritic scaly disorder, common in young adults, with seasonal peaks in the spring and fall. The rash often begins with a solitary scaly oval plaque (mother lesion or herald patch) followed by crops of similar, smaller lesions accentuated in the lines of the trunk, hence the characteristic "Christmas-tree pattern." Inverse patterns, involving the face and intertriginous areas are more common in patients of African-American descent. The differential diagnosis includes secondary syphillis and a drug reaction.

Although the etiology is unknown, pityriasis rosea almost always remits spontaneously after an 8- to 12-week course. Repeat episodes are uncommon. Minimal therapy, if any, is required with the exception of deeply pigmented patients in whom more aggressive treatment may be indicated to prevent secondary hyperpigmentation. Cases that persist longer than 3 months should be reevaluated to exclude parasporiasis or other relatively rare disorders that may mimic pityriasis rosea.

▶ SKIN INFECTIONS

Fungal Infections

Fungal infections are common and categorized primarily by body location. The lay term for many fungal infections is "ringworm" although no worm or similar parasite is involved.

Tinea Capitis

Tinea capitis is usually a disease of children, with a higher incidence among African-Americans. Mild cases present with scale suggestive of dandruff. Increased diagnostic suspicion is raised by the presence of occipital lymph nodes, rare in seborrhea. The alopecia associated with tinea capitis is called "black dot" because of the black remaining stubble of hair. A local inflammatory reaction to the fungus in some individuals produces a pronounced inflammatory mass with suppurative drainage called a *kerion.* Kerions may have secondary bacterial infection, necessitating treatment for both bacterial and the underlying fungal infection. In addition, a brief course of steroids is indicated in some cases to limit the inflammation and to prevent permanent scarring.

Tinea Pedis

Tinea pedis usually presents as a dry scaly pattern on the periphery of the foot, known as *moccasin scale.* Infection is more common in men than women, particularly premenopausally. Complications include intertriginous tinea, which can result in moist erosions, and bullous tinea which is a hypersensitivity to the fungus, resulting in bullae on the soles of the feet, particularly in the summer months. Severely hypersensitive patients may develop an *id* reaction of vesicles or blisters on the palms. Id reactions are due to generalized allergic reaction to a local phenomenon.

The fissures resulting from tinea infections of the feet can be a source of secondary bacterial infection leading to cellulitus, especially in diabetics.

Tinea Corporis

This is the prototypical "ringworm" due to the round, scaly shape of most lesions. Classical tinea corporis lesions are centrally clear with a rim of scale; it is this scaly rim or edge that can be scraped to examine for hyphae. A drop of potassium hydroxide (KOH) is added to a slide containing superficial scale, allowed to dissolve for a few minutes after gently heating, and examined for the characteristic branching, *septate hyphae.* Experience is required to exclude false–positives and artifact development. Immunocompromised patients and those who have liberally used topical steroids have an increased risk of widespread tinea corporis, suggesting psoriasis, eczema, or an exanthem.

Tinea Cruris

Fungal infections of the inguinal crease can be confusing, especially if a classic expanding scaly ring is not present. The area is often slightly moist and may have underlying irritation or intertrigo. True fungal infections of the inguinal creases are much more common in adult men, with women more prone to candidal infection. Infection of the inguinal crease may coexist with tinea pedis or onychomycosis.

Onychomycosis

Fungal infections of the toenails begin most often distally, with yellow debris accumulating under the nail and progressing slowly over years, to wider nail involvement. Infection starts earlier in men than in women—late adolescence or early adulthood in men, postmenopausally in women. Complications include ingrown toenails and difficulty in cutting the nails. Psoriatic nail disease can closely mirror fungal disease; therefore, no patient should be started on systemic therapy for fungus without a culture or smear confirming tinea.

Tinea Versicolor

Tinea versicolor is caused by a normal cutaneous yeast, Malassesia furur, which proliferates in the sebaceous areas in warm, humid climates. Tinea versicolor is not seen in childhood, as the yeast apparently requires mature sebaceous gland development. The rash is macular (flat, nonpalpable) and scaly, affecting primarily the trunk, with an increased prevalence on the face in African-American patients. The yeast produces a chemical, azealic acid, which triggers a range of color change from pink to beige, as well as hyper- and hypopigmentation in patients. The color changes induced by tinea versicolor may persist for months after the yeast is controlled.

Treatment of fungal infections has improved dramatically over the past two decades with a multitude of topical antifungals available to control most mild to moderate infections. Tinea versicolor often responds to mild keratolytics such as topical selenium or zinc washes.

Widespread cutaneous, hair, scalp, and nail disease usually require oral therapy. All of the commonly available systemic antifungals—including griseofulvin, ketoconozole, sporonox, and lamisil—have the potential for drug-induced side effects including allergic hepatitis; therefore, therapy must be properly monitored.

Bacterial Infections

Impetigo

Impetigo produces fragile blisters and/or honey- or yellow-colored crusts over superficial erosions. *Staphlococcus aureus* is responsible for most bullous lesions and *Streptococcus* classically causes deeper erosions called *ecthyma.* However, the majority of lesions are combined infections with both organisms present. Spread of infection is common from close personal contact and insect bites. Treatment consists of either topical therapy with mupirocin (Bactroban) for localized disease, or oral medication effective against both organisms; regular penicillin is generally ineffective.

Folliculitis and Furunculosis

Folliculitis is infection of one or more single hair follicles, while furunculosis is infection of multiple adjacent follicles. The offending organism is usually *S aureus.* The primary lesion of *Staphylococcus* is a central pin-head white pustule surrounded by a red or pink circular flare. Recurrent episodes of *Staphylococcus* may occur in "Staph carriers"—those individuals who harbor infectious strains of *Staphylococcus* (aureus in place of epidermis), particularly in the nose, axillae, or groin.

Gram-negative folliculitis may also occur. A sudden crop of papules or pustules in an area previously treated long term with antibiotics—such as the face or trunk for acne or the axillae for hidradenitis suppuritiva—should trigger suspicion of gram-negative organism overgrowth. Culture of recalcitrant lesions or fresh lesions while on antibiotics is indicated to rule out a change in flora to a gram-negative organism with different antibiotic coverage indicated. Widespread folliculitis secondary to *Pseudomonas* is not rare following prolonged submersion in hot tubs. It should be remembered that mupirocin (Bactroban) is ineffective against a gram-negative organism.

Cellulitus

Cellulitus is an infection of soft tissue and is associated with the potential for increased systemic toxicity. Cellulitus is most common on the lower extremity, usually in the setting of underlying diabetes or vascular disease, especially chronic venous stasis. Infection begins with small breaks in the cutaneous barrier, as in severe xerosis, marked edema, or tinea pedis with fissuring between the toes. Cellulitus of the face, appearing as clinically asymmetrical red–purple swelling of the cheek and periorbital area with fever and sometimes sepsis, is called *erysipelas.*

Most episodes of cellulitus begin rapidly with a warm red streak or swelling, are associated with fever, and are due to *Streptococcus.* Initial episodes respond quickly to appropriate antibiotic therapy but continued infection can lead to fibrosis and lymphedema, predisposing the patient to recurrent episodes. Patients with severe fibrosis and scarring may have chronic, low-grade infection, recalcitrant to conventional courses of antibiotics. Gram-negative cellulitus, more common in diabetics, usually emanates from the toe web space and may be bullous, with foul-smelling green or brown pus. Any blister or open area should be cultured to maximize antibiotic efficacy.

Lyme Disease

Lyme disease is a bacterial infection transmitted to humans by a tick. The tick vectors include mice and deer and human exposure to the tick predominates along the edge of woods. The highest incidence occurs in the Northeast, upper Midwest, and Northwestern United States.

Lyme disease has early, intermittent, and late manifestations, but the skin manifestations occur relatively early. The classic lesion of Lyme is an expanding pink or red plaque at the site of the tick bite (Color Plate 14), often on the breast, lateral abdomen, or upper thigh. The lesion typically expands greater than 4 cm and may be confluent or centrally clear. Lesions last days or weeks and may be accompanied by fever, arthralgias, and malaise. Untreated disease may progress to disseminated lesions, which are multiple smaller, round or oval plaques, some of which may be centrally clear or confluent. Secondary and tertiary Lyme disease has the potential for serious cardiac, central nervous system, and arthritic complications.

Viral Infections

Herpes Simplex

Clustered blisters on an erythematous base characterize herpes simplex infections (Color Plate 15). These blisters are fragile and break readily to form superficial erosions. Primary herpes simplex infections occur most commonly in the mouth or lip area and on the genitalia but can occur anywhere the virus is inoculated. Fever, malaise, and lymphadenopathy can accompany the initial infection. Primary perioral infections can include gingivostomatitis mimicking "trench mouth," but recurrences rarely affect the oral mucosa.

Recurrences are due to reactivation of latent infection of the sensory root ganglion. Approximately one third of patients with herpes simplex infections never experience recrudescence, one third develop rare recurrences, and one third experience relatively frequent episodes of the disease. Illness, fever, and ultraviolet light may precipitate attacks, hence the phrases "fever blister," "cold sore," and sometimes mistakenly "sun poisoning" for severe blistering of the labial areas after sun exposure. Recurrences generally become less frequent with time. Complications of recurrent infection include secondary impetiginization with *Staphlococcus* or *Streptococcus* and scarring of the cornea if the periorbital area is involved.

Treatment of primary herpes infections includes acyclovir (Zovirax), or one of the newer acyclovir metabolites, as well as supportive care for severe disease. Recurrent infection may be treated with topical or oral antiviral medication for 5 to 7 days; those patients with multiple recurrences can receive suppressive doses of acyclovir to minimize the number of outbreaks.

Varicella Infections

The most common manifestation of the varicella virus is chickenpox, usually a childhood viral exanthem of 2 to 3 weeks' duration. The classic lesions of chickenpox appear as a "dew-drop on a rose petal," a small vesicle on a pink base (Color Plate 16). The lesions first appear on the trunk and scalp, then spread in a centrifugal pattern to the extremities. Sequela include depressed or pitted scars, usually from secondary infection of the primary lesions. Immunocompromised children and some healthy adults with primary varicella infections may have significant morbidity, including liver and lung involvement, and may die of respiratory failure or sepsis.

Herpes zoster or *shingles* is a recrudescence of the varicella virus that has remained dormant in the ganglion, usually for many years, The virus manifests itself as clustered blisters on erythematous bases, usually grouped along one (or two adjacent) dermatomes. Frequently affected areas are the thorax and face, particularly the trigemminal distribution of the forehead, but extremity, sacral, and lower facial presentations occur.

The diagnosis of shingles can be obscured by the fact that pain can precede the eruption for up to a week and thus can present as atypical chest pain, headache, gall bladder disease, or bursitis until the characteristic blisters appear. Complications include disseminated disease, scarring of the affected site, secondary infection of the blisters, and postherpetic neuralgia.

Anticipate disseminated disease by examining the entire patient at the initial presentation, as numerous lesions outside the dermatome suggest viremia and may require systemic therapy.

Scarring of the affected site is especially common for trigemminal zoster as the cornea may become permanently scarred. Patients with eyelid or forehead lesions, particularly if the tip of the nose is affected, should be referred to an opthalmologist for evaluation of orbital disease.

Impetiginization of the blisters is more common in chronically ill patients such as those with malignancies or diabetes, and may require both topical and systemic treatment.

Postherpetic neuralgia is the most feared complication of zoster. In these patients, the rash resolves but the pain does not. Postherpetic pain is more common in those over 50 and can range from mild to debilitatingly severe. Early treatment with systemic antiviral therapy, while widely acknowledged to modestly shorten the duration of acute lesions, has not eliminated all cases of postherpetic pain.

Papilloma Viruses

The papilloma virus is a large group of closely related viruses, producing warty lesions in various clinical manifestations. Currently, location and appearance classify warts, but identifying the viral subtype may become important in predicting which lesions confer a potential for malignant transformation. It is recognized that at least several subtypes, notably HPV 16 and 18 in the genitalia, are associated with a significant rate of malignant degeneration of the affected cells, conferring an increased risk of cervical malignancy.

The most common clinical lesions of the papilloma virus include common warts, plane warts, plantar warts, and genital warts.

Common Warts. These warts are typically found on the hands, especially fingers and periungual spaces. There is a peak incidence in middle childhood and lesions are raised, rough, hyperkeratotic, or "verrucous."

Plane or Flat Warts. These warts are much smaller, flatter lesions, each lesion measuring 1 to 3 mm, but they can become confluent. Flat warts are mainly found on the bearded area of the face, especially in men, the dorsae of the hands, and legs, particularly in women, perhaps due to nicks in the skin from shaving.

Plantar Warts. Plantar warts or warts on the soles of the feet can be painful. Punctate areas of hemorrhage in the debrided wart may be helpful in distinguishing plantar warts from calluses.

Genital Warts. Genital warts are often the most troublesome warts because of the concern about the increased rate of abnormal Pap smears and cervical cancer in women who have genital warts. While they may be numerous, genital warts are often discrete, small, and hyperkeratotic in men, but in women may be flat, skin colored, confluent, and more difficult to detect clinically. Any woman suspected of having genital warts should be closely followed with regular Pap smears by her gynecologist. As with any sexually transmitted disease (STD), patients with genital warts should be evaluated for the concomitant acquisition of other STDs.

Treatment of papilloma viral infections remains inelegant and imprecise. Warts can be cut off, cauterized, frozen, or treated with a variety of acid preparations. None of these modalities are completely satisfying for either the patient or provider and caution must be exercised not to induce a permanent scar for a condition to which most patients develop spontaneous resistance.

Molluscum Contagiosum

Molluscum produce a type of wart unrelated to the papilloma virus. Lesions are typically pearly, discrete and umbilicated, with a central dimple or core. Molluscum occur in two age spikes—children and sexually active adults—and are thought to spread from direct skin contact. Each lesion is 1 to 5 mm in size and peak sites of involvement are the face in children and upper inner thighs in young adults. Lesions may develop in areas of trauma, such as an abraded knee.

Widespread molluscum contagiosum is uncommon except in atopics or those who are immunocompromised, particularly with HIV infection. Molluscum in HIV patients are especially prevalent on the face, presumably due to the small breaks in the skin induced by shaving. With advanced AIDS, solitary lesions can become large and nodular, mimicking basal-cell carcinoma, and multiple lesions can become confluent.

There is no specific therapy for molluscum and no vaccination to prevent infection. Fortunately, most patients spontaneously develop immunity to the virus, although this may take months or even years. No serious systemic effect is recognized from molluscum infection. Patients who desire treatment can have individual lesions treated with liquid nitrogen, mechanical expression, or removal but it must be remembered that the treatment can leave scars for a condition that usually resolves spontaneously. Recent treatment of advanced HIV infection with protease inhibitors has resulted in regression of molluscum in some patients.

Scabies

Scabies is an infection with a human mite, transmitted person to person by close human contact. Itch is the chief symptom of scabies and there is no characteristic rash other than excoriations, typically worse in the intertriginous or web space areas (i.e., between the fingers). A diagnostic clue is pruritus that awakens or keeps the patient awake at night. Other family members or bed partners may be affected.

Scabies is treated by the topical application of a pyremethrin cream (Elimite) applied from the neck to the toes and left on 8 to 14 hours. Reapplication is generally not necessary but patients should be advised that the itch resolves slowly over days or weeks, not immediately after treatment. It is important that all clothing and linens with which the patient has had contact be washed to kill the mites and eggs. Family members should also be treated.

Head Lice

Head lice are a contagious human parasite, spread by person-to-person contact and from contact with fomites such as combs or hats. Outbreaks occur primarily in schools and day care centers, with a greater prevalence among caucasian children. Infection presents with itch and sometimes secondary infection from scratching. Live lice or eggs can be best detected visually at the occipital region. Treatment with pyremethrin shampoo usually eradicates the infection. Patients are generally no longer contagious after one treatment. As with scabies, it is important that all clothing and linens with which the patient has had contact be washed to kill the parasite. Family members should also be evaluated.

▶ DRUG REACTIONS

Allergic reactions to medications remain common, yet frequently unpredictable. It is important to think of a potential drug reaction in any rash of uncertain etiology as drug reactions can mimic many other cutaneous disorders. A good drug history includes asking not only "What drugs do you take?" but "What medications have been prescribed for you? What over-the-counter medications do you take? Have you tried anything to treat the rash? Do you use any medications for your eyes, headache, allergy or sinus problems, dental antibiotics, laxatives, or sleeping pills?" It is sometimes helpful to have the patient bring in all the medications taken in the last few months, sometimes a shopping bag full.

First-time allergic reactions to medications usually develop 5 to 14 days after the medication is initiated; repeat exposure may induce a reaction much faster. Patients may develop allergy to a medication they have taken repeatedly in the past without incident. Some groups of medications stimulate allergic phenomenon more frequently, notably sulfa- and penicillin-based antibiotics, seizure medications, pain medications, and nonsteroidal antiinflammatory agents, but it remains an axiom that "any drug can cause any reaction."

Drug reactions are classified by the type of cutaneous reaction they produce. These are hypersensitivity reactions, however, that can also be triggered by other allergic phenomenon such as viral infections or autoimmune disease.

Urticarial Reactions

Urticarial reactions can occur with medications, food, environmental, or unknown antigens. Urticarial reactions wax and wane over a 24-hour period and are marked by prominent dermatographism. Patients should be questioned about tongue or lip swelling, difficulty swallowing or breathing, and wheezing. Patients with these findings merit closer evaluation and more aggressive treatment.

Some drugs are direct histamine releasers and induce urticarial reactions without requiring an immunologic response from the host. These include aspirin, morphine, codeine, demerol, and nonsteroidal antiinflammatories.

Morbilliform Reactions

This is the classic, diffuse, macular or slightly palpable "salmon pink" or "drug red" rash. The rash typically begins on dependent areas, the back, or buttocks in hospitalized patients, frequently mistaken initally as a reaction "to the sheets."

Fixed-Drug Eruption

This relatively unusual reaction consists of erythematous plaques with dusky or erythematous centers on discrete asymmetrical locations. Lesions are sparse, one to several in number, and one to several centimeters in diameter. Lesions appear irregularly and can occur on the genitalia or oral mucosa. The sporadic and asymmetrical nature of the lesions makes the diagnosis easily confused with nummular eczema, a patch of psoriasis, or fixed urticarial reaction such as an insect bite. Drugs most often associated with fixed-drug reactions include phenolphthalein in laxatives and tetracyclines.

Erythema Multiforme

This is a reaction spectrum due to a variety of drugs and viruses as well as unknown causes. Erythema multiforme lesions are focal plaques with central or erythematous centers called "bull's eye" or "targetoid" lesions (Color Plate 17). These lesions are classically on the palms and soles, although they can be located anywhere.

Stevens–Johnson syndrome implies oral, ocular, or genital lesions, usually presenting as blisters or erosions, with or without the cutaneous targetoid lesions of erythema multiforme. These sites are at increased risk of scarring, resulting in blindness or urethral obstruction.

Toxic Epidermal Necrolysis

This generalized sloughing of the skin presents with erythema that rapidly blisters (Color Plate 18). Light rubbing of the skin produces erosions (Nikolsky sign) due to epidermal separation from the dermis. The result is the absence of an effective cutaneous barrier—similar to second- or third-degree burns. There is substantial morbidity due to scarring of mucous membranes and mortality from infection and septic shock. The use of systemic steroids for treatment of toxic epidermal necrolysis remains controversial; transfer to a burn unit optimizes local care.

▶ PHOTOSENSITIVITY REACTIONS

Enhanced sensitivity to ultraviolet light can be the result of genetic predisposition, connective tissue disease, or allergic phenomenon. Photosensitivity reactions are divided into phototoxic and photoallergic categories.

Phototoxic Reactions

Any agent that in sufficient quantity can produce an enhanced photosensitivity in any person is known as phototoxic. Drugs such as doxycycline and psoralen that lower the minimal erythema dose (MED) do not require an immune reaction on the part of the host, but will make any person photosensitive, given sufficient exposure to the drug.

Photoallergic Reactions

Photoallergic reactions require the host to process and react to the chemical before lowering the MED; thus, reactivity is selective and generally unpredictable. Photosensitive reactions can be to topical or systemic agents. Examples of potentially photosensitive topical chemicals include fragrances, pre-servatives, and, ironically, some sunscreen ingredients. Systemic photosensitizers include most frequently thiazide diuretics and nonsteroidal antiinflammatory medications, but many others have been implicated. Photosensitivity to a medication may take months or years to develop and likewise months or years for the photosensitivity to wane after the drug is withdrawn.

▶ VASCULITIS

Vasculitis is a hypersensitivity reaction that causes an inflammation around the blood vessels. Vasculitic reactions can be caused by drugs, infection, or autoimmune disease, and are classified clinically as small- or large-vessel disease.

Small-vessel disease produces "palpable purpura" or leukocytoclastic vasculitis (Color Plate 19). Palpable lesions imply inflammation around the blood vessels; in leukocytoclastic vasculitis, around the small postcapillary venules. Clinically, nonpalpable purpuric lesions are due to bleeding into the skin, such as ecchymoses (bruises), petechiae, or large infiltration from a clotting disorder vasculitic. Lesions begin acrally, or on the buttocks in dependent patients, and are symmetrically distributed. The differential diagnosis of this reaction pattern must first exclude a serious infectious etiology such as meningococcemia or Rocky Mountain spotted fever, but other causes include allergic reactions to drugs or autoimmune disease such as lupus erythematosus or Sjogren's disease.

Large-vessel disease produces inflammation around medium- to large-sized vessels, usually arteries. Clinically, large-vessel vasculitis presents as livedo reticularis, a mottled, lacy, dusky purple or blue pattern of vascular accentuation, usually beginning acrally and progressing centrally. Livedo can be a benign process or imply an underlying connective tissue disorder such as cardiolipin antibody syndrome or polyarteritis nodosa. Advanced inflammation of the blood vessels can result in nodular lesions, skin breakdown, and ulceration, such as in cases of calciphylaxis (seen rarely in end-stage renal failure patients).

▶ CUTANEOUS TUMORS

Benign and malignant tumors of the skin represent a significant percentage of visits to health-care providers. Both types of tumors can be proliferations of vascular, pigmented, or appendage cells. The most common types of benign lesions include cherry angiomas, acrochordons (skin tags), cysts, seborrheic keratosis, nevi, and dermatofibroma.

Benign Tumors

Cherry Angiomas

These discrete red or pink papules commonly develop in early adulthood on the trunk. They range from pinpoint to 4 to 5 mm in size. They are predominantly asymptomatic and require no treatment unless the lesions get caught on clothing, bleed, or if the diagnosis is in doubt.

Acrochordons (Skin Tags)

Acrochordons are fleshy polypoid lesions located in flexural folds such as the neck, axillae, inframammary, or inguinal creases. Skin tags develop in adulthood and are frequently familial. No treatment is required unless lesions get caught on clothing, jewelry, or seatbelts. Simple excision usually suffices. Individual lesions rarely recur but patients typically develop further crops of skin tags over their lifetime. Any atypical lesion should be biopsied.

Cysts

Cysts are localized collections or sacs of oily material and are generally classified as (1) *pilar cysts* or *wens* when they develop on the scalp and (2) *sebaceous cysts* when located on the trunk or face. Cysts are generally semi-soft and freely moveable, and many have a central opening or comedone. They are often familial, particularly on the scalp, and can recur after excision. Complications include rupture and infection.

Seborrheic Keratosis

The word *keratosis* implies a rough or warty lesion. *Seborrheic keratoses* are raised, rough, "stuck on," or warty papules or plaques (Color Plate 20). The lesions feel as though they can be scraped off with a fingernail due to the fact that they are epidermal proliferations without a dermal component. Seborrheic keratoses can be beige, brown, or black, and can be few to numerous in number. They are located primarily on the non sun-exposed areas of the trunk, although they can also occur on the legs and scalp perimeter. Seborrheic keratoses are benign but any atypical lesion should be biopsied to rule out skin cancer.

Nevi

Nevi, also known as *moles,* are a collection of pigmented cells. One to 2% of the population has congenital nevi, meaning nevi clinically present at birth. Almost everyone acquires some nevi in childhood or young adulthood. Nevi go through their own natural evolution throughout life, beginning as flat macules, progressing to raised papules with an even distribution of pigment, and a symmetrical border. Benign nevi often have obvious normal hair growth. Nevi range in color from nearly white to dark black, but in general, most nevi are consistent with the patient's overall coloring, in that it is unusual to find very dark nevi in very light patients. Nevi out of character with the rest of a patient's mole pattern should raise clinical suspicion for dysplasia or malignancy.

Dermatofibroma

A dermatofibroma is a localized firm papule, usually located on the lower leg in women, one to few in number, and less than 5 mm in diameter. These lesions often feel like a small pea in the skin and have an overlying hyperpigmented dimple when compressed. Rarely, these lesions develop a basal-cell carcinoma over the surface, so any changing or atypical lesion should be biopsied.

Precancerous Skin Lesions

Actinic keratoses are localized, flat, scaly, and erythematous lesions of abnormal epidermal proliferation. Actinic kertoses are common in fair individuals with a history of extensive photoexposure. They are located primarily on the face, dorsae of the hands, extensor forearms, ears, and scalp (in men without hair). Histologically, actinic keratoses have abnormal cells confined to the epidermis.

Actinic keratoses have a low rate of conversion to squamous-cell carcinoma; approximately 4% of lesions progress to squamous cell carcinoma. However, actinic keratoses are markers for individuals who may be at increased risk of other skin cancer, including basal-cell carcinoma and melanoma; therefore, these patients should use photoprotection and have regular skin cancer screenings.

Treatment of actinic keratoses includes cryotherapy, local removal, or topical 5-flourouracil cream. Any atypical lesion should be biopsied prior to removal.

Malignant Tumors

Basal-Cell Carcinoma

Basal-cell carcinoma is the most common skin cancer. Fortunately, most lesions have a low metastatic potential. They are malignant chiefly in the sense that they are locally invasive and nonhealing. The risk of development of basal-cell carcinoma rises with photoexposure, particularly with a history of sunburns, occupational exposure, and sun tanning parlor use.

Most basal-cell carcinomas have a pearly, shiny, or

translucent hue, especially at the margin. Developed lesions typically have telangiectasias on the surface. Basal-cell carcinomas are classified by their morphology.

Nodular Basal-Cell Carcinoma. Nodular basal-cell carcinoma is the most frequent variety of the basal-cell carcinomas. They are evenly raised papules, which later umbilicate or ulcerate. Patients often complain of a "pimple that does not heal" or that bleeds when washing or shaving.

Pigmented Basal-Cell Carcinoma. Pigmented basal-cell carcinoma can be brown, black, gray, or blue and may be relatively flat. These lesions may be clinically confused with pigmented nevi or melanoma, and require histologic confirmation.

Bowenoid Basal-Cell Carcinoma. These scaly lesions may be multiple and mimic actinic keratoses or Bowen's disease (intraepidermal squamous-cell carcinoma). These lesions must also be differentiated from plaques of nummular eczema or psoriasis (Color Plate 21).

Morpheaform or Sclerosing Basal-Cell Carcinoma. These occult lesions may present as scaly or atrophic plaques that centrally scar, thus appearing to heal, only to advance at the edges. These lesions may obtain substantial size before being clinically obvious to either the patient or provider. Lesions may be extensively locally invasive, especially if they occur in facial plane lines such as the nasal crease, behind the ear, or the periorbital area.

Melanoma

Melanoma is a cancer of melanocytes or pigment-forming cells. Melanoma typically arises in preexisting nevi, but some tumors develop *de novo.* Most melanoma take months or years to become invasive and develop a metastatic potential; thus, many evolving melanomas can be detected early by carefully monitoring nevi for change by both the patient and health-care provider.

Normal nevi are evenly raised and pigmented, with a symmetrical perimeter, and most are 6 mm or less in diameter. Changes that should prompt closer attention or removal include:

- Asymmetry of color or size
- A mole "out of character" with the rest of the patient's nevi; that is, larger, darker, or more irregular
- Darkening or lightening of a preexisting mole: black discoloration or loss of color should raise suspicion
- Growth or symptoms in a mole, such as itch, burning, tenderness

Superficial Spreading Melanoma. The most common type of melanoma, superficial spreading melanoma, undergoes gradual malignant degeneration. The lesions spread laterally (radially) at first, later vertically, acquiring metastatic potential (Color Plate 22). Most lesions detected in the radial growth phase are curable with adequate excision.

Nodular Melanoma. Nodular melanoma begins as a raised lesion with an initial vertical growth phase, and thus is at much greater risk of early metastatic spread.

Lentigo Maligna. Lentigo maligna is a slowly evolving lesion that has an extremely long radial growth phase and is generally found on the face of elderly patients who have a history of chronic sun exposure. Because of the long radial growth phase, vertical growth and metastases are rare.

Acral Melanoma. Acral melanoma occur on the palms, soles, nail beds, and mucosal surfaces. Acral melanoma are uncommon but found in patients of all races. These lesions may escape clinical detection because of the relatively obscure locations and slow growth; patients may attribute a discolored or black toenail, for example, to past trauma. Any changing, pigmented streak of a nail should be biopsied to rule out atypical change of a nail bed nevus.

Nevi

There are several variants of nevi that warrant special mention: congenital nevi, halo nevi, and dysplastic nevi.

Congenital Nevi

Congenital nevi are present at birth, can range in size from minute to extremely large plaques, and often contain hair. Congenital nevi have a small but real lifetime risk of malignant degeneration and thus need to be followed over time for change.

Halo Nevi

Halo nevi are nevi surrounded by a "halo" formed by an area of hypopigmentation that develops around one or several moles, particularly after extensive photoexposure. These nevi need to be evaluated for dysplasia and malignancy and certainly any atypical or solitary halo nevus should be considered for removal and biopsy.

Dysplastic Nevi

Moles with irregular pigmentation, radial growth, and asymmetrical edges—but not irregular enough to be malignant—are called "funny looking moles" or dysplastic nevi. One form of dysplastic nevi is the "fried egg mole," meaning darker or lighter in the center compared with the perimeter. Individuals with a family history of melanoma and a personal history of dysplastic nevi have an extremely high rate of development of melanoma. The risk for those with few dysplastic nevi and no family history of melanoma is unknown but thought to be higher than the overall population's and, therefore, these individuals should be followed more carefully and use photoprotection.

V

Approach to the Patient with Specialized Needs

52

The Hospitalized Child

Sandra L. Gomberg
Sally Boyle Quinn
Leonard Friedland

Children are physiologically, developmentally, and anatomically different than adults (Ball & Bindler, 1995; Thomas, 1996). These differences require unique approaches in the assessment, care, and treatment of a child and his or her family.

FAMILY-CENTERED CARE

Children must rely on family members to assure that their basic needs are met. Health care for children is typically organized in a framework called family-centered care. Family-centered care models strive to organize health-care services in a respectful and supportive approach that fully involves family members (Letourneau & Elliot, 1996). The assessment, care, and treatment of children must be provided in ways that recognize the inseparability of the child and family.

Families, however, represent diverse groups of people who provide the ongoing care for children. Traditional family units may include the child's parents and other siblings. Other families may include extended relatives or friends who provide care for the child on a continuous basis.

To assure that health-care services are provided to meet the needs of the child while continuously including the family members, the clinician must first identify the members of the family and their relationship to the child.

It is imperative to determine that the adults presenting with the child are, in fact, either the parents or legal guardians. Guardianship is a legal status and differs from informal custody situations where the child lives with, and is cared for by, a family friend or relative. Relatives without legal custody or guardianship may not have the ability to provide consent for medical care and treatment. Determination of parental or legal guardianship status is necessary to assure that proper consents are obtained for necessary medical care. When parental or guardianship questions arise, hospital personnel in social work, risk management, and the legal department can provide necessary guidance.

ASSESSMENT

Assessment of a pediatric patient must include the child and the parents/guardians (Callery, 1997). Key subjective data will be obtained during interviews with the parent/guardian as well as from the child. Key objective data will be obtained from the clinician's direct observation and examination of the child.

The Interview

General principles of conducting a patient interview are the same: introduce yourself, provide privacy, explain the purpose of the interview, use varying questioning techniques, and demonstrate empathetic listening (Bates, Bickley, & Hoekelman, 1995). Key variations in conducting a patient interview with a child and parents/guardians include privacy, asking questions, and honesty.

Privacy

Provide an environment where parents/guardians feel free to speak candidly. This may be with or without the child present. Eliminate distractions for both the child and the parents/guardians. Parents/guardians will struggle to focus on your interview if their child is anxious, crying, having a procedure performed, or is distracted by the environment (lights, people, equipment) (Callery, 1997). Infants and children can benefit from strategies used to provide privacy to adult patients. Close the door of the exam room or pull the privacy curtain around the child and/or parent/guardian prior to beginning the assessment. This minimizes environmental distractions and provides a focus for your interaction with the family. Children of all ages deserve privacy when being examined or undressed. Older children may prefer to answer questions or be examined without the parent/guardian present.

Asking Questions

Asking one question at a time allows the parents/guardians to focus on the specific piece of information you want. Young children can be asked questions as well (Bates et al., 1995). By first asking questions that demonstrate your interest in the child, you can build a rapport for later discussions about the illness or treatment (Ball & Bindler, 1995; Wong, 1993). For example, asking a young child about a favorite toy can be as informative and helpful to your assessment as asking "Where does it hurt." Use a language level and style that both the parent and the child can understand.

Honesty

Being honest with a child helps build his or her trust in you. For example, it is inappropriate to tell a child "this won't hurt" if, in fact, it will hurt. When preparing a child for a painful or unpleasant experience, such as receiving an injection, use descriptive words that are within the child's knowledge base, experience, and vocabulary, such as: "This will feel like a pinch" (Ball & Bindler, 1995; Wong, 1993). It is important to verbally prepare and warn infants and children of all ages prior to performing a painful procedure, regardless of how quickly the procedure may be completed. It is unacceptable to perform a painful procedure without this preparation, such as when the infant or child is asleep. Finally, children often ask questions that appear complicated and mature. Consider the child's knowledge base, life experiences, and developmental level before formulating your answer to assure that you provide honest information the child will understand (Ball & Bindler, 1995; Mellick & Lau, 1994; Wong, 1993). Rely on parents/guardians to provide insight in how to "honestly" communicate with the child. Parents/guardians can offer words, analogies, and guidance that are critical in the success of your communication with the child. Table 52–1 describes strategies for communicating with children.

TABLE 52–1. Strategies for Communicating with Children

- Get down to the child's eye level to make eye contact
- Speak slowly and gently, using simple words and sentences
- Speak directly to the child, not just to the parents
- Acknowledge the presence of special items such as a doll or stuffed toy and include them in your conversation
- Clearly identify yourself and what your interaction with the child and family will be
- Encourage questions
- Be honest
- Identify, allow, and respect normal expressions of emotions
- Give realistic choices only when one exists
- Support the relationship between parents/guardians and the child
- Respect the child's right to privacy
- Watch for signs of information overload such as frequent interruptions, fidgeting, and long periods of silence
- Allow children to communicate through play, such as drawing and storytelling
- Use nonverbal strategies, such as charts and stickers, to praise the child's participation or cooperation. Reward positive behaviors

From Ball & Bindler (1995); Mellick & Lau (1994); Wong (1993).

The Physical Examination

Understanding a child's expected growth and developmental stages and age-specific characteristics can guide the clinician's approach to assessment and care delivery (Ball & Bindler, 1995; Mellick & Lau, 1994; Wong, 1993). A fundamental knowledge base of developmental stages and normal physical characteristics, including vital signs, is essential in the care of children. Recognize that children may regress at times of crisis, fear, or uncertainty, making it difficult to identify age-appropriate behaviors and coping skills. This causes an additional stress for parents who may grow frustrated by regression and changes in behavior, such as bed wetting in the previously potty-trained child. Clinical departments are well served by maintaining up-to-date pediatric reference materials that include normal variations in developmental and physiological parameters in children of all age groups. Tables 52–2 through 52–6 highlight developmental and age-related considerations in approaching the assessment and care of a child.

The physical assessment of the child begins as you observe the child from a distance prior to actually approaching the bedside (Mellick & Lau, 1994; Thomas, 1996). Focus on the child's general appearance, position of comfort, color, expression, activity level, respiratory effort and rate, interaction with parents, and vital sign parameters obvious from monitors. The way the child "looks," particularly at rest and when not distracted, is an important indicator of the child's status. Compare these initial observations with the same clinical parameters once the child has been disturbed and is awake and alert. The differences in the child's status when asleep or at rest versus when awake and disturbed can indicate important clinical information. For ex-

TABLE 52–2. Unique Considerations in Approaching the Assessment of the Care of the Child

Infants (Birth to 12 months)

- Keep parents with the child
- Perform exam with child in parents' lap, being held in position of comfort
- Use a gentle voice, make eye contact, and smile
- Perform distressing procedures last
- Avoid abrupt movements
- Determine nap, sleep, and feeding times; plan care and treatment accordingly
- Never use needle-to-needle connections. Avoid using needles taped to insertion caps or IV sites. Use direct connections, such as tubing to catheter hub, for all IVs. (A disconnected needle could seriously hurt an infant.)
- Obtain weight. Medication dosages and fluid requirements are calculated using weight
- Be alert to blood volumes needed for lab tests
- Place IV in nondominant extremity to promote comfort and use of dominant extremity
- Never leave an infant unattended
- Side rails should always be in full upright position
- Minimize noise and bright lights
- Offer pacifier if parent consents
- Recognize opportunities to provide anticipatory guidance:
  - ▶ Car seat safety
  - ▶ Toy safety
  - ▶ Immunizations
  - ▶ Home child-proofing

From Ball & Bindler 1995); Bates, Bickley, & Hoekelman (1995); Mellick & Lau (1994); Wong (1993).

ample, a child with an upper airway obstruction may breathe comfortably when asleep but will demonstrate severe distress when awake. Any child observed to be in distress when asleep, at rest, or during an initial observation should be immediately evaluated and necessary emergency care implemented.

Parents/guardians are important components of the physical examination. Infants and young children often cooperate best when examined in the lap of their parent (Ball & Bindler, 1995; Bates et al., 1995; Wong, 1993). Plan to perform the least invasive parts of the examination first, moving towards the most invasive last. For example, plan to evaluate the child's respiratory rate and heart rate prior to performing a rectal or oral temperature. Plan to complete all key elements of the assessment prior to beginning procedures, as the child's ability to cooperate will diminish rapidly.

If performing physical assessments in urgent and unexpected situations, such as in an emergency room setting or during an unexpected medical emergency, focus on airway, breathing, and circulation (American Heart Association, 1997; Bates et al., 1995). Tables 52–7 and 52–8 outline key anatomic and physiologic considerations in the evaluation and management of the airway, breathing, and circulation of a child.

TABLE 52–3. Unique Considerations in Approaching the Assessment of the Care of the Child

Toddler (12–36 Months)

- Keep parents with the child
- Privacy becomes important
- Have parents and child remove clothing as needed
- Exam one body area at a time
- Mimick parents—find out what works for them
- Provide legitimate choices. ("Do you want me to listen to the right side or the left side first?")
- Be honest
- Give child permission to cry
- Explain to parents that difficult behavior during examinations and hospitalization can be normal and expected and is not a correlation to bad parenting
- Allow security items (blankets, dolls, stuffed toys) to stay with the child at all times. Include these items in explanations and care
- Allow child to play with equipment (stethoscope, pulse oximeter) with staff supervision
- Give child a job, particularly during minor procedures or during the examination (holding the reflex hammer or Band-aid)
- Praise good behavior. Provide rewards
- Determine the child's usual routines. Recognize illness often interferes with daily routines. Child may sleep longer and nap erratically. Recognize parental frustration caused by disrupted routines
- Meal times may require additional staff supervision. Watch for age-appropriate meal selections and utensils
- Recognize regression. Be supportive of child and parents
- Maintain safe environment and increased surveillance
- Explain procedures to both parents and child
- Recognize opportunities to provide anticipatory guidance:
  - ▶ Accident prevention
  - ▶ Poisoning prevention
  - ▶ Immunization
  - ▶ Toy safety
  - ▶ Rewards and discipline strategies

From Ball & Bindler (1995); Bates, Bickley, & Hoekelman (1995); Mellick & Lau (1994); Wong (1993).

There are normal variations in vital-sign and laboratory test-result ranges for infants, children, and adolescents. It is recommended that up-to-date references be made available in clinical departments that care for children, no matter how infrequently. Helpful strategies include documenting the normal vital signs or lab test results anticipated for the child along with the actual values as part of your clinical assessment. Normal ranges for individual pediatric patients could be posted for reference on the front of the chart to provide ease in comparison. Children with chronic illnesses, such as congenital heart disease or cystic fibrosis, will have individual "normals" in their vital signs or laboratory test results that are often outside of typical ranges. Parents/guardians as well as older children are often very articulate in sharing what is normal for the child and relaying typical treatment strategies that have worked and that do

TABLE 52–4. Unique Considerations in Approaching the Assessment of the Care of the Child

Preschool (Ages 3–6 Years)

- Keep parents with the child
- Privacy is important
- Language skills developing quickly
- Allow the child to undress independently. Allow child to wear underpants
- Communicate in simple terms. Use 1- and 2-step directions and explanations
- Provide explanations using descriptions that the child will see, feel, smell, hear, touch; for example, "The room will be dark." "The medicine will feel cold"
- Have child participate—hold hand, hold supplies, help open packages
- Make use of child's interest in fantasy—popular characters and superheroes
- Set limits; offer choices that are reasonable
- Be alert to hospital vocabulary ("CAT SCAN," "ICU," "STICK") that can confuse the child's literal understanding of these words
- Pain is often perceived as punishment
- Provide explanations prior to all procedures
- Recognize opportunities to provide anticipatory guidance:
  - Accident prevention
  - Poisoning prevention
  - Immunizations
  - Toy safety
  - Friendships and peers
  - Growing independence

From Ball & Bindler (1995); Bates, Bickley, & Hoekelman (1995); Mellick & Lau (1994); Wong (1993).

TABLE 52–5. Unique Considerations in Approaching the Assessment of the Care of the Child

School Age (6–11 Years)

- Still need parents when stressed
- Allow child to undress. Provide cover gown
- Privacy needed
- Peer pressure becomes evident
- Communication skills improve
- Perceives pain as a result of bad behavior. May refuse pain relief in fear of an injection
- Do not reinforce stoic behavior
- Fears loss of control. Use simple explanations to provide information. Anticipate concerns
- Fantasy still evident
- Offer opportunities for reasonable choices
- Have child describe problem in his or her own words. Assist parents in allowing the child to do so
- Provide explanations in terms of senses. Be alert to hospital language that can be confusing
- Use opportunities to discuss the child's likes and dislikes to minimize anxiety or provide distraction
- Set limits
- Use the child's understanding of time to plan care, and offer the child choices in scheduling, if possible
- Avoid hospital vocabulary that can cause confusion and anxiety
- Recognize opportunities to provide anticipatory guidance:
  - Bike safety
  - Immunizations
  - Accident prevention
  - Peer relationships

From Ball & Bindler (1995); Bates, Bickley, & Hoekelman (1995); Mellick & Lau (1994); Wong (1993).

work for this child. Tables 52–9, 52–10, and 52–11 provide normal ranges for pediatric vital signs.

Medical plans of treatment for the sick or injured child should be developed in consultation with physicians with expertise in the care of children. While there are often many similarities in the treatment plans for children and adults with the same illness or injury, there are important and unique considerations in how the plan of treatment and related interdisciplinary care is actually implemented.

The differences in the care and treatment of the hospitalized child can be discussed in terms of the environment where the child receives the care and the types of services that the child will receive.

THE CHILD IN THE HOSPITAL

Physical Environment

The unfamiliar hospital environment can be a dangerous place for a child. Children are inquisitive and adventurous even when sick. It is important to survey the area where the child will be receiving care and treatment. Just as at home,

TABLE 52–6. Unique Considerations in Approaching the Assessment of the Care of the Child

Adolescent (12 Years and Older)

- Can be a good historian
- Provide child choice of parental presence for explanations, examinations, and procedures
- Respect privacy and confidentiality
- Allow child to undress in private or provide a cover gown
- Avoid language that sounds juvenile
- Provide feedback to reinforce normal physical development throughout physical examination
- Fears loss of control. Do not encourage stoic behavior
- Recognize opportunity for providing anticipatory guidance:
  - Drug or alcohol use
  - Motor vehicle safety
  - Sexual development
  - Peer relationships

From Ball & Bindler (1995); Bates, Bickley, & Hoekelman (1995); Mellick & Lau (1994); Wong (1993).

TABLE 52–7. Anatomic and Physiologic Considerations: Child Compared with Adult

	Anatomy and Physiology	Clinical Consequences
Airway and Breathing	Infant's and child's upper airway are smaller	Small amounts of mucous and airway swelling can occlude the small airway diameter, and greatly increase the work of breathing
	Infant's tongue is larger	The tongue can displace posterior and occlude the airway; can also interfere with tracheal intubation
	Infant's and child's head are larger in proportion to body size	Difficulty in exposing the vocal cords during tracheal intubation
	Infant's and child's epiglottis are short, narrow, and thick	Difficult to control the epiglottis with a curved laryngoscope blade
	Vocal cords attach lower anteriorly	Difficulty in exposing the vocal cords during tracheal intubation
	Infant's and child's larynx are positioned higher	Difficult with a curved laryngoscope blade to control the line of vision between the tongue and vocal cords
	Infant's and child's larynx are funnel shaped (compared with cylinder shape) and subsequently the narrowest portion of the airway is at the nondistensible cricoid cartilage	Cuffed endotracheal tubes are not used in children below age 8 years
	In infants the ribs and intercostal cartilage are highly compliant	If the airway is obstructed, the ribs and intercostal cartilage may not support the lungs and the sternum, and intercostal areas may move during respiration rather than the chest and lungs (paradoxical respiration) Upper airway obstruction (croup, extrathoracic foreign bodies) may cause tracheal collapse during inspiration Intrathoracic foreign bodies and lower airway disease (bronchiolitis, asthma) may cause lower airway obstruction during expiration Opposing these dynamics with positive end-expiratory pressure (PEEP) may improve gas exchange
	Oxygen demand in the child is 6–8 mL/kg/minute (3–4 mL/kg/minute in the adult)	Hypoxemia develops more rapidly in the setting of inadequate ventilation
Circulation	In children and adults the normal hemodynamic response to blood loss is tachycardia and vasoconstriction early, with hypotension occurring as a late sign of shock	Assess indirect signs of cardiac output and systemic vascular resistance *Pulses:* Weak or narrow peripheral pulses may indicate low cardiac output; bounding and wide peripheral pulses may be a sign of decreased systemic vascular resistance *Skin:* Cold skin and delayed capillary refill may indicate low cardiac output; delayed capillary refill, pallor, mottling, and peripheral cyanosis may indicate increased systemic vascular resistance *Kidneys:* Urine output below 1 mL/kg/hour implies hypovolemia; insert an indwelling urinary catheter to best assess urine output *Brain:* Early clinical signs of brain hypoperfusion include subtle alterations in level of consciousness. These may include agitation, lethargy, poor concentration, irritability, confusion, poor response to painful stimuli. Often the child's parents will notice that "something is wrong" with their child. Listen carefully to what the parents say
	Infant and children have higher resting HR than adults	Important to recognize normal values, as sinus tachycardia commonly occurs as a response to anxiety, pain, fever, hypoxemia, hypovolemia; thus, the presence of true tachycardia merits further investigation
	Infant's and child's normal BP values vary by age	Median systolic BP estimated as: 90 mm Hg + (2 × age in years) Lower limit systolic BP can be estimated as: 70 mm Hg + (2 × age in years)
	Cardiac output in the infant and child is affected more by heart rate than stroke volume	The development of bradycardia in children with cardiorespiratory distress signifies decreasing cardiac output
	Circulating blood volume in infants is 80 mL/kg; children, 75 mL/kg; and adults, 70 mL/kg	Hypotension is usually not observed until 25% blood volume is acutely lost
Fluids	Water is based on the following daily caloric requirements: First 10 kg = 100 calories/kg/day Next 10 kg = 50 cal/kg/day 20 kg and beyond = 20 cal/kg/day	Example: a 25 kg 6-year-old's daily maintenance caloric requirement is: (10 kg × 100 cal/kg) + (10 kg × 50 cal/kg) + (5 kg × 20 cal/kg) = 1600 cal/day
	In the acute period (1–2 days) to remain in a nonketotic state the child must receive at least 20% of his/her daily fluid requirement	In a 25 kg 6-year-old whose daily maintenance caloric requirement is 1600 cal/day: 20% of 1600 cal/day = 320 cal/day; therefore, 320 cal is the minimum necessary for this child to remain in a nonketotic state in the first 1–2 days of an acute illness

(Continued)

TABLE 52–7. Anatomic and Physiologic Considerations: Child Compared with Adult *(Continued)*

Anatomy and Physiology	Clinical Consequences
D5 saline has 5 grams of dextrose/100 mL of saline Carbohydrates have 4 cal/gram Therefore, every 1000 cc of D5 saline supplies 200 cal	To provide all of the 320 calories required in the first day of an acute illness using D5 $^1/_2$ NS, give: $\frac{1000\text{ cc D5 } ^1/_2\text{ NS}}{200\text{ cal}} = \frac{X\text{ cc D5 } ^1/_2\text{ NS}}{320\text{ cal}}$ $X = 1600$ cc/day Analysis of the above calculations shows that maintenance calories = maintenance fluids when using D5 $^1/_2$ NS. In the example of the 25 kg 6-year-old, maintenance calories in the first 24 hours are 1600 calories, and maintenance fluids are 1600 cc Therefore, a commonly used method to calculate daily fluid requirements is first 10 kg = 100 cc/kg/day next 10 kg = 50 cc/kg/day 20 kg and beyond = 20 cc/kg/day The 25 kg 6-year-old's daily fluid requirement of 1600 cc: (10 kg × 100 cc/kg) + (10 kg × 50 cc/kg) + (5 kg × 20 cc/kg) = 1600 cc/day = 66 cc/hour

From American Academy of Pediatrics (1995).

it may be helpful to bend down or kneel on the floor to see what the environment looks like from the eye level of the child. Loose hanging cords from monitors or equipment may be pulled, causing the equipment to fall, break, and/or cause injury. Supplies left at the bedside or in bathrooms, such as small caps from syringes or medicine containers that could be mistakenly ingested or plastic bags and rubber tourniquets that could be placed over the head or other body parts, could cause severe injury. Electrical outlets left uncovered could cause risk to the investigating child. Automatic controls for beds or the buttons on the IV pump can be inviting to the child yet pose serious safety risks. Cribs with properly working side rails should be used for infants and toddlers who are not able to be placed in a bed. Cribs should be regularly evaluated to assure that the width of the slats in the side rails meets current guidelines and that siderail mechanisms are in proper working order. Typically, if children sleep in a bed at home, they should be considered appropriate to sleep in a bed in the hospital. Use of side rails is important especially during sleep for children of all ages.

Be aware of excess environmental stimulation such as a bright light, loud conversations, and alarms from equipment like monitors and pumps (Wong, 1993). This is particularly important in clinical areas where the child will remain for extended periods of time while receiving care. If possible, perform such procedures as IV insertions, blood tests, and spinal taps in treatment rooms rather than in the child's bed. This promotes a sense of security when in their bed or crib and helps reduce anxiety. Plan ahead when completing painful procedures to assure ample opportunity to prepare the child and parent/guardian and to implement pain-relief strategies.

Visiting and Supervision

Parents and guardians are the best translators for their children (Ball & Bindler, 1995; Wong, 1993). Most children use special words and phrases to refer to common things in their environment. Allowing flexible visiting privileges, including overnight accommodations for at least one parent/guardian, is imperative for the child's rest and recovery and for providing direct supervision to assure that the child remains safe while in the hospital. Parents/guardians are not always able to stay with their hospitalized child 24 hours a day. Hospital staff must utilize direct supervision and creative use of the call-bell system to assure the child's safety. Infants and young toddlers are unable to use the call bell to alert the staff that they need help. These children require frequent visual monitoring and may be best placed in rooms near the nurse's station. Children of preschool age

TABLE 52–8. Endotracheal Tube Sizes

Full-term newborn	3.0–3.5 ET tube
First year of life	3.5–4.0 ET tube
After age 2	$\frac{16 + \text{Age in Years}}{4}$ = Size of ET tube

From Ball & Bindler (1995).

TABLE 52–9. Normal Pediatric Heart Rate

Age	Heart Rate
Newborn	100–170
6 months–1 year	90–130
3 years	80–120
5 years	70–110
10–14 years	60–100

From Ball & Bindler (1995).

TABLE 52–10. Normal Pediatric Respiratory Rate

Age	Respiratory Rate
Newborn	30–80
6 months	24–36
1 year	20–40
3 years	20–30
6 years	16–22
10 years	16–20
17 years	12–20

From Ball & Bindler (1995).

and older children can use the call bell if properly instructed and supervised. Some young children may benefit from using the call-bell devices that are typically used with disabled adult patients because they do not require manual dexterity.

Food and Nutrition

Parents/guardians are best able to assist the staff in choosing meal selections that meet the child's medical needs and are consistent with the child's likes and dislikes. Be alert to known allergies as young children may not be able to make appropriate food choices relative to allergies. Paper plates and cups are easier for young children to use without fear of harm if dropped. Staff should be alert to food that is very hot or very cold in temperatures. Staff must provide increased assistance to cut and prepare food and to feed or supervise young children. Snacks are both nutritionally and developmentally an important part of the child's day (Ball & Bindler, 1995; Wong, 1993). Collaboration with the dietician will be helpful in identifying nutritionally appropriate snacks.

There are a wide variety of infant formulas available. Typical formulas used by parents at home are 20 calories per ounce, but other concentrations—such as 27 calories per ounce—are commercially available. Infant formulas come in the following preparations: "ready to feed," "concentrated liquid," and "powdered." Infants are usually maintained on the formula used at home unless the child's medical condition requires that the baby remain NPO or that the formula be changed to a different type. Staff preparing the formula must be careful to assure that the correct type and calorie concentration of formula is chosen. Formula that must be prepared from either liquid concentrate or powdered preparations must be done so in proportions directed by the manufacturer. Improperly prepared formulas can cause the infant additional medical problems, such as severe diarrhea and dehydration (Ball & Bindler, 1995; Wong, 1993).

TABLE 52–11. Normal Pediatric Blood Pressures

Age	Systolic (mm Hg)	Diastolic (mm Hg)
Newborn	73	55
1 month	86	52
6 months	90	53
1 year	90	56
3 years	92	55
6 years	96	57
9 years	100	61
12 years	107	64
15 years	114	65
18 years	121	70

Adapted from the Normal Blood Pressure Readings for Boys from the Second Task Force on Blood Pressure Control in Children. National Heart, Lung, and Blood Institute (1987), Bethesda, MD. Normal blood pressure readings for girls are very similar to those for boys at all age groups.

Median Systolic and Diastolic Blood Pressure Values for Children of Different Ages (Readings show 50th percentile.)

From Ball & Bindler (1995).

Medications and Fluids

Medication dosages for children are calculated on the child's weight in kilograms (Jew, Gordin, & Lengetti, 1997). All medication dosages, dilutions, and routes of administration for an infant or child should be verified by referring to an accepted pediatric drug dosage guide. It is recommended that each hospital adopt a standard pediatric drug reference guide for use by all departments that may care for children, even if infrequently. Utilization of a standard reference guide will allow for consistency and familiarity with typical drugs and dosage ranges. Medication dosages for children can be prepared in varying concentrations. Medication orders should be written in actual dosages, such as in milligrams, micrograms and grams, and *not* in milliliters to prevent drug dosage or concentration errors. Medications should not be mixed in meals or in bottles of formula or juice as the flavor of the medication can cause the child to reject all or part of the mixture causing unreliable medication and nutritional intake. If necessary, medications may be mixed in small portions of a liquid or food, such as in a tablespoon of applesauce or in an ounce of juice. This allows for more reliable assessment of the medication intake without compromising nutritional intake.

Several researchers state that children have fluid requirements that are also based on their weight in kilograms (Ball & Bindler, 1995; Jew et al., 1997; Wong, 1993). All maintenance fluids should be calculated according to standard fluid guidelines for children. Extreme caution must be used when administering IV maintenance fluids and regular IV medications. The amount of fluid used in the administration of the IV medication should be included in the ongoing calculation of maintenance fluid requirements. The proper dilution of IV medications is as critical to the safe care of the child as is assuring that the dosage of the medication is correct. Table 52–12 provides guidelines for calculating fluid requirements for children.

TABLE 52–12. Pediatric Fluid Requirements

Weight (kg)	Fluid Requirements
0–10	100 mL/kg/24 hr
10–20	1000 mL + 50 mL/kg/24 hr for each kg between 11 and 20
20–70	1500 mL + 20 mL/kg/24 hr for each kg between 21 and 70
Over 70	2500 mL/24 hr (adult requirement)

From Ball & Bindler (1995).

Supplies and Equipment

Standardization of supplies and equipment used in the care of children is important, particularly in hospitals where the admission or treatment of children occurs infrequently. Most supplies must be ordered in a wide range of sizes to assure that the correct age- and weight-specific size is available for each child; this is particularly important for emergency supplies such as ambu bags and masks, nasogastric tubes, and chest tubes (American Academy of Pediatrics, 1995). However, to prevent harm, seemingly simple items such as pacifiers also come in different sizes to meet the safety needs of infants and older babies and toddlers. It is never recommended to "make shift" items needed in the care of a child. For example, making a pacifier out of a rubber nipple stuffed with a gauze pad and covered with tape can directly cause a life-threatening choking hazard. The American Academy of Pediatrics (1995) recommends basic supplies including: pacifiers, diapers, linens, slippers, formulas, bottles, and nipples; and medical supplies including: ambu bags, endotreacheal tubes, resuscitation masks, nasogastric tubes, chest tubes, IV catheters, buretrol IV tubing, arm boards, butterfly needles, and blood tubes in microtainer sizes.

Laboratory Services

Blood tests can be processed on different volumes of specimen (Ball & Bindler, 1995; Wong, 1993). Both small volume and micro-volume blood specimen tubes are commercially available. It is imperative to verify what volumes the hospital laboratory can utilize in the lab processing equipment. Development of a list of typical blood tests used in the care of children and the associated minimum volumes of blood required to process the test would be helpful to the clinical staff. If the hospital regularly cares for children in either an emergency or a surgical setting, it is helpful to work with the blood bank to arrange for split or quartered units of blood to obtain small volumes without wasting unnecessary blood. Phlebotomy in children takes skill, patience, and experience. Development of procedures and policies for obtaining blood specimen in infants and children is needed. In the critically ill or injured child, or in the child receiving very frequent blood draws, it is imperative to maintain a record of the volumes of blood withdrawn from the child. Due to the smaller circulating blood volume in infants and children, these patients can become anemic due to frequent blood tests (Ball & Bindler, 1995; Wong, 1993).

Approaching the care of children requires consideration of their unique physiological developmental and anatomic difference. Clinicians must recognize that the role of the family is paramount in providing a level of clinical care that meets the special needs of the young child. Both the parents/guardians and the child can be considered valuable participants in providing a detailed history during the physical examination. Understanding normal growth and development, physiologic parameters, and causes of regressions at times of stress are imperative to approaching the care of the child.

Finally, the hospital environment itself must be carefully considered to assure that the clinical and support departments are able to provide standardized services based on accepted pediatric references and resources. Children are not small adults. However, by recognizing some of the unique differences about children, clinicians can creatively approach the assessment and development of a plan of care that best meets the needs of the child and his or her family.

REFERENCES

American Academy of Pediatrics, Committee on Pediatric Emergency Medicine (1995). Guidelines for Pediatric Emergency Care Facilities.

American Heart Association (1997). *Pediatric Advanced Life Support.* Dallas, TX: AHA.

Ball, J. & Bindler, R. (1995). *Pediatric nursing.* Norwalk, CT: Appleton and Lange.

Bates, B., Bickley, L. S., & Hoekelman, R. A. (1995). *Physical examination and history takings* (6th Ed.). Philadelphia: J. B. Lippincott.

Callery, P. (1997). Caring for parents of hospitalized children: A hidden area of nursing work. *Journal of Advanced Nursing, 26,* 992–998.

Jew, R. A., Gordin, P., & Lengetti, E. (1997). Clinical implications of IV drug administration in infants and children. *Critical Care Nurse, 17* (4), 62–69.

Letourneau, N. L. & Elliot, M. R. (1996). Pediatric health care professionals' perceptions and practices of family-centered care. *Children's Health Care, 25* (3), 157–174.

Mellick, L. B. & Lau, K. L. (1994). Pearls and pitfalls of pediatric assessment: Secrets for approaching children in the emergency department. *Emergency Medicine Reports, 15* (3), 19–30.

Thomas, D. (1996). "Assessing children—It's different." *RN,* April, 38–44.

Wong, D. L. (1993). *Essentials of pediatric nursing* (4th Ed.). St. Louis: Mosby.

53

The Hospitalized Older Adult

Kay Huber

Older adults are the largest group of consumers of health-care services in the United States. Although most of their health care is provided outside the hospital, persons age 65 and older account for 31% of acute care hospital admissions and 45% of hospital expenditures for adults (Hahn & Lefkowitz, 1992). In 1993, persons 75 years of age and older had the longest average length of stay (8.4 days), the most days of care per 1000 persons (3665), and the highest number of discharges per 1000 (6310) of all age groups (U.S. Bureau of the Census 1996).

Older adults are often admitted to the hospital—and, frequently into intensive care units—by way of the emergency department. Prior to arrival in the emergency department they may have experienced a catastrophic episode, such as a cerebrovascular accident or a hip fracture, that started a sequence of events, both physiological and psychological, that are beyond their knowledge and control. In addition to being acutely ill and at risk for physiologic complications, they are often overwhelmed, frightened, separated from assistive devices that enhance their functional ability, and isolated from familiar surroundings.

More than 80% of people age 65 or older have at least one chronic illness, 85% of people over age 65 have no disability, and many of the chronic illnesses that manifest in old age can be successfully managed while maintaining an active lifestyle (U.S. Senate Special Committee on Aging, 1991). When an acute disease results in hospitalization, however, it can often be related to a chronic disease process. The effects of chronic illness on older adults, coupled with usual age-related physiologic changes, place this age group at high risk for a myriad of problems when they are hospitalized.

With the fastest growing segment of the population those persons over 85 years of age, advanced practice nurses who care for adults will be increasingly challenged by the number and complexity of those who are hospitalized. The focus should be on treating the reason for their admission while doing them no harm.

The primary focus of this chapter is on the risks of hospitalization for older adult patients, the predisposing factors, clinical assessment, and intervention strategies that can be employed. Consideration will be given to discharge planning and special age-related concerns in this population.

CLINICAL AND MANAGEMENT CONSIDERATIONS

Rowe and Schneider (1995) make the distinction between *successful* and *usual* aging. Successful, or pure, aging is the changes due solely to the aging process that are uncomplicated by damage from the environment, lifestyle, or disease. Usual, or average, aging reflects changes due to the combined effects of aging itself and of disease and adverse environmental and lifestyle factors. Important considerations about age-related changes include:

- The manifestations of aging are unique to each person, since advancing age results in increasing differentiation and biologic uniqueness.
- Biologic systems minimally affected by age may be profoundly influenced by lifestyle circumstances such as physical activity, nutritional intake, eco-

nomic advantage, or cigarette smoking (Williams, 1994).
- Many age-related decreases in physiologic functions reduce compensatory reserve. This reduction is often compounded by a variety of losses in other aspects of an older adult's life.
- Many age-related decreases in physiologic functions may never produce clinical symptoms or illness until other factors affect an older adult.
- The impact of aging and disease combined can produce severe dysfunction in one person and minimal evidence of compromise in another.
- There are no successful (pure) age-related changes in cognition that should impair or affect function.
- Age-related changes combined with disease and other factors influence the presentation of symptoms in older adults.

Many clinicians have never learned to differentiate between usual age-related changes and pathological processes (Walker, 1992). It is critically important that these distinct entities are not confused. This may be very difficult because of individual variability in physiological and psychological functioning and the interplay between acute and chronic diseases. Expected physiological changes of aging are incorporated throughout the chapter as they relate to the topics discussed.

Presentation of Illness in Older Adults

Three factors that influence the presentation of illness in older adults are: the underreporting of illness, changes in the pattern of illness, and altered responses to illness (Williams, 1994). Any one or a combination of these factors may confound clinical findings in the older adult.

Underreporting of significant symptoms of illness, while likely to occur more often in primary care settings, may happen in acute care as well. The older adult patient may be reluctant to report subtle and subjective changes because of fear of lengthening the hospital stay, fear of discharge to another institutional setting, or belief that such changes are part of aging itself. Other older adults may underreport because of depression, denial, or isolation.

The pattern or distribution of illness may influence its presentation in some older persons. This may occur because some disease processes are more prevalent in old age and clinicians must understand the epidemiological implications in the interpretation of signs and symptoms. Examples of health problems more prevalent in the older adult population are hip fracture, congestive heart failure, pneumonia, and malignancy.

Another pattern unique to the older population is the accumulation of multiple chronic diseases where symptoms of one condition may exacerbate or mask symptoms of another (Williams, 1994). An example of this would be masking of cardiovascular disease because degenerative joint disease has limited physical activity and the heart is not subjected to stress.

The final dimension, and one most likely to cause the greatest concern in acute care, is the atypical or blunted presentation of signs and symptoms in older adults. One of the greatest challenges for clinicians may be recognizing and diagnosing problems presented in an atypical manner. Also, the older adult's perception of illness may be modified by sensory impairments, changes in the central nervous system, social and cultural factors, or health beliefs. Atypical clinical presentation of illness may involve modification of signs and symptoms, complete absence of expected signs and symptoms, or presentation of symptoms from one organ system that reflect abnormalities in another. Nonspecific manifestations that occur abruptly without pointing to specific pathology, such as acute confusion, warrant immediate attention on the part of clinicians. Establishing baseline information at the time of admission is necessary to compare new clinical findings with acute changes. Table 53–1 shows examples of some common atypical presentations of illness.

TABLE 53–1. Common Atypical Presentations of Illness in Older Adults

Problem	Classic Presentation	Presentation in Older Adult
Acute myocardial infarction	Crushing substernal pain, diaphoresis, hypotension	Dyspnea, confusion
Bacteremia	Fever	General malaise, unexplained change in mental status, febrile or afebrile
Urinary tract infection	Dysuria, frequency, urgency, voiding small amounts, low back and/or suprapubic pain	Dysuria may be absent, frequency/urgency present or absent, dizziness, confusion, anorexia, fatigue, recent onset incontinence
Pneumonia	Fever, chills, pleuritic chest pain, sweats, cough, sputum production, hemoptysis, dyspnea, headache, fatigue	Malaise, anorexia, confusion, fever and sputum may be absent, tachypnea, tachycardia, cough may be mild
Congestive heart failure	Cough, dyspnea on exertion, orthopnea, paroxysmal nocturnal dyspnea	Confusion, agitation, weakness, anorexia, insomnia
Hypothyroidism	Sensitivity to cold, dry skin/hair, lethargy, weight gain, depression	Weight loss, changes in cognition, constipation, vague changes generic to other disease processes
Hyperthyroidism	Agitated, irritable, hand tremor at rest, weight loss, increased temp/pulse/BP	Subtle signs/symptoms, apathetic rather than hyperkinetic, tremor, atrial fibrillation

The clinical management of older adult patients involves what Kavesh (1996) calls the "incessant collection of evidence" (p. 55) wherein the collection often ranges far afield from the usual realms of information gathering. Because of the complexity of these patients, advanced practice nurses need to involve other disciplines from the health-care team to participate in the ongoing assessment and interventions that will help decrease the risks of hospitalization.

RISKS OF HOSPITALIZATION FOR OLDER ADULTS

Older adult patients, especially the frail old, have a decreased ability to adapt to what is an unfamiliar, and for them, frequently hostile, environment. Hospitalization constitutes a major risk for this population as it is often followed by an apparently irreversible decline in function and a change in their quality and style of life (Carty & Day, 1993; Creditor, 1993).

The Physical Environment

The physical environment, while functional for the staff, is often not conducive to either function or orientation of the older adult. There are many environmental modifications that can be made to reduce risks and enhance the safety and functioning of older adults (Table 53–2).

TABLE 53–2. Modifications of Physical and Functional Environment

Orientation	
Clocks with large numbers and nonglare glass	Large-print calendars
Television/telephones with large numbers	Baseboard in contrast color to floor covering
Doors/door frames in contrast with wall color	Clear, easily-readable signage
Sensory	
Nonglare, nonskid floor wax	Carpeting with low pile
Eliminate glossy surfaces (wall, furniture, pictures)	Avoid fluorescent lights
Light switches reachable from wheelchairs	Amplification available for telephones
Decrease irrelevant noise	Nightlights
Consistent, nonglare lighting intensity	Polarized window glass
Mobility/Function	
Beds that lower so patient's feet are flat on floor when sitting on edge/no rails or recessible rails	Firm chairs of proper height with armrests
Rounded, contrasting color handrails in hallways	Lever-type faucets, doorknobs
Elevated toilet seats available/grab bars at toilets and in bathing areas	Accessible/easily usable call bells
Contrasting color on step edges	Dressing aids available
	Modified eating utensils available

Iatrogenic Illness

Iatrogenic illnesses are another hazard faced by hospitalized older adults. These illnesses—medical treatments intended to be therapeutic, but instead cause additional problems—are common events for older adults (Dugan, Deane, & Mosel, 1996). Older adults are at increased risk for iatrogenic illness, and some of the predisposing factors are: (1) age-related declines in cardiovascular, renal, pulmonary, hepatic, and neurological function; (2) an increased prevalence of multisystem and comorbid diseases; (3) polypharmacy and increased physiological sensitivity to various drugs; (4) increased sensitivity to the adverse consequences of bed rest; and (5) the tendency of older adults to manifest atypical disease presentations, often resulting in more extensive diagnostic workups (Rich, Shah, Vinson, Freedland, Kuru, & Sperry, 1996). Older adults may not report early signs and symptoms of adverse events, especially if cognitively impaired or depressed. The totality of these factors means not only that iatrogenic illnesses are more common, but the consequences are more likely to be severe or life-threatening (Gorbien, Bishop, Beers, Norman, Osterweil, & Rubenstein, 1992).

Some common iatrogenic problems include incontinence, complications from surgery, effects from bed rest and reduced mobility, adverse effects from medications, and nutritional and fluid disturbances. Nosocomial infections, which continue to be a major complication of hospitalization, are often considered to be iatrogenic diseases. These infections result in major increases in morbidity and mortality and often contribute to increased length of stay. Frail older adults have an increased risk for most common nosocomial infections including pneumonia, urinary tract infection, bacteremia, toxin-induced diarrhea, and wound infection (Gorbien et al., 1992; Stolley & Buckwalter, 1991). The risk of nosocomial infection increases with length of hospitalization; however, the age-associated increase is not due solely to increased length of stay. The declining immunocompetence that accompanies aging, physiologic changes in skin integrity, and changes within the respiratory system and urinary tract all make the older adult more susceptible to infection (Fraser, 1993).

Frail and debilitated hospitalized older adults are also at increased risk for developing iatrogenic heart failure, even in the absence of left ventricular contractile dysfunction or a previous history of cardiac disease (Rich et al., 1996). Factors that may precipitate heart failure in hospitalized older adults include nosocomial infection, medication-induced renal failure, side effects of drugs, overhydration, dysrhythmias, and myocardial infarction or ischemia. Rich et al. (1996) found excessive intravenous fluid administration to be the predisposing factor for almost all of the older patients in their study who developed iatrogenic heart failure.

Functional Decline

Approximately 75% of adults age 75 years and older who are functionally independent when admitted from their homes are not functionally independent at time of discharge (Creditor, 1993). Older adults who have experienced declines in functional ability prior to acute hospitalization have a higher risk for additional losses and complications. Functional decline, defined as a deterioration in self-care skills (Inouye, Wagner, Acampora, Horwitz, Cooney, Hurst, & Tinetti, 1993), has been shown to occur as early as the second day of hospitalization. This common problem is associated with a prolonged hospital stay, increased mortality, increased rates of institutionalization, and greater health-care costs. Functional decline is frequently unrelated to the older adult patient's primary diagnosis (Creditor, 1993; Hirsch, Sommers, Olsen, Mullen & Winograd, 1990).

Predisposing Factors

Impaired physical mobility is one of the predisposing factors for functional decline in hospitalized older adults. Mobility may be affected by biological health, sensory–perceptual capacity, motor skills, cognitive capacity, environmental features, medical regimens, and patterns of nursing care (Mobily & Kelley, 1991). Impaired mobility can have negative physiological and psychological consequences for older adults.

A number of authors have described factors associated with hospitalization and bed rest (Hamilton & Lyon, 1995; Harper & Lyles, 1988; Hoenig & Rubenstein, 1991; Mobily & Kelley, 1991), but Creditor (1993, 1995) has combined them, along with aging changes, into what he describes as a cascade of events (Fig. 53–1). In older adults—especially those who are sedentary—muscle mass, muscle strength, and aerobic capacity decline, resulting in progressive loss of reserve capacity for physical activity. Changes in joint structure, which may occur after as few as five days of immobilization (Mobily & Kelley, 1991), and muscle shortening contribute to limitation of motion and contractures. Even a few days of bed rest may result in deconditioning and loss of independent function.

Baroreceptor insensitivity combined with age-related decreases in body water and plasma volume results in a tendency toward orthostatic hypotension and syncope. Ortho-

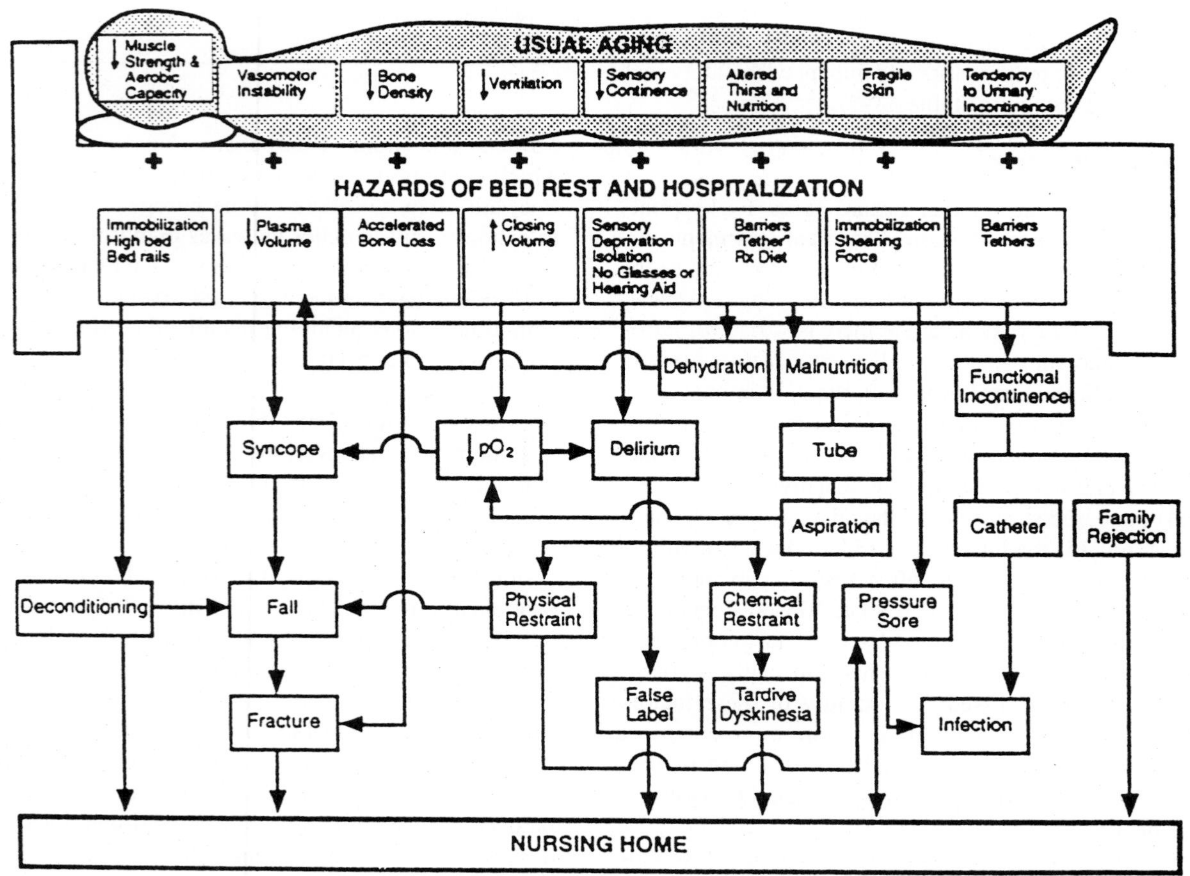

Figure 53–1. Hazards of bed rest and hospitalization. *(Used with permission from Creditor. [1993].)*

static hypotension can occur in younger persons who are immobilized for as little as one week, whether they are supine or sitting (Mobily & Kelley, 1991). Older adults deteriorate more quickly and take longer to recover from a period of immobility. The combination of immobility and orthostatic hypotension significantly increases the older adult's risk for falls.

Age-related changes in respiratory function increase closing volume, affect pulmonary ventilation, and reduce arterial oxygen tension (PaO_2); changes that seldom have consequences for healthy older adults. In the supine position, vital capacity is decreased; ventilation is further reduced, causing a further reduction in PaO_2; secretions increase; and expectoration decreases or becomes inadequate. The further reduction in PaO_2 may produce confusion or drowsiness and may contribute to syncope. An altered level of awareness or alertness, pooled secretions in the lungs, and age-related respiratory changes place older adults at risk for pneumonia. The risk escalates if they are receiving medications that further compromise respiratory function.

Progressive skeletal bone loss occurs with aging, more so in women than in men, with the loss accelerated after menopause. Creditor (1993, 1995) points out that vertebral bone loss accelerates to 50 times the involutional rate in healthy men on bed rest. While some bone loss occurs because of lack of weight bearing, the remainder is probably from the general negative nitrogen balance associated with immobility. With ambulation, bone mineral is restored at a rate of only 1% per month (Mobily & Kelley, 1991). Therefore, it is important to prevent the initial loss of bone calcium. Hospitalization may accelerate osteoporosis, and increase fracture risk both in the hospital and after discharge.

Although age-related changes in the genitourinary system increase the potential for incontinence, most older adults in the community are continent. Hospitalization interferes with their usual strategies to avoid incontinence because of environmental barriers, treatment regimens that make going to the bathroom either impossible or very difficult, mobility restrictions for a variety of reasons, or medications that reduce the perception of the need to void. Immobility may result in the development of renal calculi and/or a urinary tract infection.

Impaired skin integrity and the development of pressure sores can occur within hours after hospitalization, especially in frail, debilitated older adults. Age-related changes in the integument combined with factors such as nutritional deficiency, peripheral neuropathy, and incontinence interact with pressure and shearing forces to produce tissue injury.

Sensory deprivation or overstimulation, particular predisposing factors in critical care units, lead to an increased risk for acute confusional states. Age-related changes in the gastrointestinal and sensory systems—coupled with immobility, significant changes in diet or type of food available, and barriers to obtaining food and fluid—may lead to dehydration, malnutrition, and constipation. The consequences of the interactions between aging and hospitalization are likely to be both additive and cumulative with the end result being significant loss of functional ability.

Assessment

Assessment of the risk for functional decline following hospitalization can occur in a variety of ways. Comprehensive geriatric assessment is usually performed by a core team consisting of a geriatrician, an advanced practice nurse with specialization in gerontology, and a social worker, with other disciplines and medical specialties added as needed. Advanced practice nurses or geriatricians may serve as consultants who assess older adult patients admitted to designated units or to any location in the hospital. Some assessments are done by nursing staff who receive special training in the identification and management of older adult patients at risk for functional decline during hospitalization (Inouye, Wagner, et al., 1993). Less formal assessments are done by staff nurses during their observations of patient function and behavior. Regardless of the approach used, going beyond the medical model is critical because illness may present as a nonspecific deterioration in functional status (Gallo, Reichel, & Andersen, 1995). Because of the potential of functional decline occurring within the first 48 hours of admission, assessment of function to establish baseline risk information should occur within this time period.

Several instruments are commonly used, in differing combinations, to assess functional ability. The most widely used, the Katz Index of Activities of Daily Living (ADL) (Katz, Ford, Moskowitz, Jackson, & Jaffee, 1963) and the Scale for Instrumental Activities of Daily Living (IADL) (Lawton & Brody, 1969) are discussed here. Instruments used to assess mental status are presented in the next section of the chapter.

The Katz Index of ADL (Katz et al., 1963) covers bathing, dressing, toileting, transfer, continence, and feeding. The functions are rated in order of decreasing dependency based on the older adult's actual performance of them. The hierarchical order of the functions implies a pattern of recovery from a disabling illness in older age similar to the order of development of primary functions in children. Lekan-Rutledge (1996) points out that loss of function begins with complex activities while the most basic and least complex are retained the longest.

Lawton and Brody's (1969) Scale for IADL includes a range of more complex activities such as using the telephone, traveling, shopping, preparing meals, doing housework, taking medicine properly, and managing money. Inability to perform these tasks is correlated with mortality, and when the items are in vertical order, performance of one activity indicates the person can probably perform all the activities listed below it on the scale but not above it (Gallo et al., 1995). Measurement of these items in the hospital setting is necessarily dependent on verbal reports from both the patient and most knowledgeable caregiver or a person who lives with the patient.

The Hospital Admission Risk Profile (HARP) (Fig. 53–2) has been developed and validated to identify older adult patients at risk of functional decline following hospitalization (Sager, Rudberg, Jalaluddin, Franke, Inouye, Landefeld, Siebens, & Winograd, 1996). This instrument is a product of the Hospital Outcomes Project for the Elderly (HOPE) conducted in six hospitals where clearly delineated nursing care models were used. The study population did not include older adults who were living in nursing homes prior to admission, those admitted for surgery, or those admitted to intensive care units. The authors indicate that the most valid use for HARP would be to identify patients for comprehensive discharge planning, geriatric assessment, special inpatient care, and both inpatient and posthospital rehabilitation (Sager et al., 1996).

Interventions

Although interventions to improve the outcomes of hospitalized older adults have not all been successful, some of the most effective approaches have included the direct involvement of nurses and advanced practice nurses (Fulmer & Mezey, 1994; Hamilton & Lyon, 1995; Huber & Kennard, 1991; Inouye, Acampora, et al., 1993; Inouye, Wagner, et al., 1993; Landefeld, Palmer, Kresevic, Fortinsky, & Kowal, 1995; Meissner, Andolsek, Mears, & Fletcher, 1989).

Specific interventions include modification of the physical and functional environment (refer to Table 53–2); provision of patient-centered care; use of specially-trained primary nurses and gerontological nurse specialists or practitioners; development of specific protocols to stabilize or improve continence, skin integrity, mental status, nutrition, mobility, ADLs, and sleep as well as protocols to minimize the adverse effects of specific procedures such as urinary catheterization; and recommendations on use of or adjustment of medications, for involvement of multiple disciplines, and for early and comprehensive discharge planning.

Acute Confusion

Acute confusion is a commonly recognized and serious problem for hospitalized older adults with a range of occurrence between 14 and 56% and associated mortality rates of 10 to 65%, increased length of stay, costlier hospitalization, and increased rates of long-term care facility placement (Inouye & Charpentier, 1996; O'Keeffe & Lavan, 1997). Persons with acute confusion are more likely to experience an adverse effect of a diagnostic or therapeutic intervention; more frequently experience falls, pressure ulcers, infections, and adverse reactions to therapeutic doses of medications; and frequently exhibit unsafe behaviors (Foreman, 1996). Additionally, confusion is often a presenting feature of an acute physical illness such as myocardial infarction, pneumonia, heart failure, or a serious adverse drug event, and failure to recognize and treat could have serious, perhaps fatal, consequences. Acute confusion in persons with no previous history of cognitive impairment may serve as an early marker of cognitive decline that may

Hospital Admission Risk Profile (HARP)

1. Scoring range 0–5
   a) Age

Age category	Risk score	
<75	0	
75–84	1	
≥85	2	score = ________

   b) Cognitive function (abbreviated MMSE)*

MMSE score	Risk score	
15–21	0	
0–14	1	score = ________

   c) IADL function prior to admission**

Independent IADL's	Risk score	
6–7	0	
0–5	2	score = ________

Total = ________

2. Risk categories

Total score	Risk of Decline in ADL function
4 or 5	high risk
2 or 3	intermediate risk
0 or 1	low risk

* Abbreviated Mini Mental State Exam includes only the orientation (10 items), registration (3 items), attention (5 items) and recall (3 items) portions of the original 30 item test.

** A person is judged independent in an activity if he/she is able to perform the activity without assistance. A person is scored dependent if he/she either does not perform an activity, requires the assistance of another person or is unable to perform an activity. IADL activities include telephoning, shopping, cooking, doing housework, taking medications, using transportation and managing finances.

Figure 53–2. Hospital Admission Risk Profile (HARP). *(Used with permission from Sager, et al. [1996].)*

reflect low cerebral and neurologic reserves (Murray, Levkoff, Wetle, Beckett, Cleary, Schor, Lipsitz, Rowe, & Evans, 1993).

The term *acute confusion* has also been called delirium, transient cognitive impairment, and acute confusional state. It can be defined as an acute organic brain syndrome encompassing a broad spectrum of psychophysical manifestations, ranging from mild disorientation to agitated delirium, altered consciousness, and physiological deterioration (Neelon, Champagne, Carlson, & Funk, 1996). The term *acute confusional state* means an organic brain syndrome characterized by transient, global cognitive impairment with an abrupt onset and relatively brief duration that is accompanied by daily fluctuation of simultaneous disturbance of the sleep–wake cycle, psychomotor behavior, attention, and affect (Foreman, 1986). Foreman considered this state to be an acute and reversible syndrome. Delirium has also been succintly defined as an acute disorder of cognition and attention (Inouye & Charpentier, 1996).

Acute confusion has been consistently underrecognized or underreported by both physicians and nurses (Foreman, 1993; Francis, Martin, & Kapoor, 1990; Pompei, Foreman, Rudberg, Inouye, Braund, & Cassel, 1994). Most investigators concluded that underdetecting occurred because clinicians did not use standardized methods of cognitive assessment. Also, in many studies observations and assessments were conducted only once a day or less often; therefore, acute confusion may have gone unrecognized because of fluctuations in clinical signs. Nurses have been more likely than physicians to detect acute confusion because of its fluctuating nature.

The pathophysiology of acute confusion is poorly understood partly because of its fluctuating and transient presentation and partly because underlying physical illness, drugs, and dementia confound diagnosis. Current knowledge about acute confusion depends on indirect evidence from biochemical and electrophysiological studies. One mechanism responsible for confusion appears to be a failure of cerebral oxidative metabolism, because interventions such as administering oxygen to hypoxic patients and providing glucose to hypoglycemic patients can reverse the clinical and electroencephalogram (EEG) manifestations (Francis, 1992). There is a correlation between EEG slowing and cognitive impairment, and both hypo- and hyperactive variants of acute confusion show similar patterns of EEG change. There is considerable evidence to support the hypothesis that acute confusion is mediated by a failure of cholinergic transmission (Francis, 1992). Acute confusion related to infections or inflammatory conditions may be due to central nervous system effects of lymphokines, one of the chemical factors produced and released by T lymphocytes.

Predisposing Factors

The onset of acute confusion in hospitalized older adults has been reported to range from within the first 24 hours to the ninth day after admission. Although researchers have examined factors present at the time of admission and factors that occurred after admission, there has been little investigation of the relationships among them, and no definite conclusions reached about the relationships. Baseline vulnerability factors that may be present at time of admission and precipitating factors that may occur during hospitalization are presented in Table 53–3.

Assessment

Clinicians must be able to differentiate acute confusion from dementia, depression, and acute functional psychosis in hospitalized older adults. The clinical features of acute confusion appear in Table 53–4.

Methods for the systematic assessment of acute confusion have been slow to enter bedside practice (Neelon et al., 1996). The standard mental status screening instruments requiring a patient to respond to specific questions or commands are now known to be limited for use in the bedside assessment of ill older adults. Traditionally, the instruments known as mental status questionnaires, or bedside cognitive screening instruments, were preferred by physicians (Foreman, 1993). The most familiar and most often used were Pfeiffer's (1975) Short Portable Mental Status Questionnaire (SPMSQ) and the Mini-Mental State Examination (MMSE) by Folstein, Folstein, and McHugh (1975). The only discriminations available with these screening devices is between impaired or not impaired, so their diagnostic precision is limited. Other concerns about mental status questionnaires are that (1) performance is influenced by age, amount of formal education, ethnicity, and language; (2) distinction cannot be made between acute and chronic impairment; (3) all facets of acute confusion cannot be measured by these instruments; and (4) because responses are heavily verbal, they cannot be used with persons unable to speak (Foreman, 1993).

Newer instruments, designed to detect acute confu-

TABLE 53–3. Probable Risks and Predisposing Factors for Acute Confusion in Hospitalized Older Adults

Baseline Vulnerability Factors Present at Admission
- Age of 80 years or over
- Dementia (chronic cognitive impairment)
- Severe illness
- Prior functional decline/disability
- Multiple comorbid conditions

Precipitating Factors During Hospitalization
- Immobility (e.g., physical restraints, other "tethers")
- Environmental extremes (e.g., sensory deprivation or overload)
- Pharmacologic agents (e.g., anticholinergics, psychoactives)
- Any iatrogenic event (e.g., volume overload, unintentional injury, new pressure ulcer)
- Infection (especially urinary tract and pneumonia)
- Fluid and electrolyte imbalances (especially sodium and potassium)
- Metabolic disturbances (e.g., azotemia, changes in pH, low serum albumin)

TABLE 53–4. Clinical Features of Acute Confusion

***Note:* All symptoms are worse when patient is fatigued**

Acute onset/subacute onset—cause dependent	Transient
Short course—several hours to less than a month	Diurnal (daily) fluctuations of symptoms
Worse at night and on awakening (nocturnal increase called "sundowning")	Reduced awareness
Impaired attention span; easily distracted	Fluctuating levels of awareness
Disorganized thinking; distorted perceptions	Impaired short-term memory/orientation
	Disturbed or reversed sleep–wake cycle

Hyperalert/hyperactive—hyperarousal of autonomic nervous system, psychomotor hyperactivity, marked excitability, rapid speech, tendency toward hallucinations and illusions, restlessness, agitation, irritability

OR

Hypoalert/hypoactive—reduced psychomotor activity, lethargy, drowsiness, apathy, reduced arousal, slowed response to questions, initiates hardly any action, may be misdiagnosed as depressed or overlooked completely

OR

Mixed Presentation—unpredictable fluctuation between hypo- and hyperactive states

Modified from Foreman. (1993); Lipowski. (1989).

sion, that depend on observations rather than testing have been developed. The first, the Clinical Assessment of Confusion–B (CAC–B) (Vermeersch, 1992) was inductively developed to measure confusion in hospitalized adults by using behaviors nurses used to describe confusion. The instrument takes approximately 10 minutes to complete and requires no training beyond the written directions. The CAC–B can be used to assess cognition, general behavior, motor activity, orientation, behaviors that threaten patient safety, psychotic/neurotic behaviors, and the ability of the patient to perform ADLs. An earlier version, the CAC–A, can be used as a screening instrument.

Another tool, the Confusion Assessment Method (CAM) enables nonpsychiatrically trained clinicians to identify acute confusion in both clinical and research settings (Inouye, vanDyck, Alessi, Balkin, Siegal, & Horwitz, 1990). The CAM includes an instrument and standardized diagnostic algorithm shown to have high sensitivity, high specificity, and high interrater reliability. The diagnosis of acute confusion is based on four features: (1) acute onset and fluctuating course; (2) inattention; (3) disorganized thinking; and (4) altered level of consciousness. The diagnosis of acute confusion requires the presence of (1) and (2) and either (3) or (4). The instrument can be completed in about five minutes.

The NEECHAM Confusion Scale (Neelon, Champagne, McConnell, Carlson, & Funk, 1992) is used for systematic assessment and monitoring of acute confusion in hospitalized older adults. The validity of the use of the NEECHAM as a reliable instrument for assessing acute confusion, particularly in the early stages, is now supported (Neelon et al., 1996). The scale can be scored in approximately 10 minutes using information derived during routine clinical assessment of older adults hospitalized for acute medical illness.

The preceding instruments, and others that are similar, cannot measure all aspects of acute confusion, nor can they be used to make a distinction between acute and chronic conditions.

Interventions

Few intervention studies have been conducted to examine ways of preventing or managing acute confusion (Cronin-Stubbs, 1996; Foreman, 1993). Lack of ability to prevent acute confusion, or to effectively intervene to reduce or eliminate it, often results in a prognosis of progressive functional decline on discharge from the hospital (Francis, 1992; Murray et al., 1993; O'Keeffe & Lavan, 1997). The treatment of acute confusion has been based primarily on clincial experience for centuries, and these empirical principles can be divided into three phases: prevention, indentification and treatment of underlying problems, and supportive care. Although there is always some integration and overlap of these phases, Table 53–5 is an attempt to categorize them as treatment. Funded studies are currently in progress to assess the impact of following preventive protocols in the acute care setting.

TABLE 53–5. Treatment of Acute Confusion

Prevention

Identify persons at high risk	Complete systematic assessment
Eliminate/minimize/monitor all medications	Environmental modifications
Maintain/accomplish early mobility	Adequate hydration/oxygenation
Decrease/eliminate restraints	Ongoing, consistent orientation

Interventions

Prompt recognition is critical

Identify/eliminate and/or correct underlying pathophysiological condition	Correct environmental extremes
Correct fluid/electrolyte imbalance	Treat infection
Identify/treat/correct iatrogenic factors	Correct metabolic disturbances
	Pharmacologic measures, if necessary

Supportive Care

Best if multidisciplinary team is used

Conserve reserves (e.g., balance rest with activity)	Clear, concrete communication
Maintain skin integrity	Ensure safety
Caregiver continuity; enlist family to "sit"	Orientation to environment
Nonpharmacologic pain management if possible	Maintain nutrition
	Regular elimination, especially bowel
	Mobility

Dehydration

Dehydration (decrease in total body water) is the most common fluid and electrolyte problem accompanying acute illnesses in older adults, and is associated with significant mortality (Davis & Minaker, 1994; Wilson & Morley, 1996). Early clinical recognition is important as diminished functional reserves may hamper the older adult's compensatory ability. Consequences of dehydration may include decreased functional ability, predisposition to falls and for infection, constipation, fecal impaction, and acute confusion.

Age-related changes are associated with a decline in total body water, a decrease in thirst perception, a reduction in voluntary fluid intake, a reduced response to antidiuretic hormone that affects the ability of the kidneys to concentrate urine, and a decreased response to aldosterone in the kidney tubules that causes an increase in sodium excretion. The hospitalized older adult may have isotonic dehydration (normal plasma osmolarity and serum sodium levels), hypertonic dehydration (elevated plasma osmolarity and hypernatremia), or hypotonic dehydration (low plasma osmolarity and hyponatremia).

Predisposing Factors

Risk factors for dehydration can be divided between increased fluid loss and decreased fluid intake (Tables 53–6 and 53–7). Chronic or acute infections, such as urinary tract infections and pneumonia, are the most common cause of dehydration in older adults. The fever associated with acute infection results in insensible water loss from tachypnea, sweating, and increased cellular catabolism. Upper urinary tract infection may result in reduction of the renal concentrating ability and may persist for weeks following resolution (Davis & Minaker, 1994). Excessive urinary losses of water and sodium occur due to diruetic therapy, often continued in the presence of dehydration; the diuresis associated with diseases such as diabetes mellitus and chronic renal failure; and gastrointestinal losses that occur with vomiting, nasogastric drainage, diarrhea, and bleeding. Older adults may lose significant amounts of fluid because of aggressive bowel cleansing regimens prior to diagnostic studies. Intravascular dehydration without clinically obvious fluid loss may occur due to compartment fluid shifts from problems such as acute pancreatitis, hypoalbuminemia, and congestive heart failure.

Hospitalized older adults are at risk for dehydration when their access to fluids is limited from restricted mobility (physical restraints or disease-related) or when they cannot see or locate fluids. Davis and Minaker (1994) point out that patients presenting with deteriorating mobility, vision, or level of consciousness who were independent in accessing fluids prior to becoming ill are among the most underrecognized as being at risk for fluid access problems. Fluid deprivation may be iatrogenic because of nothing by mouth (NPO) restrictions prior to diagnostic or surgical procedures or because fluid is restricted, sometimes inappropriately, in hyponatremia or edema. Patients who are cognitively impaired, but physically able to manage their own fluid intake and vice versa, are at high risk for inadequate fluid intake. Intestinal obstruction may be complicated by occult sequestration of large volumes of intraabdominal fluid (Wilson & Morley, 1996). Other gastrointestinal problems, including the side effects of medications—such as nausea, vomiting, anorexia, and further decreases in thirst perception—affect fluid intake.

TABLE 53–6. Causes of Increased Fluid Loss in Older Adult Patients

Excessive blood losses
Chronic or acute infections
Excessive urinary losses
Diuretic misuse, glycosuria, hypercalciuria, mannitol, radiographic contrast agents, elevated blood urea nitrogen (BUN), diabetes insipidus (central [pituitary]; nephrogenic), hypoaldosteronism (Addison's disease; hyporeninemic hypoaldosteronism), suppressed vasopressin (Alzheimer's disease; phenytoin; ethanol; postatrial tachyarrhythmia), postobstructive diuresis
Gastrointestinal losses
Upper GI (vomiting; nasogastric drainage)
Lower GI (diarrhea)—laxative abuse or bowel preps, infectious or secretory
Surgical bypass or fistulas, ischemic bowel, colectomy
Environment-related fluid loss
Heat wave, hypothermia
Compartmental fluid shifts
Hypoalbuminemia, pancreatitis, ascites, anaphylaxis, burns, hypertonic peritoneal dialysate

Used with permission from Davis & Minaker. (1994).

TABLE 53–7. Causes of Decreased Fluid Intake in Older Adult Patients

Limited access to fluids
Physical restraints, mobility restriction, poor visual acuity
Fluid restriction
Preprocedure, prevention of incontinence or nocturia or aspiration, therapy for edema or hyponatremia
Altered sensorium
Decreased consciousness level (sedatives, neuroleptics, narcotics; structural and metabolic CNS insults; febrile illness)
Decreased level of awareness (dementia, delirium; mania, psychosis, depression)
Gastrointestinal disorders
Swallowing disorders
Bowel obstruction (mechanical, metabolic, ischemic)
Anticholinergic medication
Alteration in thirst mechanism
Primary adipsia, medication-related (cardiac glycosides, amphetamines)
Associated with focal CNS pathology

Used with permission from Davis & Minaker (1994).

Assessment

Clinical indicators of dehydration and self-reported perceptions of thirst are unreliable in older adults. Loss of skin turgor may be nothing more than a reflection of age-related decrease in elasticity; however, if assessment of skin turgor occurs, it should be done over the sternum and forehead where age-related skin changes are less pronounced. Other skin and soft-tissue changes—such as a dry, furrowed tongue; dry oral mucosa; decreased salivation; and dry, warm skin—may be indicative of dehydration. Clinicians must review medications because similar changes may be produced by anticholinergics. Other signs and symptoms to be considered during assessment are confusion; disorientation; scanty or concentrated urine, with marked ammonia odor; weak, rapid pulse; and altered respirations (Burke & Walsh, 1997).

The most reliable index of dehydration, but one that mandates prior knowledge of the patient's weight, is a sudden reduction in baseline body weight. Loss of lean body mass resulting from hypercatabolism in acute illnesses may interfere with the predictive value of this figure, but those losses rarely exceed 300 to 500 grams, so weight loss exceeding this can be considered secondary to fluid depletion (Wilson & Morley, 1994).

The most sensitive index of significant vascular volume depletion is orthostatic hypotension; however, between 10% and 30% of older adults may have chronic postural hypotension (Wandel, 1990). Additionally, certain diseases, medications, and disorders—such as diabetes-induced autonomic neuropathy and pernicious anemia—may produce postural hypotension. In the dehydrated older adult, the presence of impaired autonomic reflexes may result in orthostatic hypotension even if the dehydration is relatively mild. Pulse and blood pressure should be done with the older adult in a standing position. Older adults experiencing profound dehydration, from events such as hypovolemic shock, will have an altered sensorium; cold, clammy skin; tachycardia; and hypotension with urine flow rates of less than 30 mL/hour.

Interventions

Interventions should be preceded by an objective assessment of clinical severity and serum osmolarity. Obtaining serum sodium levels helps to classify the extent of dehydration in older adults. In dehydration the serum sodium is usually 148 mmol/L (SI Units) or 148 mEq/L (conventional units) or higher (normal reference values are 136-145 mmol/L) and the serum BUN/creatinine ratio is generally 25 or higher (Hoffman, 1991). Therefore, a sodium concentration greater than 150 mmol/L indicates hypertonic dehydration, a situation usually resulting from restricted access to fluid or a diminished thirst response.

Serum osmolarity can be calculated by the following equation:

$$\text{Serum osmolarity} = 2 \cdot [\text{Na}^+] \left[\frac{\text{Glucose}}{18}\right]\left[\frac{\text{BUN}}{2.8}\right]$$

where sodium level is measured in mEq/L and glucose and BUN levels are in mg/dL (Davis & Minaker, 1994; Wilson & Morley, 1996). If measured osmolarity is significantly greater than the calculated value, an accumulation of a nonphysiological substance such as ethanol, mannitol, methanol, or lactic acid exists.

Rehydration of persons with predominantly free water loss (hypertonic dehydration) can be guided by calculating the net fluid deficit with the following equation:

$$\text{Fluid deficit (Liters)} = \text{Expected TBW} - \text{Current TBW}$$

$$\text{Current TBW (Liters)} = \text{current body weight (kg)} \times 0.5^*$$

$$\text{Desired TBW} = \frac{\text{serum Na}^+ \times \text{current TBW}}{140}$$

*Value for older adult men (use 0.45 for older adult women)

The TBW is total body water; this constitutes only about 50% in older adult men and 45% in older adult women of total body weight (Davis & Minaker, 1994; Wilson & Morley, 1996). Use of this formula should be limited to patients without grossly abnormal serum sodium levels.

Several methods of fluid replacement may be used singly or in combination, with oral rehydration being the preferred method. A minimum water intake of approximately 1500-2500 mL/day should be given in the absence of contraindicating circumstances such as cirrhosis, heart failure, and nephrotic syndrome where reductions in intake may be necessary (Hoffman, 1991; Zauderer, 1996). Absolutely accurate intake and output from all sources must be maintained.

In instances of significant hypernatremia, the first step in therapy is correction of hemodynamic collapse which is manifested by hypotension, orthostasis, and decreased urine output (Davis & Minaker, 1994). Initial treatment is rapid infusions of isotonic saline until hemodynamic parameters stabilize. Following stabilization, the patient should have replacement of one-half of the fluid deficit over the next 24 hours with the remaining deficit replaced, by using 5% dextrose in half-normal saline, over the next 48 to 72 hours. In addition to correcting the fluid deficit, there must be replacement of ongoing fluid losses (two to three liters/day in healthy persons and possibly higher during illnesses). Assessment of fluid status, including intake and output, weight, blood pressure, pulse, serum chemistries, and osmolarities must be ongoing.

Complications of fluid replacement therapy may occur in older adults because they are particularly vulnerable to circulatory overload from aggressive fluid replacement. When plasma hyperosmolarity is corrected too rapidly, an osmotic gradient may be generated that results in rapid migration of free water into neurones, resulting in cerebral edema. This may be manifested by acute confusion or significant alterations in level of consciousness with the potential of transient or permanent neurological deficits or death as a result. Iatrogenic congestive heart failure, mentioned earlier in the chapter, may also result from overzealous intravenous fluid therapy.

The possibility of hyponatremia (serum sodium less than 135 mEq/L) increases with age, and may also occur with fluid overload or hypovolemia. Clinical manifestations of hyponatremia include nonspecific symptoms such as lethargy, anorexia, nausea, acute confusion, and a decline in functional ability as well as muscle cramps and seizures. Most older adults with hyponatremia have a defect in the capacity of the kidneys to excrete free water; however, some have normal renal water excretion.

Pseudohyponatremia, low sodium levels associated with normal or elevated serum osmolarity, may occur because of high levels of substances such as glucose, triglycerides, or plasma proteins. When the underlying problem is treated, serum sodium levels return to normal. Therefore, the diagnosis of true hyponatremia requires a detailed history of diseases, medications, and fluid intake as well as a physical examination.

Discussion of all facets of hyponatremia with altered normal water excretion is beyond this chapter. However, clinicians need to monitor use of diuretics because they are frequently associated with hyponatremia in older adult patients as they alter free water excretion. Thiazide diuretics (e.g., hydrochlorothiazide) cause hyponatremia more often than loop diuretics (e.g., furosemide, bumetanide). The syndrome of inappropriate antidiuretic hormone (SIADH) secretion may also occur in older adult patients who have normal volume control. A few of the common causes of SIADH are drugs (e.g., haloperidol, amitriptyline, thioridazine, NSAIDs), pulmonary disease (e.g., pneumonia, chronic obstructive pulmonary disease), and neurological disease (e.g., cerebrovascular disease, neoplasms). Persons with SIADH excrete relatively concentrated urine when they should be excreting dilute urine. Diagnosis is made based on a variety of serum and urine laboratory results. Therapy for SIADH involves identifying and treating the underlying disease and/or discontinuing implicated medications, as well as reversing the physiologic abnormality by either restricting free water intake or administering intravenous sodium replacement depending on the acuity of the situation.

Falls

A fall may be defined as "an unintentional event that results in a person coming to rest on the ground or other lower level" (Hogue, 1992, p. 45). Falling is one of the leading causes of morbidity and mortality in the older adult population. It is also one of the three health conditions, in addition to urinary incontinence and acute confusion, often referred to as geriatric syndromes (Tinetti, Inouye, Gill, & Doucette, 1995). Falling, as is true for acute confusion, increases in frequency with the number of predisposing impairments possessed by the older adult. Therefore, most falls can be predicted. Falls are not accidents, they are not part of successful aging, and they can be prevented.

The rate of falls in long-term care facilities is especially high, and falls in hospitals are also frequent. Although about 90% of persons who are known to fall suffer no substantial physical injury, complications caused by falls are the leading cause of death from injury in adults over age 65 (King & Tinetti, 1995). Older adults admitted to the hospital following falls may have been lying on the floor for long periods of time after the fall and are at risk for dehydration, pressure sores, pneumonia, the breakdown of skeletal muscle, and decline in functional ability at the time of admission.

Predisposing Factors

Most falls by older adult patients are multifactorial in origin, resulting from an interaction between impaired stability characteristics of the person and hazards or demands of the environment (Tinetti, 1994). Attempts have been made to classify falls by etiology and to identify the factors that make older adults susceptible to falling (King & Tinetti, 1995). Determination of exactly who is at risk and under what circumstances continues to be investigated.

Predisposing factors for falling can be classified as intrinsic (related to the person) and extrinsic (related to the environment), although the multifactorial nature of falls belies this simple distinction. Intrinsic factors include age-related changes in gait and balance and vision and visual perception; vestibular dysfunction; chronic disease processes that impair sensory, cognitive, neurologic, or musculoskeletal function; acute illnesses; postural hypotension; and medications. The liklihood of falling increases as the number of intrinsic factors increase.

Extrinsic factors create challenges to balance, and the degree to which they are a threat depends on the vulnerability of older adults and the frequency of their exposure to a potentially destabilizing situation. Examples of extrinsic factors are environmental hazards (e.g., slippery floors, poor lighting), ordinary activities (e.g., climbing stairs), and movements that may lead to the older adults' loss of control of their center of gravity, such as when turning the neck or transferring from bed to chair (King & Tinetti, 1995).

Hospitalized older adults are likely to have an increased risk of falling because they are experiencing an acute illness, often in conjunction with one or more chronic diseases, and are receiving multiple medications. Their risk for falling increases if they experience the predisposing factors, and subsequent development, of functional decline, acute confusion, or dehydration. There appears to be less contribution from environmental factors in the hospital than in the community, although hazards such as furniture, cluttered pathways, slippery floors, and walking aids do exist (Tinetti, 1994).

Assessment

The initial comprehensive assessment should focus on the known risk factors for falling such as cognitive impairment, type and amount of medications, presence of visual deficit, impaired mobility, impaired muscle strength, and the presence of chronic disease that has resulted in functional impairment. The history should include whether or not the patient has had any previous falls, the circumstances surrounding the fall, any premonitions, dizziness, recent use of medications, or postural hypotension. A precise description of the patient's activity at the time the fall occurred is also important so that appropriate interventions can be done.

Direct observation and evaluation of balance and gait can be done using the Tinetti Scale (Tinetti, 1986) which permits the clinician to estimate the risk of falling. Special attention needs to be given to direct observation of the patient during performance of daily activities (Tinetti & Speechley, 1989). A careful balance-and-gait assessment may identify both older adults at risk of falling and the situations, such as getting up from a chair, when falls are most likely to occur.

Medications need to be carefully assessed, paying special attention to any drugs that impair mental alertness such as antidepressants and neuroleptics. Antihypertensives may increase the risk of falling by enhancing or causing orthostatic hypotension, and diuretics may contribute to electrolyte imbalance, cause fluid volume deficit, or increase the number of times the patient needs to void. Assessment of fall risk for patients taking diuretics must include toileting, mobility, and ability to get in and out of bed.

An environmental assessment should focus on potential hazards in light of identified age-related changes and known disabilities.

A comprehensive and systematic assessment conducted on admission and throughout the hospital stay is essential to attempt to reduce the risk of falling of hospitalized older adults.

Interventions

The advanced practice nurse can play a crucial role in educating nursing staff about risk factors, assessment, and prevention for falls.

Following assessment, the first priority should be to prevent the occurrence of a fall. Protocols can be developed and institutued for older adult patients who fit specific risk profiles based on knowledge of predisposing factors. Intrinsic risk factors need to be identified and modifications made where possible. Environmental modifications, beyond those carried out in an institutional sense, may need to be specific to individual patients. For instance, if a patient has diminished proprioception, manifested by unsteady gait, decreased step height, and dizziness when turning the head, an appropriate walking aid, wearing low-heeled shoes with firm soles for walking, and ensuring adequate lighting with removal of tripping hazards is essential (Tinetti & Speechley, 1989).

Environmental prevention measures include ensuring adequate glare-free lighting; dry, nonslippery floors; paths free of obstacles; high, firm chairs and beds at appropriate levels; and raised toilet seats. Patients who use canes and walkers must be measured for appropriate height, taught correct use, and have ambulation closely monitored. Wearing shoes or sneakers for walking is always safer than wearing slippers or hospital-supplied foot coverings. Also, older adults should be oriented to their immediate environment on admission and as often thereafter as warranted based on ongoing and systematic assessment of cognitive function.

Prevention of falls is the most common reason for use of physical restraints in acute care settings. Most patients who fall are physically restrained, and serious injuries from falls are greater when physical restraints are used (Mion, Strumpf, & NICHE faculty, 1994). Restraints limit activity, increase risks associated with immobility, increase the possiblity of acute confusion, cause psychological distress, and often result in complications, severe or permanent injuries, and even death. Rather than use restraints, interventions may include (1) using alternative and adaptive seating; (2) using a restorative nursing approach where maintaining function is the focus; (3) encouraging and assisting mobility; (4) making environmental modifications; and (5) facilitating closer observation by moving certain patients closer to the nursing station, enlisting family or friends to visit, using sitters or volunteers, and using electronic warning devices to alert personnel of persons getting out of bed or out of a chair. The advanced practice nurse is a valuable resource for ways to manage agitation and disruptive behavior of confused patients that do not include the use of restraints.

The side effects and interactions of medications represent a major source of iatrogenic falls (King & Tinetti, 1995; Liu, Topper, Reeves, Gryfe, & Maki, 1995; Ross, 1991; Tinetti & Speechley, 1989). Medication use is potentially the most modifiable predisposing factor for falls. Although specific drug classifications, such as antidepressants, sedatives, neuroleptics, diuretics, and antihypertensives, are easily identified as increasing the risk for falls, individual responses to medications and interactions among medications not generally implicated must always be considered.

Adverse Drug Events

Older adults take about one-third of all the prescription drugs and purchase over 40% of all the over-the-counter (OTC) drugs in the United States. These same adults average 4.5 or more prescription medicines daily and probably double that number when they are hospitalized (DeMaagd, 1995; French, 1996; Gleason, 1996). Drug use in older adults occurs primarily because of multiple chronic health problems. The use of multiple drugs combined with disease and age-related changes puts the older adult at high risk for adverse drug reactions and interactions. The number of medications prescribed in the hospital tends to increase in proportion to the patient's age and length of stay (Johnson, 1996). It is estimated that approximately 75% of older adult patients have one or more medicines discontinued and new ones started during hospitalization (McConnell, Linton, & Hanlon, 1996). The potential for adverse drug reactions is even higher when older adults are acutely or critically ill.

Predisposing Factors

The relationship between aging and adverse drug reactions remains ambiguous, and age does not seem to be the major determinant of adverse drug events (Schwartz, 1994). It is more likely that the number of drugs administered is directly related to the risk of adverse drug reactions. In the older adult patient the risk is, once again, multifactorial involving altered pharmacokinetics, altered pharmacodynamics, the presence of multiple diseases, and the complexities of the drug regimen, especially polypharmacy.

Pharmacokinetic changes involve the way drugs are absorbed, distributed, metabolized, and eliminated in older adults. Changes in the gastrointestinal tract include a reduced number of acinar cells in the salivary glands, a decrease in the production of gastric acid, a reduction in intestinal blood flow, a decrease in gastric emptying and motility, some impairment in active transport mechanisms, and some reduced activity of enzymes. Although these changes may affect drug absorption, they are usually insignificant and may be offset by a general decrease in motility and the large surface area of the gastrointestinal tract.

Body composition changes affect the way drugs are distributed in older adults. Drug distribution can be affected by a decrease in total body water that results in a decrease in the volume of distribution of water-soluble drugs. Volume of distribution may be defined as the amount of drug in the body divided by the serum drug concentration in plasma (Planchock & Slay, 1996). The consequence is higher initial concentration unless the drug dose is reduced. A decrease in lean body mass, coupled with an increase in body fat, results in an increase in the volume of distribution of fat-soluble drugs. This prolongs the half life and action of lipid-soluble drugs such as diazepam, barbiturates, antidepressants, and most other psychotropic drugs. Therefore, water-soluble drugs may require lower loading doses, and fat-soluble drugs may require higher doses.

With aging, serum albumin concentration may decrease, especially in the presence of disease or malnutrition, and this may result in decreased protein binding and a higher circulating serum concentration of highly protein-bound drugs. Warfarin, for example, is highly protein-bound, and small changes in albumin levels result in significant increases of free drug available to inhibit clotting factors and produce an anticoagulant effect (Schwartz, 1994). Nonsteroidal antiinflammatory drugs (NSAIDs) are also highly bound to albumin.

Structural and functional changes occur in the liver, the major organ responsible for drug metabolism. There is a reduction in liver mass, as the number of functional hepatocytes decreases, and reduced hepatic blood flow. Decreased hepatic blood flow results in decreased hepatic drug clearance of high-clearance drugs (those usually efficiently and rapidly metabolized by the liver). The "first-pass effect" occurs when orally administered drugs are initially transported through the portal circulation. Older adults tend to have a decrease in first-pass metabolism, so there is higher bioavailability of drugs that have first-pass metabolism, such as nitroglycerin, morphine, verapamil, furosemide, and propranolol. Decreased hepatic size results in declines in phase I and II oxidative pathways, but conjugation pathways are generally unaffected in aging. The clinical implications are that, in general, drug dosage of hepatically metabolized drugs should be reduced in older adult patients since decreases in hepatic clearance can be anticipated, but the exact extent cannot be precisely quantified (Schwartz, 1994). Acutely ill older adults with congestive heart failure or sepsis may experience a decrease in hepatic perfusion and function.

The most significant and best understood age-related changes occur in renal function which affects total body drug clearance or elimination. Older adults have decreased renal blood flow, renal mass, glomerular filtration rate, and tubular secretion, all of which contribute to decreased creatinine clearance. Serum creatinine concentrations alone do not accurately reflect creatinine clearance in older adults, because of decreased muscle mass that reduces the rate of formation of creatinine. Calculation of creatinine clearance, which offers a more accurate estimation of glomerular filtration rate, can be done by using an equation developed by Cockcroft and Gault (as cited in Schwartz, 1994):

$$\text{Creatinine clearance} = \frac{(140 - \text{age}) \times \text{lean body weight}}{72 \times \text{serum creatinine}}$$

For females, multiply by 0.85

Age-related physiological decreases in renal drug elimination are enhanced by the effects of renal insufficiency. Disease processes such as hypertension, diabetes, and atherosclerosis, common in older adults, can produce further decreases in renal function. Critically ill older adults may experience compromised renal function as a result of reduced perfusion, accumulated toxins, or intrinsic injury (Gleason, 1996).

Pharmacodynamics, what the drug does to the body, involves the effect of a particular drug on its receptor site or the end-organ responsiveness to the drug. A major determinant of the type of response is serum drug concentration (Planchock & Slay, 1996). Changes that occur with aging are not well defined, the physiologic responsiveness of older adults is quite variable, and responses may be exaggerated or diminished. Homeostatic mechanisms that may change with aging include a decrease in autonomic nervous system response to postural challenge, autonomic-mediated changes in bladder and bowel function, impairment in thermoregulation, glucose intolerance, and reduced immune response. Planchock and Slay also indicate that alteration in homeostatic mechanisms may lessen the body's ability to adjust to or counteract the effects of drugs. The response to psychotropic medications, especially benzodiazepines, may be greatly altered by a change in the concentration of various neurotransmitters.

The problem of polypharmacy, often existent on admission, or the cause of admission, occurs for a variety of reasons. Multiple diseases, multiple health-care providers, copious prescribing, increasing age, increasing accessibility of OTC drugs with serious potential side effects for older adults, and other problems seen primarily in the community all contribute to polypharmacy. The complications of polypharmacy include increased problems with side effects of medications; adverse drug events; drug–drug interactions; drug–food interactions; both direct and indirect drug costs, with the latter resulting from hospitalization for iatrogenic illness; and potential increased length of stay and increased cost of hospitalization from iatrogenic illness.

Assessing the clinical significance of a drug interaction depends on the therapeutic index of the affected drug, the magnitude of hepatic enzyme induction or inhibition, the clinical status of the patient, the timing of drug administration, and patient variability in clinical response to a drug interaction (Johnson, 1996).

Additional predisposing factors to be considered are the appropriateness of prescribing and the possibility of medication errors. Although inappropriate prescribing may not independently be a risk factor for adverse outcomes, it does occur. In one study nurse practitioners achieved a higher level of appropriate prescribing for older adults than physicians when a model was tested to determine the effect of legalized prescriptive authority for practitioners (Mahoney, 1994). Medication errors include prescribing, dispensing, and administering drugs.

Assessment

Assessment of the medication regimen of an older adult patient must take into account age-related changes, disease processes, severity of illness, pharmacokinetic and pharmacodynamic changes, the drug history, the drugs and dosages prescribed, the appropriateness of the drugs, the frailty of the individual, and the possibility of medication errors. Prevention of adverse drug reactions is the goal; however, it is probable that the indepth assessment is more likely to occur when and if there is an adverse drug event. Advanced practice nurses who work in acute care settings can serve as advocates for greater caution in prescribing practices. Suggested questions to ask when assessing the drug regimen are contained in Table 53–8.

The possibility of interpatient variability in drug responses is always a clinical consideration. On a patient-by-patient basis the response to each drug must be assessed. To do this effectively, clinicians must have a working knowledge of the classifications of drugs, the common drugs within the classifications, and the individual drugs and classifications most likely to have gerontologic considerations.

Interventions

The advanced practice nurse may be prescribing drugs; monitoring drug use; problem-solving after adverse drug events; serving as a consultant for staff; or educating nursing staff, physicians, patients, and families about drugs. The focus of this content will be on thoughtful drug prescribing and monitoring drug regimens for older adult patients.

Because geriatric pharmacology is so complex, the principal concerns include not only efficacy and safety but also the complexity of the drug regimen, the number of medications and their dosages, costs, and whether the patient can comply with the regimen after discharge. Ways to simplify the drug regimen include eliminating therapeutic duplication, decreasing the dosing frequency, and reviewing the drug regimen on a regular basis (Colley & Lucas, 1993). Eliminating therapeutic duplication may occur by consolidating therapy whenever possible. For example, use medications to manage multiple diseases, such as an angiotensin-converting enzyme inhibitor to treat a patient with congestive heart failure and hypertension. Avoid combinations that duplicate therapy or increase the potential for augmented side effects, such as prescribing two antianxiety agents for two different problems. When one medication fails, whenever possible replace it with another drug rather than adding a second one. Try to avoid any medication that may exacerbate another problem the patient has, such as using beta blockers for hypertension in a patient who also has reactive airway disease. Begin therapy with the lowest rea-

TABLE 53–8. Questions to Ask in Assessing the Drug Regimen

Is there a documented and appropriate indication for the medication?
Is the dose appropriate for the patient's age, weight, renal or liver function, etc.?
Does the patient have a documented drug allergy to a medication?
Is the dose being scheduled appropriately?
Is the duration of treatment appropriate?
Is the chosen medication the best one (most effective with least side effects) for the patient?
Are two or more similar drugs prescribed (therapeutic duplication)?
Is the patient experiencing an adverse drug reaction?
Is there a drug–drug interaction?
Is there a medical indication for use of a medication but none is prescribed?
Is the patient using over-the-counter medications inappropriately?
Is the patient compliant?

Adapted from Johnson. (1996). Used with permission.

sonable dose and slowly increase the dose in an attempt to achieve therapeutic levels or goals (French, 1996).

Decreasing the dosing frequency may help simplify the drug regimen as well as increase compliance after discharge. Try to avoid regimens that include twice-a-day, three-times-a-day, and four-times-a-day dosing frequencies together (Colley & Lucas, 1993). Consider using sustained-release dosage forms as a way of reducing the complexity of the drug regimen.

Review the drug regimen on a daily basis when the older adult is hospitalized. This involves not only chart review but also examining the patient, discussing observations made by nursing staff, and communicating with others on the team who are writing orders. Prioritize medications in order of relative importance to achieve therapeutic goals. Weigh the risks versus the benefits of whether certain diseases and symptoms are worth treating with medications. Unless absolutely necessary, don't attempt to treat an adverse effect from one drug with another drug. Always maintain a high index of suspicion when patients experience changes in cognition, affect, or behavior. A potentially useful mnemonic for using medications in older adults is presented in Table 53–9.

Finally, always consider the posthospitalization ability of patients and families to manage the drug regimen. Compliance may be affected by all the preceding factors and many clinicians do not know about, or even consider, ability to pay for drugs, literacy level, ability to monitor for side effects and adverse events, psychosocial and cultural factors, and ability to understand and follow complex regimens when they prescribe medications.

Transient Urinary Incontinence

Urinary incontinence is defined as the involuntary loss of urine sufficient to be a problem (Fantl, Newman, Colling, et al., 1996). It is classified as either transient (acute or reversible) or chronic (established). Urinary incontinence is a symptom rather than a disease, and when it is transient, it is generally secondary to a causative or contributing condition. In the acute care setting, about 35% of patients over age 65 experience urinary incontinence (Gray & Burns, 1996). Transient incontinence may account for half of the incontinence that occurs in acutely ill hospitalized older adults (Resnick, 1990). Clearly, some older adults, especially those admitted from nursing homes, are incontinent at the time of admission to the hospital, but the focus of this content is on the development of incontinence following admission.

TABLE 53–9. The MASTER Rules for Rational Drug Therapy

Minimize number of drugs used. Use the fewest number of drugs possible.
Alternatives should be considered. Alternative therapy, drugs, and dosage forms should be considered for older adult patients.
Start low, and go slow. Start with lowest dosage and increase gradually.
Titrate therapy. Adjust initial dosage according to individual characteristics and readjust dosage to optimize the monitored plasma levels and/or clinical response.
Educate the patient. To increase compliance and to decrease side effects, instruct patient or family about the need for and potential problems of therapy.
Review regularly. Monitor response regularly, and reevaluate need periodically.

Used with permission from Johnson. (1996).

Predisposing Factors

Aging alone does not cause urinary incontinence, but age-related changes in the genitourinary tract do make the older adult more susceptible to factors that may cause incontinence. Bladder capacity decreases and involuntary bladder contractions increase, which can lead to urgency and frequency. More urine is produced at night leading to nocturia. In older men, prostatic hypertrophy is nearly universal and can interfere with bladder emptying. Older women may experience relaxation of pelvic musculature and thinning and increased friability of the urethral mucosa, both contributors to urinary frequency and urgency.

Age-related changes in gait and balance as well as other musculoskeletal and body composition changes may affect mobility. When these changes are coupled with urgency and frequency, the older adult is at increased risk for incontinence due to increased travel time to the bathroom.

As pointed out earlier in the chapter, the hospital environment may be a risk factor, because older adults may have difficulty implementing their habitual strategies to avoid incontinence (Creditor, 1993). Patients who were previously independent find themselves in an unfamiliar room with different equipment, different clothing, different furniture, and obstacles on the way to the bathroom. The bed may serve as a type of restraint due to its height from the floor and the use of siderails.

Older adults may be on bed rest, or have other forms of immobilization such as traction, restraints, braces, casts, or neuromuscular conditions that require new ways of voiding. Before being able to void they must find a call light and wait for someone to respond. Then, they must adjust to the unusual position and discomfort of a bedpan, given and removed by a stranger, that is used with only the questionable privacy of a curtain.

Other predisposing factors for transient incontinence include acute confusion, symptomatic urinary tract infection, atrophic urethritis or vaginitis, psychological alterations (although cause and effect remain controversial), excessive urine production, stool impaction, and a variety of medications (Table 53–10).

Assessment

At the time of admission the nursing staff generally determine whether or not patients are continent by asking both patients and family about patterns and frequency of void-

TABLE 53–10. Predisposing Factors for Transient Urinary Incontinence

Potential Causes	Comment
Delirium (confusional state)	In the delirious patient, incontinence is usually an associated symptom that will abate with proper diagnosis and treatment of the underlying cause of confusion.
Infection (e.g., symptomatic urinary tract infection)	Dysuria and urgency from symptomatic infection may defeat the older person's ability to reach the toilet in time. Asymptomatic infection, although more common, is rarely a cause of incontinence.
Pharmaceuticals	
Sedatives/hypnotics	Benzodiazepines, especially long-acting agents such as flurazepam and diazepam, may accumulate in elderly patients and cause confusion and secondary incontinence. Alcohol, frequently used as a sedative, can cloud the sensorium, impair mobility, and induce a diuresis, resulting in incontinence.
Diuretics	A brisk diuresis induced by loop diuretics can overwhelm bladder capacity and lead to polyuria, frequency, and urgency, thereby precipitating incontinence in a frail older person. The loop diuretics include furosemide, ethacrynic acid, and bumetanide.
Anticholinergic agents	Nonprescription (over-the-counter) agents with anticholinergic properties are commonly taken by older patients for insomnia, coryza, pruritus, and vertigo, and many prescriptions medications also have anticholinergic properties. Anticholinergic side effects include urinary retention with associated urinary frequency and overflow incontinence. Besides anticholinergic actions, antiphychotics such as thioridazine and haloperidol may cause sedation, rigidity, and immobility.
Alpha–adrenergic agents	Sphincter tone in the proximal urethra can be decreased by alpha antagonists and increased by alpha agonists. An older woman, whose urethra is shortened and weakened with age, may develop stress incontinence when taking an alpha antagonist for hypertension. An older man with prostate enlargement may develop acute urinary retention and overflow incontinence when taking multicomponent "cold" capsules that contain alpha agonists and anticholinergic agents, especially if a nasal decongestant and a nonprescription hypnotic antihistamine are added.
Calcium channel blockers	Calcium channel blockers can reduce smooth muscle contractility in the bladder and occasionally can cause urinary retention and overflow incontinence.
Psychological	Severe depression may occasionally be associated with incontinence but is probably less frequently a cause in older patients.
Excessive urine production	Excess intake, endocrine conditions that cloud sensorium and induce a diuresis (e.g., hypercalcemia, hyperglycemia, and diabetes insipidus), and expanded volume states such as congestive heart failure, lower extremity venous insufficiency, drug-induced ankle edema (e.g., nifedipine, indomethacin) and low albumin states cause polyuria and can lead to incontinence.
Restricted mobility	Limited mobility is an aggravating or precipitating cause of incontinence that can frequently be corrected or improved by treating the underlying condition (e.g., arthritis, poor eyesight, Parkinson's disease, or orthostatic hypotension). A urinal or bedside commode and scheduled toileting often help resolve the incontinence that results from hospitalization and its environmental barriers (e.g., bedrails, restraints, and poor lighting).
Stool impaction	Patients with stool impaction present with either urge or overflow incontinence and may have fecal incontinence as well. Disimpaction restores incontinence.

From Agency for Health Care Policy and Research. (1992b).

ing. This initial assessment establishes the baseline against which future problems with continence can be evaluated. A functional assessment can determine the need for environmental modifications to prevent incontinence. Additionally, a cognitive assessment is done as the cognitive function of the older adult is important for the development of strategies for maintaining continence (Lincoln & Roberts, 1989).

If incontinence occurs, investigation of all the previously identified predisposing factors must be done with special attention to the environment, including restricted mobility, medications, and the presence of acute confusion. Additionally, a physical examination, including neurologic assessment to detect lower extremity problems; an abdominal examination to determine the presence or absence of bladder distention, suprapubic tenderness, or costovertebral angle tenderness; a rectal examination; sitting and standing blood pressures; and, if warranted, a pelvic examination should be done. A urinalysis and postvoid residual (PVR) should be ordered. The estimation of PVR can be made by abdominal palpation and percussion and/or on bimanual examination. If specific measurement of PVR is needed, it can be done by catheterization or pelvic ultrasound.

Interventions

The interventions for transient urinary incontinence are dependent on the outcome of the assessment. If medication, or some combination of medications, appears to be a contributing factor, therapy should be discontinued or changed if it is clinically possible. Symptomatic urinary tract infections should be treated with antibiotics. Asymptomatic urinary tract infections are generally not treated in the absence of renal disease or clinical signs of sepsis. Atrophic vaginitis or urethritis may be treated with estrogen replacement therapy. Stool disimpaction will restore continence in most instances of fecal impaction, and if this was the cause, a bowel regimen should be implemented. Underlying conditions causing excess urine production or endocrine conditions that cloud the sensorium and induce diuresis (e.g., hypercalcemia and hyperglycemia), expanded volume states such as congestive heart failure, and low serum albumin can cause polyuria and should be treated. Older adult patients with acute confusion may experience incontinence that may subside once the underlying problem is treated. Problems involving restricted mobility may be treatable or amenable to environmental modification or use of assistive devices. Indwelling bladder catheters, especially those used for long periods of time, should be avoided because of the substantial morbidity associated with them (Ouslander, 1997).

Pressure Ulcers

The Agency for Health Care Policy and Research (AHCPR) (1992a) pointed out that the incidence of pressure ulcers in hospitals ranges from nearly 3% to as high as 60% with a prevalence rate as high as nearly 30%. More than 50% of pressure ulcers occur in older adults over age 70, and increased death rates have been observed in older adults who do develop them (Allman, 1994).

Pressure ulcers (also known as bedsores or decubitus ulcers) are lesions caused by unrelieved pressure that results in damage of underlying tissue (AHCPR, 1992a). They develop when the external tissue pressure on the skin covering bony prominences exceeds capillary hydrostatic pressure. The most common bony prominences susceptible to pressure ulcer development are the sacrum, ischial tuberosity, ears, lateral malleolus, trochanter, and heels (Burke & Walsh, 1997; Sanders, 1996). Tissue anoxia, ischemia, edema, and tissue necrosis occur because of intense pressure, compounded by the duration of pressure and tissue tolerance, that leads to capillary closure. Pressure, shearing forces, friction, and moisture have all been implicated in the development of pressure ulcers.

Predisposing Factors

Age-related changes in the integument result in decreased elasticity and skin strength, decreased vascularity of the dermal skin, greater vascular fragility, a slower rate of repair, decreased subcutaneous fat tissue, and dryer skin. Additionally, age-related changes in the cardiovascular and pulmonary systems affect the oxygenation and nutrition of tissues (Shannon & Lehman, 1996). Alone, these age-related changes place the older adult at risk for skin breakdown, and the addition of chronic and/or acute illness markedly increases the risk.

Immobility and inactivity are important risk factors. Acutely ill older adults spend more time in bed or sitting in a chair, both situations that predispose them to intense and prolonged pressure on specific body parts.

Nutritional status influences the development of pressure ulcers because protein deficiency weakens tissue tolerance and hypoproteinemia changes osmotic equilibrium leading to edema (Sanders, 1996). Poor nutritional status also negatively affects the cardiovascular, respiratory, gastrointestinal, renal, neuromuscular, and immune systems. Older adults with albumin levels below 2.5 g/dL are at particularly high risk for skin breakdown (Shannon & Lehman, 1996).

Bowel and bladder incontinence create moisture that alters the resilience of the skin to external forces; however, recent literature suggests that urinary incontinence may not be so significant in pressure ulcer development as previously thought (Sanders, 1996). Stool, when mixed with urine, contributes to skin breakdown because stool pH is converted into the alkaline range, reactivating enzymes that begin to break down intact skin.

Other risk factors for skin breakdown are medications that affect the delivery of oxygen to the tissues (e.g., narcotic analgesics, sedatives), physical restraints that create immobility and friction, infection, low blood pressure, dehydration, emotional stress, elevated body temperature, and altered level of consciousness.

Assessment

Systematic, consistent, and accurate assessment of the hospitalized older adult is essential to prevent the development of pressure ulcers. There should be written protocols specifying the exact use of any risk-assessment tool. Risk assessment should be conducted on all patients who are bedbound, chairbound, incontinent, frail, disabled, nutritionally compromised, or who have altered cognition (AHCPR, 1992a). All older adults should be assessed for risk factors on admission, and those identified as high risk should be reassessed every 48 hours (Braden & Bryant, 1990). Reassessment should be done whenever there is a change in the patient's condition.

The Braden Scale for Predicting Pressure Sore Risk (Fig. 53–3) is the most rigorously tested risk assessment tool (AHCPR, 1992a). The scale identifies critical factors in the formation of pressure ulcers, and is highly sensitive and reliable. Facilities that use the Braden Scale must decide on a cut-off point (numerical value) at which patients are determined to be at risk (Vandenbosch, Montoye, Satwicz, Durkee-Leonard, & Boylan-Lewis, 1996). The orginators of the scale suggest a cut-off score of 16 or less to predict risk and institute preventive protocols. Another study indicates that the functional concepts measured by the Braden Scale are better predictors of risk than any single medical diagno-

FOR PREDICTING PRESSURE SORE RISK

Patient's Name ____________ Evaluator's Name ____________ Date of Assessment

SENSORY PERCEPTION ability to respond meaningfully to pressure-related discomfort	**1. Completely limited:** Unresponsive (does not moan, flinch, or grasp) to painful stimuli, due to diminished level of consciousness or sedation. OR limited ability to feel pain over most of body surface.	**2. Very Limited:** Responds only to painful stimuli. Cannot communicate discomfort except by moaning or restlessness. OR has a sensory impairment which limits the ability to feel pain or discomfort over 1/2 of body.	**3. Slightly Limited:** Responds to verbal commands, but cannot always communicate discomfort or need to be turned. OR has some sensory impairment which limits ability to feel pain or discomfort in 1 or 2 extremities.	**4. No Impairment:** Responds to verbal commands. Has no sensory deficit which would limit ability to feel or voice pain or discomfort.	
MOISTURE degree to which skin is exposed to moisture	**1. Constantly Moist:** Skin is kept moist almost constantly by perspiration, urine, etc. Dampness is detected every time patient is moved or turned.	**2. Very Moist:** Skin is often, but not always moist. Linen must be changed at least once a shift.	**3. Occasionally Moist:** Skin is occasionally moist, requiring an extra linen change approximately once a day.	**4. Rarely Moist:** Skin is usually dry, linen only requires changing at routine intervals.	
ACTIVITY degree of physical activity	**1. Bedfast:** Confined to bed	**2. Chairfast:** Ability to walk severely limited or non-existent. Cannot bear own weight and/or must be assisted into chair or wheelchair.	**3. Walks Occasionally:** Walks occasionally during day, but for very short distances, with or without assistance. Spends majority of each shift in bed or chair.	**4. Walks Frequently:** walks outside the room at least twice a day and inside room at least once every 2 hours during waking hours.	
MOBILITY ability to change and control body position	**1. Completely Immobile:** Does not make even slight changes in body or extremity position without assistance.	**2. Very Limited:** Makes occasional slight changes in body or extremity position but unable to make frequent or significant changes independently.	**3. Slightly Limited:** Makes frequent though slight changes in body or extremity position independently.	**4. No Limitations:** Makes major and frequent changes in position without assistance.	
NUTRITION usual food intake pattern	**1. Very Poor:** Never eats a complete meal. Rarely eats more than 1/3 of any food offered. Eats 2 servings or less of protein (meat or dairy products) per day. Takes fluids poorly. Does not take a liquid dietary supplement. OR is NPO and/or maintained on clear liquids or IV's for more than 5 days.	**2. Probably Inadequate:** Rarely eats a complete meal and generally eats only about 1/2 of any food offered. Protein intake includes only 3 servings of meat or dairy products per day. Occasionally will take a dietary supplement. OR receives less than optimum amount of liquid diet or tube feeding.	**3. Adequate:** Eats over half of most meals. Eats a total of 4 servings of protein (meat, dairy products) each day. Occasionally will refuse a meal, but will usually take a supplement if offered. OR is on a tube feeding or TPN regimen which probably meets most of nutritional needs.	**4. Excellent:** Eats most of every meal. Never refuses a meal. Usually eats a total of 4 or more servings of meat and dairy products. Occasionally eats between meals. Does not require supplementation.	
FRICTION AND SHEAR	**1. Problem:** Requires moderate to maximum assistance in moving. Complete lifting without sliding against sheets is impossible. Frequently slides down in bed or chair, requiring frequent repositioning with maximum assistance. Spasticity, contractures or agitation leads to almost constant friction.	**2. Potential Problem:** Moves feebly or requires minimum assistance . During a move skin probably slides to some extent against sheets, chair, restraints, or other devices. Maintains relatively good position in chair or bed most of the time but occasionally slides down.	**3. No Apparent Problem:** Moves in bed and in chair independently and has sufficient muscle strength to lift up completely during move. Maintains good position in bed or chair at all times.		
				Total Score	

Figure 53–3. Braden Scale. Copyright Barbara Branden and Nancy Bergstrom, 1988. *(Used with permission of copyright holder.)*

sis or disease process (Bergstrom, Braden, Kemp, Champagne, & Ruby, 1996). All individual risk factors, such as decreased mental status, moisture, incontinence, and nutritional deficiency, must be identified to direct specific preventive treatments.

Interventions

The first line of defense for pressure ulcers is prevention. The advanced practice nurse has an important role as a consultant and educator concerning both prevention of skin breakdown and interventions for the treatment of pressure ulcers. Clinical guidelines for the prevention of pressure ulcers in patients identified as being at risk (AHCPR,1992a) are outlined in Table 53–11, and guidelines for mechanical loading and support surfaces are outlined in Table 53–12.

Staging or classification systems are used to describe the severity of skin breakdown. The following classification (AHCPR, 1992a) offers an objective way to describe the degree of tissue breakdown:

- *Stage I:* Nonblanchable erythema of intact skin
- *Stage II:* Partial-thickness skin loss involving epidermis and/or dermis. The ulcer is superficial and presents clinically as an abrasion, blister, or shallow crater.
- *Stage III:* Full-thickness skin loss involving damage or necrosis of subcutaneous tissue that may extend down to, but not through, underlying fascia. The ulcer presents clinically as a deep crater with or without undermining of adjacent tissue.
- *Stage IV:* Full-thickness skin loss with extensive destruction, tissue necrosis, or damage to muscle, bone, or supporting structures (e.g., tendon, joint capsule, etc.). Undermining and sinus tracts may also be associated with ulcers in this stage.

TABLE 53–11. Guidelines for Skin Care and Early Treatment

Daily inspection with close attention to bony prominences
Cleanse skin at the time of soiling and at routine intervals with a mild, nonirritating cleanser using warm—not hot—water
Use moisturizers immediately after bathing to prevent skin dryness
Minimize skin drying due to low humidity and exposure to cold
Avoid massage over bony prominences
Minimize skin exposure to moisture from incontinence, wound drainage, or perspiration
Minimize skin injury due to friction and shear by using proper positioning, transferring, and turning; friction injuries may be reduced by using lubricants (such as cornstarch), protective films, protective dressings, and protective padding
Ensure adequate dietary intake and correct nutritional deficiencies
Institute rehabilitation for improvement of mobility and activity status if consistent with therapeutic goals; maintain current activity level, mobility and range of motion if adequate
Document and monitor interventions and outcomes

From Agency for Health Care Policy and Research. (1992a).

TABLE 53–12. Guidelines for Mechanical Loading and Support Surfaces

Use written repositioning schedule
Turn and reposition bed-bound persons every two hours; chairbound persons, every hour
Use positioning devices to keep bony prominences from direct contact with one another
Relieve pressure on heels by raising them off the bed (e.g., pillows under calves)
When using side-lying position in bed, avoid positioning directly on trochanter (use 30-degree lateral inclined position)
Maintain head of bed at lowest degree of elevation consistent with condition and any restrictions; limit amount of time head of bed is elevated
Use lifting devices to move persons in bed
Place persons at risk on pressure-reducing mattress/chair cushions
Avoid use of donut-type devices to relieve pressure
Avoid uninterrupted sitting in any chair/wheelchair
Teach chair-bound persons who are able to shift weight every 15 minutes
Consider postural alignment, distribution of weight, balance and stability, and pressure relief when positioning persons in chairs or wheelchairs

From Agency for Health Care Policy and Research. (1992a).

Basic principles of pressure ulcer management include eliminating or minimizing precipitating factors identified during risk assessment; monitoring and supporting nutritional status; and wound management that creates and maintains a clean, moist environment. Specific wound care management protocols differ from one institutional setting to another.

Clinicians are encouraged to obtain educational materials and guidelines on pressure ulcers directly from AHCPR or by accessing the AHCPR web site at http://www.ahcpr.gov.

▶ DISCHARGE PLANNING

Discharge planning for older adult patients must begin at the time of admission to the hospital. Planning should take into account the reasons why older adults are at high risk for poor postdischarge outcomes as well as the unique and complex needs of this population and their families (Naylor, 1992). A major factor in discharge planning is that acutely ill older adults may experience a sustained loss of functional independence as a result of hospitalization (Hirsch, Sommers, Olsen, Mullen, & Winograd, 1990). The goal should be to assist older adults and their families in finding the best solutions to handling health-care problems in the most appropriate location from the most appropriate source to meet their needs.

Hospitalized older adults need early discharge planning to avoid inappropriate placement after hospitalization. This early intervention may occur in a variety of ways. Interdisciplinary geriatric teams may do comprehensive assessment, serve as consultants for nursing staff and other disciplines, provide direct care, focus on patients identified as high risk, or focus on patients with specific medical diagnoses. Nurse or social work case managers or multidisciplinary case management teams are becoming common models as the length of stay decreases, older adults have a higher acuity level at the time of discharge, and the time for planning transition to posthospital care is compacted. Several innovative nursing models to enhance health outcomes, such as the Geriatric Resource Nurse Model at Yale–New Haven, the Acute Care of the Elderly Medical Surgical Nursing Unit at University Hospitals of Cleveland, and the Comprehensive Discharge Planning for the Elderly Model at the University of Pennsylvania School of Nursing are currently in place (Fulmer & Mezey, 1994). These nursing models incorporate advanced practice nurses in roles such as educators and consultants for staff nurses, as resource persons for intervention protocols, and as care and program coordinators. Despite existing models that effectively decrease the incidence of functional decline and structured discharge planning teams, some barriers still interfere with expeditious discharge.

Four categories of barriers to discharge planning have been identified: (1) patient care issue; (2) structural and administrative issues; (3) community-related issues; and (4) financial and legal issues (Girard, 1996). Multidisciplinary

Blaylock Discharge Planning Risk Assessment Screen

Admission Date: Transfer to Floor Date:

CIRCLE ALL THAT APPLY AND TOTAL
REFER TO RATING SCALE FOR RISK FACTOR INDEX AND INSTRUCTIONS*

Age:
0 = 55 or younger
1 = 56-64 years
2 = 65-79 years
3 = 80+ years

Living Situation/Social Support:
0 = Lives with spouse only
1 = Lives with family
2 = Lives alone with family support
3 = Lives alone with friends support
4 = Lives alone—no support
5 = Nursing home/Residential Care

Functional Status:
0 = ADL&IADL Independent
Dependent In:
1 = Eating/Feeding
1 = Bathing/Grooming
1 = Toileting
1 = Transferring
1 = Incontinent of bowel function
1 = Incontinent of bladder function
1 = Meal preparation
1 = Responsible for own medication admin.
1 = Handling own finances
1 = Grocery shopping
1= Transportation

Cognition:
0 = Oriented
1 = Disoriented—some spheres some time
2 = Disoriented—some spheres all time
3 = Disoriented—all spheres some time
4 = Disoriented—all spheres all time
5 = Comatose
Spheres (Person, place, time, self)

Behavior Pattern:
0 = Appropriate
1 = Wandering
1 = Agitation
1 = Confusion
1 = Other

Mobility:
0 = Ambulatory
1 = Ambulatory with mechanical assistance
2 = Ambulatory with human assistance
3 = Non-ambulatory

Sensory Deficits:
0 = None
1 = Visual deficits or hearing
2 = Visual and hearing deficits

Number of Previous Admission/ER Visits:
0 = None in the past 3 months
1 = 1 in the past 3 months
2 = 2 in the past 3 months
3 = More than 2 in the past 3 months

Number of Active Medical Problems:
0 = 3 medical problems
1 = 3-5 medical problems
2 = More than 5 medical problems

Number of Drugs:
0 = Less than 3 drugs
1 = 3 to 5 drugs
2 = More than 5 drugs

Total Score:

*Risk Factor Index
Score of 10: At risk for home care resources
Score of 11 to 19: At risk for extended discharge planning
Score of more than 20: At risk for placement other than home

If patient's score is 10 or greater, refer Patient to Discharge Planning Coordinator Discharge Planning Team

Nurse Signature:

Figure 53–4. Blaylock discharge planning risk assessment screen. *(From Blaylock & Cason. [1996]. [pp. 275–282].)*

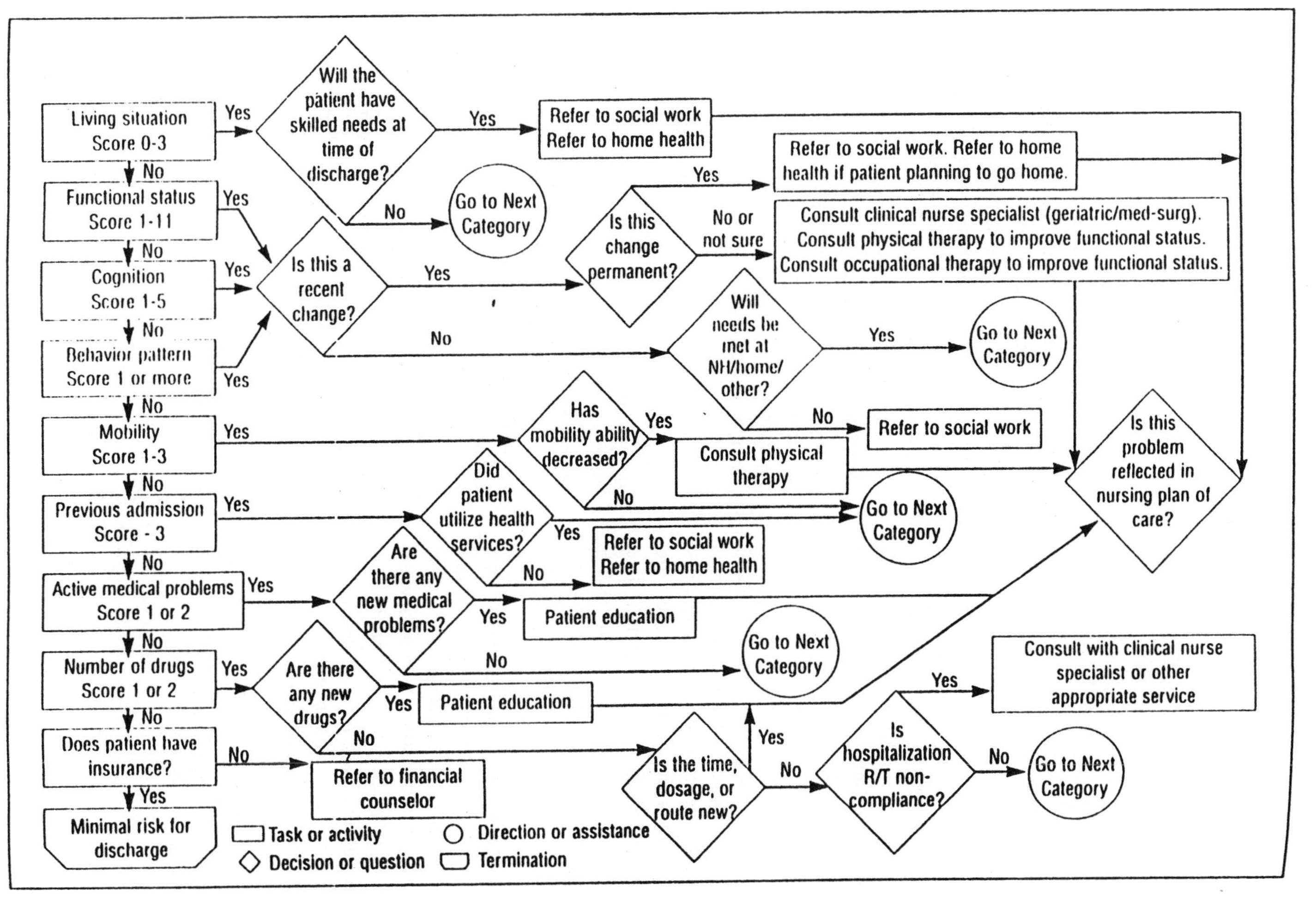

Figure 53–5. Decision Tree for use with BRASS. *(Used with permission from Blaylock & Cason. [1996].)*

case management seems to be an effective model for overcoming these diverse barriers.

There are variables helpful in predicting the postdischarge outcomes of hospitalized older adults as well as their need for some type of transitional care (Naylor, 1992). Long-term health outcomes and needs are often related to the patient's own assessment of general health. A second class of variables involves the complexity of the medical condition, such as the number of chronic illnesses, the medication regimen, and the severity of the acute illness. A third group of variables that can predict outcomes include those that suggest a prior history of patients who are unable to be responsible for their own health, such as cognitive impairment, functional deficits, a history of repeated hospitalizations in the past 12 months, and the use of community agencies for health and social services. Finally, a group of variables correlated with positive postdischarge outcomes include the presence of family or social networks that can provide needed support.

The Blaylock Risk Assessment Screen (BRASS) was developed as part of a discharge planning program to meet the needs of hospitalized older adults (Blaylock & Cason, 1996). This instrument, to be included as part of the admission assessment, identifies patients at risk for prolonged hospital stay and in need of discharge planning resources. As seen by the tool (Fig. 53–4), there are ten patient characteristics assessed. Each option under the characteristics has a numerical value that represents the degree to which the characteristic affects the need for discharge planning. The validity and reliability of the instrument have been established (Blaylock & Cason, 1992). An accompanying decision tree (Fig. 53–5) assists in organizing data and deciding on interventions.

Comprehensive discharge planning may help decrease the rehospitalization of many older adults by putting into place services that enable them to function in their own homes, by assessing the need for transition to a sub-acute care setting for rehabilitation, or by helping older adults and their families with making the decision for long-term care placement. As the number of older adults increases, the number of them who will need and can benefit from systematic planning also grows. Despite increasing better health and activity levels, with better outcomes following hospitalization, institution-based discharge planning needs to become as sophisticated as possible.

Older adults account for 31% of hospital admissions, with those persons over age 75 having the longest average length of stay, the most days of care, and the highest number of discharges of all age groups in the United States. Even though the general health and activity level of older adults is better now than ever before in history, more than 80% of persons age 65 or older have at least one chronic illness, and when hospitalization occurs, it is often related to a chronic disease process.

A distinction can be made between successful aging and usual aging in terms of the changes that occur. Important age-related information about older adults includes the knowledge that the manifestations of aging are unique to each person, a reduction of compensatory reserve is related to age-related decreases in physiologic function, that there are no age-related changes in cognition that should impair or affect function, and that the presentation of symptoms in older adults is often atypical.

Hospitalization poses many risks for older adults as they attempt to adapt to an unfamiliar, and often hostile, environment. Major risks for hospitalized older adults are functional decline, iatrogenic illnesses, such as incontinence, effects from bed rest and reduced mobility, adverse effects from medications, nosocomial infections, and nutritional and fluid disturbances.

This chapter specifically focused on the risks during hospitalization for functional decline, acute confusion, dehydration, falls, adverse drug events, transient urinary incontinence, and pressure ulcers by addressing the predisposing factors, assessment, and interventions for each risk.

Discharge planning was discussed because of its importance in the early identification of the needs of older adults and their families in order to find the best solutions to handling health-care problems in the most appropriate location from the most appropriate sources.

Care of the hospitalized older adult will continue to be a challenge for advanced practice nurses and all members of the health-care team. The particular complexities and needs of this population represent an opportunity for nurses to use advanced knowledge and clinical decision-making skills to enhance positive outcomes and decrease the risks of hospitalization.

REFERENCES

Abrams, W., Beers, M., & Berkow, R. (Eds.). (1995). *The Merck manual of geriatrics* (2nd ed.). Whitehouse Station, NJ: Merck Research Laboratories.

Agency for Health Care Policy and Research. (1992a). *Pressure ulcers in adults: Prediction and prevention.* Clinical Practice Guideline, No. 3 (AHCPR Pub. No. 92-0047). Rockville, MD: U.S. Department of Health and Human Services, Public Health Service.

Agency for Health Care Policy and Research. (1992b). *Urinary incontinence in adults.* Clinical Practice Guideline (AHCPR Pub. No. 92-0038). Rockville, MD: U.S. Department of Health and Human Services, Public Health Service.

Allman, R. (1994). Pressure ulcers. In W. Hazzard, E. Bierman, J. Blass, W. Ettinger, & J. Halter (Eds.), *Principles of geriatric medicine and gerontology* (3rd ed.). (pp. 1329–1336). New York: McGraw-Hill.

Bergstrom, N., Braden, B., Kemp, M., Champagne, M., & Ruby, E. (1996). Multi-site study of incidence of pressure ulcers and the relationship between risk level, demographic characteristics, diagnoses, and prescription of preventive interventions. *Journal of the American Geriatrics Society, 44,* 22–30.

Blaylock, A. & Cason, C. (1992). Discharge planning, predicting patients needs. *Journal of Gerontological Nursing, 18* (7), 5–10.

Blaylock, A. & Cason, C. (1996). Predicting discharge planning needs. In V. Burggraf & R. Barry (Eds.), *Gerontological nursing, current practice and research* (pp. 275–282). Thorofare, NJ: Slack.

Braden, B. & Bryant, R. (1990). Innovations to prevent and treat pressure ulcers. *Geriatric Nursing, 11,* 182–186.

Burke, M. & Walsh, M. (1997). *Gerontologic nursing, wholistic care of the older adult* (2nd ed.). St. Louis: Mosby.

Carty, A. & Day, S. (1993). Interdisciplinary care, effect in acute hospital setting. *Journal of Gerontological Nursing, 19*(3), 22–32.

Colley, C. & Lucas, L. (1993). Polypharmacy: The cure becomes the disease. *Journal of General Internal Medicine, 8,* 278–283.

Creditor, M. (1993). Hazards of hospitalization of the elderly. *Annals of Internal Medicine, 118,* 219–223.

Creditor, M. (1995). Hospitalization. In W. Abrams, M. Beers, & R. Berkow (Eds.), *The Merck manual of geriatrics* (2nd ed.). (pp. 314–320). Whitehouse Station, NJ: Merck Research Laboratories.

Cronin-Stubbs, D. (1996). Delirium intervention research in acute care settings. *Annual Review of Nursing Research, 14,* 57–73.

Davis, K. & Minaker, K. (1994). Disorders of fluid balance: Dehydration and hyponatremia. In W. Hazzard, E. Bierman, J. Blass, W. Ettinger, & J. Halter (Eds.), *Principles of Geriatric Medicine and Gerontology* (3rd ed.). (pp. 1183–1190). New York: McGraw-Hill.

DeMaagd, G. (1995). High-risk drugs in the elderly population. *Geriatric Nursing, 16,* 198–207.

Dugan, J., Deane, D., & Mosel, L. (1996). Acute care. In A. Lueckenotte (Ed.), *Gerontologic nursing* (pp. 899–912). St. Louis: Mosby.

Fantl, J., Newman, D., Colling, J., et al. (1996). *Urinary incontinence in adults: Acute and chronic management.* Clinical Practice Guideline, No. 2 (AHCPR Pub. No. 96-0682). Rockville, MD: U.S. Department of Health and Human Services, Public Health Service, Agency for Health Care Policy and Research.

Folstein, M., Folstein, S., & McHugh, P. (1975). Mini-mental state: A practical method for grading the cognitive status of patients for the clinician. *Journal of Psychiatric Research, 12,* 189–198.

Foreman, M. (1986). Acute confusional states in hospitalized elderly: A research dilemma. *Nursing Research, 35* (1), 34–38.

Foreman, M. (1989). Confusion in the hospitalized elderly: Incidence, onset, and associated factors. *Research in Nursing and Health, 12,* 21–29.

Foreman, M. (1993). Acute confusion in the elderly. *Annual Review of Nursing Research, 11,* 3–30.

Foreman, M. (1996). Nursing strategies for acute confusion in elders. *American Journal of Nursing, 96* (4), 44–51.

Francis, J. (1992). Delirium in older patients. *Journal of the American Geriatrics Society, 40,* 829–838.

Francis, J., Martin, D., & Kapoor, W. (1990). A prospective study of delirium in hospitalized elderly. *Journal of the American Medical Association, 263,* 1097–1101.

Fraser, D. (1993). Patient assessment, infection in the elderly. *Journal of Gerontological Nursing, 19* (7), 5–11.

French, D. (1996). Avoiding adverse drug reactions in the elderly patient: Issues and strategies. *Nurse Practitioner, 21,* 90–105.

Fulmer, T. & Mezey, M. (1994). Nurses improving care to the hospitalized elderly. *Geriatric Nursing, 15,* 126.

Gallo, J., Reichel, W., & Andersen, L. (1995). *Handbook of Geriatric Assessment* (2nd ed.). Gaithersburg, MD: Aspen Publishers.

Girard, N. (1996). Gerontological nursing in acute care settings. In M. Matteson, E. McConnell, & A. Linton (Eds.), *Gerontological Nursing* (2nd ed.). (pp. 855–895). Philadelphia: W. B. Saunders.

Gleason, M. (1996). Pharmacologic issues in aging. *Critical Care Nursing Quarterly, 19* (2), 7–12.

Gorbien, M., Bishop, J., Beers, M., Norman, D., Osterweil, D., & Rubenstein, L. (1992). Iatrogenic illness in hospitalized elderly people. *Journal of the American Geriatrics Society, 40,* 1031–1042.

Gray, M. & Burns, S. (1996). Continence management. *Critical Care Nursing Clinics of North America, 8* (1), 29–38.

Hahn, B. & Lefkowitz, D. (1992). *Annual expenses and sources of payment for health care services: National medical expenditure surevey: Research findings 14.* (AHCPR Pub. No. 93-0007). Rockville, MD: Department of Health and Human Services, Public Health Service, Agency for Health Care Policy and Research.

Hamilton, L. & Lyon, P. (1995). A nursing-driven program to preserve and restore functional ability in hospitalized elderly patients. *Journal of Nursing Administration, 25* (4), 30–37.

Harper, C. & Lyles, Y. (1988). Physiology and complications of bedrest. *Journal of the American Geriatrics Society, 36,* 1047–1054.

Hirsch, C., Sommers, L., Olsen, A., Mullen, L., & Winograd, C. (1990). The natural history of functional morbidity in hospitalized older patients. *Journal of the American Geriatrics Society, 38,* 1296–1303.

Hoenig, H. & Rubenstein, L. (1991). Hospital-associated deconditioning and dysfunction. *Journal of the American Geriatrics Society, 39,* 220–222.

Hoffman, N. (1991). Dehydration in the elderly: Insidious and manageable. *Geriatrics, 46* (6), 35–38.

Hogue, C. (1992). Managing falls: The current bases for practice. In S. Funk, E. Tornquist, M. Champagne, & R. Wiese (Eds.), *Key aspects of elder care. Managing falls, incontinence, and cognitive impairment* (pp. 41–57). New York: Springer.

Huber, M. & Kennard, A. (1991). Functional and mental status outcomes of clients discharged from acute gerontological versus medical/surgical units. *Journal of Gerontological Nursing, 17* (7), 20–24.

Inouye, S. & Charpentier, P. (1996). Precipitating factors for delirium in hospitalized elderly persons. *Journal of the American Medical Association, 275,* 852–857.

Inouye, S., Acampora, D., Miller, R., Fulmer, T., Hurst, L., & Cooney, L. (1993). The Yale Geriatric Care Program: A model of care to prevent functional decline in hospitalized elderly patients. *Journal of the American Geriatrics Society, 41,* 1345–1352.

Inouye, S., vanDyck, C., Alessi, C., Balkin, S., Siegal, A., & Horwitz, R. (1990). Clarifying confusion: The Confusion Assessment Method. *Annals of Internal Medicine, 113,* 941–948.

Inouye, S., Wagner, D., Acampora, D., Horwitz, R., Cooney, L., Hurst, L., & Tinetti, M. (1993). A controlled trial of a nursing-centered intervention in hospitalized elderly medical patients: The Yale Geriatric Care Program. *Journal of the American Geriatrics Society, 41,* 1353–1360.

Johnson, J. (1996). Pharmacologic management. In A. Lueckenotte (Ed.), *Gerontologic Nursing* (pp. 452–483). St. Louis: Mosby.

Katz, S., Ford, A., Moskowitz, R., Jackson, B., & Jaffee, M. (1963). Studies of illness in the aged. The Index of ADL: A standardized measure of biological and psychosocial function. *Journal of the American Medical Association, 185,* 94–98.

Kavesh, W. (1996). The practice of geriatric medicine: How geriatricians think. *Generations, 20* (4), 54–59.

King, M. & Tinetti, M. (1995). Falls in community-dwelling older persons. *Journal of the American Geriatrics Society, 43,* 1146–1154.

Landefeld, C., Palmer, R., Kresevic, D., Fortinsky, R., & Kowal, J. (1995). A randomized trial of care in a hospital medical unit designed to improve the functional outcomes of acutely ill older patients. *New England Journal of Medicine, 332,* 1338–1344.

Lawton, M. & Brody, E. (1969). Assessment of older people: Self-maintaining and instrumental activities of daily living. *The Gerontologist, 9,* 179–186.

Lekan-Rutledge, D. (1996). Functional assessment. In M. Matteson, E. McConnell, & A. Linton (Eds.), *Gerontological Nursing* (2nd ed.). (pp. 75–121). Philadelphia: W. B. Saunders.

Lincoln, R. & Roberts, R. (1989). Continence issues in acute care. *Nursing Clinics of North America, 24* (3), 741–754.

Lipowski, Z. (1989). Delirium in the elderly patient. *New England Journal of Medicine, 320,* 578–582.

Liu, B., Topper, A., Reeves, R., Gryfe, C., & Maki, B. (1995). Falls among older people: Relationship to medication use and orthostatic hypotension. *Journal of the American Geriatrics Society, 43,* 1141–1145.

Mahoney, D. (1994). Appropriateness of geriatric prescribing decisions made by nurse practitioners and physicians. *Image: Journal of Nursing Scholarship, 26* (1), 41–46.

McConnell, E., Linton, A., & Hanlon, J. (1996). Pharmacological considerations. In M. Matteson, E. McConnell & A. Linton (Eds.), *Gerontological Nursing* (2nd ed.). (pp. 739–763). Philadelphia: W. B. Saunders.

Meissner, P., Andolsek, K., Mears, P., & Fletcher, B. (1989). Maximizing the functional status of geriatric patients in an acute community hospital setting. *The Gerontologist, 29,* 524–528.

Mion, L., Strumpf, N., & the NICHE faculty. (1994). Use of physical restraints in the hospital setting: Implications for the nurse. *Geriatric Nursing, 15,* 127–131.

Mobily, P. & Kelley, L. (1991). Iatrogenesis in the elderly, factors of immobility. *Journal of Gerontological Nursing, 17* (9), 5–10.

Murray, A., Levkoff, S., Wetle, T., Beckett, L., Cleary, P., Schor, J., Lipsitz, L., Rowe, J., & Evans, D. (1993). Acute delirium and functional decline in the hospitalized elderly patient. *Journal of Gerontology, 48,* M181–186.

Naylor, M. (1992). The implications of discharge planning for hospitalized elders. In T. Fulmer & M. Walker (Eds.), *Critical care nursing of the elderly* (pp. 331–347). New York: Springer.

Neelon, V., Champagne, M., Carlson, J., & Funk, S. (1996). The NEECHAM Confusion Scale: Construction, validation, and clinical testing. *Nursing Research, 45,* 324–330.

Neelon, V., Champagne, M., McConnell, E., Carlson, J., & Funk, S. (1992). Use of the NEECHAM Confusion Scale to assess acute confusional states of hospitalized older persons. In S. Funk, E. Tornquist, M. Champagne, & R. Wiese (Eds.), *Key Aspects of Elder Care. Managing Falls, Incontinence, and Cognitive Impairment* (pp. 278–289). New York: Springer.

O'Keeffe, S. & Lavan, J. (1997). The prognostic significance of delirium in older hospital patients. *Journal of the American Geriatrics Society, 45,* 174–178.

Ouslander, J. (1997). Geriatric urinary incontinence. *Generations, 20* (4), 33–38.

Pfeiffer, E. (1975). A Short Portable Mental Status Questionnaire for the assessment of organic brain deficit in elderly patients. *Journal of the American Geriatrics Society, 23,* 433–441.

Planchock, N. & Slay, L. (1996). Pharmacokinetic and pharmacodynamic monitoring of the elderly in critical care. *Critical Care Nursing Clinics of North America, 8* (1), 79–89.

Pompei, P., Foreman, M., Rudberg, M., Inouye, S., Braund, V., & Cassel, C. (1994). Delirium in hospitalized older persons: Outcomes and predictors. *Journal of the American Geriatrics Society, 42,* 809–815.

Resnick, N. (1990). Initial evaluation of the incontinent patient. *Journal of the American Geriatrics Society, 38,* 311–316.

Rich, M., Shah, A., Vinson, J., Freedland, K., Kuru, T., & Sperry, J. (1996). Iatrogenic congestive heart failure in older adults: Clinical course and prognosis. *Journal of the American Geriatrics Society, 44,* 638–643.

Ross, J. (1991). Iatrogenesis in the elderly, contributors to falls. *Journal of Gerontological Nursing, 17* (9), 19–23.

Rowe, J. & Schneider, E. (1995). Aging process. In W. Abrams, M. Beers, & R. Berkow (Eds.), *The Merck Manual of Geriatrics* (2nd Edition), (pp. 419–424). Whitehouse Station, NJ: Merck Research Laboratories.

Sager, M., Rudberg, M., Jalaluddin, M., Franke, T., Inouye, S., Landefeld, S., Siebens, H. & Winograd, C. (1996). Hospital Admission Risk Profile (HARP): Identifying older patients at risk for functional decline following acute medical illness and hospitalization. *Journal of the American Geriatrics Society, 44,* 251–257.

Sanders, S. (1996). Integumentary function. In A. Lueckenotte (Ed.), *Gerontologic Nursing* (pp. 767–812). St. Louis: Mosby.

Schor, J., Levkoff, S., Lipsitz, L., Reilly, C., Cleary, P., Rowe, J., & Evans, D. (1992). Risk factors for delirium in hospitalized elderly. *Journal of the American Medical Association, 267,* 827–831.

Schwartz, J. (1994). Clinical pharmacology. In W. Hazzard, E. Bierman, J. Blass, W. Ettinger, & J. Halter (Eds.), *Principles of geriatric medicine and gerontology* (3rd ed.). (pp. 259–275). New York: McGraw-Hill.

Shannon, M. & Lehman, C. (1996). Protecting the skin of the elderly patient in the intensive care unit. *Critical Care Nursing Clinics of North America, 8* (1), 17–28.

Stoehr, G. (1995). Pharmacology and the elderly: The problem of polypharmacy. In M. Stanley & P. Beare (Eds.), *Gerontological Nursing,* (pp. 522–534). Philadelphia: F. A. Davis.

Stolley, J. & Buckwalter, K. (1991). Iatrogenesis in the elderly, nosocomial infection. *Journal of Gerontological Nursing, 17* (9), 30–34.

Tinetti, M. (1986). Performance oriented assessment of mobility problems in elderly patients. *Journal of the American Geriatrics Society, 34,* 119–126.

Tinetti, M. (1994). Falls. In W. Hazzard, E. Bierman, J. Blass, W. Ettinger, & J. Halter (Eds.), *Principles of Geriatric Medicine and Gerontology* (3rd Ed.). (pp. 1313–1320). New York: McGraw-Hill.

Tinetti, M. & Speechley, M. (1989). Prevention of falls among the elderly. *New England Journal of Medicine, 320,* 1055–1059.

Tinetti, M., Inouye, S., Gill, T., & Doucette, J. (1995). Shared risk factors for falls, incontinence, and functional dependence. *Journal of the American Medical Association, 273,* 1348–1353.

U.S. Bureau of the Census. (1996). *Statistical Abstract of the United States: 1996* (116th ed.). Washington, DC: U.S. Bureau of the Census.

U.S. Senate Special Committee on Aging. (1991). *Aging America: Trends and Projections.* Washington, DC: U.S. Department of Health and Human Services.

Vandenbosch, T., Montoye, C., Satwicz, M., Durkee-Leonard, K., & Boylan-Lewis, B. (1996). Predictive validity of the Braden Scale and nurse perception in identifying pressure ulcer risk. *Applied Nursing Research, 9,* 80–86.

Vermeersch, P. (1992). Clinical assessment of confusion. In S. Funk, E. Tornquist, M. Champagne & R. Wiese (Eds.), *Key aspects of elder care. Managing falls, incontinence, and cognitive impairment* (pp. 251–262). New York: Springer.

Walker, M. (1992). The physiology of normal aging: Implications for nursing management of critically compromised adults. In T. Fulmer & M. Walker (Eds.), *Critical care nursing of the elderly,* (pp. 32–47). New York: Springer.

Wandel, J. (1990). The use of postural vital signs in the assessment of fluid volume status. *Journal of Professional Nursing, 6,* 46–54.

Williams, M. (1994). Clinical management of the elderly patient. In W. Hazzard, E. Bierman, J. Blass, W. Ettinger, & J. Halter (Eds.), *Principles of geriatric medicine and gerontology* (3rd ed.). (pp. 195–201.). New York: McGraw-Hill.

Wilson, M. & Morley, J. (1996). Thirst and hydration. In J. Birren (Ed.), *Encyclopedia of Gerontology,* Vol. 1. (pp. 573–581). New York: Academic Press.

Zauderer, B. (1996). Age-related changes in renal function. *Critical Care Nursing Quarterly, 19* (2), 34–40.

54

The Hospitalized Patient's Psychological Response to Illness

Susan L. W. Krupnick

Coping with illness and/or injury—whether acute, chronic, or a combination—produces emotional upheaval for the patient, family, designated caregivers, and sometimes their appointed health-care professionals. Periodically serious conflict emerges within the patient, family system, and even within the context of the health-care system. When personal, cultural, and religious values do not complement each other, a conflictual situation may arise that at least in the short term affects everyone's ability to cope with the situation. These conflicts often require some mediation and opportunity to listen to each other and understand the source of the conflict. The acute care nurse practitioner (ACNP) is well accustomed to "being in the middle" of colliding value systems that can generate anxiety, anger, frustration, and sometimes open hostility from all participants in the conflict. This chapter is devoted to assessment and intervention strategies that hopefully will lessen some of these occurrences when they are a function of the patient's difficulty in coping due to emotional, psychological, and/or psychiatric disturbances. Additionally, included will be information about when it is time to refer the patient for additional psychiatric–mental health consultation and focused mental health care.

Most individuals possess specific coping strategies, and can marshal them when they are facing a stressful and anxiety-producing event. Hospitalization in an acute care center certainly qualifies as an anxiety-producing event. Many patients are fortunate to be resilient and can cope effectively and in an adaptive manner with an illness or injury. However, emotional disturbances and psychiatric illness often accompany medical illness and can become a significant health-care problem in addition to their preexisting problem. Also, the patient in the acute care environment might be experiencing a preexisting acute psychiatric disorder or a chronic mental illness. Chronic mental illness in medically ill patients usually requires more attention to the interrelationship of physical and mental health assessments; therefore, it is necessary to foster collaborative partnerships with the patient, family, psychiatric provider(s), and the acute care providers (Lambdan, Ramchandani, & Schindler, 1997).

The most common emotional and psychological responses to illness and injury are anger, anxiety, denial, depression, fear, and withdrawal from the environment and responsibilities. The majority of primary and associate nurses in acute care are accustomed to managing these common emotional responses. However, they may need to marshal resources to assist them and their patients when their usual repertoire of interventions cease to be effective. Often the ACNP is the first resource to be summoned. Generally, the ACNP is looked to for focused, efficient, and workable solutions because he or she may have an established relationship with the patient and family members. Therefore, it is important to have specific assessment tools and intervention strategies to meet these frequent challenges. The focus of this chapter is to address the predominant emotional, psychological, and psychiatric disturbances that may go undetected and often complicate the acute care and early recovery of the hospitalized patient. The identified emotional responses and psychiatric disturbances that will be discussed include the most commonly exhibited in acute care and include: anxiety, depression, delirium, and substance abuse. These four disorders are the most prevalent in acute care, and pose the most significant risk to the patient and health-care providers. Additionally, they are the most costly to an already-vulnerable health-care system, and produce suffering for the patient, family, and caregivers.

PREVALENCE AND IMPACT OF EMOTIONAL DISTURBANCES AND PSYCHIATRIC ILLNESS ON MEDICALLY ILL PATIENTS

Individuals with chronic medical illness(es) have about a 40% higher rate of psychiatric disorders with the onset corresponding to the beginning of the illness/injury or treatment regimen. Additionally, chronic medical illness is associated with a 28% higher lifetime prevalence rate of psychiatric disorders (Cassem, 1990). The overall affect of these disturbances has been examined and the outcomes include: increased complexity of illness trajectory, treatment course, and response; diminution of their functional capacity; retardation of early recovery; lengthening of hospital stay; impairment in long-term coping ability; and contribution in the patient's morbidity and mortality (Blanchard & Hickling, 1997; Bostwick & Masterton, 1998; Frasure-Smith et al., 1995; Jorge et al., 1994; Morris et al., 1992; Roach et al., 1998; Vingerhoets, 1998).

The ACNP working in concert with the psychiatric clinical nurse specialist, primary psychiatric nurse practitioner, or psychiatrist can have a direct and positive impact on the mental health and coping ability of the patient in an acute care environment. A collaborative and integrated approach to the patient and his or her family may be the first time that the patient's suffering from a mental illness or psychiatric disturbance has been addressed. This may also be an opportunity to provide both the patient and the family with guidance about specific strategies and resources to assist them in managing a new onset psychiatric disturbance that has emerged because of the patient's physical illness, injury, or as a result of treatment.

ANXIETY AND ANXIETY-RELATED DISORDERS IN THE ACUTE CARE PATIENT

Anxiety accompanies any type of illness and injury, especially when hospitalization, pain, disability, possible economic loss, or a threat to life is perceived or realized. Anxiety is a subjective feeling of apprehension and tension that is manifested by autonomic arousal and a wide array of psychophysiologic symptoms. The common presenting feature of all anxiety-related disorders is that affected patients experience a level of anxiety that in some manner interferes with functioning in personal, occupational, social, and psychophysiologic well-being. Hopelessness often accompanies anxiety, especially in the patient who feels a loss of control over his or her environment, situation, and events associated with the illness/injury, treatment, and recovery. Usually that is a portrait of an acute care environment for the newly hospitalized patient who is naive to the "ways of the health-care system," and is just beginning to understand his or her lack of knowledge in negotiating this maze. That in itself could spawn anxiety in a patient!

There are several clinical challenges in the diagnosis and treatment of anxiety, including: differentiating normal/expected anxiety from pathological, potentially debilitating anxiety; differentiating psychiatric from medical (illnesses, medication, other treatments) causes of anxiety; choosing effective and nonharmful treatments; and measuring treatment outcomes. Sometimes in acute care the importance of early recognition and aggressive treatment of the patient suffering with anxiety escapes the acute care practitioner because the response is so universal.

Epidemiology of Anxiety Disorders in the Medically Ill Patient

Pathological anxiety results in the development of an anxiety disorder. Anxiety disorders are among the most prevalent psychiatric disorders in the general population. Approximately 25% of the population in the United States experience an anxiety disorder in their lifetime (Kessler et al., 1994). Numerous investigators have conducted various types of studies to determine the prevalence of anxiety disorders in the medical patient. These reports have estimated rates from 10% to 30%. Comparisons have been extrapolated from the Epidemiologic Catchment Area (ECA) data that show 18% of the group with a chronic medical condition had a significantly higher adjusted lifetime prevalence of an anxiety disorder in comparison with 12% of those without a chronic medical condition. Specific patient populations have recently received further investigation to identify prevalence rates and signal high-risk patient populations.

Chest pain is common in patients with panic. Panic disorder occurs in 10 to 20% of patients who present to emergency departments complaining of chest pain. Katon and colleagues (1988) discovered that 40-60% of patients diagnosed with atypical chest pain who had normal cardiac catheterization findings had panic disorder. In some studies, between 15 to 20% of patients who had been referred for an evaluation of dizziness were diagnosed with panic disorder (Stein et al., 1994). Walker and colleagues (1995) discovered that 20 to 40% of patients diagnosed with irritable bowel syndrome had panic disorder. Additionally, irritable bowel symptoms are frequently discovered with panic disorder. Several studies have detailed the interrelationship of chronic obstructive pulmonary disease, asthma, and anxiety disorders. (Janson et al., 1994; Karajgi et al., 1990; Kellner et al., 1992; Smoller, 1996). Research studies have reported that effective anxiety-reduction strategies have positive effects on perceived dyspnea and overall functional capacity of patients with chronic pulmonary disease.

Etiology of Anxiety Disorders

The development of anxiety disorders involves multiple factors, including neurobiological abnormalities, current and previous psychological stressors, along with environmentally conditioned behaviors. The abnormalities in the central nervous system (CNS) associated with anxiety disorders are related to the gamma–aminobutyric acid (GABA) receptor and the locus ceruleus. GABA is an inhibitory neurotransmitter located throughout most of the CNS. It is believed to decrease anxiety by inhibiting locus ceruleus activity and modulating the reticular activating system (RAS). The reticular activating system is an area of the brain that controls alertness and fear. Also, genetic factors are thought to have a role in the development of anxiety disorders.

Stressful and/or catastrophic life events are also critical factors in the development of an anxiety disorder, particularly in acute stress disorder (ASD), posttraumatic stress disorder (PTSD), and adjustment disorder with anxiety.

Clinical Presentation of Anxiety Disorders

The major primary and secondary anxiety disorders that can affect acute care patients are described in Table 54–1.

Diagnostic Assessment of the Anxious Patient

- Is the patient's anxiety a primary psychiatric disorder or secondary to either organic or situational causes
- Assessment includes evaluation of patient's knowledge of medical illness, complication(s), and treatments
- Anxiety associated with organic causes is likely to present with physical symptoms and is less likely to be associated with avoidance-escape behaviors, or the onset with emotionally traumatic events
- Focus the diagnostic evaluation toward the somatic system most closely related to the reported anxiety symptoms (pulmonary system in patients complaining of shortness of breath, cardiac system in patients complaining of chest pain, dizziness, or syncope)
- Consider factors that are associated with organic anxiety syndrome to help distinguish it from a primary anxiety disorder; several factors have been identified by Rosenbaum and colleagues (1996), including:
  - Age onset of anxiety symptoms: after 35 years
  - Personal and family history are negative for anxiety disorder(s)
  - No childhood history of increased anxiety, phobias, or noticeable separation anxiety
  - No significant life events generating or exacerbating the anxiety symptoms
  - No avoidance behavior
  - Poor response to antipanic medications

Assessment and Measurement of Anxiety by Rating Scales

Clinician-Conducted Rating Scales

Hamilton Anxiety Rating Scale (HARS)
Anxiety Status Inventory
Yale Brown Obsessive–Compulsive Scale

Patient Self-Report Rating Scales

Beck's Anxiety Inventory (BAI)
Maudsley Obsessive–Compulsive Inventory
Self Rating Anxiety Scale (SRAS)

General Medical Evaluation of the Anxious Patient

- Thorough history and physical including neurological screening examination
- Evaluate and determine the axiogenic (anxiety-causing) effects of medications (Table 54–2)
- Identify possible medication(s) as causative agent and make adjustments (if possible) in the medication regimen
- Evaluate and determine contribution of medical illness to the development of anxiety (Table 54–3)
- Evaluate and determine effects of substance use/intoxication (caffeine, nicotine, amphetamine, cocaine) or withdrawal (alcohol, sedative–hypnotics)

Laboratory Studies

Albumin
BUN with creatinine
Electrolytes (especially calcium, magnesium, phosphorus, sodium)
Liver function tests
Thyroid function tests

TABLE 54–1. DSM IV Anxiety Disorders and Associated Screening Questions

DSM IV Diagnosis	Clinical Presentation	Screening Question
300.01 Panic Disorder with agoraphobia 300.21 Panic Disorder without agoraphobia	Recurrent, unexpected anxiety attacks, sudden onset with intense apprehension, and dread. Concern about future attacks. Symptoms include: chest discomfort, diaphoresis, dizziness, dyspnea, fear of losing control, going crazy or dying, hot/cold flashes, tingling of limbs, palpitations, trembling, feelings of unreality	Have you ever had a sudden attack of fast heart beat? Have you ever felt very fearful, anxious, or nervous? Did you notice that something triggered these feelings? Have you started to avoid going out or engaging in usual activities because you are afraid that it might happen again?
300.22 Agoraphobia (without history of panic disorder)	Fear that the occurrence of incapacitating or embarrassing panic-like symptoms or limited symptom attacks will occur	Have you ever avoided activities (i.e., social, work) because you were afraid about having a sudden "anxiety attack"? If YES: How often do you recall this happening?
300.23 Social Phobia	Fear of situations in which one might be seen and embarrassed or criticized; fear of eating in public, public speaking, or performance	Some individuals are uncomfortable and become fearful of being watched or evaluated by others: Have you ever experienced being uncomfortable or fearful in a public situation, such as eating in a restaurant or giving a speech to a small group? If YES: Please tell me about a particular time when this has occurred.
300.29 Specific Phobia	Fear of a single object, activity, or situation (i.e., needles, closed spaces, germs, bugs, snakes)	Some individuals have intense fears or phobias about things like flying, snakes, bugs, being in closed areas. Do you have any intense fears or phobias that we need to know about to keep you safe and comfortable in the hospital? If YES: Tell me what they are. What happens if you come in contact with this object/situation?
300.3 Obsessive–Compulsive Disorder (OCD)	Preoccupation with persistent, intrusive thoughts (obsessions), and/or repeated performance rituals designed to prevent some event (compulsion). Both obsessions and compulsions may be experienced by the same time. Anxiety is increased if obsessions or compulsions are resisted	Some individuals are bothered by persistent ongoing thoughts, such as a family member being harmed or wanting to hurt someone else even though you don't really want to do so. Have you ever had any thoughts like that? Would they not go away? Have you ever engaged in repeated rituals (i.e., handwashing, checking light switches or gas stoves)? If YES: Tell me about it.
308.3 Acute Stress Disorder	Development of characteristic anxiety, dissociative, and other symptoms that occurs within one month after exposure to a traumatic event. Duration is 2 days–1 month	Have you ever been involved in a traumatic event when you thought your life was in danger? Have you ever witnessed another person in serious danger? If YES: Tell me about the incident. What happened to you?
309.81 Post Traumatic Stress Disorder (PTSD)	Persistent reexperiencing a traumatic event outside the range of usual experience (i.e., rape, combat, kidnapping, being a hostage, gunshot wound, stabbing from gang violence, motor vehicle crash). Symptoms include recurrent dreams, nightmares, flashbacks, emotional numbness, detachment, and withdrawal	Have you ever been involved in a traumatic event when you thought your life was in danger? Have you ever witnessed another person in serious danger? If YES: Tell me about the incident. What happened to you?
300.02 Generalized Anxiety Disorder (GAD)	Persists for at least 6 months: excessive anxiety and worry about several areas of life. Symptoms include motor tension with autonomic hyperactivity, hypervigilance, and marked apprehensiveness	How would you describe yourself? Are you a "worrier," or fretful? Do you feel nervous or tense most of the time?
293.89 Anxiety Disorder due to a General Medical Condition	Clinically significant anxiety that is determined to be due to the direct physiological effects of a general medical condition. Symptoms include generalized anxiety symptoms, panic attacks, or obsessions/compulsions	Review other screening questions with the patient to rule out primary anxiety disorder. When did you first notice these symptoms? Does your "anxiety" or "bad nerves" worsen when you are feeling physically bad? Does your anxiety lessen when you feel physically better? When are the symptoms the worst? the least? What makes you feel better?
291-292 Substance-Induced Anxiety Disorder	Prominent anxiety symptoms that are determined to be the direct physiological effects of a substance. Symptoms include anxiety, panic attacks, obsessions/compulsions. Develops within one month of substance ingestion, intoxication, withdrawal. Significant distress or impairment in social and occupational functioning	Review other screening questions with patient to rule out a primary anxiety. Would you tell me what medications you are currently taking? Probe about: prescribed, OTC, herbal preparations, dietary supplements, anabolic steroids, and illicit drugs. Have you noticed any difference in your anxiety symptoms in relation to any of the above medications, herbs, or preparations? Does anything make it better?

Compiled from Krupnick & Wade. (1999); and Krupnick. (1996). (pp. 1423–1427).

TABLE 54–2. Medications Associated with Anxiety

- Amphetamines
- Analgesics
- Anesthetics
- Anticholinergics
- Antidepressants (tricyclics, SSRIs, bupropion)
- Antihistamines
- Antihypertensives
- Antimicrobials
- Appetite suppressants
- Asthma medications (bronchodilators)
- Caffeine preparations
- Calcium-blocking agents
- Cholinergic-blocking agents
- CNS depressants (withdrawal syndrome)
- Cocaine
- Digitalis
- Estrogen
- Ethosuximide
- Heavy metals
- Hydralazine
- Insulin
- Levodopa
- Muscle relaxants
- Nasal decongestants
- Neuroleptics
- Nonsteroidal antiinflammatory drugs (NSAIDs)
- Procaine
- Procarbazine
- Steroids
- Sympathomimetics
- Theopylline
- Thyroid preparations
- Tranylcypromine

Compiled from: Preston, O'Neal, & Talaga. (1997); Rundell & Wise. (1996); and Reichman & Katz. (1996).

Toxicology screen: serum and urine (even though a patient may have been hospitalized for several days, he or she may have recently used an illicit drug or taken some of his or her own medications and is experiencing an intoxication from too much medication)

Diagnostic Studies/Procedures

- Brain imaging (CT, MRI): to rule out structural lesion, hydrocephalus
- CSF: to rule out CNS infection, hemorrhage, demyelinating or inflammatory processes
- ECG: to rule out cardiac disturbances
- EEG: to rule out seizure origin

Differential Diagnosis

It is not uncommon to have to consider several different diagnoses as you are trying to definitively diagnosis the patient with anxiety. The following represents an overview of the differential diagnoses for several of the primary anxiety disorders. It is important to always rule out a physiological basis for the medically ill patient who is experiencing anxiety.

TABLE 54–3. Medical Conditions Presenting with Anxiety

Anxiety may result from medical conditions or exacerbate preexisting medical conditions. The following are commonly associated with anxiety, and should be considered when making the diagnosis of anxiety.

Cardiovascular disorders
- Arrhythmias (i.e., supraventricular tachycardia, ventricular tachycardia)
- Cardiomyopathies
- Congestive heart failure
- Coronary insufficiency
- Mitral valve prolapse
- Myocardial infarction or angina

Endocrine disorders
- Adrenal insufficiency
- Carcinoid syndrome
- Cushing's syndrome
- Hyperparathyroidism
- Hyperthyroidism or hypothyroidism
- Hypoglycemia, hyperinsulinemia
- Thyroiditis

Gastrointestinal disorders
- Colitis
- Irritable bowel syndrome
- Peptic ulcer disease

Metabolic disorders
- Hypocalcemia or hypercalcemia
- Hypokalemia
- Hyponatremia

Neurologic disorders
- CNS infections/masses
- Essential tremor
- Huntington's chorea
- Multiple sclerosis
- Parkinson's disease
- Postconcussion syndrome
- Seizure disorders (i.e., temporal lobe epilepsy, complex partial seizures)
- Vestibular dysfunction

Pulmonary disorders
- Asthma
- Chronic obstructive pulmonary disease
- Hyperventilation syndrome
- Pneumothorax
- Pneumonia
- Primary pulmonary hypertension
- Pulmonary edema
- Pulmonary embolism

Compiled from: Colon & Popkin. (1996). (p. 409); and Sheikh. (1994). (p. 284).

Disorder	Differential Diagnoses
Panic Disorder	Asthma, bowel/bladder disorders, caffeine, cardiac dysrhymia, coronary ischemia, esophageal spasm, hypoglycemia, Meniere's syndrome (vestibular neuronitis), mitral valve prolapse, pheochromocytoma, pulmonary embolism, temporal lobe epilepsy, thyroid disease
Specific Phobia	Panic disorder with agoraphobia, PTSD with phobic avoidance
Social Phobia	Panic disorder
Acute Stress Disorder/ Post Traumatic Stress Disorder	Generalized anxiety disorder (GAD), Adjustment disorder with anxiety
Generalized Axiety Disorder	Adjustment reactions of adult life, major depressive disorder, reactive anxiety, substance abuse

Treatment of the Patient with Anxiety

General Principles in Managing the Anxious Patient

- A reassuring, supportive, and unhurried approach is important. The patient will probably require more of your time to begin to trust the health-care providers (especially if the patient is new to the health-care system or is a "novice" to hospitalization). The patient will benefit from several methods of explanation (verbal, written, drawings, and reviews).
- After a definitive diagnosis has been made, the patient and family will need education about the disorder, what the treatment options are, how effective they are, and what is the responsibility of the patient in the treatment process. Additionally, a discussion of the availability of the treatment options will be needed.
- If pharmacotherapy is one of the chosen treatment options, the patient needs to be monitored closely until a dosage has been reached that produces symptom relief. Vigilance by the ACNP and nursing staff is imperative in the early identification of side effects. Aggressive side-effect management is important; otherwise, the patient's chances of medication adherence after discharge will be diminished.

Effective (Evidence-Based) Treatments of the Anxiety Disorders

See Table 54–4.

Indications for Referral to a Specialist in Psychiatric–Mental Health

- Diagnostic uncertainty, increased complexity of clinical situation
- Complex, refractory anxiety disorders (i.e., OCD, PTSD)
- Treatment has not improved patient's symptomatology within the expected time frame
- Treatment options involve intensive behavior therapy (i.e., specific phobia, social phobia, agoraphobia)

TABLE 54–4. Treatments of the Anxiety Disorders

Disorder	Effective Treatments
Panic disorder	Cognitive–behavioral therapy (CBT) Tricyclic antidepressants Imipramine (Tofranil) Desipramine (Norpramin) Clomipramine (Anafranil) Selective Serotonin Reuptake Inhibitors (SSRI) Fluoxetine (Prozac) Fluvoxamine (Luvox) Paroxetine (Paxil) High-potency benzodiazepines Clonazepam (Klonopin) Alprazolam (Xanax) MAO inhibitors Phenelzine (Nardil)
Agoraphobia	Initially treat panic disorder Exposure therapy Support group
Social phobia (circumscribed type)	Exposure therapy Adjunctive beta blockers Propranolol (Inderal) Atenolol (Tenormin) Adjunctive benzodiazepines Lorazepam (Ativan)
Social phobia (generalized type)	Selective Serotonin Reuptake Inhibitor's (SSRI) Fluoxetine (Prozac) High-potency benzodiazepines Clonazepam (Klonopin) MAO inhibitor Phenelzine (Nardil) Cognitve–behavioral therapy
Specific phobia	Exposure therapy Adjunctive benzodiazepines Lorazepam (Ativan) Chlordiazepoxide (Librium) Oxazepam (Serax)
Obsessive–compulsive disorder	Selective Serotonin Reuptake Inhibitors (SSRI) Fluoxetine (Prozac) Fluvoxamine (Luvox) Sertraline (Zoloft) Paroxetine (Paxil) Tricyclic antidepressant (TCA) Clomipramine (Anafranil) Exposure with responsive prevention Support groups Stereotactic surgery (for extremely severe OCD that is a threat to the physical and mental health)
Generalized anxiety disorder	Buspirone (BuSpar) Antidepressants: Tricyclic antidepressants Imipramine (Tofranil) Selective serotonin–norepinephrine reuptake inhibitor (SSNRI) Venlafaxine (Effexor) Benzodiazepines (not a first-line choice due to

(Continued)

TABLE 54–4. Treatments of the Anxiety Disorders *(Continued)*

Disorder	Effective Treatments
	abuse potential and other more efficacious choices)
Stress disorders:	Exposure therapy
Acute stress disorder	Brief use of benzodiazepine (acute care period)
Posttraumatic stress disorder	Exposure therapy Individual and group support Adjunctive antidepressants SSRIs MAO inhibitors

Compiled from: Stahl. (1996). (pp. 167–248); Gelenberg & Bassuk. (1997). (pp. 213–264); and Schatzberg & Nemeroff. (1998). (pp. 775–789).

- Concurrent substance abuse
- High level of suicidal ideation exhibited by verbalization of wanting to die, discussion of a potentially lethal plan, and/or discussion of ending the pain with the "tools" to do so
- Question of—or actual—psychosis is present
- Prior to initiating long-term (chronic) benzodiazepine treatment or discontinuance of benzodiazepine treatment

Nursing Care Consultation

The primary nurse and nursing colleagues may find it necessary to consult the ACNP about the patient who is anxious and is not responding to their usual nursing interventions. Specific interventions that you might employ as the expert consultant includes:

- Identify and utilize consultants in the system for yourself and for the nurses caring for this patient (i.e., Psychiatric Consultation Liaison Nurse, Psychiatric Consultation Physician, Pastoral Counseling, Psychiatric Social Worker, Pharmacist)
- Assist the nurses in clearly identifying the behavior(s) that are of concern to them
- Meet with the staff (especially primary nurse or associate nurse) to gain a clear understanding about the patient's anxiety
- Set up a patient care conference in collaboration with the primary nurse, invite the patient to join in if he or she is physically stable and can participate in a behavior focused discussion
- Remind everyone (including yourself) that the patient is probably doing the best he or she can at coping, and the entire team (including the patient) are going to work together to begin anxiety reduction and try to make the patient more comfortable; this strategy aims at "getting everyone on the team" to assist and not blame the patient or the nurses
- Try to negotiate with the patient, family, and nursing staff to establish a daily routine (especially if the patient will be hospitalized for many days/weeks); this can assist the patient by decreasing his or her possible boredom and uncertainty (not knowing what is coming next)
- Collaborate with nursing and other services to decrease the "surprise" element in the area of tests/procedures, surgeries; do not surprise this patient with a quick discharge plan

DEPRESSION AND DEPRESSIVE DISORDERS IN THE ACUTE CARE PATIENT

Depression is common, disabling, often undetected, minimized, and inadequately treated in the acute care environment. Depression is a period of impaired functioning associated with depressed mood and related symptoms that include sleep and appetite changes, psychomotor changes, impaired concentration, anhedonia (lack of pleasure), fatigue, feelings of hopelessness and helplessness, and frequent thoughts of suicide. A depressive illness is painful, can become psychophysiologically debilitating, and often significantly complicates treatment and impedes recovery of the medically ill patient (Carney et al., 1988; Frasure-Smith et al., 1995; Morris, 1993; Silverstone, 1990). It is apparent that depression in medically ill patients is an important clinical condition to be assessed, recognized early, and treated appropriately and adequately.

Epidemiology of Depressive Disorders in the Medically Ill Patient

Depression is one of the most frequently occurring of all medical illnesses. Approximately 10% of the general population is affected sufficiently enough to seek out professional guidance and treatment. Depressive disorders, including episodic major depression, and dysthymia have a reported lifetime prevalence of up to 15% for males and is twofold greater in women than in men. (Kessler et al., 1994; Kaplan, Sadoch, & Grebb, 1994; WPA Dysthymia Working Group, 1995). Depression in later life is all too common and debilitating. Approximately 5 million of the 31 million adults age 65 years and older suffer from depression (Schneider, Reynolds, & Lebowitz, 1994). Several prevalence studies of elders report dramatic rates of combined minor and major depression in various environments: acute care (30%), medical outpatients (24%), long-term care facilities (nursing homes) (43%), and in-community dwelling (13%) (Blazer, 1993).

The presence of one or more chronic medical conditions and/or devastating injury increases both the recent and lifetime prevalences of mood disorders. Generally, the more severe the medical illness, the more likely depression will complicate it (Cassem, 1990; Elliott, & Frank, 1996). Moreover, evidence from several sources suggests that the age of onset has decreased, and the overall risk of suffering from a depressive disorder has markedly increased over each of the past several generations. Therefore, the public health significance of depressive disorders has proportionately increased (Cross National Collaborative Group, 1992; Robins and Regier, 1991). Although depression occurs commonly in medically ill patients, as well as in the general population, it is underdiagnosed and inadequately treated (Hirschfeld et al., 1997; Perez-Stable et al., 1990; Slimon et al., 1992). The following information about assessment and treatment will assist in diminishing that unfortunate trend.

Etiology of Depressive Disorders

Brain Dysregulation

Major depressive disorders and bipolar disorder are neurobiologcal ("brain disorders") that have genetic predisposition. They are attributed to dysregulation (an imbalance) of certain central nervous system networks that control and mediate pain, pleasure, motivation, reward and reinforcement, biologic rhythms, sexuality, psychomotor function, and cognition. Patients experiencing depression or mania have changes in brain neurotransmitters, neuroendocrine and neuropeptide hormones, second messenger systems, and/or gene expression. Additionally, research evidence has demonstrated by using positron emission tomography (PET), single photon emission computed tomography (SPECT), and sleep electroencephalography that patients with depression and mania have changes in brain metabolism and regional cerebral blood flow.

Role of Stress in Depressive Disorders

It is common for depressive episodes to be precipitated by major stressful or traumatic life events and losses (i.e., death in the family, separation, divorce, assault, life-threatening illness of self or loved one). Some neuroscientists have postulated that each new episode of depression sensitizes the brain, which produces possible changes in gene expression and increases the chance that less intense stressors might initiate a future episode. They further hypothesize that depressive episodes may then develop in the absence of any stressful event.

Differential Psychiatric Diagnoses for Major Depressive Disorder

- Anxiety disorders
- Bipolar depression
- Dementia
- Hypoactive delirium
- Medical conditions (Table 54–5)
- Premenstrual dysphoric disorder
- Psychotic disorders
- Somatoform disorders

Diagnostic Assessment of the Depressed Medically Ill Patient

- Is the patient's depression a primary psychiatric disorder or secondary to organic or situational causes (Table 54–6)
- Assess presence of both physical and psychological

TABLE 54–5. Medical Conditions Associated with Depression

Cardiovascular–Pulmonary disorders
- Arrhythmias (especially life-threatening ventricular tachycardia)
- Chronic Obstructive Pulmonary Disease (COPD, end-stage lung disease)
- Congestive heart failure (end-stage heart disease)
- Myocardial infarction

Endocrine Disorders
- Adrenal insufficiency
- Cushing's disease
- Diabetes
- Hyperparathyroidism or hypoparathyroidism
- Hyperprolactinemia
- Hypothyroidism or hyperthyroidism
- Menopause

Gastrointestinal Disorders
- Chronic abdominal pain
- Colitis
- Islet cell adenoma
- Hepatitis

Infectious and Inflammatory
- Acquired immune disorder syndrome (AIDS)
- Chronic fatigue syndrome
- Mononucleosis
- Pneumonia (bacterial and viral)
- Rheumatoid arthritis
- Sjogren's arteritis
- Systemic lupus erthymatosus
- Temporal arteritis
- Tuberculosis

Metabolic Disorders
- Electrolyte imbalance
- Gout
- Hypercalcemia
- Pernicious anemia
- Porphyria
- Uremia (and other renal diseases)

Neurologic Disorders
- Cerebrovascular disease
- Chronic pain
- CNS tumors
- Dementias (including Alzheimer's type)
- Hydrocephalus
- Migraine headache
- Multiple sclerosis
- Narcolepsy
- Parkinson's disease
- Progressive supranuclear palsy
- Seizure disorders
- Sleep apnea

(Continued)

TABLE 54–5. Medical Conditions Associated with Depression *(Continued)*

Nutritional Disorders
- Dehydration
- Iron deficiency
- Obesity
- Vitamin deficiencies (vitamins B_{12} and C, folate, niacin)

Miscellaneous Disorders
- Alcoholism
- Bilateral cataracts
- Cancer (especially pancreatic and other GI)
- Hypertension
- Influenza

Compiled from Kaplan & Sadock. (1996). (p. 222); and Rundell & Wise. (1996). (p. 318).

signs and symptoms that have occurred at least one month before hospitalization
- Onset, duration, and course of symptoms
- Present and past psychiatric history; especially probe for anxiety and substance abuse disorders
- Family history of depression
- Recent loss(es), often cumulative
- What is the impact of these symptoms; probe about difficulties at home, work, school, and in patient's personal relationships

Assessment and Measurement of Depression by Rating Scales

Beck Depression Inventory (BDI)
Carroll Self Rating Scale
Center for Epidemiologic Studies/Depressed Mood Scale (CES–D)
Hamilton Depression Scale
Raskin Severity of Depression Scale
Yeasavage Geriatric Depression Scale
Zung Self Rating Depression Scale

General Medical Evaluation of the Depressed Patient

- Thorough history and physical including mental status examination; mental status findings in major depression are usually unremarkable, may demonstrate decreased ability to concentrate and attend, which can alter patient's performance on the Folstein Mini-Mental Status Examination
- Medical history including medications (prescribed, OTC, dietary supplements, herbal preparations)
- Evaluate and determine the effects of medication (Table 54–7)
- Identify possible depressogenic medication(s) as the causative or contributory agents and make adjustments (when possible) in their medication regimen
- Evaluate and determine contribution of medical illness to development of depression (refer to Table 54–5)
- Assess patient's risk factors for suicidality (Table 54–8)
- Assess and monitor patient for suicidal ideation (Table 54–9)

TABLE 54–6. Characteristics of (Secondary) Depression Due to Medical Illness

- Later age (older) at onset
- Increased chance to respond positively to electroconvulsive therapy (ECT)
- Increased chance to exhibit "organic" features in the mental status examination
- Increased chance of improvement by time of discharge
- Decreased incidence of family history of depression and alcoholism
- Decreased incidence of having suicidal thoughts and committing suicide

Laboratory Studies

General

B12
CBC with differential
Cortisol
Electrolytes
Folate
Renal function tests
Thyroid function tests
Toxicology screen: serum and urine
Urinalysis

Focused

ABGs
Oxygen saturation levels (oximetry)

Diagnostic Studies

General

Chest x-ray
ECG

Focused

CT scan
MRI

Treatment of the Patient with Depression

Clinical management of the patient with depressive symptoms and/or a depressive disorder should generally include:

- Openly acknowledging the patient's distress
- Discuss relevant interpersonal and social issues that may provide you with contributing factors to patient's depressive symptoms

TABLE 54–7. Medications Associated with Depression

Analgesics
- Ibuprofen
- Indomethacin
- Opioids
- Phenacetin

Antibacterials and antifungals
- Ampicillin
- Cycloserine
- Ethionamide
- Griseofulvin
- Metronidazole
- Nitrofurantoin
- Streptomycin
- Sulfamethoxazole
- Sulfonamides
- Tetracyclines

Antihypertensives
- Beta blockers: propranolol (Inderal)
- Clonidine (Catapres)
- Digitalis
- Guanethidine (Ismelin)
- Hydralazine (Apresoline)
- Lidocaine
- Methyldopa (Aldomet)
- Propranolol (Inderal)
- Reserpine (Serpasil)
- Veratrum

Antiparkinsonians
- Amantadine
- Levodopa

Cancer chemotherapeutics
- Amphotericin B
- Bleomycin
- Interferon
- L-asparaginase
- Procarbazine
- Trimethoprim
- Vinblastine, Vincristine
- Zidovudine

Hormones
- Contraceptives (oral)
- Estrogen (Premarin)
- Progesterone (Gesterol)

Pychoactives
- Antipsychotics (butyrophenones, phenothiazines, oxyindoles)
- Bromocriptine
- Carbamazepine (Tegretol)
- Sedative/hypnotics (barbiturates, benzodiazepines, chloralhydrate)

Steroids
- Cortcosteroids (including ACTH)
- Dexamethasone (Decadron)
- Prednisone

Stimulants
- Amphetamines (fenfluramine)
- Cocaine
- Methylphenidate (Ritalin)

Miscellaneous drugs
- Acetazolamide
- Choline
- Cimetidine (Tagamet)
- Cyproheptadine
- Diphenoxylate
- Disulfiram
- Methylsergide

Compiled from Feldman & Christensen. (1997). (p. 182); Rundell & Wise. (1996). (p. 318); and Kaplan & Sadock. (1996). (p. 222).

- Reassure the patient by normalizing his or her experience and clearly stating that you expect the patient to improve with some focused treatment
- After a diagnosis has been made, the patient and family will need education about the disorder, what the treatment options are, how effective those treatments are, and what is the patient's responsibility in the treatment process; also, in the current health care of managed cost and regulation it is important to discuss the availability and insurance coverage/approval process for these treatments
- Pharmacotherapy is often a treatment option considered for the acute care patient (Table 54–10)
- If pharmacotherapy is one of the chosen treatment options, the patient needs to be monitored closely until a dosage has been reached that produces symptom relief; both the ACNP and nursing staff must collaborate to identify (early) side effect symptoms and treat them adequately (not just tell the patient that they will adjust to them)
- Close monitoring for adverse effects, such as serotonin syndrome, is important (Table 54–11)
- Discussion about depression with patient and family—framework that depression is a medical illness, with focused signs and symptoms; describe depression as a neurobiological illness that is caused by neurochemical disturbances or changes in the brain chemistry
- Review and clearly state that depression is not a fault or weakness and that it is a treatable disease that requires patient's and family's participation in the treatment

Indications for Referral to a Specialist in Psychiatric–Mental Health

- Patient presents a significant suicidal risk or is actively suicidal
- Patient is debilitated and disabled by depression
- Patient is pregnant or is considering pregnancy
- Diagnosis uncertainty; increased complexity of clinical situation

TABLE 54–8. Risk Factors for Suicide

Disinhibition

- Alcohol and/or drug use
- Impulsivity: tumultuous early family life, chaotic lifestyle, violence-focused coping
- Isolation: divorced, separated, widowed, or living alone with decreased social supports
- Psychotic thoughts

Intent

- Inability to agree with a no-harm or suicide contract or safety plan
- Loss: recent personal loss, financial and/or legal difficulties
- Suicidal ideation, organized suicide plan, plan and "tools" to carry it out (a straightforward, highly lethal plan place the patient at very high risk, i.e., jumping into highway traffic, shootings)
- Plan that involves killing others (i.e., children, spouse) so they won't suffer
- Unrelenting, chronic, and/or painful illness(es)
- Availability or possession of firearms

Vulnerability

- Family member(s) has completed suicide
- Elderly >65 years (especially if physical health is failing)
- Presence of psychiatric disorder
- Previous suicide attempt(s) by the patient (especially of concern if attempts demonstrate an increasing pattern of lethality)
- Sense of overwhelming hopelessness

Adapted from Boyd & Nihart. (1998). (p. 1091).

TABLE 54–9. Assessing Suicidality

Components of the Suicide Evaluation

- Evaluate suicidal ideation, intent, and plan:
  How does the future look to you?
  Have you ever felt that life was not worth living?
  Do you ever wish or pray that you would not wake up?
  Have you ever thought about hurting or killing yourself?
- Evaluate and examine details of suicide plan, degree of planning:
  Is the plan simple and straightforward with minimal margin for rescue or complex with several areas for rescue
  Does the patient have the "tools" to implement the plan (i.e., hanging—rope with a sturdy and isolated place to hang it with something to climb onto, or several types of highly lethal pills in combination at home; shooting—have a gun, knowledge about how to use it and bullets)
  Location of the plan (a remote location where there is little probability of being rescued or at home close to the time when family members are usually coming home)
- Who will discover or find you?
- Evaluate the degree of hopelessness
- Identify precipitants
- Identify available social supports
- Conduct mental status evaluation
- Evaluate patient's risk factors for suicide (refer to Table 54–8 for review of risk factors)

- Patient has comorbid conditions (i.e, dementia, OCD, panic disorder, substance abuse)
- Refractory, resistant depression fails to respond to first-line treatment or is worsening

Nursing Care Consultation

The primary nurse and his or her colleagues may find it necessary to consult the ACNP about the patient who is depressed and not responding to their interventions, or is beginning to "fail" and not respond to medical treatments, or beginning the process of failure to thrive and recover. Specific interventions you might employ as the expert consultant include:

- If nurses/family are concerned about suicidality or the patient simply "giving up or giving in" to the disease, arrange for a psychiatric–mental health consultation as soon as possible
- Utilize and collaborate with consultants to assist in managing the patient with depression (i.e., psychiatric–mental health specialists, nutrition specialists, pharmacist, activity therapist (if available), social worker or case manager, and relevant medical consultants to advance their medical treatment, especially geriatricians)
- Organize a patient care conference with the collaboration of the primary nurse to include all health-care providers invested in the patient's care, with the patient and family (if patient's functional status permits participation) to identify causative factors and develop a focused and adequate plan of care
- Encourage primary nurse to work with patient and family to establish a structured daily routine (with appropriate rest cycles) that gives back some control to the patient for how the "things" he or she has to participate in are done (this is particularly helpful in a patient who may have a protracted stay in the acute care environment)
- If patient is not eating due to depression and "hospital food," then work with family and the dietician to incorporate favorite and "comfort" foods from home that are within the patient's dietary plan
- Collaborate with nursing to arrange for diversional activities (if protracted stay or significant boredom contributes to depressive feelings) within functional status
- Collaborate with the primary nurse to determine if going outside on a deck or protected area would make the patient feel less trapped and confined; if so, try to assist the nursing staff in arranging this activity

▶ DELIRIUM IN THE ACUTE CARE PATIENT

Delirium was one of the first mental disorders described in medicine. Delirium is an acute state of cerebral dysfunc-

TABLE 54–10. Mood Disorders: Clinical Presentation and Associated Treatments

DSM IV Disorder	Clinical Presentation	Treatments
296.xx Major Depressive Disorder (MDD)	Characterized by one month or more major depressive episodes without a history of manic, mixed, or hypomanic episodes. Symptoms include: depressed mood, appetite and sleep disturbances, ↓ interest/pleasure in activities, fatigue, psychomotor agitation or retardation, ↓ energy, feelings of worthlessness, ↓ concentration, indecisiveness, suicidal ideation	*Pharmacologic* *First line:* SSRIs: Fluoxetine (Prozac) Sertraline (Zoloft) Paroxetine (Paxil) SSNRIs: Venlafaxine (Effexor) Nefazodone (Serzone) *Second line:* Bupropion (Wellbutrin) Desipramine (Norpramin) Nortriptyline (Aventyl, Pamelor) Augmenting agents: Lithium, T3/T4 Pindolol (Visken) Divalproex (Depakote) *Maintenance:* Continue full dose of antidepressant and augmenting agents if necessary (at least one year) *Psychotherapy:* Individual Group Marital/Family Electroconvulsive therapy (ECT) for psychotic depressed patient not responding to first- and second-line medications
300.4 Dysthymic Disorder	A chronically depressed mood that occurs for most of the day, more days than not for at least 2 years. Describe their mood as sad or "down in the dumps," appetite and sleep disturbances, difficulty making decisions, fatigue, ↓ energy, ↓ concentration	*First line:* SSRI: Fluoxetine (Prozac) Sertraline (Zoloft) Paroxetine (Paxil) Venlafaxine (Effexor) Desipramine (Norpramin) *Second line:* Bupropion MAOI Phenelzine (Nardil) Nortriptyline (Aventyl, Pamelor) *Augmenting agents:* Lithium T3/T4 Pindolol (for SSRIs) *Psychotherapy:* Individual Group Marital/Family
296.0 Bipolar I Disorder	A recurrent disorder that is characterized by the occurrence of one or more manic or mixed episodes, may have experienced one or more major depressive episodes	*First line:* Lithium Divalproex (Depakote) SSRIs (Fluoxetine, Sertraline, Paroxetine)
Bipolar II Disorder	Clinical course is characterized by the occurrence of one or more major depressive episodes accompanied by at least one hypomanic episode	Venlafaxine (Effexor) *Second line:* Bupropion (Wellbutrin) Desipramine (Norpramin)

(Continued)

TABLE 54–10. Mood Disorders: Clinical Presentation and Associated Treatments *(Continued)*

DSM IV Disorder	Clinical Presentation	Treatments
		Nortriptyline (Aventyl, Pamelor) *Augmenting agents:* Divalproex (Depakote) Carbamazepine (Tegretol) T3/T4 Pindolol (for SSRIs) *Maintenance:* Lithium Divalproex (Depakote) Carbamazepine (Tegretol) Targeted combinations
301.13 Cyclothymic	A chronic fluctuating mood disturbance, involves several periods of hypomanic symptoms and depressive symptoms. Symptoms are insufficient to meet criteria for manic or major depressive episode	Lithium Valproate (valproic acid) Psychotherapy
293.83 Mood Disorder due to a General Medical Disorder	Prominent and persistent disturbance in mood that is determined to be the direct physiological effects of a medical condition. Symptoms include depressed mood, or an expansive, elevated or irritable mood, ↓ interest or pleasure in activities	Identify and remove the offending factor (when possible) Consider pharmacotherapy SSRIs *Psychostimulants:* Methylphenidate (Ritalin) Pemoline (Cylert) Psychiatric consultation Single-session therapy while in acute care setting Brief, solution-focus therapy
292.84 Substance Induced Mood Disorder	Prominent and persistent disturbance in mood that is determined to be the direct physiological effects of a substance (i.e., drug abuse, toxic exposure, medication, treatment related). Symptoms are dependent on the context in which the symptoms occur (intoxication vs. withdrawal states)	Identify and remove the offending agents (when possible) Switch medication—consult pharmacist to assist in choice Consider pharmacotherapy Psychiatric consultation to assist in early diagnosis and definitive treatment

Compiled from American Psychiatric Association. (1994); and Nathan & Gorman. (1998).

tion, commonly referred to as an acute confusional state. More than 30 diagnostic terms and/or labels have been used to describe this clinical syndrome (Francis, 1992). Delirium is a transient, usually reversible dysfunction in cerebral metabolism that has an acute or subacute onset and is manifested clinically by a wide array of neuropyschiatric abnormalities (Wise & Gray, 1994).

Delirium involves alterations in cognition, mood, perception, thinking, and sleep. Symptom manifestation fluctuates in intensity over the 24-hour period. The usual pattern has periods of relative lucidity interspersed with periods of increased impairment. Levels of consciousness and awareness also fluctuate. Additionally, the sleep–wake cycle in delirium is disturbed by fragmentation over the 24-hour period; this alteration in sleep physiology may affect level of awareness and consciousness.

Several studies report that delirium as a comorbid condition increases the length of stay during acute care hospitalizations (Francis, Martin, & Kapoor, 1990; Marcantonio et al., 1994; Thomas, Cameron, & Fahs, 1988). Additionally, there is substantial evidence that reveals patients with delirium have higher mortality rates (Folstein et al., 1991; Pompei et al., 1994; van Hemert et al., 1994), will experience further cognitive decline (Francis & Kapoor, 1992), have increased frequency of major postoperative complications (Marcantonio et al., 1994), experience poor functional capacity recovery (Cole & Primeau 1993; Marcantonio et al., 1994; Murray et al., 1993), and have increased hospital resource utilization (Kane et al., 1993). The outcome studies provide a powerful argument for prevention and/or early recognition of delirium in the acute care patient. Delirium costs everyone: the patient suffers needlessly, his or her family members are often frightened, health-care workers can be physically hurt while trying to keep the patient safe from inadvertent injury, and the health-care system suffers increased costs.

TABLE 54–11. Serotonin Syndrome: Identification and Treatment

Identification

Phase	*Characteristics*
Early	Agitation
	Confusion
	Diaphoresis
	Diarrhea
	Flushing
	Lethargy
	Myoclonic jerks
	Restlessness
	Tremors
Middle	Hypertension
	Hypertonicity
	Increased myoclonus
	Rigor
Late	Acidosis
	DIC
	Respiratory failure
	Renal failure
	Rhabdomyolysis

Treatment

Early identification!

Discontinue serotonergic medications: switch to another class of agents after recovery

Emergency medical treatment: middle–late phase (support physiological recovery)

Cooling blankets for hyperthermia
Clonazepam for myoclonus
Chlorpromazine IM for hyperthermia and sedation
Nifedipine for hypertension
5HT1a antagonists and beta blockers

Adapted from Krupnick & Wade. (1999).

Epidemiology of Delirium in the Acute Care Patient

Delirium occurs in approximately 15 to 20% of the acute care patients. The prevalence is increased in certain high-risk populations including 30% of patients who are post-coronary artery bypass graft (CABG) (Smith & Dimsdale, 1989), and 50% of posthip surgery patients (Gustafson et al., 1988). Delirium is the most common psychiatric syndrome found in the general medical hospitals (Lipowski, 1990).

Delirium: An Overview of DSM IV Categories and Clinical Presentation

DSM IV Categories

- Delirium due to a general medical condition
- Delirium due to a substance

Clinical Presentation

Prodrome phase—manifested symptoms prior to evident onset of delirium:

- Anxiety
- Irritability
- Restlessness
- Sleep-pattern disruption

Characteristics of Delirium

- *Fluctuating Course:* variability and fluctuations in clinical findings; this can lead to diagnostic confusion and uncertainty
- *Attentional Deficits:* core feature of delirium; patient is easily distracted by activities in the environment (decreased ability to focus on you and your interview questions)
- *Arousal Disturbance and Psychomotor Abnormalities:* the reticular activating system of the brain may be either hypoactive or hyperactive, which produces the alertness and arousal changes evident in a delirious patient (apathetic, somnolent, and "quietly confused" or agitated, hypervigilant and psychomotor hyperactivity, and "actively confused"); another grouping that leads to diagnostic confusion is the patient who has a "mixed" presentation, vacillating between hypoactive and hyperactive
- *Sleep–Wake Disturbance:* symptomatic of delirium and sleep deprivation may worsen the confusion; generally, the sleep–wake cycle of the delirious patient is reversed—the patient is somnolent during the day, restless in the evening, and agitated and hypervigilant at night time
- *Impaired Memory:* registration of information and events into memory is significantly impaired; attentional deficits, perceptual disturbances, and malfunction of the hippocampus contribute to the patient's recent and immediate memory deficits; it is common for patients recovering from delirium to be amnestic for the entire episode or to have fragmented memory for events during the delirium
- *Disorganized Thinking and Impaired Speech:* disorganized thought patterns with impaired reasoning ability; with increasing severity of delirium, spontaneous speech increases and develops into incoherent ramblings
- *Disorientation:* usually disoriented to time, often place but rarely to person (his or her own person, not you the health-care provider); often the patient reports being in a familiar place such as home; disorientation also fluctuates with severity of the delirium
- *Altered Perceptions:* frequently experiences misperceptions, that can be illusions, delusions (often persecutory), and/or hallucinations; visual hallucinations occur more frequently than auditory; they can be simple distortions or very complex, intricate scenes
- Neurologic abnormalities demonstrated in delirium:
  Asterixis
  Change in reflex and muscle tone

Difficulty naming objects
Dysgraphia (difficulty writing can be an indicator of delirium)
Myoclonus
Tremor

- Emotional disturbances demonstrated in delirium:
  Anger to rage
  Apathy
  Emotional fluctuation/lability
  Euphoria (usually steroid induced)
  Fearful
  Sadness

Risk Factors for Developing Delirium

Adults

Brain damage (preexisting)
Low serum albumin
Multiple medical problems
Polypharmacy
Substance intoxication
Thiamine deficiency

Elderly

Advanced age > 80
Dementia
Fever or hypothermia
Few social interactions/supports
Fractures
Infections (especially UTI, URI)
Low serum albumin
Metabolic disturbances
Polypharmacy (frequently found in elders)
Substance abuse (underrecognized in the elderly)
Visual impairment

Specific Patient Populations at High Risk for Delirium

AIDS
Burns
Postlung transplant
Postcardiotomy
Preexisting brain damage (dementia, stroke, Down syndrome)

Etiology of Delirium

Several medical and especially neurological problems, as well as medications and substances, can cause delirium. Some causes of delirium are life threatening and require early identification and immediate intervention There are several other causes of delirium that are less threatening to the patient's life; however, they are still critical causes of delirium. The reader is referred to the book *Delirium* for a clear and well-developed discussion (Lipowski, 1990). Many medications can be delirogenic alone or—in combination with other medications.

Foreman (1993) identifies the most common causes of delirium in order of frequency as medications, infections (especially UTI and URI), fluid and electrolyte imbalances, and metabolic disturbances (i.e., nutritional, pH derangement).

Lipowski (1990) categorizes etiologies of delirium according to predisposing factors, facilitating factors, and precipitating factors. The predisposing factors are identified in the earlier section on risk factors for adults and elderly. There is some research evidence that the following conditions can facilitate the onset of delirium, increase its severity, and prolong its course: immobilization, psychosocial stress, sensory overstimulation or understimulation, and sleep deprivation. Lipowski (1990) further groups the causative factors into four general classifications:

- Primary cerebral disease (focal, widespread, or both)
- Systemic diseases affecting the brain
- Intoxication with exogenous substances (i.e, prescribed, illicit, OTC, poisons of animal origin, industrial, or plant)
- Withdrawal from substances of abuse (generally alcohol or hypnosedative agents)

The presence of cerebral dysfunction due to one or more of the identified organic factors is necessary for the development of delirium. Although specific etiologies have not been linked with different subtypes or patterns of delirium, Liptzin & Levkoff (1992) propose that pattern variation is a function of etiology.

Diagnosis of Delirium in the Acute Care Patient

- Differentiate between delirium from dementia and/or depression (Nicholas & Lindsey, 1995)
- Identify pattern of delirium: is it linked to particular medication administration time, part of the day (better or worse)
- Has this patient ever experienced anything like this before

General Medical Evaluation of the Delirious Patient

- Conduct a complete physical examination; examine the patient for focal neurological signs (suggesting CNS event), fever, (infection[s]), increased BP and HR (possible withdrawal state or infection)
- Conduct a mental status examination (Table 54–12); document the areas of cognitive impairment and level of psychomotor activity
- Obtain focused consultations early (preferably in the prodrome phase or early onset of delirium): Neurology, Infectious Disease, Psychiatry, Geriatrics
- If cause(s) are identified, work aggressively to reverse them (untreated delirium can lead to death)
- If the delirium seems to be medication related, list all of the patient's medications and have family and/or

friends bring in all the medications from patient's residence (especially if the patient has been admitted in a delirious state)

Assessment and Measurement of Delirium by Rating Scales

The Confusion Assessment Method (CAM)
Confusion Rating Scale
Delirium Symptom Interview
Delirium Rating Scale (DRS) (translated into six languages and most widely used)
High Sensitivity Cognitive Screen (HSCS)
Memorial Delirium Assessment Scale (MDAS)
NEECHAM Confusion Scale
Cognitive Test for Delirium (CTD)

Laboratory Studies

General for All Patients with Delirium

ABGs
Albumin
Ammonia
BUN with creatinine

TABLE 54–12. Folstein Mini-Mental State Examination

The Folstein Mini-Mental State Examination is an easy and portable tool for assessing the mental status of a patient with suspected cognitive impairment. To perform the examination, ask the patient to follow a series of simple commands that test the ability to understand and perform cognitive functions. Award a designated point value for successful completion of each instruction; then total the scores to determine the client's mental status. Scores of 26 to 30 indicate that the patient is within normal cognitive functioning; 22 to 25, mildly impaired; and less than 22, significantly impaired.

Patient Instructions	Maximum score	Actual score
Orientation		
• Ask the client to name the year, season, date, day, and month. (Score one point for each correct response.)	5	___
• Ask the patient to name his state, city, street, and house address, and the room in which he is standing. (Score one point for each correct response.)	5	___
Comprehension		
• Name three objects, pausing 1 second between each name. Then ask the patient to repeat all three names. (Score one point for each correct response.) Repeat this exercise until the patient can correctly name all three objects (the client will be tested on his ability to recall this information later in the examination).	3	___
Attention and calculation		
• Ask the patient to count backward by sevens, beginning at 100; have him stop after counting out five numbers. Alternatively, ask the client to spell "World" backward. (Score one point for each correct response.)	5	___
Recall		
• Ask the patient to restate the name of the three objects previously identified in the examination. (Score one point for each correct response.)	3	___
Language		
• Point to a pencil and a watch. Ask the patient to identify each object. (Score one point for each correct response.)	2	___
• Ask the patient to repeat "No ifs, ands, or buts." (Score one point for a correct response.)	1	___
• Ask the patient to take a paper in the right hand, then fold the paper in half, then put the paper on the floor. (Score one point for each correct response to this three-part command.)	3	___
• Ask the patient to read and obey the written instruction "Close your eyes." (Score one point for a correct response.)	1	___
• Ask the patient to copy the following design. (Score one point for a correct response.)	1	___

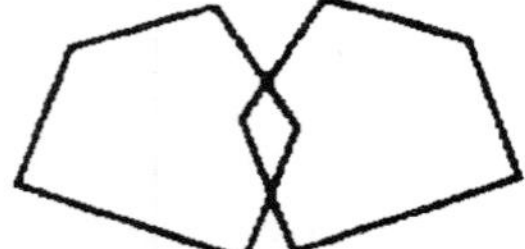

Adapted from Folstein et al. (1975). (196–197).

Calcium
CBC with differential
Drug levels (toxicology screens, medication blood levels)
Electrolytes
ESR (sedimentation rate)
Glucose
LFTs
Urinalysis, C & S (culture and sensitivity)
VDRL, FTA–ABS (fluorescent treponemal antibody absorption)

Focused Studies

Antinuclear antibodies (ANA)
Folate (especially in alcohol-related delirium)
Glycol levels (if on medications with glycol diluent)
Heavy metals
HIV
Lupus erythematosus preparation
Thiamine
Thiocynate levels (if on long-term nitroprusside)
Thyroid function tests (TFTs)
Urinary porphobilinogen

Diagnostic Studies/Procedures

General for All Patients with Delirium

Chest x-ray
EKG

Focused Studies

CT scan
EEG
Lumbar puncture
MRI

Treatment of the Patient with Delirium

General Principles in Managing the Delirious Patient

- Focus on prevention!
- Identify patients at high risk: avoid delirogenic medications especially in the elderly and patient with preexisting brain injury
- Reassure, support, and acknowledge the patient's fears
- Encourage and support family involvement (especially members that have a calming effect on the patient)
- Educate the patient and family about delirium (define it, describe what is thought to be causing it, and what the focused plan of care is to alleviate it)
- Do not minimize it—"they are a little confused today"; if the patient was cognitively intact when he or she arrived in the acute care center and isn't now, it becomes a "big deal" to the family and the patient (especially a patient who has periods of lucidity and knows that something is wrong with him or her)

Focused Treatment of the Delirious Patient

Primary goal is to identify and treat the underlying condition
Secondary goal is to reduce psychiatric symptoms of delirium with medications and environmental manipulation
Focused treatment is further divided into when the etiology is known and unknown

Treatment with Known Etiologic Factor(s)

- Reverse causative factor(s)

  Examples

  A patient with hypertension, papilledema, confusion and agitation

  Address the hypertension with antihypertensive medication and monitor the patient's mental status, the patient may still require additional medication for agitation and confusion

  A patient with alcohol or hypnosedative withdrawal who is agitated, incoherent, incontinent, with increased autonomic signs (increased heart rate, BP & RR); further assessment of drinking history, especially quantity and last drink, the focused treatment includes benzodiazepine sedation and close monitoring, folate, MVI and thiamine along with hydration and a low stimulation environment
- Sometimes agitation persists even after focused treatment has been initiated. If agitation persists, haloperidol (haldol) has been demonstrated to have efficacy in the treatment of agitation due to delirium (even before focused treatment has been initiated) (Lipowski, 1990; Platt et al., 1994). Haldol is a potent antipsychotic medication with a safe side-effect profile, and can be administered by several routes.

Treatment of Delirium with Unknown or Multiple Etiologies

This patient requires a multifocal approach to his or her delirium management, including medical, pharmacological, psychosocial, and environmental interventions to achieve a positive outcome.

Medical

- Discontinue all nonessential medications after conducting a medication review.
- Increase monitoring and surveillance of patient (increase VS checks, careful I/O monitoring, laboratory assessments, daily thorough physical assessment).
- If possible, try to examine patient more than once in the 24-hour cycle (morning and early evening to determine cyclic pattern changes).

Pharmacological

- No perfect pharmacologic agent exists!
- Sometimes a combination of pharmacologic agents is necessary to provide targeted symptom relief (avoid polypharmacy: more than two medications with no focused plan)
- Haloperidol can be administered through several routes: oral, intramuscular, and parenterally. (Gelfand, Indelicato, & Benjamin, 1992; Levenson, 1995; Nicholas & Lindsey, 1995; Riker, Fraser, & Cox, 1994; Sanders, Murray, & Cassem, 1991; Stern 1994). However, the FDA has not approved the intravenous route of administration. Its potency intravenously is twice that of oral doses.
- If intravenous haloperidol is considered, it can be given by IV bolus or continuous drip. When a patient requires intravenous haldol, additional consultation with a specialist who is experienced in prescribing, titrating, and managing potential side effects represents safe and deliberate practice with a patient who is probably experiencing a severe delirium.
- Prolonged QT interval (torsades de pointes—multifocal ventricular tachycardia) has been demonstrated with the use of intravenous haldol (Kriwisky et al., 1990; Metzger & Friedman, 1993; Wilt et al., 1993). However, Wilt and colleagues (1993) found only 4 out of 1100 ICU cases of haldol-induced torsades over a 3-year period in the largest survey of this particular side effect.
- If intravenous drip haldol is utilized, the patient needs to have cardiac monitoring and close observation.
- Combination therapy of lorazepam (ativan) and haloperidol (haldol) may be particularly beneficial in the critically ill patient (haldol 5 mg every 30 minutes with lorazepam 1-2 mg every 30 minutes before the haldol). This regimen is given until the patient is quiet and calm.
- Each patient must be individualized in his or her doses in relation to his or her response; initial dose of haldol:

  Young to Middle Adult Patient
  0.5-1.0 mg for mild agitation
  2.0-5.0 mg for moderate agitation
  5.0-10.0 mg for severe agitation

  Frail Elderly Patient
  0.5 mg for mild agitation
  1.0 mg for moderate agitation
  2.0 mg for severe agitation

  Doses are repeated at regular intervals (not closer than every 30 minutes) until patient is calm. Then continue at dose it took to obtain calmness (total amount in equally divided doses over the next 24 hours). Then begin to taper over the next 1-5 days with close monitoring of the patient's responses to the titration process. Often a nighttime dose of haloperidol (haldol) with lorazepam (ativan) may be beneficial in the patient with a sleep cycle that is still disrupted and has not responded sufficiently to just haldol.
- Additional pharmacologic choices:
  —Droperidol (Inapsine) IM or IV can offer quicker relief; however, it is more sedating than haldol and can produce hypotension.
  —Propofol (Diprivan) is an excellent agent for sedating critically ill patients for a short duration. It has been demonstrated to be effective in calming agitation (Barr & Donner, 1995). However, propofol has several drawbacks for prolonged management of agitation due to delirium: fat overload syndrome, higher doses are required after 4-7 days, seizures after discontinuance, increased expense (El-Ebiury, 1995; Mirenda, 1995; Valenti et al., 1994).
- Risperidone (Risperdal) (not yet available in parenteral formulation) has some demonstrated efficacy in treating delirium. Olanzapine (Zyprexa) has recently been reported to have efficacy in delirium management (Sipuhimalani & Masard, 1998).
- Buspirone (BuSpar) and Carbmazepine (Tegretol) have been effective in controlling agitation in patients with traumatic brain injury (Pourcher et al., 1994).
- Close monitoring for side effects and adverse effects especially for neuroleptic malignant syndrome (Table 54–13).

Nursing Care Consultation

The nurses caring for the patient who is delirious may have several consultation questions. The following guidelines have positive effects when coupled with medical and pharmacologic management. These are the environmental management strategies that are often overlooked in delirium management.

- Encourage (teach) the nurses to utilize a bedside cognitive screening tool such as the Folstein Mini-Mental Status Examination (MMSE) to assist in understanding the patient's cognitive changes and to better delineate alterations (refer to Table 54–12).
- Identify safety risks (falls, aggression) and utilize safety precautions, side rails, padding (especially if the patient is at risk for seizing), use of constant companion or sitter, family involvement at nighttime (might have a calming effect).
- Room close to nurses' station for increased observation ability.
- Physical restraints as a last resort; can actually increase agitation, requiring more medications.
- Keep environment harm free, lessen clutter at the bedside, technology (pumps with drips, oximetry) behind the patient and not in his or her line of vision.
- Make certain the proper ID bracelet is on the patient

TABLE 54–13. Neuroleptic Malignant Syndrome

Neuroleptic malignant syndrome is a potentially fatal syndrome. It is an idiosyncratic reaction either to the use of dopamine blocking or depleting agents, or to the withdrawal of dopamine agonists.

Symptoms

Early	*Middle*	*Late*
Fever Mild–Moderate rigidity	Catatonia (mute to stupor) Delirium High fever (≥ 102°) Marked and generalized rigidity Tremor (coarse)	Autonomic instability: BP labile Diaphoresis Tachycardia Tachypnea Chest wall rigidity Increased CPK (> 15,000) Increased WBC (> 15,000) Increased LDH, SGOT Alkaline phosphatase Pallor

Complications

Acute renal failure from myoglobinuria
Disseminated intravascular coagulation (DIC)
Respiratory failure
Rhabdomyolysis

Treatment

Dantrolene 1–2 mg/Kg IV Repeated if necessary. Dose not to exceed 10 mg/Kg/day
Bromocriptine 2.5–20 mg TID po or NGT
Cooling blanket for temperature reduction
Hydration
Ventilatory support

Compiled from Schatzberg & Neineroff. (1995). (p. 626); and Moore & Jefferson. (1996). (pp. 284–285).

(who probably will not be the most reliable person to tell anyone who he or she is).

- Use environmental cues (clocks, calendars, pictures that are familiar).
- Try not to frequently quiz the patient who is delirious about orientation; instead inquire how safe he or she feels and gently reintroduce patient to the location, who you are and how you and all the health-care providers are trying to help him or her.
- Reassure patient that "we" are going to keep him or her safe until he or she feels better.
- Maintain appropriate lighting that reflects the time of day.
- Provide a low stimulation environment for the patient, especially when stimulation increases their confusion and disorientation (i.e., delirium tremens).
- Collaborate with the nursing and medical staff to arrange for consistency in the patient's health-care providers.
- When speaking with the delirious patient, speak slowly; don't yell—patient is delirious, not deaf—increased voices may signal a threat and produce increased agitation.
- Reintroduce yourself to the patient with each subsequent contact.
- Provide information to the patient in small portions and ask for his or her understanding of what has been told to him or her.
- Schedule frequent rest breaks in patient's daily schedule.

▶ SUBSTANCE ABUSE IN THE ACUTE CARE PATIENT

Substance use and abuse-related problems in the United States have reached epidemic proportions. Substance abuse has been identified as one of the major health issues in this nation, and it has become the focus of social, legal, and political concerns. Substance abuse inflicts a significant toll in relation to the social, medical, and emotional health of individuals, families, and communities at large. It is one of the primary health and social issues currently confronting our society. Presently, substance abuse threatens to affect the overall welfare of our already burdened health-care system.

Health-care professionals, especially nurses, are crucial to implementing evidence-based screening and assessment techniques, and to promoting early diagnosis and corresponding early treatment. Nurses have an integral role in educating individuals, families, and communities about the impact and trajectory of substance abuse. The overriding message is that substance abuse and related disorders are treatable diseases that require daily maintenance, just like any other chronic illness.

The related social and health issues are well described in the literature and include: the rise of criminal and illegal activities; violence associated with the distribution/sale of illicit drugs in neighborhoods and school areas jeopardize the safety and well being and general health of communities. Younger age groups are being exposed to and are experimenting with drugs. Additional health issues include the increased risk to exposure and transmission of the human immunodeficiency virus (HIV), as well as other communicable diseases among intravenous drug users; and major developmental and medical problems of babies born to "crack" and/or "ice" addicted mothers. There is a direct connection between the number of premature deaths and/or traumatic injury (motor vehicle crashes, swimming/diving and boating accidents while drinking) due to drug overdoses or engaging in unsafe activities or practices while under the influence of substances.

The extent of substance-related illnesses in the acute care environment is overwhelming. Alcohol and nicotine use contribute to several chronic and often life-threatening medical illnesses. There has been a steady increase in overdoses seen in our nation's emergency departments.

Epidemiology of Substance Abuse in Acute Care

Substance abuse and dependence affect between 17 and 27% of Americans over their lifetime. Approximately 20% of outpatients in primary care services have alcohol disorders. There is a higher rate of substance abuse in hospitalized and emergency room patients. However, many cases of substance abuse remain undiagnosed or undetected, which contributes to the hidden diagnosis phenomenon.

The use/abuse of alcohol and other drugs (AOD) has been recognized as a significant, independent risk factor in unintentional fatal and nonfatal injuries, as well as intentional injuries such as physical assaults, homicides, and suicides. Some clinicians have proposed that traumatic injury is a marker of alcohol abuse (Clark et al., 1985, Maull, 1982). Alcohol-intoxicated individuals are involved in 40 to 50% of fatal motor vehicle crashes and 25 to 30% of nonfatal crashes. Additionally, alcohol has been identified in more than 50% of homicides and more than 50% of burns, 48% of frostbite and hypothermia, and 40% of falls (NIAAA, 1989). Waller (1988) estimated that 20 to 25% of all patients hospitalized for injury are alcoholics or have a drinking problem. Even more concerning is evidence has been found that in some samples three-quarters of trauma patients are experiencing chronic alcoholism (Rivara et al., 1993). Several studies have shown that cocaine, amphetamines, and marijuana—in combination with alcohol—play a significant role in all types of traumatic injuries, especially motor vehicle crashes (Bailey, 1990, 1993; Brookoff et al., 1993; Clark & Harchelroad, 1991; Marzuk et al., 1990). Cleary and colleagues (1988) and Moore (1989) further illuminated the impact of alcohol-related disorders in the general hospital population. Both conservatively estimated reports that 25% of general hospital inpatients and 20% of medical outpatients have alcohol-related disorders. A truly unfortunate finding is that only 20 to 50% of the acute care populations problems are diagnosed (Moore et al., 1989).

The ACNP and his or her colleagues are integral in the process of early identification of alcohol and other drug problems in their practice environments. Earlier identification of substance-related disorders is important in decreasing the comorbidity and overwhelmingly negative impact on the patient, family, and health-care system.

Impact of Substance Abuse on the Patient in Acute Care

The United States Department of Health and Human Services's 7th Special Report to the United States Congress on Alcohol (1990) estimated that 200,000 deaths per year are alcohol related. Annually 25,000 people die and 150,000 are permanently disabled because of alcohol-related traffic crashes. Additionally, there is a strong association between alcohol use and violent crime including assault, rape, child molestation, attempted murder, and murder.

The alcohol and drug abusers who sustain burns have longer treatment times with more complications (Kelly & Lynch 1992). Additionally, alcoholism is strongly associated with suicide and increased rates between 60 to 120 times that of the nonalcoholic population. Murphy & Wetzel (1990) estimated that the lifetime risk of suicide in alcoholic patients is 2 to 3.4%. It has been reported that alcoholic patients who attempt suicide may have more severe alcohol problems and increased comorbidity than those who do not attempt suicide (Murphy et al., 1992; Roy et al., 1990).

Etiology of Substance Abuse

Several etiologic factors have been proposed as contributing to substance abuse. However, the primary determinants are genetics and envrionmental influences. Genetic evidence indicates that there is a familial predisposition toward addiction, and that children of alcoholics have a 3-4 times greater chance of having this disorder than children of nonalcoholics (Anthenelli & Schuckit, 1997).

The ongoing search for a genetic marker for alcoholism has led to investigation into the link of the A1 allele at the D2 dopamine receptor gene (Blum et al., 1990; Gelernter et al., 1993). The A1 allele is associated with an overall reduction in the number of D2 receptors, and a decrease in the number of D2 receptors has been correlated with a number of pleasure-seeking behaviors. Additionally, the B1 allele is associated with severe alcoholism.

The neurobiology of substance abuse is another area of

important research. Some studies suggest that alcohol and drug abuse reinforce dependency by stimulating future use through a biologic brain reward mechanism (Gold, 1994; Miller & Gold, 1993; Winger et al., 1992). Biochemical and behavioral studies have demonstrated an interaction between alcohol and opioid receptors. Opioid anatagonists, such as naltrexone, have been shown to decrease alcohol craving and days of alcohol consumption in some alcohol-dependent patients (Volpicelli et al., 1995). Additionally, serotonin deficiency has been examined whereby Naranjo and colleagues (1992) revealed that the selective serotonin reuptake inhibitors (SSRIs) decrease alcohol intake in (moderately dependent) alcoholic patients.

The environmental factors that increase the risk to develop a substance-abuse disorder are numerous. The primary factors that have been demonstrated to increase the risk include: children modeling adult/parental behaviors, children attempting to conform to peer pressure, job stress, marital discord, poverty, and underemployment.

Diagnosis of Substance Abuse in the Acute Care Patient

For specific substance-related disorders described in an overivew form, see Table 54–14. It includes the DSM IV diagnosis with code and the related diagnostic criteria.

General Recommendations for the ACNP

- Screen all patients for alcohol and other drug use.
- Intervene to facilitate the patient's action to change pathologic substance use.

General Medical Evaluation of Substance Abuse

It is often helpful to identify possible medical conditions that are closely associated with alcohol or other drug abuse, because often the patient is trying to minimize or hide his or her substance use/abuse from health-care providers, family, and him- or herself. Identification of these associated medical conditions allows you an entry point to begin a discussion with your patient about the relationship between alcohol or another drug and the medical condition. Tables 54–15 and 54–16 will assist in this identification process.

Additionally, there are several psychiatric and social problems associated with substance abuse including: antisocial personality disorder, anxiety disorders, attention deficit hyperactivity disorder (ADHD), conduct disorder, major depressive disorder, mania, posttraumatic stress disorder, and schizophrenia.

Screening and Assessment Scales

Alcohol or Drug Screening Tools

AUDIT (Alcohol Use Disorders Identification Test)—10-item questionnaire developed by the World Health Organization (WHO)

CAGE/CAGE–AID—four simple questions to screen the potential for alcohol and/or drug abuse (see Table 54–17 for details); tested and validated in several populations including medical/surgical patients in acute care and primary care environments

DAST (Drug Abuse Screening Test)—28 questions to determine drug use

MAST (Michigan Alcoholism Screening Test)—25 questions to determine alcoholism

Brief MAST (revised and shortened MAST)—10 questions

MAST–G—geriatric version of MAST

CHARM—elderly population tested

RAFFT—adolescent population tested

T–ACE—prenatal population tested

TWEAK—ob/gyn population tested

Trauma Scale Screening Tool—trauma patients tested

Assessment (Quantification) of Withdrawal Syndrome Scales

Clinical Institute Withdrawal Assessment—Alcohol (revised) (CIWA–Ar)—10-item questionnaire to assess severity of alcohol withdrawal by quantifying the overt symptoms (see Table 54–18 for a description)

Clinical Institute Withdrawal Assessment–Benzodiazepine (CIWA–B)—22-item questionnaire to assess the severity of benzodiazepine withdrawal by quantifying the overt symptoms

Objective Opiate Wthidrawal Scale (OOWS)

Subjective Opiate Withdrawal Scale (SOWS)

Physical Assessment of Substance Abuse in the Acute Care Patient

A thorough and focused physical assessment may provide clues to intoxication, withdrawal, and long-term (chronic) substance abuse. Although the physical examination is not so sensitive as a screening test for substance abuse, all positive findings require attention and focused exploration that may lead to an underlying substance-abuse problem. In the acute care environment, the physical findings may be evident; however, the patient is often a master at concealing, denying, and/or justifying the substance-related findings. Be prepared to spend more time with the patient to review the importance of your findings and listen to the patient's explanations with frequent reminders of the facts and the linkages to substance abuse. The ACNP must remain persistent and focused on "facts" rather than assuming a confrontative stance. The substance-abusing patient has had to practice and develop incredible skills to remain active so it will take time and persistence to begin to chip away at defenses that are almost as firm as concrete. Remember, these defenses protect the patient from a truth he or she may not yet be prepared to accept and deal with in a constructive manner.

TABLE 54–14. Overview: Key Diagnostic Criteria of Substance-Related Disorders

DSM IV Substance-Related Disorder	Diagnostic Criteria
Substance Abuse Disorders 305.00 Alcohol abuse 305.70 Amphetamine abuse 305.20 Cannabis abuse 305.30 Hallucinogen abuse 305.90 Inhalant abuse 305.50 Opioid abuse 305.90 Phencyclidine abuse 305.40 Sedative, hypnotic or anxiolytic abuse	Maladaptive pattern of substance use that leads to clinically significant impairment or distress. Impairment is manifested by at least three or more of the following symptoms within the last 12-month period: failure to fulfill role responsibilities and obligations (work, school, home); recurrent use in physically dangerous situations (driving under the influence, working machinery under the influence, boating/swimming under the influence); recurrent substance-related legal problems; continued use despite recurrent social or interpersonal problems
Substance Dependence Disorders 303.90 Alcohol dependence 304.40 Amphetamine dependence 304.30 Cannabis dependence 304.50 Hallucinogen dependence 304.60 Inhalant dependence 305.10 Nicotine dependence 304.00 Opioid dependence 304.90 Phencyclidine dependence 301.10 Sedative, hypnotic, or anxiolytic dependence	Maladaptive pattern of substance use leading to clinically significant impairment or distress. Impairment is manifested by three or more of the following symptoms within a 12-month period: tolerance, withdrawal, use in larger amounts, or for longer periods than atttended; unsuccessful efforts to cut down or control use; increasing time spent in obtaining and/or using the substance; reduction or cessation of important social, occupational and/or recreational activities; continued use despite acknowledgment of psychological, physical, and/or legal problems
Substance Intoxication Disorders 303.00 Alcohol intoxication 291.0 Alcohol intoxication delirium 292.89 Amphetamine intoxication 292.81 Amphetamine intoxication delirium 305.90 Caffeine intoxication 292.89 Cannabis intoxication 292.81 Cannabis intoxication delirium 292.89 Cocaine intoxication 292.0 Cocaine intoxication delirium 292.89 Hallucinogen intoxication 292.81 Hallucinogen intoxication delirium 292.89 Opioid intoxication 292.81 Opioid intoxication delirium 292.89 Inhalant intoxication 292.81 Inhalant intoxication delirium 292.89 Phencyclidine intoxication 292.81 Phencyclidine intoxication delirium 292.89 Sedative, hypnotic, or anxiolytic intoxication 292.81 Sedative, hypnotic, or anxiolytic intoxication delirium	Reversible substance-specific syndrome due to recent ingestion/exposure to a substance. Clinically significant maladaptive behavioral, psychological, and/or physiological changes due to effect of substance on central nervous system, during or after use of substance. Symptoms are not a direct effect of a medical conditon or another mental disorder
Substance Withdrawal Disorders 291.8 Alcohol withdrawal 291.0 Alcohol withdrawal delirium 292.0 Amphetamine withdrawal 292.0 Cocaine withdrawal 292.0 Nicotine withdrawal 292.0 Opioid withdrawal 292.0 Sedative, hypnotic, or anxiolytic withdrawal 292.81 Sedative, hypnotic, or anxiolytic withdrawal delirium	Development of substance-specific syndrome due to cessation or the reduction in the substance use that had been large in quantity and/or prolonged. Syndrome causes significant distress and/or impairment in social, occupational, and functional status. Maladaptive pattern of substance use leading to clinically significant impairment or distress. Impairment is manifested by three or more of the following: tolerance, withdrawal; using an increased amount; increased time in substance-seeking behavior; reduction or cessation of involvement in important activities; persistent desire and lack of success in attempts to reduce or cease use; continued use of substance despite knowledge of problems caused by substance use

Adapted from American Psychiatric Association. (1994).

TABLE 54–15. Medical Conditions Related to Alcohol Abuse

Cardiovascular
- alcoholic cardiomyopathy
- increased systolic and pulse pressure
- tissue damage, weakened heart muscle, and heart failure

Gastrointestinal
- abdominal distention, pain, belching, and hematemesis
- acute and chronic pancreatitis
- alcoholic hepatitis leading to cirrhosis
- cancer of the esophagus, liver, or pancreas
- esophageal varices, hemorrhoids, and ascites
- gastritis, colitis, and enteritis
- gastric or duodenal ulcers
- gastrointestinal malabsorption
- hepatorenal syndrome
- swollen, enlarged fatty liver

Genitourinary
- hypogonadism, hypoandrogenization, hyperestrogenization in men
- increased urinary excretion of potassium and magnesium (results in hypomagnesemia, hypokalemia)
- infertility, decreased menstruation
- prostate gland enlargement, leading to prostatitis and interference with urination
- prostate cancer
- sexual dysfunction: decreased libido, decreased sexual performance, impotency

Metabolic
- hypoglycemia, hyperlipidemia, hyperuricemia
- ketoacidosis
- osteoporosis

Hematologic
- abnormal red blood cells, white blood cells, and platelets
- anemia and increased risk of infection
- bleeding tendencies, increased bruising, and decreased clotting time
- mineral and vitamin deficiencies (folate, iron, phosphate, thiamine)

Neurologic
- Wernicke–Korsakoff syndrome, Marchiafava–Bignami disease, cerebellar degeneration
- peripheral neuropathy, polyneuropathy
- seizures
- sleep disturbances
- stroke (increased risk of hemorrhagic stroke)

Respiratory
- cancer of the oropharynx
- impaired diffusion, chronic obstructive pulmonary disease, infection, and tuberculosis
- respiratory depression causing decreased respiratory rate and cough reflex and increased susceptibility to infection and trauma

Trauma related
- burns, smoke inhalation injuries
- injuries from motor vehicle crashes and falls

Adapted from Miller. (1997). (pp. 144–154).

TABLE 54–16. Medical Consequences of Parenteral Drug Use

Infectious complications
- brain abcesses
- cellulitis
- cutaneous abscesses
- epidural abscess
- endocarditis
- gas gangrene
- hepatitis A, B, C, and D viruses
- HIV (AIDS)
- infected pseudoaneurysm
- malaria
- septic arthritis
- subdural abscess
- sexually transmitted diseases
- tetanus
- tuberculosis

Noninfectious complications
- amenorrhea
- arrhythmia
- constipation with possible impaction
- gastrointestinal motility disturbances
- glomerulonephritis
- mycotic aneurysm
- myositis
- necrotizing angiitis
- needle embolus
- nephrotic syndrome
- overdose with possible coma and death
- pneumomediastinum
- pneumothorax
- pulmonary edema (flash)
- pulmonary fibrosis
- pulmonary hypertension
- renal failure (acute to chronic)
- stroke (cerebrovascular accident)
- talc granuloma (from talc used to cut the "street narcotic")
- thrombocytopenia
- trauma (unisystem or multisystem trauma, from falls, jumps, burns, and vehicle crashes)

Adapted from Miller. (1997). (p. 148); and Novick, Haverkos, & Teller. (1997). (p. 536).

General Appearance

Weight loss and emaciated or "wasting" appearance seen in alcoholics from poor nutrition; in chronic stimulant/cocaine abusers, it is from the anorexic effects of the substances

Muscular hypertrophy/"athletic" appearance—consider anabolic steriod use

Shivering/huddling/seeking blankets may be indicative of opioid withdrawal

Alcohol on the breath is highly suggestive of impaired control over drinking

TABLE 54–17. Alcohol and Drug Screening Test

It is important in these hectic days to choose an assessment tool that has been tested in a variety of clinical settings and is "user friendly," easy to use, and portable. We have chosen to instruct you in the CAGE–AID for all of those reasons. To use this test, ask your patient the following questions. For each positive response, score one point and then total the points. Generally, a score of two or more points indicates an individual who needs further evaluation of his or her drinking and definitive assessment for possible alcohol withdrawal syndrome.

Questions

1. Have you ever felt you should *cut down* on your drinking and/or drugging?	Yes	No
2. Have people *annoyed* you by criticizing your drinking and/or drugging?	Yes	No
3. Have you ever felt bad or *guilty* about your drinking and/or drugging?	Yes	No
4. Have you ever had a drink or a drug first thing in the morning to steady your nerves, get rid of a hangover (*eye-opener*), or get your day started?	Yes	No

Scoring: Two or more positive answers to these questions strongly suggest alcohol dependence, physical dependence in relation to their inability to cut down, and the need for an awakening drink. Additional exploration of the quantity of the alcohol, the frequency, and in what circumstance do they drink. It is important to know if they think they have experienced some form of alcohol and/or drug withdrawal any time during a period of reduced drinking or abstinence.

Adapted from Mayfield, McLeod, & Hall. (1974). (p. 1121) (original CAGE questions); Sdao-Jarvie, Berolzheimer, Rounds, & Janowsky. (1993). (pp. 28–34).

Vital Signs

Increased autonomic signs (elevated HR, RR, BP) associated with stimulant, cocaine, hallucinogen, PCP, ketamine intoxication

Elevated HR only associated with marijuana

Lowered RR can be associated with opioid intoxication

Elevated BP (mild) associated with anabolic steroids

Increased autonomic signs (elevated HR, RR, BP) associated with withdrawal syndrome from alcohol, sedatives, and opioids

Elevated HR/lowered BP associated with acute ingestion of nitrite inhalants (duration of changes only 5 minutes)

Integumentary

Needletracks along forearm, hands, feet, leg veins associated with intravenous drug abuse with heroin and/or cocaine

Thrombosed or hardened veins associated with intravenous drug use

Abscesses and cellulitis associated with intravenous drug abuse and subcutaneous injections (skin popping); also circumscribed "pock-like" depression in the skin from skin popping

Diaphoresis associated with stimulant/cocaine/hallucinogen intoxication, and withdrawal from alcohol, marijuana, and sedatives or opioids

Piloerection ("gooseflesh") associated with opioid withdrawal

Self-inflicted excoriations associated with cocaine/stimulant induced formincation (sense of bugs) crawling under the skin)

Abnormal vascularization of facial skin associated with chronic alcoholics including spider angiomas when liver disease is present

Jaundice associated with alcohol-related liver disease, steroid-related liver disease, or viral hepatitis from contaminated needles

Acne associated with anabolic steroid use

Hirsutism in females and male pattern baldness in males associated with anabolic steroid use

Fingertip burns and/or nasal burns associated with smoking drugs (crack, ice, nicotine)

Bruises, falls, accidents, fights while intoxicated with alcohol

Facial/neck flushing associated with alcohol, hallucinogen, and opioid intoxication

Eyes

Dilated pupils associated with cocaine/stimulant and hallucinogen intoxication and withdrawal from opioids

Pinpoint pupils associated with opioid intoxication

Lacrimation associated with opioid withdrawal

Conjunctival erythema associated with marijuana or inhalant intoxication and chronic alcoholism

Nystagmus associated with intoxication with alcohol, sedatives, some inhalants, Wernicke's encephalopathy (thiamine-deficient alcoholic)

Vertical nystagmus is more specific for PCP intoxication

Jaundiced eyes associated with substance-related liver disease

Nose, Mouth, and Throat

Infected, ulcerated, or perforated nasal septum associated with intranasal cocaine use

Nasal and mouth rash associated with glue sniffing ("glue sniffers" rash)

Rhinorrhea associated with opioid withdrawal

Yawning associated with cocaine/stimulant and opioid withdrawal

Dry mouth associated with marijuana use

Excessive salivation associated with PCP intoxication

TABLE 54–18. Clinical Institute Withdrawal Assessment–Alcohol (revised)

Temp_____ **BP_____** **Pulse_____** **Resp_____** **BAL_____** Score

Nausea and Vomiting

0 None
1 Mild nausea with no vomiting
4 Intermittent
7 Nausea, dry heaves, vomiting

Tremor (*arms extended, fingers spread*)

0 No tremor
1 Not visible—can be felt fingertip to fingertip
4 Moderate with arms extended
7 Severe, even arms not extended

Sweating (*observation*)

0 No sweat visible
1 Barely perceptible, palms sweats
4 Beads of sweat visible
7 Drenching sweats

Tactile Disturbances

0 None
1 Very mild itching, pins and needles or numbness
2 Mild itching or pins and needles, burning or numbness
3 Moderate itching, pins and needles, burning or numbness
4 Moderately severe hallucinations
5 Severe hallucinations
6 Extremely severe hallucinations
7 Continuous hallucinations

Visual Disturbances - Ask "Does the light appear to be too bright? Is its color different? Does it hurt your eyes? Are you seeing anything that is disturbing to you? Are you seeing things you know are not there?"

0 Not present
1 Very mild sensitivity
2 Mild sensitivity
3 Moderate sensitivity
4 Moderately severe hallucinations
5 Severe hallucinations
6 Extremely severe hallucinations
7 Continuous hallucinations

Auditory Disturbances - Ask "Are you more aware of sounds around you? Are they harsh? Do they frighten you? Are you hearing anything that is disturbing to you? Are you hearing things you know are not there?"

0 Not present
1 Very mild harshness or ability to frighten
2 Mild harshness or ability to frighten
3 Moderate harshness or ability to frighten
4 Moderately severe hallucinations
5 Severe hallucinations
6 Extremely severe hallucinations
7 Continuous hallucinations

Orientation and Clouding of Sensorium (What day is this? What is this place?)

0 Oriented and can do serial additions
1 Cannot do serial additions or is uncertain about dates
2 Disoriented for date by no more that 2 calendar days
3 Disoriented for date by more than 2 calendar days
4 Disoriented for place and/or person

Anxiety (Observation, "Do you feel nervous?")

0 No anxiety, at ease
1 Mildly anxious
4 Moderately anxious or guarded, anxiety inferred
7 Equivalent to panic states as seen in severe delirium, acute schizophrenic reactions

Agitation (Observation)

0 Normal activity
1 Somewhat more than normal activity
4 Moderately fidgety and restless
7 Pacing, or thrashing about constantly

Headache, fullness in head. Ask, "Does your head feel different? Does it feel like a band around your head?" Do not rate for dizziness or lightheadedness. Otherwise, rate severity.

0 Not present
1 Very mild
2 Mild
3 Moderate
4 Moderately severe
5 Severe
6 Very severe
7 Extremely severe

Name: **Last Drink Date:** **Time:** **Total Score**
Assessment date: **Day #:** **Maximum Score** 67

Scoring, Monitoring, and Medication Recommendations

(0–7) No overt evidence of active withdrawal symptoms: continue to monitor with regular vital signs
(8–14) Stage 1: Early stage of withdrawal: monitor with increased frequency and begin medication
(15–19) Stage 2: Moderate signs of withdrawal: monitor with CIWA–Ar hourly and medicate until score is < 8 for three hours
> 20 Stage 3: Severe withdrawal: at risk for developing delirium tremens and/or seizures—increased monitoring and medications every 30 minutes until CIWA–Ar score < 8 for two hours

Scoring and monitoring recommendations reference: Adapted from Krupnick, Grunwald, Fischel, Gavryck, & Ryzewicz. (1998).
CIWA–Ar assessment tool reference adapted from Sullivan, Sykora, Schneiderman, Naranjo, & Sellers. (1989). (pp. 1353–1357).

Pharyngeal erythema associated with smoking drugs (nicotine, marijuana, cocaine, PCP)
Oral cancers associated with heavy nicotine and alcohol abuse
Coated tongue associated with chronic alcoholism
Poor dentition associated with several different types of substance abuse (general health neglect)

Chest

Breath sounds, rhonchi, and coughing associated with long-term nicotine use, marijuana, and cocaine
Gynecomastia associated with alcoholics with severe liver disease
Gynecomastia with painful lumps associated with anabolic steroids

Abdomen

Diffuse abdominal tenderness associated with withdrawal from alcohol, opioids, and sedatives
Hepatomegaly and right upper quadrant tenderness associated with alcohol-related liver disease and anabolic steroids
Ascites, dilated periumbilical veins, and venous hum associated with late signs of alcoholic cirrhosis

Genitourinary

Clitoral hypertrophy associated with anabolic steroids
Prostatic hypertrophy associated with anabolic steroids
Testicular atrophy associated with chronic heavy alcohol or anabolic steroids

Neurological

Ataxia and uncoordination associated with alcohol, sedatives, marijuana, opioids, hallucinogens, PCP, and inhalant intoxication
Depressed reflexes associated with inhalant intoxication
Diminished response to pain and numbness associated with PCP intoxication (due to anesthetic properties), alcohol, sedatives, and opioid intoxication
Hyperreflexia associated with cocaine, PCP, stimulant, and hallucinogen intoxication and during withdrawal from alcohol and sedatives
Persistent ataxia and uncoordination associated with alcohol or inhalant-related cerebellar degeneration
Slurred speech associated with intoxication from alcohol, cocaine, stimulants, hallucinogens, and inhalants, and withdrawal from alcohol, sedatives, and opioids

Laboratory Studies

General Studies

Bilirubin
Blood alcohol level (BAL) (Table 54–19)
B_{12} level
BUN with creatinine
Calcium
CBC with differential
Electrolyte panel
Folate level
FBS
Hepatitis B surface antigen
Liver function tests (GGT most sensitive blood test for screening long-term heavy drinking), AST (SGOT), ALT (SGPT)
Magnesium
Stool for guiaic
Thiamine level
Urinalysis
Urine toxicology screen

Focused Studies

Albumin with total protein
Alkaline phosphatase
Cholesterol/triglycerides
HIV screen (especially if untested IV drug abuse)
Prothrombin time
TB skin test

Table 54–20 provides additional information about the effect of alcohol on selected laboratory studies.

Diagnostic Studies

General Studies

Chest x-ray
EKG

TABLE 54–19. Amount of Alcohol Intake, Blood Alcohol Levels, and Behavioral Manifestations: In Nonphysiologically Tolerant Individuals

Alcohol Intake	Blood Alcohol Levels	Behavioral Manifestations
1–2 drinks	0.05 mg%	Mood and behavioral changes: judgment is impaired.
5–6 drinks	0.10 mg%	*Legal level of intoxication in most states.* Psychomotor action response time is slowed, voluntary motor action becomes clumsy.
10–12 drinks	0.20 mg%	Motor function area of the cerebral cortex is depressed: produces ataxia and staggering. Emotional liability occurs.
15–18 drinks	0.30 mg%	Confusion, marked difficulty problem solving and thinking; can become stuporous.
20–24 drinks	0.40 mg%	Coma, respiratory depression can become a problem.
25–30 drinks	0.50 mg%	Death due to respiratory depression due to brainstem depression. Arrhythmias often develop.

TABLE 54–20. Characteristic Laboratory Findings Associated with Alcohol Abuse

Laboratory Test	Associated Findings
Albumin	Decreased
Amylase	Elevated
Blood Alcohol Level (BAL)	Positive and significantly elevated ≥ 200 mg/100 mg (200 mg/dL = 0.2 g/dL = 200 mg%) **CAUTION:** A negative or 0 alcohol level in a known chronic alcoholic can signal impending alcohol withdrawal syndrome
Breathalyzer	Positive
Folic Acid and Thiamine	Decreased
MCV	Elevated (indicator of heavy drinking); direct toxic effect and indirect alcohol-induced megaloblastic changes
SGOT (AST)	Elevated
SGPT (ALT)	Elevated
SGGT (GGT)	Elevated
Uric Acid	Increased

Focused Studies

CAT scan (CT)
EEG
MRI

Treatment of the Substance Abuse Patient in the Acute Care Environment

General Principles

Objectives in Managing Intoxication

- Decrease external stimulation in the environment
- Interrupt ingestion of substance
- Protect patient from harming self and others until toxic effects dissipate
- Attempt to obtain a history of substance(s) and quantity from patient or family/friends
- Ascertain if patient previously experienced any form of withdrawal (if yes, what were the signs and symptoms; how was it treated; and did that treatment work)

Objectives in Managing Withdrawal

- Prevent complications of withdrawal (delirium tremens, oversedation, patient or staff injury)
- Increase patient comfort (pharmacologic management)
- Provide explicit instructions to staff regarding signs and symptoms of withdrawal and method to be used to provide comfort during acute withdrawal process
- Avoid masking medications (clonidine and propranolol) if possible; these will mask the true symptoms of withdrawal (they may be needed if the patient has increased autonomic stimulation)
- Identify and treat metabolic alterations (dehydration, electrolyte, glucose, magnesium, phosphate)
- Provide nutritional supplementation by increasing calories (when appropriate); add vitamins, minerals, and vitamin K (if prothrombin time is decreased)
- Maintain a quiet and harm-free environment

Tables 54–21 and 54–22 present more detail on the physiological and behavioral effects of intoxication and withdrawal syndromes.

Managing Detoxification in the Acute Care Patient

This discussion will primarily focus on alcohol and benzodiazepine withdrawal since they are currently the most common presentations in acute care.

Choosing an Effective and Safe Sedation Medication

Benzodiazepines are the preferred medications because of their reduced side-effect profile and diverse routes of administration. The short- to intermediate-acting benzodiazepine called lorazepam (Ativan) is recommended for patients with liver disease, cognitive impairment, unstable medical problems, or individuals age ≥ 65 years. This describes the majority of acute care patients! Therefore, this medication has recently been utilized in sedation protocol development by several sources rather than the longer-acting benzodiazepines (chlordaizepoxide and diazepam) (Krupnick et al., 1998; Patch et al., 1998) to avoid oversedation in the medically ill patient.

Although no clear evidence supports the use of one benzodiazepine over another, lorazepam (Ativan) has an appealing profile for safe and effective use. Lorazepam demonstrates good bioavailability in oral, intramuscular, and intravenous forms. Additionally, it is stable in a continuous intravenous drip unlike the long-acting diazepam (Valium), has rapid and complete absorption from intramuscular injection in an agitated patient with no intravenous access, and has an intermediate half life, which is an important consideraton in avoiding oversedation. It also has a smaller increase in its half life in patients with cirrhosis or liver failure than other benzodiazepines. Finally, lorazepam (Ativan) is metabolized to the glucoronide form and therefore is excreted by the kidney rather than through the liver.

Symptom-Triggered Sedation Management

Symptom-triggered sedation management is a dosing system based on the utilization of withdrawal severity scales to guide the medication management of the patient in withdrawal. Refer to Table 54–18 for additional information. The CIWA–Ar quantifies the overt symptoms of alcohol

TABLE 54–21. Central Nervous System Depressants: Clinical Syndromes

Drug Category/Drug	Abuse/Intoxication	Signs and Symptoms of Withdrawal
Barbiturates		
amobarbital (Amytal)	Distorted mood	Anxiety
butabarbital (Butisol)	Impaired judgment	Cardiovascular collapse
pentobarbital (Nembutal)	Impaired motor skills	Delirium, hallucinations
phenobarbital (Luminal)	Residual sedation (hangover)	Insomnia
secobarbital(Seconal)		Muscle twitching
		Nausea and vomiting
		Postural hypotension
		Seizures
		Weakness
		Weight loss
Benzodiazepines		
alprazolam (Xanax)	Ataxia	Anorexia
chlorazepate (Tranxene)	Drowsiness	Anxiety
chlordiazepoxide (Librium)	Slurred speech	Ataxia
clonazepam (Klonopin)	Vertigo	Diaphoresis
diazepam (Valium)		Diaphoresis
flurazepam (Dalmane)		Diarrhea
lorazepam (Ativan)		Dysphoria
oxazepam (Serax)		Hallucinations
prazepam (Centrax)		Insomnia
temazepam (Restoril)		Irritability
triazolam (Halcion)		Memory impairment
		Muscle cramps
		Psychosis
		Seizures
		Tremors
		Vomiting
Narcotics		
Natural	Behavioral changes	Initial phase (0–24 hrs)
morphine		
Semi-synthetics		
heroin	Constipation	Diaphoresis
Synthetics	Decreased sexual drive	Excessive yawning
codeine	Miosis	Gooseflesh
fentanyl (sublimaze)	Urine retention	Increased lacrimation
hydromorphone (Dilaudid)		Mydriasis
meperidine (Demerol)		Restlessness
methadone (dolophine)		Rhinorrhea
oxycodone (percodan)		Active abstinence withdrawal phase
		(After 24 hours–72 hours)
		Anorexia
		Acid–base imbalance
		Dehydration
		Hot and cold flashes
		Hypertension
		↑ body temperature
		Insomnia
		Involuntary kicking
		Leukocytosis
		Muscle twitching and spasms
		Nausea, vomiting, and diarrhea
		Severe back, abdominal, and leg pain
		Severe sneezing
		Spontaneous ejaculation and orgasm
		Tachycardia, tachypnea

Compiled from Gelenberg & Bassuk. (1997). (pp. 293–317); and Miller, Gold, & Smith. (1997). (pp. 97–110).

TABLE 54–22. Central Nervous System Stimulants: Clinical Syndromes

Drug	Signs and Symptoms Abuse/Intoxication	Signs and Symptoms of Withdrawal
Amphetamines (long acting) dextroamphetamine (Dexedrine) methamphetamine (Methadrine) Ice (synthesized for illicit use)	**Physiological:** ↑ HR, BP dialted pupils, nausea/vomiting twitching **Behavioral/Perceptual:** assaultive, euphoric→manic grandiose, ↑energy, impaired judgment, impaired social functioning, impaired work functioning, violence	agitation, apathy, depression, disorienttation fatigue lethargy sleepiness
Cocaine/crack (short acting) injectable nasal (snorted) smokable	**Physiological:** ↑ HR, BP, anorexia, dilated pupils insomnia **Behavioral/Perceptual:** disturbed concentration elation, grandiosity, impaired judgment, paranoid thinking, psychosis, resisting fatigue, violent, angry outburst	anxiety, apathy, craving, depression fatigue, use of CNS depressants to ↓ anxiety and symptoms of withdrawal
Nicotine cigarettes smokeless tobacco nicotine gum nicotine patch	No clear, well-documented symptoms of nicotine intoxication syndrome	anxiety, constipation, craving (nicotine fits), ↓concentration fatigue, GI problems, headaches, ↑eating, irritability
Xanthines caffeine	**Physiological:** arrhythmia, diuresis excitement, flushed face, GI complaints nervousness, periods of inexhaustibilty, psychomotor agitation, rambling speech, restlessness	No well-documented symptoms of a withdrawal syndrome have been consistently substantiated, although many complaints by patients depict a "flu-like" syndrome during the first week after totally stopping caffeine intake

Compiled from Miller, Gold, & Smith. (1997).

withdrawal and has been used in developing sedation protocols (Sullivan et al., 1989). Symptom-triggered sedation management has been demonstrated to have more effective outcomes than prn or straight order dosing methods of medication management in alcohol withdrawal. Symptom-triggered treatment does require frequent monitoring and overall education for both the nurses and physicians.

This method accomplishes several objectives in detoxification: provides effective symptom control, avoids overmedication, and shortens the period of detoxification treatment (Mayo-Smith, 1997; Patch et al., 1997; Saitz et al., 1994; Sullivan et al., 1991). Studies have demonstrated that the CIWA–Ar can be used by nursing staff on general hospital medical/surgical and orthopedic units to monitor and treat patients with coexisting alcohol withdrawal and medical and/or surgical problems (Foy et al., 1988; Patch et al., 1997). In the symptom-triggered sedation method, the patient is assessed using a structured assessement scale, often the CIWA–Ar, and administered medication only when the symptoms move across a chosen threshold of predetermined severity (Krupnick et al., 1998; Patch et al., 1997; Sullivan, et al., 1991; Wartenberg et al., 1990). See Table 54–23 for additional information on the process of conducting and monitoring a symptom-triggered sedation model of treatment in the patient experiencing withdrawal.

Adjunctive Medications for the Substance-Abusing Patient

Generally, the substance-abusing patient suffers from nutritional deficiencies. Therefore, daily doses of either oral or intravenous thiamine 100 mg, folate 1 mg, and multivitamin (one) can decrease the development of Wernicke's disease and Wernicke–Korsakoff Syndrome (Marcus & Coulston 1996).

Criteria for Referral

Consider **early** consultation with patients who have the following conditions to assist in safely and efficiently managing sedation treatment:

- Active/unstable angina
- Active GI bleed
- Cerebrovascular accident
- Elderly patient (≥ 65 years)
- Head injury
- Hepatic failure (PT > 15 seconds)
- Pneumonia (especially if hypoxemia)
- Recent MI (in last 3 months)
- Sepsis
- Any patient being treated who continues to require increasing doses and is resistant

TABLE 54–23. Example of Symptom-Triggered Sedation Management

CAGE Questions: Any one positive answer →Institute the CIWA–Ar Assessment Scale

Stage	CIWA–Ar score	Medication Recommendation
0 (At Risk)	(0–7)	Continue to monitor CIWA–Ar every 2 hours × 2 if remains < 8, then monitor every 4 hours × 24hrs **If at any interval score** ≥ **8** go to stage 1 interventions
1 (Early Withdrawal)	(8–14)	Administer lorazepam 2 mg po IV Remonitor CIWA–Ar every 2 hrs Give medication each time until the CIWA–Ar is <8 for 3 intervals If CIWA–Ar remains >8 or is ↑, then double the dose (4 mg po IV) and remonitor in 1 hr; if score continues to be ↑ then go to stage 2 treatment
2 (Moderate Withdrawal)	(15–19)	Administer lorazepam 4 mg po IV Remonitor in 1 hr. If same score give same dose (4 mg). If score is ↑, then give 6 mg po IV and remonitor in 1 hr. If score is remaining stable at any interval, then give the same dose until score is stable <8 for 3 hrs. If score is ↑ then go to stage 3 treatment
3 (Severe Withdrawal) (Delirium tremens)	≥ 20	Adminisiter 6 mg of lorazepam IV. Remonitor in 30 minutes. If score same or ↑ then administer 8 mg IV. Remonitor in 30 minutes and give same dose if score is < 15. If score is same or increasing, consider further consultation; patient may require continuous drip or larger doses with increased nursing monitoring, may require step down or high-technology monitoring in ICU

Adapted from Krupnick, Grunwald, Fischel, Gavryck, & Ryzewicz. (1998).

Consultation to Assist with Treatment Referral(s) Decision Process

- Inpatient vs. outpatient detoxification program
- Psychiatric vs. addiction treatment
- Dual diagnosis treatment
- Physical medicine rehabilitation vs. addiction rehabilitation

Referral Resources

Acute Care Addiction Consult Team (find out if your institution has this type of team; if so, establish a relationship with it)
Consult to inpatient detoxification unit (especially if Level IV unit)
Psychiatric consultation service
Psychiatric consultation liaison nurse
Addiction social worker
Clinical resource coordinator

Referral for Inpatient Detoxification

Often the patient's medical or surgical condition is improving and warrants dicharge from the acute care environment; however, the patient is not completely tapered of all his or her sedation and may require additional detoxification. There are certain variables to consider when placing the patient for continued detoxification. If you become the decision maker, here are some general guidelines to assist you in the decision-making process.

Inpatient Detoxification Criteria

- History of unsuccessful outpatient detoxification identified by multiple relapses
- History of delirium tremens
- History of withdrawal-related seizures
- Comorbid medical problems requiring frequent daily monitoring during detoxification
- High doses of several substances
- Still on high doses of benzodiazepine started in the acute care sedation management

Nursing Care Consultation

Just as you will often discover how challenging patients with substance-abuse disorders can be, so too will your nurse colleagues in direct patient care. The nursing staff may experience several competing and paradoxical reactions to the patient with a substance-abuse disorder and may need, request, and benefit from your guidance. The consultations usually focus on specific issues of behavioral, medication, and delirium management. The section discussing delirium provides the ACNP with effective strategies for substance-related delirium, so the reader is referred to that section for review.

Medication Management Issues

Generally the nurses, family, and sometimes the patient complain about not receiving enough medication (sedation, pain) and often the underlying issue is concern for making or contributing to the patient's addiction. The first point to remember is that the patient is already addicted; you will not cause that! The second point is that if the patient does not receive enough sedation medication or the patient's tolerance has not been factored into the pain-management equation, then the patient will begin to withdraw or suffer increasing pain from underdosing. You then have a patient who is starting withdrawal and who also may be undermedicated for his or her pain problem.

If you are not a pain specialist or have expert knowledge in substance abuse, call in the consultants to help you in assisting the patient and plan a collaborative education program to instruct your nursing and physician colleagues in sedation management of the withdrawing patient. This may help to decrease the patient's "drug seeking" behaviors because the patient will actually receive medication to decrease both sets of symptoms.

Wandering Off the Unit

These patients can be at risk for leaving the hospital property and using illicit substances, especially if their treatment has provided them with direct intravenous access. It is helpful to establish a written contract with the patients about when and with whom they may leave the unit and for what reasons (e.g., smoking is always a significant request). Additionally, if they leave the unit in an unescorted manner, they will be assessed—which may include a toxicology screen—for alcohol or drug use during their absence.

Agitation, Aggression, and Threatened Violence

The substance-abuse patient in the acute care environment can be agitated and become increasingly aggressive to health-care workers and possibly threaten to harm them. It is not uncommon for a patient with increasing aggressiveness to threaten violence toward staff members. Generally, each institution does have some type of policy to manage verbal threats or acts of violence from patients toward staff members. If you are being consulted about one of your patients becoming verbally or physically aggressive, then be knowledgeable about the institution's policy. Overall, it is important for all health-care providers to take either verbal or written threats of violence very seriously and activate the standing policy. It may be useful to have security involved (if they are skillful in defusing techniques used in potentially violent situations), and have a discussion with the patient and/or family that allows them to be upset and express those feelings without threatening harm to anyone. If the patient/family responds to this level of intervention, then having a patient care conference to discuss how to effectively defuse the verbally escalating patient would be helpful. Encourage the staff to de-escalate the verbal or physical aggression by focusing on what prompted it and try to enlist the patient in problem-solving with them. Remove any staff member who further escalates the situation until patient and staff member regain composure. An honest discussion among staff members may be necessary if a staff member or several staff members are in some way contributing to the patient's escalation.

Also, it is important to enlist the assistance of relevent resources (primary nurse, unit manager, clinical nurse specialists, security, patient advocate service, pastoral counseling, supportive and calming family and/or friends). The overall goal is to determine what is driving the aggression (acute reaction or a chronic pattern of behavior) and develop focused strategies to keep the patient, yourself, colleagues, and family safe.

REFERENCES

Aakerlund, L. & Rosenberg, J. (1994). Writing disturbances: An indication of postoperative delirium. *International Journal of Psychiatry in Medicine, 24,* 245–257.

American Psychiatric Association. (1994). *Diagnostic and statistical manual of mental disorders* (4th ed.). Washington, DC: American Psychiatric Press.

Anthenelli, R. M. & Schuckit, M. A. (1997). Genetics. In J. H. Lowinson, P. Ruiz, R. B. Millman, & J. G. Langrod (Eds.), *Substance Abuse: A Comprehensive Textbook* (3rd ed.). Baltimore: Williams and Wilkins, pp. 41–50.

Arieff, A. & Griggs, R. (Eds.) (1992). *Metabolic brain dysfunction in systemic disorders.* Boston: Little Brown.

Armstrong, S. C., Cozza, K. L., & Watanabe, K. S. (1997). The misdiagnosis of delirium. *Psychosomatics, 38* (5), 433–439.

Bailey, D. N. (1990). Drug use in patients admitted to a university trauma center; results of limited (rather than comprehensive) toxicology screening. *Journal of Analytical Toxicology, 14,* 22–24.

Bailey, D. N. (1993). Plasma cocaethylene concentrations in patients treated in the emergency room or trauma unit. *American Journal of Clinical Pathology, 99,* 123–127.

Barr, J. & Donner, A. (1995). Optimal intravenous dosing strategies and analgesics in the intensive care unit. *Critical Care Clinics, 11,* 827–847.

Beck, A. T., Brown, G., Epstein, N., et al. (1988). An inventory for measuring clinical anxiety: Psychometric properties. *Journal of Consulting and Clinical Psychiatry, 56,* 893–897.

Blanchard, E. B., & Hickling, E. J. (1997). *After the crash: Assessment and treatment of motor vehicle accident surviviors* Washington, D. C. American Psychological Association.

Blazer, D. G. (1993). *Depression in Late Life* (2nd ed.). St. Louis: Mosby.

Blum, K., Noble, E. P., Sheridan, P. J., et al. (1990). Allelic association of human dopamine D_2 receptor gene in alcoholism. *Journal of the American Medical Association. 263,* 2055–2060.

Blumenfield, M. & Schoeps, M. M. (1993). *Psychological care of the burn and trauma patient.* Baltimore: Williams and Wilkins.

Bostwick, J. M., & Masterton, B. J. (1998). Pharmacological treatment of delirium to restore mental capacity. *Psychosomatics, 39* (2), 112–117.

Boyd, M. A. & Nihart, M. A. (1998). *Psychiatric nursing: Contemporary practice.* Philadelphia: Lippincott-Raven.

Bradley, B. P., Gossop, M., Phillips, G. T., & Legarda, J. J. (1987). The development of an opiate withdrawal scale (OWS). *British Journal of Addiciton, 82,* 1139–1142.

Breitbart, W. & Holland, J. (Eds.) (1993). *Psychiatric aspects of symptom management in cancer patients.* Washington, DC: American Psychiatric Press.

Brookoff, D., Campbell, E. A., & Shaw, L. M. (1993). The underreporting of cocaine-related trauma: Drug abuse warning network reports vs. hospital toxicology tests. *American Journal of Public Health. 83,* 369–371.

Buckley, P. F. & Hutchinson, M. (1995). Neuroleptic malignant syndrome. *Journal of Neurology, Neurosurgery, and Psychiatry, 58,* 271.

Burns, M. & Eisendrath, S. (1994). Dextroamphetamine treatment for depression in terminally ill patients. *Psychosomatics, 35,* 80–83.

Busto, U. E., Sykora, K. & Sellers, E. M. (1989). A clinical scale to assess benzodiazepine withdrawal. *Journal of Clinical Psychopharmacology, 9* (6), 412–416.

Carney, R. M., Rich, M. W., Freedland, K. E., et al. (1988). Major depressive disorder predicts cardiac events in patients with coronary artery disease. *Psychosomatic Medicine, 50,* 627–633.

Cassem, E. H. (1990). Depression and anxiety secondary to medical illness. *Psychiatric Clinics of North America, 13,* (4), 597–612.

Cavanaugh, S. (1995). Depression in the medically ill: Critical issues in diagnostic assessment. *Psychosomatics, 36,* 48–59.

Clark, R. F. & Harchelroad, F. (1991). Toxicology screening of the trauma patient: A changing profile. *Annals of Emergency Medicine. 20,* 151–153.

Clark, D. E., McCarthy, E. & Robinson, E. (1985). Trauma as a symptom of alcoholism (editorial). *Annals of Emergency Medicine, 14,* 274.

Cleary, P. D., Miller, M., Bush, B. T., et al. (1988). Prevalence and recognition of alcohol abuse in a primary care population. *American Journal of Medicine. 85,* 466–471.

Cole, M. G. & Primeau, F. J. (1993). Prognosis of delirium in elderly hospital patients. *Canadian Medical Association Journal, 149,* 41–46.

Colon, E. A. & Papkin, M. K. (1996). Anxiety and panic. In J. R. Rundell & M. G. Wise (Eds.), *Textbook of consultation liaison psychiatry.* Washington, DC: American Psychiatric Press.

Cross National Collaborative Group. (1992). The changing rate of major depression. *Journal of the American Medical Association, 268,* 3098–3105.

Dube, C., Goldstein, M. G. & Lewis, D. C. (1989). Project ADEPT volume 1: *Core Modules.* Providence, RI: Brown University.

El-Ebiury, M., Torres, A., Ramirez, J., et al. (1995). Lipid deposition during long-term infusion of propofol. *Critical Care Medicine, 23,* 1928-1930.

Elliott, T. R. & Frank, R. G. (1996). Depression following spinal cord injury. *Archives of Physical Medicine and Rehabilitation, 77,* 816–823.

Ewing, J. (1984). Detecting alcoholism: The CAGE questionnaire. *Journal of the American Medical Association, 252* (14), 1905–1907.

Faust, D. & Fogel, B. S. (1989). The development and initial validation of a sensitive bedside cognitive screening test. *The Journal of Nervous and Mental Disease, 177,* 25–31.

Feldman, M. D. & Christensen, J. E. (1997). *Behavioral medicine in primary care: A practical guide.* Stamford, CT: Appleton & Lange.

Folstein, M. F. et al. (1975). Mini-mental state: A practical method for grading the cognitive state of patients for the clinician. *Journal of Psychiatric Research, 12,* 196–197.

Folstein, M. F., Bassett, S. S., Romanoski, A. J. et al. (1991). The epidemiology of delirium in the community: The eastern Baltimore mental health survey. In N. E. Miller, Z. J. Lipowski & Lebowitz (Eds.), *International Psychogeriatrics.* New York: Springer.

Foreman, M. (1993). Acute confusion in the elderly. *Annual Review of Nursing Research, 11,* 3–30.

Foy, A., March, S., & Drinkwater, V. (1988) Use of an objective clinical scale in the assessment and management of alcohol withdrawal in a large general hospital. *Alcohol Clinical Experimental Research. 12,* 360–364.

Francis, J. (1992). Delirium in older patients. *Journal of American Geriatric Society, 40,* 829–838.

Francis, J., Martin, D., & Kapoor, W. (1990). A prospective study of delirium in hospitalized elderly. *Journal of American Medical Association. 263,* 1097–1101.

Francis, J. & Kapoor, W. N. (1992). Prognosis after hospital discharge of older medical patients with delirium. *Journal of American Geriatrics Society. 40,* 601–606.

Frasure-Smith, N., Lesprance, F. & Talajic, M. (1995). Depression and 18 month prognosis after myocardial infarction. *Circulation, 91,* 999–1005.

Freedland, K., Carney, R., Rich, M., et al (1991). Depression in elderly patients with congestive heart failure. *Journal of Geriatric Psychiatry, 24,* 59–71.

Gelfand, S. B., Indelicato, J., & Benjamin, J. (1992). Using intravenous haloperidol to control delirium. *Hospital and Community Psychiatry. 43,* 215.

Gelenberg, A. J. & Bassuk, E. L. (1997). *The Practitioner's Guide to Psychoactive Drugs.* (4th ed.). New York: Plenum Medical Books.

Gold, M. S. (1994). Neurobiology of addiction and recovery: The brain, the drive for the drug and the 12 step fellowship. *Journal of Substance Abuse Treatment, 11,* 93–97.

Green, B. L., Rowland, J., Krupnick, J. L., Epstein, S. A. et al (1998). Prevalence of post traumatic stress disorder in women with breast cancer. *Psychosomatics, 39* (2), 102–111.

Gustafson, Y., Berggren, D., Brannstrom, B., et al (1988). Acute confusional states in elderly patients treated for femoral neck fracture. *Journal of American Geriatrics Society, 36,* 525–530.

Hamilton, M. (1959). The assessment of anxiety states by rating. *Journal of Medical Psychology, 32,* 50–55.

Hart, R. P., Levensen, J. L., Sissler, C. N., et al. (1996). Validation of a cognitive test for delirium in medical ICU patients. *Psychosomatics, 37* (6), 533–546.

Heiman-Patterson, T. D. (1993). Neuroleptic malignant syndrome and malignant hyperthermia: Important issues for the medical consultant. *The Medical Clinics of North America, 77,* 477.

Hirschfeld, R. A., Keller, M. B., Panico, S., Aron, B. S., Barlow, D., et al. (1997). Consensus Statement on the Undertreatment of Depression. *Journal of the American Medical Association, 277* (4), 333–340.

Holmes, T., Sabaawi, M. & Fragala, M. (1994). Psychostimulant suppository treatment for depression in the gravely ill (letter). *Journal of Clinical Psychiatry, 55,* 265–266.

Inouye, S. K., vanDyck, C. H., Alessi, C. A., et al (1990). Clarifying confusion: The confusion assessment method. *Annals of Internal Medicine, 113,* 941–948.

Inouye, S., Viscoli, C., Horwitz, R., et al (1993). The dilemma of delirium: Clinical and research controversies regarding diagnosis and evaluation of delirium in hospitalized elderly medical patients. *American Journal of Medicine, 97,* 278–288.

Janson, C., Bjornsson, E., Helt, J., et al (1994). Anxiety and depression in relation to respiratory symptoms and asthma. *American Journal of Respiratory and Critical Care Medicine, 49* (4, pt 1), 930–934.

Jorge, R. E., Robinson, R. G., Starkstein, S. E., & Arndt, S. V. (1994). Influence of major depression on one year outcome in patients with traumatic brain injury. *Journal of Neurosurgery, 81,* 726–733.

Jorge, R. E., Robinson, R. G., Starkstein, S., et al (1993). Secondary mania following traumatic brain injury. *American Journal of Psychiatry, 150,* 916.

Kane, F. J., Remmell, R., & Moody, S. (1993). Recognizing and treating delirium in patients admitted to general hospitals. *Southern Medical Journal. 86,* 985–988.

Kaplan, H. I., & Sadock, B. J. (1996). *Pocket handbook of primary care psychiatry.* Baltimore, MD: Williams & Wilkins.

Kaplan, H. I., Sadock, B. J., Grebb, J. A. (1994) Mood disorders in Cancrow, R., Gabhard, G. O., Jones, R. M. et al. (ed.). Baltimore, MD: Williams & Wilkins.

Karajgi, B., Rifkin, A., Dodd, S., et al. (1990). The prevalence of anxiety disorders in patients with COPD. *American Journal of Psychiatry, 147,* 200–201.

Katon, W., Hall, M. L., Russo, J., et al. (1988). Chest pain: The relationship of psychiatric illness to coronary arteriography results. *American Journal of Medicine, 84,* 1–9.

Katon, W. J. (1991). *Panic Disorder in the Medical Setting.* Washington, DC: American Psychiatric Press.

Kellner, R. & Uhlenhuth, E. H. (1991). The rating and self rating on anxiety. *British Journal of Psychiatry, 159* (suppl), 15–22.

Kellner, R., Samet, J., & Pathak, D. (1992). Dyspnea, anxiety, and depression in chronic respiratory impairment. *General Hospital Psychiatry, 14,* 20–28.

Kelly, D. & Lynch, J. B. (1992). Burns in alcohol and drug users result in longer treatment times with more complications. *Journal of Burn Care Rehabilitation, 13*(2, pt 1), 218–220.

Kessler, R. C, McGonagle, K. A., Zhao, S., et al (1994). Lifetime and 12 month prevalence of DSM III-R psychiatric disorders in the US: Results from the National Co-Morbidity Survey. *Archives of General Psychiatry, 51,* 8–19.

Klein, R. (1995). The role of methylphenidate in psychiatry. *Archives of General Psychiatry, 52,* 429–433.

Kriwisky, M., Perry, G. Y., et al (1990). Haloperidol-induced torsades de pointes. *Chest. 98,* 482–484.

Krupnick, S. (1996). Psychiatric disorders. In S. Nettina (Ed.). *The Lippincott manual of nursing practice.* (6th ed.). Philadelphia: Lippincott.

Krupnick, S., & Wade, A. (1999). *Psychiatric care planning.* (2nd ed.). Springhouse, PA: Springhouse Corporation.

Krupnick, S., Grunwald, E., Fischel, S., Gavryck, W., & Ryzewicz, S. (1998). Alcohol Abstinence Withdrawal Syndrome: An evidence-based collaborative assessment and intervention guideline for the acute care patient. Baystate Medical Center Medical QI Team: Substance Abuse in the Medical Patient. Springfield, MA: Baystate Healthcare System.

Kurlowicz, L. (1997). Nursing standard of practice protocol: Depression in elderly patients. *Geriatric Nursing, 18* (5), 192–200.

Lambdan, R. M., Ramchandani, D., & Schindler, B. A. (1997). The chronically mentally ill on a general hospital consultation–liaison service: Their needs and managment. *Psychosomatics, 38* (5), 472–477.

Levenson, J. (1995). High-dose intravenous haloperidol for agitated delirium following lung transplantation. *Psychosomatics, 36,* 66–73.

Levkoff, S., Liptzin, B., Cleary, P., et al. (1991). Review of research instruments and techniques used to detect delirium. *International Psychogeritatrics, 3,* 253–270.

Lipowski, Z. (1990). *Delirium: Acute Confusional States.* New York: Oxford University Press.

Liptzin, B. & Levkoff, S. E. (1992). An empirical study of delirium subtypes. *British Journal of Psychiatry, 161,* 843–845.

Lydiard, R., Fossey, M., Marsh, W., et al. (1993). Prevalence of psychiatric disorders in patients with irritable bowel syndrome. *Psychosomatics, 34,* 229–234.

Marcantonio, E. R., Goldman, I., Mangione, C. M., et al. (1994). A clinical prediction rule for delirium after elective noncardiac surgery. *Journal of the American Medical Association, 271,* 134–139.

Marcus, R. & Coulston, A. M. (1996). Water soluble vitamines. In J. G. Hardman, A. G. Goodman, L. E. Limbird (Eds.), *Goodman's and Gilman's: The Pharmacologic Basis of Therapeutics* (9th ed.). New York: McGraw-Hill, pp. 1550–1572.

Marzuk, P. M., Tardiff, K., Leon, A. C., Stajic, M., et al. (1990). Prevalence of recent cocaine use among motor vehicle fatalities in New York City. *Journal of the American Medical Association. 263,* 250–256.

Masand, P., Pickett, P., & Murray, G. (1995). Hypomania precipitated by psychostimulant use in depressed medically ill patients. *Psychosomatics, 36,* 145–147.

Masand, P. S. & Tesar, G. E. (1996). Use of psychostimulants in the medically ill. *The Psychiatric Clincs of North America, 19* (3), 515–547.

Maull, K. (1982). Alcohol abuse: Its implications in trauma care. *Southern Medical Journal, 75,* 794–798.

Mayfield, D., McLeod, G., & Hall, P. (1974). The CAGE questionaire: Validation of a new alcoholism screening instrument. *American Journal of Psychiatry, 131,* 1121.

Mayo-Smith, M. F. (1997). Pharmacological management of alcohol withdrawal: A meta-analysis and evidence based practice guideline. *Journal of the American Medical Association, 278* (2), 144–151.

McCartney, J. & Boland, R. (1994). Anxiety and delirium in the intensive care unit. *Critical Care Clinics, 10,* 673–680.

McDaniel, J. & Johnson, K. (1995). Obsessive–compulsive disorder in HIV disease: Response to fluoxetine. *Psychosomatics, 36,* 147–150.

McDaniel, J., Musselman, D., Porter, M., et al. (1995). Depression in patients with cancer: diagnosis, biology, and treatment. *Archives of General Psychiatry, 52,* 89–99.

Metzger, E. & Friedman, R. (1993). Prolongation of the corrected

QT and torsades de pointes cardiac arrhythmia associated with intravenous haloperidol in the medically ill. *Journal of Clinical Psychopharmacolocy, 13,* 128–132.

Miller, N. S. (1997). *Principles and practices of additions in psychiatry.* Philadelphia, PA: W. B. Saunders.

Miller, N. S. & Gold, M. S. (1993). A neurochemical basis for alcohol and other drug addiction. *Journal of Psychoactive Drugs, 25* (2), 121–126.

Miller, N. S., Gold, M. S., & Smith, D. E. (1997). *Manual of therapeutics of additions.* New York: Wiley-Liss.

Mirenda, J. (1995). Prolonged propofol sedation in the critical care unit. *Critical Care Medicine, 23,* 1304-1305.

Moore, R. D., Bone, L. R., Geller, G., et al. (1989). Prevalence, detection and treatment of alcoholism in hospitalized patients. *Journal of the American Medical Association. 261,* 403–407.

Moore, D. P. & Moore, J. W. (1996). *Handbook of Medical Psychiatry.* St. Louis: Mosby.

Morris, P. L., Raphael, B., & Robinson, R. G. (1992). Clinical depression is associated with impaired recovery from stroke. *Medical Journal of Australia, 157,* 239–242.

Morris, P. L., Robinson, R. G., & Rzejewski, P. et al. (1993). Association of depression with 10 year post stroke mortality. *American Journal of Psychiatry, 150,* 124–129.

Munster, A. M. (1993). *Severe Burns: A family guide to medical and emotional recovery.* Baltimore: Johns Hopkins University Press.

Murphy, G. E. & Wetzel, R. D. (1990). The life time risk of suicide in alcoholism. *Archives of General Psychiatry, 47,* 383–392.

Murphy, G. E., Wetzel, R. D., Robine, E., et al. (1992). Multiple risk factors predict suicide in alcoholism. *Archives of General Psychiatry, 49,* 459–463.

Murray, A. M., Levkoff, S. E., & Wetle, T. T. (1993). Acute delirium and functional decline in the hospitalized elderly patient. *Journal of Gerontology, 48,* M181-M186.

Nadler, J., Richardson, E., & Malloy, P. (1994). Detection of impairment with the mini-mental state examination. *Neuropsychiatry, Neuropsychology, and Behavioral Neurology, 7,* 109–113.

Naranjo, C. A., Poulos, C. X., Bremmer, K. E., et al. (1992). Citalopram decreases desirability, liking, and consumption of alcohol in alcohol-dependent drinkers. *Clinical Pharmacologic Therapy, 51,* 729–739.

Nathan, P. E. & Gorman, J. M. (1998). *A guide to treatments that work.* New York: Oxford University Press.

National Institute on Alcohol Abuse and Alcoholism (1989). *Alcohol Alert.* No 3. Rockville, MD: NIAAA.

Nicholas, L. & Lindsey, A. (1995). Delirium presenting with symptoms of depression. *Psychosomatics, 36,* 471–479.

Novick, D. M., Hauerkos, H. W., & Teller, D. W. (1997). In Lowinson, J. H., Ruiz, P., Millman, R. B. & Langrod, J. G. (eds). *Substance abuse: a comprehensive textbook* (3rd ed.). Baltimore, MD: Williams & Wilkins. p. 536.

Patch, P. B., Phelps, G. L., & Cowan, G. (1997). Alcohol withdrawal in a medical–surgical setting: The "too little, too late" phenomenon. *MED/SURG Nursing, 6* (2), 80–90.

Perez-Stable, E. J., Miranda, J., Munoz, R. F., et al. (1990). Depression in medical outpatients: Underrecognition and misdiagnosis. *Archives of Internal Medicine, 150,* 1083–1088.

Platt, M. M., Breitbart, W., Smith, M., et al. (1994). Efficacy of neuroleptics for hypoactive delirium (letter). *Journal of Neuroscience, 6,* 66–67.

Pokovny, A. D., Miller, B. A., & Kaplan, H. B. (1972). The brief MAST: A shortened version of the MAST. *American Journal of Psychology, 129,* 342–345.

Pompeii, P., Foreman, M., Ridber, M. A., et al (1994). Delirium in hospitalized older persons: Outcomes and predictors. *Journal of American Geriatric Society, 42,* 809–815.

Pourcher, E., Filteau, M. J., Bourchard, R. H., et al. (1994). Efficacy of the combination of buspirone and carbamazepine in early post traumatic delirium (letter). *American Journal of Psychiatry, 151,* 150–151.

Preston, J. D., O'Neal, J. H., & Talaga, M. C. (1997). *Handbook of psychopharmacology for therapists.* Oakland, CA: New Harbinger Press.

Reichman, W. E. & Katz, P. R. (1996). *Psychiatric care in the nursing home.* New York: Oxford University Press.

Riker, R. R., Fraser, G. L., & Cox, P. M. (1994). Continuous infusion of haloperidol controls agitation in critically ill patients. *Critical Care Medicine, 22,* 433–440.

Rivara, F. P., Jurkovich, G. J., Gurney, J. G., Seguin, D., et al (1993). The magnitude of acute and chronic alcohol abuse in trauma patients. *Archives of Surgery, 128,* 907–913.

Roach, M. J., Connors, A. F., Dawson, N. V., et al. (1998). Depressed mood and survival in seriously ill hospitalized adults. *Archives of Internal Medicine, 158,* 397–404.

Robins, L. N. & Regier, D. A. (Eds.) (1991). *Psychiatric Disorders in America: The Epidemiologic Catchment Area Study.* New York: Free Press.

Rosen, J., Sweet, R., Mulsant, B., et al (1994). The delirium rating scale in a psychogeriatric inpatient setting. *Journal of Neuropsychiatry and Clincal Neurosciences, 6,* 30–35.

Rosenbaum, J. F., Pollack, M. H., Otto, M. W., et al (1996). Anxiety. In N. H. Cassem, T. A. Stern, J. F. Rosenbaum, M. S. Jellinek, (eds.), *Massachusetts General Hospital: Handbook of General Hospital Psychiatry* (4th ed.). St. Louis: Mosby.

Rostenberg, P. O. (1995). *Alcoholic and Other Drug Screening of Hospitalized Trauma Patients.* Treatment Improvement Protocol (TIP) Series (16). Rockville, MD: U.S. Department of Health and Human Services, Public Health Service, Substance Abuse and Mental Health Services Administration.

Rounsaville, B., Tims, F., Horter, A., & Sowder, B. (1993). *Diagnostic Source Book on Drug Abuse Research and Treatment* NIH publication No 93–3508. Rockville, MD: National Institutes of Health.

Rovner, B. W. & Folstein, M. F. (1987). Mini-mental status exam in clinical practice. *Hospital Practice,* January, 99.

Roy, A., Lampanski, D., DeJong, J., et al. (1990). Characteristics of alcoholics who attempt suicide. *American Journal of Psychiatry, 147,* 761–765.

Rundell, J. R. & Wise, M. G. (1996). *Textbook of consultation-liaison psychiatry.* Washington, DC: American Psychiatric Press.

Russell, M., Martier, S. S., Sokol, R. J., Jacobson, S, Jacobson, J., & Bottoms, S. (1991). Screening for pregnancy risk drinking: TWEAKING the tests. *Alcoholism Clinical Experimental Research, 15* (2), 638.

Saitz, R., Mayo-Smith, M., Roberts, M., Redmond, H., Benard, D., & Calkins, D. (1994). Individualized treatment for alcohol withdrawal: A randomized double-blind controlled trial. *Journal of the American Medical Association, 272* (7), 519–523.

Sanders, K., Murray, G., & Cassem, N. (1991). High-dose intravenous haloperidol for agitated delirium in a cardiac patient on an intra-aortic balloon pump. *Journal of Clinical Psychopharmacology, 11,* 146–147.

Sanders, K., Stern, T., O'Gara, P., et al (1992). Delirium during intra-aortic balloon pump therapy: Incidence and management. *Psychosomatics, 33,* 35–44.

Saravay, S. M. (1996). Psychiatric interventions in the medically ill: Outcomes and effectiveness research. *The Psychiatric Clinics of North America, 19* (3), 467–480.

Schatzberg, A. F. & Neineroff, C. B. (1995). *Textbook of psychopharmacology.* Washington, DC: American Psychiatric Press.

Schatzberg, A. F. & Neineroff, C. B. (1998). *Textbook of psychopharmacology* (2nd ed.) Washington, DC: American Psychiatric Press, pp. 775–789.

Sdao-Jarvie, K., Berolzheimer, N., Rounds, J. & Janowsky, D. S. (1993). Substance abuse screening of hospitalized patients and its effects on physician behavior. *Substance Abuse, 14* (1), 28–34.

Selzer, M. L. (1971). The Michigan Alcoholism Screening Test (MAST): The quest for a new diagnostic instrument. *American Journal of Psychiatry, 127,* 1653–1658.

Sheikh, J. (1994). Anxiety disorders. In C. E. Caffey & J. L. Cummings (Eds.). *Textbook of geriatric psychiatry.* Washington, DC: American Psychiatric Press.

Silverstone, P. H. (1990). Depression increases mortality and morbidity in acute life threatening medical illness. *Journal of Psychosomatic Research, 34,* 651–657.

Sipuhimalani, A. & Masard, P. S. (1998) Olanzapine in the treatment of delirium. *Psychosomatics, 39* (5), 422–430.

Skinner, H. A. (1982). The drug abuse screening test (DAST). *Addictive Behaviors, 7* (4), 363.

Skinner, H. A., Holt, S., Schuler, R., Roy, J., & Israel, Y. (1984). Identification of alcohol abuse using laboratory tests and a history of trauma. *Annals of Internal Medicine, 101,* 847–851.

Sliman, R. J., Donahue, T. A., Jarjoura, D., et al. (1992). Recognition of depression by internal medicine residents. *Journal of Community Health, 17,* 143–152.

Smith, M. J., Breitbart, W. S., Passik, S., et al. (1994). The Memorial Delirium Assessment scale (MDAS): Psychometric characteristics. *Psychosomatics, 35,* 192–193.

Smith, M., Breitbart, W., & Platt, M. (1995). A critique of instruments and methods to detect, diagnose and rate delirium. *Journal of Pain and Symptom Management, 10,* 35–77.

Smith, L. & Dimsdale, J. (1989). Postcardiotomy delirium: conclusions after 25 years? *American Journal of Psychiatry, 146,* 452–458.

Smoller, J. W., Pollack, M. H., Rosenbaum, J. F., et al. (1996). Panic, anxiety, and pulmonary disease: Theoretical considerations. *American Journal of Respiratory Critical Care Medicine, 154,* 6–17.

Soderstrom, C. A., Smith, G. S., Dischinger, P. C., McDuff, D. R., et al. (1997). Psychoactive substance abuse disorders among seriously injured trauma center patients. *Journal of the American Medical Association, 277* (22), 1769–1774.

Sokol, R., Martier, S., & Ager, J. (1989). T–ACE questions: Practical prenatal detection of risk-drinking. *American Journal of Obstetrics and Gynecology, 160* (4), 863–870.

Stahl, S. M. (1996). *Essential phamacology: Neuroscientific basis and practical application.* Cambridge, United Kingdom: Cambridge Press.

Stein, M. D., Asmundson, J. G., Ireland, D., et al (1994). Panic disorder in patients attending a clinic for vestibular disorders. *American Journal of Psychiatry, 151,* 1697–1700.

Stein, M. B., Asmundson, J. G., Ireland, D., et al. (1994). Panic disorder in patients attending a clinic for vestibular disorders. *American Journal of Psychiatry, 151,* 1697–1700.

Stern, T. A. (1994). Continuous infusion of haloperidol in agitated critically ill patients. *Critical Care Medicine, 22,* 378–379.

Stoudemire, A. & Fogel, B. (1993). *Psychiatric Care of the Medical Patient.* New York: Oxford University Press.

Stoudemire, A. (Ed.) (1995). *Psychological factors affecting medical conditions.* Washington, DC: American Psychiatric Press.

Stoudemire, A. (1996). New antidepressant drugs and the treatment of depression in the medically ill patient. *The Psychiatric Clinics of North America, 19* (3), 495–514.

Stuppaceck, C. H., Barnas, C., Falk, M., Guenther, V., Hummer, M., et al. (1994). Assessment of the alcohol withdrawal syndrome: Validity and reliability for the translated and modified Clinical Institute Withdrawal Assessment for Alcohol Scale (CIWA–A). *Addiction, 89* (10), 1287–1292.

Sullivan, J. T., Sykora, K., Schneiderman, J., et al. (1989a). Assessment of alcohol withdrawal: The revised Clinical Institute Withdrawal Assessment for Alcohol Scale (CIWA–Ar). *British Journal of Addiction, 84,* 1353–1357.

Sullivan, J. T., Swift, R. M., & Lewis, D. C. (1991b). Benzodiazepine requirements during alcohol withdrawal syndrome: Clinical implications of using a standardized withdrawal scale. *Journal of Clinical Psychopharmacology, 11* (5), 291–295.

Thomas, R. I., Cameron, D. J., & Fahs, M. C. (1988). A prospective study of delirium and prolonged hospital stay. *Archives of Psychiatry, 45,* 937–940.

Trzepacz, P. T., Baker, R. W., & Greenhouse, J. (1988). A symptom rating scale for delirium. *Psychiatry Research, 23,* 89–97.

Trzepacz, P. (1994). A review of delirium assessment instruments. *General Hospital Psychiatry, 16,* 397–405.

U.S. Department of Health and Human Services. (1990). *Seventh Special Report to the United States Congress on Alcohol and Health.* Rockville, MD. NIAAA

Valenti J. F., Anderson, G. L., Branson, R. D., et al. (1994). Disadvantages of propofol sedation in the critical care unit. *Critical Care Medicine, 22,* 710-712.

van Hemert, A. M., van der Mast, R. C., Hengeveld, M. W., et al. (1994). Excess mortality in general hospital patients with delirium: A five year follow up study of 519 patients seen in psychiatric consultation. *Journal of Psychosomatic Research, 38,* 339–346.

Vingerhoets, G. (1998). Perioperative anxiety and depression in open heart surgery. *Psychosomatics, 39* (1), 30–37.

Volpicelli, J. R., Watson, N. T., King, A. C., et al (1995). Effect of naltrexone on alcohol "high" in alcoholics. *American Journal of Psychiatry, 152,* 613–615.

Walker, E. A., Gelfand, A, N., & Gelfand, M. D. (1995). Psychiatric diagnoses, sexual and physical victimization, and disability in patients with irritable bowel syndrome or inflammatory bowel syndrome. *Psychological Medicine, 25,* 1259–1267.

Waller, J. A. (1988). Diagnosis of alcoholism in the injured patient. Paper presented at an NIAAA conference on post-injury treatment of patients with alcohol-related trauma. Washington, DC: Department of Health and Human Services.

Wartenberg, A., Nirenberg, T., Liepman, O., et al (1990). Detoxification of alcoholics: improving care by symptom triggered sedation. *Alcohol Clinical and Experimental Research. 13,* 71–75.

Williams, M. A., Ward, S. E., & Campbell, E. B. (1988). Confusion: Testing versus observation. *Journal of Gerontological Nursing, 14* (1), 25–30.

Wilt, J., Minnema, A., Johnson, R., et al. (1993). Torsades de pointes associated with the use of intravenous haloperidol. *Annals of Internal Medicine, 119,* 391–394.

Winger, G., Hofman, F. G., & Woods, J. H. (1992). *A Handbook on Drug and Alcohol Abuse.* New York: Oxford University Press.

Wise, M. G. & Gray, K. F. (1994). Delirium, dementia and amnestic disorders. In R. E. Hales, S. C. Yudofsky & J. A. Talbott (eds.), *Textbook of Psychiatry* (2nd ed.), Washington, DC: American Psychiatric Press.

Woodman, C. L., Breen, K., Noyes, R., Moss, C., et al. (1998). The relationship between irritable bowel and psychiatric illness: A family study. *Psychosomatics, 39* (1), 45–54.

WPA Dysthymia Working Group. (1995). Dysthymia in clinical practice. *British Journal of Psychiatry,* 166, 174.

Zung, W. K. W. (1971). A rating instrument to measure anxiety disorders. *Psychosomatics, 12,* 371–379.

Index

Page numbers followed by *f* indicate figures and page numbers followed by *t* indicate tables.